VOLUME 90 - JAN-FEB, 1981
No. 1, Part 1 (Issued in 4 Parts)

THE ANNALS OF OTOLOGY RHINOLOGY & LARYNGOLOGY

ANNALS OF HEAD & NECK MEDICINE & SURGERY

Adductor Spastic Dysphonia: 1½ Years after Recurrent Laryngeal Nerve Resection
A.E. Aronson, PhD; L.W. DeSanto, MD

Influence of Adenoid Hypertrophy on Secretory Otitis Media
H.H. Elverland, MD; I.W.S. Mair, MD, FRCSG; O.K. Haugeto, MD; K.E. Schrøder, MD

Reciprocal Synapses at the Base of Outer Hair Cells in the Organ of Corti of Man
J.B. Nadol, Jr., MD

Effect of Voice Therapy on Contact Granuloma of the Vocal Fold
C.S. Bloch, MA; W.J. Gould, MD; M. Hirano, MD

Second Louis H. Clerf Lecture. Vestibular Neuritis
H.F. Schuknecht, MD; K. Kitamura, MD
Supplement 78

Measurement of Optokinetic Nystagmus for Otoneurological Diagnosis
S.M. Abel, PhD; H.O. Barber, MD, FRCS(C)
Supplement 79

ANNALS PUBLISHING COMPANY
SAINT LOUIS, MISSOURI 63108

ANNALS OF OTOLOGY, RHINOLOGY AND LARYNGOLOGY

ANNALS OF HEAD AND NECK MEDICINE AND SURGERY

VOL. 90 JANUARY-FEBRUARY 1981 NO. 1

CONTENTS

PART I

Editorial 1

Adductor Spastic Dysphonia: 1½ Years after Recurrent Laryngeal Nerve Resection. A.E. Aronson, PhD; L.W. DeSanto, MD 2

Influence of Adenoid Hypertrophy on Secretory Otitis Media. H.H. Elverland, MD; I.W.S. Mair, MD, FRCSG; O.K. Haugeto, MD; K.E. Schrøder, MD 7

Reciprocal Synapses at the Base of Outer Hair Cells in the Organ of Corti of Man. J.B. Nadol, Jr., MD 12

Vasculature of the Anterior Commissure. M. Andrea, MD 18

Electronystagmography in Congenital and Acquired Syphilitic Otitis. W.R. Wilson, MD; M. Zoller, MD 21

Elemental Composition of the Developing Inner Ear. M. Anniko, MD; R. Wroblewski, PhD 25

Quantitative Histology of the Mucous Membrane of the Accessory Nasal Sinus and Mastoid Cavities. M.J. Harris, PhD; R.A. Schlenker, PhD 33

Protease Inhibitors in Middle Ear Effusions. B. Carlsson, MD; C. Lundberg, MD; K. Ohlsson, MD 38

Carcinoid Tumor of the Larynx. B. Gapany-Gapanavicius, MD, DSc; S. Kenan, MD 42

Effect of Voice Therapy on Contact Granuloma of the Vocal Fold. C.S. Bloch, MA; W.J. Gould, MD; M. Hirano, MD 48

Chondrosarcoma at the Skull Base. I. Gay, MD; J. Elidan, MD; J. Kopolovic, MD 53

Study of Ventilation Testing with Electronystagmography. W.R. Wilson, MD; J.W. Kim, MD 56

Familial Multiple Glomus Tumors and Pheochromocytomas. J. L. Parkin, MD, MS 60

Parotolymphatic Backflow: A New Sign of Malignancy. P.M. Som, MD; J.M.A. Shugar, MD 64

Aberrant Internal Carotid Artery in the Middle Ear. R.S. Goodman, MD; N.L. Cohen, MD 67

Use of the CO_2 Laser in Otology. D.J. Williams, MB, FRACS; I.M. Hunter-Duvar, PhD; D.P. Mitchell, MD 70

Pneumococcal Otitis Media Following Middle Ear Deflation. W.L. Meyerhoff, MD, PhD; G.S. Giebink, MD; D. Shea, MD 72

Idiopathic Endolymphatic Hydrops and the Vestibular Aqueduct. S.S. Rizvi, MD, FRCS; L.E. Smith, MD 77

Temporal Bone Findings in a Patient with Möbius Syndrome. H. Saito, MD; S. Kishimoto, MD; M. Furuta, MD 80

Eye-Head Coordination during Optokinetic Stimulation in Squirrel Monkeys. T. Kubo, MD; M. Igarashi, MD; D.W. Jensen, PhD; J.L. Homick, PhD 85

Objective Evaluation of Earplugs for the Control of Water-Borne Infection. D.W. Johnson, MS, MA; R.H. Maisel, MD 89

Book Reviews 94

Programs: Combined Otolaryngological Spring Meetings
- American Broncho-Esophagological Association 95
- American Laryngological Association 95
- American Laryngological, Rhinological and Otological Society, Inc. 96
- American Otological Society, Inc. 96

Program: Combined Meeting
- Society for Head and Neck Surgeons and American Society for Head and Neck Surgery 98

Index to Advertisers xxvi

PART II

Second Louis H. Clerf Lecture. Vestibular Neuritis. H.F. Schuknecht, MD; K. Kitamura, MD .... Supplement 78

PART III

Measurement of Optokinetic Nystagmus for Otoneurological Diagnosis. S.M. Abel, PhD; H.O. Barber, MD, FRCS(C) ..... Supplement 79

PART IV

Tumors of the Parapharyngeal Space. Preoperative Evaluation, Diagnosis and Surgical Approaches. P.M. Som, MD; H.F. Biller, MD; W. Lawson, MD ..... Supplement 80

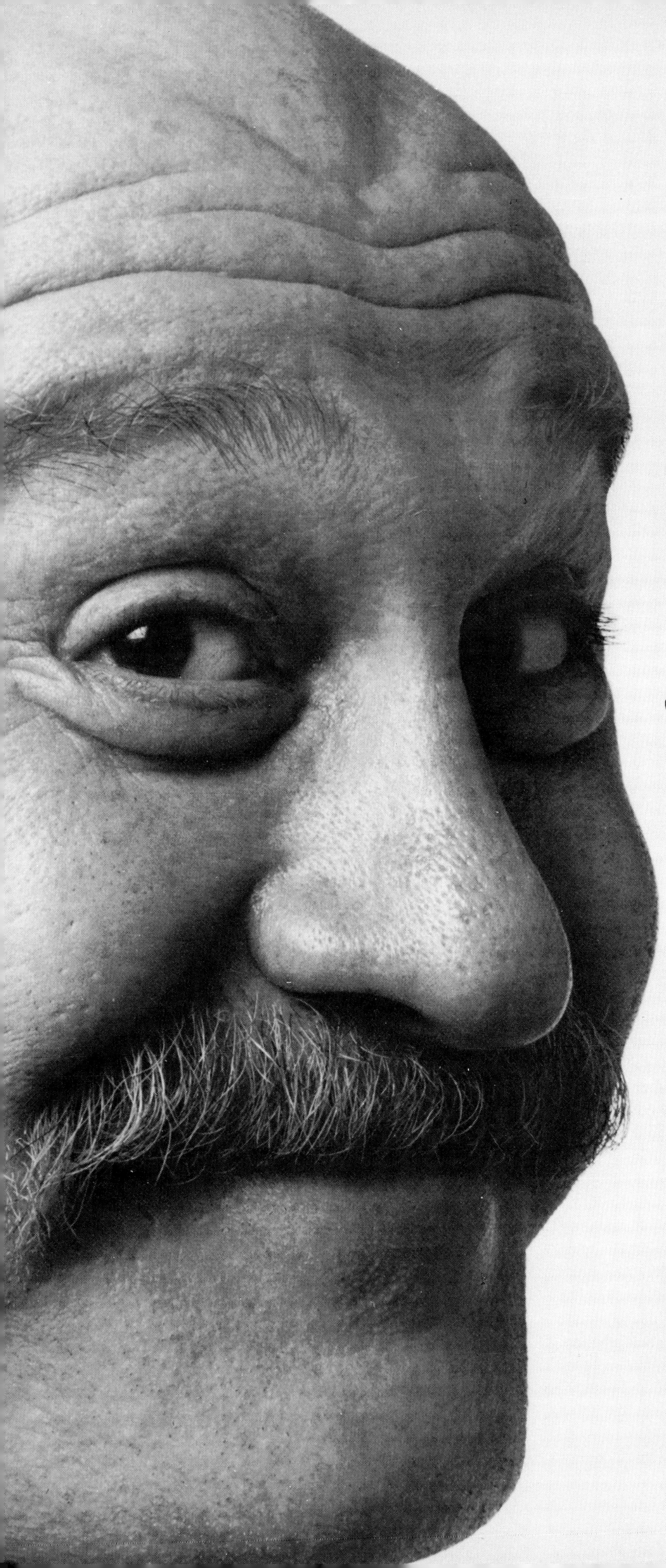

ANNALS OF OTOLOGY, RHINOLOGY AND LARYNGOLOGY
ANNALS OF HEAD AND NECK MEDICINE AND SURGERY
VOL. 90 MARCH-APRIL 1981 NO. 2

CONTENTS

PART I

Leaking Labyrinth Lesions, Deafness, Tinnitus and Dizziness. V. Goodhill, MD, FACS ... 99

Radiation-Associated Carcinoma of Salivary Glands. A Controlled Study. H.R. Maxon, MD; E.L. Saenger, MD; C.R. Buncher, ScD; S.R. Thomas, PhD; J.G. Kereiakes, PhD; M.L. Shafer, RN; C.A. McLaughlin ... 107

Temporal Bone Histopathology of Necrotizing External Otitis. A Case Report. I. Sando, MD, DMS; T. Harada, MD; Y. Okano, MD; R. Saito, MD; R.J. Caparosa, MD ... 109

Prosthetic Vocal Rehabilitation Following Laryngectomy. The Voice Button. W.R. Panje, MD ... 116

Quantitative Study of Scarpa's Ganglion and Vestibular Sense Organs in Endolymphatic Hydrops. E. Richter, MD ... 121

Ultrasonic Analysis of Head and Neck Neoplasms. Correlation with Surgical Findings. S.R. Baker, MD; C.J. Krause, MD ... 126

Complications of CO_2 Laser Surgery of the Larynx. A. Meyers, MD, FACS ... 132

Nature of Blood-Labyrinth Barrier in Experimental Conditions. S.K. Juhn, MD; L.P. Rybak, MD, PhD; S. Prado, MD, PhD ... 135

Medical Management of Menière's Disease. C.G. Jackson, MD; M.E. Glasscock III, MD, FACS; W.E. Davis, MD, FACS; G.B. Hughes, MD; A. Sismanis, MD ... 142

Lysosomal Hydrolases in Middle Ear Effusions. W.F. Diven, PhD; R.H. Glew, PhD; C.D. Bluestone, MD ... 148

Eye-Head Coordination and Lateral Canal Block in Squirrel Monkeys. T. Kubo, MD; M. Igarashi, MD; D.W. Jensen, PhD; W.K. Wright, MD ... 154

Efferent Innervation of the Cochlea. J. Strutz, MD ... 158

Sarcoidosis and Fluctuating Hearing Loss. R.A. Jahrsdoerfer, MD; E.G. Thompson, MD; M.M.E. Johns, MD; R.W. Cantrell, MD ... 161

Velocity of Rapid Eye Movements and Vertigo of Central Origin. I. Pyykkö, MD; N-G. Henriksson, MD; C. Wennmo, MD; L. Schalén ... 164

Myositis Ossificans Following Radical Neck Dissection. M.A. Shugar, MD; A.L. Weber, MD; T.J. Mulvaney, MD ... 169

Myringoplasty with Fascial Stakes. H. Rediano, MD; M. Englender, MD ... 172

Microfissure in the Oval Window Area. T. Harada, MD; I. Sando, MD, DMS; E.N. Myers, MD, FACS ... 174

Association of a Thyroglossal Duct Cyst and a Dermoid Cyst in the Neck. A Case Report. J.G. Haar, DDS, MD; E.J. Boulos, MD; M.H. Sadeghi, MD; J. Sheffer, MD ... 181

Perineural Metastases from Squamous Cell Carcinoma of the Face. Therapeutic Considerations. N. Green, MD; M. Landman, MD ... 183

Prehistoric Trephination of the Frontal Sinus. R.F. Canalis, MD; F. Cabieses, MD; W.G. Hemenway, MD; R. Aragon, MD ... 186

Pathology Consultation. Nasal (Schneiderian) Papillomas. J.G. Batsakis, MD ... 190

X-Ray of the Month. Pleomorphic Adenoma of the Hard Palate. A.L. Weber, MD ... 192

ENG of the Month. Vestibulo-Ocular and Oculomotor Responses Following Brainstem Cerebrovascular Accident. P. Kileny, PhD; A.F. Wilson, MD ... 194

Information for Authors ... 197

Book Reviews ... 198

Index to Advertisers ... 198

PART II

Vitamin A-Induced Ear Malformations in Rats as a Model for Analysis of Atresia Auris Congenita. A Microsurgical and Histological Study. M. Weidenbecher, MD ... Supplement 81

PART III

Proceedings of the West Coast Cochlear Prosthesis Conference ... Supplement 82

ANNALS OF OTOLOGY, RHINOLOGY AND LARYNGOLOGY
ANNALS OF HEAD AND NECK MEDICINE AND SURGERY
VOL. 90 MAY-JUNE 1981 NO. 3

CONTENTS

PART I

Osteogenesis Imperfecta Tarda and Otosclerosis. A Temporal Bone Histopathology Report. I. Sando, MD, DMS; D. Myers, MD; T. Harada, MD; R. Hinojosa, MD; E. N. Myers, MD 199

Changes of Nasal Epithelial Cells and Mucus Layer After Challenge of Allergen. K. Watanabe, MD; I. Watanabe, MD 204

Ear Deformities Associated with the Klippel-Feil Syndrome. P. C. Windle-Taylor, FRCS; P. J. Emery, FRCS; P. D. Phelps, FRCS, FRCR 210

Total Laryngectomy with Tracheopharyngeal Fistula (Neoglottis). C. V. Calearo, MD; A. Caroggio, MD 217

Analysis of Factors Affecting Complications of Carotid Ligation. A. Konno, MD; K. Togawa, MD; K. Iizuka, MD 222

A Multiple-Channel Cochlear Implant: An Evaluation Using Nonsense Syllables. G. M. Clark, PhD, FRCS; Y. C. Tong, BE, PhD; L. F. Martin, BSc, DipAud; P. A. Busby, MA; R. C. Dowell, BSc, DipAud; P. M. Seligman, BE, PhD; J. F. Patrick, MSc 227

Wegener's Granulomatosis. Long-Term Results of Treatment. P. Illum, MD; K. Thorling, MD 231

Auditory Brainstem and Middle Latency Evoked Response Sensitivity Near Threshold. F. E. Musiek, PhD; N. A. Geurkink, MD 236

Compensatory Eye Movement and Gaze Fixation During Active Head Rotation in Patients with Labyrinthine Disorders. M. Takahashi, MD; T. Uemura, MD; T. Fujishiro, MD 241

In Vitro Cultivation of the Fetal Guinea Pig Inner Ear. G. L. Davis, MD; M. M. Hawrisiak, ScM 246

Alternaria Sinusitis. M. A. Shugar, MD; W. W. Montgomery, MD; N. E. Hyslop, Jr., MD 251

Ototoxicity of Intracisternal Gentamicin in Cats. K. L. Parrish, PhD; M. Tachibana, MD, PhD; F. R. Domer, PhD; C. H. Norris, PhD; P. S. Guth, PhD 255

Aerobic and Anaerobic Bacteria in Tonsils of Children with Recurrent Tonsillitis. I. Brook, MD, MS; P. Yocum, BS; E. M. Friedman, MD 261

Effect of Increased Perilymphatic Pressure on Endocochlear Potential. T. Nakashima, MD; A. Ito, MD 264

Common Migraine and Vestibular Function. Electronystagmographic Study and Pathogenesis. J. U. Toglia, MD; D. Thomas, DO, PhD; A. Kuritzky, MD 267

Discrimination of Purulent from Nonpurulent Maxillary Sinusitis. Clinical and Radiographic Diagnosis. O. Berg, MD; H. Bergstedt, MD; C. Carenfelt, MD; M. G. Lind, MD; O. Perols, MD 272

New Neurotological Test for Detecting Cerebellar Dysfunction. Vestibulo-Ocular Reflex Changes with Horizontal Vision-Reversal Prisms. T. Yagi, MD; M. Shimizu, MD; S. Sekine, MD; T. Kamio, MD 276

Chronic Effects of Phasic Middle Ear Pressure Changes. J. M. Miller, PhD; A. Axelsson, MD; W. Potter, BA 281

Customized Dilator for the Treatment of Subglottic Stenosis in Children. N. R. T. Pashley, MB, FRCS(C) 287

Otolaryngic Osteopathology in 14th Century Mid-America. The Crow Creek Massacre. J. B. Gregg, MD; J. P. Steele, MD; L. Zimmerman, PhD; H. Ferwerda, RTR; P. S. Gregg, RN 288

Surgical and Radiological Effects upon the Development of Speech after Total Laryngectomy. J. L. Richardson, DrPH 294

Obituary. Sir Alexander Ewing 298

Letters to the Editor 299

Book Reviews 300

Index to Advertisers xxiv

PART II

Upper Respiratory Tract Ciliary Ultrastructural Pathology. F. S. Herzon, MD .... Supplement 83

PART III

Recent Advances in Antimicrobial Therapy for Infections of the Ear, Nose, and Throat—Head and Neck .. Supplement 84

ANNALS OF OTOLOGY, RHINOLOGY AND LARYNGOLOGY

ANNALS OF HEAD AND NECK MEDICINE AND SURGERY

VOL. 90 — MAY-JUNE 1981 — NO. 3

CONTENTS

PART I

Osteogenesis Imperfecta Tarda and Otosclerosis. A Temporal Bone Histopathology Report. I. Sando, MD, DMS; D. Myers, MD; T. Harada, MD; R. Hinojosa, MD; E. N. Myers, MD 199

Changes of Nasal Epithelial Cells and Mucus Layer After Challenge of Allergen. K. Watanabe, MD; I. Watanabe, MD 204

Ear Deformities Associated with the Klippel-Feil Syndrome. P. C. Windle-Taylor, FRCS; P. J. Emery, FRCS; P. D. Phelps, FRCS, FRCR 210

Total Laryngectomy with Tracheopharyngeal Fistula (Neoglottis). C. V. Calearo, MD; A. Caroggio, MD 217

Analysis of Factors Affecting Complications of Carotid Ligation. A. Konno, MD; K. Togawa, MD; K. Iizuka, MD 222

A Multiple-Channel Cochlear Implant: An Evaluation Using Nonsense Syllables. G. M. Clark, PhD, FRCS; Y. C. Tong, BE, PhD; L. F. Martin, BSc, DipAud; P. A. Busby, MA; R. C. Dowell, BSc, DipAud; P. M. Seligman, BE, PhD; J. F. Patrick, MSc 227

Wegener's Granulomatosis. Long-Term Results of Treatment. P. Illum, MD; K. Thorling, MD 231

Auditory Brainstem and Middle Latency Evoked Response Sensitivity Near Threshold. F. E. Musiek, PhD; N. A. Geurkink, MD 236

Compensatory Eye Movement and Gaze Fixation During Active Head Rotation in Patients with Labyrinthine Disorders. M. Takahashi, MD; T. Uemura, MD; T. Fujishiro, MD 241

In Vitro Cultivation of the Fetal Guinea Pig Inner Ear. G. L. Davis, MD; M. M. Hawrisiak, ScM 246

Alternaria Sinusitis. M. A. Shugar, MD; W. W. Montgomery, MD; N. E. Hyslop, Jr., MD 251

Ototoxicity of Intracisternal Gentamicin in Cats. K. L. Parrish, PhD; M. Tachibana, MD, PhD; F. R. Domer, PhD; C. H. Norris, PhD; P. S. Guth, PhD 255

Aerobic and Anaerobic Bacteria in Tonsils of Children with Recurrent Tonsillitis. I. Brook, MD, MS; P. Yocum, BS; E. M. Friedman, MD 261

Effect of Increased Perilymphatic Pressure on Endocochlear Potential. T. Nakashima, MD; A. Ito, MD 264

Common Migraine and Vestibular Function. Electronystagmographic Study and Pathogenesis. J. U. Toglia, MD; D. Thomas, DO, PhD; A. Kuritzky, MD 267

Discrimination of Purulent from Nonpurulent Maxillary Sinusitis. Clinical and Radiographic Diagnosis. O. Berg, MD; H. Bergstedt, MD; C. Carenfelt, MD; M. G. Lind, MD; O. Perols, MD 272

New Neurotological Test for Detecting Cerebellar Dysfunction. Vestibulo-Ocular Reflex Changes with Horizontal Vision-Reversal Prisms. T. Yagi, MD; M. Shimizu, MD; S. Sekine, MD; T. Kamio, MD 276

Chronic Effects of Phasic Middle Ear Pressure Changes. J. M. Miller, PhD; A. Axelsson, MD; W. Potter, BA 281

Customized Dilator for the Treatment of Subglottic Stenosis in Children. N. R. T. Pashley, MB, FRCS(C) 287

Otolaryngic Osteopathology in 14th Century Mid-America. The Crow Creek Massacre. J. B. Gregg, MD; J. P. Steele, MD; L. Zimmerman, PhD; H. Ferwerda, RTR; P. S. Gregg, RN 288

Surgical and Radiological Effects upon the Development of Speech after Total Laryngectomy. J. L. Richardson, DrPH 294

Obituary. Sir Alexander Ewing 298

Letters to the Editor 299

Book Reviews 300

Index to Advertisers xxiv

PART II

Upper Respiratory Tract Ciliary Ultrastructural Pathology. F. S. Herzon, MD . . . . Supplement 83

PART III

Recent Advances in Antimicrobial Therapy for Infections of the Ear, Nose, and Throat—Head and Neck . . Supplement 84

Bactrim™ succeeds
...even where

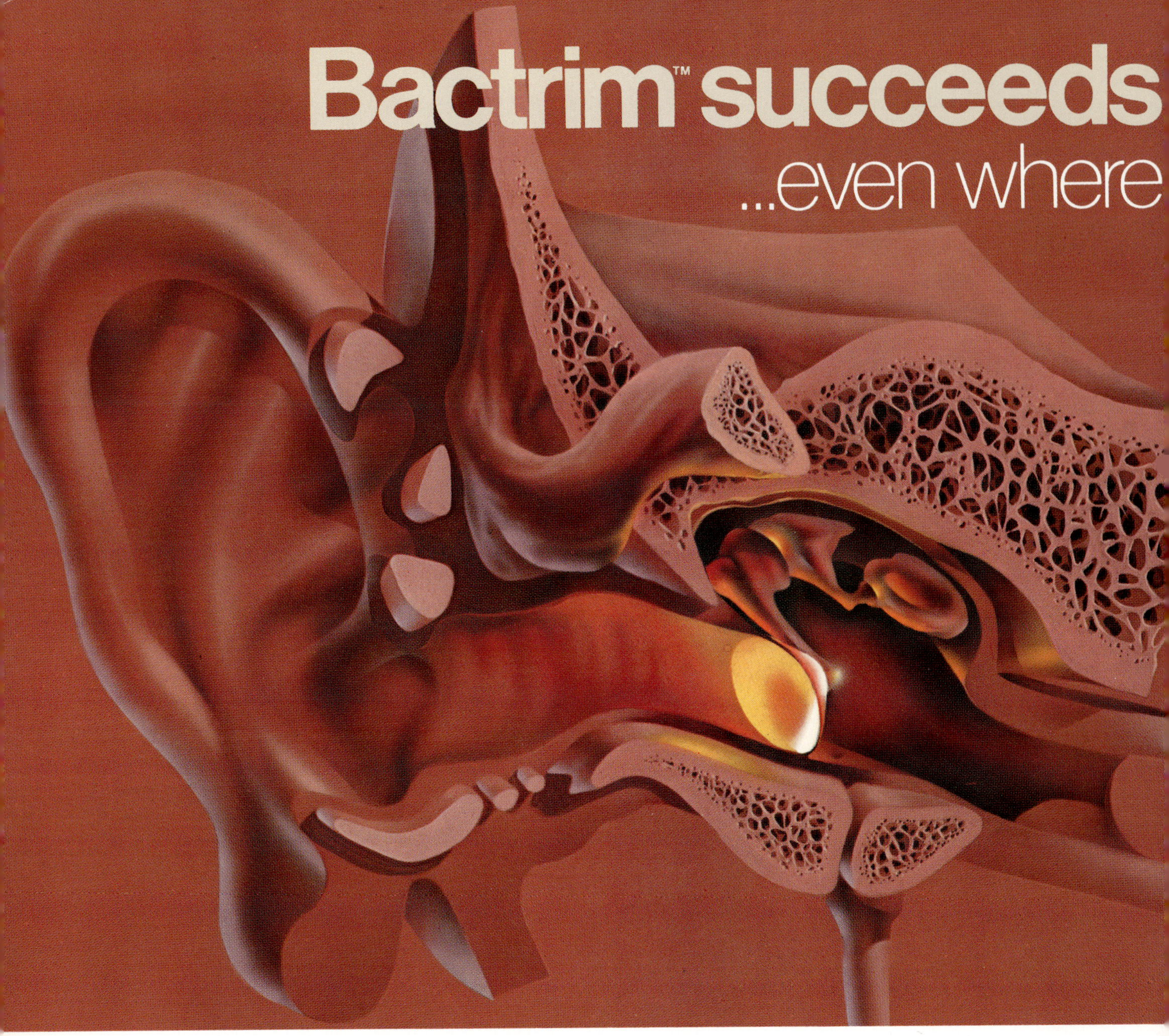

OTOSCOPIC VIEW

Tympanic membrane after 10 days of ampicillin therapy, 9/14/79	Same patient after 10 days of BACTRIM therapy, 9/24/79
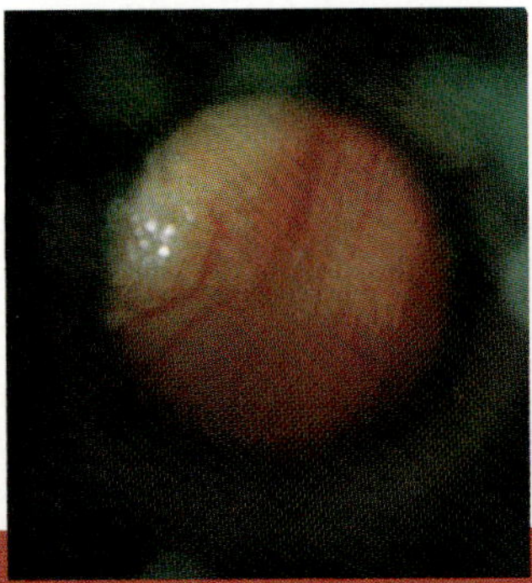	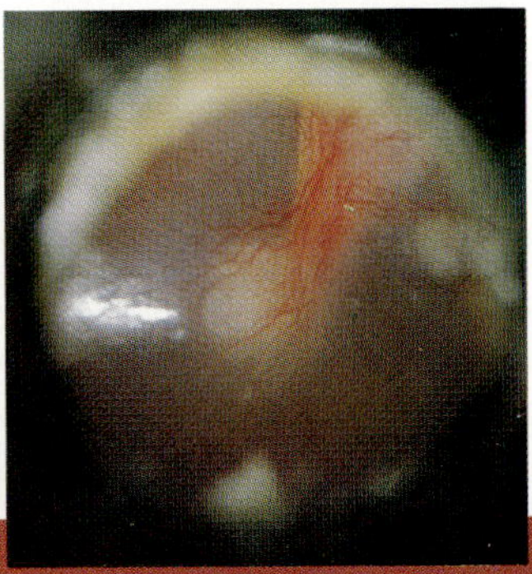

Five-year-old female presented on 9/4/79 with acute otitis media, pain, but no fever. Treated with ampicillin 250 mg P.O. *q.i.d.* On 9/14/79 tympanic membrane still bulging and yellow; no fever or pain but decreased energy and appetite. Bioassay to confirm compliance was positive for ampicillin. Case was considered an ampicillin treatment failure. Deep nasopharyngeal culture revealed heavy growth of *H. influenzae* resistant to ampicillin by disc sensitivity and beta-lactamase tests. On 9/14 therapy switched to Bactrim Pediatric Suspension 1½ teaspoonfuls (7.5 ml) *b.i.d.* Tympanic membrane no longer bulging by 9/18; movable, with normal architecture, on 9/24.

ANNALS OF OTOLOGY, RHINOLOGY AND LARYNGOLOGY
ANNALS OF HEAD AND NECK MEDICINE AND SURGERY
VOL. 90 JULY-AUGUST 1981 NO. 4

CONTENTS

PART I

Tracheomalacia in an with Infant Multiplex Congenita (Larsen's) Syndrome. K. M. Grundfast, MD; A. Mumtaz, MD; R. Kanter, MD; M. Pollack, MD 303

Flexible Fiberoptic Endoscopy in Difficult Intubations. E. T. Edens, MD; R. L. Sia, MD 307

Carbon Dioxide Laser Treatment of Metastatic Melanoma of the Trachea and Bronchi. A. H. Andrews, Jr., MD; D. D. Caldarelli, MD 310

Sputum Cytologic Diagnosis of Upper Respiratory Tract Cancer. Second Report. H. B. Neel III, MD, PhD; D. R. Sanderson, MD; R. S. Fontana, MD; W. F. Taylor, MD; L. B. Woolner, MD 312

Unusual Presentations and Problems Created by Mismanagement of Foreign Bodies in the Aerodigestive Tract of the Pediatric Patient. S. R. Cohen, MD 316

Esophageal and Hypopharyngeal Injuries in Patients with Cervical Spine Trauma. R. A. Pollock, MD; J. M. Purvis, MD; D. F. Apple, Jr., MD; H. H. Murray, MD 323

Incendiary Characteristics of Endotracheal Tubes with the Carbon Dioxide Laser. An Experimental Study. E. Treyve, MD; C. T. Yarington, Jr., MD; G. E. Thompson, MD 328

Effect of Total Laryngectomy on Esophageal Motility. J. B. Hanks, MD; S. R. Fisher, MD; W. C. Meyers, MD; K. C. Christian, BA; R. W. Postlethwait, MD; R. S. Jones, MD 331

Histopathology of Acquired Subglottic Stenosis. A Documented Case Report. G. F. Tucker, Jr., MD; L. Newton, MD; R. J. Ruben, MD 335

Endoscopic Findings in Sarcoidosis. Characteristics and Correlations with Radiographic Staging and Bronchial Mucosal Biopsy Yield. J. R. Armstrong, MD; J. R. Radke, MD; P. A. Kvale, MD; M. S. Eichenhorn, MD; J. Popovich, Jr., MD 339

A New Universal Bivalved Speculum Direct Laryngoscope. G. Berci, MD; P. H. Ward, MD 344

Video Laryngoscopy Using a Rigid Telescope and Video Home System Color Camera. A Useful Office Procedure. E. Yanagisawa, MD; J. R. Casuccio, MD; M. Suzuki, MD 346

Flexible Fiberoptic Bronchoscopy and Pulmonary Cytology in the Evaluation of Patients with Head and Neck Malignancies. T. J. Garfinkle, MD; R. A. Weisman, MD; J. C. Denneny III, MD 351

Bronchoscopic Cryotherapy. D. R. Sanderson, MD; H. B. Neel III, MD, PhD; R. S. Fontana, MD 354

Esophageal Cancer Research in the People's Republic of China. W. Huan-Hsing, MD, DMR 359

Congenital Tracheal Stenosis. B. Benjamin, FRACS; J. Pitkin, FRACS, FRCS; D. Cohen, MS, FRACS 364

Surgical Repair in Hypopharyngeal and Cervical Esophageal Cancer. Analysis of 162 Patients. D. F. N. Harrison, MD, MS 372

Endoscopy in Esophageal Atresia and Tracheoesophageal Fistula. B. Benjamin, FRACS 376

Abnormal Esophageal Manometry in Globus Hystericus. T. C. Flores, MD; R. S. Cross, MD, PhD; R. D. Jones, PhD 383

Esophageal Hiatal Hernia in Infants and Children. B. Fearon, MD; I. Brama, MD 387

Duplication of the Esophagus. D. O. Mikaelian, MD; J. J. O'Keefe, MD; S. Simonian, MD 392

Horseradish Peroxidase Studies in Animals with Neuromuscular Transpositions. G. D. Neal, MD; G. Duncan, BS; D. Sutton, PhD; C. W. Cummings, MD 396

Use of Videotape in Diagnosis and Treatment of Cancer of the Larynx. H. R. Konrad, MD; D. M. Hopla, MD; J. Bussen; F. C. Griswold 398

Management of Laryngotracheoesophageal Cleft. R. T. Cotton, MD; J. T. Schreiber, MD 401

Grassheads in the Tracheobronchial Tree: Two Different Outcomes. M. J. Spencer, MD; V. E. Millet, MD; J. P. Dudley, MD; J. L. Sherrod, MD; Y. J. Bryson, MD 406

Epiglottic Laryngoplasty for Complicated Laryngeal Stenosis. S. M. Sobol, MD; H. Levine, MD; B. Wood, MD; H. M. Tucker, MD 409

Book Reviews 412

Index to Advertisers xxxiv

PART II

Labyrinthine Segment and Geniculate Ganglion of Facial Nerve in Fetal and Adult Human Temporal Bones. Xian-Xi Ge, MD; G. J. Spector, MD ..... Supplement 85

PART III

Proceedings of the Seminar on Sinusoidal Harmonic Acceleration and Computerized Optokinetic Tracking Tests ..... Supplement 86

ANNALS OF OTOLOGY, RHINOLOGY AND LARYNGOLOGY

ANNALS OF HEAD AND NECK MEDICINE AND SURGERY

VOL. 90 SEPTEMBER-OCTOBER 1981 NO. 5

CONTENTS

PART I

Surgical Approach to the Medial Orbital Wall. D. F. N. Harrison, MD 415

Juvenile Nasopharyngeal Fibroma. R. Tapia Acuña, MD 420

Histochemical Characteristics of Muscle Fiber Types in the Posterior Cricoarytenoid Muscle. L. T. Malmgren, PhD; R. R. Gacek, MD 423

Observations on Central Neurologic Etiology for Laryngeal Dysfunction. P. H. Ward, MD; D. G. Hanson, MD; G. Berci, MD 430

Treatment of Carcinoma of the Epiglottis. J. B. Nadol, Jr., MD 442

Hypothyroidism following Treatment for Head and Neck Cancer. D. P. Vrabec, MD; T. J. Heffron, MD 449

Significance of Positive Bronchial Cytology in Presence of Squamous Cell Carcinoma of Upper Aerodigestive Tract. J. T. Johnson, MD; J. Turner, MD; A. Dekker, MD; E. N. Myers, MD, FACS 454

Laryngeal Reinnervation for Unilateral Vocal Cord Paralysis: Long-term Results. H. M. Tucker, MD; M. Rusnov, MA 457

Panendoscopy for Second Primaries in Head and Neck Cancer. R. H. Maisel, MD; H. Vermeersch, MD 460

Laryngeal Complications of Nasogastric Tubes. R. A. Sofferman, MD; R. N. Hubbell, MD 465

Laryngeal Injuries Secondary to Nasogastric Tubes. M. Friedman, MD; H. Baim, MD; V. Shelton, MD; M. Stobnicki, MD; T. Chilis, MD; T. Ferrara, MD; E. Skolnik, MD 469

Anesthesia for Laryngeal Laser Surgery in the Infant and Child. W. M. Brummitt, MD; B. Fearon, MD; I. Brama, MD 475

Documentation in Pediatric Laryngology. B. Benjamin, FRACS 478

Pseudolaryngeal Paralysis: A Postintubation Complication. S. R. Cohen, MD 483

Bilateral Vertical Partial Laryngectomy for Bilateral Vocal Cord Carcinoma. H. F. Biller, MD; W. Lawson, DDS, MD 489

Tracheoesophageal Puncture for Alaryngeal Voice Restoration. B. G. Wood, MD; M. G. Rusnov, MA; H. M. Tucker, MD; H. L. Levine, MD 492

Limitations of the Blom-Singer Technique for Voice Restoration. J. O. Donegan, MD; J. L. Gluckman, MD; J. Singh, MD 495

Further Experience with Voice Restoration after Total Laryngectomy. M. I. Singer, MD; E. D. Blom, PhD; R. C. Hamaker, MD 498

Voice Button Prosthesis Rehabilitation of the Laryngectomee. Additional Notes. W. R. Panje, MD; D. VanDemark, PhD; B. F. McCabe, MD 503

Role of Chemotherapy in the Multidisciplinary Approach to Advanced Head and Neck Cancer: Potentials and Problems. T. J. Ervin, MD; D. D. Karp, MD; R. R. Weichselbaum, MD; M. R. Posner, MD; R. L. Fabian, MD; D. Miller, MD 506

Treatment of Laryngeal Stenosis. A Conservative New Approach. S. A. Peerless, MD; H. R. Pillsbury III, MD; A. G. Peerless, MD 512

Laryngotracheal Reconstruction in Children. Five-year Follow-up. R. T. Cotton, FRCS(C), FACS; J. N. G. Evans, FRCS 516

Books Received 521

X-Ray Study of the Month. Laryngeal Cyst. N. C. Goldman, MD 522

ENG of the Month. Periodic Alternating Nystagmus. R. W. Babin, MD 524

Index to Advertisers xxxvii

Information for Authors .... See March-April 1981 issue, p. 197

PART II

Third Louis H. Clerf Lecture. Legacies of Jefferson Men to Japanese Medicine. J. Ono, MD .... Supplement 87

ANNALS OF OTOLOGY, RHINOLOGY AND LARYNGOLOGY

ANNALS OF HEAD AND NECK MEDICINE AND SURGERY

VOL. 90 NOVEMBER-DECEMBER 1981 NO. 6

CONTENTS

PART I

Otology in Today's Medical Setting. H.F. Schuknecht, MD 527

Panel on Experiences with Middle Ear Ventilating Tubes 529
 Tympanostomy Tubes: The Conservative Approach. R.F. Naunton, MD
 Chronic Nonsuppurative Otitis Media. Comparison of Tympanostomy Tubes and Medication with Ventilation. B.W. Armstrong, MD; R.B. Armstrong, MD
 Comment. R.J. Caparosa, MD

Use of Tympanostomy Tubes in Otitis Media. W.L. Meyerhoff, MD, PhD 537

Auditory Processing Abilities in Children with Previous Middle Ear Effusion. K. Hoffman-Lawless, MA; R.W. Keith, PhD; R.T. Cotton, MD 543

Recurrent Middle Ear Effusion in Childhood: Implications of Temporary Auditory Deprivation for Language and Learning. R.J. Sak, MA; R.J. Ruben, MD 546

Panel on Experiences with Testing Eustachian Tube Function 552
 Current Clinical Methods, Indications and Interpretation of Eustachian Tube Function Tests. C.D. Bluestone, MD; E.I. Cantekin, PhD
 Testing Eustachian Tube Function. J.L. Sheehy, MD
 Comment. J. Jerger, PhD

Neural Connections Between the Middle Ear, Eustachian Tube and Brain. Implications for the Reflex Control of Middle Ear Aeration. A.R. Eden, MD 566

Panel on Treatment of Bell's Palsy 570
 Early Decompression of the Facial Nerve in Bell's Palsy. J. L. Pulec, MD
 Pathomechanisms in Cell Metabolism: A Key to Treatment of Bell's Palsy. E. Stennert, MD
 Comment. R.R. Gacek, MD

Total Energy and Critical Intensity Concepts in Noise Damage. W.D. Ward, PhD; P.A. Santi, PhD; A.J. Duvall III, MD; C.W. Turner, MS 584

Neural Generators of Brainstem Evoked Potentials. Results from Human Intracranial Recordings. A.R. Møller, PhD; P.J. Jannetta, MD; M.B. Møller, MD, PhD 591

Panel on Tinnitus Control 597
 Management of the Tinnitus Patient. J.W. House, MD
 Medical Treatment of Tinnitus. J.J. Shea, MD; J.R. Emmett, MD; D.J. Orchik, PhD; K. Mays, MD; W. Webb, MD
 Comment. V. Goodhill, MD, FACS

Panel on Menière's Disease 610
 Endolymphatic Sac Enhancement Surgery for Menière's Disease. An Extension of Conservative Therapy. M.M. Paparella, MD; M. Goycoolea, PhD, MD
 Metabolic Management in Menière's Disease. B. Proctor, MD; C. Proctor, MD
 Comment. H. Schuknecht, MD

Endolymphatic Duct Obstruction from a Jugular Bulb Diverticulum. R.A. Jahrsdoerfer, MD; W.S. Cail, MD; R.W. Cantrell, MD 619

Central Vestibular Signs, Posterior Fossa Pathology and Computerized Tomography-Regional Blood Brain Circulation. A. Kumar, MD, FRCS; N. Torok, MD; G. Valvassori, MD 624

Panel on Stapes Surgery 630
 Total Footplate Extraction in Stapedectomy. M. Robinson, MD
 Comparison of Small Fenestra and Total Stapedectomy. T.M. McGee, MD
 Contraindications to the Small Hole Stapedectomy. B. Farrior, MD

Bioinert Ceramic Implants in Middle Ear Surgery. K. Jahnke, MD; D. Plester, MD 640

Comparative Study Using Computed Tomographic Thin-Section Zoom Reconstructions and Anatomic Macrosections of the Temporal Bone. C.W. Beatty, MD; K.W. Suh, MD; L. D. Harris, PhD; D.F. Reese, MD 643

Author Index 650

Subject Index 652

Information to Authors xx

Statement of Ownership 656

Index to Advertisers xlii

PART II

Development of the Hypotympanum in the Human Fetus and Neonate. G.J. Spector, MD; Xian-Xi Ge, MD ..... Supplement 88

EDITORIAL

The publishers, editors and staff of the ANNALS hope that you like the new format and have found the larger size page and new typography pleasing. During the past year we began to utilize the newest advances in computerized photocomposition to produce our journal and have had a great deal to learn. The changes in ANNALS size and the new technology produce a more readable page, clearly delineated illustrations, and in addition, allow us to publish more papers in each issue.

In keeping with the present thinking of a majority of the members of our specialty, the ANNALS OF OTOLOGY, RHINOLOGY AND LARYNGOLOGY has acquired a subtitle, ie, the ANNALS OF HEAD AND NECK MEDICINE AND SURGERY. The ANNALS Editors are desirous of remaining responsive to the needs of the members of our profession. As otolaryngology expands its horizons so shall the ANNALS.

With this first issue of the year we welcome to the Board of Editors I. Sando, MD, Pittsburgh; A.J. Duvall III, MD, Minneapolis; and S.K. Juhn, MD, Minneapolis. We thank L.W. Pratt, MD, Waterville and J.M. Frederickson, MD, Canada, for their past help and guidance; we are pleased that they have agreed to be part of the Emeritus Board. We look forward to continued productive interaction with members of both the Board of Editors and the Emeritus Board.

The ANNALS supplement program has been expanding, and in 1980 we published 13 supplements with a total of 782 pages. Our supplement program makes it possible to publish papers which are too long for inclusion in the conventional issue; it also allows for quicker publication, since the preparation of a single supplement can be performed at varied and unpredictable work intervals which occur in our printing schedule.

We are grateful to the many clinicians, investigators and teachers of otolaryngology throughout the world who entrust us with the publication and distribution of their manuscripts. We appreciate every subscriber without whom the ANNALS would lose its reason for being. We pray that such intelligent interaction and understanding will bring us all closer together and in some way will contribute to making a happier and more peaceful world.

Ben H. Senturia, MD
Brian F. McCabe, MD

Ann Otol 90:1981

ADDUCTOR SPASTIC DYSPHONIA: 1 1/2 YEARS AFTER RECURRENT LARYNGEAL NERVE RESECTION

ARNOLD E. ARONSON, PhD LAWRENCE W. DESANTO, MD

ROCHESTER, MINNESOTA

After recurrent laryngeal nerve resection for adductor spastic dysphonia, the voices of 37 patients (ages 39 to 79 years) were assessed 24 hours, 1 month, 6 months, and 1 year after surgery, and those of 33 patients up to 1 1/2 years after surgery. By 24 hours after surgery, 97% of patients had improved and 3% had failed; by 1 month, 97% were still improved while 3% had failed; by 6 months, 92% had maintained improvement while 8% had failed; by 1 year, 68% were still improved but 32% had failed; and by 1 1/2 years, 61% were still improved while 39% had failed. The patients whose voices improved varied from one another in both type and degree of residual dysphonia. The typical postsurgical voice was free of spasm, with some breathiness, hoarseness, and reduced volume being present. The voices of some patients approached normalcy. To most patients, relief from the physical effort to phonate was as important as the improved voice. Continued long-term follow-up studies and careful, collaborative selection of surgical candidates are needed.

Adductor spastic dysphonia is a strained, hoarse, groaning, effortful, or staccato voice without other physical signs or symptoms. The dysphonia results from hyperadduction of the true and false vocal folds and laryngeal elevation, reminiscent of involuntary effort closure of the larynx, during volitional speech. The disorder most often starts during the fourth decade of life and is more frequently seen in females. Once the spasms occur, they tenaciously persist, resisting psychotherapy, voice therapy, drug therapy, hypnosis, relaxation techniques, or biofeedback. What begins as a mild, strained hoarseness develops, as the months and years pass, into a more intensely strained voice. Severe, massive spasm of the true and false vocal folds can arrest phonation virtually completely. Sensitive to adverse listener reactions, these patients become withdrawn and depressed. Those who depend on their voices for a livelihood have to find other work. Severe spastic dysphonia can have catastrophic life consequences.

Spastic dysphonia may have more than one cause. One type is attributed to psychoneurosis, specifically, conversion reaction.[1] Recent evidence suggests that another type may be a sign of severe essential (voice) tremor[2,3] or of a focal laryngeal dystonia.[4] The peripheral nervous system also has been implicated. Histopathologic studies of recurrent laryngeal nerves by Dedo et al[5] and by Bocchino and Tucker[6] have noted demyelination of the recurrent laryngeal nerve, but Ravits et al[7] were unable to find any evidence of such demyelination.

From the first description of spastic dysphonia more than 100 years ago by Traube[8] until recently, no clinical or surgical specialty — laryngology, speech pathology, neurology, or psychiatry — was able to help the voice disorder. But Dedo[9] obtained immediate relief from the dysphonia in 34 patients after sectioning the right recurrent laryngeal nerve, thus paralyzing the corresponding vocal fold. Despite various degrees of postsurgical dysphonia, virtually all patients were well satisfied with the result and resumed more normal everyday communication.

Several hundred operations have been performed, with favorable results reported.[10,11] However, systematic studies at postsurgical intervals to determine the long-term fate of such patients are lacking. A longitudinal study was reported by Levine et al,[12] who noted immediate postsurgical success in 22 patients with spastic dysphonia. Improvement was defined as clear, unhalting speech with relief of spasmodic quality and improved ease of sound production. However, five patients (22%) had "some recurrence" of the disorder, one 4 months, one 7 months, one 8 months, one 11 months, and one 22 months after surgery. These five patients underwent ipsilateral superior laryngeal nerve division; two noted improvement, while three did not. Injection of Teflon® was done in one patient nine months after surgery because of persistent breathiness.

After crushing the left recurrent laryngeal nerve, Biller et al[13] noted satisfactory results in three of four patients; at 20 months in one patient, 29 months in another, and 30 months in the third. The spastic dysphonia of the fourth patient had returned within six months after surgery.

The present study was done to determine 1) the percentage of patients who benefited from recurrent laryngeal nerve surgery at successive postsurgical intervals extending to 1 1/2 years after surgery, and 2) the pattern of postsurgical voice change with the passage of time. The study did not concern voice refinements; judgments were made on the basis of whether the voice as a whole was improved, remained the same, or worsened.

From the Mayo Clinic and Mayo Foundation, Rochester, Minnesota.

REPRINTS — Arnold E. Aronson, PhD, Mayo Clinic and Mayo Foundation, Rochester, MN 55901.

TABLE 1. POSTOPERATIVE VOICE STATUS OF PATIENTS WITH SPASTIC DYSPHONIA

Time Postop	Patients No.	Patients %
24 hr		
Better than preop	36	97
Same as preop	1	3*
1 mo		
Better than 24 hr postop	28	76
Same as 24 hr postop	7	18
Worse than 24 hr postop	1	3
Same as preop	1	3*
6 mo		
Better than 1 mo postop	6	16
Same as 1 mo postop	18	49
Worse than 1 mo postop	10	27
Same as preop	2	5*
Worse than preop	1	3*
1 yr		
Better than 6 mo postop	6	16
Same as 6 mo postop	9	25
Worse than 6 mo postop	10	27
Same as preop	7	19*
Worse than preop	5	13*
1 1/2 yr		
Better than 1 yr postop	4	12
Same as 1 yr postop	11	34
Worse than 1 yr postop	5	15
Same as preop	8	24*
Worse than preop	5	15*

*Total failed.

SUBJECTS

From 1976 through 1978, 61 patients were seen with severe adductor spastic dysphonia. All 61 underwent lidocaine injection of the right recurrent laryngeal nerve to predetermine their potential for surgery. Of this group, 17 patients did not undergo surgery because they or we were dissatisfied with the voice result from the injection. The remaining 44 underwent resection of the right recurrent laryngeal nerve. Of that group, 37 were followed for 1 year and 33 for 1 1/2 years.

Of the 37 patients, 11 (30%) were males, and 26 (70%) were females. The males had a mean age of 63 years and a range of 45 to 79 years, with a mean duration of their disorder of 10 years. The females had a mean age of 60 years and a range of 39 to 77 years, with a mean duration of their disorder of 7 years.

PROCEDURES

Audiotape and videotape recordings were made of each patient immediately before and 24 hours after surgery. Audiotape recordings were then received by mail from each patient 1 month, 6 months, 1 year, and 1 1/2 years after surgery. In each recording, the patient read a standard paragraph, sustained the vowed /a/, coughed as sharply as possible, sang up and down the scale, and subjectively evaluated his or her voice. No patient had had corrective laryngeal surgery or systematic postsurgical voice therapy.

The tape recordings were analyzed by the speech pathologist in the study (A.E.A.), who listened to the contextual speech portions at each presurgical and postsurgical interval and rated the voice as 1) improved, 2) the same, 3) worse, or 4) failed, as compared with the recording of the previous period. Improvement was defined as reduced severity of strained hoarseness, smoother voice flow, and fewer audible signs of phonatory struggle or effort. Worse was defined as an increase in the above parameters. Failed was defined as either no change from the presurgical recording, voice decline to the patient's presurgical level of spastic dysphonia, or worse. At 1 1/2 years after surgery, the patients were sent a questionnaire to sample their attitudes about the effects of surgery.

RESULTS

Twenty-four Hours After Surgery. Twenty-four hours after surgery, 36 (97%) patients had improved and 1 (3%) had failed (Table 1). The voice characteristics of the improved patients varied considerably in both degree of improvement and type. No patient's voice was normal, but a few of the patients had voices so mildly dysphonic that their voices approached normality. The most frequent voice quality defect at this stage was breathiness. Hoarseness and diplophonia were other findings. Severely breathy voices lacked tonal quality and were weak. A few of the patients had inspiratory stridor. Still others had voices that had an unprecedented high pitch.

These voice aberrations did not obscure the fact that all patients in the improved group had reduction or elimination of the presurgical strained hoarseness and all had smoother, more audible voices. All volunteered that they were relieved of the physical effort to phonate, and although they were aware that their voices were not normal, they preferred their postsurgical dysphonias to the spastic dysphonia. Our impression was that relief from the aggravating fatigue of phonation was at least as important as achievement of a more normal voice. The improved patients had a weaker than normal cough. All patients could sing up and down the scale without compromise of their pitch range.

Videotape recordings after surgery as compared with those before surgery disclosed a dramatic alteration in facial expression from a frowning and grimacing and depressive turning down at the angles of the mouth to the disappearance of these features and the assumption of a generally happier facial expression. In summary, the 24-hour postsurgical period was one of patient and clinician optimism, relief, and satisfaction.

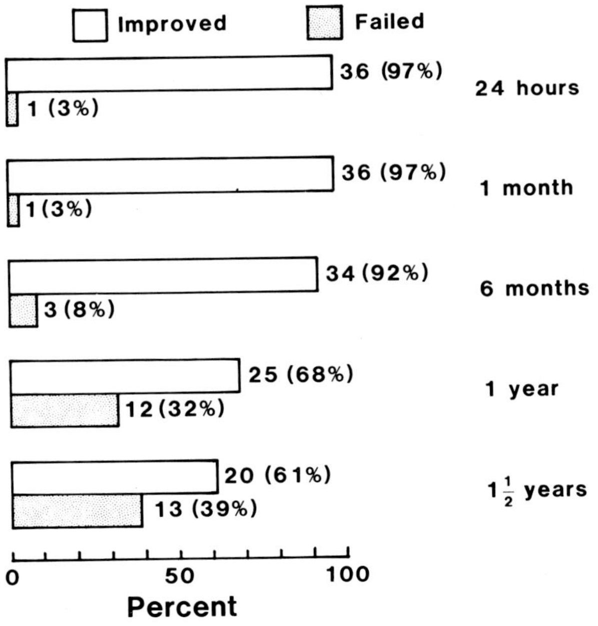

Fig. 1. Postsurgical voice status of patients with spastic dysphonia.

One Month After Surgery. One month after surgery, 28 (76%) patients had further voice improvement, compared with voice parameters noted at the 24-hour period, 7 (18%) remained the same, 1 (3%) had worsened, and 1 (3%) remained in the failed category (Table 1). The voice improvement in the 28 patients consisted of 1) reduced breathiness and more audible tonal or musical quality in patients who had predominantly breathy voices at the 24-hour period, 2) reduced strained hoarseness in those who had residual strained hoarseness, 3) lower pitch in those who had a noticeably high pitch or falsetto voice, 4) higher pitch in those who had an unusually low pitch, and 5) reduction or disappearance of falsetto pitch breaks and diplophonia.

The voice of the patient who had worsened since the 24-hour period changed from a mildly breathy, smoothly textured voice to a harsh, lower pitched and less tonal one.

In summary, the one-month postoperative period, similar to the 24-hour one, was marked by more patients with better voices than at any time in the study. Not only was 97% of the group improved from the surgery but 76% had better voices, as compared with voice quality in the previous period.

Six Months After Surgery. The first signs of group decline began at this period (Table 1). Although 6 (16%) patients had improved since the 1-month recheck, 18 (49%) had remained the same, and 10 (27%) had worsened. At this time, two (5%) had regressed to their presurgical status and one (3%) was worse than before surgery, for a total of 8% failure.

The voices of the six patients who had continued

TABLE 2. PATIENTS WITH SPASTIC DYSPHONIA WHO HAD RECURRENT LARYNGEAL NERVE RESECTION

	Females (N=26)	*Males (N=11)*
Age at surgery (yr)		
Mean	60	63
Range	39 to 77	45 to 79
Duration of dysphonia (yr)		
Mean	7	10
Range	1 to 24	2 to 43
Status at 1 1/2 yr follow-up		
No. failed	12 (46%)	2 (18%)
No. improved	14 (54%)	9 (82%)

to improve were less strained, hoarse, or stridorous; they were clearer and more tonal and had a better pitch level. The ten worsened voices were more strained, harsh, breathy, and lower pitched and had more falsetto pitch-breaks. The trend of the worsened group was toward return of the spastic dysphonia.

In summary, at the six-month postsurgical period, 92% of the group still had better voices than before surgery, but there was a trend toward return of the strained, harsh, spastic dysphonia quality. More patients were in the failed category, and for the first time, one patient had spastic dysphonia that was worse than before surgery.

One Year After Surgery. By one year, 6 (16%) patients had further improved, compared with the status at the six-month period, 9 (24%) had remained the same, and 10 (27%) were worse (Table 1). At this time, seven (19%) had regressed to their presurgical spastic dysphonia and five (14%) were worse than before surgery. In summary, by one year, 67% of the patients were still better than they were before surgery, although 27% had declined from their six-month levels and 33% had failed to their presurgical levels or worse.

One and One-Half Years After Surgery. Of the 33 patients with 1 1/2-year follow-up, 4 (12%) had further improvement over that seen at the one-year period, 11 (34%) were the same, and 5 (15%) were worse (Table 1). At this time, eight (24%) had returned to their presurgical spastic dysphonia and five (15%) were worse than before surgery. At 1 1/2 years after surgery, 61% were still improved from surgery and 39% had failed (Fig. 1). Females had a higher proportion of failures (46%) than did males (18%) (Table 2).

Questionnaire Results. Of the 33 patients 1 1/2 years after surgery, 27 (82%) considered themselves to be better than before surgery, although only 20 (61%) were judged to be so by the clinician; thus 7 patients misperceived their voice status as better than it was. None of the patients considered their voices to be worse than before surgery; this also was at variance with the clinician's judgment of five

(15%) patients whose voices were judged to be worse than before surgery.

Six (18%) patients reported that their voices were unimproved, 5 (15%) mildly improved, 15 (46%) moderately improved, and 7 (21%) greatly improved. None of the patients considered their voices to be normal.

Six (18%) patients reported that they were unimproved in their physical effort to phonate (the same patients who reported no voice improvement), 6 (18%) mildly improved, 13 (40%) moderately improved, 7 (21%) greatly improved, and 1 (3%) was normal.

In response to whether the sound of the voice or the physical ease of phonation was more important, 6 (18%) patients reported that the voice was more important, 4 (12%) reported that ease of phonation was more important, and 17 (52%) reported both were of equal importance. Six (18%) said neither had improved.

Patients were asked when, after surgery, they noticed voice improvement beyond the initial postsurgical improvement. Of 24 patients who reported such an increment, 16 (67%) said it had occurred between 1 and 3 months after surgery, 2 (8%) between 3 and 6 months after surgery, 3 (13%) between 6 and 9 months after surgery, 1 (4%) between 9 and 12 months after surgery, and 2 (8%) between 12 and 15 months after surgery.

Estimation of maximal voice improvement yielded the following results: of the 24 patients who responded, 5 (20%) said this point occurred between 1 and 3 months after surgery, 5 (20%) between 3 and 6 months, 3 (13%) between 6 and 9 months, 3 (13%) between 9 and 12 months, 5 (20%) between 12 and 15 months, and 3 (13%) between 15 and 18 months after surgery.

Of 12 patients who responded to the question about initial voice worsening, none said this occurred between 1 and 3 months, 6 (50%) reported worsening between 3 and 6 months, 1 (8%) between 6 and 9 months, 1 (8%) between 9 and 12 months, 1 (8%) between 12 and 15 months, and 3 (25%) between 15 and 18 months.

One (8%) of 12 patients said maximal voice worsening occurred between 3 and 6 months, 3 (25%) between 6 and 9 months, 1 (8%) between 9 and 12 months, 1 (8%) between 12 and 15 months, and 6 (50%) between 15 and 18 months.

Concerning the optimism and feeling of well-being after surgery, of the 33 patients responding, 25 (76%) described improvement, 8 (24%) said they felt the same; no patient reported feeling worse. Asked about the effects of the surgery on their social participation, 18 (55%) said they had become more socially active and 15 (45%) said no change had taken place. No patient became less socially active after the surgery.

TABLE 3. INCIDENCE OF TRANSIENT SIDE EFFECTS FROM SURGERY

Side Effect	*No. of Patients*
Feeling of tightness in throat	1
Sore throat	4
Shortness of breath	3
Choking on liquids and solids	5
Congestion on awakening	1
Difficulty in swallowing	6
Run out of air while speaking; inhale more often	1
Coughing spells	1
Dry throat	2
Lump in throat	1
Phlegm	2
Neck and chest pain	2

Asked if they would have the surgery again, 32 (97%) said "yes" and 1 (3%) said "no." Of the 13 patients who had failed at 1 1/2 years postoperatively, 12 (92%) said they would have done it again in spite of their eventual failure while 1 (8%) said "no."

Although transient in most cases, the most frequent postsurgical complaint was choking on liquids or solids, followed in frequency by sore throat, shortness of breath, dry throat, phlegm, neck and chest pain, tightness in the throat, congestion, coughing, and a feeling of a lump in the throat (Table 3).

DISCUSSION

This study revealed several points about clinician and patient perception of surgical treatment for spastic dysphonia. First, the surgery is not a panacea for all patients who have adductor spastic dysphonia. Despite excellent voice during the first few months after surgery, an increasing number of failures accrued with time, and many patients who were still improved after 1 1/2 years were not doing as well as on previous examinations. Females, for reasons unknown, experience a higher percentage of failures than males. It is not possible now to predict who will retain improvement and who will fail.

Second, patients failed because the normal vocal fold vigorously overcompensated. Laryngologic examinations of several patients who had failed indicated that their spastic dysphonia had returned because the normal vocal fold had hyperadducted against the still-paralyzed fold, at times with hyperadduction of the accompanying ventricular fold.

Third, the degree of voice improvement from surgery varies widely among patients, and the voices of virtually all patients change with time. Voices ranged from severe breathiness to near normal. Breathy quality and reduced volume can be expected immediately after surgery. With time, the breathiness tends to disappear and to be replaced by a more tonal, louder voice. These changes probably occur because of increasing adductor compensation by the normal vocal fold.

Fourth, despite the considerable variations in voice effects and a moderate number of failures by 1 1/2 years postoperatively, the group was not displeased. We attribute this attitude to at least two factors: 1) the patients had severe spastic dysphonia and were willing to try anything that might help, and 2) patients were thoroughly briefed on the experimental nature of the surgery and given no guarantees as to the result. Even those who had failed, despite their deep disappointment, took their failure with equanimity and said that at least they had had a brief respite from their spastic dysphonia. The 61% who at 1 1/2 years were still better than before surgery were grateful despite residual dysphonia and transient laryngeal discomforts. Their universal complaint about not being heard in high ambient noise was, in their opinion, relatively unimportant in comparison with the benefits obtained.

Fifth, relief from effortful phonation is as much a benefit from surgery as is voice improvement. A disproportionate emphasis has been placed on the sound of the voice as the essence of spastic dysphonia. We have long believed that a considerable handicap is the utterly fatiguing, aggravating physical effort to force voice through the constricted glottis. This study supports the importance of that component.

CONCLUSION

Recurrent laryngeal nerve resection as a treatment for adductor spastic dysphonia is still experimental. Data of the above type beyond the 1 1/2 -year period need to be obtained, and those who are performing corrective surgery on patients who fail need to determine the long-term effectiveness of those procedures. Finally, we are concerned about the ever-present hazard of misdiagnosis of spastic dysphonia. Not all patients who have strained hoarseness have the intractable spastic dysphonia for which this surgery was designed. Patients with varying degrees of breathy dysphonia, misperceived as spastic dysphonia, can suffer severe breathiness or aphonia from the surgery. Because proper patient selection is a critical determinant of success, we advocate a collaborative approach to treatment of such patients in which the speech pathologist is integral in decision making as to the nature of the dysphonia under consideration and in the measurement of its parameters both before and after surgery.

REFERENCES

1. Bloch P. Neuro-psychiatric aspects of spastic dysphonia. Folia Phoniatr (Basel) 1965; 17:301-64.

2. Aronson AE, Brown JR, Littin EM, Pearson JS. Spastic dysphonia. II. Comparison with essential (voice) tremor and other neurologic and psychogenic dysphonias. J Speech Hear Disord 1968; 33:219-31.

3. Aronson AE, Hartman DE. Adductor spastic dysphonia as a sign of essential (voice) tremor. J Speech Hear Disord (in press).

4. Aminoff MJ, Dedo HH, Izdebski K. Clinical aspects of spasmodic dysphonia. J Neurol Neurosurg Psychiatry 1978; 41:361-5.

5. Dedo HH, Izdebski K, Townsend JJ. Recurrent laryngeal nerve histopathology in spastic dysphonia: a preliminary study. Ann Otol Rhinol Laryngol 1977; 86:806-12.

6. Bocchino JV, Tucker HM. Recurrent laryngeal nerve pathology in spasmodic dysphonia. Laryngoscope 1978; 88:1274-8.

7. Ravits JM, Aronson AE, DeSanto LW, Dyck PJ. No morphometric abnormality of recurrent laryngeal nerve in spastic dysphonia. Neurology (Minneap) 1979; 29:1376-82.

8. Traube L. Gesammelte Beiträge zur Pathologie und Physiologie. Vol 2. Berlin: August Hirschwald, 1871:677.

9. Dedo HH. Recurrent laryngeal nerve section for spastic dysphonia. Ann Otol Rhinol Laryngol 1976; 85:451-9.

10. Izdebski K, Shipp T, Dedo HH. Predicting postoperative voice characteristics of spastic dysphonia patients. Otolaryngol Head Neck Surg 1979; 87:428-34.

11. Barton RT. Treatment of spastic dysphonia by recurrent laryngeal nerve section. Laryngoscope 1979; 89:244-8.

12. Levine HL, Wood BG, Batza E, Rusnov M, Tucker HM. Recurrent laryngeal nerve section for spasmodic dysphonia. Ann Otol Rhinol Laryngol 1979; 88:527-30.

13. Biller HF, Som ML, Lawson W. Laryngeal nerve crush for spastic dysphonia. Ann Otol Rhinol Laryngol 1979; 88:531-2.

INFLUENCE OF ADENOID HYPERTROPHY ON SECRETORY OTITIS MEDIA

HANS H. ELVERLAND, MD
OLAV K. HAUGETO, MD
IAIN W. S. MAIR MD, FRCSG
KNUT E. SCHRØDER, MD

TROMSØ, NORWAY

The prognostic influence of adenoidectomy on the clinical course of chronic secretory otitis media (SOM) is reported after an observation period of five years in 166 children. Adenoidectomy was performed in connection with the first tubulation on the basis of concurrent symptoms of nasal obstruction, and resulted in a significant reduction in the need for repeated insertion of tympanostomy tubes in patients younger than eight years of age. The tubulation rate was also significantly reduced when adenoidectomy was performed in association with the first recurrence of SOM. This effect was, however, absent when the operation was performed at later stages, and both the otoscopic and audiological findings after five years revealed no significant differences between the adenoidectomy and nonadenoidectomy groups. Possible pathogenetic mechanisms leading to the development of SOM in the presence of large adenoids are discussed.

The clinical value of adenoidectomy has been much disputed throughout the years. Although this operation is often highly appreciated by the lay public, a better scientific documentation of its health benefits is badly needed in order to justify the prominent position of adenoidectomy in national health budgets.[1] However, randomized clinical studies of the possible advantages of adenoidectomy are difficult to perform since ethical considerations frequently lead to the withdrawal of those cases subjectively deemed to be in the greatest need of operation.[1,2] Another possible approach to this problem is to estimate the influence of adenoidectomy on other disease states with well-established diagnostic criteria, thus avoiding the ethical problems associated with randomization in clinical investigations.

Many authors have reported favorable effects of adenoidectomy on disease states in the middle ear cleft, but no statistical evidence for this opinion has been provided with the exception of the work of McKee.[3] On the other hand, Rynnel-Dagöö et al[2] have demonstrated no significant difference in the prognosis of secretory otitis media (SOM) between an adenoidectomy and a nonadenoidectomy group. The present report is part of a long-term study of SOM designed to investigate the possible association between nasal obstruction and the development of persistent middle ear fluid, and the influence of adenoidectomy on the latter. A short overview has been given in a previous interim report.[4]

METHODS

A prospective study of surgically treated SOM in children was initiated in our department in 1972. In the course of that year, 242 patients were admitted for surgery, but 76 who had received their primary treatment for SOM prior to this date have been excluded in order to ensure uniformity of treatment and follow-up protocols. The age and sex distributions of the 166 patients in the study cohort are shown in Figure 1.

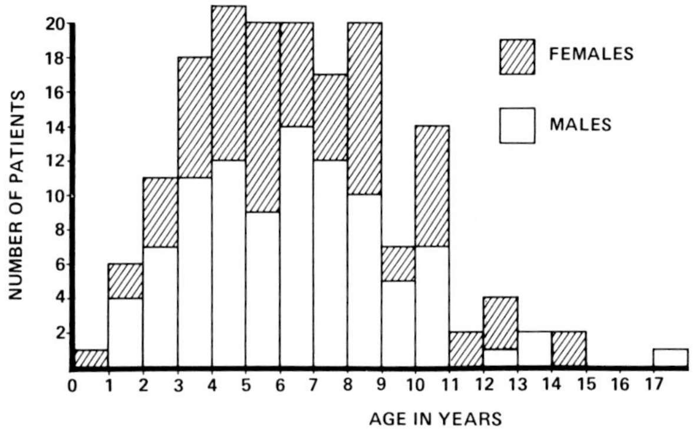

Fig. 1. Age and sex distribution of the 166 patients with mean age 6.1 years. The 71 girls and 95 boys have a mean age of 6.3 and 5.9 years respectively.

The majority of patients were first treated in the out-patient department with nose drops or oral decongestants. Only those cases in which normalization of the otoscopic and audiometric findings had not occurred within six to eight weeks were admitted for surgery. The anamnestic duration of SOM amounted to about four months before any kind of surgery was performed. A few seriously hearing-handicapped children were admitted after a shorter observation period.

The standard otosurgical procedure was tubulation following myringotomy in the lower anterior quadrant and thorough aspiration of middle ear effusion. Fluid in the middle ear cleft was found in 303 of the 332 ears, the secretion being mucus in 69% and serous in 31%. Patients with normalized otoscopic findings and hearing tests had their tympanostomy tubes removed three months after the first otosurgical procedure. In recurrent cases tubes were left in place until they were extruded spontaneously. Follow-up examinations were discontinued after an observation period of at least three months without recurrence of SOM.

Adenoidectomy was performed at the time of the first myringotomy only in cases with both symptoms and signs of nasal obstruction and x-ray confirmation of large adenoids. However, subsequent recurrence of middle ear effusion was regarded as a relative indication for adenoidectomy, although only in cases with x-ray evidence of enlargement of the adenoid tissue. Ade-

From the Department of Otorhinolaryngology, University of Tromsø, Institute of Clinical Medicine, Tromsø, Norway.
REPRINTS — Hans H. Elverland, MD, Department of Otorhinolaryngology, N-9012 Regionsykehuset i Tromsø, Norway.

TABLE 1. NUMBER OF TUBULATIONS PER PATIENT DURING THE FIVE-YEAR-PERIOD AS FUNCTION OF ADENOIDECTOMY/READENOIDECTOMY

Number of Adenoidectomies	Number of Tubulations 1	2	3	4	5	6	7	8	Total
0	38	4	6	1	1	0	0	0	50
1	58	22	9	4	2	3	3	1	102
2	2	2	3	3	1	1	0	1	13
3	0	0	1	0	0	0	0	0	1
Total	98	28	19	8	4	4	3	2	166

noidectomy was performed with a curette in the midline, no specific attempt being made to clear tissue from the fossa of Rosenmüller. Only one patient had had this operation performed three years earlier. Tonsillectomy was also performed in patients with frequent febrile sore throats, but SOM did not influence the decision for this procedure.

All patients were requested to attend for control examination five years later, in 1977, and the otoscopic findings, pure tone audiogram and tympanogram were recorded in 144 or 86.7% of the cases. Mean hearing thresholds poorer than 20 dB for the frequencies 500, 1000, and 2000 Hz and tympanograms showing greater negative middle ear pressures than −100 mm water were considered abnormal.

Relevant information from the patients' records was stored in a microcomputer system for later statistical treatment, significance being calculated according to the Fisher-Irwin method.

RESULTS

The adenoids were removed in connection with the first otosurgical procedure in 81 (49%) of the 166 patients. However, adenoidectomy has been performed a total of 131 times in 116 patients (70%) in the course of the five-year observation period. The relationship between numbers of adenoidectomies and tubulations is given in Table 1. Comparison of patients with only one tubulation and those requiring two or more otosurgical procedures, shows that adenoidectomy was performed in 61% of the former group and in 82% of the latter. This could apparently indicate an association between adenoidectomy and failure of the primary otosurgical treatment. However, the prognostic effect of adenoidectomy in the treatment of SOM can be more accurately assessed by comparing the need for further otosurgery in patients in whom primary adenoidectomy has or has not been performed.

Table 2 shows that the majority of patients in whom adenoidectomy was performed at the time of their first otosurgical procedure did not need a further otological procedure, while the opposite occurred in the nonadenoidectomy group, thus demonstrating a very significant improvement in prognosis for the adenoidectomy group ($P = 0.00003$). When the material is split into different age groups, the prognostic influence of adenoidectomy on SOM was significant in the age group below eight years, while the difference was not significant in the older children. Although the incidence of adenoidectomy was equal in both sexes, the beneficial effect of the operation was more pronounced in males than in females.

TABLE 2. NUMBER OF TUBULATIONS IN PATIENTS WITH AND WITHOUT ADENOIDECTOMY AT FIRST OTOSURGICAL PROCEDURE

	Number of Tubulations 1	2 and More	Total
Adenoidectomy	60	21	81
No adeoidectomy	38	47	85
Total	98	69	166

$P = 0.00003$.

Follow-up examination revealed that 47 patients in whom adenoidectomy was not performed at the time of the first otosurgical procedure, had recurrent or persistent SOM. The adenoids were removed in 24 of these patients in connection with the second myringotomy and insertion of tympanostomy tubes. Table 3 shows that this adenoidectomy produced a significant reduction ($P = 0.00008$) in the need for subsequent tubulations in the age group 0-7 years. The total number of patients in the older age group was low, only 12, and removal of adenoids had no statistically significant effect on SOM. These patients serve as their own controls since they all have one earlier treatment failure. There is no reason to believe that the second episode of SOM implies a better prognosis per se.

Extensive tests have been performed to see whether there are any inherent differences between SOM in patients with and without large adenoids which could indicate a less severe form of the disease in the former. The proportions of serous and mucus middle ear effusions were equal in both groups. The prognosis of SOM did not show any difference between males and females, and the sex distribution was similar in the adenoidectomy and nonadenoidectomy groups. The pure tone threshold in patients younger than eight years in whom adenoidectomy was performed at the first admission for SOM, was significantly poorer than for those who underwent otosurgery only. The highest rate of adenoidectomies was found in the age group four to five years, and this is coincident with the highest rate of myringotomies. There is therefore no tendency toward a generally good prognosis of SOM in the age group most likely to have adenoid tissue removed. Postoperative drainage from myringostomy tubes occurred in 13.6% of all cases, but with equal frequency in the adenoidectomy and nonadenoidectomy groups.

TABLE 3. PROGNOSTIC EFFECT OF ADENOIDECTOMY IN CONNECTION WITH THE SECOND TUBULATION AFTER INITIAL TREATMENT FAILURE WITHOUT EARLIER ADENOIDECTOMY (AGE 0-7 YR)

	Number of Tubulations 2	3 and More	Total
Adenoidectomy	10	8	18
No adenoidectomy	1	16	17
Total	11	24	35

$P = 0.00008$.

Five years after the initial treatment, there was a tendency toward a higher rate of ongoing follow-up consultations of the adenoidectomy patients at our out-patient department compared with those without earlier adenoidectomy. To illustrate our nonliberal practice of adenoidectomy in connection with SOM, it may be mentioned that the operation has since been performed in three patients in this series who have subsequently developed signs and symptoms of nasal obstruction.

There was no difference in pure tone thresholds between adenoidectomy and nonadenoidectomy patients at the five-year control. The proportions of normal and pathological tympanograms were also equal in both groups. However, the acoustic middle ear reflex could be more frequently elicited in the nonadenoidectomy group, and this difference was marginally significant. Calcified scars in the tympanic membrane were prevalent in the adenoidectomy group at the control in 1977, while atrophic scarring was found more frequently in the nonadenoidectomy patients. The presence of SOM, attic cup formation, atelectasis, and chronic suppurative otitis media showed no systematic difference between the two test groups five years after the primary treatment.

DISCUSSION

The prevalence of lowered intratympanic pressure and middle ear effusion found by acoustic impedance screening procedures in children is surprisingly high,[5-8] particularly in the younger age groups.[5] Brooks[9] reported longitudinal impedance studies during a six-year observation period of 104 school children, and found persistently normal middle ear parameters throughout this period in only 53%. In 222 children investigated four times during the second year of life, Tos and Poulsen[10] found unchanged type A tympanograms throughout the period in only 23.4% of the ears. A considerable tendency toward spontaneous normalization of impedance patterns has been demonstrated in follow-up examinations of children with abnormal tympanograms.[6,11] It is therefore conceivable that middle ear effusion occurs one or more times in the majority of people during childhood. The frequent occurrence of transient middle ear effusion necessitates an observation period of at least three to four months before surgical treatment for secretory otitis media (SOM) should be considered.[10] With the exception of the work of Stevens[12] and Dawes,[13] this fact is generally neglected throughout the literature on SOM, and probably contributes to the very variable treatment results. In the current study, clinical findings of SOM had been present for six to eight weeks. In addition comes a symptomatic interval of at least two months due to referral delays from primary care doctors and waiting lists at our outpatient department, thus ensuring chronicity of the middle ear condition prior to surgical treatment.

In the present series, 49% of the patients had symptoms and both clinical and radiological signs of nasopharyngeal obstruction at the time of primary admission for surgical treatment of SOM. The total number of adenoidectomies performed in our department in 1972 was 193, of which 116, or 60% were combined with otosurgery for SOM. These two conditions, hypertrophy of the adenoids and SOM, therefore show a high degree of coincidental occurrence in the pediatric population, a conclusion which is also supported by the study of Rynnel-Dagöö et al,[2] who found that 30 of 76 children admitted for adenoidectomy on the basis of nasal symptoms also had SOM. The adenoidectomy rate in the area of northern Norway served by our department is only 35.9/10,000 inhabitants in the age group below 16 years, and this low incidence[1] also shows a striking association with concomitant SOM. In this context the study of Hibbert and Tweedie[14] is of interest; these authors reported that the weight of tissue removed at adenoidectomy was similar for patients in whom the indications for operation were either nasal or aural symptoms.

Although the overall incidence of adenoidectomy in our material is fairly high (70%), we do not regard SOM as an indication for routine performance of this operation since many cases of SOM are obviously not associated with large adenoids. Bluestone et al[15] have even suggested that adenoid tissue may protect against SOM in some cases of abnormal patulence of the eustachian tube. Although their investigational technique is not applicable for routine use in a busy clinic, it is a very common experience that many cases of SOM are extremely therapy resistant after adenoidectomy. We would contend that the latter has been performed on inadequate and incorrect indications, and that other etiological factors account for the persistence of SOM.

Adenoidectomy patients in this material had initially a more severe hearing loss, with an increased need for follow-up consultations. These patients would thus appear to have a clinically more severe form of SOM, although other tested parameters indicated that SOM is a unimodal disease at the chronic stage at which we instituted surgical treatment. A closer scrutiny of Table 1 demonstrates a higher average rate of otosurgery in the adenoidectomy group as compared to the nonadenoidectomy group, 2.2 and 1.5 myringotomies per patient respectively. This would appear to be due to the tendency toward performing adenoidectomy, both primary and reoperations, late in the course of therapy resistant SOM, without proper indications. Adenoidectomy should therefore not be used as a last resort in recurrent SOM.

The mechanism by which the hypertrophied adenoid tissue influences the eustachian tube and middle ear ventilation is not yet settled. Mechanical obstruction of the eustachian orifice is very rarely observed,[16] and is not a valid explanation. Bluestone et al[15] found predominantly preoperative retrograde obstruction with postoperative normalization of eustachian tube function following adenoidectomy in patients with otitis media. Further investigations in tubulated middle ears by the same group,[17] with assessment of the ability to equilibrate positive and negative middle ear pressures, showed improved eustachian tube ventilatory function in 42% of the patients after adenoidectomy. Hypertrophied adenoid tissue may lead to increased tension in the adjacent nasopharyngeal tissue with extrinsic compression of the cartilaginous part of the eustachian tube as a result. Adenoidectomy may increase the pliability of the eustachian tube, leading to improved middle ear ventilation.

Experience from patients with tracheotomy or nasotracheal intubation has shown a tendency to lowered pressure and development of effusion in the middle ear.[18,19] The maintenance of atmospheric middle ear pressure probably depends on a ventilated nasopharyngeal space. Although the nasal passage is very seldom blocked due to enlarged adenoids, mouth-breathing is often found to be predominant, even in daytime. It is therefore conceivable that the nasopharyngeal space is poorly ventilated in these children, thus impairing eustachian tube function.

A further prominent feature in some children with enlarged adenoids is the feeling of a stuffed nose with stagnant nasal secretion leading to habitual sniffing. This transient lowering of nasopharyngeal pressure may be transmitted to the middle ear in cases with different degrees of closing failure of the eustachian tube.[20] It is probable that swallowing in the presence of adenoid enlargement results in an involuntary Toynbee maneuver[21] which, in combination with the sniffing habit, will perpetuate the processes producing SOM. We have observed striking disappearance of SOM in some patients when the sniffing habit was discontinued and replaced with proper nasal hygiene and nasal respiration.

Although infections in the middle ear cleft may be of importance in the pathogenesis of SOM,[22] evidence points to an indirect influence of infectious agents via nasopharyngeal infections facilitated by the presence of enlarged adenoid tissue. Tos et al[16] found a preponderance both of pathogenic bacteria in the nasopharynx and of previous acute otitis media in children with abnormal tympanograms; the latter had also a history of more frequent catarrhal infections. A recent study by Ruokonen et al[23] showed a significant increase in positive cultures of *Haemophilus influenzae* and of virus isolates from adenoid tissue removed from patients with middle ear effusions, as compared to adenoids from patients with simple hypertrophy and no ear disease. Rynnel-Dagöö et al[2] have also found a significant reduction of positive nasopharyngeal cultures of *Diplococcus pneumoniae* following adenoidectomy as compared with a nonoperated control group. Adenoidectomy may thus improve the eustachian tube function both by a reduction of upper respiratory tract infections due to a normalizing of the nasopharyngeal microflora and by reinstitution of respiratory ventilation of the nasopharyngeal space.

REFERENCES

1. Bluestone CD. Status of tonsillectomy and adenoidectomy: 1977. Laryngoscope 1977; 87:1233-43.

2. Rynnel-Dagöö B, Ahlbom A, Schiratzki H. Effects of adenoidectomy. A controlled two-year follow-up. Ann Otol Rhinol Laryngol 1979; 87:272-8.

3. McKee WJE. The part played by adenoidectomy in the combined operation of tonsillectomy with adenoidectomy. Second part of a controlled study in children. Br J Prev Soc Med 1963; 17:272-8.

4. Haugeto OK, Elverland HH, Schrøder KE, Mair IWS. Chronic secretory otitis media. Acta Otolaryngol (Stockh) 1979; Suppl 360:192-4.

5. Brooks DN. The use of electro-acoustic impedance bridge in assessment of middle ear function. Int Audiol 1969; 8:563-9.

6. Renvall U, Lidén G, Jungert S, Nilsson E. Impedance audiometry in the detection of secretory otitis media. Scand Audiol 1975; 4:119-24.

7. Fiellau-Nikolajsen M, Lous J, Vang Pedersen S, Schousboe HH. Tympanometry in three-year-old children. I. A regional prevalence study on the distribution of tympanometric results in a non-selected population of 3-year-old children. Scand Audiol 1977; 6:199-204.

8. Tos M, Poulsen G, Borch J. Tympanometry in 2-year-old children. Alterations of tympanograms at reevaluation. ORL 1978; 40:77-85.

9. Brooks DN. Middle ear effusion in children. J Otolaryngol 1976; 5:453-8.

10. Tos M, Poulsen G. Tympanometry in 2-year-old children. Seasonal influence on frequency of secretory otitis and tubal function. ORL 1979; 41:1-10.

11. Fiellau-Nikolajsen M, Lous J. Prospective tympanometry in 3-year-old children. Arch Otolaryngol 1979; 105:461-6.

12. Stevens DM. Long-term effects of serous otitis. Lancet 1962; 2:216-8.

13. Dawes JDK. The aetiology and sequelae of exudative otitis media. J Laryngol Otol 1970; 84:583-610.

14. Hibbert M, Tweedie MCK. The value of signs and symptoms in the diagnosis of enlarged adenoids. Clin Otolaryngol 1977; 2:297-304.

15. Bluestone CD, Wittel RA, Paradise JL, Felder H. Eustachian tube function as related to adenoidectomy for otitis media. Trans Am Acad Ophthalmol Otolaryngol 1972; 76:1325-39.

16. Tos M, Poulsen G, Borch J. Etiologic factors in secretory otitis. Arch Otolaryngol 1979; 105:582-8.

17. Bluestone CD, Cantekin EI, Beery QC. Certain effects of adenoidectomy on Eustachian tube ventilatory function. Laryngoscope 1975; 85:113-27.

18. Brookler KH, Birken EA, Blaugrund SM, Osserman KE.

Nonsuppurative otitis media in myasthenia gravis. Arch Otolaryngol 1972; 96:535-7.

19. Tos M, Bonding P. Middle ear pressure during and after prolonged nasotracheal and/or nasogastric intubation. Acta Otolaryngol (Stockh) 1977; 83:353-9.

20. Magnuson B. Tubal closing failure in retraction type cholesteatoma and adhesive middle ear lesions. Acta Otolaryngol (Stockh) 1978; 86:408-17.

21. Lamp CB. Chronic secretory otitis media: etiologic factors and pathologic mechanisms. Laryngoscope 1973; 83:276-91.

22. Lim DJ, Lewis DM, Schram JL, Birck HG. Otitis media with effusion. Cytological and microbiological correlates. Arch Otolaryngol 1979; 105:404-12.

23. Ruokonen J, Sandelin K, Mäkinen J. Adenoids and otitis media with effusion. Ann Otol Rhinol Laryngol 1979; 88:166-71.

≈

CANADIAN OTOLARYNGOLOGICAL SOCIETY

The annual meeting of the Canadian Otolaryngological Society will be held in London, Ontario, June 15-17, 1981. Inquiries may be sent to Dr. William Crysdale, c/o Hospital for Sick Children, 555 University Avenue, Toronto, Ontario.

≈

DEAFNESS RESEARCH FOUNDATION

The DRF invites applications for 1982 grant support of research projects directed to any aspect of the ear: e.g., investigator of function, physiology, biochemistry, genetics, anatomy or pathology. Grant support is given for one year, in an amount that cannot exceed $10,000, but can be renewed for one or two additional years.

The deadlines for applications for 1982 grant support are as follows: first-year applications postmarked by July 15, 1981; renewal applications postmarked by August 15, 1981.

For applications and for any information please contact: Director of Medical Affairs, The Deafness Research Foundation, 55 East 34th Street, New York, NY 10016.

RECIPROCAL SYNAPSES AT THE BASE OF OUTER HAIR CELLS IN THE ORGAN OF CORTI OF MAN

JOSEPH B. NADOL, JR., MD

BOSTON, MASSACHUSETTS

Reciprocal synapses have been found between nerve terminals and the outer hair cells in the human organ of Corti. A single nerve ending of the nonvesiculated type may possess two types of synaptic specialization of opposite polarity. The first is typical of the "afferent" synapse with a presynaptic body in the hair cell and pre- and postsynaptic membrane thickening. The second consists of a small collection of presynaptic vesicles in the neural cytoplasm near the plasma membrane facing the hair cell and a subsynaptic cisterna within the hair cell cytoplasm. The second type of specialization is similar to the synapses seen in "efferent" endings. This suggests that both an afferent (hair cell to neuron) and efferent (neuron to hair cell) synaptic relationship may exist between an outer hair cell and a single nerve terminal.

INTRODUCTION

Two types of nerve endings, differentiated in part by their synaptic specialization, have been described at the base of the outer hair cells of the organ of Corti. Engstrom[1] first recognized this dual innervation which he designated as "type 1" and "type 2" endings. These observations have been confirmed in a number of animal species.[2-5] The type 1 or nonvesiculated ending is recognized by the presence of pre- and postsynaptic membrane thickening and, in most species, a presynaptic ribbon or body surrounded by synaptic vesicles in the hair cell. The type 2 or vesiculated ending on the outer hair cell is characterized by the presence of many presynaptic vesicles which fill the nerve terminal

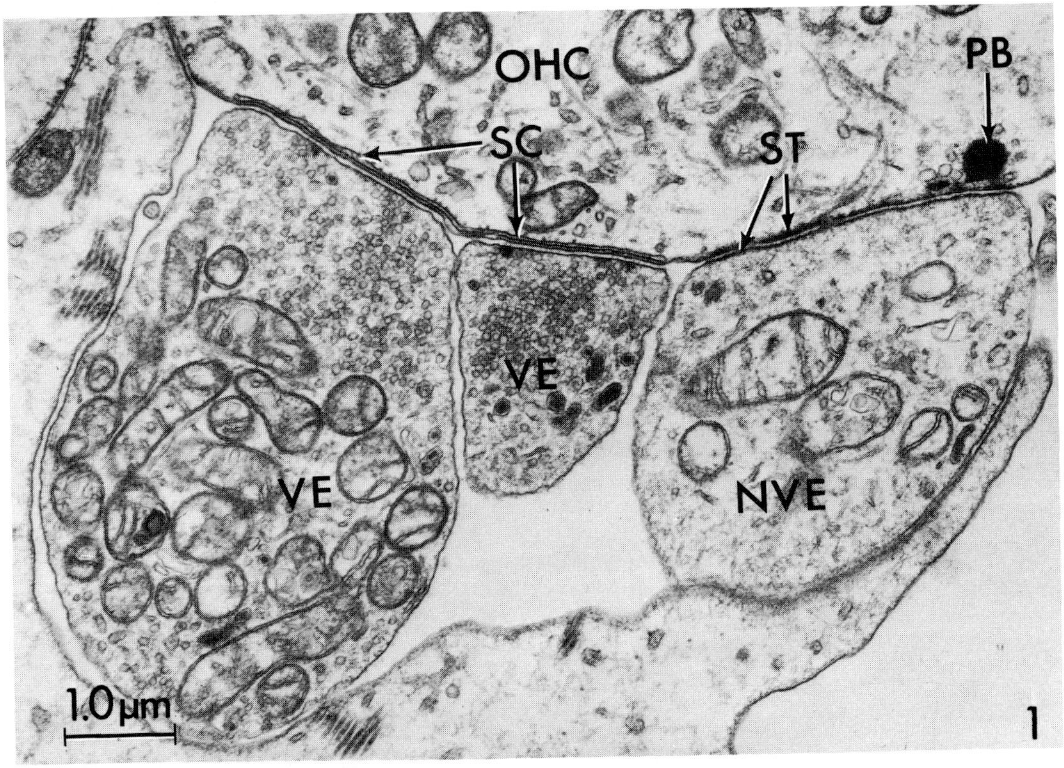

Fig. 1 Synapses at the base of a human outer hair cell (OHC) in the first row of the basal turn. The type 1 or nonvesiculated ending (NVE) is characterized by presynaptic and postsynaptic membrane thickening (ST) and a presynaptic body (PB) and vesicles. The type 2 or vesiculated ending (VE) is characterized by many presynaptic vesicles in the nerve terminal and a subsynaptic cisterna (SC) in the outer hair cell.

From the Department of Otolaryngology, Harvard Medical School and the Massachusetts Eye and Ear Infirmary, Boston, Massachusetts. Supported by the National Institutes of Health Teacher-Investigator Award No. 5 K07 NS00174-04, a grant from the American Otological Society, and Grant No. 1 R01 NS15840-01 from the National Institutes of Health.

REPRINTS — Joseph B. Nadol, Jr., MD, Department of Otolaryngology, Massachusetts Eye and Ear Infirmary, 243 Charles Street, Boston, MA 02114.

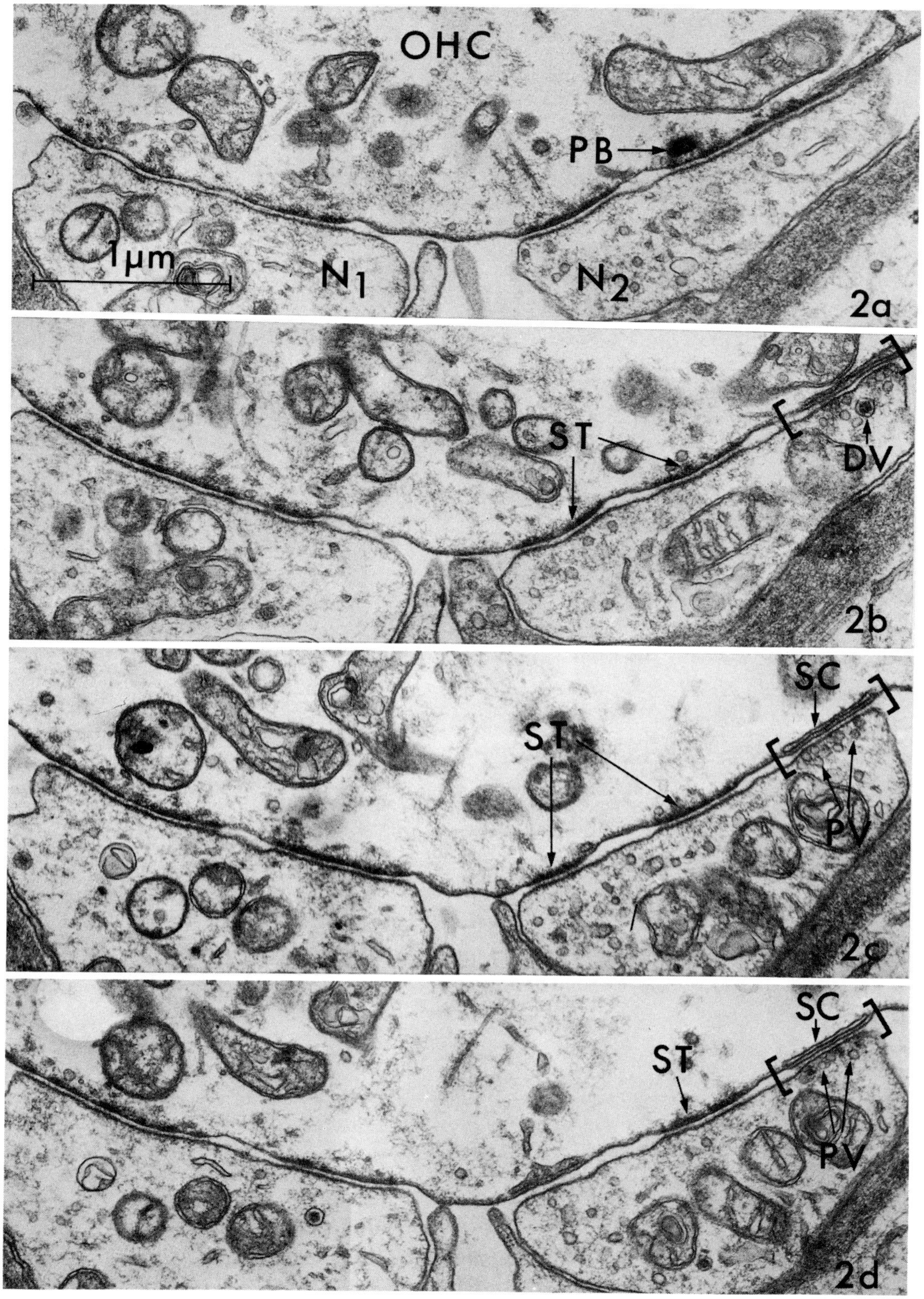

Fig. 2. a-d) A portion of a series of serial sections of nerve terminals at the base of an outer hair cell (OHC) in the third row of the middle turn of the human organ of Corti. Two nerve terminals (N_1 and N_2) of the nonvesiculated type demonstrate presynaptic and postsynaptic membrane thickening (ST) and a presynaptic body (PB). In addition, in one nerve terminal (N_2) a second type of specialization is seen (bracket). This consists of presynaptic vesicles (PV) in the cytoplasm of N_2 and a postsynaptic subsurface cisterna (SC) in the cytoplasm of the outer hair cell. An occasional dense core vesicle (DV) was seen among the presynaptic vesicles. Three sections between Figure 2a and 2b, three sections between Figure 2b and 2c, and one section between Figure 2c and 2d are not shown.

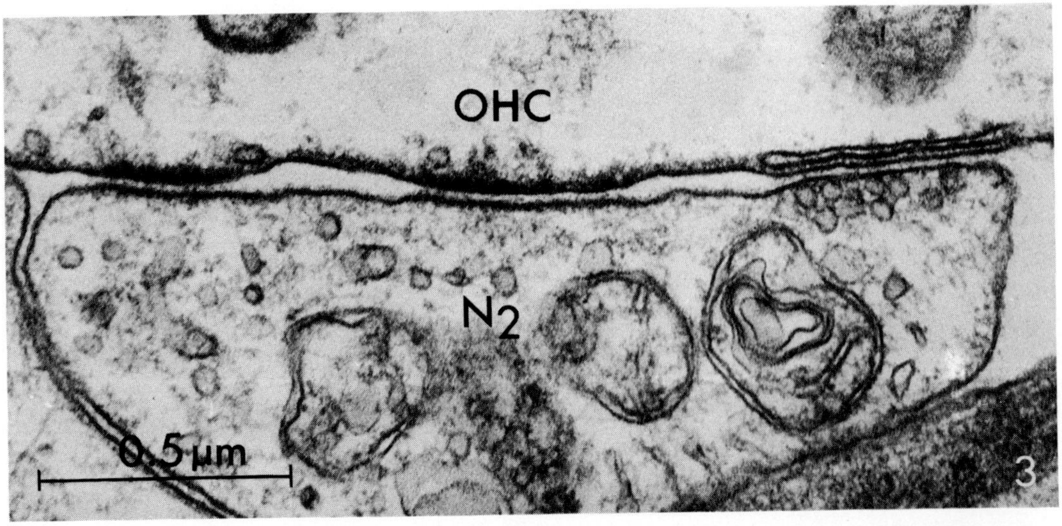

Fig. 3. Higher magnification of Figure 2c showing reciprocal synapses between one nerve terminal (N_2) and an outer hair cell (OHC).

and a subsynaptic cisterna within the outer hair cell cytoplasm. As a result of a variety of observations,[3,6,7] the type 2 endings are considered to be the terminals of the olivocochlear bundle and efferent in nature, whereas the type 1 endings are considered to be afferent dendritic processes of cell bodies in the spiral ganglion.

Electron microscopy of serial sections of the human organ of Corti has revealed a synaptic relationship not previously reported. This consists of two synapses of opposite polarity, or reciprocal synapses, between an outer hair cell and a single nerve terminal.

MATERIAL AND METHODS

The inner ears of a 64-year-old male who died of cardiomyopathy were fixed two hours after death. Although no audiogram was available, this man had no auditory or vestibular complaints and was said by his family to have had normal hearing throughout his life. Additional observations were made on the inner ears of another individual who died at age 66 of ventricular rupture. This patient was said to have had normal hearing throughout life. There had been loud noise exposure in the military, but in the absence of any subjective hearing loss, no audiogram was ever performed. Temporal bones were fixed 2.5 hours after death. Details of the method of fixation and tissue preparation have been reported elsewhere.[8] The fixative was 2% glutaraldehyde and 2% paraformaldehyde in 0.1 M phosphate buffer. After thinning the otic capsule with a power drill, the specimens were decalcified in 0.1 M disodium ethylenediamine tetra-acetic acid (EDTA) with 2% glutaraldehyde in 0.1 M phosphate buffer and postfixed in 2% osmium tetroxide in 0.1 M phosphate buffer. The tissue was stained en bloc with aqueous uranyl acetate, dehydrated in graded alcohols, exchanged with propylene oxide and embedded in Epon®. Serial sections of the middle and basal turns were cut in a radial orientation. The neural poles of several inner and outer hair cells were examined in their entirety.

FINDINGS

Nerve terminals of both type 1 (nonvesiculated) and type 2 (vesiculated) were found at the base of outer hair cells of the human organ of Corti (Fig. 1). The type 1 ending demonstrated pre- and postsynaptic membrane thickening, and often a presynaptic body surrounded by vesicles in the hair cell. The postsynaptic neuronal cytoplasm of the type 1 ending contained a paucity of vesicles compared to the type 2 ending which contained a large collection of presynaptic vesicles filling the nerve terminal. The type 2 ending also demonstrated a postsynaptic subsurface cisterna in the outer hair cell cytoplasm.

Some nonvesiculated nerve terminals on outer hair cells demonstrated two distinct types of synaptic specialization in adjacent areas of the same nerve terminal. The first was typical of an "afferent" synapse, with pre- and postsynaptic membrane thickening and a presynaptic body in the hair cell. The second consisted of a small collection of vesicles within the nerve terminal and a subsynaptic cisterna within the apposed hair cell cytoplasm (Figs. 2-5). The second synaptic specialization was very similar to the synapse seen in the classic type 2 or "efferent" ending. However, it differed from the type 2 ending in that the area of synaptic specialization was much smaller and it contained fewer presynaptic vesicles. This type of nerve terminal with reciprocal synapses between neuron and hair cell was found in all three rows of outer hair cells and in both basal and middle turns. Not every ending with afferent synapses possessed this reciprocal synaptic specialization but it was frequently seen. Eleven reciprocal synapses were found in 888 serial sections from the first human specimen, and three were found in 50 serial sections from the second specimen. However, because of the small size of the synaptic specialization of the efferent type within terminals with reciprocal synapses, this feature would be easily missed unless serial sections of the nerve terminals were studied. No reciprocal synapses were found at the base of inner hair cells.

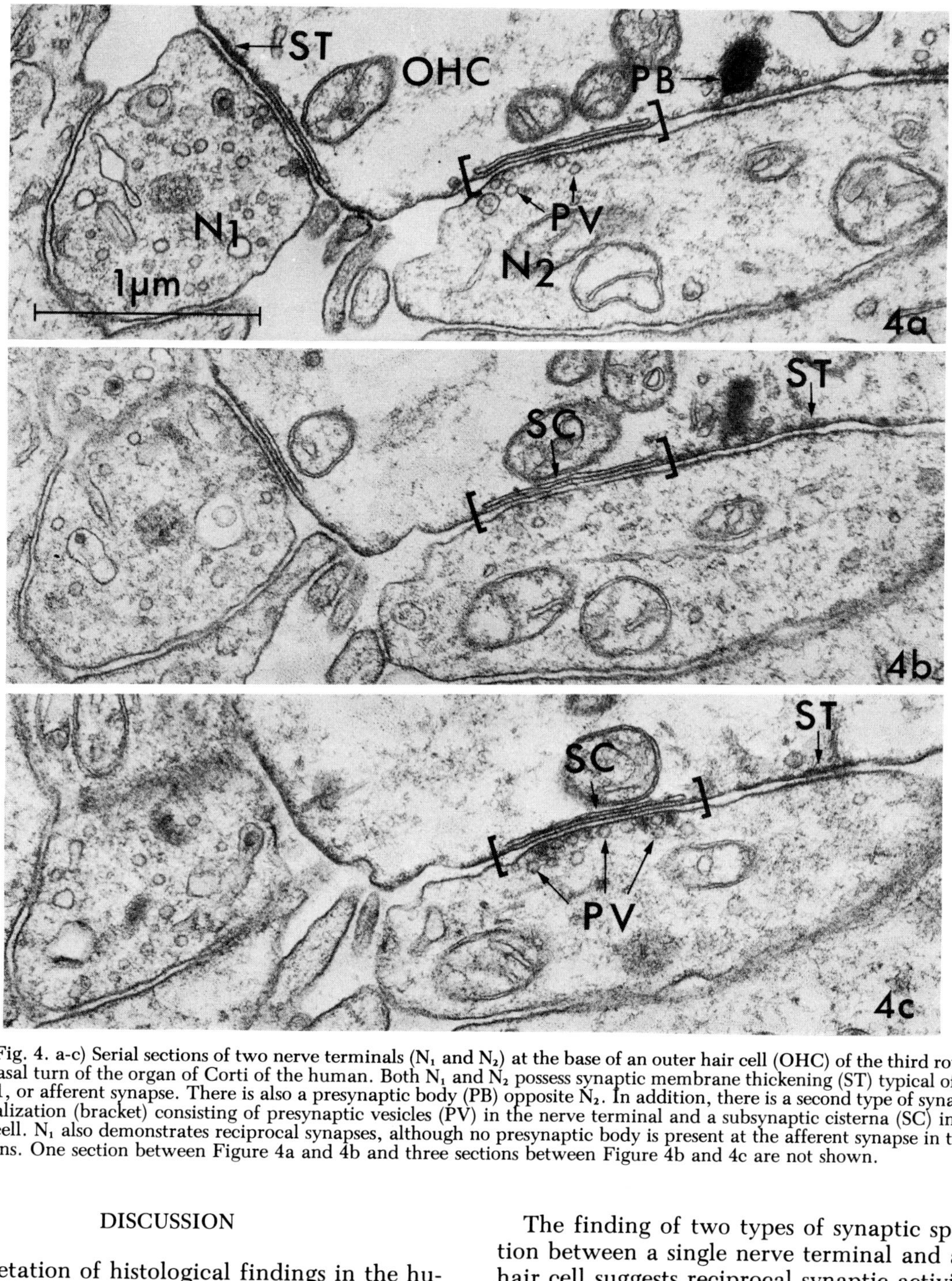

Fig. 4. a-c) Serial sections of two nerve terminals (N_1 and N_2) at the base of an outer hair cell (OHC) of the third row in the basal turn of the organ of Corti of the human. Both N_1 and N_2 possess synaptic membrane thickening (ST) typical of the type 1, or afferent synapse. There is also a presynaptic body (PB) opposite N_2. In addition, there is a second type of synaptic specialization (bracket) consisting of presynaptic vesicles (PV) in the nerve terminal and a subsynaptic cisterna (SC) in the hair cell. N_1 also demonstrates reciprocal synapses, although no presynaptic body is present at the afferent synapse in these sections. One section between Figure 4a and 4b and three sections between Figure 4b and 4c are not shown.

DISCUSSION

Interpretation of histological findings in the human must include consideration of postmortem autolysis. In the organ of Corti of the guinea pig, Wersall et al[9] described rupture of limiting membranes, vacuolization of cytoplasm, and eventual lysis of synaptic vesicles as typical changes due to postmortem autolysis. It is unlikely that a subsynaptic cisterna in one cell and a collection of vesicles in an apposed portion of a second cell are due to autolysis. The possibilities that the reciprocal synapses may represent a pathological change in the human, or may be species-specific, require further investigation.

The finding of two types of synaptic specialization between a single nerve terminal and an outer hair cell suggests reciprocal synaptic activity. This finding requires careful attention to terminology. That is, "endings" and "synapses" cannot be considered equivalent terms. Nonvesiculated, or type 1 endings, have been equated with afferent function, and vesiculated, or type 2 endings, have been equated with efferent function.[3,7] However, the morphological characteristics of the reciprocal synapses suggest that both afferent, or hair cell to neuron transmission, and efferent, or neuron to hair cell transmission, may occur between an outer hair cell and the same nerve terminal. Therefore it is probably best to refer to specific synaptic specializa-

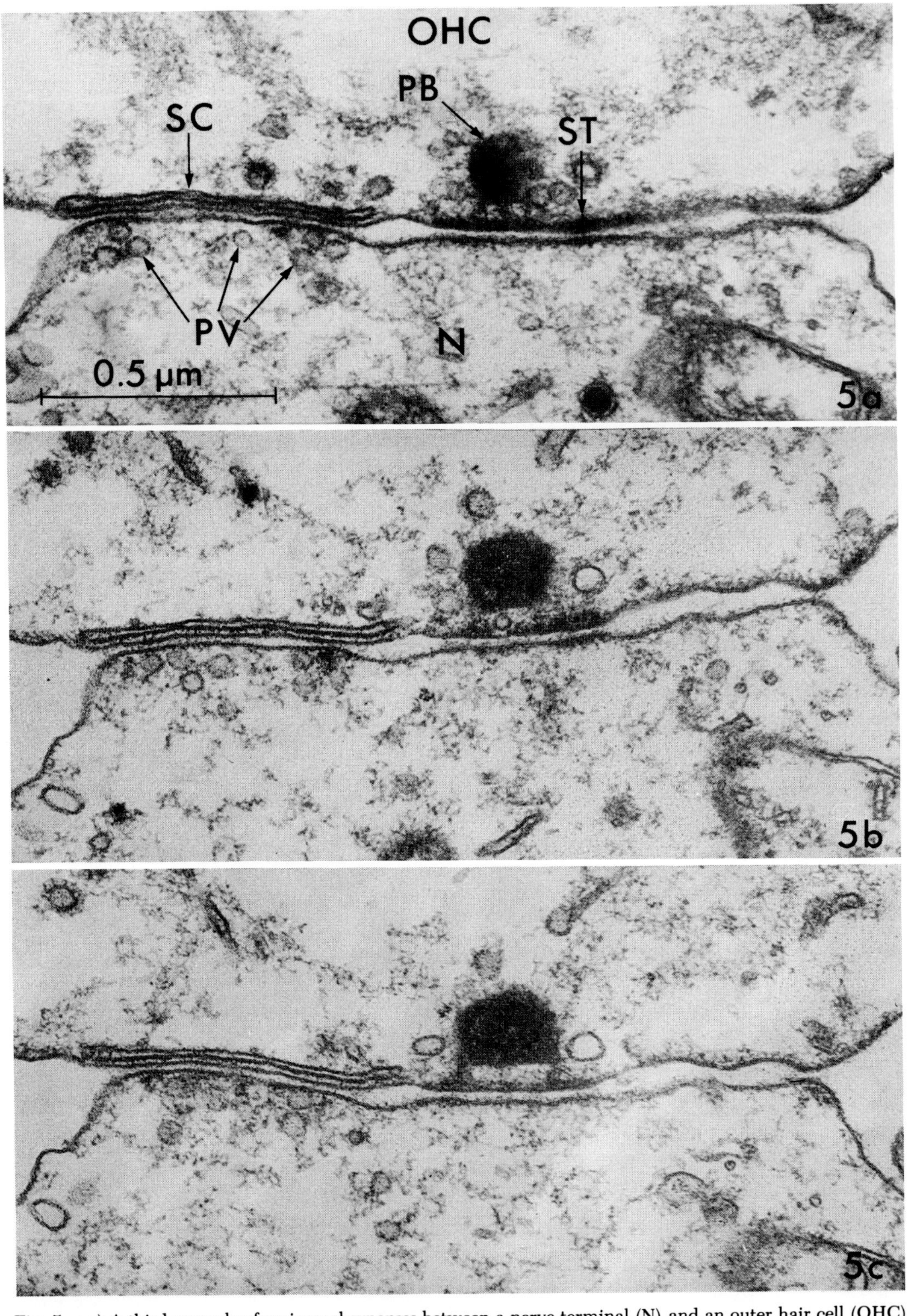

Fig. 5. a-c) A third example of reciprocal synapses between a nerve terminal (N) and an outer hair cell (OHC) of the third row of the middle turn of the organ of Corti of the human in three sequential serial sections. The afferent synapse consists of a presynaptic body (PB) and synaptic membrane thickening (ST). The efferent synapse consists of presynaptic vesicles (PV) in the neural cytoplasm and a subsurface cisterna (SC) in the hair cell.

tion rather than to type 1 or type 2 nerve endings. The following nomenclature is suggested. A synapse suggestive of afferent transmission may be called the "type 1 synapse." The classic synapse seen in terminals of the olivocochlear bundle and considered to be efferent may be called the "type 2 synapse." The third type of synapse, which is similar to, but smaller than, the classic efferent synapse may be called the "type 3 synapse." Using these terms, nerve terminals with reciprocal synapses can be redefined as nerve terminals demonstrating both type 1 and type 3 synapses with the outer hair cell.

The role of such reciprocal synaptic activity can only be speculative since the ganglionic origin of such terminals is not known. However, with the exception of the small areas of synaptic specialization of type 3, the nerve terminals with reciprocal synapses are identical to the classic type 1 endings, which are thought to be peripheral dendritic processes of cell bodies in the spiral ganglion. Reciprocal synapses have also been found in the central nervous system[10-12] and retina[13] between apposed dendrites. In addition, they have been found in the carotid body receptor[14] and the frog crista ampullaris[15,16] between neuroepithelial cells and neurons. In these systems reciprocal synapses are thought to serve as part of a feedback loop. Tanaka and Smith[17] and Thorn et al[18] mention the possibility of reciprocal synapses in the organ of Corti based on the observation of presynaptic bodies near type 2 endings but do not demonstrate distinct reciprocal synaptic specialization between a hair cell and a single nerve terminal. If, in fact, these terminals are part of the afferent pathway from outer hair cells, then the presence of reciprocal synapses within the same nerve terminal suggests the possibility of a local feedback mechanism which could influence afferent synaptic activity. This could occur within the nerve terminal at the base of the same hair cell or between many hair cells innervated by the dendritic aborization of the same afferent neuron. The apparent absence of such reciprocal synapses at the base of inner hair cells may reflect different functions of inner and outer hair cells.

ACKNOWLEDGMENT — The assistance of Ms. Barbara Burgess in tissue preparation and of Ms. Jean Dinon in manuscript preparation is gratefully acknowledged.

REFERENCES

1. Engstrom H. On the double innervation of the sensory epithelia of the inner ear. Acta Otolaryngol (Stockh) 1958; 49:109-18.

2. Smith CA, Sjostrand FS. Structure of the nerve endings on the external hair cells of the guinea pig cochlea as studied by serial sections. J Ultrastruct Res 1961; 5:523-56.

3. Kimura R, Wersall J. Termination of the olivocochlear bundle in relation to the outer hair cells of the organ of Corti in guinea pig. Acta Otolaryngol (Stockh) 1962; 55:11-32.

4. Smith CA, Rasmussen GL. Recent observations on the olivocochlear bundle. Ann Otol Rhinol Laryngol 1963; 72:489-506.

5. Kimura R. The ultrastructure of the organ of Corti. Int Rev Cytol 1975; 42:173-222.

6. Rasmussen GL. Further observations of efferent cochlear bundle. J Comp Neurol 1953; 99:61-74.

7. Spoendlin HH, Gacek RR. Electronmicroscopic study of the efferent and afferent innervation of the organ of Corti in the cat. Ann Otol Rhinol Laryngol 1963; 72:660-86.

8. Nadol JB Jr. Electron microscopic observations in a case of long-standing profound sensorineural deafness. Ann Otol Rhinol Laryngol 1977; 86:507-17.

9. Wersall J, Kimura RS, Lundquist P-G. Early postmortem changes in the organ of Corti (guinea pig). Z Zellforsch Mikrosk Anat 1965; 65:220-37.

10. Andres KH. Der Feinbau des Bulbus olfactorius der Ratte unter besonderer Berucksichtigung der synaptischen Verbindungen. Z Zellforsch Mikrosk Anat 1965; 65:530-61.

11. Famiglietti EV Jr. Dendro-dendritic synapses in the lateral geniculate nucleus of the cat. Brain Res 1970; 20:181-91.

12. Yamauchi A, Fujimaki Y, Yokota R. Reciprocal synapses between cholinergic postganglionic axon and adrenergic interneuron in the cardiac ganglion of the turtle. J Ultrastruct Res 1975; 50:47-57.

13. Dowling JE, Boycott BB. Organization of the primate retina: electron microscopy. Proc R Soc Lond [Biol] 1966; 166:80-111.

14. McDonald D, Mitchell RA. The innervation of glomus cells, ganglion cells and blood vessels in the rat carotid body: a quantitative ultrastructural study. J Neurocytol 1975; 4:177-230.

15. Dunn RF. Reciprocal synapses in the crista ampullaris of the bullfrog, abstracted. Neuroscience 1975; 1:221.

16. Dunn RF. Reciprocal synapses in the crista ampullaris: a possible mechanism for hair cell interaction. ORL 1976; 82:188-9.

17. Tanaka K, Smith CA. Structure of the chicken's inner ear: SEM and TEM study. Am J Anat 1978; 153:251-72.

18. Thorn L, Schinko I, Wetzstein R. Synaptic bar in the efferent part of a synapse in the organ of Corti. Experientia 1972; 28:835.

Ann Otol 90:1981

VASCULATURE OF THE ANTERIOR COMMISSURE

MARIO ANDREA, MD

LISBON, PORTUGAL

Results of a study of the vasculature of the anterior commissure, part of a larger study of the larynx, are presented. The vasculature of the anterior commissure is dependent on the medial branch of the anteroinferior laryngeal artery. The techniques used, postmortem angiography, dissection, cleared method, microangiography and histological sections, made it possible to follow the course of the artery and determine its configuration. The results reveal separation of the supraglottis and the glottis between the thyroepiglottic ligament and the anterior commissure; the study also establishes that a separation does not exist between the glottis and the subglottis in the anterior larynx. Particular emphasis is placed on ossification of the thyroid cartilage and the relationship between the vascular network of the glottic and subglottic mucosa and the tissues immediately in front of the larynx.

Of the various regions of the larynx, the anterior commissure provides perhaps the greatest challenge to the investigator; there is no agreement concerning its boundaries and its morphology also is controversial.

In 1979 we published a paper about the anterior commissure[1] in which we emphasized the existence of a small zone designated as "plane zero," which separates the supraglottis from the glottis at the most anterior portion of the larynx. The existence of this plane has been demonstrated by serial horizontal sections of normal human larynges.

Although the anterior commissure tendon and the thyroepiglottic ligament have a similar constitution (fibers, glands and vessels) it is important to note that of all these elements only the fibers provide true continuity. These facts suggested the hypothesis that there is a small zone immediately above the anterior commissure in the midline larynx where the glands are absent and where the mucosa is separated from the thyroid cartilage only by fibers. The designation of this small zone as "plane zero" was preferred to a more general label such as "interglottic-supraglottic plane" because the concept of "plane zero" is only valid at the anterior midline of the larynx and not at other locations.

Plane zero, which constitutes the histologic separation between the supraglottis and the glottis at the most anterior portion of the larynx, has a macroscopic expression. In fact if we follow the superior face of one of the vocal cords with a stylet we can pass to the opposite side without difficulty. In this way we hypothesized a separation between the supraglottis and the glottis at the most anterior portion of the larynx. We do not separate the glottis from the subglottis because there is no possible separation at the anterior portion of the larynx. For us the anterior commissure constitutes not only the most anterior part of the glottis but also the anterosuperior limit of a more vast region, the glottic-subglottic region, where the conus elasticus is significant. For several years we were attracted by the arterial vasculature of the larynx,[2-4] and we decided to study the macrovasculature and microvascular distribution of arterial blood to the anterior commissure.

METHODS

The results[3] concerning the vasculature of the anterior commissure were obtained by the study of 95 human larynges obtained at necropsy. In 57 specimens the macrovasculature was studied using portmortem angiography. Micropaque® (Damancy Co.) usually was injected into the right primitive carotid. In 34 specimens the arteriograms were then controlled by the anatomic dissection and in 23 specimens the cleared method was used for this purpose.

In 38 specimens angiography was used to study the microvasculature also. Micropaque in a dilute form was used, and sections 400-500μ thick were obtained at several levels of the larynx.

We obtained a specific angiographic pattern for each part of the larynx, and found a clear correlation between histological structure and microvascular configuration. In this study cross sections were compared with angiograms.

RESULTS

Since we were unable to find a uniform taxonomy of laryngeal arteries in the literature,[3,5,6] we consider a simple classification in which the name corresponds to the site where the artery enters the larynx, as suggested by Terracol and Guerrier.[6] Three major arteries are identified (Fig. 1A,B): the superior laryngeal artery usually penetrates the larynx through the thyrohyoid membrane; the anteroinferior laryngeal arteries perforate the cricothyroid membrane; the posteroinferior laryngeal artery enters the larynx posteriorly.

While on each side there is only one superior laryngeal and one posteroinferior laryngeal artery, the anteroinferior laryngeal arteries may differ in number; usually there are three, one medial and two paramedial (right and left).

The anteroinferior laryngeal arteries seem to be the most controversial with respect both to their

From the Department of Otolaryngology, Faculdade de Medicina, Lisbon, Portugal.

REPRINTS — Mario Andrea, MD, Serviço O.R.L., Faculdade de Medicina, Av. Egas Moniz-1600, Lisbon, Portugal.

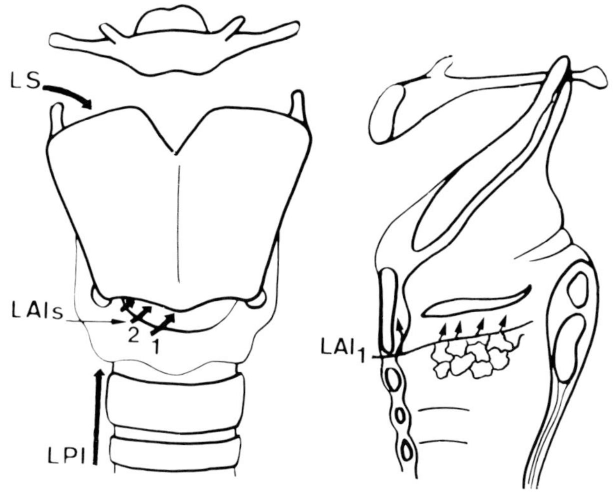

Fig. 1. A, B) The laryngeal arteries. LS - Superior laryngeal artery; LAIs - Anteroinferior laryngeal arteries: medial (1), paramedial (2); LPI - Posteroinferior laryngeal artery.

number and importance. If observed only at the level of the cricothyroid membrane, the short courses suggest that they are vessels of secondary importance. If, however, we follow these arteries within the larynx their role is more readily apparent.

The paramedial anteroinferior laryngeal arteries join to form a longitudinal intralaryngeal arcade;[3] and the medial anteroinferior laryngeal artery supplies the subglottic mucosa and the anterior commissure.[3]

We verified the existence of the medial anteroinferior laryngeal artery in 97% of the larynges examined; in 60% of these, there was only one artery which either divided before reaching the middle part of the cricothyroid membrane, or remained as a single vessel; in 40% there were two separate arteries at origin.

In order to observe the course of arteries after they perforate the cricothyroid membrane, the cleared method is useful. In this method the vascular system is injected and the extravascular tissues are homogenized chemically, or "cleared." If we then open the larynx posteriorly and view the anterior larynx from behind, it is possible to see the distribution of the medial anteroinferior artery (Fig. 2).

We verified that this artery(ies) follows an ascending course toward the anterior commissure. One branch of this vessel supplies the subglottic mucosa; thus we named it the transverse branch of the vocal cord mucosa.[3]

In the cases where there was only one medial anteroinferior laryngeal artery, the vessel bifurcated to form a right and left branch before reaching the anterior commissure (Fig. 2); in other cases these two arteries have a longer course, being separate at the point of origin, the cricothyroid ligament. In both cases we observed the existence of two arteries

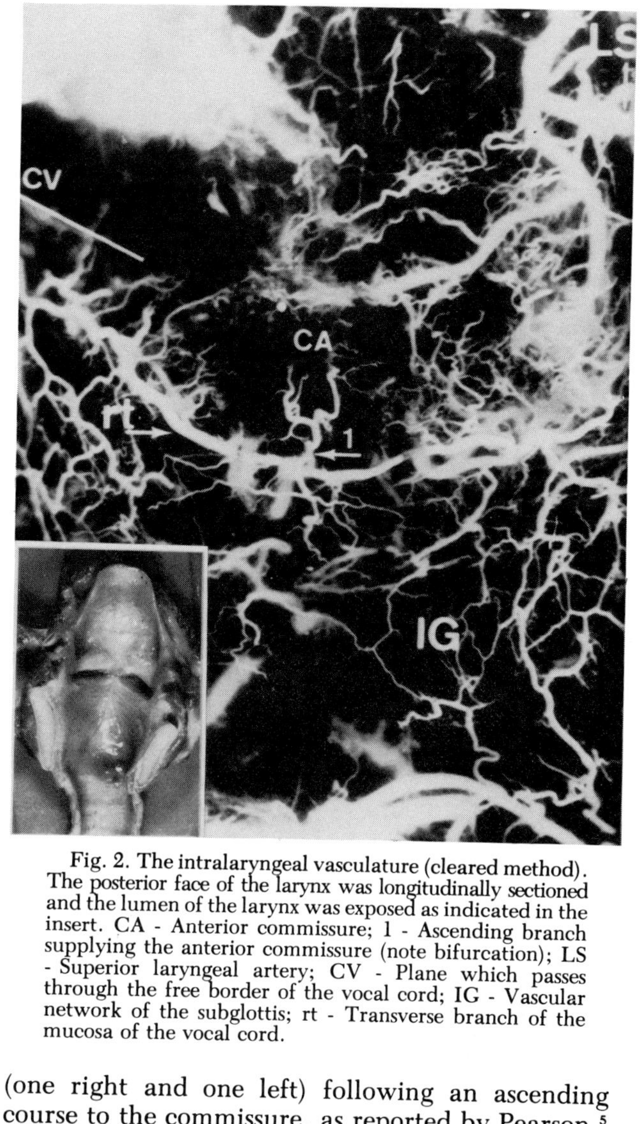

Fig. 2. The intralaryngeal vasculature (cleared method). The posterior face of the larynx was longitudinally sectioned and the lumen of the larynx was exposed as indicated in the insert. CA - Anterior commissure; 1 - Ascending branch supplying the anterior commissure (note bifurcation); LS - Superior laryngeal artery; CV - Plane which passes through the free border of the vocal cord; IG - Vascular network of the subglottis; rt - Transverse branch of the mucosa of the vocal cord.

(one right and one left) following an ascending course to the commissure, as reported by Pearson.[5] These arteries assume a particular importance because we have not observed the existence of other vessels specifically supplying the anterior commissure, coming from either the supraglottic or the glottic vasculature. These observations are not in agreement with those of other authors.[7,8]

Concerning the vessels of the supraglottis, we do not observe any supplying the anterior commissure. The vessels existing at the level of the thyroepiglottic ligament were not related with those of the anterior commissure. This fact confirms the notion of "plane zero" referred to previously.[1]

Microangiography permitted us to observe the configuration of the two arteries of the anterior commissure. Figure 3 shows cross sections of these arteries. The arteries of the anterior commissure are situated inside the fibers of the conus elasticus, and branch arteries supply the numerous glands and the mucosa existing at this level.

In microangiograms the vocal ligament appears as an avascular shadow situated between the vascu-

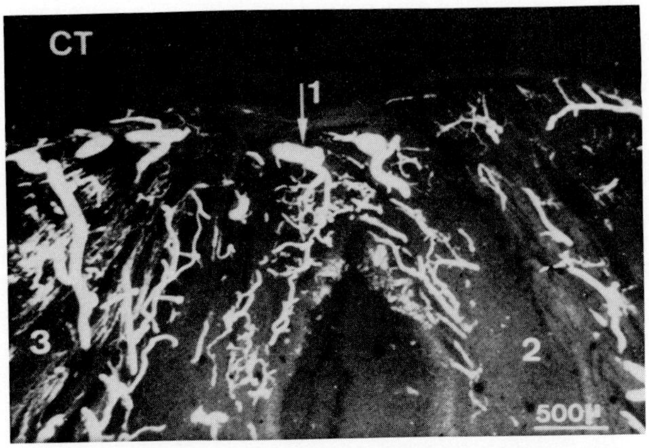

Fig. 3. Microangiography of a horizontal section at the level of the anterior commissure. Note the interruption of the vascular network of the internal perichondrium of the thyroid cartilage. CT - Thyroid cartilage; 1 - Arteries of the anterior commissure; 2 - Vocal ligament; 3 - Thyroarytenoid muscle.

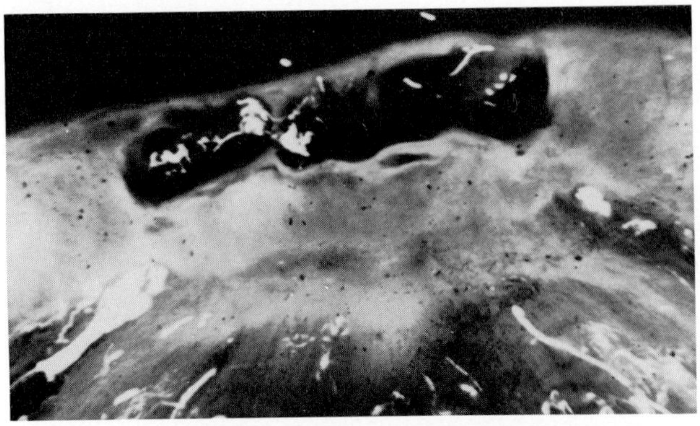

Fig. 4. Microangiography of a horizontal section at the anterior commissure. Notice the interruption of the vascular network of the internal perichondrium of the thyroid cartilage and the alterations due to the ossification of the thyroid cartilage (See Fig. 3).

lature of the muscles outside the conus elasticus and the vascular network of the mucosa. Inside the conus elasticus, vascular configuration corresponds to that of the glands (Fig. 3).

The relationship of the anterior commissure to the thyroid cartilage was also evident in the microangiograms. The vasculature of the internal perichondrium of the thyroid cartilage is interrupted at the anterior commissure (Figs. 3 and 4), and there appears to be an avascular zone at the origin of the vocal cords in the thyroid cartilage. These findings agree with those of other authors.[5,7,9]

Microangiography provided further information on the ossification process (Figs. 3 and 4). The segment of the thyroid cartilage situated in front of the anterior commissure ossifies early in the developmental process. The microangiograms show no homogeneous radiologic density characteristic of the cartilaginous tissue (Fig. 3), and the "cartilage" appears as heterogeneous shadows (Fig. 4). This reflects the replacement of cartilaginous tissue with bony tissue which is accompanied by the appearance of vessels inside the "ossified cartilages" (Fig. 4).[3,4,10] Differences between the cartilage zones still in the cartilaginous phase and those where the ossification process has already started can be seen in Figure 4.

SUMMARY

This study of the vasculature of the anterior commissure included macroscopic examination of the laryngeal arteries as well as microvascular analysis at various levels of the larynx.

The results indicate a separation of the anterior commissure from the supraglottis between the anterior commissure and the thyroepiglottic ligament. These facts are relevant to the assessment of tumors originating in or spreading to the anterior commissure.

The study also revealed that there is no separation at the most anterior part of the larynx between the glottis and the subglottis. In this glottic-subglottic region the glands and vessels are continuous.

We think that is important to emphasize that the vasculature of the anterior commissure as well as that of the mucosa and submucosa of the subglottis derives from the medial anteroinferior laryngeal artery. This fact suggests a close relationship between the anterior commissure and the tissues immediately in front of the larynx at the level of the cricothyroid ligament. The significance of these results for local and regional spread of subglottic tumors is an important subject for further research.

REFERENCES

1. Guerrier Y, Andrea M. La commissure anterieure du larynx-nouveaux aspects. In: Arnette, ed. Comptes Rendus des Seances du 76° Congres Français. Paris: ORL (in press).

2. Santos Ferreira A, Andrea M. Contribution to the study of the arterial blood supply of the larynx (preliminary note). Verhandlungen der Anatomishen Gesellschaft 1972; 120:569-73.

3. Andrea M. Vascularizaçao arterial da laringe, distribuçao macro e micro vascular. Arq Anat Antropol 1977; 37:111-337.

4. Guerrier Y, Andrea M. La vascularization des cartilages du larynx-son importance clinique. Ann Otol Laryngol 1977; 94:273-89.

5. Pearson BW. Laryngeal micro circulation and pathways of cancer spread. Laryngoscope 1975; 85:700-13.

6. Terracol J, Guerrier Y. Le système artérial du larynx. Étude anatomique. Montpellier Médicale 1951; 41-2:340-65.

7. Kirchner JA. Anterior commissure cancer. In: Centennial conference on laryngeal cancer. New York: Appleton-Century-Crofts, 1976:679-81.

8. Speiden LM, Tucker G, Soulen R. Angiography of the larynx: an anatomic study in cadaver larynges. J Otolaryngol 1972; 1:219-23.

9. Freeland AP. Microfil angiography: a demonstration of the microvasculature of the larynx with reference to tumor spread. In: Centennial conference of laryngeal cancer. New York: Appleton-Century-Crofts, 1976:279-95.

10. Olzewski E. Vascularization of ossified cartilage and the spread of cancer in the larynx. Arch Otolaryngol 1976; 102:200-3.

ELECTRONYSTAGMOGRAPHY IN CONGENITAL AND ACQUIRED SYPHILITIC OTITIS

WILLIAM R. WILSON, MD
BOSTON, MASSACHUSETTS

MICHAEL ZOLLER, MD
SAVANNAH, GEORGIA

This study is an analysis of the electronystagmogram (ENG) changes in 17 patients with luetic vestibular disease with early and late acquired syphilis and congenital syphilis. Vestibular disturbances occurred in 80% of patients with luetic otitis. Among these patients the ENG gives signs of peripheral rather than central vestibular injury, and reduced vestibular response to caloric stimulation is the most common finding. Congenital syphilis patients have the greatest dysfunction, both in degree of ENG changes and incidence of bilaterality. We found no correlation between FTA-ABS levels and the amount of hearing impairment or vestibular injury. Treatment with penicillin and steroids had a beneficial subjective effect upon the symptoms of vertigo in over half the patients.

Luetic vestibular disease is a frequent concomitant of syphilitic hearing loss. Among our patients 80% with serum FTA-ABS-confirmed luetic otitis had complaints of dizziness sometime during the course of their illness.[1] In a few this was the presenting complaint. Vestibular dysfunction secondary to syphilis is not a rare disorder. Even though a positive FTA-ABS test does not prove the presence of luetic ear disease, a positive FTA-ABS test is found in 6.5% of patients with otherwise unexplained sensorineural hearing loss[2] and in 7% of patients with cochleovestibular disorders diagnosed as Menière's disease.[3]

It is well known that the inner ear is one site of predilection for long-term progressive spirochetal injury, and this fact is at least partly due to the failure of earlier penicillin dosage schedules to achieve spirocheticidal penicillin levels in cerebrospinal fluid[4-6] and the fluids of the inner ear.[7,8] The otologic symptoms of hearing loss and vertigo of late congenital syphilis or tertiary syphilis are often indistinguishable from Menière's disease.[9] The reason for this can be best understood from the otopathology. A luetic infection of the inner ear progresses from a mononuclear leukocytic infiltration, with advancing obliterative endarteritis and osteitis, to increasing fibrosis that results in an end stage characterized by endolymphatic hydrops and progressive degeneration of the membranous labyrinth.[10]

The purpose of this study is to gain further insight into the vestibular injury that results from acquired and congenital syphilitic otitis, and the effects of our treatment upon symptoms of vertigo and vestibular abnormalities as measured by electronystagmogram (ENG).

SUBJECTS AND METHODS

The authors examined the ENGs of 17 patients previously evaluated and treated at the Massachusetts Eye and Ear Infirmary and in the Genito-urinary Infectious Disease (GID) Clinic maintained by the Department of Dermatology, Massachusetts General Hospital. Many were included as patients in a previously reported study of hearing improvement following combined penicillin and steroid therapy.[1]

This group of patients all have serologically confirmed luetic cochleovestibular disease. There are 12 males and five females who range in age from 21 to 68 years, with a mean age of 46.4 years. By careful review of the hospital records, seven patients could be confirmed as having late congenital syphilis. Of the remainder, two patients had secondary acquired syphilis manifest by a luetic skin rash and simultaneous otologic involvement, and the remaining eight patients had tertiary acquired syphilis with progressive sensorineural hearing loss that often fluctuated (Table 1). All patients had a positive FTA-ABS or *Treponema pallidum* immobilization test as specific evidence of spirochetal antibodies. All patients had suffered hearing loss of some degree during the course of their illness (Table 2), however only 12 patients had known vertigo. Both the degree of hearing loss and symptoms of vertigo were most severe in the congenital luetic patients (Table 3).

The ENGs were performed using D-C recording equipment in a darkened room. The testing included calibration, head shaking,

TABLE 1. COMPARISON OF PATIENTS STUDIED FOR AGE, TYPE OF SYPHILITIC INVOLVEMENT, AND YEARS WITH THE DISEASE (N = 17)

	No. Pts.	*M*	*F*	*Age* (yr)*	*No. Years with Lues* *Range*	*Mean*
Secondary	2	2	0	30	<1	<1
Tertiary	8	6	2	49	1-38	16
Congenital	7	4	3	45	33-63	46
Totals	17	12	5			

M - Male; F - Female.
*Mean - 46.4 years.

From the Department of Otolaryngology, Harvard Medical School and the Massachusets Eye and Ear Infirmary, Boston, Massachusetts.
REPRINTS — William R. Wilson, MD, Massachusetts Eye and Ear Infirmary, 243 Charles Street, Boston, MA 02114.

TABLE 2. SUMMARY OF HEARING LEVELS IN PATIENTS STUDIED (N = 17)*

	No. Pts.	Mean SRT (dB) AS	Mean SRT (dB) AD	Mean Discrimination Score (%) AS	Mean Discrimination Score (%) AD
Secondary	2	35	45	70	72
Tertiary	8	44	54	70	60
Congenital	7	70	54	20	50

SRT - Speech reception threshold.

*Among the patients studied, the hearing became progressively worse with each succeeding type of syphilis, from secondary to congenital.

pendulum tracking, gaze tests, optokinetic tests, and hyperventilation tests. The patients were studied for spontaneous horizontal and vertical nystagmus. Positional tests included cervical positioning tests, right and left lateral and supine-positioning tests, and right, left and midline head hanging, each followed by an abrupt return to the erect sitting position. Classic Hallpike water calorics were used as a measure of lateral canal function. If no response was obtained, 10 cc of ice water were used to confirm the absence of vestibular function. Five patients, four with acquired and one with congenital syphilis, had ENG evaluations prior to and subsequent to penicillin and/or steroid therapy.

TABLE 3. SUMMARY OF PATIENTS WITH PRESENCE OF VERTIGO (N = 17)

	No.	Vertigo*	%	
Secondary	2	0/2	0	50 (Secondary + Tertiary)
Tertiary	8	5/8	60	
Congenital	7	7/7	100	

*All patients with congenital syphilis suffered vertigo while only half the acquired syphilitics were affected.

TABLE 4. SUMMARY OF ENG INTERPRETATIONS* (N = 17)

	Secondary	Tertiary	Congenital
Normal	2	2	0
Unilateral PVSD	0	3	1
Bilateral PVSD	0	1	4
Nonlocalizing	0	2	0
PVSD + central signs	0	0	0
Central	0	0	0
Totals	2	8	7

PVSD - Peripheral vestibular system dysfunction.

*All the ENGs were interpreted as peripheral, although there were central signs on two tracings among the congenital syphilis patients.

Treatment consisted of a three-month course of benzathine penicillin G, 2.4 million units administered intramuscularly each week, and when not contraindicated, 80 mg of prednisone orally every other morning.

TABLE 6. SUMMARY OF POSITIONAL TESTS (N = 17)

	No. Pts.	None	Nystagmus* Directional Fixed	Nystagmus* Directional Changing
Secondary	2	1	1	0
Tertiary	8	4	3	1
Congenital	7	1	4	2

*Positional nystagmus was another common finding on the ENGs.

RESULTS

The ENGs demonstrate that congenital and acquired syphilis patients suffer primarily from a peripheral vestibular injury. There is an increasing magnitude of vestibular dysfunction, beginning with the secondary lues patients who have few, to the congenital syphilis patients who have the greatest number of ENG abnormalities. There was very little indication of central vestibular system dysfunction, except among the congenital syphilis patients, who had an occasional feature on the tracings of possible central pathology (Table 4). However, in most instances, these findings were attributed to the fact that many of the congenital patients suffer from reduced vision secondary to interstitial keratitis, which affects performance on the tests of central vestibular function such as the pendulum test (slow pursuit test), optokinetic and gaze tests.

Ten of 12 patients with complaints of vertigo had an abnormal ENG with an abnormal caloric test. Of those patients with no complaints of vertigo, the ENGs were normal or had minor changes, principally directional preponderance.

The most common feature of the ENG abnormality associated with syphilitic otitis is a unilateral or bilateral reduced vestibular response (Table 5). Directional fixed spontaneous nystagmus, or direction-fixed nystagmus evoked by positional testing, were also common features of these ENGs (Table 6). Direction-changing nystagmus was seen on only three of the ENGs, despite the prevalence of bilateral vestibular disease, especially among the patients with congenital syphilis. Five of seven of the congenital syphilis patients had eye disease. Only one patient with presumed acquired syphilis had

TABLE 5. SUMMARY OF CALORIC* RESPONSES IN PATIENTS STUDIED (N = 17)

	No. Pts.	No. Ears	Normal	Reduced Vestibular Response†	Canal Paresis§	Absent∮	Directional Preponderance	Bilateral Abnormal Caloric Response
Secondary	2	4	3	1	0	0	0	0
Tertiary	8	16	12	2	1	1	2	0
Congenital	7	14	1	0	9	4	0	6

*Hallpike calorics 30 and 44C, and 10 cc ice water.

†The reduced vestibular response was the most common finding on the ENGs. There were 5 abnormally functioning horizontal canals among 10 patients with acquired syphilis, and 13 among the 7 congenital syphilis patients.

§Canal paresis - Response of 7°/sec or less, but having response to ice water.

∮Absent - No response to ice water.

TABLE 7. SUMMARY OF FTA-ABS LEVELS: CORRELATION* TO HEARING LOSS AND VESTIBULAR INJURY (N = 17)

Level FTA-ABS	*No. Pts.*	*Secondary*	*Tertiary*	*Congenital*	*Mean SRT AU*	*Hallpike Calorics No. Normal*
Bdln.	1			1	40	0
1 +	6		2	4	66	0
2 +	3	1	1	1	63	1
3 +	4		4		40	1
4 +	3	1	1	1	43	2

SRT - Speech reception threshold; AU - Both ears; Bdln. - Borderline.

*There is no direct correlation between FTA/ABS levels and type of syphilis or degree of hearing loss. In general, the patients with acquired syphilis have the higher titers. The FTA/ABS once positive, remains positive, and is unaffected by treatment; however, the titer levels tend to diminish with time. Therefore, the patients with congenital syphilis have lower titers associated with greater hearing loss and a 100% incidence of vertigo.

keratitis. This patient stated that the syphilis was contracted during World War II.

The relationship of reagin tests to specific antibody tests in luetic hearing loss, and the response of patients with syphilitic hearing loss to treatment, have been discussed in our previous papers.[1,2] It is clear that hearing loss and ENG abnormality do not correlate directly with FTA-ABS levels. Nonetheless, the degree of hearing loss is paralleled by the vestibular symptomatology, and the vestibular abnormality as measured by ENG. The poorest hearing is found among the congenital syphilis patients who have the most abnormal ENGs.

All the congenital syphilis patients in this study suffered from vertigo, while only half or less of the patients with acquired lues had complaints of dizziness or imbalance (Table 7). The ENGs reflect this difference. Two of the eight patients with acquired tertiary syphilis had normal ENGs, two had changes other than caloric test abnormalities. Only half had peripheral vestibular system dysfunction marked enough to produce a reduced vestibular response with Hallpike testing. On the other hand, all seven of the congenital luetic patients had reduced canal function, and three patients had absent caloric response in both ears. The congenital luetic patients have increased bilaterality and also more severe vestibular disease.

Table 8 illustrates the changes in symptoms and ENG findings in five patients who had ENGs prior to and following treatment. Three of the five ENGs of patients treated with our regime of penicillin and steroids demonstrated objective evidence of improved peripheral vestibular system function. Four of five patients noted subjective improvement in vertigo.

Table 9 illustrates the subjective improvement of symptoms in 12 vertiginous patients treated. All the congenital syphilis patients in this study suffered from vertigo, while only half or less of the acquired syphilis patients had complaints of dizziness or imbalance. The response to this therapy was satisfactory in a majority of the patients with vertigo.

DISCUSSION

At this time we are not certain that syphilitic

TABLE 8. ENG READINGS BEFORE AND AFTER LUETIC THERAPY* (N = 9)

Patient No.	*Type of Lues*		*ENG Data*	*Rx*	*Comment*
1	A-3	ENG 1:	Absent caloric,† AS; paresis,‡ AD.	S	ENG: unchanged.
		ENG 2:	Absent caloric,† AS; paresis,‡ AD.		Symptoms: continued hearing loss, vertigo improved
2	A-3	ENG 1:	PN-C, normal caloric, AD; AS responds to ice water only.	P/S	ENG: improved Symptoms: improved.
		ENG 2:	PN-F, normal caloric, AD; AS responds to cool water, but not to warm.		
3	A-3 (reinfection)	ENG 1:	PN-F, LDP on calorics.	P/S	ENG: improved.
		ENG 2:	No PN, normal calorics.		Symptoms: patients had no vertigo pre or post Rx.
4	A-3	ENG 1:	Pend T:§ II; RSHN, PN-F, unilateral RVR.∮	P/S	ENG: probably improved.
		ENG 2:	Pend T:§ III; no RSHN, no PN, unilateral RVR∮		Symptoms: improved vertigo.
5	C	ENG 1:	Pend T:§ III; RVR,∮ AU.	P/S	ENG: unchanged.
		ENG 2:	Pend T:§ III; RVR,∮ AU.		Symptoms: improved vertigo.

RSHN - Right spontaneous horizontal nystagmus; PN-C - Direction changing postitional nystagmus; PN-F - Direction fixed positional nystagmus; Pend T - Pendulum test; RVR - Reduced vestibular response; P - Penicillin; S - Steroids; Rx - Treatment; LDP - Left directional preponderance.

*The effect of treatment on the ENG findings is not clear-cut. Three tracings were thought to be improved.

†Absent caloric is no response to 10 cc ice water.

‡Canal paresis is a response to 7°/sec or less but having a response to ice water.

∮RVR indicates there is a 15% or greater reduction in the maximum speed of the slow phase in the most affected ear, unless that response is 7°/sec or less.

§Pendulum test is scored I-IV according to method of Benitez;[11] type I is sinusoidal curves, type II is superimposed nonnystagmic movements, type III is superimposed nystagmic or saccadic movements, type IV is ataxic eye movements.

TABLE 9. SUBJECTIVE RESPONSE TO THERAPY FOR VERTIGO OF LUETIC ORIGIN (N = 12*)

	No. Pts.	Treatment P	S	P/S	Unknown	Vertigo Unchanged	Inproved†
Tertiary	5	1	1	3	2	0	3
Congenital	7	0	0	6	0	3	4

P -Benzathine penicillin G 2.4 million units parenterally q week x 12; S - Prednisone 80 mg/q o AM/30 days.

*One patient was treated earlier.

†There was better than 50% subjective improvement in vertigo among all patients treated.

otitis can be arrested. Previous dosage schedules for penicillin were too low to produce spirocheticidal doses of drug in the CSF and inner ear fluids of syphilis patients. As a result, patients who received penicillin injections years ago are returning with luetic otologic or ophthalmic disease without other evidence of the syphilis.[2,8,12,13] Reagin antibody studies involving serum and cerebral spinal fluid from these patients are too frequently negative to be reliable. The serum FTA-ABS must be used routinely to confirm syphilitic otitis in unexplained hearing loss or vertigo, despite the otherwise negative history. We have found that a majority of previously treated patients will tell you they have never had syphilis.[1] Only by proper identification of patients, appropriate treatment, and long-term follow-up can the pathophysiology of this disease be understood.

From the data in this study, it appears that congenital syphilis has a more injurious effect upon the inner ear than acquired syphilis. There may be two factors involved. First, the fetus is exposed to the circulating spirochete without the benefit of a developed intrinsic immune response or treatment for nine months.[14] This probably ensures that both eyes and both ears become seeded with the bacteria. All seven of our congenital syphilis patients had bilateral hearing loss, and of 14 ears, only one lateral canal was functioning within the normal range. On the other hand, the acquired syphilis patient may receive some treatment prior to complete dispersal of the infection. Second, time elapsed from the onset of infection is certainly important. While the mean age of the congenital syphilitic is 45 years, and that of the acquired tertiary syphilitic is 49 years, the average congenital patient has probably had the disorder at least 15-20 years longer than the acquired patients in this study.

It has been our clinical impression, confirmed by this chart review, that symptoms of vertigo secondary to luetic cochlear-vestibular disease do respond to penicillin and steroid therapy. The follow-up on these patients ranges up to four years and the results to date appear long lasting. As permanent hearing improvement occurred in only 15% of patients treated, improved vertigo in a higher percentage was a further welcomed benefit of 12 weeks of treatment.

CONCLUSIONS

1. Late congenital and acquired syphilis results in a peripheral rather than central vestibular injury, as measured by ENG. The most common feature of the ENG abnormality is a unilateral or bilateral reduced vestibular response.

2. Congenital syphilis patients have the greatest vestibular system dysfunction, both in degree and incidence of bilaterality. There is a high correlation between symptoms and ENG findings.

3. FTA-ABS levels do not correlate with degree of hearing loss or vestibular injury. The latter are related to the length of infection and most probably also the timing and dosage of proper treatment.

4. Penicillin and steroids in the dosages described have a beneficial subjective effect upon the symptoms of vertigo in over half the patients treated.

REFERENCES

1. Zoller M, Wilson WR, Nadol JB Jr. Treatment of syphilitic hearing loss: combined penicillin and steroid therapy in 29 patients. Ann Otol Rhinol Laryngol 1979; 88:160-5.

2. Zoller M, Wilson WR, Nadol JB Jr, Girard KF. Detection of syphilitic hearing loss. Arch Otolaryngol 1978; 104:63-5.

3. Pulec JL. Meniere's disease: results of a 2 1/2 year study of etiology, natural history, and results of treatment. Laryngoscope 1972; 82:1703-15.

4. Yoder FW. Penicillin treatment of neurosyphilis: are recommended dosages sufficient? JAMA 1975; 232:270-1.

5. Tramont EC. Persistence of *Treponema pallidum* following penicillin G therapy: report of 2 cases. JAMA 1976; 236:2206-7.

6. Dunlop EMC, Al-Egaily MB, Houang ET. Penicillin levels in blood and CSF achieved by treatment of syphilis. JAMA 1979; 241:2538-41.

7. Mack LW, Smith JL, Walter EK, Rios-Montenegro EN, Nichol WG. Temporal bone treponemes. Arch Otolaryngol 1969; 90:11-5.

8. Weit RJ, Milko DA. Isolation of the spirochetes in the perilymph despite prior antisyphilitic therapy: a case report. Arch Otolaryngol 1975; 101:104-6.

9. Karmody CS, Schuknecht HF. Deafness in congenital syphilis. Arch Otolaryngol 1966; 83:18-28.

10. Schuknecht HF. Pathology of the ear. Cambridge: Harvard University Press, 1974:262-6.

11. Benitez JT. Eye-tracking and optokinetic tests: diagnostic significance in peripheral and central vestibular disorders. Laryngoscope 1970; 80:834-48.

12. Smith JL, Isreal CW. The presence of spirochetes in late seronegative syphilis. JAMA 1967; 199:126-30.

13. Hendershot EL. Luetic deafness. Laryngoscope 1973; 83:865-70.

14. Musher DM, Schell RF. The immunology of syphilis. Hosp Pract 1975; 10:45-50.

ELEMENTAL COMPOSITION OF THE DEVELOPING INNER EAR

MATTI ANNIKO, MD ROMUALD WROBLEWSKI, PhD

STOCKHOLM, SWEDEN

The elemental composition of the inner ear fluid-filled compartments has been analyzed using the x-ray energy dispersive technique (CBA mouse). Special attention has been focused on the maturation of endolymph. A few days before and after birth the relative peak intensity of potassium (R_K) in the vestibular endolymphatic compartment was slightly surpassing that in the cochlear part of the labyrinth. From the fourth day after birth (DAB) a rapid increase occurred concerning the R_K. The highest R_K was found in the endolymphatic space in the basal part of the cochlea followed by that in the vestibular endolymph. The lowest R_K was measured in endolymph of the apical part of the cochlea. These obvious differences were abandoned already on the sixth DAB. A mature composition of endolymph was reached on the eighth DAB. The present technique does not allow analyses of differences between cochlear and vestibular endolymph with regard to minimal shifts.

INTRODUCTION

During the embryologic development, the inner ear undergoes dramatic changes. Morphologically it passes from the otocyst stage organogenesis to cytodifferentiation. Physiologically, there is the development of the specific inner ear fluids and maturation of cochlear and eighth nerve potentials. Little, however, is known of the elemental distribution in the inner ear under development and especially the time for the development of endolymph.

The latter question is of special interest because of the introduction of in vitro techniques for the culture of the mammalian inner ear.[1-3] While complete maturation of, eg, vestibular hair cells can be obtained in vitro[4] except for their innervation,[5] the explantation of newborn or adult inner ears is not successful with regard to specialized hair cell structure[6] although the hair cell itself can survive for a considerable time.[7] Also the postnatal secretory epithelium reveals cytological changes in vitro.[8]

The present study is the first to analyze the elemental distribution of the developing inner ear which follows when the specific composition of endolymph is reached. According to the reports of Anniko and Wroblewski,[9] a mature ionic distribution was found in the endolymph of the eight-day-old CBA/CBA mouse.

METHODS

Material. Inner ears from the 13th, 16th and 19th gestational day fetuses of the CBA/CBA mouse were analyzed together with labyrinths from newborn, 2, 4, 6 and 8-day-old animals. Each group consisted of three serial sectioned inner ears.

The 13th gestational day inner ear anlage is still cystic but has begun its organogenesis which is completed on the 16th gestational day, except for a slight elongation of the cochlear end. Cytodifferentiation of most vestibular hair cells is ended on the 19th gestational day, but for the maturation of their innervation which takes place mainly postpartum. Cochlear hair cells are present at birth but the organ of Corti is still immature, as is also the stria vascularis which completes its morphological maturation during the first week postpartum.[1,3,10,11]

Methods. The preparation of sections for the x-ray energy dispersive analyses and the analytical equipment has been described in detail by Wroblewski et al[12] and Anniko and Wroblewski.[9] In addition to the semithick cryostat sections for analysis of the elemental distribution, ordinary histological sections of the inner ear were prepared, stained with hemotoxylin and eosin. All inner ears have been serial sectioned. In some cases, one ear from the fetus was taken for immediate freezing in liquid propane cooled with liquid nitrogen to −190 C while the other ear was fixed either in a solution of 3% glutaraldehyde in 0.133 M sodium phosphate buffer and prepared for electron microscopy (embedding in Epon® mixture) or fixed in 4% formaldehyde, embedded in paraffin and serial sectioned for light microscopy.

The analyses were performed by measuring specific counts for each element detected according to $P_x + B_x$, $P_x - B_x$, B and by calculating the relative peak intensity (R_X) for each detected element using the formula $R_x = (P\text{-}B)_x/B$. The symbols are designed as follows: P_x -energy quanta counts for the element x, B_x -background counts for the element x, B -background counts in general, R_x -relative peak intensity for the element x.

In addition to these calculations measurements were also made of the weight and atomic percentage in the analyzed areas via a standardless analysis computorized program including the precision of 3 sigma. All these measurements were performed three to five times giving the average values of these repeated measurements. The K alpha line was used in the calculations of detected elements.

RESULTS

EMBRYOLOGIC DEVELOPMENT OF THE INNER EAR OTOCYST (TABLES 1 AND 2)

Gestational Day 13. The elemental distribution in the cystic space was compared with that measured at the adjacent cells. The living otocyst is illustrated in Figure 1 as also a section through this area. A corresponding semithick cryostat section is shown in Figure 2. Analysis of the material in the otocyst lumen gives a distinct peak for Cl but peaks

From the Department of Otorhinolaryngology, Karolinska Hospital and King Gustaf V Research Institute, the Karolinska Institute, and the Wenner-Gren Institute, University of Stockholm, Stockholm, Sweden. Supported by grants from the Swedish Medical Research Council (grant no. 12X-720), Ragnar and Torsten Söderbergs Stiftelse and funds from Tysta Skolan.

REPRINTS — Matti Anniko, MD, Department of Otolaryngology, Karolinska Hospital, S-104 01 Stockholm, Sweden.

TABLE 1. ENERGY QUANTA RATIO BETWEEN DIFFERENT ELEMENTS IN ENDOLYMPHATIC SPACE DURING EMBRYOLOGIC AND EARLY POSTNATAL DEVELOPMENT*

Age (days)	*Cl:Na + K*	*Cl:K*	*Cl:Na*	*K:Na*
Gestational				
13	1.37:1	2.4:1	3.06:1	1.31:1
16	1.05:1	1.53:1	2.31:1	1.62:1
19	0.78:1	1.21:1	2.21:1	1.84:1
Birth	0.65:1	0.97:1	2.02:1	2.08:1
Postpartum				
2	1.14:1	1.41:1	3.82:1	2.30:1
4	–†	0.71:1	–†	–†
6		0.69:1		
8		0.73:1		

*The values indicated are means based on at least three measurements at different regions. The analyses were performed by using the P - B value for each measurement.

†Sodium could not be identified in the basal coil. In the apical coil of the cochlea the ratio K:Na was 3.2:1.

for K, P and Na are also indicated (Fig. 3). As a comparison, Figure 4 illustrates the intracellular/cytoplasmic elemental distribution showing distinct peaks for Na, S, P, Cl and K.

Gestational Day 16. The vestibular organs and the cochlea were easily identified (Fig. 5 A, B). The material in the endolymphatic space gave distinct but relatively small peaks for Cl and K and peaks were indicated for Na, S and P in the vestibular part of the inner ear (Fig. 6). In contrast, measurements from the apical part of the cochlear endolymphatic space resulted in a peak for Cl while the peak for K hardly could be identified (Fig. 7). A slight difference in the levels of the relative peak intensities was obvious in some measurements between the vestibular and cochlear partitions of the endolymphatic space. The ratio of Cl/K approximated 3: 1 for the cochlea while this ratio was only approximately 1.5: 1 in the vestibular part.

As compared with the 13th gestational day inner ear/otocyst, the relative peak intensity for K was slightly increased (Table 2). The ratios of K versus Cl and Na, respectively, changed, indicating a higher amount of K in the 16th gestational day inner ear, than at the earlier stage of embryologic development (Table 1).

Gestational Day 19. The elemental distribution in the endolymphatic space revealed distinct peaks for Na, S, P, Cl and K (Fig. 8). The relative peak intensity in the endolymphatic space had increased with regard to K (R_K = 2.23) while that of Cl was

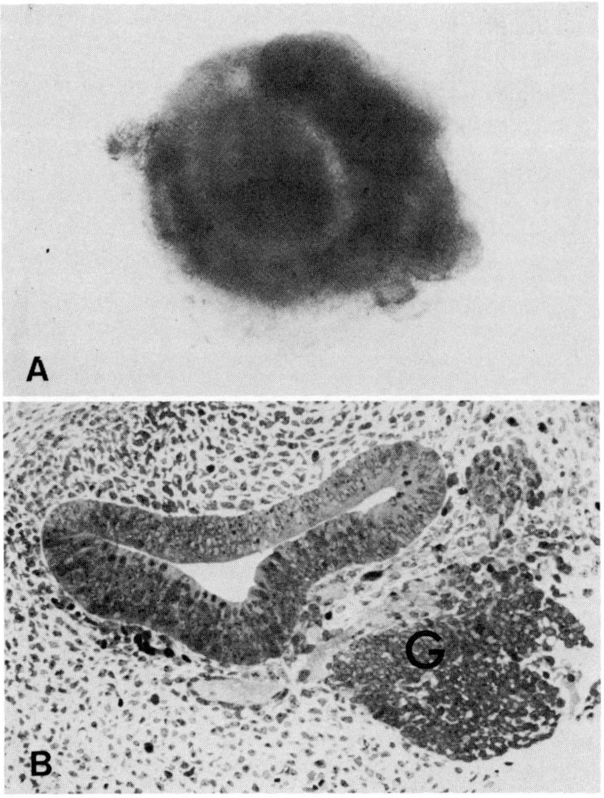

Fig. 1. A) Light microscopy of the 13th gestational day inner ear (otocyst). B) Cross section of otocyst in A. The inner ear anlage is still cystic but has now several layers of cells in the epithelium. The adjacent ganglion (G) can be identified easily.

TABLE 2. RELATIVE PEAK INTENSITY IN ENDOLYMPHATIC SPACE FOR ELEMENTS K, Na and Cl DURING EMBRYOLOGIC DEVELOPMENT AND POSTNATAL MATURATION*

Age During Development	*K*	*R_X* *Na*	*Cl*
Gestation period			
13th day	1.07	1.31	1.81
16th day	1.75	2.02	2.72
19th day	2.23	1.90	2.60
Birth	2.48†	1.22†	2.94†
Postnatal maturation			
2 DAB	2.30	1.24	3.66
4 DAB	4.55	0 ∫	4.20
6 DAB	6.05	0	6.35
8 DAB	7.10	0	7.00

*The indicated values are means based on measurements from at least three different regions. DAB - Days after birth.

†Cochlea only.

∫No detectable peak for Na.

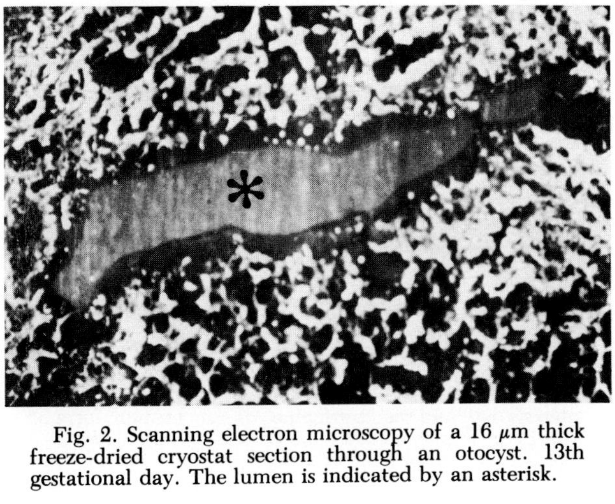

Fig. 2. Scanning electron microscopy of a 16 μm thick freeze-dried cryostat section through an otocyst. 13th gestational day. The lumen is indicated by an asterisk.

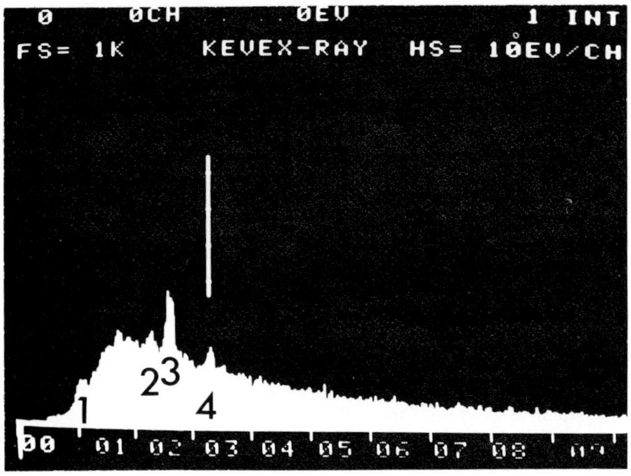

Fig. 3. Emitted energy histogram (EEH). Full scale (FS) 1 K. The elemental analysis of the specimen illustrated in Fig. 2 gives peaks for sodium (1), sulphur (2), chloride (3) and potassium (4). The vertical line above the histogram gives the location for potassium.

approximately the same as compared with the 16th gestational day (R_{Cl} = 2.60) (Table 2). Also the ratio K/Na in this compartment had changed from 1.31:1 on the 13th gestational day, 1.62:1 on the 16th to 1.84:1 on the 19th gestational day (Table 1).

POSTNATAL INNER EAR

Newborn Animals. The maturation process of the ionic composition of endolymph continues. The ratio of K/Cl is approximately 1:1. There occurs twice as much of K as of Na. With regard to the relative peak intensities of Na, Cl and K, obvious differences are found between the endolymphatic and perilymphatic spaces. It has to be noted that such differences were not present in the 19th gestational day inner ear. In both the endolymphatic and perilymphatic compartments distinct peaks were identified for S and P (Figs. 9 and 10).

TWO DAYS AFTER BIRTH. The relative peak intensity of K in the endolymphatic space has increased as compared with the newborn animal (Fig. 11). The

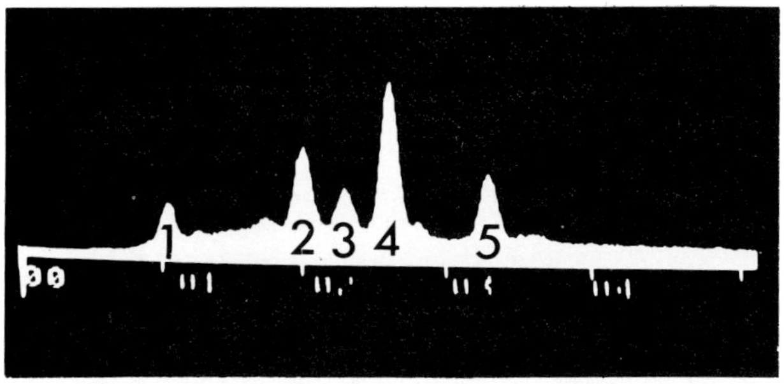

Fig. 4. EEH. FS 2 K. The elemental analysis has now been performed on cells adjacent to the otocyst lumen. The relative peak intensities (R_x: x = element analyzed) for chlorine (4) and phosphorus (2) are distinctly exceeding those for sodium (1), sulphur (3) and potassium (5). X-ray microanalysis of biological material gives the elemental analysis only and the interference of the chemical form or activity of the elements or the compounds that they may represent has to be based on other independent information.

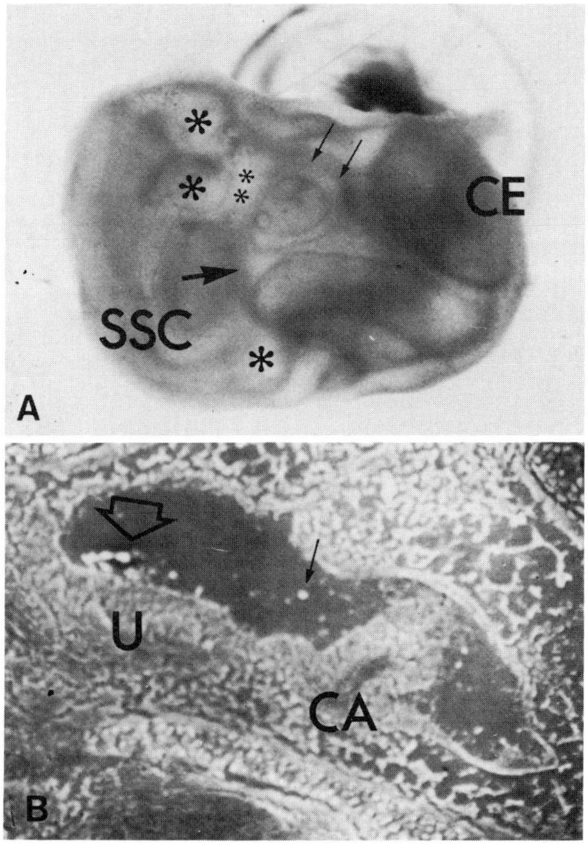

Fig. 5. A) Light microscopy of 16th gestational day inner ear. At this stage morphogenesis is ended while cytodifferentiation of inner ear organs is in progress. The cristae ampullares are indicated by large asterisks. The utricle is marked with two small asterisks. Large arrow - Saccule near the base of the cochlea; Double arrows - Endolymphatic duct; SSC - Semicircular canals; CE - Cochlear end. B) Scanning electron microscopy. A 16 μm thick freeze-dried cryostat serial section through the vestibular part of the inner ear. The outlines of a crista ampullaris (CA) and the utricle (U) are indicated. Above the surface of the utricle otoconia can be observed (unfilled arrow). During sectioning one otoconia has been removed from its normal location as indicated by the small arrow. Elemental analysis of these otoconia already gives extremely high peaks for calcium.

R_{Cl} too has increased; Na is still identified. The ratios Cl/Na and K/Na have increased to 3.82:1 and 2.30:1, respectively (Table 1). S and P are still identified as having rather high relative peak intensities.

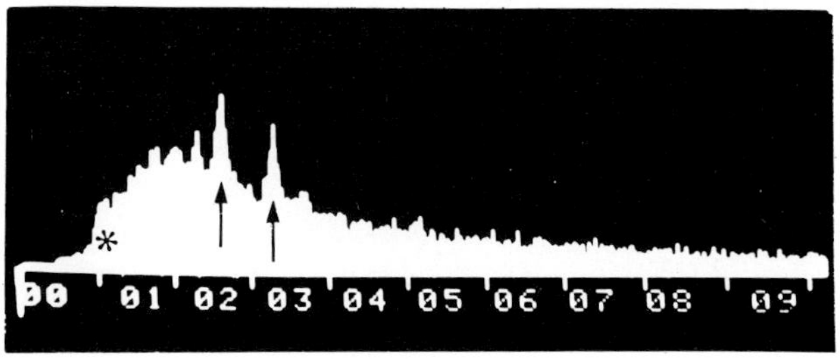

Fig. 6. EEH. FS 1 K. 16th gestational day inner ear. Analysis of the elemental content in the endolymphatic space of the vestibular labyrinth reveals the identification of several elements among other sodium (asterisk), chlorine (arrow to the left) and potassium (arrow to the right).

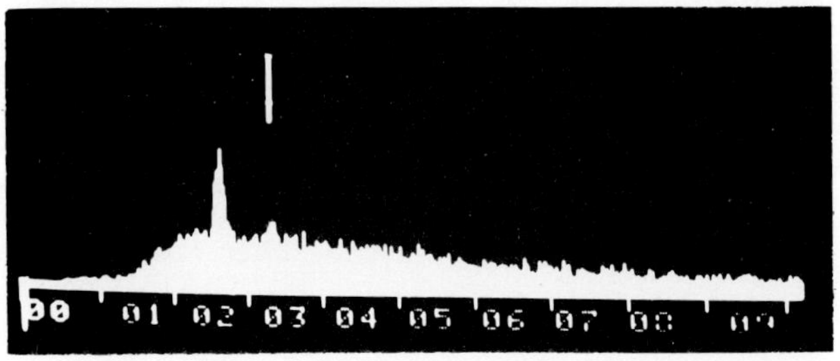

Fig. 7. EEH. FS 2 K. 16th gestational day inner ear. Apical coil of the cochlea. A distinct peak for chlorine can be observed. The location for the potassium peak is indicated by the vertical line.

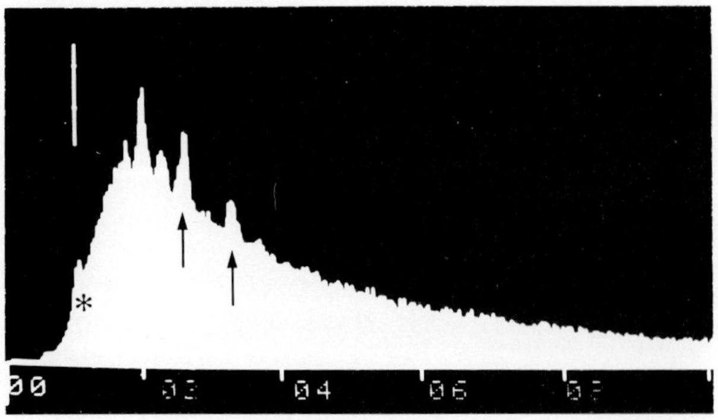

Fig. 9. EEH. FS 500. Day of birth. Basal coil of the cochlea. Endolymphatic space. There is still no specific elemental composition of endolymph. Sodium (asterisk), chlorine (arrow to the left), potassium (arrow to the right). A high relative peak intensity can be found concerning phosphorus (R_p) (second peak to the left of that for chlorine). Also sulphur (between phosphorus and chlorine) is identified.

FOUR DAYS AFTER BIRTH. This day indicates an important stage in the maturation process of endolymph. First, Na can no longer be identified (Fig. 12). Second, the ratio Cl/K has changed to 0.71:1, ie, the concentration of K has increased more than that of Cl which it now exceeds. In one animal, the ratio K/Na was 3.2:1 in the apical coil of the cochlea. In contrast no Na could be detected in the basal coil. The relative peak intensities for S and P remained rather unchanged. In the perilymphatic space the relative peak intensity of Na was slightly increased while those for S and P decreased to approximately half of the values noted at birth (Fig.13).

When analyzing the elemental mapping of sodium, potassium and chlorine in the tectorial membrane, no obvious difference could be found between different regions of the membrane. The control mapping of background counts confirmed that these elements were confined mainly to the tectorial membrane and only a considerably lower content, according to this method, was found in the endolymphatic space concerning potassium and chlorine.

SIX DAYS AFTER BIRTH. A considerable increase of K concentration in endolymph occurred. A slight difference was found between the apical and the basal parts of the cochlea, the former having a lower concentration of K. In elemental distribution no obvious difference occurred between the vestibular endolymph and that in the basal coil of the cochlea. P and S were still identified in relative high concentrations both in the endolymphatic and perilymphatic spaces. Elements identified during this stage of development were determined also with regard to weight and atomic percentage including the precision of 3 sigma (Table 3). Except the expected differences in K concentration between the endolymphatic and perilymphatic spaces, the weight percentage of Ca (K_{alpha} line) was 5.09 in the endolymphatic space in contrast to 17.46 in the perilymphatic compartment of the inner ear (basal coil of the cochlea). The weight percentages of S were 12.60 and 17.71, respectively, and for P 16.75 and 16.32, respectively.

EIGHT DAYS AFTER BIRTH. The endolymph now comprised mature conditions. Both the relative peak intensities and the weight/atomic percentage of elements identified were determined (Fig. 14 and Table 4). It has to be noted that the concentrations of P, S and Ca (weight and atomic percentage) had decreased to very low levels as also Na (Table 4). These elements can no longer be distinctly identified when analyzing the relative peak intensities (Fig. 14). The perilymphatic space revealed a mature elemental composition (Fig. 15).

DISCUSSION

The present study of the CBA/CBA mouse reveals

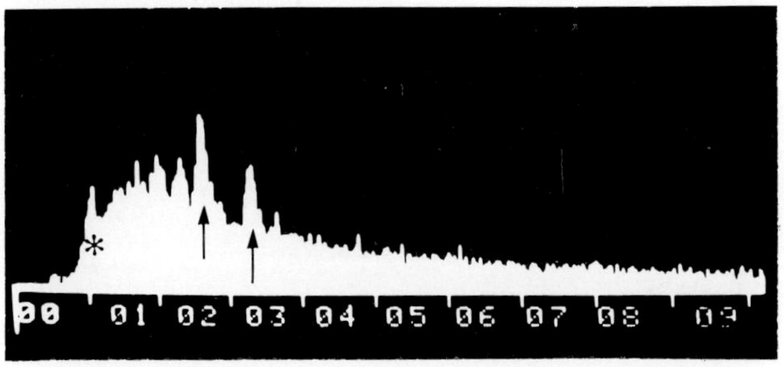

Fig. 8. EEH. FS 1 K. 19th gestational day. The elemental analysis reveals elements similar to those found in an extracellular fluid environment. Sodium (asterisk), chlorine (arrow to the left), potassium (arrow to the right). Also phosphorus and sulphur are identified (peaks to the left of that for chlorine).

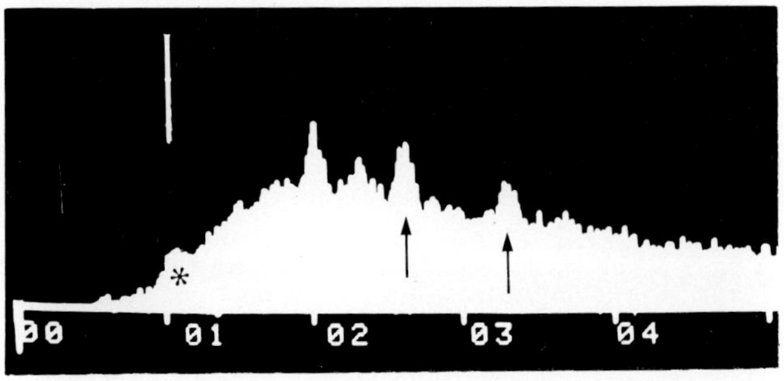

Fig. 10. EEH. FS 1 K. Day of birth. Perilymphatic space of the basal coil of the cochlea (scala vestibuli). Sodium (asterisk), chlorine (arrow to the left), potassium (arrow to the right).

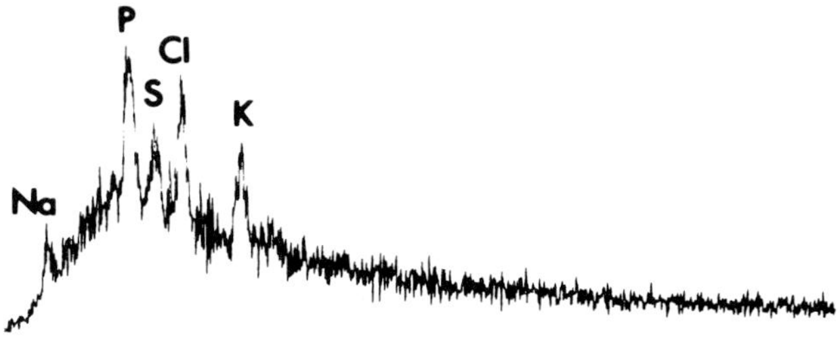

Fig. 11. EEH. FS 500. Two days after birth (DAB). Endolymphatic space in the basal coil of the cochlea. Although the R_K is increasing and the R_{Na} is decreasing the elemental composition with regard to identified elements still shows a rather extracellular type. P - Phosphorus; Cl -Chlorine; S - Sulphur; K - Potassium; Na - Sodium.

that the maturation process of inner ear fluids occurs postpartum. The unique composition of endolymph is reached six to eight days after birth. The maturation of the ionic/elemental composition of endolymph occurs largely parallel to the morphological maturation of the cochlea, especially the development of the stria vascularis but before the development of electrical potentials (Table 5).

Cochlear hair cells are evident at birth. Fluid spaces occur in the organ of Corti by the sixth day. By the 14th day the organ of Corti appears morphologically well developed.[13]

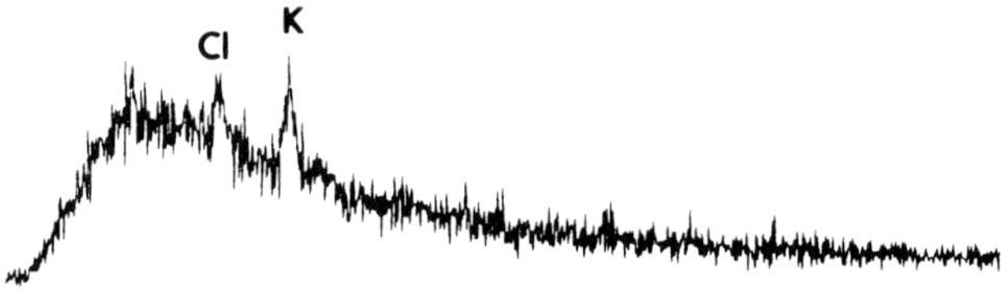

Fig. 12. EEH. FS 1 K. Four DAB. Endolymphatic space in the basal coil of the cochlea. Maturation of the endolymph has started. Sodium is no longer identified. Cl -Chlorine; K - Potassium.

Cochlear potentials occur in the mouse first on the eighth day after birth and increase gradually to adult values by the 14th day.[14] On the 9th day N_1 N_2 recordings can be obtained from the round window membrane; also observed is a Preyer reflex. It has been suggested that neural activity may develop later than hair cell activity since the eighth nerve action potential, R_1 R_2, was recorded only in 10-day-old animals.[15]

The comparison of electrophysiological and electron microscopical findings on inner ear synapses

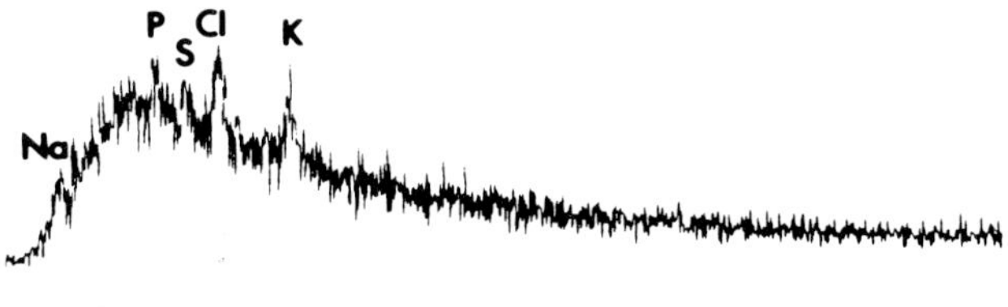

Fig. 13. EEH. FS 1 K. Four DAB. Perilymphatic space in the basal coil of the cochlea (scala vestibuli). Sodium (Na), phosphorus (P), sulphur (S), chlorine (Cl) and potassium (K) are easily identified.

TABLE 3. WEIGHT PERCENTAGE OF ELEMENTS IDENTIFIED IN THE APICAL COIL OF THE COCHLEA SIX DAYS AFTER BIRTH* (ENDOLYMPHATIC SPACE)

Element	*Weight %*	*Atomic %*	*Precision 3 Sigma*
Na	8.62	12.65	3.21
P	16.75	18.25	4.10
S	12.60	13.26	3.78
Cl	27.44	26.11	6.05
K	29.50	25.45	6.89
Ca	5.09	4.29	4.05
Total	100.00	100.00	

*Measurements are made in the K_{alpha} line.

from a variety of species reveals that morphological maturation of both the afferent and the efferent innervation precede functional capability by two to three days, eg, in the rabbit.[16] The cochlear function with regard to electrophysiology is likely to be dependent on a mature composition of inner ear fluids.

A morphological maturation of the inner ear secretory epithelia should precede the formation of the mature composition of endolymph. Anniko[11] reported a mature ultrastructure in the dark cell region of the vestibular labyrinth at birth except for an increase in the number of interdigitations toward the basal membrane during the first days after birth. In contrast, the cells of the stria vascularis pass their terminal mitosis postpartum.[17] From the studies of Kikuchi and Hilding,[18] although not detailed, it can be concluded that the stria vascularis reaches a rapid maturation within the first week after birth with regard to main structures while, eg, kinocilia on marginal cell surfaces are sometimes not lost until the tenth day.[10]

Anatomical, electrophysiological and behavioral correlates of the development of the inner ear functions may vary in different species in the time-course relationship. Bosher and Warren[19] analyzed the electrochemistry of cochlear fluids of the 8th-18th day neonatal rat, ie, during the development of the endocochlear potential (EP). The ionic composition of endolymph remained unchanged during the rapid increase of EP indicating that these two processes arise largely independently during cochlear maturation. Thus, in the rat, too, the develop-

TABLE 4. WEIGHT PERCENTAGE OF ELEMENTS IDENTIFIED ON THE EIGHTH DAY AFTER BIRTH IN THE BASAL COIL OF THE COCHLEA (ENDOLYMPHATIC SPACE).*

Element	*Weight %*	*Atomic %*	*Precision 3 Sigma*
Na	3.99	6.28	2.05
P	0.58	0.67	0.77
S	8.99	10.15	2.96
Cl	30.87	31.50	6.07
K	54.62	50.54	9.44
Ca	0.95	0.86	1.43
Total	100.00	100.00	

*The measurements are made in the K_{alpha} line.

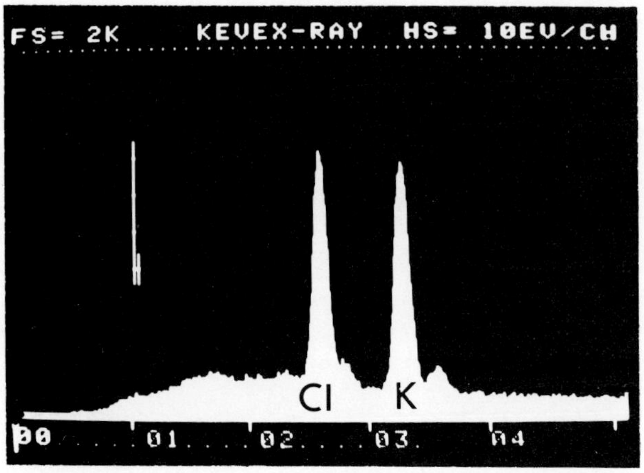

Fig. 14. EEH. FS 2 K. Eight DAB. Endolymphatic space of the basal coil in the cochlea. Very high R_{Cl} and R_K are identified whereas other elements cannot be detected. The location for sodium in the emitted energy scale is indicated by the vertical line.

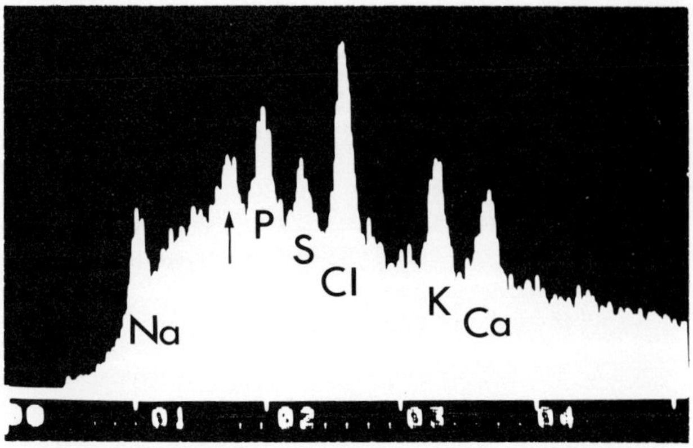

Fig. 15. EEH. FS 2 K. Eight DAB. Scala vestibuli of the basal coil of the cochlea. Normal distribution of elements. The arrow indicates a peak for Si (silicon) which is considered an artifact due to the analytical equipment using a crystal made of silicon.

ment of the ionic composition of endolymph had occurred prior to the development of the EP. Histological analyses revealed that the cochlea was morphologically fully mature before the rapid change in the EP. However, it was indicated that some degree of hypo-osmolality was present in cochlear fluids during this period. In the opossum[20] and the rabbit[16] the stria vascularis has gained its main morphology before the onset of the endocochlear potential.

These comparative morphological and electrophysiological observations in combination with our present study strongly indicate that the stria vascularis is the main source to reach the unique ionic composition of endolymph during maturation.

The maturation process is in general slightly more advanced in the vestibular part of the inner ear as compared with the cochlear portion of the labyrinth. Curthoys[21,22] demonstrated that a certain function does in fact occur in the vestibular system at birth in the rat. Anatomical evidence has appeared confirming the appearance of vestibular receptors and some innervation (mainly afferents) at this stage of development (mouse).[23,24] The development of the inner ear in mouse and rat has been reported to be rather parallel.[20]

TABLE 5. MORPHOLOGIC, ELECTROPHYSIOLOGIC AND ELEMENTAL MATURATION OF THE INNER EAR IN THE MOUSE*

Age	*Morphological Feature*	*Elements in the Endolymphatic Space (Present Study)*	*Electrophysiological Recording*	*Reference*
7 DBB	First vestibular HC			23, 24
5-4 DBB	First vestibular afferent NE	Extracellular composition		4
5-3 DBB	Differentiation of HC type 1, and type 2; Synapse formation; First cochlear HC	Minimal increase of K (vestibular part)		4, 10
3 DBB	First vestibular efferent NE (?)			4
2-1 DBB	Onset cochlear afferent NE	R_K: Vestibular surpassing cochlear (minimal changes)		18, 35
Birth	Mature dark cells except interdigitations		Onset of EP	20
2-4 DAB	Mature dark cells. Onset maturation of stria vascularis			18
4-5 DAB	Many mature nerve calyces (vestibular HC)	Na cannot be identified. Increasing conc. of K. R_K similar in vestibular and cochlear part		5
6 DAB	Fluid spaces in the organ of Corti	High conc. of K		18
8 DAB	Mature stria vascularis	Mature composition	Onset of CM	14
9 DAB			Onset of N1 N2 Onset of Preyer's reflex	14
10 DAB	Efferent NE in contact with cochlear HC		Onset of R1 R2	18 14
11 DAB			Mature Preyer's reflex	14
14 DAB	Mature organ of Corti		Mature cochlear potentials	14, 18

*The gestational period is 21 days when the day for visualization of the vaginal plug is encountered as day 1. DBB - Days before birth; DAB - Days after birth; HC - Hair cell; NE - Nerve ending; R_K - Relative peak intensity for potassium (K).

Conc. - Concentration.

In correlation with the present findings on the formation of endolymph the immature recordings of vestibular function at birth[21] might be connected with the increasing potassium content of endolymph during the first days postpartum. A certain difference in potassium content of endolymph, measured as relative peak intensity of potassium, did in fact occur during a few days before and after birth between vestibular and cochlear endolymph, the former containing slightly more potassium.

A description of the maturation process of the vestibular EP has not so far been published. Concerning the mature animal there is no general agreement regarding the magnitude of the vestibular EP[25] though it is clearly smaller[26,27] (+5 mV) than the corresponding cochlear potential showing approximately +80 mV relative to perilymph.[28] Whether or not this reflects the volume of the secretory epithelia, the functional capacity of these tissues, or both in the cochlear and vestibular parts of the inner ear, respectively, remains to be further analyzed.

On the fourth postnatal day the relative peak intensity for Na had decreased so much that measurements of its energy quanta became most uncertain and were in some instances not possible to perform. This phenomenon is one of the first signs of the maturation process to reach the final elemental composition of endolymph. At this stage of postnatal development a difference was observed in the endolymphatic space between the basal and the apical parts of the cochlea: at apex distinct peaks were observed for P and S while these two elements were lacking in the first coil. The ratios of Cl : Na + K varied – 0.54:1 at apex and 0.73:1 at the base. These observations are likely to point at differences in the maturation of the stria vascularis between the two ends of the cochlea. Structural and physiological maturation in general start in the basal part of the cochlea and successively progress apicalward.[29]

The formation of endolymph occurs between the fourth and eighth days after birth. According to the measurements of the weight percentage of elements in endolymph, the potassium concentration had increased to approximately 55% of the mature level on the sixth day after birth (50% if measured with regard to atomic weight). At this stage both phosphorus and sulphur were present in high concentrations (16.75% and 12.60% of total weight, respectively) but had decreased to one thirtieth and three fourths, respectively, of these concentrations on the eighth postnatal day, concentrations which are also found in mature endolymph.

The decrease of sulphur can be interpreted as being due to a decrease in the concentration of total proteins. It is a well-known fact that the most important primary valence bond between side chains of amino acids is the disulphide bond formed by dehydrogenation.[30] As the potassium concentration increases the protein content might decrease to maintain the same osmotic concentration in toto.

According to Rauch[31] the total protein content of mature endolymph in cat, guinea pig and man is only one third of that in perilymph. This ratio was also found in the present study of the mouse on the eighth day after birth, a fact that furthermore confirms that adult conditions are reached on this day. The drastic changes in phosphorus concentrations between the sixth and eighth day after birth indicate that the maturation process of the ionic composition of endolymph is ended and has reached a steady state. In the mature endolymph the turnover of both sulphur and phosphorus is a very slow process.[31] The time relation in the development of endolymph is unknown in man. Rauch[31] has reported the analyses of human embryos aged four to eight months. A high concentration of potassium was found in endolymph on the fourth to fifth embryonic month (1 case) and adult levels had been reached in the seventh gestational month embryo (3 cases).

Ethacrynic acid has been shown to act on the stria vascularis (ultrastructural and electrophysiological alterations and measurements of ion changes in endolymph)[32,33] while the dark cell region has been morphologically unaffected as also concerning ototoxic agents in general except for atoxyl.[34] A certain difference in physiological function between these two areas is therefore indicated, a fact that may furthermore emphasize the importance of the stria vascularis for the initial production of endolymph for the whole labyrinth.

REFERENCES

1. Van De Water TR, Ruben R. Organ culture of the mammalian inner ear. Acta Otolaryngol (Stockh) 1971; 71:303-12.

2. Van De Water TR. Effects of removal of the statoacoustic ganglion complex upon the growing otocyst. Ann Otol Rhinol Laryngol 1976; 85 Suppl 33:1-32.

3. Anniko M, Van De Water TR, Nordemar H. Organ culture of the 16th gestation day mouse labyrinth. A model suggestion for pre- and post partum development. Acta Otolaryngol (Stockh) 1978; 86:52-5.

4. Anniko M, Nordemar H, Van De Water TR. Embryogenesis of the inner ear. I. Development and differentiation of the mammalian crista ampullaris *in vivo* and *in vitro*. Arch Otorhinolaryngol 1979; 224:285-99.

5. Nordemar H, Anniko M. Post natal maturation of vestibular hair cells. Paper presented at the 16th Workshop on Inner Ear Biology, Bern, 1979.

6. Anniko M, Wersäll J. The inner ear and the *in vitro* system. Arch Otorhinolaryngol 1979; 224:25-30.

7. Anniko M. Extracorporal preservation. Organ culture of the post natal mammalian inner ear. Acta Otolaryngol (Stockh) 1979; 88:211-9.

8. Anniko M. The post natal mammalian labyrinthine secretory epithelium *in vitro*. Acta Otolaryngol (Stockh) 1980 (in press).

9. Anniko M, Wroblewski R. Elemental composition of the mature inner ear. Acta Otolaryngol (Stockh) 1980 (in press).

10. Sher AE. The embryonic and postnatal development of the inner ear of the mouse. Acta Otolaryngol (Stockh) 1971; Suppl 285:1-77.

11. Anniko M. Embryologic development *in vivo* and *in vitro* of the dark cell region of the mammalian crista ampullaris. Acta Otolaryngol (Stockh) 1980 (in press).

12. Wroblewski R, Roomans GM, Jansson E, Edström L. Electron probe x-ray microanalysis of human muscle biopsies. Histochemistry 1978; 55:281-92.

13. Kikuchi K, Hilding D. The development of the organ of Corti in the mouse. Acta Otolaryngol (Stockh) 1965; 60:207-22.

14. Mikaelian D, Ruben RJ. Development of hearing in the normal CBA-J mouse. Correlation of physiological observations with behavioral responses and with cochlear anatomy. Acta Otolaryngol (Stockh) 1965; 59:451-61.

15. Alford BR, Ruben RJ. Physiological, behavioral and anatomical correlates of the development of hearing in mouse. Ann Otol Rhinol Laryngol 1976; 72:237-47.

16. Änggård L. An electrophysiological study of the development of cochlear functions in the rabbit. Acta Otolaryngol (Stockh) 1965; Suppl 203:1-64.

17. Ruben RJ. Development of the inner ear of the mouse: a radioautographic study of terminal mitoses. Acta Otolaryngol (Stockh) 1967; Suppl 220:1-44.

18. Kikuchi K, Hilding D. The development of the stria vascularis in the mouse. Acta Otolaryngol (Stockh) 1966; 62:277-91.

19. Bosher SK, Warren RL. A study of the electrochemistry and osmotic relationships of the cochlear fluids in the neonatal rat at the time of the development of the endocochlear potential. J Physiol (Lond) 1971; 212:739-61.

20. Schmidt RS, Fernandez C. Development of mammalian endocochlear potential. J Exp Zool 1963; 153:227-36.

21. Curthoys IS. The vestibulo-occular reflex in newborn rats. Acta Otolaryngol (Stockh) 1979; 87:484-9.

22. Curthoys IS. The development of function of horizontal semicircular canal primary neurons in the rat. Brain Res 1980. In press.

23. Van De Water TR, Anniko M, Nordemar H, Wersäll J. Embryonic development of the sensory cells in macula utriculi of mouse. 1977; INSERM Symposium 68:25-36.

24. Anniko M, Nordemar H, Wersäll J. Comparative embryologic development *in vivo* and *in vitro* of mammalian hair cells of the crista ampullaris. Proceedings 3rd Ordinary Meeting of Bárány Society, Uppsala 1978; 4-5.

25. Goldberg JM, Fernandez C. Vestibular mechanisms. Annu Rev Physiol 1975; 37:129-62.

26. Gannon RP, Eldridge DH, Smith CA, Davis H. DC potentials of the semicircular canals. Physiologist 1958; 1:4.

27. Eldridge DH, Smith CA, Davis H, Gannon RP. The electrical polarization of the semicircular canals (guinea pig). Ann Otol Rhinol Laryngol 1961; 70:1024-36.

28. Békésy G von. DC resting potentials inside the cochlear partition. J Acoust Soc Am 1952; 24:72-6.

29. Rubel EW. Ontogeny of structure and function in the vertebrate auditory system. In Jacobsen M, ed. Handbook of sensory physiology, vol 9. Development of sensory systems. Berlin: Springer Verlag, 1978; 135-237.

30. Karlsson P. Introduction to modern biochemistry. 4th ed. New York: Academic Press, 1975.

31. Rauch S. Biochemie des Hörorgans. Stuttgart: Georg Thieme Verlag, 1964.

32. Bosher SK. Ethacrynic acid ototoxicity as a general model in cochlear pathology. Adv Otorhinolaryngol 1977; 22:81-9.

33. Bosher SK, Smith C, Warren RL. The effects of ethacrynic acid upon the cochlear endolymph and stria vascularis. Acta Otolaryngol (Stockh) 1973; 75:184-91.

34. Anniko M, Wersäll J. Experimentally (atoxy-induced ampullar degeneration and damage to the maculae utriculi. Acta Otolaryngol (Stockh) 1977; 83:429-40.

35. Weibel ER. Zur Kenntnis der Differenziersvorgänge in Epithel des Ductus cochlearis. Acta Anat (Basel) 1957; 29:53-90.

≈

ERRATUM

The *Annals* regrets the publication of an error in the article, "Foreign Bodies in the Airway: Five-Year Retrospective Study with Special Reference to Management," by Seymour R. Cohen, MD, Wayne I. Herbert, MD, George B. Lewis, Jr., MD, and Kenneth A. Geller, MD, which appeared on page 440 of the September-October 1980 issue. In column two, the last sentence in the first full paragraph reads as follows. "One milligram [1 mg] doses of atropine are sufficient and may be repeated as necessary." The sentence should read, "One-tenth milligram [0.1 mg] doses of atropine are sufficient and may be repeated as necessary."

QUANTITATIVE HISTOLOGY OF THE MUCOUS MEMBRANE OF THE ACCESSORY NASAL SINUS AND MASTOID CAVITIES

MICHAEL J. HARRIS, PhD ROBERT A. SCHLENKER, PhD

ARGONNE, ILLINOIS

The mucous membranes of the accessory nasal sinuses and of the mastoid labyrinth were measured in undecalcified, plastic-embedded specimens from nonpathologic postmortem cases. Epithelial thicknesses, lamina propria thicknesses and the ratio of nuclear to total cell area of the epithelia are presented for these organs to provide a quantitative basis for dosimetric calculations of alpha-emitting radionuclides. These data will be of value for studies in populations at risk for head carcinomas from the intake of radium and related nuclides.

This study began from a need to support dosimetric investigations on persons who have received occupational or medical exposures to radium. When taken into the body, radium lodges principally in the skeleton and produces a variety of effects[1-3] of which the most severe are neoplasms of bone and of the membranes lining the paranasal sinuses and air cells of the temporal bone.[4] The latter tumors are thought to arise from the cells of the mucosal epithelium or from the cells of the serous glands present in the lamina propria of certain of the paranasal sinuses (Fig. 1).

We consider it important to determine accurately the dose received by the epithelial cells. For this, we need quantitative information on the locations, sizes and microscopic anatomy of the cell populations at risk. Up to now, the literature dealing with microscopic features of the accessory nasal sinuses has been concerned primarily with the physiology and pathology of these structures,[5-10] and the observations in these reports have been mostly descriptive. The present study provides the quantitative data needed for radiation dosimetry.

The data were collected in a light microscopic study of undecalcified bone from persons with clinically nonsignificant body burdens of radium and from persons with no known exposure to radionuclides. There was no evidence of sinus or mastoid pathology in the subjects studied. Measurements were made of the thicknesses of the epithelium and of the lamina propria and also of the percentage of the epithelium occupied by cell nuclei. We believe these variables to be among the important morphological determinants of radiation dose and risk.

Relationship to Dose and Risk. There are two sources of radioactivity in the organs studied, the bone, where radium is deposited, and the air space, where radon gas accumulates. Alpha particles are the biologically significant radiations bombarding the epithelium. For neoplasia to occur, we believe that an alpha particle must strike nucleoplasm. Intervening tissue affects the chance of this occurring. If the tissue is thick, most particles stop before reaching the region of target nucleus concentration. If it is thin, such shielding is minimal and most particles reach the nuclear region causing the dose and the chance for nuclear damage to be high. In addition, the more nuclear material there is, the greater the risk that some of it will be altered in a way which may lead to the production of a tumor. Our data on the percentage of epithelium occupied by cell nuclei provides one of the factors needed to estimate the amount of nuclear material in the sinuses or in the air cell system (the other factor being the amount of epithelium present).

In summary, tissue thickness affects dose and risk through its ability to shield the radiosensitive nuclei from alpha particles. The percentage of epithelium occupied by cell nuclei affects dose and risk through

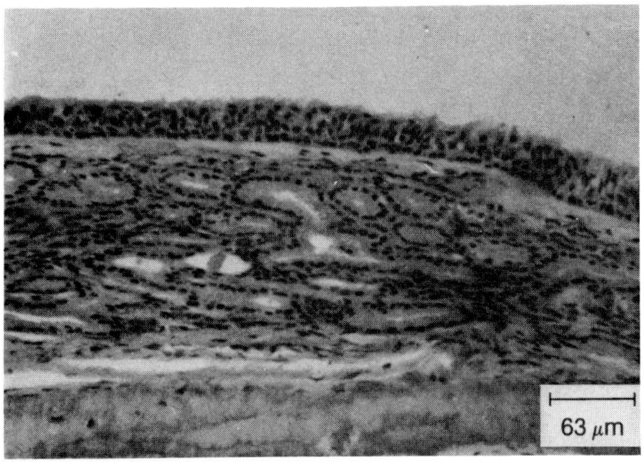

Fig. 1. Mucous membrane from the ethmoid sinus showing the general features of soft tissue in paranasal sinuses. Both the surface and glandular epithelia would be effectively shielded from α - particles emitted from bone. (H&E stain)

From the Center for Human Radiobiology, Radiological and Environmental Research Division, Argonne National Laboratory, Argonne, Illinois. Work performed under the auspices of the US Department of Energy.

REPRINTS — Michael J. Harris, PhD, Center for Human Radiobiology, Argonne National Laboratory, 9700 South Cass Avenue, Argonne, IL 60439.

TABLE 1. THICKNESSES OF PARANASAL SINUS AND MASTOID AIR CELL MUCOSA FROM NORMAL POSTMORTEM SPECIMENS OF THE CHR COLLECTION

Case No.	*Age/Sex*	*Site*	*Sample No.*	*Epithelial Thickness μm**	*Lamina Propria Thickness μm**
01-141†	92y/M	Frontal sinus	1	37.6± 8.1	38.6± 4.8
			2	43.5± 0.8	36.6± 2.4
			3	11.0± 1.5	13.6± 1.8
			4	12.4± 1.7	26.1± 3.2
		Ethmoid sinus	1	24.8± 2.0	112.0± 9.0
			2	29.1± 1.4	170.0± 2.0
		Sphenoid sinus	1	29.8± 2.8	341.0±77.0
			2	34.2± 2.9	224.0±28.0
		Maxillary sinus	1	17.2± 2.8	29.2± 2.9
			2	15.4± 1.5	61.6± 2.8
05-044†	80y/M	Frontal sinus	1	54.7± 7.5	207.0±20.0
			2	77.9± 6.4	—
		Sphenoid sinus	1	29.9± 4.0	140.0±18.0
			2	37.5± 2.0	155.0± 2.0
			3	46.8± 4.4	140.0± 5.0
			4	34.0± 6.2	133.0± 4.0
			5	36.4± 3.2	111.0± 9.0
		Maxillary sinus	1	136.0±17.0	541.0±68.0
			2	133.0±21.0	528.0±40.0
10-247†	61y/M	Mastoid air cell	1	3.1± 0.6	19.6± 2.4
A78 120∫	42y/M	Mastoid air cell	1	5.0± 1.4	76.5± 8.7
			2	5.4± 1.2	98.6± 4.7
A78 132∫	37y/M	Mastoid air cell	1	3.6± 0.9	18.7± 6.6
			2	3.9± 0.6	32.4± 3.1
			3	6.4± 1.9	89.8±18.6
			4	7.9± 2.7	73.2± 3.2
			5	4.0± 0.6	59.7± 4.4
			6	14.2± 7.0	120.3±51.2
			7	4.8± 2.1	56.1± 6.3
			8	4.9± 1.2	55.1± 7.6
			9	9.7± 3.9	111.4±46.7
A78 226∫	78y/F	Mastoid air cell	1	6.9± 2.3	25.3± 5.0
			2	7.0± 2.6	30.4± 3.1

*Based on 10 measurements within a 200 μm span on a photographic enlargement of the slide. Mean and standard deviation.

†/∫Multiply thickness by 1.4 (†) or 1.1 (∫) to correct for shrinkage.

its influence on the amount of nuclear material irradiated.

METHODS

Specimens of paranasal sinus and of temporal bone were removed at autopsy, usually within 24 hours of expiration. Fixation was in either 10% buffered neutral formalin or in 3% buffered glutaraldehyde. The specimens were refrigerated at 4 C prior to histological processing.

Two methacrylate embedding procedures were used, a nonaqueous one modified from Woodruff and Norris[11] and an aqueous method modified from Leduc and Bernhard[12] and from Bennett et al.[13] Five micrometer sections were cut from the resulting blocks on a Jung model K sledge microtome. The sections were floated onto glass slides from the surface of a water bath, affixed by heating at 60-70 C on a slide warmer and then stained with aqueous hematoxylin and alcoholic eosin. Care was taken to minimize folding and wrinkling of the thin sections.

The sections were next photographed with Polaroid® type 55 P/N film and the negative was enlarged in a positive format. Measurements of epithelial and lamina propria thicknesses were made with a ruler at several locations in several sections. A planimeter was used to measure the cross-sectional areas of nuclei and of the epithelial cells at the same locations, and all dimensions were later converted to their unmagnified values. The ratio of total nuclear cross-sectional area to total cell area was computed to provide the data on the percentage of the epithelium occupied by nuclei.

Tissue distortions are introduced by fixation and embedding. We established a criterion for their estimation. If one assumes that the mucosal tissue behaves in processing as do red blood cells (RBC), it is possible to determine size changes under the conditions of fixation and embedding which were used in this work. By measuring the average diameter change of RBCs in the two embedding media, it was determined that RBC diameter was reduced by 30% in the nonaqueous system. In the aqueous system, the reduction was 13%. The former percentage is based on 25 measurements of diameter whose mean and standard deviation (not standard error) are 5.96±1.44 μm. The latter percentage is based on 56 measurements of diameter whose mean and standard deviation are 7.45±0.86 μm. Westerman et al[14] reported the diameter of single flat cells in wet preparations to be 8.56±0.21 μm. We have adopted this value as the standard for undistorted RBC diameter.

We determined, on the basis of 160 measurements, that no significant diameter reduction occurred during fixation. A value of 8.76±0.77 μm, based on 80 RBCs, was established as normal diameter in this test. The corresponding value for glutaraldehyde fixed RBCs, also based on 80 measurements, was 8.53±0.93 μm.

In the tables below, we report the actual tissue dimensions measured. The data must be corrected upward by appropriate factors to account for tissue shrinkage. The correction factors are indicated in footnotes to the tables.

RESULTS

Thickness data are presented in Table 1. The variability of sample means among sinuses and within the mastoid air cells is great, especially for the lamina propria. This may reflect the limited

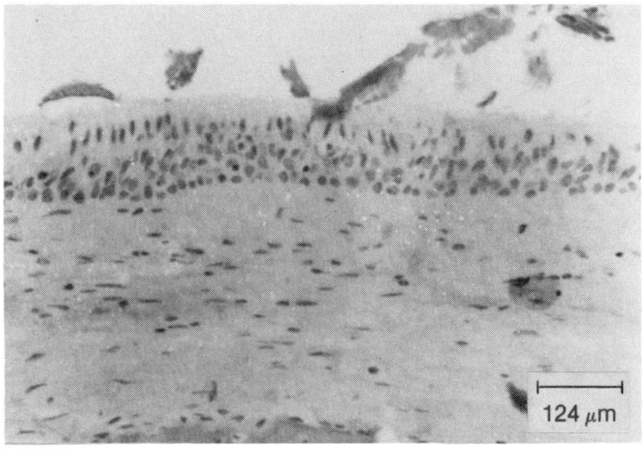

Fig. 2. Mucous membrane from a frontal sinus showing pseudostratified columnar epithelium. Note the thickness of the lamina propria.

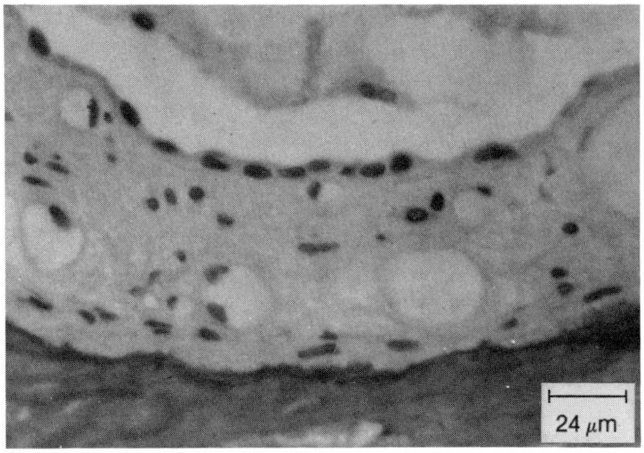

Fig. 4. Low cuboidal epithelium from a mastoid air cell.

sample size or the irregular morphology of the air spaces.[15-20]

In spite of the variability, we can make two generalizations from the data: 1) the lamina propria is thicker than the eithelium and 2) the paranasal sinus epithelium is thicker than the mastoid air cell epithelium. The first derives from the fact that the mean thickness of the lamina propria exceeds the mean epithelial thickness in every sample, save one, where both layers were measured and the thickness difference in the exceptional case is small. The second stems from the fact that the thickness range for the paranasal sinuses is 11.0 to 136.0 μm, and for the mastoid air cells, it is 3.1 to 14.2 μm with only one sample mean exceeding 11.0 μm. These observations quantitatively reflect the different histological characteristics of these regions. The paranasal sinus epithelium is cuboidal to pseudostratified columnar (Figs. 1-3) while the mastoid air cell epithelium is squamous to cuboidal (Fig. 4) and generally unstratified. This agrees with the observations reported in other investigations.[5-8] Cell height and arrangement result, therefore, in thicker or thinner epithelial layers.

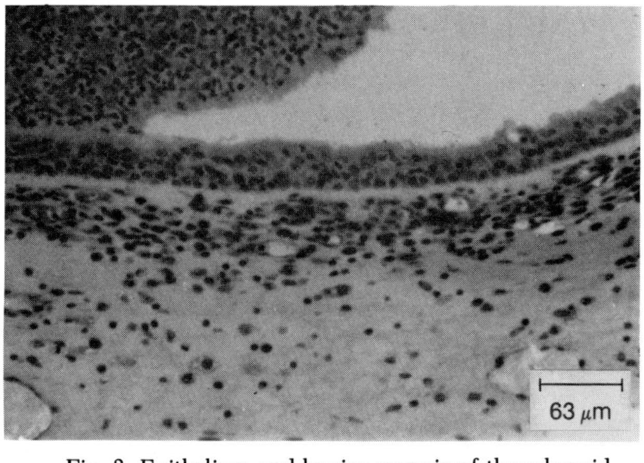

Fig. 3. Epithelium and lamina propria of the sphenoid sinus showing clearly the basement membrane, moderate vascularity and lymphocyte infiltration of the lamina.

Table 1 also shows the lamina propria to be thicker, as a rule, in the paranasal sinuses than in the mastoid air cells. It may not be valid to draw a general conclusion from this because of the limited sampling and the wide variation in thickness of the lamina even in a restricted area. Such an objection does not apply to our statement about epithelial thicknesses since the quantitative comparison is consistent with the established histology of these sites, and the epithelium varies much less widely than does the lamina propria, especially in the mastoid air cells.

Table 2 contains data on the percentage of the total cell area occupied by nuclei and the data from which this value was computed. The percentage appears to be greater in the mastoid air cells (range: 19.4 to 46.7%; midrange: 33.0%) than in the paranasal sinuses (range: 9.7 to 38.0%; midrange: 23.8%). We have applied statistical analyses to determine whether or not the difference is significant. The details are presented in the Appendix and lead to the conclusion that it is highly significant.

DISCUSSION

Carcinomas of the mastoid air cells in our study population outnumber paranasal sinus carcinomas among 5,058 radium-exposed persons by two to one.[4] The anatomical differences reported here may help to explain this. The mastoids have thin epithelia with no cilia (Fig. 4) and provide the nuclei with relatively little shielding against alpha particles from the air space. A typical paranasal sinus (Figs. 1 and 2), on the other hand, has a relatively thick epithelium which is ciliated[8,15] and provides better shielding. This suggests less radiation and fewer alpha particles striking the epithelial nuclei of the sinuses than striking those of the mastoid air cells and, consequently, a low tumor risk, other factors being equal.

Before interpreting the apparent differences between the paranasal sinuses and mastoid air cells in

TABLE 2. DATA ON POPULATION OF TARGET NUCLEI IN PARANASAL SINUS AND MASTOID AIR CELL EPITHELIUM IN NORMAL POSTMORTEM SPECIMENS FROM CHR COLLECTION

Case No.	*Age/Sex*	*Site*	*Sample No.*	*Total Cell Area* Studied μm²*	*Avg. Area† of a Cell Nucleus, μm²*	*No. of Nuclei in Area Studied*	*Total Nuclear Area, μm²*	*Area of Nuclei / Total Cell Area X100 %*
01-141∫	92y/M	Frontal sinus	1	6768	16.7± 4.0	54	902	13.3
			2	3833	14.0± 4.7	33	462	12.1
			3	1730	13.0± 5.3	37	481	27.8
			4	2508	13.8± 4.3	62	856	34.1
		Ethmoid sinus	1	4310	20.1± 5.7	69	1387	32.2
			2	5467	17.0± 4.7	89	1513	27.7
		Sphenoid sinus	1	4413	41.4±15.8	23	952	21.6
			2	9516	36.2± 8.4	100	3620	38.0
		Maxillary sinus	1	3716	15.1± 4.7	70	1057	28.4
			2	2536	18.9± 5.1	39	737	29.1
		Mastoid air cell	1	5765	45.6±11.3	59	2692	46.7
05-044∫	80y/M	Frontal sinus	1	6451	23.4± 8.0	89	2085	32.3
			2	7572	49.8±11.0	42	2090	27.6
		Sphenoid sinus	1	4963	30.2±16.2	24	725	14.6
			2	5687	30.6± 3.7	18	551	9.7
			3	5511	45.2±11.0	24	1085	19.7
			4	6003	36.2±12.3	32	1158	19.3
10-247∫	61y/M	Mastoid air cell	1	46	1.4± 0.5	8	11	24.3
A78 120∮	42y/M	Mastoid air cell	1	262	8.5± 2.8	6	51	19.4
			2	888	10.7± 3.8	24	256	28.8
A78 132∮	37y/M	Mastoid air cell	1	51	2.4± 0.8	9	22	42.4
			2	62	2.1± 0.5	10	21	34.5
			3	86	3.0± 1.3	10	30	34.8
			4	48	2.1± 0.7	6	12	25.8
			5	722	3.5± 1.1	78	270	37.3
			6	49	2.2± 0.9	10	21	44.0
			7	65	2.3± 1.0	11	26	39.5
			8	725	4.6± 1.9	57	262	36.1
			9	610	13.4± 4.9	13	174	28.5
A78 226∮	78y/F	Mastoid air cell	1	1974	25.9±11.3	22	569	28.8
			2	867	14.4±10.3	17	245	28.2

*Measured on a photographic enlargement using a planimeter; 3 repetitions.

†Based on planimeter measurements of photographically enlarged nuclei; 5 or 10 repetitions. Mean and standard deviation.

∫,∮Multiply areas by 2.04 (∫) or 1.32 (∮) to correct for shrinkage.

the percentage of total cell area occupied by nuclei, data on the amount of epithelium present in each region must be collected. Since epithelial thickness is greater in the sinuses but epithelial surface area would be greater in the mastoids, it is difficult to guess which region would have the greater epithelial volume.

The lamina propria is generally wider than the range of a typical radium alpha particle in soft tissue, roughly 50 μm. In fact, at most sites sampled, an alpha particle emitted from bone could not reach the epithelium. Therefore, the dose from radionuclides in bone appears to be quite small.

Wider sampling throughout the paranasal sinuses and mastoid air cells is needed to obtain more precise data on thickness and on the amount of nuclear material present. There is, additionally, a need for data on the submucosal glands and their cellular components. These structures occur infrequently, but quantitative information about them is required before they can be ruled out as significant factors in the problem of radiation risk in the paranasal sinuses.

The effects of age, sex and race of the subjects, as well as any prior history of radiation damage, need to be analyzed. It is expected that data from future cases will help in clariflying these issues.

REFERENCES

1. Evans RD. The effect of skeletally deposited alpha-ray emitters in man. Br J Radiol 1966; 39:881-95.

2. Finkel AJ, Miller CE, Hasterlik RJ. Radium-induced malignant tumors in man. In: Mays CW, Jee WSS, Lloyd RD, Stover BJ, Dougherty JH, Taylor GN, eds. Delayed effects of bone-seeking radionuclides. Salt Lake City: University of Utah Press, 1969: 195.

3. Sharpe WD. Chronic radium intoxication: clinical and autopsy findings in long-term New Jersey survivors. Environ Res 1974; 8:243-383.

4. Littman MS, Kirsh IE, Keane AT. Radium-induced malignant tumors of the mastoid and paranasal sinuses. Am J Roentgenol 1978; 131:773-85.

5. Schaeffer JP. The mucous membrane of the nasal cavity and the paranasal sinuses. In: Cowdry EV, ed. Special cytology. 2nd ed. New York: Hoebner, 1928: 47-68.

6. Ojala L. Contribution to the physiology of mastoid air cell formation. Acta Otolaryngol (Stockh) 1950; Suppl 86.

7. Hentzer E. Histologic studies of the normal mucosa in the

middle ear, mastoid cavities and eustachian tube. Ann Otol Rhinol Laryngol 1970; 43:825-33.

8. Latta JS, Schall RF. The histology of the epithelium of the paranasal sinuses under various conditions. Ann Otol Rhinol Laryngol 1934; 43:945-71.

9. Messerklinger W. Über die Drainage der menschlichem Nasennebenhöhlen unter normalen und pathologischen Bedingungen. Monatsschr Ohrenheilkd Laryngo-Rhinol 1966; 100:56-68.

10. Messerklinger W. Über die Drainage der menschlichem Nasennebenhöhlen unter normalen und pathologischen Bedingungen. Die Stirnhohle und ihr Ausfuhrungssystem. Monatsschr Ohrenheilkd Laryngo-Rhinol 1967; 101:313-26.

11. Woodruff LA, Norris WP. Sectioning of undecalcified bone: with special reference to radioautographic applications. Stain Technol 1954; 30:179-88.

12. Leduc EH, Bernhard W. Recent modifications of the glycol methacrylate embedding procedure. J Ultrastruct Res 1967; 19:196-9.

13. Bennett HS, Wyrick AD, Lee SW, McNeil JW. Science and art in preparing tissues embedded in plastic for light microscopy, with special reference to glycol methacrylate, glass knives and simple stains. Stain Technol 1976; 51:71-97.

14. Westerman MP, Pierce LE, Jensen WN. A direct method for the quantitative measurement of red cell dimensions. J Lab Clin Med 1961; 57:819-24.

15. Van Alyea OE. Nasal sinuses. An anatomic and clinical consideration. 3rd ed. Baltimore: Williams and Wilkins, 1951: 1-9; 31-4; 78-96; 117-38; 155-75.

16. Alberti PW. Applied surgical anatomy of the maxillary sinus. Otolaryngol Clin North Am 1976; 9:3-20.

17. van Nostrand AW, Goodman WS. Pathologic aspects of mucosal lesions of the maxillary sinus. Otolaryngol Clin North Am 1976; 9:21-34.

18. Yanagisawa E, Smith HW. Radiology of the normal maxillary sinus and related structures. Otolaryngol Clin North Am 1976; 9:55-81.

19. Shambaugh GE. The construction of the ethmoid labyrinth. Ann Otol Rhinol Laryngol 1907; 16:771-6 + plates.

20. Wittmaack K. Über die normale und pathologische Pneumatisation des Schläfenbeines. Jena: Gustav Fischer, 1918.

APPENDIX

The objective of this appendix is to determine whether or not statistically significant differences exist between the paranasal sinuses and mastoid air cells in the percentage of total cell area occupied by nuclei.

To arrive at a conclusion, data for the two regions are compared using a nonparametric or distribution-free method, the Wilcoxon two-sample test for unpaired, ranked observations.* The null hypothesis, H_0, is that the two samples come from populations having the same distribution (Table 3).

The Wilcoxon statistic is computed as

$$C = n_1 n_2 + \frac{n_2(n_2+1)}{2} - \Sigma R$$

$$= 16(15) + \frac{15(15+1)}{2} - 306$$

$$= 240 + 120 - 306 = 54$$

Comparing this value with $C' = n_1 n_2 - C$, which is 186, we choose the latter value as a test statistic U_S. Referring to appropriate tables and using a two-tailed test, we find that the critical value for this statistic is greater than the computed value at $P < 0.01$. The difference is significant when the computed value exceeds the critical value. Therefore, the null hypothesis is provisionally rejected and we conclude that the samples come from populations with different distributions. Since the statistic U_S, exceeds its expected value, we may regard this as evidence that the means of the two groups are unequal.

*Sokal RR, Rohlf FJ. Biometry. San Francisco: WH Freeman, 1969:387-95.

TABLE 3. WILCOXON TWO-SAMPLE TEST TO DETERMINE EQUALITY OF LOCATION OF PERCENTAGE OF TOTAL CELL AREA OCCUPIED BY NUCLEI IN MUCOSA OF PARANASAL SINUS AND MASTOID AIR CELL

Paranasal Sinus		*Mastoid Air Cell*	
Variate %	*Rank*	*Variate %*	*Rank*
9.7	1	19.4	6
12.1	2	24.3	9
13.3	3	25.8	10
14.6	4	28.2	14
19.3	5	28.5	16
19.7	7	28.8	17
21.6	8	28.8	17
27.6	11	34.5	23
27.7	12	34.8	24
27.8	13	36.1	25
28.4	15	37.3	26
29.1	19	39.5	28
32.2	20	42.4	29
32.3	21	44.0	30
34.1	22	46.7	31
38.0	27		
	n_1		n_2
	$190 = \Sigma R$		$306 = \Sigma R$

PROTEASE INHIBITORS IN MIDDLE EAR EFFUSIONS

BRITT CARLSSON, MD
STOCKHOLM, SWEDEN

CHRISTER LUNDBERG, MD
STOCKHOLM, SWEDEN

KJELL OHLSSON, MD
MALMÖ, SWEDEN

As the presence of granulocytes in middle ear fluid in serous otitis media implicates a potential risk of extracellular release of granulocyte proteases, the main protease inhibitors in serum, α_1-antitrypsin, α_1-antichymotrypsin and α_2-macroglobulin, were immunochemically quantitated in such effusions. The mean concentration of α_1-antitrypsin was found to be higher in middle ear effusion and the mean concentration of α_1-antichymotrypsin slightly lower than in plasma. On comparison with albumin, however, lower values than expected were found in the middle ear fluid for the two inhibitors. The high molecular weight α_2-macroglobulin was significantly lower than in plasma. Furthermore a low molecular weight protease inhibitor, which is thought to be locally produced in the respiratory epithelium, was demonstrated in the effusion.

INTRODUCTION

Studies of middle ear effusions (MEE) in serous otitis media (SOM) have demonstrated several characteristics of inflammation such as the presence of inflammatory cells,[1] chemotaxis for neutrophils,[2] elevated levels of lysosomal enzymes[3] and LDH,[4] and evidence of complement activation.[2,3] These observations imply an inflammatory etiology of SOM.

One of the main occurrences in an inflammatory process is phagocytosis. During this process, the granulocytes can release proteolytic enzymes extracellularly.[5-7] If not inactivated, the proteolytic enzymes will then attack healthy as well as diseased tissues.

So far, a number of proteins are known having the ability to inactivate proteolytic enzymes derived from granulocytes. In serum, the main inhibitors are α_1-antitrypsin, α_1-antichymotrypsin and α_2-macroglobulin.[8-10] In human bronchial secretion, the main elastase inhibitor is a low molecular weight acid stable protein not found in serum.[11,12] This has also been demonstrated in nasal secretion, in tracheal and sinus mucosa, and in fluid of chronic otitis media.[13-15] In the present study, MEE in SOM were analyzed with respect to inflammatory cells and the presence of inhibitors of granulocyte proteases.

METHODS

Patients with SOM over a period exceeding two months and without signs or symptoms of active ear infection were selected for this study. Diagnosis was established by morphologic findings of a pale, retracted tympanic membrane and the presence of fluid in the middle ear cavity. The patients varied in age from 1-20 years, mean age 5.9 years. Under general anesthesia, middle ear fluid was aspirated through the eardrum in connection with therapeutic myringotomy. Analysis was confined to macroscopically nonpurulent fluid varying in viscosity from serous to seromucoid. High viscosity mucoid fluids that were nonpipettable, or macroscopically blood-contaminated fluids were excluded from the study. Specimens were studied from a total of 22 ears from 17 patients.

Inflammatory Cells. In 13 ears, 20 μl of the middle ear specimen were taken for white cell count in a Bürker chamber after staining with gentian violet solution. Smears were prepared from the same specimens and examined for differential counts after staining with May-Grünwald-Giemsa stain. In another four specimens, only fluid sufficient for smear analysis was obtained.

Protein Analyses. Fifty microliters of the middle ear fluid were obtained from 22 ears of 17 patients. The samples were immediately diluted 1:10 with 0.9% NaCl solution containing ethylenediaminetetraacetic acid (EDTA) and centrifuged at 1,000 gm for five minutes. The clear supernatants were recovered and stored at –18 C until studied.

Blood specimens were obtained from the same patients at the time of myringotomy. Venous blood (5 ml) was collected in test tubes containing 0.04 ml EDTA solution. After centrifugation at 1,000 gm for five minutes, the plasma was recovered and stored at –18 C until analyzed.

Albumin was tested for reference purposes. Since a local production of albumin in the middle ear mucosa is highly improbable, the ratio of middle ear fluid albumin to plasma albumin was assumed to reflect the passage of albumin through the mucous membrane. Corresponding ratios of substances with molecular weights similar to that of albumin, such as α_1-antitrypsin (55,000) and α_1-antichymotrypsin (69,000), were then compared with the albumin ratio. Provided neither of the two inhibitors are locally produced, the amount of each inhibitor in MEE (protein X_{mee}) ultrafiltrated through the mucosa should then equal the obtained ratio of albumin ($albumin_{mee}/albumin_{plasma}$) multiplied by the plasma concentration of the inhibitor in question (protein X_{plasma}).[16]

$$\text{Protein } X_{mee} = albumin_{mee}/albumin_{plasma} \times \text{protein } X_{plasma} \quad \text{(formula 1)}$$

From the Department of Otolaryngology, Södersjukhuset, Stockholm, and the Department of Clinical Chemistry, Malmö General Hospital, Malmö, Sweden. This investigation was supported by grants from the Swedish Medical Research Foundation (project No. B80-17X-03910-08B), and Medical Faculty, University of Lund, the Swedish Association against Chest and Lung Diseases, the Swedish Association against Rheumatism, the Swedish Society of Medical Sciences, the Foundation of Alfred Österlund, the Foundation of Greta and Johan Kock, the Foundation of King Gustav Vth, the Foundation of Eir, and the Foundation of Malmö General Hospital.

REPRINTS — Britt Carlsson, MD, Sturevägen 1, 182 74 Stocksund, Sweden.

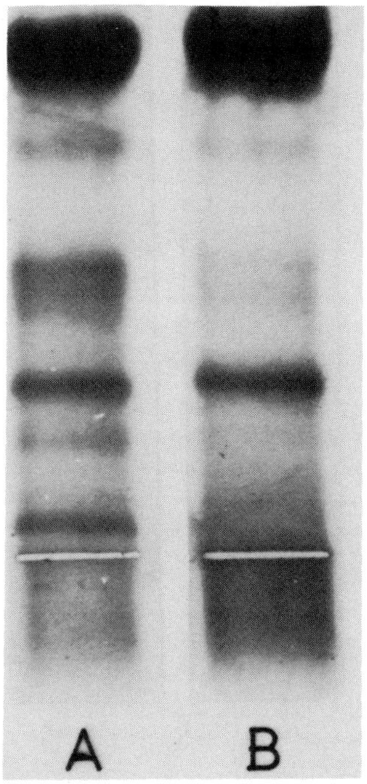

Fig. 1. A) Electrophoresis patterns of undiluted plasma and B) middle ear effusion diluted 1:10 in saline demonstrating the high protein content of middle ear effusion.

In screening for protein patterns of MEE, agarose* gel electrophoresis was performed using 0.8% (w/v) agarose gel, otherwise as described by Johanson.[17] The MEE specimens were thus diluted 1:10, while the corresponding plasmas were undiluted.

Quantitative analyses of albumin, α_1-antitrypsin, α_1-antichymotrypsin and α_2-macroglobulin were performed with the electroimmunoassay technique described by Laurell,[18] except that the agarose gel was prepared with 0.8% (w/v) agarose. Analyses of MEE and corresponding plasmas were run with identical standards achieved from a blood pool of healthy adult donors.

Qualitative analyses of albumin in MEE were studied with crossed immunoelectrophoresis according to Ganrot.[19]

Quantitative assay of the low molecular weight protease inhibitor in MEE was performed with the single radial immunodiffusion plate technique of Mancini et al,[20] using 1 mm thick 1% (w/v) agarose gel containing 3% (w/v) polyethyleneglycol. A purified inhibitor with known concentration was used as standard.

Specific antisera against the low molecular weight protease inhibitor were prepared at the laboratory.[21] Rabbit antisera against human α_1-antitrypsin, α_1-antichymotrypsin, α_2-macroglobulin and albumin are routinely prepared at the laboratory.

RESULTS

Inflammatory Cells. In 13 ears, material was obtained for white cell count and smear. The total number of white cells ranged from 0.5 to 6.6 x 10^9/liter. The neutrophils varied from 0.03 to 5.02 x 10^9. The neutrophils predominated in 10 of 17 examined smears. In the remainder, the lymphocytes were in the majority.

Proteins. A high protein content in MEE was suggested on comparison of the screen electrophoresis patterns of undiluted plasma and the effusions diluted 1:10 (Fig. 1).

*Miles-Seravac, Maidenhead, Berkshire, England.

TABLE 1. PROTEASE INHIBITORS IN MIDDLE EAR EFFUSION IN RELATION TO PATIENT'S OWN PLASMA CONCENTRATION (MEE/PLASMA x 100)

	α_1-*Antitrypsin*	α_1-*Antichymotrypsin*	α_2-*Macroglobulin*
Range	22 - 224	47 - 143	20 - 100
Mean	115 ± 12.2*	97 ± 5.1 *	61 ± 5.1*
Number	22	20	22

*Standard error.

Albumin. In 22 MEE, albumin ranged from 58-267% of the patient's own plasma value, with a mean value of 171±12.4. The albumin content exceeded that of the corresponding plasma in 17 middle ear fluids. Crossed immunoelectrophoresis showed homogeneity of the albumin fraction.

α_1-*Antitrypsin.* The α_1-antitrypsin concentration in plasma of the patients ranged from 56-125% as compared to the pool. The concentration of α_1-antitrypsin in MEE in relation to the patient's own plasma value showed a variation of 22-224% with a mean value of 115% (Table 1). In 14 of 22 middle ear effusions, the value exceeded that of the patient's plasma. A positive correlation was seen between the ratio $albumin_{mee}/albumin_{plasma}$ and the ratio α_1-$antitrypsin_{mee}/\alpha_1$-$antitrypsin_{plasma}$ ($r = 0.95$) (Fig. 2). In all studied middle ear effusions, the observed value of α_1-antitrypsin was lower than the value calculated according to formula 1.

α_1-*Antichymotrypsin.* The concentration of α_1-antichymotrypsin in plasma, with one exception (the oldest patient), fell below that of the pool. The range was 36-102% with a mean value of 63%. The concentration of α_1-antichymotrypsin in MEE in relation to the patient's own plasma concentration ranged from 47-143% with a mean value of 97% (Table 1). Due to a technical mishap, α_1-antichymotrypsin was tested in only 20 middle ear specimens from 15 patients. A positive correlation was seen between the ratio $albumin_{mee}/albumin_{plasma}$ and the ratio α_1-$antichymotrypsin_{mee}/\alpha_1$-$antichymotrypsin_{plasma}$ although weaker than for α_1-antitrypsin ($r = 0.68$) (Fig. 2). The observed value of α_1-antichymotrypsin was lower in all middle ear specimens than the value calculated according to formula 1.

α_2-*Macroglobulin.* The plasma concentration of α_2-macroglobulin in all specimens exceeded the concentration of the serum pool from adult donors. The range was 132-312%, the lowest value emanating from the oldest patient (20 years). The concentration of α_2-macroglobulin in the 22 middle ear effusions in relation to the patient's plasma concentration varied from 20-100% with a mean value of 61% (Table 1). In all but one middle ear specimens, the value fell below the plasma concentration. A positive though weak correlation was seen between the ratio $albumin_{mee}/albumin_{plasma}$ and the ratio α_2-$macroglobulin_{mee}/\alpha_2$-$macroglobulin_{plasma}$ ($r = 0.46$) (Fig. 2).

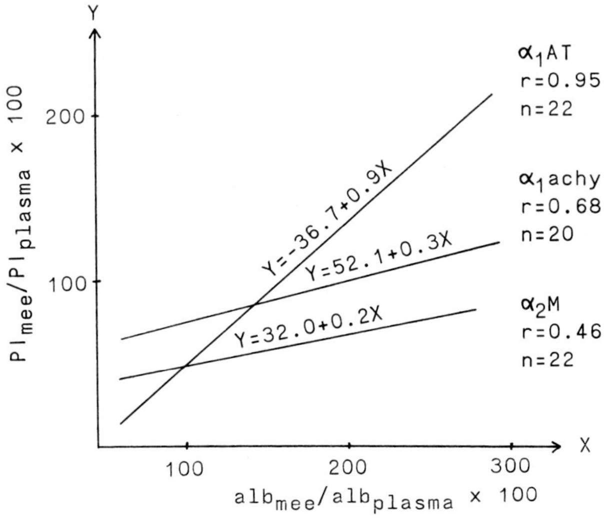

Fig. 2. Correlation between the ratio protease inhibitor concentration in middle ear effusion (PI_{mee}) and protease inhibitor in plasma (PI_{plasma}) and the ratio albumin concentration in middle ear effusion (alb_{mee}) and albumin in plasma (alb_{plasma}). α_1AT - α_1-antitrypsin; $\alpha_1$achy - α_1-antichymotrypsin; α_2M - α_2-macroglobulin; r - Correlation coefficient; n - Number of samples.

Low Molecular Weight Protease Inhibitor. The low molecular weight protease inhibitor tested with the Mancini et al[20] technique was detected in 21 of 22 middle ear fluids. The range was 12-33 μg/ml with a mean value of 24 μg/ml.

DISCUSSION

The fluids investigated in our study consisted of serous to seromucoid specimens. The highly mucoid fluids had to be discarded owing to difficulties in obtaining an accurately measured quantity and dilution. However, the different types of effusion seen during the natural course of otitis media with effusion reflect different stages in a continuous process taking place in the middle ear cavity. The mucoid effusions with a high glucoprotein content[22] and high concentrations of SIgA[23] reflect an inflammatory stage in the mucosa with functioning goblet cells and mucous glands.[24] The low viscosity fluids represent a higher degree of inflammation as its major constituents are emanating from plasma.[23,25] Thus, our material represents a stage in otitis media with effusion where the inflammatory reaction is pronounced, though yet not to such a degree as to cause a clinical manifestation of infection. The majority of specimens in our study contained leukocytes in such number as to be classified as seropurulent effusions according to Senturia's classification.[26]

The main protease inhibitors in serum, α_1-antitrypsin, α_1-antichymotrypsin and α_2-macroglobulin were measurable in all MEE studied (Table 1). In the majority of specimens, α_1-antitrypsin was found in accordance with Bernstein[2] to exceed the patient's own plasma concentration of α_1-antitrypsin. In the MEE, α_1-antichymotrypsin showed a mean value of 97% of the patient's plasma value. No other report of the presence of this inhibitor in MEE is to be found in the literature. In accordance with a previous study,[2] the α_2-macroglobulin concentration in the effusions was below that of the corresponding plasma value. This is probably explained by the high molecular weight of α_2-macroglobulin (725,000) which prevents simple diffusion from plasma to the middle ear cavity. However in young individuals, as all but one of our patients were, the plasma concentration of α_2-macroglobulin is high as compared to adults.[27] Thus, the concentration of α_2-macroglobulin in the MEE of our patients was equal or above that of the normal α_2-macroglobulin concentration in plasma of adults. The low molecular weight protease inhibitor was demonstrated in 21 of 22 specimens. This inhibitor is not found in serum and is assumed to be locally produced in the respiratory epithelium. In bronchial secretion, it is responsible for the major inhibiting capacity against granulocyte elastase. In noninfected bronchial lavage fluid, Tegner[12] found a mean concentration of 15 mg/liter. Our study showed a mean concentration in the undiluted MEE of 24 mg/liter. However, the importance of this inhibitor in serous otitis media has yet to be quantified.

In the present study, the albumin concentration in MEE varied considerably with a mean value of 171% of the patient's own plasma value. The concentration of α_1-antitrypsin showed a similar pattern. Crossed immunoelectrophoresis showed homogeneity of the albumin, and the presence of albumin split products as a cause of false high values could be ruled out. Determination of the osmolality in MEE in SOM has shown the existence of higher osmolality than in plasma.*† This supports the accuracy of the high albumin concentrations in MEE in the present study, since it is reasonable to assume albumin in serous middle ear fluid to be the major regulator of colloid-osmotic pressure, as it is in plasma. Previous studies of the albumin concentration in MEE of SOM have shown varying results of mean concentrations in relation to plasma concentrations.[28-31] The wide range of the individual values is a general feature. This probably reflects the differences in inflammatory condition of the middle ears investigated, and thus the difference in plasma leakage. This in turn illustrates in each individual the different phases of inflammation that are found in the natural course within the defined group of SOM. Another reason for the divergence in results between investigators can be the difference in methods of analysis.

Assuming our data obtained for albumin to be correct, they can serve as reference values for

*Juhn SK. Personal communication.

†Carlsson B. Unpublished data.

evaluating the passage over the biological membrane from plasma to the middle ear cavity for other nonlocally produced substances with similar molecular weights, such as α_1-antitrypsin and α_1-antichymotrypsin. Positive correlations were found when comparing the individual MEE/plasma ratios of albumin and the two inhibitors respectively. The covariations are however more complicated than what can be described as a straight line, characterized as y = x. Furthermore, when applying formula 1 for ultrafiltration, and as illustrated in Figure 2, the observed values of α_1-antitrypsin and α_1-antichymotrypsin in MEE were lower than the calculated values. An explanation for this can be that degradation of the inhibitors has occurred in the effusions, or more probably, that the inhibitors have formed complexes with proteases, thereby reducing the antigenic sites necessary for detection with the immunochemical technique used. In clinical terms complex formation between protease inhibitors and proteases would indicate a protective role of the protease inhibitors in the middle ear cavity. Further analyses of the extent of complex formations and remaining inhibitory capacity of protease inhibitors in MEE are in progress in our laboratory.

REFERENCES

1. Palva T, Holopainen E, Karma P. Protein and cellular pattern of glue ear secretions. Ann Otol Rhinol Laryngol 1976; 85 Suppl 25:103-9.

2. Bernstein JM. Biological mediators of inflammation in middle ear effusions. Ann Otol Rhinol Laryngol 1976; 85 Suppl 25:90-6.

3. Veltri RW, Sprinkle PM. Secretory otitis media. An immune complex disease. Ann Otol Rhinol Laryngol 1976; 85 Suppl 25:135-9.

4. Juhn SK, Huff JS, Paparella MM. Lactate dehydrogenase activity and isoenzyme patterns in serous middle ear effusions. Ann Otol Rhinol Laryngol 1973; 82:192-5.

5. Wright DG, Malawista SE. The mobilization and extracellular release of granular enzymes from human leukocytes during phagocytosis. J Cell Biol 1972; 53:788-97.

6. Ohlsson K. Collagenase and elastase released during peritonitis are complexed by plasma protease inhibitors. Surgery 1976; 79:652-7.

7. Ohlsson K, Olsson I. The extracellular release of granulocyte collagenase and elastase during phagocytosis and inflammatory processes. Scand J Haematol 1977; 19:145-52.

8. Ohlsson K, Olsson I. Neutral proteases of human granulocytes. III. Interaction between human granulocyte elastase and plasma protease inhibitors. Scand J Clin Lab Invest 1974; 34:349-55.

9. Ohlsson K, Olsson I. Neutral proteases of human granulocytes. IV. Interaction between human granulocyte collagenase and plasma protease inhibitors. J Lab Clin Med 1977; 89:269-77.

10. Ohlsson K, Åkesson U. Alpha$_1$-antichymotrypsin interaction with cationic proteins from granulocytes. Clin Chim Acta 1976; 73:285-91.

11. Hochstrasser K, Reichert R, Schwarz S, et al. Isolierung und Charakterisierung eines Proteaseninhibitors aus menschlichem Bronchialsekret. Hoppe Seylers Z Physiol Chem 1972; 353:221-6.

12. Tegner H. Quantitation of human granulocyte protease inhibitors in non-purulent bronchial lavage fluids. Acta Otolaryngol (Stockh) 1978; 85:282-9.

13. Hochstrasser K, Haendle H, Reichert T, et al. Über Vorkommen und Eigenschaften eines Proteaseninhibitors im menschlichem Nasensekret. Hoppe Seylers Z Physiol Chem 1971; 352:954-8.

14. Tegner H, Ohlsson K. Localization of a low molecular weight protease inhibitor to tracheal and maxillary sinus mucosa. Hoppe Seylers Z Physiol Chem 1977; 358:225-9.

15. Kastenbauer ER, Hochstrasser K, Reichert R, et al. Der Nachweis eines niedermolekularen säurestabilen Proteaseninhibitors im Ohrsekret bei chronischer Mittelohreiterung. J Laryngol Otol 1977; 56:201-6.

16. Deutschl H, Johansson SGO. Immunoglobulins in tracheobronchial secretion with special reference to IgE. Clin Exp Immunol 1974; 16:401-12.

17. Johansson BG. Agarose gel electrophoresis. Scand J Clin Lab Invest 1972; 29 Suppl 124:7-19.

18. Laurell C-B. Electroimmuno assay. Scand J Clin Lab Invest 1972; 29 Suppl 124:21-37.

19. Ganrot PO. Crossed immunoelectrophoresis. Scand J Clin Lab Invest 1972; 29 Suppl 124:39-41.

20. Mancini G, Carbonara AO, Heremans JF. Immunochemical quantitation of antigens by single radial immunodiffusion. Immunochemistry 1965;2:235-54.

21. Ohlsson K, Tegner H. Inhibition of elastase from granulocytes by the low molecular weight bronchial protease inhibitor. Scand J Clin Lab Invest 1976; 36:437-45.

22. Vered J, Eliezer N, Sadé J. Biochemical characterization of middle ear effusions. Ann Otol Rhinol Laryngol 1972; 81:394-400.

23. Mogi G, Honjo S, Maeda S, Yoshida T, Watanabe N. Quantitative determination of secretory immunoglobulin A (SIgA) in middle ear effusions. Ann Otol Rhinol Laryngol 1974; 83:239-46.

24. Lim D, Birck H. Ultrastructural pathology of middle ear mucosa in serous otitis media. Ann Otol Rhinol Laryngol 1971; 80:838-53.

25. Mogi G, Yoshida T, Honjo S, Maeda S. Middle ear effusions: quantitative analysis of immunoglobulins. Ann Otol Rhinol Laryngol 1973; 82:196-202.

26. Senturia BH. Classification of middle ear effusions. Ann Otol Rhinol Laryngol 1970; 79:358-70.

27. Weiss WA. Normalwerte spezifischer Serumproteine im Kindes und Erwachsenenalter. Klin Wochenschr 1965; 43:273-7.

28. Carlson LA, Lökk T. Protein studies of transudates of the middle ear. Scand J Clin Invest 1955; 7:43-8.

29. Juhn SK, Huff JS, Paparella MM. Biochemical analyses of middle ear effusions. Preliminary report. Ann Otol Rhinol Laryngol 1971; 80:347-53.

30. Mogi G, Honjo S. Middle ear effusions. Analysis of protein components. Ann Otol Rhinol Laryngol 1972; 81:99-105.

31. Tönder O, Gundersen T. Nature of the fluid in serous otitis media. Arch Otolaryngol 1971; 93:473-8.

Ann Otol 90:1981

CARCINOID TUMOR OF THE LARYNX

BORIS GAPANY-GAPANAVIČIUS, MD, DSc
SAMUEL KENAN, MD
JERUSALEM, ISRAEL

Primary carcinoid of the larynx is an unusual neoplasm. Only one case could be traced in the literature so far. Another case, a 55-year-old male patient, is presented and discussed. The tumor proved to be malignant, showing histological, histochemical and electron microscopical characteristics of a carcinoid. Initially there was a striking discrepancy between the scanty findings in the larynx and the wide metastatic spread of the tumor into the cervical lymph nodes along the internal jugular vein, and the progression of the process was markedly slower than that of laryngeal carcinoma. Despite the massive dose of radiotherapy that had been administered after radical neck dissection in an attempt to preserve the larynx, the tumor continued to expand, infiltrating the laryngeal tissues and causing stenosis that necessitated total laryngectomy, thus again proving that the treatment of choice in laryngeal carcinoid should be wide surgical excision.

INTRODUCTION

Carcinoid tumor of the larynx is an unusual clinical entity, although cases of tracheal carcinoids have been reported.[1-3] Primary carcinoid tumor of the larynx, however, has, to the best of our knowledge, been previously described only once.[4] Another case is presented herein.

Our case and the one previously reported[4] clearly demonstrate that carcinoid of the larynx is a malignant neoplasm, which deeply infiltrates the laryngeal tissues and widely metastasizes into the cervical lymph nodes, though the growth of the tumor is markedly slower than that of laryngeal carcinoma. It does not respond to radiotherapy, and the treatment of choice should be wide surgical excision.

CASE REPORT

A 55-year-old Armenian male patient from Iran, a nonsmoker, but with a history of abuse in alcohol consumption, was first examined by one of the authors in the ENT Clinic of the Hadassah-Hebrew University Hospital in mid-June 1978. He presented with a 3 1/2 years' history of intermittent hoarseness. A year after the onset of hoarseness, a biopsy was taken from the larynx, and the histological examination did not reveal any malignancy. Two months before his present examination, enlarged lymph nodes in the right side of the neck were noticed by his doctor, and a repeat biopsy from the larynx was performed and reported to be papillary carcinoma. Total laryngectomy with radical neck dissection had been suggested, but the patient refused.

Indirect laryngoscopy revealed only a small bulge in the anterior portion of the right ventricular fold. The mucous membrane in this area looked smooth, with no signs of erosion of the epithelium. There were no other noticeable changes in the larynx. Both vocal cords were perfectly mobile. In the right side of the neck there was a chain of markedly enlarged lymphatic nodes along the internal jugular vein. Three of them were the size of an olive and the rest smaller ones. The nodes were firm, but mobile. The nasopharynx looked normal and there were no changes in the other ear, nose, and throat organs. The first impression was that of a laryngeal cancer with metastases in the cervical lymph nodes, but clinically there was a striking discrepancy between the scanty findings in the larynx and the wide spread of the tumor into the right internal jugular chain.

A biopsy was taken from the bulging anterior portion of the right ventricular fold, and one cervical lymph node was excised simultaneously for histopathological examination. The report of the histopathological examination was not unequivocal. The findings in the cervical lymph node were reported as metastatic carcinoma, but there was doubt as to the type of carcinoma. It was suggested that the site of primary lesion might not have been the larynx, since in the laryngeal specimen several foci of anaplastic carcinoma were found only in the submucous layer, while in the mucosa there were no traces of tumor. The consulting pathologist assumed that the primary tumor might be in the thyroid gland or in the lungs.

A thorough clinical examination that included tomography of the chest, radioactive iodine (I^{131}) uptake, and scanning of the thyroid gland did not confirm the above assumption. Since the clinical facts indicated that the primary tumor most probably originated in the larynx, it became evident that ex-

From the Department of Otolaryngology and the Department of Pathology, Hadassah University Hospital, and Hebrew University Hadassah Medical School, Jerusalem, Israel.

REPRINTS — Prof. B. Gapany-Gapanavičius, MD, Department of Otolaryngology, Hadassah-Hebrew University Medical Center, Jerusalem, Israel.

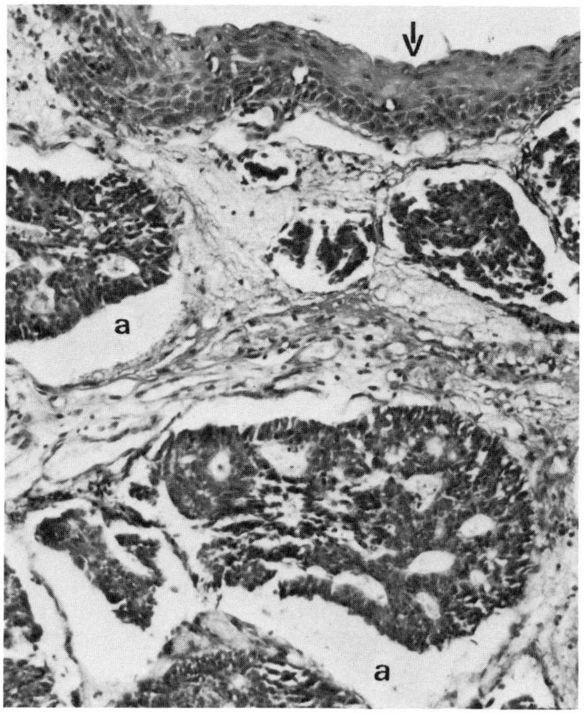

Fig. 1. Primary carcinoid tumor of the larynx. The neoplastic tissue consists of masses of relatively small cells with large hyperchromatic nuclei. The cells are arranged in an acinar pattern with cribriform areas (a). The tumor is covered by a lining of normal squamous cell epithelium (arrow). (H & E, x125)

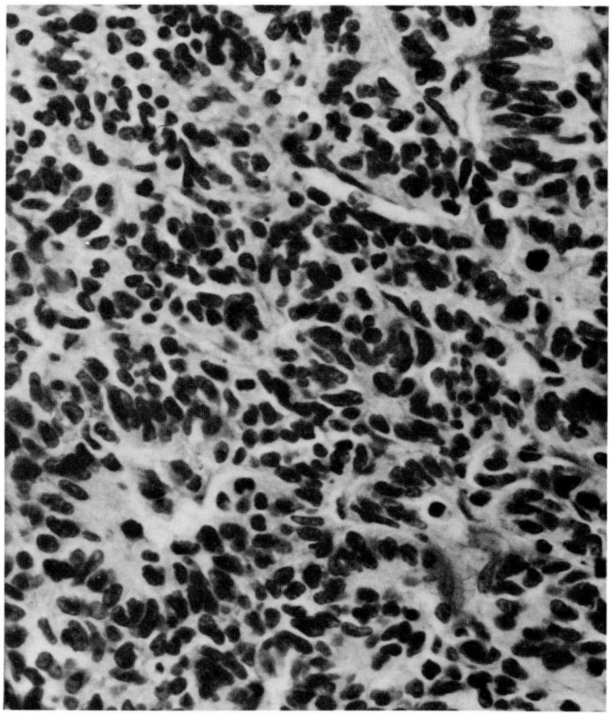

Fig. 2. Metastatic carcinoid tumor within a cervical lymph node. Note the acinar pattern of the tumor, similar to that found in the laryngeal specimen. (H & E, x400)

ploration of the larynx would be reasonable before making any decision concerning laryngectomy.

A laryngofissure was performed under general anesthesia and the larynx explored. The laryngeal mucosa looked smooth, without evident signs of neoplasm. In a repeat biopsy, taken from the somewhat thickened anterior portion of the right ventricular fold, no tumor had been recognized in the frozen section, only fibrosis and chronic inflammation were noticed. It was therefore decided to preserve the larynx, and the operation was confined to right radical neck dissection. Frozen section examination of the latter specimen showed metastatic carcinoma of the cervical lymph nodes. Since there still were doubts as to the site of origin of the tumor, biopsies were also taken from the thyroid gland and from the nasopharynx, but both proved to be negative.

The postoperative period was uneventful. The incision healed by first intention, and the patient was successfully decannulated on the fifth postoperative day. The mobility of both vocal cords, as seen by indirect laryngoscopy, was good, but the bulge in the right ventricular fold still covered the anterior portion of the vocal cord.

Examination of the serial sections, prepared from the laryngeal specimen taken during laryngofissure, revealed the same kind of malignant cells as in the cervical lymph nodes.

At our request, the slides of the first laryngeal biopsy were brought by the patient from Iran and reexamined. It became quite evident that it was not a papillary carcinoma, as reported.

Pathological Findings. A thorough histopathological and histochemical examination and comparison of the serial sections of all biopsies taken from the larynx and of the excised cervical lymph nodes was undertaken.

Review of the hematoxylin and eosin-stained paraffin sections of all biopsy specimens taken from the larynx (including those performed in Iran) revealed that in all specimens the neoplastic tissue consisted of relatively small epithelial cells, with large, hyperchromatic, round nuclei and a small amount of cytoplasm. The cells were arranged in solid sheets, and in some areas the tumor had a trabecular-acinar pattern, with cribriform appearance (Fig. 1). Stains for argentaffin and argyrophil granules were negative, as were the special stains for mucus.

Sections of the excised cervical lymph nodes showed partial replacement of the nodes by metastatic tumor. In hematoxylin and eosin-stained slides the tumor had the same appearance as the laryngeal biopsy specimens, although the acinar pattern was less evident (Fig. 2). Special stains for mucus were negative. Stains for argentaffin and argyrophil granules, however, were strongly positive in many groups of the tumor cells within the lymph nodes (Figs. 3 and 4).

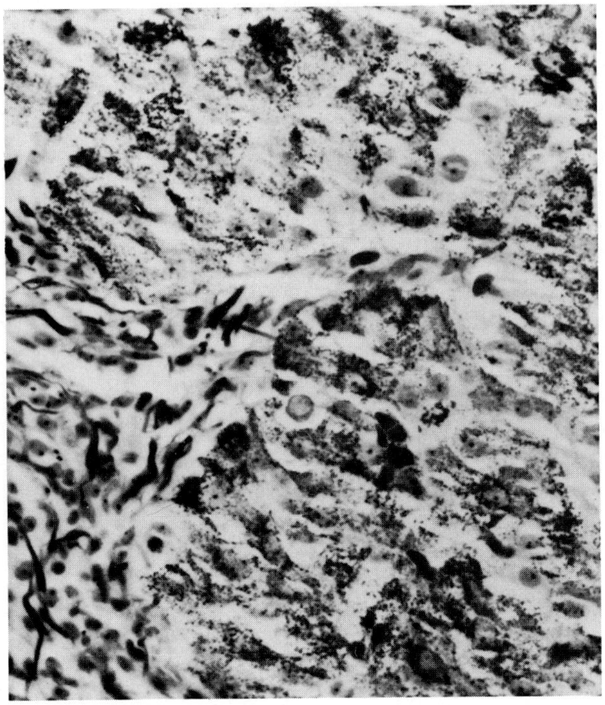

Fig. 3. Metastatic carcinoid tumor within a cervical lymph node showing dispersion of argyrophil granules. (Sevier-Munger stain, x500)

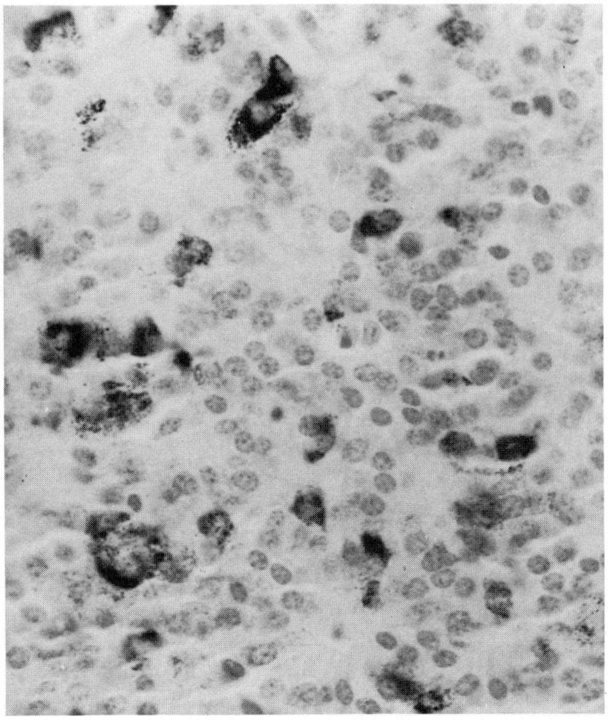

Fig. 4. Metastatic carcinoid tumor within a cervical lymph node showing argentaffin granules. (Fontana-Masson stain, x500)

In addition, an electron microscopic study was subsequently made of specimens that had previously been fixed in formalin and embedded in paraffin. Neurosecretory granules in large numbers could easily be recognized in most of the tumor cells (Figs. 5 and 6).*

The above findings led to the diagonsis of primary malignant carcinoid tumor of the larynx with metastases in the cervical lymph nodes.

Postoperative Course. The patient was subjected to a thorough clinical examination that ruled out any distant metastases. He did not exhibit the well-known carcinoid syndrome,[5,6] and the amount of hydroxy-indol-acetic acid (5-HIAA) daily excretion in the urine was normal (5.8 mg/day).

Since the laryngoscopic findings were insignificant, a course of radiotherapy was administered in an attempt to preserve the larynx, though irradiation is usually not the recommended treatment for carcinoids. The patient received a total dose of 8000 rads, delivered over a period of three months, to the larynx, neck, right supraclavicular area and superior mediastinum. Mild edema of the arytenoids that developed towards the completion of radiotherapy subsided under treatment with steroids (prednisone) and antibiotics. By the end of November 1978, the patient was permitted to leave for home, having been instructed to return for a follow-up examination and evaluation of the condition in two to three months' time.

*The electron microscopic study was performed by Dr. Itzhak S. Levij, Professor of Pathology.

Due to the situation in Iran, the patient arrived six months later, being extremely hoarse, and his breathing becoming labored on physical exertion. Indirect laryngoscopy revealed a gross infiltrating tumor that involved the right ventricular and ary-epiglottic folds and the right arytenoid area, where a smooth-surfaced swelling, bulging into the laryngeal lumen, could be seen. The infiltration extended into the posterior laryngeal wall, causing immobility of both vocal cords and severe stenosis of the larynx. Tomography showed marked narrowing of the larynx by a large infiltrating tumor, and a contrast x-ray study of the esophagus revealed a well-defined filling defect indenting the esophagus posteriorly at the C_6-C_7 level.

All these signs attested that the carcinoid of the larynx had failed to respond to radiation treatment, as anticipated, and had significantly grown and expanded since its completion, but there were no palpable lymph nodes in the neck, and the area of the radical neck dissection seemed to be free of recurrent regional metastases. The amount of 5-HIAA daily excretion in the urine was at the upper limits of normal (9 mg/day), nor were there any signs of the carcinoid syndrome. No signs of distant metastases could be detected by a complete clinical work-up that, inter alia, included x-ray examination and tomography of the chest, a contrast study of the upper and lower gastrointestinal tract, and bone and liver scan. Cardiac examination and all routine and biochemical blood tests were within normal range.

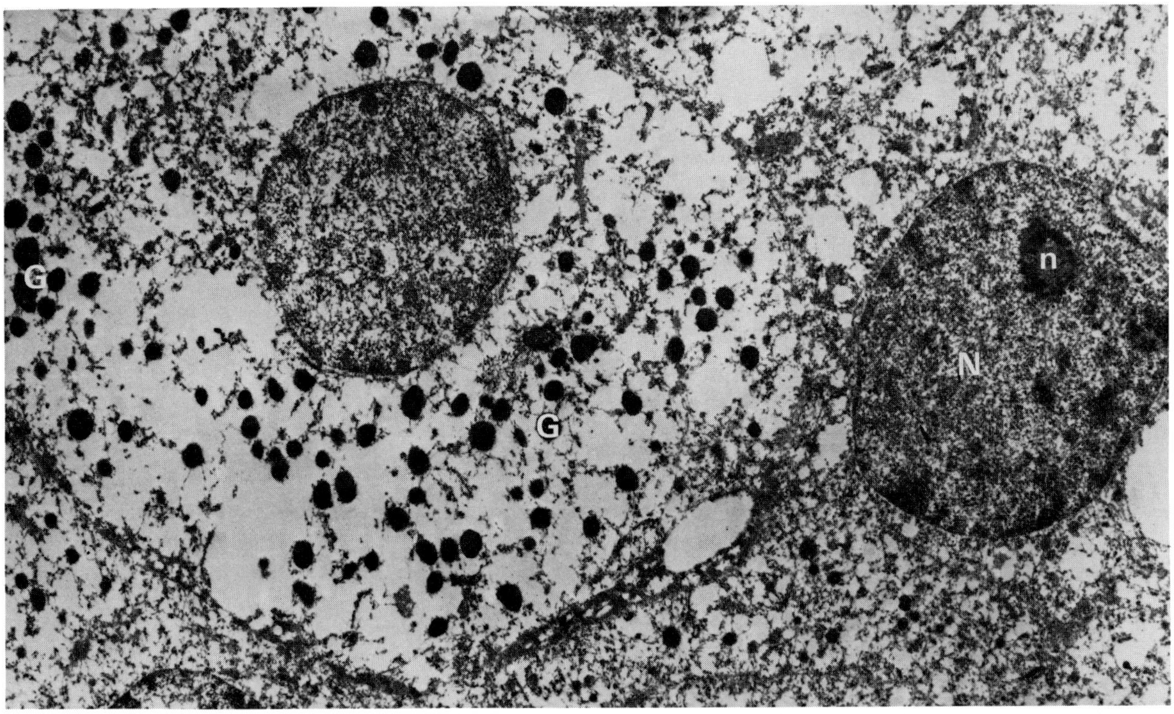

Fig 5. Transmission electron micrograph showing numerous round and oval granules (G) in the tumor cells. N - Nucleus; n - Nucleolus. (x8,600)

Total laryngectomy was recommended. The patient consented, but because of family and other circumstances, this time he preferred to be operated on in his home country. A repeat biopsy was not done at this stage, as that might have led to an emergency tracheostomy, which was not desirable. The patient left for home with instructions to his otolaryngologist.

In October 1979 we were informed that the patient underwent total laryngectomy. His general condition was reported as satisfactory except for loss of weight.

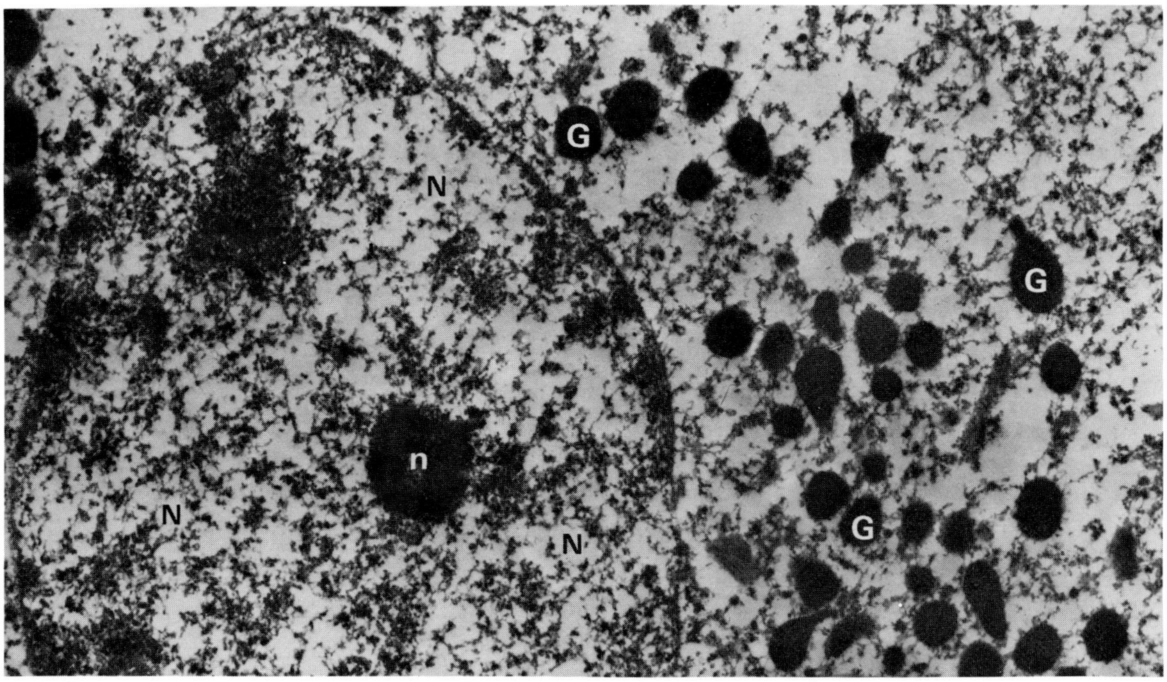

Fig. 6. Transmission electron micrograph at higher magnification (x19,200) showing the granules as having a homogenous electron-dense appearance, compatible with that of neurosecretory granules as described in carcinoid tumors. G - Oval granules; N - Nucleus; n - Nucleolus.

DISCUSSION

The term carcinoid was introduced by Oberndorfer,[7] who described tumors of the small intestine which were less aggressive than most carcinomas. Carcinoid tumors arise from the enterochromaffin or the so-called Kulchitsky cells, that include a number of cell types which are differently distributed throughout the primitive gut. They tend to correspond cytologically to the type of enterochromaffin cell which is preponderant in the given region. Williams and Sandler[8] classified carcinoid tumors according to the embryology of the site of origin of the neoplasm: carcinoid of foregut (bronchi, stomach, biliary tract and pancreatic ducts), midgut (lower duodenum, jejunum, ileum, cecum, and appendix) and hindgut (descending colon and rectum) derivation.

Midgut carcinoids contain argentaffin granules which are relatively large and pleomorphic. The granules contain serotonin (5-hydroxytryptamine) and usually give a positive argentaffin reaction.[9] Foregut carcinoids contain relatively small, uniformly rounded granules. These granules do not contain serotonin, but instead 5-hydroxytryptophan, its immediate precursor, and usually give a negative argentaffin reaction. In hindgut carcinoids, the argentaffin reaction is rarely positive. Despite the fact that carcinoids of foregut and hindgut origin are often negative in the histochemical argentaffin reaction, the term *argentaffinoma* is commonly used as a synonym for all carcinoid tumors. Such argentaffin-negative carcinoids, however, may give a positive argyrophil reaction.[9]

One of the methods of demonstrating argentaffin-positive carcinoids is the Fontana-Masson stain. Argyrophil-positive carcinoids are well demonstrated by the Sevier-Munger technique. Both these histochemical methods have been used in our case, and proved the stains for argentaffin and argyrophil granules in many groups of the metastatic tumor cells within the cervical lymph nodes to be strongly positive.

In biopsies taken from the larynx, the stain for argentaffin and argyrophil granules were negative, but this could be explained by the presence of only a few small groups of tumor cells in these specimens. Some of the metastatic tumor cells in the cervical lymph nodes were also negative in the above stains, while the rest were strongly positive.

It should, however, be noted that the demonstration of a positive argentaffin or argyrophil histochemical reaction only does not yet prove the tumor to be a carcinoid, since the diagnosis is made on the histological appearance of the tumor. Histologically, most foregut carcinoids resemble argentaffinomas of the alimentary tract. The typical carcinoid tumor is composed of solid trabeculae or nests and clusters of relatively small, fairly uniform polygonal cells with large hyperchromatic nuclei and moderate amounts of cytoplasm. The cells are in an orderly arrangement, with only few mitotic figures. The cytoplasm often contains eosinophilic granules, and the stroma is usually delicate. Tumors of foregut derivation tend to become more trabecular, as demonstrated by Goldman et al[4] and by our case.

The carcinoid nature of the tumor was also corroborated by an electron microscopic study of the specimens that revealed large numbers of typical neurosecretory granules in most of the tumor cells.

The malignancy potential of foregut carcinoids has generally been accepted as low. Bronchial carcinoids tend to be locally invasive, but grow slowly and may be present for years before evidence of dissemination occurs,[6,10,11] though a much higher malignancy potential was also described, with metastases in 44% of the patients.[12] An 87% five-year survival rate has been reported for bronchial and lung carcinoids in an extensive statistical study by Godwin.[13] In a recent study on tracheal carcinoids by Briselli et al[3] metastatic spread was recorded only in 1 out of 14 cases reported in the English literature. Carcinoid tumors of the larynx, on the other hand, showed a higher degree of malignancy, as clearly demonstrated in our case and by the one previously reported.[4] These proved to be locally infiltrative and spread extensively via the lymphatics to the regional cervical lymph nodes, where their histological appearance was identical to that of the primary tumor. In carcinoids, the metastatic lymph nodes very frequently are larger than the primary tumor.[14] This is very well illustrated in the presented case.

Carcinoid tumors may spread by the blood stream to cause distant metastases in various organs, including the skin and subcutaneous tissue.[4,14] In our case, a year after radical neck dissection for extensive cervical metastases, there still were no signs of distant spread, but such a possibility cannot be ruled out in the future. In the only reported case of laryngeal carcinoid by Goldman et al,[4] distant skin metastases appeared ten months after total laryngectomy with bilateral neck dissection.

Our patient did not demonstrate the well-known carcinoid syndrome. The latter is frequent with carcinoids of foregut origin, but is rarely present in carcinoids of its respiratory diverticulum. The amount of 5-HIAA daily excretion in the urine was also within normal range. It was not until the laryngofissure and the radical neck dissection that the diagnosis of carcinoid tumor was made. All previous biopsies were reported as carcinomas (papillary, anaplastic, adenocarcinoma).

Radiotherapy has again proved to be ineffective in the treatment of carcinoids. Despite the massive dose of local irradiation (8000 rads) that had been administered after radical neck dissection in an attempt to preserve the larynx, the primary tumor continued to grow and expand. It is, therefore, reasonable to conclude that the treatment of choice in laryngeal carcinoids should be wide surgical excision of the primary lesion and of all accessible metastases.

ACKNOWLEDGMENTS — We are indebted to Dr. Itzhak S. Levij, Professor of Pathology, Hadassah-Hebrew University Medical School, for the electron microscopic study of the specimens.

REFERENCES

1. Kononov EP. Carcinoid of the trachea. Zh Ushn Nos Gorl Bolezn 1967; 27:104.

2. Habal MB, Murray JE. Argentaffin adenoma of the trachea. Am J Surg 1973; 125:336-7.

3. Briselli M, Mark GJ, Grillo HC. Tracheal carcinoids. Cancer 1978; 42:2870-9.

4. Goldman NC, Hood CI, Singleton GT. Carcinoid of the larynx. Arch Otolaryngol 1969; 90:64-7.

5. Thorson A, Biörck G, Björkman G, Waldenstrom J. Malignant carcinoid of the small intestine with metastases to the liver, valvular disease of the right side of the heart (pulmonary stenosis and tricuspid regurgitation without septal defects), peripheral vasomotor symptoms, bronchoconstriction, and an unusual type of cyanosis. A clinical and pathologic syndrome. Am Heart J 1954; 47:795-817.

6. Brindley GV, Bonnet GD. Bronchial adenoma and the carcinoid syndrome. Ann Surg 1967; 165:670-80.

7. Oberndorfer S. Karcinoid Tumoren des Dünndarms. Frankf Z Pathol 1907; 1:426-32.

8. Williams ED, Sandler M. The classification of carcinoid tumor. Lancet 1963; 1:238-9.

9. Lillie RD, Glener GG. Histochemical reaction in carcinoid tumors of the human gastrointestinal tract. Am J Pathol 1960; 36:623-51.

10. Donahue JK, Weichart RF, Ochsner JL. Bronchial adenoma. Ann Surg 1968; 167:873-85.

11. Salyer DC, Salyer WR, Eggleston JC. Bronchial carcinoid tumor. Cancer 1975; 36:1522-37.

12. Goodner JT, Berg JW, Watson WL. The nonbenign nature of bronchial carcinoids and cylindromas. Cancer 1961; 14:539-46.

13. Godwin JD. Carcinoid tumors. An analysis of 2837 cases. Cancer 1975; 36:560-9.

14. Welling RE, Taggart JP. Carcinoid tumor metastatic to the neck. Arch Surg 1975; 110:111-3.

≈

LURIE LIBRARY FUND

Many inquiries have been made about a memorial fund to which friends and colleagues of Dr. Moses Hyman Lurie could contribute. Shortly before his death Dr. Lurie established a modest fund for the purchase of books in Otolaryngology for the Library at the Massachusetts Eye and Ear Infirmary. The Library Committee of the Infirmary has verified that donations can be made in memory of Dr. Lurie to this fund. Contributions may be sent to the "Lurie Library Fund," in care of Mr. Charles Snyder, Librarian, Massachusetts Eye and Ear Infirmary, 243 Charles St., Boston, MA 02114.

Ann Otol 90:1981

EFFECT OF VOICE THERAPY ON CONTACT GRANULOMA OF THE VOCAL FOLD

CAROLE S. BLOCH, MA
NEW YORK, NEW YORK

WILBER J. GOULD, MD
NEW YORK, NEW YORK

MINORU HIRANO, MD
KURUME, JAPAN

Contact granuloma of the vocal folds caused by physical trauma secondary to voice abuse has traditionally been treated by surgical removal. This mode of handling can be frequently disappointing since these lesions have a strong tendency to recur and may require additional operative procedures. This paper describes 17 patients in whom treatment of the primary problem was approached through voice therapy. Treatment consisted of a comprehensive history and voice evaluation, stress reduction, relaxation methods, auditory and kinesthetic feedback, pitch change and elimination of voice abuse. Patients were closely followed by the speech pathologist and laryngologist who worked together as a team. The results of voice therapy were evaluated by the laryngologist, the speech pathologist and the patient himself. As a result of voice therapy, the granuloma disappeared in 9 patients, was reduced in size in 4 and remained unchanged in 1. For the remaining three patients, posttherapeutic laryngoscopic findings were not available. The speech pathologist found voice and manner of phonation returned to normal in 4 patients, improved in 7 and remained unchanged in 6. Four patients felt that complete recovery had taken place, 10 felt that some improvement was noted, and 3 felt no change had taken place. Based on the assessments of all three evaluators, the success rate of treatment with voice therapy can be stated as 71% (12 of 17 cases) or 100% (eliminating 5 of 17 cases who terminated treatment very early).

Granuloma of the larynx can be classified into two major groups: specific and nonspecific. The former, which is considered somewhat rare, includes granulomas caused by tuberculosis and syphilis. Nonspecific granulomas include three typical entities: contact granuloma, intubation granuloma, and granuloma secondary to gastroesophageal reflux. This paper deals with contact granuloma which is basically caused by trauma related to phonation. It has also been termed posterior hypertrophic pachydermia or contact ulcer. This clinical entity was first identified by Chevalier Jackson in 1928.[1] He had collected 127 cases as far back as 1888.

Indirect laryngoscopy reveals a unilateral or bilateral lesion at or near the tip of the vocal process of the arytenoid cartilage. The primary etiologic factor is trauma. It is the forceful meeting of the vocal process of the arytenoid cartilages which initially causes an ulcerative lesion. Later, excessive granulation tissue and eventually fibrous tissue may form. It is because of the abusive manner in which the patient uses his vocal folds that he inflicts the trauma.

Traditional treatment for contact granuloma has been surgical removal through direct laryngoscopy. In some cases, removal by indirect laryngoscopy as an office procedure has been the method of choice. Surgical treatment can be disappointing since these lesions have a strong tendency to recur and may require repeated operative procedures.[2-4] Furthermore, the healing process often takes longer as the number of surgical interventions increases.[5]

Other recommended modes of treatment include a regimen of silence,[6,7] change of occupation,[4] aerosol therapy with penicillin,[6] persuading the patient to change his manner of speaking and eliminating excessive consumption of alcohol.[5,6] Many of these modalities, however, appear impractical and unrealistic in terms of the average patient's lifestyle.

Thorough voice evaluation followed by voice therapy has been recommended as a means of treatment either in conjuntion with surgery to prevent recurrence, or in lieu of surgery.[8-16] The important principle here is that if the presence of the granuloma is the end result of a complex pathological process, removal of tissue would not necessarily affect the underlying pathological process, in spite of any temporary palliation it might offer. Surgical removal may have only temporary value and does not alter the basic etiologic factors.[8,9,12]

Before 1947 there was no definitive plan of voice therapy in general use and patients were placed for long periods on absolute voice rest and occasional local excision. Many of these patients were disturbed because of the long time it took to establish good results.[9,13,15,16]

Peacher and Holinger[16] in 1947 were the first to describe the effects of voice therapy for contact granuloma. They reported 16 patients, 6 who received voice therapy and 10 controls. All individuals who had undergone vocal reeducation showed definitive curative results. Six of the 10 not receiving treatment suffered from continuance of symptoms. Thus, after 1947 the direction of treat-

From the Center for Communication Disorders, Lenox Hill Hospital, New York.

REPRINTS — Carole S. Bloch, MA, Lenox Hill Hospital, Center for Communication Disorders, 100 E. 77th Street, New York, NY 10021.

ment for contact granuloma changed. Baker reviewed 19 patients. Twelve were seen before 1947, were placed on complete voice rest and had occasional local excisions. Seven patients were seen after 1947 and received voice therapy with good results. Speech therapy was begun once the diagnosis of the ulceration was made. The patients found speech therapy, which didn't involve lost time from work, more economical than voice rest. In addition, the tendency for the lesion to recur was less with voice therapy.[13] Holinger and Johnston reviewed 92 patients, 50 of whom had voice therapy,[14] Brodnitz reviewed 26 patients in voice therapy[11] and Peacher studied 12-year follow-ups of 70 patients with voice therapy;[15] all reported excellent results with this mode of treatment for contact granuloma.

The main purpose of this paper is to reacquaint the laryngologist with voice therapy as a primary consideration in his treatment of contact granuloma of the vocal folds. While there has been much evidence of the success of voice therapy in the literature, it dates back to before the early 1960s. This may be the reason that we have seen many patients in the past few years in whom surgery was the first choice of treatment. We also wish to emphasize the efficacy of voice therapy in this age of technological change in which new techniques such as endolaryngeal microsurgery have become available.

METHODS

Subjects. During the period from June 1972 to June 1979, 17 patients with contact granuloma were seen at our center for voice evaluation and therapy by our speech pathologist. Patients who had a history of intratracheal intubation preceding the development of the granuloma were not included in the investigation. All of the subjects were male, ranging from 30 to 74 years of age. The majority of these patients (11), were in the age range 30-49 years; three were in the group 50-59 years, 2 in the 60-69 age group, and 1 was 74 years of age. Eight patients had not undergone surgery for contact granuloma at any point. Nine patients were referred for voice therapy following surgery and recurrence of the granuloma. One of these 9 had had surgery on three separate occasions for granulomas which occurred on each vocal fold. In most of the patients, diagnosis was based on history and laryngoscopic findings. In those few cases in which there was doubt as to the nonspecific character of the lesion, a biopsy was performed.

All patients were in demanding careers, either as leaders within companies or in occupations in which the patients reported rigorous self-imposed standards. They were all in the upper-middle socioeconomic class. With few exceptions, all patients were able to correlate job-related tensions with the onset of their laryngeal problems.

Patients complained of mild-to-severe hoarseness, laryngeal and vocal fatigue, mild-to-sharp laryngeal pain, or pain elsewhere in the head and neck, coughing up blood or a foreign-body sensation in the throat. Twelve of 17 patients reported having had one or more of the following gastrointestinal difficulties: hiatus hernia, peptic ulcer, acidity, heartburn, or stress reaction in the abdomen. (It was, however, unlikely that the gastrointestinal difficulties could be related to the granuloma of the vocal folds.)

Voice Evaluation and Therapy. All 17 patients underwent indirect laryngoscopic evaluation prior to referral to the speech pathologist. The pretherapeutic laryngologic findings were typical in all cases. The lesion was located at or near the tip of the vocal process of the arytenoid cartilage. Most patients were followed by the laryngologist at various intervals throughout the duration of the voice treatment plan. Prior to therapy, each patient underwent a thorough diagnostic evaluation by a speech pathologist. This included a careful and comprehensive history of the patient's complaint, associated medical and psychologic factors, analysis of voice usage and a surface assessment of personality dynamics. In addition, pretherapeutic and posttherapeutic tape recordings were made in order to note changes in the patient's voice.

Patients were seen for voice therapy once a week or less. The scheduling depended upon time availability and progress in therapy. As the patient improved, the number of sessions decreased; total sessions ranged from two to 24. One patient underwent two series of six sessions, discontinuing prematurely and then having additional sessions the next year. Follow-up was from six months to seven years.

Voice therapy was conventional, encompassing work directly aimed at changing the manner of vocal fold vibration and taking into account the psychological aspects of the patient's complaint. The methods varied according to each patient's needs. What was important for all patients, however, was an attempt to establish rapport and gain the patient's respect and confidence.

The patient was instructed to eliminate such vocally abusive habits as coughing, excessive throat clearing and shouting. None of the patients were instructed to institute complete voice rest or reduction in the amount of time spent talking. Voice use was critical to the occupation of most of these patients. Preventing the individual from speaking or even suggesting less speech would have been financially as well as morally detrimental. Patients were advised to curtail or reduce activities that might increase pressure or tension on the larynx and affect its function as a valving system, ie, weight lifting, excessive pushing or pulling, strained anal elimination. When necessary, they were taught the essentials of adequate breathing for voice production, or given relaxation exercises, for the total body or for specific areas of the head and neck. Many of our patients used an excessively low pitch during conversation which sometimes dropped as low as glottal fry. In such cases, we instructed the patient to raise his pitch slightly. When there was evidence of excessive hard glottal attacks, the patient was made aware of this in an effort to eliminate them. All patients were instructed in the need for auditory discrimination for constant feedback and the continuous monitoring of conversational voice.

The psychological aspect of voice treatment focused on the interrelationship between voice and emotional state. While many patients appeared relatively calm initially, a nonthreatening discussion of their emotional, professional and domestic lifestyles often aided in bringing various problems to the forefront. Helping the individual gain some awareness of and insight into his problems was often enough to assist in reducing some of the tension associated with voice production.

RESULTS OF VOICE THERAPY

The results of voice therapy were judged by the laryngologist who followed the case, the speech pathologist involved in the treatment and the patient himself. Evaluations of the results are categorized in the following manner.

Laryngoscopic findings (with symbols used in Table 1).

- \+ + Complete disappearance of granuloma
- \+ Reduction in size of granuloma
- – No change in appearance of granuloma
- ? Not seen again

TABLE 1. RESULTS OF VOICE THERAPY IN PATIENTS WITH CONTACT GRANULOMA (N = 17)

Case	*Age*	*Previous Surgery*	*Number of Voice Therapy Sessions*	*Laryngoscopic Findings*	*Speech Pathologist's Findings*	*Patient's Subjective Evaluation*
1.	41	0	7	+ +	+	+
2.	47	0	11	+ +	+	+
3.	43	1	12	+ +	+ +	+ +
4.	41	3	23	+ +	+	+
5.	61	0	2	?	–	+
6.	31	1	2	+	–	–
7.	47	0	13	+ +	+	+
8.	54	1	8	+	–	+
9.	74	0	3	?	–	+
10.	40	0	5	–	–	–
11.	63	1	3	+	+	+
12.	56	0	11	+ +	+ +	+ +
13.	38	0	4	?	–	–
14.	46	1	17	+ +	+ +	+ +
15.	30	1	24	+ +	+ +	+ +
16.	52	1	7	+	+	+
17.	39	1	12 (6 + 6)	+ +	+	+

For explanation of symbols, see test.

Evaluation by speech pathologist:

+ + Voice recovery and manner of phonation within normal limits

+ Voice and manner of phonation improved

– No change in voice or manner of phonation

Patient's subjective evaluation:

+ + Completely free of symptoms

+ Symptoms improved

– No change in symptoms.

Nine patients treated were successful in eliminating all laryngoscopic evidence of the lesion (Table 1). In four patients the laryngologist observed that the size of the granuloma was significantly reduced. One patient showed no change in the size of the growth and the remaining three patients discontinued treatment before it was completed.

The speech pathologist felt that in 4 patients, voice and manner of phonation improved to within normal limits; the laryngologist noted disappearance of the growth in 5 patients and marked improvement in 2. For the remaining 6 patients, there was felt to be no significant change in voice or manner of phonation; the laryngologist saw improvement in 2 patients and no change in 1; 3 patients were not seen again.

Four patients felt that all symptoms had disappeared and were in agreement with the laryngologist, who no longer saw evidence of the growth, and the speech pathologist who diagnosed complete voice recovery. The majority, ten patients, felt that they had made some progress in symptom alleviation. Of these 10, 7 were found to have made progress by the speech pathologist and 3 showed no change. For the laryngologist 5 of these 10 patients showed complete disappearance of the growth, 3 had some reduction in size of the granuloma and 2 did not return for a second visit. Three patients felt that the symptoms were not alleviated and the speech pathologist concurred that there had been no change. For the laryngologist, 1 patient did improve, 1 showed no change and 1 was not seen again.

It should be noted that in many cases where the otolaryngologist no longer saw evidence of the growth, the speech pathologist thought more could be done with the patient. The patient was also a severe critic in terms of evaluating symptoms when the growth had disappeared. This was believed to have been a result of the therapeutic process in which the patient was taught to monitor the auditory and kinesthetic feedback aspects of his sound production constantly; in doing so he became his own severest critic.

Looking at the results in terms of all three evaluators, voice therapy was successful in 12 of 17 cases, or 71%. The remaining five patients (Nos. 5, 6, 9, 10 and 13) had five or fewer sessions before discontinuing therapy. If we exclude these five patients the success rate would be 11 of 11, or 100%.

Nine patients had undergone surgery for removal of contact granuloma, suffered a recurrence, and then sought voice therapy. Of these patients, eight showed significant improvement with voice therapy. For another 8 patients voice therapy was the primary mode of treatment; of these patients, 4 showed improvement, and the remaining 4, who discontinued after five or fewer sessions, showed little or no improvement. The fact that therapy was more successful with the patients who had undergone surgery can be attributed to the fact that these patients were more concerned with continuing treat-

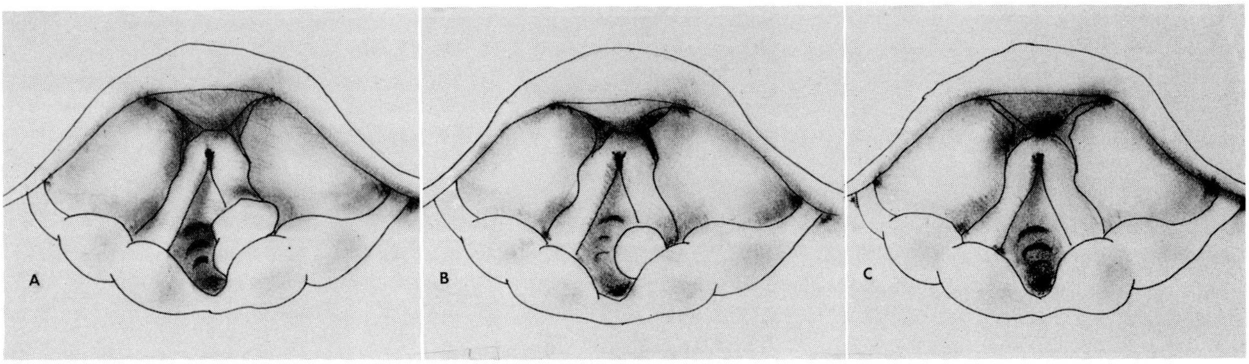

Fig. 1. Line drawings of photographs obtained by indirect laryngoscopies of patient with contact granuloma treated with voice therapy. A) Larynx prior to initiation of voice therapy; B) larynx midway through therapy; C) larynx after completion of voice therapy.

ment and showed more persistence in the therapeutic process.

Indirect laryngoscopy provided evidence of the efficacy of voice therapy in patient 3 (Table 1 and Fig. 1). Details of this patient's progress have been reported by Bloch and Gould.[8]

COMMENT

The results of the present investigation demonstrate that voice therapy is an effective mode of treatment in many cases of contact granuloma of the vocal fold. Voice therapy can be utilized as the single treatment method for elimination of the lesion and of the symptoms. It is applicable both to early and to fairly extensive lesions. It is also valuable postsurgically as a means of preventing recurrence. For two additional patients voice therapy was instituted following surgical removal of contact granuloma as a means to prevent recurrence. In both cases, therapy was successful in preventing recurrence, in effecting a positive manner of phonation and in providing symptom relief.

The importance of the team approach to management of this disease must be emphasized. The laryngologist and the speech pathologist should work together for successful management. Ongoing discussion of changes in symptoms as treatment proceeds is important to insure adequate patient care. Ideally, when a patient presents with symptoms of contact granuloma, he should be seen by both the laryngologist and the speech pathologist. The laryngologist should see the patient initially to diagnose and describe the lesion. Biopsy may be indicated in doubtful cases. The patient should be referred to a speech pathologist for diagnostic evaluation and a trial period of voice therapy. Periodic discussions between specialists help to assess the patient's progress from the viewpoint of both disciplines. The decision to continue voice therapy or attempt surgery also should be made jointly. If surgery is necessary, then speech therapy should be continued postoperatively to prevent recurrence.

The question of when voice therapy might be discontinued may be based not only on evidence of normal vocal fold appearance, but on complete remission as assessed by the patient, laryngologist and speech pathologist. Laryngologic information of complete disappearance of granuloma does not necessarily imply a complete resolution of the patient's problems. It might be that remaining symptoms are experienced by the patient, and the assessment of voice and the manner of phonation by the speech pathologist are the only means of determining realistically the resolution of underlying problems.

ACKNOWLEDGMENTS — The authors are greatly indebted to Dr. Hugh Biller for his encouragement and valuable suggestions for this paper.

Minoru Hirano, MD, is on leave of absence from the Department of Otolaryngology, Kurume University, Kurume, Japan.

REFERENCES

1. Jackson C. Contact ulcer of the larynx. Ann Otol Rhinol Laryngol 1928; 37:227-30.

2. Ellis M. Chronic laryngitis. In: Ballantyne J, Groves J, eds. Scott-Brown's diseases of the ear, nose and throat. Philadelphia: JB Lippincott, 1971:361-2.

3. Miglets AW Jr. ENT case of the month: contact granuloma of the larynx. Ohio State Med J 1973; 69:364.

4. Jackson C. Larynx and hypopharynx. In: Jackson C, Jackson CL, eds. Diseases of the nose, throat and ear. Philadelphia: WB Saunders, 1959:600-1.

5. Ballantyne J. Occupational disorders of the larynx. In: Ballantyne J, Groves J, eds. Scott-Brown's diseases of the ear, nose and throat. Philadelphia: JB Lippincott, 1971:541-57.

6. DeWeese DD, Saunders WH. Textbook of otolaryngology. St. Louis: CV Mosby, 1973.

7. Peacher G. Contact ulcer of the larynx. I. history. J Speech Hear Disord 1947; 12:67-76.

8. Bloch CS, Gould WJ. Vocal therapy in lieu of surgery for contact granuloma: a case report. J Speech Hear Disord 1974; 39:478-85.

9. Brodnitz FS. Post-operative vocal rehabilitation in benign lesions of the vocal cords. Folia Phoniatr (Basel) 1955; 7:193-200.

10. Brodnitz FS. Vocal rehabilitation in benign lesions of the vocal cords. Speech Hear Disord 1958; 23:112-17.

11. Brodnitz FS. Contact ulcer of the larynx. Arch Otolaryngol 1961; 74:70-80.

12. Von Leden H, Moore P. Contact ulcer of the larynx. Arch Otolaryngol 1960; 72:746-52.

13. Baker DC Jr. Contact ulcers of the larynx. Laryngoscope 1954; 64:73-8.

14. Holinger PH, Johnston KC. Contact ulcer of the larynx. JAMA 1960; 172:511-55.

15. Peacher GM. Vocal therapy for contact ulcer of the larynx: a follow-up of 70 patients. Laryngoscope 1961; 71:37-47.

16. Peacher G, Holinger P. Contact ulcer of the larynx II. the role of vocal re-education. Arch Otolaryngol 1947; 46:617-23.

≈

NINCDS NOTES*

OTITIS MEDIA RESEARCH CENTER FUNDED

NINCDS is stepping up efforts to improve recognition and treatment of otitis media. Latest in a series of actions toward this end is a 5-year grant to the University Health Center of Pittsburgh for an otitis media research center. To be headed by Dr. Charles D. Bluestone, Professor of Otolaryngology at the University of Pittsburgh, the center will conduct basic and clinical research into every aspect of middle ear infections, the most common childhood illness diagnosed by physicians in the United States.

Studies that center scientists will undertake include comparing the effectiveness of different treatments of otitis media, such as myringotomy and removal of tonsils and adenoids.

Even when diagnosed and controlled before any complications occur, otitis media costs the Nation some $1.5 billion in yearly medical bills. The new center is expected to make important contributions toward settling some of the controversies surrounding treatment of otitis media, ultimately reducing its human and economic costs.

REYE'S SYNDROME CONFERENCE SET FOR MARCH

"The Diagnosis and Treatment of Reye's Syndrome" will be the subject of an NIH Consensus Development Conference March 2-4, 1981, at NIH.

For information, contact: Dr. Joseph S. Drage, Chief, Developmental Neurology Branch, NDP, NINCDS, Rm. 816, Federal Building, Bethesda, MD 20205, (301) 496-6701.

TENTATIVE CONSENSUS REACHED ON BRAIN DISSECTION ISSUES

An NINCDS-NIMH sponsored workshop on human brain dissection was held in Cambridge, England, September 4-6, as part of a continuing effort to develop international standards for the collection, dissection, and chemical analysis of human nervous system specimens. Methods currently used are extremely diverse, complicating comparisons of data between laboratories and impeding attempts to map transmitter systems in the brain.

HEAD AND SPINAL CORD INJURY SURVEY PUBLISHED

A survey sponsored by NINCDS scientists is considered to be the first reliable statistical picture of the incidence and costs of head and spinal cord injury in the United States. A limited number of copies of the survey report, published as a supplement to the *Journal of Neurosurgery* (Volume 53, November 1980), are available from the Office of Scientific and Health Reports, NINCDS.

*This information is prepared monthly by the Office of Scientific and Health Reports, National Institute of Neurological and Communicative Disorders and Stroke, National Institutes of Health, Bldg. 31, Rm. 8A06, Bethesda, MD 20205, (301) 496-5751.

CHONDROSARCOMA AT THE SKULL BASE

I. GAY, MD

J. ELIDAN, MD

J. KOPOLOVIC, MD

JERUSALEM, ISRAEL

A rare case of chondrosarcoma at the skull base is presented. Computerized tomography scan was very helpful in delineating the exact extent of the tumor. Chondrosarcoma is a slow growing malignant tumor which metastasizes very late. Usually it is radioresistant, but when surgery is not feasible, irradiation treatment is worth a trial.

Chondrosarcomas arising in the base of skull are very rare. The incidence of all kinds of sarcomas is no more than 1% of all malignant tumors of head and neck.[1] Gaisford and Hanna[2] found two cases of chondrosarcomas among 36 cases of head and neck sarcomas. In the series of Ketchan et al,[1] out of 19 cases of head and neck sarcomas, 2 were classified as chondrosarcomas. Arlen et al,[3] found 18 cases of chondrosarcomas of the head and neck, over a period of 36 years (excluding lesions of the larynx). None of these tumors was reported to originate from the basicranium, although death usually occurred as a result of extension into the cranial cavity. Jones[4] estimated that only 10% of chondrosarcomas occur in the head and neck regions. He described seven cases, one of which originated in the ethmoid complex, and another one arose from the nasopharynx. Coats and his associates in 1977[5] presented the largest series of sarcomas of the nasal cavity, paranasal sinuses, and nasopharynx. Out of 82 patients who were seen at the Mayo Clinic during a period of 25 years, with sarcomas of those regions, 13 (16%) were classified as chondrosarcomas. In all the cases which arose in the region of the nasal cavity, the clinical picture was predominated by nasal symptoms.

We present here a case of chondrosarcoma which was unusual in its clinical symptomatology.

CASE REPORT

A 50-year-old male tourist from Iran was admitted to Hadassah University Hospital for evaluation of severe headache and complete blindness in his left eye. His complaints had started about six months before admission with slow deterioration of vision in this eye. He was examined and treated in Iran by retrobulbar injections (of steroids?) but without any effect.

On admission, his general condition was good. The ophthalmological examination revealed proptosis of 4 mm of the left globe, and advanced optic atrophy was noticed. The eye movements were normal. The ears were normal. The inferior concha was markedly hypertrophied on the left side, but no sign of tumor was seen either in the nose or in the nasopharynx. The rest of the physical examination was within normal limits.

Regular x-ray pictures and anterior-posterior tomography of the nasal sinuses demonstrated a large mass with increased density (between soft tissue and bone density) involving the left ethmoid and the sphenoid sinuses, with extension into the posterior part of the left orbit, into the cranial cavity, and to the roof of the left nasal fossa (Fig. 1).

Computerized tomography (CT) scan confirmed the above findings (Fig. 2) and showed the tumor penetrating into the left orbit. The optic nerve was displaced laterally, and the globe was pushed forward.

On the third hospitalization day diagnostic antrotomy, through a Caldwell-Luc approach was done. The left maxillary sinus was found to be normal. The ethmoid sinuses were entered and a hard, pale tumoral tissue was encountered.

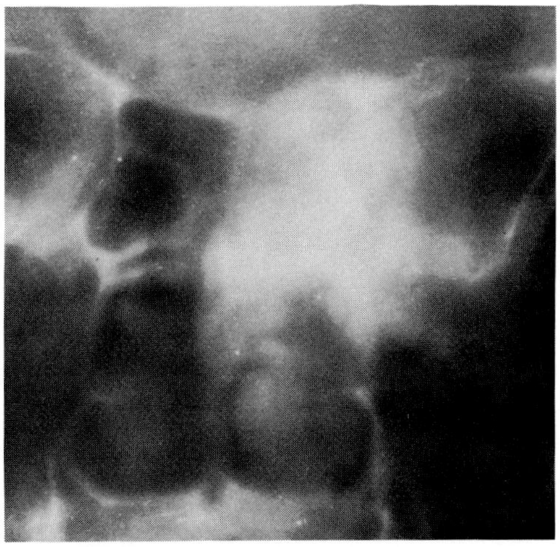

Fig. 1. Anterior-posterior tomography of the paranasal sinuses. The tumor is demonstrated by the markedly dense mass, involving the left ethmoid sinus, the posterior part of the left orbit, and the upper part of the left nose.

From the Departments of Otolaryngology and Pathology, Hadassah University Hospital, Jerusalem, Israel.

REPRINTS — I. Gay, MD, Department of Otolaryngology, Hadassah University Hospital, Jerusalem, Israel.

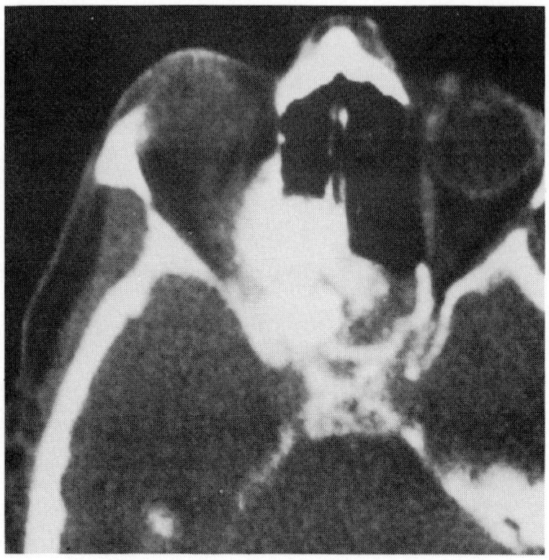

Fig. 2. Computerized tomography scan of the skull. The tumor is well shown by the dense mass in the left ethmoid and sphenoid sinuses, penetrating into the left orbit, pushing the optic nerve and the globe. The density of the tumor is almost equal to that of bone.

The biopsied material consisted of fragments of upper respiratory tract epithelium, fibrovascular tissue, bone with fibrosis and fragments of cartilage. The cartilage showed areas of hypercellularity with binucleated and multinucleated chondrocytes (Figs. 3 and 4). The nuclei of the chondrocytes were hyperchromatic and pleomorphic. The stroma was myxomatous hyalinized and with some areas of calcification. The histological diagnosis was chondrosarcoma, well-differentiated.

It was obvious that no definite surgical treatment

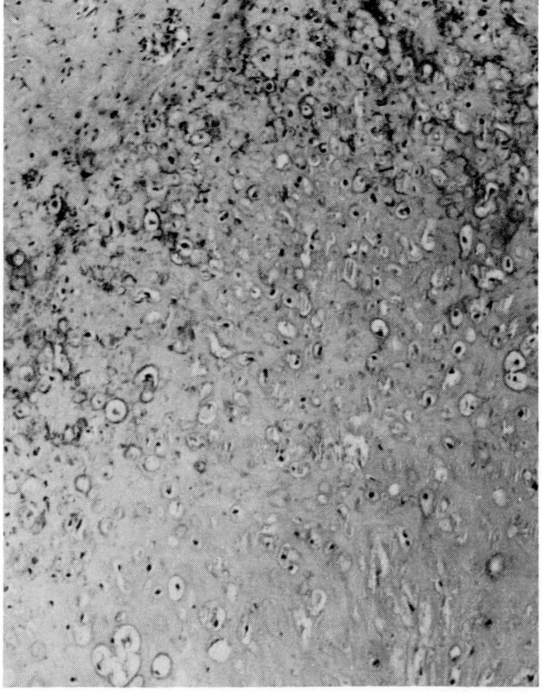

Fig. 3. Malignant cartilage with areas of calcification and hyalinization. (H&E, x100)

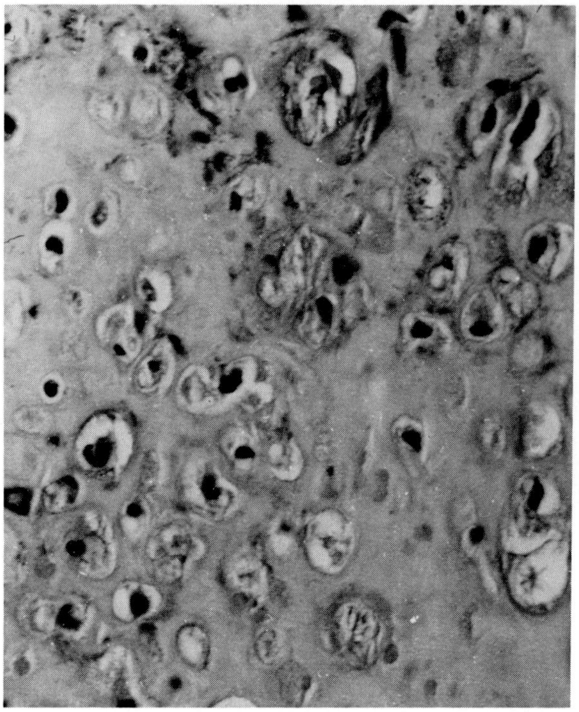

Fig. 4. Cellular area with pleomorphic and hyperchromatic chondrocytes. (H&E, x400)

was possible. The patient was referred to Oncology Department for irradiation treatment.

DISCUSSION

Chondrosarcoma of the head and neck can be divided into three groups:[4] 1) those arising from the base of the skull and from the nasal cavity regions; 2) those arising from the larynx; and 3) miscellaneous.

The tumor in this case arose from the sphenoethmoidal region. It is very difficult usually to decide where the exact site of origin of these tumors is, because they are in an advanced stage when first diagnosed.

Fifty-seven cases of chondrosarcomas originating in the sphenoid region are reported in the literature till 1973.[4] In most of them the presenting symptom was some nasal disturbances, eg, obstruction and bleeding, and in almost all of them nasal or nasopharyngeal examination revealed a tumor mass.[4,5] The present case was unusual and marked by the lack of any nasal symptomatology, although the radiological study showed extension to the roof of the nasal fossa. The source of cartilaginous tumors in this region is believed to be from "cartilaginous cell rests"[4] in the basicranium, which is preformed in cartilage.

The roentgenological manifestations of chondrosarcoma include bony destruction, mass or opacity involving one or more of the paranasal sinuses,[5] usually with motling calcification. The high density of the tumor mass shown by tomographs in the present case is remarkable. The CT scan picture, one of the first published of chondrosarcoma was very helpful in delineating the exact extent of the tumor.

Chondrosarcoma at the sphenoid region should be differentiated from chondroma, chordoma, meningioma, craniopharyngioma, or even with arterial aneurysm.[6] Among these, chordoma is the most difficult to differentiate clinically, radiologically and pathologically.

The clinical course of osteosarcoma is usually much more aggressive.[3] Whereas the osteocartilaginous neoplasms generally arise in a parasellar location and later may destroy the clivus or sella turcica, chordomas are typically found in the midline, near the clivus, and are not parasellar until relatively large.

The histological diagnosis of chondrosarcoma may present difficulties. Well-differentiated chondrosarcoma may resemble benign chondroma with differentiated chondrocytes. Only in some foci the chondrocytes may show cytologic characteristics of malignancy such as increased cellularity, binucleated and multinucleated chondrocytes with hyperchromatic, pleomorphic and plump nuclei; biopsy material may contain only the well-differentiated areas and the diagnosis of malignancy may be postponed until recurrence and adequate biopsy is performed.

The histologic diagnosis may be particularly difficult in the case of "chondroid chordoma" described by Heffelfinger et al[7] as mixture of chordoma with chondroid component that has the features of chondroma or chondrosarcoma. Other diagnostic difficulty may arise in differentiation of chondrosarcoma from osteogenic sarcoma. Chondrosarcoma may show areas of calcification and ossification. However, chondrosarcoma does not show neoplastic osteoid, nor osseous tissue nor sarcomatous connective tissue stroma.

Chondrosarcoma are slow-growing malignant tumors which metastasize very late and usually cause death by local extension and intracranial involvement.[1,3,4] The tumor is radioresistant,[1,8] but there are few reports in the literature of good response to irradiation.[9,10]

The only effective curative treatment is wide radical excision, if feasible.[1,4] This treatment is contraindicated in cases where the tumor originates from or spreads to the base of the skull.

REFERENCES

1. Ketcham AS, Chretien PB, Pilch YH. Sarcomas of the head and neck. In: Gaisford GC, ed. Symposium on cancer of the head and neck. vol 2. St. Louis: CV Mosby, 1969:337.

2. Gaisford JC, Hanna DC. Sarcomas of the head and neck. Plast Reconstr Surg 1962; 29:250-8.

3. Arlen M, Tollefsen HR, Huvos AG, Marcove RC. Chondrosarcomas of the head and neck. Am J Surg 1970; 120:456-60.

4. Jones HM. Cartilaginous tumors of the head and neck. J Laryngol Otol 1973; 87:135-51.

5. Coates MB, Pearson BW, Devine KD, Unni KK. Chondrosarcoma of the nasal cavity, paranasal sinuses and nasopharynx. Trans Am Acad Ophthalmol Otolaryngol 1977; 84:919-26.

6. Berkman YM, Blatt ES. Cranial and intracranial cartilaginous tumors. Clin Radiol 1968; 19:327-33.

7. Heffelfinger MJ, Dahlin DC, MacCarty CS, Beabout JW. Chordomas and cartilaginous tumors at the skull base. Cancer 1973; 32:410-9.

8. Wirth JE, Shimkin MB, Chondrosarcoma of the nasopharynx simulating juvenile angiofibroma. Arch Pathol 1943; 36:83-8.

9. Padison GM, Hanks GE. Chondrosarcoma of the maxilla: report of case responding to supravoltage irradiation, and review of the literature. Cancer 1971; 28:616-9.

10. Lott S, Bordley JE. A radiosensitive chondrosarcoma of the sphenoid sinus and base of skull — report of a case. Laryngoscope 1972; 82:57-60.

Ann Otol 90:1981

STUDY OF VENTILATION TESTING WITH ELECTRONYSTAGMOGRAPHY

WILLIAM R. WILSON, MD JIN W. KIM, MD

BOSTON, MASSACHUSETTS

Provocation tests such as head shaking and positional tests, as well as hyperventilation, have been used routinely by many laboratories to elicit nystagmus during an electronystagmogram. We added oxygen testing to this routine battery and compared the results with hyperventilation and other forms of provocative testing. Hyperventilation and oxygen testing are unique in that they probably affect the vestibular system by changing the levels of oxygen and carbon dioxide supplied. Hyperventilation in theory would decrease available oxygen, while oxygen testing would cause an increase. In a study of two groups totaling over 700 patients, we found that oxygen testing is only occasionally positive (2.5%) and is of little practical value. Hyperventilation testing is positive 8% of the time but rarely alone, and has no localizing value. When hyperventilation and oxygen tests are both positive, the nystagmus may be in opposite directions. In 6 of 18 patients with acoustic neurinomas, hyperventilation produced transitory direction-changing nystagmus.

INTRODUCTION

Vertigo and disequilibrium are the symptomatic complaints associated with dysfunction of the vestibular system. One of the objective counterparts of these complaints is nystagmus. In many patients nystagmus associated with nonacute vestibular injury can be detected only by electronystagmographic (ENG) recordings made with the subject's eyes closed. On an ENG, latent nystagmus (LN) may be present, but often nystagmus must be evoked by the use of any of several provocative testing maneuvers such as head shaking (HS), positional testing (PT), and hyperventilation (HV).

To this group of provocative testing maneuvers we have added oxygen testing in order to study its effects, along with that of hyperventilation, upon the vestibular system. Hyperventilation and oxygen testing together we call ventilation testing (VT). These tests are unique in that they might affect the vestibular system by altering the arterial partial pressure of carbon dioxide ($PaCO_2$) or oxygen (PaO_2).

METHODS

Seven hundred ENGs from patients examined at the Massachusetts Eye and Ear Infirmary with vestibular complaints were studied. The recording method utilized skin electrodes for direct-current recordings of nystagmus throughout all tests. No attempts were made to assess patients for the presence of pulmonary or cardiovascular disease and no preselection of the patients was made on the basis of the presumed vestibular system diagnosis in this group.

The test consisted of a pretest tracing taken in the erect-sitting, eyes-closed position in a darkened room. At this time, it was established if nystagmus was present or absent. The patient was then asked to hyperventilate as rapidly as possible for three minutes, and a tracing was taken. Some of the patients were unable to complete this task as they became lightheaded or vertiginous before the allotted time, and tracings were taken at the point when they became unable to continue. After a five-minute rest period the oxygen test was performed. Oxygen was administered with a McKesson anesthesia machine employing a semiclosed-circle system with a CO_2 absorber. This apparatus was used to ensure a stable $PaCO_2$ for the duration of the test. The patients wore a tightly fiting rubber face mask and received 100% oxygen at the flow rate of six liters per minute. Patients were asked to breathe spontaneously for four minutes. At the end of this time, an ENG tracing was taken. No attempts were made to measure the arterial PaO_2 or $PaCO_2$ nor were exhaled gasses measured.

Definition of a Positive Response. There were several forms of positive response to VT. First, enhancement of nystagmus; this is defined as the onset of nystagmus when it was not present immediately prior to HV or O_2 testing (Fig. 1), or an increase of 100% or more in the slope of the slow phase nystagmus compared to the pretest slope (Fig. 2), or the establishment of regularly beating nystagmus when the pretest spontaneous nystagmus merely consists of occasional scattered beats. Second, reduction of spontaneous nystagmus; this positive finding was noted when brisk nystagmus observed immediately prior to testing was absent following HV or O_2. Third, direction-changing nystagmus; this was observed when HV and oxygenation tests produced nystagmus in directions opposite to one another, or when direction-changing nystagmus was noted during one of these tests (Figs. 3 and 4).

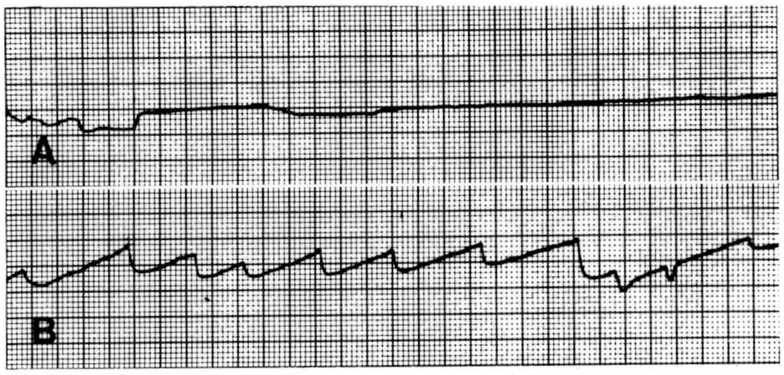

Fig. 1. Hyperventilation test. A) Before hyperventilation no nystagmus is present. B) Following hyperventilation left-beating nystagmus is present.

From the Departments of Otolaryngology and Anesthesiology, Massachusetts Eye and Ear Infirmary, Boston, Massachusetts.

REPRINTS — William R. Wilson, MD, Department of Otolaryngology, Massachusetts Eye and Ear Infirmary, 243 Charles Street, Boston, MA 02114.

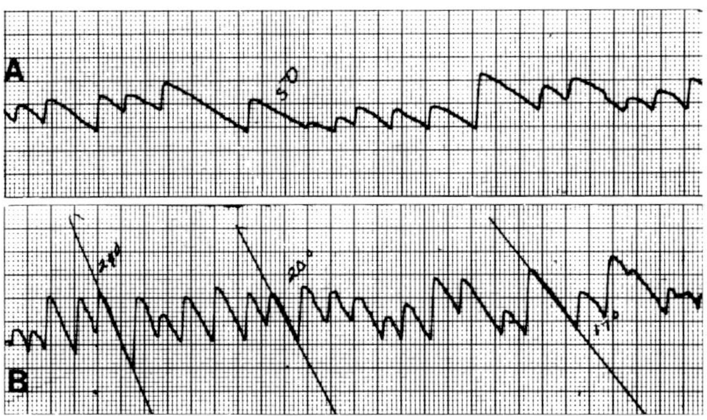

Fig. 2. Slope of the slow phase of spontaneous nystagmus present prior to hyperventilation was increased by this test. A) Before hyperventilation; B) After hyperventilation.

RESULTS

A group of 500 randomly selected ENGs were reviewed to establish the incidence of positive VTs (Table 1). The mean age of the 500 patients was 45.0 years. Of this group, 54 patients (11%) with a mean age of 48.5 years had positive VTs.

Forty-one patients had positive HV tests alone and three patients were positive for both HV and O_2 testing. Two patients, both with acoustic neurinomas, had transient direction-changing nystagmus produced by HV.

Only 13 of 500 patients (2.5%), with a mean age of 55.9 years, had positive oxygen tests. While the sample is too small to be significant, there is a tendency for these patients to be older. As mentioned above, three of these patients had positive HV tests as well. In two instances nystagmus induced by O_2 was in a direction opposite to that induced by HV (Fig. 3).

In the majority of patients nystagmus was not produced de novo by HV or O_2 but could be found elsewhere on the ENG as LN, or could be evoked by HS and PT. The effect of HV and O_2 testing was to enhance nystagmus over 90% of the time rather than reduce spontaneous nystagmus or cause a change in direction. Also, it was found that HV testing provides a much stronger stimulus than O_2 testing as it was positive four times more frequently.

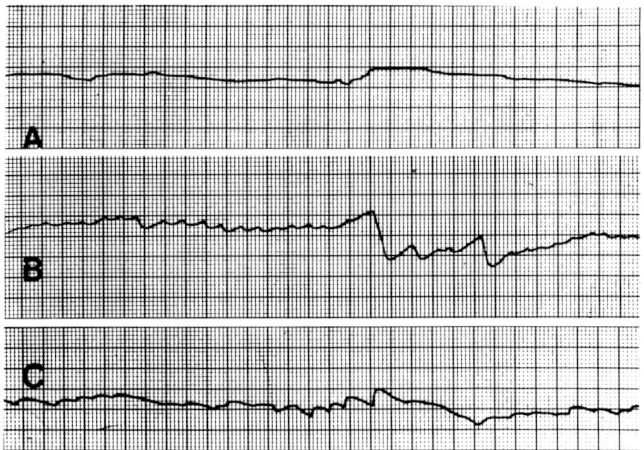

Fig. 3. Hyperventilation and oxygen testing can induce nystagmus in opposite directions. This finding occurred in two patients reported in this study. A) Before hyperventilation; B) After hyperventilation; C) After 100% oxygen.

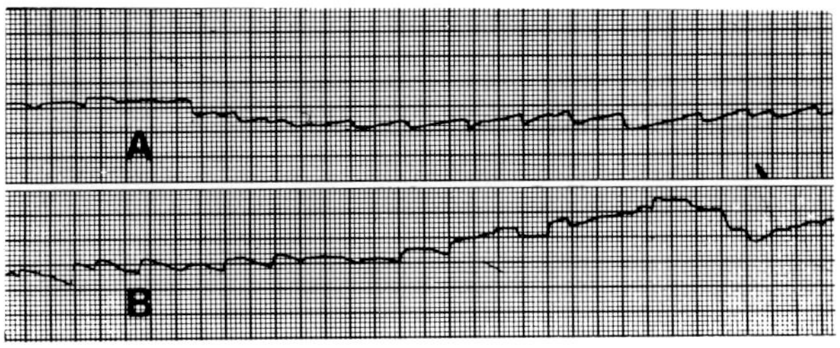

Fig. 4. Hyperventilation test. A) B) Direction-changing nystagmus in a patient with acoustic neurinoma.

Because of the impression from the first 100 charts reviewed that the mean age of patients with positive VTs is greater than the group mean, a second group of 200 charts was reviewed. The charts were taken at random and included 100 patients under 40 years of age and 100 patients 40 years or older. We found no age difference between the incidence of LN or provoked nystagmus as manifested by HS or PT (Table 2). However, there was a tendency for the VTs to be positive more often in the 40 and over group ($P = 0.07$). There was no difference among the age groups in the number of normal ENGs or those with readings of central or peripheral vestibular dysfunction.

The records of 18 patients with acoustic neurinomas, who represent all those seen in the ENG laboratory from 1974 to present, were reviewed. Of this group, six patients (33%) were found to have transient (lasting less than one minute) direction-changing (D-C) nystagmus during the HV test (Fig. 4). The incidence of D-C nystagmus in the total population was 2 in 500 or 0.04%; this difference was significant to the $P < 0.001$ level.

Audiograms of the six patients with acoustic neurinomas and positive D-C hyperventilation tests demonstrate relatively good hearing when compared with the group of 12 patients who did not have D-C hyperventilation tests. All six had sloping high-frequency hearing losses with sufficient residual hearing to perform tone decay and recruitment tests in five of the six patients. Among the 12 patients with acoustic neurinomas without a positive

TABLE 1. POSITIVE ENG RESULTS IN 500 PATIENTS

Test Results	Patients No.	Patients %	Mean Age* (yr)
Positive for HV or O_2	54	11.0	48.5
Positive for HV alone	41	8.0	—
Positive for HV and O_2 combined	3	0.5	—
Positive for O_2 alone	10	2.0	55.9

*Mean age of the 500 patients reviewed: 45.0 yr.
HV - Hyperventilation; ENG - Electronystagmogram.

TABLE 2. COMPARISON OF PATIENTS BY PROVOCATIVE TESTS AND AGE GROUP (N = 200)

	LN	HS	PT	VT
100 patients under 40 years	9	29	53	9
100 patients over 40 years	10	32	65	18
% increase over 40 years	5	5	9	33

LN - Latent nystagmus; HS - Head shaking; PT - Positional tests; VT -Ventilation tests.

D-C hyperventilation test, only 5 of 12 patients had sufficient hearing to perform both these tests. In the D-C group, the speech reception threshold (SRT) ranged from 25 to 70 dB, and discrimination from 88 to 0%. The tone decay test, suggesting neural dysfunction, was positive in five of six patients; and recruitment, generally considered to be a test of cochlear injury, was positive in half of these patients. There was no correlation noted between the degree of reduced vestibular response on the Hallpike caloric tests and the amount of hearing loss in this small group of patients. By reviewing operative notes and radiology reports, no difference could be found between groups in tumor size or the incidence of widening the internal auditory canals or meatuses.

It seems reasonable to assume that the hearing loss and vestibular changes from acoustic neurinomas are due, in part, to vascular compression and changes in perfusion of the involved nerve and end-organ. The above data are consistent with the concept that a positive D-C hyperventilation test is found during an earlier stage of neurovascular compression by injury due to the effect of HV on the partial pressures of O_2 and CO_2.

DISCUSSION

Hyperventilation has been used as a provocative test for eliciting vertigo and nystagmus. Drachman and Hart[1] analyzed 104 patients with complaints of vertigo and found that a patient's complaint of chronic dizziness could be reproduced by HV in nearly 25% of those patients studied. Although some of these patients were felt by the authors to have self-induced psychogenic dizziness, it was HV that produced that patient's symptoms of dizziness and nystagmus. In addition, they described a syndrome of positional vertigo that occurred only after HV in two of their patients and thereby thought that these methods of eliciting symptoms might be additive.

The effects of HV upon a locus of vestibular dysfunction are complex. First, VT requires the active participation of the test subject which may serve to increase nystagmus through an alerting response. Second, the physiologic effect of HV is to decrease $PaCO_2$ by blowing air off through the lung. Hyperventilation causes little or no change in the partial pressure of oxygen or oxygen saturation of hemoglobin because the relatively low partial pressure of oxygen in room air becomes a limiting factor. Since hypocapnia, which in this instance results from HV, is a strong stimuli for cerebral vasoconstriction, there is a subsequent reduction of cerebral blood flow in conscious man.[2] It is likely, therefore, that a reduction in available O_2 as well as CO_2 to the vestibular and neural tissue occurs during the HV test.

On the other hand, breathing 100% oxygen over four minutes will increase the PaO_2 from 95 mm Hg to over 600 mm Hg in a normal, young individual.[3] Aging factors such as chronic pulmonary disease, pulmonary shunts, and cardiovascular disease would all serve to reduce the PaO_2 achieved in elderly people. One hundred percent oxygenation for a short period of time is a relatively benign procedure that results in increased oxygen tension throughout the body including the vestibular system. The effect of this test in terms of available oxygen would be the opposite to HV.[4,5]

Hyperventilation testing amounts to a stronger stimulus in the younger age groups because of greater cardiovascular reactivity. It has been demonstrated that HV causes EEG slowing that is closely correlated to a reduction in cerebral venous oxygen and these changes are more marked in young patients.[6] Therefore, a paradox exists. Vascular disease as it exists in an older population probably causes symptomatic ischemic vestibular injuries, but the same disease process makes the results of HV or breathing 100% oxygen less dramatic in the affected individuals.

Bruner and Norris[7] studied age-related changes in ENG. They found, as we, that ENG did not vary greatly with age. Our study demonstrated a tendency for increased incidence for positive oxygen testing in a patient group over 40 years of age that may be related to increased vascular disease with advancing age.

Following acute cerebral infarction, unexpected responses to HV and subsequent hypocapnia can occur. The vasoconstriction of hypocapnia can, at times, displace blood toward an ischemic zone, "inverse intracerebral steal."[8] This special situation is unlikely to occur in our patient population.

The effects of changes in both oxygen and carbon dioxide tension on those patients studied were to increase nystagmus in the majority of cases. That HV and O_2 testing work in opposing manners is supported by the fact that two patients that we examined had a vestibular disorder that responded differently to hypocapnia and reduced oxygen tension than to increased oxygen tension. These theories, however, require further corroborating neurophysiological and anatomical data.

CONCLUSIONS

1. Hyperventilation tests are positive 8% of the

time and are useful for provocative testing of the vestibular system. However, they are rarely found as isolated findings on an ENG.

2. Oxygen testing is positive only 2.5% of the time and was determined not to be a practical screening test.

3. It is likely that HV and O_2 tests have opposite effects upon the oxygenation of the vestibular end-organ.

4. Transient direction-changing nystagmus was found to occur with acoustic neurinomas in about one third of cases.

ACKNOWLEDGMENT — The authors extend their sincere appreciation to Mrs. Elizabeth McHugh who performed the electronystagmograms used for this study and to Mrs. Geraldine Marion who typed the manuscript.

REFERENCES

1. Drachman DA, Hart CW. An approach to the dizzy patient. Neurology (Minneap) 1972; 22:323-34.

2. Alexander SC, Wollman H, Cohen PJ, et al. Cerebral-vascular response to $PaCO_2$ during halothane anesthesia in man. J Appl Physiol 1964; 19:561-5.

3. Wood EH. Normal oxygen saturation of arterial blood during inhalation of air and oxygen. J Appl Physiol 1949; 1:567-74.

4. Meyer JS, Gotah F, Akiyama M, Joshitake S. Monitoring cerebral blood flow, oxygen, and glucose metabolism. Analysis of cerebral metabolic disorder in stroke and therapeutic trials in human volunteers. Circulation 1967; 36:197-211.

5. Meyer JS, Ryu R, Toyoda M, et al. Evidence for a Pasteur effect regulating cerebral oxygen and carbohydrate metabolism in man. Neurology (Minneap) 1969; 19:954-62.

6. Gotah F, Meyer JS, Tagaki Y. Cerebral effects of hyperventilation in man. Arch Neurol 1965; 12:410-23.

7. Bruner A, Norris TW. Age related changes in caloric nystagmus. Acta Otolaryngol (Stockh) 1971; Suppl 282.

8. Meyer JS. Medical and surgical treatment of cerebral-vascular disease. In: Meyer JS, ed. Modern concepts of cerebrovascular disease. New York: Spectrum Publications, 1975:158-77.

≈

AFIP TRAINING PROGRAM IN HEAD AND NECK PATHOLOGY

A three-month fellowship is available to residents in training in otolaryngology as well as postgraduate fellows. This fellowship is designed to provide a broad-based understanding of pathology of the head and neck in one of the institutions with the most expertise and experience in this country. The curriculum consists of daily lecture periods discussing the pathology of the head and neck area, examination and discussions of interesting consultation cases, self study material and encouragement to undertake a publishable research project. Facilities for temporal bone dissection are available.

Interested candidates may contact Vincent J. Hyams, MD, Chief, Otolaryngic Pathology, Armed Forces Institute of Pathology, Washington, DC 20306.

Ann Otol 90:1981

FAMILIAL MULTIPLE GLOMUS TUMORS AND PHEOCHROMOCYTOMAS

JAMES L. PARKIN, MD, MS
SALT LAKE CITY, UTAH

Isolated cases of cervical cranial glomus tumors have been reported in association with pheochromocytoma. Two family pedigrees are presented and four individual cases discussed indicating a hereditary syndrome of pheochromocytoma associated with multiple glomus tumors of the head and neck. The hereditary potential has not previously been described. In three of the patients, the pheochromocytomas were asymptomatic at the time of initial presentation. These pheochromocytomas were discovered by arteriography after one of the patients developed a hypertensive crisis with the induction of anesthesia. The silent presence of pheochromocytoma in patients with multiple glomus tumors should be considered in the evaluation of these patients.

In 1957 Haller first reported an anatomical structure in the carotid bifurcation region termed the carotid body.[1] This structure consists of cells which fail to give a histological chromaffin reaction and are structurally similar to the neuroectodermal paraganglion cells found in the adrenal medulla. Similar histological tissue has subsequently been described in various anatomical areas, mainly in the head and neck regions.[2,3]

Neoplastic growth originating in this specialized tissue has generated much interest resulting in a large number of contributions to the medical literature of the past 30 years. In 1956, because of the theoretical chemoreceptor activity of the glomus tissue, Mulligan suggested the term chemodectoma to describe the tumors which originate from these cells.[4] Conley and Clairmont state that the tumor should be called nonchromaffin paragangliomas, which they believe more accurately indicates their cellular origin.[5] Others prefer to call these neoplasms glomus tumors with the additional anatomical terminology indicating the tumor location, ie, glomus jugulare, glomus vagale, and glomus tympanicum, etc.[6] The term glomus tumors will be used in this paper recognizing that other authors prefer different terminology.

The carotid body tumor is the most common form of cervical cranial glomus tumors. The first carotid body tumor removal was accomplished in 1880 by Riegner.[7,8] In 1945, Rosenwasser[7] first described the removal of a vascular middle ear tumor and associated this tumor etiologically with the glomus structure described by Guild.[9] Glomus tumors have been described in other locations including the trachea, periaortic area, mandible, ciliary ganglion of the eye, retroperitoneal region, and in association with the cervical vagus nerve and with the laryngeal branches of the vagus nerve.

Glomus tumors most frequently present in the fifth and sixth decades of life; however, they have been reported in patients as young as six months and over 80 years of age. Carotid body glomus tumors usually present as painless, firm, pulsatile neck masses. Glomus tympanicum and glomus jugulare tumors present most commonly with hearing loss and tinnitus. The presenting symptoms may be from the tumor bulk itself, or from tumor extension to adjacent vital structures. Cranial nerve paralysis is a frequent sign seen at patient presentation.

Patient evaluation must include a careful history and physical examination. The probable diagnosis of glomus tumor and the anatomic extent are best determined by radiographic evaluations including skull films, temporal bone polytomography, carotid arteriography, retrograde jugulography, and computerized axial tomography. Selective arteriography is, in the author's opinion, the most helpful radiographic technique for diagnosis and delineation of glomus tumors. Careful attention to the venous phase of the arteriography will often allow assessment of the patency of the jugular venous system without submitting the patient to retrograde jugulography.

A familial incidence of glomus tumors in some patients indicates a hereditary factor. The hereditary pattern in familial glomus tumors appears to be autosomal dominant.[10] Multiplicity of these tumors occurs in approximately 25 to 35% of the hereditary variety, but in less than 5% of the nonhereditary variety.[5,8,9]

The association of cervical cranial glomus tumors with pheochromocytomas has been reported.[11,12] No hereditary factor was evident in these reports. Pheochromocytomas have also been reported in association with neurofibromatosis, hemangioblastomas, medullary carcinoma of the thyroid, ependymoma, astrocytoma and carcinoid tumors.[11] Some of these associations do occur in hereditary patterns.

From the Division of Otolaryngology, Department of Surgery, College of Medicine, University of Utah, Salt Lake City, Utah.
REPRINTS — James L. Parkin, MD, MS, Division of Otolaryngology, 3B326 University Medical Center, Salt Lake City, UT 84132.

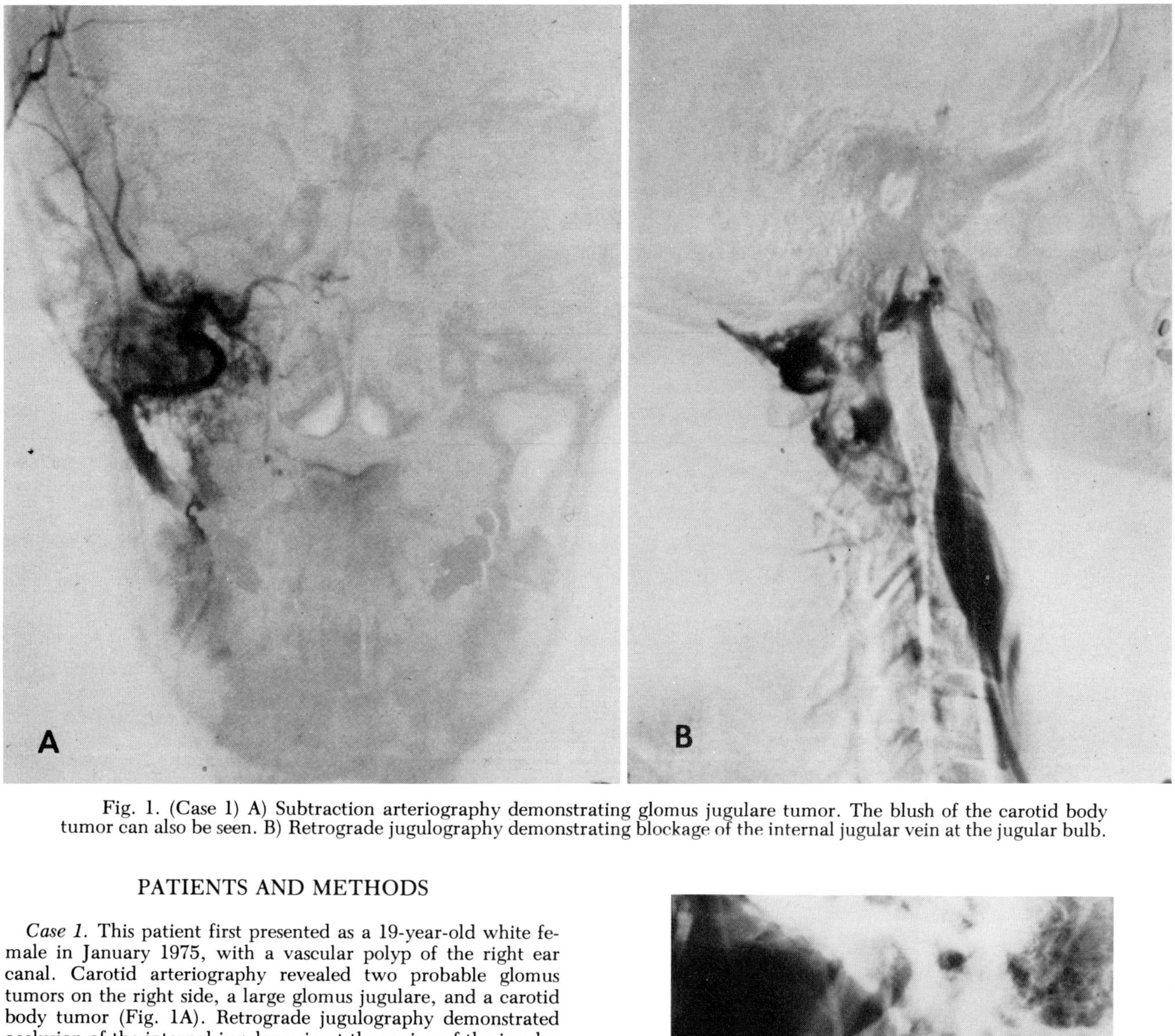

Fig. 1. (Case 1) A) Subtraction arteriography demonstrating glomus jugulare tumor. The blush of the carotid body tumor can also be seen. B) Retrograde jugulography demonstrating blockage of the internal jugular vein at the jugular bulb.

PATIENTS AND METHODS

Case 1. This patient first presented as a 19-year-old white female in January 1975, with a vascular polyp of the right ear canal. Carotid arteriography revealed two probable glomus tumors on the right side, a large glomus jugulare, and a carotid body tumor (Fig. 1A). Retrograde jugulography demonstrated occlusion of the internal jugular vein at the region of the jugular bulb (Fig. 1B). The patient was normotensive and gave no history of hypertension.

Surgical excision of the glomus jugulare was accomplished through an extended radical mastoidectomy and high cervical dissection. The carotid body tumor was excised at the same time. It was necessary to mobilize the facial nerve from the geniculate ganglion to the extratemporal segment in order to achieve excision of the glomus jugulare tumor. Postoperatively the patient had moderately good facial function which deteriorated over a three-day period. A wound infection developed in the mastoid area which was successfully treated with antibiotics. The patient had no significant recovery of facial nerve function at eight months following her surgery.

At ten months postoperatively, it was elected to perform a facial nerve graft. During induction of anesthesia, a hypertensive crisis developed and surgery was deferred. The hypertensive crisis was managed without complication. Additional medical workup revealed elevated urinary metanephrine and vanillylmandelic acid levels. Arteriography was performed revealing a suprarenal pheochromocytoma which was subsequently successfully excised. The facial nerve graft was accomplished at a later date with good results.

Case 2. This 34-year-old white male, brother of patient of case 1, presented in October 1977 with bilateral anterior cervical masses. These masses were firm and pulsatile. The patient had a

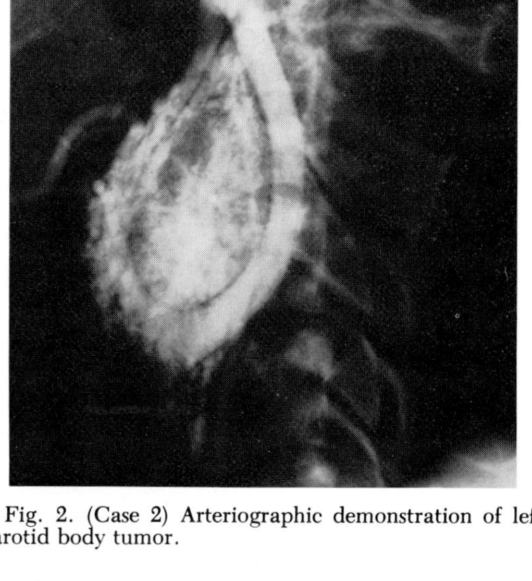

Fig. 2. (Case 2) Arteriographic demonstration of left carotid body tumor.

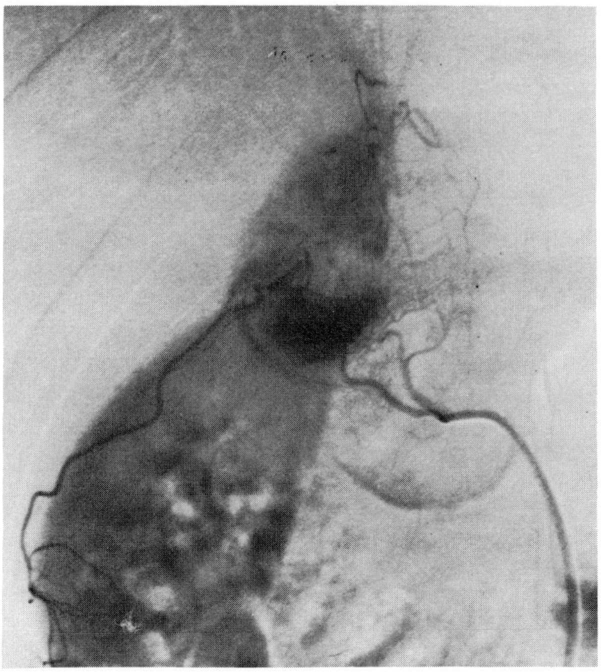

Fig. 3 (Case 3) Demonstration of asymptomatic pheochromocytoma discovered with abdominal arteriography.

history of hypertension and had undergone a full hypertensive workup within the year prior to admission. Urinary metanephrine levels and vanillylmandelic acid levels were normal. An intravenous pyelogram had also been normal within the year prior to admission.

Arteriography was performed revealing bilateral carotid body tumors (Fig. 2). Abdominal arteriography revealed no evidence of pheochromocytoma. The right carotid body tumor was excised in October 1977. During surgery a tear developed high in the internal carotid artery. A graft could not be placed so the internal carotid artery was ligated. Postoperatively the patient was carefully monitored, blood pressure maintained, and oxygen administered. He recovered without sequelae.

Six months later, repeat arteriography revealed the left carotid body tumor to be increasing in size. Again, abdominal arteriography was performed with the presence of a suprarenal pheochromocytoma now being confirmed. This later tumor was successfully excised. The patient was allowed to return home and was readmitted in August 1978 for excision of the left carotid body tumor. This excision was undertaken with apprehension because of the complication encountered on the opposite side. A cardiovascular surgeon assisted with the second excision which was accomplished without complication and with an estimated blood loss of 250 cc. Postoperatively the patient has done well. However, he continues to have mild hypertension.

Case 3. This 23-year-old male brother of patients of cases 1 and 2 presented in October 1977 during a visit to his brother in the hospital. Bilateral asymptomatic neck masses were discovered. The patient was normotensive. He was admitted to the hospital and selective bilateral carotid arteriography and abdominal arteriography were performed (Fig. 3). These studies revealed bilateral glomus tumors of the carotid bodies and an asymptomatic pheochromocytoma. The patient's urinary catecholamine tests were all normal. Excision of the pheochromocytoma was accomplished on this hospital admission.

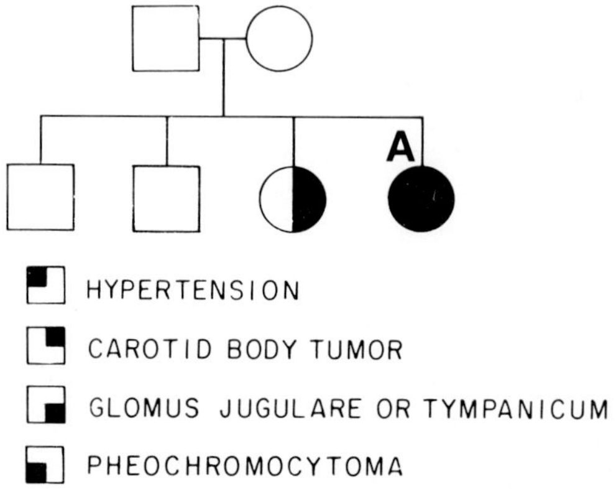

Fig. 5. (Case 4) Pedigree. There is no other known history of chemodectoma in family lines.

Following recovery from the abdominal surgery the patient was readmitted in January and February 1978 for the uneventful excision of the right and then the left carotid body tumors. His postoperative course has been without complications and he remains normotensive.

Case 4. This 33-year-old white female with a history of multiple pheochromocytomas of the bladder and retroperitoneum was first evaluated by the author in October 1977. She also had a history of surgical removal of a right glomus tympanicum, bilateral carotid body glomus tumors and a left glomus jugulare tumor. She has had a total of 14 glomus tumors and pheochromocytomas. The patient was referred to our institution for irradiation of the glomus jugulare tumor. The other cervical cranial glomus tumors had been surgically treated at another institution.

This patient's family history indicated that her sister has had bilateral carotid body tumors and a glomus jugulare tumor removed. The sister has had no evidence of pheochromocytoma. Two brothers are reportedly without evidence of glomus tumors or hypertension. This patient was presented by Bogdasarian at the 1978 Annual Meeting of the American Academy of Otolaryngology.[13]

Figure 4 demonstrates the pedigree of patients of cases 1, 2, and 3. Figure 5 demonstrates the pedigree of patient of case 4. There is no additional history of glomus tumors or pheochromocytomas in more distant relatives of either familial group.

DISCUSSION

It is noteworthy that in the first three presented cases, the diagnosis of pheochromocytoma was not evident at the time of initial presentation. The pheochromocytoma became evident in case 1 only after a hypertensive crisis developed with induction of general anesthesia. Case 2 was mildly hypertensive on presentation; however, his urinary catecholamine studies were normal and his initial ab-

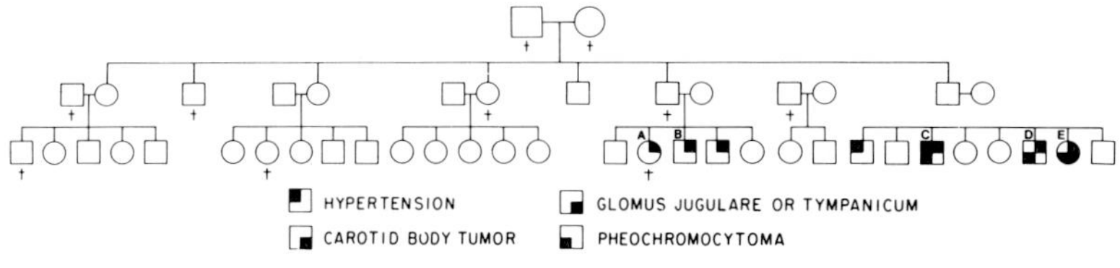

Fig. 4 (Cases 1-3) Pedigree including case 1 (E), case 2 (C), and case 3(D). Patient A had two carotid body tumors and subsequently died of carcinoma of the lung. Patient B had two large neck tumors in childhood which were irradiated. Exact diagnosis is not available.

dominal arteriography failed to demonstrate a pheochromocytoma. It was demonstrated on repeat arteriography six months later. Case 3 also had normal urinary catecholamine values and an asymptomatic pheochromocytoma was discovered during arteriography because of the family history.

Pheochromocytomas have been described in association with many different tumors.[11] Some of these associations have occurred in a hereditary pattern. Pheochromocytoma has previously been described in association with glomus tumors of the head and neck.[11,12] A hereditary relationship has not been previously described. The patients presented in this paper strongly indicate a hereditary factor in the association of multiple cervical cranial glomus tumors and pheochromocytomas.

It is suggested that in evaluation of patients with multiple cervical cranial chemodectomas, abdominal arteriography should be accomplished at the time of cervical arteriography to evaluate for the possibility of occult pheochromocytomas. This should be accomplished with little additional risk to the patient. Ruijs et al recently described the use of radionuclide scintiangiography for the screening of asymptomatic family members. They screened 59 relatives of patients with familial chemodectomas. Three new chemodectomas were discovered and confirmed with standard angiography. Four false positives were not confirmed with angiography. Technetium-99 was utilized as the radionuclide.[14] This technique may be useful in the evaluation of asymptomatic family members.

REFERENCES

1. Haller A. Elementa physiologiae corporis humani. Lausanne: 1757-1763; Berne: 1764-6.
2. Palacios E. Chemodectomas of the head and neck. Am J Roentgenol 1979; 110:129-40.
3. Guild SR. A hitherto unrecognized structure, the glomus jugularis in man. Abstract. Anat Rec 1941; 79 Suppl 2:28.
4. Mulligan RM. Chemodectoma in dog. Am J Pathol 1950; 26:680-1.
5. Conley JJ, Clairmont AA. Glomus intravagale. Laryngoscope 1977; 87:2096-100.
6. Alford BR, Guilford FR. A comprehensive study of tumors of the glomus jugulare. Laryngoscope 1962; 72:765-87.
7. Marchand F. Beitraege zur kenntniss der normalen und pathologischen anatomie der glandula carotica an der nebennieren. Internat Beitr Wissensch Med Festschr Berlin: Vershow 1891; 1:535-81.
8. Fletcher WE, Arnold JH. Carotid body tumor: review of the literature and report of an unusual case. Am J Surg 1954; 87:617-23.
9. Rosenwasser H. Carotid body tumor of the middle ear and mastoid. Arch Otolaryngol 1945; 41:64-7.
10. Chedid A, Jao W. Hereditary tumors of the carotid bodies and chronic obstructive pulmonary disease. Cancer 1974; 33:1635-41.
11. Sato T, Saito H, Yoshinaga K, Shibota Y, Susano N. Concurrence of carotid body tumor and pheochromocytoma. Cancer 1974; 34:1787-95.
12. Revak CS, Morris SM, Alexander GH. Pheochromocytoma and recurrent chemodectomas over a 25-year period. Radiology 1971; 100:53-4.
13. Bogdasarian RS, Lotz PR. Multiple simultaneous paragangliomas of the head and neck in association with multiple retroperitoneal pheochromocytomas. Otolaryngol Head Neck Surg 1979; 87:648-52.
14. Ruijs JHJ, Van Waes PFGM, de Haas G, Hockstra A, Mulder PH, Veldman JE. Screening of family for chemodectoma. Radiologica Clin 1978; 47:114-23.

≈

AMERICAN BOARD OF OTOLARYNGOLOGY
SPECIAL ANNOUNCEMENT

This is to announce that the written examination of the American Board of Otolaryngology will be given Sunday, September 27, 1981 at the Palmer House in Chicago, Illinois. Registration will be on Saturday, September 26, 1981 at 5:00 p.m. at the Palmer House. It is estimated that the examination will conclude at 6:00 p.m. on Sunday.

Deadline for application is May 1st. Please contact Walter P.Work, MD, Secretary-Treasurer, at the American Board of Otolaryngology, 220 Collingwood, Suite 130, Ann Arbor, MI 48103 for the new application forms.

This is the official announcement. Please disregard any previous announcements concerning this examination.

Ann Otol 90:1981

PAROTOLYMPHATIC BACKFLOW: A NEW SIGN OF MALIGNANCY

PETER M. SOM, MD JOEL M. A. SHUGAR, MD

NEW YORK, NEW YORK

The embryology and anatomy of the parotid lymphatics are reviewed. Instances where intraparotid adenopathy can be confused with a parotid tumor are cited. Added to the roentgen signs of parotid malignancy, a new finding, parotolymphatic backflow, is described for what we believe is the first time. Its pathogenesis is discussed.

In the clinical setting of a noninflammatory lesion, sialography is an aid to the clinician in evaluating the benign or malignant nature of a tumor.[1-3] The sialographic criteria for malignancy are abrupt ductal cutoff, lack of parenchymal filling and irregular pooling of the contrast material. We present a case in which a sialogram demonstrated parotolymphatic backflow. To our knowledge this is the first such case presented. We feel that this is an additional criterion of malignancy and probably correlates with a highly destructive tumor. The probable pathogenesis is discussed.

CASE REPORT

This 64-year-old male presented with a one year history of a right parotid mass and a progressive right seventh nerve paralysis. Physical examination revealed a 2.5 cm rock-hard nontender mass in the right parotid gland. In addition, there was a right ninth and tenth nerve paralysis.

A sialogram revealed a round mass in the superficial lobe which was characterized by the absence of ductal architecture and the lack of parenchymal filling. Areas of irregular pooling of contrast material were also seen within the mass. Posteriorly, there was some ductal displacement around the contours of the tumor. Thin duct-like structures were seen extending from the mass into the soft tissues of the neck. They did not appear as extravasation into the muscle planes of the neck, nor was subcapsular contrast seen in the parotid gland (Fig. 1A, B).

At surgery, a tumor of the superficial lobe was found without extension into the deep lobe or to the base of the skull. Histology revealed a highly anaplastic tumor. No explanation for the right ninth and tenth paralysis was found, however, metastases were suspected.

DISCUSSION

The parotid gland is unique among the salivary glands in its embryonic development.[4,5] Although the parotid anlage is the first to form, it is the submaxillary and sublingual glands that first become arranged into encapsulated organ structures. The parotid gland develops in a loose cellular arrangement which contains aggregates of lymphoid tissue. Since the capsule of the gland forms late in ontogeny, these developing lymph nodes become entrapped both within the substance of the gland as well as on the surface of the gland under the capsule.

In the adult, there are two separate layers of lymph nodes that lie in relationships to the parotid gland: a superficial group which is under the outer parotid fascia, and a deep group both in the substance of the gland as well as on its undersurface.[6,7] In all, there are approximately 20 nodes in the system.[8] The afferent vessels drain the root of the nose, cheeks, eyelids, frontotemporal scalp, external auditory canal and pinna as well as the posterior palate and nasal cavity. The efferent vessels drain into the superior deep cervical nodes.

Of particular interest in this report are the intraparotid lymph nodes. These nodes, imbedded within the substance of the gland can be rarely visualized on a sialogram. The adjacent parotid ducts are smoothly displaced around the node and the appearance is similar to that of a benign mixed tumor or a parotid cyst.

Conditions which cause lymph node enlargement will increase the chances of confusing an intraparotid node with a parotid tumor. This is particularly true in children where the high incidence of infections in the ear and nasal cavity frequently can cause intraparotid lymphadenopathy.[8] Acute infections cause enlarged nodes which are tender to palpation, whereas chronic infectious and reactive hyperplasias cause nontender adenopathy. Rarely an acute suppurative nodal necrosis will occur which may result in draining sinuses to the adjacent skin.[9] Alternately, a parotid gland abscess may secondarily necrose into an intraparotid node. This may be the only inflammatory condition in which the lymph node capsule is broken and there is free communication with the adjacent parotid tissues. The chronic granulomatous diseases evoke a peripheral fibrotic reaction which continuously acts as a barrier to the surrounding tissues. In these instances the clinical settings are characteristic and a sialogram in the presence of infection is contraindicated.

During sialography the contrast material is in-

From the Department of Radiology, and the Department of Otolaryngology, The Mount Sinai Hospital and The Mount Sinai School of Medicine of the City University of New York.

REPRINTS — Peter M. Som, MD, Department of Radiology, The Mount Sinai Hospital, One Gustave Levy Place, New York, NY 10029.

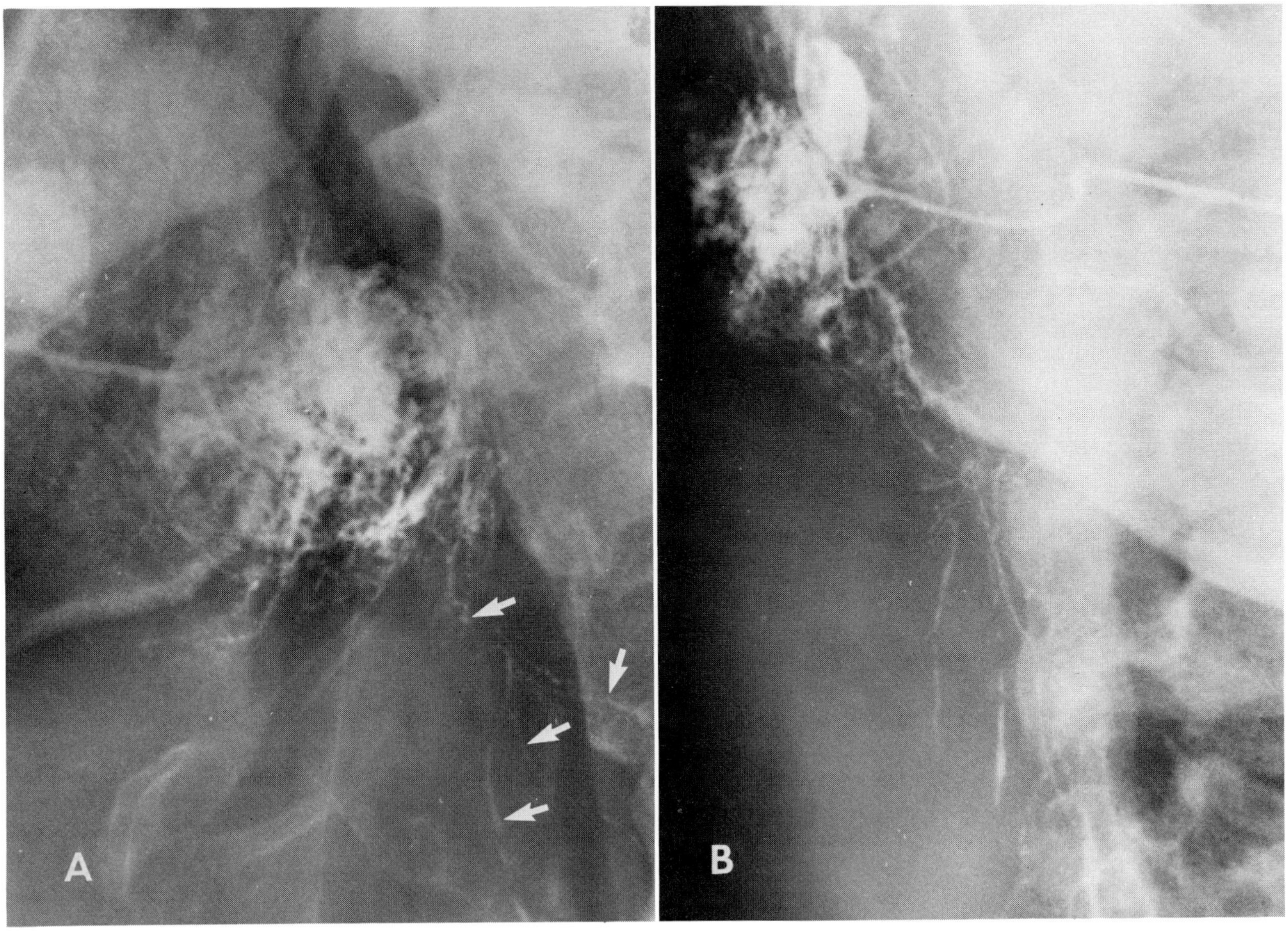

Fig. 1. A) Lateral sialogram reveals a circular parotid mass characterized by loss of ductal architecture and irregular pooling of the contrast material. Some ductal displacement is present at the margins of the lesion. Thin duct-like structures are seen extending from the mass into the soft tissues of the neck (arrows). B) AP sialogram reveals the lymphatic ducts leading from the parotid mass into the deep cervical lymph chains.

jected under hand pressure. This pressure is reflected back into the gland and the patient will complain of discomfort in the parotid region. This sensation is more intense the narrower the ductal caliber being filled. This reflects the increased pressure necessary to overcome the ductal resistance. When the injection pressure is held constant or released completely, the parotid gland adapts and usually within a few minutes the discomfort abates. If extravasation occurs, there is usually a sudden sharp pain experienced at the moment of extravasation followed by a rapid decrease in parotid discomfort as the pressure within the system vents via the extravasation. Radiographically, this is seen as irregular extraductal collections of contrast in the cheek, layering under the parotid capsule, or globular collections usually following tissue planes in the neck.

However, in the case of malignancy, the neoplasm may destroy sufficient tissue to allow a potential parotolymphatic communication to occur. This is possible with either an aggressive parotid malignancy which engulfs and destroys the lymph node or a nodal metastasis which breaks out to invade the parotid gland. In both cases, clinically there is a nontender hard mass and indications for a sialogram can be justified.

If an open pathway exists between the ductal system and the lymphatics, then the low resistance lymphatic ducts could fill via the parotid ducts. The roentgen appearance in our case not only is unlike reported instances of extravasation, but is the same as seen in examples of cervical lymphangiographic early filling films.[10] This belief is further attested to by the visualization of cervical lymph nodes with the sialographic contrast material (Ethiodol®) three weeks postoperatively. The initial scout films for the sialogram showed no abnormal nodal calcifications and these follow-up films (Fig. 2A, B) are essentially delayed lymphangiographic pictures.

Cervical lymphangiography has been of limited clinical usefulness.[10] It is not only technically difficult to perform, but more importantly it has proven unreliable in detecting malignant disease.[10,11] This probably reflects the extensive lymph node changes resulting from the numerous infections that drain to these nodes.

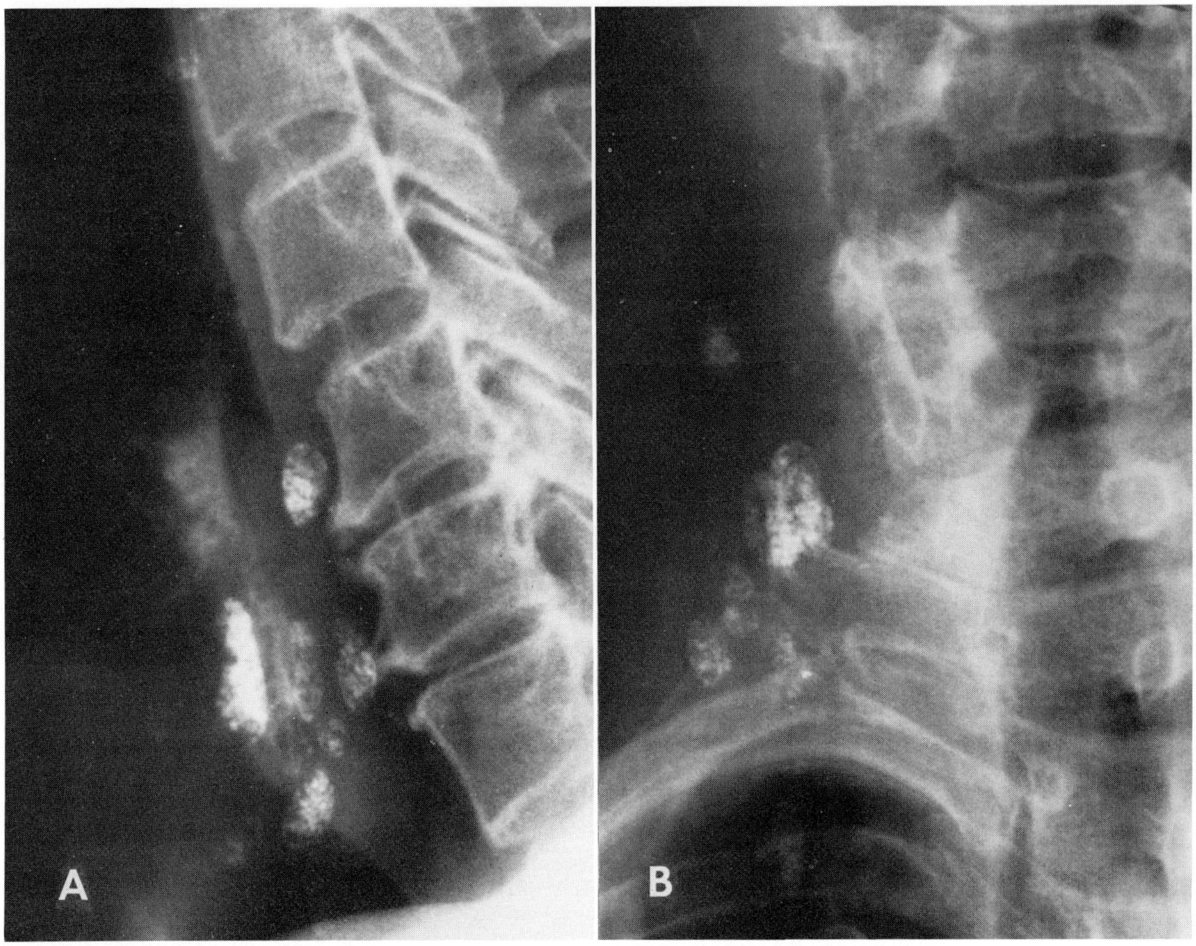

Fig. 2. A) Lateral soft tissue film taken three weeks postoperatively visualizes the cervical lymph nodes by the Ethiodol used in the sialogram. B) AP soft tissue film confirms that the lymph nodes visualized by means of the sialogram are in the deep cervical chain.

As further evidence of the integrity of the normal parotolymphatic barrier, even in cases where acinarization has occurred on a sialogram, delayed filming does not show cervical lymph node visualization. This parotolymphatic pathway can be created apparently only if the local tumor process is highly destructive. Most of the parotid neoplasms pathologically displace or encase but do not break into an intraparotid node. Thus the visualization of lymphatic channels on a parotid sialogram implies a highly aggressive neoplasm which has created the situation for parotolymphatic backflow.

REFERENCES

1. Calcaterra TC, Hemenway WG, Hansen GC, Hanafee WN. The value of sialography in the diagnosis of parotid tumors. Arch Otolaryngol 1977; 103:727-9.

2. White IL. Sialoangiography: x-ray visualization of major salivary glands. Laryngosocpe 1972; 82:2032-48.

3. Meine FJ, Woloshen HJ. Radiologic diagnosis of salivary gland tumors. Radiol Clin North Am 1970; 8:475-85.

4. Mason DK, Chisholm DM. Salivary glands in health and disease. Philadelphia: WB Saunders, 1975: 3-17.

5. Batsakis JG. Tumors of the head and neck. Clinical and pathological considerations. 2nd ed. Baltimore: Williams and Wilkins, 1979: 54-6.

6. Johns ME. The salivary glands: anatomy and embryology. Otolaryngol Clin North Am 1977; 10:261-71.

7. Gray H. Anatomy of the human body. Goss CM, ed. 27th ed. Philadelphia: Lea & Febiger, 1959.

8. Schuller DE, McCabe BF. Salivary gland neoplasms in children. Otolaryngol Clin North Am 1977; 10:399-412.

9. Robbins SL. Pathologic basis of disease. Philadelphia: WB Saunders, 1974.

10. Fisch U. Lymphography of the cervical lymphatic system. Philadelphia: WB Saunders, 1968.

11. Clouse ME, ed. Clinical lymphography. Baltimore: Williams and Wilkins, 1977: 55.

Ann Otol 90:1981

ABERRANT INTERNAL CAROTID ARTERY IN THE MIDDLE EAR

ROY S. GOODMAN, MD
GREAT NECK, NEW YORK

NOEL L. COHEN, MD
NEW YORK, NEW YORK

Aberrant internal carotid artery in the middle ear is a rare anomaly. Myringotomy in a patient with this anomaly caused violent hemorrhage, requiring immediate packing and eventual ligation of the artery. The anomaly may represent the artery bulging through a dehiscent bony canal, or it may be due to traction on the developing carotid by a persistent stapedial artery. Various middle ear symptoms have been reported in earlier cases. Diagnosis is by angiography, and therapy is surgical.

The course of the internal carotid artery normally passes close to the mesotympanum, and on rare occasions the artery may present in the middle ear as a normal vessel of aberrant course or as an aneurysm. The first of these anomalies was described in the German literature in 1899[1] and in 1903,[2] but then none were reported again until the 1960s.

CASE HISTORY

Seven weeks prior to admission, a 24-year-old female developed acute tonsillitis with pain, dysphagia, and painful cervical adenopathy. At that time she also complained of fullness in her right ear. She was seen by a local otolaryngologist who treated her with Keflex®. Four weeks later she again developed tonsillitis, again with fullness in the right ear and this time with a vague feeling of dysequilibrium but not vertigo, tinnitus, or hearing loss. The otolaryngologist noted what appeared to be a blood clot behind the right eardrum and treated her with decongestants, an antibiotic, and self-insufflation. Her past medical history was otherwise unremarkable.

The dysequilibrium and the apparent blood clot persisted, and on the evening of admission a myringotomy was performed in the doctor's office under local anesthesia. There was an immediate gush of bright red blood, and bleeding could be controlled only by packing the ear very firmly and applying a tight mastoid dressing.

On arrival at University Hospital, physical examination was normal except for the presence of the mastoid dressing and Weber test lateralizing to the right. There was no bleeding, no nystagmus, no facial nerve weakness, and no other neurologic deficits; hematocrit was 34.5.

Due to a failure of communications, the dressing was inadvertently removed the next day with immediate rapid bleeding. This was controlled by repacking the ear and reapplying the dressing, and the work-up proceeded.

Tomograms of the temporal bone showed the carotid canal to be posterior to its normal location, with dehiscence into the middle ear space (Figs. 1 and 2). Carotid angiography demonstrated the right internal carotid artery in the middle ear; there was a small pseudoaneurysm of the artery (Fig. 3 A, B).

The dressing was left in place for one week. Then the mastoid dressing was removed but the packing left undisturbed. After several hours blood began to

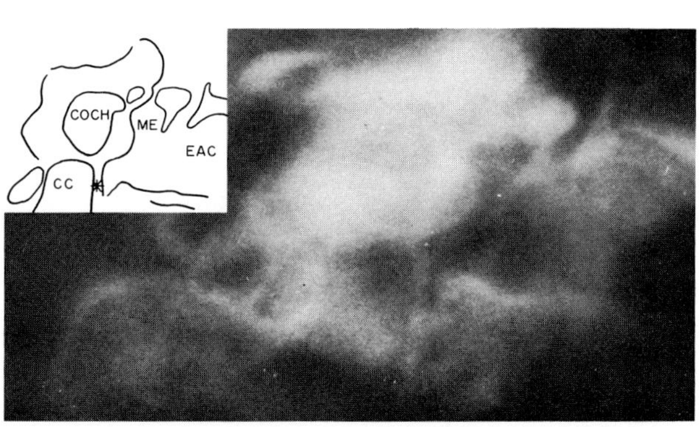

Fig. 1. Tomogram of left (normal) ear. Insert) Anterior location of carotid canal (CC) is evident from relation to cochlea (coch). Bony partition between carotid canal and middle ear (ME) is clearly visible (asterisk). EAC - External auditory canal.

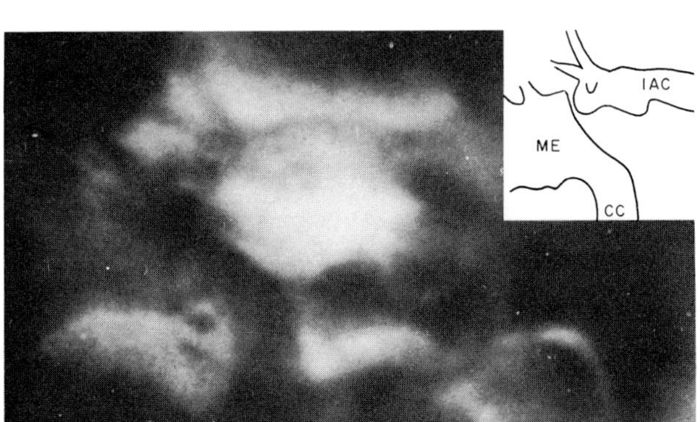

Fig. 2. Tomogram of right ear. Insert) Carotid canal (CC) is posterior to normal location as shown by relation to vestibule (V). There is no bony partition between carotid canal and middle ear (ME). IAC - Internal auditory canal.

From the New York University Medical Center, New York.

REPRINTS — Roy S. Goodman, MD, Barstow Medical Center, 29 Barstow Road, Great Neck, NY 11021.

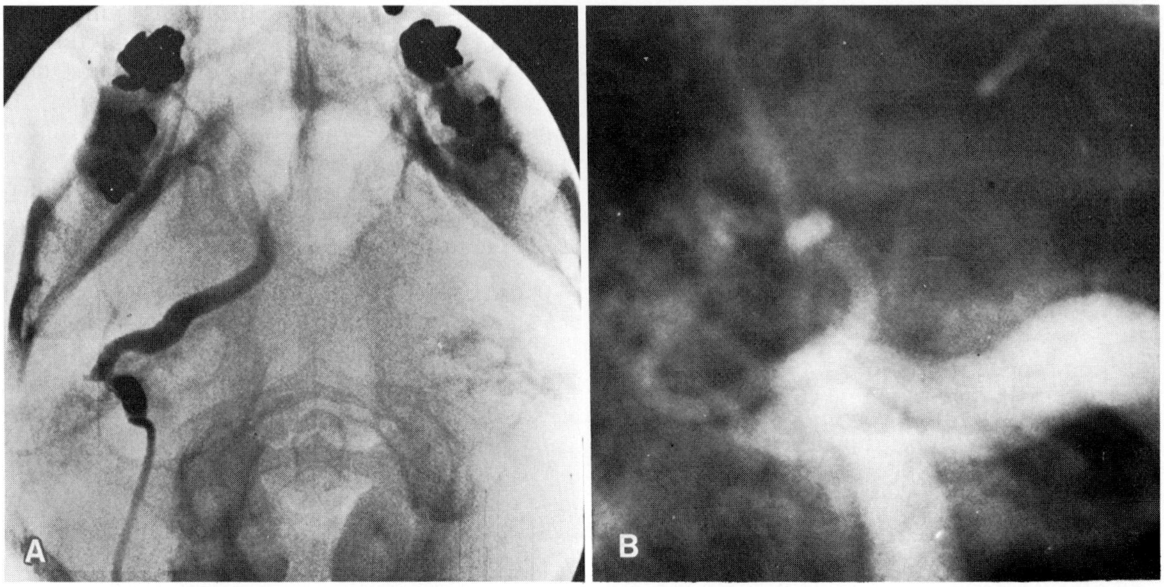

Fig. 3. A) Base view of angiogram. Lateral course of internal carotid artery is visible. Irregularity of most lateral portion of the artery represents a pseudoaneurysm. B) Anterior-posterior view of angiogram. Internal carotid artery can be seen to course lateral to the lateral aspect of the vestibule.

well up from the ear; this could be controlled only by packing more tightly and applying a tight mastoid dressing.

Repeat angiography was performed and the left carotid system studied while the right was compressed. This demonstrated excellent cerebral cross-circulation. The following day the patient was taken to the operating room. Under cervical plexus block, the internal carotid artery was isolated in the neck and secured with vessel loops. It was temporarily occluded with a bulldog clamp, and there were no ill effects. The ear packing was removed, and under local anesthesia the middle ear was entered through a postauricular incision, the plan being to patch or pack the vessel in the middle ear. The skin of the canal was found to be lacerated in places. No normal structures could be identified in the middle ear, which was filled with vessel, aneurysm, and clot. Muscle grafts from the sternocleidomastoid were packed firmly between the artery and the posterior wall of the middle ear, but this did not control bleeding; therefore the internal carotid artery was ligated in the neck with immediate control of bleeding. The ear canal was packed, all incisions closed, and a tight mastoid dressing applied. There was no further bleeding.

The packing was removed on the 11th postoperative day, and no bleeding ensued. The external canal and tympanic membrane were swollen, but this gradually resolved. When last seen, the patient's tympanic membrane was intact, with some opacification but no discoloration. There was faint pulsation noted in the middle ear and no tinnitus; hearing had returned to normal (Fig. 4).

DISCUSSION

It is rare for the internal carotid artery to appear in the middle ear as either an aneurysm or as a normal artery of aberrant course. A list of malformations and anatomical variants does not include these, in a series of 500 stapes operations or in a review of 169 articles.[3] Two articles on the complications of myringotomy, one of which reviews 838 cases, do not mention the possibility that the internal carotid artery might be lurking behind the eardrum.[4,5]

The causes of these anomalies are unknown. The internal carotid artery is separated from the middle ear by a plate of bone often less than 0.5 mm in thickness,[6] so that occasional dehiscences could well be expected; in fact one source gives the rate of dehiscence as one percent.[7] An aneurysm could bulge through such a dehiscence, or a normal artery could do so as it elongates with aging.[8] Conley and Hildyard[9] argue against these theories by pointing out the lack of published cases in which carotid

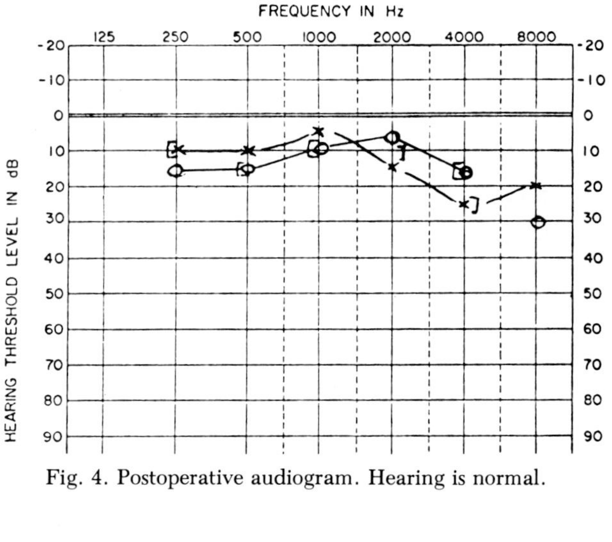

Fig. 4. Postoperative audiogram. Hearing is normal.

aneurysm or aberrant artery in the middle ear has resulted from skull fracture or chronic infection, but in fact there is one reported case in which an aneurysm apparently resulted from surgical trauma,[10] and two unpublished cases of aneurysm following skull fracture.* Steffen,[11] in a major review of vascular anomalies, suggests several possibilities involving the embryonic stapedial artery. This transitory artery could leave a permanent pathway in the bony wall of the carotid canal, or it may persist long enough to tether the developing carotid in an abnormal position. Persistence of a short segment of the stapedial artery might contribute to the formation of an aneurysm, since these most commonly arise at arterial bifurcations.

Nearly all reported cases have presented with middle ear symptoms. Most had hearing loss,[7,8,12] many had pain,[12] and other cases were noted to have tympanic membrane retraction with granulation tissue and cholesteatoma[6] and a bluish mass resembling middle ear fluid.[6] Though the normal carotid artery is white, the aberrant arteries were said to look blue or red.[6,7] In some but by no means all cases the mass appeared pulsatile.

As might be expected, myringotomy in a patient with an aberrant internal carotid artery may lead to immediate profuse bleeding. Only two such cases have been reported previously;[7,13] myringotomy had been planned in a third patient, but his physicians had just returned from a conference where the anomaly was reported![6] Fortunately, packing with firm pressure controls the bleeding and is the appropriate emergency treatment.

Differential diagnosis in these cases includes

*Ruben R. Personal communication.

aberrant jugular bulb and glomus tumor. Usually the jugular bulb lies posteriorly and the carotid anteriorly,[14] but when a major vascular structure is violated and the ear packed, diagnosis depends on special radiographic studies. The jugular bulb or glomus tumor can be seen on jugular venograms; carotid angiography will demonatrate these in the venous phase and show the blood supply of a glomus tumor (usually the ascending pharyngeal artery). Angiography displays the aberrant internal carotid artery to advantage. Lapayowker et al[8] describe the vestibular line, a vertical drawn through the lateral aspect of the vestibule on anterior-posterior views (Fig. 3 B). This approximates the medial limit of the middle ear, and the internal carotid artery normally courses medial to it. In the present case, tomography showed the carotid canal to be displaced laterally and posteriorly.

Treatment is not well established. In this case it was hoped that the pseudoaneurysm, most likely caused by injury at myringotomy, would be filled and sealed by thrombus. When this did not occur, surgery was performed with the precautionary step of gaining control of the internal carotid artery in the neck before removing the packing in the ear. Ligation was found to be necessary. The damaged artery was heavily packed with muscle to close the leak, as bleeding from retrograde blood flow might have been a threat without this step. Ruggles and Reed[12] were able to reposition an aberrant artery, and Ruben* repaired an aneurysm while leaving the artery intact. (Access for this was at the expense of surrounding normal structures.) In this case such procedures were unnecessary due to excellent collateral circulation.

*Ruben R. Personal communication.

REFERENCES

1. Gruber, Tollak. Osterreichesche Otologische Gesellshaft. Monatsschr Ohrenheilk 1899; 33:248-57.

2. Hansen E. Ein Fall Von Verlauf der Carotis Interna Durch die Paukenhohle. Munchen Med Wochenschr 1903; 50:949.

3. Hough JVD. Malformations and anatomical variations seen in the middle ear during the operation for mobilization of the stapes. Laryngoscope 1958; 68:1337-79.

4. Hughes LA, Warder FR, Hudson WR. Complications of tympanostomy tubes. Arch Otolaryngol 1974; 100:151-4.

5. Pratt LL, Murray J. The placement of middle ear ventilating tubes: some indications and complications. Laryngoscope 1973; 83:1022-6.

6. Glasgold AI, Horrigan W. The internal carotid artery presenting as a middle ear tumor. Laryngoscope 82:2217-21.

7. Goldman NC, Singleton GT, Holly EH. Aberrant internal carotid artery. Arch Otolaryngol 1971; 94:269-73.

8. Lapayowker MS, Liebman EP, Ronis ML, Safer JN. Presentation of the internal carotid artery as a tumor of the middle ear. Radiology 98:293-7.

9. Conley J, Hildyard V. Aneurysm of the internal carotid artery presenting in the middle ear. Arch Otolaryngol 1969; 90:61-4.

10. Barrett JH, Lawrence VL. Aneurysm of the internal carotid artery as a complication of mastoidectomy. Arch Otolaryngol 1960; 72:366-8.

11. Steffen TN. Vascular anomalies of the middle ear. Laryngoscope 1968; 78:171-97.

12. Ruggles RL, Reed RC. Treatment of aberrant carotid arteries in the middle ear. Laryngoscope 1972; 82:1199-205.

13. Stallings JO, McCabe BF. Congenital middle ear aneurysm of internal carotid. Arch Otolaryngol 1969; 90:65-9.

14. West JM, Bandy BC, Jafela BW. Aberrant jugular bulb in the middle ear cavity. Arch Otolaryngol 1974; 100:370-2.

Ann Otol 90:1981

USE OF THE CO_2 LASER IN OTOLOGY

DAVID J. WILLIAMS, MB, FRACS
ADELAIDE, SOUTH AUSTRALIA

IVAN M. HUNTER-DUVAR, PhD
TORONTO, ONTARIO, CANADA

DAVID P. MITCHELL, MD
TORONTO, ONTARIO, CANADA

There are conflicting reports of the effect on the inner ear of the use of a carbon dioxide (CO_2) laser. In four cats, we made middle ear lesions with a CO_2 laser. Subsequent evaluation by inverted-phase and scanning electron microscopy revealed no inner ear pathology attributable to the CO_2 laser. Apparently, appropriate use of the CO_2 laser does not harm the inner ear.

The CO_2 laser produces an intense, focused, coherent, highly collimated, highly monochromatic beam of infrared radiation which can destroy biological tissue. The infra-red waves heat materials which absorb it but do not ionize the molecules of these substances. The radiation (10.6 μ wavelength) is absorbed within 30 μ by water. However, bone has a high level of thermal conductivity; thus there is serious risk of vitrification and devascularization of regions adjacent to the target site.

The CO_2 laser has an important role in surgery of the aerodigestive tract, but is still experimental in otologic surgery. In early experiments the laser was able to destroy vascular stria or sensory epithelium of the cochlea by transmitting energy through the otic capsule without perforating it.[1] More recent studies give conflicting results.[2-5] Therefore, we deliberately produced laser lesions in the middle ear of cats and determined the degree of middle and inner ear damage by evaluation with light and scanning electron microscopy.

METHODS

From four adult cats we removed the pinna and the tortuous portion of the external canal, permitting an unobstructed view of the middle ear through the tympanic membrane. Each cat was anesthetized with ketamine (Ketalar®) and if necessary, the cat's tympanic membrane was reflected to gain access to the middle ear. In each cat one middle ear was irradiated with a CO_2 laser system for microsurgery (Cavitron model A0300) with a stereoscope microscope and micromanipulator (Zeiss OPMI 1). The exposure was at 8 W for 50 msec. The cat's other ear acted as a control. The surgical procedures were posterior myringotomy (required two applications in cat 1), and posterior myringotomy after instillation of 1.5 ml saline into the middle ear (two applications in cat 2). In cat 3, the subiculum near the round window was irradiated twice and in cat 4 the promontory five times.

Postoperatively, the cats were maintained for two to three months and middle ears were inspected routinely. Then the cats were sacrificed and both cochleas removed and processed for evaluation by inverted-phase and scanning electron microscopy (SEM).[6,7] The evaluations were made by one author (I.H-D) who had no knowledge of the experimental treatment.

FINDINGS

Gross examination revealed visible burns of the medial wall and promontory of the middle ear immediately after the procedures in cats 1, 3 and 4. Fluid in the middle ear cavity apparently prevented any microscopically visible promontory burn in cat 2.

There were no lesions in the control ears. In the "treated" ears all tympanic membrane lesions were healed within three weeks. In cat 1 the crus of the stapes was still charred (Fig. 1) but the cochlea was normal throughout (Fig. 2). In cat 2 the organ of Corti was normal at light microscopy. Some disturbance was noted in the cuticular plates of the pillar

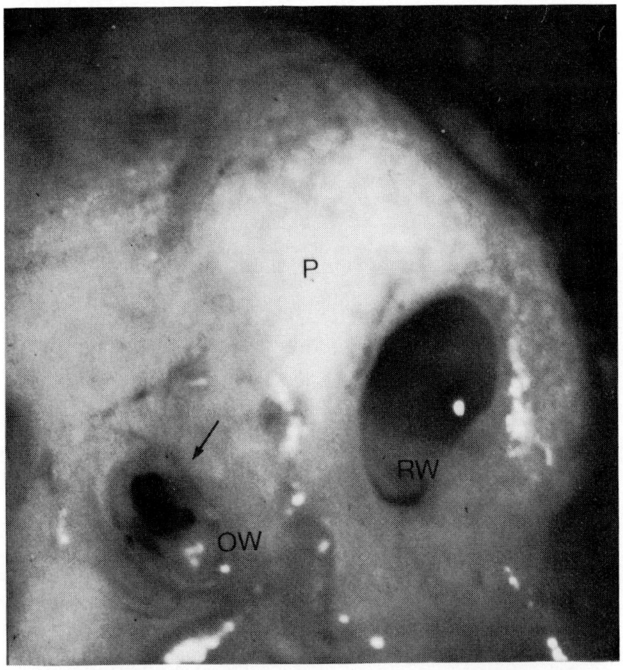

Fig. 1. (Cat 1) Charred anterior crus of the stapes. OW - Oval window with posterior crus of stapes and charred anterior half of stapes footplate (arrow). RW - Round window; P - Promontory.

———

From the Department of Otolaryngology, The Hospital for Sick Children, Toronto, Ontario, Canada.
REPRINTS — D. J. Williams, MB, FRACS, 341 Glynburn Rd., Kensington Park 5066, South Australia.

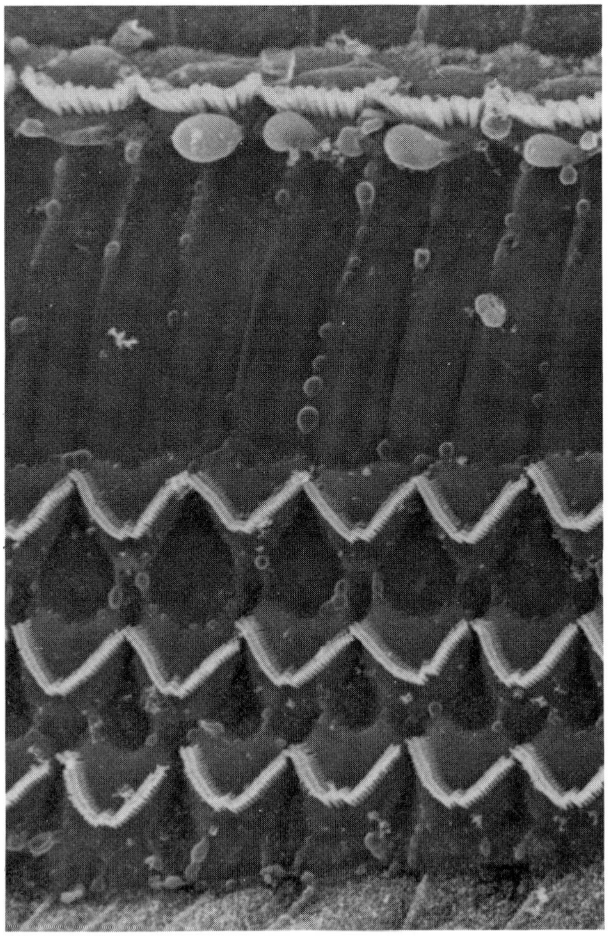

Fig. 2. (Cat 1) Scanning electron micrograph of the sensory cells of the basal turn beneath the promontory. There is no abnormality and this is typical of the hair cell condition in all irradiated ears. The bubbles are fixation artifacts.

cells in the basal areas, a shrinkage artifact resulting from the secondary osseous spiral lamina in this area. In cat 3 all turns were inspected with the light microscope and were judged normal. In cat 4 the stapes was fixed, the cochlea had a full population of inner and outer hair cells and there was a large number of giant cilia on the outer hair cells of the upper apical turn.

DISCUSSION

In experimental middle ear surgery on squirrel monkeys which involved myringotomy and ossicular surgery as well as deliberate attempts to damage the cochlea, Wilpizeski noted no loss of sensorineural function at any postoperative interval as measured by bone conduction.[2] More recently, Lima and Wilpizeski[3] obtained a similar result in experimental laser tympanic neurectomy. Goode[4] recently reported a series of laser myringotomies, including data on human subjects who apparently suffered no postoperative loss in bone conduction thresholds.

In contrast, Lyons et al[5] reported that even the lowest available intensities and duration (0.4 W, 50 msec) resulted in damage to the inner ear of guinea pigs. Stahle et al,[1] using an argon laser, found that lack of a visible lesion of the optic capsule at the time of irradiation did not preclude a lesion of the organ of Corti.

We attempted no specific surgical procedures, but deliberately exposed the cochlea to varying doses of irradiation at higher output than the 5 W Wilpizeski[2] suggested for crurotomy. We produced obvious immediate surface lesions in three of the four animals; the fourth (cat 2) was apparently protected by the presence of middle ear fluids. One stapes was charred in one procedure but there was no evidence of cochlear damage. These results are totally contradictory to those of Lyons et al.[5]

The CO_2 laser appears to be safe to the inner ear during middle ear surgery; however, further investigation and experimentation are necessary to determine its role in clinical otology.

ACKNOWLEDGMENTS — We are grateful to the Department of Surgical Research, Otologic Research Division, the Research Institute, and the Medical Publications Department at The Hospital for Sick Children, Toronto, and to Miss Debbie Baker for typing the manuscript.

REFERENCES

1. Stahle J, Högberg L, Engström B. The laser as a tool in inner-ear surgery. Acta Otolaryngol (Stockh) 1972; 73:27-37.

2. Wilpizeski CR. Otological applications of lasers. In: Wolbarsht ML, ed. Laser applications in medicine and biology, vol 3. New York: Plenum Press, 1977:289-328.

3. Lima JA, Wilpizeski CR. Effectiveness of the CO_2 laser in experimental tympanic neurectomy. Presented at the American Triological Society Meeting, Los Angeles, April 3-5, 1979.

4. Goode RL. Laser myringotomy. Presented at the American Triological Society Meeting in Los Angeles, April 3-5, 1979.

5. Lyons GD Jr, Webster DB, Mouney DF, Lousteau RJ. Anatomical consequences of CO_2 laser surgery of the guinea pig ear. Laryngoscope 1978; 88:1749-54.

6. Hunter-Duvar IM. Electron microscopic assessment of the cochlea: some techniques and results. Acta Otolaryngol (Stockh) 1978; Suppl 351.

7. Hunter-Duvar IM, Bredberg G. Effects of intense auditory stimulation: hearing losses and inner ear changes in the chinchilla. J Acoust Soc Am 1974; 55:795-801.

PNEUMOCOCCAL OTITIS MEDIA FOLLOWING MIDDLE EAR DEFLATION

WILLIAM L. MEYERHOFF, MD, PhD
G. SCOTT GIEBINK, MD DONALD SHEA, MD
MINNEAPOLIS, MINNESOTA

Temporal bone histology has been studied in chinchillas following middle ear deflation in the presence of nasopharyngeal colonization with *S pneumoniae*. All animals sacrificed within one hour following deflation had similar middle ear hsitology regardless of whether or not the animals had been colonized with *S pneumoniae*. All animals with negative nasopharyngeal culture for *S pneumoniae* sacrificed from 3-24 days following – 30 mm Hg negative middle ear pressure had negative middle ear cultures and normal morphology. During the same time period, however, nearly 60% of animals colonized with *S pneumoniae* developed acute otitis media with positive middle ear cultures for *S pneumoniae*. Histologic changes in the middle ear included the presence of effusion, leukocytes, granulation tissue, osteoneogenesis, mucosal metaplasia, and hemorrhage. Changes in the inner ear were much less frequent and included some leukocyte infiltration with hyperemia in the scala tympani and endolymphatic hydrops.

INTRODUCTION

Sudden changes in the relationship between middle ear pressure and atmospheric pressure may result in morphologic alterations of the middle ear mucosa, middle ear space, or inner ear with an associated decrease in hearing.[1] The hearing loss may be conductive or sensorineural depending on the site of the lesion. Generally, the middle ear equilibrates positive pressure better than negative pressure with fewer sequelae since positive middle ear pressure is equalized passively while equalization of negative middle ear pressure requires active eustachian tube opening.[2]

Clinically, negative middle ear pressure can be seen with eustachian tube dysfunction or with descent in air or water. During descent in air and water, the middle ear pressure is negative relative to the atmospheric pressure and the eustachian tube may fail to open in spite of contraction of the tensor veli palatini muscle. The eustachian tube is especially prone to failure if descent is rapid or if eustachian tube physiology is impaired. Resulting otologic injuries include middle ear effusion, tympanic membrane rupture, or perilymph fistula.[3]

Animal studies have been performed to help understand eustachian tube physiology as well as the pathophysiological processes associated with sudden changes in middle ear pressure.[4-7] The effect of nasopharyngeal bacterial or viral pathogens on these events, however, is not known. This relationship is quite important since the frequency of nasopharyngeal carriage of *Streptococcus pneumoniae* in children is 20-50% and since children are susceptible to negative middle pressure.[8,9] A study of the effects of negative middle ear pressure in animals with pneumococcal colonization of the nasopharynx was undertaken.

METHODS

Twenty-two healthy chinchillas, each weighing approximately 500 gm, were used for study. Encapsulated, recently mouse-passed type 7F *S pneumoniae* (type 51 by American nomenclature) were grown to early stationary-phase and were frozen in aliquots in a glycerol-buffered albumin suspension at –70 C. An aliquot of the frozen pneumococcal suspension was thawed and diluted in sterile saline to contain 2×10^5 pneumococci/ml immediately prior to each experiment. The chinchillas were anesthetized using 15 mg ketamine HCl administered intramuscularly and 0.5 ml of the diluted pneumococcal suspension was gently inoculated intranasally by passive inhalation.

Three days postinoculation, under ketamine anesthesia, gentle deflation of the chinchilla middle ear cavity was undertaken. Immediately prior to the application of negative pressure, 0.5 ml of sterile saline was gently introduced into the nares of the chinchilla for culture. The saline wash was collected for culture directly on 5% sheep blood agar containing 3 μg gentamicin/ml. The skin overlying the middle ear bulla was aseptically prepared with Betadine®. A 23 gauge needle, attached to a mercury manometer via firm plastic tubing, was inserted into the bulla, and negative pressure was applied to the middle ear at a rate of – 15 mm Hg/3 sec while visualizing the tympanic membrane with an otoscope. Continuous recordings of middle ear pressure revealed that tran-

TABLE 1. ANIMAL SUBGROUPS

Group No.	*No. Ears*	*Applied Pressure (mm Hg)*	*Interval to Sacrifice*	*Ears Cult. Pos.*
1	3	0	1 hr	0
2	3	–15	1 hr	0
3	3	–30	1 hr	0
4	3	–50	1 hr	0
5	7	–30	3 days	4/7
6	6	–30	7 days	3/6
7	9	–30	14 days	4/9
8	10	–30	28 days	2/10

Cult. Pos. - Culture positive.

From the Departments of Otolaryngology and Pediatrics, University of Minnesota Hospitals, and the Department of Otolaryngology, Hennepin County Medical Center, Minneapolis. This work has been supported in part by NIH Grant No. NS14538.

REPRINTS — William L. Meyerhoff, MD, Department of Otolaryngology, University of Minnesota, Box 396 Mayo Memorial Bldg., 420 Delaware St. SE, Minneapolis, MN 55455.

TABLE 2. MIDDLE EAR SPACE PATHOLOGY

Group No.	Ears with Effusion	Middle Ear Space: Ears with Leukocytes PMN	Mono	Ears with Granulation Tissue	Ears with Osteoneo-genesis	Ears with Hemorrhage
1	0	0	0	0	0	0
2	0	0	0	0	0	1/3
3	0	0	0	0	0	0
4	0	0	0	0	0	3/3
5	4/7	0	4/7	0	0	3/7
6	3/6	0	3/6	1/16	0	0
7	6/9	2/9	5/9	4/9	3/9	5/9
8	2/0	2/10	4/10	4/10	4/10	0

PMN - Polymorphonuclear.
Mono - Mononuclear.

sient failure of eustachian tube opening persisted for at least 15 minutes following the nasal rinse. Moderate retraction of the membrane confirmed application of negative pressure. Pressure was maintained for five minutes with continuous manometric recording before removing the needle.

The tympanic membranes of anesthetized animals were examined at regular intervals following middle ear deflation. Evidence of otitis media defined as visualization of middle ear effusion was sought. Samples of middle ear effusion were obtained by perforating the tympanic membrane with a sterile capillary glass tube (0.7 mm diameter) on days 2, 3, 7, 14 and 28. After the effusion rose within the tubing by capillary action, it was inoculated on sheep blood agar for culture. Tympanic membrane perforations healed within 48 hours.

Animals were randomized for sacrifice at one hour and on days 3, 7, 14 and 28 after middle ear deflation. The temporal bones were harvested, fixed in 10% formalin, followed by 5% trichloracetic acid and dehydrated in a graded series of alcohol. Specimens were embedded in celloidin and sectioned at a thickness of 20 μ; every tenth section was stained with hematoxylin and eosin for histologic study. The ears from 11 control animals not inoculated with *S pneumoniae* were subjected to the same manipulation, pressure changes, and method of study.

RESULTS

From the total of 22 animals with positive nasopharyngeal cultures for *S pneumoniae* used in this experiment, all 44 ears were available for histologic study. The ears were divided into eight groups based on the amount of middle ear deflation and the interval between the deflation and sacrifice (Table 1). One hour following deflation none of the ears harvested had effusion or inner ear changes and none exhibited middle ear pathological changes until −50 mm Hg deflation was reached. With −50 mm Hg pressure, middle ear hyperemia, edema, and hemorrhage was an almost universal finding (Tables 2-4, Figs. 1 and 2). The control animals without nasopharyngeal *S pneumoniae* also were free from effusion and inner ear changes and demonstrated normal middle ear histology until middle ear deflation exceeded −30 mm Hg. At −50 mm Hg pressure control animals, like the animals colonized with pneumococci, consistently showed hyperemia, hemorrhage, and edema of the middle ear mucosa.

Forty-four percent of the ears from animals with positive nasopharyngeal cultures harvested between day 3 and day 28 demonstrated purulent middle ear effusion which yielded *S pneumoniae* on culture. Middle ear changes of granulation tissue, mucosal metaplasia (from flat squamous epithelium to tall ciliated pseudocolumnar epithelium with goblet cells), and osteoneogenesis were apparent by day 14 (Tables 2 and 3, Figs. 3 and 4). Labyrinthitis was observed in 11% of the 32 ears harvested between day 3 and day 28 and endolymphatic hydrops was observed in 34% (Table 4, Fig. 5). All ears demonstrating labyrinthitis and 64% of those ears with endolymphatic hydrops showed purulent otitis media.

Four of the seven ears studied three days following the application of −30 mm Hg pressure demonstrated purulent middle ear effusion and all four yielded *S pneumoniae* on culture. These four ears also demonstrated edema, hyperemia, and hemorrhage in the middle ear mucosa. All four of the ears

TABLE 3. MIDDLE EAR MUCOSA PATHOLOGY

Group No.	Middle Ear Mucosa: Ears with Hyperemia	Ears with Edema	Ears with Leukocytes PMN	Mono	Ears with Metaplasia	Ears with Hemorrhage
1	0	0	0	0	0	0
2	1/3	0	0	0	0	0
3	0	0	0	0	0	0
4	3/3	3/3	0	0	0	3/3
5	3/7	4/7	3/7	0	0	4/7
6	1/6	2/6	0	0	2/6	1/6
7	1/9	6/9	6/9	2/9	6/9	2/9
8	2/10	2/10	2/10	2/10	2/10	2/10

PMN - Polymorphonuclear.
Mono - Mononuclear.

TABLE 4. INNER EAR PATHOLOGY

Group No.	Ears with Ppt	Inner Ear Ears with Leukocytes PMN	Mono	Ears with Hyperemia	Ears with Hydrops
1	3/3	0	0	0	0
2	3/3	0	0	0	0
3	3/3	0	0	0	0
4	3/3	0	0	0	0
5	7/7	2/7	0	4/7	2/7
6	6/6	1/6	0	3/6	3/6
7	9/9	0	0	0	4/9
8	10/10	0	0	0	2/10

Ppt - Precipitate.

PMN - Polymorphonuclear.

Mono - Mononuclear.

with purulent otitis media had inner ear findings of hyperemia of the lining of the scala tympani while two showed purulent labyrinthitis and endolymphatic hydrops. No other middle ear or inner ear abnormalities were identified and the three noninfected ears were normal from all parameters studied (Tables 2-4).

Three of the six middle ears studied seven days following the application of −30 mm Hg pressure contained purulent effusion and three ears were culture positive for *S pneumoniae*. Two of these middle ears showed mucosal edema and one demonstrated hyperemia and hemorrhage in the middle ear mucosa. Two of the three middle ears with purulent effusion manifested mucosal metaplasia and granulation tissue (Tables 2 and 3). All three of the ears with purulent middle ear effusion demonstrated hyperemia of the scala tympani lining and endolymphatic hydrops. One of these latter ears had purulent labyrinthitis. No additional middle ear or inner ear abnormalities were noted and the three noninfected ears were normal for all parameters studied (Table 4).

Six of the nine ears studied 14 days following the application of −30 mm Hg pressure contained purulent middle ear effusion, five of which were culture positive for *S pneumoniae*. These six ears also demonstrated mucosal edema and metaplasia of the middle ear epithelium. Five of these latter ears demonstrated hemorrhage into the middle ear space, four had middle ear granulation tissue, three had osteoneogenesis, and one contained hyperemic mucosa (Tables 2 and 3). Endolymphatic hydrops occurred in four of the six ears with purulent middle ear effusion and was the only inner ear abnormality identified. The three noninfected ears were normal from all parameters studied (Table 4).

Two of the 10 ears studied 28 days following the application of −30 mm Hg had purulent middle ear effusion and both were culture positive for *S pneumoniae*. These ears also demonstrated hemorrhage and mucosal edema, hyperemia, and metaplasia. Middle ear granulation tissue and osteoneogenesis were present in both infected ears and in two ears that failed to demonstrate active infection (Tables 2 and 3). Endolymphatic hydrops was the only inner ear abnormality and was present in two

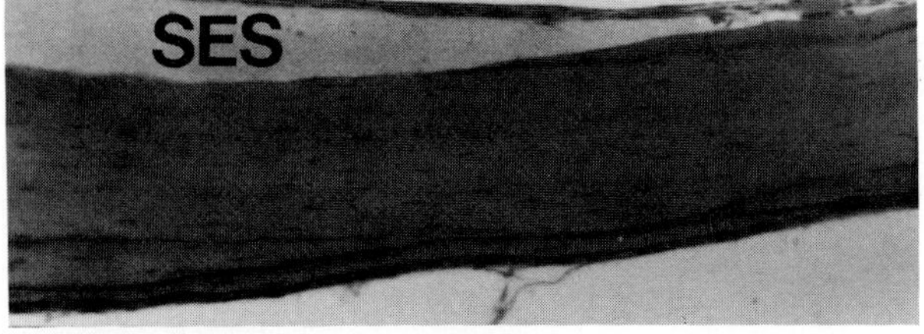

Fig. 1. Bulla of a chinchilla with positive nasopharyngeal culture for *S pneumoniae* that was subjected to −50 mm Hg middle ear deflation. Fluid can be identified in the subepithelial space (SES). Arrow - Middle ear mucosa. (x130)

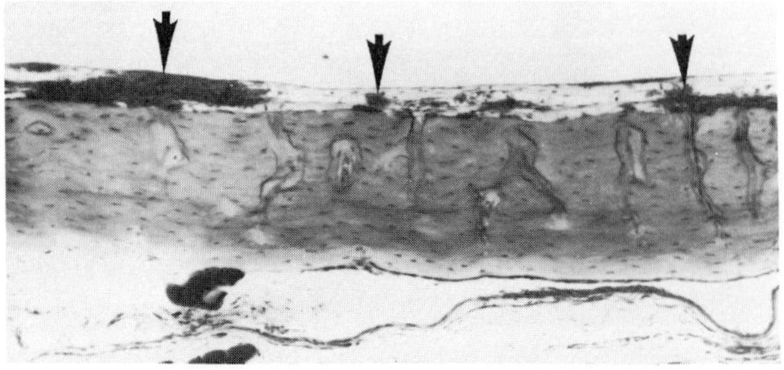

Fig. 2. Bulla from a chinchilla with positive nasopharyngeal culture for *S pneumoniae* that was subjected to −50 mm Hg middle ear deflation. Arrows -Hemorrhage in the subepithelial space. (x130)

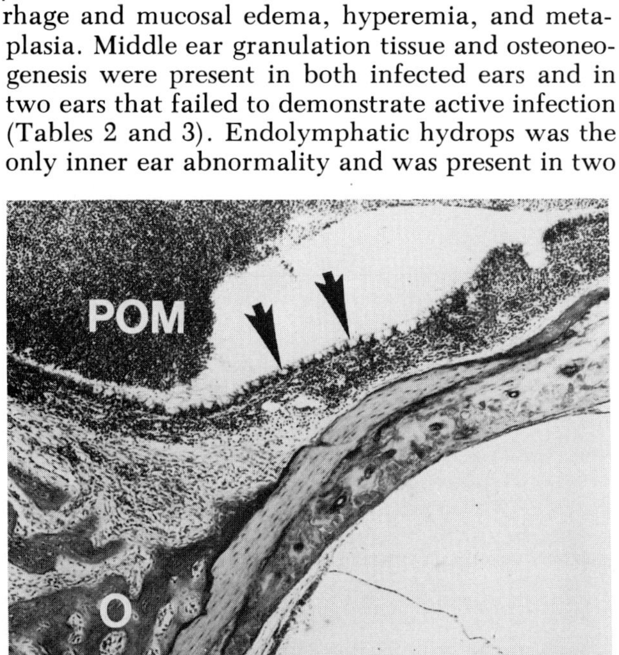

Fig. 3. Middle ear at the level of the cochlear apex in a chinchilla with positive nasopharyngeal culture for *S pneumoniae* that was subjected to −30 mm Hg middle ear deflation and allowed to survive for 14 days. Purulent exudate (POM) can be identified in the middle ear space as can osteoneogenesis (O). Arrows - Metaplasia of the middle ear mucosa. (x50)

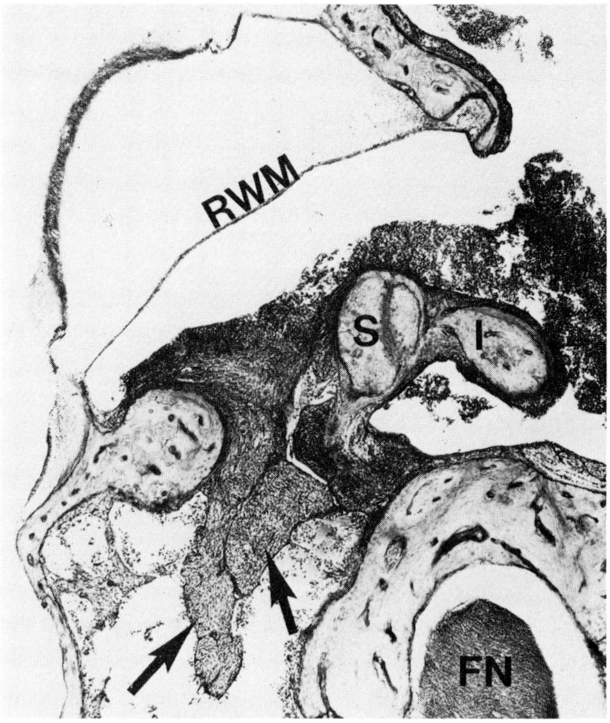

Fig. 4. Round window membrane (RWM) of the same animal in Figure 3. The stapes (S), incus (I), and facial nerve (FN) can be identified. Arrows - Granulation tissue in the middle ear cleft. (x35)

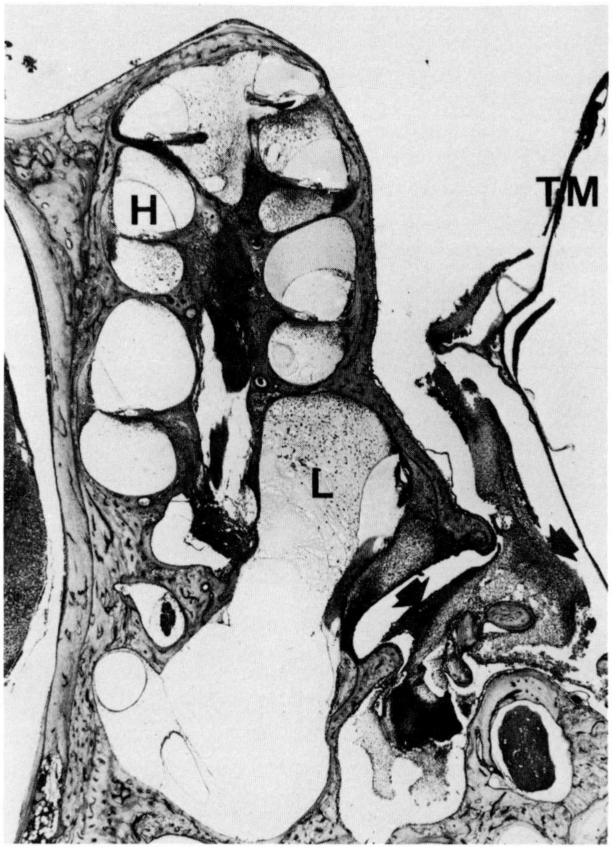

Fig. 5. Midmodiolar section from a chinchilla with positive nasopharyngeal culture for *S pneumoniae* that was subjected to –30 mm Hg middle ear deflation and allowed to live for seven days. The tympanic membrane (TM), endolymphatic hydrops (H), and labyrinthitis (L) can be identified. Arrows - Granulation tissue within the middle ear cleft. (x15)

ears both of which were without middle ear changes. The remaining four noninfected ears were normal for all parameters studied (Table 4).

DISCUSSION

Negative middle ear pressure is frequently observed early in acute otitis media with effusion with pressures as low as – 60 cm HOH (– 5 mm Hg).[10] Compromised middle ear ventilation and negative middle ear pressure may actually precede the onset of acute otitis media.[11] Accordingly, chinchillas were used to study the relationship between negative middle ear pressure and otitis media. Since a majority of episodes of acute otitis media in humans are caused by *S pneumoniae* and since an appreciable number of children harbor *S pneumoniae* in their upper respiratory tract, chinchillas were inoculated intranasally with *S pneumoniae* prior to the application of negative middle ear pressure.

Nearly 60% of chinchillas colonized with *S pneumoniae* developed pneumococcal otitis media within the first week following middle ear deflation while otitis media developed in less than 15% of colonized chinchillas that were not subjected to middle ear deflation.[12] The present investigation was performed to describe the histopathology of pneumococcal otitis media following middle ear deflation and to compare these results with the pathology of pneumococcal otitis media following direct inoculation of *S pneumoniae* into the middle ear cavity.[13]

In this investigation the negative middle ear pressure was applied slowly (– 15 mm Hg/3 sec) in a uniform manner. Otherwise unmolested, the chinchilla demonstrated excellent ability to equalize this pressure by active eustachian tube opening. This problem was fortuitously overcome by instilling 0.5 ml sterile saline into the chinchilla nares as a means for obtaining nasopharyngeal culture prior to the application of negative middle ear pressure as it rendered the chinchilla incapable of equalizing middle ear pressure for at least 15 minutes. The explanation for this alteration in eustachian tube physiology is currently under investigation.

During the acute phase of this experiment, the presence of nasopharyngeal *S pneumoniae* made little recognizable difference in the histologic effects of negative middle ear pressure. It was only in those animals allowed to survive for three days and beyond that the effect of colonizing the nasopharynx with *S pneumoniae* was observed. The histologic changes appeared, therefore, not to be an effect of the pressure change itself but rather the effect of infection made possible by the milieu created by the pressure change. By day three, 57% of the ears from animals with positive nasopharyngeal cultures demonstrated purulent otitis media with positive middle ear cultures for *S pneumoniae*. This finding persisted through day 14 and did not occur in animals not colonized with *S pneumoniae*. By day 28, 20% of the animals had persistent purulent otitis media. The histologic findings in animals sacrificed on days 3, 7, 14, and 28 were similar but less severe than following direct inoculation of *S pneumoniae* into the middle ear. With direct inoculation, all animals developed severe otitis media, and the majority demonstrated middle ear exudate, mucosal edema, submucosal hemorrhage, osteoneogenesis, mucosal metaplasia, and granulation tissue. Suppurative labyrinthitis, which occurred in 44% of animals in that study with associated endolymphatic hydrops, and inner ear osteoneogenesis and granulation tissue were less frequent findings in this study.

Others have studied the effect of negative middle ear pressure on middle ear morphology.[6,7] In guinea pigs, the application of only −5 mm Hg for five minutes following the intravenous injection of a colloid suspension of carbon particles led to serous otitis media and leakage of the carbon particles through the mucosal capillaries, venules, and small veins. Slight edema of the middle ear mucoperiosteum was also noted in those animals. Increasing negative pressure resulted in increased leakage, increased edema, and hemorrhage similar to the findings in our investigation.[6] Greater and more rapid alterations in middle ear pressure from −6000 mm H_2O to +6000 mm H_2O led to serous otitis media, hemorrhage, and tympanic membrane perforation with distortion of the round window membrane and air in the scala tympani. In general the severity of the changes was related to the magnitude of the pressure applied.[7]

Mechanical obstruction of the eustachian tube in guinea pigs, squirrel monkeys, cats, and chinchillas also leads to serous otitis media. Morphologic changes in the middle ear include widening of the subepithelial space and histologic and biochemical evidence for the passive transfer of this serous middle ear fluid from the subepithelial vessels. Small vessel leakage is first identified 12 hours following eustachian tube obstruction. By 24 hours, leakage increases and an acellular effusion develops. The mucoperiosteum in these animals becomes edematous and small mucosal hemorrhage is developed by two days, presumably due to the negative middle ear pressure. With prolonged eustachian tube obstruction, metaplasia of the middle ear mucosa occurs, the effusion becomes more mucoid, and a round cell infiltrate appears in the subepithelial space.[4,5,14]

In this current investigation the route of middle ear infection with *S pneumoniae* from the nasopharynx is not known. Gram stains were performed on selected temporal bone sections but due to previous celloidin embedding it was not possible to localize bacteria. The organisms might have reached the middle ear by direct ascent up the eustachian tube lumen or by infiltration through the subepithelial lymphatics. Regardless of the route of contamination, the occurrence of negative middle ear pressure during nasopharyngeal colonization with *S pneumoniae* resulted in purulent otitis media with all of the previously described histologic sequelae. Although cross species assumptions must be regarded with care, negative middle ear pressure in children whose nasopharynx is colonized with *S pneumoniae* may lead to acute otitis media.

REFERENCES

1. Miller J, Donaldson J. Primate model for studies of clinical problems of middle ear function. Ann Otol Rhinol Laryngol 1976; 85 Suppl 25:194-201.

2. Brookler KH. Otitic barotrauma. Laryngoscope 1973; 83:966-8.

3. Curtis AW, Clemis JD. Middle ear effusions. Part I — Pathophysiology. J Cont Educ ORL Allergy 1979; 41:13-25.

4. Hiraide F, Paparella MM. Vascular changes in middle ear effusions. Arch Otolaryngol 1972; 96:45-51.

5. Paparella MM, Juhn SK, Hiraide F, Kaneko Y. Cellular events involved in middle ear fluid production. Ann Otol Rhinol Laryngol 1970; 79:766-81.

6. Hiraide F, Eriksson H. The effects of the vacuum on vascular permeability of the middle ear. Acta Otolaryngol (Stockh) 1978; 85:10-6.

7. Axelsson A, Miller J, Silverman M. Anatomical effects of sudden middle ear pressure changes. Ann Otol Rhinol Laryngol 1979; 88:368-76.

8. Loda RA, Collier AM, Glezen WP, Strangert K, Clyde WA Jr, Denny FW. Occurrence of *Diplococcus pneumoniae* in the upper respiratory tract of children. J Pediatr 1975; 87:1087-93.

9. Perrielo VA, Ford RF, McLean WC, Schoeny ZG, Sande MA. Otitis media: a review. Va Med 1977; 104:319-28.

10. VanDishoeck HAE. Negative pressure and loss of hearing in tubal catarrh. Acta Otolaryngol (Stockh) 1941; 29:303-12.

11. Groothius JR, Sell SH, Wright PF, Thompson JM, Altenmeier WA III. Otitis media in infancy: tympanometric findings. Pediatrics 1979; 63:435-42.

12. Giebink GS, Berzins IK, Schiffman G, Quie PG. Experimental otitis media following nasal colonization with *Streptococcus pneumoniae*: prevention after vaccination with pneumococcal capsular polysaccharide. J Infect Dis (in press).

13. Meyerhoff WL, Shea D, Giebink GS. Experimental pneumococcal otitis media: a histopathological study. Otolaryngol Head Neck Surg (in press).

14. Paparella MM, Goycoolea MV, Meyerhoff WL. Inner ear pathology and otitis media. Ann Otol Rhinol Laryngol 1980; 89 Suppl 68:249-53.

IDIOPATHIC ENDOLYMPHATIC HYDROPS AND THE VESTIBULAR AQUEDUCT

SYED S. RIZVI, MD, FRCS

LEE ELIOTT SMITH, MD

BOSTON, MASSACHUSETTS

The vestibular aqueduct (VA) and endolymphatic sac were examined topographically in 29 human ears with idiopathic endolymphatic hydrops. When compared with 34 control ears, there was found to be a slight but statistically significant reduction in the width ($P < 0.005$) and length ($P < 0.05$) of the vestibular aqueduct. A small hypoplastic endolymphatic sac was found in three of the ears with hydrops but was also present in one control ear. It would appear that a marked reduction in sac size is not a consistent feature in ears with endolymphatic hydrops.

INTRODUCTION

The endolymphatic duct and/or sac have been increasingly implicated as the site of alterations leading to endolymphatic hydrops (Menière's disease). The evidence is somewhat conflicting and inconclusive. In an attempt to shed further light on this possible relationship we have studied the 29 temporal bones with idiopathic endolymphatic hydrops which are available in this laboratory utilizing the method of Egami et al.[1] This two-dimensional method of reconstruction provides information on the size and configuration of the vestibular aqueduct (VA) and the endolymphatic duct and sac.

METHODS

Included in this study were 29 ears with idiopathic endolymphatic hydrops and 34 control ears without endolymphatic hydrops. They were deemed idiopathic because except for the significant endolymphatic hydrops, no other pathology was found that could explain the membranous distension. The technique of graphic reconstruction of the VA was a modification of the one used by Egami et al.[1] Figure 1A represents the projection of a temporal bone slide through a Bausch and Lomb projector. The junction of pillars (A) is identified as is the sinus (F). The distance of AF is measured and plotted as A′F in Figure 1B which outlines the reconstructed cochlear duct and where A′ corresponds to A. This system marks the exact position of the VA in a serial order from the sinus to the foveate sulcus until an outline of the aqueduct is obtained as in Figure 1B. The length of the VA was measured along F′G, a line joining the midpoints of the aqueductal lumina. The anterior-posterior (A-P) diameter (HI) was measured across the largest lumen of the reconstructed aqueduct as was the lateral diameter (width) (JK).

RESULTS

The values for the various parameters measured are summarized in Table 1. The mean length of the VA in cases of endolymphatic hydrops was 5.65 mm with a standard deviation of ±1.85. This measurement

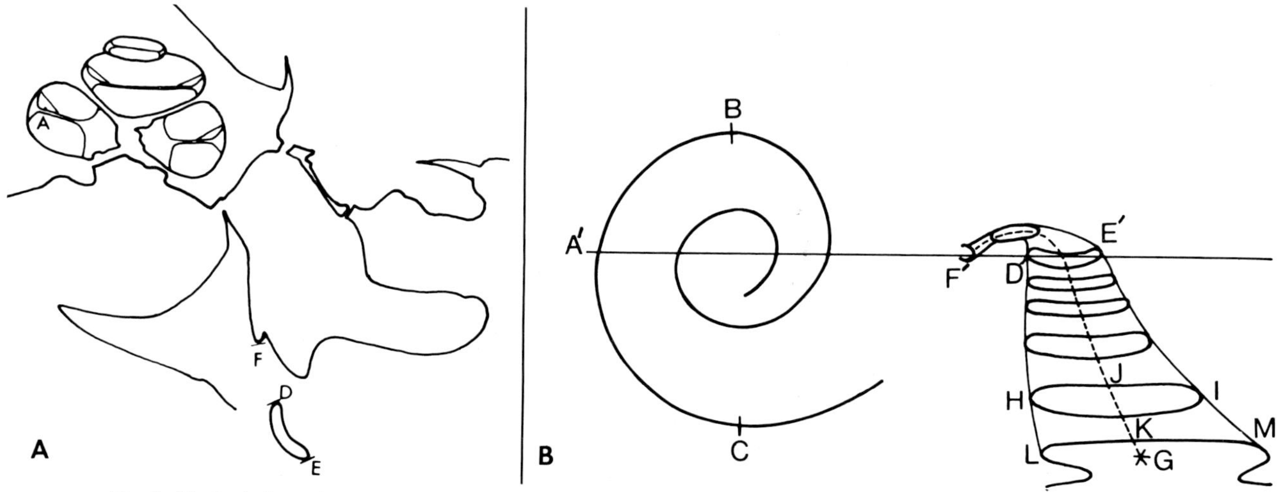

Fig. 1. Method of graphic reconstruction of the vestibular aqueduct (VA) and foveate fossa. A) Outline of inner ear from rear midmodiolar horizontal section. A - Junction of pillars; F - Sinus of VA; DE - VA. B) Graphic reconstruction of the vestibular aqueduct and foveate fossa after the method of Egami et al.[1] A,F,D,E in Fig. 1A correspond to A′, F′, D′, E′ in Fig. 1B. The broken line F′G is located in the middle of the vestibular aqueduct and foveate fossa.

From the Department of Otolaryngology, Harvard Medical School and Massachusetts Eye and Ear Infirmary, and the University Hospital, Boston, Massachusetts.

REPRINTS — Syed S. Rizvi, MD, Massachusetts Eye and Ear Infirmary, 243 Charles St., Boston, MA 02114.

TABLE 1. DIMENSIONS OF VESTIBULAR AQUEDUCTS

	No.	Length (mm)	A-P Diam (mm)	Lat Diam (mm)
Hydrops	29	5.65±1.85 SEM 0.35	3.23±2.04 SEM 0.39	0.42±0.19 SEM 0.03
Control	34	6.95±1.61 SEM 0.28	3.88±1.82 SEM 0.28	0.59±0.21 SEM 0.03

SEM - Standard error of the mean; A-P - Anterior-posterior; Lat - Lateral; Diam - Diameter.

was less than the mean value for the length in the control series which was 6.95±1.61 mm. Statistically, this difference was considered marginally significant ($P<0.05$). The lateral diameter of the VA in ears with endolymphatic hydrops showed a mean of 0.42 mm with a standard deviation of ±0.19. This was significantly different from the control group which indicated a mean of 0.59±0.21 ($P<0.005$). The mean A-P diameter of the VA in ears with endolymphatic hydrops was 3.23 mm with a standard deviation of ±2.04, while in the control group it was 3.88 mm with a standard deviation of ±1.82. This difference was not statistically significant. The overlapping distribution of the values for length and lateral diameter of the VA for ears with and without endolymphatic hydrops are shown in Figure 2. In the ears with endolymphatic hydrops 21 of 29 aqueducts showed a gradual flaring towards the foveate impression. Twenty-five of 34 control ears showed a similar flaring of the aqueduct distally. Of the 29 ears with endolymphatic hydrops 4 were extensively pneumatized, 6 were sclerotic and 19 were minimally pneumatized. Of the 24 control ears 2 were extensively pneumatized, 3 were sclerotic and 29 were minimally pneumatized.

The anatomical characteristics of the endolymphatic sacs are summarized in Table 2. Three of the endolymphatic sacs from ears with endolymphatic hydrops were markedly reduced in size and were tubular rather than racemose in configuration. All three had scant rugae. Their aqueducts were correspondingly reduced in size and were the smallest in the series. There was one diminutive sac in the control group. All the other sacs demonstrated a racemose pattern of branching with varying degrees of rugosity of the epithelium. The epithelial cells lining the sacs appeared identical in both groups.

TABLE 2. ANATOMICAL CHARACTERISTICS OF THE ENDOLYMPHATIC SACS

	No.	Racemose	Simple Tubular	Diminutive
Hydrops	29	26	3*	3*
Control	34	34	0	1

*Same sacs.

There was fibrous occlusion of the endolymphatic duct and sac in two ears with endolymphatic sac nearly filling the lumen which might have caused obstruction. The amount of perisaccular fibrous tissue appeared identical in the two groups.

DISCUSSION

The evidence for a causal relationship between the endolymphatic duct and sac on the one hand and endolymphatic hydrops on the other derives principally from three sources:

1. Nonvisualization of the vestibular aqueduct on radiologic studies of ears exhibiting Menière's disease.[2-5]

2. Observation of histological alterations in the endolymphatic ducts and sacs of ears with Menière's disease.[6-10]

3. Creation of endolymphatic hydrops in the experimental animals by ablating the endolymphatic sac.[11-16]

Several authors have measured the dimensions of the vestibular aqueduct in normal ears and ears with endolymphatic hydrops and these are compared in Table 3. Although the series of Egami et al[1] comprised a very small number of ears with endolymphatic hydrops, these sacs and aqueducts showed a dramatic reduction in size. Plantenga and Browning,[17] on the other hand, found no significant difference in the lengths of the VA in normal and diseased bones. The lengths of the aqueducts for normal bones in their series and ours is the same, but we note a slight reduction in their lengths in the ears with endolymphatic hydrops. This difference could be explained by the fact that Plantenga and Browning included cases of secondary hydrops whereas we confined our study to those ears show-

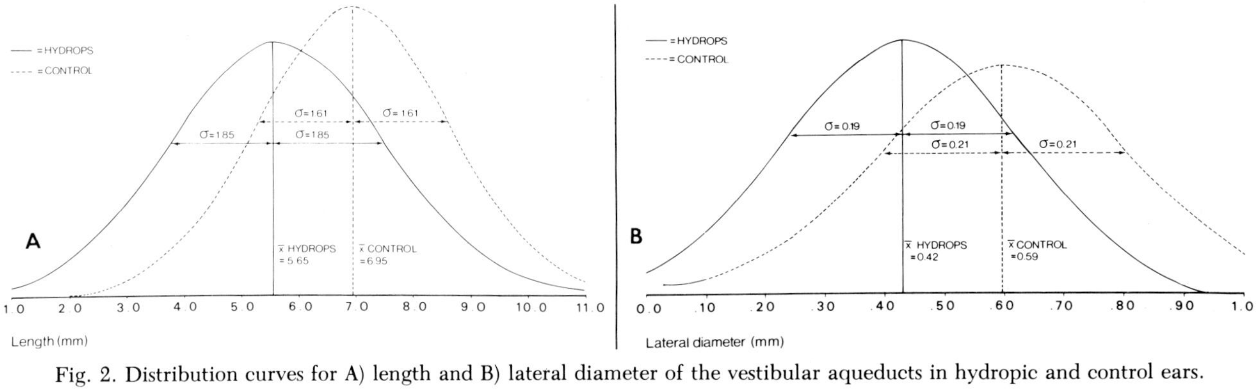

Fig. 2. Distribution curves for A) length and B) lateral diameter of the vestibular aqueducts in hydropic and control ears.

TABLE 3. DIMENSIONS OF THE VESTIBULAR AQUEDUCT

	Normal		*Hydrops*	
	Length	*Lat Diam*	*Length*	*Lat Diam*
Anson et al[18] (1965)	7.1	0.35	—	—
Ogura & Clemis (1976)[19]	7.3	0.2	—	—
Stahle & Wilbrand (1974)[4]	8.7	—	6.8	—
Egami et al (1978)[1]	—	—	2.3	0.45
Plantenga & Browning (1977)[17]	6.9	—	6.7	—
Rizvi & Smith (1980)	6.95	0.59	5.56	0.42

ing idiopathic endolymphatic hydrops. Also, they did not compare the widths of the aqueducts where we note a more significant reduction in size. Although these findings may be read as suggesting a smaller and therefore inadequate resorptive surface for endolymph, there is no compelling evidence to believe that a slightly smaller sac is necessarily inadequate and will inevitably lead to hydrops. It is possible that the failure of the resorptive mechanism is one of many causes for hydrops. The inability to find a consistent pathological basis for its origin lends credence to the concept that this disease may be multifactorial.

CONCLUSION

There is a wide variation in the individual dimensions of the VA in normal ears and ears with endolymphatic hydrops. However, there is a statistically significant reduction in the mean lengths and lateral diameters of ears showing endolymphatic hydrops. Although this is suggestive of a smaller and perhaps "inadequately functioning" sac, the arguments are not conclusive and lead us to believe that endolymphatic hydrops may be produced in more ways than a simple reduction in the resorptive surface of the sac.

ACKNOWLEDGMENT — We would like to express our gratitude to Dr. H. F. Schuknecht for his advice and guidance in this study. We also wish to thank Dr. N. Laird for her help in the statistical analysis of our data and Mrs. D. Arnold and Miss E. Safe for their help in the preparation of this manuscript.

REFERENCES

1. Egami T, Sando I, Black FW. Hypoplasia of the vestibular aqueduct and endolymphatic sac in endolymphatic hydrops. ORL 1978; 86:327-41.

2. Clemis JD, Valvassori GE. Recent radiographic and clinical observations on the vestibular aqueduct (a preliminary report). Otolaryngol Clin North Am Oct 1968; 339-46.

3. Valvassori GE. Tomographic findings in Meniere's disease. IX International Congress ORL Mexico City Excerpta Medica (International Congress Series) 1969; 189:50 (112).

4. Stahle J, Wilbrand H. The vestibular aqueduct in patients with Meniere's disease. Acta Otolaryngol (Stockh) 1974; 78:36-48.

5. Oigaard A, Thomsen J, Jensen J, Dorph S. The vestibular aqueduct in Meniere's disease. Acta Otolaryngol (Stockh) 1976; 82:279-81.

6. Hallpike LS, Cairns H. Observations on the pathology of Meniere's syndrome. J Laryngol Otol 1938; 53:625-54.

7. Altman F, Fowler EP Jr. Histological findings in Meniere's symptom complex. Ann Otol Rhinol Laryngol 1943; 52:52-80.

8. Shambaugh GE Jr, Clemis JD, Arenberg IK. Endolymphatic duct and sac in Meniere's disease. Arch Otolaryngol 1969; 89:816-25.

9. Arenberg IK, Marovitz WF, Shambaugh GE. The role of the endolymphatic sac in the pathogenesis of endolymphatic hydrops in man. Acta Otolaryngol (Stockh) 1970; 76 Suppl 75.

10. Saito H, Kitahara M, Yazawa Y, Matsumoto M. Histopathological findings in surgical specimens of endolymphatic sac in Meniere's disease. Acta Otolaryngol (Stockh) 1977; 83:465-9.

11. Portmann G. Recherches sur la physiologie du sac et du canal endolymphatic valeur fonctionelle de l'organ endolymphatic des selaciens. C R Soc Biol 1921; 85:1070

12. Kimura RS, Schuknecht HF. Membranous hydrops in the inner ear of the guinea pig after obliteration of the endolymphatic sac. Pract Otorhinolaryngol 1965; 27:343-54.

13. Kimura R. Experimental blockage of the endolymphatic duct and sac on the inner ear of the guinea pig: a study on endolymphatic hydrops. Ann Otol Rhinol Laryngol 1967; 76:664-87.

14. Schuknecht H, Northrop C, Igarashi M. Cochlear pathology after destruction of the endolymphatic sac in the cat. Acta Otolaryngol (Stockh) 1968; 65:479-87.

15. Beal D. Effect of endolymphatic sac ablation in the rabbit and cat. Acta Otolaryngol (Stockh) 1978; 66:333-46.

16. Kimura RS, Schuknecht HF, Ota CY, Jones DD. Experimental study of sacculotomy in endolymphatic hydrops. Arch Otolaryngol 1977; 217:123-37.

17. Plantenga KF, Browning GG. The vestibular aqueduct and endolymphatic sac and duct in endolymphatic hydrops. Arch Otolaryngol 1979; 105:546-52.

18. Anson BJ, Donaldson JA, Warpeha RL, Winch TR. The vestibular and cochlear aqueducts: their variational anatomy in the adult human ear. Laryngoscope 1965; 55:1203-23.

19. Ogura J, Clemis JD. A study of the topographic anatomy of the human vestibular aqueduct. Auris Nasus Larynx 1974; 1:19-31.

Ann Otol 90:1981

TEMPORAL BONE FINDINGS IN A PATIENT WITH MÖBIUS SYNDROME

HARUO SAITO, MD
OTSU, JAPAN

SEIJI KISHIMOTO, MD
KYOTO, JAPAN

MUTSUHIRO FURUTA, MD
KYOTO, JAPAN

Temporal bone findings in a case of Möbius syndrome are presented. The most striking pathological feature of the case is that the facial nerves ended in the horizontal segment in the temporal bones on both sides. This finding gives direct evidence that the site of nerve lesion in Möbius syndrome is in the peripheral nerve. Despite the disappearance of the facial nerve in the horizontal segment, a neural element reappeared in the vertical segment of the fallopian canal, and moreover, the chorda tympani was found to cross the tympanic cavity in the normal position. This finding suggests that fibers of the chorda tympani sometimes take an alternative pathway via Arnold's nerve.

The aim of this paper is to report some additional evidence of the site of neural lesion in Möbius syndrome and on "distal excess" of the facial nerve.

Möbius syndrome is a nonprogressive congenital anomaly complex, having as major characteristics bilateral facial paralysis and unilateral or bilateral loss of the abductors of the eye. The etiology of the neurological defect of the syndrome complex still remains obscure. Theories suggest central nervous system hypoplasia,[1-4] primary peripheral muscle defect with secondary nerve degeneration,[4] or lower motor neuron involvement.[5] None of the previous reports studied the facial nerve in its temporal bone course, except Pitner and others[6] and only in subserial sections.

From the anatomical point of view, the facial nerve still has some obscure points. The number of fibers in the facial nerve distal to the geniculate ganglion was reported as always greater than that in the proximal part of the nerve.[7-9] This has been called "distal excess."

We have studied the temporal bones from a baby with bilateral facial and abducent paralysis. The facial nerves in both temporal bones showed identical findings revealing the etiology of the facial palsy of Möbius syndrome to be of peripheral nerve origin; in addition nerve components other than facial joined the facial canal in the vertical segment.

CASE REPORT

An 83-day-old female was the product of a 37-gestational-week premature birth from a 25-year-old mother. The delivery was atraumatic, with birth weight 2,150 gm and height 44.5 cm. The mother had a trouble-free pregnancy.

At birth, holoprosencephaly, right microphthalmus, hypertelorism, double nose, and bilateral cleft lip and palate were noted. She was hospitalized for feeding difficulties. In her hospital course, convulsions and episodes of apnea related to congenital hydrocephalus necessitated repeated ventricular taps and finally permanent drainage by a silicone tube. *Pseudomonas* infection followed after the last procedure and she died of uncontrolled meningitis after 83 days of life. During her 81 days of hospitalization, she had no noticeable facial movements except around the mouth attributed to movements of the tongue. It was noted that she could gaze upwards but her eyes did not move laterally. She had lacrimal flow when crying and salivation from profuse drooping from the mouth. Her record showed that she responded to sound stimuli.

Due to the presence of such multiple anomalies, a chromosomal evaluation was performed which failed to show any pathological type.

The autopsy examination demonstrated the following abnormalities: severe encephalomeningitis, subarachnoidal hemorrhage, severe hydrocephalus, cleft palate, bilateral hare lip, absence of the ethmoidal plate, absence of the bulbus olfactorius, accessory spleen, interstitial pneumonia and pulmonary atelectasis.

HISTOPATHOLOGY OF TEMPORAL BONES

Both temporal bones were removed eight hours after death, fixed in 10% formaldehyde solution, decalcified with 5% trichloracetic acid and embedded in celloidin. Serial 20 μ thick sections were made and tracer sets of every 10th section were stained with hematoxylin and eosin.

RIGHT EAR

The middle ear was partially damaged by the saw in removal. The internal auditory canal was slightly wider than normal, but other structures were almost normal in configuration.

Cochlea. Although there were some postmorten changes, hair cells were present in the whole length of the organ of Corti. The cochlear spiral had normal configuration and was fully developed, having normal length of the basilar membrane (Fig. 1).

From the Department of Otolaryngology, Shiga University of Medical Science, Otsu, Japan; the Department of Otolaryngology, Kyoto University, Faculty of Medicine, Kyoto, Japan; and the Department of Pathology, Kyoto National Hospital, Kyoto, Japan.

REPRINTS — H. Saito, MD, Department of Otolaryngology, Shiga University of Medical Science, Otsu, Japan 520-21.

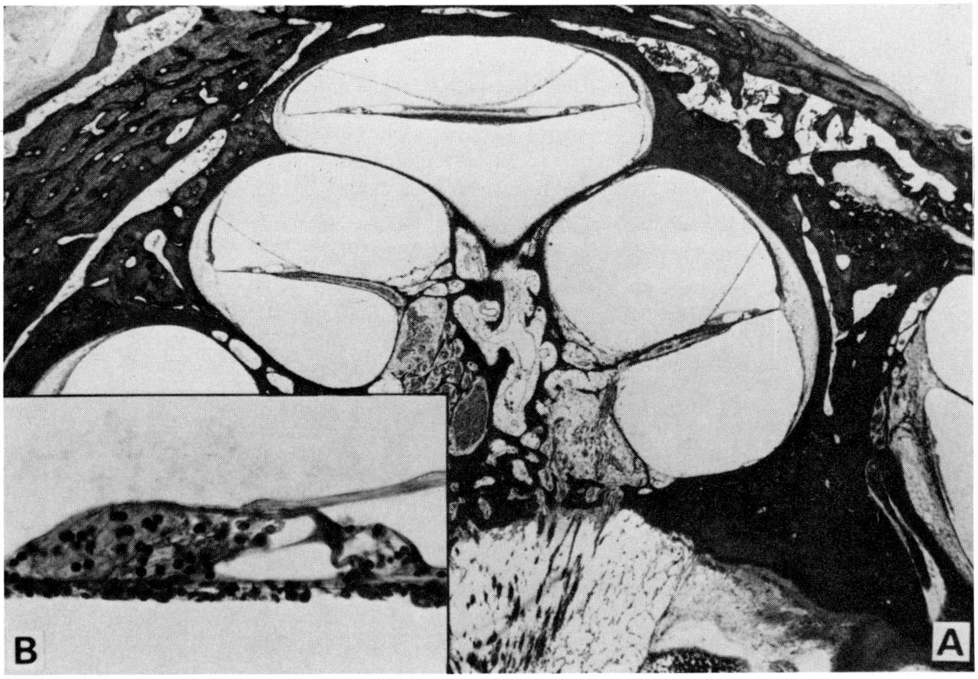

Fig. 1. A) The cochlea has normal configuration and is fully developed (x27.5). B) Fine inner ear structure such as hair cells is present in the whole length of the organ of Corti (x75).

The spiral ganglion population was slightly reduced in the basal turn. Although there was massive infiltration of the inflammatory cells around the cochlear nerve in the internal auditory canal, the nerve fibers remained unchanged.

Vestibule. The sensory epithelia on the saccular and utricular maculae and ampullar cristae were found to be normal.

Facial Nerve. The most dominant pathological feature of this specimen was the change in the facial nerve. The facial nerve appeared to be normal in size and in its course in the internal auditory canal. At the geniculate ganglion, it formed an obtuse angle. However, the ganglion cells, normal in population, were scattered towards the internal auditory canal (Fig. 2). At midsection within the horizontal segment, the nerve abruptly diminished

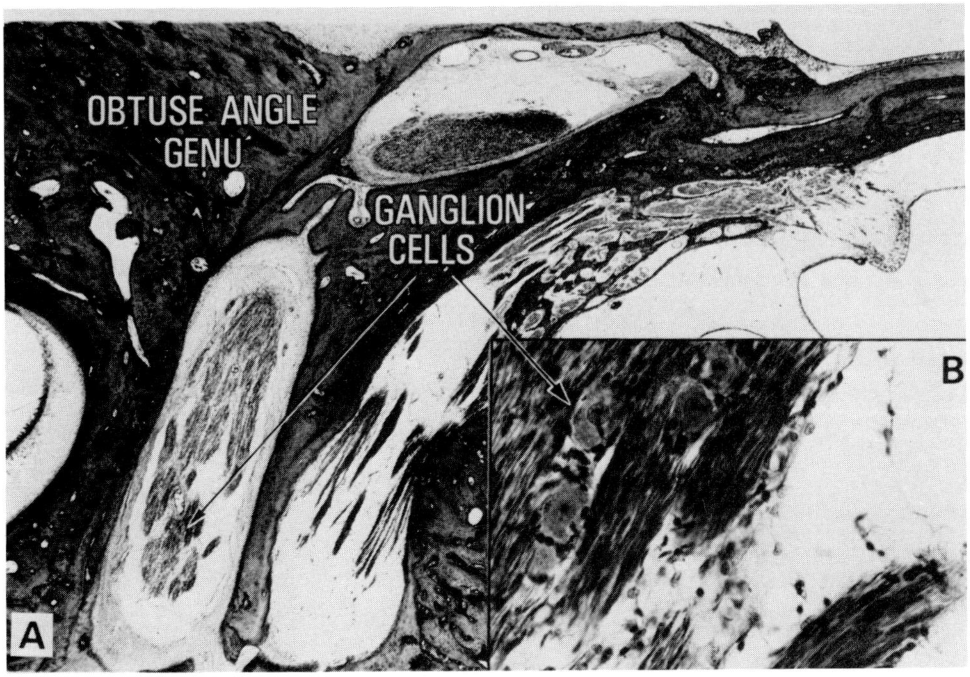

Fig. 2. A) The genu forms an obtuse angle. The ganglion cells are normal in population, somewhat scattered towards the internal auditory canal (x30). B) Higher magnification of the proximally located ganglion cells (x145).

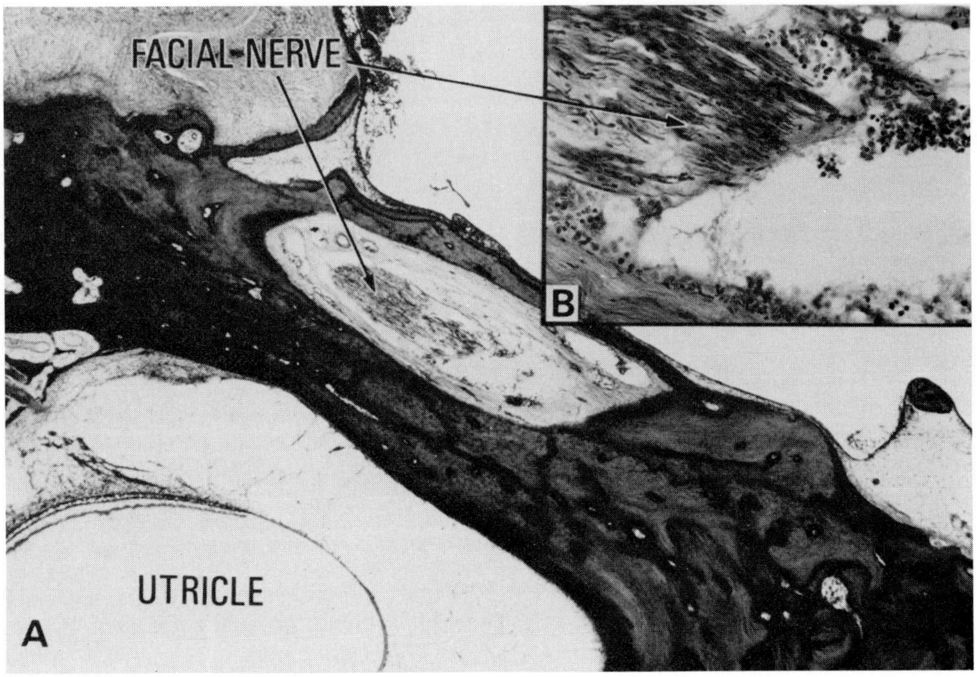

Fig. 3. A) At midway section within the horizontal segment, the facial nerve abruptly disminishes in size and disappears (x25). B) Loose connective tissue and sparse inflammatory cells are left within the epineural sheath (x75).

in size and disappeared, leaving loose connective tissue and sparse inflammatory cells within the epineural sheath (Fig. 3). The posterior half of the horizontal segment of the fallopian canal was normal in width, but there was a lack of neural elements, the canal being filled with loose connective tissue and sparse inflammatory cell infiltration. At the pyramidal segment, a small nerve bundle reappeared within the canal. This nerve bundle continuously increased in size within the vertical segment of the facial canal, but was considerably smaller than the normal facial nerve at this level. The stapedius muscle, situated in normal anatomical position near the facial nerve, appeared normal (Fig. 4). In spite of the interruption of the facial nerve in the horizontal segment, a chorda tympani of normal size was identifiable crossing the tympanic cavity. The junction between the small vertical segment and the chorda tympani could not be traced due to the limitation of the specimen (Fig. 5).

LEFT EAR

Pathological findings were similar to those in the right ear. The identical anomalous findings of the

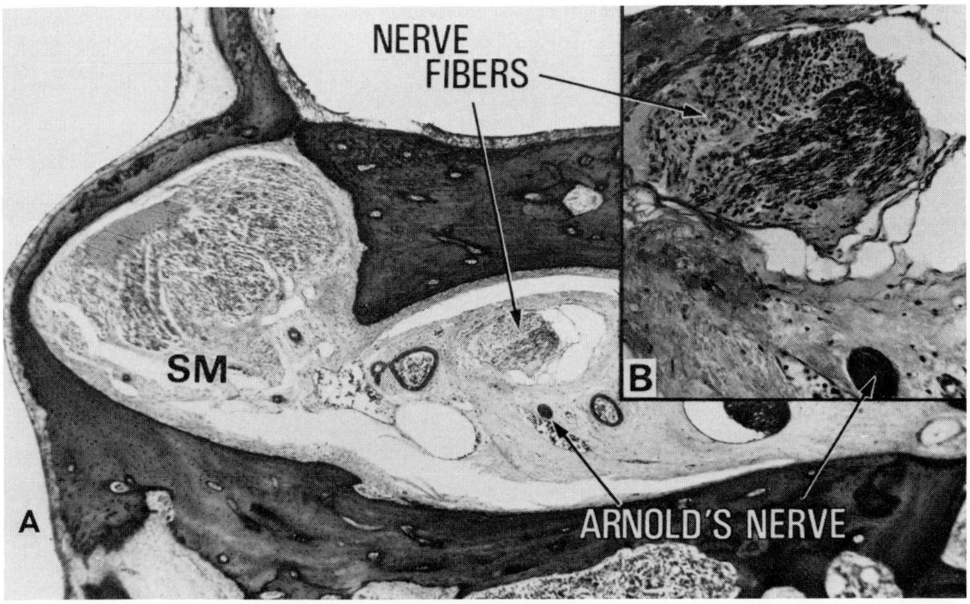

Fig. 4. At the pyramidal segment, a small nerve bundle reappears into the vacant canal. A) x22. B) x75.

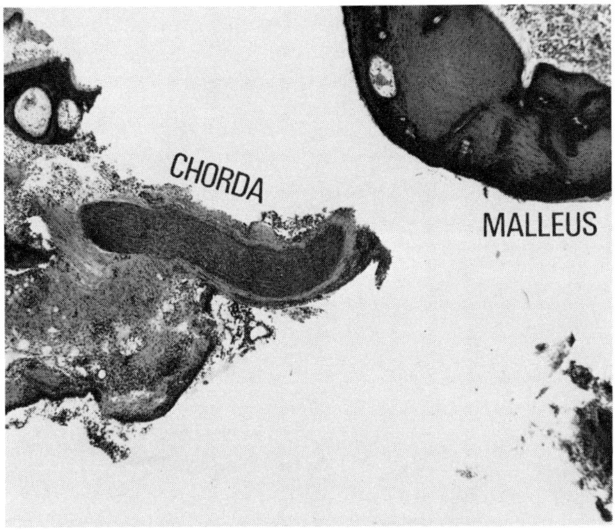

Fig. 5. In spite of the interruption of the facial nerve at the horizontal segment, a normal size chorda tympani is identifiable crossing the tympanic cavity. (x22)

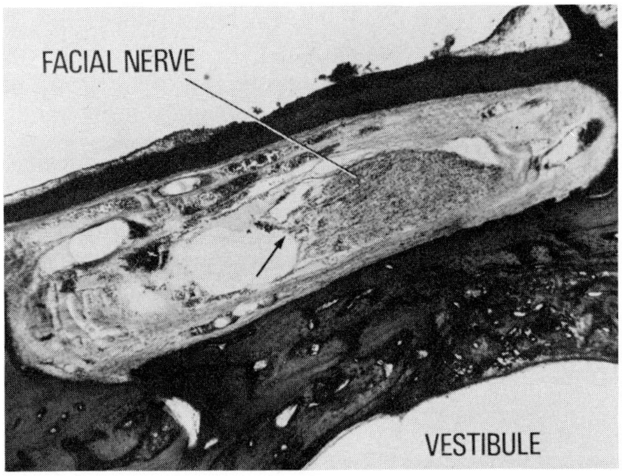

Fig. 6. The identical findings of the facial nerve on the opposite side. The facial nerve abruptly disappears at its horizontal segment (arrow). (x55)

facial nerve should be mentioned on this side as well.

Facial Nerve. An obtuse angle of approximately 120° was demonstrated at the geniculate ganglion. The great petrosal nerve was normal. In the horizontal segment immediately distal to the cochleariform process, the facial nerve disappeared exactly in the same manner as in the opposite side (Fig. 6). Still further distally, the facial canal was filled with epineural connective tissue and with vascular structures. No identifiable nerve bundle was in it. In the vertical segment, a small bundle of nerve fibers reappeared in the canal (Fig. 7). The chorda tympani on this side was not included in the specimen due to removal artifact.

DISCUSSION

The prominent finding of the temporal bones in this report was the disappearance of the facial nerves in their course in the horizontal segment of the fallopian canals.

Although there have been many reports on Möbius syndrome, the divergent views as to pathogenesis constitute an indirect challenge and therefore have led to confusion. Findings on the facial nerve in its temporal bone course have been reported on only one occasion, by Pitner and others.[6] They reported that examination of the subserial sections of the petrous portions of the temporal bones revealed no significant abnormalities. Autolytic and embalming artifacts had prevented a detailed evaluation of the fine structure of the facial nerves in the temporal bones.

In our temporal bones, the abnormal findings of the facial nerves cannot be attributed to postmortem and autolytic artifacts. The membranous labyrinth was fairly well preserved and the facial nerve is always less affected by this process. There were some inflammatory cells in the facial canals, but not to the extent to dissolve the nerve fibers. Moreover, the nerve fibers were not swollen as in a degenerative process. It is very unlikely that the facial nerves would end in identical abnormal positions on both sides as a result of artifact. Igarashi and others[10] reported identical findings on the facial nerve in a case of conjoined twins, although there was no description on facial and eye movements in the case history. The facial nerves in their case gradually diminished in size within their horizontal and vertical segments similar to the present case. Thus, it may be postulated that the disappearance of the facial nerves in their horizontal segments in our report can be attributed to a teratogenic process initiated in embryonic life.

The number of fibers in the facial nerve distal to the geniculate ganglion has been reported as always greater than that in the proximal part of the nerve. Foley and DuBois[11] carefully eliminated the motor component of the facial nerve, vagal and sympathetic components, and still found a significant num-

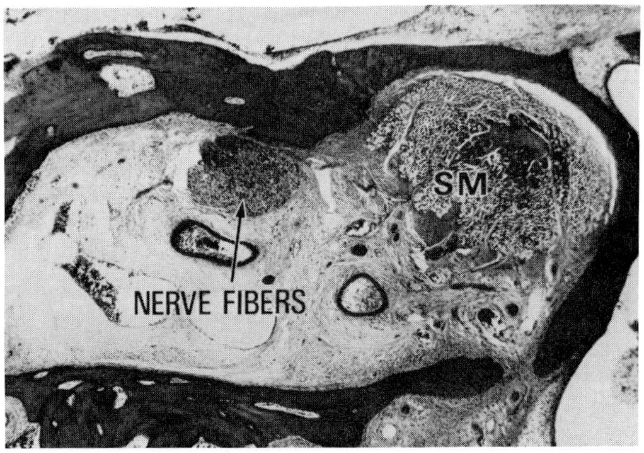

Fig. 7. The identical findings of the horizontal segment of the fallopian canal on the opposite side. (x22)

ber of axons at the stylomastoid foramen. Bruesch[9] also showed an excess of fibers between the geniculate ganglion and the junction of the auricular branch of the vagus. Vidić[12] supposed the origin of the distal excess to be from the auricular branch of the vagus. Saito[13] described aberrant neurons in the pyramidal and vertical segments of the facial nerve trunk, and pointed out that these neurons furnished additional source of the distal excess.

In both temporal bones in this report, a considerable number of nerve fibers reappeared in the empty facial canals at the level of the lower part of the pyramidal segment. Moreover, despite the interruption of the facial nerves in the horizontal segment, a normal size chorda tympani was seen crossing the tympanic cavity in normal position.

Yntema[14] made an experimental ablation in chick embryo and found that in early embryonic life the nerve used alternative pathways via other than the seventh in cases of destruction of the neuromere. The newly joined nerve element was supposed to be as Arnold's nerve from their anatomical position and was suspected to give an alternative pathway at the chorda tympani.

ACKNOWLEDGMENT — The authors would like to thank Andrew Baxter, FRCS(Ed), to whom the English of this article owes much.

REFERENCES

1. Möbius PJ. Ueber angeborene doppelseitige Abducens-Facialis-Lähmung. Münch Med Wochenschr 1888; 35:91-4.

2. Henderson JL. The congenital facial diplegia syndrome: clinical features, pathology and aetiology. Brain 1939; 62:381-403.

3. Heubner O. Ueber angeborenen Kernmangel. Charite-Annalen 1900; 25:211-43.

4. Richards RN. The Möbius syndrome. J Bone Joint Surg 1953; 35:437-44.

5. Olson WH, Bardin CW, Walsh GO, et al. Moebius syndrome. Neurology 1970; 20:1002-8.

6. Pitner SM, Edwards JE, McCormick WF. Observations on the pathology of the Moebius syndrome. J Neurol Neurosurg Psychiatry 1965; 28:362-74.

7. Foley JO. A quantitative study of the functional components of the facial nerve. Am J Anat 1960; 107:237-44.

8. Van Buskirk C. The 7th nerve complex. J Comp Neurol 1945; 82:303-33.

9. Bruesch SR. The distribution of myelinated afferent fibers in the branches of the cat's facial nerve. J Comp Neurol 1944; 81:169-91.

10. Igarashi M, Singer DB, Alford BR, et al. Middle and inner ear anomalies in a conjoined twin. Laryngoscope 1974; 84:1188-201.

11. Foley JO, DuBois FS. An experimental study of the facial nerve. J Comp Neurol 1943; 79:79-105.

12. Vidić B. The origin and the course of the communicating branch of the facial nerve to the lesser petrosal nerve in man. Anat Rec 1968; 162:511-6.

13. Saito H. Aberrant neurons in the facial nerve trunk. Arch Otorhinolaryngol (NY) 1973; 206:69-76.

14. Yntema CL. Experiments on the origin of the sensory ganglia of the facial nerve in the chick. J Comp Neurol 1944; 81:147-67.

≈

REPORT OF THE PANEL ON COMMUNICATIVE DISORDERS

Single copies of the *Report of the Panel on Communicative Disorders to the National Advisory Neurological and Communicative Disorders and Stroke Council* (NIH publication no. 79-1914) may be obtained from: Chief, Office of Scientific and Health Reports, National Institute of Neurological and Communicative Disorders and Stroke, Bldg. 31, Rm 8A08, 9000 Rockville Pike, Bethesda, MD 20205.

Ann Otol 90:1981

EYE-HEAD COORDINATION DURING OPTOKINETIC STIMULATION IN SQUIRREL MONKEYS

TAKESHI KUBO, MD
OSAKA, JAPAN

MAKOTO IGARASHI, MD
HOUSTON, TEXAS

DAVID W. JENSEN, PhD
HOUSTON, TEXAS

JERRY L. HOMICK, PhD
HOUSTON, TEXAS

Head and eye movements in the yaw plane were recorded during and after optokinetic stimulation in squirrel monkeys. 1) Phasic or tonic head deviations to the side of the ocular quick phase occurred in 94% of total recordings (n = 50) during the perstimulus period, and in 75% of recordings (n = 49) during the poststimulus period. Magnitude of mean head deviation was significantly different between perstimulus and poststimulus periods. 2) Head nystagmus associated with eye nystagmus was consistently observed in seven of nine squirrel monkeys during optokinetic stimulation. Squirrel monkeys are thereby less prone to display head nystagmus than either guinea pigs, pigeons or chickens. 3) Slow phase speeds of coupled head and eye nystagmus were subjected to statistical analysis. A highly significant negative correlation was found between slow phase head and eye speeds. The correlation coefficient was −0.81 at 60°/sec stimulus (n = 119) and −0.72 at 100°/sec stimulus (n = 131). The gaze speed, calculated by summing the head and eye speeds, was 59.1 ± 6.8/sec at 60°/sec and 92.2 ± 11.4 at 100°/sec stimulus. There was no significant difference between the gaze speed in a free head condition and the eye speed when the head was fixed.

INTRODUCTION

Previous experiments dealing with eye-head coordination in man and rhesus monkeys have demonstrated that during saccades and smooth pursuits, head movements are generated to position an object at a center of visual field condition.[1-4] Stabilization of the retinal image during head movements can be accomplished by reflex control of the oculomotor system by visual, vestibular and neck proprioceptive inputs in normal subjects. Quantitative studies on oculomotor control during active head turning have been done only in humans and rhesus monkeys at present, since techniques used in these experiments are not applicable to other vertebrates.

Dunlop and Mowrer[5] and Huizinga and van der Meulen[6] reported predominance of head nystagmus over ocular nystagmus in pigeons during vestibular and optokinetic stimulations. Head nystagmus with regular rhythm was also observed in guinea pigs.[7] In the course of pilot studies in squirrel monkeys, we have found that a considerable number of monkeys showed distinctive head nystagmus when the speed of optokinetic stimulus (OKS) was from 40 to 120°/sec. In this report, the slow phase speeds of ocular nystagmus during optokinetically induced head nystagmus are subjected to quantitative analysis in squirrel monkeys. Head deviations occurring during and after OKS are also described.

METHODS

Experimental animals were squirrel monkeys (*Saimiri sciureus*) randomly assigned from a colony. Amphetamine sulfate (0.5 mg/kg) was injected intramuscularly 15 minutes prior to recording to maintain a constant level of alertness.

Head movements in the yaw plane were measured using a lightweight aluminum shaft which extended upward from a chronically implanted pedestal of top of the monkey's skull. This shaft was mechanically coupled to a potentiometer that registered a voltage dependent on head position. The aluminum shaft was constructed such as to minimize head movements in the roll and pitch planes. Thus the monkey was allowed to turn the head about the vertical axis while its body was restrained.

A pair of platinum needle electrodes was inserted into the lateral canthi in order to record horizontal eye movements. Recorded activity was passed through a high-cut filter; thus the activities ranging between direct current (DC) to 25 Hz were amplified.

Eye and head movements were recorded by a Beckman dynograph recorder. Eye speed was calibrated using the slow phase speed of ocular nystagmus while the head was stable, which was induced by 30°/sec OKS given at the beginning and end of the recording. Slow phase speeds of head and eye nystagmus were calculated manually from the recordings on an oscillographic paper. Gaze speed was calculated by summing the slow phase speed of coupled head and eye nystagmus.

The animal was restrained in a laboratory-built chair that was placed on the turntable located within and coaxial to a surrounding vertically striped drum. The drum was a white cylinder 0.6 m in diameter with 1.5° wide black stripes that were evenly distributed at 22.5° intervals. OKS could be given either by drum rotation or by constant velocity table rotation. The inside of the drum was illuminated before and during OKS and darkened immediately at the cessation of the stimulus.

From the Department of Otorhinolaryngology and Communicative Sciences, Baylor College of Medicine, Houston, Texas, and the Neurophysiology Laboratory, Medical Research Branch, NASA Johnson Space Center, Houston, Texas. This study was supported by McFadden Trust Research Fund, NINCDS grants NS-7237 and NS-10940, and NASA contract NAS-9-14546.

Presented at the Midwinter Meeting of the Association for Research in Otolaryngology, St. Petersburg, Florida, January 24, 1979.

REPRINTS — Makoto Igarashi, MD, Department of Otorhinolaryngology and Communicative Sciences, Baylor College of Medicine, 1200 Moursund Avenue, Houston, TX 77030.

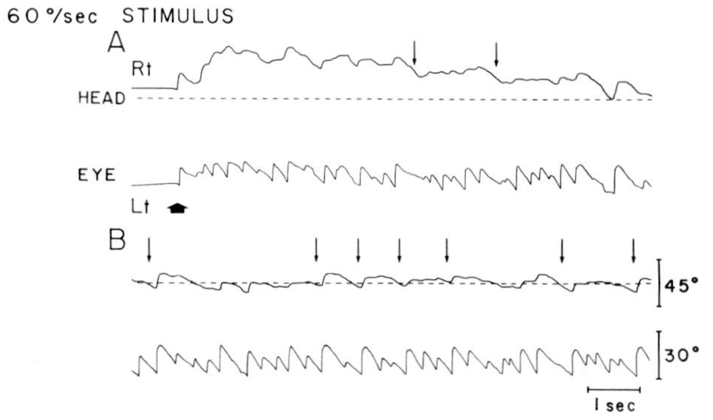

Fig. 1. A, B) Continuous head- and eye-movement recordings induced by 60°/sec counterclockwise optokinetic stimulation. Upward arrow in A indicates the onset of stimulus. Downward arrows show head nystagmus subjected to slow phase speed measurement. Upward deflection in eye and head movement recordings indicates deviation to right. Dashed line in head movement recording shows a straight forward head position in this and Fig. 2. Note that the head immediately deviates to the side of ocular quick phase after stimulus onset.

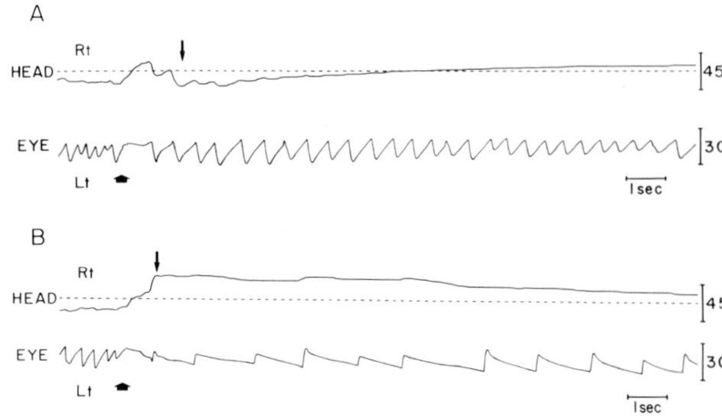

Fig. 2. A, B) Head deviations occur after the end of stimulus in association with the ocular nystagmus. Upward arrows in A and B indicate the end of optokinetic stimulus. Optokinetic stimulus is induced by drum rotation at 60°/sec and optokinetic after-nystagmus follows after the end of stimulus in A. In B the optokinetic stimulus is produced by a table rotation at 60°/sec and postrotational nystagmus follows. Records A and B were obtained from the same animal on the same day. Downward arrows in A and B show poststimulus head deviation in the dark. Note that the direction of head deviation is opposite in A and B.

RESULTS

Head Deviation. A representative recording of head and eye movements induced by 60°/sec OKS is shown in Figure 1. When the stimulus starts, the head immediately deviates to the side opposite to the nystagmus quick phase. This head deviation is transient and gradually returns to the center taking about nine seconds. Head deviation which occurred at the beginning of the stimulus to the side of the ocular quick phase was observed in 47 of 50 recordings, although head deviation was not apparent in three other recordings. Head deviation to the side of the slow phase was never found. Head deviation was transient in 55.3% (26/47) of the recordings and the time required to return to the straight forward position was 11.6 ± 4.8 sec (mean ± SD). In the remaining 44.7% (21/47), head deviation lasted for as long as the stimulus was continued.

Head deviation to the side of the ocular quick phase was also observed during the poststimulus period. When optokinetic eye nystagmus (OKN) was elicited by drum rotation (Fig. 2A), optokinetic after-nystagmus (OKAN) appears immediately after the cessation of the stimulus (indicated by upward arrow) in the dark. The head again deviates to the quick phase side, though at the stimulus offset it moves momentarily to the slow phase side.

On the other hand, when OKN was elicited by constant velocity table rotation (Fig. 2B), postrotational nystagmus (PRN) directed opposite to OKN appears after the stimulus in the dark. The direction of the head deviation associated with PRN again is toward the side of the ocular quick phase. Since PRN is directed toward the side opposite to that of OKAN, the direction of head deviation is now reversed. Head deviations appearing during the poststimulus period were, as expected, always phasic, and occurred in 75.5% (37/49) of the trials. The head did not necessarily return to the straight forward position after initial deviation; however, it reached final position after an average period of 11.2 ± 4.5 sec (n = 37). The duration of poststimulus head deviation was usually shorter than either OKAN or PRN.

The amplitudes of maximum head deviations are summarized in Table 1 as a function of stimulus factors. Values show the means and standard deviations of maximum head deviations which occurred during the first five seconds after stimulus onset and offset. The overall difference between perstimulus and poststimulus groups was significant according to the F test ($P < 0.05$). However, no significant difference was found across other stimulus factors, ie, 60 vs 100°/sec and drum vs table rotation. This means that the magnitude of head deviation is not linearly related to the frequency or speed of ocular nystagmus.

Head Nystagmus. Head movements consisting of slow and quick phases (indicated by downward arrows in Figure 1) show certain correlations with ocular nystagmus: 1) the direction of slow and quick head movements are the same as those of ocular nystagmus; and 2) the occurrence of the quick phase of head nystagmus is almost always associated with that of ocular nystagmus. These correlations between head and eye movements were also confirmed when the animals were exposed to impulsive acceleration in the dark (vestibular stimulation). As these features of slow and quick head movements were similar to the head nystagmus described in birds,[5,6] this kind of movement in the monkey will also be named "head nystagmus." Nine squirrel monkeys were repeatedly tested by OKS and seven showed head nystagmus consistently. However, only small and intermittent head nystagmus was observed in the remaining two animals.

TABLE 1. HEAD DEVIATIONS AS A FUNCTION OF STIMULUS FACTORS (n≥12)

	60°/sec Stimulus		*100°/sec Stimulus*	
	Drum Rotation ($\bar{X}\pm 1SD$)	*Table Rotation* ($\bar{X}\pm 1SD$)	*Drum Rotation* ($\bar{X}\pm 1SD$)	*Table Rotation* ($\bar{X}\pm 1SD$)
Perstimulus	22.1±11.6°	15.5±12.5°	25.7±11.8°	18.8± 5.8°
Poststimulus	11.6± 8.6°	11.3±12.0°	17.0± 8.8°	10.8±11.7°

Eye-Head Coordination. If slow phase speeds of coordinated head and eye nystagmus are compared (Fig. 1), one sees a negative correlation between head and eye speeds. That is, when the head speed increases, the eye speed decreases and vice versa. Representative beats of head and eye nystagmus were selected according to the following criteria: 1) head nystagmus is not interrupted by random head movements, 2) head and eye nystagmus occur simultaneously and 3) slow phase head and eye speeds are nearly constant over a certain period. Eye speeds during random head movements were not subjected to data analysis in this report because of technical difficulty in measuring the speed. Slow phase speeds of coupled head and eye nystagmus collected from 12 recordings of three squirrel monkeys are plotted in Figure 3. Although a highly significant negative correlation can be seen between head and eye speeds in Figure 3A, B, the negative correlation coefficient is slightly lower in B than in A. The correlation coefficients were −0.81 (n = 119) in A and −0.72 (n = 131) in B. As the eye speed starts to lag behind the stimulus speed (when the latter becomes about 100°/sec),[8] it may be speculated that as the stimulus speed increases an ability of eye-head coordination decreases. This is the result of negative oculomotor control performed by the visual, vestibular and neck proprioceptive systems. Therefore, the gaze speed, which is the sum of head and eye speed, would be maintained at a constant level irrespective of the magnitude of head speed. Thus retinal image slip is minimized and clear vision is possible.

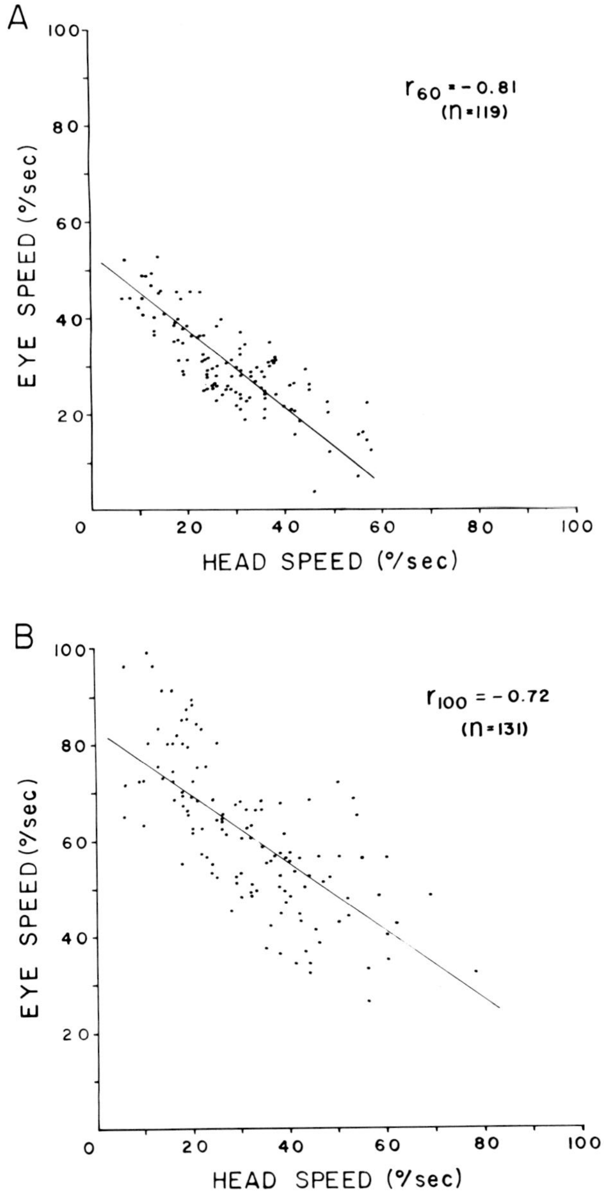

Fig. 3. A, B) Slow phase speeds of coupled head and eye nystagmus were plotted. The data in A were obtained by 60°/sec stimulus and in B by 100°/sec stimulus. Abscissa and ordinate indicate the slow phase head and eye speed, respectively. Straight lines in A and B show the regression lines calculated from the samples. Significant negative correlations can be seen between the head and eye speeds.

Slow phase speed of head, eye and gaze movements are summarized in Table 2. The mean gaze speeds at 60 and 100°/sec are close to the stimulus speed. The mean errors of gaze are less at 60°/sec stimulus speed than at 100°/sec stimulus where there is a 7.8% error. Slow phase eye speeds under the *fixed head* condition were calculated from two recordings from each of eight squirrel monkeys. The means and standard deviations were 57.5±3.0°/sec at 60°/sec and 95.7±6.0°/sec at 100°/sec stimuli (not shown in Table 2). A *t* test showed no significant difference between gaze speed in a *free head* condition and eye speed in a *fixed head* condition. It can be concluded that under the experimental conditions employed the presence of head movements did demonstrate equal accuracy of gaze performance with that obtained when the head was fixed.

TABLE 2. SLOW PHASE SPEEDS OF HEAD, EYE AND GAZE MOVEMENTS

	Stimulus Speed	
	60°/sec (n = 119)	*100°/sec (n = 131)*
Head speed	28.9±11.8°/sec	31.3±14.8°/sec
Eye speed	30.2± 9.4°/sec	60.9±15.6°/sec
Gaze speed	59.1± 6.8°/sec	92.2±11.4°/sec
Mean error of gaze	−0.9°/sec	−7.8°/sec

DISCUSSION

Head Deviation. Head deviation during OKS occurring in man seems to be uncertain; however, OKS invariably causes a head deviation to the side of ocular *slow* phase in lower vertebrates (eg, birds, guinea pigs and rabbits).[5-7,9] In the present study, squirrel monkeys showed tonic or phasic head deviation to the side of ocular quick phase during and after OKS. Although the magnitude of head deviation varied, its direction did not. We suspect that optokinetic influence on neck muscles is stronger in rabbits, guinea pigs, pigeons and chickens than in man and squirrel monkeys. Volitional factors such as the intent to fixate moving stripes as fast as possible may cause head deviation to the side of ocular quick phase in squirrel monkeys.

Fukuda[9] reported that the head deviation in chickens gradually decreased when they were exposed to OKS daily. After two weeks of trials the animals started to turn their heads toward the side of the quick phase. He suggested that animals gained the ability to maintain head and body equilibrium or otherwise they would fall toward the slow phase. Since squirrel monkeys showed head deviation toward the quick phase from the first exposure to OKS they may possess the type of ability that was seen in trained chickens, even without any training.

Head Nystagmus and Oculomotor Control. Outerbridge and Melvill Jones[10] reported that of seven human subjects tested by impulsive acceleration in the dark, only three showed head nystagmus. Of nine squirrel monkeys tested by OKS in the present study, seven showed clear head nystagmus; the same result was obtained by using impulsive angular acceleration in the dark. Therefore, head nystagmus in squirrel monkeys is more frequent and of larger amplitude than in humans; however, it is smaller than in birds, guinea pigs and rabbits. The fact strongly suggests a species difference in visual and vestibular influence on neck motoneurons.

Visual stimuli were given in two different modes (ie, predictive vs unpredictive) in previous papers.[1,3,4,11] Some differences in eye and head movement patterns were found between these two stimulus paradigms. However, the subjects achieved essentially the same performance, ie, fixation of retinal image into the fovea. The visual stimulus used in this experiment is quite different in nature. It is noteworthy that although a different type of visual stimulus and a different species of animal were used in this experiment, nearly perfect eye-head coordination was demonstrated. Among three oculomotor negative control systems, the cervico-ocular reflex has the lowest gain, hence seems to play a secondary role.[12,13] The visual-oculomotor feedback loop has no functional role during saccadic gaze shift because of its slow operation time;[14] however, during the slow phase of nystagmus, it probably plays some significant role. The compensatory vestibular reflex seems to be most important for eye-head coordination because the gain of this system is close to unity and also because the reflex arc is a feedforward system instead of feedback system.[15,16] The significance of the vestibulo-ocular reflex on eye-head coordination has been confirmed by several studies including ours[3,4,15,17] which demonstrate gaze overshoot after interruption of the vestibulo-ocular reflex.

ACKNOWLEDGMENT — We are indebted to Mark Simon, Ronald DeWitt, Ermastine Marbley, June Brown and Jeanmarie Amend for their technical assistance. Gratitude is extended to Joel Levy for his assistance in statistical evaluation.

Dr. Kubo's present address is: Department of Otolaryngology, Osaka University Medical Center, Osaka 553, Japan.

REFERENCES

1. Bartz AEL. Eye and head movements in peripheral vision: nature of compensatory eye movements. Science 1966; 152:1644-5.

2. Bizzi E, Kalil RE, Tagliasco V. Eye-head coordination in monkeys: evidence for centrally patterned organization. Science 1971; 173:452-4.

3. Kasai T, Zee DS. Eye-head coordination in labyrinthine defective human beings. Brain Res 1978; 144:123-41.

4. Lanman J, Bizzi E, Allum J. The coordination of eye and head movement during smooth pursuit. Brain Res 1978; 153:39-53.

5. Dunlop K, Mowrer OH. Head movements and eye functions of birds. J Comp Psychol 1930; 11:99-112.

6. Huizinga E, van der Meulen P. Vestibular rotatory and optokinetic reactions in the pigeon. Ann Otol Rhinol Laryngol 1951; 60:927-47.

7. Gresty MA. Eye, head and body movements of the guinea pig in response to optokinetic stimulation and sinusoidal oscillation in yaw. Pfluegers Arch 1975; 353:201-14.

8. Takahashi M, Igarashi M. Comparison of vertical and horizontal optokinetic nystagmus in the squirrel monkey. ORL 1977; 39:321-9.

9. Fukuda T. Stato-kinetic reflexes in equilibrium and movement. In Japanese. Tokyo: Igaku Shoin, 1957:92-6.

10. Outerbridge JS, Melvill Jones G. Reflex vestibular control of head movement in man. Aerosp Med 1971; 42:935-40.

11. Bizzi E, Kalil RE, Morasso P. Two modes of active eye-head coordination in monkeys. Brain Res 1972; 40:45-8.

12. Thoden U, Wirbitzky J. Influence of passive neck movements on eye position and brain stem neurones. Pfluegers Arch 1976; 362;R37.

13. Barlow DE, Freeman W. The cervico-ocular reflex in normal human adults. Neurosci Abstract 1978; 291.

14. Morasso P, Bizzi E, Dichgans J. Adjustment of saccade characteristics during head movements. Exp Brain Res 1973; 16:492-500.

15. Dichgans J. Bizzi E, Morasso P, et al. Mechanisms underlying recovery of eye-head coordination following bilateral labyrinthectomy in monkeys. Exp Brain Res 1973; 18:548-62.

16. Robinson DA. Adaptive gain control of vestibuloocular reflex by the cerebellum . J Neurophysiol 1976; 39:954-69.

17. Kubo T, Igarashi M, Jensen DW, et al. Eye-head coordination and lateral canal block in squirrel monkeys. Ann Otol Rhinol Laryngol (in press).

OBJECTIVE EVALUATION OF EARPLUGS FOR THE CONTROL OF WATER-BORNE INFECTION

DAVID W. JOHNSON, MS, MA
ROBERT H. MAISEL, MD
MINNEAPOLIS, MINNESOTA

Eighty-two cotton, foam, and solid core stock and custom earplugs were evaluated objectively for water absorption and water penetration characteristics in order to determine their efficacy for control of water-borne infection in ears having open middle ear cavities. Cotton plugs, even when saturated with petroleum jelly, had poor consistency in resisting even minimal water pressure. Polymeric foam plugs, especially when saturated with petroleum jelly, appeared to inhibit water flow in conditions approximating actual ear protection use. No plugs evaluated, including custom elastomeric solid core plugs, inhibited water penetration in conditions approximating shallow surface dives. A clinical protocol for evaluation of potential earplugs for patient use is proposed on the basis of this study.

INTRODUCTION

The middle ear cleft may become contaminated in individuals with tympanostomy tubes, with perforated tympanic membranes, or with open mastoid bowls exposed to water-borne infection. Occlusion of the external auditory canal either with a custom earplug[1,2] or with various stock earplugs[1] has been suggested for the management of water-borne infection during high risk activities such as showering, bathing, or even swimming. Custom made plugs satisfactorily occlude the external canal in close to 100% of patients using them, while some stock type earplugs are satisfactory in about 90% of the patients. A myriad plugs purported to protect the ear from water are available in the marketplace at this time.[3]

The success of an earplug in controlling water-borne infection is directly related to the occluding ability of the earplug. Factors such as comfort and ease of insertion and removal have been of additional importance. In previous work[1] rejection of the stock type earplug by some youngsters resulted in the children's ears being unprotected in high risk activities. Stock plugs of cotton or soft flexible polymeric foam can solve this type of complication in fitting and are readily available. The polymeric foam plug can be collapsed between the fingers and inserted into the external auditory canal. The foam earplug swells to its original volume within a minute while seating itself within the canal.

The effect is for the plug to fully occlude all irregularities of the external auditory canal so that occlusion is complete. This particular plug was designed for use in hearing conservation programs and was not designed for control of water-borne infection. Because of previous success using noise control earplugs for the control of water-borne infection, however, it was decided to evaluate this sponge-like earplug for infection control purposes by comparing it to other plugs of the soft variety already in use or to other plugs previously reported.[1,2,4]

METHODS

Cotton sponges and earwicks were obtained from a local medical supply house while the polymeric foam, the triple flange synthetic rubber, and the elastomeric silicone polymeric plugs and mold materials were obtained from a local industrial hearing conservationist. The earplugs were evaluated under a two-part study protocol under several conditions. The porous plugs were analyzed for water absorption characteristics and water occluding ability with and without petroleum jelly saturation.

Water Absorption (Fig. 1). Earwicks (plugs 1, 2) were submerged under 200 cc of water. Cotton sponges were divided into plugs (3-8) with diameters of 1.5, 2.0, and 3.0 cm and were compressed once and allowed to fully expand before being submerged under 200 cc of water. Polymeric foam plugs were treated in a different manner because of their compression/expansion characteristics.

One set of polymeric foam plugs (9, 10) was collapsed completely one time and allowed to swell to original volume. The plugs were submerged under 200 cc of water then removed at the end of a 30-minute soaking period and the amount of absorbed water was determined. The plugs were collapsed and allowed to fully expand 15 more times before again being placed under 200 cc of water for an additional 30 minutes. They were removed a second time and residual water retention was determined. They were compressed and allowed to fully expand an additional 30 times and were again submerged under 200 cc of water and allowed to soak an additional 30 minutes before determining for a third time what amount of water had been absorbed.

Additional polymeric plugs (11, 12) were initially compressed and expanded 15 times before initial immersion and water absorption determination after 30 minutes submersion. These plugs were compressed and allowed to expand an additional 30 times before another 30 minutes of submersion and determination of water absorption. A third set of polymeric plugs (13, 14) was compressed and expanded 30 times before initial immersion under 200 cc of water and evaluation for water absorption.

From the Department of Otolaryngology, University of Minnesota Medical School, and the Department of Otolaryngology, Hennepin County Medical Center, Minneapolis, Minnesota.

REPRINTS — David W. Johnson, MS, MA, Department of Otolaryngology, Hennepin County Medical Center, 701 Park Avenue South, Minneapolis, MN 55415.

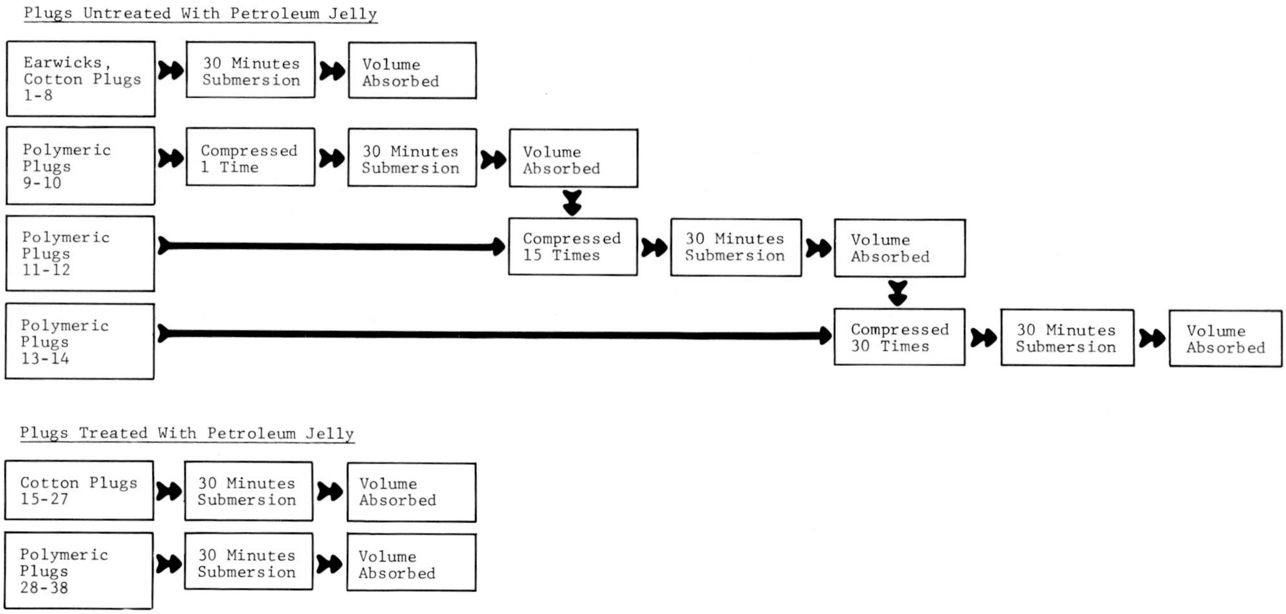

Fig. 1. Water absorption evaluation protocols.

Cotton plugs with diameters of 1.5 cm (15-20), 2 cm (21-25) and 3 cm (26, 27) were saturated with petroleum jelly by placing them in hand and working the jelly well into the fibers. The petroleum jelly compressed the respective plugs to a size .5 cm less than the original diameter. Petroleum jelly was worked into the polymeric foam plugs (28-38) in a similar manner. All plugs treated with petroleum jelly (15-38) were evaluated with water soaking in a manner similar to that of plugs 1-8 outlined above.

Water Penetration Rate (Fig. 2). Water could pass plugs used to seal an experimental ear canal model by either going through the plugs or around them. The rate at which water would flow through or around each variety of earplug was evaluated under three conditions. Condition 1 was designed to be easy enough for the individual clinician to use in his own practice for evaluation of plugs prior to patient use. Condition 2 was a validation study of condition 1, essentially an attempt to evaluate the plugs experimentally in an occluding condition where a 2-cc volume, approximating the volume of the external auditory canal, was coupled to the tube holding the respective plugs. This condition would approximate surface swimming, showering, shampooing, etc. Condition 3 was designed to approximate conditions of a surface dive while swimming. To evaluate occluding ability during submersion, condition 3 used portions of conditions 1 and 2 for evaluation. Of the three conditions, only condition 1 was suitable for clinician use on a regular basis.

In condition 1, plugs without petroleum jelly (39-43) were evaluated by inserting them into an .8 cm (inside diameter) tube, and 1.5 cc water was placed in the upper portion of the tube. The amount of time it took for water to penetrate the length of the plug was determined. Plugs saturated with petroleum jelly (44-50) were evaluated in a similar manner. A number of plugs utilized in the absorption part of our protocol (plugs 3, 12, 14, 16, 20, 21, 26, 29, 34, 38) were used a second time (as plugs 39, 40, 41, 44-50, respectively).

Condition 2 was more complex because the plugs were evaluated in a similar manner to condition 1, except that the extruding end of the plug was surrounded by a 2 cc cavity to approximate external auditory canal volume with plug in place. Again, some plugs (51-54) were evaluated without petroleum jelly saturation and the other plugs (55-58) were evaluated with petroleum jelly saturation for rate of water penetration.

In condition 3, the column of water exerting pressure on the respective plugs evaluated was increased from 1.5 cc used in condition 1 to 162 cc in order to simulate the depth reached in a shallow 180 cm surface dive while swimming. Again, we used plugs untreated with petroleum jelly (59-63) and plugs treated with petroleum jelly (64-68). A second subset of untreated plugs (69-73) and petroleum jelly-treated plugs (74-78) were evaluated in the same manner except for placement of the 2 cc cavity at the extruding end of the tube.

Stock synthetic rubber plugs (79, 80) and clinic fabricated plugs (81, 82) of the elastomeric silicone polymeric variety (ie, custom

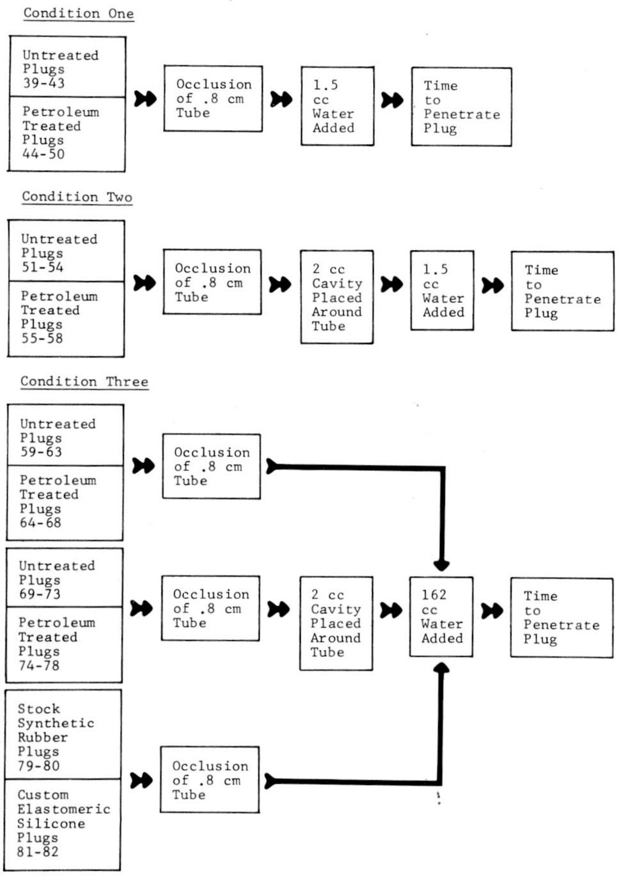

Fig. 2. Water penetration rate.

TABLE 1. WATER ABSORPTION OF COLLAPSIBLE EARPLUGS

	Earplug No.	*Mean Absorption (ml)*	*Range (ml) Min.-Max.*
Untreated earplugs			
Earwicks	1,2	18.0	18.0-18.0
Cotton	3,4	10.8	7.5-14.0
Cotton	5,6	31.5	29.0-34.0
Cotton	7,8	80.0	77.0-83.0
Polymeric foam	9-14	4.6	2.0- 9.0
Petroleum-treated plugs			
Cotton	15-20	1.8	1.5- 2.0
Cotton	21-25	3.6	1.8- 4.8
Cotton	26-27	4.0	2.0- 6.0
Polymeric foam	28-38	.5	.3- .5

plugs) were evaluated similarly. The extruding portion of each plug (79-82) precluded evaluation with our 2 cc volume container coupled to the end of the test tubing.

FINDINGS

Water Absorption. All collapsible earplugs did absorb water (Table 1). Earwicks (plugs 1, 2) and 1.5 cm cotton plugs (3, 4) absorbed small amounts of water (less than 18 ml). The amount of water absorption did not appear to be related to the amount of time under water. Polymeric foam plugs which were squeezed considerably before submersion in water (13, 14) appeared to absorb more water than plugs receiving less compression and expansion before submersion (9-12). The earwick plugs (1, 2) absorbed three to six times as much water as did the polymeric foam plugs (9-14).

Plugs saturated with petroleum jelly (15-38) performed more efficiently than did the untreated plugs (1-14) in resisting water absorption (Table 1). Cotton plugs impregnated with petroleum jelly demonstrated considerable variability in the amount of water absorbed (1.5 ml to 6.0 ml) independent of the diameter of the respective plugs while the polymeric foam plugs impregnated with petroleum jelly appeared to resist water absorption with more uniformity (.3 ml to .5 ml absorbed).

TABLE 2. RAPIDITY OF WATER PENETRATION THROUGH A .8 cm DIAMETER ORIFICE WITH 1.5 cc WATER PRESSURE FOR COLLAPSIBLE EARPLUGS

	Earplug No.	*Mean Minutes Before Penetration*	*Range in Minutes Min.-Max.*
Untreated earplugs			
Presoaked			
Cotton-polymeric	37-41	.03	.01- .06
New			
Polymeric	42-43	3.50	2.80- 4.20
Petroleum-treated plugs			
Presoaked			
Cotton	44-47	7.50	.03-30.00
Polymeric	48-50	14.30	10.00-18.00

TABLE 3. RAPIDITY OF WATER PENETRATION THROUGH A .8 cm DIAMETER ORIFICE WITH 1.5 cc WATER PRESSURE FOR COLLAPSIBLE EARPLUGS SURROUNDED BY A 2 cc CAVITY

	Earplug No.	*Mean Minutes Before Penetration*	*Range in Minutes Min.-Max.*
Untreated earplugs			
Cotton	51-52	.02	.02- .02
Polymeric	53-54	11.75	8.00-15.50
Petroleum-treated plugs			
Cotton	55-56	45.75	1.50-90.00*
Polymeric	57-58	58.50	27.00-90.00*

*Portion of study terminated at end of 90 minutes.

One variety of stock plug (79, 80) and one variety of custom plug (81, 82) were not evaluated for water absorption because each of these types of plugs had a solid nonwater-absorbing core.

Water Penetration Rate. Water rapidly penetrated past untreated earplugs when they had been previously soaked in water (plugs 39, 40, 41) but not when used without previous soaking (plugs 42, 43) (Table 2). Water was able to penetrate the presoaked plugs in .5 to 3.5 seconds with the very minimal pressure of 1.5 cc of water of condition 1. Dry, new plugs required 2.8 to 4.2 minutes for penetration.

Rapidity of water absorption in condition 1 changed dramatically with most plugs (15-38) when impregnated with petroleum jelly (Table 2). Small diameter cotton plugs continued to pass water through their length very rapidly (plugs 44-46), but the large diameter cotton plug with petroleum jelly saturation (47) sealed our .8 cm diameter orifice very effectively. Polymeric foam plugs impregnated with petroleum jelly (48-50) also performed well in condition 1, effectively sealing the orifice for 10 to 18 minutes.

TABLE 4. RAPIDITY OF WATER PENETRATION THROUGH A .8 cm DIAMETER ORIFICE WITH 162 cc WATER PRESSURE FOR COLLAPSIBLE EARPLUGS

	Earplug No.	*Mean Minutes Before Penetration*	*Range in Minutes Min.-Max.*
Not surrounded by 2 cc cavity condition			
Untreated earplugs			
Polymeric	59-63	.01	.01-.01
Petroleum-treated plugs			
Polymeric	64-68	.08	.03-.18
Surrounded by 2 cc cavity condition			
Untreated earplugs			
Polymeric	69-73	.02	.02-.02
Petroleum-treated plugs			
Polymeric	74-78	.34	.08-.88

TABLE 5. RAPIDITY OF WATER PENETRATION THROUGH A .8 cm DIAMETER ORIFICE WITH 162 cc WATER PRESSURE FOR SOLID CORE STOCK AND CUSTOM EARPLUGS

Earplugs	*Earplug No.*	*Mean Minutes Before Penetration*	*Range in Minutes Min.-Max.*
Synthetic rubber	79-80	7.58	.16-15.00*
Elastomeric	81-82	.03	.02- .05

*Portion of study terminated at end of 15 minutes.

In condition 2 where the space between an earplug and the tympanic membrane was approximated, untreated cotton plugs (51, 52) continued to have very poor occluding ability (Table 3). Untreated polymeric foam plugs (53, 54) appeared about twice as effective when the 2 cc volume cavity was coupled to the tube serving as our synthetic external auditory canal (Table 3) as opposed to condition 1 where no cavity was used (plugs 42-43) (Table 2).

Plugs treated with petroleum jelly and evaluated with the 2 cc cavity resisted water absorption. Treated cotton plugs (55, 56) were able to withstand water penetration for 1.5 minutes (Table 3). Polymeric foam plugs treated with petroleum jelly in condition 2 were able to withstand penetration for about half an hour (Table 3).

When the column of water exerting pressure through the .8 cm diameter tube was increased from 1.5 cc to 162 cc (condition 3) water rapidly penetrated past the occluding device whether or not the 2 cc cavity was coupled to the tubing holding the plugs (59-78), regardless of petroleum jelly saturation (Table 4). Solid stock and custom plugs (79-82) were not universally successful either (Table 5). In condition 3 water did not appear to penetrate any of the plugs, but rather appeared to pass in the space between the plugs and the walls of the tube, especially when the plugs were petroleum jelly saturated or when the plugs were solid.

DISCUSSION

All varieties of earplugs evaluated will occlude the external auditory canals of most people with the exceptions of the earwicks which do not fully occlude the canals unless moist. Absorption characteristics of cotton and earwick plugs were three to six times poorer than those of the polymeric foam plugs when the respective plugs were not saturated with petroleum jelly. When any plugs (including polymeric) had been "presoaked," the plugs similarly absorbed water within several seconds. The implication was that each plug could occlude the external auditory canals of appropriate patients, but would tend to absorb water quickly unless it was polymeric and being used for the first time. The polymeric foam plugs were slightly better than standard cotton when they were presoaked if they were not compressed many times before use.

All plugs absorbed considerably less water when saturated with petroleum jelly. The polymeric plugs tended to absorb about one fourth the volume of water that the 1.5 cm diameter cotton plugs did, one eighth the volume of the 2 cc diameter cotton plugs, and less than one twelfth the volume of 3 cm diameter cotton plugs. The 1.5 and the 2 cm diameter cotton plugs saturated with petroleum jelly did not substantially inhibit the water absorption through our .8 cm orifice. Perhaps this occurred because these plugs did not expand as well as the other plugs and thus perhaps expanded more fully in water than did the others. The 3 cm cotton saturated plug and the polymeric saturated plugs did better in inhibiting water absorption when petroleum jelly had been worked into the plug. The cotton, however, was too large to fit the external auditory canals of many people and actually protruded from the experimental canal. This allowed considerable air contact area, perhaps inhibiting rapid absorption by surface tension or air absorption during the study period. The petroleum jelly-saturated foam plugs did well, inhibiting water flow for ten or more minutes in condition 1 or even up to half an hour or more in condition 2. These data suggest that the polymeric foam plugs treated with petroleum jelly could be most useful in protecting from middle ear contamination in appropriate patients, although untreated polymeric plugs could be of some help. Cotton plugs treated with petroleum jelly may be useful, but their water inhibition predictability would appear poor based on this study.

No plugs evaluated in this study in condition 3 were able to withstand substantial water pressure for any significant amount of time. Neither stock plugs of soft polymeric material or synthetic rubber, nor custom plugs of elastomeric polymer would appear efficacious for middle ear protection with head submerged at shallow depth (180 cm). Occluding ability of the plugs appeared not to be measured by condition 3, but rather by the outward force of the respective plugs against our synthetic external auditory canal. Again, the problem is not the material from which the plug is made but the adhesion characteristics of the respective plugs to the experimental canal walls.

Of the plugs evaluated, the polymeric foam plug, when saturated with petroleum jelly, would appear best in selected patients for swimming on the surface or for bathing and showering for brief periods of time. Untreated polymeric plugs would appear adequate for brief showers or shampooing purposes. Cost economies suggest the use of such plugs (about $.50 a set without petroleum jelly) in place of more expensive custom plugs necessitating clinican time in taking impressions and manufacturing the earplug.[4] Because a number of foam type plugs are on the market, it would be appropriate for the individual clinician to evaluate the locally available foam plugs before implementing prosthetic use. The test protocol using 1.5 cc water through a .8 cm diameter orifice without a 2 cc cavity would appear to be a reasonable method for evaluation (ie, condition 1) for predicting success.

REFERENCES

1. Johnson DW, Mathog RH, Maisel RH. Tympanostomy protection with earplugs. Arch Otolaryngol 1977; 103:377-80.

2. Kasten SD, Robinson M. Fabrication of custom-made earplugs for swimming. Arch Otolaryngol 1974; 100:68.

3. Annual directory of hearing health care products and services. Hearing Instruments 1978; 29:48.

4. Johnson DW, Mathog RH. Protection of the ear from waterborne infection. Soc Med Audiol Newsletter 1977; 4:28, 30, 32.

ADDENDUM

TABLE 6. EVALUATION OF EARPLUGS USED BY ADULT MALES WHILE SWIMMING

Swimming Protocol Prior to Ear Canal Examination	*Custom Elastomeric Plugs*	*Stock Synthetic Rubber Plugs*	*Stock Polymeric Foam Plugs*	*Stock Polymeric Foam Plugs Impregnated with Petroleum Jelly*	*Controls Without Plugs*
	No. and Percentage of Ears Showing No Penetration by Water After Swimming Protocol				
Submersion under 162 cm of water with bathing cap over plugs	6 (100%)	10 (100%)	6 (100%)	8 (100%)	10 (0%)
Submersion under 162 cm of water with bathing cap over plugs and five-minute swim	2 (100%)	2 (100%)	8 (87.5%)	2 (100%)	10 (0%)

Further studies relating to actual human in-use evaluation of earplugs are ongoing as we develop another paper, but our very preliminary data may be of interest. The plugs used in the experimental model study (except for the cotton plugs which we excluded on the basis of data from our model) were evaluated in young adult males. The protocol was to inspect the external auditory canals of the subjects, insert the earplugs, and place a bathing cap on the subject. The subject would then jump into a swimming pool and submerge to a depth approximately 162 cm (ie, touch the bottom of the pool at 270 cm), return to the surface, dry off the external ear while the plugs were still in place, and remove the plugs. A second inspection of the external auditory canals was made and any water penetration was noted. Studies of one surface dive to a depth of 162 cm and swimming for a period of five minutes were carried out; one subject did not cover his ears with the bathing cap during this part of the study.

Preliminary results from this ministudy are summarized in Table 6. The results demonstrate that the plugs appear to work equally well for the short term occlusion (jumping into the pool and jumping out), and indeed appear to work better than our experimental model might have predicted. For longer periods of time, the model would appear to have prospective validity (jumping into the pool and swimming for five minutes) since the untreated polymeric foam plugs failed with time.

It appears that the experimental model proposed in our manuscript can predict those plugs which are likely to fail in vivo. Studies in vivo suggest that plugs will be resistant to water penetration for a longer period than the model might have projected. However, a poorly occluding plug will be identified by the proposed experimental model and the plugs showing promise on evaluation experimentally are likely to be safe for actual use.

BOOK REVIEWS

Classics in Modern Otology

By *Luis García-Ballester, Guillermo Olagüe,* and *Miguel Ciges.* Illustrated, 354 pp, 1978. Granada University Press, Barcelona. Price $18.00.

Few practicing physicians realize that otology is a very old specialty and it was only a fairly recent development that combined it with rhinology and laryngology. Indeed, otology has a rich, although infrequently documented, history. The medical specialties underwent rapid evolution in the latter part of the 18th and early 19th centuries. This was due to a number of factors such as development of concepts relating pathologic changes to symptoms and signs and the use of instruments which would permit physicians to describe in the living patient what the pathologist would discover by autopsy. Social economic changes which occurred with the development of large urban communities permitted a physician to become interested in one organ system. An added spur to the development of specialties was the evolution of specialized journals, which were a tremendous aid to communication.

This book, which was published for the meeting of the *Collegium Otorhinolaryngologicum Amicitiae Sacrum* Congress in Granada in 1978 is a compilation of articles that the authors felt were of special importance in the evolution of otology as a specialty. The Introduction offers a review of the emergence of medical specialties and concentrates on the development of otology. The selected readings are divided into four sections on the position of otology and its changes throughout the nineteenth century; methods of examination; the middle ear, which includes a group of articles on mastoid surgery and otosclerosis; and diseases of the inner ear. These articles provide examples of the clinical and anatomic observations made by pioneers in the specialty. It is a humbling experience to peruse an article by Toynbee, who dissected 2000 temporal bones, and to realize that his article might have been published in the present decade. The description of the tympanic membrane by Politzer has not been surpassed. The arguments regarding indications for and techniques of mastoid surgery are a revelation when one considers that "in 1873 Dr. A. H. Buck could record 31 operations with 23 good results," and "in the remaining 8 fatal cases, death could not be attributed to the operation directly or indirectly in more than one case."

The articles are written in their original language. Since much of the work was in German and French with occasional Spanish articles, it is necessary to translate them. This is not always an easy task. Biographical sketches of the authors are included for the reader which adds much interest to the text. These biographies reveal the efforts that this group of men made to obtain an education which would prepare them to make such significant contributions.

The text is published by the University of Granada Press and, with the exception of some typographical errors, it is presented in a very readable manner. This book should be in the library of every student of otology and should be used as an introduction in all training programs.

SYLVAN E. STOOL, MD
Pittsburgh, Pennsylvania

Diseases of the Ear: A Textbook of Otology, Fourth Edition

By *Stuart R. Mawson* and *Harold Ludman.* Hard cover, black and white illustrations, indexed, 580 pp, 1979. Year Book Medical Publishers, Chicago. Price $69.95.

This text is written primarily for the postgraduate student who is studying for his qualifying examinations. The basic science sections, Embryology, Anatomy and Physiology, are presented in a concise manner. The chapters on diseases reflect the authors' wide clinical experience and are written in a very readable manner. References are not included in the text but a short bibliography is available at the end of each chapter. This method of presentation permits the authors to write authoritatively, which is an advantage to the student who does not wish to explore the controversies in otology. It is a disadvantage to the reader who desires to evaluate the pros and cons of various therapeutic methods. Since there are divergent methods for therapy, a less authoritarian approach or more complete documentation of the results of a suggested method would be helpful to this reader.

The illustrations are line drawings and therefore not as interesting as they might be; however, they are adequate.

The book is certainly recommended for the audience the authors wish to address and for the student or resident who needs a concise, easy-to-read review of contemporary basic science, diagnosis, and therapy in otology.

SYLVAN E. STOOL, MD
Pittsburgh, Pennsylvania

Secretory Otitis Media and Its Sequelae

By *Jacob Sadé.* Hard cover, black and white and color illustrations, 314 pp, 1979. Churchill Livingstone, New York. Price $35.00.

Dr. Sadé states that "secretory otitis is both a fascinating and important subject." It is fascinating because it enhances our understanding of otitis media and is related to various fundamental biological and pathological processes. Its importance lies in its prevalence in the general population and its high incidence in children.

This text, which is the first in a proposed series of clinical otolaryngology monographs, is devoted to the many aspects of this disease as interpreted by the center which has been studying secretory otitis for 20 years. There are 17 chapters, each of which is virtually a unit in itself. Of most interest are those which summarize basic research in the field. While much of this information has been published elsewhere, it is collated and evaluated in several excellent chapters by the author. Other chapters on mucosa, mucus, immunology, audiology and pneumatization are written by carefully chosen contributors from other institutions and demonstrate how difficult it is to have one center that can investigate all aspects of this very complex disease.

The chapters devoted to clinical management are not as lucid and integrated; the clinical information is scattered throughout the text, a fact the author recognizes in the foreword. The text also suffers from the introduction of terminology such as "the semi-hot ear," "metula" and "herodium;" while Dr. Sadé acknowledges there is nothing sacred about nomenclature, this does not add to the clarity of the book.

This text is not for the casual reader, and it must be approached in a critical manner because there are so many areas of controversy. For instance, the author makes a statement that children with cystic fibrosis have an increased incidence of acute otitis media. However, the reviewer was unable to find the documentation that substantiates this observation. While this may be considered "nit-picking," in a text devoted to a single condition one should expect documentation of such a potentially controversial statement.

With the above caveats, I recommend this text to the serious student of otology. As the author states in the foreword (which is very good and alone is worth the price of the text), most of this information was unknown 20 years ago and 20 years hence it may be obsolete. This book represents the state of the art in several centers which are devoted to understanding this fascinating and important disease.

SYLVAN E. STOOL, MD
Pittsburgh, Pennsylvania

COMBINED OTOLARYNGOLOGICAL SPRING MEETINGS

The Bayshore Inn, Vancouver, British Columbia

1981 Preliminary Programs
(Subject to change and Council approval)

AMERICAN BRONCHO-ESOPHAGOLOGICAL ASSOCIATION
May 11-12, 1981

Airway Compromise Due to an Abnormally Compliant Trachea in a Neonate with Multiplex Congenita (Larsen) Syndrome. Kenneth M. Grundfast, MD, Anwar Mumtaz, MD, Robert K. Kanter, MD, Murray M. Pollack, MD.

Flexible Fiber-Optic Endoscopy in Difficult Intubations. Enje Th. Edens, MD, Roberto Sia, MD.

Laser Treatment of Metastatic Melanoma of the Trachea and Bronchus. Albert H. Andrews, Jr., MD, David D. Caldarelli, MD.

Sputum Cytologic Diagnosis of Upper Respiratory Cancer — II. H. Bryan Neel III, MD, David R. Sanderson, MD, Robert S. Fontana, MD, Lewis B. Woolner, MD.

Unusual Presentations of Foreign Bodies in the Air and Food Passages. Seymour R. Cohen, MD.

Hypopharyngeal and Proximal Esophageal Injuries in Patients with Cervical Trauma. Richard A. Pollock, MD, John M. Purvis, MD, Herndon Murray, MD.

A Simple ENT Problem with Dire Complications. Harry R. Morse, MD.

The Incendiary Characteristics of Endotracheal Tubes with the Carbon Dioxide Laser: An Experimental Study. Ed Treyve, MD, Gale E. Thompson, MD, C. Thomas Yarington, Jr., MD.

Management of the Laser Ignited Explosion Injury of the Tracheobronchial Tree. Victor L. Schramm, Jr., MD, Peter Ferson, MD, Douglas E. Mattox, MD.

Endoscopic Findings in Sarcoidosis: Characteristics and Correlation with Radiographic Staging and Bronchial Biopsy Yield. John Armstrong, MD, Jan R. Radke, MD, Paul A. Kvale, MD.

Flexible Fiberoptic Bronchoscopy and Chest Roentgenogram in the Evaluation of Patients with Head and Neck Malignancies. Terry Garfinkle, MD, Robert A. Weisman, MD, James C. Denneny, III, MD.

Bronchogenic Cryotherapy. David R. Sanderson, MD, H. Bryan Neel III, MD, Robert S. Fontana, MD.

Congenital Tracheal Stenosis. Bruce Benjamin, MD, D. H. Cohen, MD, J. Pitkin, MD.

Histopathology of Acquired Subglottic Stenosis — A Documented Case Report. Gabriel F. Tucker, Jr., MD, Leonard Newton, MD, Robert J. Ruben, MD.

Televising and Videotaping of Microsurgery of the Larynx. Eiji Yanagisawa, MD.

A New Universal Bi-valved Speculum Direct Laryngoscope. George Berci, MD, Paul H. Ward, MD.

Epidemiology of Esophageal Cancer in Lin Xian. George Wu, MD.

Surgical Repair in Hypopharyngeal and Cervical Esophageal Cancer — Analysis of 164 Patients. D. F. N. Harrison, MD.

Abnormal Esophageal Manometry in Globus Hystericus. Toribio C. Flores, MD, Frederick S. Cross, MD, Richard D. Jones, PhD.

Esophageal Hiatal Hernia in Infants and Children. Blair Fearon, MD, Israel Brama, MD, Roman Dykun, MD.

Disorders of Swallowing. John E. Rayl, MD.

Duplication of the Cervical Esophagus. Diran O. Mikaelian, MD, John J. O'Keefe, MD, Simon K. Simonian, MD.

Horseradish Peroxidase Studies in Animals with Neuromuscular Transpositions. G. David Neal, MD, Dwight Sutton, PhD, Charles W. Cummings, MD.

The Role of Videotaping in the Diagnosis and Management of Laryngeal Cancer. Horst R. Konrad, MD, John Bussen, Skip Griswold, Dan Hopla, MD.

Management of Laryngotracheoesophageal Cleft. Robin T. Cotton, MD.

Grassheads in the Tracheobronchial Tree: Two Different Outcomes. Mary J. Spencer, MD, Victoria E. Millet, MD, James P. Dudley, MD.

Epiglottic Laryngoplasty for Severe Glottic Stenosis. Harvey M. Tucker, MD, Steven M. Sobol, MD.

AMERICAN LARYNGOLOGICAL ASSOCIATION

May 10-11, 1981

Surgical Approach to the Medial Orbital Wall: 527 Patients. Donald N. F. Harrison, MD.

Histochemical Studies on the Human Intrinsic Laryngeal Muscles and Their Innervation. Leslie T. Malmgren, MD, Richard R. Gacek, MD.

Laryngeal Paresis and Paralysis of Central Origin. Paul H. Ward, MD, David G. Hanson, MD, George Berci, MD.

Nasopharyngeal Juvenile Fibroma: 321 Cases. Ricardo Tapia Acuna, MD.

Daniel C. Baker, Jr., Memorial Lecture. The Chinese Health System. Dr. George Wu.

The Treatment of Carcinoma of the Epiglottis: An Update. Joseph B. Nadol, MD.

Hypothyroidism Following Treatment for Head and Neck Cancer. Donald P. Vrabec, MD.

The Significance of Positive Bronchial Cytology in the Presence of Squamous Cell Carcinoma of the Upper Aerodigestive Tract. Jonas T. Johnson, MD, Joseph Turner, MD.

Laryngeal Reinnervation for Unilateral Vocal Cord Paralysis: Long-Term Results. Harvey M. Tucker, MD.

Metachronous Second Primaries in Head and Neck Cancer. Robert H. Maisel, MD, Hubert Vermeersch, MD.

Laryngeal Complications of Nasogastric Tubes: A Prospective Clinical Study. Robert A. Sofferman, MD, Richard Hubbell, MD.

Laryngeal Injuries Secondary to Nasal Gastric Tubes. Michael Friedman, MD, Emanuel Skolnik, MD.

Anesthesia for Laryngeal Surgery in the Infant and Child. William Brumitt, MD, Blair Fearon, MD, Israel Brama, MD.

Documentation in Pediatric Laryngology. Bruce Benjamin, OBE, DLO, FRACS.

Pseudo-Laryngeal Paralysis: A Post Intubation Complication. Seymour R. Cohen, MD, Kenneth A. Geller, MD, Jeffrey W. Birns, MD.

Vertical Partial Laryngectomy for Bilateral Glottic Carcinoma with Fixation. Hugh F. Biller, MD, William Lawson, MD.

The Cleveland Clinic Foundation's Experience with Post Total Laryngectomy Voice Restoration Following Tracheal-Esophageal Puncture. Benjamin G. Wood, MD, Melinda H. Rusnov, MA, Harvey M. Tucker, MD, Howard L. Levine, MD.

Limitations of the Blom-Singer Technique for Voice Restoration. Jagdev Singh, MD, Jack L. Gluckman, MD, J. Oliver Donegan, MD.

Further Experiences with Vocie Restoration After Total Laryngectomy. Mark I. Singer, MD, Eric D. Blom, PhD.

Prosthetic Vocal Rehabilitation Post Laryngectomy with Voice Button. Brian F. McCabe, MD, William R. Panje, MD.

Voice Restoration After Laryngectomy — Where Do We Stand in 1981? Jerome C. Goldstein, MD.

The Status of Chemotherapy in the Multi-Disciplined Treatment of Advanced Head and Neck Cancer: Progress Report 1981. Thomas J. Ervin, MD, Daniel Miller, MD, Richard L. Fabian, MD, Ralph Weichselbaum, MD, Marshall Posner, MD.

Laryngeal and Subglottic Stenosis — Conservative Approach. Sidney A. Peerless, MD, Alter G. Peerless, MD.

Laryngotracheoplasty in Children. John N. G. Evans, MD, Robin T. Cotton, MD.

AMERICAN LARYNGOLOGICAL, RHINOLOGICAL AND OTOLOGICAL SOCIETY, INC.

May 12-14, 1981

Chemotherapy for Salivary Gland Cancer. J. Y. Suen, MD, M. E. Johns, MD.

Respiratory Distress after Recurrent Laryngeal Nerve Sectioning for Adductor Spastic Dysphonia. J. R. Salassa, MD.

Simultaneous Video Recording of Airway and Polysomnograph During Obstructive Sleep Apnea. T. E. Rojewski, MD.

Test Battery Assessment of Auditory Perceptual Dysfunction in Children. F. E. Musiek, PhD.

Otosclerosis, I.R.P. and T.O.R.P. J. L. Sheehy, MD.

Proximal Facial Nerve Exposure in Bell's Palsy Surgery. D. W. Goin, MD.

Panel Discussion: Pathogenesis of Otitis Media. M. M. Paparella, MD.

The Nasal Acilia Syndrome. James P. Dudley, MD.

The Mechanical Basis of Septoplasty. T. M. Davidson, MD.

The "Light Reflex" Tip Plasty Surgical Application of a New Theory in Tip Esthetics. N. Fanous, MD.

Long-Term Evaluation of the Use of Systemic Estrogen in Familial Hemorrhagic Telangectasia. D. F. N. Harrison, MD.

Pyriform Sinus Carcinoma. H. Goepfert, MD.

Lymphoma and the Parotid Gland. R. D. Nichols, MD.

Ludwig's Angina, an Update. James H. Kelly, MD.

The Argon Laser in Reconstructive and Otologic Surgery. J. R. Di Bartolomeo, MD.

Rhinologic Surgery with the Carbon Dioxide Laser. G. T. Simpson, MD.

Experimental Skin Incisions Made with the Laser. C. W. Norris, MD.

Microprobe Analysis of Intracochlear Fluids. R. C. Bone, MD.

A Ten-Year Statistical Follow-Up of 1142 Consecutive Cases of Cholesteatoma: The Closed vs the Open Technique. James S. Brown, MD.

Malignant External Otitis. Melvin Strauss, MD.

Regional Flap Reconstruction During "Extended" Supraglottic Laryngectomy. B. G. Wood, MD.

Prosthetic Management of Oral Commissure Burns. G. R. Holt, MD.

Transseptal Dacryocystorhinostomy. Bruce H. Berryhill, MD.

Lateral Tarsal Strip for Correction of Paralytic Ectropion. F. F. Becker, MD.

Panel Discussion: Expectations from Single Channel Cochlear Implants. Blair Simmons, MD, William F. House, MD, Donald Eddington, PhD, Earl Schubert, PhD, Robin P. Michelson, MD.

AMERICAN OTOLOGICAL SOCIETY, INC.

May 9-10, 1981

Mini-panel on Experiences with Middle Ear Ventilating Tubes. Ralph F. Naunton, MD, Beverly W. Armstrong, MD, Ralph J. Caparosa, MD.

The Use of Tympanostomy Tubes in Otitis Media. William L. Meyerhoff, MD, G. Scott Giebink, MD, Donald Shea.

Auditory Processing Abilities in Children with Previous Middle Ear Effusion. Kimberley Hoffman-Lawless, MA, Robert W. Keith, PhD, Robin T. Cotton, MD.

Recurrent Middle Ear Effusion in Childhood: Implications of Temporary Auditory Deprivation for Language and Learning. Robert J. Sak, MA, Robert J. Ruben, MD.

Mini-panel on Experiences with Testing of Eustachian Tube Function. Charles Bluestone, MD, James L. Sheehy, MD, James Jerger, PhD.

Neural Connections Between the Middle Ear, Eustachian Tube and Brain: Implications for the Reflex Control of Tubal Function. Avrim R. Eden, MD.

Mini-panel on Menière's Disease. Michael M. Paparella, MD, Bruce Proctor, MD, Harold F. Schuknecht, MD.

Endolymphatic Duct Obstruction from a Jugular Bulb Diverticulum. Robert Jahrsdoerfer, MD, Wayne S. Cail, MD, Robert W. Cantrell, MD.

Central Vestibular Signs, Posterior Fossa Pathology and CT Regional Blood Brain Circulation. Arvind Kumar, MD, Nicholas Torok, MD, Galdino Valvassori, MD.

Mini-panel on Control of Tinnitus. John W. House, MD, John J. Shea, MD, Victor Goodhill, MD.

The Total Energy Concept of Noise Trauma and its Limitations — an Update. W. Dixon Ward, PhD, Arndt J. Duvall, III, MD, Christopher W. Turner.

Mini-panel of Treatment of Bell's Palsy. Jack L. Pulec, MD, Eberhard Stennert, MD, Richard R. Gacek, MD.

Neural Generators of the Brainstem Evoked Responses: Results from Human Intracranial Recordings. Aage R. Moller, PhD, Peter Jannetta, MD, Margareta B. Moller, MD, PhD.

Mini-panel on Stapes Surgery. Mendell Robinson, MD, T. Manford McGee, MD, J. Brown Farrior, MD.

The Use of Bio-Inert Ceramic Implants in Middle Ear Surgery. Klaus Jahnke, MD, Dietrich Plester, MD.

A Pattern of Hearing Loss Originating in the Cochlea Associated with Hypoxia or Anoxic Anoxia at Birth. Gretchen Probst, MAT, Nigel R. T. Pashley, MD, BS.

COMBINED MEETING
SOCIETY OF HEAD AND NECK SURGEONS AND AMERICAN SOCIETY FOR HEAD AND NECK SURGERY
Hyatt Regency, Phoenix, Arizona
March 9-11, 1981

Scientific Program Summary

Extracapsular Spread of Tumors in Cervical Node Metastasis. J. Johnson, L. Barnes, E. Myers, V. Schramm, D. Borochovitz.

Prostaglandin Synthesis Inhibitor Produces Marked Regression of Head and Neck Epidermoid Carcinoma. W. Panje.

Can Vocal Cord Carcinoma in Situ Be Managed by a Watchful Waiting Policy? B. Hintz, A. Kagan, P. Chan, H. Nussbaum, H. Gilbert, A. Rao.

Erythrocyte Polyamine Determinations in Head and Neck Cancer Patients. M. Johns, C. Shideler, J. Shipe, M. Wills, J. Savory, R. Cantrell.

Singer-Blom Voice Restoration Procedure. S. Wetmore, M. Johns, S. Baker.

Selective Myotomy for Voice Rehabilitation After Total Laryngectomy. M. Singer, E. Blom.

Retropharyngeal Implantable Voice Box for Vocal Restoration. J. Fredrickson, G. Lafond.

Contralateral Laryngoplasty Following Supraglottic Laryngectomy with Vertical Extension. W. Friedman, G. Katsantonis.

Immediate Reconstruction of Mandibular Defects with a Composite Sternocleidomastoid Musculo-clavicular Graft. D. Barnes, R. Ossoff, G. Sisson, B. Pecaro.

Pectoralis Major Myocutaneous Flap for a Single Stage Reconstruction Following Laryngopharyngectomy. R. Hayden, T. Briant, D. Bryce.

Comparative Study of Conservation vs. Resection and Reconstruction of the Mandible. P. Caracciolo.

Pharyngoesophageal Reconstruction with Gastric Transposition. M. Bains, R. Spiro, J. Shah, E. Strong.

Surgical Treatment of Recurrent Benign Mixed Tumors. R. Piorkowski, O. Guillamondegui.

New Technique for Wide-field Exposure of the Base of the Skull. H. Biller, J. Shugar, Y. Krespi.

Prospects for Improved Survival in Head and Neck Cancer Using a Kinetically Based Adjuvant Chemotherapy Protocol. H. Shaw, V. Dalley, B. Hill, L. Price.

Cisplatinum Therapy of Adenoid Cystic Carcinoma. V. Schramm, C. Schrodes, E. Myers.

Radiotherapy for Melanomas of the Head and Neck. A. Harwood, V. Lawson.

Cis-Platinum and 5-Fluorouracil as Initial Therapy for Advanced Epidermoid Cancer of the Head and Neck. A. Weaver, S. Flemming, H. Vandenberg, M. Al-Sarraf.

Society of Head and Neck Surgeons: The Hayes Martin Lecture. Dr. Richard Jesse.

Preoperative CIS-Platinum (DDP) and Bleomycin (BLM) in Patients with Head and Neck Squamous Carcinoma (HNSCC): Prognostic Factors for Tumor Response: The Head and Neck Contracts Program. S. Baker, R. Makuch, G. Wolf.

Preoperative Chemo-radiotherapy for Advanced Head and Neck Cancer. N. Pearlman, A. Meyers, F. Johnson, N. DiBella.

Comparative Study of Complications Following Planned Post-operative and Pre-operative Radiation Therapy in Head and Neck Cancer. R. Mantravadi, E. Skolnik, E. Applebaum.

Panel: Reconstruction in Head and Neck Cancer Surgery. Dr. M. Jurkiewicz (Moderator), Dr. J. Fredrickson, Dr. W. Panje, Dr. S. Ariyan.

Carcinoma of the Base of Tongue. M. Razack, K. Sako, J. Patel.

Management of Advanced Carcinoma of the Tongue by Total Glossectomy Without Laryngectomy. M. Effron, J. Johnson, E. Myers, H. Curtin, O. Beery, B. Sigler.

Survival Rate of 100 Patients with Carcinoma of Floor of Mouth Treated by Monobloc Resection. R. Barton.

Epidermoid Carcinoma of the Palate. J. Evans, J. Shah.

Role of Initial Modality in Treatment of Squamous Cell Carcinoma of the Tongue. M. Razack, K. Sako, J. Patel.

Esthesioneuroblastoma. J. Shah, J. Feghali.

Management of Carotid Body Tumors with Special Reference to Vascular Problems. I. Rosen, J. Palmer, W. Lougheed, M. Goldberg, R. Mustard.

Auricular Malignancies: When is Chemosurgery (Mohs' Technique) Necessary? R. Bumsted, R. Ceilley, R. Crumley.

Role of Parotidectomy for Skin Cancer of the Head and Neck. G. Jackson, A. Ballantyne.

Regional Lymph Node Management and Outcome in 100 Head and Neck Melanoma Patients. R. Olson, J. Woods, E. Soule.

Thyroid Cancer — Some Basic Considerations. H. Wanebo, W. Andrew.

Locally Invasive Well Differentiated Carcinoma of the Thyroid. H. Cody, J. Shah.

Pre-operative Selective Venous Catheterization — A Basis for Conservative Parathyroidectomy. E. Shannon, Y. Rapoport, D. Ayalon, H. Miller.

Parathyroid Autotransplantation in Parathyroid Disease and in Total Thyroidectomies: Indications in 100 Cases. A. Katz.

Association of Fibrous Tumors of the Facial Skeleton with Hyperparathyroidism — New Clinical Syndrome. I. Rosen, J. Palmer.

Sarcoidosis, Hypercalcemia and Primary Hyperparathyroidism: The Vicissitudes of Diagnosis. V. Schweitzer, R. Nishiyama, N. Thompson.

Ann Otol 90:1981

BEN H. SENTURIA LECTURE

LEAKING LABYRINTH LESIONS, DEAFNESS, TINNITUS AND DIZZINESS

VICTOR GOODHILL, MD, FACS

LOS ANGELES, CALIFORNIA

The remarkable integrity of the finely balanced membranous labyrinth is occasionally disrupted, resulting in fistulae of various types in a number of locations. Such leaking labyrinth lesions can be of congenital origin, due to various types of malformations. They may be caused by destructive diseases such as syphilis, by many variants of acute and chronic otomastoiditis, and sequelae of otosclerosis surgery, and finally, as results of a variety of traumatic disruptions of labyrinthine integrity. Deafness, dizziness, and tinnitus are frequent symptoms and sequelae may include meningitis and other intracranial complications. The clinical consideration of leaking labyrinth lesions must always be considered in otologic diagnoses.

INTRODUCTION

Labyrinthine fistulae, or "leaking labyrinth lesions," can occur both internally and externally. Internal leaks are defined as occurring within the labyrinth and can occur between the various components of the membranous endolymph-perilymph labyrinthine system. External leaks are defined as occurring between the labyrinthine membranous components and the middle ear and/or mastoid pneumatic air spaces, as well as between these membranous components and cerebrospinal fluid spaces (Fig. 1). Complex fistulae of intralabyrinthine and extralabyrinthine forms have been shown to cause a number of symptom complexes including deafness, dizziness and tinnitus.

Leaking labyrinth lesions can be caused by congenital malformations, syphilis, otomastoiditis of various types, otosclerosis surgery, and trauma.

CONGENITAL MALFORMATIONS

The "fissula ante fenestram" anterior to the oval window is open in the fetus.[1] It extends from the middle ear to the labyrinthine vestibule through the otic capsule and has been observed partly open and partly closed as late as the second year of infancy, and may persist in the adult.

Congenital round window and oval window malformations of various types with or without fistulae can occur in utero and may persist into infancy, childhood and adult life.

Mayer[2,3] first described a variety of microfissures in adult temporal bones including 1) a fissure between the posterior canal ampulla and the round window niche, and 2) a fissure superior to the oval window between the tympanum and the vestibule.

A number of years ago, prior to the stapes surgery era, I found congenital round window fistulae on tympanic explorations in two children with slowly progressive bilateral mixed sensorineural/conductive hearing losses. Normal mobile ossicles were present. In both patients clear fluid was seen in the round window niche. I considered the fluid to be due to infiltration of local anesthetic solution into the middle ear. However, the fluid repeatedly welled up in the niche after aspiration. The fluid was undoubtedly perilymph coming from small bony fistulae in the inferior portion of the round window niche.

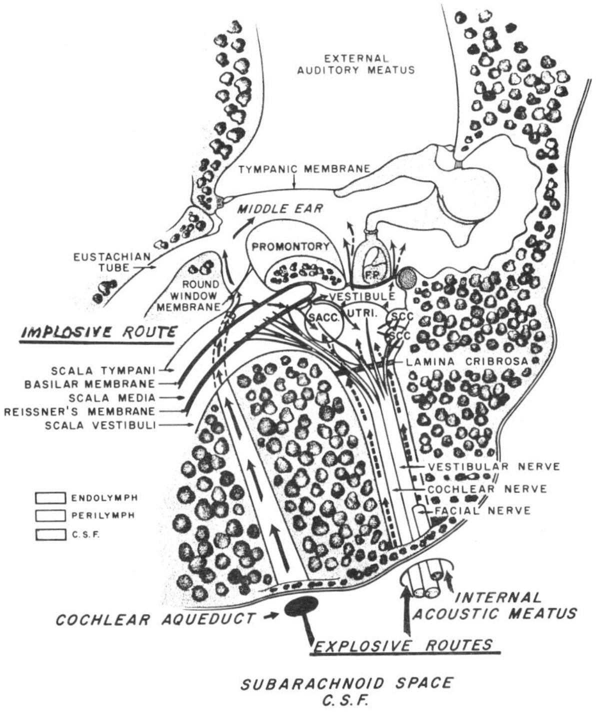

Fig. 1. Possible pathways of implosive and explosive forces in inner ear. (Reprinted with permission.[21])

From the Department of Surgery, Head and Neck Division, University of California at Los Angeles.

Presented under the auspices of the St. Louis Otological Foundation before the St. Louis Ear, Nose and Throat Club, November 15, 1978.

REPRINTS — Victor Goodhill, MD, Otosurgical Group Medical Clinic, Inc., 469 North Roxbury Drive, Beverly Hills, CA 90210.

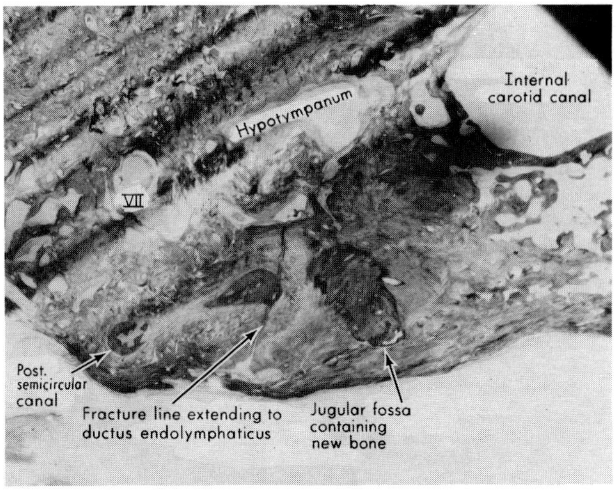

Fig. 2. Hypotympanum. The two limbs of posterior semicircular canal solidly cast in new bone, from which fracture line diverges, extending to ductus endolymphaticus. Superior level of jugular fossa also contains new bone. VII - Seventh nerve. (Reprinted with permission.[7])

As my awareness of window fistulae increased, I also found fistulae in several adults with combined cochlear-conductive hearing losses preoperatively attributed to mixed cochlear-conductive otosclerosis. In one such patient whose anomalous monopod nonotosclerotic fixed footplate was mobilized on one side, I subsequently found a mobile anomalous monopod stapes on the other side, accompanied by a round window niche abnormality. The round window membrane was widely exposed, larger than average, with an excellent reflex on stapes palpation. However, clear fluid welled up in the bottom of the round window niche, following repeated aspiration. This small leaking defect in the bony margin at the inferior aspect of the round window membrane insertion was sealed with a perichondrial graft, followed by closure of a 20 dB air-bone gap.

In a study of congenital cerebrospinal otorrhea recently reported by Gacek and Leipzig[4] it was noted that leaks can occur through the round window membrane into the middle ear as a result of a large cochlear aqueduct. This mix of CSF and perilymph can also leak into the middle ear via Hyrtl's fissure, a bony cleft inferior to the round window.

A congenital cyst of the oval window recently reported by Lahovary[5] in a child with recurrent pneumococcal meningitis was identified by scintigraphy as a middle ear CSF leak. At surgical exploration clear fluid was seen coming from a stapedial footplate cyst. The cyst actually represented a congenital malformation between the stapedial footplate and the labyrinthine perilymph pool.

Dufour et al[6] described a patient with recurrent meningitis and unilateral deafness in whom surgical exploration revealed a similar CSF leak through the stapedial footplate. These reports enrich an already significant literature on the subjects of recurrent meningitis and congenital oval window or round window leaking labyrinths.

SYPHILITIC LESIONS

In an otopathologic study of 16 luetic temporal bones which I reported in 1939[7] I described a fracture line in one temporal bone between the hypotympanum and the endolymphatic duct (Fig. 2).

The "syndrome of Hennebert" a term coined by Buys[8] refers to eye deviations and/or dizziness which result from transcanal pneumatic tympanic compression and rarefaction. Pathological openings between the middle ear and the labyrinth have been clinically suspected for some time in patients with Hennebert's sign (positive fistula sign). In the past, a positive Hennebert's sign was considered to be diagnostic of labyrinthine syphilis, but this is now disputed. Kohut et al[9] have reported positive Hennebert's signs in cases of minute perilymph fistulae associated with vertigo without hearing loss. Nadol[10] has reported several cases of positive fistula signs with intact tympanic membranes.

At the present time, relationships between a positive Hennebert's sign and temporal bone lues remain unclear.

Recently, at surgical exploration of an ear in a patient who had fluctuating hearing loss, tinnitus and vertigo with a positive luetic serology, I found a perilymph leak from several bony dehiscences inferior to the round window membrane attachment. These dehiscences were sealed with perichondrium resulting in a 15 dB improvement in hearing, and a 50% air-bone gap closure.

OTOMASTOIDITIS FISTULAE

Fistulae of the labyrinth in acute and chronic otomastoiditis have long been known clinically. Vertigo, tinnitus and sudden or gradual deafness still occur as complications of otitis media and mastoiditis.[11]

Labyrinthine fistula is uncommon during the course of acute otomastoiditis. It may occur with acute fulminating *β-Streptococcus hemolyticus* infections and may accompany other complications, such as seventh nerve paralysis.

The most common sign of fistula is vertigo accompanied by spontaneous nystagmus, which may be manifest or which may be detected only on electronystagmographic vestibular examination. Dry calorization electronystagmography (ENG) will usually show a hypoactive response, and occasionally a hyperactive response.[12]

Labyrinthine fistula as a complication of otomastoiditis is most commonly the sequel of ker-

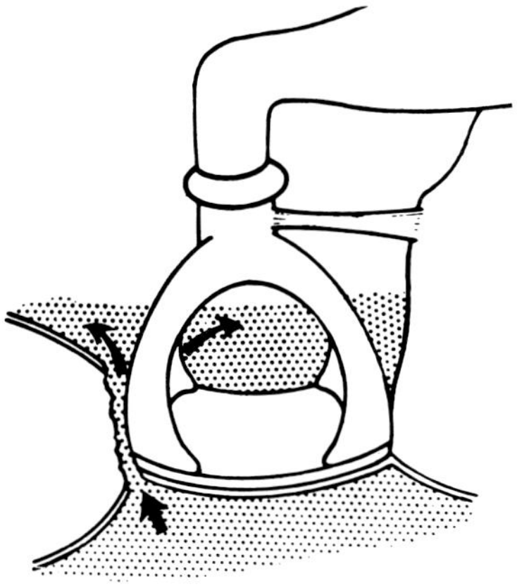

Fig. 3. Peribasal mobilization. The chronic perilymphatic fistula may follow a simple peribasal mobilization. Cross-hatched area - Perilymph; arrows - Direction of flow. This has been observed in several cases, in one case almost 10 years after operation. (From English, GM, ed. Otolaryngology, Vol II. Hagerstown: Harper and Row, 1976. Reprinted with permission.)

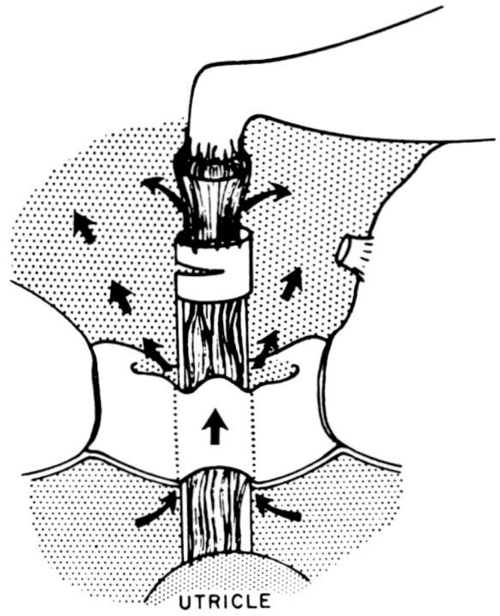

Fig. 4. Displaced polyethylene prosthesis that has perforated a tissue graft and is now in contact with the utricle, producing a positional type of equilibrium disturbance along with a conductive hearing loss. Cross-hatched area - Perilymph pooling at site of penetration of the prosthesis. Arrows - Direction of flow. There is scar tissue between the top of the prosthesis and the lenticular process of the incus, also extending down along the lumen of the tube into the vestibule in current contact with the utricle. This is a common type of perilymphatic fistula and can be seen not only with polyethylene prostheses, but also with various types of Teflon® pistons and other plastic prostheses. (From English GM, ed. Otolaryngology, Vol II. Hagerstown: Harper and Row, 1976. Reprinted with permission.)

atoma (cholesteatoma) or tympanosclerosis although it may be due to granulomatous or polypoid disease. The most common location for such a fistula is in the dome of the horizontal semicircular canal. The fistula may be total, with complete exposure of the perilymphatic space, or subtotal, with bone erosion and only marginal exposure of the perilymphatic space endosteum.

A fistula may occur through the oval window following necrosis of the stapedial arch and footplate, or through the bony cochlear wall. With such a fistula, there will be a slow, but occasionally rather sudden hearing loss due to cochlear involvement, with vertigo, and/or tinnitus as a concomitant. Comparable lesions occur occasionally in the round window niche, with rupture through the round window membrane and fistulization into scala tympani.

The management of a surgically encountered fistula requires delicate microsurgical removal of the specific etiologic lesion and closure of the fistulous area in the otic capsule by a tissue graft of either tragal perichondrium or fascia temporalis.

OTOSCLEROSIS SURGERY FISTULAE

Kessel, in 1878[13] in making the first deliberate oval window opening in extracting the stapes in otosclerosis, certainly created a temporary or, in some cases, a permanent leaking labyrinth. Thus, for more than a century we should have been aware of oval window leaks produced iatrogenically by surgeons in otosclerosis surgery. Clinical awareness came much later.

Miot[14] performed many stapes operations for otosclerosis. These were undoubtedly accompanied by some unhealed leaking labyrinths, since no attempt was made to seal the surgically created labyrinthine fistula. Such persistent surgically created fistulae may have been related to the condemnation of his work which stopped otosclerosis surgery for half a century.

In the early rare promontory and later common Lempert semicircular canal fenestration operations, leaking labyrinths were deliberately created surgically, hopefully as only temporary surgical leaks. Lempert type fenestrations probably resulted in fewer "dead ears" proportionately than stapedectomy procedures, because the technique always required that the surgically created fistula was deliberately sealed with the tympanomeatal flap.

In modern stapes surgery, surgical oval window fistulae (leaks) are also deliberately created, but the term "fistulization" has rarely been used to describe the essential part of the operation. When an otosclerotic stapes was mobilized in early mobilization techniques by transincudal pressure or by fracturing footplate margins, thus restoring mobility to a previously fixed stapes arch, a temporary fistula in the oval window was created (hopefully temporary) (Fig. 3). We now know that perilymph leaked out, but it was considered an incidental part of the procedure. No attempts were made to seal the leak.

Following the introduction of prostheses in stapedectomy surgery, otologists were rudely shaken into an awareness that such iatrogenic leaking labyrinths might continue to leak indefinitely with a variety of possible sequelae including irreversible labyrinthopathies, with deafness, dizziness and even meningitis (Fig. 4). Fistulae were found as we began to explore postoperative stapes cases with poor results. Not only did some primary fistulae continue to leak

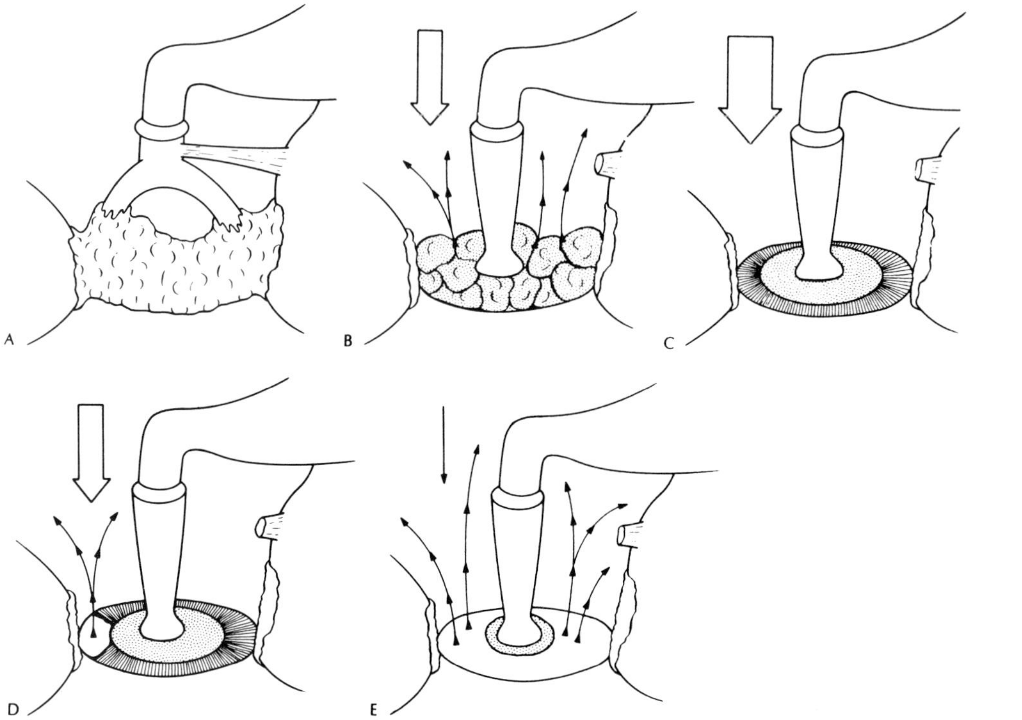

Fig. 5. Sequence of events from A) preoperative otosclerotic state (fixed stapes) to B) first postoperative day, in which a fistula is always present, to C) final ideal result with completely hermetically sealed oval window-to-incus strut. D) Partial and major perilymph leaks, causing backsplash and partial conductive loss, and E) major backsplash with major conductive loss, indicate relationship between size of fistula and extent of conductive hearing loss. (From English GM, ed. Otolaryngology, Vol II. Hagerstown: Harper and Row, 1976. Reprinted with permission.)

indefinitely, but in many successful stapes cases with primary healing and excellent hearing, secondary fistulae began to occur and finally were recognized. Such clinical recognition however continues to evade the attention of some surgeons even today.[15]

A variety of poststapedectomy problems related to fistulae were reported.[16-18] The early reports placed much emphasis on partial or complete cochlear damage resulting in dead ears. We later learned that the partial or complete *conductive loss phenomena* which occur in stapes surgery (which I called the "backsplash phenomenon") is really due to unhealed fistulization and is the sign of a simple leaking labyrinth without sensorineural hearing loss indicative of cochlear damage (Fig. 5). Thus, otosclerosis surgery has been and still is a major cause of leaking labyrinths.

TRAUMATIC LESIONS

Traumatic labyrinthine fistulae can result from a number of varieties of temporal bone injuries.[19]

Blunt blows or penetrating temporal bone trauma can cause cerebrospinal fluid fistulae accompanying tegmen fractures, with or without accompanying labyrinthine perilymph fistulae from fractures through oval window, round window, cochlear promontory and/or semicircular canals (Fig. 6). Cerebrospinal fluid and perilymph fistulae can coexist. Two potential mechanisms, *explosive* and

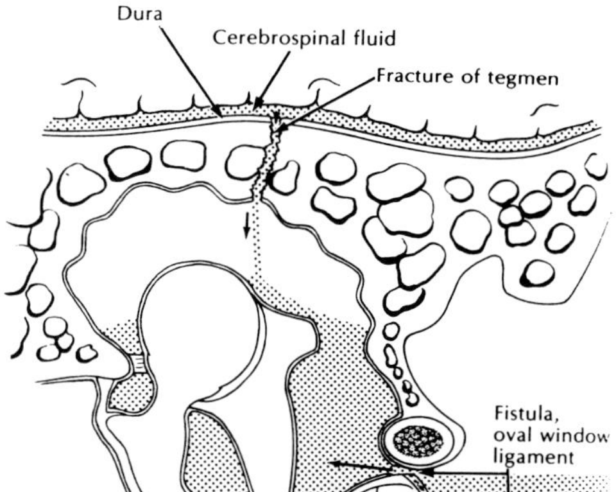

Fig. 6. Diagrammatic representation of the most common potential pathways for posttraumatic CSF otorrhea: through a tegmental fracture, OW or RW rupture. (From Shulman J. Traumatic diseases of the ear and temporal bone. In: Goodhill V, ed. Ear diseases, deafness and dizziness. Hagerstown: Harper and Row, 1979. Reprinted with permission.)

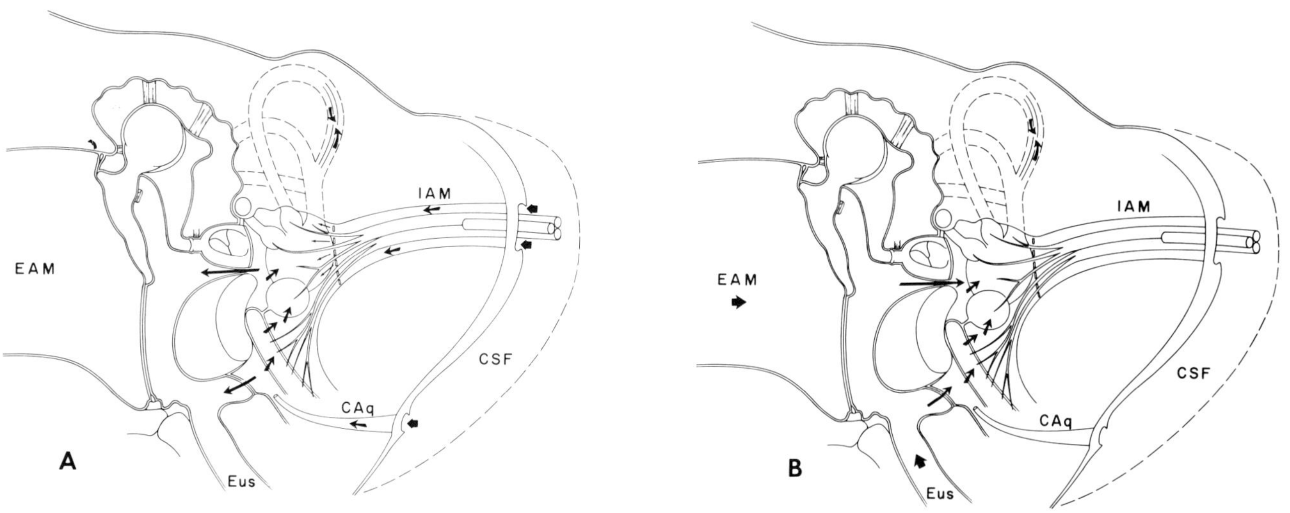

Fig. 7. A) Explosive routes for labyrinthine membrane ruptures from CSF system via cochlear aqueduct or internal auditory meatus. B) Implosive routes for labyrinthine membrane ruptures from middle ear, eustachian tube, and external ear. (Reprinted with permission.[22])

implosive, can explain perilymphatic fistulae due to trauma.

Traumatic events which can produce fistulae are: 1) head trauma; 2) blunt ear trauma; 3) penetrating ear trauma; 4) acoustic/blast trauma; 5) tubotympanic compression trauma; and 6) flying and diving barotrauma.

Surgically encountered perilymph fistulae as seen in the middle ear via promontory fractures, or from oval window and/or round window membrane breaks are frequently accompanied by surgically invisible intralabyrinthine perilymph-endolymph fistulae due to internal membrane breaks. The latter can occur alone.

Hydrodynamic (CSF) or *aerodynamic* (tubotympanic) routes can be responsible for such membrane breaks and they can coexist in some cases.

Hydrodynamic Explosive Fistula Mechanisms via the Cerebrospinal Fluid System. Labyrinthine perilymph-endolymph systems are linked to arterial, venous and cerebrospinal fluid hydrodynamic forces. The most crucial CSF-perilymph relationships function either through the cochlear aqueduct or through internal auditory canal neural foramina. Sudden CSF pressure surges to the perilymph system can cause explosive fistulae.

Variations in patency between perilymph-CSF connections, cochlear aqueduct and internal auditory canal can be significant.[20-27]

Explosive fistulae can result from either self-induced diaphragmatic splinting stresses or from other Valsalva forces, environmental barotrauma or head trauma.

The *cochlear aqueduct route* to *scala tympani* can cause leaks from round window membrane and/or internal breaks and leaks through Reissner's basilar, saccular, utricular or semicircular canal membranes (Fig. 7A).

The *internal auditory canal route* to *scala vestibuli* can cause leaks from oval window via footplate or through oval window ligament especially anterior to the footplate margin and/or similar internal labyrinthine membrane breaks producing explosive fistulae resulting in hearing loss, vertigo and tinnitus.

Aerodynamic Implosive Fistula Mechanisms. Aerodynamic pressure surges via the tubotympanic system communicate with both round window membrane and oval window footplate and ligament areas as routes for *implosive fistulae* (Fig. 7B). Self-induced forceful eustachian tube inflation forces or tubotympanic Valsalva forces in flying and diving can cause implosive round window and/or oval window leaks, with chain reaction internal labyrinth membrane breaks producing implosive fistulae with resulting hearing loss, vertigo and tinnitus.

PERILYMPH LEAKS DUE TO HEAD TRAUMA

Both closed and open head injuries can produce perilymph leaks, a number of which have been reported.[20,28-30] If fractures occur they may also result in CSF fistulae, via explosive and/or implosive routes. I reported three such cases as examples.[31]

PERILYMPH LEAKS DUE TO BLUNT EAR TRAUMA

Blunt blows to the auricle can produce perilymph fistulae. Open hand slaps to the auricle which usually produce large tympanic membrane perforations can also produce accompanying perilymph fistulae. Two illustrative cases were reported by me.[31]

LABYRINTHINE LEAKS PRODUCED BY PENETRATING EAR TRAUMA.

Gunshot wounds, slag injuries and iatrogenic injuries in attempts to remove external ear canal and middle ear foreign bodies can be causes of penetrating perilymph leaks accompanying tympanic membrane-ossicular injuries. Oval window, round window, and intralabyrinthine lesions frequently occur due to labyrinthine capsule fractures.

DOUBLE WINDOW LEAKS AND INTERNAL MEMBRANE BREAKS DUE TO ACOUSTIC/BLAST TRAUMA

High intensity acute acoustic trauma (not related to ordinary noise induced hearing loss) and/or blast from explosives can produce perilymph fistulae with or without tympanic membrane ruptures. A previously reported case followed a single shot from a magnum revolver fired at a firing range. It caused severe right otalgia, tinnitus, deafness and violent dizziness. At surgery, an extensive friable fibrous network surrounded oval window and round window leaks. The fibrous compartments were all filled with perilymph. Following repair of the fistulae there was immediate relief of dizziness and a marked diminution of tinnitus but there was no return of hearing.[31]

LEAKS DUE TO TUBOTYMPANIC COMPRESSION TRAUMA

Forced "tubal clearing" done voluntarily by violent closed nose blowing can produce perilymph leaks.

LEAKS DUE TO FLYING AND DIVING BAROTRAUMA

Round window leaks in aviators have been recently described in a report by Tingley and MacDougall.[32] They described two patients. In one there is an example of a susceptible individual, namely, a person flying with an upper respiratory infection which jeopardizes middle ear pressure equalization. Their second case dramatically describes a potential catastrophe due to disorientation in a pilot on night or instrument flying when he is being bombarded with misleading vestibular information created by a round window membrane leak.

PROBLEMS OF SUDDEN HEARING LOSS AS IT RELATES TO LABYRINTH LEAKS

Sudden hearing loss, an otologic emergency, can occur as a result of lesions of the external ear, middle ear, inner ear, internal auditory meatus and canal, cerebellopontine angle and lesions of the central nervous system. Although sudden hearing losses may be conductive or sensorineural, mild or moderate in degree, the emphasis here relates to moderate, severe or total cochlear losses. Tinnitus and vertigo are frequent concomitants.

Differential diagnosis must include Menière's disease, labyrinthine complications of previous ear surgery, ear or cranial trauma. In addition, one must consider acoustic trauma, barotrauma, ototoxicity, labyrinthogenic diseases such as syphilis, sudden edema in an eighth nerve tumor,[33] multiple sclerosis, Cogan's syndrome, encephalitis, metastatic carcinoma, and a number of cerebrovascular lesions. Malingering and psychogenic hearing losses must always be considered in the differential diagnosis.

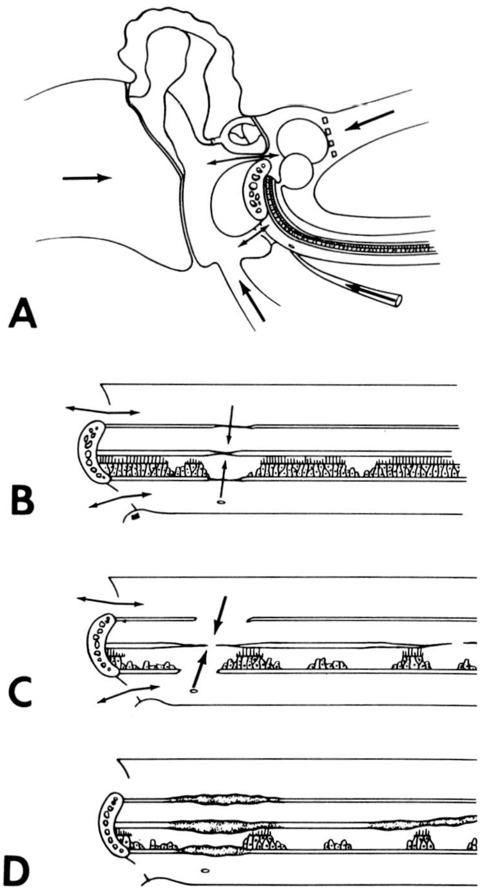

Fig. 8. Potential labyrinthine sequelae: theoretic possibilities. A) Diagram of explosive-plus-implosive rupture routes. B) Minor intralabyrinthine lesion with minimal damage to organ of Corti. C) Major ruptures with persistent intracochlear fistulas. D) Healed intracochlear lesions. (Reprinted with permission.[22])

The term "idiopathic" has been used classically in discussing the lesion of sudden sensorineural hearing loss occurring in a previously presumably normal ear. Various hypotheses and speculations have characterized management based on presumptive viral, vascular, endocrine, allergic, and/or other causes. Thus, therapy has been purely empirical in the past, and continues to be so today in most clinics.

Since the surgical demonstration of perilymphatic leaks from round window membrane and/or oval window ligament breaks[17,22,23,34] in cases either associated with barotrauma and physical exertion or without clear-cut physical stress histories, we must now, therefore, divide all sudden sensorineural hearing losses into 1) a "labyrinthine membrane rupture" group due to verifiable oval window or round window (or both) fistulae, and/or to associated presumptive intralabyrinthine membrane ruptures, due to sudden barotrauma, physical exertion, or to stresses from tubotympanic and/or cerebrospinal fluid systems; and 2) an "idiopathic" group which may be presumptively based in viral, vascular, endocrine, allergic, or other systemic lesions.[35]

The suggested explosive and implosive pathways for membrane ruptures, oval window and round window fistulae and associated intralabyrinthine membrane breaks (Fig. 8), and my clinical findings have been confirmed.[35]

A systemic approach to the management of labyrinth leaks in sudden hearing loss has been described.

The diagnostic criteria for perilymph fistula exploration have been ably summarized by Singleton et al,[36] in a study using discriminant analysis techniques. They point out the importance of consideration of bed rest for the first five days before surgical intervention. In their report surgical intervention with repair of the fistula by perichondrial grafts provided effective control of vertigo very frequently, more frequently than restoration of hearing. This finding is in agreement with my experience.

SOME FINAL CONSIDERATIONS REGARDING MANAGEMENT OF LEAKING LABYRINTHS

Appearance of a Fistula. It is not usually a "rapidly running stream." It appears as a slow limpid clear fluid collection. In the oval window niche it tends to "puddle" anterior to the anterior crus. There is rarely a distinct bony opening either in the footplate or in the circumferential ligament. It is more of a recurrent seepage following gentle suction. In the round window niche it most commonly is seen at the inferior margin of the round window membrane. One does not usually see a "hole" in the round window membrane. Recurrent seepage is seen in the inferior portion of the round window niche.

"Plugging" the Labyrinth Leak. Fistulae are almost always surrounded at least partly by fibrous bands requiring microdissection. Following delicate dissection of fibrous compartments in the window area, very gentle fine suction in anterior oval window area and in round window area is necessary. The extent of fluid leaks may vary from a very rare "gusher" to a very minute, slow, but persistent fluid flow, which may be increased by gentle incudostapedial joint palpation. Jugular compression may give improved visualization by temporarily increasing perilymph flow. The round window membrane is rarely completely visualized. A persistent or recurrent perilymph flow is usually seen from the region of the round window membrane margin, and/or from the anterior pericrural (fissula ante fenestram) oval window region. Endosteum is elevated from the superior and/or inferior round window niche bony margins and/or from the anterior stapedial margin to furnish a base for anchorage of a tragal perichondrium or temporalis fascia graft. Gelfoam® is not a seal. I do not drill away promontory bone overhang in the round window niche. In spite of careful persistent searches there may be no fistula. Obviously this concludes the procedure.

Some Future Concerns. It is desirable that clinical awareness of leaking labyrinthine fistulae will increase. However, it is important that such awareness will *not necessarily* be accompanied by unwarranted dramatic increases in urgent surgery in patients with relatively minor audiovestibular changes, many of which may be temporary and self-limited. Most labyrinth leaks probably heal spontaneously. A trial with bed rest in head elevated position should precede surgery decisions. Final answers to these leaking labyrinth problems will only come from temporal bone pathology studies.

REFERENCES

1. Wolff D, Bellucci RT, Eggston AA. Microscopic anatomy of the temporal bone. Baltimore: Williams & Wilkins, 1957.

2. Mayer O. Uber die Entstehung der spontanfrakturen der labyrinthkapsel und ihre Bedeutung fur die Otosklerose. Z Hals Nasen Ohrenheilkd 1930; 26:261-79.

3. Mayer O. Die Ursache der Knochenneubildung bei der Otosklerose. Acta Otolaryngol (Stockh) 1931; 15:35-7.

4. Gacek R, Leipzig B. Congenital cerebrospinal otorrhea. Ann Otol Rhinol Laryngol 1979; 88:358-65.

5. Lahovary A. Congenital cysts of the oval window. HNO 1978; 26:419-20.

6. Dufour JJ, Wurtele P, Charest Y. Meningite recidivante et fistule de L.C.-R. A travers la platine de l'etrier. J Otolaryngol 1978; 7:119-24.

7. Goodhill V. Syphilis of the ear: a histopathologic study. Ann Otol Rhinol Laryngol 1939; 48:676-707.

8. Buys X. Un nouveau cas de labyrinthite heredo-syphilitique presentant le syndrome de Hennebert. J Med Bruxelles 1911; 16:297-9.

9. Kohut R, Waldorf RA, Haenel JL, Thompson JN. Minute perilymph fistulas: vertigo and Hennebert's sign without hearing loss. Ann Otol Rhinol Laryngol 1979; 88:153-9.

10. Nadol JB. Positive "fistula sign" with an intact tympanic membrane. Arch Otolaryngol 1974; 100:273-8.

11. Goodhill V. Ear diseases, deafness and dizziness. Hagerstown: Harper & Row, 1979, chap 18.

12. Eviatar A, Goodhill V. A dry calorization method for vestibular function. Laryngoscope 1968; 78:1746-55.

13. Kessel J. Uber das mobilisieren des steigbugels durch ausschneiden des Trommelfelles, Hammers und Ambosses bei undurchgangigkeit der Tube. Arch Ohren Nasen Kehlkopfheilkd 1878; 13:69.

14. Miot C. Die la mobilisation de l'etrier. Rev Laryngol 1890; 10:49.

15. Goodhill V. Ear diseases, deafness and dizziness. Hagerstown: Harper & Row, 1979, chap 19.

16. Goodhill V. Conductive loss phenomenon in post stapedectomy perilymphatic fistulae. Laryngoscope 1967; 77:1179-90.

17. Goodhill V. Stapedectomy revisions and "commandments," posterior arch stapedioplasty. Trans Pac Coast Otol Ophthalmol Soc Annu Meet 1974:35-9.

18. Goodhill V. Complications of surgical treatment of otosclerosis. In English G, ed. Otolaryngology. Hagerstown: Harper & Row, 1980: chap 49.

19. Simmons FB. Theory of membrane breaks in sudden hearing loss. Arch Otolaryngol 1968; 88:41-8.

20. Althaus SR. Spontaneous and traumatic perilymphatic fistulas. Laryngoscope 1977; 87:364-71.

21. Goodhill V. Sudden deafness and round window rupture. Laryngoscope 1971; 81:1462-74.

22. Goodhill V. Labyrinthine membrane ruptures in sudden sensorineural hearing loss. Proc R Soc Med 1976; 69:565-72.

23. Goodhill V, Brockman SJ, Harris I, Hantz O. Sudden deafness and labyrinthine window ruptures. Ann Otol Rhinol Laryngol 1973; 82:2-12.

24. Palva T. Cochlear aqueduct in infants. Acta Otolaryngol (Stockh) 1970; 70:83-94.

25. Palva T, Dammert K. Human cochlear aqueduct. Acta Otolaryngol (Stockh) 1969; Suppl 246.

26. Stroud MH, Calcaterra TC. Spontaneous perilymph fistulas. Laryngoscope 1970; 80:479-87.

27. Tonkin JP, Fagan P. Rupture of the round window membrane. J Laryngol Otol 1975; 89:733-56.

28. Fee GA. Traumatic perilymphatic fistulas. Arch Otolaryngol 1968; 88:477-80.

29. Fernandes CMC. Labyrinthine membrane rupture: a cause of post traumatic vertigo. S Afr J Surg 1977; 15:71-4.

30. Healey GB, Friedman JM, Strong MS. Vestibular and auditory findings of perilymphatic fistula. A review of 40 cases. Trans Am Acad Ophthalmol Otolaryngol 1976; 82:44-9.

31. Goodhill V. Traumatic fistulae. J Laryngol Otol 1980; 94:123-8.

32. Tingley DR, MacDougall JA. Round window tear in aviators. Aviat Space Environ Med 1977; 48:971-5.

33. Higgs WA. Sudden deafness as the presenting symptom of acoustic neurinoma. Arch Otolaryngol 1973; 98:73-6.

34. Goodhill V. Ear diseases, deafness and dizziness. Hagerstown: Harper & Row, 1979, chap 37.

35. Goodhill V. The idiopathic group and the labyrinthine membrane rupture group approaches to sudden sensorineural hearing loss. In Snow JB, ed. Controversy in otolaryngology. Philadelphia: WB Saunders, 1980.

36. Singleton GT, Karlan MS, Post KN, Bock OG. Perilymph fistulas: diagnostic criteria and therapy. Ann Otol Rhinol Laryngol 1978; 87:797-803.

≈

CANADIAN OTOLARYNGOLOGICAL SOCIETY

The annual meeting of the Canadian Otolaryngological Society will be held in London, Ontario, June 15-17, 1981. Inquiries may be sent to Dr. William Crysdale, c/o Hospital for Sick Children, 555 University Avenue, Toronto, Ontario.

RADIATION-ASSOCIATED CARCINOMA OF THE SALIVARY GLANDS
A CONTROLLED STUDY

HARRY R. MAXON, MD

EUGENE L. SAENGER, MD
STEPHEN R. THOMAS, PhD
MARGARET L. SHAFER, RN

C. RALPH BUNCHER, ScD
JAMES G. KEREIAKES, PhD
CAROLYN A. MCLAUGHLIN

CINCINNATI, OHIO

Five hundred fifty-four persons were evaluated who had received external radiation therapy for benign diseases of the head and neck in childhood and whose salivary glands were presumably included in the radiation field. A significant excess of salivary gland cancers were noted when they were compared to 958 nonirradiated control subjects.

INTRODUCTION

An association between external radiation therapy to the head and neck and subsequent salivary gland cancer has been noted over the last several years in Japanese survivors of the atomic bomb[1] and in Israeli children irradiated for tinea capitis.[2] We have completed the data analysis from a large, controlled study of individuals in the midwestern United States who received external radiotherapy for benign diseases in childhood and have observed the same findings in an American population.

TABLE 1. PREVALENCE OF SALIVARY GLAND MALIGNANCIES

	No. of Subjects	*No. of Cancers*	*Level of Significance**
Irradiated probands	554	3	$P = 0.0490$
Nonirradiated controls	958	0	

*Using a one-tailed Fisher's exact test of significance.

METHODS

In 1960 we reported a follow-up study of children who had received external radiotherapy for benign disease of the head, neck, or chest.[3] Between 1963 and 1967 a more extensively controlled follow-up survey was initiated which will be referred to in this report as the "survey."

The irradiated probands all had received external radiation therapy in childhood for benign disease. A total of 1,266 subjects of 2,230 listed in the radiation therapy records of four Cincinnati hospitals could be located and were willing to submit to an interview. After receiving their radiation therapy records, we found that 554 of the 1,266 subjects received therapy to areas of the head and neck which had a high probability of including one or more of the salivary glands directly in the radiation field. These 554 subjects were classified as "probable salivary gland irradiated probands" and form the basis for this report. The majority of the remaining irradiated subjects appeared to have been treated in such a way that their salivary glands probably were not included directly in the radiation field. The nonirradiated controls included age, race, and sex group-matched subjects who had received medical or surgical treatment for similar diseases in childhood. Family members of both populations were also evaluated. All reviews of radiation therapy records and decision-making were "blinded" with respect to subsequently detected disease.

The evaluation consisted of interviews which were conducted by four registered nurses, each of whom was familiar with the field of radiation therapy and had special training in the public health aspects of nursing.

Subsequent to the survey, we continued to follow up the irradiated probands and the nonirradiated control population through May 1978, using our regional Edward A. Gall Neoplastic Disease Registry. These results will be referred to as "registry" data.

In all of our subjects, the reason for medical intervention was clinically evident salivary gland disease. All neoplasms were verified either by review of the microscopic sections, or by inspection of the report of the pathologist and/or the hospital records.

TABLE 2. REASON FOR RADIATION THERAPY, PREVALENCE OF SALIVARY GLAND CANCER, AND MEAN TOTAL EXPOSURE

Reason for Radiation	*Number of Subjects*	*No. Who Developed Salivary Gland Cancer*		*Mean Total Exposure (roentgens)*
Otitis/mastoiditis	84	0 (0.0%)		349
Cervical adenitis	391	2 (0.5%)		448
Tonsillitis/adenoiditis	79	1 (1.3%)		739
Total	554	3 (0.5%)	Weighted mean:	475

From the Eugene L. Saenger Radioisotope Laboratory, Department of Radiology, The Metabolism Division, Department of Internal Medicine, The Division of Epidemiology and Biostatistics, Department of Environment Health, The University of Cincinnati College of Medicine and the University of Cincinnati Computing Center, Cincinnati. This work was supported in part by grant C6500 from the National Cancer Institute of the United States Public Health Service.

REPRINTS — Harry R. Maxon, MD, Eugene L. Saenger Radioisotope Laboratory, Cincinnati General Hospital, Cincinnati, OH 45267.

TABLE 3. MALIGNANT SALIVARY GLAND NEOPLASMS FOLLOWING EXTERNAL RADIOTHERAPY

Source	Estimated Parotid Dose (rads)	No. irradiated	No. of Salivary Gland Cancers Found	Expected
Hempelmann et al[4]	< 20*	2,872	0 (0.00%)	< 1
Modan et al[2]	140†	10,902	4 (0.04%)	< 1
Belsky et al[1]	> 300	1,340	2 (0.15%)	< 1

*Our calculation, assuming that the parotid glands were at least 2 cm beyond the edge of the thymic irradiation field.

†Assuming that the parotid dose approximately equals the brain dose.

RESULTS

Based on the combined survey and registry data, we found significantly more ($P < 0.05$) salivary gland cancers in the irradiated probands than in the nonirradiated controls (Table 1). This finding could not be explained on a familial basis, since there was no significant difference between the prevalence of salivary gland malignancies in the families of the irradiated probands (none found) and in the families of the nonirradiated controls (one found).

Three salivary gland cancers were found in the "probable salivary gland irradiated probands," two during the survey and one during the registry follow-up. Two of the carcinomas were mucoepidermoid in type, and the third was a mixed carcinoma with local invasion. The parotid gland was the primary site for two of the cancers, and a submandibular gland was the primary site for the third. No salivary gland cancers were found in the 712 irradiated subjects whose salivary glands had been previously judged to have a low probability of having been included directly in the radiation field.

The primary conditions for which the irradiated probands received treatment and their mean total radiation exposure in roentgens are indicated in Table 2. Estimates made from records of two of the three subjects with salivary gland cancer showed salivary gland radiation doses in the range of 500 ± 200 rads.

The mean age of the probands at the time of irradiation was 5.1 years. The mean time from irradiation to survey follow-up was 21.5 years, and the registry follow-up extended to a mean of 36.5 years postirradiation.

DISCUSSION

Our survey information is limited to the extent that data collection was terminated with a mean follow-up of 21.5 years. During the survey we did not clinically examine each irradiated subject for salivary gland cancer. Although we assumed that underestimation of the prevalence of such cancers which did not cause individuals to seek medical care would be the same in the irradiated and in the control groups, we elected to follow these groups in our Neoplastic Disease Registry for the continued appearance of previously undiscovered salivary gland cancers.

The registry data were limited by the necessary but unproven assumption that equal portions of each population still lived in the Cincinnati area and would be included in the registry. We believe that the registry data provide a minimum estimate of the number of additional excess cases which might have been found if all subjects still lived in this area.

In spite of these limitations, our data indicate that there is an increased risk of salivary gland cancers following external radiotherapy to the head and neck for benign diseases in childhood. The prevalence of such radiation-associated salivary gland cancers in our series appears to increase with the radiation dose (Table 2), a finding consistent with previous reports in the literature (Table 3). Although the risk appears to be quite small, especially at radiation doses below 100 rads, a careful evaluation of the salivary glands during the routine examination of previously irradiated persons would seem prudent.

ACKNOWLEDGMENTS — The authors wish to thank Dr. T.D. Sterling for assistance in designing the original survey, Dr. Paul Herget for assistance in the Neoplastic Disease Registry follow-up, Mr. Ismail Kaya for assistance in the data analysis, and Miss Jill Peters for assistance in preparation of the manuscript.

REFERENCES

1. Belsky JL, Takeichi N, Yamamoto T, et al. Salivary gland neoplasms following atomic radiation: additional cases and reanalysis of combined data in a fixed population, 1957-1970. Cancer 1975; 35:555-9.

2. Modan B, Baidatz D, Mart H, Steinitz R, Levin SG. Radiation-induced head and neck tumors. Lancet 1974; 1:277-9.

3. Saenger EL, Silverman FN, Sterling TD, Turner ME. Neoplasia following therapeutic irradiation for benign conditions in childhood. Radiology 1960; 74:899-904.

4. Hemplemann LH, Hall WJ, Phillips M. Neoplasms in persons treated with x-rays in infancy: fourth survey in 20 years. J Natl Cancer Inst 1975; 55:519-30.

Ann Otol 90:1981

TEMPORAL BONE HISTOPATHOLOGY OF NECROTIZING EXTERNAL OTITIS

A CASE REPORT

ISAMU SANDO, MD, DMS
PITTSBURGH, PENNSYLVANIA

TAKEHIKO HARADA, MD
TOKYO, JAPAN

YASUMASA OKANO, MD
SAITAMA, JAPAN

REISUKE SAITO, MD
PITTSBURGH, PENNSYLVANIA

RALPH J. CAPAROSA, MD
PITTSBURGH, PENNSYLVANIA

Histopathological examination of the temporal bone of an individual with necrotizing external otitis revealed severe inflammation with necrosis in the subcutaneous granulation tissue in the external auditory canal. Erosion of the bony walls of the canal had created a defect in the anterior wall, through which infection spread to the preauricular region. The lateral part of the middle ear cavity was also filled with granulation tissue and purulent exudate. A dehiscence of the horizontal portion of the facial canal had apparently allowed spread of an inflammatory round cell infiltrate along the facial nerve up to the fundus of the internal auditory canal. The only evidence of inner ear pathology was the presence of eosinophilic fluid material in the perilymphatic spaces of the labyrinth. A review of other reports of cases of necrotizing external otitis seems to show that this is the only instance of this disease in which infection spread from the external canal through the tympanic membrane to the middle ear and thence to the internal auditory canal.

Necrotizing (malignant) external otitis* was first introduced by Chandler[2] in 1968 to describe a particularly severe form of external otitis which primarily affects elderly diabetics. The causative organism in this disease is uniformly the bacterium *Pseudomonas aeruginosa*. Chandler[2] described the disease as "malignant" because of its resistance to treatment, the destruction of the temporal bone and the base of the skull characteristic of the disease, the multiple cranial nerve palsies associated with this destruction, and the overall poor prognosis for individuals with this disease. Subsequently, many other authors have described their clinical experiences in treating patients with this disease.

In 1959, before necrotizing external otitis was introduced, Meltzer and Kelemen[3] reported the histopathological findings in a case of osteomyelitis of the temporal bone, mandible, and zygoma. The individual so affected was an elderly male with severe diabetes, and *Pseudomonas* was repeatedly isolated from the exudate. In 1971, Morgenstein and Seung[4] presented a temporal bone histopathology case report on a patient who was mildly diabetic and suffered from *Pseudomonas* mastoiditis. Wilson et al[5] in 1971 and Shanon et al[6] in 1972 reported on the clinical findings in cases of necrotizing external otitis and made reference to histologic examinations of the temporal bones in these cases; however, they did not describe the histological findings in full detail. Recently, Kohut and Lindsay[7] described histopathologic alterations in the temporal bone of a diabetic patient who died of a brain abscess secondary to necrotizing external otitis which was pseudomonous in origin.

This is the fourth report to describe fully the temporal bone histopathology associated with *Pseudomonas* ear infection in a diabetic. Furthermore, it is only the second report to describe completely the temporal bone histopathology in a case of what is now known at necrotizing external otitis.

CASE REPORT

A 79-year-old white male was admitted to the Eye and Ear Hospital of Pittsburgh on October 2, 1972, because of a "clogged" feeling and severe hearing loss in his left ear. For three months prior to admission, he had had persistent and progressive pain in the left external ear and temporal region. He complained not only of a metallic taste on the left side of his tongue but also of intermittent dizziness, and he had had some trismus for several weeks. He had been a diabetic, but well controlled, for 20 years prior to admission. His past history was otherwise unremarkable.

On admission, a physical examination revealed a

*It is the authors present opinion as suggested by Evans and Richards[1] that the term "necrotizing external otitis" rather than "malignant external otitis" is appropriate since the word "necrotizing" describes more precisely the pathology, and patients will not be mislead by the word "malignant" because it is suggestive of a neoplastic etiology.

From the Departments of Otolaryngology and Pathology, University of Pittsburgh; the Eye and Ear Hospital and the Veterans Administration Hospital, Pittsburgh; and the Departments of Otolaryngology of the University of Tokyo Faculty of Medicine, and the Josai Dental College, Saitama, Japan. Supported by Research Grant NS13787 from the National Institute of Neurological and Communicative Disorders and Stroke.

REPRINTS — Isamu Sando, MD, Department of Otolaryngology, Eye and Ear Hospital, 230 Lothrop Street, Pittsburgh, PA 15213.

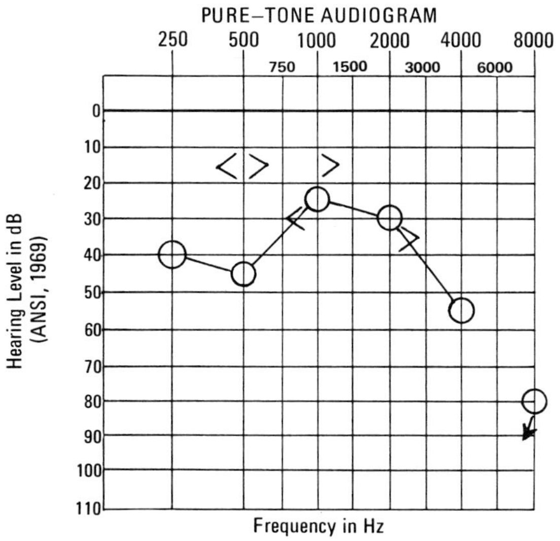

Fig. 1. Audiogram of a patient with necrotizing external otitis, obtained 18 days prior to his death. Right ear: average hearing loss — 33 dB, hearing level for speech — 26 dB, discrimination score — 100%. Left ear: could not test due to packing in the ear canal.

purulent discharge and a large amount of aural granulation tissue filling the left external auditory canal. Swelling of the external auditory canal, the auricle, and the entire parotid gland and preauricular area was also observed.

It was impossible to test the left ear for air conduction because of the occlusion of the external auditory canal; however, there was a high frequency hearing loss for bone conduction (Fig. 1). The right ear showed a moderate sensorineural hearing loss combined with a slight conductive component. No evidence of facial weakness, nystagmus, or of other cranial nerve deficits was noted. A culture of the exudate in the patient's left ear showed *P aeruginosa* and coagulase-negative *Staphylococcus epidermidis*.

During the course of his hospital stay, the patient underwent two operations which confirmed the diagnosis of necrotizing external otitis. These operations revealed the left mastoid to be completely normal; the left middle ear was partly filled with granulation tissue and there was a defect in the anterior wall of the left external auditory canal. Additionally, the left parotid gland showed inflammatory changes. The patient was treated with gentamicin 80 mg three times a day for seven days and carbenicillin 1 g every hour for five days, as well as with Garamycin®* applied topically to the left ear canal. On October 22, 1972, the patient died as a result of cardiac arrest.

The postmortem examination revealed a myocardial infarction which was considered to be the cause of death. At this time, both temporal bones were removed and fixed in 10% formalin. After decalcification and dehydration they were embedded in celloidin and sectioned horizontally at 20 μ. Every tenth section was stained with hematoxylin and eosin, and studied under a light microscope.

*Schering Corp, Kenilworth, NJ.

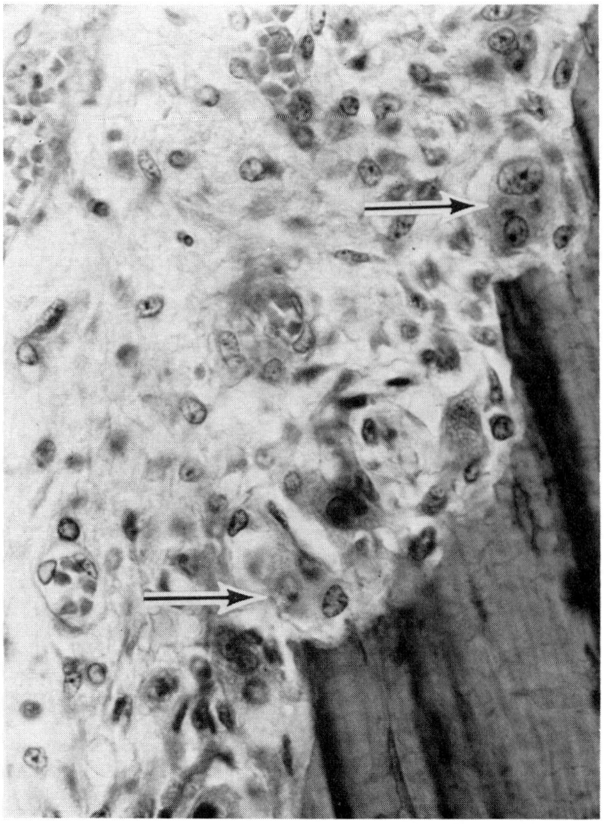

Fig. 2. Left ear. Osteoclasts (arrows) destroying the posterior wall of the external auditory canal. (H & E, x600)

TEMPORAL BONE HISTOPATHOLOGY

LEFT EAR

External Ear. The inflammation of the external auditory canal was evidenced by fibroblastic and capillary proliferation in stages from granulation to fibrosis and by the presence of a mixture of acute and chronic inflammatory cells. There were remaining focal necrosis and hyperplasia of the skin of the canal wall. The inflammation was most striking in the medial portion of the external auditory canal where it became widely confluent with the inflammation of the middle ear through most of the tympanic membrane. Both the anterior and posterior bony walls were eroded by osteoclastic activity (Fig. 2). In particular, total destruction of the bony matrix of the anterior wall medially had permitted the inflammation to spread to the preauricular region (Fig. 3).

Middle Ear.

TYMPANIC MEMBRANE. The tympanic membrane had been completely destroyed as a result of the severe inflammation in the external and middle ears.

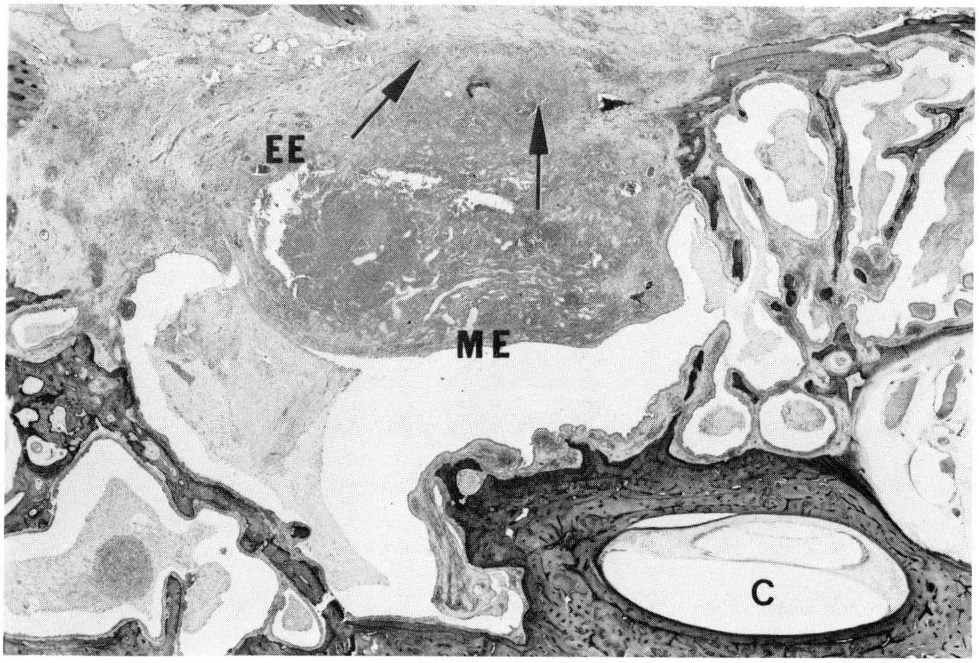

Fig. 3. Left ear. Note the bony defect in the anterior wall of the external auditory canal (arrows) and severe inflammation in the external ear (EE) and the middle ear (ME) with granulation tissue and purulent exudate evident. C - Cochlea. (H & E, x11.5)

MIDDLE EAR CAVITY. The inflammation present in the middle ear cavity was continuous with that of the external auditory canal. The mucous membrane was hyperplastic with conspicuous inflammatory round cell infiltration, and the lateral part of the middle ear cavity was filled with granulation tissue and purulent exudate (Fig. 3). The lateral portion of the anterior wall of the middle ear cavity was so severely eroded by inflammation in the area adjacent to the external auditory canal that it was totally destroyed. Numerous osteoclasts and osteoblasts gave evidence of active bone resorption and new bone formation in this area. Erosion of the posterior and medial walls was much less pronounced than that noted in the anterior walls.

OSSICLES. The malleus was almost completely destroyed (Fig. 4). The erosion of the incus was less marked, a large part of the body, the short process, and the long process having been spared. The stapes had been thinned by surface erosion, and the crura had been displaced inwardly by the granulation tissue to form a narrowed foramen obturatum.

EUSTACHIAN TUBE. The inflammation extended anteriorly into the eustachian tube, destroying the bony portion and filling the tube with granulation tissue.

FACIAL NERVE. There was a dehiscence of the facial canal in its horizontal portion through which the submucosal inflammatory round cells had invaded the canal and surrounded the facial nerve. This round cell infiltration was observed also in the trunk of the facial nerve itself, being most pronounced near the genu (Fig. 5). Such infiltration was also seen along the greater superficial petrosal nerve near the facial hiatus. The round cells in the areas mentioned above were mostly lymphocytes and polymorphonuclear leukocytes.

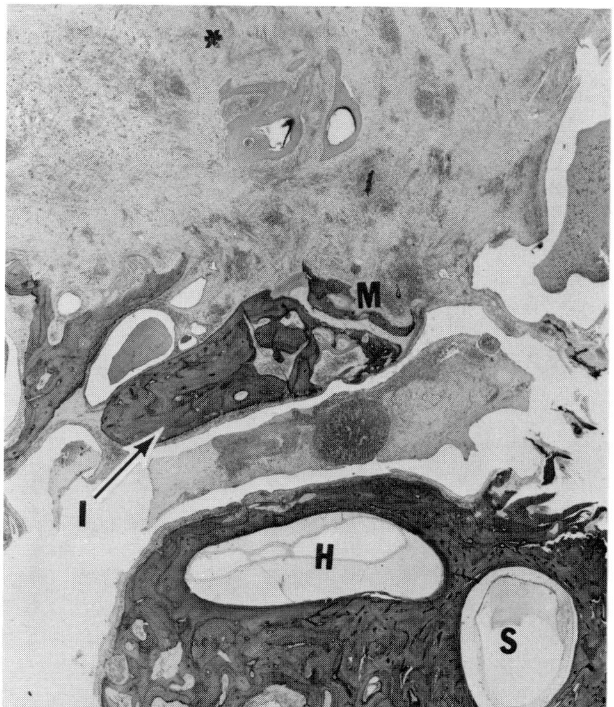

Fig. 4. Left ear. Conspicuous erosion of the malleus (M) as a result of inflammatory process (*). I - Incus; H - Horizontal canal; S - Superior canal. (H & E, x13)

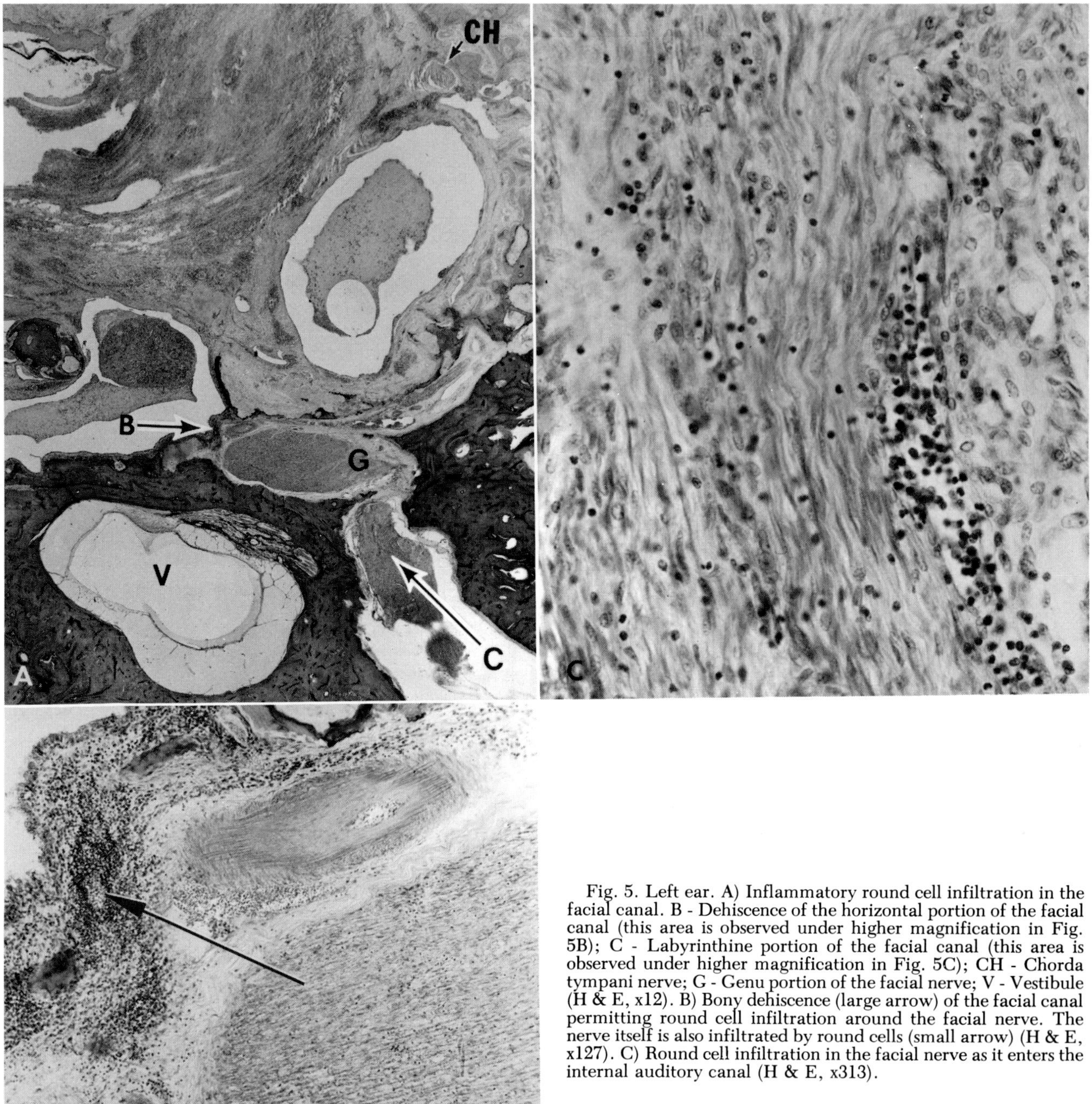

Fig. 5. Left ear. A) Inflammatory round cell infiltration in the facial canal. B - Dehiscence of the horizontal portion of the facial canal (this area is observed under higher magnification in Fig. 5B); C - Labyrinthine portion of the facial canal (this area is observed under higher magnification in Fig. 5C); CH - Chorda tympani nerve; G - Genu portion of the facial nerve; V - Vestibule (H & E, x12). B) Bony dehiscence (large arrow) of the facial canal permitting round cell infiltration around the facial nerve. The nerve itself is also infiltrated by round cells (small arrow) (H & E, x127). C) Round cell infiltration in the facial nerve as it enters the internal auditory canal (H & E, x313).

CHORDA TYMPANI NERVE. The chorda tympani nerve was not seen in most of its course in the middle ear cavity where there was a marked amount of inflammation, but faintly stained fibers of this nerve were seen to approach the bony canaliculi itae chordae anterior (Fig. 5A) and itae chordae posterior.

MASTOID. The mastoid cavity had been drilled out in previous operations. There was no evidence of destruction of the remaining trabeculae by osteoclasts or osteoblasts. A lesser degree of round cell infiltration was present in the mastoid mucosa than was found in the middle ear mucosa, which seems to indicate that the inflammation had spread to the mastoid from the middle ear.

Inner Ear. No inflammatory round cell infiltrate was present in the inner ear.

COCHLEA. In the scala vestibuli and scala tympani, homogeneous eosinophilic fluid was present in a layer in contact with the basilar membrane. Neither hydrops nor collapse of the cochlear duct was observed. The organ of Corti seemed free of pathologic changes. The population of spiral ganglion cells as well as that of cochlear nerve fibers was considered to be normal.

VESTIBULE. Homogeneous eosinophilic fluid, presumably of the same character as that seen in the cochlea, was observed to fill the perilymphatic space uniformly. The maculae of the saccule and utricle and the cristae of the three semicircular canals were considered to be normal as were the nerve fibers.

ENDOLYMPHATIC SAC. The rugose portion of the endolymphatic sac was lined with cuboidal cells and contained protein-rich eosinophilic material.

Internal Auditory Canal. Inflammatory round cell infiltration, although of mild degree, was observed in the fundus of the internal auditory canal. The presence of those inflammatory round cells along the course of the facial nerve in its labyrinthine portion indicated that the inflammation had spread from the middle ear into the internal auditory canal (Fig. 5). The cochlear nerve, the vestibular nerve, and the facial nerve seemed to be normal.

Other Findings. Some evidence of osteomyelitis with new bone formation, although not severe, was noted in the petrous apex. There was no particular osteoclastic activity observed.

RIGHT EAR

In contrast to the severe changes in the left ear characteristic of necrotizing external otitis the right ear showed virtually no pathology and was regarded as being essentially normal.

DISCUSSION

Reports and studies on the association of hearing impairment with diabetes have been accumulating for over 100 years. Before the advent of insulin therapy for diabetes, ear infections in individuals suffering from this disorder were dreaded because of the rapidity with which the inflammatory process destroyed hearing. Raynaud[8] (1881) drew attention to this problem, which he called diabetic otitis. Steinbrugge[9] (1891) and Manasse[10] (1904) also reported on the histopathology of diabetic ear infections.

Although *Pseudomonas aeruginosa* was originally described as being of low virulence, the general role that this microorganism plays in the development of ear disease was elucidated by Voss[11] (1906), and Stanley[12] reported that it could cause an extremely invasive type of infection. The significance of *Pseudomonas* as an etiologic factor in external otitis was thoroughly discussed by Senturia[13] (1957).

It was Chandler[2] (1968), however, who first drew attention to a particularly severe type of external otitis which tended to affect elderly diabetic patients and in which the causative agent was uniformly *Pseudomonas.* He used the term "malignant external otitis" to describe this serious infection since the term "malignant" accurately describes the typical clinical course. Several clinical case reports describing this entity were subsequently published,[1,5,6,14,15] and other investigators discussed the neurologic complications.[16,17] and radiologic findings[18] which may be associated with necrotizing external otitis. In 1973, Evans and Richards[1] suggested the use of the term "necrotizing otitis externa" rather than "malignant otitis externa" which may be misleading to the patient since it is suggestive of neoplastic etiology. It was then reported that this ailment could affect not only elderly diabetic patients, but also children under certain circumstances.[19,20]

Kohut and Lindsay[7] reported temporal bone histopathological findings in a patient with necrotizing external otitis. They suggested the following mechanism of inflammatory invasion of this disease: The invasion of the external auditory canal is due to local bone necrosis. This in turn extends to the submucosal vasculature of the pneumatic spaces. The infectious process extends submucosally, establishing one or several sites of bone destruction.

Recently, some interesting findings concerning the site of the lesion were made. Cohn[21] observed that the *Pseudomonas* infection might take a similar rapidly progressive course in patients when the initial site of the infection was the middle ear and mastoid, and proposed the term "progressive necrotizing otitis" for this process. Badrawy et al[22] suggested that "necrotizing external otitis" is due to a masked middle ear infection extending to the mastoid process and bulging toward the floor of the external auditory canal.

The two operations performed on this patient succeeded in excluding the presence of a neoplasm and confirmed the presence of the inflammation that extended beyond the confines of the external ear, thus establishing the diagnosis of necrotizing external otitis. Chandler[2] stated that the tympanic membrane was extremely resistant to this particular inflammatory process, and that the middle ear, if involved at all, became so only late in the course of the disease by way of the mastoid process. A case reported histopathologically by Kohut and Lindsay[7] demonstrated no evidence of active bone destruction in the middle ear cavity, whereas the bone adjacent to the pneumatic spaces was severely involved. In the present case, however, it was demonstrated that the mastoid was normal, while the lateral portion of the middle ear was found to be filled with granulation tissue. Histopathologic examination of this temporal bone revealed the presence of pronounced changes: there was necrotic granulation tissue in the external and middle ears with the changes being least severe in the mastoid region. From the clinical history it appears that the external auditory canal was the original site of infection and that the infection atypically took a direct course into the middle ear through the tympanic membrane rather than through the mastoid. This middle ear infection might have been the cause of destruction of the chorda tympani nerve in the middle ear cavity and may explain the clinical complaint of "a metallic taste on the left side of the tongue."

The pathologic changes observed were severe in the present case, as evidenced by extension of the inflammation to the preauricular region through the defect in the anterior wall of the bony external auditory canal, which was continuous with the anterior bony defect of the middle ear cavity. In most cases such infection gains access to the surrounding tissues through an area where the cartilage and bone are absent or through the incisura Santorini. Trismus, one of this patient's complaints, might have been secondary to extensive inflammatory lesions in the preauricular area.

Chandler[23,24] has described several ways in which an infectious process in the external auditory canal might reach the facial nerve. One of the most likely of these is involvement of the nerve at its exit from the stylomastoid foramen, while some reports have confirmed infectious involvement of the facial nerve in this area associated with necrotizing external otitis.[16-18] Morgenstein and Seung[4] found the nerve disrupted in its entire horizontal portion where dehiscence of the facial canal had permitted the massive invasion of inflammatory cells.

Joachims,[20] during an operation for necrotizing external otitis, observed destruction of the fallopian canal in its horizontal portion and the superior third of its descending portion, as well as atrophy and/or absence of the facial nerve in the middle ear. In the case reported by Meltzer and Kelemen[3] the facial palsy was attributed to edema of the sheath which had occurred as a result of osteitis. Shanon et al[6] observed perineural inflammatory infiltration in the vicinity of the vertical portion of the facial nerve in the case they studied. In the present case, submucosal inflammatory round cells entered the facial canal through a bony dehiscence in the horizontal portion of the fallopian canal and invaded the facial nerve in its horizontal and genu portions.

This round cell infiltration of the facial nerve which had spread to the fundus of the internal auditory canal is the significant finding in our case. To our knowledge such a spread of infection from the middle ear to the internal auditory canal has not been reported previously. In the reports presented by Meltzer and Kelemen[3] and by Morgenstein and Seung[4] there was no evidence of infection in the internal auditory canal, and in the cases reported by Wilson et al[5] the infection was observed to have invaded from the posterior cranial fossa, rather than from the middle ear.

In contrast to the severe inflammation present in the external and middle ears of the present case, no particular inflammatory cell infiltration was noted in the inner ear. Again, while Wilson et al[5] observed purulent labyrinthitis which had seemingly spread from the posterior cranial fossa, neither Meltzer and Kelemen[3] nor Morgenstein and Seung[4] found infection in the inner ear. The inner ear thus appears to be resistant to the spread of inflammation from the middle ear through the facial canal and the cribriform plate. However, in this case the presence of homogeneous eosinophilic material in the perilymphatic space may be evidence for a reaction to the inflammation of the fundus of the internal auditory canal and middle ear. Such a reaction could have caused the clinical symptoms of high frequency sensorineural hearing loss and dizziness which our patient experienced.

ACKNOWLEDGMENTS — The authors are extremely grateful to Eugene N. Myers, MD, Professor and Chairman, Department of Otolaryngology, University of Pittsburgh School of Medicine, for giving helpful criticism during the preparation of the paper. Appreciation is also expressed to Dr. Joanne Dunn, Mrs. Ellie Lee, and Mrs. Ruth Anderson for their kind assistance in this study.

REFERENCES

1. Evans ITG, Richards SH. Malignant (necrotizing) otitis externa. J Laryngol Otol 1973; 8:13-20.

2. Chandler JR. Malignant external otitis. Laryngoscope 1968; 78:1257-94.

3. Meltzer PE, Kelemen G. Pyocyaneous osteomyelitis of the temporal bone, mandible and zygoma. Laryngoscope 1959; 69:1300-16.

4. Morgenstein KM, Seung HI. Pseudomonas mastoiditis. Laryngoscope 1971; 81:200-15.

5. Wilson DF, Pulec JL, Linthicum FH. Malignant external otitis. Arch Otolaryngol 1971; 93:419-22.

6. Shanon E, Bialystock G, Schujman E, et al. Pseudomonal granulomatous external otitis. Acta Otolaryngol (Stockh) 1972; 73:374-8.

7. Kohut RI, Lindsay JR. Necrotizing ("malignant") external otitis histopathologic processes. Ann Otol Rhinol Laryngol 1979; 88:714-20.

8. Raynaud M. De l'otite diabetique. Ann Mal Oreille Larynx 1881; 7:63-73.

9. Steinbrugge H. Die pathologische Anatomie des Gehororganes. In: Orth J. Lehrbuch der Speciellen Pathologischen Anatomie. Berlin: August Hirschwald, 1891.

10. Manasse P. Zur pathologischen Anatomie des inneren Ohres and des Hornerven: III. Mitteilung. Z Ohren 1904; 49:109-36.

11. Voss O. Der Bacillus pyocyaneous im Ohr. Veroeff Geb Militaer-Sanitaetswesens 1906; 34:1-197.

12. Stanley MM. Bacillus pyocyaneous infections. A review, report of cases and discussion of newer therapy including streptomycin. Am J Med 1947; 2:253-77, 347-67.

13. Senturia BH. Diseases of the external ear. Springfield: Charles C. Thomas, 1957.

14. Aldous EW, Shinn JB. Far advanced malignant external otitis: report of a survival. Laryngoscope 1973; 83:1810-5.

15. Zaky DA, Bentley DW, Lowy K, et al. Malignant external otitis: a severe form of otitis in diabetic patients. Am J Med 1976; 61:298-302.

16. Schwarz GA, Blumenkrantz MJ, Sundmaker WLH. Neurologic complications of malignant external otitis. Neurology 1971; 21:1077-84.

17. Dinapoli RP, Thoman JE. Neurologic aspects of malignant external otitis: report of three cases. Mayo Clin Proc 1971; 46:339-43.

18. Kim BH. Roentgenographic findings of malignant external otitis. Am J Roentgenol 1971; 112:366-72.

19. Giguere P, Rouillard G. Otite externe maligne bilaterale chez une fillette de 10 ans. J Otolaryngol 1976; 5:159-66.

20. Joachims HZ. Malignant external otitis in children. Arch Otolaryngol 1976; 102:236-7.

21. Cohn AM. Progressive necrotizing otitis. Malignant external otitis. Arch Otolaryngol 1974; 99:136-9.

22. Badrawy R, Abou-Bieh A, Taha A. Masked diabetic mastoiditis. J Laryngol Otol 1975; 89:815-21.

23. Chandler JR. Pathogenesis and treatment of facial paralysis due to malignant external otitis. Ann Otol Rhinol Laryngol 1972; 81:648-58.

24. Chandler JR. Malignant external otitis and facial paralysis. Otolaryngol Clin North Am 1974; 7:375-83.

≈

PAN AMERICAN ASSOCIATION OF OTORHINOLARYNGOLOGY AND BRONCHOESOPHAGOLOGY

The XVIII Congress of the Pan American Association of Otorhinolaryngology and Bronchoesophagology will be held November 2-6, 1982, in San Juan, Puerto Rico. Dr. Hans von Leden has been elected President of the Association.

Ann Otol 90:1981

PROSTHETIC VOCAL REHABILITATION FOLLOWING LARYNGECTOMY

THE VOICE BUTTON

WILLIAM R. PANJE, MD

IOWA CITY, IOWA

The Voice Button is a simple biflanged silicone device placed in the tracheoesophageal wall which has been found to enable speech without aspiration in approximately 80% of unselected laryngectomy patients. A simple surgical outpatient procedure provides the necessary tracheoesophageal fistula for insertion of the Voice Button. Indications, results, advantages, disadvantages and complications are discussed.

Prosthetic restoration of speech dates back to the time of the first laryngectomy performed by Billroth in 1873. The early technique of laryngectomy was to create a fistula in the gullet through the neck. In order to prevent aspiration of saliva into the trachea a tubular device with a vibrating reed, similar to the present day fenestrated tracheostomy tube, was made by one of Billroth's students. The device not only prevented aspiration, but restored the patient's voice. Subsequent modifications of the laryngectomy operation in which the trachea was brought out through the neck and the gullet closed resulted in design changes of the prosthetic device used for vocal rehabilitation. The devices in general became more complicated, with variable patient and surgeon satisfaction.[1]

Most recently Blom and Singer[2] and Singer and Blom[3] have developed an inexpensive, miniature, valved prosthesis that allows for rapid voice rehabilitation with minimal complications. The prosthesis is inserted approximately two days following an endoscopic procedure in which a midline tracheoesophageal "puncture" is performed. The device projects through the upper part of the tracheostoma and is taped to the neck. The patient is hospitalized for approximately 5-7 days. Drawbacks of the device appear to be minimal with a success rate approaching 90%.

Because of the problems encountered with the various tracheoesophageal (TE) fistula operations, a silicone device (Voice Button, U.S. Patent No. 156,177) was developed that could be inserted through the previously formed fistula tract that would prevent aspiration and stenosis and allow vocalization. Because of the success of the Voice Button in overcoming "neoglottic" operative failures and the encouraging reports by Singer and Blom with their prosthesis, placement of the Voice Button was utilized as a primary procedure in 24 laryngectomized patients. The present report confirms that a high rate of success with minimal complications can be expected with the TE fistula-prosthetic technique for voice rehabilitation.

Advantages of the Voice Button compared with the Blom-Singer device are: placement is accomplished with an outpatient surgical procedure requiring no special instrumentation, the prosthesis is self-contained within the tracheostoma, it cannot be dislodged unintentionally, and no sizing is needed.

Specifications of the Voice Button. The Voice Button is a biflanged silicone tube (No. 14 French) with a one-way valve at one end and open at the other end (Fig. 1). The device is 1.5 cm long and the largest flange (tracheal side) is 13 mm in diameter. The inner flange (esophageal side) measures 10 mm and is located 7 mm or 12 mm from the larger flanges. A 30.5 cm string attached to the large-flange side of the prosthesis is used to dislodge and prevent aspiration of the device.

Since the device is self-contained within the tracheostoma an inserter must be used in order to place the Voice Button. The inserter is made of wire and comes in various handle lengths to accommodate patient dexterity, which is variable, especially among arthritics.

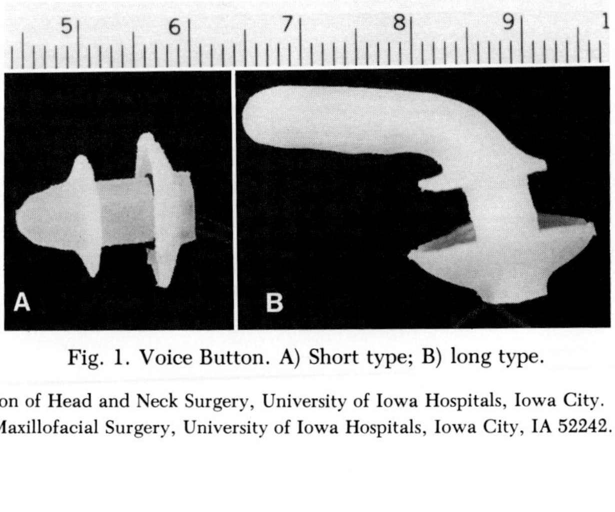

Fig. 1. Voice Button. A) Short type; B) long type.

From the Department of Otolaryngology and Maxillofacial Surgery, Division of Head and Neck Surgery, University of Iowa Hospitals, Iowa City.
REPRINTS — William R. Panje, MD, Department of Otolaryngology and Maxillofacial Surgery, University of Iowa Hospitals, Iowa City, IA 52242.

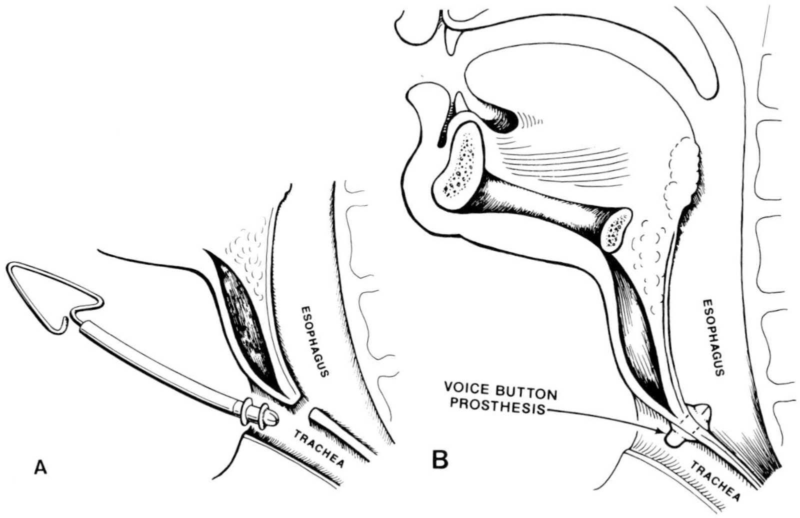

Fig. 2. Voice Button. A) On inserter being put into fistula; B) in place.

The Voice Button valve tip is of two types; the short type (Fig. 1A), which emanates 6 mm from the inner flange, has a four-flutter flap, one-way valve; this model has been the most frequently used. The long-type Voice Button (Fig. 1B) was developed for patients who cannot generate sufficient lung pressure for good long-term vocalization, and is for some patients easier to insert than the short type.

SURGICAL PROCEDURE

In preparation for placement of the Voice Button a tracheoesophageal fistula is created, a procedure that can be done easily on an outpatient basis. Instrumentation should include a headlight, air suction equipment, soft-tissue surgical instruments, 5% cocaine solution, 2% Viscus Xylocaine®, 1% Xylocaine with 1:100,000 epinephrine for injection, and Nos. 32 and 34 French thick-walled rubber tubes* for females, and Nos. 38 and 40 for males.

The patient's pharynx and esophagus are anesthetized with Viscus Xylocaine. The tracheal tree is copiously sprayed with 5% cocaine. The tracheostoma must measure at least 1.5 cm diameter. An appropriately sized esophageal tube is passed with visualization of the posterior wall of the tracheostoma. As the esophageal tube passes the area of the tracheostoma a bulge will be seen to develop. It is *crucial* to ascertain the point of maximum bulge because this is the anterior midpoint of the esophagus. This midpoint can vary depending upon the extent of the original surgical resection and whether a neck dissection has been performed. The patient is placed in the supine position and the midpoint of the esophagus is injected through the membranous tracheal wall with 0.5 cc of 1% Xylocaine with epinephrine. A No. 22-gauge spinal needle is then inserted through the intended fistula site into the rubber esophageal tube. The fistula site should be made just above the level of the lower verge of the tracheostoma. Note: the fistula is usually placed approximately 1 cm from the upper verge of the tracheostoma. The site is more inferiorly located than that of the puncture site suggested by Singer for placement of his valve. Trying to use the Voice Button in the Singer puncture site is not suggested since the tracheosophageal wall has varying degrees of thickness in this area, unlike the area suggested for the Voice Button. It is important that the patient be able to see the opening for easier prosthetic insertion. An incision is then made with a No. 15 or 11 Bard-Parker blade at the midpoint site. The incision is made vertically, approximately 7-10 mm in length from the spinal needle down to the esophageal tube. The tracheoesophageal wall varies in thickness between 5 and 10 mm. The esophageal mucosa may be attached to tracheal mucosa with 4-0 absorbable sutures. A No. 14 rubber catheter, previously cut to approximately 10 cm, is then inserted toward the stomach through the TE fistula upon slow withdrawal of the esophageal tube. The catheter is tied with a string to the neck similar to the placement of a tracheostomy tube. It is important to occlude the catheter by either tying the string tightly or plugging the cut end of the catheter in order to avoid regurgitation of fluids through the catheter.

The patient is instructed not to remove the catheter. If the catheter comes out it should be immediately reinserted. The patient can do this and should be instructed on how to do it before leaving the office. There may be some leakage of liquids around the catheter upon drinking for the first 4-25 hours. This leakage is reduced by taking solid foods at the same time liquids are consumed. Patients are given a 5-day course of penicillin or erythromycin. In approximately 7-14 days the patient returns to

*If Hurst or Maloney dilators are used for this purpose the mercury must be emptied. Weight is not needed since the tube is acting to mildly expand (not dilate) the esophagus so that the membranous tracheal wall will be made evident, and also to protect the posterior esophageal wall from injury.

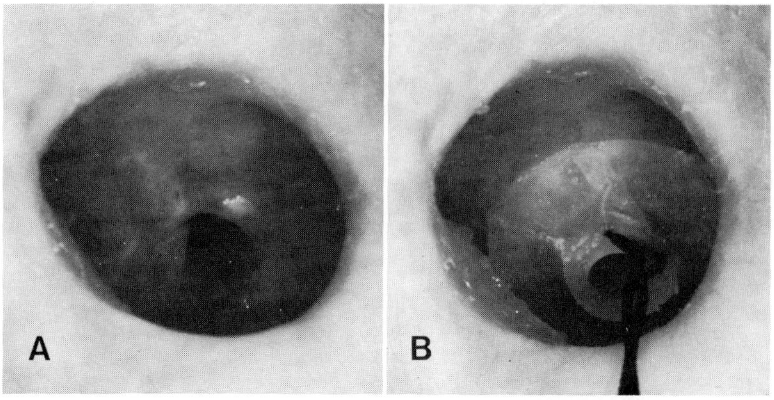

Fig. 3. A) Tracheoesophageal fistula as seen through stoma two weeks postoperatively. B) Voice Button as seen through tracheostoma of patient.

the office. The Voice Button is inserted through the TE fistula site and the patient given instructions on insertion and removal (Figs. 2 and 3). The device is cleaned once a day. The patient is then encouraged to consult a speech pathologist for training in respiratory muscle control, stomal capping methods, and muscle relaxation techniques.

RESULTS

Twenty-four patients have undergone prosthetic vocal rehabilitation since December 1978. Ages ranged from 42-67 years, 21 of 24 were male, and occupations were varied. Approximately a third of the patient population was drawn from the ENT Service of the Iowa City VA Hospital. All had had a wide-field total laryngectomy. Seventeen had a unilateral neck dissection and two a bilateral neck dissection. Twenty had received radiation therapy, 12 preoperatively and 8 postoperatively. Six patients had been irradiation failures. Two patients had TE fistulas created at the time of the total laryngectomy, with stenting of the fistula with a No. 14 French feeding catheter. They were fed through this tube during the postoperative period, thus avoiding nasal intubation.

There have been four failures to date. Two patients were unable to achieve speech although one was able to speak under Valium® sedation. Both patients had undergone postoperative irradiation within one year of placement of the prosthesis. Two patients have been failures because of inability to efficiently insert the short type of prosthesis because of irritation and subsequent thickness of the tracheoesophageal parting wall. Their fistula sites were allowed to heal spontaneously. Two other patients who were initial failures because of inability to place the short-type Voice Button became successes with the advent of the long-type Voice Button. One of these patients was a moderately severe arthritic who had sufficient dexterity problems to preclude satisfactory use of the short-type prosthesis.

Four patients had developed some esophageal speech before placement of the Voice Button. These patients requested the prosthesis because of lack of voice volume, intelligibility, or inability to carry on a sustained conversation. All of these patients have been very successful with the Voice Button. They are able to use esophageal speech for 2-4 syllable phrases such as "Good Day," "Hi," "Stop," without having to occlude their tracheostomas. When they desire increased volume or extended conversation they occlude the stoma and use prosthetic neolaryngeal speech. There were no surgical or infectious complications. Improper positioning of the TE fistula in several early cases was corrected by allowing the fistula to spontaneously close and redoing a more centrally located opening as described above.

All patients have been successful in not having aspiration of liquids or foods (Fig. 4). If aspiration did occur it was because the prosthetic valve had not been properly inserted or had deteriorated. Instructing the patient to gently pull on the valve's strings after insertion will aid in insurance of proper placement. Simple replacement with a new Voice Button allowed resumption of deglutition without aspiration in those patients who were properly inserting the valve. Deterioration rate has been variable to date, ranging anywhere from several weeks to eight months. This is probably related to variability of custom making of the device and how well the patient inserts the device.

There have been no extrusions or inadvertent dislodging of the Voice Button prosthesis, even during vomiting and excessive coughing. The biflange feature of the prosthesis allows the patient to test for positioning by gently tugging on the dislodging string. A popping sensation after insertion is frequently felt by the patient when the Voice Button has been properly inserted.

The external neck surface does not influence use of the Voice Button since nothing is needed to fix the prosthesis to the stoma. The one drawback that must be overcome is the size of the tracheostoma, which must be at least 1.5 cm in diameter.

Patient Selection. As with most treatment plans, patient selection can significantly bias the end results to the point of misleading the observer as to the

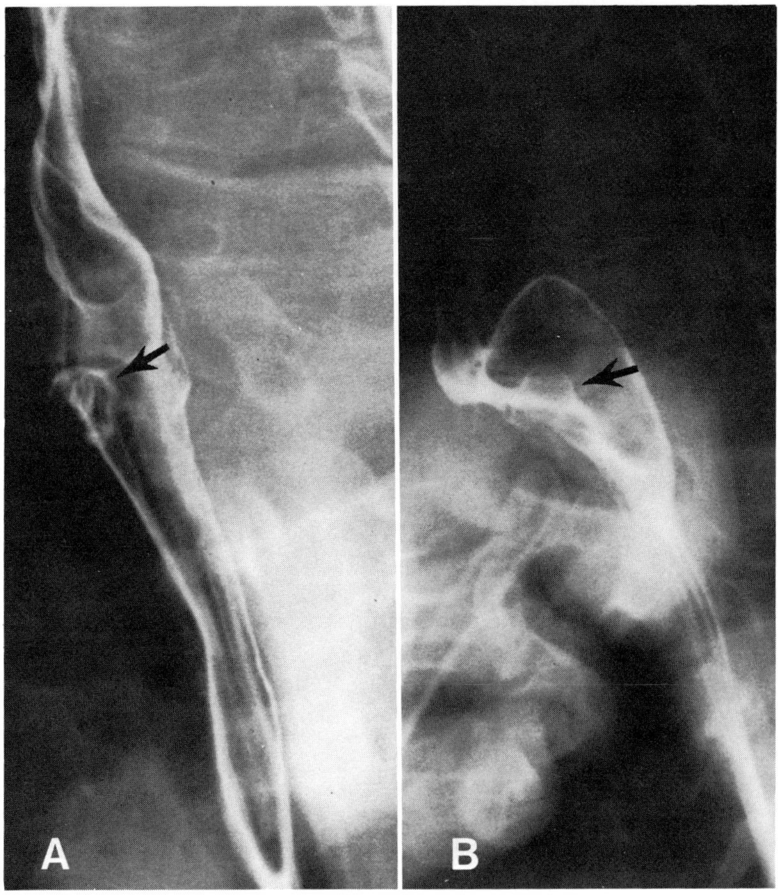

Fig. 4. Barium swallow film with Voice Button in place. A) No aspiration; arrow indicates location of Voice Button. B) Patient forcing air through Voice Button producing sound. Note ballooning of esophagus at level of button.

effectiveness of the treatment or technique. Just as the attainment of esophageal speech is markedly influenced by patient anatomy, interest, intelligence and habits, so might these factors influence the success of prosthetic vocal rehabilitation. Although these factors were not specifically analyzed in this study, patient selection was limited by the following physical characteristics: stomal diameter, dexterity of the patient, and thickness of the tracheoesophageal wall. If the stoma was too large for finger or thumb coverage, a sponge pad acted as an effective occlusive device. The sponge device also minimized stomal irritation following irradiation. (There was at least a 6-month delay between irradiation and prosthetic replacement.)

Patients with impaired manual dexterity are not good candidates for the type of prosthetic devices described herein. Severe arthritics and persons with parkinsonism are definitely not suitable candidates.

Thickness of the tracheoesophageal wall can be a problem in insertion of the Voice Button. Usually the wall is < 1 cm in thickness. However, frequent removal and reinsertion of the device can cause irritation of the fistula with concomitant thickening of the tracheoesophageal wall. The patient should not remove and reinsert the prosthesis more than once a day to avoid irritation, and should be so instructed. The best method for avoiding irritation at the fistula site is to have the patient remove the valve at night before going to bed. The catheter used for original stenting of the fistula is then worn overnight. Upon arising the catheter is removed and the Voice Button inserted. If granulation tissue develops at the fistula site simple chemical cauterization and returning to the catheter for a 2-4 day continuous wearing period will allow for easier insertion of the valve.

Patients with excessive lung disease who cannot generate moderate stomal pressure against the surgeon's thumb, asthmatics, or patients who cough excessively with stomal capping do not appear to be good candidates for this or any other type of TE fistula procedure.

The air insufflation test has been advocated by some as a determinant of those patients who will do best with TE fistula sound production. This specific test was not done in this study. However, both patients who failed to develop speech with Voice Button placement had had sound production on the administration of air into the esophagus via a small catheter, which seems to demonstrate the capricious nature of the test and the variability among patients.

Twenty-two patients achieved speech following fistula site maturation regardless of the Voice Button's presence. Of these "successful" patients five could not achieve sustained connected speech. They could produce only 3-5 syllables. These patients acted as if they were tightening their pharyngeal muscles. Valium helped two to increase the number of syllables produced in one breath; however the others were unaffected.

DISCUSSION

The Voice Button prosthesis technique appears to be an acceptable method for vocal rehabilitation of the laryngectomy patient who has not achieved satisfactory esophageal speech. Although the initial results with prosthetic TE fistula speech production have been encouraging, the primary use of this technique at the time of laryngectomy does not appear, at this time, to be in the best interest of the patient or the surgeon. This conclusion is based on experience with a number of TE fistula patients, both prosthetic and surgery-only, in whom appreciation, self-management, reduced physician-patient contact time, and, in general, overall success appeared better with a delayed fistula operation.

The question of doing the surgical-only method versus the prosthetic-fistula method appears to need further investigation. However, the excellent results of Singer's prosthesis-puncture technique and the results obtained with the Voice Button prosthesis would suggest the superiority of the prosthetic technique. This is especially true for the head and neck surgeon who occasionally encounters the laryngectomy patient needing voice rehabilitation. The TE fistula-prosthesis procedure offers a technique that is reproducible, highly successful, inexpensive, and reversible. Additional advantages of the TE fistula-Voice Button procedure over those using other presently available prosthetic valves are that placement of the Voice Button can be done on an outpatient basis, requires no adhesives or sizing, and literally cannot dislodge accidentally. Finally the Voice Button provides two different valve systems that effectively preclude aspiration while reducing lung pressure for sound production.

REFERENCES

1. Shed D, Weinberg B, eds. Surgical and prosthetic approaches to speech rehabilitation. Boston: GK Hall, 1980.

2. Blom ED, Singer MI. Surgical-prosthetic approaches for postlaryngectomy rehabilitation. In: Keith RL, ed. Laryngectomee rehabilitation. Houston: College Hill Press, 1979.

3. Singer MI, Blom ED. Tracheoesophageal puncture: a surgical prosthetic method for postlaryngectomy speech restoration. Read before the Third International Symposium on Plastic and Reconstructive Surgery of the Head and Neck, New Orleans, April 29-May 4, 1979.

≈

INTERNATIONAL CONGRESS OF AUDIOPHONOLOGY & GERONTOLOGY

A Congress entitled "Aging and Communication" devoted to the communicative problems of the aged will be held in Besançon, France, November 11-14, 1981. Organizational committee: Audiophonology & Gerontology, Faculté de Médicine, 25030 Besançon, France.

Ann Otol 90:1981

QUANTITATIVE STUDY OF SCARPA'S GANGLION AND VESTIBULAR SENSE ORGANS IN ENDOLYMPHATIC HYDROPS

ERNST RICHTER, MD
INNSBRUCK, AUSTRIA

The density of vestibular hair cells and the number of neurons in Scarpa's ganglion were estimated for 11 temporal bones with endolymphatic hydrops. The ten subjects from which these bones were taken all exhibited decreased caloric response (when tested), fluctuating hearing loss, and episodic vertigo. The degeneration of vestibular sense organs was found within the "normal" range for all except one case, which showed total degeneration of the posterior crista ampullaris. Ganglion cell counts in all cases were low. In three of the ten subjects, counts fell below the lowest values seen in a sample of "normal" ears. These three subjects exhibited fluctuating hearing loss and episodic vertigo for more than six years prior to death. In cases of unilateral endolymphatic hydrops there was no significant difference between counts in the affected and unaffected ear. Thus, the apparent ganglion cell degeneration may be due to ear disease other than endolymphatic hydrops.

INTRODUCTION

Most studies of temporal bones from individuals exhibiting the symptoms characteristic of Menière's disease report the presence of endolymphatic hydrops.[1-6] In one case with a short symptomatic period, endolymphatic hydrops was not seen.[7] When present, the extent of the hydrops varies from involvement of the apical turn only[8] to distention of the cochlear duct in all turns with outpouchings or ruptures.[9] Other studies have reported changes of the vestibular sensory epithelia[10-15] in material from individuals with Menière's disease, but appropriate normal material was not examined. Degeneration of Scarpa's ganglion has also been reported, but in these cases the presence or absence of endolymphatic hydrops could not be determined.[16,17]

The purpose of the present study was to quantify the sensory cell and ganglion cell populations of ears with clear endolymphatic hydrops. These data

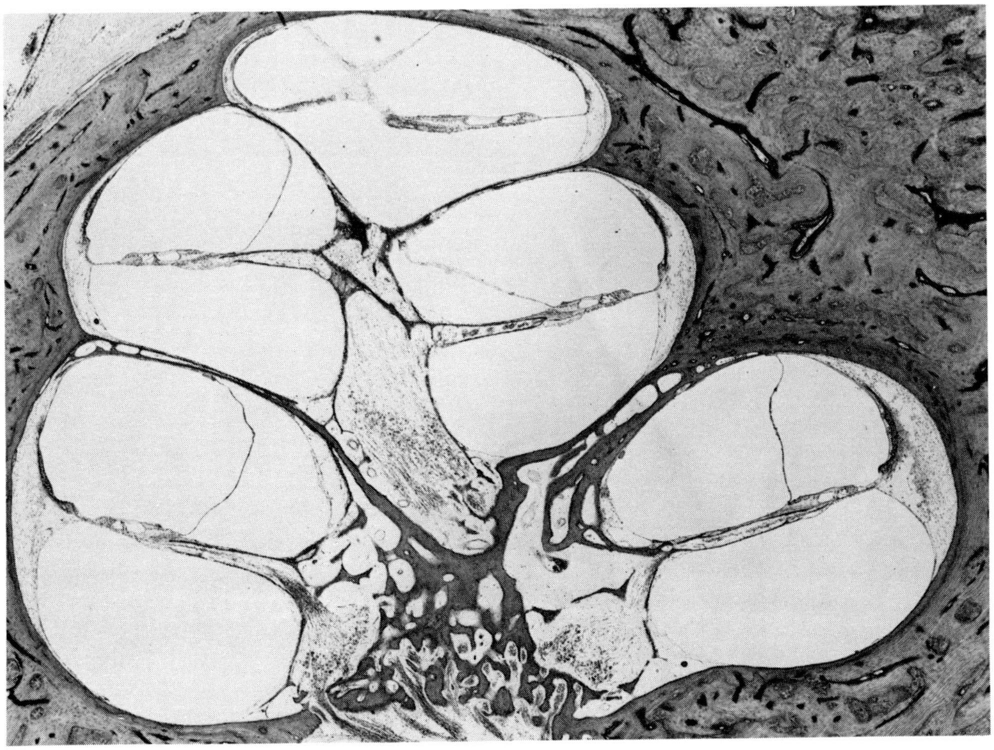

Fig. 1. Photomicrograph of a midmodiolar section through the cochlea of the 78-year-old female (Table 1). In the basal turn, scala media appears to have swollen to about twice its normal volume, while in the middle turn it is roughly three times normal. (x22)

From the Department of Otolaryngology, Harvard Medical School, and the Massachusetts Eye and Ear Infirmary, Boston.
REPRINTS — Harold F. Schuknecht, MD, Massachusetts Eye and Ear Infirmary, 243 Charles Street, Boston, MA 02114.

TABLE 1. CLINICAL DATA AND GANGLION CELL COUNTS (N = 10)

Age (yr)	Sex	Cause of Death	Side	Hy-drops	First Attack	Last Attack	Last Test	Clinical Tests: Calorics*	Hearing Loss	Discrim. (%)	Cell Counts in Scarpa's Ganglia†
					(yr before death)						
58	M	Cardiac arrest (anesthesia)	R	+	3	< 1	< 1	Decreased	Flat, 70 dB	44	12,600
			L	−			< 1	Normal	No loss	100	12,700
59	F	Peritonitis, septicemia	R	+	7	< 1	< 3	Decreased	Flat, 30 dB	90	12,800
			L	−			< 3	Normal	No loss	100	14,800
62	F	Bronchopneumonia	R	+	4	< 1	< 1	—	Flat, 90 dB	16	14,300
			L	+	4	< 1	< 1	—	Flat, 70 dB	48	13,800
66	M	Cerebral infarction	R	+	7	< 1	< 1	Decreased	Low freq loss	88	13,900
67	M	Myocardial infarction	R	−			< 5	Normal	High freq loss	90	14,700
			L	+	5	< 1	< 5	No response	Flat, 50-80 dB	78	13,900
68	F	Subdural hematoma	R	+	6	> 2	< 1	No response	Flat, 75-80 dB	—	9,700
			L	−			< 1	No response	Flat, 75-80 dB	—	10,200
74	M	Rupture of abdominal aorta aneurysm	R	+	12	> 2	< 3	—	Low freq loss	—	9,400
			L	−			< 3	—	No loss	—	11,100
78	F	Cerebral infarction	R	+	5	< 1	< 2	—	Flat, 60 dB	4	13,800
78	M	Intestinal carcinoma	L	+	13	< 1	< 1	Decreased	Flat, 70-80 dB	60	11,200
87	M	Rupture of abdominal aorta aneurysm	R	+	10	?	—	—	—	—	10,300
			L	−			—				11,700

\+ - Presence of endolymphatic hydrops; − - Absence of endolymphatic hydrops; Freq - Frequency.

*Used Kobrak's minimal test for measurement.

†Corrected for split nucleoli.

could be compared to similar counts made in "normal" material from individuals ranging in age from 1 to 91 years.[18,19] The relations between the clinical symptoms, the degree of cellular degeneration and the presence of hydrops could then be investigated.

METHODS

Selection of Temporal Bones. The temporal bone collection of the Massachusetts Eye and Ear Infirmary was screened for cases of endolymphatic hydrops. Ten cases, four with bilateral hydrops, were selected. In three ears of the four bilateral cases the vestibular nerve had been lost during temporal bone removal. Thus, a total of 11 hydropic and 6 nonhydropic ears could be evaluated. Since the scope of this study was limited to idiopathic endolymphatic hydrops, temporal bones from cases with known disorders which could elicit hydrops (leukosis, syphilitic neurolabyrinthitis, temporal bone fracture) were excluded. Temporal bones were also excluded if the subject had a history of diabetes mellitus, radiation treatment, cytotoxic or ototoxic treatment on tumors of the ear since any of these could cause degeneration of the vestibular epithelia or their innervation.

Processing of Temporal Bones. The procedure for tissue processing has been described by Schuknecht.[6] Temporal bones were removed between 1 and 23 hours postmortem. After fixation in Heidenhain-susa solution, they were decalcified, embedded in celloidin and sectioned in the horizontal plane at 20 μm. Sections were stained with hematoxylin and eosin, and every tenth section was mounted for microscopic examination.

Cell Counts. Counts were performed as described in previous papers.[18,19] For the ganglion cells the nucleoli were counted in every tenth section of Scarpa's ganglion. Counts were multiplied by the sampling period and corrected to account for split nucleoli. The densities of hair cells and inclusion bodies were determined separately for each macula and crista by analysis of those slides in which the epithelia appeared in cross section.

RESULTS

In 7 of 11 ears, endolymphatic hydrops could be described as severe. In at least one cochlear turn, Reissner's membrane seemed to make contact with the entire bony wall of scala vestibuli. In these cases the volume of scala media was estimated to be three to four times normal. In the remaining four ears the hydrops of the cochlea was more moderate. Scala media was at most about two times the normal volume (Fig. 1). The saccular membrane was found distended in all cases with cochlear hydrops. In most cases the saccular membrane was found to make contact with the footplate of the stapes. Volume changes in the saccule, utricle and semicircular canals were more difficult to estimate.

In Table 1, the relevant clinical data from each of the subjects can be compared to the numbers of vestibular neurons estimated for each case. The hearing loss was fluctuating in all cases. Note that the individuals who did not report episodes of vertigo

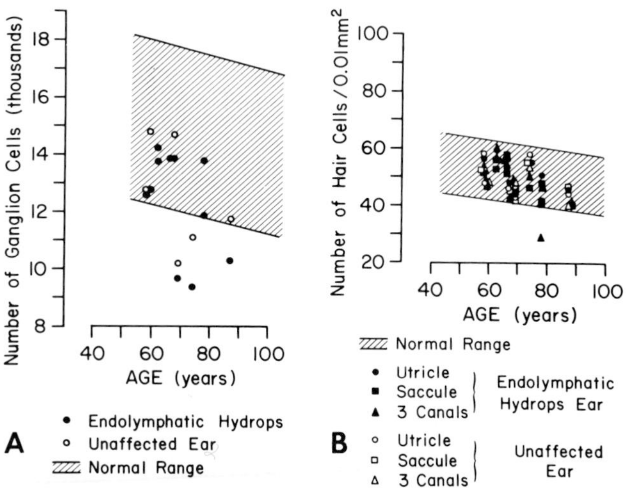

Fig. 2. A) Number of ganglion cells and B) vestibular hair cell densities plotted as a function of age.

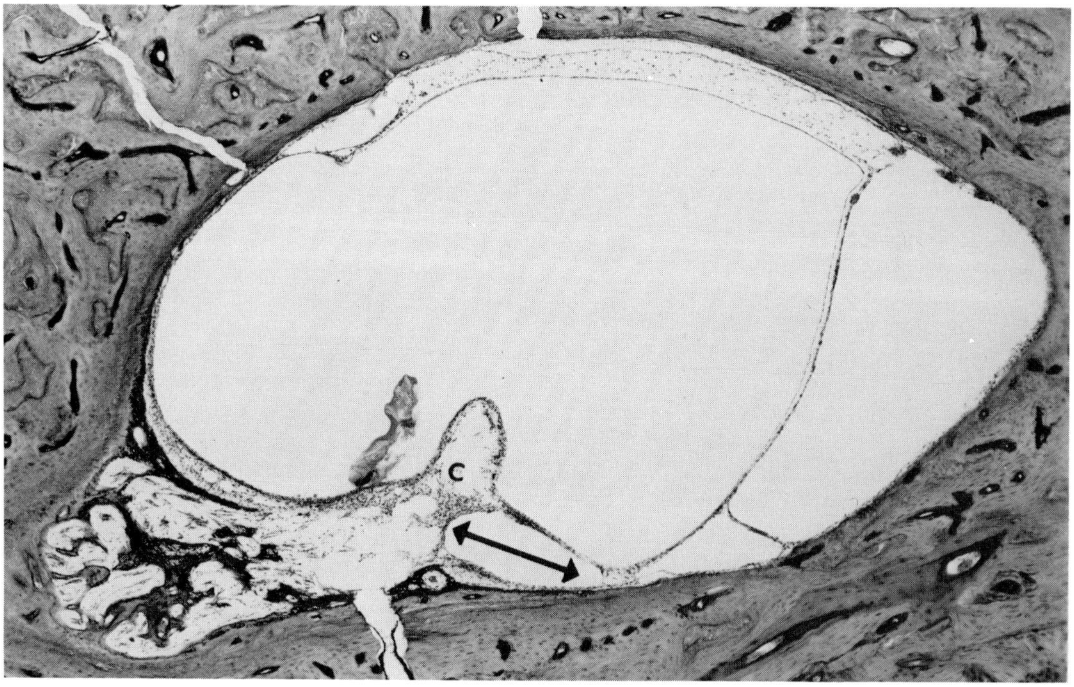

Fig. 3. Photomicrograph of section through the posterior crista of 78-year-old male (Table 1). Supporting structures (C) appear atrophied. The arrow shows a vacuole within the supporting structures. (x30)

during at least the last two years of life had the lowest neuronal counts. Caloric responses are decreased or absent in all ears with endolymphatic hydrops. No correlation between decreased caloric responses and low neuronal counts can be seen.

Ganglion cell counts are plotted as a function of age at death in the left panel of Figure 2. Most of the data fall in the low normal range. In three cases the number of neurons in Scarpa's ganglion appears to be lower than normal. In all three cases, the counts of the nonhydropic side were within 20% of those on the affected side. Right-left differences on the order of 20% were not uncommon in ears from "normal" individuals.[18,19] Values for hair cell densities are shown in the right panel. In the cases of

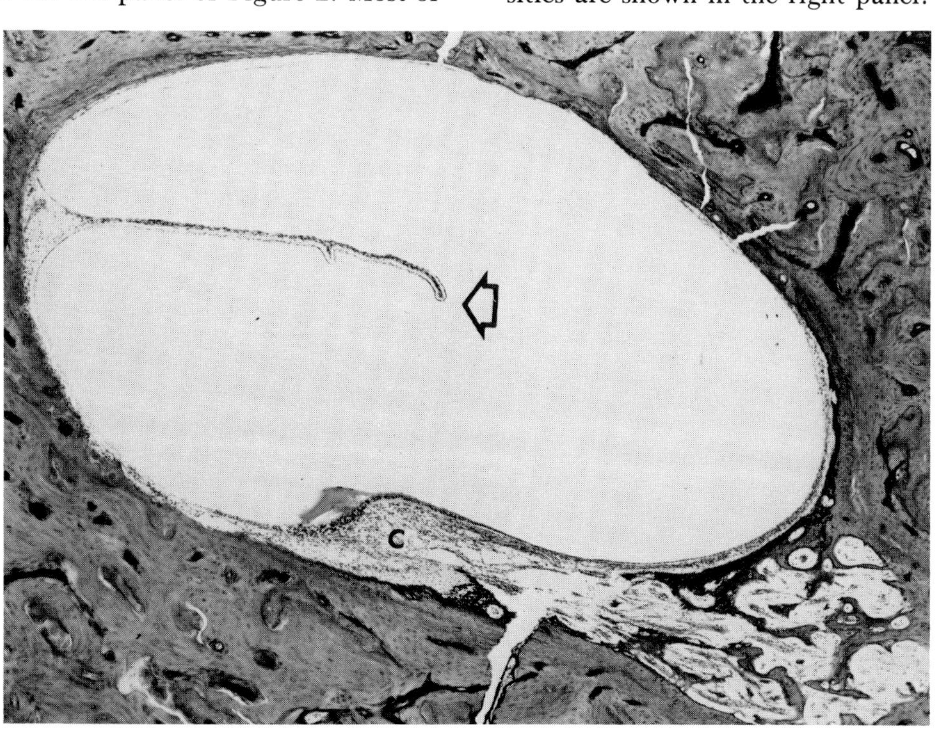

Fig. 4. Photomicrograph of section through the posterior crista of 78-year-old female (Table 1). The arrow points to the ruptured epithelium where it has folded back on itself. (x30)

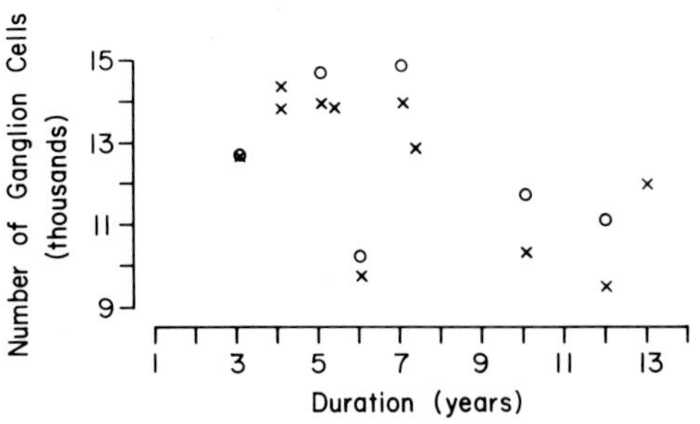

Fig. 5. Number of ganglion cells as a function of time from the first episodes of vertigo to time of death. X - Endolymphatic hydrops; O - Normal ear.

unilateral hydrops, hair cell densities were not significantly lower in the affected ears. In ears from aged "normal" individuals, the densities of intraepithelial inclusion bodies seem to rise with increasing degeneration of vestibular sensory epithelia.[18,19] Densities of inclusion bodies in all cases of this study were within "normal" limits.

The density of hair cells in one posterior crista was clearly below the normal range. A photomicrograph of a section of this crista is shown in Figure 3. It is interesting that this one case with low hair cell density did not show a rupture of the ampullary membrane (at least in the sections available for study, ie, every tenth section at 20 μm), whereas four cases with clear epithelial ruptures showed normal hair cell population. One such case is shown in Figure 4.

In Figure 5, vestibular ganglion cell counts are plotted as a function of the number of years between the first episodes of vertigo and the time of death. Counts are lower with longer durations. This tendency is evident in both the hydropic and the unaffected ear in cases of unilateral hydrops.

DISCUSSION

The observation that almost all of the vestibular sensory epithelia in these cases had normal hair cell densities is in agreement with earlier studies reporting that degeneration of sensory epithelia represents a rare finding in hydropic ears.[1-6] Even ruptures of membranes did not seem to affect the hair cell density of the sense organ. In one case with clear degeneration of the sensory epithelium in the posterior crista an outpouching or rupture of the ampullary membrane could not be demonstrated. The cause of this isolated instance of degeneration remains unclear.

Ultrastructural changes, such as loss of sensory hairs, vesiculation and laminated inclusions of hair cells and long-spaced collagen underneath the basement membrane of the sensory epithelium, have been observed in vestibular sensory epithelia from patients with Menière's syndrome.[10-15] It is not clear however, to what extent such "abnormalities" are present in normal human ears of similar age.

The cell counts of Scarpa's ganglion indicated that neuronal degeneration was more pronounced in three of ten cases than in "normal" individuals of similar age. Counts seemed to be lower in both hydropic and unaffected ears, suggesting that the hydrops was not the direct cause of the degeneration. Each of these cases had exhibited episodes of vertigo for more than six months prior to death. The bilateral neuronal degeneration in these cases may have preceded the onset of endolymphatic hydrops. Several authors have suggested a type of "delayed endolymphatic hydrops" due to secondary damage to the endolymphatic sac caused by previous disease of the ear.[20-22] It is possible that the neuronal degeneration in our cases was caused by a previous disease, also affecting the vestibular nerve.

In view of our findings it is interesting that fibrosis of the vestibular nerve has been detected in specimens removed at operations from individuals with Menière's syndrome.[17]

REFERENCES

1. Hallpike CS, Cairns H. Observations on the pathology of Meniere's syndrome. Proc R Soc Med 1938; 31:1317-36.

2. Lindsay JR. Labyrinthine dropsy and Meniere's disease. Arch Otolaryngol 1942; 35:853-67.

3. Altmann F, Fowler EP. Histological findings in Ménière's symptom complex. Ann Otol Rhinol Laryngol 1943; 52:52-80.

4. Schuknecht HF, Benitez JT, Beekhuis J. Further observations on the pathology of Menière's disease. Ann Otol Rhinol Laryngol 1962; 71:1039-53.

5. Altmann F, Kornfeld M. Histologic studies of Menière's disease. Ann Otol Rhinol Laryngol 1965; 74:915-43.

6. Schuknecht HF. Pathology of the ear. Cambridge: Harvard University Press, 1974.

7. Seymour JC. The etiology, pathology and conservative surgical treatment of Meniere's disease. J Laryngol Otol 1960; 74:599-627.

8. Lindsay JR, von Schulthess G. An unusual case of labyrinthine hydrops. Acta Otolaryngol (Stockh) 1958; 49:315-29.

9. Altmann F, Zechner G. The pathology and pathogenesis of endolymphatic hydrops. New investigations. Arch Klin Exp Ohren Nasen Kehlkopfheilkd 1968; 192:1-19.

10. Pietrantoni L, Iurato S. Some initial electron-microscope investigations of a case of Meniere's syndrome. Acta Otolaryngol (Stockh) 1960; 52:15-26.

11. Litton WB, Lawrence M. Electron microscopy in Meniere's disease. Arch Otolaryngol 1961; 74:52-9.

12. Ireland PE, Farkashidy J. Electron microscopic studies of Meniere's disease: twelve fresh specimens taken at operation. Trans Am Acad Ophthalmol Otolaryngol 1963; 67:28-36.

13. Hilding DA, House WF. An evaluation of ultrastructural findings in the utricle in Meniere's disease. Laryngoscope 1964; 74:1135-48.

14. Friedmann I. Electron microscope studies of the diseased macula of the utricle of the human inner ear with particular reference to Meniere's disease. In: Iurato S, ed. Submicroscopic structure of the inner ear. Oxford: Pergamon Press, 1967:261.

15. Ylikoski J, Collan Y, Palva R. Vestibular sensory epithelium in Meniere's disease. Arch Otolaryngol 1979; 105:486-91.

16. Ylikoski J, Palva T, Virtanen I. The morphology of the vestibular nerve in a patient with normal vestibular function and in patients with Meniere's disease. Arch Otorhinolaryngol 1977; 215:45-54.

17. Helms J, Steinbach E. The vestibular nerve in Meniere's disease: findings from light microscopy. Abstracts 2nd Midwinter Meeting of the Association for Research in Otolaryngology, St. Petersburg, Florida, January 1979:69.

18. Richter E. Counts of neurons in Scarpa's ganglion from human temporal bones. Abstracts 2nd Midwinter Meeting of the Association for Research in Otolaryngology, St. Petersburg, Florida, January 1979:28.

19. Richter E. Quantitative study of human Scarpa's ganglion and hair cell densities in vestibular sensory epithelia. Acta Otolaryngol (Stockh). In press.

20. Wolfson R, Leiberman A. Unilateral deafness with subsequent vertigo. Laryngoscope 1975; 85:1752-66.

21. Nadol J, Weiss A, Parker S. Vertigo of delayed onset after sudden deafness. Ann Otol Rhinol Laryngol 1975; 84:841-6.

22. Schuknecht HF. Delayed endolymphatic hydrops. Ann Otol Rhinol Laryngol 1978; 87:743-9.

LURIE LIBRARY FUND

Many inquiries have been made about a memorial fund to which friends and colleagues of Dr. Moses Hyman Lurie could contribute. Shortly before his death Dr. Lurie established a modest fund for the purchase of books in Otolaryngology for the Library at the Massachusetts Eye and Ear Infirmary. The Library Committee of the Infirmary has verified that donations can be made in memory of Dr. Lurie to this fund. Contributions may be sent to the "Lurie Library Fund," in care of Mr. Charles Snyder, Librarian, Massachusetts Eye and Ear Infirmary, 243 Charles St., Boston, MA 02114.

Ann Otol 90:1981

ULTRASONIC ANALYSIS OF HEAD AND NECK NEOPLASMS
CORRELATION WITH SURGICAL FINDINGS

SHAN R. BAKER, MD CHARLES J. KRAUSE, MD

ANN ARBOR, MICHIGAN

Ultrasonography of head and neck neoplasms is useful in the preoperative evaluation of patients. Inflammatory masses demonstrate high reflectivity in a homogeneous pattern and have diffuse borders. Similarly, lipomas show medium to high reflectivity and have a homogeneous pattern, but are well outlined. Mixed tumors of the major salivary glands have a characteristic heterogeneous pattern and are well outlined. Malignant lesions demonstrate low reflectivity in a homogeneous or heterogeneous pattern and have poorly outlined or diffuse borders. Cysts of the head and neck are well outlined and devoid of interior echoes.

The echo technique, which is used in all areas of modern medicine today, was first developed by Langevin during World War I for detection of submarines.[1] Since that time, the principle has been expanded to include sophisticated applications for the diagnosis and treatment of a variety of diseases.

Ultrasound consists of sound waves with a frequency above the audible range. For this study, a frequency of 8 million cycles per second (8 MHz) has been used. The sound waves are produced by a piezo-electric crystal that changes its thickness under the influence of an electrical field. Short, high voltage electric pulses are sent by a transmitter to the crystal, which then oscillates at its own resonant frequency of 8 MHz, emitting ultrasonic waves into the tissues being analyzed.

Ultrasound energy is reflected whenever the sound beam passes from one medium into another having a different acoustic impedance. The amount of energy reflected is dependent upon the difference in acoustic impedance of the two substances and the angle between the reflecting interface and the sound beam.[2]

Reflected acoustic energy is picked up by the same crystal which emits the initial sound beam, and is converted into electrical signals which are amplified and fed into an oscilloscope. A-Scan ultrasonograms* are one way to display the echographic information on the oscilloscope screen.

Figure 1 represents a diagram of an A-Scan ultrasonic analysis of a parotid neoplasm. The first several echo peaks are referred to as the "initial bang" and correspond to the emission of an ultrasonic pulse. As the sound beam is propagated through the tumor, interfaces within the tumor cause reflection of portions of the beam producing interior echoes. When the sound beam meets the deep interface between tumor and surrounding tissue, a tall border echo is produced in circumscribed neoplasms. The more superficial tumor border near the skin surface is obscured by the initial bang.

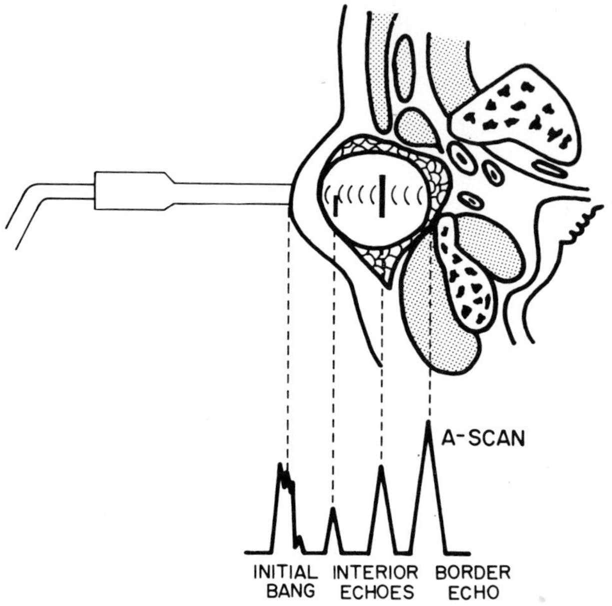

Fig. 1. Diagrammatic demonstration of an A-Scan analysis of a parotid neoplasm. The initial bang corresponds to the emission of an ultrasonic pulse which obscures the superficial tumor border. Interfaces within the tumor cause reflection of portions of the sound beam producing interior echoes. In circumscribed neoplasms a tall discrete border echo is seen at the deep interface between tumor and surrounding tissue.

Ultrasound analysis of head and neck diseases is known as diagnostic echography and is discussed in terms of quantitative, topographic and kinetic properties. Reflectivity refers to the intensity of echoes produced in the interior of the tumor (inner reflectivity) and is influenced by the size, number and distribution of interfaces which are struck simultaneously by the sound beam, each participating in the production of individual echo spikes. Assessment of reflectivity is known as quantitative echography. For the purpose of head and neck masses, inner reflectivity may be divided into five divisions by comparing the average spike height or

*The unit 7200 MA of Kretztechnik® (Rohe Scientific Corporation), found to be most effective for tissue diagnosis in ophthalmology, was used in the preoperative analysis of our patients.

From the Department of Otorhinolaryngology, University of Michigan, Ann Arbor.

REPRINTS — Shan R. Baker, MD, Department of Otorhinolaryngology, Box 61 — Outpatient Building, University Hospital, Ann Arbor, MI 48109.

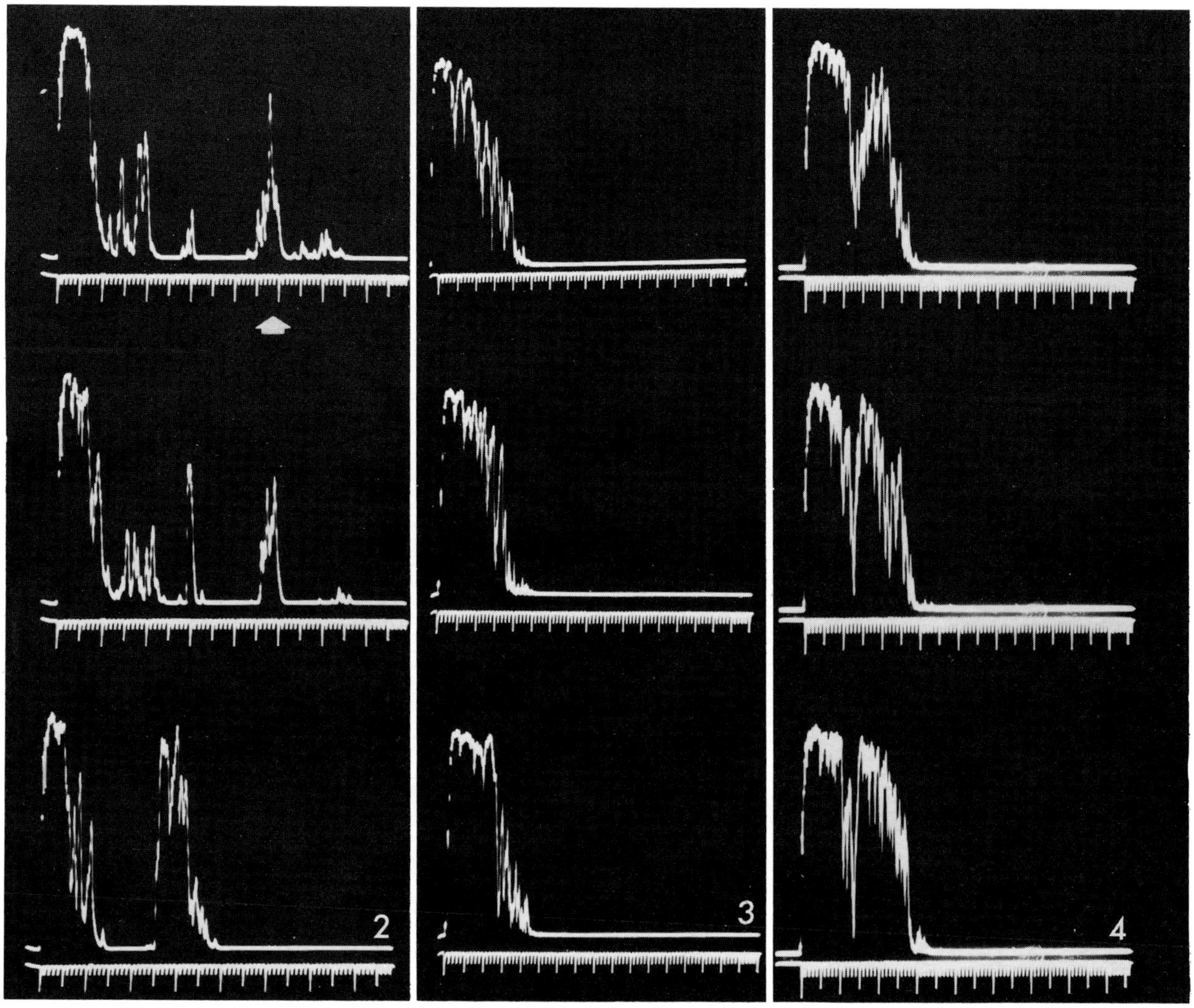

Fig. 2. Ultrasonograms of a varix. A few medium to high echo spikes make up the interior echo pattern. Upper A-Scan demonstrates a steeply rising, narrow, high echo spike (arrow) from the deep border of the mass. Bottom A-Scan demonstrates a change in the configuration of the echo pattern on compression of the varix with the probe.

Fig. 3. Ultrasonograms of three normal parotid glands. High reflectivity and a homogeneous pattern are present because of evenly distributed fibrous septa that appear as large interfaces to the sound beam. The parotid gland is not well circumscribed from surrounding structures, thus discrete border echoes are not observed.

Fig. 4. Ultrasonograms of sialadenitis of the submandibular gland. The lack of a well-defined border echo suggests a diffuse disease process. The V-shaped interior echo pattern is produced by heavy inflammatory cell infiltration which causes local tissue destruction.

amplitude of the reflected echo pattern expressed in percent of the initial spike height in the tissue echogram (Table 1).

The classification of head and neck tumors into one of five categories as outlined in Table 1 requires the use of a standardized system sensitivity setting, the so-called tissue sensitivity. Tissue sensitivity is established once for each instrument-probe combination using a standard tissue model of citrated blood.[3,4]

TABLE 1. QUANTITATIVE ECHOGRAPHY: REFLECTIVITY

Degree	*Interior Echo Amplitude % of Initial Spike*
Extremely high	95-100
High	60-95
Medium	40-60
Low	5-40
Extremely low	0-5

In addition to the intensity of the interior echo pattern, the arrangement of the pattern is important in tumor differentiation. Inner reflectivity is considered homogeneous when the majority of echoes are of the same amplitude. This pattern is seen when similar-sized interfaces predominate within the substance of the tumor. Heterogeneous patterns occur when interior echoes vary widely in their amplitude, suggesting interfaces of variable size within the substance of the tumor. Heterogeneous patterns are considered regular when there is a consistent relationship between the higher and lower spikes within the tissue echogram, and irregular when there is a random relationship in spike heights.

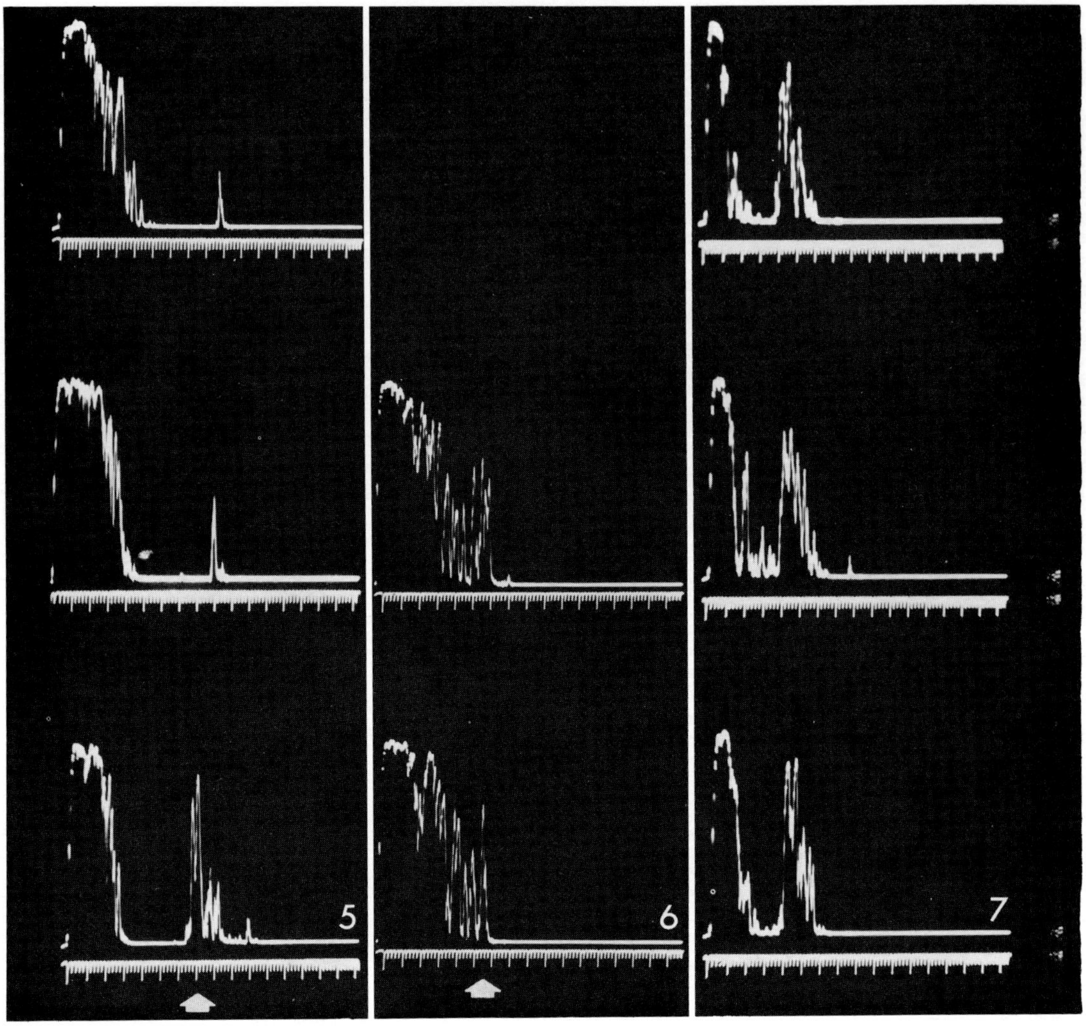

Fig. 5. Ultrasonograms of a submandibular gland abscess. No interior echoes are seen. Bottom A-Scan shows a double-peaked border echo (arrow) representing sound reflection from the inner and outer surfaces of the abscess wall. When this finding is present the lesion is considered to be encapsulated.

Fig. 6. Ultrasonograms of a lipoma of the parotid gland. Medium to high echo spikes occur in a homogeneous pattern. A discrete border spike (arrow) demonstrates that this lipoma is well circumscribed from the parotid gland.

Fig. 7. Ultrasonograms of a dermoid cyst of the parotid gland. Low to extremely low reflectivity is seen. The double peaked border echo demonstrates encapsulation of the lesion. The fine-textured sebaceous material filling the cyst presents few interfaces to the ultrasound beam, thus low reflectivity is seen.

Topographic echography is the use of ultrasound for determining the size, shape and borders of head and neck masses. A three-dimensional measurement may often be obtained by placing the ultrasound probe over the lateral, anterior, and inferior aspect of the lesion. At the same time, borders are evaluated by angling the probe in various directions over the surface of the tumor. Using this method, borders are determined to be well outlined, poorly outlined (diffuse), or cyst walls. Border echoes are important in helping to differentiate tumor types.

Kinetic echography is the use of ultrasound in assessing the consistency of a mass lesion. This is accomplished by pressing the probe against the skin overlying the tumor while observing changes in its size and characteristics of its borders. Lymphangiomas, hemangiomas and arteriovenous fistulae are amenable to this form of echography. In such cases, compression with the probe may change the nature of the interior echo pattern as well as surface border signals due to the softness of their internal structure. Pulsating borders can be easily observed with this technique and warn that tumors are resting against major arteries.

Diagnostic ultrasound has been used extensively in ophthalmology to detect orbital masses and to differentiate these masses into various histological types with an accuracy of 87%.[5] Ultrasound has been applied as a diagnostic tool in otolaryngology;[6-8] however, only recently has quantitative, topographic and kinetic echography been utilized for the diagnosis of head and neck disorders.[9] A multitude of head and neck disease processes have been analyzed and representative cases are presented to demonstrate the applicability of this procedure.

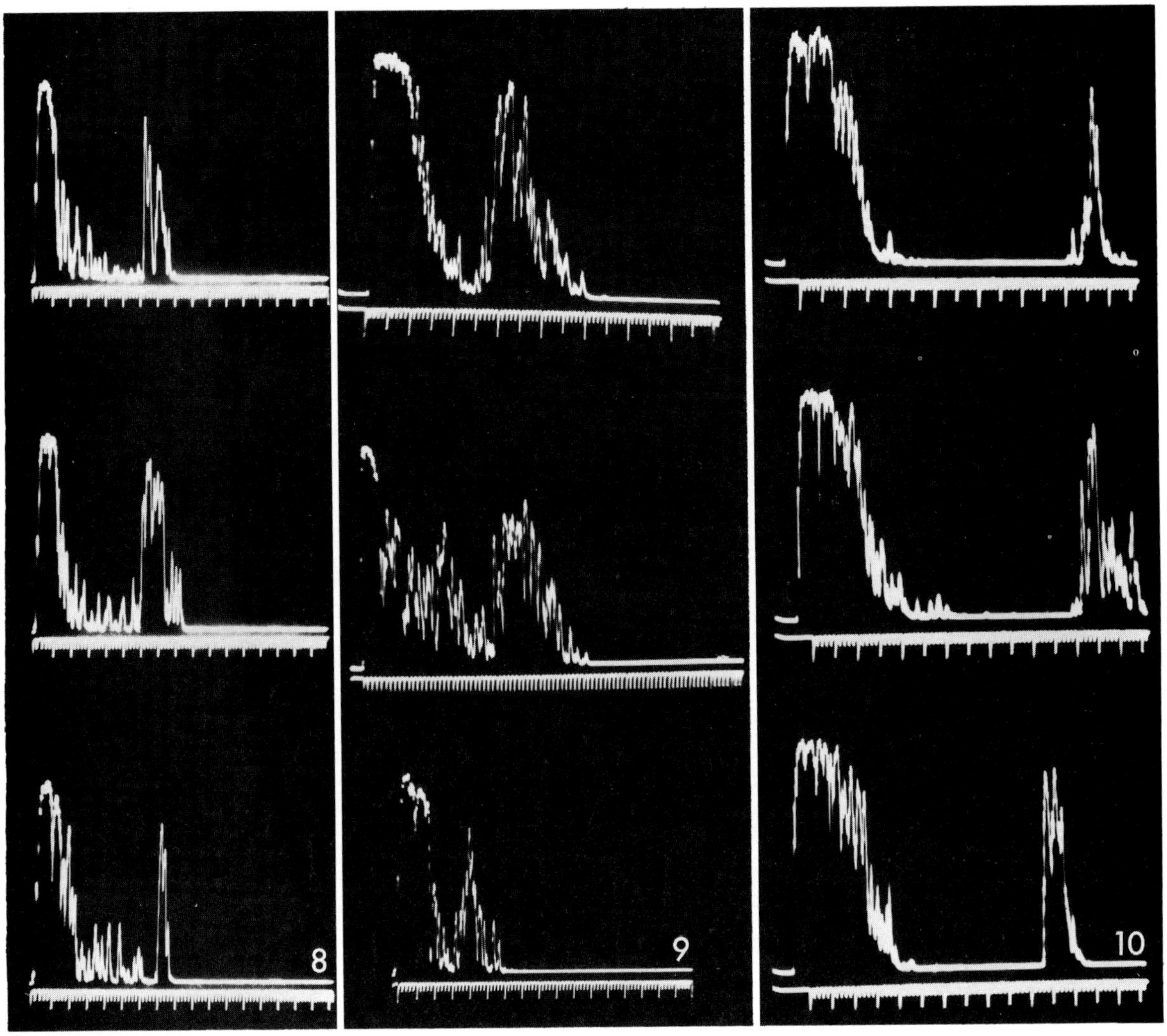

Fig. 8. Ultrasonograms of a benign mixed tumor of the parotid gland. A well-outlined tumor of medium to low reflectivity with a regular heterogeneous interior echo pattern is seen. Low to medium high echo spikes separated by zones relatively free of echoes are characteristic of benign mixed tumors.

Fig. 9. Ultrasonograms of three malignant head and neck tumors. Top) Lymphoma of the neck. Middle) Undifferentiated carcinoma of the parotid. Bottom) Melanoma of the neck. Medium to low reflectivity is seen in the three ultrasonograms. Due to the infiltrating nature of these tumors, no discrete border echo can be seen.

Fig. 10. Ultrasonograms of three cysts of the head and neck. Top) Thyroglossal duct cyst. Middle) Large parotid gland cyst. Bottom) Branchial cleft cyst of the neck. The double-peaked border echo of the branchial cleft cyst suggests encapsulation.

CASE REPORTS

Case 1. A 54-year-old female presented with a slowly enlarging parotid mass over a two-year period. Examination revealed a 4 x 6 cm soft cystic-appearing lesion involving the right parotid gland. Pathological examination following surgical removal revealed a partially thrombosed varix. The echogram of this lesion is seen in Figure 2. A mass with relatively few interior echoes of medium to high reflectivity is seen. Interior echoes represent reflection of sound from interfaces between thrombus and unclotted blood. The upper A-Scan demonstrates a steeply rising, narrow, high echo spike from the deep border of the mass. Smooth, well-circumscribed tumor surfaces produce sharp discrete border echo spikes and suggest a well-outlined lesion. The bottom echogram demonstrates the importance of kinetic echography. A change in the configuration of the echo pattern on compression of the mass with the probe is noted, suggesting a vascular lesion. During compression, the deep border spike was noted to pulsate with the heartbeat. At the time of surgical resection the varix was found to lie adjacent to the superficial temporal artery and was well delineated from surrounding parotid tissue.

Case 2. A 65-year-old male was treated for chronic sialadenitis of the left submandibular gland. Histological examination of the gland after surgical excision revealed chronic inflammation.

Normal major salivary glands have high reflectivity and a homogeneous pattern because of multiple, evenly distributed fibrous septa that appear as large interfaces to the sound beam. The major salivary glands are not well circumscribed from surrounding structures, therefore a discrete border echo is not observed (Fig. 3). Early sialadenitis provides a similar echogram because the main architecture of the gland is not destroyed. However, when heavy infiltration by lymphocytes occurs in inflammation of the gland, these fibrous septa are destroyed and one finds a decreased reflectivity in the area. This local tissue destruction produces a dip or "V" in the echo pattern. Figure 4 represents the preoperative ultrasonograms of this patient's submandibular gland. A V-shaped echo pattern is produced in the area of heaviest inflammatory cell infiltration. A lack of well-defined border echoes suggests a diffuse disease process, as is characteristic of inflammation.

As inflammation progresses, more and more tissue in the area of inflammatory infiltration is destroyed, and eventually abscess

TABLE 2. ULTRASONIC PATTERNS OF HEAD AND NECK DISEASES

Histology	*Echographic Pattern*	*Reflectivity*	*Topography*
Normal salivary gland	Homogeneous	High	Diffuse
Inflammation	Homogeneous	High	Diffuse
Lipoma	Homogeneous	Medium to high	Well-outlined
Mixed tumor	Heterogeneous	Low to medium	Well-outlined
Malignancy	Homogeneous or Heterogeneous	Low	Poorly outlined or Diffuse
Cyst	No interior echoes	No interior echoes	Well-outlined or Encapsulated (double-peaked border spike)

formation occurs. The necrotic materials within the abscess are rather homogeneous to ultrasound and cause only weak echo signals. Figure 5 illustrates ultrasonograms of an abscess involving the submandibular gland of another patient. In this case, no interior echoes were recorded from the abscess. This is explained by the strong sound attenuation of the overlying normal tissue layers represented by the high spikes on the left side of the echogram. A well-outlined border echo is seen because the abscess is walled off from surrounding tissue. A double-peaked surface spike is seen in the bottom A-Scan and represents reflections from inner and outer surfaces of the thick abscess capsule. When a double-peaked border echo is present, the mass is considered to be encapsulated.

Case 3. A 36-year-old female presented with a mass involving the left parotid gland which had been noted for several months. Palpation of the lesion revealed a soft, cyst-like, 3 x 4 cm mass. Ultrasonography suggested that the mass was a lipoma. Figure 6 shows the preoperative ultrasonograms of this lesion. Medium to high interior echo spikes occur in a homogeneous pattern. These spikes represent reflections from large fibrous septa separating lobules of fat. A tall, narrow border spike demonstrates that lipomas are well circumscribed from the parotid gland. Surgical resection confirmed the ultrasonic diagnosis of lipoma.

Case 4. A 39-year-old female presented with a seven-year history of a slowly enlarging mass involving the parotid gland. The examining physician's initial impression was that of a lipoma. Ultrasonography, however, did not suggest such a lesion. It revealed a well-circumscribed tumor with low to extremely low reflectivity (Fig. 7). A double-spiked border echo pointed to a moderately thick capsule encompassing the tumor. Surgical resection revealed a thick-walled dermoid cyst filled with sebaceous material. The homogeneous, fine-textured sebaceous material presented few interfaces to the sound beam and thus inner reflectivity was low.

Case 5. A 26-year-old female presented with a rapidly enlarging parotid neoplasm. A preoperative diagnosis of adenoidcystic carcinoma was made because of the history of rapid growth and tenderness to palpation. Ultrasonography, however, demonstrated an echo pattern characteristic of a benign mixed tumor. Pathological examination of the mass following parotidectomy confirmed this diagnosis. Preoperative ultrasonograms of the tumor are seen in Figure 8. A well-outlined tumor of medium to low reflectivity with a regular heterogeneous interior echo pattern is seen. Low to medium high spikes separated by zones relatively free of echoes is the most common echographic pattern of benign mixed tumors. These zones represent myxomatous areas, or densely cellular areas, whereas the echo spikes represent interfaces between the zones and fibrous septa.

Case 6. A 67-year-old female presented with a three-month history of a rapidly enlarging mass in the upper neck. Biopsy of the tumor revealed malignant lymphoma. Ultrasonography revealed a tumor of low reflectivity and diffuse borders (Fig. 9, top). No distinct high border surface spike could be seen. Malignant tumors such as lymphomas and carcinomas consist mainly of densely packed cells. These tumors have little intercellular substance, and thus lack acoustic interfaces that would produce high echo spikes. Therefore, malignant tumors can be expected to have low to medium reflectivity. Figure 9, middle, is an ultrasonogram of an undifferentiated carcinoma of the parotid gland. Medium reflectivity is seen. Figure 9, bottom, is an A-Scan of a neck mass which, on removal, revealed a malignant melanoma. Low reflectivity is noted.

Due to the infiltrating nature of malignant tumors, they are poorly outlined and do not demonstrate discrete border signals. For comparison, the mixed tumor surface spikes seen in Figure 8 are steeply rising with only a few high spikes composing the surface signal. In contrast, the border spikes of the malignant tumors in Figure 9 are rising slowly with several peaks appearing along the ascending left limb; thus, the surface signal of malignant neoplasms is not as distinct as the surface signal from benign mixed tumors.

Case 7. An 18-year-old male presented with a large cystic mass in the upper neck at the left of the midline. Ultrasonography demonstrated a cyst (Fig. 10, top). Surgical removal of the mass revealed a thin-walled thyroglossal duct cyst. The cyst was filled with fluid and therefore no interior echoes were seen on A-Scan. The thin wall of the cyst produced only a single border spike. Figure 10, middle, is an A-Scan of a parotid cyst and Figure 10, bottom, is an ultrasonogram of a branchial cleft cyst of the neck. The wall of the latter lesion was sufficiently thick to produce a double-peaked border spike. Cysts of the head and neck are perhaps the easiest masses to diagnose with ultrasound because of the consistent echographic pattern they produce. Large echo-free central areas are noted with discrete, well-defined border echoes. Since many of these cysts are soft and compressible, kinetic echography could be helpful. Changes in the reflectivity and shape of borders are usually observed in kinetic echography of head and neck cysts.

DISCUSSION

Ultrasonography of head and neck neoplasms has been useful in the preoperative evaluation of patients. The study of many benign and malignant lesions has enabled us to ascribe certain ultrasonic patterns to certain disease processes (Table 2). Inflammatory masses tend to demonstrate high reflectivity in a homogeneous pattern and have diffuse borders. Lipomas show medium to high reflectivity, have a homogeneous pattern and are well outlined. Mixed tumors of the major salivary glands tend to have low to medium reflectivity and are well outlined. A typical heterogeneous echo pattern is often produced, characterized by medium echo spikes, separated by echo-free zones. This may occur in either a regular or irregular fashion. Malignant lesions demonstrate low to medium reflectivity in a homogeneous or heterogeneous pattern and have poorly outlined or diffuse borders. Cysts of the head and neck produce an A-Scan devoid of interior echoes unless hemorrhage and thrombosis have occurred within the interior of the cyst. These masses are well outlined and may show a double-peaked border spike when the wall of the cyst is sufficiently thick.

Diagnostic ultrasound offers a new frontier in noninvasive evaluation of head and neck diseases. The technique enables the surgeon to determine preoperatively whether a tumor is solid or cystic, encapsulated or nonencapsulated. It accurately determines the size and extension of disease into the interior of the anatomical area involved. It may, in the future, allow preoperative knowledge of the histology of a tumor as derived from the echographic pattern produced.

REFERENCES

1. Kitamura T, Kaneko T, Asano H, Muira T. Ultrasonic diagnosis in otorhinolaryngology. Eye Ear Nose Throat Mon 1969; 48:329-37.

2. Kelsey CA, Minifie FD, Hixon TJ. Applications of ultrasound in speech research. J Speech Hear Res 1969; 12:546-65.

3. Ossoinig K, Till P. Clinical standardization in ophthalmology. I. Proc Conf Ultrasonics Biol Med 1970; 70:175-82.

4. Till P, Ossoinig K. Clinical standardization in ophthalmology. II. Proc Conf Ultrasonics Biol Med 1970; 70:233-8.

5. Ossoinig KC. Preoperative differential diagnosis of tumors with echography. In: Blodi F, ed. Current concepts in ophthalmology. Vol 4. St. Louis: CV Mosby, 1974: chap 17.

6. Brzezinska H. Application of the ultrasonic echo method for laryngological diagnostics in children. Proc Conf Ultrasonics Biol Med 1970; 70:29-33.

7. Neiman HL, Phillips JF, Jaques DA, Brown TL. Ultrasound of the parotid gland. J Clin Ultrasound 1976; 4:11-3.

8. Abramson DH, Abramson AL, Coleman DJ. Ultrasonics in otolaryngology: an aid in the diagnosis of middle ear fluid. Arch Otolaryngol 1972; 96:146-50.

9. Baker S, Ossoinig KC. Ultrasonic evaluation of salivary glands. Trans Am Acad Ophthalmol Otolaryngol 1977; 84:750-62.

≈

REPORT OF THE PANEL ON COMMUNICATIVE DISORDERS

Single copies of the *Report of the Panel on Communicative Disorders to the National Advisory Neurological and Communicative Disorders and Stroke Council* (NIH publication no. 79-1914) may be obtained from: Chief, Office of Scientific and Health Reports, National Institute of Neurological and Communicative Disorders and Stroke, Bldg. 31, Rm 8A08, 9000 Rockville Pike, Bethesda, MD 20205.

Ann Otol 90:1981

COMPLICATIONS OF CO_2 LASER SURGERY OF THE LARYNX

ARLEN MEYERS, MD, FACS
DENVER, COLORADO

Since the introduction of CO_2 laser surgery, surgeons have stressed the importance of protecting nontarget structures from errant irradiation. Although striking areas outside the intended field may inflict little or no damage, irradiating an exposed endotracheal tube may result in an endotracheal fire. Recent experience with a case of endotracheal tube ignition led to a reevaluation of those factors associated with this serious complication. In an attempt to determine the best endotracheal tube to use during laser surgery of the larynx, the flammability of polyvinyl chloride and red rubber endotracheal tubes was compared. Several factors were noted to contribute to the potential hazard of endotracheal tube ignition. Since red rubber tubes are less flammable, they should be used during laryngeal CO_2 laser surgery.

INTRODUCTION

Since its introduction, the surgical CO_2 laser has come to be recognized as an extremely valuable adjunct in the management of laryngeal problems.[1,2] The unique properties of nonionizing radiation, however, present specific anesthetic hazards. Birch[3] outlined some precautions that need to be taken. He stressed the importance of protecting the endotracheal tube from the laser beam, cautioned the operator about the possibility of endotracheal fire, and restated the need to protect the patient and operating room personnel from the effects of stray infrared radiation.

Despite the expanded use of the laser, only a few reports have emerged describing endotracheal tube ignition. Snow et al[4,5] reported four cases of tube ignition and outlined a plan of management. Burgess and LeJeune[6] documented an additional case. Recent experience with a case of endotracheal tube ignition led to a reevaluation of those factors associated with this serious complication. In addition, in an attempt to determine the best endotracheal tube to use during laser surgery of the larynx the flammability of two commonly used tubes, polyvinyl chloride and red rubber, was compared.

CASE REPORT

A 28-year-old white male welder was admitted to the hospital for elective direct laryngoscopy and removal of residual papillomas of his right vocal cord with a CO_2 laser. The patient had undergone direct laryngoscopy and microsurgical removal of papillomas from his left vocal cord four months previously. Admission urinalysis, complete blood cell count, electrocardiogram, and chest x-ray were normal. Physical examination revealed papillomas of the right true vocal cord along its entire length, covering the vocal process of the arytenoid.

The patient was anesthetized with sodium penthothal, a succinylcholine drip and intubated with a cuffed aluminum foil-wrapped No. 6 polyvinyl chloride endotracheal tube. The tube was carefully wrapped in an overlapping fashion with a single strip of tape, and the tip of the tube, distal to the balloon, was likewise covered. Following intubation the balloon in the subglottis was inflated and covered with saline-soaked neurosurgical cottonoids. The patient's eyes were covered with moistened eye pads.

Following biopsy of the mass, the papillomas were removed with intermittent CO_2 laser bursts (0.1 second at 20 W). During the procedure, it was noted that the endotracheal tube balloon was deflated and additional cottonoids were placed subglottically to assure an adequate seal, and to protect the tube from stray laser radiation. Papillomas were removed from the anterior and middle third of the vocal cord without problem. While removing papillomas from the vocal process of the arytenoid, however, the endotracheal tube ignited. The laryngoscope was immediately removed, the patient extubated, and reintubated with a No. 6.5 tube. The patient was immediately given 8 mg Decadron® IV, 1 gm ampicillin IV, and a 7x40 ventilating bronchoscope was introduced over the endotracheal tube. A piece of charred neurosurgical cottonoid (1 cm above the carina) was removed from the distal trachea. Examination of the tracheobronchial mucosa showed only mild erythema. The endotracheal tube was left in place with the cuff deflated for 24 hours. The patient received 1 gm ampicillin IV for 24 hours, and 100 mg hydrocortisone daily IV.

The patient remained afebrile, blood gases were normal, and his chest x-ray was normal. The morning following surgery, a fiberoptic bronchoscope was placed through the lumen of the endotracheal tube and the distal trachea visualized and seen to be normal. While visualizing the subglottis, the patient was extubated and the area below the vocal cord showed only mild edema and erythema. Copious secretions made complete visualization difficult.

Following extubation, the patient had no evidence of stridor or airway obstruction. He made an uneventful recovery and was discharged on the second hospital day. A repeat chest x-ray prior to discharge was normal. Follow-up examination three weeks later showed a few residual papillomas on the vocal process of arytenoid. His voice was much improved, however.

TABLE 1. POLYVINYL CHLORIDE TUBE

		Power	
Time (sec)	*5 W (mm)*	*10 W (mm)*	*20 W (mm)*
50% Oxygen			
0.1	1.8	2.0 (f)	
0.2	2.0	3.0	
0.5	3.0 (f)	3.0	
1.0	3.0 (f, hole)	3.0 (fire)	
100% Oxygen			
0.1	1.0	1.5 (f)	1.5
0.2	2.0 (f)	2.0	2.0 (f)
0.5	3.0 (f)	2.5	
1.0	3.0 (f, crater)	2.0 (f, through)	

f - Flame.

From the Department of Otolaryngology, University of Colorado Health Sciences Center, Denver.

TABLE 2. RED RUBBER TUBE

	Power			
Time (sec)	*5 mm W*	*10 mm W*	*20 mm W*	*20 mm W (100%)*
0.1	1.0	1.0	2.0	2.0
0.2	1.5	1.5	2.5	2.5
0.5	2.0	2.0	2.5	2.5
1.0	2.5	2.5	3.0	3.0

METHODS

To determine the relative flammability of endotracheal tubes, red rubber tubes and polyvinyl chloride tubes were exposed to doses of CO_2 laser radiation from 5 W to 20 W, and at time intervals of 0.1 second, 0.2 second, 0.5 second, and 1 second. Test runs were made while 50% and 100% oxygen were passed through the tube. In an attempt to simulate clinical conditions, a balloon was tied to the endotracheal tube so that the oxygen flow would be as constant as possible. Oxygen was insufflated with a standard anesthesia machine. The resultant craters on the tubes were measured, the presence or absence of flame was noted, and the resultant integrity of the tube wall was assessed.

RESULTS

Irradiating polyvinyl chloride tubes resulted in crater formation with or without the production of a flame. The use of 10 W or greater produced a flame at all time exposures. In addition, when 100% oxygen was flowing through the tube, the polyvinyl chloride tube flamed at 5 W/0.2 sec, whereas it did not when 50% oxygen was used. The size and depth of the resultant craters were proportional to increasing time and power exposures (Table 1).

A correlation was likewise found between the size of the burn crater and the time/dose when using red rubber tubes (Table 2). In no instance, however, did the red rubber tubes flame. In addition, there was no difference in crater size or flaming when 50% or 100% oxygen was used.

DISCUSSION

Although the CO_2 laser is being used increasingly for the management of airway problems in patients of all ages,[1,2] relatively few reports have detailed the potential complications associated with its use. Our experience with endotracheal tube ignition prompted a review of the operative pitfalls associated with this serious complication.

Complications of CO_2 laser microlaryngoscopy are generally associated with striking unprotected materials in the airway or unprotected tissues of the patient or operating room personnel (Table 3).

To reduce the risk of ocular damage, the patient's eyes should be covered by moistened eye pads and all personnel in the operating room should wear plastic protective glasses. In addition, while the laser is in use, the flow of traffic in and out of the operating room should be minimized, and windows facing halls should be blocked. Unlike other forms of laser energy, the radiation emitted by the CO_2 laser is predominantly absorbed in the cornea, not the retina, and heat is generated in the epithelial layers. As the intensity and duration of the beam is enlarged, the resultant temperature rise within the cornea is sufficient to produce thermal denaturation and coagulation of proteins, and gross corneal opacification results. Should higher doses strike the unprotected cornea, then corneal perforation occurs.[7]

TABLE 3. COMPLICATIONS OF CO_2 LASER SURGERY OF THE LARYNX

- Exposure hazards to patient or OR personnel
  - Corneal burns[7]
  - Skin exposure
  - Postoperative dysgeusia
- Anesthetic hazards
  - Endotracheal ignition[6]
  - Inadequate ventilation (tube kink, balloon rupture, increased CO_2 gas escape)
  - Intraoperative airway obstruction secondary to foreign body (aluminum foil, cottonoids)
- Complications of microlaryngoscopy
  - Tooth trauma
  - TM joint dislocation
  - Arrhythmia or acute myocardial infarction
  - Airway obstruction secondary to tongue swelling
- Complications of inadvertent CO_2 irradiation
  - Misdirected burns from direct or reflected energy
  - Tracheal perforation
  - Endotracheal tube ignition
  - Acquired glottic web
  - Subglottic stenosis
  - Vocal cord fibrosis
  - Arytenoid perichondritis
- Other
  - Bleeding
  - Infection
  - Delayed healing
  - Postoperative airway obstruction
  - Otalgia
  - Dysphagia and/or odynophagia
  - Papilloma implantation on lips, nasopharynx, oropharynx, or oral cavity
- Complication of aluminum foil wrapped ET tube
  - Airway obstruction from displaced aluminum foil
  - Trauma to vocal cord during intubation
  - Limited flexibility of tube

OR - Operating room; ET - Endotracheal.

The anesthetic management of patients undergoing CO_2 laser has recently been reviewed.[8] Several points should be stressed, however. Of primary importance is the need to protect the endotracheal tube and balloon from laser energy. To accomplish this, most authors recommend the use of aluminum foil tape, metal endotracheal tubes,[9] or saline-soaked adhesive tape. The entire tube should be covered, particularly the end distal to the balloon, since its location in the subglottis puts it in precarious proximity to the beam. Unfortunately, there is no acceptable means of covering the balloon with reflective tape. Consequently, the balloon is usually covered with neurosurgical cottonoids. Recent experience has taught us that, when used, the cottonoids should be large enough to cover the entire balloon (usually 2.5 x 2.5 cm) and that both the string attached to the cotton and the pledget itself be moistened frequently during the procedure. Despite these precautions, however, errant laser radiation will periodically strike the balloon and deflate it. Most of the time, cottonoids can be added to protect the exposed tube and seal any anesthetic leak. Should there be any problem in doing this, or if the balloon and unprotected tube are close to the target, as while working near the posterior commissure or vocal process of the arytenoid, then the endotracheal tube should be removed and replaced with a new functioning tube.

Despite taking the necessary precautions, endotracheal tube ignition still occurs. The surgeon should be prepared to deal with this eventuality ahead of time and be sure that the necessary instruments and equipment are available. Management includes several steps. The patient should be paralyzed while the damaged endotracheal tube is removed. This prevents laryngospasms and makes subsequent reintubation possible quickly. The tube should be removed since the distal tip can collapse and make ventilation difficult or impossible. In addition, fumes from the burned polyvinyl chloride may contribute to pulmonary damage or further injure the subglottic mucosa. Intravenous antibiotics and steroids are given, as in treating a tracheal or pulmonary burn, and intraoperative bronchoscopy should be performed. In addition to enabling the surgeon to remove charred debris from the tracheal lumen, any foreign bodies can be removed, as was the cottonoid in our case, and the extent of any damage to the tracheobronchial mucosa can be assessed. Delayed extubation may be necessary and reexamination of the subglottis and trachea at frequent intervals is important to assess the extent of any long-term airway compromise. The appearance of granulation tissue or stenosis should be treated aggressively in its early stages.

Results of irradiating polyvinyl chloride and red rubber tubes indicate that red rubber is less flammable and, therefore, safer to use in conjunction with the CO_2 laser. Despite this fact, the balloon can still be damaged by as little as 10 W at 0.1 second. It's clear that a new endotracheal tube equipped with a balloon capable of withstanding usual doses of laser irradition is needed.

An additional risk factor in endotracheal ignition is high oxygen flows and, of course, flammable anesthetic agents. Whereas a polyvinyl chloride tube will flame at lower doses of irradiation with higher oxygen flows within it, red rubber tubes are relatively impermeable to laser radiation at usual doses. Oxygen concentration seems to be a less critical factor, therefore, when using them.

Finally, additional care is needed when lasering near the endotracheal tube at any point. Whereas most pathology is at the anterior two thirds of the vocal cords or the anterior commissure, problems at the vocal process of the anterior or posterior commissure require that the laser energy be delivered closer to the endotracheal tube. These "danger zones" require additional concentration on the surgeon's part and meticulous protection of the endotracheal tube.

CONCLUSIONS

1. Several factors contribute to the potential hazard of endotracheal tube ignition.

2. Polyvinyl chloride endotracheal tubes tend to burn more than red rubber tubes. When exposed to doses of irradiation customarily used in laser laryngoscopy, polyvinyl chloride flamed, and the lumen of the endotracheal tube was routinely exposed. At no time was the lumen of the red rubber tube exposed and the material did not ignite.

3. Since the walls of red rubber tubes are not violated at usual doses, the use of high oxygen concentrations through the tube is less of a hazard.

4. If the balloon of an endotracheal tube is accidently deflated, the tube should be replaced or extreme care should be taken to protect the exposed portion of the tube.

5. When neurosurgical cottonoids are used to protect the balloon in the subglottis, they should be moistened frequently.

6. The endotracheal tube balloon should be placed as far from the undersurface of the vocal cords as possible.

7. Adhesive tape-wrapped red rubber tubes are safer than polyvinyl chloride tubes when the CO_2 laser is used in the aerodigestive system.

8. Extra care should be taken when lasering near the vocal process of the arytenoid or the posterior commissure.

REFERENCES

1. Strong MS, Jako GJ, Vaughn CW, Healy GB, Polanyi T. The use of CO_2 laser in otolaryngology; a progress report. Trans Am Acad Ophthalmol Otolaryngol 1976; 82:595-602.

2. Simpson GT, Healy GB, McGill T, Strong MS. Benign tumors and lesions of the larynx in children: surgical excision by CO_2 laser. Ann Otol Rhinol Laryngol 1979; 88:479-85.

3. Birch AA. Anesthetic considerations during laser surgery. Anesth Analg (Cleve) 1973; 52:53-8.

4. Snow JC, Kripke BJ, Strong MS, Jako GJ, Meyer MR, Vaughan CW. Anesthesia for carbon dioxide laser microsurgery on the larynx and trachea. Anesth Analg (Cleve) 1974; 53:507-12.

5. Snow JC, Morton ML, Saluja TS, Estanislao AF. Fire hazard during CO_2 laser microsurgery on the larynx and trachea. Anesth Analg (Cleve) 1976; 55:146-7.

6. Burgess GE, LeJeune FE. Endotracheal tube ignition during laser surgery of the larynx. Arch Otolaryngol 1979; 105:561-2.

7. Leibowitz HM, Peacock GR. Corneal injury by CO_2 laser radiation. Arch Ophthalmol 1969; 81:713-21.

8. Oliverio RM, Ferman CM. Carbon dioxide laser surgery on the larynx: anesthetic technique. NY State J Med 1979; 79:1235-6.

9. Vourch G, Tannieres ML, Freche G. Anesthesia for microsurgery of the larynx using a carbon dioxide laser. Anaesthesia 1979; 34:53-7.

NATURE OF BLOOD-LABYRINTH BARRIER IN EXPERIMENTAL CONDITIONS

S. K. JUHN, MD

L. P. RYBAK, MD, PhD   S. PRADO, MD, PhD

MINNEAPOLIS, MINNESOTA

The blood-labyrinth barrier is a concept that has evolved based on marked difference in chemical composition between perilymph and blood. Studies reported here have been designed to manipulate physiologic, metabolic, and pharmacologic conditions in experimental animals in order to determine the characteristics of this regulatory mechanism. Tracer studies of uptake of sodium, calcium, and albumin from blood into perilymph showed that these substances penetrate into inner ear fluids quite slowly. Injections of ototoxic substances (kanamycin, furosemide) show limited transport of these agents into perilymph. Another ototoxic agent, ethacrynic acid, was found to transiently reduce the transport of sodium into perilymph. Administration of an osmotic agent (urea) resulted in a parallel but delayed elevation of perilymph concentration. The possible role of alteration of blood-labyrinth barrier in inner ear disorders has been discussed.

INTRODUCTION

Fluid compartments within the inner ear each have a characteristic composition. These unique characteristics of each type of fluid seem to be maintained by homeostatic mechanisms, so that hearing in the normal individual remains within narrow limits. The maintenance of a constant ionic environment in the labyrinth appears to depend upon energy-dependent ion pumps, constant blood circulation, and a blood-labyrinth barrier mechanism.[1]

The nature of the blood-labyrinth barrier has not yet been fully documented. This concept is based on marked differences in the chemical composition of blood, cerebrospinal fluid (CSF), and other fluids under physiological conditions. The blood-labyrinth barrier may include all processes which prevent, reduce, delay, or even actually facilitate the penetration of any substance into the inner ear fluid system. This penetration might be mediated by simple diffusion, ultrafiltration, osmosis, lipid solubility, special tissue affinity, or metabolic activity of inner ear tissues for certain substances.

The blood-labyrinth barrier certainly contributes to the maintenance of constant composition of inner ear fluids. Because the inner ear fluids are in contact with the surrounding tissues and are connected directly or indirectly with CSF and blood, it is very likely that there is a continuous exchange of ions and metabolites between these various body fluids. Even so, there are marked differences between the chemical composition of perilymph and that of blood or CSF (Table 1).

In experimental hyperglycemia the glucose concentration in perilymph parallels the blood glucose concentration; however, a time lag before attainment of maximum concentration has been observed.[2] Glucose-loading studies in streptozotocin-diabetic chinchillas revealed that the glucose concentration of perilymph also paralleled the blood glucose concentration, but there was much less of an increment of glucose in perilymph than in serum.[1] In experimental hypoglycemia induced by insulin administration, glucose concentration in perilymph decreased proportionately with the blood glucose concentration.[2]

The concept of a barrier system that limits the access of certain blood-borne substances to the inner ear fluids has been derived by analogy to the blood-brain barrier which was first described by Ehrlich.[3] Since the concept of a blood-labyrinth barrier has just evolved in the past decade or so, its function has not yet been as fully documented or characterized as has the blood-brain barrier. To characterize the blood-labyrinth barrier, a number of studies have been carried out in this laboratory in recent years, utilizing physiologic, metabolic, and pharmacologic conditions. Various test substances have been employed to study this blood-labyrinth barrier (Fig. 1).

METHODS

Chinchillas of either sex weighing 400-500 g were used for all the studies reported here. Animals were anesthetized using either pentobarbital sodium (30 mg/kg) or urethane (0.7 ml/100 g of a 25% solution) intraperitoneally. Blood samples were drawn from the jugular vein. Perilymph from the scala tympani was obtained by opening the auditory bulla and inserting a clean glass capillary tube through the round window membrane and removing fluid by capillary action. Cerebrospinal fluid was withdrawn from the subarachnoid space beneath the membrana atlantooccipitalis, using a tuberculin syringe. Aqueous humor was taken from the anterior chamber of the eye by inserting a needle through the cornea and withdrawing the fluid with a tuberculin syringe.[4] Care was taken to avoid blood contamination of perilymph, CSF, and aqueous humor samples. Samples that were contaminated with

From the Department of Otolaryngology, University of Minnesota Medical School, Minneapolis. This research was supported by USPHS Grants NS-12125-01 and K07 NS-00492.

Presented at the meeting of the American Neurotology Society, Los Angeles, March 30, 1979.

REPRINTS — S. K. Juhn, MD, Department of Otolaryngology, University of Minnesota Medical School, Minneapolis, MN 55455.

TABLE 1. CERTAIN CHEMICAL PARAMETERS OF NORMAL CHINCHILLA BODY FLUIDS

	Serum	CSF	Perilymph	Aqueous humor
Sodium (mEq/l) (mEq/l)	153.4 ± 4.4* (15)**	165.1 ± 2.5 (10)	171.3 ± 6.4 (15)	161.6 ± 4.4 (10)
Potassium (mEq/l)	3.8 ± 0.4* (15)	2.9 ± 0.3 (10)	4.7 ± 0.8 (15)	3.5 ± 0.5 (10)
Chloride (mEq/l)	105.1 ± 4.2 (18)	139.7 ± 6.0 (9)	153.3 ± 8.9 (9)	113.4 ± 5.8 (10)
Calcium (mg/dl)	7.2 ± 1.4 (15)	5.0 ± 0.92 (10)	4.9 ± 0.76 (10)	6.4 ± 1.4 (10)
Total protein (mg/dl)	3,999 ± 360 (15)	25.5 ± 2.8 (10)	191.2 ± 34.6 (15)	53.3 ± 8.2 (10)
Glucose (mg/dl)	125.7 ± 18.8 (10)	128.7 ± 8.5 (10)	162.2 ± 16.3 (15)	163.5 ± 27.7 (10)
LDH*** (mU/ml)	521.1 ± 115.4 (15)	29.6 ± 9.6 (10)	98.6 ± 26.0 (15)	35.3 ± 15.0 (8)
MDH*** (mU/ml)	416.5 ± 109.0 (15)	34.9 ± 12.7 (10)	99.8 ± 34.0 (15)	46.8 ± 11.1 (10)

*Values are expressed as mean ± standard deviation
**Number in parenthesis indicates number of samples
***International Units

LDH - Lactic dehydrogenase; MDH - Malic dehydrogenase. (From Lab Anim Sci 1974; 24:691-5. Copyright 1974, American Association for Laboratory Animal Science. Published with permission.)

blood were discarded. Only single samples of each body fluid were used per animal.

Sodium Study. For the sodium study, each control animal received intravenously 20 μCi/kg ^{22}Na in physiological saline with an activity of 10 μCi/ml. Samples of blood and perilymph were taken 15, 30, 60 and 90 minutes after injection. Five microliters of each sample were diluted with 50 μl of distilled water and counted using a spectrometer.* Animals treated with ethacrynic acid were treated in the same way as controls, except that they were given sodium ethacrynate (30 mg/kg) intravenously just prior to ^{22}Na administration.

Calcium Study. Animals in the calcium study were anesthetized as above; ^{45}Ca (10 mCi/mg) was diluted with physiological saline to an activity of 100 μCi/ml. Chinchillas then were injected with 40 μCi/kg intravenously. Samples of serum, perilymph, CSF, and aqueous humor were collected at 30 minutes, 2, 6, 12, 18 and 24 hours after injection. Five microliters of each body fluid were diluted with 50 μl of distilled water and counted with a spectrometer.*

RISA Study. For the radioiodinated ^{125}I serum albumin (RISA) study, animals were anesthetized in a similar manner. RISA was diluted to an activity of 100 μCi/ml in normal saline. Each animal was injected with 70 μCi/kg and samples of serum, perilymph, CSF, and aqueous humor were obtained at 30 minutes, 2, 6, 12 and 24 hours after injection. Five-microliter samples were diluted

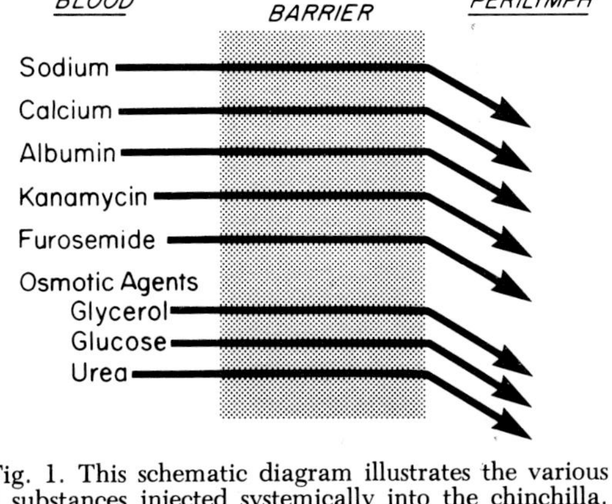

Fig. 1. This schematic diagram illustrates the various test substances injected systemically into the chinchilla. These substances were subsequently retrieved by collection and analysis of perilymph.

*Packard Autogamma Spectrometer, Model 3003.

with 50 μl distilled water and counted with a Beckman gamma counter.

Kanamycin Study. Chinchillas were injected with 200 mg/kg kanamycin intramuscularly. Samples of blood, perilymph, CSF, and aqueous humor were obtained one hour after injection under anesthesia induced by sodium pentobarbital (30 mg/kg).

Kanamycin concentration was measured using a radioimmunoassay kit that is commercially available.* This technique uses the double antibody technique with ^{125}I as the tracer. The concentration of unknowns is extrapolated from a standard curve.

Furosemide Study. The next group of chinchillas was anesthetized with pentobarbital (30 mg/kg intraperitoneally) and injected with furosemide, 100 mg/kg intravenously. Samples of serum and perilymph were obtained 5, 15, 30 and 60 minutes after injection. Furosemide concentrations were determined using high-pressure liquid chromatography separation with ultraviolet detection at 235 nm.

Concentrations were extrapolated from standard curves, prepared from known concentrations of furosemide, which are linear from 0.050 to 500 μg/ml. Samples prepared from untreated animals showed no interfering substances.[5]

Urea Study. Chinchillas anesthetized with urethane were injected with urea 2 g/kg intravenously. Samples of blood, perilymph, and CSF were obtained from individual animals 30, 60, 90, 120 and 180 minutes after injection. Samples were analyzed by a colorimetric method with urease and the Bertholet reaction. A detailed description of the method has been published previously.[6]

RESULTS

Sodium Study. A plot of the ratio of ^{22}Na activity of perilymph, CSF, and aqueous humor to that in serum (Fig. 2) shows that the net transport of sodium ions into the perilymphatic space is a slow process compared to that of CSF or aqueous humor. The sodium exchange time (SET) is about 190 minutes for perilymph, but is much shorter for CSF and aqueous humor. Sodium exchange time represents the time to reach 50% of serum activity.

Animals injected with ethacrynic acid at the same time as ^{22}Na was injected showed an interesting pattern (Fig. 3). Fifteen minutes after in-

*Monitor Science Corporation, Newport Beach, Calif.

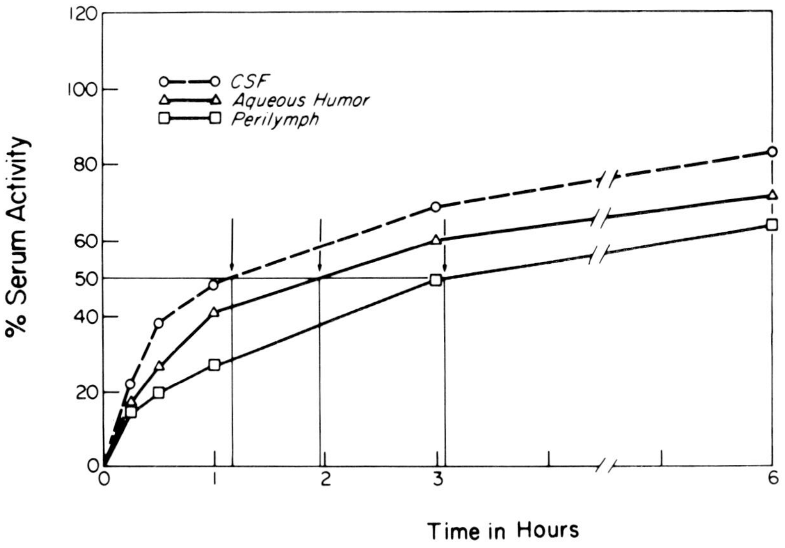

Fig. 2. Ratio of perilymph, CSF, and aqueous humor activities to that of serum after intravenous administration of ^{22}Na in chinchillas. (From Arch Otorhinolaryngol 1976; 212: 213-4. Copyright 1976, Springer Verlag. Published with permission.)

jection, the perilymph of the ethacrynic acid-treated animals had the same ratio of ^{22}Na activity to that of serum as the control animals. However, 30 and 60 minutes after injection, ^{22}Na activity of diuretic-treated animals was substantially reduced. By 90 minutes, the ^{22}Na activity in the perilymph of both groups was equal.

Calcium Study. The calcium activity measurement (Fig. 4) showed that calcium uptake into aqueous humor was considerably more rapid than its entry into CSF or perilymph. Only two hours were required for the activity of ^{45}Ca in aqueous humor to reach 50% of serum values. On the other hand, perilymph uptake of ^{45}Ca rose even more slowly, requiring more than 20 hours to attain 50% of serum activity. The rate of uptake of calcium tracer into CSF was intermediate between that of serum and perilymph.

RISA Study. The relative activity of RISA in perilymph (Fig. 5) gradually increased with time, reaching a peak at 12 hours after injection. The activity of RISA in CSF was considerably lower than that in perilymph. It is clear that only a very minute amount of albumin is transported into the perilymph, but even less seems to penetrate into CSF. This may be a reflection of the low ratio of protein content in CSF to that of perilymph under normal conditions. The small degree of penetration of albumin into CSF compared with transport into perilymph may reflect the normal tendency of perilymph protein concentration to be maintained about eight times that of CSF (200 mg/100 ml compared to 25 mg/100 ml).[4]

Kanamycin Study. Kanamycin concentrations in serum and perilymph one hour after intramuscular

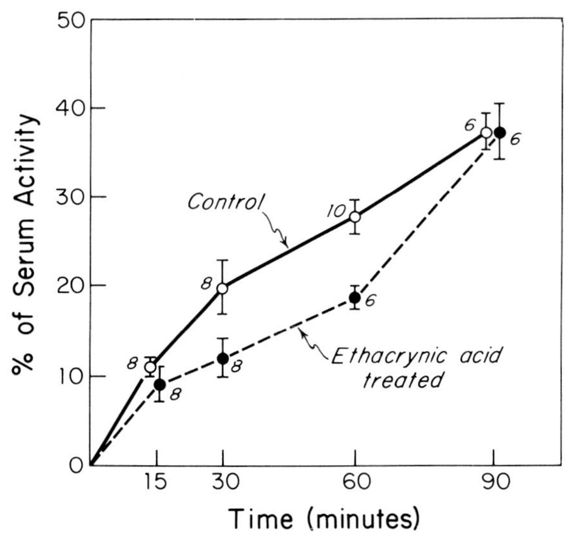

Fig. 3. Comparison of ratio of perilymph ^{22}Na activity to that of serum in control and ethacrynic acid-treated (30 mg/kg) chinchillas.

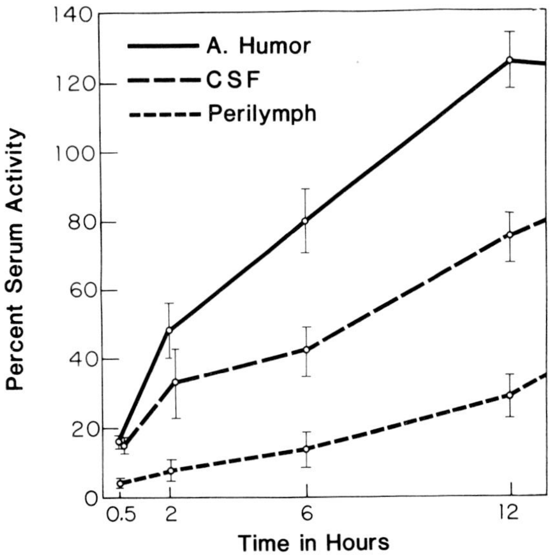

Fig. 4. Ratio of perilymph, CSF, and aqueous humor activities to that of serum after intravenous administration of ^{45}Ca in chinchillas.

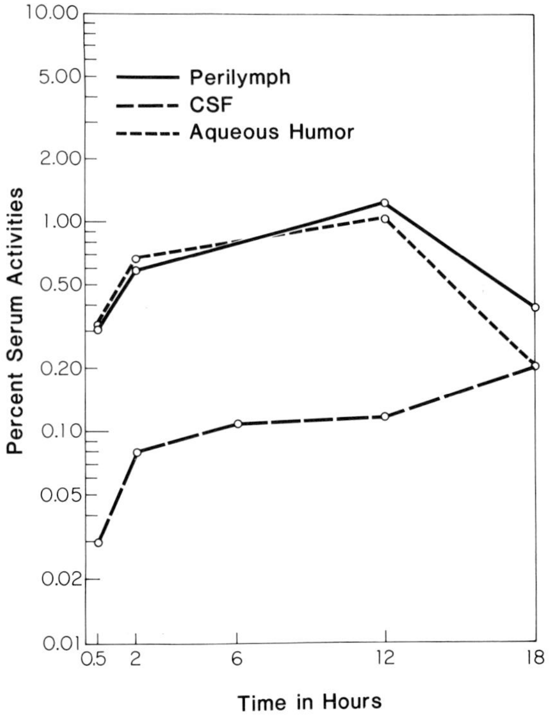

Fig. 5. Ratio of perilymph, CSF, and aqueous humor activities to that of serum after intravenous administration of RISA in chincillas.

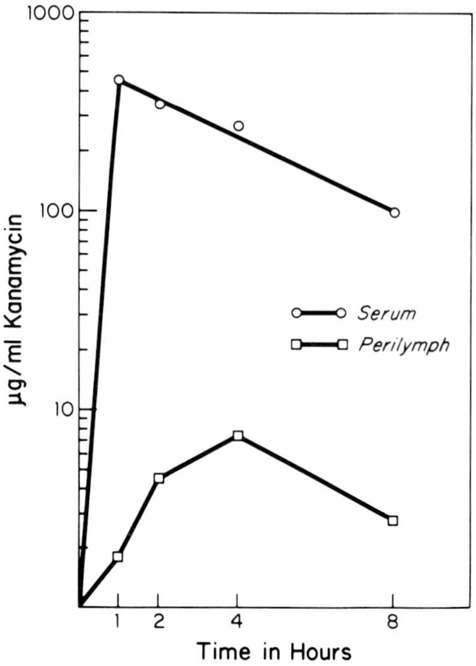

Fig. 6. Kanamycin concentration in perilymph and serum after injection of 200 mg/kg intramuscularly in chinchillas.

injection show a distinct difference between serum and perilymph, with a ratio of about 45:1 (Fig. 6). In contrast with furosemide, this ratio does not remain constant over time. It is interesting to observe that the peak serum concentration occurs one hour after infection, but perilymph concentration does not reach a maximum until four hours after injection.

Furosemide Study. Furosemide concentrations in serum (Fig. 7) were highest at the earliest time of sampling (495 μg/ml), as expected. The half-life was calculated to be 33.6 minutes in serum. Perilymph, on the other hand, was found to have a much lower peak concentration (5.2 μg/ml) than serum. Furthermore, the rate of decline of furosemide concentration in perilymph, as reflected in the half-life of 131 minutes, was slightly longer than that of serum. Protein binding studies with furosemide added to chinchilla serum (500 μg/ml) showed that about 86% of the drug was bound to plasma proteins (data not shown). Perilymph to serum ratios were calculated for furosemide. These values were found to approximate a constant value of 0.015 at each time point.

Urea Study. When a hyperosmotic agent (urea) was injected into blood, peak serum concentration was reached within 15 minutes after infection (Fig. 8). Perilymph, however, did not reach a peak concentration of urea until 120 minutes after injection.

DISCUSSION

A previous report from this laboratory[7] demonstrated that CSF, aqueous humor, and perilymph each had distinct rates of uptake of ^{22}Na after intravenous injection. This observation and the results reported here suggest the presence of a blood-labyrinth barrier, since an ion of small radius (Na^+) seems to slowly exchange with Na^+ ions that were already present in perilymph before injection.

It is interesting to observe that ethacrynic acid administration reduces the rate of ^{22}Na entrance into perilymph. Assuming that there are dynamic Na^+ fluxes between perilymph and blood[8] these data suggest that the transport of sodium ions from blood into perilymph is inhibited by ethacrynic acid. Although the exact site of this inhibition is not revealed by these experiments, a direct effect of ethacrynic acid on the cellular lining of the perilymphatic space is quite possible. Because reduced membrane transport of sodium into the CNS due to ethacrynic acid has been suggested by Miner and Reed[9] a similar mechanism can be invoked to account for the reduced rate of sodium transport revealed by this study. Sequential changes in ion composition caused by ethacrynic acid may be responsible for the changes in endocochlear potential observed by other investigators. The results of the present study also demonstrate that certain ototoxic drugs can alter the Na^+ flux through the blood-labyrinth barrier.

The results of the calcium study are not surprising, at least with regard to the rate of uptake into

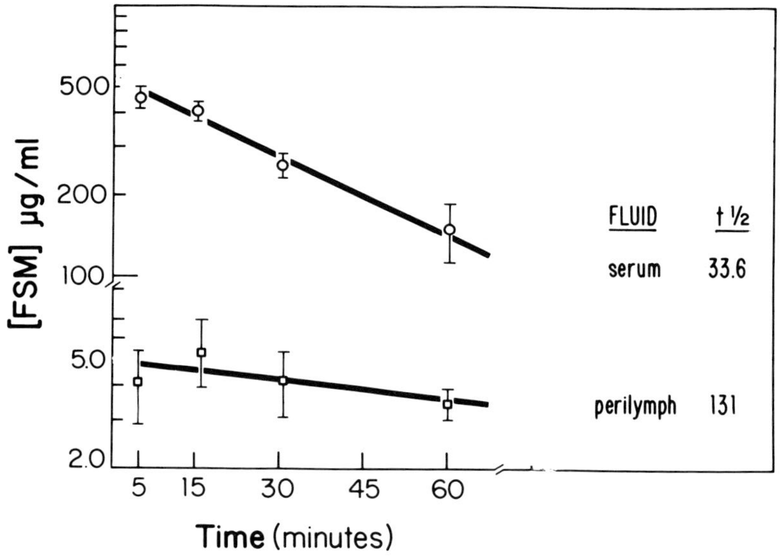

Fig. 7. Furosemide kinetics in serum and perilymph after intravenous injection (100 mg/kg). FSM - Furosemide.

the CSF. Oppelt et al[10] reported that a period of 5-6 hours was required before a CSF/plasma ratio of 0.5 was achieved in dogs who were injected with ^{45}Ca intravenously. This agrees quite well with our value in the chinchilla (7 hours). The calcium concentrations in CSF appear to be regulated by an active transport mechanism, rather than by diffusion or ultrafiltration.[10,11]

Previous studies from the laboratory[2] demonstrated that the concentration of calcium in perilymph did not change significantly three hours after induction of hypocalcemia by injection of thyrocalcitonin.

The importance of a barrier system limiting the quantity of calcium entering the CSF and perilymphatic space seems obvious, since the calcium plays such an important role in neural transmission and in membrane permeability. Ionic homeostasis in the brain has been related to the fact that the function of the CNS is in general resistant to disturbances of calcium and other ionic composition of blood, whereas excitable tissues without effective blood-interstitial fluid barriers may manifest considerable dysfunction. Therefore, in the face of altered circulating ion concentration in blood, cardiac muscle, smooth muscle, skeletal muscle, peripheral nerves, or neuromuscular junctions are affected before the brain or the spinal cord.[12]

Koide et al[13] reported that calcium ions can affect the metabolism of labyrinthine tissues by inhibiting oxidative phosphorylation.

Moscovitch and Gannon[14] demonstrated that an increase in calcium concentration in perilymph caused an augmentation of the cochlear microphonic and summation potential while depressing the action potential. They attributed these electrophysiological changes to the effects of the calcium on the olivocochlear bundle transmitter release and polarization of the hair cell membrane.

Albumin is an ellipsoid protein molecule. The filtration of albumin through the glomerular capillaries of the kidney is normally quite limited.[15]

Therefore, it is not surprising to find a slow rate of RISA uptake into body fluid compartments. It is interesting to observe, however, the marked difference between penetration of RISA into perilymph and into CSF. The barrier to penetration of RISA into perilymph is consistent with the observations of Winther[16] who found that the capillaries of the guinea pig spiral prominence and spiral ligament were impermeable to horseradish peroxidase (a protein of 40,000 molecular weight).

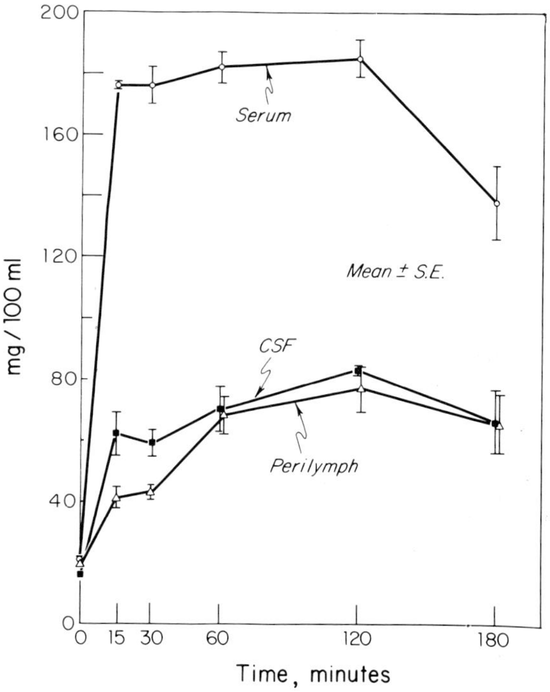

Fig. 8. Concentration of urea (mg/100 ml) in serum, CSF, and perilymph at various times after intravenous administration (2 g/kg) in chinchillas. SE - Standard error. (From Arch Otolaryngol 1979; 105:538-41. Copyright 1979, AMA. Published with permission.)

Furosemide is very highly protein-bound — about 90-95% in normal patients[17] and 86% in the present study at the maximum serum concentration. Therefore, one would expect only about 14% of the drug concentration in plasma to be free for diffusion. The degree of transfer of drug across the blood-perilymph interface probably depends on the relative affinity of drug in plasma for plasma water, plasma proteins, membrane lipid and membrane carrier protein, as suggested by Oldendorf's model for brain permeability to drugs.[18] Perhaps more than just the free plasma fraction of furosemide is potentially able to enter the perilymphatic space. However, we found that the perilymph concentrations of furosemide were only about 1.5% of serum concentrations, a value one tenth as great as would be expected by passive diffusion of the free fraction alone. This suggests a process controlling the net penetration of furosemide into perilymph. The elimination of furosemide from perilymph also occurs at a slower rate than the rate of excretion from serum.

An organic acid efflux transport system within the choroid plexus of the fourth ventricle transfers weak acids from CSF to blood. Such materials as Diodrast®, phenolphthalein, salicylic acid, and penicillin are transported from CSF into blood faster than from blood to CSF. Efflux can be blocked by probenecid.[19] A similar efflux transport system may exist in the inner ear. Since furosemide is a weak acid that is transported by the organic acid transport system in the kidney,[20] it is possible that the rate of efflux from perilymph exceeds the rate of influx, thereby limiting perilymph concentration.

Kanamycin is a relatively polar molecule which is not significantly bound to serum proteins.[21] However, it is slowly taken up into perilymph and is very slowly removed from this compartment. The half-life of kanamycin in blood has been shown to be about 85 minutes, whereas in perilymph the half-life is about 15 hours.[22]

The fact that kanamycin penetration into perilymph is limited in spite of the low fraction of protein binding suggests a barrier that tends to exclude this relatively small positively charged drug from the perilymph.

The study of an osmotic agent, namely urea, demonstrates that osmotic pressure in the perilymph does parallel changes in serum but with a distinct lag period as was demonstrated in previous studies with glycerol.[23]

Urea is a diffusible molecule that is readily filtered by the kidney glomerulus.[15] Although urea has been shown to enter perilymph after systemic administration[6,24] its peak concentration is limited and occurs two hours after injection. The slow accumulation of urea suggests a blood-labyrinth barrier that regulates the net concentration of urea in perilymph.

Osmotic relationships between the body fluids and inner ear fluids have been studied in the past. Bosher and Warren[25] reported that alterations in body fluid osmolality (induced by the intraperitoneal injection of water or hypertonic glycerol) were accompanied by changes in the osmotic pressure of the inner ear fluids in neonatal rats. Juhn et al[6,23] also demonstrated that perilymph osmolality changes in the chinchilla and guinea pig parallel changes in serum; however, a time lag was observed.

These studies demonstrate that perilymph osmolality responds to variations of serum osmolality and that water is transported in either direction through the blood-labyrinth barrier when serum osmolality is either increased or reduced. Therefore, the blood-labyrinth barrier appears to be freely permeable to water, but less permeable to other substances such as glucose,[6] glycerol[23] and urea.[24]

The investigations reported here support the existence of mechanisms that regulate the concentrations of certain substances in inner ear fluids. The distinct concentration differences from serum and the slow and incomplete equilibration over prolonged periods of observation implicate a blood-labyrinth barrier. This barrier apparently can be altered by experimental manipulations, as shown by the reduction of ^{22}Na transport into perilymph produced by administration of ethacrynic acid.

The delayed transfer of substances from blood into perilymph may represent a slow diffusion of the material from the capillaries through the extracellular space of the spiral ligament, and through the layers of connective tissue between the vessels and the perilymphatic space.[26] Capillaries of brain,[18] the ciliary process of the eye[27] and the spiral ligament[16] demonstrate a lack of fenestration. This anatomic feature would tend to prevent high molecular weight substance from passing between capillary endothelial cells and would require penetration through these cells.[18] Such structural factors could form part of the basis by which certain substances are restricted from entering the labyrinthine fluids. Thus, the blood-labyrinth barrier, defined as the sum of various special transport mechanisms between blood and labyrinth, appears to be an essential system for maintaining the ultrastable environment of the inner ear necessary for proper function. Better understanding of the nature of the blood-labyrinth barrier will certainly enhance the clarification of the pathogenesis of various inner ear disorders such as Menière's disease, or metabolic disturbance resulting in cochleovestibular dysfunction. Additional morphologic, physiologic and biochemical studies are warranted to further characterize this blood-labyrinth barrier.

ACKNOWLEDGMENTS — The authors gratefully acknowledge the helpful advice of Drs. W. Fowlks and D. W. Ward. Mr. Darryl Emery and Ms. Jean Braunworth provided excellent technical assistance. Furosemide was kindly provided by Hoechst-Roussel Pharmaceuticals, Inc. Dr. Don Frascella of that company provided helpful suggestions for the handling of furosemide.

REFERENCES

1. Juhn SK. Experimental alteration of physiological state of inner ear fluids. Ann Otol Rhinol Laryngol 1977; 86:689-98.

2. Juhn SK, Youngs JN. The effect on perilymph of the alteration of serum glucose or calcium concentration. Laryngoscope 1976; 86:273-9.

3. Ehrlich P. Das Sauerstoff Bedürfness des Organismus eine Farbanalytische Studie. Berlin, 1885.

4. Juhn SK, Haugen J, Steven L. Some chemical parameters of serum, cerebrospinal fluid and aqueous humor of the chinchilla. Lab Anim Sci 1974; 24:691-5.

5. Rybak LP, Green TP, Juhn SK, Moiizono T, Mirkin DL. Elimination kinetics of furosemide in perilymph and serum of the chinchilla: neuropharmacologic correlates. Acta Otolaryngol (Stockh) 1979; 88:382-7.

6. Juhn SK, Prado S, Rybak L. The effect of urea on osmolality of perilymph. Arch Otolaryngol 1979; 105:538-41.

7. Juhn SK, Pearce J, Guzowski J. Sodium exchange time of perilymph. Arch Otorhinolaryngol 1976; 212:213-4.

8. Schnieder EA. A contribution to the physiology of the perilymph. I. The origins of perilymph. Ann Otol Rhinol Laryngol 1974; 83:76-83.

9. Miner LC, Reed DJ. The effect of ethacrynic acid on sodium uptake into the cerebrospinal fluid of the rat. Arch Int Pharmacodyn Ther 1971; 190:316-20.

10. Oppelt WW, Owens ES, Rall DP. Calcium exchange between blood and cerebrospinal fluid. Life Sci 1963; 2:599-605.

11. Bradbury MWB, Wong RPK. Entry of 45-calcium from blood into brain and cerebrospinal fluid of normal and adrenalectomized rats. J Physiol (Lond) 1972; 225:65P-66P.

12. Bradbury MWB, Sarna GS. Homeostasis of the ionic composition of the cerebrospinal fluid. Exp Eye Res 1977; 25 Suppl: 249-57.

13. Koide Y, Tajima S, Yoshida M, Konno M. Biochemical changes in the inner ear induced by insulin in relation to cochlear microphonics. Ann Otol Rhinol Laryngol 1960; 69:1083-97.

14. Moscovitch DH, Gannon RP. Effects of calcium on sound-evoked cochlear potential in the guinea pig. J Acoust Soc Am 1966; 40:583-90.

15. Pitts RF. Physiology of the kidney and body fluids. 3rd ed. Chicago: Year Book Medical Publishers, 1974.

16. Winther FO. The permeability of the guinea pig cochlear capillaries to horseradish peroxidase. Z Zellforsch Mikrosk Anat 1971; 114:193-202.

17. Rane A, Villeneuve WJ, Stone AS. Plasma binding and disposition of furosemide in the nephrotic syndrome and uremia. Clin Pharmacol Ther 1978; 24:199-207.

18. Oldendorf WH. Certain aspects of drug distribution to brain. Adv Exp Med Biol 1976; 69:103-9.

19. Lorenzo AV. Factors governing the composition of cerebrospinal fluid. Exp Eye Res 1977; 25 Suppl: 205-28.

20. Hirsch GH, Pakuts AP, Bayne AJ. Furosemide accumulation by renal tissue. Biochem Pharmacol 1975; 24:1943-6.

21. Jackson GG. Present status of aminoglycoside antibiotics and their safe, effective use. Clin Ther 1977; 1:200-15.

22. Stupp HF, Rauch S, Sous M, Brun JP, Lagler F. Kanamycin dosage and levels in ear and other organs. Arch Otolaryngol 1967; 86:515-21.

23. Juhn SK, Prado S, Pearce J. Osmolality changes in perilymph after systemic administration of glycerin. Arch Otolaryngol 1976; 102;683-5.

24. Youngs JN, Juhn SK. Perilymph findings after intravenous urea administration. ORL 1972; 34:140-4.

25. Bosher SK, Warren RL. A study of the electrochemistry and osmotic relationships in the neonatal rat at the time of development of the endocochlear potential. J Physiol (Lond) 1971; 212:739-61.

26. Takahashi T, Kimura RS. The ultrastructure of the spiral ligament in the rhesus monkey. Acta Otolaryngol (Stockh) 1970; 69:46-60.

27. Vegge T. An epithelial blood-aqueous barrier to horseradish peroxidase in the ciliary process of the vervet monkey (cercopithecus aethiops). Z Zellforsch Mikrosk Anat 1971; 114:309-20.

MEDICAL MANAGEMENT OF MENIÈRE'S DISEASE

C. GARY JACKSON, MD
NASHVILLE, TENNESSEE

MICHAEL E. GLASSCOCK III, MD, FACS
NASHVILLE, TENNESSEE

WILLIAM E. DAVIS, MD, FACS
COLUMBIA, MISSOURI

GORDON B. HUGHES, MD
NASHVILLE, TENNESSEE

ARISTIDES SISMANIS, MD
NASHVILLE, TENNESSEE

The medical management of Menière's disease appears to be a misunderstood and controversial subject. There are those physicians who state that all cases can be controlled by medical means and that surgery is never indicated. Another group of investigators now emphasizes early surgical intervention without a medical trial. These conflicting views have led the authors to review all of their cases of Menière's disease (almost 1,000) in relation to medical management. The medical regime and its rationale are presented in detail. The results of this therapy are discussed in the context of control of vertigo, relief of tinnitus and pressure, and the stabilization of hearing.

On January 8, 1861, Prosper Menière presented before the Paris Academy of Medicine his paper entitled "A Report on Lesions of the Inner Ear Giving Rise to Symptoms of Cerebral Congestion of Apoplectic Type."[1] Fomenting considerable controversy, he identified the classic triad of vertigo, deafness, and tinnitus as a disease of the inner ear. One hundred nineteen years later, the controversy which surrounds the enigma of Menière's disease persists, largely the result of a poor understanding of the basic principles of etiology. The bewildering array of therapeutic options available serves to reaffirm this confusion relative to the pathogenesis of the basic pathology of endolymphatic hydrops.

Nonsurgical regimens for the treatment of Menière's disease are effective and currently accepted as efficacious clinical management. Medical management, however, appears to be a controversial and misunderstood topic. Some physicians hold that all cases can be controlled medically alone, while other groups emphasize early surgical intervention without medical trial. The purpose of this paper is to specifically describe diuretic therapy and salt restriction as one logical approach to the necessarily empiric treatment of Menière's disease as a disease of endolymphatic hydrops. This conservative approach to initial therapy must, however, be aggressively related to the concepts of the surgical management of Menière's disease and guidelines will be presented. A large series of patients is reviewed and a reasonable approach to therapy formulated.

LITERATURE REVIEW

In 1938, Hallpike and Cairns[2] first described the histopathology of Menière's disease consistent with endolymphatic hydrops. Even prior to 1938, however, disturbances of salt and water balance were implicated in a number of diseases such as epilepsy, migraine, asthma, allergy, hypertension, and later glaucoma, as well as Menière's disease.[3]

Dederding in 1929[4] and 1931,[5] and Mygind and Dederding in 1938[6] clearly associated water retention and an aggravation of both the cochlear and vestibular symptoms in this disease.

Later, Furstenberg and his co-workers[7,8] reported "the basic disturbance in patients with Menière's disease is sodium retention . . ." Their data and Hallpike and Cairns' histologic findings served as the theoretic basis for all future medical regimens which were ultimately designed to prevent or reduce the accumulation of excess endolymph. Furstenberg et al published their regimen of strict salt restriction and ammonium chloride diuretic therapy as providing complete symptomatic relief from vertigo in 57% of 35 patients. An additional 26% were "improved." Only 9% had any improvement in hearing.

Norell and Stahle[9,10] throughout the 1960s also documented favorable responses to this therapeutic approach. More efficient diuretics in the form of thiazides proved effective in stimulating both clinical application and patient compliance.

In one of the few well-controlled studies on this subject, Klockhoff and Lindbloom[11] and Klockhoff et al[12] declared oral diuretics and dietary sodium control as "superior to any other medical treatment." In a double-blind study of 30 patients, hearing was stabilized in 69%; vertigo controlled in

From the Otology Group and the Department of Surgery (Otology and Neuro-Otology), Vanderbilt University School of Medicine, Nashville, Tennessee, and the Department of Surgery, University of Missouri, Columbia. This study was sponsored by the E.A.R. Foundation, Nashville.

Presented at the meeting of the American Neurotological Society, Dallas, Texas, October 7, 1979.

REPRINTS — C. Gary Jackson, MD, 1811 State Street, Nashville, TN 37203.

58%; and an overall improvement in "general condition" was seen in 77%. End-stage or nonfluctuating forms responded poorly and although no correlation as to degree of response was noted, glycerol-positive patients responded best to diuretic therapy. Follow-up of this group, however, revealed ". . . few patients in whom a longstanding, obviously drug-related, improvement of the *hearing* occurred." Since hearing loss, in many, continued to progress, they concluded that this form of therapy does not arrest the long-term effects of the disease but that vertigo control produced excellent functional results.

Boles et al reconfirmed the efficacy of the Furstenberg regimen in 1975.[13] In reviewing 125 patients followed at the University of Michigan, "response of the patient to treatment was determined by the degree of relief from vertiginous episodes." Good to excellent responses were identified in 86% of those whose disease was classified as severe, 94% of those moderately severe, and 100% whose disease was mild. The subject of hearing was poorly dealt with but the inference was that progression was apparently uninterrupted. It was, in fact, this study that prompted the senior author to modify his medical approach to the therapy of Menière's disease.

There has been much contradictory evidence produced, but it is this contradictory enigma which constitutes the modern concept of Menière's disease.[14-16]

THERAPEUTIC BASIS

A myriad of pharmacologic agents have been proposed as components of therapeutic approaches to Menière's disease, all based on differing theories of pathogenesis. It is beyond the scope of this communication to discuss them all. Diuretic therapy and salt restriction is one of only two medical approaches proved to be effective by double-blind study and it is this approach on which we shall concentrate.[17]

It is safe to say that the pathogenesis of Hallpike and Cairns'[2] original observation, to date, remains obscure. Nonetheless, endolymphatic hydrops is a consistent finding and of significant pathophysiologic importance in the fluctuant symptom complex of Menière's disease. The effects of glycerine are thought to reaffirm this.

Glycerine reduces CSF pressure and has been used in Europe therapeutically to control intraocular pressure in glaucoma.[18] Angelborg and Agerup[19] and Juhn et al[20] clearly demonstrated intracochlear pressure and osmolality changes in response to systemic administration of glycerine. Klockhoff and Lindbloom[21] demonstrated complete labyrinthine collapse in guinea pigs to which glycerine was given. Arenberg et al[22] and many others have, as well, clearly documented the clinical effects of glycerine on the symptom complex of Menière's disease within the format of a diagnostic evaluation. It is thought that glycerine produces an intracochlear hydrodynamic effect which is osmotic in nature and which directly and/or indirectly alters the hydropic state. On this basis, it would appear that the observed hydropic pathology is pathophysiologically crucial. It also suggests that this process is amenable to hydrodynamic treatment.

Suffice it to say that body fluid and particularly extracellular fluid (ECF) volume homeostasis is under nervous and hormonal control. Sodium restriction and diuretic therapy is based on an attack on the ECF and, consequently, endolymphatic hydrops. In order to justify this approach, certain basic assumptions must be made. First, as proposed by Naftalin,[23] endolymph is a component, albeit modified, of the ECF and is contracted and expanded in volume with the rest of the ECF, its constituents under the influence of the active hormones. Recently a second proposal has been made; that is, that the diuretic directly intervenes in the intralabyrinthine fluid-electrolyte balance, most probably at the level of the stria vascularis.[11,12] On these proposals or assumptions, salt restriction and diuretic therapy is based. Sodium restriction flattens gross fluctuations in sodium balance and consequent fluctuations in ECF volume resulting in a general dehydration. At the same time, normal movements of sodium, potassium and water between endolymph and associated fluids is allowed, possibly even facilitated directly by diuretic therapy.

There is much clinical evidence from which the importance of dietary sodium balance and body fluid homeostasis can be inferred. A significant number of patients with Menière's disease volunteer a history of attack provocation by dietary (sodium) indiscretion. Similarly, premenstrual women under the influence of fluid-retaining hormones commonly describe aural fullness occasionally associated with vertigo, both of which can clearly be eliminated by diuretic therapy. The problems associated with oral contraceptives support this line of thought in this context. Attacks are regularly precipitated by fluid overloading patients with Menière's disease in the postoperative period when they have undergone unrelated surgery. Last, and most important, is the fact that glycerol-positive patients generally respond better to this form of medical manipulation.

THE REGIMEN

Once the diagnosis of Menière's disease has been made according to the guidelines established by the American Academy of Ophthalmology and Otolaryngology (AAOO)[24] and a thorough neurotologic evaluation completed to effectively exclude the

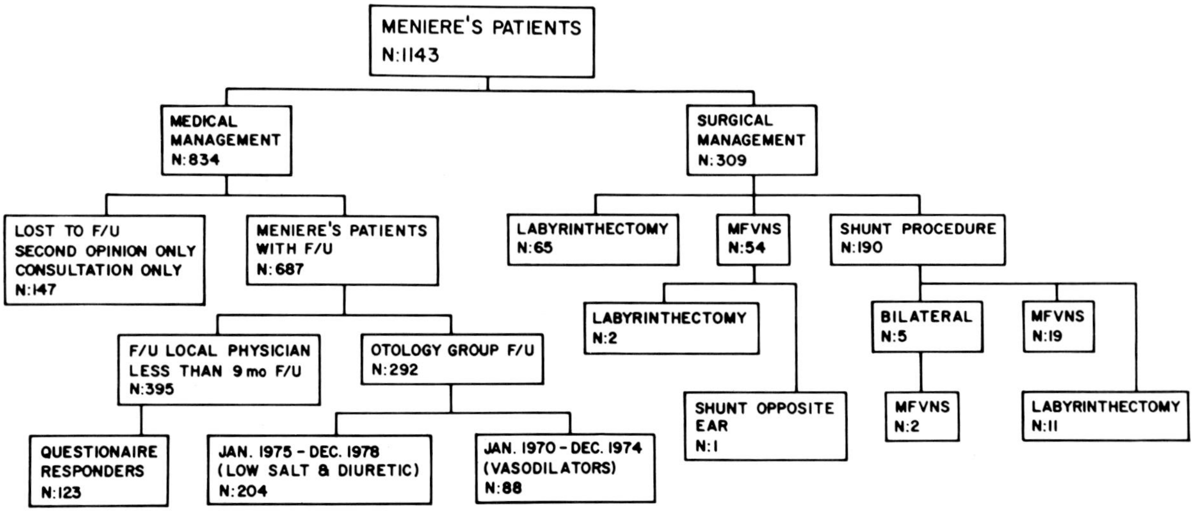

Fig. 1. This flow chart illustrates therapeutic direction for the studied patient population. F/U - Follow-up; MFVNS - Middle fossa vestibular nerve section.

possibility of acoustic tumor and any other causally treatable etiology (allergy, lues or endocrine abnormalities), a trial medical regimen is initiated. The mainstay of this conservative program is dietary salt restriction and diuretic therapy. Labyrinthine sedatives are used for ancillary support.

What is a low salt diet? How strict should it be? How long will I have to stay on it? These are all crucial questions which, in order to assure patient compliance, must be answered with clarity. Generally "low salt diets" can range from 500 mg to 4 gm sodium diets. Severe salt restriction permits 1 gm of sodium daily. It is stringent and patient compliance is poor. Moderate salt restriction allows 2 gm/day. This is practical and is used commonly to treat cardiopulmonary disease. Although practical, it is still somewhat unpalatable. The authors prefer what we refer to as a "common sense" salt restriction. Simply stated, this diet excludes heavily salted foods as well as use of the salt shaker at tableside. Salted peanuts, bacon, sausage, cured meats (pork), potato chips, pretzels, etc, are examples of excluded foods. A salt substitute is encouraged. This diet amounts to a 3 to 4 gm sodium restricted diet, is palatable and is quite effective when used in conjunction with a diuretic. Patient compliance is generally excellent.

Thiazide diuretics have been found to be effective and of the most use to us. The authors prefer hydrochlorothiazide in combination with a triamterene derivative,* the advantage being its potassium-sparing effects. The diuretic is taken daily with a glass of orange juice. Few problems are encountered that are sufficiently severe enough to warrant dosage modification, but every other day or twice daily schedules are options. Furosemide and ethacrynic acid are generally avoided.

It is strongly suggested that tobacco abuse be abrogated. As noted, labyrinthine sedatives and anticholinergics serve as ancillary support. We prefer diazepam* and glycopyrrolate.†

The patient is instructed of the importance of behavioral modification around this regimen in that, in our philosophy, compliance will be necessary for the rest of his/her lifetime. Favorable results do not permit noncompliance and regimen failure does not permit cessation even once surgical therapy is executed. Medical management in the form of salt restriction and diuretic therapy is continued even though, as an initial failure, surgical treatment was necessary. The patient with newly diagnosed Menière's disease is asked to return for an office visit in six weeks. The duration of medical trial should not exceed three months if it is apparent that symptoms are uncontrolled. Vertigo and hearing loss are viewed as equally important even though, most usually, the patient's primary concern is his incapacitating vertigo.

METHODS

This study spans a period from January 1970 to December 1978. During this time span 1,143 patients were seen, to whom the diagnosis of Menière's disease was appended. The vast majority were described as having classic Menière's disease (83%) while the remainder were composed of the more unusual varieties of cochlear hydrops (13%) and vestibular Menière's (3.6%). An overall incidence of bilaterality was seen in 28%. No unusual sexual distribution was identified. Average age of presentation was 45.9 years while mean duration of symptoms before diagnosed was 2.41 years. The classification of these patients into therapeutic categories is as demonstrated in Figure 1.

Prior to any therapeutic intervention, all patients underwent thorough neurotologic evaluation. A neurotologic historical review and physical examination were performed in all cases. Our neurotologic test battery included pure tone and speech audiometry, Olsen modification of the Carhart tone decay test, modified SISI, stapedial reflex decay, electronystagmography (ENG), petrous pyramid x-rays and brainstem electric response audiometry (BERA). Should any of these studies be suspect, com-

*Dyazide®.

*Valium®.

†Robinul®.

TABLE 1. RESULTS OF THERAPY GENERALLY EXCLUSIVE OF SALT RESTRICTION AND DIURETIC THERAPY, JAN 1970-DEC 1975 (N = 88)

Class	*No.*	*%*	*Vertigo*	*Hearing*
A	25	28.4	C	Improved (> 15 dB and/or 15% SD)
B	26	29.5	C	Unchanged
C	3	3.5	C	Worse (> 15 dB and/or 15% SD)
D	34	38.6	U	

C - Controlled; U - Uncontrolled.

TABLE 2. RESULTS OF THERAPY WITH SALT RESTRICTION AND A DIURETIC, DEC 1975-DEC 1978 (N = 204)

Class	*No.*	*%*	*Vertigo*	*Hearing*
A	77	37.7	C	Improved (> 15 dB and/or 15% SD)
B	75	36.8	C	Unchanged
C	9	4.4	C	Worse (> 15 dB and/or 15% SD)
D	43	21.1	U	

C - Controlled; U - Uncontrolled.

puterized axial tomography (CAT scan) of the head and/or posterior fossa myelography were performed. Appropriate serologic, endocrine-metabolic and allergic evaluations were applied as indicated.

Patients undergoing surgery upon initial referral had already undergone unsuccessful medical trials and were referred specifically for surgical consideration. The remainder were subjected to the medical regimen consistent with two conceptually different approaches. From January 1970 to December 1974 the medical protocol followed by the senior author included basically nicotinic acid, vitamins and histamine treatments. Labyrinthine sedatives were inconsistently applied. Between January 1975 and December 1978 these agents had been abandoned and diuretic therapy and salt restriction formulated the mainstays of our medical format.

The wide geographical distribution of the referral pattern that our Otology Group enjoys complicates greatly accurate follow-up. Of the 687 patients on whom follow-up was available, 292 were followed through the authors' practice. It is this group which comprises the bulk of this investigation. After initial diagnosis and therapeutic formulation, 395 subjects, for practical considerations, were referred back to the care of their referring otolaryngologists. A portion of this group also included a number whose duration of clinical follow-up is inadequate to allow justifiable conclusion of therapeutic outcome or had definitive etiologies otherwise established.

When a patient is referred back to his originating geography, he is also returned to the diversified therapeutic philosophies of their respective physicians. The study and resultant data thus became significantly contaminated so as to prevent analysis of data as absolute. A subjective response was then sought from this group as to whether they were still using salt restriction and diuretic therapy as well as their subjective evaluation of therapeutic efficacy. Such information was obtained on an additional 123 patients and is presented separately. Follow-up is therefore available on 415 patients in this series. Duration of follow-up ranges from nine months to eight years with a mean duration for the studied group of two years and nine months.

RESULTS

For this study all chart reviews were performed by investigators independent of the staff of the Otology Group. All results are reported according to the guidelines established by the AAOO.[24] Results are reported in three groups: the group pre-January 1975; post-January 1975; and questionnaire responses.

Results of medical therapy generally exclusive of salt restriction and diuretic therapy are summarized in Table 1.

Class A and B results can be considered as favorable and when combined, present a success rate of 57.9%. Hearing decrement and uncontrolled vertigo comprise medical failure in 42.1% of this population. Thirty-three percent of those who failed to respond did so within the first six months of the trial where 59% failed within the first year.

A medical protocol including diuretic therapy and salt restriction generated therapeutic success which is summarized in Table 2.

Again, combination of class A and B results generate a figure of favorable therapeutic efficacy of 74.5%. Twenty-five and five-tenths percent of this group represented medical failures and were managed, therefore, surgically. Medical failure occurred within six months in 66.7% of the failure group while 90% of medical failures were evident by one year.

The subjective symptoms of tinnitus and pressure could not be absolutely evaluated. When polled, the majority of patients admitted to persistent tinnitus (81.3%) and pressure (77.2%). Tinnitus was unchanged in 48% and improved in 30.9%, whereas pressure persisted unchanged in 42.3% but improved in 34.1%.

One hundred twenty-three patients responded to a questionnaire seeking their subjective responses regarding the efficacy of salt restriction and diuretic therapy for their Menière's disease. Eighty and five-tenths percent were still undergoing this protocol, 65.9% volunteering information that this regimen had helped them. Hearing could not be quantitatively evaluated but 9.8% noted hearing improvement; 19.5% reported a decrease in auditory acuity while 70.7% acknowledged no change in their hearing states.

DISCUSSION

The therapeutic attack of the salt restriction and diuretic format is based on the premise that endolymphatic hydrops is a consistent finding in Menière's disease and is of significant pathophysiologic importance. Diuretic therapy and dietary sodium control is effective and in this regard should precede surgical intervention as a medical trial.

The title of this communication may be somewhat misleading in that all forms of medical management are not equally effective. The double-blind studies of Klockhoff and Lindbloom[11,12] validate clinical studies such as ours which suggest that the emphasis of the concept of "medical therapy for Meniere's disease" holds diuretic therapy and dietary sodium control as its mainstays. This concept is clearly illustrated by the disparity in successful results generated within the two periods of our experience. Prior to January 1975, during which salt restriction and diuretic therapy was not applied, a successful outcome was noted in but 57.9%. After January 1975, when this regimen was specifically employed, class A and B results were noted in 74.5% of those treated.

Diuretic therapy and dietary salt restriction is not causal therapy such that the disease is cured by its application. The pathogenetic origin of Hallpike and Cairns'[2] observations, even today, remains at best obscure. Any therapy, by definition, then must be empiric. For this reason the safest regimen which achieves symptomatic control is indicated. Herein lies the basis of our philosophy of medical trial representing a precondition to surgical and more aggressive intervention.

Since diuretic therapy and salt restriction is not causal therapy, specific etiologic factors must be sought which, when identified, can be specifically managed as casual. Particular attention to the allergic, luetic, and endocrine-metabolic aspects of Menière's disease as treatable etiologies must not be overlooked under the blanket of "symptomatic control."

What constitutes medical failure? Under what circumstances is surgical intervention indicated? Historically, success or failure of any therapeutic protocol designed to confront Menière's disease was judged by its ability to control this disease's most disabling symptom — vertigo. It is this whirling incapacitation which originally brings the patient with Menière's disease to seek medical assistance. Torok[16] has somewhat nihilistically suggested that no matter what we do, vertigo will be controlled in 60-80% of those treated. It is time to reorient our thinking on Menière's disease to include hearing loss as well. This concept is certainly not one that is original,[17,25] but is certainly one that puts the historical view of the concepts of medical management in an entirely new perspective.

Vertigo is, of course, the patient's most distressing problem and, obviously, inability to control this symptom forthrightly indicates therapeutic failure. Vertigo control, however, should not necessarily signal conservative success. "Medical treatment is not conservative if it allows the inner ear to be lost."[26] If medical therapy is able to control vertigo while *simultaneously* preventing wide hearing fluctuation of significant (15 dB/15% SD) hearing regression, the patient's Menière's disease is being successfully managed conservatively. Apparent effective control of the patient's most disabling symptom of vertigo should not lull the otologist into a false sense of security relative to potentially irreversible progression of the auditory aspects of his disease. Medical failure therefore is inability to control vertigo and/or progressive hearing disability. Under these circumstances the patient is a candidate for endolymphatic sac (drainage) surgery.

In this regard, the authors do not wish to imply that in 204 patients treated with salt restriction and diuretics only 9 (4.4%) suffered hearing progression. Indeed, in our experience, when vertigo fails to respond to this regimen, hearing generally progresses negatively in a likewise uncontrolled fashion so that the majority of the class D results were associated with hearing loss progression.

Medical failure, when it occurs, is generally obvious within the first three months of trial while 66% declare themselves by six months. Even equivocal responders declared success or failure by one year (90%). These statistics are presented as clinical guidelines by which patients who occasionally present unclear clinical pictures can be judged. As noted the majority of failures are immediate and a decision as to surgical intervention can usually be made within three months. Equivocal responders or those patients reluctant to accept sac surgery in face of near but not quite total incapacitation will also declare their response to medical management generally within a time span short enough to preclude irreversible changes possibly prevented by more aggressive measures. The advantage of early surgery is not compromised by medical trial.

Klockhoff et al[12] as well as Arenberg and Bayer,[17] while acknowledging diuretic and sodium dietary therapy as the best of all medical formats, have suggested that medical management does not interrupt the "inexorable progression of endolymphatic hydrops and its effects on hearing."[17] At this time, the authors are not able to respond to their claim with absolute data in the form of "long-term" follow-up since our mean follow-up is but two years, nine months. For practical purposes, five to ten years will be needed. We can, however, suggest our impressions. A point to consider in this regard is therapeutic persistence. In many studies, therapeutic medical protocols are relaxed when symptoms are improved or relieved. The authors insist upon absolute compliance with their medical protocol "for life" and generally regardless of outcome or future treatment direction. We have in general been quite pleased with not only the patient's response with respect to vertigo but also the resultant stability and, in some cases, improvement in auditory ability. Repeatedly, even in times of "remission," dietary sodium indiscretion is betrayed by prompt reexacerbation of symptoms. Continued, persistent application of this regimen in an effort to control endolymphatic hydrops may well alter the "inexorable progression" attributed to this disorder when it is considered in terms of long-term effects. The concepts of early diagnosis and prompt therapeutic attack cannot, therefore, be overemphasized.

Despite the vast amount of literature which continues to document the successful management of Menière's disease, there still exists a philosophy of therapeutic nihilism. Patients continue to be told that they have Menière's disease, an incurable condition that will eventually "burn itself out." The outcome of this clinical analysis of medical therapy, as well as the surgical success which we have previously documented,[24,26] directly refutes this philosophy of therapeutic impotence. When the medical management outlined is aggressively related to surgical formats a very reasonable and effective protocol emerges.

With this information in hand, the patient can be given a very realistic picture of what is expected of him and of what he can reasonably anticipate as far as the result is concerned. Curative therapy is the mandate of the future. Nonetheless, medical concepts when appropriately related to the advantages of surgery provide the patient with Menière's disease with considerable symptomatic relief, preserving, while occasionally improving, auditory function in the process.

SUMMARY

The purpose of this communication has been to outline the efficacy of medical management of Menière's disease and to aggressively relate this to surgical protocols. Diuretic and salt restriction therapy is effective and is exhibited in an analysis of a large series of patients with Menière's disease followed through the Otology Group. Analysis of results and treatment guidelines are formulated. Relief from vertigo as well as the auditory symptoms of this disorder are viewed with equal importance when evaluating therapeutic success.

REFERENCES

1. Meniere P. Maladies de l'oreille interne offrant les symptoms de la congestion cerebrale apoplectiforme. Gaz Med Paris 1961; 16:239-40.

2. Hallpike CS, Cairns H. Observation on the pathology of Meniere's syndrome. Proc R Soc Med 1938; 31:1317-36.

3. Foldes E. A new approach to dietetic therapy. Boston: RG Badgerm, 1933.

4. Dederding D. Clinical and experimental examination in patients suffering from morbus Meniere including study of problems of bone conduction. Acta Otolaryngol (Stockh) 1929; 10 Suppl 1-123.

5. Dederding D. Our Menière treatment (principles and results). Acta Otolaryngol (Stockh) 1931; 16:404-15.

6. Mygind SH, Dederding D. Ménière's disease as indicator of disturbance in water metabolism, capillary function and body condition. Ann Otol Rhinol Laryngol 1938; 47:55-62.

7. Furstenberg AC, Lashinet FH, Lathrop FD. Meniere's symptom complex: medical treatment. Ann Otol Rhinol Laryngol 1934; 43:1035-47.

8. Furstenberg AC, Richardson G, Lathrop FD. Meniere's disease: addenda to medical therapy. Arch Otolaryngol 1941; 34:1083-92.

9. Norell I, Stahle J. Hydrochlorothiazide (Esidrex) via morbus Meniere. Nord Med 1961; 66:1652-5.

10. Norell I, Stahle J. Treatment of Menière's disease with hydrochlorothiazide. Acta Otolaryngol (Stockh) 1962; 54:447-56.

11. Klockhoff I, Lindbloom U. Meniere's disease and hydrochlorothiazide — a critical analysis of symptoms and therapeutic effects. Acta Otolaryngol (Stockh) 1967; 63:347-65.

12. Klockhoff I, Lindbloom U, Stahle J. Diuretic treatment of Meniere's disease: long term results with chlorothalidone. Arch Otolaryngol 1974; 100:262-5.

13. Boles R, Rice DH, Hybels R, Work WP. Conservative management of Meniere's disease: Furstenberg revisited. Ann Otol Rhinol Laryngol 1975; 84:513-7.

14. Perlman HP, Goldinger JM, Cales JO. Electrolyte studies in Meniere's disease. Laryngoscope 1953; 63:640-51.

15. Golding-Wood PH. Water and salt balance in Ménière's disease. J Laryngol Otol 1960; 74:480-8.

16. Torok N. Old and new in Ménière's disease. Laryngoscope 1977; 87:1870-7.

17. Arenberg IK, Bayer RF. Therapeutic opticus in Meniere's disease. Arch Otolaryngol 1977; 103:589-93.

18. Virno M, Cantore P, Bietti C, Bucci M. Oral glycerol in ophthalmology. Am J Ophthalmol 1963; 55:1133-42.

19. Angelborg C, Agerup B. Glycerol effects on the perilymphatic and cerebrospinal fluid pressure. Acta Otolaryngol (Stockh) 1975; 79:81-7.

20. Juhn SK, Prado S, Pearce J. Osmolality changes in perilymph after systemic administration of glycerine. Acta Otolaryngol (Stockh) 1976; 102:683-5.

21. Klockhoff I, Lindbloom U. Glycerol test in Meniere's disease. Acta Otolaryngol (Stockh) 1967; Suppl 224:450-1.

22. Arenberg IK, Herman LE, Swanson SN. Salt loading glycerol test in fluctuant hearing loss. In: Shambaugh GE Jr, Shea JJ, eds. Proceedings of Shambaugh Fifth International Workshop on Middle Ear Microsurgery and Fluctuant Hearing Loss. Huntsville: Strode Publishing, 1977:374-8.

23. Naftalin L. The medical treatment of fluctuant hearing loss. Otolaryngol Clin North Am 1975; 8:475-82.

24. Committee on Hearing and Equilibrium. Report of subcommittee on equilibrium and its measurement. Trans Am Acad Ophthalmol Otolaryngol 1972; 76:1462-4.

25. Glasscock ME, Miller GW, Drake FD, Kanok MM. Surgical management of Ménière's disease with the endolymphatic subarachnoid shunt: a five-year study. Laryngoscope 1977; 87:1668-75.

26. House WF. Long-term results of endolymphatic subarachnoid shunt surgery in Meniere's disease. In: Shambaugh GE Jr, Shea JJ, eds. Proceedings Shambaugh Fifth International Workshop on Middle Ear Microsurgery and Fluctuant Hearing Loss. Huntsville: Strode Publishing, 1977:441-4.

Ann Otol 90:1981

LYSOSOMAL HYDROLASES IN MIDDLE EAR EFFUSIONS

WARREN F. DIVEN, PhD
ROBERT H. GLEW, PhD CHARLES D. BLUESTONE, MD
PITTSBURGH, PENNSYLVANIA

Biochemical studies of middle ear effusions have demonstrated generally higher levels of certain hydrolytic and oxidative enzymes in mucoid fluids when compared to serous. We have extended these studies by analyzing middle ear effusions for the content of a large number of lysosomal hydrolases. The mean specific activity for α-glucosidase in mucoid fluids was found to be ten times that for serous fluids while α-mannosidase, β-glucuronidase, hexosaminidase, acid phosphatase, β-galactosidase, alkaline phosphatase, and lactate dehydrogenase were found to be three to five times greater in mucoid than serous effusions. In this study the specific enzyme activities for lysosomal hydrolases from purulent effusions were found to be intermediate between the activities in serous and mucoid effusions. No significant correlation was found between the specific activities of lysosomal hydrolases and the presence or absence of bacteria in mucoid or serous middle ear effusions. The hexosaminidase isozyme distribution was found to be identical for serous and mucoid fluids and similar to that found in human serum. However, the isozyme pattern of β-glucuronidase in mucoid effusions was significantly different than that in normal human serum as mucoid fluids contain a large amount of an anionic isoenzyme of β-glucuronidase that is barely detectable in human serum.

INTRODUCTION

Persistent middle ear effusions (MEE) are one of the characteristics of otitis media with effusion (OME) and there have been many studies attempting to learn more about the etiology and pathophysiological properties of these fluids. Obstruction of the eustachian tube is the most often cited cause of effusions.[1] It has also been suggested that both serous and mucoid MEE represent pure transudates of plasma.[2] Both types of fluids have been shown to contain inflammatory cells, polymorphonuclear leukocytes, macrophages, lymphocytes, and cell debris.[3]

Fluid accumulations could also result from morphological and functional changes in the middle ear mucosa induced by bacteria since various microorganisms have been identified as possible pathogens in ear effusions.[4,5] Analysis of the biochemical properties and nature of the components of MEE from patients with OME has been used to gain insight into the origin and mechanism of formation of these fluids. Based on measurements of total protein, alkaline phosphatase, aspartate amino transferase, and lysosomal acid phosphatase in middle ear effusions, Lupovich and Harkins[6] suggested that such fluids arise as secretions of the middle ear mucosa in an inflammatory response.

Juhn and coworkers studied the levels of certain oxidative and hydrolytic enzymes in serum and MEE from serous otitis media[7] and found consistently higher values in the effusions. These investigators suggested that the enzymes contained in MEE arise from three sources: 1) enzymes normally present in blood, 2) release from inflamed middle ear mucosa, and 3) release from inflammatory cells present in effusions. Juhn and Huff[8] extended these studies on the enzymes present in MEE to include fluids classified as mucoid MEE in order to examine biochemical differences between several effusion types. In general, mucoid MEE were reported to have higher activities than serous fluids when expressed as activity per unit volume. When specific activities were expressed (U/mg protein), several of the hydrolytic enzymes were essentially the same in both fluid types. Bernstein et al, in a study of the lysosomal enzyme hexosaminidase, concluded that lysosomal enzymes in MEE derive from cells and not from plasma.[9]

We also analyzed the content of acid lysosomal hydrolases in MEE using fluorogenic substrates that permit microassay of β-galactosidase, acid phosphatase, α-mannosidase, β-glucuronidase, hexosaminidase, β-glucosidase, and α-glucosidase. This further characterization of the biochemical nature of MEE was undertaken to compare the enzymatic composition of the three major classifications of MEE (serous, mucoid, and purulent) and to evaluate the influence of the presence of microorganisms on the enzyme content of these effusions.

METHODS

Alpha-D-glucopyranoside, β-D-galactopyranoside, α-D-mannopyranoside, β-D-glucuronide, and N-acetyl-β-D-glucosaminide derivatives of 4-methylumbelliferone were obtained from Pierce Chemical Company and 4-methylumbelliferyl phosphate from Sigma Chemical Company.

Subjects. The subjects for this study were patients receiving a myringotomy for the treatment of recurrent or chronic OME. Since the effusion obtained from each ear in a single patient can have very different properties, each ear was treated as a separate

From the Departments of Pathology, Biochemistry, and Otolaryngology, University of Pittsburgh School of Medicine, and the Children's Hospital of Pittsburgh, Pittsburgh, Pennsylvania. This work was supported in part by a grant HL 20547 from the Heart and Lung Institute of the National Institutes of Health and a grant from the National Foundation, March of Dimes.

REPRINTS — Warren F. Diven, PhD, University Health Center of Pittsburgh, 201 DeSoto Street, Pittsburgh, PA 15261.

TABLE 1. DISTRIBUTION OF SPECIMENS BY PATIENT, AGE, AND SEX

Fluid Classification	Sex Male	Sex Female	Age 0-23 mo	Age 2-6 yr	Age 7-16 yr
Serous	12	4	2	6	8
Mucoid	15	16	3	23	5
Purulent	1	3	1	3	—

specimen. Table 1 provides a summary of specimens obtained according to age and sex of the patient. A total of 51 specimens were analyzed.

Middle Ear Effusions. After swab of the external ear canal was taken for culture, the canal was washed with 70% alcohol and the middle ear aspirated as described in detail by Riding et al.[4]

Effusions (0.5-1.0 ml) were obtained by aspiration into 1 ml of sterile distilled water. At the time of aspiration, each ear was visually classified into four groups: 1) dry - no effusion; 2) serous - pale, usually yellow liquid with low viscosity; 3) mucoid - thick, tenacious, usually gray liquid; and 4) purulent - thick, yellowish pus. No further consideration was given to those ears classified as dry, but all MEE results are grouped according to these classifications. Aliquots were removed for microbiological studies, then the diluted fluids were centrifuged to remove cells and particulates. The supernatent was used without further preparation for the various assays to be described.

Enzyme Assays. All assays were carried out at 37 C and unless otherwise specified contained the following constituents in a final volume of 0.1 ml:0.2 M sodium acetate buffer adjusted to the specified pH, 1-20 μl of ear fluid, and one of the following substrates at the final concentration indicated: α-mannosidase, 4-methylumbelliferyl-α-D-mannopyranoside (1.5 mM, pH 5.0), acid phosphatase, 4-methylumbelliferyl phosphate (6.6 mM, pH 5.0), β-glucuronidase, 4-methylumbelliferyl-β-D-glucuronic acid (10 mM, pH 4.8), alkaline phosphatase, 4-methylumbelliferyl phosphate (1.5 mM, pH 9.2), α-glucosidase, 4-methylumbelliferyl-α-D-glucopyranoside (1.5 mM, pH 5.0), β-galactosidase, 4-methylumbelliferyl-β-D-galactopyranoside (5.0 mM, pH 4.0).

Hexosaminidase was measured using 4-methylumbelliferyl-N-acetyl-β-D-glucosaminide (5 mM in 0.08 M citrate-phosphate buffer, pH 4.4 containing 10 mg bovine serum albumin per 100 ml of buffer). β-glucosidase was determined under conditions specific for glucocerebrosidase[9] using 4-methylumbelliferyl-β-D-glucopyranoside (1.5 mM in presence of 0.06% sodium taurocholate). All fluorometric assays were terminated by the addition of 0.1 M ammonium hydroxide-glycine buffer, pH 10.5. The extent of hydrolysis was determined as described previously.[10]

Lactate dehydrogenase was measured spectrophotometrically by the method of Wroblewski and LaDue.[11] The unit of enzyme activity used for these studies is defined as nmoles of product formed per hour.

Protein Determination. Protein was estimated by the method of Lowry et al[12] using bovine serum albumin as standard.

Ion Exchange Chromatography. Columns (0.5 x 5.0 cm) of DEAE Sephadex® were prepared by equilibrating the resin in 0.01 M phosphate buffer, pH 6.0.

Samples of MEE were diluted one fourth with the same phosphate buffer and 1.0 ml of the diluted sample was applied to the column. The column was washed with 10 ml of equilibrating buffer and then a 40 ml linear 0-0.5 M NaCl gradient was applied. The column was finally washed with 5 ml of phosphate buffer containing 1 M NaCl. Fractions of 1 ml were collected and assayed for various enzymatic activities.

RESULTS

The results of enzyme determinations on fluids classified as serous or mucoid are presented in Table 2. The mean specific activity for each enzyme within the group is presented along with the range of activities observed. Fluids in which the protein concentration after collection into distilled water was less than 0.3 mg/ml were eliminated from the study because of the decreased accuracy of protein and enzyme determinations. It can be seen that in every case the mean enzyme activity is higher in the fluids classified as mucoid. For α-mannosidase, β-glucuronidase, and hexosaminidase the difference between the group means is statistically significant at the level of $P < 0.001$. The mean activities of these enzymes in mucoid effusions is four to five-fold elevated compared to the serous effusions. For β-galactosidase and acid phosphatase, the difference is significant at the level of $P < 0.01$ and the mean values for the enzyme activities from the mucoid fluids range from three to five times higher than the values for serous fluids. For α-glucosidase and alkaline phosphatase the difference between the mean activities for the two groups is significant at the level of $P < 0.05$. The most striking elevation is observed with α-glucosidase where there is found an 11-fold elevation of the mucoid mean value when compared to the value obtained for the serous effusions. The difference between the mean values for lactate dehydrogenase was significant only at the $P < 0.1$ level, although there was approximately a five-fold elevation. The values for alkaline phosphatase and lactate dehydrogenase can be compared to those reported by Juhn and Huff[8] who found from one to three-fold elevation of these enzymes in mucoid effusions. Table 3 presents the re-

TABLE 2. ENZYME LEVELS IN MUCOID MIDDLE EAR EFFUSION COMPARED TO SEROUS MIDDLE EAR EFFUSION

Specimen Classification	β-Galactosidase*	Acid Phosphatase	α-Mannosidase	β-Glucuronidase	Hexosaminidase	α-Glucosidase	Alkaline Phosphatase	Lactate Dehydrogenase x10^{-3}
Mucoid								
Mean	2.3 30†	194.0 31†	9.0 31†	27.0 31†	227.0 31†	6.8 15†	50.0 16†	3.4 12†
Range	0.26-13	14.0-730	1.3-38	1.1-122	22.0-650	0.68-17	6.8-123	0.32-12
Serous								
Mean	0.42 14†	63.0 16†	2.2 16†	5.2 16†	52.0 16†	0.63 7†	18.0 7†	0.71 4†
Range	0-1.7	11.0-345	0-10	0-15	1.1-150	0-2.3	0.47-47	0.34-1.3
Student's t-test	$P<0.01$	$P<0.01$	$P<0.001$	$P<0.001$	$P<0.001$	$P<0.05$	$P<0.05$	$P<0.1$

*Enzyme activity U/mg protein.

†Indicates the number of samples.

TABLE 3. ENZYME ACTIVITY IN PURULENT MIDDLE EAR EFFUSION

	β-Galactosidase	Acid Phosphatase	α-Mannosidase	β-Glucuronidase	Hexosaminidase
Mean	0.81 4*	79 4*	4.5 4*	18 4*	146 4*
Range	0.21-1.6	48-121	3.4-6.0	13-23	98-185

*Indicates the number of samples.

sults obtained with fluids classified as purulent at the time of aspiration. When the mean values found in Tables 2 and 3 are compared, in every case, activity of enzymes found in purulent effusions is intermediate between that found in serous or mucoid effusions. The difference in means between the serous and purulent fluids is significant ($P < .05$) for α-mannosidase, β-glucuronidase, and hexosaminidase, but not for β-galactosidase and acid phosphatase. When comparing the purulent effusions to the mucoid, the differences in mean activity are significant ($P < .05$) for β-galactosidase, acid phosphatase, and α-mannosidase, but not for β-glucuronidase and hexosaminidase.

The enzyme activities from serous and mucoid effusions were examined further on the basis of the microbiological findings. Middle ear effusion was considered to be culture-positive when the organism identified was not the same as that identified from the external canal. Most middle ear fluids showed no growth of microorganisms after ten days of incubation in broth, even when significant bacterial contamination was found in the external ear. The organisms identified from the culture-positive fluids were micrococci, *Moraxella* species, *Staphylococcus*, coagulation negative, and *Hemophilus influenzae*, untypable. Table 4 presents the results of this analysis. Mean enzyme activities are shown together with the standard deviation for each group. There seems to be essentially no difference between the enzyme activities of the culture-positive effusions and the culture-negative effusions.

Ion Exchange Chromatography of Ear Fluids. Most tissues and body fluids including serum, tears, and CSF contain two prominent hexosaminidase isoenzymes, designated hexosaminidases A and B.[13] Since all ear fluids exhibited significant amounts of hexosaminidase activity, we were interested in examining the isoenzyme distribution. Aliquots of ear fluids were subjected to chromatography on columns containing DEAE Sephadex under conditions of pH and ionic strength which resolve hexosaminidase A and B. The results of a typical study are presented in Figure 1. A peak of hexosaminidase activity was eluted first from DEAE Sephadex in the buffer wash followed by the elution of a second peak of hexosaminidase activity at approximately 0.3 M NaCl. The recovery of hexosaminidase activity from the ion-exchange column was always greater than 90%. The temperature stabilities of the hexosaminidase fractions were determined by incubating enzyme in the presence of citrate-phosphate buffer containing bovine serum albumin at 50 C for periods of 15, 30, and 60 minutes. The fraction eluting in the buffer wash retained greater than 90% of its enzymatic activity under these conditions, thus confirming its identity as hexosaminidase B.[10] The fraction eluting at approximately 0.1 M NaCl retained less than 10% of its initial activity after 60 minutes, and thus its identity was confirmed as hexosaminidase A.[10]

The results presented in Figure 1 suggest that the hexosaminidase isoenzymes from MEE have elution properties similar to those found for these enzymes in human serum, and that there are no significant charge differences between enzymes from mucoid or serous effusions. The ratio of the A component to the B component in both serous and mucoid cases

TABLE 4. ENZYME LEVELS IN CULTURE POSITIVE SEROUS OR MUCOID MIDDLE EAR EFFUSIONS COMPARED TO CULTURE NEGATIVE EFFUSIONS

Specimen Classification	β-Galactosidase	Acid Phosphatase	α-Mannosidase	β-Glucuronidase	Total Hexosaminidase	α-Glucosidase	Alkaline Phosphatase
Mucoid, Culture positive							
Mean	2.4* ± 2.6 7†	206 ± 197 7†	7.7 ± 3.3 7†	27 ± 19 7†	168 ± 114 7†	4.9 ± 2.3 5†	70 ± 37 4†
Mucoid, Culture-negative							
Mean	1.4 ± 1.2 14†	214 ± 212 14†	8.2 ± 7.0 14†	24 ± 19 14†	212 ± 114 14†	4.7 ± 6.2 6†	43 ± 42 6†
Serous, Culture-positive							
Value	0.70 ± 0.13 2†	32 ± 5 2†	2.6 ± 0.2 2†	5.4 ± 1.3 2†	35 ± 6 2†	ND	ND
Serous, Culture-negative							
Mean	0.45 ± 0.6 9†	73 ± 105 11†	2.0 ± 2.8 11†	4.6 ± 5.8 11†	49 ± 45 11†	ND	ND

*Values are expressed as the mean ± the standard deviation.

†Indicates the number of samples.

ND - Not determined.

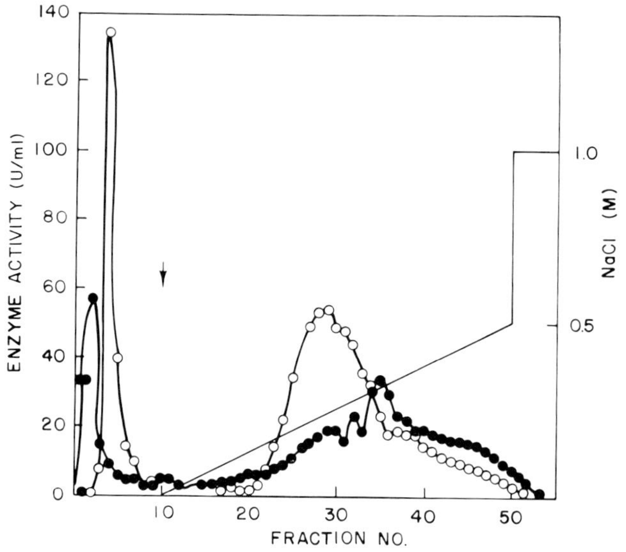

Fig. 1. DEAE Sephadex chromatography of middle ear fluid. Hexosaminidase activity of column fractions from mucoid (○-○) and serous (●-●) fluids. Conditions of chromatography and assay are as described in text. Elution of the column with a linear salt gradient was begun at the point indicated by the arrow.

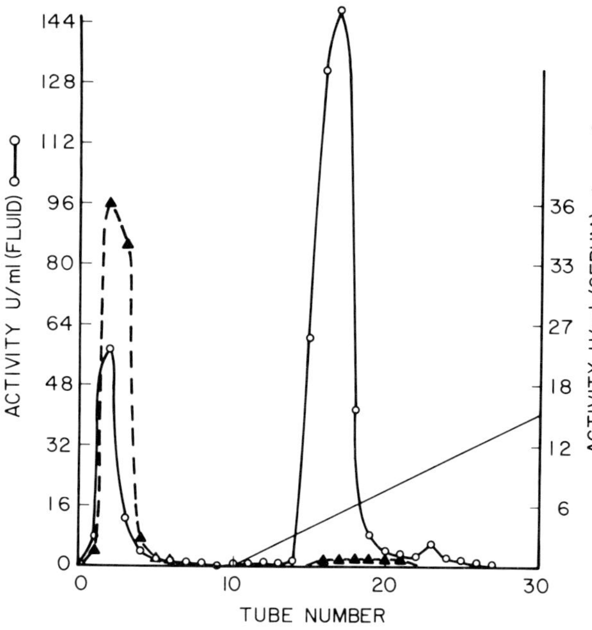

Fig. 2. DEAE Sephadex chromatography of MEE and human serum. β-Glucuronidase activity of column fractions from mucoid MEE (○-○) and normal human serum (△-△-△). Conditions of chromatography and assay are described in the text.

ranged from 3.0 to 4.0. These are values similar to that found in normal serum.[14]

These same column fractions were assayed for β-glucuronidase activity and the results of a typical experiment are shown in Figure 2. It can be seen that the conditions of chromatography separated two isozymes of β-glucuronidase in mucoid fluid: one peak appears in the initial buffer wash and a second peak of activity elutes at approximately 0.1 M NaCl. Results are shown only for an ear fluid classified as mucoid since the lower level of β-glucuronidase activity could not be detected in the DEAE fractions obtained after chromatography of serous ear fluids. The results of DEAE chromatography of a normal serum are also shown in Figure 2. The fraction of activity eluting in the gradient is only a small fraction of the total activity; however, in each case only two peaks of activity are observed and there are no unique peaks found in the MEE. Heat stability studies, conducted in a similar manner as those for hexosaminidase, resulted in the loss of all β-glucuronidase activity within 15 minutes.

Column fractions were also assayed for acid phosphatase, β-galactosidase, and α-mannosidase activities, but under these conditions of ion-exchange chromatography, which were designed for maximum separation of hexosaminidase A and B, no satisfactory resolution of isoenzymes was obtained.

Enzyme Properties. It was of interest to compare the properties of the hexosaminidase and β-glucuronidase isoenzymes obtained from middle ear fluids, particularly with respect to the pH optimum and dependence of the reaction velocity on substrate concentration.

Appropriate DEAE Sephadex column fractions were combined for these studies. The initial velocity of the enzyme catalyzed reaction was studied as a function of substrate concentration between 0.67-5 mM for hexosaminidase and between 2-10 mM for glucuronidase. Values of the Michaelis constant (Km) were estimated from the intercepts of double reciprocal plots of velocity vs substrate concentration. The Km obtained for hexosaminidase A was 3.4 mM and that for hexosaminidase B was 2.5 mM, while the Km obtained for β-glucuronidase was 2.6 mM. These values are comparable to those obtained for these enzymes from other sources and show no difference between enzyme obtained from serous or mucoid ear fluids. The Km values determined for both β-glucuronidase isoenzymes obtained from a particular MEE were indistinguishable.

The effect of buffer on the enzyme activity was studied from pH 3.0 to pH 5.5 for hexosaminidase and from pH 4.0 to 6.0 for β-glucuronidase. The pH optima was found to be at pH 4.4 for both hexosaminidase A and B. These values are comparable to those reported by others for these enzymes from other sources including serum, and again, no differences were observed between the hexosaminidases obtained from serous or mucoid ear fluids. Similarly, both isoenzymes of β-glucuronidase exhibited broad pH optima between pH 4-5.

DISCUSSION

A previous study of various oxidative and hydrolytic enzymes present in both serous and mucoid

MEE[8] found moderately higher levels in mucoid than in serous effusions. The ratio of mucoid to serous activity of the lysosomal enzymes, acid phosphatase, and lysozyme were found to be 1.6 to 1.2 respectively. We have extended those studies to include a large number of lysosomal hydrolases and find that for all of the measured enzyme activities, mucoid effusions show a much greater specific activity than serous effusions. We find the ratio of mucoid to serous activities vary from 3 to 11, depending on the particular enzyme. The differences of enzyme specific activity between serous and mucoid effusions observed in the current study cannot be attributed to merely lower protein in the mucoid effusions accompanied by constant hydrolase activity. The protein concentrations of mucoid MEE were frequently greater than that of serous effusions and thus the differences in enzyme activity would be even greater if expressed on a volume basis. The present work was undertaken, in part, to determine if the measurement of lysosomal hydrolase activity could be helpful in determining the presence of bacterial infection in the middle ear. Although the specific activities of hydrolases are markedly elevated in mucoid MEE, this higher enzymatic activity cannot be attributed to the presence of bacteria since we were unable to detect any difference in enzyme levels between fluids from which we were unable to grow bacteria and those which contained microorganisms. The same observation is true for serous effusions; we were unable to detect significant differences between mean activities from culture positive and culture negative effusions. Riding et al, in a study of the microbiology of recurrent and chronic OME,[4] found that 43.8% of the mucoid effusions and 42.4% of the serous effusions were culture positive. In the current study, only 33% of the mucoid effusions and 18% of the serous effusions tested were culture positive.

Since the specific activities of all the lysosomal hydrolases measured were significantly different in mucoid and serous MEE, it was of interest to determine the distribution of isozymes. The pattern of isozyme distribution for hexosaminidase is identical for the two fluid types and is similar to that found in human serum. Both hexosaminidase A and B exhibit the same properties of pH optima and substrate binding as is found in those isozymes from other tissues.

We were unable to measure the isozyme pattern for β-glucuronidase in serous fluids since the level of enzyme was not high enough to be accurately determined after the dilution which occurs during chromatography. The isozyme pattern obtained from mucoid effusions is different than that found in normal human serum, a finding similar to the observations of others[8,15-17] for the isozyme pattern of lactate dehydrogenase. In the MEE 17% of the total β-glucuronidase activity recovered is found in the first peak and 83% in the second peak. In normal human serum 93% of the total activity is found in the first peak and almost negligible activity in the second. Thus, the distribution of isozymes is very different in the mucoid MEE than in normal serum. This finding suggests that enzymes are probably released from the inflamed middle ear mucosa and that mucoid MEE is not simply a transudate of plasma. The specific cells which may serve as the source of the released enzyme remain unidentified. Knowledge of the lysosomal enzyme content of MEE is essential if we are to explore the origin of the constituents of these fluids. Is it possible that the elevated content of lysosomal hydrolases could contribute to the tissue destruction which often occurs in untreated cases of otitis media? β-Glucuronidase, for example, is involved in the hydrolysis of acid mucopolysaccharides found in cellular ground substance and could be acting on the tissues of the middle ear. This hypothesis could be tested in an animal model by inserting purified β-glucuronidase into the inner ear of an experimental animal under conditions known to produce MEE.

It is interesting that for every enzyme determined the mean activity in purulent effusions was intermediate between that for serous and mucoid effusions. Could these effusions represent an intermediate or transition state between serous and mucoid effusions? Further studies are in progress to attempt to answer these and other questions.

ACKNOWLEDGMENTS — We are grateful to Cathy Baca, Lorna Cropcho, Joyce Sweeney, and Patrick Coyle for their technical assistance.

REFERENCES

1. Bluestone CD. Eustachian tube obstruction in the infant with cleft palate. Ann Otol Rhinol Laryngol 1971; 80 Suppl 2:1-30.

2. Tonder O, Gunderson T. Nature of the fluid in serous otitis media. Arch Otolaryngol 1971; 93:473-8.

3. Wright I, Kapadia R. The cytology of "glue ear." J Laryngol Otol 1969; 83:367-76.

4. Riding KH, Bluestone CD, Michaels RH, Cantekin EI, Doyle WJ, Pozivak C. Microbiology of recurrent and chronic otitis media with effusion. J Pediatr 1978; 93:739-43.

5. Senturia BH, Gessert CF, Carr CD, Baumann S. Studies concerned with tubotympanitis. Ann Otol Rhinol Laryngol 1958; 67:440-67.

6. Lupovich P, Harkins M. Symposium on prophylaxis and treatment of middle ear effusions. III. The pathophysiology of effusion in otitis media. Laryngoscope 1972; 82:1647-53.

7. Juhn SK, Huff JS, Paparella MM. Certain oxidative and hydrolytic enzymes in the middle ear effusion in serous otitis media. Arch Otorhinolaryngol (NY) 1976; 212:119-25.

8. Juhn SK, Huff JS. Biochemical characteristics of middle ear effusions. Ann Otol Rhinol Laryngol 1976; 85 Suppl 25:110-6.

9. Bernstein JM, Villari EM, Rattazi MC. The significance of lysosomal enzymes in middle ear effusions. Otolaryngol Head Neck Surg 1979; 87:845-51.

10. Moffitt KD, Chambers JP, Diven WF, Glew RH, Wenger DA, Farrell DP. Characterization of lysosomal hydrolases that

are elevated in Gaucher's disease. Arch Biochem Biophys 1978; 190:247-60.

11. Wroblewski F, LaDue LS. Lactic dehydrogenase activity in blood. Proc Soc Exp Biol 1955; 90:210-3.

12. Lowry OH, Rosebrough NJ, Farr AL, Randall RJ. Protein measurement with the folin phenol reagent. J Biol Chem 1951; 193:265-75.

13. Robinson D, Stirling JL. N-acetyl-beta-glucosaminidases in human spleen. Biochem J 1968; 107:321-7.

14. O'Brien JS, Okada S, Chen A, Fillerup DL. Tay-Sachs disease: detection of heterozygotes and homozygotes by serum hexosaminidase assay. N Eng J Med 1970; 283:15-20.

15. Juhn SK, Huff JS, Paparella MM. Lactate dehydrogenase activity and isoenzyme patterns in serous middle ear effusions. Ann Otol Rhinol Laryngol 1973; 82:192-5.

16. Lotz P, Kuhl KD. Die lactaldehydrogenase des innenohres. Arch Klin Exp Ohren Nasen Kehlkopfheilkd 1968; 192:237-48.

17. Palva T, Forsen R, Raunio V, et al. Lactate dehydrogenase pattern of middle ear mucosa. Pract Otorhinolaryngol (Basel) 1970; 32:129-36.

≈

EYE-HEAD COORDINATION AND LATERAL CANAL BLOCK IN SQUIRREL MONKEYS

TAKESHI KUBO, MD
OSAKA, JAPAN

MAKOTO IGARASHI, MD
HOUSTON, TEXAS

DAVID W. JENSEN, PhD
HOUSTON, TEXAS

WILLIAM K. WRIGHT, MD
HOUSTON, TEXAS

Eye and head nystagmus during horizontal optokinetic stimulation was analyzed in squirrel monkeys. Slow phase speed of coupled head and eye nystagmus showed highly significant negative correlations in normal subjects; correlation coefficients were −0.81 at 60°/sec and −0.72 at 100°/sec stimuli. Bilateral lateral semicircular canal block resulted in a reduction of the negative correlation. The postoperative reduction of the correlation coefficient value ranged from 0.17-0.28 (significant at $P<0.01$ level) at 60°/sec stimulus and 0.06-0.13 (not significant) at 100°/sec stimulus. Gaze speed was calculated by summing slow phase speeds of coupled head and eye nystagmus. Mean error of gaze in normal subjects was 1.5% at 60°/sec stimulus and 7.8% at 100°/sec stimulus. Mean gaze speed showed an overshoot (8% at 60°/sec stimulus and 6.5% at 100°/sec stimulus) in the three to four weeks postoperative period; however, this subsided two to three months after the operation. Measurement of head-turning performance (in yaw plane) in humans may provide a clinically useful index for the assessment of certain types of vestibular function.

INTRODUCTION

It has been known that the retinal image during head turning is stabilized basically by way of the vestibular compensatory reflex in rhesus monkeys.[1,2] Two different stimuli were used in these studies for visual stimuli to command gaze shift, ie, the presentation of stationary or smoothly moving visual targets. We have used optokinetic stimulation (OKS) to induce eye and head movements in squirrel monkeys.[3] In the previous study, many squirrel monkeys showed head nystagmus of large amplitude during OKS. Slow phase speed of coupled head and eye nystagmus showed a highly significant negative correlation, ie, when head speeds increased, eye speeds decreased and vice versa. In this study, the bilateral lateral semicircular canals were surgically blocked and the effects upon gaze control were examined during a three-month postoperative period. The results show that a significant change induced by this sort of vestibular deficiency is in head-turning speed. The results may warrant further investigation as to whether the measurement of head-turning performance during a visuomotor task in humans provide clinically useful information.

METHODS

The experiments were conducted on three squirrel monkeys (*Saimiri sciureus*) weighing between 600-750 gm. Head movement in the yaw plane was recorded using a lightweight potentiometer which registered a voltage dependent on head position. Head was restricted to minimize the roll and pitch movements. When the monkey's head was restricted in the pitch plane, care was taken to leave the head as close as possible to the natural position. Subsequently, the plane of lateral semicircular canal was pitched up about 20-40° to the plane of head turning. Eye movements were recorded using the platinum needle electrodes inserted into lateral canthi, ie, ENG. Slow phase speeds of head and eye nystagmus were measured manually from the recordings on an oscillographic paper.

Optokinetic stimulus speed of 60°/sec and 100°/sec were chosen in this series of experiments. Subjects were injected with amphetamine sulfate (0.5 mg/kg) 15 minutes prior to recording, to keep the alertness level constant.

After at least two preoperative data acquisitions, bilateral lateral semicircular canals were blocked by bone chips in a one-stage operation. The canal plugging was placed a distance away from the crista ampullaris lateralis.[4] Two weeks of rest period was allowed after the operation. The blockage was expected to be more tightly established in the osseous canal during this period. Recording (twice per week) was continued over three months after the operation. The monkeys were subsequently sacrificed by transcardiac perfusion under overdose of Nembutal® anesthesia. All temporal bones were prepared for microscopic examination.

RESULTS

Morphology. Microscopic evaluation of all temporal bones proved that the lateral semicircular canal pluggings by bone were properly done. The lateral semicircular canal crista appeared normal in all cases. There was a minimal amount of the eosinophilic precipitate around the plugging site.

Functional Assessment of Canal Plugging. Squirrel monkeys were tested by vestibular stimulation, ie, 60°/sec and 100°/sec velocity step stimuli in the dark, in a fixed-head condition before and after the semicircular canal plugging. The plane of head rotation was simulated with that of active head-turning during OKS. Slow phase speed of eye nystagmus was maximum within five seconds after the onset of stimulus and then gradually declined until the nystagmus disappeared. Preoperatively, averaged

From the Department of Otorhinolaryngology and Communicative Sciences, Baylor College of Medicine, Houston. This study was supported by the McFadden Trust Research Fund, NINCDS grants NS-10940 and NS-07237, and NASA contract NAS-9-14546.

REPRINTS — Makoto Igarashi, MD, Department of Otorhinolaryngology and Communicative Sciences, Baylor College of Medicine, 1200 Moursund Avenue, Houston, TX 77030.

TABLE 1. 60°/SEC STIMULUS*

	Preop	*Postop-I*	*Postop-II*
Head speed (°/sec)	28.9±11.8	21.1±9.3	18.3±9.1
Eye speed (°/sec)	30.2± 9.4	43.7±9.5	39.9±9.1
Gaze speed (°/sec)	59.1± 6.8	64.8±9.2	58.2±7.7
Mean error of gaze (°/sec)	−0.9	+4.8	−1.8
No. of sample	119	139	146

*Mean and SD of slow phase head, eye, and gaze speeds induced by 60°/sec OKS before and after lateral semicircular canal block operation. Postoperative data were collected at three to four weeks (postop-I) and two to three months (postop-II).

maximum slow phase eye speed was 41.3 ±5.9°/sec (mean±SD, N=24) at 60°/sec stimulus, and 61.7±11.7°/sec at 100°/sec stimulus under amphetamine sulfate administration. Time constant of these decay curves (time required that slow phase eye speed reduced 63% of the maximum values) was 24.2 seconds at 60°/sec stimulus and 27.4 seconds at 100°/sec stimulus. After the operation, no response to rotation was found at either 60°/sec or 100°/sec stimuli without amphetamine injection. However, after amphetamine administration a slight horizontal component of ocular nystagmus was detected; the maximum slow phase eye speed corresponded to 17.9% of preoperative value at 60°/sec stimulus and 18.8% of that at 100°/sec stimulus. The time constant decreased to 21.1% and 18.2% of preoperative levels, respectively. Therefore, the overall postoperative reduction of the horizontal vestibular compensatory reflex was estimated to be 79-82%.

Spontaneous Nystagmus. Postoperatively, no spontaneous nystagmus was found in the dark in any of the monkeys without amphetamine, but two of three monkeys showed spontaneous nystagmus after amphetamine administration. Spontaneous nystagmus did not appear consistently in these monkeys; however, it became apparent usually after first exposure to OKS or vestibular stimulation when it occurred. Minor postoperative irritation may have existed in the vestibular labyrinth and probably may have caused slight functional imbalance which was detectable only with amphetamine administration. Data contaminated by spontaneous nystagmus were eliminated from subsequent analysis.

Eye and Head Coordination. When squirrel monkeys were exposed to OKS in a free head condition, two sorts of head movements, ie, anticompensatory head deviation and head nystagmus, could be observed. Some characteristics of such head deviation have been already described in a previous paper.[3]

60°/sec OKS. Table 1 shows mean and standard deviations of slow phase head, eye, and gaze speed at 60°/sec OKS before and after lateral semicircular canal block. The gaze speed was calculated by summing the slow phase speed of coupled head and eye nystagmus. An overshoot of mean gaze speed is seen at the three to four weeks postoperative period, ie, 64.8°/sec in the column of postop-I. However, gaze speeds are properly maintained two to three months after the operation, ie, 58.2°/sec in the column of postop-II. Therefore, the data were pooled in the two to three months postoperative period. Mean error of gaze is only −0.9°/sec which corresponds to 1.5% of stimulus speed preoperatively. However, it becomes greater at postop-I period, ie, +4.8°/sec, 8%; and then it is improved at postop-II period, ie, −1.8°/sec, 3%.

Slow phase speeds of coupled head and eye nystagmus which are shown in Table 1 are plotted in Figure 1. Preoperative data (Fig. 1A) show a highly

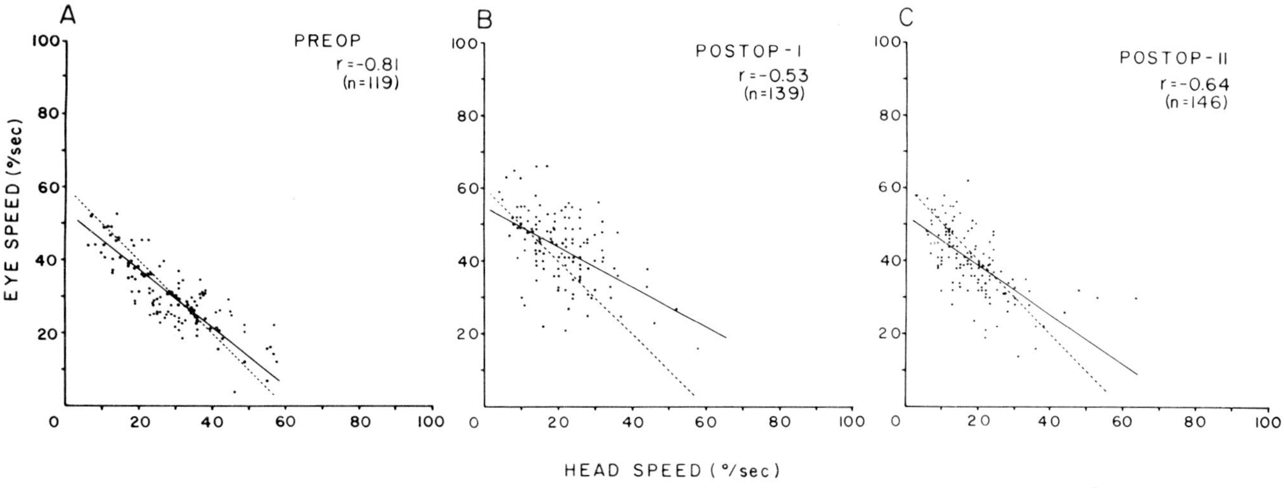

Fig. 1. Abscissa and ordinate represent slow phase speed of head and eye nystagmus, respectively. Each dot represents slow phase speed of coupled head and eye nystagmus induced by 60°/sec stimulus, A) before, and B, C) after lateral semicircular canal block operation. Data in this figure are identical with those in Table 1. Dashed and solid lines indicate experimental and −1.0 regression lines, respectively. Postoperative reduction of negative coefficient value was significant at both postop-I and -II periods (Fisher's test, <0.01). Negative correlations between head and eye speeds in A, B, and C were significant ($P<0.01$).

TABLE 2. 100°/SEC STIMULUS*

	Preop	Postop-I	Postop-II
Head speed (°/sec)	31.3± 14.8	33.9± 15.7	24.4± 11.3
Eye speed (°/sec)	60.9± 15.6	72.6± 12.8	69.9± 14.2
Gaze speed (°/sec)	92.2± 11.4	106.5± 13.6	94.4± 12.3
Mean error of gaze (°/sec)	−7.8	+6.5	−5.6
No. of sample	131	188	161

*Explanations are the same as for Table 1, but obtained by 100°/sec stimulus. Note that mean error of gaze speed at preoperative period (7.8%) is larger than that during 60°/sec stimulus.

significant negative correlation between head and eye speeds: −0.81 (N = 119), $P<0.01$. Figure 1B, C shows the data collected at postop-I and -II periods, respectively. Although the negative correlation between head and eye speed was still significant in both postop-I and -II periods ($P<0.01$), the coefficient value significantly decreased after the operation (Fisher's test, <0.01).[5]

100°/sec OKS. Table 2 shows the data obtained by 100°/sec OKS before and after lateral semicircular canal block. Mean error of gaze at preoperative period is larger at 100°/sec OKS than at 60°/sec OKS: 7.8% vs 1.5% of the stimulus speed, respectively. Since 100°/sec stimulus speed is the one where the gaze speed starts to lag behind the stimulus speed in squirrel monkeys, greater error of gaze speed is not an unexpected result. Gaze overshoot occurs at postop-I period by 100°/sec OKS as well. Later, the overshoot subsides; however, mean gaze speed is slightly higher than the preoperative level.

Slow phase speeds of coupled head and eye nystagmus which are induced by 100°/sec OKS are plotted in Figure 2. If negative correlation coefficients seen in normal subjects are compared between 60°/sec OKS and 100°/sec OKS, the value is lower at 100°/sec OKS than that at 60°/sec stimulus. It may be reasonable to consider that the coordination between eye and head movements decreases at the speed which corresponds to the upper limit of visual-oculomotor reflex induced by OKS in squirrel monkeys. A statistical test (Fisher's test) showed that postoperative reduction of the coefficient value was not significant at either postop-I or -II periods. Failure in showing significant difference between preoperative and postoperative periods may be due to rather low negative correlation between head and eye speeds at the preoperative period.

DISCUSSION

The vestibular nucleus is involved in producing optokinetic eye nystagmus and after-nystagmus.[6,7] A labyrinthine ablation causes reduction of slow phase speed of optokinetic eye nystagmus and abolishes after-nystagmus.[8,9] As the labyrinthectomy (or vestibular neurectomy) changes optokinetic response itself, such ablative procedures are not proper strategies to study the role of vestibular compensatory reflex on eye-head coordination during OKS. In our recent study[10] in squirrel monkeys, optokinetic nystagmus and after-nystagmus in yaw plane were not very much influenced by total macular ablation. Thus, changes after total elimination of labyrinthine inputs should be more reflectory to the elimination of inputs from the cristae. Static impulse originating from the crista ampullaris should be maintained at the same level to preserve the efficacy of OKS. Blockage of membranous semicircular ducts did not alter static labyrinthine input to the vestibular nuclei; whereas, it effectively eliminated the dynamic response of plugged semicircular canal to angular acceleration in the cat and squirrel monkeys.[4,11,12] Therefore, a semicircular canal block used in this study seems an appropriate approach in order to study the role of vestibular compensatory reflex.

Blockage of the lateral semicircular canal was

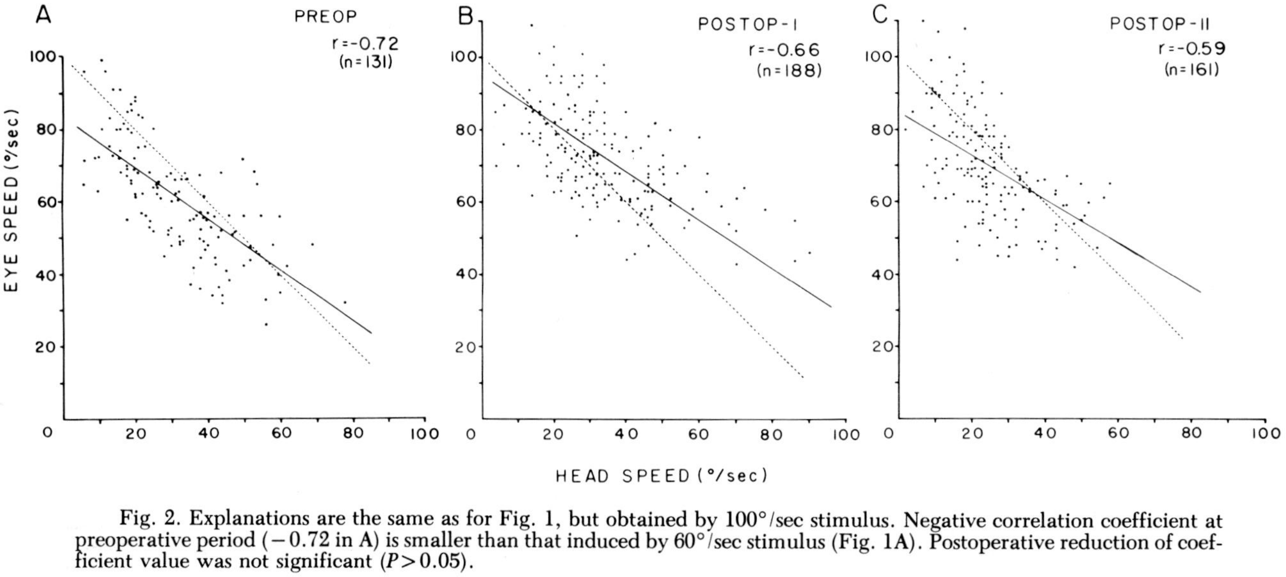

Fig. 2. Explanations are the same as for Fig. 1, but obtained by 100°/sec stimulus. Negative correlation coefficient at preoperative period (−0.72 in A) is smaller than that induced by 60°/sec stimulus (Fig. 1A). Postoperative reduction of coefficient value was not significant ($P>0.05$).

properly performed in all ears as revealed by morphological examination. However, since the plane of head turning or table rotation was not exactly parallel to that of the lateral semicircular canal, vertical semicircular canals were stimulated during head turning. Our functional assessment using vestibular stimulation showed that the horizontal component of vestibular compensatory reflex was reduced to about 18-21% of the preoperative level. A precise condition of eye movement at the postoperative period is not known, since only horizontal ENG was recorded in the present experiment. Eye movements having vertical and horizontal components probably occurred during head rotation. Even though the elimination of vestibulo-ocular reflex was incomplete, bilateral lateral semicircular canal block induced an overshoot of gaze speed at the three to four weeks postoperative period. Later, gaze overshoot subsided. The negative correlation coefficient value between head and eye speeds significantly declined after the operation, and did not recover to the preoperative level over three months when 60°/sec OKS was used.

Dichgans et al[1] reported that the vestibular compensatory reflex during active head turning recovered up to 90% of the preoperative level at one month after bilateral labyrinthectomy in rhesus monkeys. They discussed that this recovery was due to three processes: 1) enhancement of cervico-ocular gain; 2) centrally originated ocular compensatory reflex which developed after the operation; and 3) recalibration of saccade and retinal error. Since there are several differences between their experiment and ours, the compensatory process would be different. First, the vestibular nuclei activity is maintained at normal levels after semicircular canal block in this experiment. Second, the visual-oculomotor feedback system does not work during saccadic gaze performance, since the operation time of this system is slow, ie, 70-80 msec; however, during the slow phase of optokinetic nystagmus this system probably contributed to correcting the retinal error. Therefore, it is likely that the interruption of the vestibulo-ocular reflex causes less failure in the gaze adjustment in this experiment due to functioning visual-oculomotor feedback. Actually, gaze error (overshoot) occurring in the three to four weeks postoperative period was not profound. It is supposed that the three compensatory processes suggested by Dichgans and others[1] account for the recovery of gaze speed during the two to three months after the operation.

Head movements that are executed during visuomotor tasks should activate the intact vestibular system so as to stabilize the retina in space, which should facilitate clearer vision. What happens to head movements if the vestibular input is deficient? If the vestibular input is completely abolished by bilateral vestibulectomy in rhesus monkeys, the gain of head movement in gaze during smooth pursuit declines strikingly.[2] Our present study in squirrel monkeys has shown that if the portion of vestibular input signalling head movement is diminished by canal block, the slow phase speed of head nystagmus during optokinetic pursuit declines also. Given our premise, it is reasonable to consider that individuals who have deficient vestibular input reduce head movements that are normally executed in a visuomotor task. This raises the question whether the measurement of eye and head movements induced during various visuomotor tests would provide useful clinical information in the assessment of vestibular function. Furthermore, since we have shown that the optokinetic gaze speed changes with time after a canal block, repeated measurements of head and eye speeds during suitable visuomotor tasks may provide a measure of the functional compensation after a vestibular pathology or lesion.

ACKNOWLEDGMENTS — We wish to thank Mark Simon and Joel K. Levy for their assistance in data collection and analysis. Histological specimens were prepared by E. Marbley and K. Sprinkle.

REFERENCES

1. Dichgans J, Bizzi E, Morasso P, Tagliasco V. Mechanisms underlying recovery of eye-head coordination following bilateral labyrinthectomy in monkeys. Exp Brain Res 1973; 18:548-62.

2. Lanman J, Bizzi E, Allum J. The coordination of eye and head movement during smooth pursuit. Brain Res 1978; 153:39-53.

3. Kubo T, Igarashi M, Jensen DW, Homick JL. Eye-head coordination during optokinetic stimulation in squirrel monkeys. Ann Otol Rhinol Laryngol 1981; 90:85-8.

4. Takahashi M, Igarashi M, Wright WK. Damped pendular rotation nystagmus after unilateral labyrinthectomy or unilateral lateral semicircular canal block in squirrel monkeys. J Otolaryngol 1977; 6:157-65.

5. Cohen J, Cohen P. Applied multiple regression-correlation analysis for the behavioral sciences. Hillsdale: Lawrence Erlbaum Associates, 1975.

6. Waespe W, Henn V. Neuronal activity in the vestibular nuclei of the alert monkey during vestibular and optokinetic stimulation. Exp Brain Res 1977; 27:523-38.

7. Waespe W, Henn V. Vestibular nuclei activity during optokinetic after-nystagmus (OKAN) in the alert monkey. Exp Brain Res 1977; 30:323-30.

8. Cohen B, Uemura T, Takemori S. Effects of labyrinthectomy on optokinetic nystagmus and optokinetic after-nystagmus. Equilibrium Res 1973; 3:88-93.

9. Zee DS, Yee RD, Robinson DA. Optokinetic responses in labyrinthine-defective human beings. Brain Res 1976; 113:423-8.

10. Takashashi M, Igarashi M, Homick JL. Effect of otolith end organ ablation on horizontal optokinetic nystagmus, and optokinetic afternystagmus in the squirrel monkey. ORL 1977; 39:74-81.

11. Money KE, Scott JW. Functions of separate sensory receptors on non-auditory labyrinth of the cat. Am J Physiol 1962; 202:1211-20.

12. Abend WK. Response to constant angular accelerations of neurons in the monkey superior vestibular nucleus. Exp Brain Res 1978; 31:459-73.

EFFERENT INNERVATION OF THE COCHLEA

JÜRGEN STRUTZ, MD
FREIBURG, FEDERAL REPUBLIC OF GERMANY

The origin of the efferent innervation of the cochlea was investigated in the guinea pigs. Horseradish peroxidase (HRP) was injected into the cochlea and transported to the brainstem by retrograde axonal transport of the efferent fibers, showing the origin of the crossed and uncrossed olivocochlear bundles of Rasmussen. HRP-labeled neurons were found in various nuclei of the superior olivary complex bilaterally. Ipsilateral to the injected cochlea there were three times more cells than on the contralateral side. About 40% of the total number of labeled neurons, a remarkable quantity, occurred in the ipsilateral lateral superior olivary nucleus. Moreover, extraolivary origin of the efferent innervation of the cochlea could be demonstrated bilaterally in the ventral nucleus of the lateral lemniscus.

The efferent innervation of the cochlea was first described by Rasmussen[1,2] who discovered the crossed and uncrossed olivocochlear bundles (OCB). Churchill and Schuknecht[3] differentiated these efferent fibers from the afferent by their content of acetylcholinesterase (AchE). AchE-positive neurons in the superior olivary complex (SOC) were assumed to be the cells of origin of the OCB.[4-6] Warr[7] substantiated in kittens the conformity of AchE-positive neurons and those labeled by retrograde axonal-transported horseradish peroxidase (HRP) from the cochlea to the SOC. He found the cells of origin of the crossed and uncrossed OCB restricted to the nuclei of the SOC bilaterally with more cells ipsilateral to the injection side. In another HRP study of the labyrinth, Gacek and Lyon[8] demonstrated the origin of the efferent vestibular neurons to be lateral to the abducens nuclei. Ross et al,[9] however, have doubts about Warr's findings because of the use of young kittens, which do not have a mature auditory system. Ross et al[9] failed to duplicate Warr's results[7] using a modified HRP technique in guinea pigs. They concluded that labyrinthine centrifugal fibers are parasympathic neurons. More recently, Warr and Guinan[10] were able to demonstrate the origin of the OCB by means of anterograde axonal transport of radiolabeled tracers injected into the SOC.

METHODS

Twelve healthy guinea pigs ranging from 300 to 350 g were anesthetized with pentobarbital. After surgically opening the bulla tympanica, 0.3-0.5 μl of a 50% HRP solution in 1% poly-L-ornithine[11] was injected unilaterally into the scala tympani through the round window, without any spillage into the middle ear. The animals were perfused 40-48 hours later with saline transcardially and then fixed with a mixture of 1.5% glutaraldehyde and 1% paraformaldehyde in 0.1 M phosphate buffer (pH 7.2). Frozen frontal sections of the brain were cut from the region of the cochlear nuclei to the superior colliculi and were treated for the demonstration of HRP according to the o-dianisidine[12] or tetramethylbenzidine (TMB) technique.[13] The nomenclature of Morest[14] was used for the auditory nuclei of the SOC.

RESULTS

In all animals, we found cells in the SOC bilaterally labeled by the granular reaction product of retrograde-transported HRP,[15] and in ten animals in the ventral nucleus of the lateral lemniscus (VLL). In total, up to 500 neurons per animal were labeled. Generally, three times more neurons were labeled ipsilateral to the injected cochlea as the contralateral side. The ipsilateral cochlear nerve was labeled by anterograde-transported HRP entering the cochlear nucleus. No other structures exhibited HRP reaction product and no indication for HRP diffusion was found.

In the SOC ipsilateral to the injected cochlea (Fig. 1B), a large number of labeled cells occurred in the dorsal hilus and on the surface or directly next to the periolivary region of the lateral superior olivary nucleus (LSO). This population of labeled cells (Fig. 2) was about 40% of the total number of labeled neurons. The ventral (VTB), medial (MTB) and lateral (LTB) nuclei of the trapezoid body exhibited considerably fewer HRP-labeled neurons. Only a few labeled cells were found in the dorsomedial periolivary nucleus (DMPO). We could not detect any labeled cells in the medial superior olivary nucleus (MSO). In the SOC contralateral to the injected cochlea, the VTB exhibited the highest number of labeled neurons (Fig. 2), where 15% of all labeled cells were found. In comparison to the VTB, a smaller number of cells were labeled at the dorsal hilus of the LSO, fewer in the MTB and DMPO, and only a few cells were stained in the LTB. As in the ipsilateral SOC, no labeled cells appeared in the MSO contralaterally.

In ten specimens we also found HRP-labeled cells in the ventral nucleus of the lateral lemniscus (VLL, Fig. 1C), located ipsilaterally and contralaterally to the injection site. Approximately 10% of the total number of labeled cells occurred in this nucleus. Most of these cells were located in the ven-

From the Department of Oto-Rhino-Laryngology, University of Freiburg, Federal Republic of Germany. This work was supported by grants of the Deutsche Forschungsge-meinschaff, SFB 70.

REPRINTS — Jürgen Strutz, MD, University of Freiburg, Department of Oto-Rhino-Laryngology, Killianstrasse 5, D-7800 Freiburg, Federal Republic of Germany.

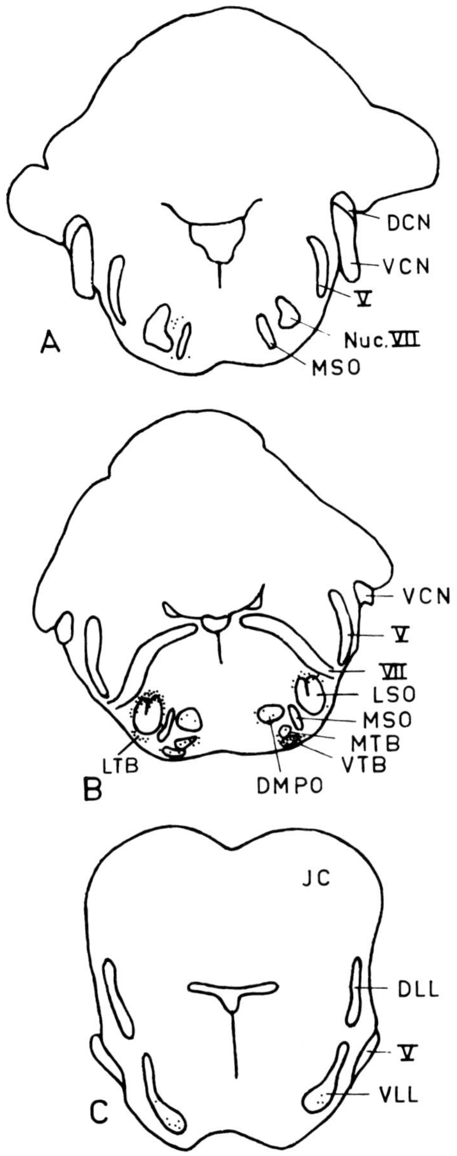

Fig. 1. Reconstructed drawings of transverse sections of the brainstem at three levels in a guinea pig. Each dot represents one labeled cell. The cochlea of the left side was injected with HRP. A) Most caudal findings at the level of the cochlear nuclei. B) Section through the SOC. C) Section through the midbrain at the level of the lateral lemniscus. DCN - Dorsal cochlear nucleus; DLL - Dorsal nucleus of lateral lemniscus; DMPO - Dorsomedial periolivary nucleus; LSO - Lateral superior olivary nucleus; LTB - Lateral nucleus of trapezoid body; MSO - Medial superior olivary nucleus; MTB - Medial nucleus of trapezoid body; Nuc. VII - Facial nucleus; VCN - Ventral cochlear nucleus; VLL - Ventral nucleus of lateral lemniscus; VTB -Ventral nucleus of trapezoid body; V - Trigeminus; VII -Facialis.

tral and caudal part of the VLL and no cells occurred at the rostral border of this nucleus. Twice as many neurons were labeled ipsilateral to the injection site as compared to the contralateral side (Fig. 3).

DISCUSSION

In contrast to Ross et al[9] we were able to demonstrate the retrograde transport of HRP from the cochlea to the SOC and the VLL in guinea pig. This animal is known to have a mature auditory system and blood-brain barrier from birth. In general, our results were in agreement with Warr's results[7] in the cat. Like Warr we found that the crossed OCB originates from neurons situated chiefly in the LSO and the VTB. The uncrossed OCB originates mainly from neurons situated in the dorsal hilus and on the surface of the LSO. Anterograde degeneration studies have shown the DMPO and the VTB as sources of the crossed and uncrossed fibers of the OCB.[16] Rasmussen[2] estimated that three fourths of the OCB arises from the contralateral SOC. Similar to Warr[7] and Firbas[17] we found that there are many more neurons of the uncrossed OCB in the SOC than of the crossed component. Possibly the uncrossed component may be unmyelinated and therefore not sensitive to silver degeneration studies. In contrast, Rossi and Cortesina[4] showed in an AchE study many more neurons of the crossed than of the uncrossed OCB.

Furthermore, we found the origin of the efferent innervation of the cochlea bilaterally in the ventral nucleus of the lateral lemniscus.[18] Warr, in his Figure 7H,[7] described in one kitten two labeled neurons which he included in the VTB at the most rostral level of the SOC, although in his discussion he referred to these cells as occurring in the VLL. According to our findings, these cells lie in the VLL. Therefore, there are two separate systems of the efferent innervations of the cochlea: the crossed and uncrossed olivocochlear bundles and the crossed and uncrossed lemniscocochlear bundles.

In contrast to Ross et al,[9] we could not detect any indication for extracellular diffusion of HRP from the cochlea into the brainstem, neither into the region of the cochlear nuclei nor to the SOC or other regions. Anterograde transport of HRP was found in the ipsilateral cochlear nerve and in the ipsilateral cochlear nuclei without any labeled neurons. Therefore we conclude that the neurons of the SOC and VLL, which contain granular HRP reaction product,[15] are labeled by retrograde axonal transport from the cochlea. These neurons seem to be the origin of the crossed and uncrossed olivocochlear and lemniscocochlear bundles. We cannot, however, demonstrate the site of termination of these efferent fibers in the cochlea with the present method of HRP application because of the retrograde axonal transport.

Anterograde axonal transport of radiolabeled

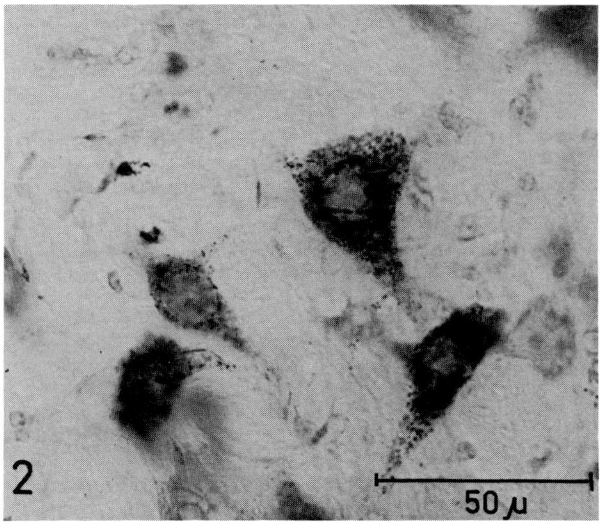

Fig. 2. Transverse section through the ipsilateral SOC. Cells in the hilus of LSO are labeled by retrograde axonal transport of HRP. TMB reaction, neutral red counterstain)

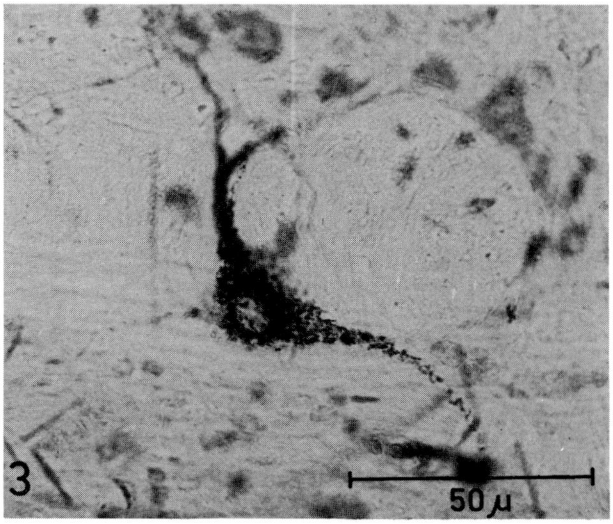

Fig. 3. Transverse section through the ipsilateral VLL, showing one HRP-labeled cell, giving off three dendrites. (TMB reaction, neutral red counterstain)

amino acids were used by Warr and Guinan[10] to demonstrate the targets of the OCB in the organ of Corti: outer and inner hair cells. They injected ^{35}S methionine into the LSO, effecting grain accumulation under inner hair cells, predominantly to the ipsilateral cochlea, while injections into MTB and DMPO effected grain accumulation under outer hair cells in the contralateral cochlea. Therefore, the existence of the efferent innervation of the cochlea could be demonstrated by use of modern neuroanatomical techniques with anterograde and retrograde axonal transported proteins.

REFERENCES

1. Rasmussen GL. An efferent cochlear bundle, abstracted. Anat Rec 1942; 82:441.

2. Rasmussen GL. The olivary peduncle and other fiber projections of the superior olivary complex. J Comp Neurol 1946; 84:141-219.

3. Churchill JA, Schuknecht HF. The relationship of acetylcholinesterase in the cochlea to the olivocochlear bundle. Henry Ford Hosp Med J 1959; 7:202-10.

4. Rossi G, Cortesina G. Research on the efferent innervation of the inner ear. J Laryngol Otol 1963; 77:202-32.

5. Osen KK, Roth K. Histochemical localization of cholinesterases in the cochlear nuclei of the cat with notes on the origin of acetylcholinesterase-positive afferents and the superior olive. Brain Res 1969; 16:165-85.

6. Brown JC, Howlett B. The olivo-cochlear tract in the rat and its bearing on the homologies of some constituent cell groups of the mammalian superior olivary complex: a thiocholin study. Acta Anat (Basel) 1972; 83:505-26.

7. Warr WB. Olivocochlear and vestibular efferent neurons of the feline brain stem: their location, morphology and number determined by retrograde axonal transport and acetylcholinesterase histochemistry. J Comp Neurol 1975; 161:159-82.

8. Gacek RR, Lyon M. The localization of vestibular efferent neurons in the kitten with horseradish peroxidase. Acta Otolaryngol (Stockh) 1974; 77:92-101.

9. Ross MD, Nuttall AL, Wright CG. Horseradish acute ototoxicity and the uptake and movement of the peroxidase in the auditory system of the guinea pig. Acta Otolaryngol (Stockh) 1977; 84:187-201.

10. Warr WB, Guinan JJ Jr. Efferent innervation of the organ of Corti: two separate systems. Brain Res 1979; 173:152-5.

11. Hadley RT, Trachtenberg MC. Poly-L-ornithine enhances the uptake of horseradish peroxidase. Brain Res 1978; 158:1-14.

12. de Olmos JS. An improved HRP method for the study of central nervous connections. Exp Brain Res 1977; 29:541-51.

13. Mesulam MM. Tetramethylbenzidine for horseradish peroxidase neurohistochemistry: a non carcinogenic blue reaction product with superior sensitivity for visualization of neural afferents and efferents. J Histochem Cytochem 1978; 26:106-17.

14. Morest DK. The collateral systems of the medial nucleus of the trapezoid body of the cat, its neural architecture and relation of the olivo-cochlear bundle. Brain Res 1968; 9:288-311.

15. Kristensson K, Olsson Y. Retrograde axonal transport of protein. Brain Res 1971; 29:363-5.

16. van Noort J. The structure and connections of the inferior colliculus: an investigation of the lower auditory system. The Netherlands: Van Gorcum & Co, 1969.

17. Firbas W. The efferent innervation in the region of inner hair cells in the organ of Corti. Acta Otolaryngol (Stockh) 1978; 86:309-13.

18. Strutz J, Spatz WB. Superior olivary and extraolivary origin of centrifugal innervation of the cochlea in guinea pig: a horseradish peroxidase study. Neurosci Lett 1980; 17:227-30.

SARCOIDOSIS AND FLUCTUATING HEARING LOSS

ROBERT A. JAHRSDOERFER, MD
MICHAEL M. E. JOHNS, MD
EDWARD G. THOMPSON, MD
ROBERT W. CANTRELL, MD
CHARLOTTESVILLE, VIRGINIA

Neurological manifestations of sarcoidosis occur in 5% of affected patients. Of the cranial nerves, the eighth nerve is the fourth most frequently involved. The central nervous system lesion is presumed to be a granulomatous meningitis that directly infiltrates the cranial nerves or causes them to be compressed from involvement of adjacent intracranial structures. Sensorineural hearing loss and vertigo usually occur in concert with other neurological findings, but may be the only presenting complaint. Sarcoidosis is not generally recognized as a cause of fluctuating sensorineural hearing loss. The fluctuating quality of the hearing loss has been noted by other investigators, but no patient has been previously reported with hearing fluctuation as the initial complaint. A chest radiograph and eye examination are mandatory. The diagnosis may be suspected from hilar adenopathy and uveitis, and confirmed by node biopsy. The hearing will usually improve on steroid therapy. Sarcoidosis represents yet another disease entity the otolaryngologist must consider in the differential diagnosis of fluctuating hearing loss.

Sarcoidosis is not generally recognized as a cause of fluctuating sensorineural hearing loss. Neurological manifestations of sarcoidosis occur in only 5% of patients affected with this disease. However, neurological dysfunction may often be the presenting complaint. The central nervous system is often involved earlier in the course of neurological sarcoidosis than is the peripheral nervous system and carries a poorer prognosis.[1] The central nervous system lesion is presumed to be a granulomatous meningitis that directly infiltrates the cranial nerves or causes them to be compressed from involvement of adjacent intracranial structures. Of the cranial nerves, the eighth cranial nerve is the fourth most frequently involved while the facial nerve is most frequently involved. Indeed, facial paralysis is the most common neurological disorder.[2] In a large review series of 118 patients, facial paralysis occurred in over 50% of cases.[3] The optic nerve is the second most affected cranial nerve while cranial nerves IX and X combined are third. Multiple cranial nerve palsies may be found.

The fluctuating quality of the hearing loss in sarcoidosis has been noted previously by others.[1,2,4-8] Hearing fluctuation has occurred in almost one half of all reported cases linking hearing loss with sarcoidosis.[4-8] Vestibular dysfunction often fluctuates with the hearing. These disturbances in balance and audition may mimic those found in other diseases. Engberg and Jepsen[4] reported on four patients with sarcoidosis who were admitted for vestibuloacoustic system disease in whom two of four were tentatively diagnosed as having bilateral acoustic neurinoma. The differential diagnosis should include lues, multiple sclerosis, Cogan's syndrome, acoustic neuroma, endolymphatic hydrops, Vogt-Koyanagi syndrome, and other intracranial tumors.

Uveitis is a common companion of neurologic sarcoidosis. It is stated to be four times more common in patients with neurological sarcoidosis than in sarcoidosis patients without neurological symptoms.[5] Uveitis was seen in 11 of 12 patients with hearing loss and sarcoidosis as reported by Gristwood,[8] and in 56% of 118 patients with sarcoidosis of the nervous system as reported by Colover.[3]

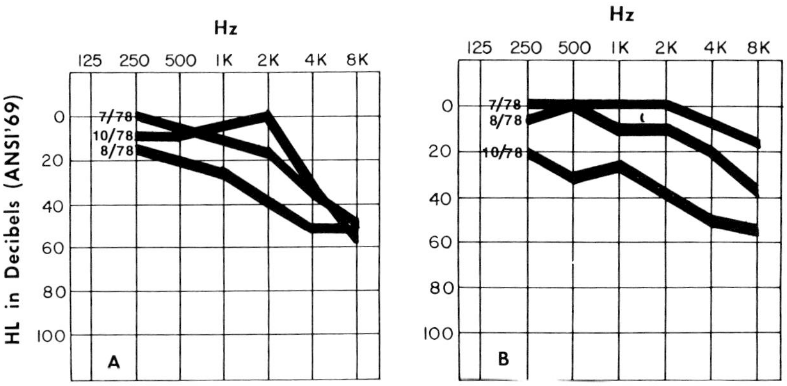

Fig. 1. Composite audiograms showing fluctuating in hearing over a period of four months. A) Left ear. B) Right ear.

From the Department of Otolaryngology and Maxillofacial Surgery, University of Virginia Hospital, Charlottesville.

Presented at the meeting of the American Neurotology Society, Dallas, Texas, October 7, 1979.

REPRINTS — Robert A. Jahrsdoerfer, MD, Department of Otolaryngology and Maxillofacial Surgery, Box 430, University of Virginia Hospital, Charlottesville, VA 22908.

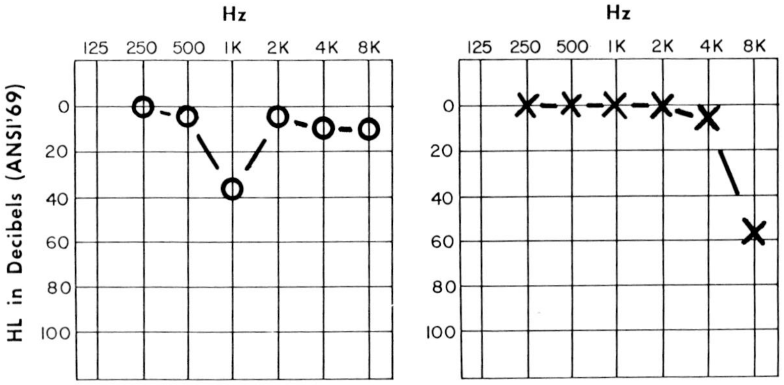

Fig. 2. Air conduction audiogram following treatment with prednisone for five months. O - Right, X - Left.

The frequent finding of uveitis in neurological sarcoidosis makes an eye examination imperative. A chest roentgenogram is mandatory and will often show hilar adenopathy. On occasion, the chest roentgenogram may be normal and delay the diagnosis.[9] Hypercalcemia, a positive Kveim test, increased serum globulins, anergy, and uveoparotid fever may be found. The typical histopathologic lesion on lymph node biopsy is an epitheloid-cell granuloma, similar to that seen in tuberculosis, but lacking central necrosis and with absent tubercle bacilli. The epitheloid tubercle is not pathognomonic for sarcoidosis but its presence contributes greatly to the diagnosis.

CASE REPORT

The patient is a 35-year-old white female who, while attending an outdoor concert on July 10, 1978, experienced fullness and tinnitus in her left ear. There was no vertigo. The following day she was seen in consultation by an otolaryngologist who confirmed a mild sensorineural hearing loss in the left ear. The otolaryngologic examination was otherwise negative. The left-sided hearing loss was slightly progressive over one month's time and she was referred to the University of Virginia for further evaluation.

Her past medical history revealed that she was under the care of an ophthalmologist since February 1978 because of iritis with blurred vision, photophobia, tearing and redness of both eyes.

Physical examination revealed both ears to be normal in appearance. An audiogram showed a mild to moderate high frequency sensorineural hearing loss in the left ear. Discrimination scores were 100% in each ear. Acoustic reflex was normal and there was no acoustic reflex decay.

A vestibular function test was performed using 1 cc ice water. There was no response on the left. Ten cubic centimeters of ice water were then used in the left ear and again there was no response. The right ear responded well to caloric stimulation. One week later an electronystagmogram showed that both ears responded comparably to 33 C water while the left ear responded very little to 44 C water.

Temporal bone polytomography was normal. Computerized axial tomography of the head was also normal. Tests for syphilis including rapid plasma reagin (RPR) and FTA/ABS were negative.

On September 19, 1978, the patient returned complaining that the hearing in her right ear, her good ear, was now impaired. An audiogram confirmed a worsening of the hearing in the right ear while the left ear was improved.

She was seen in consultation by the neurology service and admitted in October 1978 for a diagnostic workup. Hearing tests continued to show a fluctuation of hearing in both ears (Fig. 1 A,B). Her hospital workup revealed a positive anergy panel, a serum calcium of 9.3 mg%, and a chest roentgenogram showed hilar adenopathy. An ophthalmology consultant found granulomatous iritis consistent with sarcoidosis. A biopsy of a prescalene lymph node showed noncaseating granulomas.

Prednisone therapy was begun at a dose of 80 mg per day, and then gradually decreased to 35 mg every other day. The patient's hearing has improved since beginning the prednisone and her course has otherwise stabilized (Fig. 2).

COMMENT

The early signs and symptoms of neurological sarcoidosis may be subtle and easily overlooked. The only cranial nerve affected in this case was the eighth nerve. Recognition that hearing loss and vestibular function may fluctuate in sarcoidosis should alert the otolaryngologist to this disease.

The purpose of this paper is to focus attention on sarcoidosis as yet another disease entity the otolaryngologist must consider in the differential diagnosis of fluctuating hearing loss.

REFERENCES

1. Delaney P. Neurologic manifestations in sarcoidosis. Ann Intern Med 1977; 87:336-45.

2. Hybels RL, Rice DH. Neuro-otologic manifestations of sarcoidosis. Laryngoscope 1976; 86:1873-8.

3. Colover J. Sarcoidosis with involvement of the central nervous system. Brain 1948; 71:451-75.

4. Engberg J, Jepsen O. Hearing impairment and dizziness in sarcoidosis. Dan Med Bull 1962; 9:28-32.

5. Hook O. Sarcoidosis with involvement of the nervous system. Arch Neurol Psychiatry 1954; 71:554-75.

6. Pinel J, Hugon G, Trotoux J, Hadjean E. Manifestation oto-neurologique de la maladie de Besnier-Boeck-Schaumann. Ann Otolaryngol Chir Cervicofac 1973; 90:457-61.

7. Hooper R, Holden H. Acoustic and vestibular problems in sarcoidosis. Arch Otolaryngol 1970; 92:386-91.

8. Gristwood RE. Nerve deafness associated with sarcoidosis. J Laryngol Otol 1958; 72:479-91.

9. Israel RH. Diagnosing sarcoidosis. JAMA 1979; 241:1791.

≈

EUROPEAN DEVELOPMENTS IN AUDIOLOGY

During an exchange of letters with the Editor, Ronald Hinchcliffe, Professor of Audiological Medicine at the Institute of Laryngology and Otology in London, discussed the growth of audiologic professional groups in Europe. He wrote, "It is true that there have been recent developments in the organization of audiological health services in Europe. There is now a definite career structure for both Audiological Science and Audiological Medicine in the British National Health Service. We have also not only a British Society of Audiology but a British Association of Audiological Scientists and the British Association of Audiological Physicians.

"An international association of audiological physicians was founded in Krakow, Poland, in the first week of September (symptomatic of other occupational organizations trying to find an identification at that time!). The first conference of this international association took place in Wiesbaden on November 1-2, 1980. Professor W. Niemeyer of Marburg, West Germany, was elected the first President and Dr. S.D.G. Stephens, London, UK, was elected Honorary Secretary. The agreed name of the association is the International Association of Physicians in Audiology.

"No doubt otolaryngological surgeons will be eager to reap the benefits of this new specialty. Just as neurosurgical and cardiosurgical practice has been enhanced by the neurologist and the cardiologist respectively, otolaryngological surgery will be advanced by the contributions which the otological physician can provide. Indeed perhaps the term 'otolaryngological physician' instead of 'audiological physician' would have been a better term. However, since the major part of their work at the moment is concerned with auditory disorders, this has been chosen.

"The President of the Royal College of Physicians in London, Sir Douglas Black, has said that he considers a specialty has been established when it has already started to subspecialize. This was indeed the case with audiological medicine at the Royal National Throat, Nose & Ear Hospital, where there is a Division of Audiology with five departments. Although one is a science department (Audiological Physics), the other four are specialist audiological medical departments. One of these is concerned with Communication Disorders of Children, the second with Auditory Electrophysiology, the third with Diagnostic Neurootology and the fourth with Adult Auditory Rehabilitation.

"It would seem not a bad idea if, at some future world congresses of otolaryngology, the physicians and the surgeons could get together to discuss ways in which they can forge ahead with their mutual cooperation."

Ann Otol 90:1981

VELOCITY OF RAPID EYE MOVEMENTS AND VERTIGO OF CENTRAL ORIGIN

ILMARI PYYKKÖ, MD
CARSTEN WENNMO, MD
NILS-GUNNAR HENRIKSSON, MD
LUCYNA SCHALÉN
LUND, SWEDEN

Peak velocities of voluntary saccades and fast phases of different qualities of nystagmus were studied in 20 normal subjects, 5 patients with pontine lesions and 5 patients with lesions in the frontal cortex. The peak velocity of saccades was related to the amplitude of the eye movement, the alertness of the subject and whether the subject could see the target or not. The effect of the age was not significant. The quick phases of caloric, optokinetic and angular acceleration induced nystagmus were equally rapid but somewhat slower than that of vestibular nystagmus recorded in standardized visual surrounding. In the same visual condition saccades were always faster than quick phases of nystagmus. Patients with cortical lesions had normal velocities in saccades and quick phases of nystagmus. Patients with pontine disorders had significantly reduced saccadic and quick phase velocity, and some of the patients exhibited dissociations between velocity pattern of rapid eye movements. The velocity difference between saccades and quick phases probably reflects different pontine mechanisms while the somewhat higher velocity in quick phase of vestibular nystagmus recorded in light is probably related to higher attention evoked by vestibular-visual interaction.

The rapid eye movements consist of saccades and quick phases of nystagmus. Saccades are scanning motions of the eye. They can be triggered either by volition, eg, when we search an object in the horizon; or reflexively, eg, by sudden noise or when an unexpected object interferes with our visual field. The peak velocity of saccades is dependent on several factors like the amplitude of the eye movements,[1] visual conditions,[2] alertness,[3] and medication,[4] among others. A decrease in the peak velocity of saccades has been reported in diseases involving the CNS,[5] and especially in the posterior fossa lesions.[6,7] Similar evidence has not been evinced for the quick phase of nystagmus.

According to the currently accepted hypothesis saccadic eye movements use the same gate neurons in the paramedian pontine reticular formation (PPRF) as quick phases of nystagmus.[8,9] This gives reason to assume that the velocities of rapid eye movements are closely related to each other. Ron et al[10] reported that in monkeys the quick phase of vestibular nystagmus is faster than a saccade. Nauck et al[11] indicated that in man saccades and quick phases of OKN are equally rapid and faster than the quick phase of vestibular nystagmus. Contrary to this Sharpe et al[12] reported that all rapid eye movements share the same peak velocity.

The aim of this paper is to study in normals, as well as in patients with selected disorders, the velocity of different types of rapid eye movements. A part of the results have been published earlier in two separate papers considering normative values,[13] and pathologic values.[14]

METHODS

In the present study the peak velocities of rapid eye movements were examined in 20 normal subjects and in 10 patients. Five of the patients had pontine lesions and five had lesions in the frontal cortex involving Broca's speech area and the frontal eye field. The mean age, diagnosis and duration of the symptoms of the subjects was determined (Table 1).

The usual ENG technique with infinite time constant and upper cutoff frequency of 15 Hz was used. The paper was fed at 10 cm/sec to ensure accuracy in the analysis of the recordings for events occurring within 10 ms and for angular deviation of eyes of 1°. Horizontal eye movements were recorded binocularly and vertical eye movements from both eyes separately.

The subject was sitting in the chair, the head supported and looked at light diodes mounted at angles of 5°, 10°, 20°, and 30°

TABLE 1. CLASSIFICATION OF SUBJECTS ACCORDING TO DIAGNOSIS, AGE AND DURATION OF SYMPTOMS

Group	*No.*	*Age (years) Mean*	*Age (years) Range*	*Symptom/Diagnosis*	*No.*	*Duration of Symptoms (range)*
Normal subjects	20	48.4	23-72	Healthy		
Pontine disorders	5	42.8	17-61	Vascular ischemia	3	14-21 days
				Tumor of IVth ventricle	1	2 yr
				Progress. supranucl. palsy	1	1 yr
Cortical disorders (apraxia)	5	52.6	26-73	Head injury	2	2-9 mo
				Vascular ischemia	2	2-6 mo
				Presenile dementia	1	5 yr

Progress. - Progressive; Supranucl. - Supranuclear.

From the Department of Otolaryngology, University Hospital of Lund, Lund, Sweden.

Presented at the meeting of the American Neurotological Society, Palm Beach, Florida, April 12, 1980.

REPRINTS — Ilmari Pyykkö, MD, Department of Otolaryngology, University Hospital of Lund, Lund 22185, Sweden.

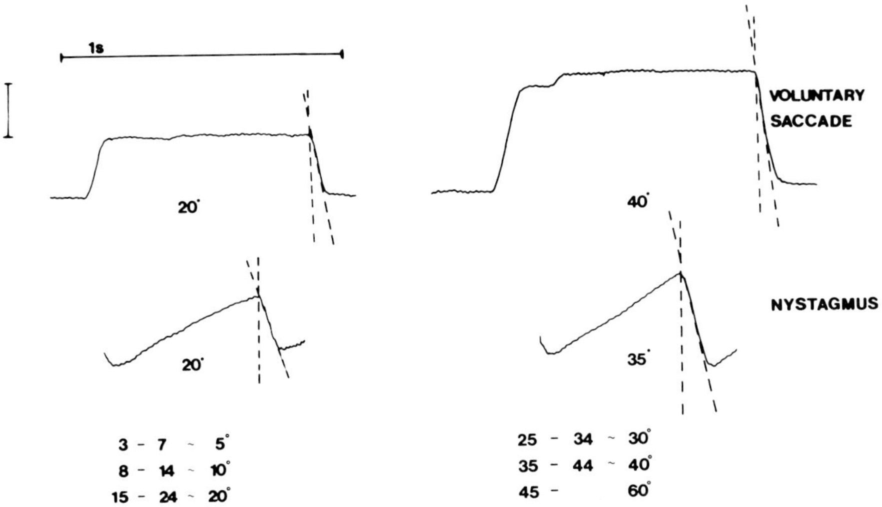

Fig. 1. Method by which peak velocities of saccades and quick phases of nystagmus were calculated: Tangent for the steepest slope of the recording was visually estimated and the peak velocity was calculated by using duration and amplitude of the tangent. The peak velocities were thereafter classified according to amplitudes into six classes.

on both sides of the midline. At least ten saccades were recorded for each amplitude. After that the light diodes were turned off and the subjects were asked to look in the darkness according to their own estimation at the amplitudes of 5°, 10°, and 30° off center.

A routine bithermal caloric test was performed in darkness with eyes open.[15] The acceleration of the chair in the rotatory test was $120°/s^2$ for one second to a constant velocity of 120°/s. The chair was brought to a stand-still by corresponding deceleration. This test also was carried out in total darkness with eyes open. To evoke vestibular nystagmus in standardized visual conditions the subjects were rotated in light within a whole field optokinetic drum. For the optokinetic test the drum, consisting of black and white stripes, was accelerated during ten seconds up to a constant velocity of 90°/s.

The peak velocities for the rapid eye movements were measured manually. For calculation they were classified according to amplitudes into five different classes (Fig. 1).

RESULTS

Normal Subjects. The peak velocities of the saccades tested in two laboratories on comparable but different equipment were the same (Fig. 2) in 20 normal subjects when they were tested within an interval of one hour. Further, same peak velocities of saccades were displayed by 12 additional subjects with comparable age range.

The peak velocity of a saccade was dependent upon amplitude of the eye movement and whether the target was visible or not (Fig. 3). The peak velocity increased with the growth of the amplitude, but this relationship was not linear. The mean peak velocity at the amplitude of 60° was about 500°/s. In the darkness the peak velocity of the sac-

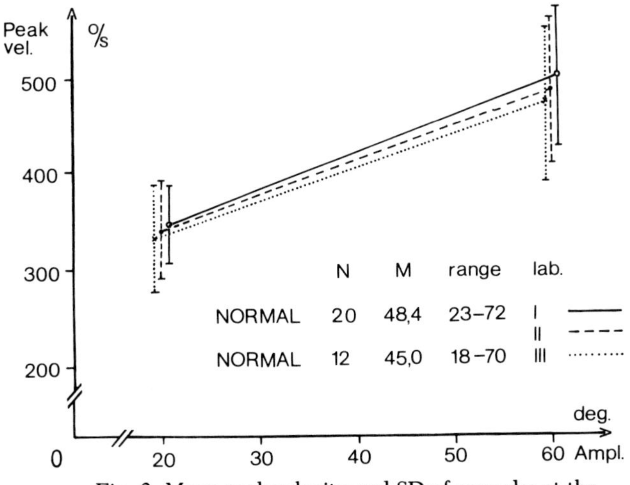

Fig. 2. Mean peak velocity and SD of saccades at the amplitudes of 20° and 60° in two groups of normal subjects and within one group when recorded in two different laboratories.

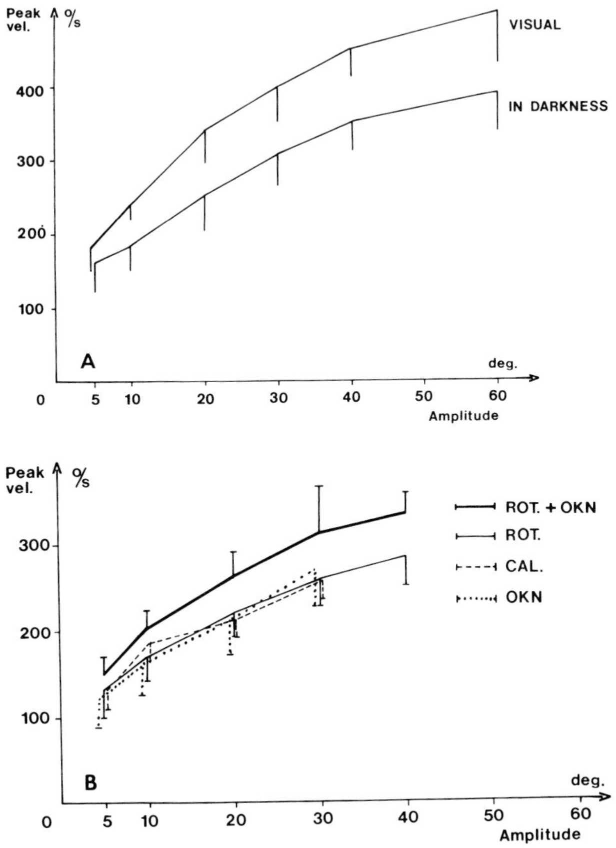

Fig. 3. A) Peak velocity curve of saccades and B) quick phases of nystagmus in normal subjects. SD are shown only in one direction.

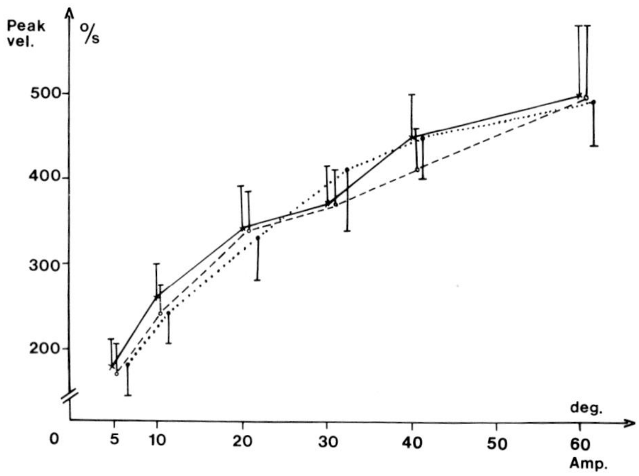

Fig. 4. Peak velocity curve of saccades at different age groups. Solid line (x———x) age group 23-39 years (N = 7), broken line (o - - - - o) age group 40-49 years (N = 7), and dotted line (. . . .) age group 60-74 years (N = 6). SD are shown in one direction.

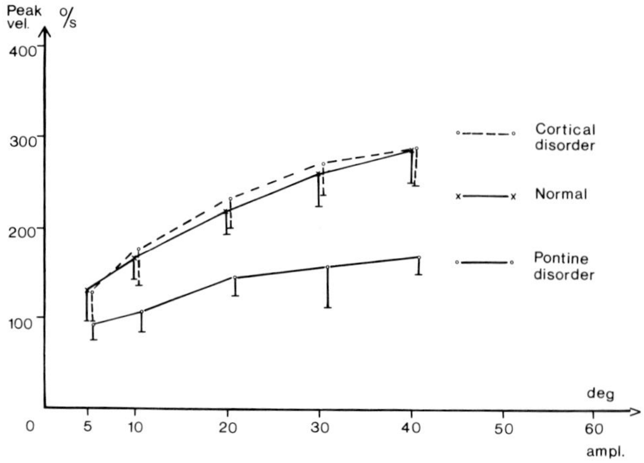

Fig. 6. Peak velocity curve of quick phase of vestibular nystagmus in the same subjects as in Fig. 5.

cades decreased significantly and was at the amplitude of 60° about 400°/s (Student's *t*-test, $p<0.01$). A similar decrease as in darkness was noticeable in drowsy subjects. We were not able to show (Fig. 4) that the peak velocity of the visual saccades is dependent upon age (up to 72 years).

The peak velocity curves of the quick phases of caloric nystagmus are caused by stimulation of one labyrinth while rotatory nystagmus is produced by activation of both labyrinths (Fig. 3). Further, these velocities were equal to those of the quick phases of optokinetic nystagmus. However, if the subjects were rotated in light within an optokinetic drum the peak velocities of the quick phases of the resulted optovestibular nystagmus increased and were statistically significantly higher than quick phases of vestibular nystagmus in the darkness (Student's *t*-test, $p<0.01$). The peak velocities of the fast phases of optovestibular nystagmus were 260°/s at an amplitude of 20° compared to 215°/s in the rotatory nystagmus. The peak velocities of saccades were always faster than quick phase of nystagmus in similar visual conditions.

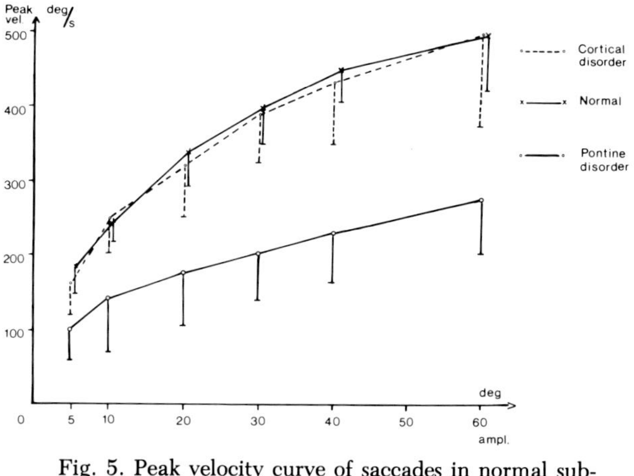

Fig. 5. Peak velocity curve of saccades in normal subjects in five patients with cortical lesion and in five patients with brainstem lesion. Mean and SD.

Patients. Patients with dyspraxia of speech indicating a disturbance in Broca's speech area in the left frontal cortex presented an interesting saccadic pattern. Their saccades were characteristically split into small saccades and they reached the target step by step by making several correction saccades. However, the peak velocity of the split saccades was normal in both directions. The patients with pontine lesions exhibited both accurate and split saccades, but their saccades showed strongly reduced peak velocities (Fig. 5).

The peak velocity of quick phase of vestibular nystagmus was normal in patients with dyspraxia of speech while reduced in patients with a pontine lesion (Fig. 6). However, the fact that the reduction of peak velocity in the quick phase of nystagmus was not as constant a finding as in saccadic test indicates that these two rapid eye movements can be injured separately. An analysis (Fig. 7) of rapid eye movements in a patient with brainstem infarction demonstrates this. Saccades, quick phases of vestibular nystagmus, and optovestibular nystagmus exhibited strongly reduced peak velocities while the quick phase of optokinetic nystagmus was still within normal values.

DISCUSSION

A velocity analysis of rapid eye movements indicates that the mechanism adapting velocity to amplitude in eye saccades is somewhat different from that of the quick phase of nystagmus. Further, the mechanism by which the visual input enhances peak velocity differs in saccades from that of fast phases of nystagmus. The results from our patients indicate that lesions in the frontal visual field (Brodmann's area 8) do not decrease the velocity of rapid eye movements while the velocity adaptation frequently seems to be disturbed in patients with lesions in the pontine reticular formation. In brainstem lesions dissociation of quick phases of nystagmus and of saccades can occur.

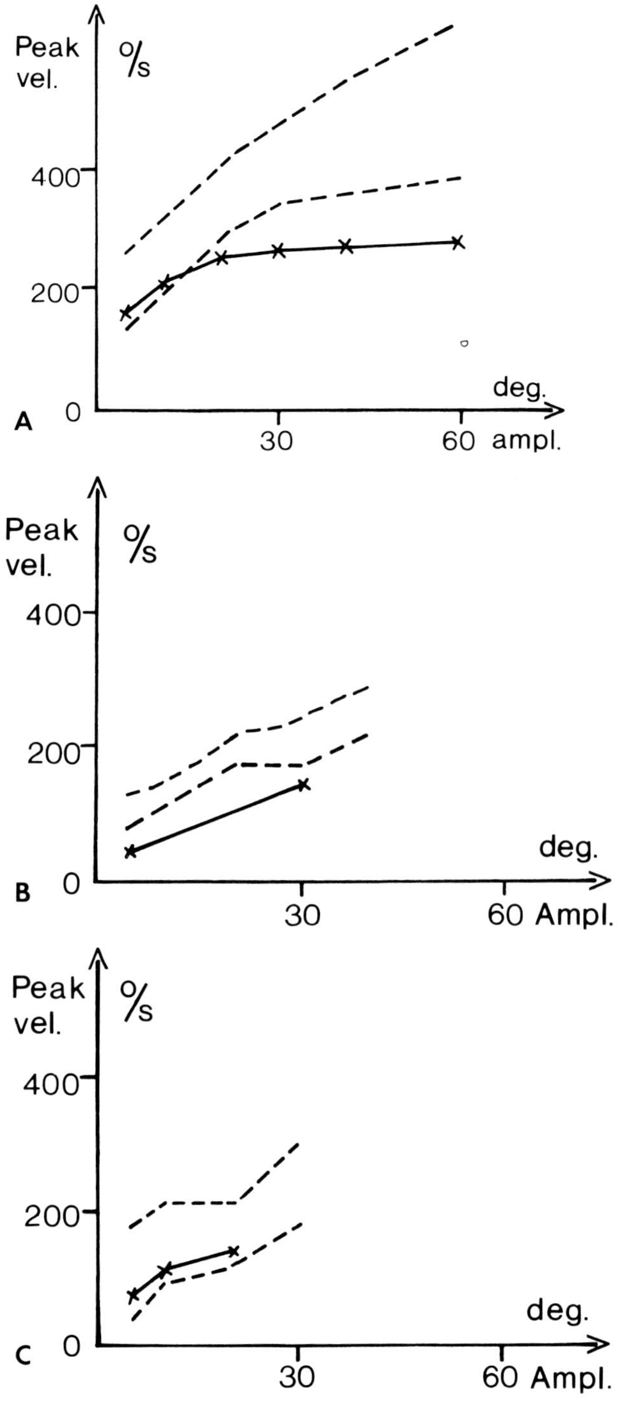

Fig. 7. A) Peak velocity curve of saccades, B) quick phase of vestibular nystagmus, and C) quick phase of optokinetic nystagmus in a subject with brainstem infarction. Normal ranges are exhibited with dotted lines.

The reason why the saccadic velocity is greater than in the fast phases of nystagmus is still not quite understood. Neuronal activity during rapid eye movement is composed of two phenomena taking place simultaneously: facilitation of agonistic extraocular muscles and inhibition of the antagonistic extraocular muscles.[16-18] Identical activity has been recorded in the very same neurons of PPRF during quick phases of nystagmus as during voluntary saccades.[8,9] Thus facilitation steered by PPRF seems to be similar.[19]

Hikosaka and Kawakami,[20] Hikosaka et al,[21] and Shimazu[22] have recently given insight into the origin of quick phase of nystagmus. During the quick phase of nystagmus four types of premotor neurons are involved in the activation of abducens neurons; two of the neurons display facilitation and two inhibition. The abducens motoneuron is facilitated monosynaptically and disynaptically from the contralateral vestibular nerve while axons mediating inhibition arise monosynaptically from the ipsilateral vestibular nerve and from the pontine reticular formation. During ipsilateral quick phase the abducens motoneurons display facilitation and disinhibition and during contralateral quick phase they display disfacilitation and inhibition. Even though all four of these neurons show burstlike activity, the duration, the timing and the intensity of the burst is different and varies. Hence the output of abducens neurons during the quick phase of nystagmus is characterized in the mathematical sense in an integrated form of facilitation and inhibition. Saccades, on the contrary, are believed to operate entirely by PPRF[19] making the output in the motoneuron simpler. The mechanisms of facilitation and disinhibition of motoneurons in the quick phase of nystagmus and saccades might provide a basis for velocity differences of these eye movements.

Further, concomitantly with the alerting effect by light, volition itself during the test can be a facilitating factor through a special pathway, increasing saccadic velocity. Because nystagmus is a reflexive eye movement, the facilitation by volition is lacking in the fast phases of nystagmus even in light. However, somewhat contradictory to this idea was the finding that the return eye movements after smooth pursuit had the peak velocity of the saccade and not of the fast phase of nystagmus.[13] Attention, as a nonspecific factor, is probably not important here in terms of explaining the difference between the two types of eye movements.

The effect of attention on the quick phase of nystagmus can be best explained as an increase of peak velocity during vestibular-visual interaction when subjects were rotated in light.

The peak velocities of rapid eye movements in the patients with pontine lesions exhibited a pronounced decrease of velocity. In most subjects the decrease took place equally in saccades and quick phases of nystagmus, even though in some subjects dissociation in the rapid eye movement pattern existed. In a larger group of subjects[23] it was shown that dissociation existed most commonly between saccades and quick phases of nystagmus. These findings, therefore, may support the idea that the mechanism triggering quick phases of nystagmus might be somewhat different from saccades.

In accordance with the lesion experiments in animals[24] our results in the patients with pontine disorders indicate that the supranuclear organization which determines the velocity of rapid eye movements is located in the brainstem. The process of velocity amplitude adaptation was unaffected in patients with dysfunction of frontal cortex. This supports the earlier findings that the brainstem mechanisms for quick phase of nystagmus[24] and saccades[6] are rather independent of higher order functions of the CNS.

Clinical analysis of rapid eye movements may then help to discriminate cortical lesions from those located in the pons. It may often be sufficient to determine the velocity of the saccades, but since a dissociation between the two types of eye movements sometimes does occur, additional information may be achieved by also analyzing the quick phases of nystagmus.

REFERENCES

1. Westheimer G. Mechanism of saccadic eye movements. Arch Ophthalmol 1954; 52:710-23.
2. Körner FH. Non-visual control of human saccadic eye movements. In: Lennerstrand G, Bach-y-Rita P, eds. Basic mechanisms of ocular motility and clinical implications. Oxford: Pergamon Press, 1975:565-9.
3. Bahill AT, Stark L. Overlapping saccades and glissades are produced by fatigue in the saccadic eye movement system. Exp Neurol 1975; 48:95-106.
4. Aschoff JC, Becker W. Der Einfluss von Sulpirid auf die Vigilans. Arzneim Forsch 1974; 24:2058-62.
5. Sharpe JA, Lo AW, Rabinovitch HE. Control of the saccadic and smooth pursuit systems after cerebral hemidecortication. Brain 1979; 102:387-403.
6. Baloh RW, Honrubia V, Sills A. Eye-tracking and optokinetic nystagmus. Results of quantitative testing in patients with well-defined nervous system lesions. Ann Otol Rhinol Laryngol 1977; 86:108-15.
7. Troost BT, Daroff RB. The ocular motor defects in progressive supranuclear palsy. Ann Neurol 1977; 2:397-403.
8. Keller EL. Participation of medial pontine reticular formation in eye movement generation in monkey. J Neurophysiol 1974; 37:316-32.
9. Henn V, Cohen B. Activity in eye muscle motoneurons and brainstem units during eye movements. In: Lennerstrand G, Bach-y-Rita P, eds. Basic mechanisms of ocular motility and their implications. Oxford: Pergamon Press, 1975:303-24.
10. Ron S, Robinson DA, Skavenski AA. Saccades and the quick phase of nystagmus. Vision Res 1972; 12:2015-22.
11. Nauck B, Dichgans J, Jung R. Different peak velocities of rapid phases in optokinetic and vestibular nystagmus. Pfluegers Arch 1969; 312:R 142.
12. Sharpe JA, Troost BT, Dell'Osso LF, Daroff RB. Comparative velocities of different types of fast eye movements in man. Invest Ophthalmol 1975; 14:689-92.
13. Henriksson NG, Pyykkö I, Schalén L, Wennmo C. Velocity pattern of rapid eye movements. Acta Otolaryngol (Stockh) 1980; 89:504-12.
14. Henriksson NG, Hindfelt B, Pyykkö I, Schalén L. Rapid eye movements reflecting neurological disorders. Ann Clin Otolaryngol (in press).
15. Henriksson NG, Pfaltz CR, Torok N, Rubin W. A synopsis of the vestibular system. Switzerland: Sandoz, 1972.
16. Shimazu H. Organization of the commissural connections: physiology. In: Brodal A, Pompeiano O, eds. Basic aspects of central vestibular mechanisms. Progress in brain research 37. Amsterdam: Elsevier, 1972:177-90.
17. Collins CC, O'Meara D, Scott A. Muscle tension during unrestrained human eye movements. J Physiol 1975; 245:351-69.
18. Precht W. Cerebellar influences on eye movements. In: Lennerstrand G, Bach-y-Rita P, eds. Basic mechanisms of ocular motility and their clinical implications. Oxford: Pergamon Press, 1975:261-80.
19. Robinson DA. Oculomotor control signals. In: Lennerstrand G, Bach-y-Rita P, eds. Basic mechanisms of ocular motility and their clinical implications. Oxford: Pergamon Press, 1975:337-74.
20. Hikosaka O, Kawakami T. Inhibitory reticular neurons related to the quick phase of nystagmus — their location and projection. Exp Brain Res 1977; 27:377-96.
21. Hikosaka O, Maeda M, Nakao S, Shimazu H, Shinoda Y. Presynaptic impulses in the abducens nucleus and their relation to postsynaptic potentials in motoneurons during vestibular nystagmus. Exp Brain Res 1977; 27:355-76.
22. Shimazu H. Excitatory and inhibitory premotor neurons related to horizontal vestibular nystagmus. In: Asanuma H, Wilson VJ, eds. Integration in the nervous system. Tokyo: Igakushoin, 1979:123-42.
23. Wennmo C, Hindfelt B. Rapid eye movements in brainstem lesions. Acta Otolaryngol (Stockh) 1980; 90:230-6.
24. McCabe BF. The quick component of nystagmus. Laryngoscope 1965; 75:1619-46.

Ann Otol 90:1981

MYOSITIS OSSIFICANS FOLLOWING RADICAL NECK DISSECTION

MARTIN A. SHUGAR, MD
CHICAGO, ILLINOIS

ALFRED L. WEBER, MD
BOSTON, MASSACHUSETTS

THOMAS J. MULVANEY, MD
BOSTON, MASSACHUSETTS

Myositis ossificans traumatica is an uncommon disorder in which there is posttraumatic bone formation in muscle and other soft tissues near bone. The lesion is exceedingly rare in the head and neck. A case is presented in which myositis ossificans of the platysma occurred following radical neck dissection. Because recurrence may follow excision of the abnormal bone, removal is recommended only if there are significant symptoms associated with the lesion. If surgery is indicated, it should be delayed for 6 to 12 months following the initial trauma to allow for maturation of the lesion.

INTRODUCTION

Myositis ossificans traumatica is an uncommon disorder in which there is bone formation in muscle and other soft tissues near bone following trauma. The lesion contains actively proliferating fibroblasts and osteoblasts and may be misdiagnosed as a malignant tumor (sarcoma) early in its development.[1,2] The name is poorly descriptive in that muscle may not be directly involved, inflammation has not always been shown to be present, and osseous tissue is not demonstrable in the early stages; hence, other terms such as heterotopic nonneoplastic ossification have been suggested as more appropriate.

Traumatic myositis ossificans occurs most frequently in active young men and has been associated with certain occupations (eg, jockeys, infantrymen) or avocations (eg, fencers) in which muscle may be traumatized, eg, "riders' bone" in the jockey's thigh adductors.[2] The disorder may occur in any skeletal muscle; however, the muscles which most frequently undergo ossification are the quadriceps femoris and the brachialis anticus.[2]

There have been few reports of the disorder occurring in the head and neck. Traumatic myositis ossificans has been reported in the masseter,[3-6] buccinator,[7] diagastric,[8] and medial pterygoid[9] muscles. Pappas and Johnson[10] reported a unique case of myositis ossificans in the intrinsic muscles and adjacent mucous membrane of the immediate subglottic portion of the larynx.

In reviewing the literature, we found no report of myositis ossificans following radical neck dissection. We believe that the following report represents a case of myositis ossificans of the platysma muscle which followed radical neck dissection. The pathogenesis, differential diagnosis, and management are discussed.

CASE REPORT

A 78-year-old white male presented at the Infirmary with complaints of a right-sided sore throat, odynophagia, and otalgia for one month. Investigations revealed a $T_3N_0M_0$ squamous cell carcinoma of the right posterolateral pharyngeal and hypopharyngeal wall. This lesion was treated with ^{60}Co radiation therapy, delivered to the primary lesion and neck by parallel opposed right and left lateral fields to a dose of 4,400 rads, followed by a "boosting" dose to the primary site for a total of 6,735 rads. He tolerated the radiation therapy well, and at the conclusion, there was no residual disease. Five months later, he developed a right-sided neck node without evidence of disease at the primary site and no distant metastases. Subsequently a right radical neck dissection was carried out using the Conley modification of the Schobinger incision. The platysma was elevated with the skin flaps, and a standard block radical neck dissection was uneventfully performed. The postoperative course was uncomplicated. Histopathological examination revealed metastatic keratinizing squamous cell carcinoma to multiple jugular lymph nodes, with focal extranodal extension of tumor into fat in one of the high jugular nodes. In view of the previous radiotherapy and the radical neck dissection, it was felt no additional treatment was indicated at this time.

Two to three weeks postoperatively, the patient noted a progressively hardening mass in the right lower neck. Two months postoperatively, he was documented to have a subcutaneous bony spike arising from the superior aspect of the lateral one third of the clavicle which measured 5.5 cm long and 0.7 cm wide. The bony mass ascended the neck superomedially, transecting the previous incision line, and stopped 2.5 cm lateral to the carotid artery (Figs. 1 and 2). There was no indication of carotid artery compression or other associated symptoms. Figures

From the Departments of Otolaryngology and Radiology, Harvard Medical School and the Massachusetts Eye and Ear Infirmary, Boston.
REPRINTS — Alfred L. Weber, MD, 243 Charles Street, Boston, MA 02114.

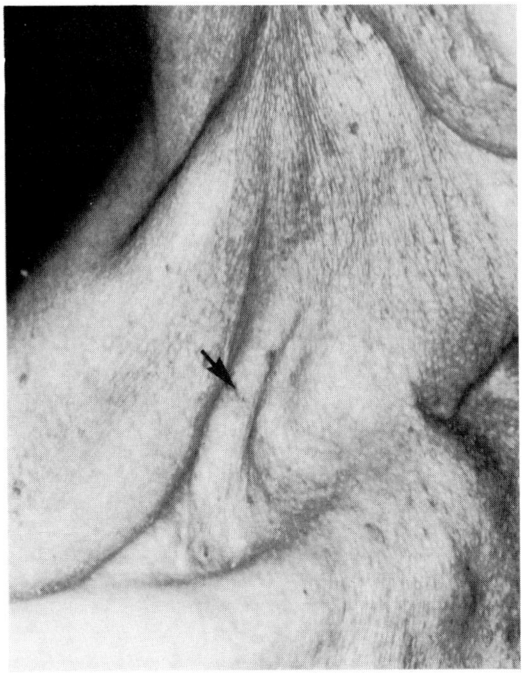

Fig. 1. Arrow points to superior end of bony lesion.

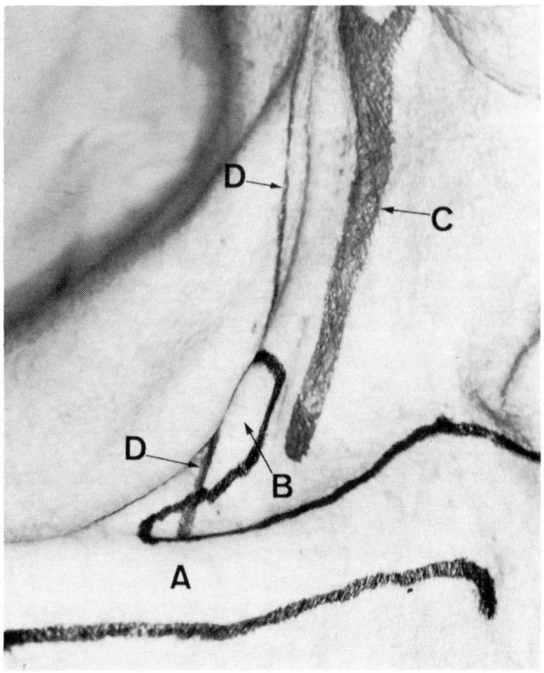

Fig. 2. Relationship of bony lesion to neck structures. A - Clavicle; B - Bony lesion; C - Carotid artery; D - Incision line of radical neck dissection.

3 and 4 show the radiographic appearance of the bony lesion six months postoperatively. There was no subsequent growth of bone or development of symptoms 12 months postoperatively.

DISCUSSION

The pathogenesis of myositis ossificans is controversial and was reviewed by Carey.[11] There are four basic theories: 1) trauma to the periosteum of an adjacent bone with displacement of osteoblasts into muscle with subsequent bone formation; 2) activation by trauma or hemorrhage of periosteal implants already present in the muscle; 3) metaplasia of pluripotential intermuscular connective tissue into bone; and 4) metaplasia of normal muscle tendon fibrocartilage into bone.

It is obvious that other unidentified factors favoring bone formation must be involved, as only a minute percentage of traumatized muscles ossify. No abnormality of calcium or phosphorus metabolism has been demonstrated.[1] Intramuscular and/or subperiosteal hemorrhage secondary to trauma is a common antecedent event, although this does not appear to be essential in all cases.[2]

The clinical presentation is usually a firm, often painful, mass appearing in the affected muscle between one and four weeks following trauma. The mass is readily palpable and may progressively limit motion depending upon its size and location.

Radiographic studies performed early in the

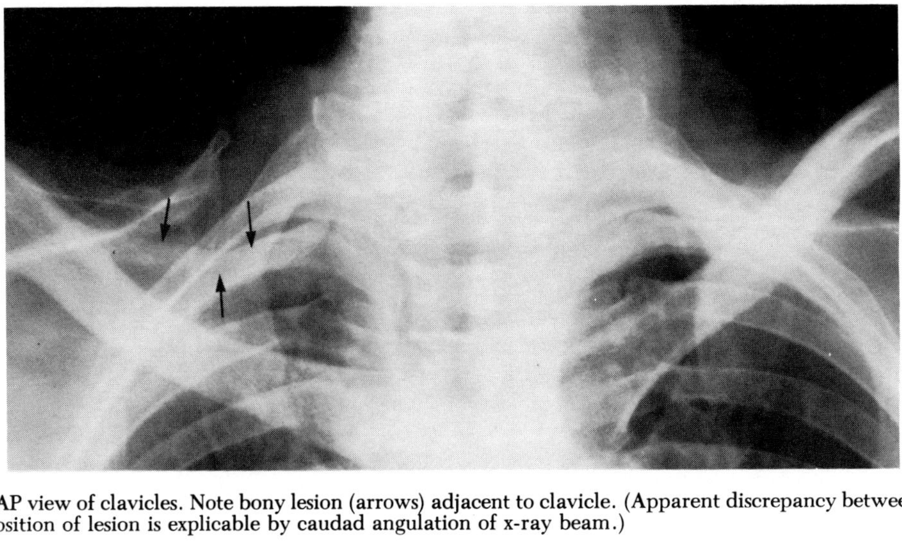

Fig. 3. AP view of clavicles. Note bony lesion (arrows) adjacent to clavicle. (Apparent discrepancy between clinical and radiologic position of lesion is explicable by caudad angulation of x-ray beam.)

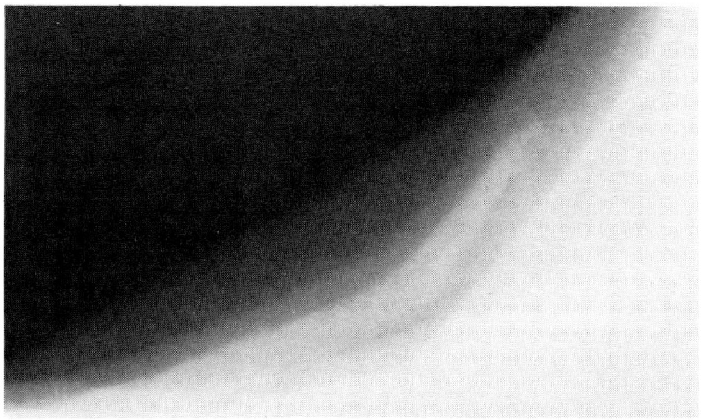

Fig. 4. Posterior oblique fluoroscopic view shows bony lesion within soft tissues.

course of this disorder may reveal no mineralization, but some ossification is usually evident by the time the lesion is observed clinically.[1] Calcification may first be detected 10-20 days after the traumatic episode, appearing as faint shadows at a variable distance from bone, which gradually increase in density.[2] The radiographic appearance correlated with the histopathology of the evolving lesion in that there is a central undifferentiated zone (histologically composed of immature mesenchymal cells), merging into an area of oriented osteoid formation. Both areas are surrounded by a peripheral zone of well-formed bone. This has been described as the "zone phenomenon."[12] Ultimately, ossification is extensive; mature bone can be identified radiographically by four to five months, at which time the benign nature of the lesion is obvious.[13] The lesion may be located near a bone and remain completely separate from it, or it may be attached to the underlying bone, the appearance sometimes resembling an osteoma with a cortex and medullary canal.[1,13]

The differential diagnosis of the lesion includes proliferative myositis, nodular fasciitis, parosteal osteoma, traumatic fibrosis and osteogenic sarcoma arising in soft tissues.[13] The diagnosis of myositis ossificans is usually evident however, based on the history, clinical presentation, and radiographic appearance. In the case presented in this report, the diagnosis of traumatic fibrosis along the incision line is excluded by the radiologic findings and the fact that the bony lesion was not in continuity, but rather transected the incision line (Fig. 2). Myositis ossificans is distinguished from sarcomas of the soft tissues by its rapid onset and growth following trauma and by its radiologic appearance.

Anatomic considerations suggest that the lesion involved the platysma muscle in this case. The platysma consists of a subcutaneous muscle sheet crossing the whole length of the lower border of the mandible above, crossing over the whole length of the clavicle below and extending downward to the level of the first or second rib and towards the acromion.[14] The bony subcutaneous spike in this case appeared to parallel the direction of platysma fibers (Fig. 1).

In general, conservative treatment of myositis ossificans is advocated. A number of these lesions reportedly disappear spontaneously after variable periods of time.[2] Surgical excision is generally reserved for cases with severe pain, limitation of motion secondary to the mass, and, in a small number of cases, to exclude malignancy.[13] Because myositis ossificans involving the muscles of mastication almost invariably results in pain and trismus, careful surgical excision has been recommended in this region.[3-6,9] Recurrence after any excision is possible[1,9] again demonstrating that removal is indicated only if symptoms are severe.[1,12] When surgery is indicated, it should not be performed for at least 6 to 12 months following the initial trauma, to allow maturation of the lesion. If an immature lesion is excised, a rapid and extensive recurrence is quite likely.[12] The absence of symptoms in our patient, coupled with his age and his primary disease excluded the need for surgical excision.

REFERENCES

1. Pitcock JA. Tumors and tumorlike lesions of somatic tissue. In: Crenshaw AH, ed. Campbell's operative orthopedics. 5th ed. St. Louis: CV Mosby, 1971: 1366-70.

2. Adams RD. Traumatic and circulatory diseases. In: Adams RD, ed. Diseases of muscle: a study in pathology. 3rd ed. Hagerstown: Harper and Row, 1975: 401-5.

3. Goodsell JO. Traumatic myositis ossificans of the masseter muscle: review of the literature and report of a case. J Oral Surg 1962; 20:116-22.

4. Parnes EI, Kinds EC. Traumatic myositis ossificans of the masseter muscle: report of case. J Oral Surg 1965; 23:245-50.

5. Vernale Ca. Traumatic myositis ossificans of the masseter muscle: report of two cases. Oral Surg 1968; 26:8-17.

6. Plezia RA, Mintz SM, Calligaro P. Myositis ossificans traumatica of the masseter muscle: report of a case. Oral Surg 1977; 44:351-7.

7. Wussow GC. Myositis ossificans of the buccinator muscle. Oral Surg 1968; 26:615-8.

8. Stafne EC. Oral roentgenographic diagnosis. Philadelphia: WB Saunders, 1958: 136.

9. Narang R, Dixon RA. Myositis ossificans: medial pterygoid muscle — a case report. Br J Oral Surg 1974; 12:229-34.

10. Pappas DG, Johnson LA. Laryngeal myositis ossificans. Arch Otolaryngol 1965; 81:227-31.

11. Carey EJ. Multiple bilateral traumatic periosteal bone and callus formations of the femurs and left innominate bone. Arch Surg 1924; 8:592-603.

12. Hait G, Boswick JA, Stone NH. Heterotopic bone formation secondary to trauma (myositis ossificans traumatica). J Trauma 1970: 10:405-11.

13. Molloy JC, McGuirk RA. Treatment of traumatic myositis ossificans circumscripta; use of aspiration and steroids. J Trauma 1976; 16:851-7.

14. Anderson JE, ed. Grant's atlas of anatomy. 7th ed. Baltimore: Williams and Wilkins, 1978, Section 9-3.

Ann Otol 90:1981

MYRINGOPLASTY WITH FASCIAL STAKES

H. REDIANO, MD M. ENGLENDER, MD

TEL-AVIV, ISRAEL

Myringoplasty reinforced by fascial stakes was performed in 87 ears. Small tongue-like fascial projections or "stakes" were used to keep the fascial graft in position. No foreign material was introduced into the middle ear cavity to support the graft and the drum. The technical details of this procedure are described and analysis of the results is presented.

The surgical principles of tympanoplasty depend largely on adequate exposure of the middle ear cavity[1] to eradicate disease and to create a functioning middle ear clinically implying a closure of the air-bone gap.

In the last few years the majority of surgeons have concluded that fascia or perichondrium are the most suitable materials for reconstructing the tympanic membrane.[2] These materials have been placed either medially or laterally to the drum.

A retrospective study by Doyle[2] of patients undergoing type I tympanoplasty demonstrated that medial grafting assures superior results with a lower incidence of complications.

In this paper we present a technique of tympanoplasty employed since 1974 on 87 ears. The technique involves medial grafting of temporal muscle fascia without the use of any supporting material in the middle ear cavity. The fascia is held in position with the help of fascial stakes. This technique has been used by Plester* for many years and was described by Bailey[3] in 1976. Recently Williams[4] reported a technique of myringoplasty by using microclips. He reported improvement of hearing in 90% of type I tympanoplastic procedures. The paucity of publications on this subject has prompted us to describe our experience.

METHODS

During the three years 1975-1978, 87 tympanoplastic procedures were performed in our department (Table 1). Thirty-five patients were females and 42 were males. The age of the patients ranged from 9-65 years with a mean age of 31.2 years.

Preoperative evaluations included assessment of eustachian tube patency, pure-tone and speech audiometry, and radiography of the mastoid. Only those patients who had postoperative follow-up for at least 12 months were included in this paper.

We prefer the postauricular approach to the middle ear because we believe that it gives a better view of the tympanic cavity and allows a more complete examination of the ossicular chain. Prior to elevation of the fibrocartilaginous rim of the anulus tympanicus and to entering the middle ear cavity, the periphery of the perforation is denuded of epithelium until a raw surface is obtained. The meatal flap and the tympanic membrane are placed forward against the anterior canal wall exposing the tympanic cavity. The fascial graft is laid on the medial surface of the tympanic membrane, and then the drum with the graft is repositioned. At this stage the cases can be divided into two groups: a) small central perforation and b) subtotal or total perforation.

Repair of a Central Perforation. Three tiny incisions are made in the anterior remnant of the drum and the fascial graft is pulled through those openings. We refer to these tongue-like fascial projections as "stakes." Three such stakes are formed superiorly, inferiorly and anteriorly to the perforation (Fig. 1 A, B). This procedure assures a firm fixation of the graft in its proper position.

Repair of Subtotal or Total Perforation. A subtotal or total perforation is more difficult to repair by the stakes technique because a limited surface of the drum is available. In most cases only the anulus tympanicus is preserved. The anulus is elevated at two points anteriorly and the fascial stakes are pulled out through these pathways. In this way the fascial graft is adequately fixed in its anterior position. An additional stake may be employed superiorly, if sufficient drum is available (Fig. 1 B). A small piece of Silastic® sheath is then put on the graft and the drum.

RESULTS

Closure of the perforation, improvement in hearing function and incidence of complications were studied for at least 12 months following surgery in all the patients. Five of the 87 eardrums were reperforated. This represents a failure rate of 5.6% (Table 2). Closure of the air-bone gap within 20 dB was noted in 75 of 87 patients. Hearing was worse in seven and unchanged in five patients (Table 3).

TABLE 1. NUMBER OF TYMPANOPLASTIES

Type of Tympanoplasty	*No. of Ears*
I	59
II	1
III	26
IV	1
Total	87

TABLE 2. REPERFORATED EARDRUMS

Type of Tympanoplasty	*Reperforated Eardrums* No. %
I	3 (3.4)
II	1 (1.1)
III	1 (1.1)
IV	—
Total	5 (5.6)

*Plester D. Personal communication, 1974.

From the Department of Otolaryngology, Ichilov Medical Center Tel-Aviv, School of Medicine, University of Tel-Aviv, Israel.

REPRINTS — M. Englender, MD, Department of Otolaryngology, Ichilov Medical Center, Tel-Aviv University Medical School, Tel-Aviv, Israel.

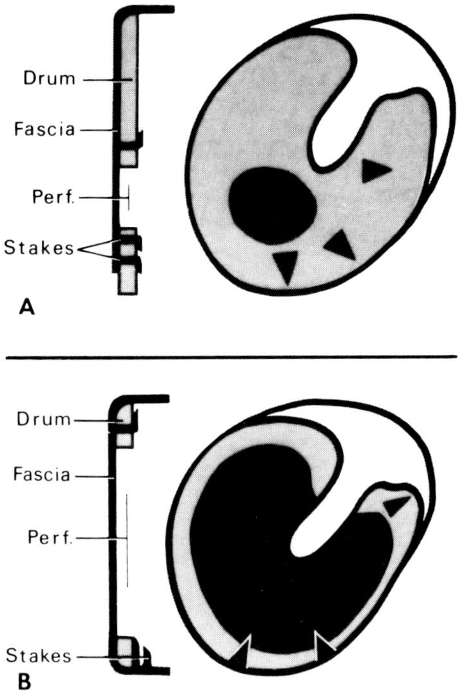

Fig. 1. A) Positioning of the stakes in a central perforation. B) Positioning of the stakes in a subtotal perforation.

TABLE 3. RESULTS

Type of Tympano-plasty	*No. of Ears*	*Improved No.*	*%*	*Hearing Worsened No.*	*%*	*Unchanged No.*	*%*
I	59	54	91.5	3	5.0	2	3.3
II	1	—		1		—	
III	26	20	76.9	3	11.5	3	11.5
IV	1	1		—		—	
Total	87	75	86.2	7	8.0	5	5.8

DISCUSSION

Diverse methods of tympanoplasty are reported in the literature associated with varying degrees of success. The method used by us differs from most reported techniques in that the fascial graft is supported by tiny fascial stakes. Foreign material is not introduced into the middle ear cavity. The use of a medially positioned graft is still debatable because it is believed to reduce the middle ear space, and to herniate towards the promontory.[5-7] Hence the need to introduce Gelfoam® or some other supporting material into the middle ear. Such materials may produce adhesive bands with medial retraction of the drum. In the pocket-like cavity which follows, cholesteatoma may develop. The stakes technique described assures that the graft remains fixed in position, eliminating the possibility of cholesteatoma formation, while preserving a relatively large middle ear cavity.

The results in our study show a hearing improvement in 92% and closure of the air-bone gap in 90% of patients who had a type I tympanoplastic procedure. A closed drum was observed in 91% of the patients. The results are similar to those reported in the literature.[8] Biological considerations support the use of natural biological material rather than metallic clips[4] for fixation of the graft. The avoidance of foreign material in the middle ear is also stressed.

REFERENCES

1. Farrior JB. Principles of surgery in tympanoplasty and mastoidectomy. Laryngoscope 1966; 76:816-41.

2. Doyle PJ, Schleuning AJ, Echevarria J. Tympanoplasty: should grafts be placed medial or lateral to the tympanic membrane? Laryngoscope 1972; 82:1425-30.

3. Bailey HAT Jr. Maintenance of the anterior sulcus — tympanic membrane relationship in tympanoplastic surgery. Laryngoscope 1976; 86:179-85.

4. Williams JD. Microclip application in tympanoplasty. Ann Otol Rhinol Laryngol 1977; 86:223-6.

5. Marquet J. Myringoplasty by eardrum transplantation. Laryngoscope 1968; 78:1329-36.

6. Sheehy JL, Glasscock ME. Tympanic membrane grafting with temporalis fascia. Arch Otolaryngol 1967; 86:391-403.

7. Storrs LA. Myringoplasty with the use of fascia grafts. Arch Otolaryngol 1961; 74:45-9.

8. Smyth GDL, Kerr AG, Hassard TH. Homograft materials in tympanoplasty. Otolaryngol Clin North Am 1977; 10:563-80.

Ann Otol 90:1981

MICROFISSURE IN THE OVAL WINDOW AREA

TAKEHIKO HARADA, MD

ISAMU SANDO, MD, DMS EUGENE N. MYERS, MD, FACS

PITTSBURGH, PENNSYLVANIA

Examination of 331 human temporal bones revealed the presence of a microfissure in the oval window area in 25%. The youngest temporal bone in which the microfissure was observed was from a child eight years old and the oldest temporal bone was from an individual 102 years old. It appears that the microfissure in this area occurs extremely rarely before 10 years of age, that it begins to be observed after the age of 10, and that the incidence of this fissure increases sharply at about age 40. In 61% of the bones in which the microfissure was observed, it was present both superior and inferior to the oval window in almost the same vertical plane. In none of the bones, however, did it extend beyond the annular ligament to the footplate. The histological appearance of the microfissure in this area was quite similar to that of the microfissure between the posterior canal ampulla and round window niche, although the latter appeared to be wider in general. The histogenesis of the microfissure is still unknown, but upon careful analysis of the results of this study and literature review, the authors consider nontraumatic spontaneous fracture by mechanical stress to be the most probable explanation for its occurrence. Possible clinical significance of the microfissure is also discussed.

INTRODUCTION

The presence of a microfissure in human temporal bone specimens has apparently been well-known for a long time. Manasse,[1] Nager,[2] and Zange[3] were among the investigators who first payed attention to the presence of a microfissure between the posterior canal ampulla and round window niche. However, it was Mayer[4,5] who first described the microfissure in various parts of the temporal bone. While he mentioned six types of microfissure in vertical sections, he described two varieties of microfissure in horizontal sections: one between the posterior canal ampulla and round window niche, and the other superior to the oval window between the middle ear and vestibule. During the years which immediately followed these investigations the presence of a microfissure in these two locations was confirmed by Meyer,[6] but only the one between the posterior canal ampulla and round window niche appears to have been discussed by others.[7-9] For some time after this period, there appears to have been no report concerning the microfissure. Recently, however, Okano et al[10] reported on the microfissure between the posterior canal ampulla and round window niche, and Saito et al[11] reported the existence of a microfissure in two locations in the temporal bone. Nomura* also noted the microfissure superior to the oval window between the vestibule and the facial canal, and called it a utriculofacial fissure. However, no detailed study focused on the microfissure superior to the oval window has apparently been undertaken.

During the examination of human temporal bones, the present authors noted that many of the bones with microfissures superior to the oval window showed the same kind of microfissure also inferior to the oval window on the promontory. These two types of microfissure appeared to be associated with each other since they were observed in almost the same vertical plane superior and inferior to the oval window. The purpose of this study is to examine in detail the microfissure in the area of the oval window and to discuss its histogenesis and possible clinical significance.

METHODS

Materials used in this study are from the temporal bone collection of the Department of Otolaryngology, University of Pittsburgh, housed in the Eye and Ear Hospital of Pittsburgh. Three hundred and thirty-one human temporal bones from 226 cases, ranging from newborn to 102 years old, were studied for the presence, location, extent, appearance, and contents of the microfissure in the oval window area. Cases showing severe anomalies of the ear or evidence of temporal bone fracture were excluded from the materials. The specimens were fixed, decalcified, dehydrated, embedded in celloidin, and sectioned horizontally at 20 μ. Every tenth section was stained with hematoxylin and eosin, and mounted for light microscopic study.

FINDINGS

The microfissure in the oval window area was observed in 84 bones (25%) of the total 331 bones studied. The age distribution of the specimens is summarized in Table 1. The youngest age at which the microfissure was observed was 8 years old, and the oldest was 102 years old. This table appears to

*Nomura Y. Personal communication.

From the Departments of Otolaryngology and Pathology, University of Pittsburgh School of Medicine, Eye and Ear Hospital of Pittsburgh, Pittsburgh, Pennsylvania. This study was supported by Research Grant NA 13787 from the National Institute of Neurological and Communicative Disorders and Stroke.

This paper was presented at the A.R.O. Research Forum in Dallas, Texas, October 6, 1979.

REPRINTS — Isamu Sando, MD, Department of Otolaryngology, Eye and Ear Hospital, 230 Lothrop Street, Pittsburgh, PA 15213.

TABLE 1. INCIDENCE OF THE MICROFISSURE IN THE OVAL WINDOW AREA WITH AGE

Age Group (yr)	No. of Bones Studied	No. of Bones with Microfissure	
0-9	174	1	0.6%
10-19	27	4	15%
20-29	11	5	45%
30-39	11	3	27%
40-49	12	8	67%
50-59	25	14	56%
60-69	33	23	70%
70-79	17	9	53%
80-89	13	12	92%
90-102	8	5	63%
Total	331	84	25%

indicate that the microfissure occurs extremely rarely before 10 years of age and that it begins to be observed after age 10, with the incidence increasing sharply at about age 40. The sex distribution of temporal bones with microfissures is summarized in Table 2. Apparently, there is no difference in distribution between the two sexes. Bilaterality of the microfissure was studied in 105 cases which permitted the study of both sides. The result is shown in Table 3, and appears to indicate that the microfissure is more commonly bilateral. Table 4 shows the location of the microfissure in relation to the oval window, and indicates that in most instances the microfissure is present both superior and inferior to the oval window (Fig. 1). In general, the microfissure superior to the oval window was larger and more distinct than that inferior to the oval window. It may be interesting to note that in each bone the fissures superior and inferior to the oval window appeared to be located in almost the same vertical plane. However, in none of the bones did the microfissure extend beyond the annular ligament to the footplate. The extent of the microfissure was studied in the horizontal plane and is summarized

TABLE 2. SEX DISTRIBUTION OF THE MICROFISSURE IN THE OVAL WINDOW AREA

	No. of Bones Studied	No. of Bones with Microfissure	
Male	169	45	27%
Female	162	39	24%
Total	331	84	

TABLE 3. BILATERALITY OF THE MICROFISSURE IN THE OVAL WINDOW AREA

No. of Cases Studied	No. of Cases with Microfissure			
105	24 (23%)	Bilateral	17	71%
		Unilateral	7	29%

TABLE 4. LOCATION OF THE MICROFISSURE IN RELATION TO THE OVAL WINDOW

Microfissure Superior to the Oval Window	Microfissure Inferior to the Oval Window	No. of Bones	
Present	Present	51	61%
Present	Absent	20	24%
Present	*	12	14%
Absent	Present	1	1.2%
Total		84	

*Could not be determined due to artifacts.

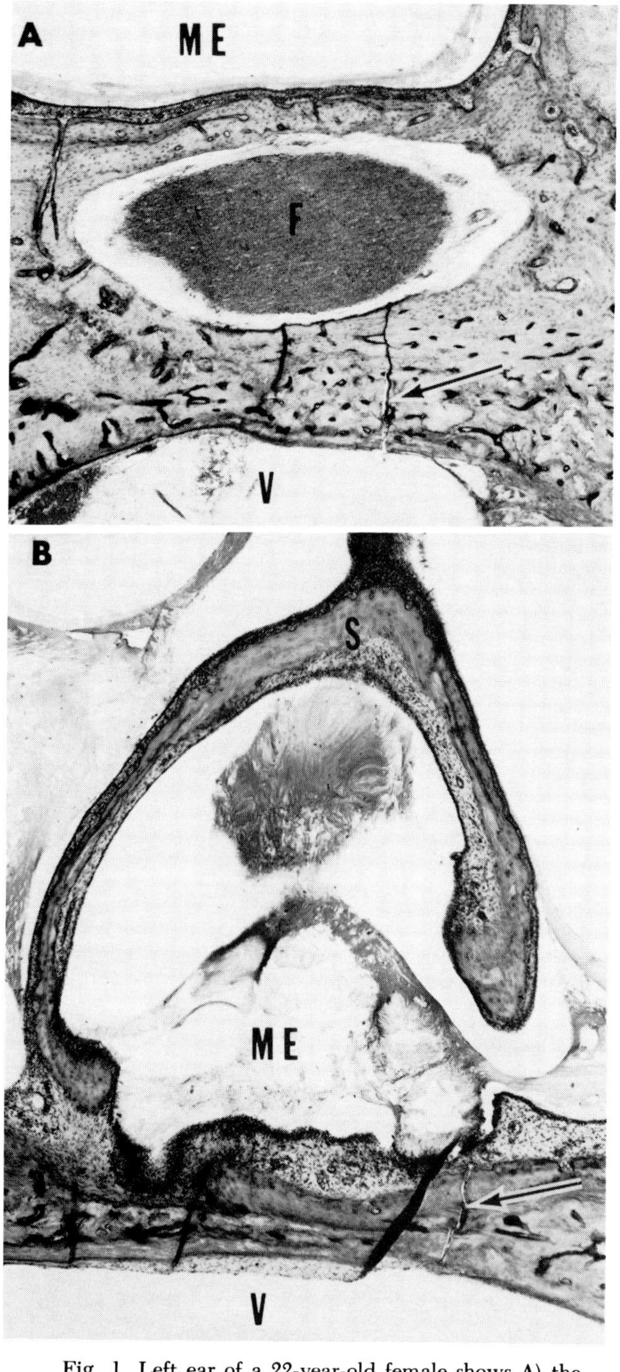

Fig. 1. Left ear of a 22-year-old female shows A) the microfissure (arrow) extending superior to the oval window, and B) also inferior to the oval window, in almost the same vertical plane. Note that the microfissure connects the facial canal (F) or middle ear (ME) with the vestibule (V). S - Stapes. (H&E, A) x37, B) x49)

TABLE 5. EXTENT OF THE MICROFISSURE IN THE HORIZONTAL PLANE

Microfissure Superior to the Oval Window	No. of Bones		Microfissure Inferior to the Oval Window	No. of Bones	
Connection: Vestibule { facial canal, middle ear	29	35%	Connection: Vestibule-middle ear	52	100%
Connection: Vestibule-facial canal	23	28%			
Connection: Vestibule-middle ear	9	11%			
No connection: Vestibular side only	22	26%			
Total	83		Total	52	

in Table 5. It should be noted that the microfissure connects the vestibule to the facial canal and/or middle ear in most instances (Fig. 1), and that when there is no connection it is present only on the vestibular side (Fig. 2). In the vertical plane, the microfissure superior to the oval window appeared to extend superiorly to the level of the lateral or superior canal ampulla, and the microfissure inferior to the oval window extended inferiorly to the level of the hook portion of the cochlea or less frequently to the round window niche. In both instances, the microfissure was most distinct in the immediate vicinity of the oval window. Another important finding was that the vertical extension was always greater on the vestibular side than on the middle ear or facial canal side. Consequently, the connection between the vestibule and the middle ear both superior and inferior to the oval window took place only in a small area immediately adjacent to the oval window, and further vertical extension of the microfissure was observed only on the vestibular side.

The histological appearance of the microfissure

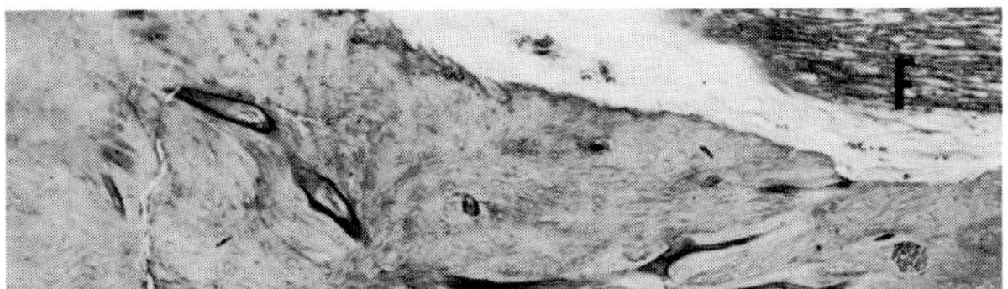

Fig. 2. Right ear of a 71-year-old female shows that the microfissure (arrow) is present superior to the oval window only on the vestibular side and does not connect with either the facial canal (F) or middle ear. V - Vestibule. (H&E, x77)

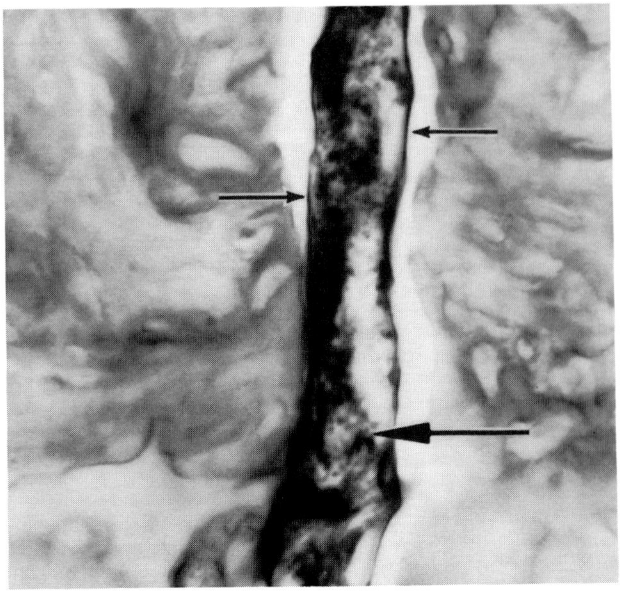

Fig. 3. Right ear of a 63-year-old female shows calcification (large arrow) in the microfissure superior to the oval window. Small arrows indicate thin lines which limit both sides of the microfissure. (H&E, x710)

in this region was identical to that of the microfissure between the posterior canal ampulla and round window niche, although the latter appeared, in general, to be wider. It was an extremely narrow space, observed in the otic capsule, filled with connective tissue-like substance, and mostly limited on both sides by thin lines which stained deeply with hematoxylin. Often the tissue showed an early stage of calcification (Fig. 3). A blood vessel was observed in the microfissures of two specimens (Fig. 4). Red blood cells without definite evidence of blood vessels were also observed in some specimens. In two other specimens, some of the nerve fibers to the lateral canal crista appeared to enter the microfissure (Fig. 5). In another specimen, inflammatory cells were observed to spread from the middle ear through the microfissure to the inner ear (Fig. 6).

Interesting findings were observed in the cases affected by otosclerosis and labyrinthitis ossificans. In some cases of otosclerosis, the microfissure observed in the normal bony tissue disappeared at the border of the otosclerotic focus which occupied the area adjacent to the oval window (Fig. 7) so that it was not observed near the oval window. In one bone affected by labyrinthitis ossificans, the microfissure was observed only in the normal bone, and did not extend into the new bone which had replaced the inner ear spaces (Fig. 8).

DISCUSSION

Although the genesis of the microfissure is uncertain, several theories have been advocated. The early investigators[1-3] believed that it represented a communication route for a blood vessel between the middle ear and the inner ear which had been first

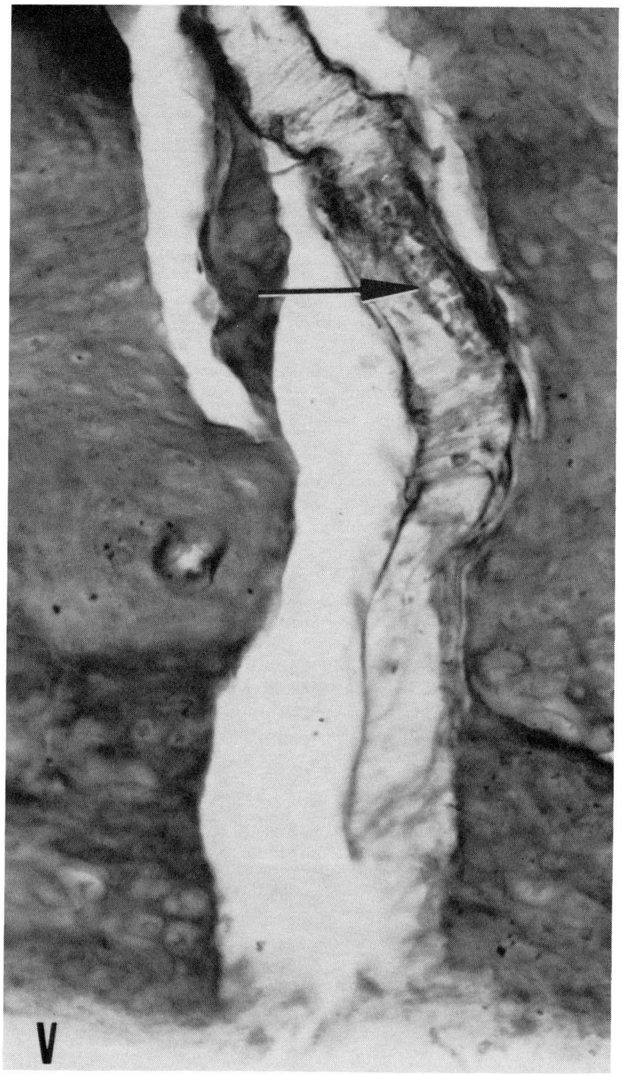

Fig. 4. Right ear of a 73-year-old female shows the presence of a blood vessel (arrow) in the microfissure superior to the oval window. V - Vestibule. (H&E, x390)

described by Politzer.[12] Then Mayer[4,5] proposed a theory which stated that the microfissure was a spontaneous fracture which resulted from mechani-

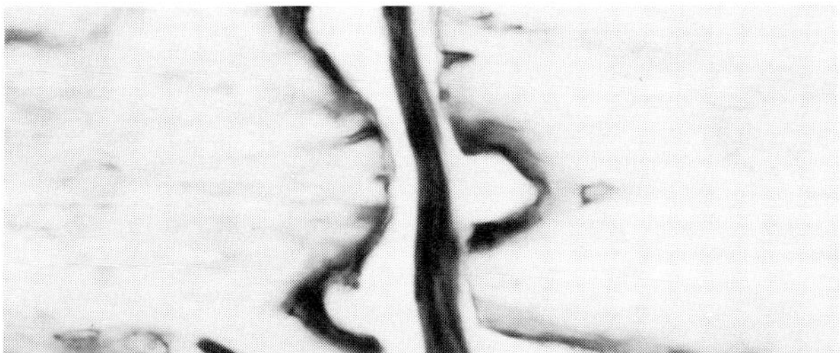

Fig. 5. Left ear of a 61-year-old male shows that some of the nerve fibers (arrow) to the lateral canal crista enter the microfissure superior to the oval window. (H&E, x900)

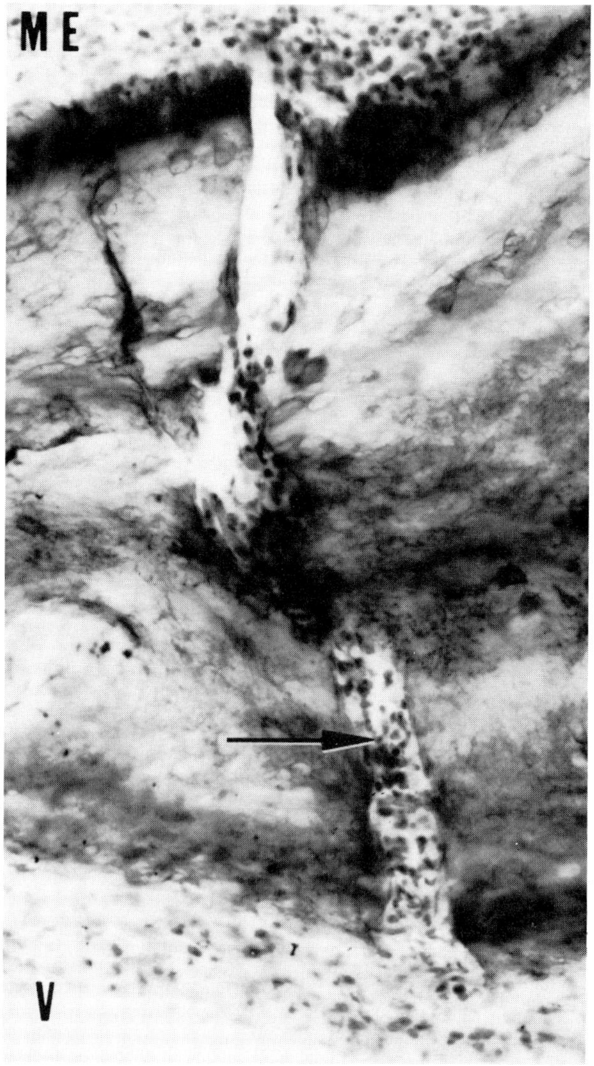

Fig. 6. Left ear of a 51-year-old male shows the presence of inflammatory cells (arrow) spreading from the middle ear (ME) to the inner ear through the microfissure inferior to the oval window. V - Vestibule. (H&E, x450)

cal stress inside the otic capsule. He further stated his hypothesis that the same mechanical stress would lead to the formation of an otosclerotic focus in individuals predisposed to otosclerosis. Meyer[6] supported Mayer's theory of spontaneous fracture, but looked with doubt upon the hypothesis concerning otosclerosis. Kelemen[7] also supported Mayer's mechanical stress theory as the cause of the microfissure. However, Wittmaack[8] strongly opposed Mayer's hypothesis, considering many of the microfissures described by Mayer to be artifacts; however, he did not consider the microfissure between the posterior canal ampulla and round window niche to be an artifact, but he failed to give a clear explanation for its occurrence. Brunner[9] expressed a similar opinion regarding the microfissures, but he thought that the communicating canal for a blood vessel was a likely explanation for those types of microfissure which were not considered to be artifacts. Brühl[13] and Eschweiler[14] considered that all

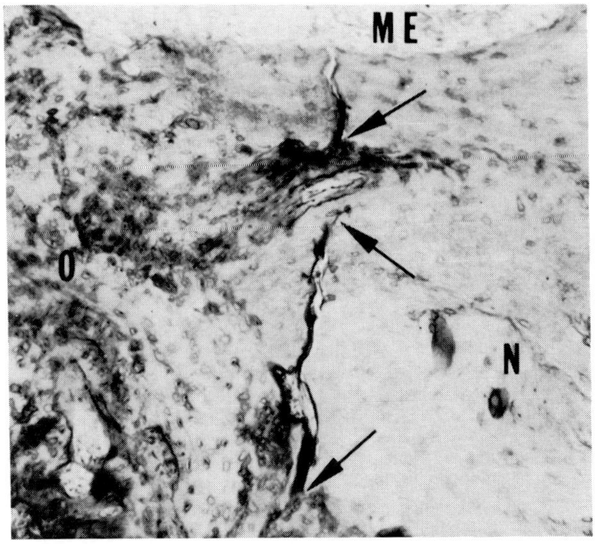

Fig. 7. Right ear of a 66-year-old male with otosclerosis shows that the microfissure superior to the oval window disappears (arrows) at the border of the otosclerotic focus (O). ME - Middle ear; N - Normal bone of the otic capsule. (H&E, x152)

microfissures were artifacts. Another theory was proposed by Szántó[15] who pointed out that a mechanical force such as increased intracranial pressure could lead to the formation of a microfissure. Okano et al[10] recently reported the presence of a communication in early fetal life between the posterior canal ampulla and round window niche and considered that the microfissure took its origin from this communication. Saito et al[11] stated that the microfissure occurred after the formation of the bony tissue was once completed; they considered that the inner ear blood flow had a collateral circulation from the external carotid artery through the microfissure.

The results of the present study show that apparently the microfissure is not an artifact, since it has been seen to contain a connective tissue-like substance, sometimes a blood vessel, red blood cells, nerve fibers, or inflammatory cells (Figs. 4-6). The present study, which demonstrates that the microfissure is not present at birth and starts to be observed with increasing frequency from a certain age (Table 1), appears to speak against the microfissure being congenital in nature or embryologic in origin. Blood vessels and red blood cells were observed only in a small number of specimens in this study. Consequently, the microfissure must not occur primarily as a communicating canal for a blood vessel, although it may be pierced by a blood vessel secondarily after its formation. At the present time, we feel that nontraumatic, spontaneous fracture by mechanical stress as first proposed by Mayer[4,5] is the most probable explanation for the occurrence of the microfissure.

The results of the present study demonstrate that the microfissure in the oval window area is a fairly common occurrence, particularly after the age of 40

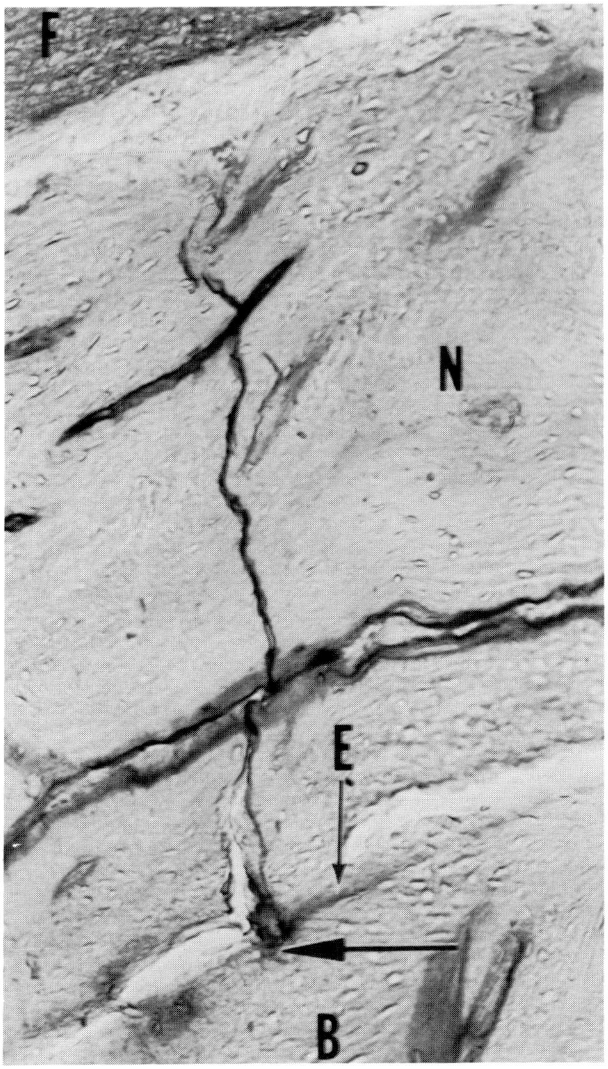

Fig. 8. Right ear of an 82-year-old male with labyrinthitis ossificans shows that the microfissure superior to the oval window does not extend (arrow) into the new bone (B), which has replaced the vestibule. E - Endosteal layer of the otic capsule; F - Facial nerve; N - Normal bone of the otic capsule. (H&E, x162)

(an average of 66% of temporal bones from individuals in this age range showed the presence of microfissures). This finding is somewhat different from the incidence of the microfissure between the

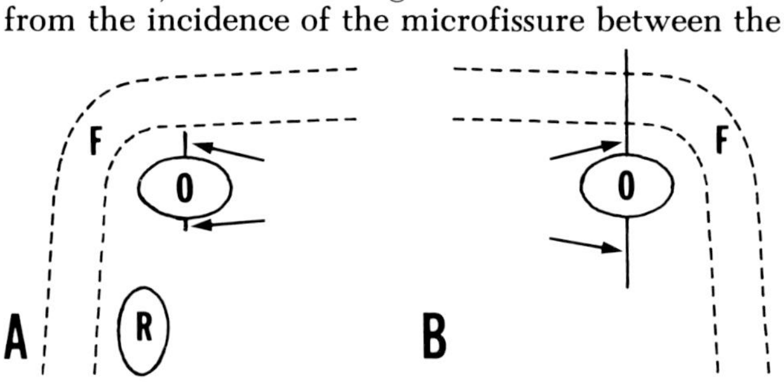

Fig. 9. Summary diagram illustrating the typical relationship of microfissures (arrows) to the oval window (O) and the facial canal (F). Both views represent the right ear viewed from the middle ear side (A), and from the vestibular side (B). Note that the vertical extension of the microfissure is greater on the vestibular side (B) than on the middle ear side (A).

posterior canal ampulla and round window niche. Okano et al[10] observed the latter microfissure in 100% of the bones over six years old. The present authors also examined this microfissure in 320 temporal bones, from individuals ranging in age from newborn to 102 years old, and found it in 100% of the bones of individuals over 8 years old. Thus, the microfissure in the oval window area is a less constant structure than that between the posterior canal ampulla and round window niche. This might reflect the difference in the mechanical stress exerted on these areas, or the difference in resistance between the two areas of the otic capsule. Our observation that the microfissure between the posterior canal ampulla and round window niche appears to be wider in general than that in the oval window area may be in accordance with more frequent and longstanding existence of the former microfissure.

One of the characteristics of the microfissure in the oval window area is that in 61% of the bones with a microfissure it was present both superior and inferior to the oval window in almost the same vertical plane (Fig. 9 and Table 4). This finding indicates that a typical microfissure in this region extends in the otic capsule vertically across the oval window, although it does not penetrate into the footplate. It is noteworthy that the microfissure was most distinct in the immediate proximity of the oval window, suggesting the possibility that the microfissure first arises at the border of the oval window and then extends either superiorly or inferiorly to it.

The microfissure was present only on the inner ear side in 26% of the bones with a microfissure, but was not present in any of the bones on the middle ear side only (Fig. 9 and Table 5). A similar observation was made with respect to the microfissure between the posterior canal ampulla and round window niche. The above findings appear to indicate that the fracture which is seen postmortem as the microfissure may start from the inner ear side, as predicted by Mayer's[4] theory of its genesis.

The disappearance of the microfissure at the border of an otosclerotic focus or ossified labyrinth is an interesting observation (Figs. 7 and 8). It cannot be determined with certainty whether the formation of the microfissure took place before or after the pathological changes began in the otic capsule or in the inner ear. The present authors consider the former possibility to be more likely, in view of the findings that the microfissure did not extend into the pathological bones and that in cases of otosclerosis the focus was observed to intervene between the microfissure and the oval window. This also appears to speak against the postmortem nature of the microfissure. However, the present authors could find no evidence to indicate such a causal relationship between the microfissure and otosclerosis as was suggested by Mayer.[4,5]

The microfissure should not be confused with histological evidence of temporal bone fracture, as pointed out by Kelemen.[7] Comparison of the microfissure findings with histopathologic reports of temporal bone fracture[16-18] reveals that the microfissure is different from this type of traumatic fracture both in site and histological appearance. In cases of temporal bone fracture, a healing process by fibrous tissue and new bone is evident in a wide fissure. It arises from the periosteal layer of the otic capsule and the enchondral and endosteal layers show minimal or no evidence of any reparative process. In cases of microfissure, the fissure is usually narrow, filled with connective tissue-like substance often with calcification but not with new bone formation, and sometimes observed only on the inner ear side. The difference between these two types of fracture may be ascribed to the supposition that on the one hand temporal bone fracture will be produced by an unusually large but momentary force exerted on the otic capsule, while on the other hand the microfissure will be due to constant stress inside the otic capsule.

The clinical significance of the microfissure has not yet been clearly determined. The possibility that it may serve as a route for the spread of inflammation from the middle ear to the inner ear was pointed out a long time ago,[1-3] and is well demonstrated in this study by Figure 6. It may also serve as a route for ototoxic ear drops to reach the inner ear.* One might also speculate that the microfissure may form the basis for certain perilymph fistulas, which have come to attract attention in relation to sudden hearing loss due to labyrinthine window rupture.[19] At the present time, however, there is no evidence to support this hypothesis, since there is no histopathologic report of such cases.

*Nomura Y. Personal communication.

ACKNOWLEDGMENTS — The authors express their deep appreciation to Harold F. Schuknecht, MD, Chairman, Department of Otolaryngology, Harvard Medical School, and Bruce W. Jafek, MD, Chairman, Department of Otolaryngology, University of Colorado Medical Center, for letting the authors include some of their cases in the series of this study. Appreciation is also expressed to Reisuke Saito, MD, for helping in the histopathological interpretations and Ruth Anderson for her kind assistance in this study.

REFERENCES

1. Manasse P. Zur pathologischen Anatomie des inneren Ohres und des Hörnerven. Z Ohrenheilkd 1905; 49:109-36.

2. Nager FR. Beiträge zur Histologie der erworbenen Taubstummheit. Z Ohrenheilkd 1907; 54:217-44.

3. Zange J. Pathologische Anatomie und Physiologie der mittelohrentspringenden Labyrinthentzündungen als Grundlage der Klinik. Wiesbaden, Bergmann, 1919:40.

4. Mayer O. Über die Entstehung der Spontanfrakturen der Labyrinthkapsel und ihre Bedeutung für die Otosklerose. Z Hals Nasen Ohrenheilkd 1930; 26:261-79.

5. Mayer O. Die Ursache der Knochenneubildung bei der Otosklerose. Acta Otolaryngol (Stockh) 1931; 15:35-73.

6. Meyer M. Die normale Anatomie der Labyrinthkapsel. Z Hals Nasen Ohrenheilkd 1933; 34:3-72.

7. Kelemen G. Über die Fissuren im knöchernen Innenohr. Arch Klin Exp Ohren Nasen Kehlkopfheilkd 1933; 137:36-49.

8. Wittmaack K. Zur dritten Otosklerose-Hypothese Otto Mayers. Arch Klin Exp Ohren Nasen Kehlkopfheilkd 1932; 131:180-207.

9. Brunner H. Über Spaltbildung in der knöchernen Innenohrkapsel. Wien Klin Wochenschr 1931; 44:173-6.

10. Okano Y, Myers EN, Dickson DR. Microfissure between the round window niche and posterior canal ampulla. Ann Otol Rhinol Laryngol 1977; 86:49-57.

11. Saito H, Kishimoto S, Suehiro S. Microfissure. Pract Otol Kyoto 1978; 71:393-7.

12. Politzer A. Über Anastomosen zwischen den Gefassbezirken des Mittelohres und des Labyrinthes. Arch f Ohrenheilk 1876; 11:237.

13. Brühl G. Bemerkungen zu O. Mayers Arbeit. Z Hals Nasen Ohrenheilkd 1930; 26:587-91.

14. Eschweiler: Über Spaltbildungen in der labyrinthkapsel. Z Hals Nasen Ohrenheilkd 1933; 34:152-65.

15. Sźantó G. Zur Pathogenese der "queren Subiculumspalte" der Innenohrkapsel. Acta Otolaryngol (Stockh) 1934; 21:228-35.

16. Druss JG. Fractures of the petrous pyramid: report of a case with histological observations eight years after injury. Arch Otolaryngol 1951; 53:540-51.

17. Fredrickson JM, Griffith AW, Lindsay JR. Transverse fracture of the temporal bone: a clinical and histopathological study. Arch Otolaryngol 1963; 78:770-84.

18. Etholm B. Non-fatal transverse fractures of the temporal bone: histopathology, late complications. ORL 1972; 34:273-80.

19. Goodhill V. Sudden deafness and round window rupture. Laryngoscope 1971; 81:1462-74.

≈

AMERICAN BOARD OF OTOLARYNGOLOGY
SPECIAL ANNOUNCEMENT

This is to announce that the written examination of the American Board of Otolaryngology will be given Sunday, September 27, 1981 at the Palmer House in Chicago, Illinois. Registration will be on Saturday, September 26, 1981 at 5:00 p.m. at the Palmer House. It is estimated that the examination will conclude at 6:00 p.m. on Sunday.

Deadline for application is May 1st. Please contact Walter P.Work, MD, Secretary-Treasurer, at the American Board of Otolaryngology, 220 Collingwood, Suite 130, Ann Arbor, MI 48103 for the new application forms.

This is the official announcement. Please disregard any previous announcements concerning this examination.

ASSOCIATION OF A THYROGLOSSAL DUCT CYST AND A DERMOID CYST IN THE NECK
A CASE REPORT

J. G. HAAR, DDS, MD
M. H. SADEGHI, MD
E. J. BOULOS, MD
J. SHEFFER, MD

BUFFALO, NEW YORK

The association of a thyroglossal duct cyst and a dermoid cyst in the neck is a very interesting pathological finding. Review of the literature could not establish any relationship between the two lesions, embryological or otherwise. To our knowledge no previous similar case has been reported in the literature.

CASE REPORT

The patient is a 39-year-old white male who presented with an asymptomatic swelling of the anterior neck discovered incidentally on routine work-up, six weeks prior to admission.

The examination of the head and neck revealed a midline cystic swelling, 2.5 x 2.5 cm in size, in the region of the thyrohyoid membrane. The mass moved along the vertical axis with deglutition and tongue movements. There was no thyromegaly or adenopathy noted. The base of the tongue was nor-

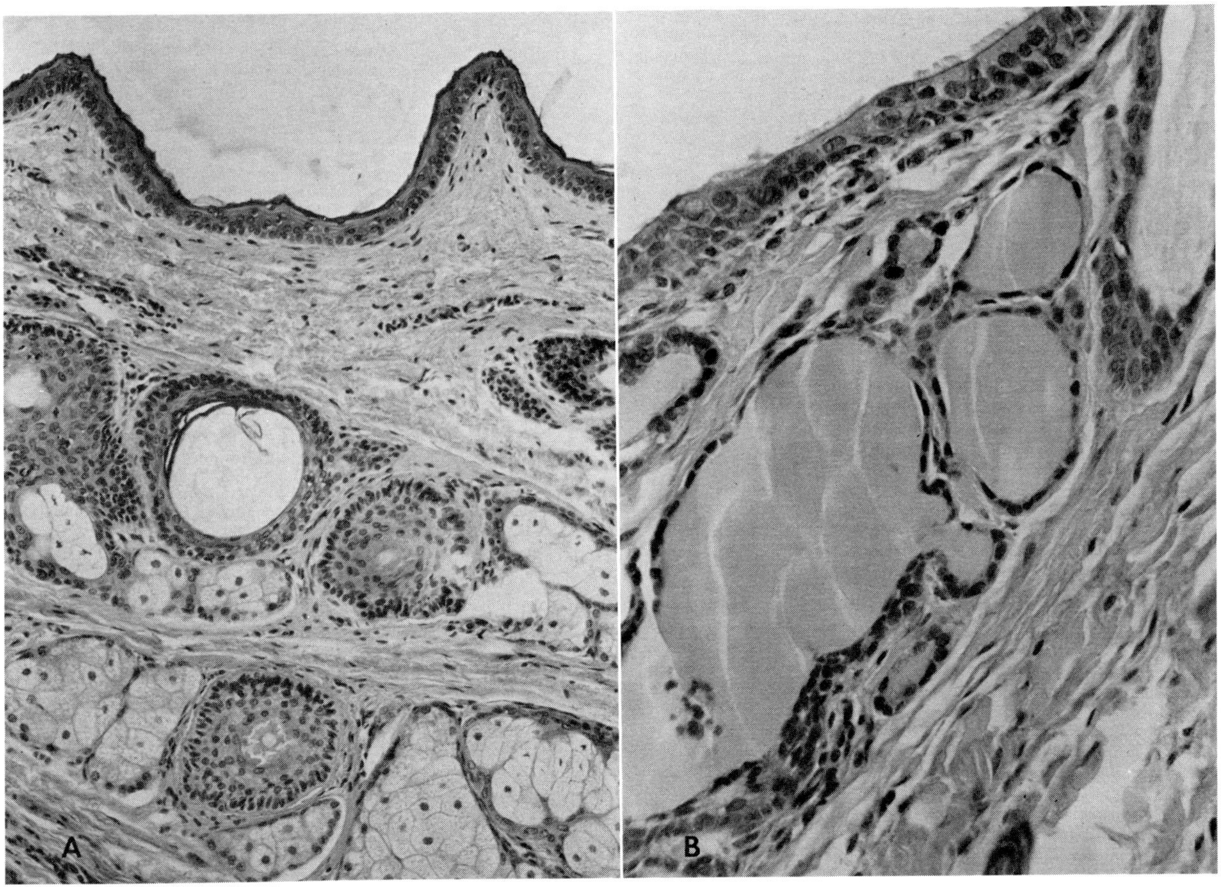

Fig. 1. A) Dermoid cyst wall showing epidermoid lining and abundant pilosebaceous structures in the stroma. B) Thyroglossal duct cyst wall lined by respiratory type ciliated epithelium with characteristic thyroid follicles in the stroma.

From the Departments of Otolaryngology and Head and Neck Surgery and Pathology, the Sisters of Charity Hospital; and the Departments of Otolaryngology and Pathology, The State University of New York School of Medicine, Buffalo.

REPRINTS — E. John Boulos, MD, 8 Center Road, Getzville, NY 14068.

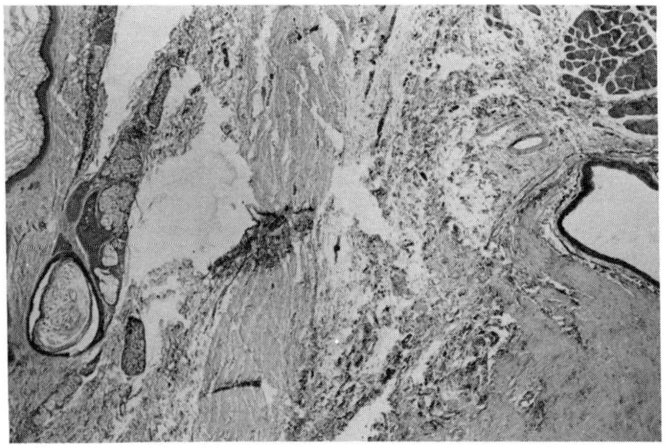

Fig. 2. Section through an area of intimate association of the two lesions shows keratin-filled dermoid cyst in upper left margin and thyroglossal cyst on right margin with metaplastic lining.

mal. The rest of the examination and work-up was within normal limits.

The patient underwent surgery for excision of the mass, a Systrunk procedure being performed. The postoperative course was uneventful.

PATHOLOGY

Multiple sections of the mass revealed features of a dermoid cyst (DC) and a thyroglossal duct cyst (TGDC) with no communication between them. The DC was lined by epidermoid stratified squamous epithelium with skin appendages (hair follicles and sebaceous glands). There were some inflammatory cells (Fig. 1A). Its cavity was filled with keratinous material (Fig. 2). The TGDC consisted of a small cystic space lined by respiratory epithelium (ciliated pseudostratified columnar) with focal squamous metaplasia. The cyst wall contained several thyroid follicles filled with colloid (Fig. 1B).

DISCUSSION

We are presenting a case report of an association of a TGDC and a DC in the neck. Talekar et al[1] have reported on the association of a teratoma and a TGDC. In the head and neck, the term dermoid cyst may apply to:[2-4]

1. Epidermoid cyst — an acquired implantation DC lined by squamous epithelium with no adnexal structures.

2. Dermoid cyst — a congenital inclusion cyst formed by displaced dermal cells around the lines of embryonic fusion. It is lined by squamous epithelium with a variable number of skin appendages.

3. Teratoid cyst — a congenital DC or teratoma arising from germ cells. It may contain any or all of the germinal structures.

Under this classification, our case is an association of a TGDC and a DC proper.

REFERENCES

1. Talekar MS, Thomas JA, Kothare SN. Teratoma of the neck in relation to thyroglossal duct cyst. Indian J Cancer 1975; 12:449-51.

2. Batsakis JG. Tumors of the head and neck: clinical and pathological considerations. Baltimore: Williams & Wilkins, 1974; 79:619-24.

4. Batsakis JG, Farber ER. Teratomas of head and neck. EENT Digest 1968; 30:67.

PERINEURAL METASTASES FROM SQUAMOUS CELL CARCINOMA OF THE FACE

THERAPEUTIC CONSIDERATIONS

NATHAN GREEN, MD MICHAEL LANDMAN, MD

VAN NUYS, CALIFORNIA

Perineural metastasis from squamous cell carcinoma of the facial skin can cause disabling pain, paresis, soft tissue tumefaction, bone destruction, impaired function and impaired vision. Two patients with perineural metastases were treated with palliative megavoltage irradiation and interstitial therapy. The meastases were controlled. Pain improved; cosmesis, function and vision were preserved.

Squamous cell carcinoma of the skin is a common malignancy often readily curable by surgery or radiation therapy.[1-3] Large or well-differentiated skin cancers have a propensity to develop lymphatic metastasis.[4-6] Less commonly observed has been spread of skin cancers along peripheral nerves. In the head and neck region perineural metastasis can cause distressing pain, paresis, soft tissue tumefaction and bone destruction.[5-8] On occasion perineural metastases are amenable to palliative surgery and have been so managed with some success.[8] Although palliative irradiation has been employed, there has been a paucity of reports describing its use. Its value has been uncertain. This report reviews the experience of two patients who developed perineural metastases following excision of a facial skin cancer with special regard to the biologic behavior and the therapeutic implications.

METHODS

Between 1968 and 1976, 118 patients were seen in the division of radiation therapy for cancer of the facial skin. One hundred sixteen patients were referred for definitive irradiation. Ninety-five patients had basal cell carcinoma and 21 patients squamous cell carcinoma. Perineural invasion was not observed in the histopathology of these skin cancers. All skin cancers were treated with 100 kV orthovoltage therapy, using a spectrum of radiation therapy techniques and time-dose factors. Three patients developed local recurrences. No patient developed perineural metastasis. Two patients were referred with perineural metastases from squamous cell carcinoma of the facial skin. Perineural invasion was observed in the original slide material of one patient and in the biopsy of a local recurrence in the other patient.

CASE REPORTS

Case 1. A 64-year-old male had skin cancer of the right temple resected on October 14, 1974. Pathology showed squamous cell carcinoma with perineural invasion (Fig. 1). Over the ensuing months, he developed right facial pain, hypalgesia of the right fifth cranial nerve, loss of right corneal reflex, right sixth nerve paresis and atrophy of the right masseter muscle. The right 8th through 12th cranial nerves were intact. X-ray tomograms of the skull showed sclerosis and erosion of the medial aspect of the greater wing of the sphenoid. An isotope brain scan, computerized axial tomograms of the brain, and carotid angiogram were normal. Perineural metastasis was thought to be the most likely explanation for these findings. The patient received 4 MV accelerator irradiation to a treatment field that included the right temple and extradural space anterior to the level of the external auditory canal and posterior to the level of the bony canthus of the right eye. The treatment field spared the right eye lens. A total dose of 6,600 rads was delivered. Facial pain, absence of the right corneal reflex, and right sixth nerve paresis persisted. A palliative neurosurgical procedure was contemplated and seemed inadvisable as the surgical risks were greater than the potential benefit. On April 8, 1976, the patient developed diplopia. Examination showed a firm, 4 cm right supraorbital mass with encroachment into the orbit and a separate firm 5 cm right hard palate mass with central ulceration. The metastasis occurred outside the radiation treatment field (Fig. 2). X-ray tomograms of the hard palate showed bony erosion. Biopsy of both sites showed squamous cell carcinoma. The location of the metastasis was uncommon for vascular or lymphatic spread. Both metastases were thought to develop from perineural spread as they occurred along the distribution of the fifth cranial nerve (Fig. 2). The supraorbital tumor was treated with ^{198}Au seed implant delivering 6,800 rads, and totally regressed. Normal vision was restored. The hard palate metastasis was initially treated with parenteral methotrexate. There was no response. Subsequently, an ^{198}AU seed implant was done delivering 7,300 rads. The metastasis totally regressed. By July 6, 1977, a painful left lung metastasis developed. Needle biopsy showed squamous cell carcinoma. The metastasis was treated with 4 MV linear accelerator delivering a total of 4,000 rads with good response. Pain was alleviated. The patient died on June 4, 1978.

Case 2. A 63-year-old male had a left temple skin cancer resected August 12, 1968. Pathology showed squamous cell carcinoma arising in a keratoacanthoma. On September 10, 1972, there was an apparent local recurrence which was excised. Histopathology showed this tumor to be a basal cell carcinoma. Neither biopsy showed perineural invasion. On May 11, 1974, the patient noted left facial pain and paresis. An electromyogram showed scattered fibrillation. Regenerative motor units were not seen. The skull x-ray was normal. A left facial nerve decompression was performed on July 29, 1974. When the nerve sheath was split, the nerve appeared thickened, but no obvious tumor was observed. The nerve was not biopsied. Postoperatively, the facial pain transiently improved. On October 4, 1974, there was a recurrence in the left temple. Biopsy showed squamous cell carcinoma with perineural invasion. A wide excision was performed. The tumor extended into the temporalis muscle. Postoperatively, the patient received 4 MV linear accelerator irradiation to a treatment field that included the right temple, temporal bone and subarachnoid space. Forty-five degree right angle wedged fields were used to deliver 6,000 rads. Facial pain improved but paresis persisted. In retrospect, the facial nerve paresis was thought to be caused by

From the Department of Radiation Therapy, Valley Presbyterian Hospital, Van Nuys, California.

REPRINTS — Nathan Green, MD, Valley Presbyterian Hospital, 15107 Vanowen Street, Van Nuys, CA 91405.

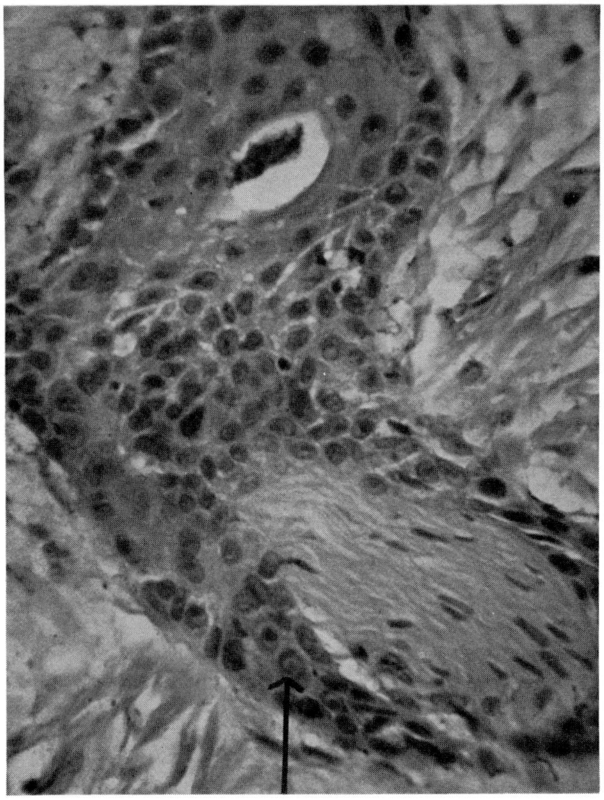

Fig. 1. Microscopy shows infiltrating squamous cell carcinoma with invasion of perineural space (arrow). (x450)

perineural metastasis. On May 8, 1975, a metastasis was noted superior to the megavoltage portal. This was thought to be a marginal recurrence and was treated with 250 kV x-ray, 3.5 cm cone delivering 5,700 rads. The tumor totally regressed. On April 5, 1976, a left forehead metastasis was noted anterior to the megavoltage portal. This was treated with a 100 kV x-ray 4 cm cone delivering 5,100 rads. The tumor totally regressed. On September 5, 1976, the patient noted diplopia and impaired left lateral gaze. Examination showed proptosis. Lumbar puncture and a computerized axial tomogram of the brain and orbit were normal. The clinical findings were thought to be caused by perineural metastasis along the fifth and sixth cranial nerves. The metastasis was treated with a 4 MV linear accelerator using a 6 cm anterior portal to deliver a total of 4,000 rads at 5 cm depth. Proptosis resolved but diplopia remained unchanged. A concurrent chest x-ray showed a left upper lobe metastasis. This was treated by 4 MV linear accelerator delivering 5,100 rads. The lung metastasis totally regressed. When last seen on March 5, 1978, the patient was clinically free of disease.

DISCUSSION

Squamous cell carcinoma of the skin has a known capacity for embolic spread through lymphatic or vascular channels.[4,5,7] Another ominous but uncommon pathway of spread is along the peripheral nerves.[8] Tumor cells can invade the perineural space and spread in a subtle and sometimes capricious fashion. Endoneural and perineural spaces extend from the smallest ramification of the peripheral nerves to the central origin.[9,10] In the head and neck region, there can be centripetal or centrifugal spread along the cranial nerves to involve the subarachnoid space, bone and soft tissue.[7-9]

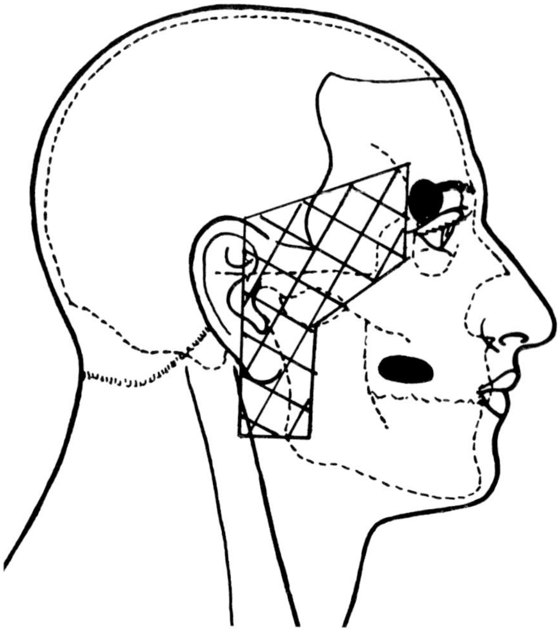

Fig. 2. Crosshatched area designates the radiation portal to the central perineural metastasis involving the fifth and sixth cranial nerves. The dark area designates subsequent perineural metastases of the right supraorbital and hard palate area.

The incidence of patients who develop perineural metastasis from facial skin cancer must be exceedingly low. In our experience perineural invasion was not observed in skin cancers of patients referred for primary irradiation. None of these patients developed perineural metastasis. However, the absence of detectable perineural invasion in the primary tumor does not preclude the development of perineural metastasis. This was illustrated by the experience of two patients referred with perineural metastases. Perineural invasion was observed in only one of the original specimens. Both patients developed perineural metastases along the central distribution of the cranial nerves. Subsequntly there was spread to involve adjacent cranial nerves with ultimate development of metastases along the peripheral distribution of the cranial nerves. Recurrences also occurred at the margins of radiation treatment portals used to palliate the initial metastasis. Both patients developed hematogenesis metastasis to the lung late in the course of their disease. Of interest is that lymphatic invasion was not observed in the microscopy of the primary tumors and neither patient developed lymphatic metastasis.

Perineural spread of facial skin cancer can cause distressing symptoms. Facial pain is an early complaint, often disabling and refractory to conservative measures.[5,10] With tumor progression patients develop cranial nerve paresis, soft tissue tumefaction, and bone destruction. Neurosurgical measures designed to alleviate pain may be of such magnitude as to preclude implementation, especially in patients who are otherwise incurable.[10,11] Multistage palliative surgical procedures are usually not justified because of the advanced stage of the disease and the likelihood of recurrence.[3,12,13] Palliative irradiation has been used. Moore et al reported it may not be effective.[10] This was not our experience. In one of our patients, facial pain was effectively palliated. In both patients, the intracranial and peripheral metastases were controlled in an expeditious manner without sequela. Vision and function were preserved. However, although disease was controlled within the treatment volume, metastasis did develop outside of the radiation portals along with ophthalmic and maxillary divisions of the fifth cranial nerve.

Ideally radiation treatment regimens should take cognizance of the potential pathways of tumor spread. Subsequent perineural metastases might be prevented if initial treatment portals would encompass the entire distribution of the involved cranial nerves. However, to do so, would require large treatment fields. In the head and neck region, this can cause inordinate morbidity. An alternative approach, which we employed, was to use treatment portals limited to the metastasis. Metastases that subsequently developed outside the treatment fields were readily controlled by additional treatment using either ^{198}AU implant or megavoltage irradition.

REFERENCES

1. Ballantyne AJ. Clinical evaluation of skin tumors. In: Cumley RW, McCay J, Aldridge D, et al, eds. Tumors of the skin. Chicago: Year Book Medical Publishers, 1964:149-73.
2. Cancer statistics. CA 1978; 28:16-32.
3. Jesse RH. Surgical management of skin cancer. In: Cumley RW, McCay J, Aldridge D, et al, eds. Tumors of the skin. Chicago: Year Book Medical Publishers, 1964:225-57.
4. Storm FK, Eliber FR, Sparkes FC, Morton DL. A prospective study of parotid metastasis from head and neck cancer. Am J Surg 1977; 134:115-9.
5. Epstein E, Epstein NN, Bragg K, Linden G. Metastases from squamous cell carcinoma of the skin. Arch Dermatol 1968; 97:245-51.
6. Lund HZ. How often does squamous cell carcinoma of the skin metastasize. Arch Dermatol 1965; 92:635-7.
7. Brownstein MH, Helwig EB. Patterns of cutaneous metastasis. Arch Dermatol 1972; 105:862-8.
8. Dodd GE, Dolan PA, Ballantyne AJ, Ibanez ML, Chan P. The dissemination of tumors of the head and neck via the cranial nerves. Radiol Clin North Am 1970; 3:445-70.
9. Ballantyne AJ, McCarten AB, Ibanez MC. The extension of cancer of the head and neck through peripheral nerves. Am J Surg 1963; 106:651.
10. Moore CE, Hoyt WF, North JB. Painful ophthalmoplegia following treated squamous carcinoma of the forehead. Med J Aust 1976; 1:657-9.
11. Freidberg SR. Neurosurgical treatment of pain caused by cancer. Med Clin North Am 1975; 29:481-94.
12. Sinclair MH. The plastic surgeon and skin cancer with special reference to the eyelid region and reconstructive procedures. In: Cumley RW, McCay J, Aldridge D, et al, eds. Tumors of the skin. Chicago: Year Book Medical Publishers, 1964:249-68.
13. Spann JL, Sandlin MD, VanWormer D. A surgical technique for resecting malignancies invading the facial nerve and petrous pyramid. J Surg Oncol 1977; 9:315-27.

Ann Otol 90:1981

PREHISTORIC TREPHINATION OF THE FRONTAL SINUS

RINALDO F. CANALIS, MD
TORRANCE, CALIFORNIA
WILLIAM G. HEMENWAY, MD
LOS ANGELES, CALIFORNIA
FERNANDO CABIESES, MD
LIMA, PERU
ROBERTO ARAGON, MD
LOS ANGELES, CALIFORNIA

Two examples of prehistoric trephination of the frontal sinus are presented. Both specimens were collected in Peru during the second decade of this century and are currently preserved at the Museum of Man in San Diego. One of the skulls represents trephining by incision and the other by scraping. Both show signs of healing indicating that the operated individuals survived the procedure. No definite clues as to the indications for surgery were found in one of the specimens. Trauma involving the frontal sinus appears to have been the reason for trephination in the other.

INTRODUCTION

Trephination of the skull is one of the most common surgical procedures attempted by ancient man. Examples of these operations are encountered in many primitive societies but are especially abundant among early Peruvian cultures. In prehistoric Peru the operation probably developed first in the more advanced Andean groups extending thereafter to those in the coastal region. Eventually several centers evolved each with a more or less characteristic surgical technique.

Examples of prehistoric Peruvian trephination are classified according to the shape of their surgical defect into three basic types: quadrilateral, round and irregular (Fig. 1A-C). In the first type trephination resulted from bony cuts made with a sharp instrument while scraping, or multiple burrholes were the methods used in the other two. It must be noted that the ultimate shape of the trephination depended not only on the technique used. Osteitis frequently altered the configuration of the surgical defect resulting in a rounded or irregular opening.[1]

Controversy exists about the instruments used for trephination in ancient Peru. Among these the crescent shaped "Tumi" (Fig. 1D) and obsidian knives have been most frequently considered. Although it is likely that an instrument such as the Tumi was used, there is no art work or other archeological finding conclusively supporting this hypothesis.

Indian surgeons attempted entrance into most regions of the skull, however, examples of trephination of the frontal sinus are rare. In fact, among over 300 specimens studied the authors have been able to find only 2 where the definite goal of the operation was to enter this cavity. They are the basis for this study and are currently preserved at the Museum of Man in San Diego.

MATERIAL

The specimens presented were collected in Peru during the second decade of this century by Hrdlicka* and have been partially described previously. In 1920, Burton[2] included them in a communication covering otolaryngological findings in prehistoric Peruvian skulls. In 1929, and again in 1931, Moodie[3,4] referred to Burton's study and included a brief description, two photographs and a radiograph of Specimen I in separate studies discussing surgery in ancient Peru. The specimens merit further discussion because they have never been studied in the light of current otolaryngological knowledge and experience. Furthermore, preceding studies are incomplete and present conclusions which cannot be supported clinically.

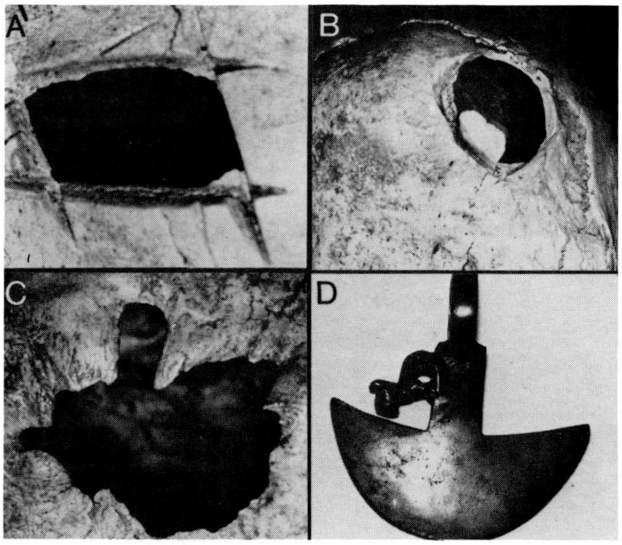

Fig. 1. A) Quadrilateral, B) round, and C) irregular types of trephination. D) Tumi knife.

*Hrdlicka A. Catalog of anthropological specimens from Peru. Unpublished data currently stored at the Museum of Man in San Diego, Calif.

From the Division of Head and Neck Surgery, U.C.L.A. School of Medicine and Harbor-UCLA Medical Center, Torrance, California; The Peruvian Museum for the Health Sciences, Lima, Peru; and the Peruvian Consulate General, Los Angeles, California.

REPRINTS — Rinaldo F. Canalis, MD, Harbor-UCLA Medical Center, 1000 W. Carson Street, Torrance, CA 90509.

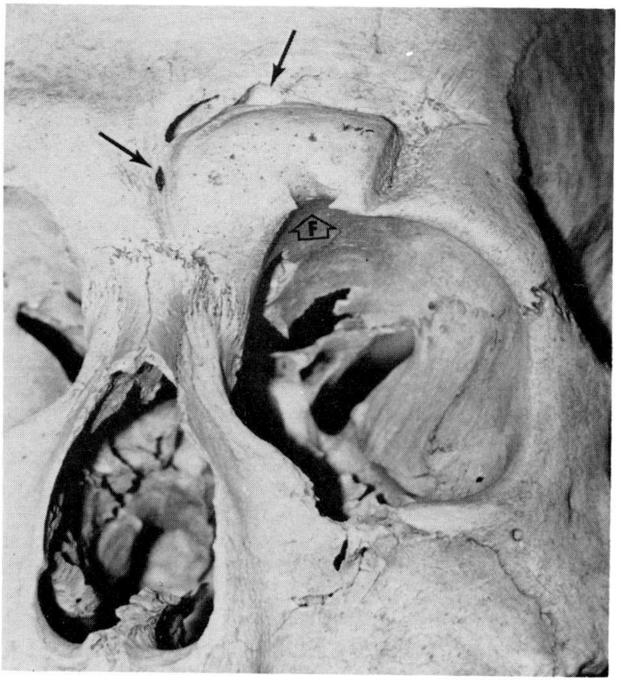

Fig. 2. (Specimen I) Frontal view showing trephination of the left frontal sinus. Arrows indicate opening into the sinus. Note widening of supraorbital foramen (F).

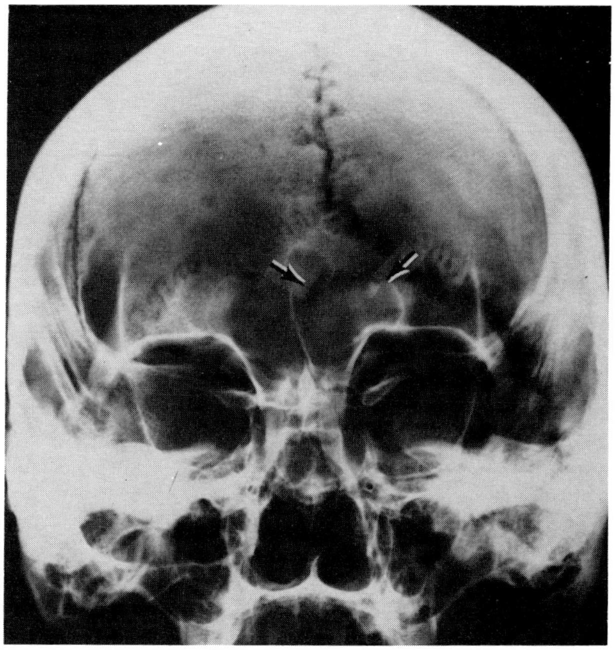

Fig. 3. (Specimen I) Radiograph. Arrows indicate superior and lateral limits of trephination. Note thickening of left lateral wall.

SPECIMEN I

Historic Background. This skull was collected in the vicinity of San Damian, a small village located on the western slope of the Andes at about 9,000 feet above sea level. Exploration of the site, which in prehistoric times was dominated by a small fortress, has yielded a large number of human remains. These include 45 trephined skulls, some of which show evidences of preoperative fracture. The one described was retrieved from the surface in an area previously disturbed by looters, a fact which prevents accurate assessment of its historical age. After exhaustive study, Hrdlicka concluded that all specimens found in this area were pre-Columbian. As there are definite indications that the practice of trephination had declined during the latter part of the Inca period,[1] approximately 1400-1532, it is likely that this specimen is at least 600 years old.

Description. The skull is that of an adult male, 30 to 40 years old. Except for postmortem fractures of the occipital bone and left infraorbital rim it exhibits little deterioration. The mandible and most of the upper teeth are missing. Surgical findings are limited to the left frontal sinus (Fig. 2). Entrance into this cavity was gained by three roughly perpendicular cuts at the medial, lateral and superior limits of the sinus. They are 1.2, 2.5 and 1.8 cm long respectively. Penetration into the sinus cavity is present at the midportion of the medial cut. These incisions exhibit smooth, rounded edges which appear partially healed. Interestingly, the superior orbital foramen also shows evidence of surgical intervention. Its inferior rim has been removed and the foramen itself is enlarged to a 0.5 cm diameter. The posterior wall of the sinus and the intersinus septum are intact.

Radiographs confirm these findings (Fig. 3). The frontal sinuses appear to be well developed and of moderate size. The appearance of the right sinus is entirely normal exhibiting sharp edges and scalloping. Examination of the left sinus demonstrates that the lateral cut was placed just outside of the sinus wall. A defect is clearly seen along the superior incision which is well within the upper extent of the sinus. The walls of the sinus show normal scalloping although thickening of the lateral bony wall is evident. The nasofrontal ducts are intact.

Comment. This skull is representative of a variant of the quadrilateral type of trephination and it presents several interesting features. It seems clear that the intent of the surgeon was to enter the sinus and that his knowledge of anatomy allowed him to do so without violating the anterior cranial fossa. Cuts were limited to the anterior bulge of the sinus wall and the usual lower incision was omitted to avoid entering the orbit.

Although it is impossible to exclude a ritual motive for this operation it is likely that it was performed for therapeutic purposes, possibly for localized pain. The ritualistic aspects of Peruvian trephination are not well known but it is generally accepted that they played a lesser role than in other civilizations.[1]

Previous authors[2-4] speculated that trephination in this skull was done to treat an infectious process. Certainly, an acute preoperative sinusitis may have

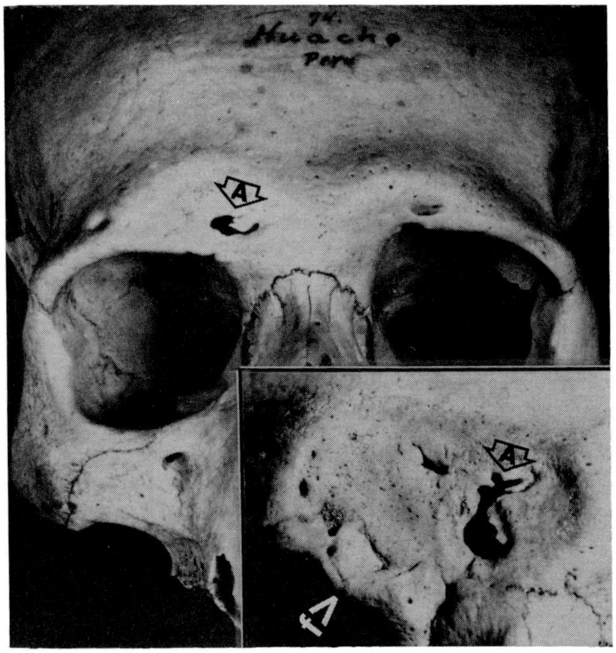

Fig. 4. (Specimen II) Frontal view showing a well-healed trephination of the right frontal sinus (A). Note orbital assymetry. Insert) Close-up view of the findings. Arrow A indicates point of entrance. Arrow f shows fracture-displacement of medial portion of the supraorbital ridge.

occurred but there is no evidence in the specimen to support this. The radiographs show normal scalloping and there are no indications of expansion or diffuse osteitis of the sinus walls. The small area of thickening in the left lateral wall is within one of the osseous cuts and it is probably related to the operation.

An interesting finding is the surgical alteration of the supraorbital foramen. This is highly suggestive that the operator severed, or in some way interfered with, the supraorbital nerve. Since this structure supplies sensation to the soft tissues and periosteum overlying the frontal sinus, such a maneuver would make the bone cuts less painful and indicates some knowledge of neural function by the surgeon. Considerable attention has been given to the use of narcotics, hallucinogens and alcohol as the possible "anesthetic" agents for these procedures.[1] This finding raises the possibility that nerve crushing or section could have been used in conjunction with such drugs to achieve some degree of pain control.

SPECIMEN II

Historic Background. The specimen was collected near Huacho, a coastal town 90 miles north of Lima. Burial sites in this location have revealed many interesting archeological findings among which craniofacial fractures are frequent. The specimen to be described is the only example of trephination discovered at this site. Again, because of looting and scattering of the remains in the area it is not possible to determine accurately the historical age of the specimen. On the basis of the reasons

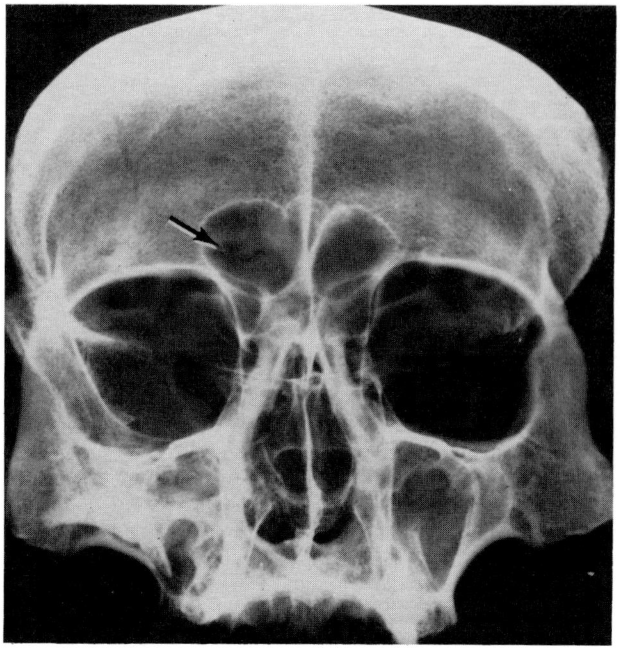

Fig. 5. (Specimen II) Radiograph. Note normal outline of frontal sinuses. Arrow indicates point of penetration into the right sinus.

previously explained for Specimen I it is probably over 600 years old.

Description. This specimen is an incomplete portion of the skull of a male over 30 years of age (Fig. 4). It consists of the fairly well-preserved maxillary and frontal portions of the face. The mandible and upper teeth are missing. Findings are limited to the right frontal sinus and orbit. The bone overlying the sinus shows an irregularly shaped, flattened area 2.7 x 1.5 cm in size. In the center of this area there is a longitudinal opening (0.7 x 0.2 cm) into the right frontal sinus. Several lines of healed fractures are noticed along the superior aspect of the orbital rim, the medial aspect of which is depressed and displaced laterally. The entire area exhibits signs of healing as evidenced by bone regrowth especially noticeable around the edges of the perforation. The inner table of the frontal bone is intact.

Plane radiographs (Fig. 5) show slight depression of the medial aspect of the superior orbital rim. In addition they demonstrate flattening of the anterior wall of the right frontal sinus and an irregular radiolucency representative of the central perforation. Otherwise the outline of the frontal sinuses is normal. The cavities are somewhat small and exhibit little natural scalloping. The nasofrontal ducts are intact.

Comment. This skull is representative of the scraping technique of trephination and it is clear that the changes altering the normal appearance of the right frontal sinus were preceded by an injury. The healed fracture of the superior orbital rim, the depression of this structure and radiographic documentation of these findings are all unrefutable evidences of trauma. It may be argued that the frontal sinus changes are secondary to post-traumatic infection, however, close examination reveals that they are almost certainly surgical. These changes are clearly limited to the anterior wall of the right sinus with avoidance of the anterior cranial fossa. In addition, there is distinct saucerization toward the center of the sinus leading directly into the opening in the anterior wall.

The fact that this is the only trephined specimen encountered in this area is intriguing, however, the possibility exists that the individual in question was operated elsewhere and eventually died at the site. Evidences of active travel during preconquest times are abundant in this valley. The most striking is the finding of seven specimens exhibiting elongation of the skull (Aymara deformation), a practice which in Peru is known to be exclusive of the Andean region. Furthermore, at least three trephination centers are within reach of this area. One, Cerro Trinidad is less than 30 miles from the site, and the important centers of Canta and Ancon are approximately 90 miles distant.

CONCLUSIONS

Three important conclusions may be derived from the study of these specimens:

1. Selective trephination of the frontal sinus was practiced in ancient Peru.

2. The procedure appears to have been directed at the correction of sinus pathology. Localized pain and the treatment of fractures are possible indications for surgery.

3. Supraorbital nerve section or crushing may have been occasionally used to aid in the control of pain during the procedure.

ACKNOWLEDGMENTS — The authors are grateful to Mrs. Rose Tyson, Curator, Physical Anthropology, and to Barton Wright, Scientific Director of the San Diego Museum of Man for their professional assistance and generous help.

REFERENCES

1. Lastres JB, Cabieses F. La trepanacion del craneo en el antiguo Peru. Lima: Universidad Nacional Mayor de San Marcos Press, 1960:123-30, 146-7.

2. Burton FA. Prehistoric trephining of the frontal sinus. Calif Med J 1920; 18:321-4.

3. Moodie RL. Surgery in precolumbian Peru. Studies in Paleophatology XXIII. Ann Med Hist 1929; 6:698-728.

4. Moodie RL. Roentgenologic studies of Egyptian and Peruvian mummies. Anthropology, memoirs vol II. Chicago: Field Museum of Natural History, 1931:31.

≈

PATHOLOGY CONSULTATION

NASAL (SCHNEIDERIAN) PAPILLOMAS

JOHN G. BATSAKIS, MD
PORTLAND, MAINE

The mucosa of the nasal cavity and paranasal sinuses differs from the remainder of the airway system in that it is embryologically derived from *ectoderm*. This uniqueness carries over into the morphogenesis of a controversial group of lesions: *papillomas* of the nasal cavity and sinuses. Controversy surrounding papillomas can be divided into problems relating to: a) nomenclature, b) histopathology, c) biologic behavior, and d) malignant potential.

Nomenclature. Perhaps no group of lesions has acquired so many names since their description.[1] Even papillomas may be inaccurate since the neoplastic nature of the lesions has not been proven. The often-used term, "transitional," carries an unwarranted implication that a histologically specific and identifiable epithelium gives rise to the papilloma. It is an ambiguous term and should be abandoned.[2]

Since the mucosa is embryologically unique, some recognition of this characteristic should be carried in the designation of its tumors. A term carrying that recognition has been used in the past and, while eponymic, clearly identifies the mucosa and lesions derived from it. Schneiderian mucosa and Schneiderian papillomas are suggested as the most suitable alternatives to the numerous synonyms being used.[3] This name honors one of the early investigators, J. V. Schneider, and cannot be confused with any other anatomically located papilloma (Fig. 1).[3]

Histopathology. Schneiderian papillomas arise from a proliferation of reserve or replacement cells of the mucosa. In its fullest expression, this proliferation assumes two basic architectural patterns: inverting, and fungiform or exophytic. Mixtures may also occur.

These two basic forms further segregate by rather specific localization in the upper airway. Fungiform papillomas are nearly restricted to the nasal septum or its environs. Lateral wall and/or sinuses are typical sites of the inverted papilloma (Fig. 2A). Why such a distribution exists is unknown but there are significant implications for biologic activity and the surgeon is cautioned to always provide localization to the pathologist for an accurate assessment of clinical course. Septal papillomas tend to remain localized to the septum and association with carcinoma is very rare. In contrast, lateral wall papillomas are often not restricted to the site, often show sinus involvement or are localized in a sinus, and have a significant association with carcinoma.

The predominant cell type in either the lateral wall or septal papilloma is epidermoid. Vestiges of the overlying epithelium may be found with variable frequency. On occasion, an entire papilloma may be composed of modified columnar epithelium. If so constituted the diagnostic term, cylindrical cell papilloma, has been used.[1]

Biologic Behavior and Malignancy. The major clinical and therapeutic problem with any form of Schneiderian papilloma is recurrence. Recurrences may be multiple and delayed. The rate of recurrence, in major series, has ranged from 28% to 67%.[2] Lateral wall lesions manifest a higher recurrence rate than those of the septum. Extension and/or metaplastic involvement occurs with lateral papillomas (Fig. 2B) but has not been documented from septal papillomas.

Left untreated, papillomas can be locally invasive, especially the lateral lesions. Erosion of bone, and death by local extension is possible.

Ascribing a premalignant quality to Schneiderian papillomas is unwarranted but a patient with a lateral wall papilloma is clearly at risk for the develop-

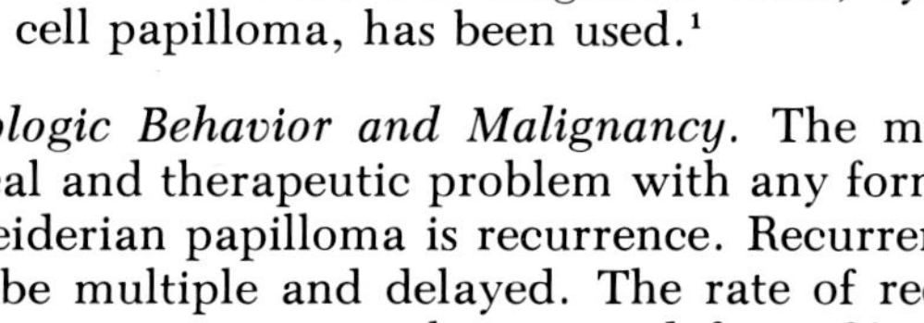

Fig. 1. Schneiderian papillomas arise from ectodermally derived mucosa and yield three histomorphologic varieties. The pure cylindrical cell papilloma is unusual and is predominantly a lateral wall or sinus lesion.

From the Department of Pathology and Laboratory Medicine, Maine Medical Center, Portland, Maine.
REPRINTS — John G. Batsakis, MD, Department of Pathology and Laboratory Medicine, Maine Medical Center, Portland, ME 04102.

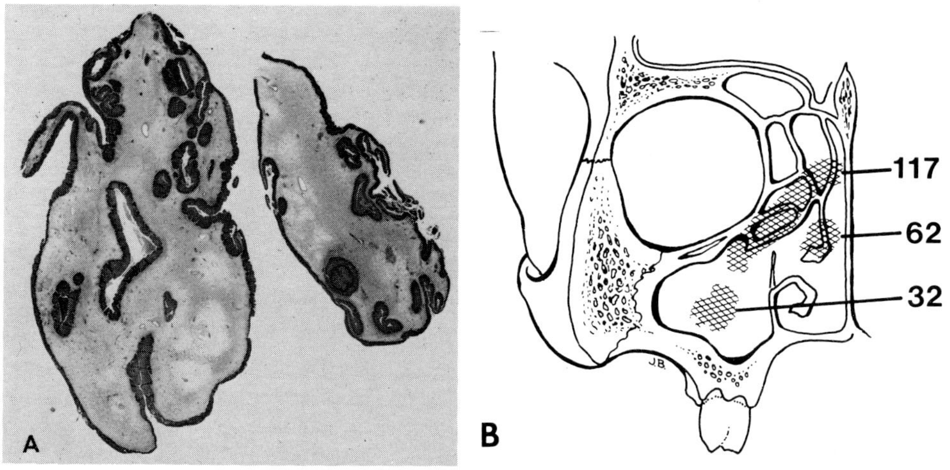

Fig. 2. A) Typical low-power light microscopic appearance of a lateral wall, inverting Schneiderian papilloma. The lack of an inflammatory reaction is typical (H & E, x10). B) Anatomic location of 211 Schneiderian nasal papillomas as derived from the literature. Note the preponderance of papillomas involving both the lateral nasal wall and adjacent sinus.

ment of associated carcinoma. Associated is to be stressed since histologic documentation of the transformation of a papilloma to carcinoma is limited. This event likely represents less than 2% of the reported cases. The usual circumstance is that of squamous cell carcinoma arising in the same anatomic region but without evidence of origin from papilloma. This event is more common and approximates a frequency of 20%.[4]

Treatment is surgical removal with a margin of normal tissue. Lateral wall lesions require inspection of adjacent sinuses. Too-conservative excision is tantamount to recurrent disease. Radiotherapy has no role in the primary management of a Schneiderian papilloma.

SUMMARY

Schneiderian papillomas are unique lesions of the nasal cavity and paranasal sinuses. Most often epidermoid in histologic appearance, the Schneiderian papilloma favors two sites: the septum and lateral wall of the nasal cavity. In both sites recurrences are frequent. Papillomas of the lateral wall, in addition, have a significant association with carcinoma.

REFERENCES

1. Hyams VJ. Papillomas of the nasal cavity and paranasal sinuses: a clinicopathological study of 315 cases. Ann Otol Rhinol Laryngol 1971; 80:192-206.

2. Batsakis JG. Tumors of the head and neck: clinical and pathological considerations. 2nd ed. Baltimore: Williams & Wilkins, 1979:131.

3. Ridolfi RL, Lieberman PH, Erlandson RA, Moore OS. Schneiderian papillomas: a clinicopathologic study of 30 cases. Am J Surg Pathol 1977; 1:43-53.

4. Yamaguchi KT, Shapshay SM, Incze JS, Vaughn CW, Strong S. Inverted papilloma and squamous cell carcinoma. J Otolaryngol 1979; 8:171-8.

X-RAY OF THE MONTH

PLEOMORPHIC ADENOMA OF THE HARD PALATE

ALFRED L. WEBER, MD
BOSTON, MASSACHUSETTS

PATIENT

This 61-year-old male complained of an enlarging palatal mass of several years duration which had been causing his dentures to fit poorly. On examination, a firm centrally ulcerated mass 3 cm in diameter was noted on the left side of the hard palate.

RADIOGRAPHS

The Waters projection (Fig. 1A) demonstrates a hemispherical density (arrow) projecting into the oral cavity on the left. A panorex view (Fig. 1B) reveals a mass (arrow) in the left alveolar ridge with bone displacement. The lateral tomographic section of the hard palate and adjacent floor of the maxillary antrum (Fig. 1C) shows biconcave cortical displacement superiorly with sharply defined bony margins. Note the homogeneous mass projecting into the oral cavity. The AP tomographic section (Fig. 1D) reveals loss of bone and irregularity in the region of the left alveolar ridge, and some loss of

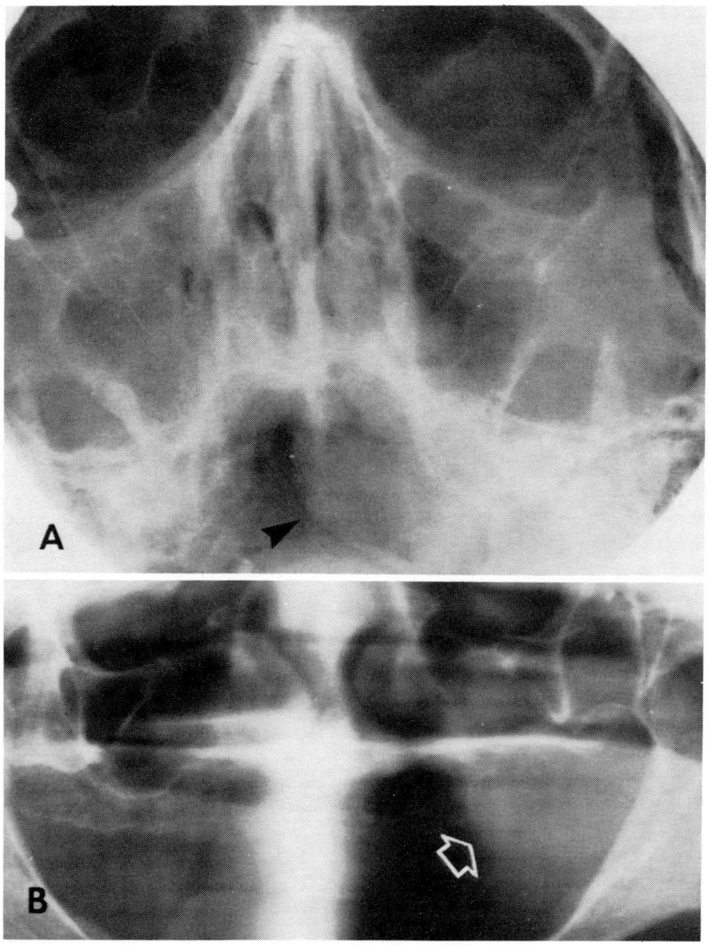

Fig. 1A & B.

From the Department of Radiology, Massachusetts Eye and Ear Infirmary, Boston, Massachusetts.
REPRINTS — Alfred L. Weber, MD, Department of Radiology, Massachusetts Eye and Ear Infirmary, 243 Charles St., Boston, MA 02114.

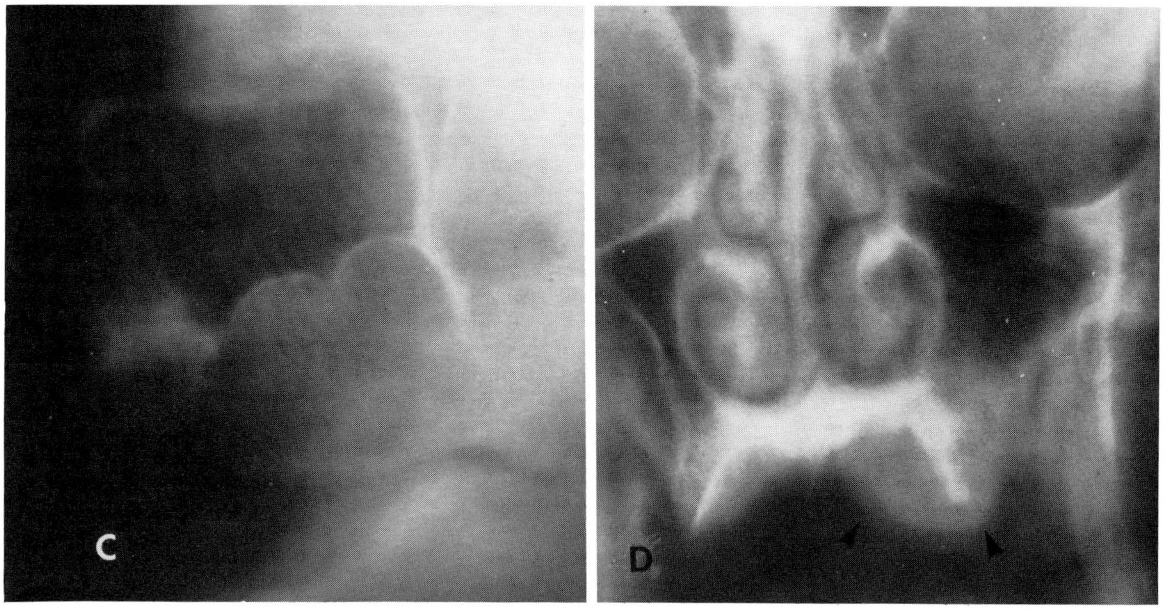

Fig. 1C & D.

bone in the floor of the left antrum. Note the slightly increased soft tissue density in the lowermost portion of the left antrum. The transverse extent projecting into the oral cavity is well delineated in this view (arrows).

DIAGNOSIS

Biopsy revealed pleomorphic adenoma. At surgery the tumor mass was found to have infiltrated the overlying mucosa and extended into the inferior portion of the left maxillary antrum. The tumor with its extension was totally excised.

DISCUSSION

Minor salivary glands are present throughout the oral cavity and adjacent structures of the head and neck. Tumors of the minor salivary glands account for approximately 18% of all salivary gland tumors.[1] The most common location of minor salivary gland tumors, either benign or malignant, is the palate.[1]

Although tumors of the palate may also originate from the oral epithelium and from the connective tissues beneath, about 44% of palatal tumors arose in the minor salivary glands in the series reported by Hjertman and Eneroth.[2] In this series, 56% of the salivary gland tumors of the palate were benign; all these were pleomorphic adenoma, also called mixed tumors. The predominant types of malignant tumors were mucoepidermoid carcinoma and adenoid cystic carcinoma.[2]

Intraoral pleomorphic adenomas appear as slow-growing, painless masses. They are usually encapsulated tumors located deep in the submucosa. Ulceration is rare and, if present, is likely to be due to denture trauma. If the mixed tumor is not completely enucleated, it may recur.[3]

Mixed tumors contain mesodermal and ectodermal elements, although they may vary greatly in histologic appearance.[3] In a small number of cases, a benign pleomorphic adenoma may degenerate into a malignant mixed tumor.[3]

Roentgenographically, benign pleomorphic adenomas may demonstrate osseous involvement of the hard palate. Benign lesions of the hard palate do not invade the bone, but the expanding tumor can cause a recess to form in the alveolar bone due to pressure resorption.[3] Radiographically, a malignant tumor shows bone erosion with poorly defined margins and lucent mottling. In the case of a mixed tumor, however, the interfacc between the normal hard palate and the region of osseous involvement by the radiolucent tumor is sharply defined by cortical bone, and the edges of the bony defect may be beveled upward.[3] On some occasions, the tumor may perforate the bone and extend into the adjacent nasal cavity or maxillary antrum. A soft tissue mass may project into the oral cavity.

ACKNOWLEDGMENT — Special thanks to Paula R. Griswold for her assistance in preparing this case.

REFERENCES

1. Frable WJ, Elzay RP. Tumors of minor salivary glands. Cancer 1970; 25:932.

2. Hjertman L, Eneroth CM. Tumors of the palate. Acta Otolaryngol (Stockh) 1970; 263:179.

3. Pinto RS, Kelly DE, George AE. Radiologic features of benign pleomorphic adenoma of the hard palate. Oral Surg 1975; 39:976.

ENG OF THE MONTH

VESTIBULO-OCULAR AND OCULOMOTOR RESPONSES FOLLOWING BRAINSTEM CEREBROVASCULAR ACCIDENT

PAUL KILENY, PhD A. F. WILSON, MD

EDMONTON, ALBERTA, CANADA

CASE REPORT

A 73-year-old female was admitted with a sudden onset of vertigo and emesis. She had collapsed with a brief loss of consciousness at the onset of the symptoms. There was no past history of blackouts, headaches, vertigo, or hearing difficulties. The patient was hypertensive on admission with a blood pressure of 230/130. Her pulse was 88 and regular. She was vertiginous with an ataxic gait. No nystagmus was evident. Diplopia was present enhanced by left lateral gaze with a paresis of abduction of the left eye. A left neck bruit was audible. Skull x-rays, EEG, ECG and CT scan of the head were considered normal. Cerebral angiography showed minimal luminal irregularities at the origins of both carotid arteries. The basilar artery appeared normal. The patient was considered to have suffered from a small brainstem pontine stroke. She was treated symptomatically for control of the vertigo. The vertigo and diplopia subsided within 24 hours of admission to the hospital.

Audiological and vestibular examinations were performed on May 17, 1979, six days following the vertiginous episode. At this time the patient reported that vertigo had not recurred since the night of admission, and it appeared that the paresis of abduction of the left eye had resolved. Audiometric examination revealed a mild symmetrical bilateral hearing loss, bilateral speech reception thresholds of 35 dB, and good speech discrimination (92%, AD; 96%, AS). Tone decay and acoustic reflex decay test results were unremarkable. Brainstem audiometry suggested normal and symmetrical I-V interwave intervals bilaterally (4.08 msec). Tympanometry suggested normal middle ear function bilaterally and acoustic reflexes were elicited bilaterally at relatively low sensation levels.

Electronystagmographic vestibular examination did not reveal any spontaneous, latent, or positional nystagmus. A slight overshoot in ocular calibration was noted (Fig. 1, top trace). Smooth pursuit eye movements (pendulum tracking) were grossly broken up and disorganized both for the right and the left eye (Fig. 1). Caloric nystagmus was absent bilaterally with eyes closed both to 5 and 10 ml ice water. With visual fixation a slight caloric nystagmus became apparent (Fig. 2).

A second vestibular examination was performed three weeks later (June 12, 1979). At this time ocular calibration was free of overshoot and a marked improvement in pendulum tracking was noted bilaterally as shown in Figure 1 (traces labelled Jun. 12/79). Caloric nystagmus was present bilaterally with eyes closed; however there was no evidence of visual fixation suppression (Fig. 2, middle trace).

The vestibular examination was repeated for a third time 5½ months following the initial vertiginous episode. None of the initial symptoms have recurred during this time. The voluntary eye movements — ocular calibration and pendulum tracking —manifested further improvement (Fig. 1, bottom trace). Visual fixation suppression of caloric nystagmus was still absent, and the caloric nystagmus was characterized by dysrhythmia (Fig. 2, bottom trace labelled Nov. 28/79).

DISCUSSION

Patients suffering from hypertensive cerebral vascular disease are known to have pathological involvement of the small intercerebral arteries and arterials in addition to accelerated atherosclerotic changes in the major vessels. This patient did not demonstrate any significant major vessel disease and by exclusion was presumed to have had small vessel disease involving the brainstem, probably in the lateral pontine region. Her clinical findings indicated a dysfunction in the brainstem with rapid recovery of the major disabling symptoms.

Failure of visual fixation suppression of postcaloric nystagmus is usually associated with CNS disease, especially posterior fossa pathology.[1,2] Thus, this phenomenon has been reported to occur with spinocerebellar degeneration, cerebellopontine angle lesions, cerebellitis, and vertebrobasilar artery insufficiency.[3] Furthermore, visual fixation suppression of vestibular nystagmus is lost following bilateral destruction of the cerebellar flocculus.[4]

From the Department of Speech Pathology-Audiology, Glenrose Hospital, Edmonton, Alberta, Canada.

REPRINTS — P. Kileny, PhD, Speech Pathology-Audiology Department, Glenrose Hospital, 10230 111th Avenue, Edmonton, Alberta, Canada T5G 0B7.

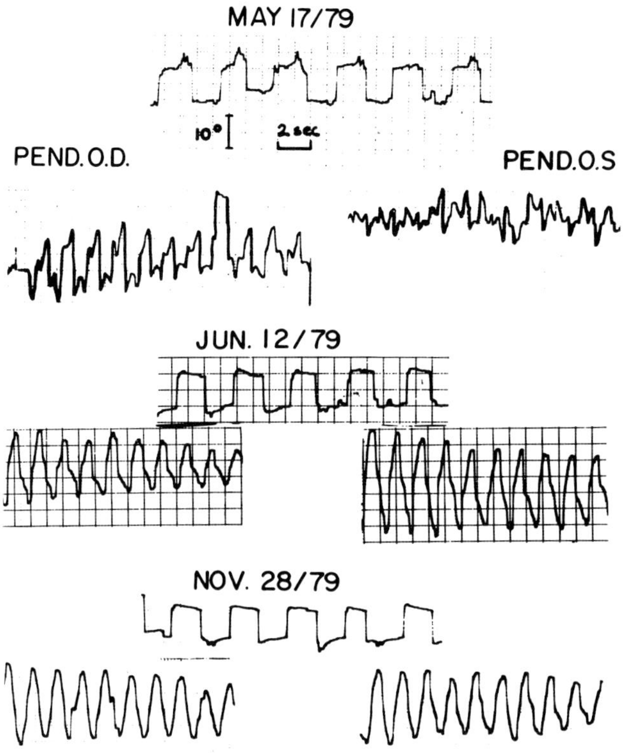

Fig. 1. Ocular calibration and pendulum tracking recordings six days (May 17/79), three weeks (Jun. 12/79) and 5½ months (Nov. 28/79) following our patient's vertiginous episode. Pend. O.D. (left hand column) - Right eye tracking; Pend. O.S. (right hand column) - Left eye tracking.

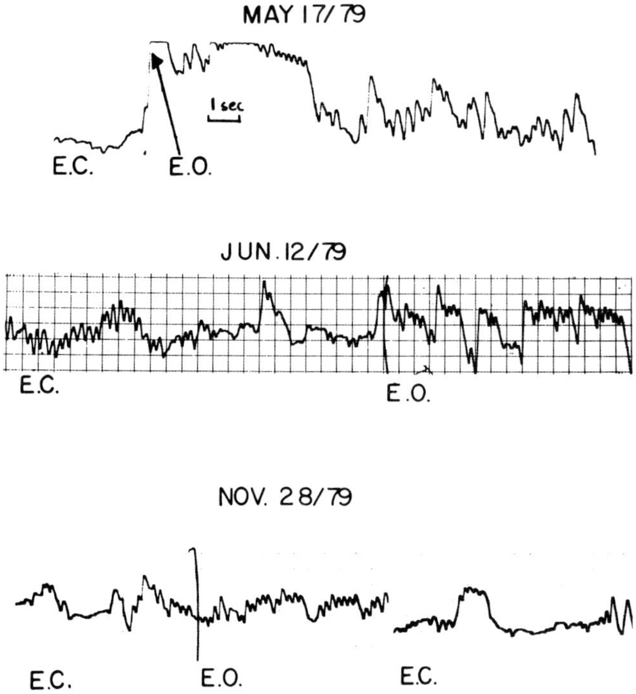

Fig. 2. Nystagmus responses to 5 cm^3 ice water calorics delivered to the left ear of the patient. Identical patterns were obtained following right ear irrigation (not shown). E.C. - Eyes closed; E.O. - Eyes open, fixating a light source.

Disorders of pursuit eye movements have also been associated with brainstem disease.[5] Smooth pursuit deficiencies are most prevalent with cerebellopontine angle tumors, cerebellar atrophy, basal ganglia disease, and vertebrobasilar insufficiency.[6] The accuracy of saccadic eye movements, as in ocular calibration, is mostly affected by cerebellar lesions.[6]

Our patient presented initially with several oculomotor and vestibuloocular phenomena commonly associated with CNS involvement: marked bilateral breakup of pendulum tracking (ie, smooth pursuit eye movements), a small but consistent calibration overshoot (ie, saccadic dysmetria) and absence of caloric nystagmus with removal of visual fixation. These aberrations were present at a time, six days following the initial episode, when the patient was essentially asymptomatic. Both ocular calibration and pendulum tracking returned to normal on subsequent examinations. The most dramatic recovery was noted in pendulum tracking. However, although caloric nystagmus was obtained on subsequent occasions with eyes closed up to 5½ months following the initial episode, visual fixation failed to suppress the postcaloric nystagmus.

Several conclusions may be derived from this case. Smooth pursuit eye movements are extremely sensitive to conditions affecting the brainstem. Although, according to the literature, there is overlap between sites of lesions documented to affect smooth pursuit eye movements and the visual fixation mechanism,[3,5] this case clearly demonstrates that one may remain impaired while the other recovers completely. Visual suppression of vestibular nystagmus probably results from the inhibitory effect of the cerebellar flocculus on vestibular nuclei.[7] This inhibitory effect appears to be activated by visual input mediated through the inferior olive[8] or the superior colliculus.[9] Our patient demonstrated lack of visual fixation in the absence of any other indication of active CNS or particularly cerebellar disease.

ACKNOWLEDGMENT — Chet DesRochers, MS, performed some of the preliminary testing on this patient.

REFERENCES

1. Hart CW. The ocular fixation index. Ann Otol Rhinol Laryngol 1973; 82:848-51.

2. Alpert JN. Failure of fixation suppression: a pathologic effect of vision on caloric nystagmus. Neurology (Minneap) 1974; 24:891-6.

3. Takemori S. Visual suppression test. Ann Otol Rhinol Laryngol 1977; 86:80-5.

4. Takemori S, Cohen B. Visual suppression of vestibular nystagmus in rhesus monkeys. Brain Res 1974; 72:203-19.

5. Correra J, Torres-Courtney G, Lopez-Rios B. Neurotological significance of alterations of pursuit eye movements and the pendular eye tracking test. Ann Otol Rhinol Laryngol 1973; 82:855-67.

6. Baloh RW, Honrubia V, Sills A. Eye tracking and optokinetic nystagmus: results of quantitative testing in patients with well-defined nervous system lesions. Ann Otol Rhinol Laryngol 1977; 86:108-14.

7. Ito M, Highstein SM, Fukuda J. Cerebellar inhibition of the vestibular-ocular reflex in rabbit and cat and its blockage by picrotoxin. Brain Res 1970; 17:524.

8. Alley K, Baker R, Simpson JI. Afferents to the vestibulocerebellum and the origin of the visual climbing fibers in the rabbit. Brain Res 1975; 98:582-90.

9. Kato I, Kawasa KT, Aoyago M, Sato Y, Mizukoshi K. Loss of visual suppression of caloric nystagmus in cats. Acta Otolaryngol (Stockh) 1979; 87:499-505.

≈

NINCDS NOTES*

Four new members were recently appointed to the National Advisory Neurological and Communicative Disorders and Stroke Council (NANCDS). The new appointees are: Dr. Guy M. McKhann, professor and chairman of the Department of Neurology at the Johns Hopkins University School of Medicine; Father Robert P. Hupp, executive director of Father Flanagan's Boys' Home in Nebraska; Dr. Michael M. Paparella, professor and chairman of the Department of Otolaryngology at the University of Minnesota Medical School; and Dr. Juan M. Taveras, radiologist-in-chief at Massachusetts General Hospital in Boston. The new appointees will serve until November 1984.

Dr. Murray Goldstein, deputy director of the Institute since 1978, will head NINCDS during the transition period between the February 1 retirement of Dr. Donald B. Tower and the appointment of a permanent director. Dr. Katherine L. Bick, previously deputy director of the NINCDS Neurological Disorders Program, will temporarily assume Dr. Goldstein's former position. Drs. Goldstein and Bick will continue in their new positions until a permanent Institute director is named. A search committee, under the guidance of NIH deputy director Dr. Thomas E. Malone, is now reviewing candidates for the position.

A Spanish-language edition of NINCDS's fact sheet on autism is now available on request from the Institute's Office of Scientific and Health Reports. The pamphlet describes possible causes, symptoms, treatments, and present areas of investigation for the developmental disability, which affects families of all racial, ethnic, and social backgrounds. The publication is the first of several new Institute pamphlets designed to inform the Hispanic community about neurological and communicative disorders. Spanish-language pamphlets on cerebral palsy and epilepsy are now in production. To obtain copies of "Autismo," contact the Office of Scientific and Health Reports, NINCDS, 9000 Rockville Pike, Bethesda, MD 20205; telephone (301) 496-5751.

*This information is prepared monthly by the Office of Scientific and Health Reports, National Institute of Neurological and Communicative Disorders and Stroke, National Institutes of Health, Bldg. 31, Rm. 8A06, Bethesda, MD 20205, (301) 496-5751.

OSTEOGENESIS IMPERFECTA TARDA AND OTOSCLEROSIS
A TEMPORAL BONE HISTOPATHOLOGY REPORT

ISAMU SANDO, MD, DMS
PITTSBURGH, PENNSYLVANIA

DAVID MYERS, MD
PHILADELPHIA, PENNSYLVANIA

TAKEHIKO HARADA, MD
PITTSBURGH, PENNSYLVANIA

RAUL HINOJOSA, MD
CHICAGO, ILLINOIS

EUGENE N. MYERS, MD
PITTSBURGH, PENNSYLVANIA

The histopathology of the temporal bones in a 59-year-old female with osteogenesis imperfecta tarda (OIT), complicated by otosclerosis, is presented. Advanced conduction and sensorineural deafness in the left ear and absence of a response to sound in the right ear had been recorded before she died and the temporal bones were acquired for histological study. Histopathological examination revealed a marked degree of porosity of the labyrinthine capsule, enlarged vascular spaces, and a deficiency in number and size of bony trabeculae in the marrow of the petrous apex. All layers of the otic capsule had been extensively replaced by otosclerotic material including the bony semicircular canals and the cochlear and vestibular walls. In the right ear, which had a profound hearing loss, the outline of the space which had been occupied by a piston prosthesis in the oval window was evident; in addition, a layer of new bone (labyrinthitis ossificans) was present in the scala tympani in the region of the round window. In the left ear the stapedial footplate was otosclerotic with the base of the crura slightly displaced but fixed in the window. The severity of the OIT in this case was demonstrated by the patient's history of repeated fractures, marked porosity of the nonotosclerotic areas of the labyrinthine capsule, and possibly by the female's relatively early death at age 59. The unique features of the otosclerosis in this case were the extensive replacement of all layers of the cochlear and vestibular capsules and the relatively large areas of an osteoporotic type of degeneration in the more central areas of the otosclerotic bone. While the etiology of otosclerosis remains unknown it is apparent that both the incidence and severity of the disorder as it occurs in association with OIT bear some as yet unknown but definite relationship to the pathologies occurring with OIT.

INTRODUCTION

Osteogenesis imperfecta (OI) is a generalized disorder of connective tissue. It involves the skeletal system, ligaments, tendons, fascia, and sclera, and in a high percentage of cases produces impairment of hearing. The first known description of the disorder has been credited to Malbranche[1] in 1694. Since then different authors have described the disease, naming it mollities ossium,[2] fragilitas ossium,[3] and osteopsathyrosis idiopathica.[4]

The term osteogenesis imperfecta was first used by Vrolik[5] in 1849. Looser[6] defended the double identity of the disease, defining that occurring in newborns as osteogenesis imperfecta congenita (OIC) and that occurring in adults as osteogenesis imperfecta tarda (OIT). The OIC type was usually fatal in utero or in early infancy, while the OIT type did not necessarily shorten the average life span.

The conductive deafness beginning usually in early adult life, which was frequently seen in association with OI, was recognized as being due to otosclerosis early in the 20th century. Adair-Dighton[7] in 1912 had described deafness in patients with blue sclera and multiple fractures. The first published report of otosclerosis associated with OI is credited to van der Hoeve and de Kleyn.[8] In addition to cases in which typical indications of otosclerosis were found in conjunction with OIT they also presented four patients who had OIT and a nonprogressive, conductive type of hearing impairment that had been present since infancy. Zajtchuk and Lindsay[9] report having seen newly fractured stapedial crura hemorrhaging into the middle ear in infants with OIC at the time of birth. These fractures apparently may occur when development of the tympanic ring is insufficient to protect the middle ear from external pressure exerted during passage through the birth canal. Such fractures probably explain moderate but nonprogressive conductive hearing impairments present since infancy.

During World War I Fraser in Edinburgh did a clinical study of the inheritance of OIT and otosclerosis which was reported by Bronson.[10] The extensive study of this disease by Bell[11] produced pedigrees of a large number of patients with blue sclera, fragile bones, and otosclerosis. The hereditary nature of OI is said to have been recognized as early as 1833 by Lobstein.[4] Accumulated evidence indicated that OIT is inherited as an autosomal dominant. However, OIC has also been found in

From the Departments of Otolaryngology and Pathology, University of Pittsburgh School of Medicine, Eye and Ear Hospital, Pittsburgh, and the Division of Otolaryngology, Department of Surgery, University of Chicago School of Medicine, Chicago. This study was supported by NS 13787-02 from the National Institute of Neurological and Communicative Diseases and Strokes.

REPRINTS — Isamu Sando, MD, Division of Otopathology, Department of Otolaryngology, University of Pittsburgh School of Medicine, 230 Lothrop Street, Pittsburgh, PA 15213.

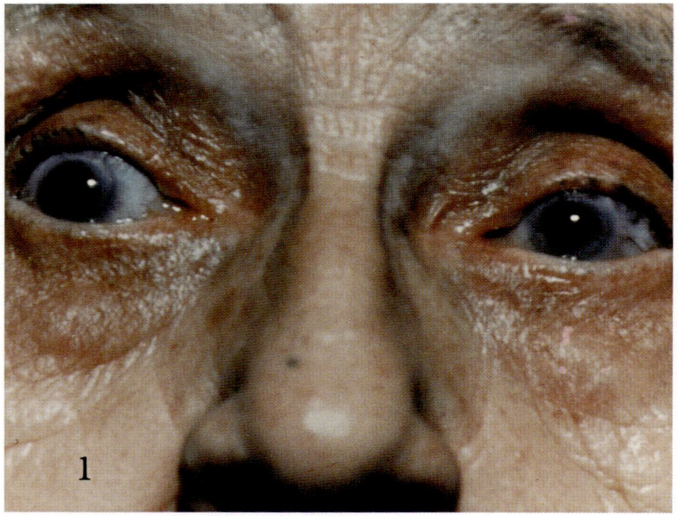

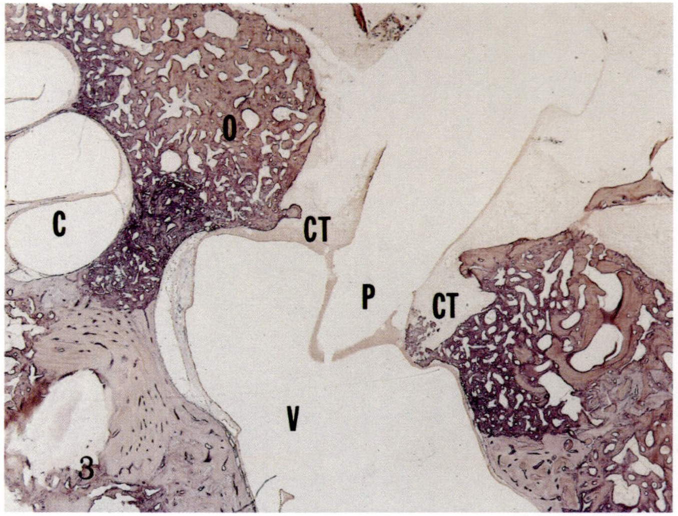

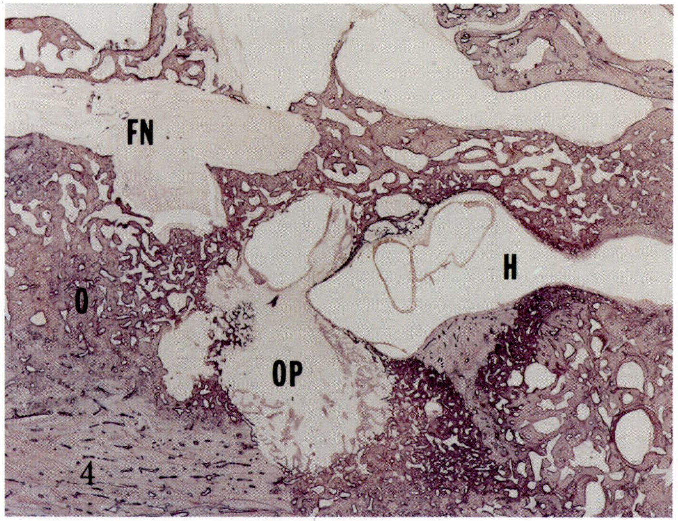

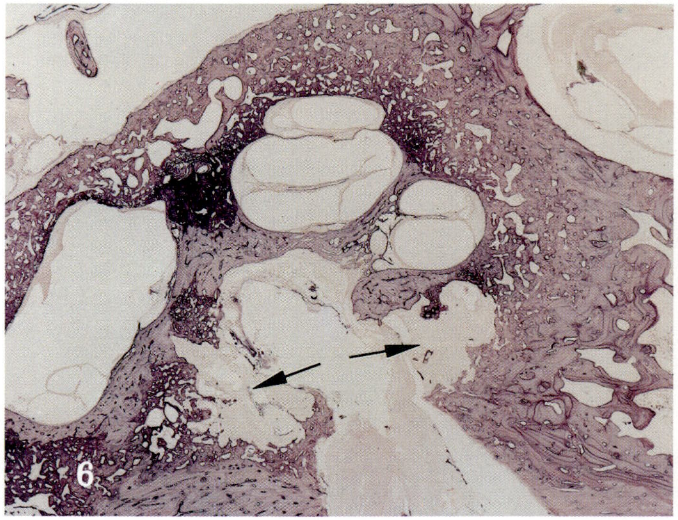

Fig. 1. Blue sclerae associated with osteogenesis imperfecta.

Fig. 3. Right ear. The oval window area is sealed by the connective tissues (CT) which surround the area of the piston prosthesis (P). Dense, homogenous, eosinophilic materials cover the surface of the top portion of the prosthesis which is protruded into the vestibule. C - Cochlea; O - Otosclerotic focus; V - Vestibule. (H & E)

Fig. 4. Right ear. Severe otosclerotic foci (O) surround osteoporotic areas (OP). FN - Geniculate ganglion of the facial nerve; H - Horizontal canal crista. (H & E)

Fig. 6. Left ear. Severe otosclerotic foci and osteoporotic areas (arrows) are seen at the fundus of the internal auditory meatus. (H & E) children of parents with no sign of the disease.[12] Otosclerosis also exhibits an autosomal dominant type of heredity with variable expressivity. McKusick[13] has pointed out that OI (OIC and OIT) is either a single entity with variations in severity and manifestations or consists of multiple distinct entities. Altmann,[14] in discussing the relationship between OIC and OIT, favored different degrees of deficiency in collagen formation as the basis for the two varieties of OI. More recent investigations have demonstrated alterations in collagen metabolism in certain heritable diseases of man, mainly the Ehlers-Danlos syndrome and OI. These have been reviewed by McKusick and Martin.[15] The estimated incidence of otosclerosis in large series of OIT cases studied has varied from 28.7%[16] to 60%.[11]

The first report of the histopathology of a temporal bone which demonstrated otosclerosis was made by Ruttin.[17] There are many histopathological reports of stapes removed at surgery which were otosclerotic. The crura have frequently been noted during surgery to be fragile. Opheim[18] has contended that fibrous degeneration of the crura may be a cause of impairment of hearing. However, in the absence of evidence that the onset of the impairment had occurred later than early childhood, fractures of the crura during birth must be considered as the cause.

The purpose of this study is to present the histopathological findings in an unusually advanced case of otosclerosis associated with OIT. The characteristics of the otosclerosis in this case are in striking contrast to those reported recently by Zajtchuk and Lindsay[9] and by Bretlau et al.[19]

CASE REPORT

A 52-year-old white female was first examined by a colleague in 1962, when she complained of bilateral hearing loss of 34 years' duration in the right ear and of somewhat shorter duration in the left ear. She also complained of tinnitus bilaterally but did not complain of vertigo. Further history revealed that she had suffered frequent fractures of the long bones. The physical examination showed that she had blue sclera (Fig. 1) but the remainder of the examination of the head and neck showed no other abnormalities. Audiologic tests revealed a profound hearing loss in the right ear with no air or bone conduction, and a severe combined loss of 80 dB (International Standards Organization) in the left ear. The diagnosis of van der Hoeve's syndrome was made.

The patient's pedigree, covering five generations, was studied (Fig. 2). Of five siblings of the patient, only one was normal. Typical stigmata of van der Hoeve's syndrome appeared in one of the patient's younger sisters.

Surgery on the patient's right ear was performed by D. Myers, MD, in October 1962. A dense, white lesion obliterating the area of the oval window was noted. An opening was drilled in the center of this abnormal stapes footplate and a piston and fat-graft prosthesis were inserted. One year after the operation the patient still had improved hearing on the operated side.

In February 1964, surgery was performed on the left ear. A thick stapes footplate was noted. This was removed; a silicone piston was inserted. Postoperatively the patient's air conduction score improved and there was closure of the air-bone gap, but the last audiogram, taken in May 1966, showed a severe bilateral sensorineural hearing loss. Three years later, in 1969, the patient died of a cerebrovascular accident at the age of 59.

The patient's temporal bones were obtained at autopsy and immediately placed in fixation solution. After decalcification and dehydration they were embedded in celloidin. Sections of 20 μ were cut in the horizontal plane, and every tenth section was stained with hematoxylin and eosin for light microscopic study. Collagen fibers of the bony tissue were studied under polarized light.

HISTOPATHOLOGIC FINDINGS

Only the outlines of the membranous labyrinths of these temporal bones could be distinguished, the nerves, vessels and most soft tissue elements having been destroyed by accidental drying of the specimens. The bony elements of both ears were preserved but the cellular contents of the marrow spaces were lost to study.

RIGHT TEMPORAL BONE

Middle Ear. The malleus and incus are present but show an excessive number of large spaces for vessels and soft tissue. The bony elements show no apparent abnormality. The stapes shows the outline of a central space which had been occupied by a piston prosthesis, the point reaching into the vestibule (Fig. 3). The margins of the footplate consist of irregular otosclerotic bone fixed to the otosclerotic margins of the oval window.

Otic Capsule. The bone of the otic capsule has been extensively replaced by otosclerosis. Diffuse otosclerotic bone occupies almost the entire cochlear capsule, including periosteal, endochondral and endosteal layers except for a few small areas where the original capsular bone remains. The inner layer of the otosclerotic bone is actively basophilic and highly cellular. This layer envelops the posterior semicircular canal extensively, replacing both the endochondral and endosteal layers. The other canals are involved to a lesser extent. The periosteal layer of the capsule is mainly occupied by acidophilic, less cellular, but more compact otosclerotic bone. In the outer layer of the capsule, beyond the dense otosclerotic bone, are many vascular spaces, the soft tissue contents of which are not clear, but some of these are lined by a layer of apparently otosclerotic bone. The basal part of the cochlear capsule surrounding the internal meatus shows a broad dehiscence of the otosclerotic bone which had apparently occupied that area. This osteoporotic area within the otosclerotic base of the cochlea shows gradual thinning of the surrounding margins by reabsorption of the remaining otosclerotic bone. A similar large, degenerated osteoporotic area is located also between the geniculate ganglion and the superior semicircular canal ampulla (Fig. 4). Surrounding margins of this otosclerotic bone show marked thinning of trabeculae.

Inner Ear. Postmortem artifacts in all soft-tissue

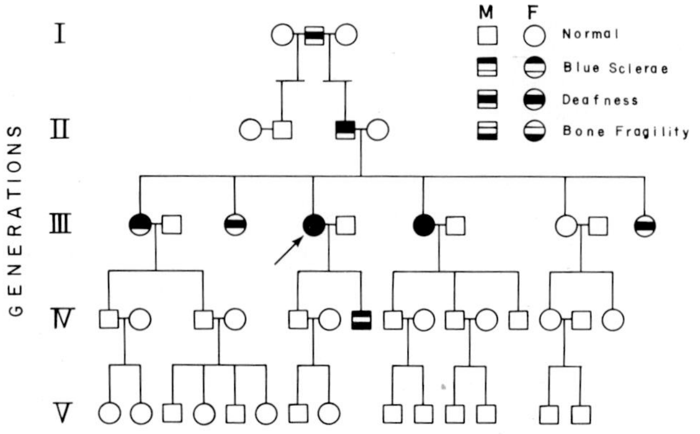

Fig. 2. Pedigree covering five generations of a female with van der Hoeve's syndrome.

structures prevented their evaluation. The only observation which can be made is that the membranous labyrinth had been present. There is a thin layer of newly formed, nonotosclerotic bone (labyrinthitis ossificans) along the posteroinferior bony wall of the scala tympani adjoining the round window. Extensive otosclerosis occupies the walls on all sides of the basal coil in the round window region, but without obstructing the round window membrane.

Internal Auditory Meatus. A broad osteoporotic area borders on the internal auditory meatus at its inner end, surrounded by otosclerotic bone. It was not possible to evaluate the state of the seventh and eighth cranial nerves because of the postmortem injury to all soft-tissue components.

LEFT TEMPORAL BONE

Middle Ear. The malleus and incus show marked porosity, similar to that seen in the right ear. The head and upper portions of the stapedial crura are absent. The footplate and approximately the lower third of each crus are present and consist of otosclerotic bone; the footplate is fixed to the otosclerotic bone surrounding the oval window. The indistinct outline of the position occupied by the prosthesis which had replaced the head and upper parts of the stapedial crura is apparent. The surgical aperture which had been made for the prosthesis is outlined in the otosclerotic footplate. A few mastoid air cells were included in the specimen; they had apparently contained fluid, but there is no evidence of infection.

Otic Capsule. The outer layers of periosteal bone show extensive development of vascular spaces (Fig. 5). The extent of otosclerotic bone in endosteal, endochondral, and deeper periosteal layers is similar to that seen on the right side. A broad area of complete degeneration of the otosclerotic bone, similar to that seen in the opposite ear, is present (Fig. 6). Within this degenerated or osteoporotic area is a fairly extensive patch of what appears to be faintly stained osteoid tissue.

Inner Ear. A few cells, apparently osteoblasts,

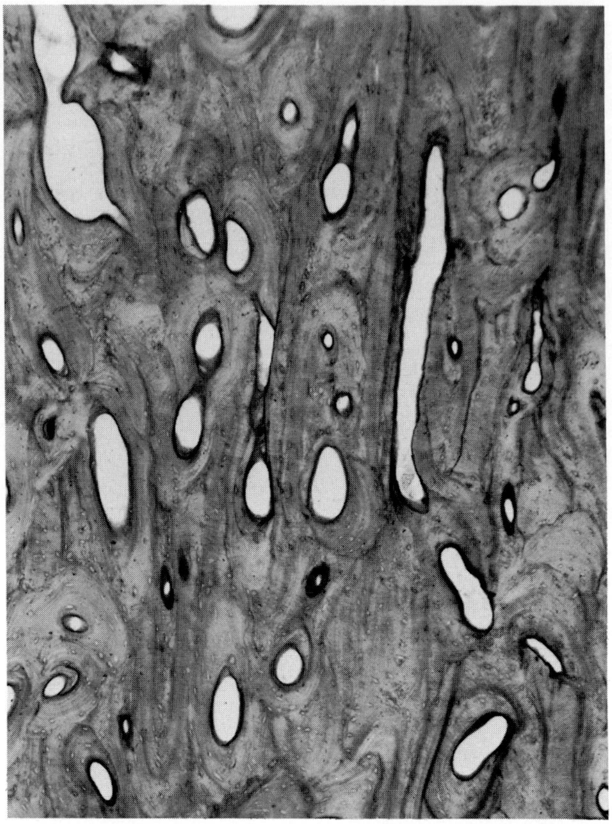

Fig. 5. Left ear. Numerous vascular spaces are seen in the periosteal bone of the otic capsule where no otosclerotic lesions are present. (H & E, x77)

were faintly observed within this tissue. The membranous labyrinth and nerves had been present and were apparently normal. The fluid spaces appear to be clear and undistorted. However, the interscalar septum between the apical and middle coils of the cochlea was fractured (premortem) (Fig. 6).

DISCUSSION

The extent and activity of the otosclerotic process in these bones was extreme bilaterally throughout both cochlear and vestibular parts of the capsules. The large osteoporotic areas in the more central parts of the otosclerotic bone are apparently unique; although small areas of this type have been seen before, even temporal bones from individuals of advanced age have not been observed to contain such large areas.

In this and in other recently reported cases[9,19] it appears that there is a direct relationship between the degree of otosclerotic change in the otic capsule and the severity of the OIT as determined by skeletal abnormalities and the frequency of fractures.

While recent investigations have indicated that variable defects in collagen are responsible for certain disorders of connective tissue, including the Ehlers-Danlos syndrome, Marfan's syndrome, and OI,[15] the etiologic factor in otosclerosis is not known. Specimens of otosclerotic bone frequently became available as a result of surgical procedures to restore hearing, but they have only been partially studied.

It is apparent that in the patient with OIT the amount of bone tissue in the temporal bone is deficient. We feel that this is due to failure of this bone to develop, as indicated by the presence of numerous enlarged vascular spaces (Fig. 5), and by the increased widths of the internal meatus and carotid canal.[9] However, this lack of bony development appears to be of less significance in the function of the ear than the decidedly brittle nature of the bony mastoid partitions, which became obvious with exenteration of the mastoid during fenestration surgery.[9] The lack of strength of the bone tissue formed in patients with OIT usually becomes most apparent in the tendency of the long bones to fracture. There are no microscopic indications that the bone formed in patients with this disorder is subject to abnormally active resorption.

In contrast to the cause of bone development characteristic of OI, otosclerosis is limited, with rare exceptions, to the otic capsule. It appears first in the deep layers of the capsule, mainly in the endochrondral layer or the closely adjoining periosteal bone. These layers are subjected to the processes involved in growth of the skull only to a minor degree.

Otosclerosis has a marked predilection for occurring in the area of the oval window or the round window, and to a lesser extent near the internal auditory meatus. It is transmitted mainly as a dominant autosomal disorder with variable expressivity. The incidence of otosclerosis is indefinite inasmuch as it is known to occur in a percentage of otherwise normal, asymptomatic temporal bones.

Both OI and otosclerosis demonstrate extreme variability in the incidence and severity of these pathologic processes. While the frequent association of the two diseases and their similarity in extent and severity in given cases suggest an etiologic relationship, there is no further evidence of a common pathologic process.

ACKNOWLEDGMENTS — The authors wish to express their deep gratitude to Professor John R. Lindsay, MD, Division of Otolaryngology, Department of Surgery, University of Chicago School of Medicine, for encouraging them to study this subject and for giving helpful criticism during the preparation of this study. The authors are also grateful to Eduardo Yunis, MD, for his consultation and Reisuke Saito, MD, Department of Pathology, University of Pittsburgh School of Medicine, for helping in the evaluation of the pathological findings; and to Ruth Anderson for her kind assistance in this study.

REFERENCES

1. Malbranche, 1694, cited by Friedman I. Pathology of the ear. Oxford: Blackwell, 1974:227.

2. Ormerod EL. An account of a case of mollities ossium. Br Med J 1859; 2:732-40.

3. Gurlt E. Handbuch der Lehre von den Knochenbrunchen, vol 1. Hamm: G Grote, 1862-1865:147-54.

4. Lobstein JF. Traité d'anatomie pathologique. Paris: FG Levrault, 1833:204.

5. Vrolik W. Tabulae ad illustrandum embryogenesium hominis et mammalium, tam naturalem quam abnormen. Lipsiae: T. O. Weigel, 1954.

6. Looser E. Zur Kenntnis der Osteogenesis imperfecta congenita und tarda (sogenanntae idiopathische Osteopsthyrosis). Mitt Granzgeb Med Chir 1906; 15:161-207.

7. Adair-Dighton CA. Four generations of blue sclerotics. Ophthalmoscope 1912; 10:188-9.

8. Van der Hoeve J, de Kleyn A. Blauwe sclera, brooscheid van het beenstelsel en gehoorstoornissen. Ned Tijdschr Geneeskd 1917; 13:1003-10.

9. Zajtchuk JT, Lindsay JR. Osteogenesis imperfecta congenita and tarda: a temporal bone report. Ann Otol Rhinol Laryngol 1975; 84:350-8.

10. Bronson E. On fragilitas ossium and its association with blue sclerotics and otosclerosis. Edinburgh Med J 1917; 18: 240-81.

11. Bell J. Blue sclerotic and fragility of bone. In: Pearson K, ed. The treasury of human inheritance, vol 2, pt 3. London: Cambridge University Press, 1928:269-324.

12. Seedorff KS. Osteogenesis imperfecta: a study of clinical features and heredity based on 55 Danish families comprising 180 affected persons. Copenhagen: Ejnar Munksgaard, 1949.

13. McKusick VA. Heritable disorders of connective tissue. 4th ed. St. Louis; C.V. Mosby, 1972:390-454.

14. Altmann F. The temporal bone in osteogenesis imperfecta congenita: a contribution to the question of the etiology of otosclerosis. Arch Otolaryngol 1962; 75:486-97.

15. McKusick VA, Martin GR. Molecular defects in collagen. Ann Intern Med 1975; 82:585-6.

16. Stoller FM. The ear in osteogenesis imperfecta. Laryngoscope 1962; 72:855-69.

17. Ruttin E. Osteopsathyrose and otosclerose. Arch Ohren-Nasen- Kehlkopfheilkd 1922-1923; 3-4:263-79.

18. Opheim O. Loss of hearing following the syndrome of van der Hoeve-de Kleyn. Acta Otolaryngol (Stockh) 1968; 65:337-44.

19. Bretlau P, Jørgensen MB, Johansen H. Osteogenesis imperfecta: light and electron microscopic studies of the stapes. Acta Otolaryngol (Stockh) 1970; 69:172-84.

Ann Otol 90:1981

CHANGES OF NASAL EPITHELIAL CELLS AND MUCUS LAYER AFTER CHALLENGE OF ALLERGEN

KENSUKE WATANABE, MD ISAMU WATANABE, MD

TOKYO, JAPAN

It has been reported that the normal epithelium of the anterior nares is covered by a mucopolysaccharide layer with a depth of approximately 0.8μ[1]. In the present study, a patient with an allergy to the Japanese cedar was found to develop a very thin mucopolysaccharide layer (0.05μ in depth) when the mucosal tissue was taken off before provocation. Adhering pollen particles could have readily come in contact with the plasma membranes of the epithelial cells. The epithelium of the nonciliated cells exfoliated in a relatively short period of time after provocation. Ten minutes after provocation, a thick mucus layer covered the exfoliated epithelial mucosa. Pollen particles could no longer be brought into contact with mucosa due to the mucus layer. On the other hand, no difference from the normal condition was seen before provocation in the middle and posterior nares where ciliated cells were located. However, at ten minutes after provocation, a large number of goblet cells appeared in place of ciliated cells, and mucus production was very much activated. Many signs appeared at this stage which suggested the impairment of ciliary beating. Specifically, there was swelling and damage of plasma membranes of cilia, bending of cilia, existence of extra cytoplasm around the microtubules in the cilia, and intrusion of mucus fluid between cilia. In the regions where ciliated cells were replaced by goblet cells, the exfoliation of epithelium could be noted, but it is generally difficult to find that ciliated cells are exfoliated even when the ciliary beating is impaired. Taking into account the above-mentioned results, it can be assumed that pollen particles penetrate the submucosa not only through the posterior nares where ciliary beating is impaired, but also through the anterior nares where epithelial cells are exfoliated.

It is known that epithelial cells do not exist in the same form throughout the nasal mucosa. In the anterior third, the nasal epithelium is nonciliated while further back the epithelium becomes ciliated.[1-4]

Under ordinary circumstances most of the inhaled pollen grains are deposited in the anterior third.[2,5] It has been demonstrated that pollen grains are able to penetrate the sensitized nasal mucosa because of cilia paralysis.[6,7] It is of interest to determine how pollen grains, which are deposited in both the nonciliated and ciliated areas, penetrate the mucosa. The purpose of the present study is to investigate whether changes in epithelial cells and the mucus layer which develops over the epithelium after pollen insufflation are different in ciliated and nonciliated areas.

METHODS

Biopsies were made of the mucosa on the inferior turbinates of 20 patients with nasal allergies who reacted to Japanese cedar pollen in skin and nasal provocation tests. The patients ranged in age from 18 to 40 years. Biopsies were taken in the pollen season. Biopsies of the nasal mucosa from five patients were taken at each of the following intervals: before provocation and 2 minutes, 10 minutes, and 20 minutes after provocation. One spray of triturated cedar pollen on the nasal mucosa was the method of provocation. Under a local anesthesia (0.5% Procaine®, 0.5 cc), biopsies were taken with small forceps from two sites: the anterior tip of the inferior turbinate and 2 cm behind the anterior tip. Small blocks were fixed for one hour by immersion in ice cold 1.5% glutaraldehyde buffered with 0.067 M cacodylate, pH 7.3, and containing 500 ppm purified ruthenium red.[8] Following fixation with glutaraldehyde-ruthenium red, the tissue blocks were immersed in 0.1 M cacodylate for ten minutes and then postfixed for three hours at room temperature, with 2% osmium tetroxide buffered with 0.067 M cacodylate, pH 7.3, and containing 500 ppm purified ruthenium red. The blocks were next dehydrated with ethanol and embedded in Epon 812®. Ultrathin sections were treated with uranyl acetate and lead to enhance contrast for electron microscopy.

RESULTS

Anterior Tip of the Inferior Turbinate. The epithelium has microvilli which were covered by a mucopolysaccharide layer (Figs. 1 and 2). In normal controls, this layer was about 0.8μ in depth, well stained by ruthenium red, had a high density, and appeared viscid[1] (Fig. 2). However, in the patients with Japanese cedar allergy the mucopolysaccharide layer which covered the nasal epithelium was very thin (0.05μ in depth), even when tissue was taken before provocation (Fig. 1). In some areas, exfoliation of the outermost one or two layers of stratified epithelium had already been observed. Shortly (two minutes) after provocation, nonciliated epithelial cells were found to be exfoliated. At ten minutes after provocation, the intercellular space among the epithelial cells was wide open and in some areas only a single layer of basal cells was still in existence. Immediately after this stage, much mucus fluid was produced and covered the mucosa. At this stage, the antigen could no longer be brought into contact with the mucosa (Fig. 3).

Two Centimeters Behind the Anterior Edge of the Inferior Turbinate. In normal controls, the ciliated cells were covered with a thick mucus layer. This layer was less stained by ruthenium red than that on the anterior tip, and did not intrude between cilia[1] (Fig. 5). At two minutes after provocation, no remarkable changes appeared. At ten min-

From the Department of Otolaryngology, Tokyo Medical and Dental University, Tokyo.

REPRINTS — Kensuke Watanabe, MD, Dept. of Otolaryngology, Tokyo Medical and Dental University, 1-5-45, Yushima Bunkyo-ku, Tokyo, Japan.

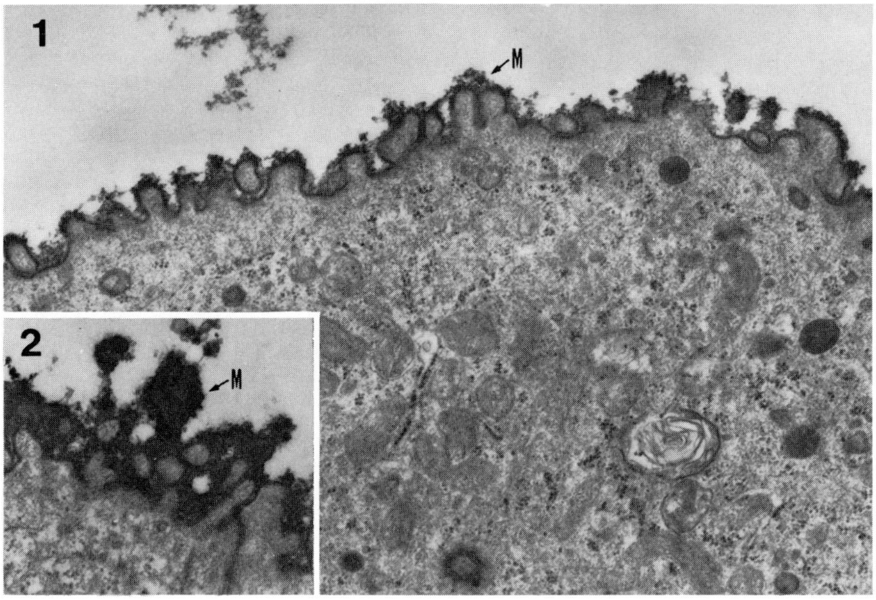

Fig. 1. In allergic patients the mucopolysaccharide layer (M) which covers the anterior nasal epithelium, is very thin even if tissue is taken before provocation. (x25,000)

Fig. 2 (Insert with Fig. 1.) In normal controls, the mucopolysaccharide layer (M) is thicker than in the allergic patient. (x25,000)

utes after provocation, the goblet cells had rapidly increased in number in many areas (Fig. 4). The mucus was found intruding between the cilia (Figs. 6 and 7, stars). This finding may mean that ciliary beating had ceased since the mucus fluid should move over the cilia and should not intrude between cilia, when the cilia are active. A variety of changes were noted in the shapes of the cilia, such as the swelling or damage of plasma membrane of cilia (Fig. 7, arrows), bending of cilia (Fig. 8), or extra cytoplasm around the microtubules in the cilia (Fig. 6, arrow). All these changes suggest that ciliary beating had slowed or ceased entirely. Despite the damage to the cilia, only rarely were the ciliated cells exfoliated. In the area where the majority of ciliated cells was replaced by goblet cells, most of the epithelial cells were exfoliated, leaving only one layer of basal cells (Fig. 9).

However, most of the exfoliated portion was goblet cells, and therefore, a large amount of mucus had already covered the mucosa. It seems unlikely that pollen particles can freely penetrate the submucosa in the exfoliated area at this stage, unlike the situation in the anterior area. At 20 minutes after provocation, no significant changes were noted from those at 10 minutes.

DISCUSSION

Any foreign particles inhaled through the nostrils and brought into contact with the nasal mucosa subsequently encounter some kind of defense. The first defensive line is the nasal mucus layer, while the second line is the ciliary beating. The third defensive line is the epithelial cells and submucosa. It has been revealed in the present study that the

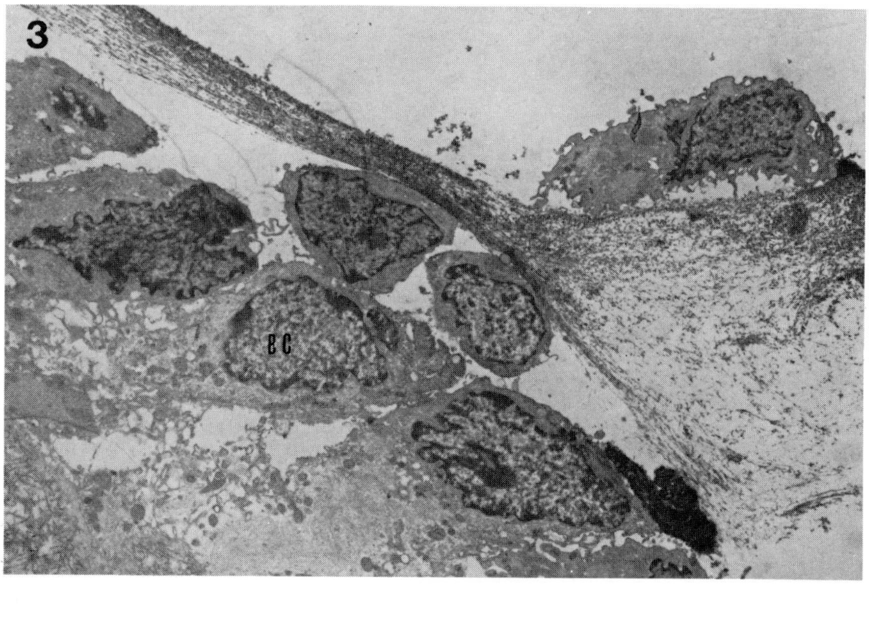

Fig. 3. Ten minutes after provocation, only one line of basal cells (BC) in the anterior nares is still in existence. The mucus layer started to cover the exfoliated epithelium. (x5,000)

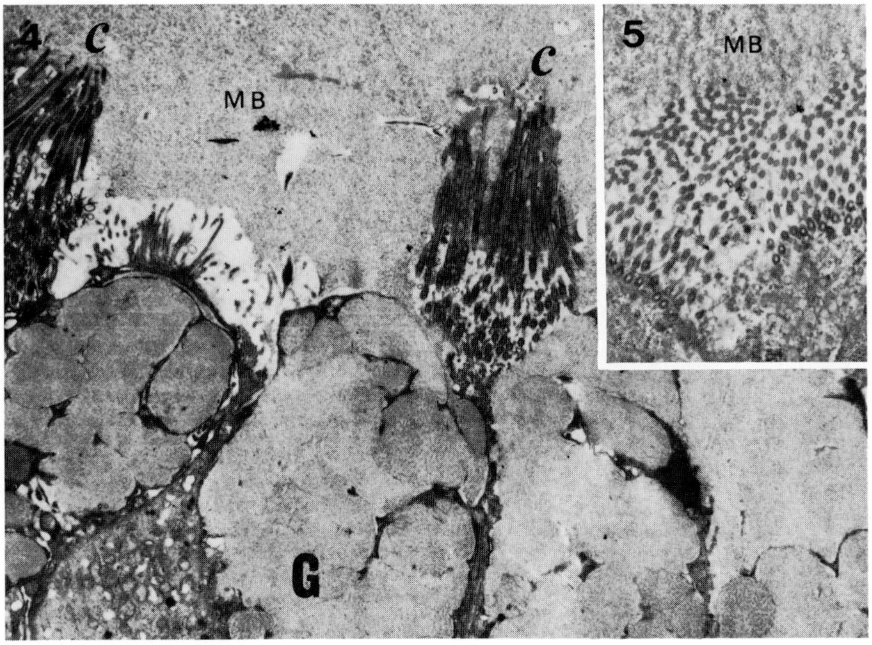

Fig. 4. Ten minutes after provocation, the goblet cells (G) were found to have rapidly increased in the posterior nares, and ciliated cells (C) were squeezed out. MB - Mucus blanket. (x5,000)

Fig. 5. (Insert with Fig. 4.) In normal controls, the ciliated cells were covered with a thick mucus blanket. This layer did not intrude between cilia. (x3,000)

mucopolysaccharide layer over the epithelium of the anterior portion is thinner in allergic patients than in normal controls, and in some areas the outermost one to two layers of stratified epithelium had exfoliated. As previously mentioned most of the inhaled pollen particles are deposited in the anterior one third of the nasal epithelium. As this epithelium is nonciliated, the flow rate of the mucus fluid is very slow.[2,9-11] Many pollen particles which are deposited in the anterior nares evidently remain there for a long time. If the mucopolysaccharide layer is thick, it is difficult for the pollen particles to come in contact with the plasma membrane of the epithelial cells. However, if this layer is thin, the pollen particles can penetrate the layer and readily attach to the plasma membrane of the epithelial cells, which may be subsequently damaged. Adamson and Bowden[12] reported that, in oxygen poisoning, the pulmonary cells with the thinner layer of mucopolysaccharide (type 1 epithelium) were highly susceptible to injury, and the cells with the thicker layer (type 2 epithelium) were more resistant. They suggested that the mucopolysaccharides served as the protectant for the lipoprotein complex of the plasma membrane.

It can be conjectured that in the anterior area the nonciliated epithelial cells with damage to their

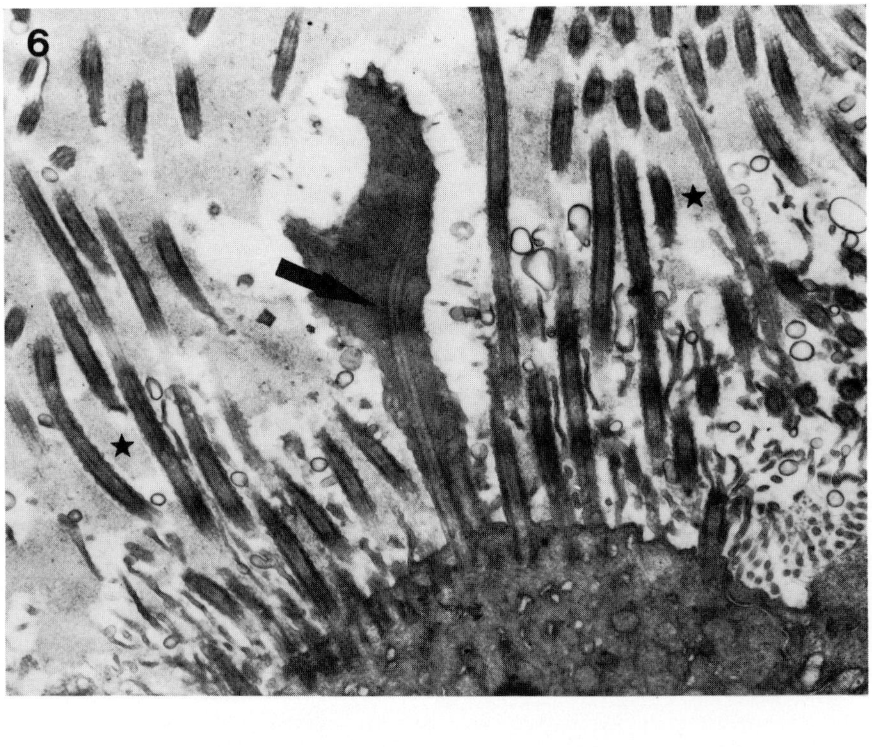

Fig. 6. Ten minutes after provocation, the cilia appeared swollen such that a large amount of cytoplasm was found around the microtubular bundles (arrow). Intrusion of mucus between cilia (stars) was also seen. These findings suggest the cessation of ciliary beating. (x17,500)

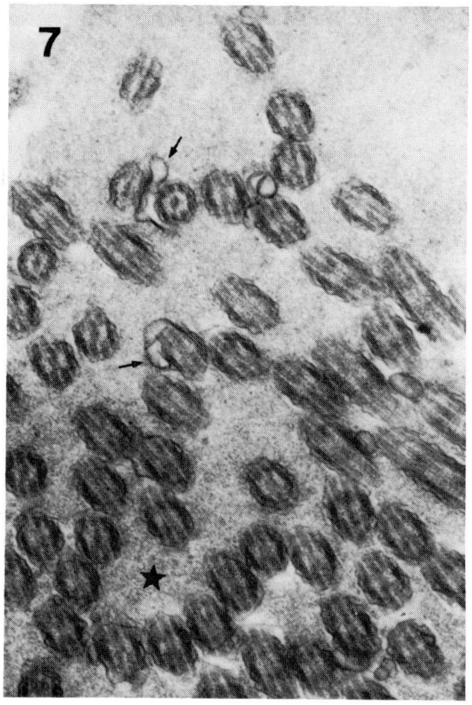

Fig. 7. Ten minutes after provocation, swelling or damage of the plasma membrane of the cilia (arrows) and intrusion of mucus between cilia (star) were found. (x25,000)

plasma membranes would be easily exfoliated. As the epithelium of the anterior area is composed of five to six layers of the epithelial cells, exfoliation of the outermost one or two layers would not exert adverse effects directly upon the submucosa. However, if there is persistent stimulation by antigens or if the amount of antigens is excessive, the majority of the epithelial cells would be exfoliated as shown in Figure 3, leaving only basal cells protecting the submucosa. It takes over ten minutes for the thick mucus layer as shown in Figure 3 to cover the mucous membrane so as to protect it from allergen.

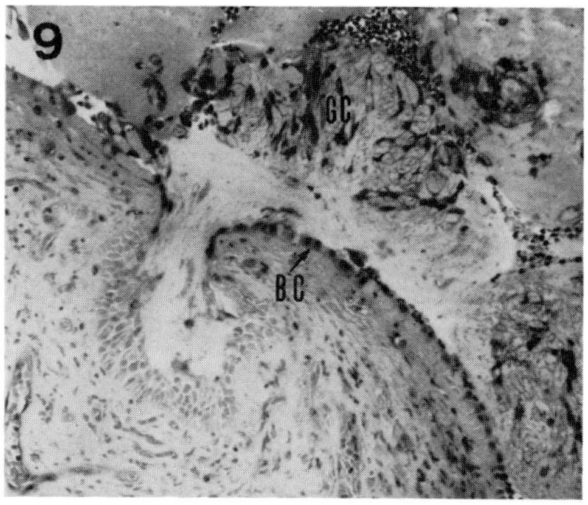

Fig. 9. Ten minutes after provocation, tissue was taken from the posterior nares. In this area, the majority of ciliated cells was replaced by goblet cells (GC). Most of these latter cells were exfoliated leaving only one layer of basal cells (BC).

In the meantime, the allergen would possibly directly penetrate the submucosa where mast cells are abundant. It is assumed that it would take several days for the exfoliated epithelium to be restored to its original condition. Therefore, it is hypothesized that once the affected epithelium is exposed to allergen, the allergen would very easily and very quickly invade the submucosa until the epithelium is restored to normal.

Chevance[6] concluded that impairment of the ciliary activity was the first manifestation of allergic shock. Indeed, the results of this study tend to indicate the cessation of ciliary beating in allergic nasal mucosa challenged by allergen. The mucus layer should move over the cilia in line with the movements of the cilia, and therefore, mucus fluid would never intrude between cilia (Fig. 5).[1] However, once ciliary beating stops, the mucus layer might easily penetrate between the cilia (Figs. 6 and 7). It remains to be determined whether Che-

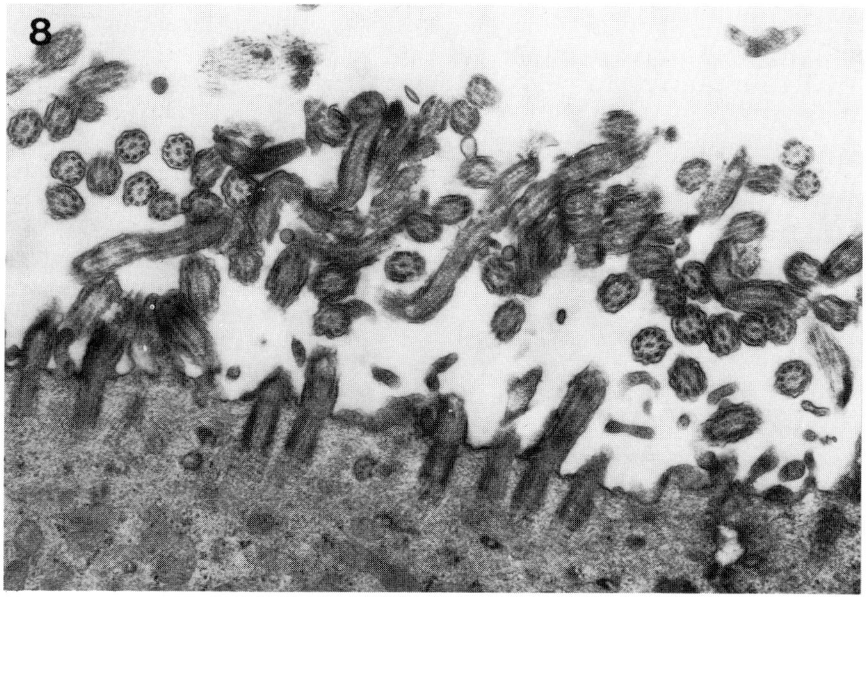

Fig. 8. Ten minutes after provocation, remarkable bendings of cilia were found. Since this tissue was not stained by ruthenium red, the mucus fluid was not visible. (x22,000)

vance's assertion is justifiable, ie, that cessation of ciliary beating is the first manifestation of allergic shock. Certainly, the ciliary beating can be terminated if a large amount of pollen particles adheres to the ciliated area and damages the cells, but it is the anterior one third of the nose where the inhaled particles are most easily deposited, and only a limited amount of pollen particles gain access to the posterior nares.[2,5] Consequently, it would be more logical to assume that changes would develop earlier in the epithelium of the anterior areas than the posterior areas. Even if ciliary impairment takes place within a very limited period, no evidence of exfoliation in the ciliated cells can be found immediately after the pollen insufflation. Occasionally at the late stage, exfoliation of the epithelium in the posterior area can be noted in the area of major replacement by goblet cells (Fig. 9). Specifically, it can be hypothesized that even if the movements of cilia cease, penetration by pollen particles into the submucosa would occur at a later stage in the posterior area. Chevance[7] also reported that destruction of the ciliary structure and epithelial cells and, consequently, penetration by pollen particles into the mucosa occurred 10-30 minutes after pollen insufflation. Therefore, it would be difficult to attribute the emergence of allergic symptoms at four to five minutes after pollen insufflation to the penetration of antigen subsequent to cessation of the ciliary beatings. Antigens may penetrate into the submucosa not only by the impairment of ciliary beatings, but also by exfoliation of the nonciliated epithelial cells in the anterior nares. Richardson et al[13] suggested that allergic symptoms appeared without penetration of the bronchial submucosa by the antigen. However, this suggestion is not accepted universally, as some workers[7,14] showed antigen in the submucosa. Richardson showed no exfoliation of the epithelial cells and no penetration of the submucosa by the antigen, but the epithelial cells filled with antigen. The authors considered the epithelial cells filling with antigen as the prestage of exfoliation. Once the epithelial cells exfoliated, the antigen would easily penetrate the submucosa.

In the pollen season, pollen particles would intrude into the nasal cavity so persistently and for such a long period that there would not be time to regenerate the epithelium in the regions of exfoliation. Consequently, the exfoliated areas would exist for some time. It is especially important to note that pollen particles would easily penetrate the submucosa within a short period because the anterior nares is the place where large amounts of pollen particles are deposited. Consequently, it would be very likely in the pollen season that allergic symptoms would take place within a short period after pollen inhalation, regardless of the cessation of ciliary beating. Wihl and Mygind[15] could not find signs of destruction of cilia or epithelium, impaired ciliary function, or pollen penetration of the mucosa following allergen challenge in hay fever patients. However, their study was conducted during the pollen-free season, when the anterior and posterior nasal epithelium was completely intact. In addition it may be very difficult for pollen to penetrate the submucosa with only one provocation.

The antigen intruding through the anterior one third of the nose would be combined with IgE antibodies on the mast cells and would release chemical mediators such as histamine from the mast cells. It can be assumed that the chemical mediators are perfused quickly into the posterior area.

Horseradish peroxidase, which passed through the blood vessels in the lamina propria of the nasal mucosa of a rat, could readily reach the subepithelium ten seconds after injection from the caudal vein.[16] As perfusion takes place very quickly in the submucosa of normal rats, it would be very likely that velocity of the perfusion of the chemical mediators would be greater if the submucosa were filled with the edematous fluid. Furthermore it would be very likely that precursor cells of the goblet cells are quickly converted to goblet cells by stimulation of the chemical mediators, and the matured goblet cells would increase within a short time. According to Tos and Morgensen,[17] goblet cells did not increase in allergic noses. The reason for such a finding may be that they examined tissues obtained before provocation.

It can be speculated that the stimulation of a large amount of antigen on the external side of the nasal cavity and the stimulation of the chemical mediators from the inner side (tissue side) would synergistically affect the ciliated cells, and cell damage would be rapidly advanced.

After secretion of mucus fluid in large amounts from both the goblet cells and nasal glands (due to stimulation by chemical mediators), the mucous membrane will be covered by a thick mucus layer which will completely protect it from pollen particles. There would be no intrusion of allergen into the submucosa after this stage.

ACKNOWLEDGMENT — The authors wish to express their thanks to Professor V. Mizuhira for his helpful suggestions and advice.

REFERENCES

1. Watanabe K, Saito Y, Watanabe I. Acid mucopolysaccharide layer of the surface nasal epithelium. Rhinology 1978; 16:215-23.

2. Hilding AC. Phagocytosis, mucous flow and ciliary action. Arch Environ Health 1963; 6:61-73.

3. Mygind N. Scanning electron microscopy of the human

nasal mucosa. Rhinology 1975; 13:57-75.

4. Lenz H. Three-dimensional surface presentation of the cilia-free nasal mucosa of men, a scanning-electron microscopical study. Acta Otolaryngol (Stockh) 1973; 76:47-57.

5. Proctor DF, Andersen I, Lundqvist G. Clearance of inhaled particles from the human nose. Arch Intern Med 1973; 131:132-9.

6. Chevance LG. The first stages of the nasal anaphylactic shock. Acta Otolaryngol (Stockh) 1957; 47:480-90.

7. Chevance LG. Experimental pollinosis: an electron microscopic study. Acta Otolaryngol (Stockh) 1971; 72:121-33.

8. Luft JH. Electron microscopy of cell extraneous coats as revealed by ruthenium red staining. J Cell Biol 1964; 23:54A-55A.

9. Bang BG, Mukherjee AL, Bang FB. Human nasal mucous flow rates. Johns Hopkins Med J 1967; 121:38-48.

10. Ewert G. On the mucous flow rate in the human nose. Acta Otolaryngol (Stockh) 1965; Suppl 200:1-62.

11. Proctor DF, Wagner HN. Clearance of particles from the human nose. Arch Environ Health 1965; 2:366-71.

12. Adamson IYR, Bowden DH. Sialomucin and pulmonary cell injury, ultrastructural and cytochemical studies in mice exposed to oxygen. Arch Pathol 1971; 92:273-8.

13. Richardson JB, Hogg JC, Bouchard T, Hall DL. Localization of antigen in experimental bronchoconstriction in guinea pigs. J Allergy Clin Immunol 1973; 52:172-81.

14. Rappaport BZ. Antigen-antibody reactions in allergic human tissues. III. Immunofluorescent study of allergic nasal mucosa. J Immunol 1964; 93:792-7.

15. Wihl JÅ, Mygind N. Studies on the allergen-challenged human nasal mucosa. Acta Otolaryngol (Stockh) 1977; 84:281-6.

16. Watanabe K, Saito Y, Watanabe I, Mizuhira V. The characteristics of the capillary permeability in nasal mucosa. Ann Otol Rhinol Laryngol 1980; 89:377-82.

17. Tos M, Morgensen C. Nasal glands in nasal allergy. Acta Otolaryngol (Stockh) 1977; 83:498-504.

≈

CORRECTION

Due to a production error, pages 6 and 7 were inadvertently numbered incorrectly and transposed in Supplement 76, Vol. 89, November-December 1980. The text reads correctly if these two pages are reordered.

Ann Otol 90:1981

EAR DEFORMITIES ASSOCIATED WITH THE KLIPPEL-FEIL SYNDROME

PAUL C. WINDLE-TAYLOR, FRCS

PAULINE J. EMERY, FRCS PETER D. PHELPS, FRCS, FRCR

LONDON, ENGLAND

Congenital spinal fusion, constituting the Klippel-Feil anomaly, has long been known to be associated with severe deafness in many patients. Ten such cases are described, with audiometric and tomographic assessment of the ear lesions. Of the 20 ears examined, 12 showed evidence of severe hearing loss and of these, 11 had evidence of significant inner ear dysplasia on tomography. Middle and external ear abnormalities were also demonstrated. The significance of these findings and the relation to other syndromes is discussed.

INTRODUCTION

Multisystem congenital defects present the clinician with many problems, and none more difficult than when hearing loss is a feature. Konigsmark and Gorlin in their treatise list 150 separate syndromes associated with hereditary deafness.[1] No system in the body was exempt from involvement with hearing loss in these patients. These authors estimated that of the children born deaf in the United States each year (2000-4000) up to one half may be classified as genetic and probably over one third of these cases are syndromal. Despite the work of such researchers, the assessment of congenital deafness has not always been as full as possible, especially with regard to the relationship between structure and function. The purpose of this paper is to present a series of ten cases of the Klippel-Feil syndrome who had associated deafness, and to show a clinicoradiological correlation which may be of significant use to the clinician. Comparison will also be made with other syndromes of the head and neck which feature in the differential diagnosis, and which may be used to show a pattern in the maldevelopment of the region.

CASE DATA

The seven females and three males whose ages at presentation ranged from 1½ to 10 years, were assessed clinically, audiometrically and radiologically. Apart from the presence of the Klippel-Feil anomaly, there were no shared defects which constituted a known syndrome. The results of pure tone audiometry were collected and found to fall into a small number of simple categories; normal, moderate conductive, mild mixed, moderate sensorineural, and severe sensorineural. In two cases it was not possible to obtain satisfactory results, so severe were the handicaps. Radiological assessment was by polytomography, with sections in the coronal plane. In some cases these were supplemented by other views.

CASE REPORTS

Case 1. A 4-year-old male with a bilateral conductive hearing loss (Fig. 1) was shown by tomography to have major external and middle ear abnormalities, with anteriorly placed facial nerves. The labyrinths were normal. Surgical intervention was not considered in view of the child's excellent academic progress at a normal school using a postaural aid.

Case 2. A 3-year-old female had a severe bilateral sensorineural hearing loss (Fig. 2). The inner ear on the right displayed a Mondini type of cochlear deformity with dilated lateral and superior semicircular canals. The left labyrinth appeared normal. The middle ear on this side had a sloping attic with deformed ossicles. The right external meatus sloped upwards. Her progress at a school for the deaf was described as slow, using a bodyworn aid with a bone conductor.

Case 3. A 9-year-old male had a unilateral severe sensorineural hearing loss, the affected ear having a very narrow internal auditory meatus. No hearing aid was thought necessary, and his progress at a normal school was good.

Case 4. An 18-month-old male had a severe bilateral sensorineural loss. Tomography revealed grossly dysplastic labyrinths with no internal meatus on the left. The middle ear cavities were sloping though the ossicles appeared normal. He was making satisfactory progress at a school for the deaf with a bodyworn aid and a "Y" lead, though his speech remained unintelligible to strangers.

Case 5. A 4½-year-old female had a moderately severe sensorineural loss (Fig. 3). Tomography showed a sloping right internal meatus: the cochlea was normal but the vestibule and canals were absent. On the left the inner ear was normal, but the middle ear had a small attic with deformed ossicles. She attended a partially hearing unit attached to a normal school, and was making good progress with a postaural aid.

Case 6. An 18-month-old male with a severe sensorineural hearing loss and total aplasia of both labyrinths had middle ear cavities and ossicles grossly abnormal. A wide variety of aids were tried and much supportive care given. Speech production was good, considering the defects which precluded any auditory perception, the child relying exclusively upon visual cueing, speech rhythms, and intonation.

Case 7. A 9-year-old female had severe sensorineural loss. Bilateral Mondini defects of the cochlea were shown on tomography, with abnormally distended semicircular canals on the

---

From the Royal National Throat, Nose and Ear Hospital, London.

REPRINTS — Paul C. Windle-Taylor, FRCS, The Royal National Throat, Nose and Ear Hospital, Gray's Inn Road, London, WC1X 8DA, England.

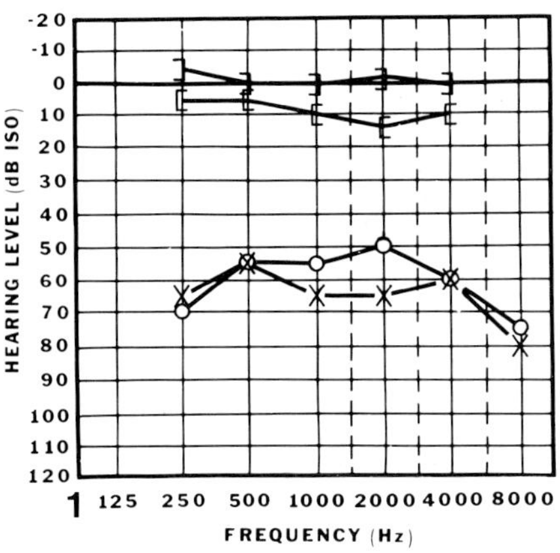

Fig. 1. (Case 1) Audiogram showing moderate bilateral conductive loss.

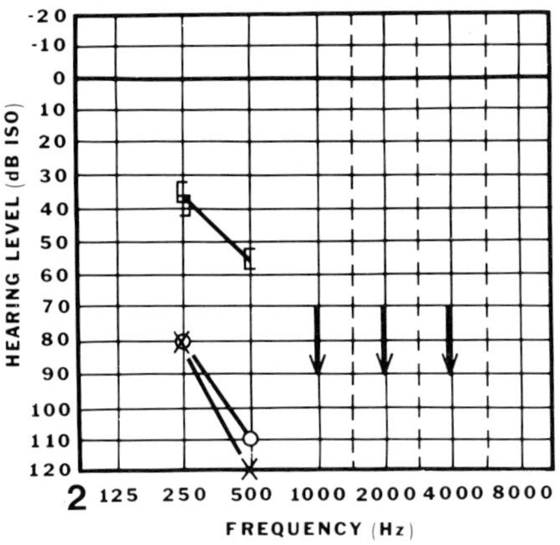

Fig. 2. (Case 2) Audiogram showing a severe sensorineural loss.

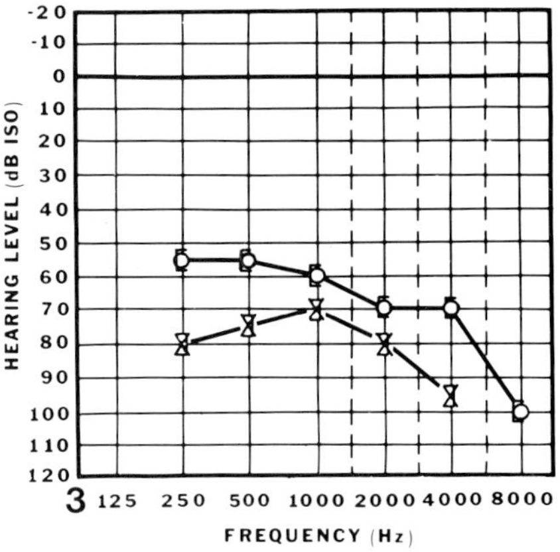

Fig. 3. (Case 5) Audiogram showing a moderate sensorineural hearing loss.

right side (Fig. 4). Both middle ear clefts were small, and the ossicles irregular, fused masses. Speech was absent. (The patient came from an underdeveloped country).

Case 8. A 10-year-old female (previously described by Livingstone and Delahunty[2]) had a severe sensorineural hearing loss. Tomography revealed no obvious inner ears and the middle ear clefts were conical (Fig. 5). The ossicles appeared normal. A tympanotomy was performed revealing almost normal ossicles, but no sign of the oval window.

Case 9. A 10-year-old female had a bilateral conductive hearing loss. Other defects were a right hemifacial dysplasia, with microphthalmos, and decreased facial movements. Tomography showed normal labyrinths, but abnormal middle ears. The right facial nerve was displayed anteriorly with no ossicles visible. The right external meatus was replaced by a large bony atretic plate. With a postaural aid, good progress was made, though other malformations, including an atrial septal defect, pulmonary hypertension and an irritable hip, imposed considerable restrictions.

Case 10. A 6-year-old female had a unilateral severe sensorineural hearing loss on the right side and a mild mixed hearing loss on the left. Tomography showed a form of Mondini deformity on the right with a deficient modiolus but the basal turn of the cochlea was also dilated (Fig. 6). The cochlea on the left was more normal but did appear to have a reduced number of turns. No hearing aid was thought necessary, and her progress at a normal school was good.

Table 1 is a compilation of the major ear abnormalities with composite impressions of the polytomographic appearances.

DISCUSSION

The series presented demonstrates the variety of anomalies found in association with Klippel-Feil syndrome. As will be seen later, some of these associations occur with enough frequency to become separate syndromes in their own right. The predominance of females in this condition has been seen before, but is usually marked in Wildervanck's syndrome[3-5] which has the Klippel-Feil anomaly as a clinical feature.

Conductive hearing loss in the Klippel-Feil syndrome has been noted before. In the present series, two of the ten cases had conductive losses with positive radiological findings. Stark and Borton,[6] reviewing four cases of the anomaly with confirmed deafness, considered three to have a mixed or conductive loss, while the fourth had a sensorineural loss in one ear and a mixed loss in the other. Bilateral exploratory tympanotomies in one case revealed ossicular abnormalities (absent ossicles on the left side; malformed incus and an absent stapedial footplate on the right). They reviewed the literature and commented on the lack of audiological and radiological detail.[6] Singh et al reported a case of a conductive loss in which both tomography and tym-

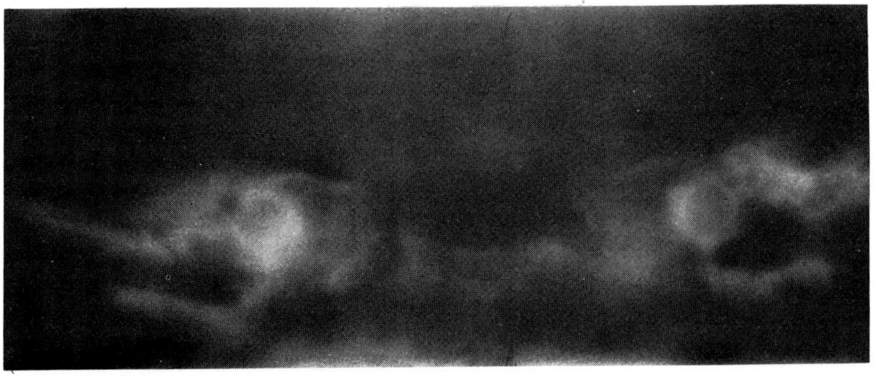

Fig. 4. (Case 7) Frontal tomograph showing bilateral Mondini defects. The cochleae appear empty due to deficiency of the modiolus in the distal part.

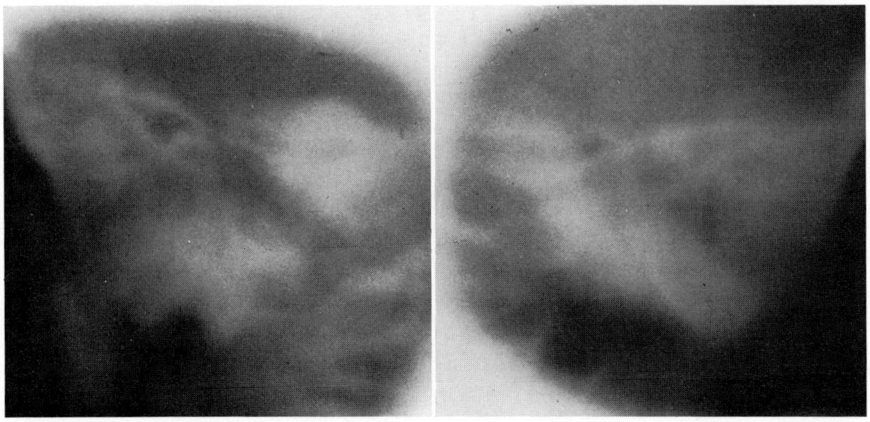

Fig. 5. (Case 8) Frontal tomograph showing inner ear aplasia and abnormal middle ear clefts.

panotomy failed to reveal any abnormality. No hypothesis was advanced to explain this finding.[7] It is possible to conjecture on the presence of chronic low-grade inflammation, though this may not explain the latter case. In gonadal dysgenesis, the high incidence of secretory otitis media has been explained in terms of abnormal eustachian tube function secondary to the skull base abnormalities found in the syndrome.[8] This may be a factor in the Klippel-Feil anomaly also.

Our series shows a high incidence of both external and middle ear abnormalities. Similar lesions have been reported before but not in such a high percentage of cases (16 out of 20 ears examined).[2,6,9,10] In most of the patients the sensorineural component predominates, thus reducing the clinical significance of the conduction abnormalities. The anomalies are similar to those found in other head and neck syndromes and are nonspecific.

Unilateral hearing loss, which was present in one case, has been described before, but the reason why the teratogenic influence should spare one ear is not known.[9,11,12] Ormerod classified the etiology of congenital deafness into developmental failure, interruption in development, or degeneration of parts of the auditory apparatus which have already developed in some degree or have reached maturity.[13] The pathological findings have been subdivided into a few eponymous types. In the present series, cases 2, 7 and 10 exhibited the Mondini type of defect where the cochlea is represented by a reduced number of turns. Other inner ear anomalies were found but cannot be so classified. This inability to fit the majority of cases into the existing limited and rigid framework (devised many years ago on the basis of little histopathological material) has led to a call for a more descriptive method of classification.[14] Such a system has been drawn up and may prove of value in the future.[15] An anatomical description of the cochlear deformity, the state of the modiolus, probable number of coils and whether they are dilated or smaller than normal, should be made from the tomograms.

The distinctive inner ear radiological features of the Mondini defect have been reported in the Klippel-Feil syndrome before.[16] It is not diagnostic of the condition and has been seen in a number of cases of congenital deafness, including those induced by thalidomide,[17] and in a case of gonadal dysgenesis.[18] The defect is not necessarily incompatible with some hearing, though in the cases of the present series there was no useful cochlear function.[19,20]

To produce such bony defects the teratogenic influence must act between the fifth and eighth week of gestation. Any variation in timing will arrest or modify embryogenesis at another point producing a different anomaly. In some head and neck syn-

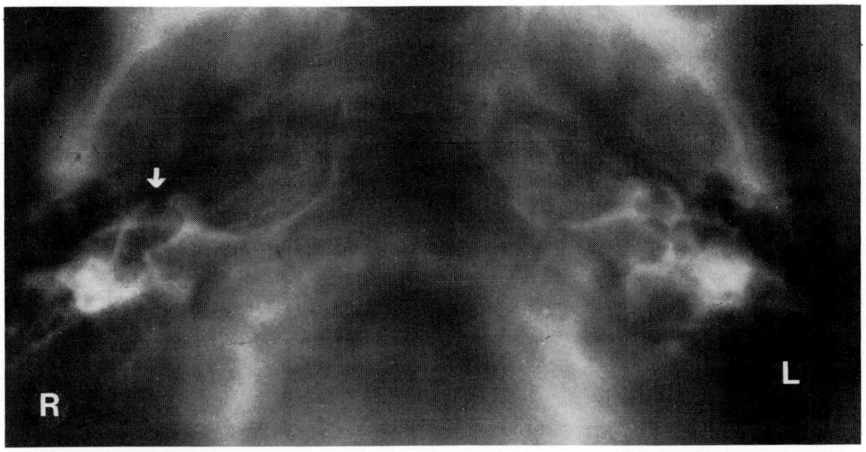

Fig. 6. (Case 10) Basal tomograph showing normal internal auditory meatus on the right. The basal turn of cochlea is significantly dilated and opens into a distal sac (arrow). On the left the cochlea appears virtually normal.

TABLE 1. SUMMARY OF SERIES WITH COMPOSITE DIAGRAMS OF EAR ANOMALIES BASED ON FRONTAL TOMOGRAMS

Age (yr)	*Radiological Abnormalities* *R*	*L*	*Diagram*	*External Ear*	*Hearing Loss* *R*	*L*
4½	AFN; no attic or ant.; descent of tegmen; no ossicles	AFN; small attic and ant.; descent of tegmen; small ossicular mass	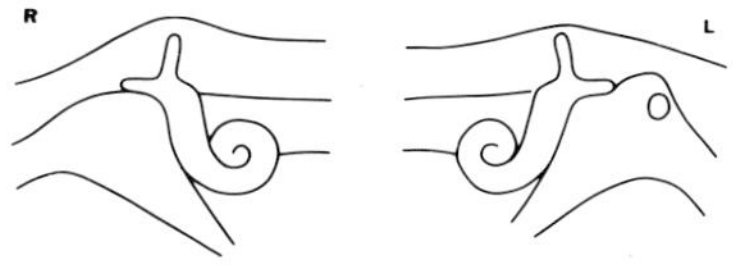	Bilateral soft tissue meatal atresia	M C	M C
3	Sloping attic; dilated canals; dys. cochlea (Mondini defect)	Ossicles fused to medial wall; small IAM	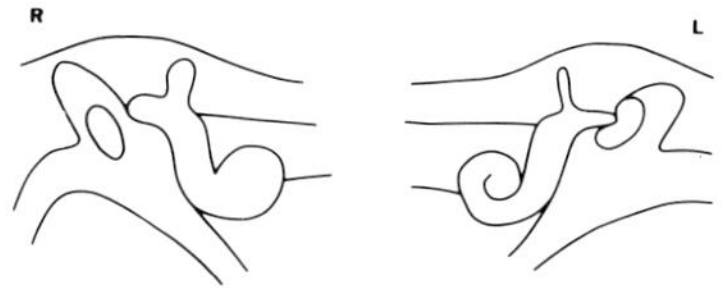	None	S SS	S SS
9	None	Small IAM	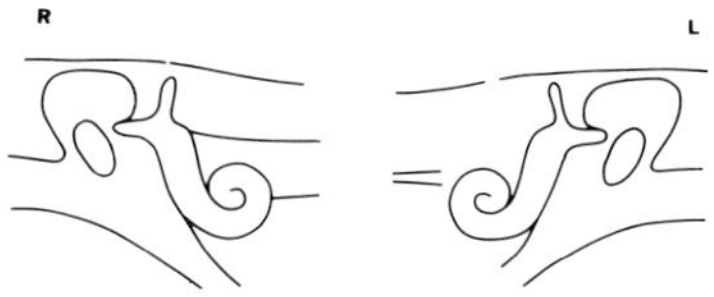	None	N	S SS
1½	Large tilted attic; dys. labyrinth; no IAM	Large tilted attic; dys. labyrinth; No IAM	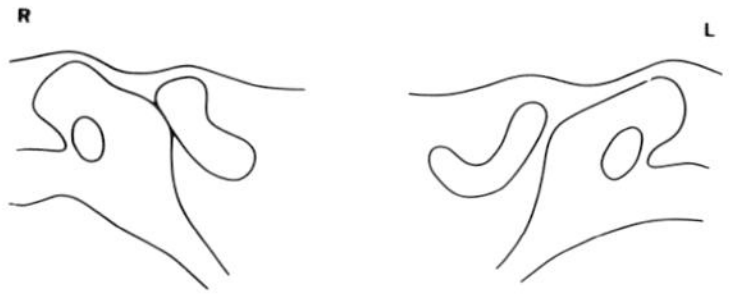	None	S SS	S SS
4½	No vestibule or canals; sloping IAM	Abnormal attic; small ossicular mass	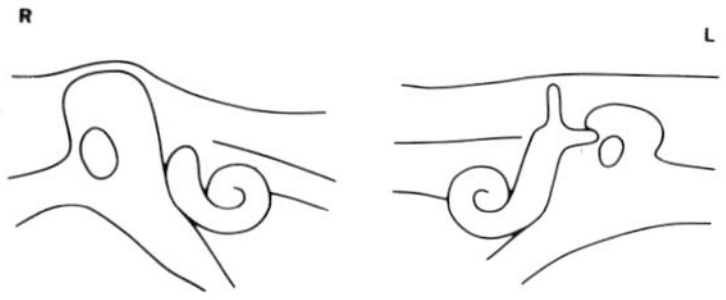	R meatal soft tissue atresia	M SS	M SS
1½	Abnormal ossicles; aplastic labyrinth; small IAM	Abnormal ossicles; aplastic labyrinth; small IAM	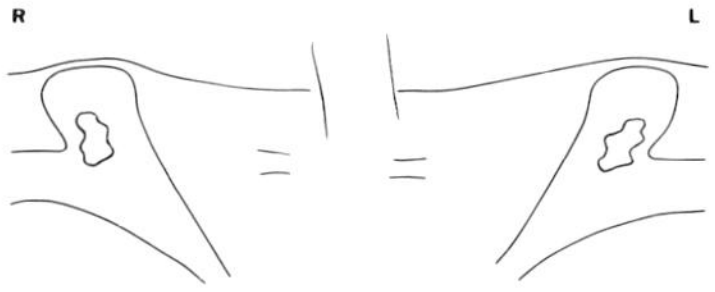	None	S SS	S SS
9	Small attic; ossicular mass fused to scutum; dilated canals; dys. cochlea (Mondini defect)	Small attic; ossicular mass fused to scutum; dys. cochlea (Mondini defect)	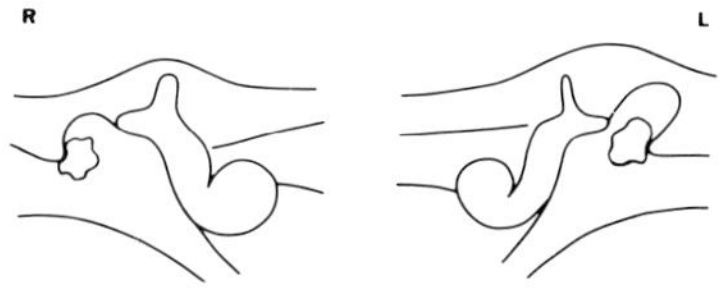	None	S SS	S SS
0	Sloping attic; dys. labyrinth; no IAM	Sloping attic; dys. labyrinth; small IAM	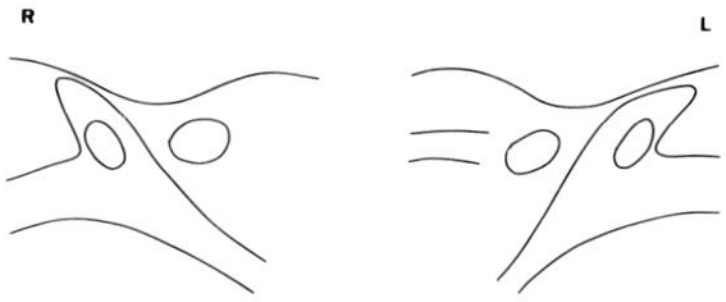	Bilateral soft tissue meatal atresia	S SS	S SS
0	AFN; bony atresia plate	Abnormal ossicles	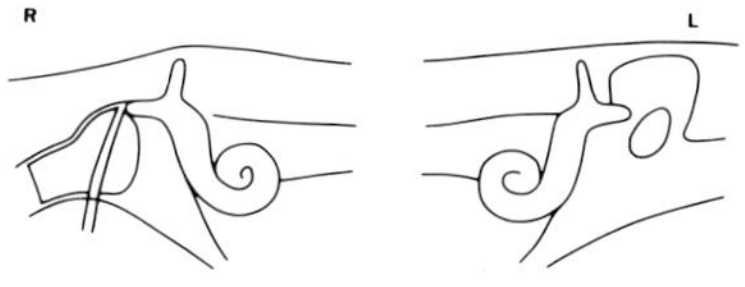	R meatal bony atresia	M C	M C
6	Dys. cochlea with dilated basal turn opening into distal sac (severe Mondini defect)	Only 2 turns of cochlea	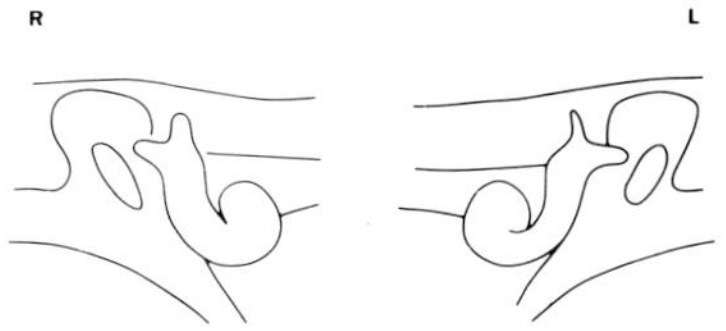	None	S SS	Mild Mixed

R - Right; L - Left; AFN - Anterior facial nerve; Ant. - Antrum; Dys. - Dysplastic; IAM - Internal auditory meatus; M - Moderate; C - Conductive; S - Severe; SS - Sensorineural; N - Normal.

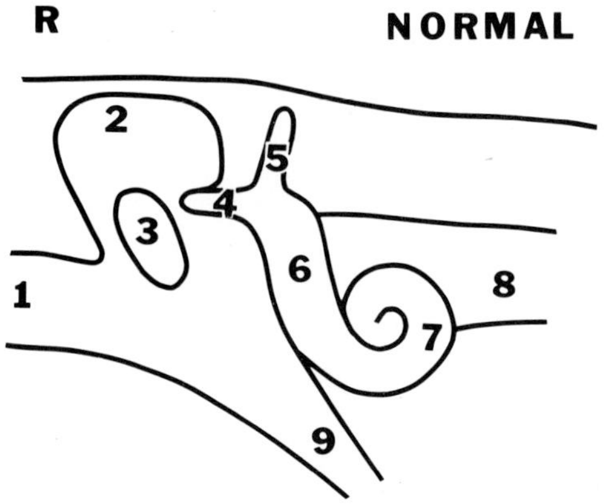

Fig. 7. Key to Table 1 diagrams. 1 - External auditory meatus; 2 - Attic; 3 - Malleus and incus; 4 - Internal semicircular canal; 5 - Superior semicircular canal; 6 - Vestibule; 7 - Cochlea; 8 - Internal auditory meatus; 9 - Eustachian tube.

dromes, for instance mandibulofacial dysostosis, the defects appear inheritable, but in others it is not certain. There is little known of the relative importance of genetic makeup, intrauterine and extrauterine factors in the normal and abnormal development of the fetus. However these factors are involved, the same structures appear vulnerable, and a variable pattern of recognizably distinct abnormalities appears.

Of the 20 ears examined, 12 showed evidence of severe hearing losses and of these, 11 had evidence of inner ear dysplasia on tomography. The validity of the audiograms obtained from the severely deaf children is open to challenge on the grounds that at the frequencies and intensities at which there is apparently a positive hearing response, there is also a marked tactile input via the headphones and a false response may be given. A corollary of this finding, if valid, is that it may not be of benefit to the patient to be taught purely auditory methods of communication learning. Hearing aids may give the child some information concerning speech rhythms and intonation patterns, but this should be supplemented with other techniques to allow early communication even if only with those closely associated, and themselves adept. There should be no insistence on using the hearing aids if they do not appear to help the child. The vocalizations of a severely deaf child are not a substitute for the spoken word, and never will be. In these days of advanced electronics, many forms of communication are available, and in many cases the child has other normal senses and a normal mentality.

Tomography not only gives valuable information regarding possible hearing function — almost to the point of being an objective investigation — but also in the case of conductive hearing loss it will allow the surgeon to assess the middle ear cavity with a view to possible corrective surgery. A report has been made of a possible hazard to stapes surgery in this syndrome, that of the stapes gusher.[21] An

TABLE 2. COMPARISON OF THE CLINICAL FEATURES OF FIVE HEAD AND NECK SYNDROMES

	W	*G*	*HM*	*MFD*	*GD*
Vertebral anomalies	+ + +	+ + +			
Pterygium colli	+				+ + +
Low hairline	+				+
Spina bibida	+	+			
Facial asymmetry	+	+	+ + +		+
Frontal bossing		+			
Microphthalmia		+	+	+	
Epibulbar dermoids	+	+ + +			
Iris and/or choroid coloboma		+	+	+	
Upper lid coloboma		+ + +			
Lower lid coloboma		+		+ + +	
Abducent nerve palsy	+ + +				+
Antimongoloid slant		+		+ + +	
External ear defects	+	+	+ + +	+ + +	+
Ear tags	+	+ + +	+	+	+
Ear pits	+	+	+	+	
Middle ear defects	+	+	+	+ + +	
Sensorineural hearing loss	+ + +		+		+
Malar hypoplasia		+	+	+ + +	
Macrostomia		+ + +	+ + +	+	
Malocclusion		+	+	+ + +	
Aplasia of mandible, ramus & condyle		+	+ + +		
High palate		+	+	+	+
Cleft palate	+	+		+	+
Abnormal karyotype					+ + +
Ovarian agenesis					+ + +
Short stature					+ + +
Digital anomalies					+ + +
Renal anomalies					+

W - Wildervanck's syndrome; G - Goldenhar's syndrome; HM - Hemifacial microsomia; MFD - Mandibulofacial dysostosis; GD - Gonadal dysgenesis; + - Recorded anomaly; + + + - Distinctive anomaly.

association between this alarming condition and inner ear anomalies has been noted previously.[17] In this series no potential communication between a dysplastic labyrinth and the subarachnoid space, as may occur via the internal auditory meatus or via a dilated cochlear aqueduct,[22] was shown on the tomograms.

The Klippel-Feil syndrome is essentially an orthopedic abnormality consisting of fusion anomalies of the cervical and upper thoracic vertebrae, with associated pectoral girdle deformities such as Sprengel's shoulder and pterygium colli. The etiology is probably due to faulty mesodermal differentiation at about the second month of gestation. The neck is short, the posterior hair line low and head movements are limited. A number of other associated anomalies may occur, including hearing loss. Some of these associations have been described as separate syndromes. There is considerable overlap and nonconformity, as well as confusion with probable unrelated syndromes. The following is a short account of the syndromes most likely to be considered in a differential diagnosis. Table 2 is a summary of the major features. A more detailed account of these syndromes may be found in the writings of Konigsmark and Gorlin,[1] Gorlin and Pindborg[3] and Goodman and Gorlin.[5]

Hemifacial microsomia consists of unilateral macrostomia, microtia, and combined mandibular ramus and condyle aplasia. Even if bilateral, there is always some asymmetry. The ear may be affected in any part and lesions are often bizarre and severe.

Goldenhar's syndrome is characterized by the Klippel-Feil anomaly with epibulbar dermoids and/or lipodermoids, preauricular appendages, and pretragal blind fistulae. The face may be asymmetrial and a relationship with hemifacial microsomia is likely. Any deafness appears secondary to the associated external ear anomalies (microtia, meatal atresia). The syndrome does not appear to be hereditary.

Wildervanck's syndrome is characterized by facial asymmetry, the Klippel-Feil anomaly, abducent nerve palsies, external ear anomalies and sensorineural hearing loss. The oculomotor anomaly is also found in isolation when it is known as Duane's syndrome. Thus it may be said that the syndrome of Wildervanck is a compound of two others, Klippel-Feil and Duane. Reference to Table 2 will serve to underline the complex interrelationship of congenital disease in the head and neck and our incomplete understanding.

Mandibulofacial dysostosis (Treacher Collins syndrome) is an anomaly of the first branchial arch and its derivatives, and does not affect the cervical vertebrae. The labyrinth is also spared save for the occasional report of lateral canal hypoplasia (an anomaly not usually associated with sensorineural hearing loss).[23] The etiology is probably due to deficient migration of neural crest cells into the branchial arches[24] with cochlear function nearly always normal. The stigmata are distinctive but variable with an antimongoloid eye slant, lower lid coloboma, hypoplastic mandibular changes, deformed external and middle ears. This is a separate syndrome and is thought to be of an autosomal dominant condition with incomplete penetrance, though new mutations appear a common occurrence. Hemifacial microsomia, once thought to be a variant, is probably not related.

Gonadal dysgenesis (Turner's syndrome) is a chromosomal abnormality with the karyotype 45,X (or a mosaic with that). The features usually found are low stature, pterygium colli, shield chest, streak ovaries and primary amenorrhea. The Klippel-Feil anomaly is not found although there have been reports of rib and cervical vertebral abnormalities.[25,26] Previous mention in this paper has been made to the ear anomalies found in this syndrome.

CONCLUSIONS

There are two major reasons for the publication of such a series of cases. The first is that the knowledge made available may help the clinician faced with a similar case, a condition with which he may never have had experience. The second is for the advancement of knowledge in a difficult and complex field of histopathology. There is a need for a dynamic, multidisciplinary approach to the problem. It is a simplification to attempt to fit cases into particular syndromes, convenient though that may be for the purposes of classification, or to classify anomalies of the inner ear into a small number of descriptive histopathological types. To do this to variations in an advancing plastic process is not logical, and serves only to confuse the inexperienced and not necessarily create order out of chaos. Every case must be recorded and then the total sum of data assessed. With regard to the present series, all that may be stated is that teratogenic influences acting upon the head and neck at about the second month of gestation produce a pattern of anomalies involving the vertebral column and the ear. More specifically, this series shows that the Klippel-Feil anomaly may be associated with deafness of any type, with variable effects on the functioning of the patient. By the medium of polytomography it is possible to demonstrate bony abnormalities of the ear and thereby give valuable information concerning the hearing status in the patient too young or too handicapped to give accurate and reliable subjective reports. Guidance may also be given as to the possibility of middle ear surgery. The clinician with such a patient should collect and analyze such investigations, and integrate them to form a balanced approach to enable the patient to acquire powers of communication not only among his fellow sufferers, but also with the normal population.

ACKNOWLEDGMENTS — The author wish to thank Dr. G. A. S. Lloyd of the Department of Radiology of the Institute of Laryngology and Otology for his advice in the preparation of this paper, and also Mr. D. Connolly of the Photographic Department.

REFERENCES

1. Konigsmark B, Gorlin RJ. Genetic and metabolic deafness. Philadelphia: WB Saunders, 1976.

2. Livingstone G, Delahunty JE. Malformation of the ear associated with congenital ophthalmic and other conditions. J Laryngol Otol 1968; 82:495-504.

3. Gorlin RJ, Pindborg JJ. Syndromes of the head and neck. New York: McGraw-Hill, 1964.

4. Fraser GR. The causes of profound deafness in childhood. London: Balliere Tindall, 1976.

5. Goodman RM, Gorlin RJ. Atlas of the face in genetic disorders. 2nd ed. St. Louis, CV Mosby, 1977.

6. Stark EW, Borton TE. Klippel-Feil Syndrome and associated hearing loss. Arch Otolaryngol 1973; 97:415-9.

7. Singh SP, Rock EH, Shulman A. Klippel-Feil syndrome with unexplained apparent conductive hearing loss. A case report. Laryngoscope 1969; 79:113-7.

8. Anderson H, Filipson R, Fluur E, Koch B, Lindsten J, Wedenberg E. Hearing impairment in Turner's syndrome. Acta Otolaryngol (Stockh) 1969: Suppl 247.

9. McLay K, Maran ADG. Deafness and the Klippel-Feil syndrome. J Laryngol Otol 1969; 83:175-84.

10. Caldarelli DD. Congenital middle ear anomalies associated with craniofacial and skeletal syndromes. In: Jaffee BF, ed. Hearing loss in children. Baltimore: Univ. Park Press, 1977.

11. Everberg G, Ratjen E, Sørensen H. Wildervanck's syndrome. Klippel-Feil's syndrome associated with deafness and retraction of the eyeball. Br J Radiol 1963; 36:562-7.

12. Fraser WI, MacGillivray RC. Cervico-oculo-acoustic dysplasia. J Ment Defic Res 1968; 12:322-9.

13. Ormerod FC. The pathology of congenital deafness. J Laryngol Otol 1960; 74:919-50.

14. Valvassori GE, Naunton RF, Lindsay JR. Inner ear anomalies: clinical and histopathological considerations. Ann Otol Rhinol Laryngol 1969; 78:929-38.

15. Suehiro S, Sando I. Congenital anomalies of the inner ear. Introducing a new classification of labyrinthine anomalies. Ann Otol Rhinol Laryngol 1979; Suppl 59.

16. Baumeister S, Terrahe K. Innenohrmissbildungen beim Klippel-Feil Syndrome. Laryngol Rhinol Otol (Stuttg) 1974; 53:120-30.

17. Phelps PD, Sheldon PWE, Lloyd GAS. Hearing in patients with congenital deformity of the inner ear. Clin Otol 1976; 1:31-8.

18. Windle-Taylor PC, Buchanan G, Michaels L. The Mondini defect in Turner's syndrome: a temporal bone report. Clin Otol 1981. In press.

19. Paparella MM, Elafiky FM. Mundini's deafness. Arch Otolaryngol 1972; 95:134-40.

20. Illum P. The Mundini type of cochlea malformation. A survey of the literature. Arch Otolaryngol 1972; 96:305-11.

21. Danilidis J, Magnaris T, Dimitriadis A, Iliades T, Manolidis L. Stapes gusher and Klippel-Feil syndrome. Laryngoscope 1978; 88:1178-83.

22. Phelps PD, Lloyd GAS. Congenital deformity of the internal auditory meatus and labyrinth associated with cerebrospinal fluid fistula. Adv Otol Rhinol Laryngol 1978; 24:51-7.

23. Phelps PD. Congenital lesions of the inner ear, demonstrated by tomography. A retrospective study of 34 cases with special reference to the lateral semicircular canal. Arch Otolaryngol 1974; 100:11-8.

24. Poswillo D. Otomandibular deformity: pathogenesis as a guide to reconstruction. J Maxillofac Surg 1974; 2:64-72.

25. Lloyd GAS, Phelps PD. Radiology of the ear in mandibulo-facial dysostosis — Treacher Collin's syndrome. Acta Radiol [Diagn] (Stockh) 1979; 20:233-40.

26. Baker DH, Berdon WE, Morishima A, Conte F. Turner's syndrome and pseudo-Turner's syndrome. Am J Roentgenol 1967; 100:40-7.

≈

HOUSE EAR INSTITUTE

The Board of Trustees of the Ear Research Institute on January 10, 1981, in its desire to honor Howard and William House for their many contributions to otology renamed the institution the House Ear Institute.

TOTAL LARYNGECTOMY WITH TRACHEOPHARYNGEAL FISTULA (NEOGLOTTIS)

CARLO V. CALEARO, MD　　ANGELO CAROGGIO, MD

FERRARA, ITALY

Our experience with the so-called "neoglottis" (according to Staffieri) after total laryngectomy is presented. The technique, described in detail, aims at giving the patient good speech by creating a tracheoesophageal fistula through which air passes. In the period from 1973-1979, 63 patients underwent the procedure. The functional results were satisfactory in 68% of the cases. The patient's voice is much more agreeable than the esophageal voice and sounds louder and less monotonous than a laryngophone voice. The spectrographic analyses confirm its resemblance to natural voice. An occasional passage of liquids into the trachea may occur, but is not prejudicial to either speech or swallowing. Some dysfunctional problems may arise early or late after the operation: they are continuous aspiration during swallowing and lack of phonatory function. In most cases, these problems are due to incorrect surgical technique; the possibilities and procedures of correction are described. In conclusion, we maintain that the "neoglottis," which may be applied to nearly all cases of total laryngectomy, represents a worthwhile "phonatory" innovation in the field of mutilating surgery of laryngeal cancer.

The treatment of laryngeal cancer today definitely tends to favor conservative, ie, functional, surgery. However, total laryngectomy still remains the only available technique in a large percentage of cases. With the aim of obviating the sequelae of this mutilating surgery, two main types of procedures have been developed.

The first type (ie, reconstructive laryngectomy), attempts to eliminate the tracheostoma.[1] The greatest obstacle encountered by this technique is the restoration of the sphincteral function, since the trachea must be fully anastomosed with the hypopharynx.

The second type, on the contrary, undertakes the less ambitious task of restoring only phonation without eliminating the permanent tracheostoma.[2,3] This is achieved by means of a small tracheopharyngeal fistula (Fig. 1), through which the flow of air from the lungs is directed toward the upper vocal resonators (pharynx, oral cavity, etc) whenever the tracheostoma is manually closed. This produces a voice of good quality with a natural-sounding timbre, while aspiration of foods into the bronchial tree is prevented by the small size of the fistula.

The present paper deals with our experience with the phonatory fistula, also called, according to Staffieri, neoglottis.

Indications. The indications for this procedure are the same as for total laryngectomy, with or without neck dissection. In fact, as stated above, the neoglottis is merely a surgical step applied after the removal of the larynx.

There are, however, some contraindications which include:

1. Hypoglottic cancers, since they make it necessary to remove some tracheal rings. In these cases a tracheal cylinder capable of trapping an adequate air volume cannot be left above the tracheostoma.

2. Posteriorly developing cancers, since large extents of pharyngoesophageal mucosa must be included in the removal. In these instances the flap of mucosa which is left is not wide enough to allow the adoption of this procedure.

3. Marginal cancers extending to the medial side of the pyriform sinus, for the same reason as in point 2.

4. Previous radiotherapy, since the alterations of

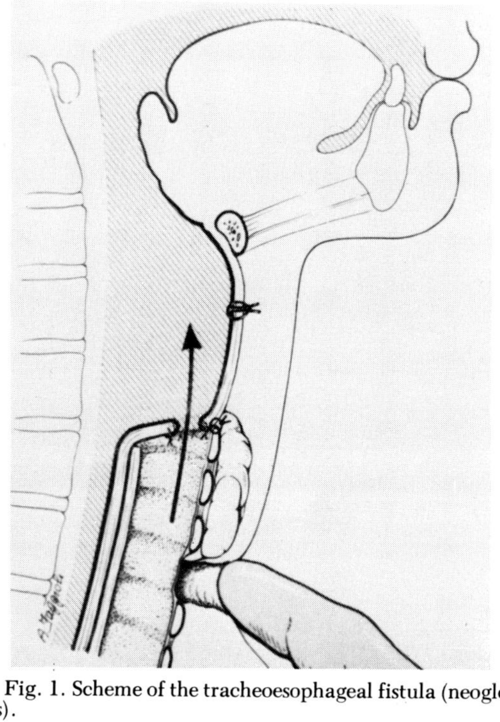

Fig. 1. Scheme of the tracheoesophageal fistula (neoglottis).

From the ENT-Clinic, University of Ferrara, Italy.

REPRINTS — Carlo V. Calearo, MD, Clinica Otorinolaringologica dell'Università, 44100 Ferrara, Italy.

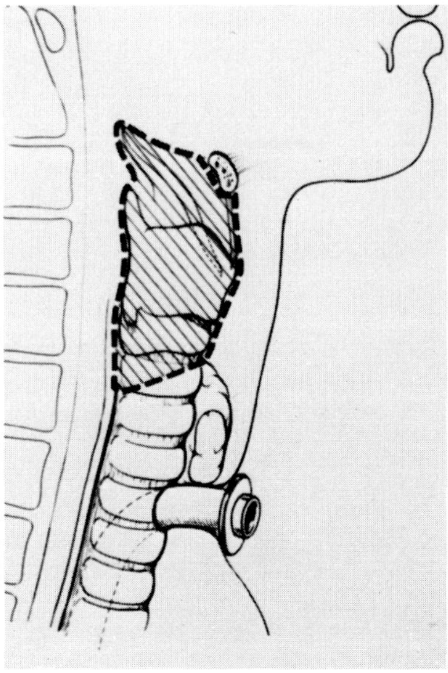

Fig. 2. When a neoglottis is planned, the removal of the larynx (shaded area) should be carried out with attention to making the tracheotomy below the thyroid isthmus and to slanting downward and backward the section of the trachea.

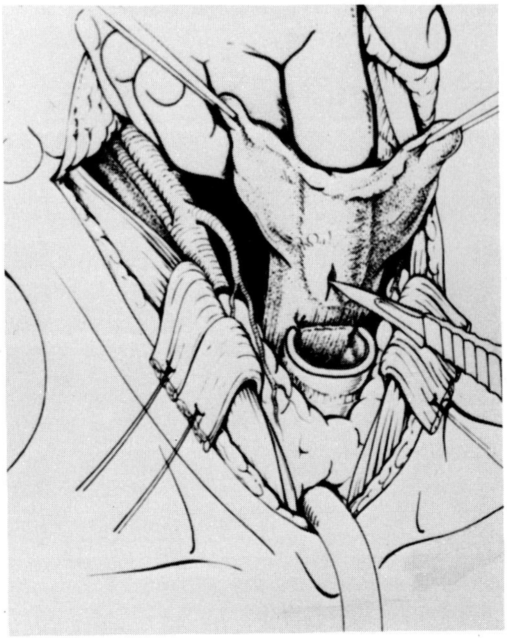

Fig. 3. After the esophagus has been anchored to the posterior ends of the tracheal rings, the fistula is made.

the tissues may prejudice a good functioning of the fistula.

5. Cancers arising in lesions of Plummer-Vinson syndrome, for the same reason as in point 4.

SURGICAL TECHNIQUE

When a phonatory fistula is planned, the total laryngectomy, with or without neck dissection, should be performed paying attention to some details. First, whenever possible, the tracheotomy should be made at the fourth or fifth ring (Fig. 2), that is, below the thyroid isthmus, in order to prevent disconnection of the gland from the trachea: this reduces the risk of cartilaginous necrosis due to deficient blood supply. Secondly, the transsection of the trachea should be carried out according to an oblique plane (Fig. 2), ie, starting anteriorly from the cricotracheal membrane, extending on both sides with a slanting cut in the first tracheal ring and ending posteriorly just below the same ring. This slope of the tracheal contour, to which the esophageal mucosa will be fastened, reduces the risk of aspiration of foods into the trachea through the fistula. Finally, the pharyngeal mucosa must be left as wide as possible, especially at the level of the pyriform sinuses and glossoepiglottic valleculae.

The construction of the phonatory fistula starts as soon as the larynx has been removed. The procedure may be divided into five steps.

1. The esophageal adventitia is anchored to the most cranial tracheal ring with two separate stitches at both posterior ends of the cartilage. Then, the fistula is created on the medial line by means of a vertical incision (8-10 mm in length) which ends 2-3 mm above the upper margin of the trachea (Fig. 3). The different layers of the visceral wall (muscular, submucosal, mucosal) should be separately transsected. The support provided by the surgeon's finger inserted into the lumen facilitates the task of identifying the successive layers.

2. Through the incision, the esophageal mucosa is pulled to the outside and sutured to the adventitia with a few separate stitches in Dexon® *4/0 (Fig. 4). When the fistula has been correctly constructed, it has a virtual opening with taut edges. It is useful to reinforce them with two anchoring stitches at each end of the fistula, passing through the muscle layer. This stretches the edges and prevents subsequent aspiration of foods.

3. A heavy silk thread is passed through the nasal cavity, the fistula and the tracheostoma (Fig. 5). It serves to keep the fistula open and will be removed after the patient has learned correct phonation. It can also be used to dilate delicately a too narrow fistula if a gauze strip with corticosteroid ointment is fastened to the thread, pulled into the fistula, and left in place for a few hours.

4. The pharyngoesophageal flap is now sutured to the tracheal opening; great care must be taken to keep the flap taut, at the same time avoiding any lateral pulling which would open the fistula. In the end, the fistula should be located approximately in the center of the tracheal lumen (Fig. 6).

5. The surgical pharyngostoma is finally closed horizontally (Fig. 6). Sometimes, when the pharyn-

*Davis-Geck, American Cyanamid Co, Pearl River, NY.

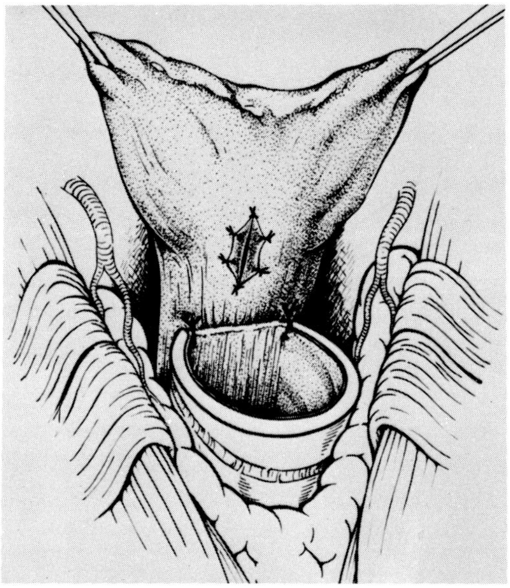

Fig. 4. The esophageal mucosa is reflected outward and sutured to the outer surface.

gostoma is very large or when the flap is irregularly shaped, it may be necessary to use a vertical or a Y-shaped suture.

RESULTS

From 1973 to 1979, 63 patients, all but one, men, ranging in age from 28 to 73, underwent this operation. As regards the tumor, 19 were primary supraglottic cancers with glottic involvement (T2-T3); 44 were primary cordal cancers with ventricular and vestibular involvement (T2-T3-T4). In 52 patients (82.5%) it was possible to perform functional neck dissection at the same time as the laryngectomy (38 bilateral, 14 unilateral). The average period of hospitalization, which includes speech rehabilitation, was 23 days. No postoperative deaths were observed.

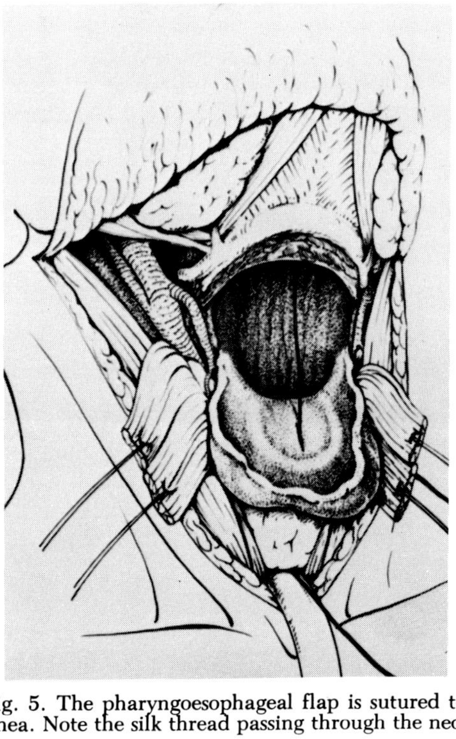

Fig. 5. The pharyngoesophageal flap is sutured to the trachea. Note the silk thread passing through the neoglottis.

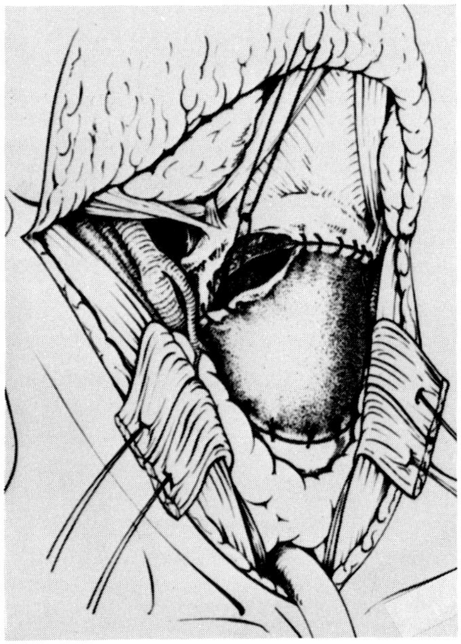

Fig. 6. Suture of the pharyngostoma.

Successful results, as regards both phonation and deglutition, were obtained in 35 patients, while in 8 other patients a good outcome was achieved after a revisional operation (see below). On the whole, the percentage of favorable results attained was 68%.

The assistance of a speech therapist is of great help in the rehabilitation which is usually begun when the wound is completely healed, ie, 8-10 days after surgery. The patient's voice is much more agreeable than the esophageal voice and sounds louder and less monotonous than a laryngophone voice. The spectrographic analysis shows its excellent qualities: it retains the harmonic structure, which clearly prevails over any residual traces of noise, and provides sufficient modulation of pitch and volume, conserving the characteristics of the personal timbre. Timing of speech is normal.

As for swallowing, it should be recalled that in most cases an occasional passage of liquids into the trachea may be seen, without any harm to the patients.

DYSFUNCTIONAL PROBLEMS AND THEIR TREATMENT

Dysfunctional problems are encountered in cases of both patulous fistula and of its occlusion. According to their appearance, they may be classified as either immediate or late. Their occurrence in our patients is listed in Table 1.

TABLE 1. DYSFUNCTIONAL PROBLEMS AND THEIR TREATMENT

	Cases	Revision Surgery	Successful
Immediate patulous	7	7	6
Immediate impermeable	12	—	—
Late patulous	6	6	1
Late impermeable	3	1	1
Total	28	14	8

Immediate Complications.

PATULOUS FISTULA. It is generally due to a faulty surgical technique. However, it can be observed when the muscle layer is very thin, as it may split when the patient resumes natural swallowing.

The symptoms of immediate patulous fistula are unmistakable: as soon as the patient attempts to swallow, foods enter the trachea, cause coughing and are expelled through the tracheostoma. A slight aspiration of liquids is admissible during the first days, as it may be due to a local edema affecting the edges of the fistula and keeping them from closing properly, but this condition must quickly disappear.

Immediate patulous fistula was observed in seven patients who underwent surgical revision. The fistula was exposed through an anterior cervical approach; it was shortened by means of stitches pulling together the edges, which had previously been scratched to cause bleeding. This procedure must be done promptly to prevent aspiration pneumonia. After revision surgery good functional results were obtained in six out of the seven cases; in the other patient, the fistula shut.

IMPERMEABLE FISTULA. Often this problem is not a question of true occlusion, but rather of the patient's initial inability to learn the new mechanism of phonation (ie, false immediate occlusion). In fact, some patients who were unable to phonate when they left the hospital, arrived at the follow-up with a satisfactory voice, either because they had learned or because the fistula was temporarily obstructed by local edema.

True immediate occlusion is always due to improper surgical technique. If the extroflexion of the mucosa on the outer pharyngeal surface is incomplete, ie, does not include the ends of the fissure, scar tissue may obstruct the lumen. More frequently, local circulatory troubles prolong the edema (contributing factors may be an excessive number of stitches and/or the use of nonabsorbable suture material), thus leading to the formation of a pseudopolyp. In this case, patients show a total inability to phonate, sometimes paradoxically accompanied by food aspiration during swallowing, as the fistula is turned into a one-way valve in the wrong direction.

Both these events, obstruction and pseudopolypoidal edema of the fistula, completely defeat the functional goals of the operation. Correcting them requires a subsequent follow-up program, first medical and then, if necessary, surgical. In some cases, when the local edema is still reversible, treatment with full dosages of corticosteroids dramatically solves the problem within a few days. In other instances, however, both medical treatment and dilations, gently performed by means of the silk thread inserted through the fistula, are ineffective, and it is necessary to adopt a surgical procedure. Once the fistula has been exposed through the anterior approach, it can be corrected or remade. Immediate occlusion was observed in 12 cases. Surgical revision was planned for these patients, but none accepted it.

Late Complications. A fistula which became patulous several months after the operation, ie, after a period during which it proved food-tight and effective in speech, was observed in five cases. This condition is presumably due to a splitting of the esophageal wall around the fistula. Thus the edges remain rigid, allowing a continuous flood of saliva and foods to the trachea.

The only solution is surgical reduction of the fistula through the anterior cervical approach. We have found this a particularly delicate situation to correct, as the atrophied esophageal wall is very fragile, and cannot easily withstand the strain of the corrective suture. Because of this difficulty, Staffieri[3] recently suggested that the surgeon should proceed in these cases as if the goal was not to reduce the fistula, but rather to close it completely.

In one out of our six cases, this corrective surgery achieved complete functional success, while in the other five patients the fistula became impermeable.

A late occlusion of the fistula was observed in only three cases, one of which was treated with radiotherapy. Surgical correction was employed in one case with good functional results.

CONCLUSIONS

Our experience allows us to state that neoglottis fully accomplishes the goal for which it was developed, ie, satisfactory speech after total laryngectomy. The construction of a fistula may conclude a total laryngectomy in nearly all cases in which this is indicated. The results are significantly good and reliable and no serious complications are to be expected.

One point should be emphasized: total laryngectomy with neoglottis remains a traditional total laryngectomy and thus requires a permanent tracheostoma. The presence of the tracheostoma is considered by common people as "the brand of the cancer" and the need to use a finger to close the tracheostoma calls even more attention to this brand. To avoid this maneuver, an effective mechanical valve to be inserted into the cannula would be required.

Nevertheless, taking into account both limitations and merits of the procedure, we feel that total laryngectomy with neoglottis represents a worthwhile "phonatory" innovation in the field of mutilating surgery for laryngeal cancer.

REFERENCES

1. Serafini I. Laringectomia totale con ricostruzione delle vie aero-digestive. Metodo personale. Arch Ital Otol 1970; 81:377-93.
2. Staffieri M. Laringectomia totale con ricostruzione di glottide fonatoria. Nuovo Arch Ital Otol 1973; 1:181-98.
3. Staffieri M. La riabilitazione chirurgica della voce e della respirazione dopo laringectomia totale. Atti XXIX Congr AOOI. Bologna, 1976:3-222.

≈

NINCDS NOTES*

CONTRACTS AWARDED FOR STUDY OF LITERATURE RETRIEVAL SYSTEM

A collaborative national study, conducted by NINCDS under contract at five evaluation centers, is under way to evaluate the usefulness of the MEDLINE literature retrieval system for communicative disorder specialists.

The two-and-a-half year project, which began in September 1980, will determine the responsiveness of the computerized retrieval system to those seeking information about communicative disorders.

WORKSHOP VOLUME EXAMINES NEUROPEPTIDES

Neurosection and Brain Peptides: Implications for Brain Functions and Neurological Disease is an extensive work involving over 100 contributors. The 700-page book examines the potential role of neuropeptides in understanding the development of neurological disease. It is based on a workshop co-sponsored by the NINCDS and held at Sea Island, Georgia, in 1980. Edited by Drs. Joseph B. Martin of Massachusetts General Hospital, Seymour Reichlin of the Tufts University School of Medicine, and Katherine L. Bick of NINCDS, the volume provides a state-of-the-art review of, and points to new directions in, an area of neurobiology that has advanced dramatically in the last decade.

The publication is available from the Raven Press, 1140 Avenue of the Americas, New York, NY 10036.

FOGARTY SCHOLAR-IN-RESIDENCE IS FIRST FROM CHINA

The first Fogarty International Scholar from China arrived at NIH on January 30, 1981. The noted visitor is Dr. Hsiang-Tung Chang, a neurophysiologist of international reputation and Professor at the Shanghai Institute of Physiology.

As a Fogarty Scholar, Dr. Chang, who is also the Director of the Brain Research Institute of the Chinese Academy of Sciences, will interact with scientists from NINCDS and the National Institute of Mental Health through lectures, seminars, and informal discussions. He will also participate in NINCDS research involving pain and the vagus nerve.

Dr. Chang is the author of nearly 80 publications, and is a member of numerous professional organizations and editorial and advisory boards. He received his undergraduate degree from the National University of Peking and his Ph.D. from Yale University. He has held positions in the United States as Assistant Professor at the Yale University School of Medicine and as an associate at the Rockefeller Institute for Medical Research.

----

*This information is prepared monthly by the Office of Scientific and Health Reports, National Institute of Neurological and Communicative Disorders and Stroke, National Institutes of Health, Bldg. 31, Rm. 8A06, Bethesda, MD 20205, (301) 496-5751.

Ann Otol 90:1981

ANALYSIS OF FACTORS AFFECTING COMPLICATIONS OF CAROTID LIGATION

AKIYOSHI KONNO, MD

KIYOSHI TOGAWA, MD KEIJI IIZUKA, MD

AKITA, JAPAN

A study of 156 patients subjected to common carotid ligation in the treatment of head and neck carcinoma was made to investigate the influence of selected factors on cerebral complications. In the analysis complications were grouped as death or coma; death, coma, hemiplegia or monoplegia; and transitory cerebral symptoms. Primary independent variables included method of occlusion (abrupt, gradual); duration of occlusion; and collateral circulation via the external carotid artery (intact, ligated external carotid artery). Death or coma occurred in 24 cases (15.4%) and complications including death, coma, hemiplegia or monoplegia occurred in 47 cases (30.1%). Although no statistically significant difference between abrupt and gradual occlusion cases was noted, the incidence of cerebral complications was significantly lower for the group with gradual carotid occlusions performed over 13 days (6.3%) than for those with abrupt occlusions or gradual occlusions performed in less than five days. The incidence of death or coma following carotid artery occlusion was 10.5% in cases with an intact external carotid artery, as against 25.5% in those with a ligated external carotid artery, a statistically significant difference. Cerebral complications occurred within 48 hours after carotid occlusion in 35 of 47 cases (74.5%) in which complications developed. In the remaining 12 cases (25.5%) complications developed after 48 hours. There was no difference between abrupt and gradual occlusion cases in the incidence of complications after 48 hours.

In surgical management of advanced head and neck carcinoma, or in the treatment of postoperative complications involving the carotid artery, it is sometimes necessary to decide whether the carotid should be ligated or grafted. Primary complications of ligation can be cerebral symptoms, ranging from death or coma to transitory symptoms, while hemorrhage due to graft failure is a major complication of transplantation. If it can be performed safely, vascular transplantation is an ideal procedure; the following disadvantages, however, need to be considered.

1. The risk of graft failure is increased in patients receiving massive preoperative radiation.

2. Grafting may interfere with complete resection of the tumor, and increase the risk of tumor dispersion.

3. Grafting necessitates delaying postoperative irradiation.

Carotid ligation, while more likely to involve cerebral complications, has the following advantages.

1. More complete resection of the tumor may be possible than with vascular transplants.

2. Postoperative irradiation can be initiated early if necessary.

3. The danger of carotid rupture is minimized, even with suppuration of the postoperative cervical wound.

The greatest problem of ligation is the possibility of death or other serious cerebral complications due to occlusion of the common carotid artery. The reported incidence of death from this cause, however, varies greatly among investigators.[1-6] Opinions also vary regarding factors influencing the safety of carotid ligation, such as whether occlusion is gradual or abrupt, and if gradual occlusion is to be used, the period of time over which it is completed. The present study is an analysis of cerebral complications in

TABLE 1. CEREBRAL COMPLICATIONS IN OCCLUSION OF COMMON CAROTID ARTERY (n = 156)

	Abrupt Occlusion		*Gradual Occlusion*		
Complications	*No.*	*%*	*No.*	*%*	*P*
Death or coma	18	17.8	6	10.9	NS
Death, coma, hemiplegia or monoplegia	35	34.7	12	21.8	NS (<0.10)
Transitory cerebral symptoms	8	7.9	8	14.6	NS
No cerebral complications	58	57.4	35	63.6	NS
Total	101		55		

P - Probability; NS - Not significant.

TABLE 2. EFFECT OF COLLATERAL CIRCULATION VIA EXTERNAL CAROTID ARTERY UPON INCIDENCE OF CEREBRAL COMPLICATIONS (N = 156)

	External Carotid Artery Intact		*Ligated*		
Complications	*No.*	*%*	*No.*	*%*	*P*
Death or coma	11	10.5	13	25.5	<0.05
Death, coma, hemiplegia or monoplegia	27	25.7	20	39.2	NS (<0.10)
Transitory cerebral symptoms	13	12.4	3	5.9	NS
No cerebral complications	65	61.9	28	54.9	NS
Total	105		51		

From the Department of Otolaryngology, Akita University School of Medicine, Akita, Japan.

REPRINTS — Akiyoshi Konno, MD, Department of Otolaryngology, Akita University School of Medicine, Akita City, Akita, Japan.

TABLE 3. EFFECT OF COLLATERAL CIRCULATION VIA EXTERNAL CAROTID ARTERY UPON CEREBRAL COMPLICATIONS (N = 156)

	Common Carotid Artery									
	Abrupt Occlusion External Carotid					*Gradual Occlusion External Carotid*				
	Intact		*Ligated*			*Intact*		*Ligated*		
Complications	*No.*	*%*	*No.*	*%*	*P*	*No.*	*%*	*No.*	*%*	*P*
Death or coma	9	13.0	9	28.1	NS (<0.10)	2	5.6	4	21.1	NS (<0.10)
Death, coma, hemiplegia or monoplegia	20	29.0	15	46.9	NS (<0.10)	7	19.4	5	26.3	NS
Transitory cerebral symptoms	7	10.1	1	3.1	NS	6	16.7	2	10.5	NS
No cerebral complications	42	60.9	16	50.0	NS	23	63.9	12	63.2	NS
Total	69		32			36		19		

cases which included ligation of the common carotid artery in the management of head and neck carcinoma; data were obtained on 156 cases from 47 institutions across Japan for the past five years.

METHODS

In this analysis cerebral complications were grouped as 1) death or coma, 2) death, coma, hemiplegia or monoplegia, and 3) transitory cerebral symptoms. Variables tested included 1) abrupt versus gradual occlusion (method of occlusion) of the common carotid artery, 2) intact versus ligated external carotid artery, and 3) reasons for common carotid ligation.

RESULTS

In 156 cases of common carotid ligation, cerebral complications of death or coma were seen in 24 cases (15.4%) and complications including death, coma, hemiplegia or monoplegia were seen in 47 cases (30.1%). Transient cerebral disturbance was observed in 16 cases (10.3%). There were no complications in 93 patients (59.3%).

Abrupt and Gradual Occlusion. The common carotid artery was abruptly ligated in 101 cases, and subjected to gradual occlusion with the use of a carotid artery clamp in 55 cases (Table 1). There were no statistically significant differences at the 5% level as determined by chi-square tests (including Fisher's exact test) in the incidence of any complications comparing abrupt and gradual carotid occlusion. The incidence of cerebral complications between the two populations when comparing death, coma, hemiplegia or monoplegia was lower in the gradual occlusion group at the 10% level.

Collateral Circulation Via External Carotid Artery. At the time of ligation of the common carotid artery, the external carotid artery remained open in 105 cases, while the external carotid artery had been ligated by a previous surgery or was ligated simultaneously with common carotid ligation in 51 cases (Table 2). The incidence of death or coma was significantly lower at the 5% level in the group with intact external carotid arteries than ligated external carotid arteries. The proportion of cerebral complications including death, coma, hemiplegia or monoplegia was lower at the 10% level in the group with intact external carotid arteries than in the ligated group.

When the subjects were subdivided into gradual or abrupt carotid occlusion groups, there were no statistically significant differences in the incidence of cerebral complications between the groups with intact and ligated external carotid arteries, with either gradual or abrupt carotid occlusion (Table 3). When complications were limited to death or coma, the incidence of complications was proportionally lower in the group with intact external carotid arteries than in the group with ligated external carotids, regardless of whether common carotid ligation was abrupt or gradual. The incidence of cerebral complications inclusive of death, coma, hemiplegia or monoplegia was proportionally lower in the intact than in the ligated external carotid artery group in cases with abrupt common carotid ligation.

In 13 cases the common carotid artery was gradually occluded with no cerebral complications and the external carotid artery was secondarily resected at the time of tumor removal. The incidence of cerebral complications of this group ranked between the gradual occlusion and the abrupt occlusion groups in cases of previously ligated external carotid arteries (Table 4).

Injury to the carotid artery due to gradual occlusion was seen in one case where hemorrhage was noted at the site of clamping eight days after initiation of the ligation, and emergency ligation of the common carotid artery was done. No serious injury to the arterial wall resulted in other cases.

TABLE 4. INCIDENCE OF CEREBRAL COMPLICATIONS ON ABRUPT OCCLUSION OF EXTERNAL CAROTID ARTERY AFTER GRADUAL OCCLUSION OF COMMON CAROTID ARTERY (n = 13)

	Cases	
Complications	*No.*	*%*
Death or coma	3	23.0
Death, coma, hemiplegia or monoplegia	5	38.5
Transitory cerebral symptoms	1	7.7
No complications	7	53.8
Total	13	100.0

TABLE 5. DAYS FOLLOWING CAROTID OCCLUSION AND INCIDENCE OF CEREBRAL COMPLICATIONS (n = 55)

	Days Spent in Ligation: Less than 7 Days (Mean 5.1±1.7)			Days Spent in Ligation: More than 8 Days (Mean 13±4.5)			
	Total No. Cases	Cases with Complications* No.	%	Total No. Cases	Cases with Complications* No.	%	p
External carotid artery intact	20	6	30.0	16	1	6.3	NS (<0.10)
External carotid artery ligated	16	5	31.3	3	0		NS
Total	36	11	30.6	19	1	5.3	<0.05

*Death, coma, hemiplegia, or monoplegia.

Duration of Ligation. The relationship between number of days spent in ligation and complications including death, coma, hemiplegia or monoplegia in gradual occlusion cases is compared in Table 5. Gradual occlusion cases were divided into two groups according to the length of time required for ligation. Average time needed for gradual occlusion was less than seven days in 36 cases (mean and SD 5.1±1.7 days), and eight days or longer in 19 cases (mean and SD 13±4.5 days). Cerebral complications were seen in 11 of 36 cases (30.6%) in the shorter duration group, and in 1 of 19 cases (5.3%) in the longer duration group. The difference was significant at the 5% level.

Reasons for Ligation. The purposes of common carotid ligation by method of occlusion (abrupt and gradual) are compared in Table 6. Common carotid ligation was performed for radical resection of a tumor that infiltrated or approached the carotid wall in 59 cases, for rupture or impending rupture of the carotid artery in terminal carcinoma in 64 cases, for treatment of postoperative complications involving the carotid artery in 29 cases, and for treatment of operative injury of the carotid artery or other purposes in 4 cases. Abrupt occlusion was used most frequently in treating rupture or impending rupture of the carotid artery in terminal carcinoma (53/64 cases, 83%) or treatment of postoperative complications involving the carotid artery (27/29 cases, 93%). Gradual occlusion, on the other hand, was more frequently performed (41/59 cases, 69%) when the purpose was resection of a tumor.

Table 7 revealed no significant correlation between cerebral complications and the purposes of abrupt occlusion of the carotid artery.

Time of Onset of Complications. In the majority of cases, cerebral complications were manifested within 24 hours of ligation. They appeared two or more days after carotid occlusion in 12 of 156 cases. These 12 cases included two cases of hemiplegia with onset 10 and 12 months after occlusion. There was no significant difference in the incidence of complications occurring after 48 hours between the groups with abrupt and gradual occlusion.

DISCUSSION

Resection of the common carotid artery is occasionally unavoidable in extirpative surgery in advanced head and neck carcinoma. The incidence of cerebral complications following common carotid occlusion varies greatly with different authors. Watson and Silverston[1] reported that the incidence of cerebral complications due to ligation of the common carotid artery was 60% and mortality 55% in cases of head and neck carcinoma. According to Moor et al[2] the incidence of cerebral complications was 40% and mortality 17% in 69 cases of elective ligation of the common carotid and/or internal carotid artery, as against 88% and 38% respectively in 87 cases of nonelective ligation for carotid rupture.

Incidence of cerebral complications of carotid ligation is generally low in surgery for cerebral aneurysm and arteriovenous fistula. Matas[3] reported a mortality rate of 3.8% in 53 cases of common carotid ligation, Dandy[4] reported 5.7% in 88 cases of internal carotid ligation, and Gurdjian[5] reported 3% in 63 cases of common or internal carotid artery ligation. According to Nishioka,[6] however, the incidence of complications of common or internal carotid ligation in 765 cases of intracranial aneurysm was 34% in abrupt occlusion, 25% in gradual occlusion, 28% in common carotid ligation, and 49% in internal carotid ligation. Such a disparity seems to have arisen from a complicated diversity of characteristics in patients subjected to carotid ligation.

In the 156 cases in the present series, the incidence of cerebral complications including death,

TABLE 6. RELATIONSHIP BETWEEN PURPOSE OF COMMON CAROTID LIGATION AND METHOD OF LIGATION (n = 156)

Reason for Procedure	Abrupt Occlusion No.	%	Gradual Occlusion No.	%	Total No.	%
Resection of tumor infiltrating around the carotid artery	18	17.8	41	74.5	59	37.8
Carotid rupture or impending rupture in terminal carcinoma	53	52.5	11	20.1	64	41.0
Carotid rupture or impending rupture as postoperative complication	27	26.7	2	3.6	29	18.6
Others	3	3.0	1	1.8	4	2.6
Total	101	100.0	55	100.0	156	100.0

TABLE 7. PURPOSE OF COMMON CAROTID LIGATION AND INCIDENCE OF CEREBRAL COMPLICATIONS IN CASES OF ABRUPT OCCLUSION OF CAROTID ARTERY (N = 101)

Complications	*Resection of Tumor Infiltrating Around the Carotid Artery* No.	%	*Carotid Rupture or Impending Rupture in Terminal Carcinoma* No.	%	*Carotid Rupture or Impending Rupture in Postoperative Complication* No.	%	*Others* No.	%	*Total*	*P*
Death or coma	4	22.2	9	17.0	5	18.5	0		18	NS
Death, coma, hemiplegia or monoplegia	7	28.9	19	35.8	9	33.3	0		35	NS
Transitory cerebral symptoms	0		4	7.6	4	14.8	0		8	NS
No cerebral complications	11	61.1	30	56.6	14	51.8	3	100	58	NS
Total	18		53		27		3		101	

NS - Not significant.

coma, hemiplegia or monoplegia was 30.1% and mortality 15.4%. While statistically significant differences in the incidence of cerebral complications between abrupt and gradual occlusion groups in the present study were not found, a significant difference was discovered between cases of abrupt occlusion and gradual occlusion performed over an average of 13 ± 4.5 days. The presence or absence of collateral circulation through the external carotid artery was also a statistically significant factor affecting the incidence of complications. This agrees with the findings of Nishioka[6] concerning differences between the incidence of complications of common carotid and internal carotid ligation, both performed for intracranial aneurysm.

After common carotid ligation, collateral circulation develops in accordance with the arterial pressure gradient. Youmans et al[7] demonstrated changes in internal carotid artery blood flow after common carotid ligation. Blood flow from the external to the internal carotid artery was recorded immediately after the common carotid ligation in one of eight cases, blood flow was not detected in the internal carotid artery in one case, and retrograde blood flow from the internal to the external carotid artery was recorded in the remaining six cases. Prolonged recording (average two hours, 36 minutes) after common carotid ligation showed blood flow from the external to the internal carotid artery in all the cases; volume of blood flow into the internal carotid artery increased with time.

The incidence of cerebral complications including death, coma, hemiplegia or monoplegia was as high as 38.5% in 13 cases in which the common carotid artery was gradually occluded and the external carotid artery was secondarily ligated abruptly and resected together with the tumor in an extended extirpative surgery. Actually cases like these are the greatest clinical problem. In such cases, it seems necessary to ligate the ipsilateral external carotid and the thyroid arteries beforehand if possible, and then perform the carotid occlusion gradually over two weeks.

Pathogenesis of cerebral complications is considered to involve insufficiency of the collateral circulation via the circle of Willis, thrombus formation following carotid ligation, and propagation of a thrombus distal to the ligation. The latter etiology was believed to be the cause of late development of cerebral complications and gradual occlusion was sometimes contraindicated due to the risk of thrombus formation.[8] In the present study, cerebral complications were manifested later than 48 hours after termination of the ligation in 12 of 156 cases (7.7%). The delayed cerebral complications occurred independently of method (gradual vs abrupt) of occlusion.

To predict cerebral complications in individual cases, various methods have been devised, such as 1) Matas' test,[3] 2) recording of electroencephalograms at the time of carotid compression,[9] 3) four-vessel angiography and visualization of collateral circulation via the contralateral internal carotid artery during carotid compression, 4) measurement of distal stump pressure and/or measurement of cerebral blood flow following temporary carotid occlusion.[10] As McCoy and Barsocchini[11] described, common carotid and internal carotid ligation probably may be safely carried out if results of these tests are normal.

To minimize development of cerebral complications, the occlusion should be done gradually over approximately two weeks, if possible. The carotid artery is constricted at a stroke by a half to two thirds of its internal diameter with a carotid artery clamp the first day; thereafter clamping is allowed to gradually increase the degree of stricture. Development of cerebral dysfunction is monitored by serial EEG recordings. Though cerebral complications may develop in the course of gradual occlusion, many cases have been reported in which paralysis was reversed by opening the carotid clamp.[6]

SUMMARY

A study of 156 surgical oncology patients with carotid ligations was made to determine the effect of selected factors on cerebral complications. The major independent variables tested were 1) method of occlusion (abrupt versus gradual), 2) collateral circulation via the external carotid artery, and 3) duration of ligation procedure.

Of 156 cases, 24 (15.4%) experienced death or coma; complications including death, coma, hemiplegia or monoplegia were seen in 47 cases (30.1%).

The incidence of cerebral complications including death, coma, hemiplegia or monoplegia varied from 6.3 - 46.9%. There was no statistically significant difference in the incidence of complications between groups with abrupt and gradual occlusion of the common carotid artery. It was significantly lower, however, in the group with gradual occlusion performed over 13$\pm$4.5 days than in the group with abrupt occlusion. In this subgroup of gradual occlusion, the incidence of cerebral complications including death, coma, hemiplegia or monoplegia was the lowest (6.3%).

The incidence of complications including death or coma was 10.5% in cases with an intact external carotid artery, as against 25.5% in those with a ligated external carotid artery. Differences between these two groups were significant at the 5% level.

Cerebral complications such as death, coma, hemiplegia or monoplegia occurred within 48 hours after occlusion in 35 of 47 cases in which complications developed. In the remaining 12 cases, complications developed after 48 hours. Complications after 48 hours appeared to occur independently of method of occlusion.

ACKNOWLEDGMENTS — The authors wish to express sincere thanks to staffs of departments of otolaryngology or head and neck services of the following 47 institutions across Japan. The data presented from each one constituted the basis of this study.

Hokkaido University School of Medicine
Sapporo Medical College
Asahikawa Medical College
Hirosaki University School of Medicine
Akita University School of Medicine
Tohoku University School of Medicine
Fukushima Medical College
National Tochigi Hospital
Jichi Medical School
Dokkyo University School of Medicine
Tsukuba University Institute of Clinical Medicine
Chiba University School of Medicine
Chiba Cancer Center Hospital
Nippon University School of Medicine
Cancer Institute Hospital
National Cancer Center Hospital
Nippon Medical School
Tokyo University Faculty of Medicine
Tokyo Medical and Dental University
Keio University Faculty of Medicine
Jikei University School of Medicine
Toho University School of Medicine
Yokohama City University School of Medicine
St. Marianna University School of Medicine
Kitasato University School of Medicine
Tokai University School of Medicine
Niigata University School of Medicine
Kanazawa University School of Medicine
Kanazawa Medical College
Aichi Cancer Center Hospital
Nagoya City University School of Medicine
Fujitagakuen School of Medicine
Mie University School of Medicine
Kyoto University School of Medicine
Kyoto Prefectural University of Medicine
Osaka University School of Medicine
Osaka City University School of Medicine
Kinki University School of Medicine
Wakayama Medical College
Kobe University School of Medicine
Hyogo Medical College
Hiroshima University School of Medicine
National Kyushu Cancer Center Hospital
Fukuoka University School of Medicine
Kumamoto University School of Medicine
Kurume University School of Medicine
Kagoshima University School of Medicine

REFERENCES

1. Watson WL, Silverstone SM. Ligature of common carotid artery in cancer of the head and neck. Ann Surg 1939; 109:1-27.

2. Moor OS, Karlan M, Sigler L. Factors influencing the safety of carotid ligation. Am J Surg 1969; 118:666-8.

3. Matas R. Personal experiences in vascular surgery, statistical synopsis. Ann Surg 1940; 112:802-39.

4. Dandy WE. Results following ligation of internal carotid artery. Arch Surg 1942; 45:521-33.

5. Gurdjian ES, Webster JE, Martin FA, et al. Carotid compression in the neck: results and significance in carotid ligation. JAMA 1957; 163:1030-6.

6. Nishioka H. Report on the cooperative study of intracranial aneurysms and subarachnoid hemorrhage: I. Results of the treatment of intracranial aneurysms by occlusion of the carotid artery in the neck. J Neurosurg 1966; 25:660-704.

7. Youmans JR, Kindt GW, Mitchell OC. Extended studies of direction of flow and pressure in the internal carotid artery following common carotid artery ligation. J Neurosurg 1967; 27:250-4.

8. Dorrance GM. Ligation of the great vessels of the neck. Ann Surg 1934; 99:721-47.

9. Sharbrough FW, Messick JM Jr, Sundt TM Jr. Correlation of continuous electroencephalograms with cerebral blood flow measurements during carotid endarterectomy. Stroke 1973; 4:674-83.

10. Jawad K, Miller JD, Wyper DJ, et al. Measurement of CBS and carotid artery pressure compared with cerebral angiography in assessing collateral blood supply after carotid ligation. J Neurosurg 1977; 46:185-96.

11. McCoy G, Barsocchini LM. Experiences in carotid artery occlusion. Laryngoscope 1968; 78:1195-210.

A MULTIPLE-CHANNEL COCHLEAR IMPLANT: AN EVALUATION USING NONSENSE SYLLABLES

GRAEME M. CLARK, PhD, FRCS
YIT CHOW TONG, BE, PhD
LOIS F. MARTIN, BSc, DipAud
PETER A. BUSBY, MA
RICHARD C. DOWELL, BSc, DipAud
PETER M. SELIGMAN, BE, PhD
JAMES F. PATRICK, MSc

EAST MELBOURNE, AUSTRALIA

A study using nonsense syllables has shown that a multiple-channel cochlear implant with speech processor is effective in providing information about voicing and manner and to a lesser extent place distinctions. These distinctions supplement lipreading cues. Furthermore, the average percentage improvements in overall identification scores for multiple-channel electrical stimulation and lipreading compared to lipreading alone were 71% for a laboratory-based speech processor and 122% for a wearable unit.

INTRODUCTION

Patients with a profound or total hearing loss do not get satisfactory help with a hearing aid. Consequently, there has been interest in producing hearing artificially by electrical stimulation of residual auditory nerve fibers, and recent studies have shown patients benefit by single channel[1-3] or multiple-channel[4-6] stimulation. This has been demonstrated by a variety of tests which have included the Utley and Norton speechreading measure,[1] the Craig lipreading inventory,[2] closed-set spondaic word lists,[2,4] vowel identification,[2,6] consonant identification,[3] phonetically-balanced word lists,[7] and everyday sentence lists.[7]

In order to evaluate the multiple-channel cochlear implant and speech processor developed at the University of Melbourne,[8,9] we have considered it desirable to use nonsense syllables with a vowel-consonant-vowel (VCV) structure as a test procedure. We have done this as these syllables have been used to evaluate and improve the speech processing strategy used with our device,[6,9] and consonant confusion tests using these syllables have been used to assess communication skills in normal and hard of hearing subjects.[10,11]

METHODS

Two patients with a total hearing loss were implanted with multiple-channel receiver-stimulator devices on August 1, 1978, and July 17, 1979, respectively. The first patient had a sudden hearing loss following a head injury 18 months prior to surgery. Pure-tone audiometry under headphones and free-field revealed no hearing at any frequency, and the patient consequently received no benefit from a hearing aid. Polytome x-rays of the temporal bone demonstrated a fracture involving the superior semicircular canal, and electrical stimulation of the promontory was positive. The second patient had a progressive hearing loss. He had interstitial keratitis at the age of 19, and was involved in a bomb blast in 1944. For 13 years prior to surgery, pure-tone audiometry had shown no residual hearing. When tested in 1978 pure-tone audiometry under headphones showed no hearing in the left or operated ear, and in the right ear a threshold of 105 dB HTL at 0.5 kHz and 90 dB HTL at 0.25 kHz. Speech audiometry under headphones at intensities of 120 dB SPL gave 0% scores. This patient received no benefit from a hearing aid. Electrical stimulation of the promontory was also positive.

The receiver-stimulator units were implanted in a bed created in the mastoid bone.[12] They provided ten channels of stimulation, with independent control of the pulse rate and current level on each channel.[13] Electrical stimulation was produced with biphasic current pulses with the leading phase negative and each phase fixed at approximately 180 μs. The current levels were varied from 70 μA in fifteen 70 μA steps to approximately 1 mA.[13] Power and data were transmitted through the skin by inductive coupling. The electrode arrays from the receiver-stimulator units were inserted into the scala tympani of the basal turn of the cochlea through the round window, and passed for a distance of 20-25 mm. The electrode arrays had 20 individual electrodes so that ten channels of stimulation could be obtained, using alternate electrodes as a common ground. The array was fabricated from Teflon®-coated platinum wires with a bare diameter of .025 mm. The wires were enclosed in a Silastic® tube (Dow Corning) with an outside diameter of 0.6 mm, and connected to 0.3 mm strips of platinum foil. These strips were then wrapped around the Silastic tube, and the free ends welded together.[14]

Following the operation on the first patient, electrical stimulus thresholds for 1000 pulse/s stimuli were obtained and these varied from 67 μA to 402 μA for the different electrodes, and there was a dynamic range of approximately 450 μA. A series of psychophysical tests was then carried out. These showed that he experienced a change in vowel color and sharpness with the position of the electrode, a variation in pitch with pulse rate, and an increase in loudness with current level.[6] It therefore appeared that a possible speech processing strategy was to transform the spectral emphasis of a speech signal to electrode position, the fundamental frequency to pulse rate, and the speech signal energy to current level.

This strategy was implemented initially using a laboratory-based speech processor.[9] In the speech processor the voicing frequency of speech (FO) and its energy (AO) were extracted using a 400 Hz low-pass filter, and an energy threshold detector of AO was used to determine whether voicing was present or not. In the presence of voicing the pulse rate on electrodes was made proportional to FO. If voicing was absent, a constant low pulse rate was used as it produced a sensation described as "rough" which was similar to a "noise" sensation previously experienced by the patients when they had hearing. In addition, the frequency of the dominant spectral peak in the midfrequency range, called the sec-

From the Department of Otolaryngology, University of Melbourne, The Royal Victorian Eye and Ear Hospital, East Melbourne, Australia.

REPRINTS — Graeme M. Clarke, PhD, FRCS, Department of Otolaryngology, University of Melbourne, The Royal Victorian Eye and Ear Hospital, East Melbourne, Vic. 3002, Australia.

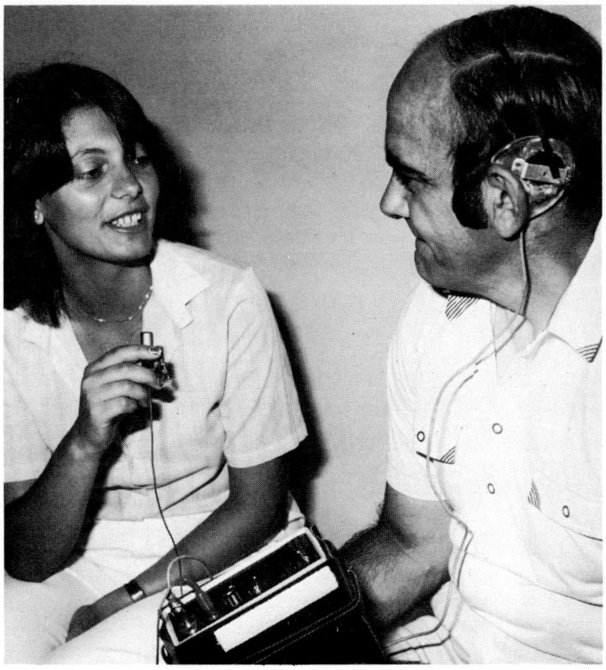

Fig. 1. Photograph of patient 1 using the wearable speech-processor.

ond formant frequency (F2) and the energy (A2) associated with this peak were estimated from the output of a 750-4000 Hz bandpass filter. For a given F2 estimate, an electrode was selected from a predetermined F2-to-electrode transformation map, which had been constructed by ranking the electrodes from dullest to sharpest, and assigning frequency subbands to these electrodes in an order from lowest to highest. Similarly, the current level was determined on the basis of an A2-to-current level map. The speech parameters were determined every 10 ms, and only one electrode was activated within a 10 ms time frame.

The laboratory-based speech processor was assessed in the two patients using nonsense syllables constructed from the consonants /b/, /p/, /m/, /d/, /t/, /n/, /g/, /k/ in a VCV structure using the vowel /a/ as in "*fa*ther." The above consonants were selected as they include important homophenous phonemes (phonemes having the same form to the eye as another). For example, /b/, /p/, /m/ look the same on the lips as do /d/, /t/, /n/ and also /g/, /k/.

The study was carried out in a well-lit room with no sound treatment in three situations: multiple-channel electrical stimulation alone (EO), vision alone (VO) and vision plus multiple-channel electrical stimulation (EV). The test material was presented by experienced audiologists using live voice at an intensity of 80 dB SPL at the microphone. The sets of nonsense syllables were spoken by both a female with a British accent, and a male with an Australian one. It was considered important to have results for both female and male voices in order to assess the capacity of the speech processor in handling both female and male speaker characteristics which can vary considerably in fundamental and formant frequencies. There was in fact quite a considerable variation in the speaker characteristics of the two testers as the female had a fundamental frequency of 230-240 Hz, and the male a frequency of 100-125 Hz.

The test results were obtained after the patients had been made familiar with each stimulus presentation situation, and the nature of the test material. Each patient was tested on four separate days. Two days were for tests with the female speaker and two for the male speaker, so that an assessment could be made of test-retest reliability. On each day the patient had three test sessions for the stimulus conditions EO, VO, EV. Each session lasted 20-25 minutes, and there was a break of 10-15 minutes between each session. Furthermore, the conditions EO, VO, EV were tested in different order to reduce the effects of learning and fatigue in

TABLE 1. IDENTIFICATION OF CONSONANTS,* LABORATORY-BASED SPEECH PROCESSOR

	Test Voice	*ES*	*Vision Alone*	*ES Plus Vision*	*Improvement† with ES plus Vision vs Vision Alone (%)*
		Proportion Correct			
Patient 1	F	.48	.36	.69	92
	M	.30	.34	.61	79
Patient 2	F	.34	.42	.70	67
	M	.35	.32	.46	44
Average		.37	.36	.62	72

*b, m, p, d, n, t, g, k.

†Improvement is defined as the difference between the implant plus vision and vision alone scores divided by the vision alone scores and expressed as a percentage.

Proportion correct - Number of phonemes correctly identified divided by number of times each phoneme was presented (20 stimuli).

ES - Electrical stimulation.

biasing the results. For patient 1 the experimental conditions were: day 1, tester 1 - EO, VO, EV; day 2, tester 2 - EV, EO, VO; day 3, tester 2 - VO, EO, EV; day 4, tester 1 - EV, VO, EO. For patient 2 the conditions were: day 1, tester 1 - EO, VO, EV; day 2, tester 2 - EV, EO, VO; day 3, tester 2 - EV, EO, VO; day 4, tester 1 - VO, EV, EO. At each session nonsense syllables were presented at random until all eight consonants had been given ten times, a total of 80 syllables.

The results of the study were recorded as confusion matrices, obtained by plotting the patients' responses to each stimulus. From the results, the overall proportion of nonsense syllables correctly identified was calculated. In addition, the proportion of voicing, manner and place distinctions correctly made was determined. It was considered important to assess the value of the implant in helping the patients to make voicing, manner and place distinctions, as this would be a measure of how effective the device is in supplementing lip reading cues. Lip reading cues are mainly based on place distinctions, for example, the bilabial plosives /p/ and /b/ have a different place of articulation from the lingua-alveolars /t/ and /d/, and this can be readily seen on the lips. Therefore, if adequate voicing distinctions are provided by electrical stimulation, this will greatly assist in communication. Furthermore, manner distinictions will be of help as these are also not readily visible on the lips, and could help distinguish the plosive /b/ from the nasal /m/.

A wearable speech-processor (Fig. 1) was also constructed to provide similar processing strategies to the laboratory-based device. It was tested in the same way although the stimulus conditions were not varied and the order was EV, VO, EO. It was considered that this would 1) maximize the fatigue effect for EO, and 2) there would be a better practice effect for VO following EV rather than for EO following EV. Presenting the conditions this way would therefore be more likely to give better results for VO rather than EO. Furthermore, due to staff changes another audiologist carried out the male voice tests. The results were also plotted as confusion matrices.

RESULTS

The results of the nonsense syllable tests for the laboratory-based speech processor are summarized in Table 1. The order of EO, VO, EV had no significant effect on the results, and test-retest reliability was good, especially for patient 1. Furthermore, it can be seen from Table 1 that when tested with female and male voices, the use of the multiple-channel cochlear implant led to a very significant improvement in both patients' abilities to speech-

TABLE 2. VOICING, MANNER AND PLACE DISTINCTIONS, LABORATORY-BASED SPEECH PROCESSOR

	Test Voice		*Proportion Correct* ES Alone	Vision Alone	ES plus Vision
Patient 1	F	Voicing	.94	.62	.98
		Manner	.75	.60	.73
		Place	.63	.78	.89
	M	Voicing	.83	.59	.86
		Manner	.66	.63	.76
		Place	.51	.71	.88
Patient 2	F	Voicing	.86	.65	.96
		Manner	.71	.64	.77
		Place	.54	.84	.93
	M	Voicing	.71	.54	.68
		Manner	.76	.66	.66
		Place	.53	.72	.84

read compared to vision alone. This improvement varied from 44 to 92%, with an average of 72%.

Furthermore, an analysis of the results to determine the proportion of voicing, manner and place distinctions correctly identified are summarized in Table 2. From this it can be seen that there was a consistent trend for the scores to be significantly better with voicing and manner distinctions for electrical stimulation alone rather than lipreading alone. There was a further improvement in the scores for voicing and manner distinctions when using electrical stimulation in combination with lipreading. Furthermore, although the place distinction results were poorer for electrical stimulation alone compared to lipreading alone, electrical stimulation was in fact a help when used in combination with lipreading as the combined scores for the place distinction were in fact better than with lipreading alone.

The results of testing the wearable speech processor on patient 1 are summarized in Table 3. The test-retest reliability was good. Table 3 shows that when the wearable speech processor was used in conjunction with lipreading, the scores were significantly better than with lipreading alone. The improvements were 156% for the female speaker and 92% for the male. When the results were analyzed

TABLE 3. IDENTIFICATION OF CONSONANTS,* WEARABLE SPEECH PROCESSOR

	Test Voice	*Proportion Correct* ES	Vision Alone	ES Plus Vision	Improvement with ES plus Vision vs Vision Alone (%)
Patient 1	F	.56	.34	.87	156
	M	.50	.36	.69	92
Average		.53	.35	.78	122

*b, m, p, d, n, t, g, k.

TABLE 4. VOICING, MANNER AND PLACE DISTINCTIONS, WEARABLE SPEECH PROCESSOR

	Test Voice		*Proportion Correct* ES Alone	Vision Alone	ES plus Vision
Patient 1	F	Voicing	.94	.64	.98
		Manner	.83	.66	.93
		Place	.71	.80	.94
	M	Voicing	.82	.62	.90
		Manner	.86	.73	.85
		Place	.62	.80	.85

to determine the proportion of voicing, manner and place distinction correctly identified it was found (Table 4) that voicing and manner distinctions were significantly better with multiple-channel electrical stimulation alone compared to lipreading alone, and the scores for electrical stimulation plus lipreading were either as good as electrical stimulation alone or better. Furthermore, although the place distinctions with electrical stimulation were not as good as those with lipreading, they were nevertheless significant, and in the combined electrical stimulation and lipreading situation they were better than with lipreading alone.

DISCUSSION

The findings in this study show that a multiple-channel cochlear implant and speech processor which extracts the voicing frequency and energy, and the frequency and energy of the dominant spectral peak in the midfrequency range are effective in providing help with voicing and manner distinctions, and to a lesser extent with place information. Help with voicing and manner distinctions should supplement lipreading cues in understanding running speech. Furthermore, it was also shown that the overall scores were significantly better when using multiple-channel electrical stimulation in conjunction with lipreading compared to lipreading alone, and the improvements varied from 44 to 92% for the laboratory-based speech processor, and from 92 to 156% for the wearable processor. The improved performance of the wearable processor may have been due to a learning effect, and the fact that a different male voice was used for the tests. The performance was nevertheless significant and indicates that the laboratory-based speech processor strategy had been adequately realized in the wearable unit. It is also of interest that the results for voicing, manner and place distinctions were slightly better in patient 1 for the wearable speech processor when compared with those for the laboratory-based speech processor.

ACKNOWLEDGMENTS — We would like to thank the Department of Productivity of the Australian government, the National Health and Medical Research Council of Australia, the Channel 10 Deafness Appeal and Lions International for providing funds for this study. We would also like to thank P. Blamey, G. Cook, L. Cole, R. Walkerden and Miss J. Maher for their help.

REFERENCES

1. House WF, Berliner K, Crary WI, et al. Cochlear implants. Ann Otol Rhinol Laryngol 1976; 85 Suppl 27.

2. Bilger RC, Black FO, Hopkinson NT, et al. Evaluation of subjects presently fitted with implanted auditory prostheses. Ann Otol Rhinol Laryngol 1977; 86 Suppl 38.

3. Fourcin AJ, Rosen SM, Moore BCJ, et al. External electrical stimulation of the cochlea: clinical, psychophysical, speech-perceptual and histological findings. Br J Audiol 1979; 13:85-107.

4. Pialoux P, Chouard CH, Meyer B, Fugain C. Indications and results of the multichannel cochlear implant. Acta Otolaryngol (Stockh) 1979; 87:189-95.

5. Simmonds FB, Mathews RG, Walker MG, White RL. A functioning multi-channel auditory nerve stimulator. Acta Otolaryngol (Stockh) 1979; 87:170-5.

6. Tong YC, Black RC, Clark GM, et al. A preliminary report on a multiple-channel cochlear implant operation. J Laryngol Otol 1979; 93:168-74.

7. Tong YC, Clark GM. Speech comprehension with multiple-channel electrical stimulation of human auditory nerve fibres. J Physiol Pharmacol Soc Aust. In press.

8. Clark GM, Tong YC, Black R, Forster IC, Patrick JF, Dewhurst DJ. A multiple-electrode cochlear implant. J Laryngol Otol 1977; 91:935-45.

9. Tong YC, Millar JB, Clark GM, Martin LF, Busby PA, Patrick JF. Psychophysical and speech perception studies on two multiple-channel cochlear implant patients. J Laryngol Otol. In press.

10. Wang MD, Reed CM, Bilger RC. A comparison of the effects of filtering and sensorinerual hearing loss on patients of consonant confusions. J Speech Hear Res 1978; 21:5-36.

11. Erber NP. Auditory, visual, and auditory-visual recognition of consonants by children with normal and impaired hearing. J Speech Hear Res 1972; 15:413-22.

12. Clark GM, Pyman BC, Bailey QR. The surgery for multiple-electrode cochlear implantations. J Laryngol Otol 1979; 93:213-23.

13. Clark GM, Tong YC, Black R, Forster IC, Patrick JF, Dewurst DJ. A multiple-electrode hearing prosthesis for cochlear implantation in deaf patients. Med Prog Technol 1977; 5:127-39.

14. Clark GM, Patrick JF, Bailey QF. A cochlear implant round window array. J Laryngol Otol 1979; 93:107-9.

≈

WEGENER'S GRANULOMATOSIS

LONG-TERM RESULTS OF TREATMENT

PETER ILLUM, MD   KAREN THORLING, MD

AARHUS, DENMARK

Seventeen patients with Wegener's granulomatosis are presented. The very complex clinical features are outlined. A recently suggested new classification (ELK-classification) is applied. Fourteen patients were treated with cytotoxic agents and steroids, 12 of these receiving 6-mercaptopurine. Of the ten patients still alive, eight are in remission with treatment withdrawn in three cases. The duration of the treatment is discussed. The results are largely satisfactory, but the course of the disease is still capricious. Progression to a higher step in the ELK-classification has been observed in several cases and a number of serious sequelae to the disease are recorded. The initial symptoms of Wegener's granulomatosis are varied and uncharacteristic, and it is important to bear this disease in mind when patients with a long course of apparently trivial infections or peculiar constellations of symptoms from several organs are encountered. Repeated biopsies from the respiratory tract are important in order to establish the diagnosis, but treatment should not be delayed in cases where only a tentative diagnosis can be made on the basis of a reasonably typical clinical picture, even with a negative histological response.

Wegener's granulomatosis (WG), described in 1936,[1] is a rare disease defined by the triad of 1) granulomatous, necrotizing processes in the upper and/or lower respiratory tract, 2) generalized vasculitis, primarily of the small arteries and veins, and 3) focal necrotizing glomerulitis. The disease was for many years considered to be invariably fatal. The average survival time was five months,[2] but spontaneous survival of up to four years has been encountered.

Subsequently, cases without renal symptoms have been described, the so-called limited Wegener's granulomatosis.[3]

A clinical picture involving only the upper respiratory tract has been termed lethal midline granuloma. This term had been used not only for patients with lesions corresponding to localized WG, but also for cases of specific infections, lymphomatoid granulomatosis, malignant lymphomas and other neoplasms. The term is unfortunately still used, but the definition has been tightened.[4]

DeRemee et al[5] suggested a new classification of WG based on the anatomical region involved by the disease: upper respiratory tract and ears (E), lungs (L) and kidneys (K). Thus, E roughly corresponds to midline granuloma, L to limited WG, while the classic pathological features are denoted as ELK. Also the combinations EL, EK, and LK may occur. Other less regular involved organ systems, such as the eyes, skin, central nervous system and heart are not included in this classification.

Steroid therapy of WG has only been able to prolong the survival time up to 12½ months,[6] and had no effect on the renal symptoms. During the last ten years or so, treatment has been improved by the use of cytotoxic drugs, usually in connection with steroid therapy. After a number of reports of treatment with chlorambucil,[7,8] methotrexate[9] and azathioprine[10,11] have appeared, the attention has lately been focused on cyclophosphamide.[12,13]

PATIENT MATERIAL

From 1959 to 1978 we encountered a total of 17 patients in whom WG was diagnosed on the basis of clinical features and histological changes in tissue obtained by biopsy or autopsy which were typical of or compatible with the diagnosis.

The series studied consisted of ten women and seven men. The average age at the onset of the disease was 47 years (range 20-67 years). As in other reports, the symptomatology was very complex with several organs involved (Table 1).

The duration of symptoms before the diagnosis varied within wide limits. Thus, 13 patients had symptoms for less than 12 months (average 4 months). The remaining four patients had symptoms for an average of 50 months.

Upper Respiratory Tract. The most common symptoms were long-standing rhinitis and sinusitis. Twenty-four percent of the patients had nasal bleeding. Nearly one half had saddle nose, and visible tumor tissue was often present.

Persistent otitis media was also a common symptom, and in some cases, this was the first manifestation of the disease. Perceptive hearing loss was found in 35% in the form of unilateral anacusis in two patients, and as severe incapacitating bilateral hearing loss in one. Several patients had undergone mastoidectomy.

Lower Respiratory Tract. One half of the patients had signs of pulmonary infection in the form

From the Department of Otolaryngology and the Department of Radiotherapy and Oncology, University Hospital of Aarhus, Aarhus, Denmark.
REPRINTS — Peter Illum, MD, ENT Department, University Hospital of Aarhus, DK-8000 Aarhus C, Denmark.

TABLE 1. SYMPTOMS AND FINDINGS IN WEGENER'S GRANULOMATOSIS (17 PATIENTS)

	During the Whole Course No.	%	At the Time of Diagnosis No.	%
Nose, paranasal sinuses	14	82	11	65
Rhinitis, sinusitis	11	65		
Bleeding	4	24		
Saddle nose	7	41		
Visible tumor tissue	5	29		
Destruction	1	6		
Crusts	2	12		
Lungs	15	88	11	65
Infection	8	47		
Hemoptysis	4	24		
Pleural pain	1	6		
Pulmonary infiltrations	12	71		
Mediastinal lymph node enlargement	3	8		
Bronchial stenosis	3	18		
Larynx, trachea	4	24	4	24
Stridor	4	24		
Hoarseness	2	12		
Thickening of vocal cords	1	6		
Subglottic or tracheal stenosis	4	24		
Ears	8	47	4	24
Otitis media	8	47		
Perceptive hearing loss	6	35		
Peripheral vestibular affection	2	12		
Kidneys, uremia	6	35	5	29
Central nervous system	5	29	1	6
Eyes	4	24	2	12
Proptosis	2	12		
Uveitis	3	18		
Keratitis, conjunctivitis	2	12		
Joints, muscles	7	41	2	12
Skin	5	29	3	18
Mouth, pharynx	3	18	3	18
Intestinal symptoms	4	24	0	0
Cardiovascular symptoms	2	12	1	6

of coughing, expectoration and periods of increased temperature. Pulmonary infiltrations were demonstrated in 71%. The infiltrations may be either well-defined or diffuse, solitary or multiple, unilateral or bilateral, sometimes with central cavitation, often fairly fleeting. Enlargement of hilar lymph nodes was demonstrated radiographically in two patients.

One patient, a woman, had no symptoms at the time of diagnosis. She was referred to us because of a juxtahilar pulmonary infiltration revealed by a health examination. During the next few months, increasing symptoms developed in spite of cytotoxic therapy.

In four patients, all women, the most conspicuous symptom was stridor caused by subglottic stenosis, in one case extending down into the trachea. Two of these patients had a permanent tracheotomy for a number of years; the other two had been subjected to tracheotomy for one and five months at the onset of the disease.

TABLE 2. HISTOLOGICAL CHANGES IN ORGANS TYPICAL OF OR COMPATIBLE WITH DIAGNOSIS OF WEGENER'S GRANULOMATOSIS

	No.	%
Nose, paranasal sinuses	8	47
Lungs	6	35
Larynx, trachea	4	24
Mediastinal lymph nodes	3	18
Kidneys	6	35
Eyes	1	6
Spleen	3	18
Heart	1	6
Muscles	1	6
Skin	4	24
Total	17	100

Kidneys. Six patients (35%) had renal affection with typical focal glomerulonephritis. Three of these patients were admitted in the terminal phase, and the diagnosis was established by autopsy. One patient had hematuria and albuminuria with slightly increased serum creatinine during the whole course, steeply increasing during the last year before death occurred, nearly six years after onset of disease. In one case, in which the disease began with facial palsy and otitis media, acute renal failure developed after a couple of months before the diagnosis was confirmed. A prompt effect of the treatment was obtained, and the renal function returned to normal. In another patient, a young man in whom the disease began with a full-defined lesion of the nasal septum, acute renal failure developed after five months of treatment with cytotoxic drugs. This patient has since been subjected to dialysis, but active disease is not present.

Other Organ Systems. Migratory arthralgias were a frequent symptom. Only one patient had previously had typical polyarthritis. Involvement of the skin was present in five patients, including three with large ulcerations. Four patients had eye symptoms; two of them had proptosis, one to such an extent that the eye had to be removed.

Occasional symptoms from the mouth and pharynx, gastrointestinal tract and the cardiovascular system have been recorded, although they were not essential features in the clinical picture.

FINDINGS

Laboratory. The most constant findings were markedly increased ESR. Before treatment only two patients had an ESR below 40 mm/hr, and the average was 88 mm/hr. As a rule, slight anemia and often slight leukocytosis were present. Tests for rheumatoid factors were occasionally slightly increased. Serum albumin was generally decreased, and the globulin fraction slightly increased. The results of the renal function tests are mentioned above.

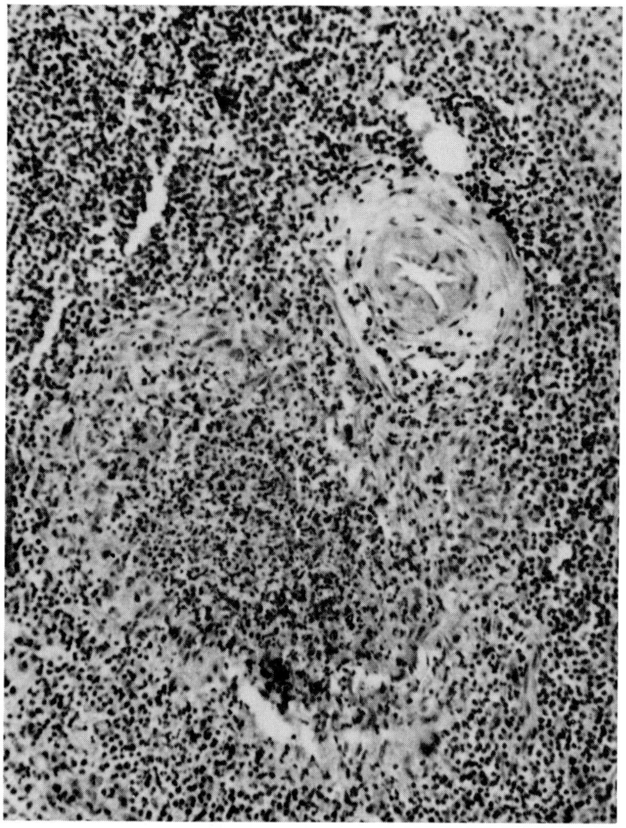

Fig. 1. Wegener's granulomatosis. Necrotizing granuloma surrounded by pale epitheloid cells. A normal artery is seen. Heavy mononuclear infiltration in the surrounding tissue (lung).

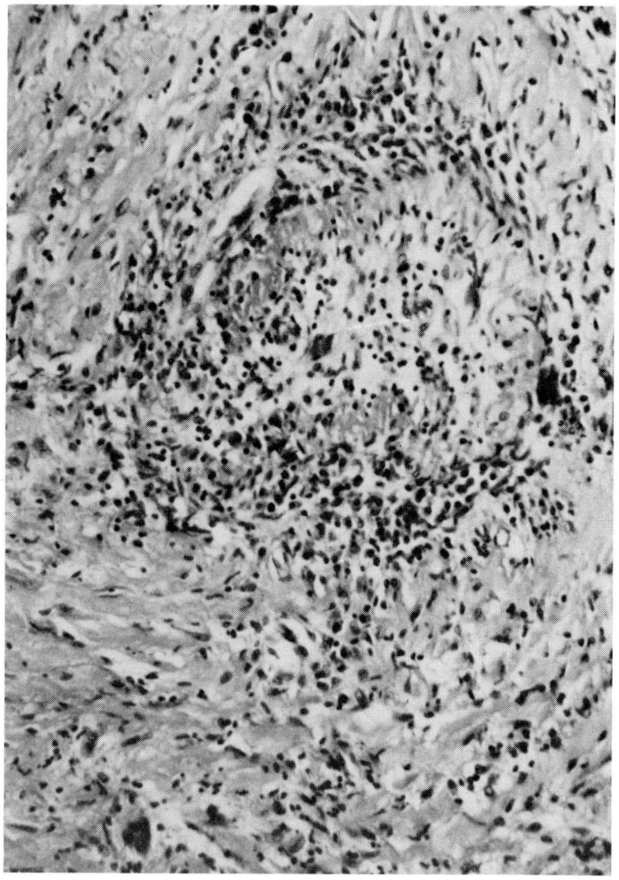

Fig. 2. Healed lesions of necrotizing arteritis. The arterial wall is hyalinized, and in the upper right part the wall fragment of the original internal elastic layer is seen. In the center new, small, intraluminar vascular channels are observed indicating revascularization (lung).

Histological. The organs in which histological changes supported or confirmed the diagnosis are listed in Table 2. Although typical lesions with granuloma formation (Fig. 1), necrosis and vasculitis of the small arteries and veins (Fig. 2) were often demonstrated, we did not require a complete histological confirmation in order to establish the diagnosis, but were content, in some cases, with less typical changes if only the clinical picture was typical. In particular, on the basis of biopsy specimens from the nose and paranasal sinuses it is difficult to make a definite histological diagnosis.

Endoscopically, lesions of the bronchial mucosa were demonstrated in three patients and of the larynx and trachea in four patients. Involvement of the mediastinal lymph nodes were revealed by mediastinoscopy in three patients. In three patients, percutaneous renal biopsies were performed, all being positive. In the other three patients with histologically verified renal affection, the diagnosis was made at autopsy (Fig. 3). We did not perform renal biopsy when the urine analysis and creatinine clearance were normal. A positive skin biopsy was obtained in four patients, including two patients who had no clinical symptoms on the skin.

ELK Classification. Table 3 shows the classification of the patients at the time of diagnosis. The classification does not consider the manifestations in other organ systems, and thus the dissemination of the disease cannot be directly read.

In four cases, a progression to a higher step of the classification occurred during the course of the disease. The disease progressed from E to EL in two cases, from L to EL in one case, and from E to ELK in another case.

TREATMENT

Three patients were admitted in a very poor general state, and the diagnosis was established only at autopsy. These patients did not receive adequate treatment and are therefore not mentioned below.

TABLE 3. ELK CLASSIFICATION AT THE TIME OF DIAGNOSIS

	No.	%
E	3	18
L	4	24
EL	5	29
ELK	5	29

E - Ear, nose, throat; L - Larynx, trachea, lungs; K - Kidneys.

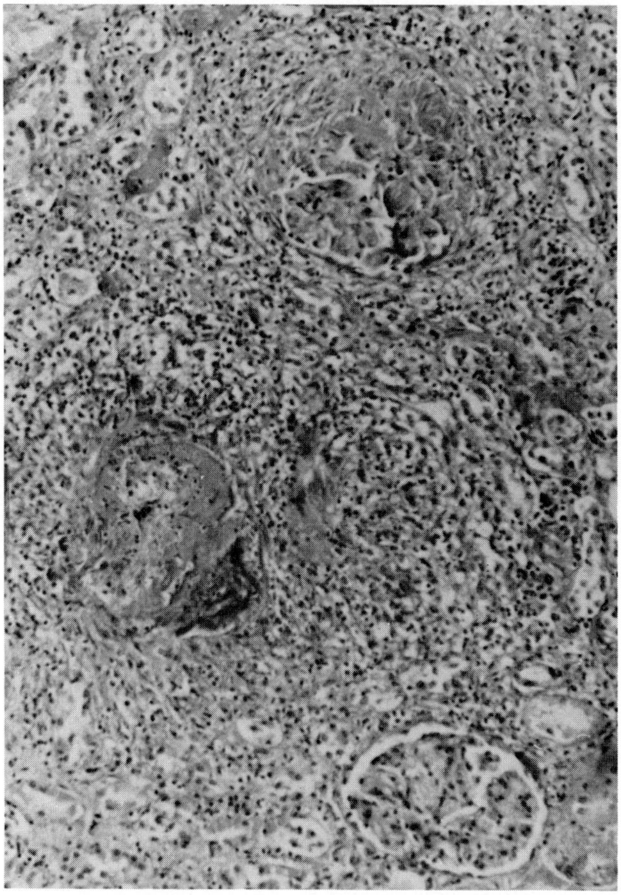

Fig. 3. Necrotizing arteritis and focal glomerulitis. A nearly normal glomerulus is seen in the lower right corner. At the top a glomerulus showing fibrinoid necrosis in most parts. Left of the center is an artery showing marked necrosis (kidney).

The remaining 14 patients were treated with cytotoxic drugs for immunosuppression. The duration of therapy varying from 5 to 138 months. Twelve patients were treated with 6-mercaptopurine. The initial dose was 100 to 150 mg daily; the maintenance dose 50 mg daily. During exacerbations, the dose was occasionally increased.

Other cytotoxic drugs were used in some cases. One patient was treated with cyclophosphamide with good effect. Another patient was first treated with azathioprine, later with cyclophosphamide. In another department, one of our patients had the treatment changed from 6-mercaptopurine to methotrexate.

Several patients had received steroid therapy before the diagnosis was established. At the start of the cytotoxic therapy, nearly all patients were given a large dose of prednisone, which was later tapered off to a maintenance dose of 15 to 30 mg daily. During exacerbations the steroid dose was increased for a short period. After 6 to 12 months, we usually tried to withdraw steroid therapy, but in many cases this was unsuccessful with symptoms reappearing. Five patients were given a small steroid dose only occasionally.

Two patients had x-ray therapy. One patient resented medical treatment and personally stopped this in spite of the fact that active disease was present in the form of a large ulceration of the breast. After treatment of the lesion with electron irradiation, a total dose of 23.00 Gray (2300 rads), she failed to appear for check-up examination. In one patient progressive symptoms developed despite medical treatment, and x-ray therapy up to a central dose of 50.00 Gray (5000 rads) was given to an ulcerating tumor process in the carina region. There was good symptomatic effect of this treatment, but subsequently irradiation pneumonitis developed, and the period of observation is as yet too short.

Withdrawal of treatment has been accomplished in four patients and one patient stopped medical treatment on her own acconut. In a number of other patients we tried to discontinue the treatment, but did not succeed because of a flare-up of symptoms.

Results of Treatment. The results of treatment appear in Table 4. Eight patients are in remission, and in three of these, all treatment has been discontinued. One patient has had several normal births since therapy was stopped seven years ago. Two patients still show active disease; both received radiation therapy a few months ago and are mentioned above. One patient died six months after therapy had been discontinued from an unrelated cause, 12 years after diagnosis and 20 years after the appearance of symptoms, and one died of hematemesis, possibly as a complication of steroid therapy; both were in remission. In one of the patients disease recurred three years after treatment had been stopped and he died one year later in spite of repeated adequate therapy.

Side Effects. The side effects were usually few. Cytotoxic treatment was given under hematological control, and in none of the cases did complications due to bone marrow depression occur. Some patients showed cushingoid features. One patient had pronounced halisteresis with a spontaneous compression fracture of the spine. One patient died of

TABLE 4. CUMULATIVE FOLLOW-UP OF PATIENTS WITH WEGENER'S GRANULOMATOSIS

	No. of Patients
Died before treatment	3
Died in spite of treatment	2
Died of complications of treatment	1
Died of unrelated cause	1
Alive, disease activity still present	2
In remission, under treatment	5
In remission, off treatment	3
Total	17

hematemesis, possibly due to steroid-induced gastric ulcer.

DISCUSSION

The etiology of WG is still unknown, but owing to the clinical features and the histological changes the disease is assumed to be due to immunological processes. The typical affection of the respiratory tract with subsequent dissemination to other organ systems including glomerulonephritis has parallels in rheumatic fever and has given rise to the hypothesis that an immunologically active, bacterial, viral or chemical agent affects the organism through the respiratory tract.

The differential-diagnostic considerations are multifarious and difficult. Biopsies from the respiratory tract must be repeated when the histological response is negative. Sometimes a skin-muscle biopsy may yield the diagnosis, also in cases with no cutaneous manifestations. On a tentative diagnosis made on the basis of a reasonably typical clinical picture, treatment should be instituted.

Our results of treatment are similar to those presented in other large-scale series published.[11-13] Although they are largely very satisfactory, the course of the disease is capricious, and like other authors[3,5] we have in several cases observed progression to a higher step in the ELK classification during treatment. Several patients had serious sequelae. Two patients have had a permanent tracheotomy for years. In one patient dialysis became necessary. In two cases, severe hearing loss was encountered, and in one case, one eye had to be removed because of proptosis, and considerable visual impairment was present in the other eye.

It has not yet been clarified which cytotoxic agent should be preferred in the immunosuppressive therapy. It seems that good effect can be obtained both by 6-mercaptopurine and cyclophosphamide. The value of steroid therapy has been the subject of discussion in the literature. We have found that steroids are a valuable supplement to the cytotoxic treatment, giving good symptomatic effect.

The duration of medical treatment cannot be definitely determined on the basis of available experience. At present, it seems to be most reasonable to try to stop treatment after one year if prompt effect has been obtained. In many patients, slower response and occasional flare-up of individual symptoms have been observed. In such patients, the treatment must be individualized and often continued for many years. In our experience, a valuable parameter in the evaluation of the patients is the ESR, which reflects the activity of the disease fairly well.

The value of radiation therapy in WG is limited. Only in completely isolated lesions might this kind of therapy be considered. Thus, results of radiation therapy in WG type E have been reported[4] which were just as good as those obtained after immunosuppressive therapy. Also a few patients with L have been given radiation, and single cases of pulmonary cases have been treated with surgical excision alone.[5,14]

WG is a rare disease. However, there is no doubt that, during recent years, the diagnosis has been established more frequently and at an earlier phase of the disease, giving better results of treatment. The rather uncharacteristic initial symptoms of the upper respiratory tract will often result in a consultation of the ENT specialist. The first condition for obtaining the proper diagnosis is that WG is borne in mind when patients with a strikingly long course of apparently trivial infections or peculiar constellations of symptoms from several organs are encountered.

ACKNOWLEDGMENT — The authors wish to express their gratitude to U. Henriques, Department of Pathology, University Hospital of Aarhus, who has provided the microphotographs.

REFERENCES

1. Wegener F. Über generalisierte, septiche Gefässerkrankungen. Verh Dtsch Ges Pathol 1936; 29:202-10.

2. Walton EW. Giant-cell granuloma of the respiratory tract (Wegener's granulomatosis). Br Med J 1958; 2:265-70.

3. Carrington CB, Liebow AA. Limited forms of angiitis and granulomatosis of Wegener's type. Am J Med 1966; 41:497-527.

4. Fauci AS, Johnson RE, Wolff SM. Radiation therapy of midline granuloma. Ann Intern Med 1976; 84:140-7.

5. DeRemee RA, McDonald TJ, Harrison EG Jr, Coles DT. Wegener's granulomatosis. Anatomic correlates, a proposed classification. Mayo Clin Proc 1976; 51:777-81.

6. Hollander D, Manning RT. The use of alkylating agents in the treatment of Wegener's granulomatosis. Ann Intern Med 1967; 67:393-8.

7. McIlvanie SK. Wegener's granulomatosis. JAMA 1966; 197:130-2.

8. Berglund G, Hansson L, Persson B, Vikgren P. Combined chlorambucil and prednisolone treatment of five patients with Wegener's granulomatosis. Acta Med Scand 1972; 191:5-9.

9. Capizzi RL, Bertino JR. Methotrexate therapy of Wegener's granulomatosis. Ann Intern Med 1971; 74:74-9.

10. Raitt JW. Wegener's granulomatosis: treatment with cytotoxic agents and adrenocorticoids. Ann Intern Med 1971; 74:344-56.

11. Thorkelsen H, Berdal P. Wegener's granulomatosis. Immunosuppressive therapy. Acta Otolaryngol (Stockh) 1976; 82:208-11.

12. Wolff SM, Fauci AS, Horn RG, Dale DC. Wegener's granulomatosis. Ann Intern Med 1974; 81:513-25.

13. Reza MJ, Dornfeld L, Goldberg LS, Bluestone R, Pearson CM. Wegener's granulomatosis. Long-term follow up of patients treated with cyclophosphamide. Arthritis Rheum 1975; 18:501-6.

14. Patchefsky AS, Israel HL. Pulmonary Wegener's granulomatosis. Ann Clin Lab Sci 1973; 3:249-58.

Ann Otol 90:1981

AUDITORY BRAINSTEM AND MIDDLE LATENCY EVOKED RESPONSE SENSITIVITY NEAR THRESHOLD

FRANK E. MUSIEK, PhD NATHAN A. GEURKINK, MD

HANOVER, NEW HAMPSHIRE

Auditory brainstem response (ABR) and middle latency evoked response (MLER) testing have been used successfully for assessing hearing sensitivity electrophysiologically. Though both procedures have their proponents, ABR seems to be the more popular of the two. However, this study shows that overall, MLER waves occur with greater frequency at low sensation levels than ABR waves. Specifically, MLER wave P_a was the most sensitive wave, followed by ABR wave V, MLER wave P_b, ABR wave III, MLER wave P_c, and ABR wave I. Latencies were more consistent and predictable for ABR than MLER. However, as expected, amplitudes for MLER waves were greater than those for ABR. Given these results, those involved in measuring hearing sensitivity electrophysiologically are encouraged to consider the potential of the MLER measure and not limit their scope of assessment to ABR.

For the past several years, auditory brainstem response (ABR) has been shown to be a valuable tool for assessing electrophysiological thresholds to sound stimuli.[1-3] In reviewing the literature, one has to wonder if ABR with its sudden popularity has overshadowed an older procedure, middle latency evoked response (MLER). Certainly, there is evidence in the literature showing MLER to be a valid and reliable auditory electrophysiological procedure.[4,5]

Recently reported experience would seem to indicate the MLER to be advantageous over ABR in regard to obtaining frequency-specific auditory information.[6-8] However, in employing clicks, a stimulus best suited for ABR, it is difficult to surmise whether ABR or MLER is better for measuring electrophysiologic responses close to threshold. To these investigators' knowledge, no such comparisons were found in a review of the literature.

Therefore, the purpose of this study was to observe middle latency and brainstem responses at low sensation levels and make comparisons along several parameters.

METHODS

Subjects. Fifteen normal-hearing subjects (ie, pure tone thresholds at 15 dB HL or better for frequencies 250-8000 Hz) between the ages of 19 and 32 volunteered for the study. This group was quite homogeneous with a mean pure tone average (PTA) of 6.9 dB HL and the range of PTAs from 11.7 to 0 dB HL. All subjects reported a history free of otologic or neurologic disease or trauma.

Procedures. Scalp electrodes were attached to the high forehead, the mastoid of the ear being tested (reference) and the opposite mastoid (ground) of each subject. Impedance was maintained below 3 kΩ for all subjects tested. Each subject was seated in a lounge-type chair located in a sound-treated room. The subjects were instructed to relax and remain as motionless as possible and to keep their eyes closed during the testing period. Responses were averaged, displayed, and measured on a Nicolet 1170.

Special effort was made to equate MLER and ABR procedures. Only one ear, which was randomly selected, was tested per subject. The stimulus was an alternating rarefaction-condensation click generated by a 100 μs rectangular electric wave delivered to a TDH-39 earphone. The clicks were presented at a rate of approximately 10/s to the test ear. There were 2,048 trials for each sensation level (SL) beginning at 5 dB and proceeding to 10, 20, and 30 dB SL. There was a brief rest period after each SL was tested. ABR and MLER testing were alternately conducted first. Filter settings, using a Nicolet 501 A amplified filter, were 150-3000 Hz at a 12 dB per octave roll-off for ABR, while MLER filtering was at 30-100 Hz with the same roll-off.

Psychophysical thresholds were established for clicks for each of the subjects, using a modified Hughson-Westlake technique[9] with decrements and increments in 2 dB steps rather than in the conventional 10 and 5 dB steps. This allowed a correlation to an actual hearing level on the subjects tested.

RESULTS

The electrophysiologic responses were determined by the consistency to established criteria (see Appendix). For the facility of direct comparison, only three ABR positive waves (I, III, and V) and three middle latency positive waves (P_a, P_b, P_c) were analyzed.

In observing the percentage of subjects with either a readable brainstem or middle latency response for the various SLs tested, there appeared to be a marked difference in the occurrence of waves. Considerably more subjects yielded middle latency waves P_a and P_b along with brainstem wave V than brainstem waves I and III and middle latency wave P_c. This was most evident at a low SL (5 dB) and this difference decreased as intensity increased (Fig. 1).

In analyzing the percentage of possible responses for each of the brainstem and middle latency waves for all SLs combined, wave P_a had the highest occurrence followed by wave V, wave P_b, wave III, wave P_c, and wave I (Fig. 2A). When combining all middle latency and brainstem waves being anal-

From the Section of Otolaryngology and Audiology, Dartmouth-Hitchcock Medical Center, Hanover, New Hampshire. This project was supported in part by Hitchcock Foundation Grant No. 65.

REPRINTS — Frank E. Musiek, PhD, Section of Otolaryngology and Audiology, Dartmouth-Hitchcock Medical Center, 2 Maynard Street, Hanover, NH 03755.

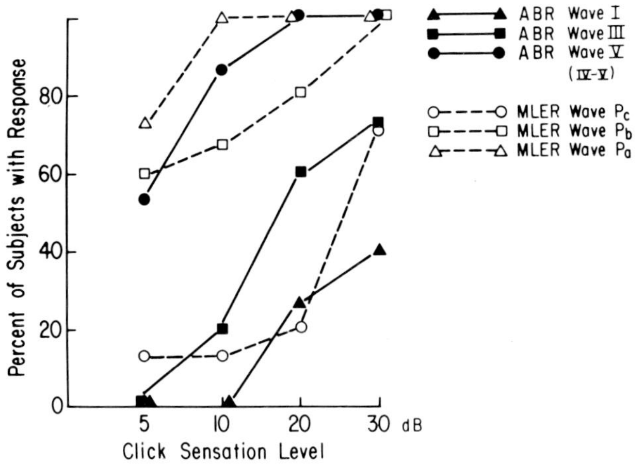

Fig. 1. Percent of subjects with an ABR or MLER response. ABR - Auditory brainstem response; MLER - Middle latency evoked response.

yzed for all SLs, MLER waves yielded a significantly higher percentage of responses than ABR waves* (Fig. 2B).

ABR latencies decreased with increases of intensity and were consistent and predictable (Fig. 3). Latencies for the middle waves were more variable and less predictable, especially wave P_c. However, there was still a systematic effect for intensity on latency for wave P_a (Fig. 4). As expected, the interwave latencies for ABR, where they could be measured, were not affected to any great extent by SL.

As expected, amplitudes for the middle latency responses were larger than those for the brainstem responses (Figs. 5 and 6). Generally, there seemed to be a systematic intensity effect on amplitude for both measures. ABR wave V was approximately twice the amplitude of either wave I or III regardless of SL. Middle latency wave P_a was consistently larger in amplitude across all SLs when compared to waves P_b and P_c.

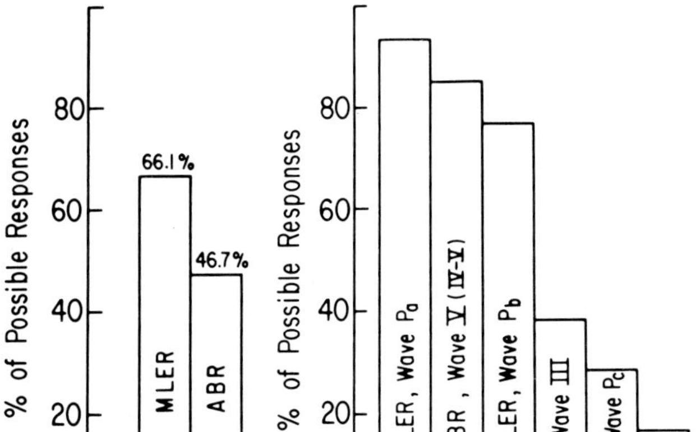

Fig. 2. A) Percent of possible responses for ABR and MLER waves for all sensation levels combined. B) Percent of possible responses for ABR and MLER for all sensation levels and waves combined.

*Statistical analysis was done employing a chi-square procedure and differences were significant beyond the 0.001 level.

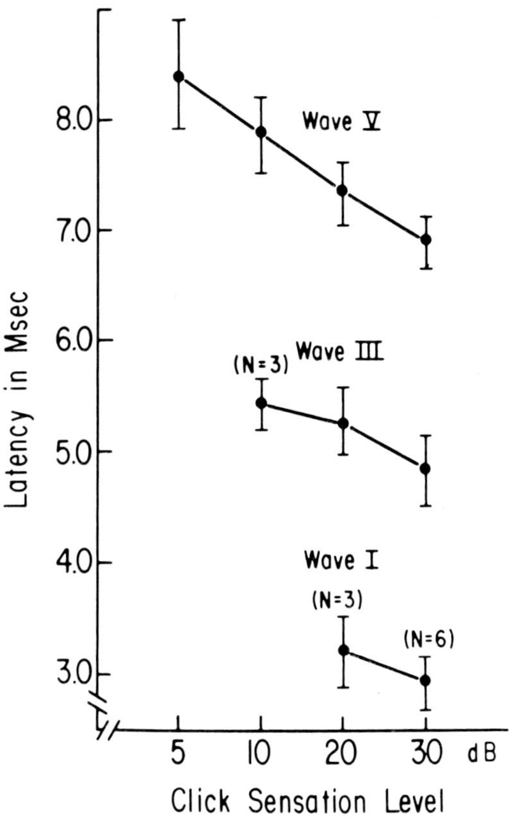

Fig. 3. Average latency of ABR waves.

DISCUSSION

Based on data obtained from this study, it appears middle latency responses seem to occur more often than ABRs at low SLs. Although no direct ABR-MLER comparisons with regard to incidence of response have been previously reported, there is evidence of good threshold approximation for both.

A number of investigators report or claim estimations of thresholds within 10 dB using the MLER,[6-8,10,11] which is comparable to our findings. Similarly, the present study shows responses at 10 dB SL and below for auditory brainstem measurement which has also been shown by others.[1,12] It is important to note that the threshold of ABR wave V is a more dependable[13] measure of auditory threshold than the latency of wave V. Latency has been shown to be affected by the type of hearing loss and can only occasionally be interpolated to provide some insight as to threshold.[13]

When observing ABR wave components, wave V was the most robust wave at low SLs, followed by wave III and wave I respectively. This information is generally consistent with observations by other investigators.[1,7,13,14]

In our data, at low SLs the most prominent middle latency positive wave was P_a followed by P_b and P_c. This is in general agreement with other findings.[2,10,15] However, not all previous studies anal-

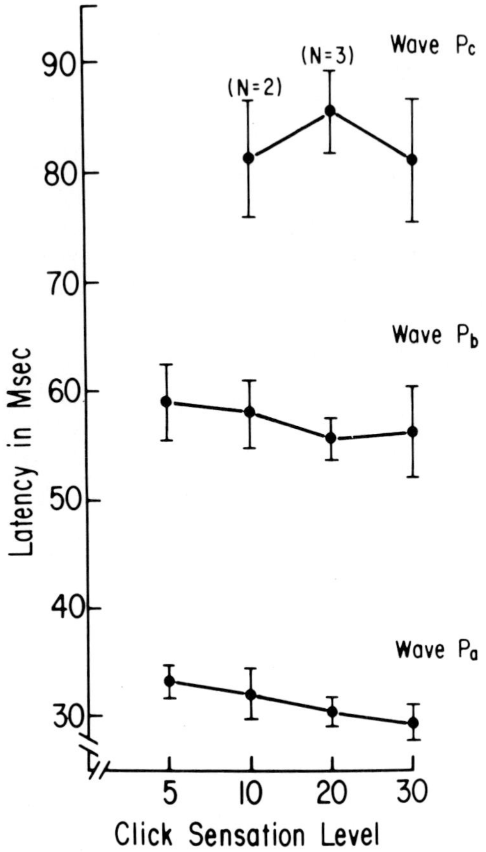

Fig. 4. Average latency of MLER waves.

yzed each of the waves mentioned in the present study.

Latencies. ABR latencies for waves I, III, and V at low SLs were similar to those reported by Chiappa et al[16] and others.[1,13] As expected, at low SLs interwave latencies (I-V, I-III, and III-V) closely approximated those obtained by other investigators at higher intensities.[13,17,18]

The mean latencies for the middle responses P_a and P_b were also in fairly good agreement with other published data.[2,10,19] However, there is less agreement in terms of the latency of wave P_c. This may be due to 1) differences in stimuli, as most studies reporting P_c waves used tone pips;[6,20] 2) only a few studies report latency findings for P_c, hence only a minimal number of comparisons could be made; and 3) this wave may be inherently more variable, as the subject's psychological state, auditory nerve fiber diffuseness, etc, may be more of a factor than with the earlier waves.

Also in our study the occurrence of P_c was very low and its latencies and amplitudes were highly variable. Hence, it is difficult to attach a great deal of meaning to our findings regarding P_c in this particular study.

Amplitudes. The greater amplitudes for the middle latencies appeared to be a chief factor in being able to read these waves more easily than the brain-

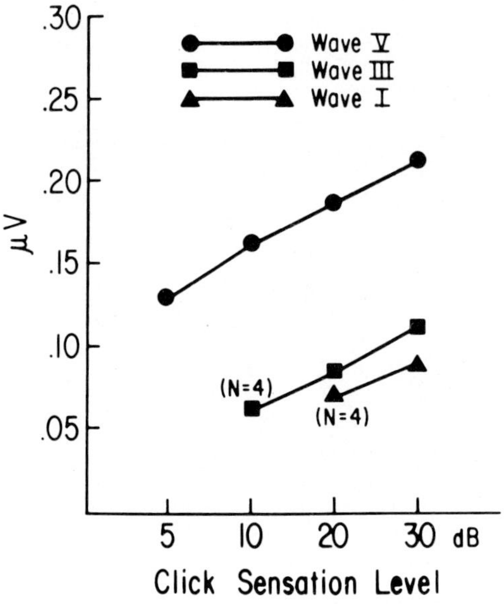

Fig. 5. Average amplitudes for ABR waves.

stem waves. This difference is especially noticed at the extremely low SLs (Fig. 7). The larger amplitude for the middle latency waves is probably attributable to a greater number of nerve fibers being involved at a higher cortical level.

Although amplitudes for ABR and MLER are highly variable, there is some general agreement with previous studies on both these measures.[21]

Implications of the Study. In comparing several major parameters, overall MLER waves occur with greater frequency than ABR waves at low SLs. In addition, the use of MLER appears clinically feasible as the only necessary alterations from an ABR setup are those of the filter settings (30 to 100 Hz) and the time window (approximately 100 ms). Most averagers used in auditory brainstem testing can easily accommodate these minor changes.

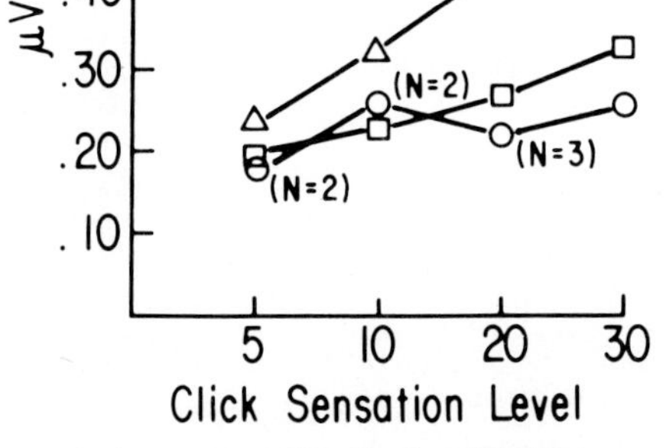

Fig. 6. Average amplitudes for MLER waves.

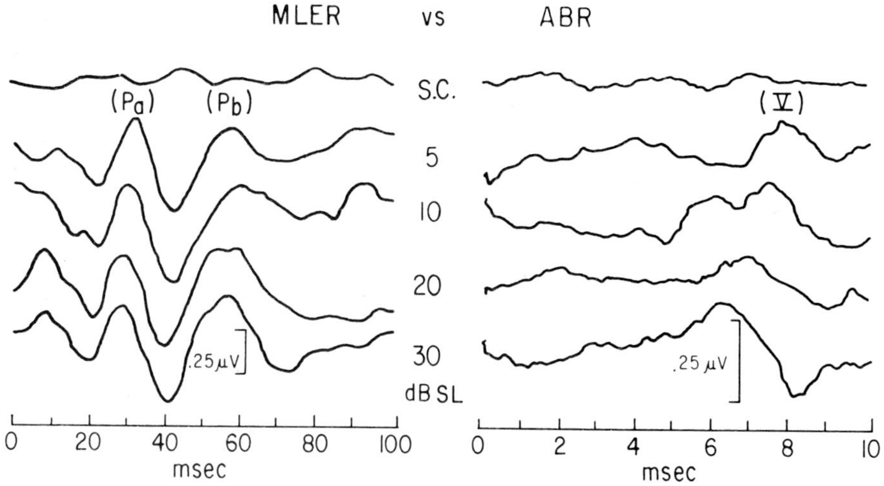

Fig. 7. Example of ABR and MLER tracings for one subject. S.C. - Silent control.

This study indicates that for measurements near auditory threshold, MLER may be as good or better a procedure than ABR. However, this view must be tempered with some reservations. It must be remembered that our population is one of adult, normal ears. Definite statements regarding MLER vs ABR with respective threshold sensitivity must be withheld until data on hearing-impaired populations are more comparable. Jerger and Mauldin[22] have reported on estimating high frequency (1,000-4,000 Hz) thresholds for a hearing-impaired population for which a 15 dB standard error was found using ABR. McFarland et al[11] using MLER also tested a hearing-impaired population. Though no standard error for threshold was reported, this study showed good responses at very low SLs. However, these two studies were considerably different in the methodologies employed and direct comparisons are impossible.

The present study does indicate MLER to be a sensitive measure near threshold. This may be of most value in pediatric testing. For example, one may be testing slightly above a given child's threshold and ABR may not yield any response while MLER may. Given our data on the frequency of subject responses for ABR and MLER, it would seem logical that if responses were not obtained by the former procedure, the latter procedure should be tried. This would seem to be a fruitful clinical strategy. It is in this manner that the use of MLER may be of most value. There is no question that further research on normals and the hearing-impaired must be conducted to determine whether ABR, MLER, or some combination of both may provide the most information about hearing thresholds.

Another consideration is that generally high repetition rates are more commonly employed with ABR than MLER. This infers a shorter test time for ABR, an important aspect of pediatric testing. However, this advantage may partially be offset by the fact that MLER often requires fewer trials to obtain a readable waveform. Hence, this is another argument that can only be resolved by clinical studies with both procedures in a similar research paradigm.

In summation, it is important for those involved in measuring auditory electrophysiological responses at low SLs not to limit their procedures to ABR testing. Rather, the potential of other electrophysiological measures such as MLER should be kept in mind. It is only by the use of these various measures clinically and experimentally that the best procedure will be realized.

ACKNOWLEDGMENT — The authors wish to thank Stephanie Keitel for her many contributions to this study.

REFERENCES

1. Hecox K, Galambos R. Brainstem auditory evoked responses in human infants and adults. Arch Otolaryngol 1974; 99:30-3.

2. Davis H. Principles of electric response audiometry. Ann Otol Rhinol Laryngol 1976; 85 Suppl 28:5-96.

3. Brackmann D. Electric response audiometry in a clinical practice. Laryngoscope 1977; 87 Suppl 5.

4. Ruhm H, Walker E, Flanigan H. Acoustically evoked potentials in man: mediation of early components. Laryngoscope 1967; 77:806-22.

5. Mendel M, Goldstein R. Stability of early components of the average electroencephalic response. J Speech Hear Res 1969; 12:351-61.

6. Thornton A, Mendel M, Anderson C. Effects of stimulus frequency and intensity on the middle components of the average auditory electrocephalic response. J Speech Hear Res 1977; 20:81-94.

7. Picton T, Woods D, Barbeau-Braum J, Healey T. Evoked potential audiometry. J Otolaryngol 1977; 6:90-119.

8. McCandless G. Neuroelectric measures of auditory function. In: Rose D, ed. Audiological assessment. Vol 2. Englewood Cliffs: Prentice-Hall, 1978.

9. Carhart R, Jerger J. Preferred method for clinical determination of pure tone thresholds. J Speech Hear Disord 1959; 24:330-45.

10. Goldstein R, Rodman L. Early components of average

evoked responses to rapidly repeated auditory stimuli. J Speech Hear Res 1967; 10:697-705.

11. McFarland W, Vivion M, Goldstein R. Middle components of the AER to tone pips in normal hearing and hearing impaired subjects. J Speech Hear Res 1977; 20:781-98.

12. Starr A, Achor L. Auditory brain stem responses in neurological disease. Arch Neurol 1975; 32:761-8.

13. Kavanagh K, Beardsley J. Brain stem auditory evoked response. Ann Otol Rhinol Laryngol 1979; 88 Suppl 58:1-28.

14. Jewett D, Williston J. Auditory evoked far fields averaged from the scalp of humans. Brain 1971; 94:681-96.

15. Wolfe K, Goldstein R. Middle component averaged electrocephalic responses to tonal stimuli for normal neonates. Arch Otolaryngol 1978; 104:508-18.

16. Chiappa K, Gladstone K, Young R. Brain stem auditory evoked responses: studies of waveform variations of 50 normal human subjects. Arch Neurol 1979; 36:81-7.

17. Gilroy J, Lynn G, Ristow G, Pellerin R. Auditory evoked brain stem potentials in case of locked-in syndrome. Arch Neurol 1977; 34:492-5.

18. Stockard J, Rossiter V. Clinical and pathological correlates of brain stem auditory response abnormalities. Neurology 1977; 27:316-25.

19. Madell J, Goldstein R. Relation between loudness and the amplitude of the early components of the averaged electroencephalic response. J Speech Hear Res 1972; 15:134-41.

20. Gutnick H, Goldstein R. Effect of contralateral noise on the middle components of the averaged electroencephalic response. J Speech Hear Res 1978; 21:613-24.

21. Zerlin S, Naunton R. Early and late averaged electroencephalic responses at low sensation levels. Audiology 1974; 13:366-78.

22. Jerger J, Mauldin L. Prediction of sensori-neural hearing level from the brainstem evoked response. Arch Otolaryngol 1978; 104:456-61.

APPENDIX

Time ranges used for judging middle latency and auditory brainstem responses:

For ABR		For MLER	
Wave I	2.4- 3.7 @ 30 dB SL	Wave P_a	27.5-33.0 @ 30 dB SL
	2.7- 4.1 @ 20 dB SL		28.0-34.5 @ 20 dB SL
	3.0- 4.5 @ 10 dB SL		28.2-36.0 @ 10 dB SL
	3.3- 4.8 @ 5 dB SL		29.8-36.5 @ 5 dB SL
Wave III	4.3- 5.8 @ 30 dB SL	Wave P_b	50.0-62.0 @ 30 dB SL
	4.6- 6.1 @ 20 dB SL		50.9-63.0 @ 20 dB SL
	4.8- 6.3 @ 10 dB SL		54.0-65.0 @ 10 dB SL
	4.9- 6.5 @ 5 dB SL		55.0-68.8 @ 5 dB SL
Wave V (IV-V)	6.4- 7.8 @ 30 dB SL	Wave P_c	75.0-92.0 @ 30 dB SL
	6.7- 8.2 @ 20 dB SL		76.9-93.0 @ 20 dB SL
	7.0- 8.6 @ 10 dB SL		76.0-94.0 @ 10 dB SL
	7.3- 9.2 @ 5 dB SL		77.0-95.0 @ 5 dB SL

The ranges shown enhanced accuracy in detecting responses. Each wave analyzed occurred within the appropriate time period designated, or it was not counted as a response. At low intensities this procedure would reduce the number of false positive interpretations due to artifact.

An additional criterion was that the wave configuration and interwave relationship were consistent with waveform shape, amplitude, and latency for higher intensities. For waveforms that were difficult to read, a replication trial was carried out. If there was good replication of peaks and troughs, the response was counted.

Statistical analysis was done employing a chi-square procedure and differences were significant beyond the 0.001 level.

COMPENSATORY EYE MOVEMENT AND GAZE FIXATION DURING ACTIVE HEAD ROTATION IN PATIENTS WITH LABYRINTHINE DISORDERS

MASAHIRO TAKAHASHI, MD

TAKUYA UEMURA, MD TAKEHISA FUJISHIRO, MD

TOKYO, JAPAN

Compensatory eye movement and gaze fixation during active head rotation were studied in patients with unilateral and bilateral loss of vestibular function. Patients with bilateral lesions were asked to perform mental arithmetic tasks in the dark. Although compensatory eye movements of these patients corresponded to 38-46% of compensatory movements in normal subjects, the ability of patients with lesions to visually fix on a stationary target was markedly impaired. Visual fixation on moving targets attached to the head (head-fixed targets) was also measured and found to be good. For patients with unilateral lesions, in the early stages of the disease, findings during rotations to the intact side resembled those for normal subjects, while results of rotations to the affected side resembled those for patients with bilateral lesions.

To investigate vestibulo-ocular reflexes and visual-vestibular interactions during active head rotation, we devised a new test in which subjects perform voluntary sinusoidal head rotations in time to an electric metronome. Our findings on normal subjects have been reported.[1] In the present study we used the same method to examine patients with unilateral or bilateral loss of labyrinthine function, and compared these findings with those on normal subjects to investigate the effects of labyrinthine disorders on compensatory eye movement and visual fixation during active head rotation.

METHODS AND MATERIALS

We used the same apparatus and methods in the present study as in the tests on normal subjects.[1] Horizontal head rotation was recorded by a head rotation detector, which functioned as a terrestial magnetic sensor, placed on the head.[2] Eye movements were recorded by DC electro-oculography through bitemporal leads. They were electrically added to the head movements in order to ascertain gaze movements in space. We asked the subjects to turn their heads alternately and smoothly to the right and left at an amplitude of 40° at three different speeds, ie, at the rates of 1, 2 and 3 cycles (0.33, 0.67, 1.0 Hz) of head rotation during a 3-second period, in time to an electric metronome. For gaze fixation, the target was either a small red lamp mounted on the wall, or a small red lamp fixed to the tip of a 30 cm rod attached to the head.

We observed eye, head and gaze movements under the following visual conditions: 1) mental arithmetic in the dark — eyes open (alert-in-dark); 2) visual fixation on a lamp on the wall (spatially fixed target); and 3) visual fixation on a lamp fixed to the head (head-fixed target). During the tests the room was completely dark. Eye movements were calibrated after the subjects had adapted to the dark by being in the dark room for at least ten minutes and whenever the test conditions were changed. Head rotation and eye speed were ascertained by measuring the maximum tangent angles of the recorded waves in which the frequency and amplitude of the head rotation were most stable.

The present study was comprised of patients with unilateral and bilateral loss of labyrinthine function (unilateral and biliateral lesions). They showed no response to ice water irrigation of the involved ear and had no CNS disorders. Of the five cases with unilateral lesions, three were male patients with vestibular neuronitis (aged 53, 58 and 33) who were examined on the 11th, 13th and 30th day after onset, respectively; one was a 27-year-old male patient with Ramsay-Hunt syndrome who was examined on the 14th day after onset, and one was a 27-year-old male patient who had sustained a temporal bone fracture one month earlier. The mean age of these 5 patients was 39.6 years; the mean interval between the time of onset and the examination was 19.8 days. Of the five cases with bilateral lesions, one was a 34-year-old female patient with bilateral vestibular neuronitis who was examined on the 21st day after onset; one was a 48-year-old female patient with acute bilateral vestibular dysfunction of unknown origin accompanied by moderate sensory hearing loss, who was examined on the 28th day; one was a 35-year-old male patient with chronic renal failure receiving dialysis therapy who became ataxic three months prior to the examination; one was a 32-year-old male patient who became ataxic five months prior to the examination during treatment for meningitis with large doses of aminoglycoside antibiotics, and one was a 39-year-old female patient with aortitis who had suffered from progressive bilateral deafness and equilibrium disturbance over a 6-year period. The mean age of these five patients was 37.6 years. As controls, results obtained on 20 individuals with normal vestibular function (mean age, 28.5 years) were used.

RESULTS

Mental Arithmetic in the Dark (Alert-in-Dark). Although head rotations induced nystagmus in the same direction in normal subjects, gaze position, ie, the summation of eye and head positions, was almost stationary in space except during the quick phases of nystagmus. In patients with unilateral lesions, nystagmus was also induced in the direction of head rotation; however, their slow-phase eye speed was lower during head rotation to the affected side than to the intact side. Therefore, while gaze recordings during head rotation to the intact side showed a stepwise or stair-like configuration similar to normal subjects, they became distorted during rotations to the affected side (Fig. 1, top, ar-

From the Department of Otolaryngology, Tokyo Women's Medical College.

REPRINTS — Masahiro Takahashi, MD, Department of Otolaryngology, Tokyo Women's Medical College, 10 Kawadacho Shinjuku-ku, Tokyo, Japan 162.

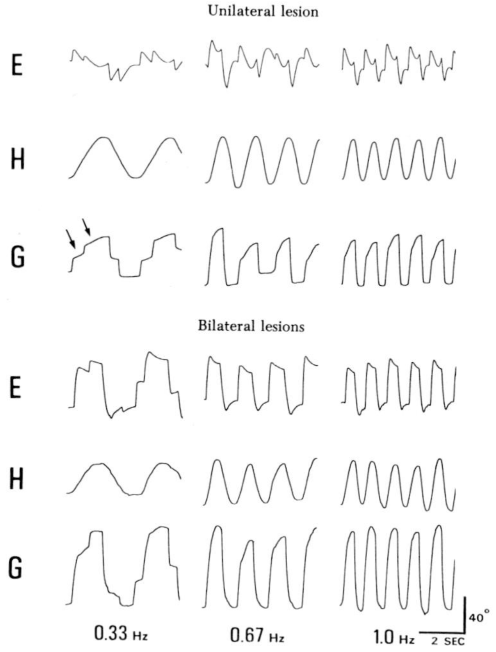

Fig. 1. Recordings under alert-in-dark conditions in a patient with a unilateral (right) lesion and a patient with bilateral lesions. From top to bottom are shown eye movements (E), head movements (H), and gaze movements (G). Upward displacements indicate movements toward the right. Arrows - See text.

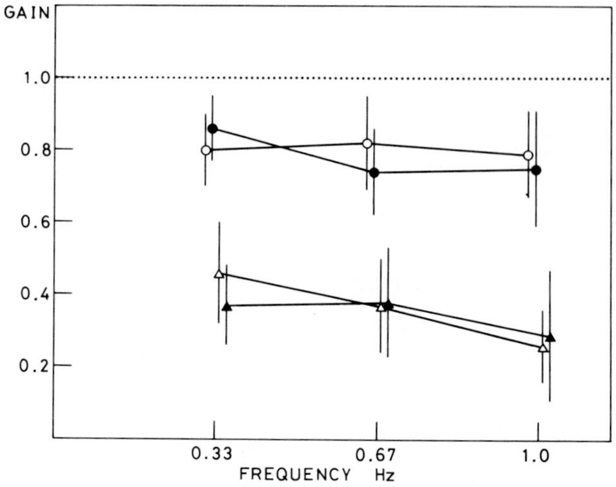

Fig. 2. The ratio (mean and SD) of maximum eye speed to head speed (gain) under alert-in-dark conditions in controls (n = 20, ○), in patients with unilateral lesions (n = 5) during rotations to the intact side (●) and to the affected side (△), and in patients with bilateral lesions (n = 5, ▲).

rows). Gaze deviation upon rotation to the affected side resulted from insufficient compensatory eye movements. Gaze deviation to the affected side became more marked with an increase in the turning speed. While compensatory eye movements were noted even in patients with bilateral lesions, the gaze recordings were remarkably distorted since the compensatory eye movements were very weak bilaterally (Fig. 1, bottom).

The ratio of the maximum eye speed to the corresponding head rotation speed (gain), except at the time of saccades, in three subject groups is shown in Table 1 and Figure 2. Variance analysis was applied to ascertain gain differences among normal subjects, patients with unilateral lesions during rotations to the intact and the affected sides, and patients with bilateral lesions. The gain of patients with unilateral lesions during rotations to the intact side (0.74-0.86 average) did not differ significantly from that of normal subjects at any head-turning frequency ($P > 0.05$). The gain in this patient group

TABLE 1. GAIN* UNDER ALERT-IN-DARK CONDITIONS (MEAN AND SD)

Subjects	*0.33 Hz*	*0.67 Hz*	*1.0 Hz*
Controls	0.80±0.10	0.82±0.13	0.79±0.12
Unilateral lesions			
Rotation to intact side	0.86±0.09	0.74±0.12	0.75±0.16
Rotation to affected side	0.46±0.14	0.37±0.13	0.26±0.10
Bilateral lesions	0.37±0.11	0.38±0.15	0.29±0.18

*Ratio of maximum eye speed to head rotation speed.

during rotations to the affected side (0.26-0.46 average) obviously differed from that during rotation to the intact side ($P < 0.01$); it was very close to the value of patients with bilateral lesions (0.29-0.38 average). We could not find any statistically significant difference between the gains of these two patient groups ($P > 0.05$). Although patients with bilateral lesions lacked vestibulo-ocular reflexes, they manifested compensatory eye movements which were 34-46% as large as those observed in normal subjects.

Visual Fixation on a Lamp on the Wall (Spatially Fixed Target). During head rotation, the eyes of normal subjects moved in a direction opposite to head movement and the gaze was fixed in space, even at 1.0 Hz. At 0.33 Hz, patients with unilateral lesions also showed spatial gaze fixation. However, fluctuations in the gaze recordings appeared and became larger as the frequency of the head rotation increased (Fig. 3, top) and saccades made up for insufficient compensatory eye movements during head rotations to the affected side (Fig. 3, top, arrows). In patients with bilateral lesions, the gaze deviated bilaterally in the direction of head rotation; therefore, the gaze recordings fluctuated more markedly than in patients with unilateral lesions (Fig. 3, bottom).

The gain in normal subjects was accurately maintained at unity (Table 2). On the average, it was also close to unity at head rotation to the intact side in patients with unilateral lesions, and showed no significant difference from the control values ($P > 0.05$, Fig. 4). Although when measured during head rotations (0.33 Hz) to the affected side, the gain was maintained relatively close to unity (0.88 average), it decreased proportionally to the increase in frequency ($r = -0.69$). Of the group with unilateral lesions, a patient with vestibular neuronitis,

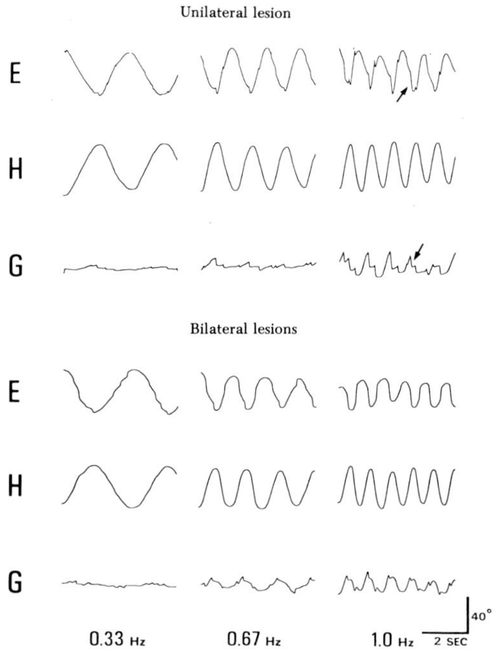

Fig. 3. Recordings with spatially fixed target in a patient with a unilateral (right) lesion and a patient with bilateral lesions. Upward displacements indicate movements toward the right. Arrows - See text.

examined on the 13th day after onset, showed the lowest gain during rotation to the affected side (Fig. 5, solid circles). His gain during rotations to the intact side and to the affected side, respectively, was 0.90 and 0.77 at 0.33 Hz, 1.00 and 0.46 at 0.67 Hz, and 1.03 and 0.33 at 1.0 Hz. Evidently, as shown in this case, visual fixation in unilateral lesion cases was well maintained during rotations to the intact side, even in patients who showed remarkable gaze fixation disturbance during rotations to the affected side. These findings confirmed the subjective sensation of patients with unilateral lesions that visual objects in the surrounding area become blurred only during head rotations toward the affected side.

While the gain of patients with bilateral lesions did not significantly differ from patients with unilateral lesions during rotations to the affected side ($P>0.05$), the mean value of the former exceeded that of the latter. In patients with bilateral lesions, there was a high correlation between the gain and the frequency of head rotation ($r=-0.66$). Of the group with bilateral lesions, the patient with acute bilateral vestibular dysfunction of unknown origin, examined on the 28th day after onset, showed the

TABLE 2. GAIN WITH SPATIALLY FIXED TARGET (MEAN AND SD)

Subjects	*0.33 Hz*	*0.67 Hz*	*1.0 Hz*
Controls	0.99±0.03	0.99±0.02	1.00±0.05
Unilateral lesions			
Rotation to intact side	1.01±0.09	1.02±0.07	1.04±0.07
Rotation to affected side	0.88±0.10	0.71±0.17	0.53±0.16
Bilateral lesions	0.94±0.09	0.81±0.12	0.65±0.17

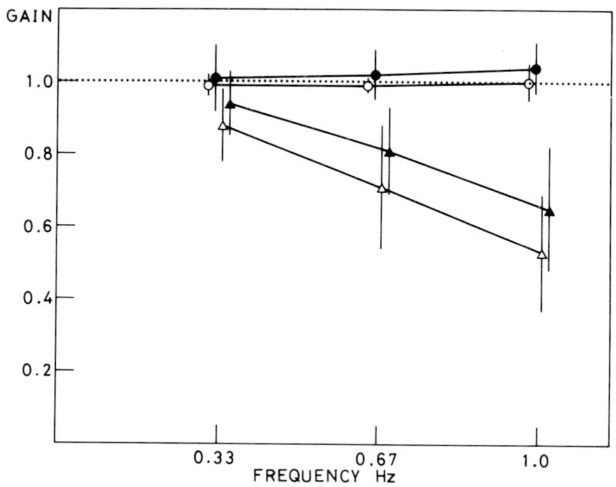

Fig. 4. Gain (mean and SD) with spatially fixed target in controls (○), in patients with unilateral lesions during rotations to the intact side (●) and to the affected side (△), and in patients with bilateral lesions (▲).

lowest value of the gain (Fig. 5, open circles). Her gain was 0.79, 0.59 and 0.39 at 0.33, 0.67 and 1.0 Hz, respectively.

Visual Fixation on a Lamp Fixed to the Head (Head-Fixed Target). Since the vestibulo-ocular reflex disturbs fixation under this test condition, normal subjects showed incomplete visual fixation. Although fixation remained fairly good at 0.33 Hz in this group, it worsened as the frequency of the head rotation increased and eye movement recordings showed a combination of compensatory eye movements and corrective saccades, ie, nystagmus in the direction of the head rotation. In patients with unilateral lesions, visual fixation during head rotations to the intact side was impaired by nystagmus in the direction of head rotation (Fig. 6, top,

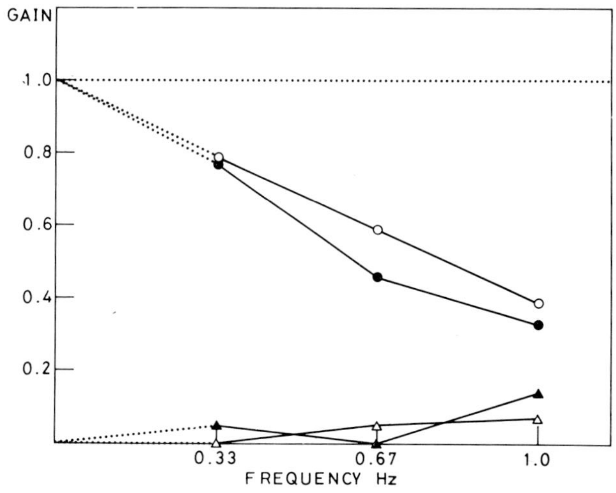

Fig. 5. Gain in a patient with bilateral lesions (○, △) and a patient with a unilateral lesion during rotations to the affected side (●, ▲). These two patients manifested the worst fixation on a spatially fixed target (circles) and the best fixation on a head-fixed target (triangles) in each group of patients.

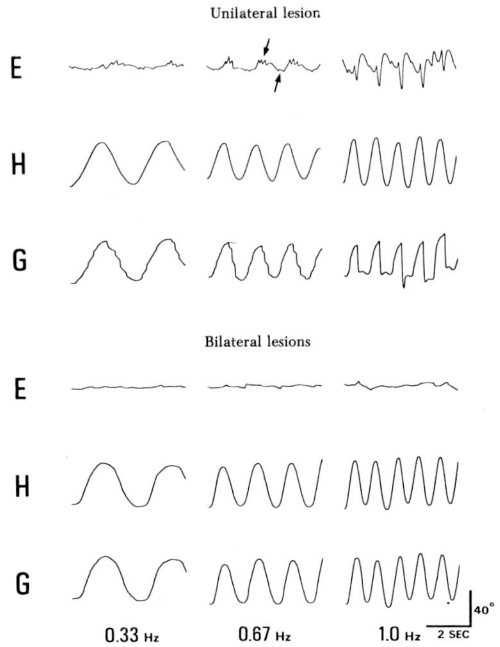

Fig. 6. Recordings with head-fixed target in a patient with a unilateral (right) lesion and a patient with bilateral lesions. Upward displacements indicate movements toward the right. Arrows - See text.

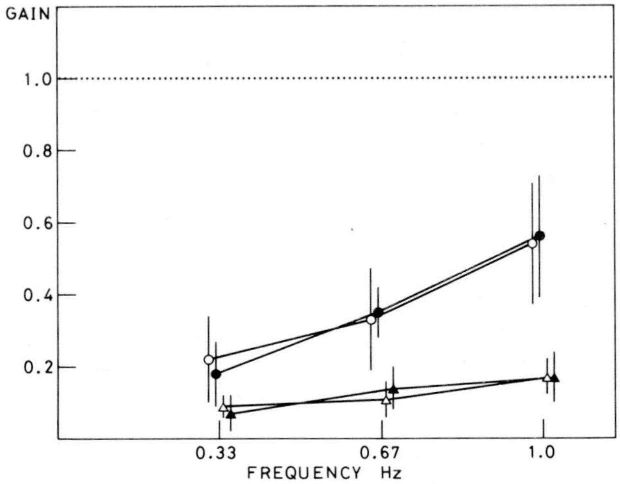

Fig. 7. Gain (mean and SD) with head-fixed target in controls (○), in patients with unilateral lesions during rotations to the intact side (●) and to the affected side (△), and in patients with bilateral lesions (▲).

downward arrow); however, fixation was relatively good during head rotations to the affected side because nystagmus was very weak (Fig. 6, top, upward arrow). The difference in the visual fixation ability between head rotations toward different directions became larger as the turning frequency increased. In patients with bilateral lesions, nystagmus was rarely induced and visual fixation was well maintained even at 1.0 Hz (Fig. 6, bottom).

As shown in Table 3, there was a high correlation between the gain and the frequency of head rotation in both normal subjects and patients with unilateral lesions during rotations to the intact side ($r = 0.65$ and 0.77, respectively, Fig. 7); no significant difference was found at any frequency between these two groups ($P > 0.05$). On the other hand, patients with bilateral lesions and patients with unilateral lesions during rotations to the affected side showed low values of gain even at high frequencies; the values did not differ significantly in these two groups ($P > 0.05$). The patient with bilateral lesions who could best fix on the head-fixed target showed the worst visual fixation on the

TABLE 3. GAIN WITH HEAD-FIXED TARGET (MEAN AND SD)

Subjects	*0.33 Hz*	*0.67 Hz*	*1.0 Hz*
Controls	0.22±0.12	0.33±0.14	0.54±0.17
Unilateral lesions			
Rotation to intact side	0.18±0.09	0.35±0.07	0.56±0.17
Rotation to affected side	0.09±0.03	0.11±0.05	0.17±0.05
Bilateral lesions	0.07±0.05	0.14±0.06	0.17±0.07

spatially fixed target (Fig. 5, open triangles). Similarly, among the cases with unilateral lesions, the patient who showed the best fixation on a head-fixed target during rotations to the affected side proved to have the poorest ability to fix on the spatially fixed target (Fig. 5, solid triangles). However, in this patient, fixation on the head-fixed target during rotations to the intact side was very poor (0.17, 0.35 and 0.45 at 0.33, 0.67 and 1.0 Hz, respectively).

DISCUSSION

Visual fixation disturbances due to a loss of vestibular function during active head rotations have been reported in bilaterally labyrinthectomized monkeys and in patients with bilateral loss of vestibular function.[3-7] Dichgans et al[4,5] showed that the severely impaired ability of visual fixation in bilaterally labyrinthectomized monkeys was recovered by means of three different mechanisms: an increase of gain in the cervico-ocular reflex, centrally-programmed compensatory eye movements, and a recalibration of the saccade. Similar compensatory mechanisms may occur in humans.[7] These findings were obtained under experimental conditions in which compensatory eye movements aided visual fixation. In the present study, to clarify the effects of a decrease in compensatory eye movements due to loss of vestibular function on the ability of visual fixation, we examined the functions of gaze fixation not only under conditions in which compensatory eye movements aided gaze fixation, but also under conditions in which they did not.

Compensatory eye movements during the alert-in-dark condition varied even among normal subjects and showed poor reproducibility in the same subject.[1] In this condition, however, we can estimate the magnitude of compensatory eye movements not affected by gaze fixation. The gain during the alert-in-dark condition in patients with bilateral lesions, which ranged from 0.2 to 0.58 at 0.67 Hz, was less than that reported by Kasai and Zee[7] (0.5-0.96 at 0.5 Hz over an amplitude of 40-50°). Since we were unable to find a patient with bilateral lesions who did not show any compensatory eye movements, compensatory eye movements in patients with bilateral loss of vestibular function may be produced by mechanisms other than the vestibulo-ocular reflex, eg, those found in labyrinthectomized monkeys.[4] Patients with unilateral lesions showed not merely a directional preponderance,[8] but a decrease of the nystagmic response confined to rotations in the direction of the affected side. In these patients, the gains showed quite different values for rotations to the intact side and to the affected side; the former resembled the values of normal subjects and the latter were similar to those of patients with bilateral lesions. The patients with unilateral lesions examined in the present study belonged in the postacute, but still early stage of the disease. Thus, it might be said that in this stage, the vestibulo-ocular reflex from the intact labyrinth scarcely affects the compensatory eye movements during rotations to the affected side.

The findings obtained under spatially fixed target conditions were highly characteristic. While fixation was well maintained, even at 1 Hz, in normal subjects and patients with unilateral lesions during rotations to the intact side, it worsened in direct proportion to an increase in the turning frequency among patients with bilateral lesions and in those with unilateral lesions during rotations to the affected side. On the other hand, while in normal subjects and patients with unilateral lesions during rotations to the intact side, visual fixation under the head-fixed target condition became impaired as the turning frequency increased, it remained good even at 1 Hz among patients with bilateral lesions and those with unilateral lesions during rotations to the affected side. These results indicate that the ability of visual fixation in patients with bilateral lesions was quite opposite that in normal subjects under these two test conditions, and that visual fixation disturbances in the early stage of unilateral lesions were confined to rotations to the affected side, resembling the disturbance noted in patients with bilateral lesions.

The present study clearly demonstrated disturbances in gaze stabilization which resulted from insufficient compensatory eye movements due to unilateral and bilateral loss of vestibular function under nearly natural circumstances of free head rotations. Therefore, our tests may be applicable in clinical situations to determine the ataxic states of the oculomotor system induced by labyrinthine diseases and other related abnormalities.

REFERENCES

1. Takahashi M, Uemura T, Fujishiro T. Studies of the vestibulo-ocular reflex and visual-vestibular interactions during active head movements. Acta Otolaryngol (Stockh) 1980; 90:115-24.

2. Uemura T, Arai Y, Shimazaki C. Eye-head coordination during lateral gaze in normal subjects. Acta Otolaryngol (Stockh) 1980; 90:191-8.

3. Atkin A, Bender MB. Ocular stabilization during oscillatory head movements. Arch Neurol 1968; 19:559-66.

4. Dichgans J, Bizzi E, Morasso P, Tagliasco V. Mechanisms underlying recovery of eye-head coordination following bilateral labyrinthectomy in monkeys. Exp Brain Res 1973; 18:548-62.

5. Dichgans J, Bizzi E, Morasso P, Tagliasco V. The role of vestibular and neck afferents during eye-head coordination in the monkey. Brain Res 1974; 71:225-32.

6. Zee DS. Disorders of eye-head coordination. In: Brooks B, Bajandas EJ, eds. Eye movements. New York: Plenum Press, 1976:9-40.

7. Kasai T, Zee DS. Eye-head coordination in labyrinthine-defective human beings. Brain Res 1978; 144:123-41.

8. Barnes GR. Head-eye coordination in normals and in patients with vestibular disorders. Adv Otorhinolaryngol 1979; 25:197-201.

IN VITRO CULTIVATION OF THE FETAL GUINEA PIG INNER EAR

GUSTAVE L. DAVIS, MD MARY M. HAWRISIAK, ScM

ST. LOUIS, MISSOURI

Fetal guinea pig inner ears, gestational age from 21 to 54 days, were cultivated in vitro and then observed with light and electron microscopes. Early 21-day gestation otocysts developed cartilaginous capsules from differentiating mesenchyme and discrete neurosensory structures from endolabyrinthine epithelium. Coiling of the cochlea occurred. Older, differentiated inner ears showed progressive increase in size and development of the labyrinth. The 26-day gestation cochlea, maintained for 12 days in vitro, doubled in size with development comparable to the 37-day gestation in vivo control. The large size of the guinea pig inner ear resulted in varying degrees of necrosis. However, the well-defined growth and development of the guinea pig fetal inner ear in vitro indicates the efficacy of the technique and suggests that similar success would be forthcoming with other animals used in audiologic research, such as chinchilla and hamster.

INTRODUCTION

During the past decade, Van de Water and Ruben successfully developed an organ culture system for the in vitro evaluation of the growth and development of the mouse fetal inner ear.[1,2] There have been few other successful efforts at this venture. Friedmann[3,4] and his associates more recently reported successful maintenance of 12-day gestational mouse otocyst in culture for 14 days.[5] Sobkowicz et al[6] studied the neural pathways of postpartum mouse organ of Corti in culture and Yamashita and Vosteen[7] have studied outgrowths of cells from explanted guinea pig inner ears. Recently, Anniko and Wersall[8] reported that "considerable difficulties occurred when explanting the guinea pig ears already on the 30th gestational day and following it in vitro thereafter."

We report herein our successful application of Van de Water and Ruben's organ culture technique[1] to the in vitro growth and development of the fetal guinea pig inner ear.

METHODS

Experimental Animals. A breeding colony of Hartley strain albino guinea pigs was established from a breeding pair obtained from Elm Hill Breeding Labs, Chelmsford, Massachusetts. Timed pregnancy was established by pairing a male guinea pig with the pregnant sow at the estimated date of delivery, since the guinea pig ovulates within 24 hours of parturition.[9] Expelled vaginal plug confirmed that copulation had taken place, and the presence of fetuses was confirmed by weekly palpation of the pregnant sow.[10]

At various times during gestation, pregnant sows were anesthetized with chloroform and, using sterile procedures, the pregnant uterus was removed and placed in prewarmed (37 C) Hanks' balanced salt solution. The embryo/fetuses were removed and crown-rump length was measured; good correlation was achieved with estimated gestational age using Draper's morphometric data.[11] At 21 days gestation, prior to the formation of the external ear, the otocyst, transilluminated from below, was visible with the dissecting microscope (Fig. 1). The fetal skin was removed with sharp forceps and the otocyst excised with a thin rim of surrounding mesenchyme (Fig. 2). By the 25th day of gestation, the external ear was visible and the inner ear was surrounded by a distinct cartilaginous capsule. These and older fetuses were therefore decapitated, the heads hemisected in the midsagittal plane, the

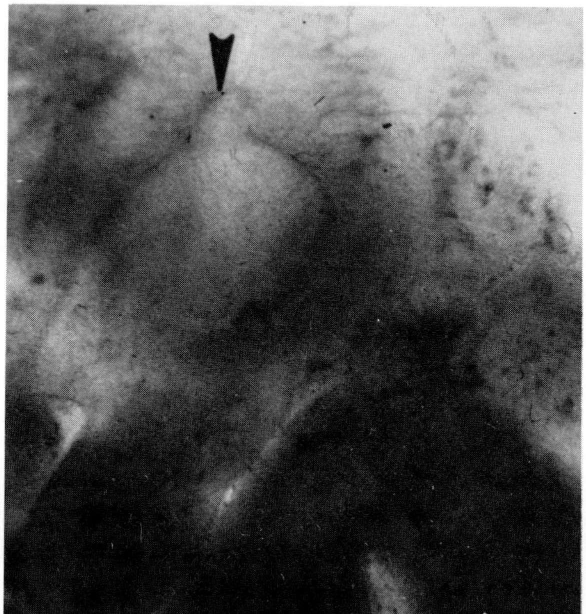

Fig. 1. Otocyst of the 21-day gestation guinea pig transilluminated in situ is roughly spherical with a dorsal endolymphatic duct outpouch (arrowhead).

From the Department of Pathology and Laboratory Medicine, The Jewish Hospital of St. Louis, Washington University School of Medicine, St. Louis, and The Institute of Laryngology and Otology, University of London. This work has been supported by Biomedical Research Funds and Endowment Funds of The Jewish Hospital of St. Louis, a Senior International Fellowship of The Fogarty International Center, National Institutes of Health (FO 6 TW00123), and the Deafness Research Foundation.

Presented at the Second and Third Annual Midwinter Meetings of the Association for Research in Otolaryngology, St. Petersburg Beach, Florida, January 23, 1979, and January 24, 1980.

REPRINTS — Gustave L. Davis, MD, Department of Pathology, The Jewish Hospital of St. Louis, 216 South Kingshighway, St. Louis, MO 63110.

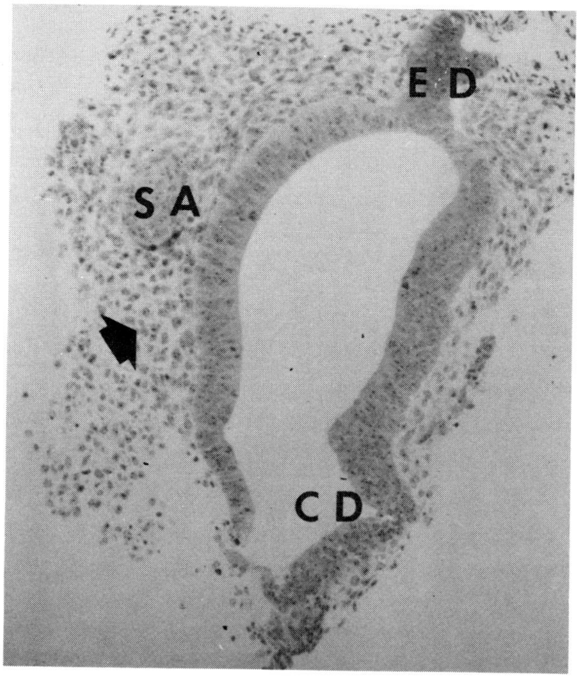

Fig. 2. Excised 21-day gestation otocyst, trimmed of much surrounding mesenchyme, shows endolymphatic duct (ED) and ventral cochlear duct outpouch (CD). The statoacoustic ganglion (SA) is present in the adjacent mesenchyme which is differentiating into cartilage (arrow). (x100)

brain removed and the cartilaginous inner ear removed intact. Otocysts and cartilaginous inner ears were separately placed in the following organ culture system both intact, and as dorsal (vestibular) and ventral (cochlear) portions.[12]

Organ Culture. The method of Van de Water and Ruben was used with little modification.[1] Excised inner ears, trimmed of the surrounding connective tissue and nerve root, were placed in the central well of a Falcon 3010 organ culture dish with 0.15 ml of Newmann and Tytell's serumless medium supplemented with 10% fetal calf serum, 1% l-glutamine with and without antibiotics. When utilized, the antibiotics were penicillin (200 units/ml) and streptomycin (100 μg/ml). Sterile distilled water was added to the bibulous paper of the outer ring of the organ culture dish to maintain humidity and the dishes were sealed with petroleum jelly and incubated at 34.5 C. The medium was changed every two days. The cultures were observed daily and photographed as desired.

Microscopy. The cultured ears were fixed in 2% glutaraldehyde, washed in 0.1 M phosphate buffer, postfixed in 1% osmium tetroxide and then dehydrated and embedded in Araldite®. Serial thick sections of the ears, cut in a horizontal plane with glass knives in an ultramicrotome, were stained with toluidine blue and observed with a light microscope. When appropriate, the next thin section was cut with a diamond knife, mounted on Formvar®-coated, slotted copper grids, stained with lead citrate and uranyl acetate and examined with a Phillips 201C electron microscope.

The morphology of the 26-day gestation inner ear cultured in vitro for 12 days was compared to noncultured controls of comparable in vivo age (26 and 37 days gestation).[13]

RESULTS

A series of explanted inner ears from 21 through 54 days gestation was studied. The inner ears were

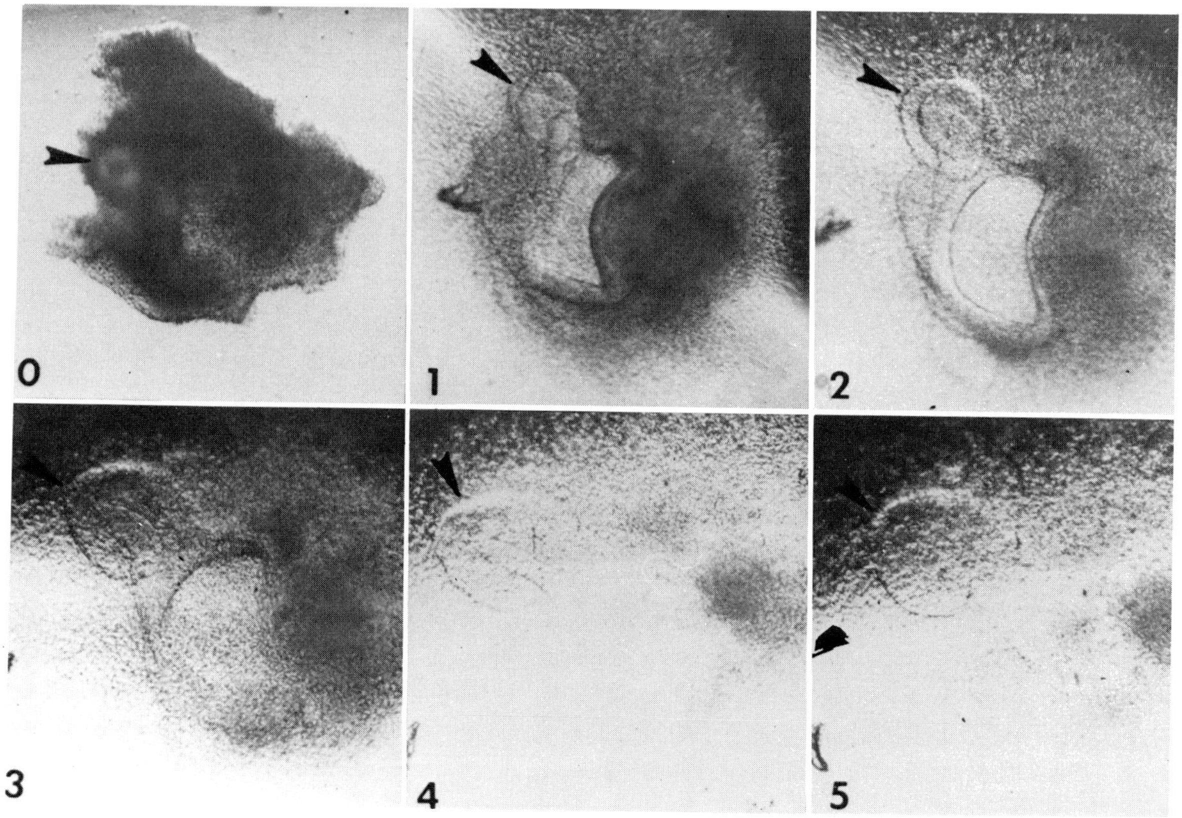

Fig. 3. Progressive coiling of the cochlear duct outpouch (arrowhead) of the explanted ventral hemiotocyst from day 0 through day 3; necrosis of the explant is apparent by day 4.

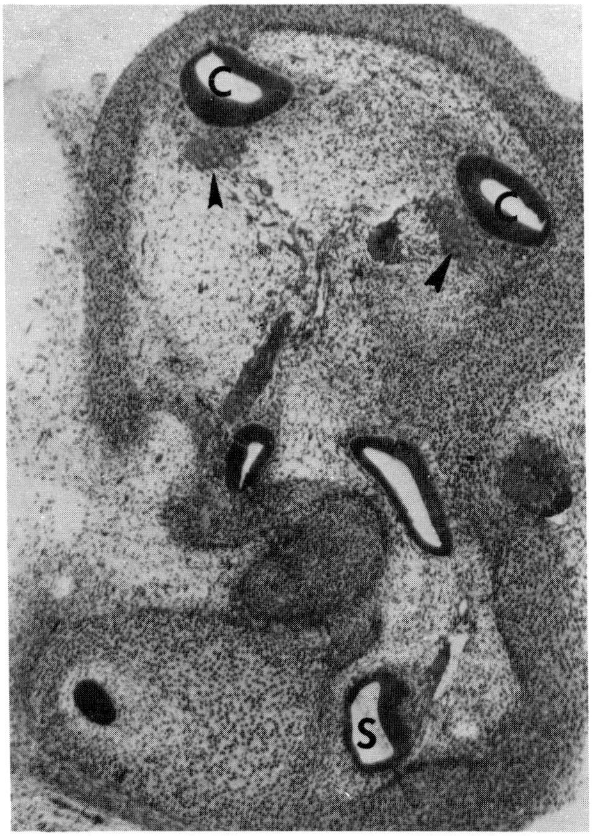

Fig. 4. Preimplantation 26-day gestation inner ear has a well-differentiated cartilaginous capsule enclosing cochlear duct (C), spiral ganglions (arrowheads), and semicircular canals (S) in perilabyrinthine connective tissue. (x40)

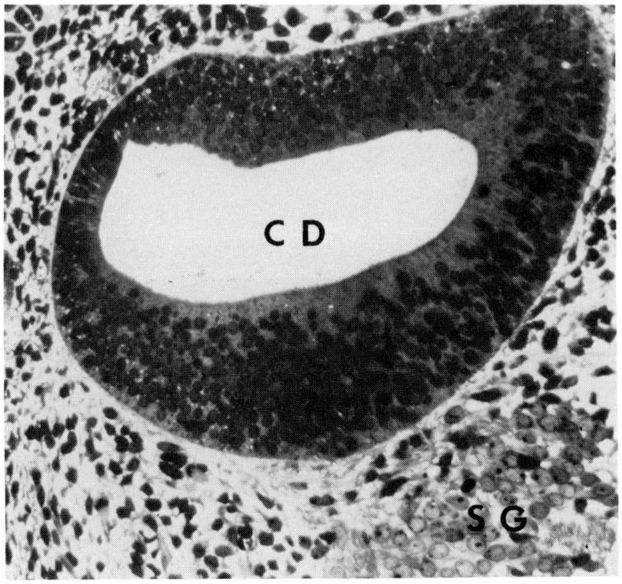

Fig. 5. Cochlear duct (CD) in Fig. 4 shows little differentiation. The thicker, ventromedian portion, adjacent to the spiral ganglion (SG) will develop into the organ of Corti. (x250)

maintained in vitro for various times up to 14 days. In virtually every experiment, gross enlargement to twice initial size occurred by eight days in vitro. Concomitant with the increase in growth was progressive development of cartilaginous and membranous labyrinth. However, various degrees of degeneration and necrosis of mesenchyme (fibroblasts, nerves and ganglia) and ultimately membranous labyrinth occurred. Cartilage rarely underwent necrosis. The degenerative changes progressed with the size of the ear and distance of tissues from the periphery, indicating a lack of diffusion of metabolites.

Nevertheless, distinct and rapid growth and differentiation of inner ear structures took place through 12 days in vitro. These changes were better appreciated and lacking necrosis in inner ears which had been divided into the ventral (cochlear) and dorsal (vestibular) portions, thus decreasing volume of tissues to be perfused. Though vestibular growth and differentiation did occur parallel to that of the cochlea, this report will concentrate on the latter.

The 21-day gestation otocyst, observed by transillumination of the fetus in situ, is round to oval with a dorsal nipple, the endolymphatic duct and sac anlage (Fig. 1). The otocyst is situated dorsally above the developing forelimb bud and immediately beneath the yet unfused neural canal. Histologic sections of the 21-day gestation otocyst prior to explantation (Fig. 2) show ventral cochlear bud and vestibular projections. The endolymphatic duct projects dorsally. The surrounding mesenchyme is condensed and differentiating into cartilage. The statoacoustic ganglion is anterodorsal and partially incorporated into the developing cartilaginous capsule. The cyst is lined by stratified columnar labyrinthine epithelium with little further differentiation.

Comparable 21-day otocysts from fetuses in the same litter as the above control were explanted in culture and observed for five days. The otocysts were divided into ventral cochlear and dorsal vestibular portions. Figure 3 shows the progressive growth and development of these "hemiotocysts"[14] over a five-day period in vitro. Cochlear development is apparent with increase in size and coiling of the cochlear bud (arrow). In this experiment, however, the tissues underwent rapid degeneration by the fourth day in vitro. Similar development of the semicircular canals takes place, but degeneration is also apparent grossly by day 3.

Better results were obtained with older inner ears. Twenty-six to 27-day gestation ears, incubated in vitro for up to 12 days, showed the most development, paralleling normal in vivo development over the same period of time.[13] Older ears, 38 and 54-day gestation, were also maintained in vitro, but showed little progressive development.

The 26-day gestation otocyst contains a distinct

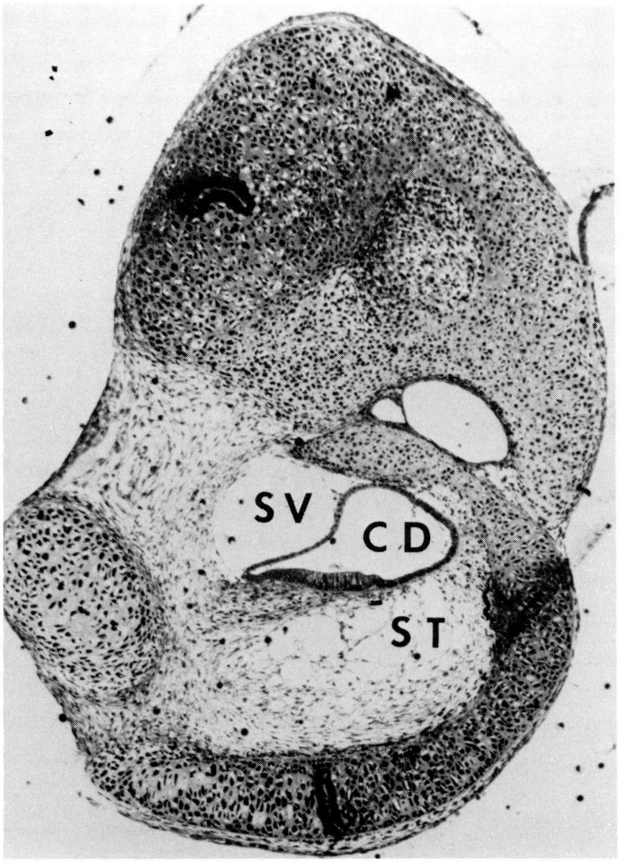

Fig. 6. Compared to the preexplantation ear (Fig. 4), the 26-day gestation cochlear portion has doubled in size following explantation for 12 days. The cartilaginous capsule is well differentiated and the cochlear duct (CD) topography is mature with separation from the scala vestibuli (SV) and scala tympani (ST). (x40)

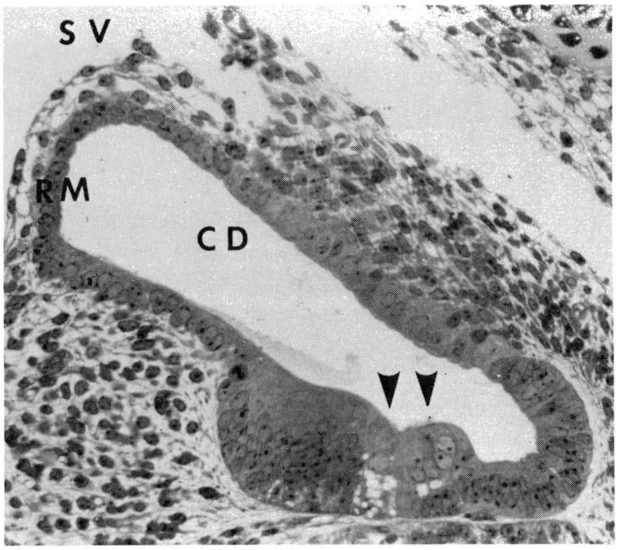

Fig. 8. Cochlear duct (CD) from a 37-day gestation guinea pig compared with that of 26-day gestation control (Fig. 5) and that explanted for 12 days (total 38 days) (Fig. 7). Reissner's membrane (RM) is not as completely developed as it is in the explant. However, spiral limbus and organ of Corti (arrowheads) development is more advanced. Though capillaries are present in the perilabyrinthine connective tissue (arrow), none yet enter the stria vascularis (SV). (x250)

cartilaginous capsule enclosing membranous labyrinth, nerves and connective tissue. Figure 4 shows basal $1^{1}/_{2}$ cochlear turns about the modiolus lacking bone or cartilage but containing cochlear nerve and spiral ganglia. A cross section of the cochlear duct (Fig. 5) shows a semblance of differentiation with relatively thick basal epithelium medially in relation to the spiral ganglion and thinner epithelial surface laterally in the region of future stria vascularis development. The degree of growth and development of the ventral portion of the 26-day gestation otocyst after 12 days in vitro is readily seen in Figure 6. The cochlear portion has increased roughly two times in size. The cartilage is quite distinct from the surrounding mesenchyme. The cochlear duct (Fig. 7) is triangular in cross section with well-developed scala vestibuli and scala tympani; Reissner's membrane is composed of a single epithelial layer on the scala media side and a single layer of mesenchymal cells on the scala vestibuli side, separated by basement membrane. The basal

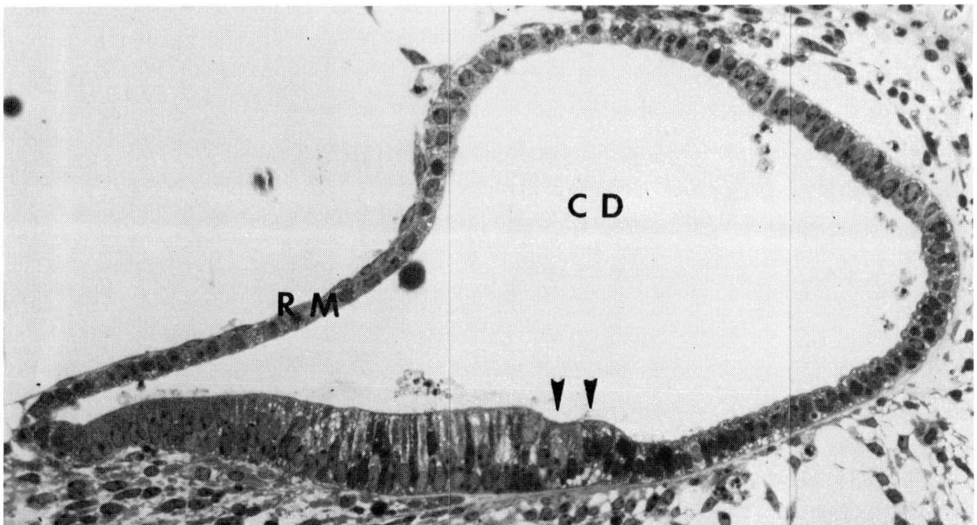

Fig. 7. Magnification of cochlear duct (CD) seen in Fig. 6 has a mature Reissner's membrane (RM) formed of single epithelial and mesenchymal layers, separated by a basement membrane. The lateral hump of the cochlear duct (arrowheads) represents the differentiating organ of Corti. (x250)

portion of the cochlear duct has a differentiated lateral hump, the site of the organ of Corti. The cochlear duct is surrounded by a basement membrane which is, however, incomplete about the stria vascularis, from the spiral ligament to the insertion of Reissner's membrane. Neurons are also present immediately adjacent to the basement membrane of the putative organ of Corti, but there is no penetration of the basement membrane by nerve growth cones.

The organ of Corti of the explant is less well developed than that of the 37-day gestation in vivo control (Fig. 8). Hair cells with stereo cilia are already present in the latter; no sensory hairs are observed in the explanted otocyst.[12]

DISCUSSION

The 26-day gestation guinea pig inner ear can grow in vitro for at least up to 12 days with development comparable to that normally occurring in vivo (to 37 days). Our results, similar to those of Van de Water and Ruben,[1] Van de Water,[2] and Anniko and Wersall[8] in mice, indicate that such success might be achieved with still other mammalian systems. The technique is simple and does not require an elaborate support system. Nevertheless, we encountered difficulties maintaining sterility and found it desirable to use antibiotics in the medium. The presence of penicillin and streptomycin, even in low doses, must be weighed against any ototoxic effects.[4] As the inner ear grows in vitro, inspite of obvious differentiation, there is concomitant central tissue necrosis. Smaller portions of the divided inner ear permit diffusion of metabolites and result in less necrosis than the intact ear. The large tissue fragments may account for Anniko and Wersall's[8] lack of success in maintaining guinea pig otocysts beyond 30 days of gestation.

In vitro organ culture of avian and mammalian inner ears have already proven useful in the study of drugs,[15,16] physical[17] and chemical[18] agents on mesenchymal-epithelial interactions, genetic predisposition to congenital deafness,[19] and viral infection[20,21] on inner ear development. For those individuals committed to guinea pig audiologic research, the in vitro system is efficacious for studies of mammalian ear development. But the long gestation period of guinea pigs (9-10 weeks vs 3 weeks for mice), relatively small litter size (an average of four fetuses for guinea pigs and eight for mice), and the relatively slower in vivo and in vitro differentiation per unit time for guinea pigs recommend the use of fetal mice as the experimental animal.

ACKNOWLEDGMENT — I (GLD) wish to thank Professor Leslie Michaels, Dean; Dr. K. E. K. Rowson, Director of Virology; and Dr. Ade Pye, Research Zoologist; and their associates for their advice and assistance in initiating this study during my tenure as Visiting Professor of Pathology at the I.L.O., 1977-1978.

REFERENCES

1. Van de Water TR, Ruben RJ. Growth of the inner ear in organ culture. Ann Otol Rhinol Laryngol 1974; 83 Suppl 14:1-16.

2. Van de Water TR. Effects of removal of the statoacoustic ganglion complex upon the growing otocyst. Ann Otol Rhinol Laryngol 1976; 85 Suppl 33:2-32.

3. Friedmann I. The ear. In: Willmer EN, ed. Cells and tissues in culture: methods, biology and physiology. Vol 2. New York: Academic Press, 1965:521-47.

4. Friedmann I. Pathology of the ear. Oxford: Blackwell Scientific Publications, 1974.

5. Friedmann I, Hodges GH, Riddle PN. Organ culture of the avian and mammalian otocyst. Acta Otolaryngol (Stockh) 1977; 83:170-4.

6. Sobkowicz HM, Bereman B, Rose JE. Organotypic development of the organ of Corti in culture. J Neurocytol 1975; 4:543-72.

7. Yamashita T,Vosteen KH. Tissue culture of the organ of Corti and the isolated hair cells from the newborn guinea pig. Acta Otolaryngol (Stockh) 1975; 30 Suppl 3:77-90.

8. Anniko M, Wersall J. The inner ear and the in vitro system. Arch Otorhinolaryngol (NY) 1979; 224:25-30.

9. Wagner JE, Manning PG, eds. Biology of the guinea pig. New York: Academic Press, 1976.

10. Matthews PJ, Jackson J. Pregnancy diagnosis on the guinea pig. Lab Anim Sci 1977; 27:248-50.

11. Draper RL. The prenatal growth of the guinea pig. Anat Rec 1920; 18:369-92.

12. Anniko M, Van de Water TR, Nordemar H. Organ culture of the 16th gestational day mouse labyrinth: a model suggestion for pre- and post-partum development. Acta Otolaryngol (Stockh) 1978; 86:52-5.

13. Chodynicki S. Embryogenesis of the auditory part of the inner ear in the guinea pig. Acta Theriol 1968; 13:219-60.

14. Li CW, Van de Water TR, Ruben RJ. The fate mapping of the eleventh and twelfth day mouse otocyst: an in vitro study of the sites or origin of the embryonic inner ear sensory structures. J Morphol 1978; 157:249-67.

15. Friedmann I, Bird ES. The effect of ototoxic antibiotics and of penicillin on the sensory areas of the isolated fowl embryo otocyst in organ culture: an EM study. J Pathol Bacteriol 1961; 81:81-90.

16. Friedmann I. The effect of sodium cyanide on the chick embryo otocyst in vitro: a tissue culture study. Acta Otolaryngol (Stockh) 1972; 73:280-9.

17. Li CW, McPhee J. Influences on the coiling of the cochlea. Ann Otol Rhinol Laryngol 1979; 88:280-7.

18. Saver J, Van de Water TR. Morphogenesis and cytodifferentiation of the mouse otocyst following exposure to trypsin. Abstracts of the Third Midwinter Research Meeting of the Association for Research in Otolaryngology, abstract 3. St. Petersburg, Florida, January 21, 1980.

19. Van de Water TR, Ruben RJ. III. Organ culture of the mammalian inner ear: a tool to study inner ear deafness. Laryngoscope 1974; 84:738-49.

20. Davis GL, Hawrisiak MM. Experimental cytomegalovirus infection and the developing mouse inner ear: in vivo and in vitro studies. Lab Invest 1977; 37:20-9.

21. Davis GL, Hawrisiak MM. Guinea pig cytomegalovirus infection of the guinea pig inner ear cultivated in vitro. Abstracts of the Third Midwinter Meeting of the Association for Research in Otolaryngology, abstract 30. St. Petersburg, Florida, January 23, 1980.

Ann Otol 90:1981

ALTERNARIA SINUSITIS

MARTIN A. SHUGAR, MD
CHICAGO, ILLINOIS

WILLIAM W. MONTGOMERY, MD
BOSTON, MASSACHUSETTS

NEWTON E. HYSLOP, JR., MD
BOSTON, MASSACHUSETTS

Alternaria is a fungus of the class Deuteromycetes and the family Dematiaceae. Fungi of this genus have generally been regarded as nonpathogenic and as contaminants when isolated from clinical specimens. Hypersensitivity to *Alternaria* spores, however, has long been recognized as a cause of allergic pulmonary disease. More recently, the organism has also been demonstrated to have potential for opportunistic invasion of immunosuppressed and debilitated patients. Presented is a case in which this organism was repeatedly isolated from naso-oral tissue specimens from an otherwise healthy patient. The organism was seen in biopsies from a granulomatous hyperplastic destructive disease of the maxilla and soft tissues of the face which extended to the ethmoid sinus and fistulized through the hard palate. The clinical course, pathophysiology and therapeutic approach are discussed. The management of this disease requires a multidisciplinary approach involving the otolaryngologist, infectious disease specialist and pathologist.

INTRODUCTION

Alternaria is a fungus of the class Deuteromycetes and the family Dematiaceae. Fungi of the genus *Alternaria* until recently were generally regarded as nonpathogenic and as specimen contaminants when isolated from culture media.[1] The natural habitat of this common plant pathogen is the soil. The organism is ubiquitous, and its spores are known to be airborne. *Alternaria* organisms are often isolated from scrapings and biopsies of normal skin,[2] which causes difficulty in determining whether it is a contaminant when found in cultures. While the organism has been considered to lack virulence factors necessary for invasion of normal tissues, hypersensitivity responses to inhalation of *Alternaria* spores have long been known as a cause of allergic pulmonary diseases such as bronchial asthma in atopics and hypersensitivity in malt workers.

Recently, *Alternaria* has been demonstrated to be an opportunistic pathogen: cutaneous alternariosis was described in two patients with primary debilitating diseases and in a patient with acute lymphocytic lymphoma.[2,3] Keratomycosis with isolation of *Alternaria* species from a corneal ulcer was described in a patient who had been on a three-month course of topical corticosteroids.[4] The first report of alternarial invasion of an apparently healthy individual described osteomyelitis involving the premaxilla, the caudal margin of the anterior nasal septum and the hard palate in a young, otherwise healthy female.[5] We present a second case in an otherwise healthy female in which *Alternaria* was repeatedly observed in biopsies of, and isolated from a sclerosing, destructive, granulomatous process in the nasal cavity and ethmoid sinus in association with fistula formation through the hard palate. The clinical course, pathophysiology and therapeutic approach are discussed.

CASE REPORT

A 50-year-old white female was referred to the Massachusetts Eye and Ear Infirmary for evaluation of a right nasal mass and palatal fistula.

In 1957, the patient moved to Florida and immediately began to experience symptoms of allergic rhinitis. As a result she became a chronic nasal spray abuser, but did not use any systemic or topical steroids. Shortly after arriving in Florida, the family acquired a horse and the patient regularly pitched hay to feed the animal.

In June 1972, the patient noted a burning sensation in the palate. Over a period of one week, a rapidly progressing ulceration developed with perforation of the hard palate into the floor of the nose. Biopsy of this lesion demonstrated inflammation and hyphal forms. Subsequent cultures revealed fungi of the genus *Alternaria*. Treatment at this time consisted of local excision of the involved area of the palate with local injections of Nystatin®; the fistula tract closed.

In November 1972, her symptoms and fistula recurred and she was referred to another physician who administered intermittent courses of amphotericin B intravenously over three months. The fistula closed and no fungal forms were found on biopsy at the completion of treatment. Subsequently, she experienced a number of recurrences, all preceded by episodic epistaxis, nasal crusting and a moldy smell which she attributed to the organism. With each recurrence, biopsy of the palate and

From the Department of Otolaryngology, Harvard Medical School and the Massachusetts Eye and Ear Infirmary; and the Infectious Disease Unit, Massachusetts General Hospital, Boston.

REPRINTS — W. W. Montgomery, MD, Massachusetts Eye and Ear Infirmary, 243 Charles Street, Boston, MA 02114.

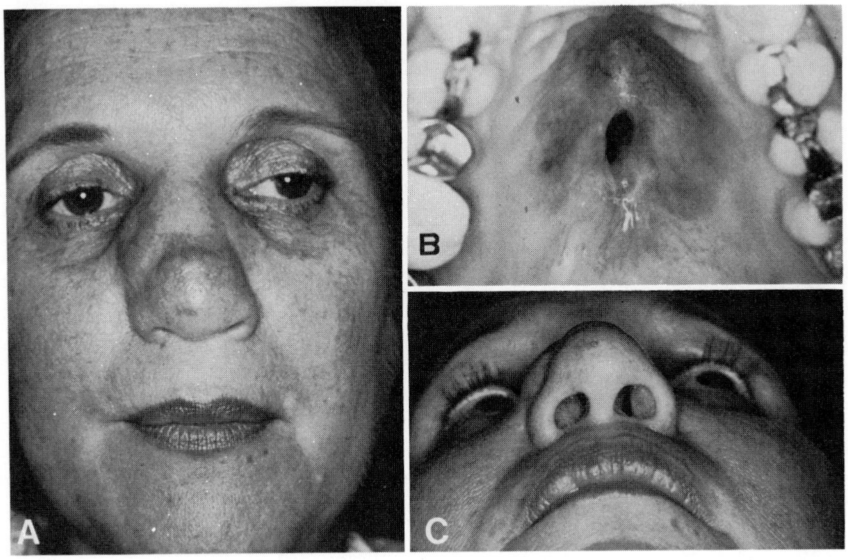

Fig. 1. A) Right nasolabial mass and supratip lesion. B) Palatal fistula. C) Note mass of right lateral nasal wall.

nasal turbinates revealed noncaseating granuloma and intracellular and extracellular branching filamentous organisms. As isolates from these early specimens underwent sporulation on culture, the organism was repeatedly identified as *Alternaria*. Subsequently, during her course, culture isolates grew only as nonsporulating mycelial mats.

Thereafter, she was administered multiple courses of amphotericin B; each time slow healing of the fistula was followed months later by relapse. The patient was referred to several institutions to undergo modifications of the amphotericin B regimen. A recurrence in December 1978 was treated with the oral antifungal agent, ketoconazole, with limited clinical response. She was also noted to have a gradually increasing mass in the right nasolabial fold and, more recently, an erythematous nodular lesion over the supratip region of the nose.

The patient was first admitted to the Massachusetts Eye and Ear Infirmary in January 1979. Examination revealed a 3 mm diameter fistula opening in the hard palate (Fig. 1B). Examination of the external nose revealed a hard, slightly erythematous mass obliterating the right nasolabial fold and an erythematous firm ridge across the supratip region (Fig. 1A). Intranasal examination showed a nonerythematous, hard mass of the right lateral nasal wall (Fig. 1C), crusting of the right inferior turbinate, and discoloration of the right anterior septum. The remainder of a complete otorhinolaryngologic and neurologic examination was within normal limits. Skin testing did not reveal anergy. Immunoglobulin and complement levels were normal.

Plain films and polytomography of the sinuses revealed only slight thickening of the right anterolateral nasal wall, and membrane thickening in the ethmoids and left sphenoid sinuses. Computerized tomography of the orbits and frontal views of the sinuses showed a focal soft tissue mass in a few ethmoid cells but no destruction of the lamina papyracae and no intraorbital mass; coronal views revealed some resorption of the inferior portion of the bony nasal septum and soft tissue swelling of the turbinates (Fig. 2). Bone scan showed no uptake in the frontal or maxillary bones. Histological exam and cultures of biopsies of the anterior tips of both middle turbinates were negative for *Alternaria*. Biopsy of the margins of the palatal fistula revealed typical hyphal forms and granulomatous inflammation; two colonies of filamentous fungi were isolated from the biopsy and from curettings of the fistula. Further identification was prevented by failure of the organism to sporulate despite subculturing on a variety of media.

Over the next eight months, the oronasal fistula tract narrowed on an increased ketoconazole dosage of 400 mg/day. However, progression of induration and erythema of the hard palate mucosa and increase of the right nasolabial fold mass dictated an attempt at surgical debulking: the objectives were to resect the advancing parameningeal ethmoid le-

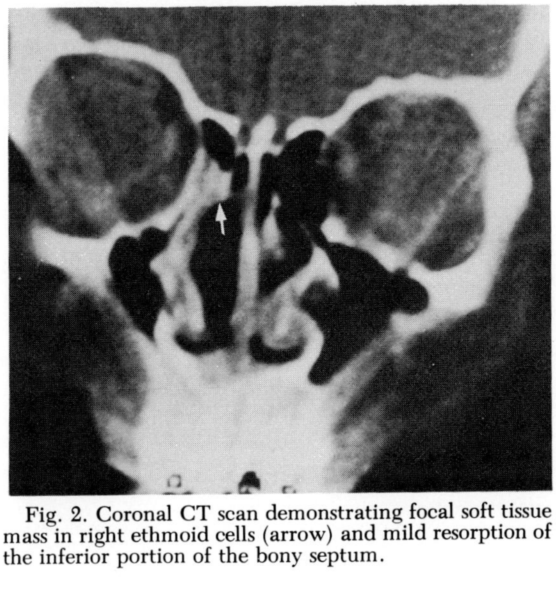

Fig. 2. Coronal CT scan demonstrating focal soft tissue mass in right ethmoid cells (arrow) and mild resorption of the inferior portion of the bony septum.

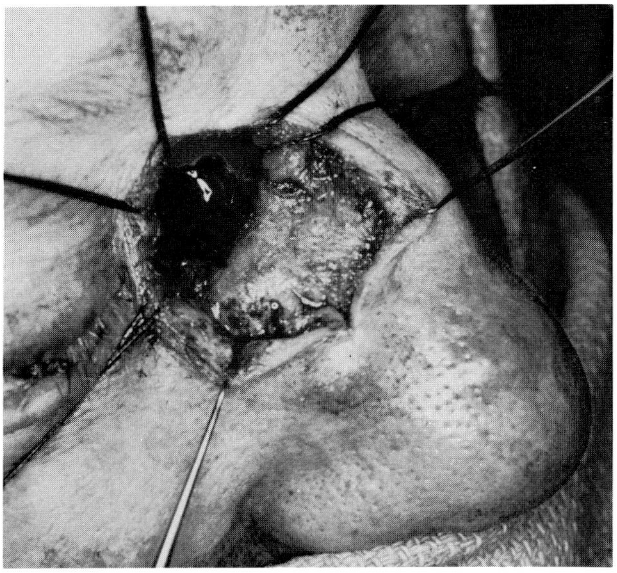

Fig. 3. Right external ethmoidectomy approach. Note the rubbery appearance of the lesion.

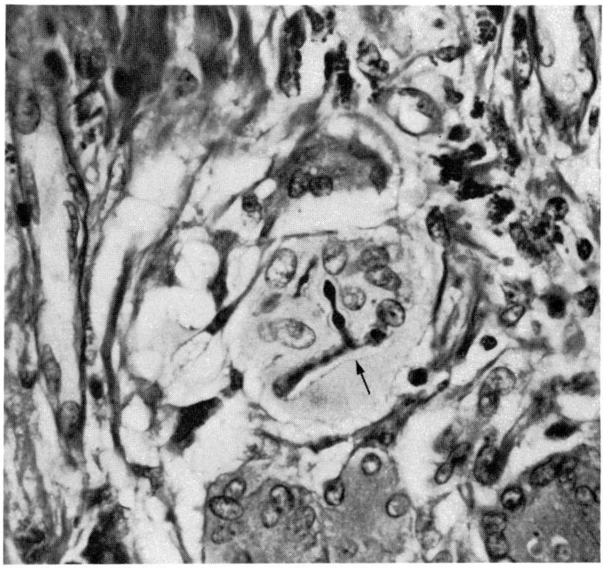

Fig. 4. Tissue section demonstrating hyphal form within giant cell (arrow). (PAS, x640)

sion and to reduce the fungal load in hopes that a further trial of amphotericin B would have a reduced chance of relapse.

The patient was readmitted in August 1979, brought up to a full amphotericin dosage of 20 mg/day over seven days, with 5-fluorocytosine at 3 gm/day, and then taken to the operating room. A right external ethmoidectomy approach was utilized to debulk the lesion over the nasolabial fold and to explore the ethmoid sinuses (Fig. 3). It was noted that the skin and immediate subcutaneous tissues appeared free of disease, the ethmoid labyrinth appeared grossly normal, and that the anterolateral nasal wall adjacent to the upper extension of the middle turbinate was moderately thickened. The incision was then extended caudad to partially debulk the nasolabial mass. The mass was avascular, extremely hard, and had replaced portions of the ascending process of the maxilla, upper lateral nasal cartilage and inferior lateral nasal bone. The right nasal cavity and ethmoid sinus were then packed with iodoform gauze impregnated with both amphotericin B cream (1%) and tetracycline ointment. The wound was closed primarily without drainage. Postoperatively the patient was maintained on amphotericin B and 5-fluorocytosine until discharge on the 14th postoperative day for continued outpatient treatment. There were no complications and healing was uneventful.

Histopathology revealed granulomatous inflammation and fibrosis involving the nasolabial lesion, ascending process of the maxilla, anterolateral nasal wall, middle turbinate, and anterior ethmoid cells. Numerous fungi were seen, occasionally branching, with septate hyphae; fungal walls did not stain with hemotoxylin and eosin but were readily seen with Grocott-methenamine-silver and periodic acid Schiff stains (Fig. 4). This morphology was consistent with the appearance in tissue sections of *Alternaria* species.[3] Cultures of the operative material at 20 C on Sabouraud's dextrose agar with chloramphenicol yielded multiple colonies of a pure growth of a dematiacious fungus (Fig. 5). Results of in vitro sensitivity studies of the susceptibility of the fungus isolated from the operative specimens to various antifungal agents are shown in Table 1. The 5-fluorocytosine was discontinued when sensitivity tests showed it to be ineffective.

DISCUSSION

The natural habitat of *Alternaria* is the soil. The organism is commonly found in grains, seeds and grasses such as wheat, barley, oats, and corn.[6] In the case reported here sinusitis and osteomyelitis of the hard palate due to *Alternaria* occurred in an otherwise healthy patient with no obvious underlying abnormality of host defense. A similar case with involvement limited to the palate has been reported elsewhere.[5] In both instances, the clinical course paralleled aspergillosis of the paranasal sinuses, which may occur as a chronic disease in an otherwise healthy person.[7]

The disease process in the present case began in the right nasal cavity, eventually fistulizing through the hard palate as the initial clinical presentation. Thereafter, the infection spread up the lateral nasal wall to the ethmoid labyrinth. The local progression of disease was marked by a noncaseating granulomatous inflammatory reaction; furthermore, certain areas showed collagen deposition and sclerosis around inflammatory sites, a feature also characteristic of paranasal sinus aspergillosis.

Important factors in the pathogenesis appeared to be the intense exposure to *Alternaria* spores in the course of pitching hay, preceded by the long period

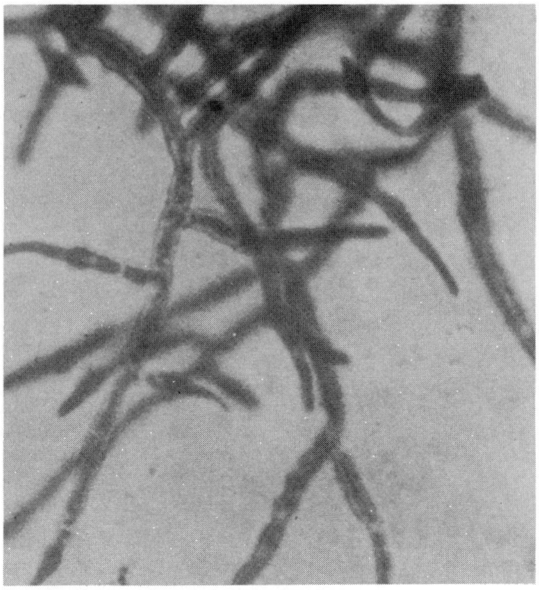

Fig. 5. Dematiaceous fungi with occasionally branching, septate hyphae (wet mount).

of allergic rhinitis and rhinitis medicamentosa. We postulate that the protective self-cleaning barrier of the nasal mucosa was impaired by the latter processes. By analogy with allergic aspergillosis, excessive mucus production may have facilitated germination of *Alternaria* spores to hyphae in the nasal mucosa; the areas of ischemic mucosa may in turn have permitted initial hyphal invasion of submucosal tissues.

It is unlikely that there was a general defect in the host defense mechanisms since the patient was not anergic, as shown by normal responses to the routine battery of skin tests and normal immunoglobulin and complement levels. It is possible that a selective defect in either intracellular killing mechanisms or in cellular immune responsiveness to *Alternaria* underlay the rarity of this entity. While incomplete intracellular killing of hyphal forms appeared to be the major host defect, it is not known whether normal macrophages are capable of fungicidal action against *Alternaria* hyphae. An important clinical fact against the hypothesis of a specific immune defect to *Alternaria* is the lack of systemic invasion over a seven-year period. However, the lack of systemic invasion could also be explained by inhibition of growth of the organism at 37 C, in which case growth would only occur in tissues adjacent to the lower temperatures of the nasal cavity and paranasal sinuses. In addition, limited and slow spread of the organism in these tissues probably also reflects some degree of effective host resistance, since organisms were seen in giant cells.

TABLE 1. IN VITRO SENSITIVITIES TO ANTIFUNGAL AGENTS OF ALTERNARIA

Agent	*MIC μg/ml*
Amphotericin B	0.8
5-Fluorocytosine	>100.00
Miconazole	0.2

MIC - Minimum inhibitory concentration.

The diagnosis of invasive fungal infection requires isolation of fungus from the area of infection and histologic confirmation of invasion of viable tissue by the putative pathogen.[5] Tissues in this case yielded pure cultures of septate filamentous fungi identical in morphology to that seen on histopathologic examination and consistent with the morphology of previous reports.[5,8] Earlier cultures had sporulated, permitting speciation of the fungus as *Alternaria*, but after repeated courses of amphotericin B therapy, isolates could not be induced to sporulate by us or by other laboratories.

The treatment we employed in an attempt to control further invasion of periorbital and parameningeal tissues consisted of a combination of chemotherapy and limited surgical removal of involved tissues with appropriate sinus drainage. These principles are similar to those in treating aspergillosis of the paranasal sinuses.[7] It should be emphasized that the clinical efficacy of the available chemotherapeutic agents used to treat *Alternaria* infections is questionable. The in vitro sensitivity studies in this case demonstrated that amphotericin B, miconazole and, by extrapolation, ketoconazole were inhibitory in vitro and that 5-fluorocytosine alone was neither inhibitory nor synergistic with amphotericin B. In vitro sensitivity studies do not allow prediction of the in vivo clinical response. A patient with *Alternaria* maxillary osteomyelitis inhibited by and treated with amphotericin B and local excision relapsed 17 months after completing therapy.[5]

Six months postoperatively, our patient experienced an exacerbation of the disease manifested by fistulization through the supratip portion of the nose and right lateral nasal wall. She is currently being treated with ketoconazole.

REFERENCES

1. Fetter BF, Klintworth GK, Hendry WS. Mycoses of the central nervous system. Baltimore: Williams & Wilkins, 1967:177-8.

2. Pederson NB, Mardh PA, Hallberg T, Jonsson N. Cutaneous alternariosis. Br J Dermatol 1976; 94:201-9.

3. Farmer SG, Komorowski RA. Cutaneous microabscess formation from *Alternaria alternata*. Am J Clin Pathol 1976; 66:565-9.

4. Azar P, Aquavelle JV, Smith RS. Keratomycosis due to an *Alternaria* species. Am J Ophthalmol 1975; 79:881-3.

5. Garat J, Diamond RD, Lagrotteria LB, Kabins SA. *Alternaria* osteomyelitis. Ann Intern Med 1977; 86:747-8.

6. Meronuck RA, Steele JA, Mirocha CJ, Christensen CM. Tenuazonic acid, a toxin produced by *Alternaria alternata*. Appl Microbiol 1972; 23:613-7.

7. Warder FR, Chikes PG, Hudson WR. Aspergillosis of the paranasal sinuses. Arch Otolaryngol 1975; 101:683-5.

8. Brinser JH. Keratomycosis due to an *Alternaria* species. Am J Ophthalmol 1976; 81:113.

Ann Otol 90:1981

OTOTOXICITY OF INTRACISTERNAL GENTAMICIN IN CATS

KATHERINE L. PARRISH, PhD
NEW ORLEANS, LOUISIANA

MASAYOSHI TACHIBANA, MD, PhD
KYOTO, JAPAN

FLOYD R. DOMER, PhD
NEW ORLEANS, LOUISIANA

CHARLES H. NORRIS, PhD
NEW ORLEANS, LOUISIANA

PAUL S. GUTH, PhD
NEW ORLEANS, LOUISIANA

The intrathecal administration of gentamicin has been used to treat bacterial meningitis. However, the influence of this route of administration on the well-known ototoxic activity of gentamicin is unknown. This route of administration should facilitate access to the inner ear and should increase the ototoxic liability. The possible ototoxic and neurotoxic effects of intrathecally administered gentamicin (0.5, 1, 2, 4, 6, 10 mg/day) in cats were evaluated. Hearing thresholds were obtained by a noninvasive technique prior to and on the 7th and 21st days after the initiation of a seven-day dosage regimen. Histological examination of the organ of Corti was routinely done. Additionally, the vestibular organs of one animal on the 4 mg/day regimen were examined. The concentrations of gentamicin in the cerebrospinal fluid were also determined. The data indicate that the 2 mg/day dose may be very close to the threshold dose for ototoxicity when gentamicin is given by intracisternal administration.

Gentamicin is of great value in the treatment of Gram-negative or tuberculous infections. It has also been used in the treatment of infections of the central nervous system (CNS) such as Gram-negative bacillary or tuberculous meningitis or ventriculitis. However, when used systemically, this drug frequently does not attain effective antibacterial concentrations in the cerebrospinal fluid (CSF). The low concentration of gentamicin in CSF has been ascribed to its poor penetration across the blood/CSF barrier. Although gentamicin has also been shown to be transported from CSF to blood via a saturable mechanism,[1] this transport is not a major factor in limiting levels of gentamicin in the CSF.

When the blood/CSF barrier is bypassed, as by intrathecal, intracisternal or intraventricular application, adequate drug levels for the treatment of infection of the CNS may be achieved. For example, Rahal[2] recommended that, for the treatment of bacillary meningitis, gentamicin be given intrathecally in a dose of 4 mg every 12-18 hours along with 5 mg/day gentamicin intravenously or intramuscularly. Successful treatment of bacterial meningitis or ventriculitis by these methods has been reported.[3-22] In these clinical reports, the reported adverse effects were mainly confined to neurotoxicities, such as grand mal seizures,[4] weakness of the lower extremities,[9] radiculopathy, cessation of respiration[4] and histological lesion in the midbrain.[22] Persistent meningeal inflammation following intrathecal gentamicin had been reported, but the causative agent could have been the preservatives in the solution rather than the gentamicin itself.[23] Molitor et al[24] revealed a direct relationship between the CSF concentration of gentamicin, brain tissue concentration of gentamicin and occurrence of brain lesions in the rabbit. Favorable clinical responses, but with some toxicity, were reported by Rahal et al[17] following intraventricular gentamicin at doses of 8 and 12 mg daily. One of Rahal's patients suffered a severe hearing loss after receiving a single intrathecal injection of 12 mg gentamicin, but this patient had a mild hearing loss before his illness. Another patient showed no ototoxicity following six intrathecal administrations of 12 mg gentamicin. Other authors employing much larger doses of gentamicin (0.5-2 mg/kg) by the intrathecal route reported no ototoxicity.[19,25]

Surprisingly, the above case of ototoxicity from gentamicin administered intrathecally is the only one that has been reported,[2] in spite of the fact that ototoxicity by systemic administration of gentamicin has been reported repeatedly in both humans and experimental animals.[26] One possible explanation for this apparent paradox is that most of the intrathecally administered gentamicin is given by lumbar puncture. It is widely accepted that substances given by lumbar puncture achieve relatively poor distribution to the cranial CSF.

Cerebrospinal fluid and cochlear perilymph are known to be continuous by way of the cochlear aqueduct.[27] In the guinea pig it is calculated that 25% of the perilymph comes from the CSF. The rest of the perilymph comes from the blood.[28] Furthermore, intracisternally injected substances have been reported to reach the perilymphatic space.[28-37] Therefore, it is most likely that when applied directly into the cisternal CSF, a water-soluble and

From the Departments of Pharmacology and Otolaryngology, Tulane University School of Medicine, New Orleans, and the Department of Otolaryngology, Kyoto Prefectural University of Medicine, Kyoto, Japan. This research was supported by the Schering Company.

REPRINTS — Katherine L. Parrish, PhD, Dept. of Pharmacology, LSU School of Medicine, 1542 Tulane Ave., New Orleans, LA 70112.

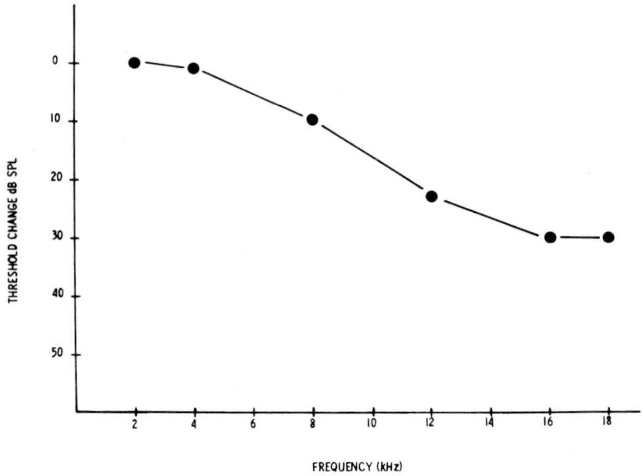

Fig. 1. Changes in VDT of hearing in the right ear of a cat which had received 2 mg gentamicin daily for seven days. The ECochG determination of VDT before drug and two weeks after drug treatment revealed increases in hearing threshold primarily at the higher frequencies tested.

small molecular weight substance (mol wt 543) may reach the perilymph of the inner ear without difficulty and cause ototoxicity. Of all the intrathecal injection sites the intracisternal route provides a maximal concentration of gentamicin in the region of the cochlear aqueduct. Thus it is of clinical importance to determine the effect of direct administration of gentamicin into the CSF upon the inner ear. The purposes of the present study are to determine 1) whether ototoxicity can be caused by the intracisternal injection of gentamicin, and 2) the threshold ototoxic dose of gentamicin by intracisternal application.

METHODS

Cats of both sexes weighing between 1.9 and 3.4 kg were given gentamicin intracisternally for seven successive days. The procedure for the intracisternal injection of gentamicin was as follows. The animal was anesthetized with ketamine hydrochloride (20 mg/kg, ip). The hair was clipped and the skin over the foramen magnum painted with Betadine®. The neck was flexed anteriorly and the cisterna magna was entered with a 20-gauge needle through the atlanto-occipital space. Location of the tip of the needle was assured by aspiration of a volume of CSF equal to the volume of solution to be injected. The test solution was composed of 1 ml of sterilized saline containing 10 or 0 (as control) mg of gentamicin sulfate (Garamycin®).

Before and on the 7th and 21st days after the start of intracisternal injections, electrocochleograms (ECochG) of both ears were obtained by a slight modification of the method of Norris et al.[38] If the animal developed a grossly observable middle ear infection either before or during the experiment, that ear was excluded from the data. For ECochG, the cats were anesthetized with ketamine (20 mg/kg ip) and placed in a sound-dampened chamber. A recording electrode (0.1 mm-diameter tungsten wire coated with vinyl enamel) was mounted on a micromanipulator and directed through the tympanic membrane (TM) to rest on the otic capsule. Tone bursts at 2, 4, 8, 12, 14, 16 and 18 kHz were presented to the cat by a Yamaha electrostatic speaker in free-field configuration. The sound pressure level near the TM was determined using a Bruel and Kjaer sound-level meter.

The electrical potentials picked up by the electrode were amplified and stored in a data retrieval computer. The intensity of each tone burst was adjusted until a compound action potential response was just visually detectable on the computer's screen after 500 stimuli had been presented and the resulting potentials summed. This intensity was then considered as the visual detection threshold (VDT) for that frequency. Ototoxicity was defined as present when the VDT was raised by more than 20 dB at two or more of the test frequencies. This criterion has been verified a number of times by histological examination. This VDT change corresponds to a decrease in the number of outer hair cells (OHC) in the organ of Corti. Before or during the experiment if the animal developed significant otitis media or massive perforation of the TM, the results were excluded from the data. Some animals were sacrificed and their cochleas examined by the surface preparation technique[39] and in one case the vestibular end-organs, eg, cristae of semicircular canals and utricle, were similarly examined. Also, in some animals the gentamicin concentration in the CSF samples obtained just prior to injection of gentamicin was measured by microbiological assay.*

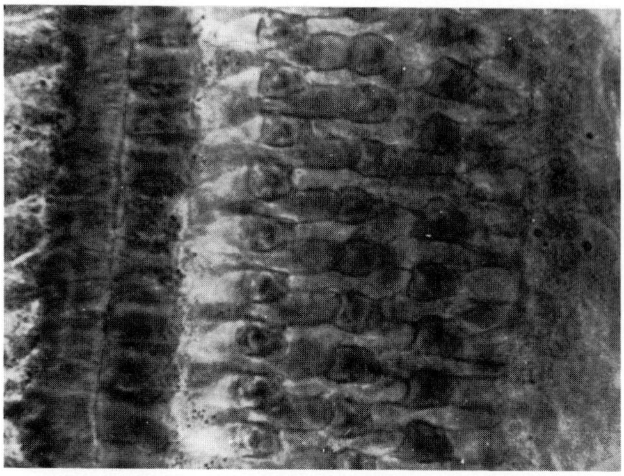

Fig. 2. Basal turn, organ of Corti, cat A (control). All three rows of OHC are intact. This photograph demonstrates the osmium tetroxide stain which allows visualization of intact hair cells. Preparation done after last ECochG.

RESULTS

In the control (saline) group, all of the animals survived throughout the experiment and showed no neurotoxicity or ototoxicity. In the experimental (gentamicin) group some animals died before the last ECochG procedure was performed. These animals usually showed signs of ataxia, prostration or

*Assays performed at Schering Company.

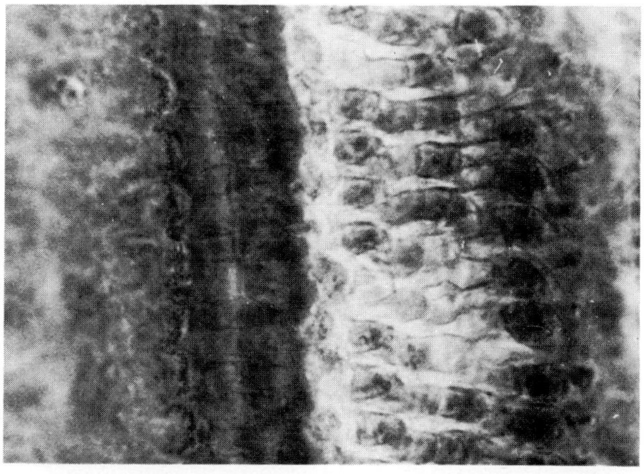

Fig. 3. Basal turn, organ of Corti, cat B, 2 mg gentamicin per day. The loss of OHC is clearly evident. Preparation done after last ECochG.

TABLE 1. SURVIVAL AND DAMAGE ACCORDING TO DOSE OF GENTAMICIN SULFATE

Dose/Day	*No. of Animals*	*No. Surviving 3 Weeks*	*Ataxia*	*Electrocochleography* *No. Ears*	*Ototoxicity**
Saline	11	11	0	17	0 (0%)
10 mg	3	0	2	—	—
6 mg	3	1	1	2	0 (0%)
4 mg	3	1	2†	2	2 (100%)
2 mg	12	8	3	14	7 (50%)
0.5 mg	2	1	1	2	2 (0%)

*Calculated from number of ears showing a greater than 20 dB increase in threshold for at least two frequencies at the three-week period.

†Surface preparations and histological examination of one of these animals revealed extensive damage in the vestibular organs.

weakness of the limbs several days before death. Deaths immediately after injection were not observed by us, although at the high doses an occasional, reversible respiratory arrest was seen.

The groups of animals receiving the larger doses of gentamicin exhibited high mortality. None of the 10 mg group survived the seventh injection. Two of the three animals died in the week between the last injection and the final ECochG in both the 6 mg and 4 mg groups. Neither surviving animal showed neurotoxicity, yet there was a bilateral hearing loss at all frequencies (40 dB SPL average loss) in the animal from the 4 mg group demonstrating ototoxicity. In the 0.5 mg group the one surviving animal was ataxic, but there was not a significant change in the ECochG indicating no ototoxicity.

Much of our effort was concentrated on the 2 mg group since we thought that this might be the threshold dose or the maximal subototoxic dose. In this group 8 of 12 animals survived. Three of the four nonsurvivors died of apparently nondrug-related causes. These included two asphyctic deaths at the time of ECochG and one death possibly related to a double intracisternal injection. Three animals within the surviving group showed ataxia but no ototoxicity by our most discriminating criterion, namely worsening of VDT by at least 20 dB at two or more frequencies.

Yet there was a 50% incidence of ototoxicity in this experimental group (Table 1). Figure 1 represents the change in thresholds across frequencies after seven daily intracisternal injections of 2 mg gentamicin. Note that the greatest loss in hearing acuity is at the higher frequencies. Concomitant alterations in the organ of Corti include extensive loss of OHC in the basal turn (Figs. 2 and 3).

Histological examination of one of the nonsurvivors from the 4 mg group revealed extensive damage in the vestibular region. The loss of sensory hairs from the crista of the superior semicircular canal can be seen by comparing Figures 4 and 5. The effect of gentamicin on the utricle is demonstrated in Figure 6. Notice the loss of hair cells as evidenced by the scarring when compared to a control animal's utricle shown in Figure 7.

A comparison of mean changes in threshold (Fig. 8) does not detect any statistically meaningful differences, except at the 4 mg dosage level. Hearing loss was usually bilateral (with one exception), but the degree of loss and the frequencies affected were not necessarily symmetrical.

Twenty-four hours after intracisternal administration of gentamicin, CSF samples were obtained for analysis. There was progressive difficulty in withdrawing CSF from experimental animals, particularly those receiving either 6 mg or 10 mg daily. The concentration of gentamicin in the CSF is shown in Figures 9 and 10, with the latter figure demonstrating a linear dose relationship. However, no direct relationship between the concentration of gentamicin in CSF and neurotoxicity or ototoxicity was observed. In many of the gentamicin-treated animals, we observed signs of infection such as run-

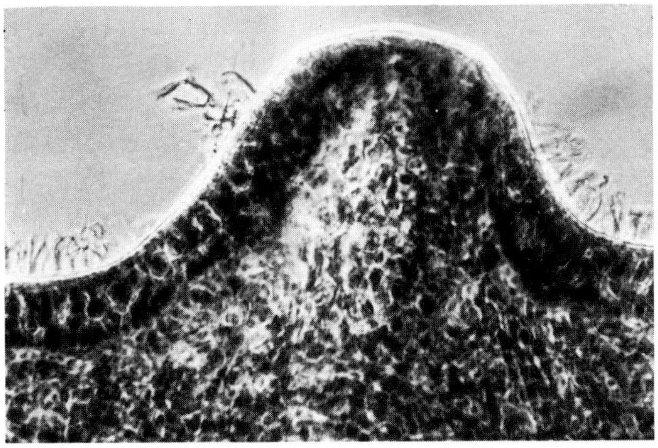

Fig. 4. Right superior crista of horizontal semicircular canal, cat A (control). The sensory hairs and intact nerve supply are evident. Preparation done after last ECochG.

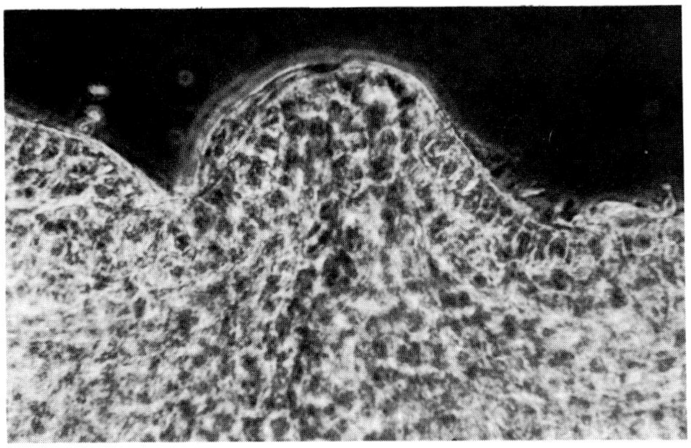

Fig. 5. Right superior crista of horizontal semicircular canal, cat C, 4 mg gentamicin per day. Note the absence of sensory hairs and the additional scarring caused by the gentamicin. Preparation done postmortem.

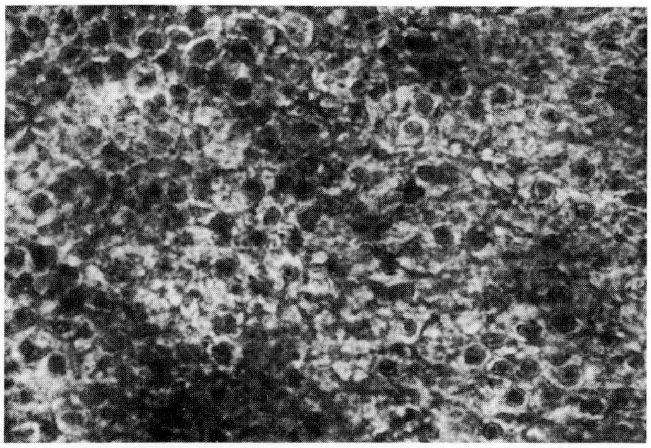

Fig. 6. Right utricle of cat C, 4 mg gentamicin per day. The loss of hair cells is evidenced by the large degree of scarring. Preparation done postmortem.

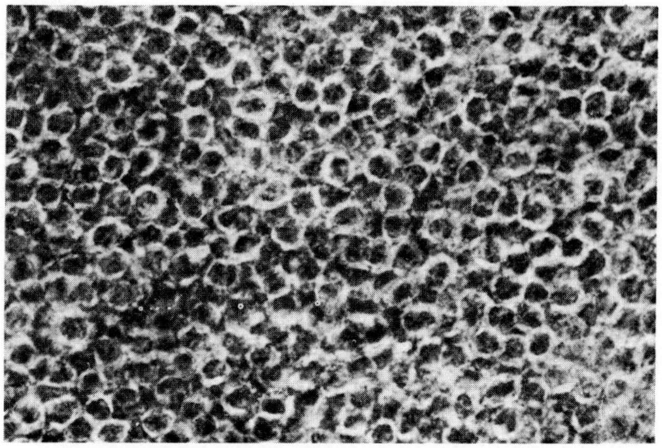

Fig. 7. Right utricle of cat A (control). The clear representation of intact hair cells is shown. Preparation done after last EcochG.

ny eyes and labored breathing during the period of the injections. These signs disappeared soon after the last injection. We observed no such signs in the control animals.

DISCUSSION

The toxic effects of intracisternal gentamicin observed in this study included cessation of respiration, ataxia and prostration. In addition, particularly at the high doses, there was great difficulty in obtaining CSF. This problem may have been due to induration of the atlanto-occipital membrane or to irritative arachnoiditis. After initial penetration, the "searching" movements with the needle which were necessitated by the difficulty in obtaining CSF could have compounded gentamicin's native neurotoxicity. For instance, hematomas were found at the autopsy of several animals. Such hematomas could explain the respiratory difficulties seen at the highest doses of gentamicin. Thus, the ataxia and prostration could have been caused by damage to the vestibular end-organs or possible cerebellar damage. We lean toward the vestibular end-organs as the more likely site of toxicity in view of the histological findings from the 4 mg per day group. The intracisternal route of administration proved innocuous of itself, since all of the control animals survived the week of injections with no obvious damage.

The change in thresholds across frequencies after seven daily injections of 2 mg gentamicin demonstrates that the greatest loss in hearing acuity is at the higher frequencies. The destruction of OHC from the basal turn of the organ of Corti corresponds to the marked attenuation of high frequency hearing.

The gentamicin concentrations in CSF must be examined with the sampling period in mind, since the samples were taken 24 hours after the injection of gentamicin during the entire seven-day regimen. Thus, the levels might be expected to be quite low. The half-life of gentamicin in CSF in man is 5.5 hours.[17] This accounts for the lack of accumulation of gentamicin in CSF. However, if the CSF levels over the seven days were averaged, there was an evident dose-concentration (CSF level) relationship. The residual gentamicin in the CSF after four half-lives (24 hours) would have to vary as a function of the initial dose. The gentamicin levels reported here are within the limits of those reported by Allison and Stach,[40] ie, 0.25 μg/ml at 24 hours.

The design of this research and analysis of these data tend to overestimate rather than underestimate the occurrence of ototoxicity. It seems likely that the intracisternal route of administration of a dose of gentamicin is more likely to produce ototoxicity than a similar dose given by lumbar puncture. Firstly, there is reduced access of drugs administered by lumbar puncture to the cranial

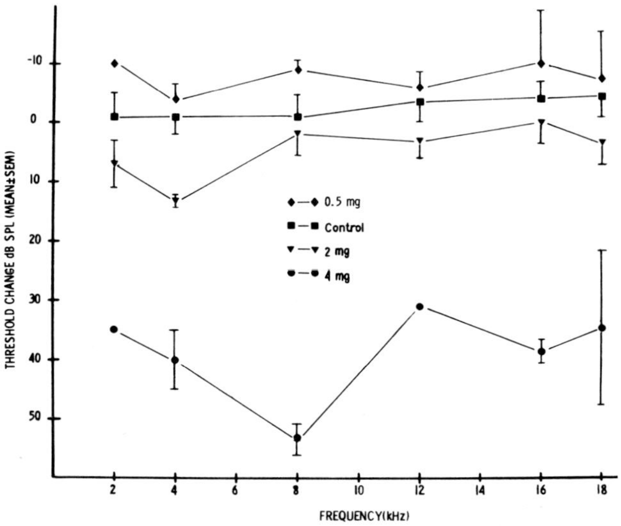

Fig. 8. Mean changes in ECochG thresholds. The differences in visual detection thresholds across frequencies, between the predrug ECochG determination and the two-week postdrug determination are expressed in dB SPL. The doses listed are the absolute amounts injected intracisternally daily for seven days. The vertical bars are the standard errors of the mean.

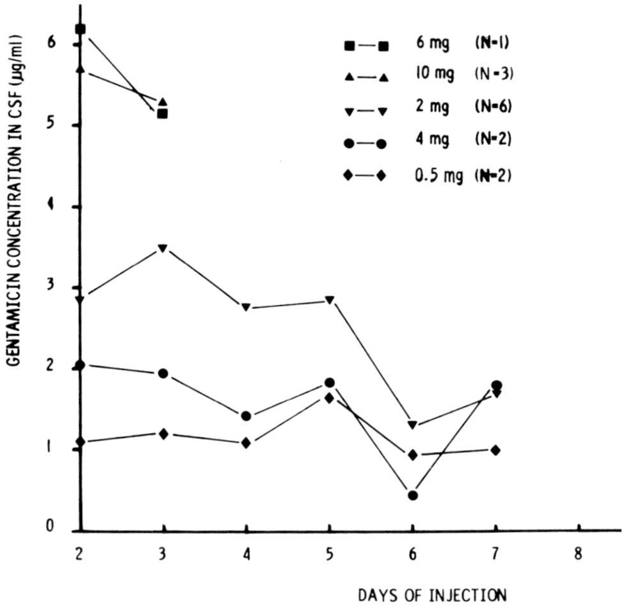

Fig. 9. Levels of gentamicin in CSF samples taken from cats 24 hours after the intracisternal injection of the drug. The points represent the means of all the determinations made.

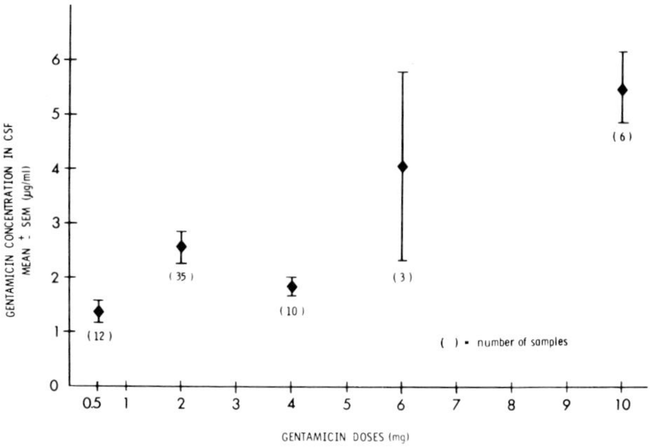

Fig. 10. Mean levels of gentamicin in CSF samples taken from cats 24 hours after the intracisternal injection of the drug. The points are means for all samples assayed from animals receiving similar doses. For instance, all the CSF concentrations of gentamicin from animals receiving 2 mg gentamicin were averaged without regard to the day of treatment. The vertical bars represent the standard errors of the mean and the numbers in parentheses are the numbers of samples assayed.

CSF spaces. Secondly, access to the cochlea from the CSF is via the cochlear aqueduct near the internal auditory meatus. This is relatively accessible from the cisterna magna. The choice of cats rather than a larger species as the experimental animals also increased the likelihood that ototoxicity would appear. Additionally, gentamicin was administered as a fixed dose, ie, not on a weight basis, and into a relatively restricted volume. Although the doses per organism employed in this study were in the range of doses employed clinically, the CSF volume of the human must be several fold larger than those in the cat. Therefore, the initial CSF concentrations achieved in the cat had to have been several fold higher than those in humans.

The results of this study indicate that ototoxicity results from the administration of 2 mg gentamicin intracisternally. However, our impression is that 2 mg may be very close to the threshold dose. Observe in Figure 1 that there is no difference between the means of threshold determinations of control and 2 mg gentamicin animals. Clinical reports using intraventricular route of administration show no ototoxicity even when administered to infants less than one month of age.[16,41] McCracken[10] reported no ototoxicities in his experience with intrathecal gentamicin, but he also stated that this route of administration did not provide a greater success in the treatment of neonatal meningitis. Using the intraventricular route of administration Lee[42] reported a greater success. Mangi et al[43] reported on the treatment of Gram-negative bacillary meningitis with either intrathecal or intraventricular injections of 2-3 mg per day of gentamicin. No vestibular or cochlear ototoxicity was observed even though the concentrations of gentamicin in the CSF 24 hours after injection had mean values of 5.9 µg/ml for intrathecal and 11.1 µg/ml for intraventricular routes. One should note that the concentration of gentamicin in this smaller CSF volume than that of man and the intracisternal route rather than lumbar puncture in this study would increase the likelihood of ototoxicity. Therefore, the extrapolation of these results to man, fraught with danger as always, may be made with less-than-usual hesitation, for if there is an error it has been on the conservative side.

ACKNOWLEDGMENTS — We wish to thank Mrs. Audria Alexander for her superb histological techniques.

REFERENCES

1. Spector R. The transport of gentamicin in the choroid plexus and cerebrospinal fluid. J Pharmacol Exp Ther 1975; 194:82-8.

2. Rahal JJ Jr. Treatment of gram-negative bacillary meningitis in adults. Ann Intern Med 1972; 77:295-302.

3. Fasano VA. Gentamicin in the treatment of infections complicating neurosurgery and neurotraumatology. In: Gentamicin, First International Symposium, January, 1967. Lucerne: Essex Chemie Act, 1967:162-8.

4. Graybill JR, Mann J, Charache P. Intrathecal gentamicin in treatment of bacterial meningitis. Johns Hopkins Med J 1973; 133:51-6.

5. Klein JO, Eickoff TC, Finland M. Gentamicin activity in vitro and observations in 26 patients. Am J Med Sci 1964; 248:528-42.

6. Lorber J, Kalhan SC, Mahgrefte B. Treatment of ventriculitis with gentamicin and cloxacillin in infants born with spina bifida. Arch Dis Child 1970; 45:178-85.

7. Marsden HB, Hyde WA. Gentamicin in childhood infections. Curr Ther Res 1970; 12:353-533.

8. Mathies AW. Gentamicin in the treatment of meningitis. J Infect Dis 1971; 124 Suppl 249.

9. McCracken GH. A controlled study of intrathecal antibiot-

ics therapy in gram-negative enteric meningitis of infancy: report of the neonatal meningitis cooperative study group. J Pediatr 1976; 89:66-72.

10. McCracken GH. Intraventricular treatment of neonatal meningitis due to gram-negative bacilli. J Pediatr 1977; 91:1037-8.

11. McCracken GH, Jones LCT. Gentamicin in the neonatal period. Am J Dis Child 1970; 120:524-33.

12. McHanry MC, Dohn DF, Tingwald FR. Meningitis due to Escherichia coli: report of a case in a young adult treated with gentamicin. JAMA 1970; 212:156-8.

13. Moellering RC Jr, Fischer EG. Relationship of intraventricular gentamicin levels to cure of meningitis: report of a case of proteus meningitis successfully treated with intraventricular gentamicin. J Pediatr 1972; 81:534-7.

14. Newman RL, Holt RJ. Intrathecal gentamicin in treatment of ventriculitis in children. Br Med J 1967; 2:539-42.

15. Newman RL, Holt FJ. Gentamicin in pediatrics: I. Report on intrathecal gentamicin. J Infect Dis 1971; 124 Suppl 254.

16. Pickering LK, Ericsson CD, Ruiz-Palacios G, Blevins J, Miner ME. Intraventricular and parenteral gentamicin therapy for ventriculitis in children. Am J Dis Child 1978; 132:480-3.

17. Rahal JJ Jr, Hyams PJ, Simberkoff MS, Rubenstein E. Combined intrathecal and intramuscular gentamicin for gram-negative meningitis: pharmacologic study of 21 patients. N Engl J Med 1974; 290:1394-8.

18. Saad AF, Farrar WE Jr. Intracisternal and intrathecal injections of gentamicin in enterobacter meningitis. Arch Intern Med 1974; 134:737-40.

19. Smilack J, McCloskey RV. Intrathecal gentamicin. Ann Intern Med 1972; 77:1002-3.

20. Van der Waarde K, Van der Wiel-Korstanje M. Treatment of ventriculitis with gentamicin in an infant born with spina bifida. Scand J Infect Dis 1972; 4:165-6.

21. Watanabe I, Hodges GR, Dworzack DL, Kepes JJ, Dvensing GF. Neurotoxicity of intrathecal gentamicin: a case report and experimental study. Ann Neurol 1978; 4:564-72.

22. Zoumboulakis D, Anagnostakis D, Arseni A, Nicolopoulos D, Matsaniotis N. Gentamicin in the treatment of purulent meningitis in neonates and infants. Acta Paediatr Scand 1973; 62:55-8.

23. Buckley RM, Watters W, MacGregor RR. Persistent meningeal inflammation associated with intrathecal gentamicin. Am J Med Sci 1977; 274:207-9.

24. Molitor H, Kuna S. The significance of neurotropic properties of commercial streptomycin. Arch Int Pharmacodyn Ther 1947; 74:334-42.

25. Mariel C, Veyssier P, Pechere SC. La gentamicine dans les meningites purulentes. Lyon Med 1972; 228:637-41.

26. Jackson GG, Arcier G. Ototoxicity of gentamicin in man: a survey and controlled analysis of clinical experience in the United States. J Infect Dis 1971; 124 Suppl 5:5130-7.

27. Lempert J, Meltzer PE, Wever EG, Lawrence M, Rombo JHT. Structure and function of the cochlear aqueduct. Arch Otolaryngol 1952; 55:134-45.

28. Kellerhals B. Perilymph production and arterial blood supply: inner ear fluids. Ann Otol Rhinol Laryngol 1977; 248:528-42.

29. Altman R, Walter JG. New investigation on the physiology of the labyrinthine fluids. Laryngoscope 1950; 60:727-39.

30. Altman F, Walter JG. The circulation of labyrinthine fluids. Ann Otol Rhinol Laryngol 1974; 56:684-708.

31. Arnold W, von Ilberg C. Verbindungswege zwischen liquor-und perilymphraum. Arch Klin Exp Ohren Nasen Kehlkopfheilkd 1971; 198:247-61.

32. Arnvig J. Relation of the ear to the subarachnoid space and absorption of the labyrinthine fluid. Acta Otolaryngol (Stockh) 1951 Suppl 96.

33. Duvall AJ III, Sutherland CR. Cochlear transport of horseradish peroxidase. Ann Otol Rhinol Laryngol 1972; 81:705-13.

34. Hughes DE, Chou JTY. The origin of the perilymph of the inner ear. Life Sci 1963; 2:107-11.

35. Jung SK. Experimental alteration of physiological state of inner ear fluids. Ann Otol Rhinol Laryngol 1977; 86:689-97.

36. Sando I, Wood RP II, Masuda Y, Hemenway WG. Perilymph communication routes in guinea pig cochlea. Ann Otol Rhinol Laryngol 1971; 80:826-34.

37. Schuknecht HG, Seifi IA. Experimental observations on the fluid physiology of the inner ear. Ann Otol Rhinol Laryngol 1963; 72:687.

38. Norris CH, Garcia-Quiroga J, Guth PS. A new and nondestructive technique for testing the cochlear toxicity of drugs. Toxicol Appl Pharmacol 1978; 43:317-26.

39. Engstrom H, Ades HW, Anderson A. Structural pattern of the organ of Corti. Stockholm; Almquist and Weksell, 1966.

40. Allison RR, Stach PE. Intrathecal drug therapy. Drug Intell Clin Pharm 1978; 12:347-59.

41. Kourtopoulos H, Holm SE. Intraventricular treatment of Seratia marcescens meningitis with gentamicin. Scand J Infect Dis 1976; 8:57-80.

42. Lee EL, Robinson MJ, Thong ML, Puthucheary SD, Ong TH, Ng KK. Intraventricular chemotherapy in neonatal meningitis. J Pediatr 1977; 91:991-5.

43. Mangi RJ, Hostein LL, Andriole VT. Treatment of gram-negative bacillary meningitis with intrathecal gentamicin. Yale J Biol Med 1977; 50:31-41.

AEROBIC AND ANAEROBIC BACTERIA IN TONSILS OF CHILDREN WITH RECURRENT TONSILLITIS

ITZHAK BROOK, MD, MS

PAULA YOCUM, BS

ELLEN M. FRIEDMAN, MD

WASHINGTON, DC

Tonsils were obtained from 50 children suffering from recurrent tonsillitis. Patients' ages ranged from 2.5 to 17 years (mean 6 years); 29 were males and 21 females. The tonsils were sectioned in half after heat searing of the surface and the core material was cultured for aerobic and anaerobic microorganisms. Mixed aerobic and anaerobic flora was obtained in all patients, yielding an average of 7.8 isolates (4.1 anaerobes and 3.7 aerobes) per specimen. There were 207 anaerobes isolated. The predominant isolates were 101 *Bacteroides* sp (including 10 *B fragilis* group, and 47 *B melaninogenicus* group), 39 *Fusobacterium* sp, 34 Gram-positive anaerobic cocci (25 *Peptococcus* sp and 9 *Peptostreptococcus* sp) and 16 *Veillonella* sp. There were 185 aerobic isolates. The predominant isolates were 41 α-hemolytic streptococci, 24 *Staphylococcus aureus*, 19 β-hemolytic streptococci (11 group A, 4 group B, and 2 each group C and F), 14 *Haemophilus* sp (including 12 *H influenzae* type B) and 5 *H parainfluenzae*. Beta-lactamase production was noted in 56 isolates recovered from 37 tonsils. These were all isolates of *S aureus* (24) and *B fragilis* (10), 15 of 47 *B melaninogenicus* (32%), 5 of 12 *B oralis* (42%), and 2 of 12 *H influenzae* type B (17%). Our findings indicate the polymicrobial aerobic and anaerobic nature of deep tonsillar flora in children with recurrent tonsillitis, and demonstrate the presence of many β-lactamase-producing organisms in 74% of the patients.

INTRODUCTION

A growing number of children with tonsillitis become refractory to therapy with penicillin. This has been attributed to the emergence of penicillin-resistant strains among the organisms belonging to the mouth flora.[1,2] Previous work related to the microbiology of recurrent tonsillitis was aimed primarily at the detection of aerobic pathogenic microorganisms such as group A β-hemolytic streptococci or *Staphylococcus aureus*.[3] The role of anaerobic microorganisms in this infectious process were rarely studied. However, anaerobes were isolated from peritonsillar and retropharyngeal abscesses,[4] and *Actinomyces* was frequently recovered from tonsillar tissue.[5]

This study was done to determine the aerobic and anaerobic flora present in the tonsil core of children with recurrent tonsillitis. Since anaerobes are normal inhabitants of the oropharynx including the surface of the tonsils, cultures taken directly from this area are difficult to interpret. To avoid this problem we obtained cultures from the core of the excised tonsils.

MATERIALS AND METHODS

The tonsils studied were removed from pediatric patients admitted for elective tonsillectomy at Children's Hospital, National Medical Center, between August 1977 and October 1979. Patients suffered from recurrent tonsillitis, defined as at least five episodes of inflammation of the tonsils within one year, during which group A β-hemolytic streptococci were recovered repeatedly. The duration of the patients' symptoms ranged from eight months to three years (average 1.5 years). They received multiple courses of antibiotics, but none received any antimicrobial therapy for at least one month prior to surgery.

Immediately after excision, the tonsils were placed in a sterile container filled with physiological saline and were promptly taken to the anaerobic microbiology laboratory. One of the tonsils was placed in a sterile Petri dish and held by forceps. One side of the tonsil was cauterized with a heated scalpel, and an incision was made through that area cutting the tonsil in half. The core of the tonsil was swabbed with a sterile cotton-tipped applicator and plated onto aerobic and anaerobic media. The time between removal of the tonsils and inoculation of the specimen was never in excess of 15 minutes.

Specimens were inoculated onto 5% sheep blood, chocolate and MacConkey's agar plates for aerobic and facultative organisms. The plates were incubated at 37 C aerobically (MacConkey's) or under 5% CO_2 (5% sheep blood and chocolate), and examined at 24 and 48 hours. For anaerobes, the material was plated onto prereduced vitamin K_1-enriched brucella blood agar, an anaerobic blood plate containing CNA and an enriched thioglycolate broth (containing hemin and vitamin K_1).[6] The anaerobic plates and thioglycolate broth were incubated in GasPak® jars (BBL, Cockeysville, Md.), and examined at 48 and 96 hours. Anaerobes were identified by techniques previously described.[6] Aerobic bacteria were identified using conventional methods.[7]

Beta-lactamase activity was determined on all organisms, utilizing the chromogenic cephalosporin analog 87/312 methodology.[8]

RESULTS

Tonsils from 50 children were studied (one tonsil from each child). Patients' ages ranged from 2 to 19 years (mean 6 years); 29 were males and 21 females.

Three hundred ninety bacteria were isolated from the tonsils, 185 aerobes and 207 anaerobes (Table 1). Mixed aerobic and anaerobic flora were present in all the tonsils yielding an average of 7.8 isolates (3.7 aerobes and 4.1 anaerobes) per specimen. No consistent pattern of combinations of the different aerobic and anaerobic bacteria was noted.

The aerobic organisms most frequently isolated

From the Department of Infectious Diseases and Otolaryngology, Clinical Microbiology Laboratories, Children's Hospital, National Medical Center, and George Washington University School of Medicine, Washington, DC.

REPRINTS — Itzhak Brook, MD, Naval Medical Research Institute, Bethesda, MD 20014.

TABLE 1. ORGANISMS ISOLATED IN 50 EXCISED TONSILS FROM PATIENTS WITH RECURRENT TONSILLITIS

Aerobic and Facultative	*No. of Isolates*		*Anaerobic*	*No. of Isolates*	
Gram-positive cocci			Gram-positive cocci		
S pneumoniae	2		*Peptococcus* sp	25	
Alpha-hem. streptococci	41		*Peptostreptococcus* sp	9	
Gamma-hem. streptococci	17				
Group A, β- hem. strept.	11		Gram-negative cocci		
Group B, β- hem. strept.	4		*V parvula*	16	
Group C, β- hem. strept.	2				
Group F, β- hem. strept.	2		Gram-positive bacilli		
S aureus	24	(24)*	*B adolescentis*	3	
S epidermidis	7		*Eubacterium* sp	9	
			Lactobacillus sp	1	
Gram-negative cocci			*P acnes*	2	
Neisseria sp	25		*Actinomyces* sp	2	
Gram-positive bacilli			Gram-negative bacilli		
Lactobacillus sp	9		*Fusobacterium* sp	11	
Diphtheroid sp	10		*F mortiferum*	1	
			F necrophorum	1	
Gram-negative bacilli			*F nucleatum*	26	
H influenzae type B	12	(2)*	*Bacteroides* sp	15	
Haemophilus sp	2		*B melaninogenicus*	7	(1)*
H parainfluenzae	5		*B melaninogenicus* ss *mel*	21	(7)*
E corrodens	4		*B melaninogenicus* ss		
P aeruginosa	1		*intermedius*	19	(7)*
E coli	1		*B oralis*	12	(5)*
			B rumin ssp *brevis*	5	
Yeast			*B biacutus*	1	
C albicans	6		*B fragilis* (*B fragilis* group)	5	(5)*
			B distasonis (*B fragilis* group)	3	(3)*
			B vulgatus (*B fragilis* group)	2	(2)*
			B corrodens	7	
			B uniformis	2	
			B ochraceus	2	
Total	185		Total	207	

*In parentheses: number of organisms producing β-lactamase.

were α-hemolytic streptococci, *S aureus*, β-hemolytic streptococci (groups A, B, C, and F), *Haemophilus* sp and γ-hemolytic streptococci. The predominant anaerobic organisms were *Bacteroides* sp (including *B melaninogenicus* and *B fragilis* group), *Fusobacterium* sp, anaerobic Gram-positive cocci, and *Veillonella parvula*.

Beta-lactamase production was detectable in 56 isolates recovered from 37 tonsils (74%). These included all isolates of *S aureus* and *B fragilis* group, 15 of the 47 *B melaninogenicus* group (32%), 5 of 12 *B oralis* (42%), and 2 of 12 *H influenzae* type B.

DISCUSSION

Anaerobes are part of the normal oropharyngeal flora and outnumber aerobes ten to one at this site.[9] Although infections of the tonsils caused by anaerobes is rare and is characterized by foul-smelling exudate,[4] potentially they can play a major role in oral infections, including tonsillitis. These organisms have also been recovered from many serious complications following tonsillitis which include peritonsillar, neck, lung and brain abscesses; thoracic empyema; purulent arthritis; and bacteremia.[4]

The anaerobic organisms recovered in our study are those commonly found in soft tissue infections adjacent to the oropharynx. Organisms belonging to group *B fragilis*, isolated from ten of our patients, are rarely recovered from the normal oropharyngeal flora.[10] However, these organisms have been isolated in few cases of aspiration pneumonia in adult[11] and pediatric[12] patients, and could conceivably colonize the oropharynx and tonsils after repeated courses of penicillin. These isolations may have clinical relevance, since *B fragilis* group and penicillin-resistant strains of *B melaninogenicus* are known to produce β-lactamase.[13]

Since we did not include in our study a control group of tonsils obtained from normal children, it is impossible to conclude that the organisms recovered are pathogens in patients with recurrent tonsillitis. Since all of these organisms are part of the oral flora[14] they might have been brought to the core via crypts penetrating from the surface, rather than representing true infection. Further studies which will include pathological documentation of the inflammatory process, quantitative cultures of the flora and analysis of a control group of normal tonsils would help on the interpretation of the clinical significance of our data.

Microbiological analysis of tonsillar flora has established β-hemolytic streptococci as the most common pathogen isolated in acute tonsillitis.[15] Penicillin has been the mainstay for tonsillar infections because of its high success in eradicating group A β-hemolytic streptococci.[16] Recently a growing number of patients develop recurrence of tonsillar infection or become carriers of group A β-hemolytic streptococci after treatment with penicillin.[1,16]

Since our patients did not receive antimicrobial therapy for at least one month prior to surgery, reinfection may explain the presence of group A β-hemolytic streptococci in 11 of them. This may also be due to inability of antimicrobial therapy to completely eradicate these organisms.

Various theories have been offered to explain the phenomena of persistent or recurrent tonsillar infection in the face of penicillin therapy. These include appearance of penicillin-resistant α-hemolytic streptococci[1,2,17] and an increased incidence of *H influenzae*[16] and *S aureus*[18] in throat culture. Other considerations include poor patient compliance with ten-day oral regimen and an inability to achieve bactericidal levels of penicillin inside the tonsillar core.[18]

Another hypothesis deserves consideration. The co-colonization of the tonsils with various β-lactamase-producing aerobic and anaerobic organisms may affect the therapeutic response to penicillin therapy. Beta-lactamase-producing organisms can limit the efficacy of penicillin therapy[19] by protecting the pathogenic streptococci by enzymatically "disarming" the penicillin, thereby allowing the infection to continue. In this study β-lactamase-producing organisms were found in 37 (74%) of our patients. These were all isolates of *S aureus* and *B fragilis*, 32% of *B melaninogenicus* group, 42% of *B oralis*, and 17% of *H influenzae* type B. The clinical significance of the isolation of these organisms may not only be due to their possible pathogenicity but also to their β-lactamase production.

Lincomycin,[20] clindamycin,[21] and oxacillin[19] have been found to be equally or more effective than penicillin in the treatment of recurrent tonsillitis, and the eradication of β-lactamase-producing organisms such as *S aureus*. It is therefore possible that their efficacy in the treatment of recurrent tonsillitis is secondary to their ability to eliminate the coexisting aerobic and anaerobic β-lactamase-producing organisms. However, most studies have not shown these drugs to be more effective than penicillin in treating acute tonsillitis or preventing rheumatic fever.

The isolation of pathogenic β-lactamase-producing organisms from three fourths of recurrently inflamed tonsils raises the question of whether the treatment of recurrent tonsillitis with penicillin is adequate in all instances and whether therapy should also be directed at the eradication of these organisms.

ACKNOWLEDGMENT — The authors gratefully acknowledge the cooperation of the staffing of the Department of Otolaryngology, the Operating Room, and Clinical Microbiology Laboratories at Children's Hospital, National Medical Center.

REFERENCES

1. Sprunt K, Redman W. Evidence suggesting importance of the role of interbacterial inhibition in maintaining balance of normal flora. Ann Intern Med 1968; 68:579-90.

2. Sprunt K, Redman W, Leidy G. Penicillin-resistant alpha streptococci in the pharynx of patients given oral penicillin. Pediatrics 1968; 42:957-68.

3. Farocki MA. Bacteriology and histology of tonsillar parenchyma in tonsillectomized specimens. Eye Ear Nose Throat Mon 1967; 46:301-12.

4. Finegold SM. Anaerobic bacteria in human disease. New York: Academic Press, 1977.

5. Gruner OPN. Actinomyces in tonsillar tissue. A historical study of tonsillectomy material. Acta Pathol Microbiol Scand 1969; 76:239-44.

6. Holdeman LV, Moore WEC. Anaerobe laboratory manual. 4th ed. Blacksburg: Virginia Polytechnic Institute, 1978.

7. Lennette EH, Spaulding EH, Truant JP. Manual of clinical microbiology. 2nd ed. Washington DC: American Society for Microbiology, 1974.

8. O'Callagham CH, Morris A, Kirby SM, Shingler AH. Novel method for detection of β-lactamase by using a chromatogenic cephalosporin substrate. Antimicrob Agents Chemother 1972; 1:283-8.

9. Rosebury T. Microorganisms indigenous to man. New York: McGraw-Hill Book Company, 1966.

10. Socransky SS, Manganiello SD. The oral microbiota of man from birth to senility. J Pediodontol 1971; 42:485-96.

11. Bartlett JG, Gorbach SL, Finegold SM. The bacteriology of aspiration pneumonia. Am J Med 1974; 56:202-7.

12. Brook I. Clindamycin in treatment of aspiration pneumonia in children. Antimicrob Agents Chemother 1979; 15:342-5.

13. Murray PR, Rosenblatt JE. Penicillin resistance and penicillinase production in clinical isolates of *Bacteroides melaninogenicus*. Antimicrob Agents Chemother 1977; 11:605-8.

14. Hallander HO, Flodstrom A, Holmberg K. Influence of the collection and transportation of specimens on the recovery of bacteria from pentosillar abscess. J Clin Microbiol 1975; 2:504-9.

15. Peter G, Smith AL. Group A streptococcal infections of the skin and pharynx. N Engl J Med 1977; 297:365-70.

16. Ross PW. Bacteriological monitoring in penicillin treatment of streptococcal sore throat. J Hyg (Camb) 1971; 69:355-60.

17. Sprinkle PM, Kirk BE, Mathias PB. Mycoplasma species found in naturally occurring adenotonsillitis. Ann Otol Rhinol Laryngol 1967; 76:503-8.

18. Kudsin RB, Miller JM. Significance of the *Staphylococcus aureus* carrier state in the treatment of disease due to group A streptococci. N Engl J Med 1964; 271:1395-7.

19. Simon HJ, Sukair W. Staphyloccal antagonism to penicillin group therapy of hemolytic streptococcal pharyngeal infection: effect of oxacillin. Pediatrics 1963; 31:463-9.

20. Breesee BB, Disney FA, Talpey WB, Green J. Beta hemolytic streptococcal infection: comparison of penicillin and lincomycin in the treatment of recurrent infections of the carrier state. Am J Dis Child 1969; 117:147-52.

21. Randolph MF, Redys JJ, Hibbard EW. Streptococcal pharyngitis: Part III — Streptococcal recurrence rates following therapy with penicillin or with clindamycin (7-chlorolincomycin). Del Med J 1970; 42:87-92.

Ann Otol 90:1981

EFFECT OF INCREASED PERILYMPHATIC PRESSURE ON ENDOCOCHLEAR POTENTIAL

TSUTOMU NAKASHIMA, MD   AKIKAZU ITO, MD

NAGOYA, JAPAN

A study was done to determine how increased fluid pressure in the inner ear influences cochlear blood flow. Hydrostatic pressure was applied to the scala vestibuli or scala tympani in guinea pigs. Endocochlear potential, which is sensitive to the lack of oxygen, was measured through the round window membrane or through the stria vascularis. Cochlear blood flow was confirmed by intravenous injection of India ink. When the perilymphatic pressure was raised to a relatively high level, endocochlear potential decreased, in a similar way as in response to anoxia, because of the cessation of the cochlear blood flow. This change was completely reversible upon applications of pressure for brief periods of time. We consider that the cochlear blood flow ceases when the fluid pressure reaches the level of intracochlear arterial pressure.

Menière's disease is closely related to the fluid pressure of the inner ear. Does increased fluid pressure interrupt the blood flow of the inner ear? Regarding the brain and eye, experimental and clinical data on the relationship between fluid pressure and blood flow are available. Increased CSF pressure reduces the cerebral blood flow and if CSF pressure reaches the level of systemic blood pressure, cerebral blood flow ceases.[1] Similarly, increased intraocular pressure interrupts retinal blood flow.[2,3]

Regarding the inner ear, McCabe and Wolsk,[4] Legouix,[5] and Butler and Honrubia[6] raised the intracochlear pressure and recorded the reduction of cochlear microphonics. These experiments were not designed to determine the effect of increased intracochlear pressure on cochlear blood flow. Therefore pressures which they applied were relatively low and compression of cochlear blood vessels was unlikely. Allen et al[7] raised the perilymphatic pressure to a relatively high level and recorded the reduction of cochlear microphonics in cats. They stated that it is possible that blood flow might be slowed to produce anoxia but it is dangerous to make this assumption without direct experimental confirmation. Our experiment was designed to determine whether increased intracochlear pressure interrupts cochlear blood flow. We raised the perilymphatic pressure and recorded endocochlear potential (EP), which is maintained by the blood flow of the stria vascularis. Pigments were injected intravenously to determine whether increased perilymphatic pressure interrupts the cochlear blood flow.

METHODS

The subjects for this investigation were guinea pigs weighing 250-500 g. They were anesthetized by intraperitoneal injection of 1.5 g/kg body weight of ethyl carbamate (urethane). Tracheostomy was performed, and the animals were paralyzed with succinylcholine chloride. Their pulmonary ventilation was maintained with an artificial respirator throughout the experiment. The right tympanic bulla of the animal was opened and the cochlea exposed. The bony wall of the scala tympani or scala vestibuli of the basal turn was drilled, and a 30 gauge needle or a glass capillary tube with a tip diameter 100-200 μ was inserted into the perilymph and fixed to the bone with dental cement to prevent leakage. The needle or the glass capillary tube was connected by a catheter and a three-way tap to a pressure transducer, with the third outlet of the tap communicating with a saline reservoir. The perilymphatic pressure could be altered by raising or lowering the reservoir along a scale calibrated in centimeters of water (cm H_2O), and the pressure was recorded continuously and controlled by the reservoir.

For recording the EP, a glass microelectrode filled with 500 mM KCl solution was used. The microelectrode was electrically connected to a DC amplifier (Nihonkoden MEZ-7101) by a wire coated with silver chloride. The indifferent electrode was placed on the neck muscles. The resistance of the microelectrodes ranged from 10 to 50 MΩ.

The relationship between the perilymphatic pressure and the EP was studied in 21 guinea pigs. In 17 cases the EP was measured through the round window membrane and in four cases through the stria vascularis at the third turn.

We injected gelatine-India ink intravenously in 20 guinea pigs, maintaining the perilymphatic pressure at a fixed level. We could observe whether or not the India ink appeared in blood vessels of the external wall of the cochlea in living animals. To know more precisely how the cochlear vascular system was perfused, 2-3 ml of air was injected intravenously and the animals were decapitated. Then both cochleas of the animals were removed and the mode of perfusion of the cochlear vascular system was examined and photographed.

RESULTS

After the pressure needle or the glass capillary tube was cemented, the average magnitude of EP, which was recorded through the round window membrane or through the stria vascularis at the third turn, was 73.9 mV or 56.5 mV respectively. As long as the perilymphatic pressure was increased smoothly, EP showed almost no change at low pressure levels. When the perilymphatic pressure

From the Department of Otorhinolaryngology, Nagoya University School of Medicine, Nagoya, Japan.

REPRINTS — Tsutomu Nakashima, MD, Department of Otorhinolaryngology, Nagoya University School of Medicine, 65, Tsurumai-cho, Showa-ku, Nagoya 466, Japan.

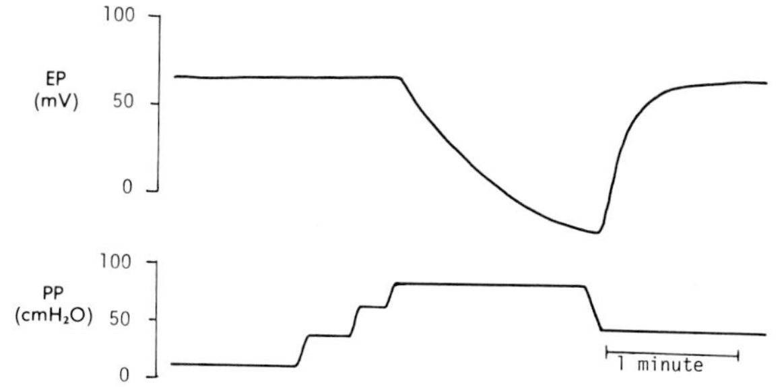

Fig. 1. Example of variations in EP and perilymphatic pressure (PP). In this case EP was recorded through the round window membrane and the pressure capillary tube was inserted into the scala tympani. The PP was raised and lowered in stages. After the third elevation of the PP, EP started to decrease within several seconds, continued to decline, and turned to negative. After the PP was lowered, EP recovered. Complete reversible changes were seen upon applications of pressure for a brief period of time.

was raised to a certain level, EP in all 21 cases decreased in a similar way as in response to anoxia (Fig. 1). This determinant level of pressure ranged from 40 to 85 cm H_2O except in one case where EP decreased at 25 cm H_2O (Table 1). Rupture of the round window membrane did not occur with this level of pressure. After having decreased in this way, the state of EP was not changed by cutting off the respirator. It was possible to maintain EP at an intermediate level with several cm H_2O smaller pressure below the lowest pressure which could decrease EP to negative.

When the perilymphatic pressure was raised and the EP showed a negative value, the injected India ink did not appear in the blood vessels of the external wall of the membranous cochlea (Fig. 2). Neither did the injected India ink appear in the blood vessels of the spiral lamina and limbus. But we did find traces of India ink in the blood vessels of the acoustic nerve after removal of the bony modiolus wall.

TABLE 1. EFFECT OF INCREASED PERILYMPHATIC PRESSURE ON ENDOCOCHLEAR POTENTIAL

Animal	*EP Before Pressure (mV)*	*Pressure to Decrease EP as in Anoxia (cm H_2O)*	*EP by Applied Pressure* (mV)*
1	80	55	−24
2	70	55	−37
3	76	75	−33
4	56	55	−18
5	50	55	−36
6	76	55	0
7	58	40	−9
8	85	50	−17
9	79	45	−20
10	80	65	−13
11	74	65	−18
12	78	40	−5
13	60	50	−21
14	60	50	−10
15	60	45	−38
16	78	60	−20
17	70	80	−3
18	60	45	0
19	76	25	−28
20	68	85	−20
21	88	65	−23

*EP by the applied pressure does not always mean the bottom of EP because the pressure was released when EP was still decreasing in some cases.

Endocochlear potential was measured in the basal turn; for animals 4, 5, 13 and 14, it was measured in the third turn.

Pressure was applied in the scala tympani; for animals 16-18 it was applied in the scala vestibuli.

DISCUSSION

Tasaki et al[8] performed experiments in which pressure was forced into the scala tympani and EP was measured simultaneously. They showed that an increase in relative pressure in the scala tympani causes a decreased electrical positivity in the scala media. Movement in the opposite direction causes the opposite change. As their experiments were designed to produce a displacement of the basilar membrane, outflow holes were made. In our exper-

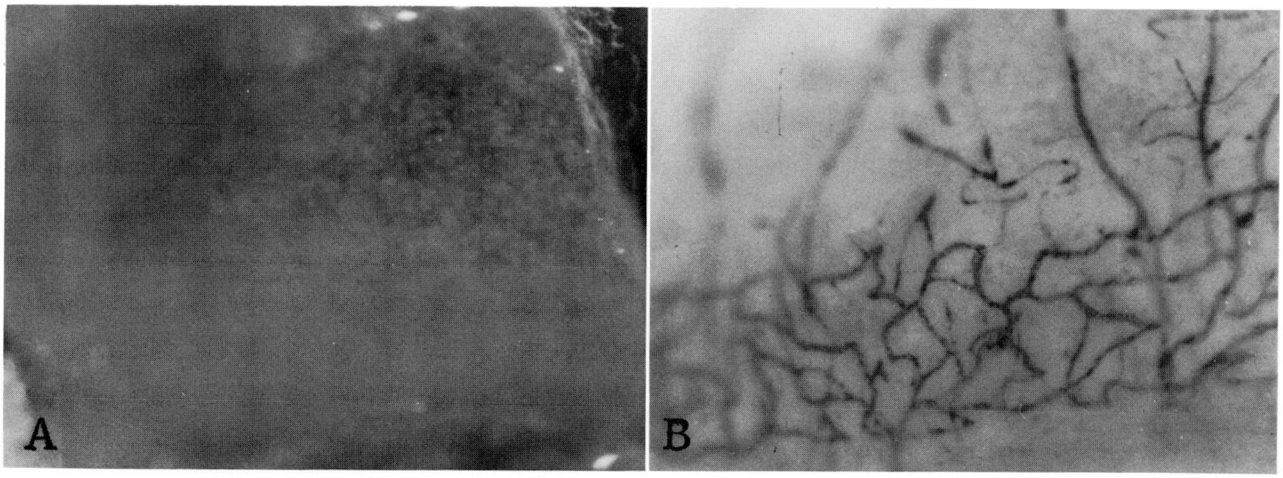

Fig. 2. External wall of the membraneous cochlea is seen from inside. The animal is the same as in Fig. 1. A) While the perilymphatic pressure was raised and EP showed negative value, the injected India ink did not appear in the blood vessels. B) Contralateral side of the cochlea, the perilymphatic pressure of which was not raised. Blood vessels were filled with the India ink.

iment no outflow holes existed and the pressure in the scala tympani and scala vestibuli was the same as long as the pressure increase was truly static. It was also assumed that the perilymphatic pressure was passed to the endolymph, probably via Reissner's membrane.[9] In these situations change in EP due to displacement of the basilar membrane was negligible so far as the perilymphatic pressure was raised or lowered smoothly. Konishi et al[10] demonstrated that EP decreased and became negative by occluding the anterior inferior cerebellar artery from which the cochlea receives its blood supply. It is considered that not only the blood flow of the membranous cochlea but also the blood flow of the acoustic nerve ceases when the anterior inferior cerebellar artery is occluded. In our experiment the blood flow of the acoustic nerve might have been preserved when the blood flow of the membranous cochlea ceased on account of the increased perilymphatic pressure. It is considered that the perilymphatic pressure is not transmitted directly to the blood vessels of the acoustic nerve because of the bony modiolus wall.

Various reports have indicated that changes in CSF pressure are reflected in the perilymphatic pressure and that pressure transmission takes place mainly via the cochlear aqueduct.[11,12] Conversely the increased perilymphatic pressure may exert influence on the CSF pressure. We observed that perilymph colored with methylene blue leaked through the cochlear aqueduct when the perilymphatic pressure was raised. But in our experiment the CSF pressure never increased enough to stop the cerebral blood flow, even if the blood flow of the membranous cochlea ceased on account of the increased perilymphatic pressure.

It has been shown that reduction of cochlear microphonics occurs when the inner ear pressure is increased by applying the pressure to the cochlea or by raising the CSF pressure.[4-7,12,13] To obtain these reductions of cochlear microphonics, compression of blood vessels is not always necessary. But it is important to consider the effect of increased inner ear pressure on cochlear blood flow when the inner ear pressure is raised to a relatively high level. We consider that the fluid pressure by which the cochlear blood vessels can be compressed is equivalent to the intracochlear arterial pressure. When the fluid pressure reaches the level of the intracochlear arterial pressure, EP decreases in the same way as in anoxia because of the cessation of blood flow. As the lowest pressure which could decrease EP to negative increased little by little during the application of pressure, it was considered that the intracochlear arterial pressure increased during the interruption of the blood flow. This elevation of arterial pressure by the increased fluid pressure is generally known in the brain and eye, and regarded as an accommodation of the living animal to the increased fluid pressure. Therefore it is difficult to measure the arterial pressure under normal conditions. But the applied pressure which could stop the cochlear blood flow was smaller than the blood pressure of the large arteries of the body because the arteries in the cochlea are small and have a pressure that is lower than that of the large arteries of the body. We measured carotid artery pressure simultaneously in two cases and confirmed this. It was thought that the one case in which EP decreased to negative with the pressure of 25 cm H_2O (18.4 mm Hg) was probably related to the decreased systemic blood pressure, though the carotid artery pressure was not measured simultaneously in this case.

REFERENCES

1. Langfitt TW, Kassel NF, Weinstein JD. Cerebral blood flow with intracranial hypertension. Neurology 1965; 15:761-73.

2. Hamasaki DI, Fujimoto T. Effect of intraocular pressure on the retinal blood flow: filling with India ink. Arch Ophthalmol 1967; 78:369-79.

3. Ffytche TJ. The effects of high intraocular pressure on the retinal circulation. In: Cant JS, ed. Vision and circulation. London: Henry Kimpton Publishers, 1974:193-200.

4. McCabe BF, Wolsk D. Experimental inner ear pressure changes: functional effects. Ann Otol Rhinol Laryngol 1961; 70:541-55.

5. Legouix JP. Changes in cochlear microphonics of guinea pigs produced by mechanical factors in inner ear. J Acoust Soc Am 1962; 34:1504-8.

6. Butler RA, Honrubia V. Responses of cochlear potentials to changes in hydrostatic pressure. J Acoust Soc Am 1963; 35:1188-92.

7. Allen GW, Dallos P, Sakamoto S, Homma T. Cochlear microphonics in cats: effects of perilymphatic pressure. Arch Otolaryngol 1971; 93:388-96.

8. Tasaki I, Davis H, Eldredge DH. Exploration of cochlear potentials in guinea pigs with a microelectrode. J Acoust Soc Am 1954; 26:765-73.

9. Beentjes BIJ. The cochlear aqueduct and the pressure of cerebrospinal and endolabyrinthine fluids. Acta Otolaryngol (Stockh) 1972; 73:112-20.

10. Konishi T, Butler RA, Fernandez C. Effects of anoxia on cochlear potentials. J Acoust Soc Am 1961; 33:349-56.

11. Kerth JD, Allen GW. Comparison of the perilymphatic and cerebrospinal fluid pressures. Arch Otolaryngol 1963; 77:581-5.

12. Allen GW, Habibi M. The effect of increasing the cerebrospinal fluid pressure upon the cochlear microphonics. Laryngoscope 1962; 72:423-34.

13. Feldman RM. Effects of increased cerebrospinal fluid pressure on CM response. J Speech Hear Res 1968; 11:18-32.

COMMON MIGRAINE AND VESTIBULAR FUNCTION

ELECTRONYSTAGMOGRAPHIC STUDY AND PATHOGENESIS

JOSEPH U. TOGLIA, MD

DAVID THOMAS, DO, PhD

ARIEH KURITZKY, MD

PHILADELPHIA, PENNSYLVANIA

Even though "classic migraine" and "complicated migraine" may be diagnosed readily, "common migraine" may be easily confused with other types of vascular headaches. This differential diagnosis is of great importance for the appropriate choice of drug therapy. It is frequently stated that family history of migraine and history of motion sickness in childhood suggest that a periodic vascular headache is most likely of migrainous origin; although this statement applies to ophthalmoplegic and hemiplegic migraine, it is doubtful that it applies to common migraine. In fact, in a pilot study of patients with common migraine, we have observed that family history and history of motion sickness in childhood did not contribute to the diagnosis. Vestibular dysfunctions are frequently associated with migraine including the common type. Utilizing labyrinthine tests with the aid of electronystagmography, abnormalities of labyrinth function were demonstrated in 80% of patients with common migraine who had no history of vertigo or of other otological and neurological disorders.

The primary motivation for this study was due to the awareness that although physicians may diagnose quite early classic and complicated migraine, there is no definite way to make an objective diagnosis of common migraine, a diagnosis indispensable for the proper choice of drug therapy.

The association of vertigo and migraine has been reported in the literature with several eponyms. "Migraine otique"[1-5] and "vestibular migraine"[6-11] imply vestibular dysfunction; "cerebellar migraine"[12-14] implies dysfunction of the cerebellum and "basilar migraine,"[15-17] irritation of the cervical sympathetic system and ischemia of the brainstem.

The association of vertigo and migraine (vertiginous migraine) may occur in several ways.[18] 1) Paroxysmal vertigo may occur in place of a migraine attack (migraine equivalent). 2) Attacks of vertigo typical of Menière's may replace, usually later in life, the attacks of migraine. 3) Attacks of Menière's and migraine may occur independently in the same subject.

The diagnosis of vertiginous migraine, whether classic or complicated, is relatively easy; it will rarely mask an underlying vascular malformation, since most patients with migraine have normal angiograms. In fact, Pearce and Foster[19] found only two vascular malformations among 40 cases of complicated migraine studied with angiography (6%); however the angiograms, except for 2 cases, did not include the vertebrobasilar system. When there is some question about the diagnosis of migraine, total angiography should be recommended, even if the patient has a normal computerized tomography of the brain, because with angiography there is less chance to miss an aneurysm.

The following case will illustrate this point. A 33-year-old nurse with a long history of migraine had recent onset of vertigo attacks which were attributed to the migraine. Since her mother, who had been diagnosed as having vertiginous migraine, died of subarachnoid hemorrhage from a ruptured basilar artery aneurysm, she specifically requested angiograms. These, indeed, revealed an aneurysm of the basilar artery (Fig. 1). The classification of migraine includes three types: classic, complicated and common.

Even though classic migraine and complicated

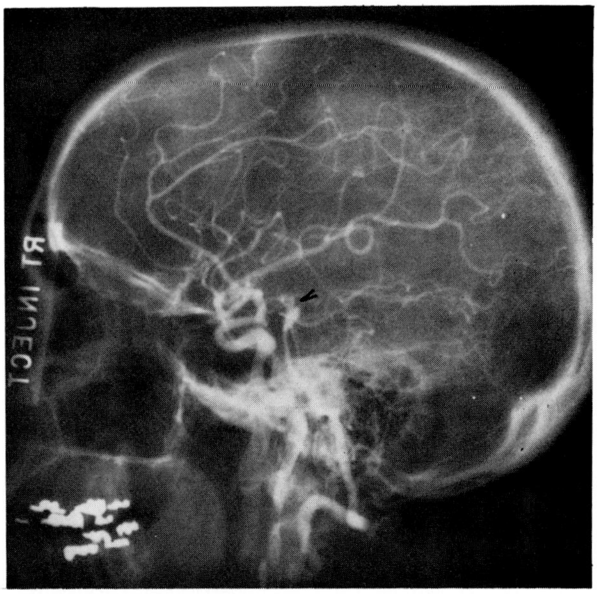

Fig. 1. Right vertebral arteriogram (lateral view). Large aneurysm at the bifurcation of the basilar artery.

From the Department of Neurology, Temple University Health Sciences Center, Philadelphia.

Presented at the meeting of the American Neurotology Society, Palm Beach, Florida, April 12, 1980.

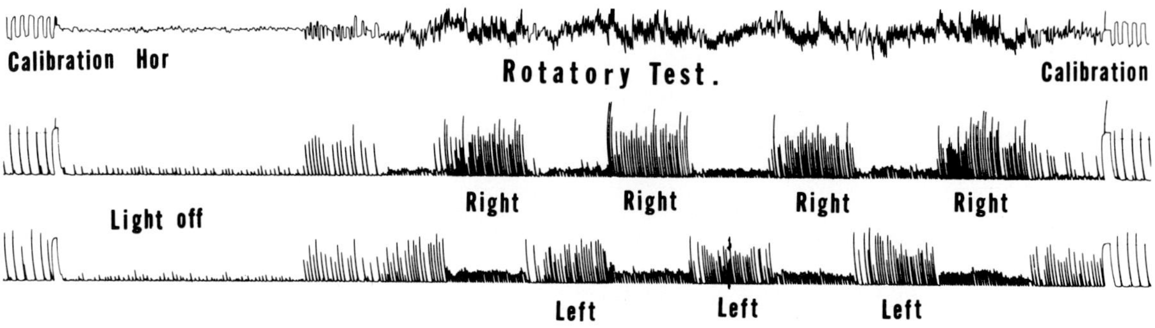

Fig. 2. Sequential alternating rotatory tests. Normal perrotatory nystagmus (see text).

migraine may be diagnosed without great difficulty, common migraine may be easily confused with other types of vascular headaches, since patients with common migraine do not have the visual prodroma of classic migraine or the neurological findings of complicated migraine. The headache is frequently unilateral, pulsating, associated with nausea, and lasts all day or several days. Patients with common migraine have no history of vertigo, but frequently have motion sickness in childhood. Pearce[20] reported that 60% of 450 migraine patients had motion sickness in childhood. He and others state that motion sickness of childhood is a forerunner of migraine, however it is not known how many children afflicted by motion sickness will not develop migraine. In our experience the history of motion sickness and family migraine does not help to diagnose common migraine. However, since vertigo and vestibular abnormalities occur in classic and complicated migraine we believe that patients with common migraine, even though having no attacks of vertigo, might have abnormal vestibular function and latent vestibular abnormalities. The following pilot study was designed to test this hypothesis.

METHODS

Twenty patients with a history of headache which had all features characteristic of common migraine were included in this study. They had no history of diseases which may cause vertigo or other vestibular symptoms. The ages ranged between 20 and 40 years with a mean of 33. Eighteen patients were female and two were male. The history of migraine varied between six months and 30 years, with an average of 16 years. Thirteen patients (65%) had histories of motion sickness. Family history of migraine was positive in 12 patients (60%). The neurological examination was normal. The patients were given vestibular tests with the aid of electronystagmography (ENG), audiological tests, tests of far field auditory evoked potentials and electroencephalography (EEG). The vestibular tests included bithermal caloric tests with a modified Hallpike technique and rotatory tests with sequential alternating rotations at a constant speed of 36°/s. The patients had not taken alcohol or drugs for one week prior to the vestibular examination. Our technique of ENG has been reported in the literature.[21] The following three figures (Figs. 2-4) are shown here to illustrate our technique. Figure 2 shows perrotatory nystagmus induced by an alternating rotation of the patient clockwise and counterclockwise at a constant speed of 36°/s, each rotation lasting ten seconds. The nystagmus is recorded by the upper line. The velocity of the fast and slow phases of the nystagmus are recorded separately by the second and third lines; the tall spikes are the fast phases and the short spikes are the slow phases.

Figure 3 shows an abnormal perrotatory response, lacking the nystagmus each time the patient is rotated leftward (counterclockwise).

Figure 4 shows two normal nystagmic responses to cold caloric stimulations of the right and left ear. The velocity of the fast and slow phases of the nystagmus are again recorded separately by the second and third lines of the graphs marked AD 30 C and AS 30 C. The vestibular tests were considered abnormal if the patient had abnormal responses to caloric tests performed with water at 30 and 40 C and/or abnormal rotatory tests. Calorics and rotatory tests were considered abnormal if there was one-third difference between the same parameters of right and left nystagmus.

The following report is limited to correlations between "common migraine" motion sickness, positive history of migraine and vestibular abnormalities.

RESULTS AND CONCLUSIONS

Caloric tests were abnormal in 16 patients (80%); 7 had canal paresis and 9 directional preponderance. *Rotatory tests* were abnormal in 15 patients; 8 had right directional preponderance, 7 left

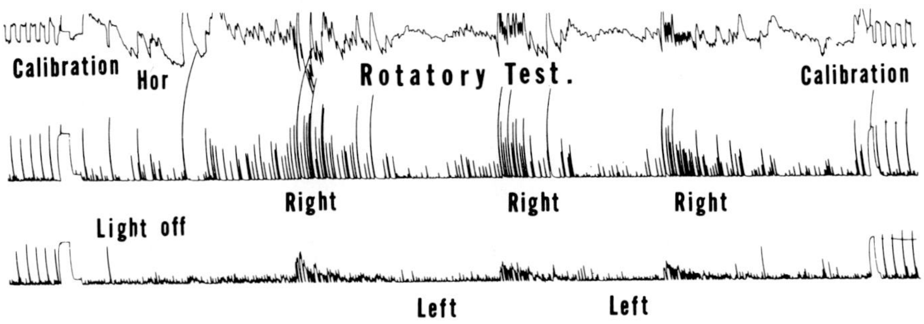

Fig. 3. Sequential alternating rotatory tests: abnormal response with directional preponderance of the right beating nystagmus (see text).

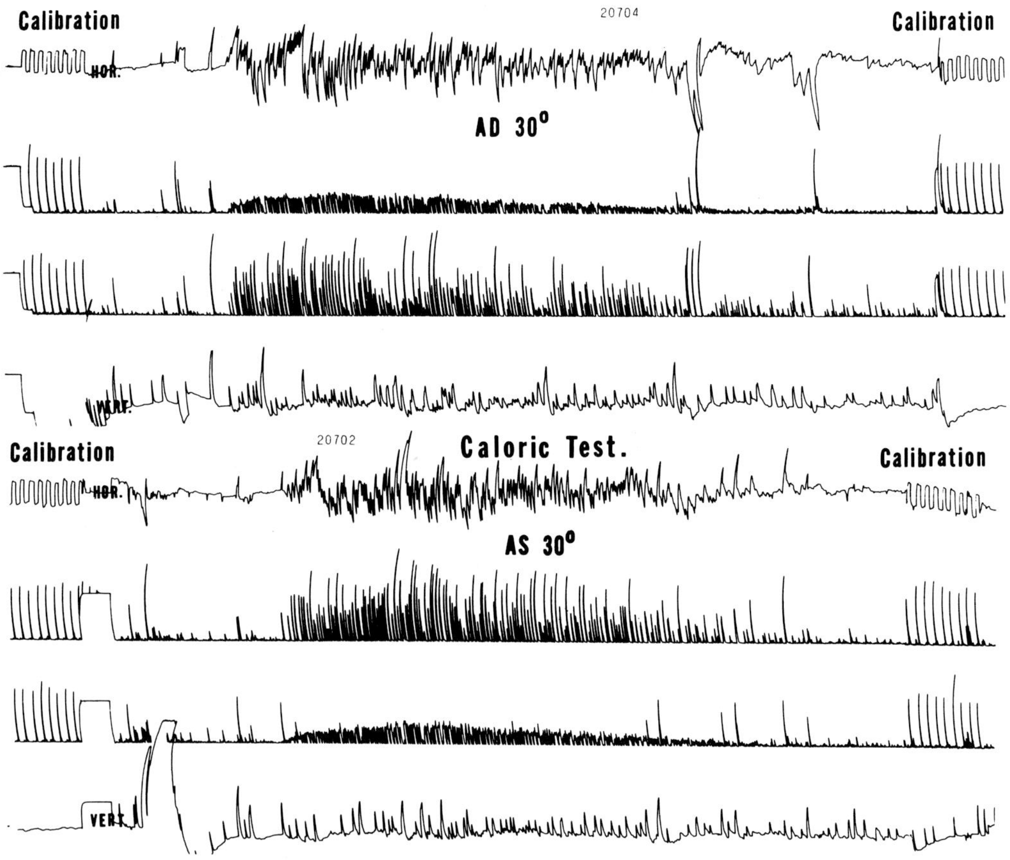

Fig. 4. Cold caloric tests of right ear (AD 30 C) and left ear (AS 30 C) (see text).

directional preponderance. These abnormalities, although not specific, occurred in a significant percentage of patients (80%) and were considered of important diagnostic value. The lower percentage (33%) of vestibular abnormalities reported by Dursteler[11] in a group of 12 patients, is perhaps due to the fact that his results were based only on the duration of nystagmus and were not recorded by ENG. Nevertheless he stated that the frequency of abnormal vestibular tests in migraine was significantly greater than in a control group.

Abnormal vestibular tests were present in 10 of the 12 patients with positive family history and in 10 of the 13 patients with history of motion sickness. However, six of eight patients with negative family history and six of seven patients with negative history of motion sickness had abnormal vestibular tests.

Of the 16 patients with abnormal vestibular tests, 10 had positive family history of migraine and 10 had positive history of motion sickness. These percentages have poor statistical levels of significance.

If we recognize that abnormal vestibular tests occur in 80% of the patients with common migraine and that there is poor statistical correlation between vestibular tests and family history of migraine or history of motion sickness we should draw a conclusion that these two historical factors (family history of migraine and history of motion sickness) are not diagnostic of common migraine; yet we know they are for classic and complicated migraine, especially the ophthalmoplegic type.

We cannot explain the occurrence of vestibular abnormalities at a time when the patients are free of headache. However, abnormal EEG and visual evoked potentials are also common between attacks of migraine.[22,23]

The high percentage of abnormal vestibular tests (80%) found in our patients with common migraine is almost twice the percentage of abnormalities found in our patients with other types of headache. In fact, in a previous study of 874 patients with headache following closed head injury and/or neck injury, we found, using the same ENG technique, caloric abnormalities only in 47% and rotatory abnormalities in 40%, even though those patients were also complaining of dizziness![24] In conclusion, this pilot investigation suggests that labyrinthine dysfunction occurs in a significant number of patients with common migraine and that vestibular tests, particularly if recorded by ENG, should help to differentiate common migraine from other types of headache.

The etiological diagnosis is indispensable for the choice of effective drug therapy; specifically analgesics are of little value in treating migraine and Cafergot® is not to be used in patients with headaches unless these are of the migrainous type.

Now some comments about the pathogenesis of vestibular abnormalities in patients with migraine.

From the review of the literature it is apparent that migraine has been attributed to dysfunction of the peripheral autonomic nervous system.[25] The prodroma of the complicated migraine and the aura of the classic migraine are attributed to vasoconstriction of arterioles and capillaries supplying brainstem and cerebral cortex. The headache is attributed to vasodilatation of extracerebral arteries accompanied by local tissue ischemia, sterile inflammation of the vessel walls and local release of vasoactive amines. The vertigo attacks are attributed to ischemia of the labyrinth or the vestibular pathways in the CNS.

The vasomotor theory is weakened by several critical observations: 1) It is not uncommon during a migraine attack to witness a variety of neurological signs and symptoms originating in several distant areas of the CNS;[26] these signs and symptoms could not be unequivocally attributed to simultaneous vasoconstriction of several independent blood vessels at distant areas of the brain. 2) Even though blood flow is increased in the occipital area during the aura of migraine[27] there is a 20% decrease of cortical blood flow in *both* cerebral hemispheres at the time when the aura is definitely *unilateral*![28] 3) Visual evoked potentials are reduced simultaneously in the occipital and parietal cortex at a time when the symptoms are confined to the occipital region.[22] These few critical observations suggest that migraine is due to dysfunction of a system, other than anatomic as defined by blood supply.

Finally it is even more difficult to understand the pathogenesis of common migraine on the basis of the vasomotor theory, since this variety of migraine characteristically lacks the vasoconstrictive phase. Therefore either common migraine should not be included in the classifications of migraine, or the vasomotor theory of migraine should be challenged.

This challenge, in fact, already exists. Several investigators agree that all clinical findings and laboratory abnormalities associated with migraine are caused by a primary metabolic disturbance of serotonin[29-33] in the CNS.

The evidence for this theory is mostly indirect and not unequivocal: during migraine attacks the concentration of serotonin in the serum and of serotonin metabolites in the urine oscillate. Since directly or indirectly serotonin is involved also in the control of emotion, sleep estrus, water retention, thermal regulation and other brainstem functions including the proprioceptive system, one may expect a variety of clinical findings including vestibular abnormalities in all types of migraine, including the common variety.

REFERENCES

1. Escat H. De la migraine otique. In: VII Congrès International d'Otologie. Bordeaux: Gounouillhon, 1904:1176.

2. Margulies A. Uber Migraine Otique. Prager Med Wochenschr 1913; 38:381-3.

3. Brunner H, Spiegel EA. Uber ohrmigraine (Hemikrania otica). Z Gesamte Neurol Psychiatr 1921; 70:18.

4. Heveroch J. La migraine vestibulaire. Rev Neurol (Paris) 1925; 33:925-9.

5. Lermoyer M. La vertige qui fait entendre (angiospasme labyrinthique). Ann Mal l'Orelle du Larynx 1929; 48:575-83.

6. Williams HL. Menière's disease. Springfield: Charles C Thomas, 1952.

7. Atkinson M. Menière's syndrome and migraine, observations on a common causal relationship. Ann Intern Med 1943; 18:797-808.

8. Fowler EP, Zeckel A. Psychophysiological factors in Menière's disease. Psychosom Med 1953; 15:127-39.

9. Federova ML. Vestibulares syndrom by migraine. Klin Med (Mosk) 1970; 48:70-6.

10. Kayan A. Migraine and related disturbances of hearing and balance. Hemicrania 1973; 4:3-4.

11. Dursteler MR. Migraine und vestibularapparat. J Neurol 1975; 210:253-69.

12. Siebert H. Uber cerebellaren Symptomen Komplex bei Migraine. Muench Med Wochenschr 1923; 70:812.

13. Phillips W, Wales MB. Cerebellar syndrome and nystagmus in migraine. Lancet 1932; 2:941-3.

14. Heidrich R. Cerebellare migraine. Psychiatr Neurol Med Psychol (Leipz) 1961; 13:42-8.

15. Barre A. Sur une syndrome sympathique cervical posterieur et sa cause frequent, l'arthrite cervicale. Rev Neurol (Paris) 1926; 55:1246-8.

16. Lieou Yong Choen. Syndrome sympathique cervicale posterieur et arthrite chronique de la colonn vertebrale cervicale, thesis. Strasbourg, 1928.

17. Bickerstaff ER. Basilar artery migraine. Lancet 1971; 1:15-17.

18. Levy I. Neurological aspects in the differential diagnosis of vertigo. In: Fields WS, Alford BF, eds. Neurological aspects of auditory and vestibular disorders. Springfield: Charles C Thomas, 1954:293.

19. Pearce J, Foster JB. An investigation of complicated migraine. Neurology (NY) 1965; 15:333-40.

20. Pearce J. General review of some aetiological factors in migraine. In: Cummings JN, ed. Background to migraine. New York: Springer Verlag, 1971:1-7.

21. Toglia JU. Electronystagmography. Technical aspects and atlas. Springfield: Charles C Thomas, 1976.

22. MacLean BA, Appenzeller O, Cordaro JT, Rhodes J. Flash evoked potentials in migraine. Headache 1975; 15:193-8.

23. Richey FT, Kooi KA, Waggoner RW. Visually evoked re-

sponses in migraine. Electroencephalogr Clin Neurophysiol 1966; 21:23-7.

24. Toglia, JU, Katinsky S. Neuro-otological aspects of closed head injury. In: Vinken PJ, Bruyn GW, eds. Handbook of clinical neurology, vol 24. Amsterdam: North-Holland, 1976:119-40.

25. Wolff HG. Headache and other head pain. New York: Oxford University Press, 1950.

26. Heyck H. Varieties of hemiplegic migraine. Headache 1973; 13:135-42.

27. Skinhoj E, Paulson OB. Regional blood flow in internal carotid distribution during migraine attacks. Br Med J 1969; 3:569-70.

28. O'Brien MP. The relationship between aura symptoms and cerebral blood flow changes in the prodoma of migraine. Headache 1971; 11:90-1.

29. Curran DA, Hinterberger H, Lance JW. Total plasma serotonin, 5-HIAA and p-hydroxy-m-methoxy-mandelic acid excretion in normal and migrainous subjects. Brain 1965; 88:997-1010.

30. Curran DA, Theaker P, Phillips B. Excretion of 5-HIAA in migraine. J Neurol Neurosurg Psychiatry 1966; 29:85-90.

31. Cumings JN. Migraine — A biochemical disorder? In: Cummings JN, ed. Background to migraine. New York: Springer Verlag, 1971:76-89.

32. Kangasniemi PJ, Sonninen V, Rinne UK. Excretion of 5-HIAA and VMA in urine and concentration of 5-HIAA and HVA in CSF during migraine attacks and the free intervals. Headache 1972; 12:64-5.

33. Sicuteri F. Headache biochemistry and pharmacology. Arch Neurobiol (Madr) 1974; 37: Suppl: 27-59.

≈

AMERICAN DIOPTER AND DECIBEL SOCIETY

A combined seminar, Ophthalmology and ENT, will be held Nov. 30 - Dec. 4, 1981, in Puerto Rico. For further information contact: Charles S. McConnell, MD, Cedar Crest Professional Park, Suite 110, 1251 South Cedar Crest Blvd., Allentown, PA 18103.

≈

INTERNATIONAL CONGRESS OF AUDIOPHONOLOGY & GERONTOLOGY

A Congress entitled "Aging and Communication" devoted to the communicative problems of the aged will be held in Besançon, France, November 11-14, 1981. Organizational committee: Audiophonology & Gerontology, Faculté de Médicine, 25030 Besançon, France.

Ann Otol 90:1981

DISCRIMINATION OF PURULENT FROM NONPURULENT MAXILLARY SINUSITIS

CLINICAL AND RADIOGRAPHIC DIAGNOSIS

O. BERG, MD

H. BERGSTEDT, MD
M. G. LIND, MD

C. CARENFELT, MD
O. PEROLS, MD

STOCKHOLM, SWEDEN

For the rational treatment of sinusitis, it is essential to distinguish sinusitis of bacterial origin from that of other etiologies. In maxillary sinusitis, antral purulence indicates a significant amount of pathogenic bacteria, whereas the presence of bacteria seems to be of less or no relevance in nonpurulent sinusitis. Hence, from a therapeutic point of view one important diagnostic goal is the differentiation of purulent from nonpurulent sinusitis. In this respect clinical examination is fairly reliable. Sinus radiography cannot distinguish purulent from nonpurulent sinusitis and offers few advantages when deciding on antibiotic therapy. Antral aspiration offers the most comprehensive information on which to base a reliable diagnosis.

Sinusitis is an inflammatory process of the mucous membrane lining the paranasal sinuses, and is either infectious or noninfectious, purulent or nonpurulent. In acute maxillary sinusitis, pneumococci, *H influenzae* and various anaerobic bacteria predominate, though sterile sinus secretions are not infrequent (15-40%).[1-3] If, however, the quality of the aspirated secretion is considered and the culture findings are related to the appearance of the secretion, the picture is quite different. Thus, in purulent antral secretion a sterile condition is extremely rare and the bacterial numbers found are significantly higher than in nonpurulent secretion.[4-6] In the sealed-off sinus, particularly in patients with lingering purulence, the sinus environment may be depleted in bacterial nutrients and rich in excretion products. Hence, sterile secretions can be expected to occur more frequently in sinusitis of extended duration. In patients with chronic maxillary sinusitis, Karma et al[7] found no bacterial growth in 12% of the purulent secretions, but heavy growth in 72% of these secretions. They established no relationship between the bacteriological characteristics and the clinical parameters, except for the quality of the sinus secretion. In purulent secretions, *H influenzae* was found significantly more often and heavy growth tended to be concentrated to these cases.

The etiologies of nonpurulent sinusitis are less well documented and the implication of bacteria in the pathogenesis is somewhat dubious. Dry sinusitis has not been subjected to accurate bacteriological studies, but heavy mucosal growth of pathogenic bacteria without a strong local inflammatory reaction and suppuration seems unlikely. In sinus polyposis etiologies other than microbial must be considered. In serous antral sinusitis vital and pathogenic bacteria can be isolated from aspirated serous secretions, but in amounts not exceeding 1% of the bacterial numbers found in purulent sinus secretions.[4,5] Furthermore, about half of the serous secretions appear to be sterile.[6] The antral inflammatory reaction associated with the serous sinusitis is slight, which is reflected by the low concentration of neutrophilic granulocytes in the secretion, ie, 1,000th of the number found in purulent sinus secretion.[4,5] This slight inflammatory reaction supports the suggestion that bacteria in serous sinus secretions merely represents a secondary bacterial occurrence or a preinfectious phase rather than a pure bacterial infection. Nevertheless, serous sinusitis is of differential diagnostic interest, as it gives rise to local symptoms and as some 20% of the patients with retained antral secretion have a serous sinusitis.[8]

The clinician has to find clinical parameters and diagnostic tools to distinguish the bacterial infection from other inflammatory disorders. In sinusitis, clinical criteria indicating a bacterial infection would facilitate the immediate choice of appropriate treatment and minimize the indiscriminate use of antibiotics. History and signs of purulence seem to be the best clinical criteria for sinus empyema. To compare the ability of the clinician to distinguish the antral empyema with the efficacy of the sinus radiography to predict such a condition, a diagnostic antral aspiration was performed. By this method it is possible to differentiate between purulent sinusitis, nonpurulent sinusitis and the healthy sinus.[8] In this paper, the results have been based on patients with a rather extended history of sinusitis.

From the Departments of Otolaryngology, Sabbatsbergs sjukhus and Karolinska sjukhuset, and the Department of Diagnostic Radiology, Karolinska sjukhuset, Stockholm.

REPRINTS — C. Carenfelt, MD, Dept. of Otolaryngology, Sabbatsbergs sjukhus, 11382 Stockholm, Sweden.

TABLE 1. CLASSIFICATION OF RADIOGRAPHIC INFORMATION

I.	No mucosal thickening; no fluid
II.	Mucosal thickening <0.5 cm or solitary polyp but no fluid
III.	Mucosal thickening ≥ 0.5 cm but no fluid
IV.	Attenuating tissue or fluid occupying the sinus or fluid level

MATERIAL AND METHODS

Selection of Patients. From patients with a suspected sinusitis or referred to us with this diagnosis, those patients were selected who fulfilled the following criteria: 1) various symptoms indicating sinusitis regardless of intensity, eg, pain, discomfort or tenderness located to the maxillary sinus, mastication pain, nasal discharge, cacosmia and nasal obstruction; 2) duration of symptoms exceeding three weeks; 3) no antibiotic medication during the previous month; 4) no decisive diagnosis other than sinusitis explaining the symptoms (eg, nasal furunculus, peridental abscess, trigeminal neuralgia, Horton's syndrome, nasal or paranasal neoplasia).

Clinical Evaluation. All patients were examined by an otolaryngologist. He had to consider not only whether the patient suffered from maxillary sinusitis, but also to specify the diagnosis in terms of purulent (empyema) or nonpurulent sinusitis. The sinusitis was considered as *definitely not purulent* when there was no history of purulent nasal discharge and no nasal or epipharyngeal pus at examination. The sinusitis was considered as *probably not purulent* when there was a history of the purulent discharge but without a finding of nasal or epipharyngeal pus. On the other hand, the sinusitis was considered as *probably purulent* when there was no history of purulence but nasal or epipharyngeal pus on examination. The combination of history of purulent discharge and the finding of nasal or epipharyngeal pus was considered to indicate that the sinusitis was *definitely purulent*. History and clinical signs were also recorded with regard to nasal allergy and vasomotor dysfunction (eg, watery nasal fluor with or without seasonal variations, pale or bluish and congested turbinates, nasal polyps).

Radiographic Evaluation. Sinus radiography was performed one to seven days following the clinical examination. Four standard projections were used: lateral, occipitofrontal, occipitomental and axial. The results as they refer to the actual maxillary sinus were classified according to the principles given in Table 1. Pronounced mucosal thickening (III) and fluid or complete opacity (IV) were considered to indicate or at least be consistent with a purulent sinusitis.

Antral Aspiration. To compare the ability of the otolaryngologist to distinguish the antral empyema with the efficacy of sinus radiography to predict such a condition, an antral aspiration was performed immediately following radiography. Unaware of the radiological results, the maxillary sinus most affected according to the clinician was selected for puncture. With a needle introduced through the inferior nasal meatus, the mucosal and bony walls were palpated and retained secretion or air was aspirated with the head in tilted position. The antral aspiration technique is described in detail elsewhere.[8] By using this technique instead of irrigation, the mucosal thickness and the ostial patency could roughly be estimated. The aspirated secretion was characterized undiluted according to its appearance as *purulent*, ie, opaque and discolored yellow or green and of various viscosity (seropurulent, mucopurulent); *serous*, ie, transparent yellow of low viscosity with the capacity to gel; or *mucous*, ie, semiopalescent grey of high viscosity. This classification has previously been shown to reflect relevant quantitative and qualitative differences of the bacterial content in the secretions and also to reflect significant differences of the inflammatory response.[4-6] The diagnoses based on antral aspiration are given in Table 2.

TABLE 2. CLASSIFICATION OF THE RESULTS OF ANTRAL ASPIRATION

No retained secretion, no mucosal thickening, patent ostium	No sinusitis
Serous or mucous secretion and/or mucosal thickening and/or ostial obstruction	Nonpurulent sinusitis
Purulent secretion	Purulent sinusitis

TABLE 3. RELATIONSHIP BETWEEN CLINICAL AND RADIOGRAPHIC EVALUATION

Clinical Evaluation	*Radiographic Evaluation* I	*II*	*III*	*IV*	*Total*
Definitely not purulent sinusitis		3	7	9	19
Probably not purulent sinusitis	3	2	1	2	8
Probably purulent sinusitis			1	4	5
Definitely purulent sinusitis			3	15	18
Total number of patients	3	5	12	30	50

RESULTS

According to the criteria given, 50 patients were selected, 22 female and 28 male with an average age of 46 years. In 14 of the patients, the duration of symptoms exceeded one year. The median duration was three months. The antral aspiration yielded purulent secretions from 25 patients, mucous from 2 and serous from 7 patients. Dry antra but with thickened sinus mucosa and/or obstructed ostium were disclosed in eight cases. In the remaining eight patients the result of the aspiration was consistent with a healthy sinus. Hence, of the 50 patients considered clinically to have maxillary sinusitis, 42 had purulent *or* nonpurulent sinusitis according to the antral aspiration.

The clinical and the radiographic evaluations are compared in Table 3. All patients considered by the clinician to have a purulent sinusitis had a pathological radiography classified as III or IV. Nevertheless the correlation between the two examinations is not particularly impressive, as 16 of 19 patients considered definitely not to have a purulent sinusitis fell into radiographic categories III or IV.

In Table 4, the specified clinical diagnoses are compared to the aspiration findings. Eight patients with a healthy antrum, according to the aspiration

TABLE 4. COMPARISON OF CLINICAL EVALUATION AND FINDINGS ON ASPIRATION

Clinical Evaluation	*Findings of Antral Aspiration* Normal Sinus	*Nonpurulent Sinusitis*	*Purulent Sinusitis*
Definitely not purulent sinusitis	3	13	3
Probably not purulent sinusitis	5	2	1
Probably purulent sinusitis		1	4
Definitely purulent sinusitis		1	17
Total number of patients	8	17	25

TABLE 5. RADIOGRAPHIC EVALUATION AND ANTRAL ASPIRATION FINDINGS

Radiographic Evaluation	*Findings of Antral Aspiration* *Normal Sinus*	*Nonpurulent Sinusitis*	*Purulent Sinusitis*
I	3		
II	4	1	
III	1	6	5
IV		10	20
Total number of patients	8	17	25

TABLE 6. OCCURRENCE OF NASAL ALLERGY OR VASOMOTOR RHINITIS IN RELATION TO DIAGNOSIS OBTAINED BY ANTRAL ASPIRATION

Diagnosis by Antral Aspiration	*Total Number of Patients*	*Nasal Allergy or Vasomotor Rhinitis*
Purulent sinusitis	25	5
Nonpurulent sinusitis	17	15
Normal sinus	8	3
Total number of patients	50	23

were considered to suffer from sinusitis, although nonpurulent. In 17 patients with nonpurulent sinusitis, this diagnosis was proposed by the clinician. In 25 patients with purulent sinusitis the clinician was correct in 21 cases.

In Table 5 the results of the radiographic evaluation are compared to the diagnoses obtained by aspiration. If classifications III and IV are considered to indicate purulent sinusitis, then all 25 patients with an empyema were identified by the sinus radiography. However, in 16 of 17 patients with nonpurulent sinusitis, the radiological suggestion of purulent sinusitis was erroneous.

History and signs of nasal allergy or vasomotor rhinitis were disclosed in 23 of the 50 patients (Table 6). In particular, allergy and vasomotor rhinitis were recognized in patients with nonpurulent sinusitis as judged from the findings of the antral aspiration, but such symptoms and signs did not exclude the occurrence of antral suppuration.

DISCUSSION

Opinions vary on the diagnostic potential of sinus radiography in maxillary sinusitis. In previous reports, the definition of sinusitis has sometimes been vague and the radiographic findings have often been compared to those of antral irrigation. Vuorinen et al found sinus radiography to be a fairly accurate diagnostic method.[9] Watt-Boolsen and Karle demonstrated that their routine radiography was affected by false positive (29-45%) and false negative (24%) results with regard to antral fluid.[10] Axelsson et al found radiography unreliable unless the examination was complemented by an occipitomental projection with the patient in a tilted position to accumulate retained secretion to the zygomatic recess.[11] On the contrary, Kalm et al found good agreement between radiography and aspiration/irrigation findings, but found no benefit of this extra projection.[1] On the basis of bacterial analyses of aspirated antral secretion, Evans et al[4] and Hamory et al[3] found radiography a reliable method in the diagnosis of acute maxillary sinusitis. By sinoscopy, Illum et al found that the presence of sinus discharge was incorrectly diagnosed by radiography in 38% of the patients.[12] Draf drew similar conclusions from sinoscopy, but he also claimed that the diagnostic antral irrigation can give false information concerning the character of the inflammation.[13]

There are few reports on the clinician's diagnostic precision in sinusitis. Evans et al found precision rather poor but their clinical routines and findings were not given.[4] Based on a detailed clinical examination, Axelsson and Runze concluded that the otolaryngologist hardly can discriminate acute maxillary sinusitis from simple rhinitis, but found sinus radiography reliable enough for therapeutic decisions.[14] Unfortunately, no attention was paid to etiological considerations and the character of the sinus inflammation was not further evaluated. Hence, the results are somewhat inconclusive, except that the ability of the otolaryngologist to predict changes within the sinuses as they appear on the radiograms is inferior to that of the radiologist.

During the viral stage of the upper respiratory infection, the paranasal mucosa may be hyperemic and the permeability of the vascular endothelium increases. Mucosal edema and exudate are formed. Goblet cells and seromucinous cells of the antral mucosa are stimulated to produce copious secretions mainly of serous character.[15] This mucosal thickening and the fluid can be seen on the radiogram. As the sinus fails to drain freely through the swollen ostium, the antral environment changes to favor bacterial replication.[16] A sinus empyema is formed and will show on the radiogram. In patients with nasal allergy or vasomotor dysfunction the nasal and paranasal mucosa may be congested and the production of serous secretion is not necessarily restricted to the nose, but will be found also within the sinus. Polyposis can engage the nasal or paranasal cavities or both. The antral cavity filled with polyps will give rise to complete opacity on the radiogram. These pathological sinus reactions can be described as sinusitis according to its definition, except possibly for the vasomotor dysfunction. All these inflammatory conditions of the sinus can have the same reflection on the radiogram, but only those of bacterial origin fulfill the criterion of antibiotic therapy.

Sinus empyema is of bacterial origin. Hence, the subjective and objective findings of nasal and epipharyngeal purulence were assumed to reflect the purulent sinusitis better than other local symptoms. The result of the clinical examinations justified this assumption, as most of the patients with purulent sinusitis were recognized. All these patients were also recognized by radiography. But, of the 17 patients with nonpurulent sinusitis 16 patients were "overdiagnosed" (Table 5), unless small volumes of pus were overlooked. The possibility of this error seems small, however, as previously demonstrated in patients who underwent antral exploration immediately following the antral aspiration.[8] The aspiration, in contrast to the irrigation, provides the secretion undiluted which will facilitate its characterization. Serous secretion and also purulent secretion of low viscosity are not easily distinguishable when diluted in a large volume of saline.

The etiological implication of bacteria in nonpurulent sinusitis without heavy inflammation is unknown, and further data are required, particularly in dry sinusitis. Hence, there is no definite answer to the question of the indication of antibiotic therapy in these cases. However, since 15 of 17 patients in this study who suffered from nonpurulent sinusitis had symptoms and signs of nasal allergy or vasomotor rhinitis, a majority of these patients would probably not benefit from antibiotic therapy. In serous sinusitis as well the indication of antibiotic treatment is questionable. The few bacteria in the serous secretion, if any, do not seem to grow exponentially.[5] Hence, their susceptibility to common antibiotics may be poor. Furthermore, serous sinusitis is usually cured by one or two antral aspirations.[8]

Irreversible lesions of the sinus mucosa with a crippling of the local host defense can be the consequence of recurrent purulent sinusitis or untreated prolonged empyema.[16] In patients with this history, the sinusitis must not remain undiagnosed. Sinus radiography is a complement to the clinical examination, but may lead to wrong conclusions. Radiography discriminates between sinusitis in its broad sense and the healthy sinus, but has per se no other diagnostic preference to the clinical examination in differentiating patients who require antibiotic therapy from those who do not. As the indication for antibiotic therapy is based on the existence of significant growth of pathogenic bacteria, and as such bacterial growth in sinusitis is closely correlated to purulence, a diagnostic distinction of purulent from nonpurulent sinus affection seems to be the most rational goal for diagnostic efforts in patients suspected of sinusitis. The clinical interpretation, especially when symptoms and signs of purulence are stressed, has a definite diagnostic value, but is not always sufficient. Antral aspiration offers comprehensive information to ensure the diagnosis and in addition is simple to perform.

REFERENCES

1. Kalm O, Kamme C, Bergström B, et al. Erythromycin stearate in acute maxillary sinusitis. Scand J Infect Dis 1975; 7:209-17.

2. Van Cauwenberge P, Verschraegen G, van Renterghem L. Bacteriological findings in sinusitis (1963-1975). Scand J Infect Dis 1975; 9:72-7.

3. Hamory BH, Sande MA, Sydnor A, et al. Etiology and antimicrobial therapy of acute maxillary sinusitis. J Infect Dis 1979; 139:197-202.

4. Evans FO, Sydnor JB, Moore WEC, et al. Sinusitis of the maxillary antrum. N Engl J Med 1975; 293:735-9.

5. Carenfelt C, Lundberg C. The role of local gas composition in pathogenesis of maxillary sinus empyema. Acta Otolaryngol (Stockh) 1978; 85:116-21.

6. Carenfelt C, Lundberg C, Nord C-E, et al. Bacteriology of maxillary sinusitis in relation to quality of the retained secretion. Acta Otolaryngol (Stockh) 1978; 86:298-302.

7. Karma P, Jokipii L. Sipilä P, et al. Bacteria in chronic maxillary sinusitis. Arch Otolaryngol 1979; 105:386-90.

8. Carenfelt C. Diagnostic and therapeutic antral aspiration. Acta Otolaryngol (Stockh) 1981 (in press).

9. Vuorinen P, Kauppila A, Pulkkinee K. Comparison of results of roentgen examination and puncture and irrigation of the maxillary sinuses. J Laryngol Otol 1962; 76:359-64.

10. Waat-Boolsen S, Karle A. The clinical use of radiological examination of the maxillary sinuses. Clin Otolaryngol 1977; 2:41-3.

11. Axelsson A, Grebelius N, Chidekel N, et al. The correlation between the radiological examination and the irrigation findings in maxillary sinusitis. Acta Otolaryngol (Stockh) 1970; 69:302-6.

12. Illum P, Jeppesen F, Langebaek E. X-ray examination and sinoscopy in maxillary sinus disease. Acta Otolaryngol (Stockh) 1972; 74:287-92.

13. Draf W. Die Endoskopie der Nasennebenhöhlen — Diagnostische und therapeutische Möglichkeiten. Laryngol Rhinol Otol (Stuttg) 1975; 54:209-15.

14. Axelsson A, Runze U. Symptoms and signs of acute maxillary sinusitis. ORL 1976; 38:298-308.

15. Van Nostrand AWP, Goodman WS. Pathological aspects of the maxillary sinus. Otolaryngol Clin N Am 1976; 9:21.

16. Carenfelt C. The pathogenesis of the sinus empyema. Ann Otol Rhinol Laryngol 1979; 88:16-20.

NEW NEUROTOLOGICAL TEST FOR DETECTING CEREBELLAR DYSFUNCTION

VESTIBULO-OCULAR REFLEX CHANGES WITH HORIZONTAL VISION-REVERSAL PRISMS

TOSHIAKI YAGI, MD
SHUJI SEKINE, MD
MOTOHIRO SHIMIZU, MD
TOMOKAZU KAMIO, MD

TOKYO, JAPAN

Adaptation of the vestibulo-ocular reflex (VOR) was studied in 26 normal subjects and 15 patients with cerebellar lesions, using horizontal vision-reversal prisms. In normal subjects, adaptation of gain after wearing prisms for one hour was approximately 50% of the VOR value in the dark. In contrast to this, patients with cerebellar lesions showed less adaptation, approximately 20% after a one-hour forced adaptation task. These cases showed three different types of abnormalities: 1) high gain before wearing prisms and normal adaptation, 2) high gain before wearing prisms and reduction of adaptation, 3) normal gain and reduction of adaptation. From these results, it is suggested that observation of the effect of vision-reversal prisms on the VOR may permit the detection of cerebellar lesions of a type or subtlety which escape established tests.

The vestibulo-ocular reflex (VOR) helps maintain a stable retinal image by generating compensatory eye movements to offset the effects of head rotation. Recent physiological experiments have revealed that the visual inputs and vestibular inputs are integrated in the vestibulocerebellum, and established that the vestibulocerebellum plays an important role in producing an adequate VOR.[1-5] Furthermore, recent observations on human subjects and animals wearing reversing prisms have clearly established that the VOR is plastic and adaptive in nature.[6-9] In the cat, Robinson[10] demonstrated that the plasticity of the VOR was abolished after removal of the vestibulocerebellum, and he concluded that the vestibulocerebellum is necessary for the plastic and adaptive process of the VOR.

On the basis of these studies, it can be expected that the observation of adaptation of the VOR to reversing prisms may lead to detection of cerebellar dysfunction. The present study was undertaken to examine clinical applications of the adaptation of the VOR to reversing prisms. Both normal subjects and patients with cerebellar lesions were tested. The test time was limited to one hour so that it would neither be too long nor too demanding for the subjects.

METHODS

Normal subjects consisted of 26 adults (12 males and 14 females), ranging in age from 19 to 34 years, who were free from vestibular and oculomotor disorders. Subjects sat on a chair which was rotated sinusoidally in a horizontal plane at 0.25 Hz and 30° angular amplitude. Eye movement (E), eye velocity ($\dot{E}$) and head movement (H) were recorded, using electronystagmography. Calibrations of E were performed before and after the experiment.

The test sequence is illustrated in Figure 1. First, the subjects were asked to watch a small, dim light fixed approximately 2 m in front of the chair in the darkened room (base line). Next, the subjects' eyes were covered by blackout goggles (initial VOR). After that, the subjects wore prisms which reversed images in the horizontal plane. During the image-reversal condition, the subjects were also asked to watch the dim light. Every 15 minutes the subjects wore the blackout goggles over the reversing prisms. E, $\dot{E}$, and H were recorded six times as indicated by the shaded areas in Figure 1. Each recording consisted of 10 to 20 sinusoidal rotations. Subjects did mental arithmetic to maintain alertness during recordings. The experiment was carried out in darkness, except

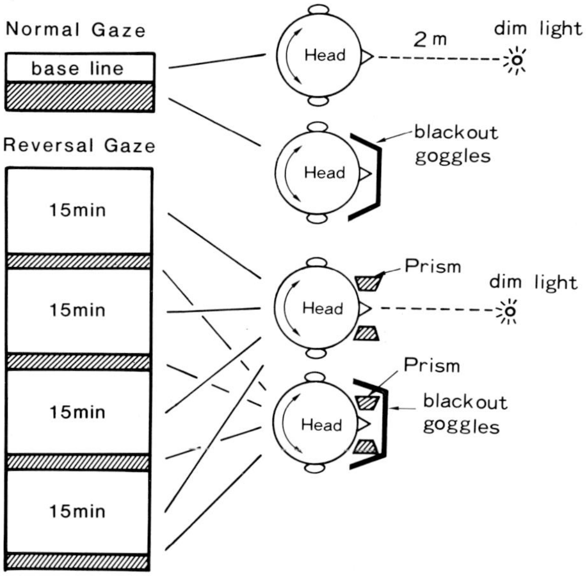

Fig. 1. Schematic diagram of experimental sequence and subject condition. VOR measurements were made in the blackout conditions (shaded areas) and expressed as gain relative to measurements in base line condition. The schemata of the subject's conditions are illustrated on the right and connected with solid lines.

From the Department of Otorhinolaryngology, Nippon Medical School, Tokyo.
REPRINTS — Toshiaki Yagi, MD, Department of Otorhinolaryngology, Nippon Medical School, Sendagi 1-1-5, Bunkyo-ku, Tokyo, Japan 113.

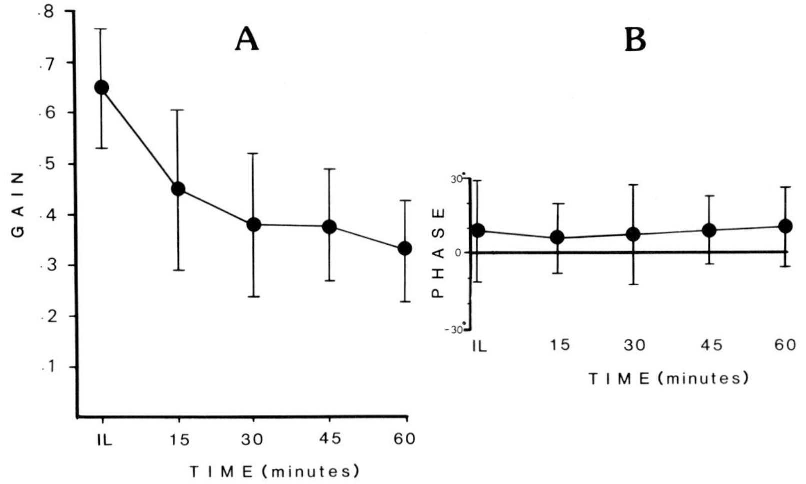

Fig. 2. Means (filled circles) and standard deviations (vertical bars) of the sequential VOR gain and phase changes during 60 minutes of forced reversal vision. A) Gradual and remarkable decreases of gain after wearing reversal prisms are noted, but B) no significant changes are observed in the phase of VOR. IL - Initial level (VOR in darkness before reversal gaze).

for the small, dim, target light used for foveal stimulation during forced adaptation, in order to avoid nausea during oscillation. Only four subjects became slightly nauseated. During forced adaptation, E, $\dot{E}$, and H were monitored to ascertain that the subjects watched the target as instructed.

Gain and phase of the VOR were calculated for each subject as follows. The relative VOR gain (G) was estimated as the ratio of $\dot{E}$ in the base line condition ($\dot{E}$gaze) to $\dot{E}$ in the eyes-covered condition (Ex), VOR gain = $\dot{E}$x/$\dot{E}$gaze. Since VOR gain in this frequency range is close to one in the base line condition ($\dot{E}$= head velocity),[7,10] this estimation of the relative value seems to be reasonable. In order to observe net adaptation, the adaptation index was also calculated. The adaptation index can be expressed as the ratio of "initial VOR" gain to gains after 15, 30, 45, and 60 minutes of wearing prisms. Phase was determined at the zero crossing. Phase was calculated as the value in each condition (θx) relative to the phase in the base line condition (θ gaze), VOR = θx - θ gaze. Gain and phase values were based on the means of at least eight cycles.

RESULTS

Means and standard deviations of VOR gain changes in darkness are illustrated in Figure 2A. VOR gains during the reversal gaze condition in the intervals between the blackout test period were the same as in the normal gaze condition, but 180° out of phase. Mean VOR gain in darkness was 0.65 before the reversal gaze period. After forced adaptation by left-right reversal, VOR gain gradually decreased as illustrated in Figure 2. Gains after 15, 30, 45, and 60 minutes of wearing reversal prisms were 0.45, 0.38, 0.38, and 0.33, respectively. The adaptation index of each subject was also calculated (VOR gain after reversal gaze/initial VOR). Mean values of the adaptation index after 15, 30, 45, and 60 minutes were 0.69, 0.58, 0.58, and 0.52, respectively.

The relative values of the VOR phases are illustrated in Figure 2B. Means and standard deviations of the VOR phases in darkness before and after wearing prisms (15, 30, 45, and 60 minutes) were 9.1 ± 19.9, 5.9 ± 14.1, 7.4 ± 20.7, 9.4 ± 13.4, and 10.5 ± 16.4, respectively. Statistically, no significant difference was found between any two pairs (*t* test).

CLINICAL APPLICATION

Fifteen subjects with cerebellar lesions confirmed

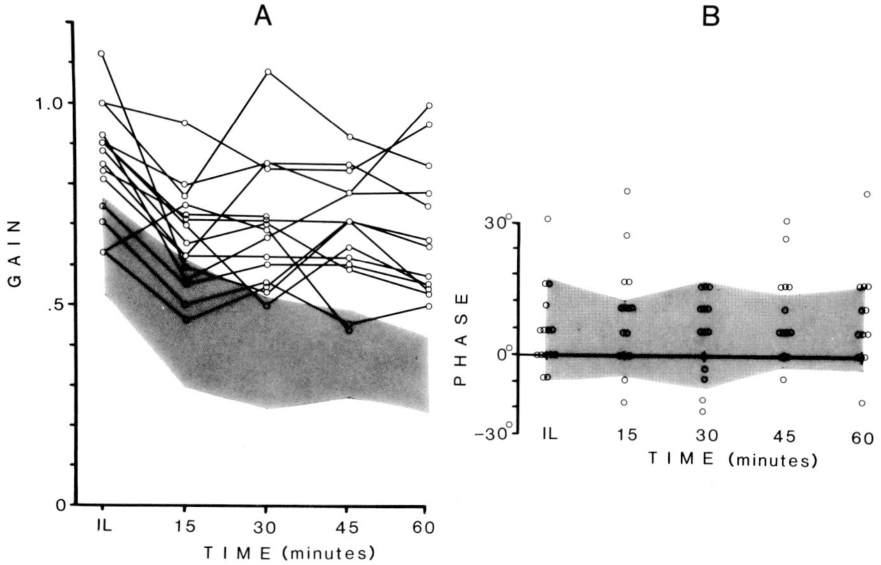

Fig. 3. Sequential changes of gain and phase of VOR in patients with cerebellar lesions. A) VOR gain changes from 15 patients. Shaded area indicates normal range (two standard deviations) from 26 normal subjects. Before wearing prisms (IL), only four patients exhibit normal values. After one-hour adaptation, all patients show higher gain than normal values. B) VOR phase changes from 15 patients. Shaded area indicates normal range. Except for a few subjects, most of patients show normal values.

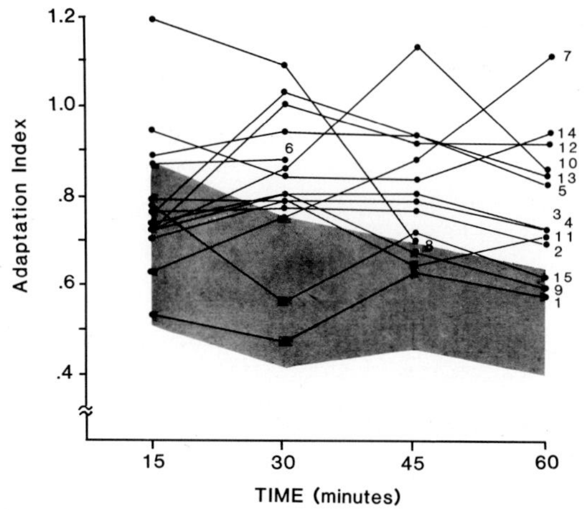

Fig. 4. Sequential changes of VOR adaptation index. Shaded area indicates normal range (two standard deviations) of adaptation index. Three cases (cases 1, 9 and 15) show normal adaptation after one hour. The other 11 cases exhibit reduction of adaptation. Numbers (1 to 15) on right indicate case numbers.

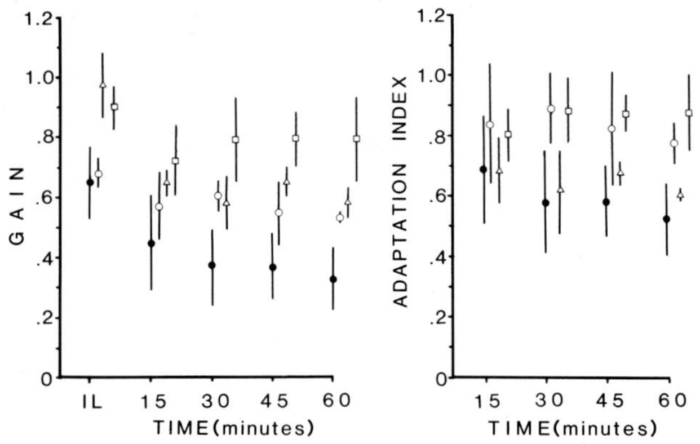

Fig. 5. Means and standard deviation of the sequential VOR gain (left) and the adaptation index (right) changes during 60 minutes of forced reversal vision. Open triangles, open squares, and open circles indicate respectively the means of the values from the cases which showed three different types of pathological responses, ie, 1) higher initial level and normal adaptation, 2) higher initial level and decreased adaptation, and 3) normal initial level and decreased adaptation. Filled circles - Means of values from 26 normal subjects; IL - Initial level.

by neurotological examinations, including nystagmus observations, optokinetic nystagmus (OKN) test and eye-tracking test, and x-ray studies, mainly CT scan, were tested. The test method was the same as for normal subjects. The diagnoses of these cases were cerebellar atrophy (6), acoustic tumor (2), vascular origin (bleeding, 1; thrombosis, 1; aneurysm, 1; and arteriovenous malformation, 1), astrocytoma (2) and metastatic tumor (1).

The VOR gain changes from the 15 cases are illustrated in Figure 3. The mean VOR gain in darkness was 0.85 before wearing reversing prisms. This value was higher than that of normal subjects (0.65). However, 4 among 15 cases showed normal values in this situation. Means and standard deviations 15, 30, 45, and 60 minutes after wearing reversing prisms were 0.66 ± 13.0, 0.70 ± 16.0, 0.69 ± 0.16, and 0.68 ± 0.17, respectively. These values were clearly higher than those of normal subjects ($p < 0.001$). Also, no abnormal subjects had a normal range value after one hour of vision reversal. This may be due to the higher value of the gain before wearing reversing prisms. To allow for this higher initial level, the adaptation index was calculated as described in the Methods section. Means and standard deviations of the adaptation index from normal subjects and those from each case of cerebellar lesion are shown in Figure 4. From the above-mentioned results, three different pathological conditions were noted. Eleven among 15 cases showed abnormally high gain before wearing reversing prisms (Fig. 3). Three of the 11 exhibited normal VOR adaptation (Fig. 4). The other 4 of 15 cases showed normal values of VOR gain in darkness before wearing prisms (Fig. 3), but reduced VOR adaptation was observed. These different conditions are summarized as 1) higher initial level and normal adaptation (cases 1, 9 and 15); 2) higher initial level and reduced adaptation (cases 2, 4-7, and 12-14); and 3) normal gain of initial level and reduced adaptation (cases 3, 8, 10 and 11). Means and standard deviations of the VOR gain changes and adaptation index changes from each pathological condition mentioned above are demonstrated in Figure 5 together with normal values.

Phase changes of VOR are illustrated in Figure 3B. Means and standard deviations of phase changes in darkness before and after (15, 30, 45, and 60 minutes) wearing reversing prisms were 9.4 ± 16.0, 14.9 ± 20.4, 7.9 ± 15.6, and 14.4 ± 19.4, respectively. No statistical difference between these values and values from normal subjects was observed.

The reports of three cases which showed three different types of gain changes, ie, 1) higher initial level and normal adaptation; 2) higher initial level and reduced adaptation; and 3) normal initial level and reduced adaptation, are described below.

CASE REPORTS

Case 1. Cerebellar Atrophy. A 39-year-old male was seen in October 1979, with a three-year history of progressive difficulty in walking. The general physical examination was normal. The neurotological examination showed a moderate degree of disturbance in balance and vertical nystagmus in the positioning nystagmus test. Caloric and optokinetic responses were normal. Smooth pursuit movements of the eye were severely disturbed. He showed normal hearing in standard pure tone audiometry and normal auditory brainstem responses. There were no abnormalities in muscle power or development. Coordination testing showed dysmetria bilaterally. His gait was wide-based and ataxic. CT scan showed mild atrophy of brainstem and cerebellum (Fig. 6A).

The gains of VOR are illustrated in Figures 3 and 4. Gains during adaptation to vision reversal were 0.59, 0.53, 0.71, and 0.65, respectively. The initial VOR gain in darkness was high (1.12) compared to normal subjects (mean 0.65), but the adaptation index after one hour of vision reversal was normal (0.58).

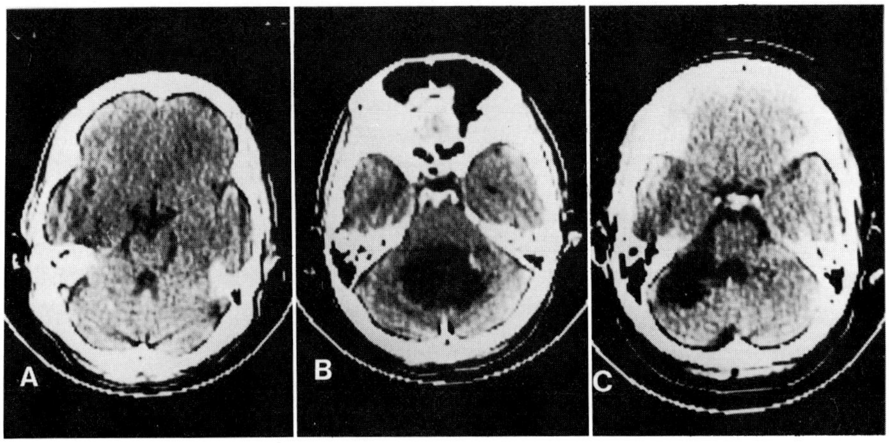

Fig. 6. A) (Case 1) CT scan shows mild atrophy of brainstem and cerebellum and moderate enlargement of the fourth ventricle. B) (Case 2) CT scan shows large, low density area in the cerebellum with small, high density area in the edge of the low density area. C) (Case 3) CT scan shows low density area in the left cerebellopontine angle and cerebellar hemisphere.

Case 2. Astrocytoma of the Cerebellum A 41-year-old male was seen in August 1979. He had noticed dizziness during head movements. This had been associated with progressive difficulty in walking. The general physical examination was normal. The neurotological examination showed a moderate degree of disturbance in balance, and gaze-directional and directional-changing nystagmus in the positional nystagmus test. OKN was almost normal but smooth eye movements were severely dysmetric. There were no abnormalities in muscle power or development. He had normal hearing on pure tone audiometry and normal auditory brainstem responses. CT scan showed a large low density area in the center of the cerebellum, slightly deviated to the left (Fig. 5B).

The gain changes of VOR are illustrated in Figures 3 and 4. The initial level was 0.81 and gains during adaptation were 0.62, 0.62, 0.62, and 0.57, respectively. The adaptation index was higher than in the normals, being increased 0.77, 0.77, 0.77, and 0.70, respectively.

Case 3. Cerebellar Bleeding. A 24-year-old male was seen in April 1979. He had a history of having injured his head while skiing one month before. He had no loss of consciousness but reported nausea, vomiting, general weakness, and oscillopsia immediately after the accident. Also, he noticed difficulty in walking and in coordinated movements of his left hand. He had a severe disturbance of balance (falling down to the right) and positional nystagmus. There was mild depression of slow phase eye velocity in left OKN but no disturbance of smooth pursuit movements. He had normal hearing on audiometry and normal caloric responses. The cranial nerve examination was normal but he had slowing of rapid alternation and dysmetria in the left hand and leg. On CT scan (Fig. 6A) there was a low density area in the cerebellum, deviated anteriorly and laterally to the left. It was smaller than in the previous case.

The VOR gain changes are demonstrated in Figures 3 and 4. The initial level was 0.75, and gains after 15, 30, 45, and 60 minutes of wearing reversing prisms were 0.55, 0.60, 0.60, and 0.55, respectively. The initial level was within the normal range and the adaptation index was higher than in the normals, being increased 0.73, 0.80, 0.80, and 0.73, respectively.

DISCUSSION

Plastic changes of cerebellar function in the vestibulo-ocular reflex from the experiments using reversal prisms have been extensively studied in human subjects,[6,7] monkeys,[9] and cats.[8,10] Gonshor and Melvill-Jones[7] reported that in the human subjects the VOR gain declined substantially during the first two days of vision reversal; reduction of gain continued, reaching a minimum by the end of one week at about 25% of normal value.

Robinson[10] reported the mechanisms of the adaptive gain control of VOR from lesion-making experiments in cats that chronically wore left-right vision reversal prisms. He observed gain increase and abolition of the plastic changes after removal of the vestibulocerebellum. From these results he concluded that the adaptation process is dependent on the vestibulocerebellum.

In the present study, normal subjects showed rapid adaptation of gain while wearing reversing prisms. The reduction was to about 50% of the normal value at the end of one hour of sinusoidal rotation stimulation. This is more rapid than the values reported by Gonshor and Melvill-Jones,[7] perhaps because in our experiment the subjects were asked to watch a target light during rotation and in their study the subjects did not receive a forced adaptation task. Furthermore, their observations of VOR gain were made daily and ours were every few minutes.

Regarding phase changes, the present study showed none within one hour. Since the phase changes are reported by Gonshor and Melvill-Jones[7] to start slowly, this finding seems reasonable.

In the present study, 11 cases among the 15 with cerebellar lesions showed high gain in the eyes-covered condition in the dark. This abnormally high gain has been already reported by Zee et al[11] and Baloh et al.[12] They speculated that the cause of this phenomenon is the lack or reduction of cerebellar inhibitory function in the VOR.

Three among these 11 cases showed normal adaptation after wearing prisms. This fact suggests that the mechanism of VOR gain control in darkness and the process of adaptation to reversal vision have different anatomical localizations. This speculation is further supported by the findings of the present study. Four cases exhibited normal VOR gain of initial level and showed decreased gain adaptation while wearing prisms. Nine other cases showed both higher initial level and decreased adaptation. The anatomical locations of the lesions in these cases were roughly identified by CT scan. Three cases which showed higher initial level and normal adaptation had mild atrophy in both brainstem and cerebellum. On the other hand, the four cases which showed normal VOR gain of initial level and decreased adaptation had lesions deviating to the one side of the cerebellum. Of the eight cases which showed higher initial level and decreased adaptation, most had widespread or midline lesions of the cerebellum.

There are several useful neurotological test methods, such as the visual suppression test[13] and VOR examination test,[11,12] for detecting cerebellar dysfunction. However, although these tests are able to detect dysfunction of the VOR arc, they cannot identify more precisely the anatomical or functional site of the cerebellar lesions. On the basis of the present study, it may be possible, by observation of the adaptation of the VOR to vision-reversal prisms, to detect cerebellar lesions which are, by their nature or subtlety, impossible to find with established tests.

REFERENCES

1. Ito M. Neural design of the cerebellar motor control system. Brain Res 1972; 40:81-4.

2. Ito M, Nisimaru N, Yamamoto M. Specific patterns of neuronal connexions involved in the control of the rabbit's vestibulo-ocular reflexes by the cerebellar flocculus. J Physiol (Lond) 1977; 265:833-54.

3. Maekawa K, Simpson JI. Climbing fiber responses evoked in vestibulocerebellum of rabbit from visual system. J Neurophysiol 1973; 36:649-66.

4. Maekawa K, Takeda T. Mossy fiber responses evoked in the cerebellar flocculus of rabbits by stimulation of the optic pathway. Brain Res 1975; 98:590-5.

5. Maekawa K, Takeda T. Electrophysiological identification of the climbing and mossy fiber pathways from the rabbit's retina to the contralateral cerebellary flocculus. Brain Res 1976; 109:169-74.

6. Gonshor A, Melvill-Jones G. Short-term adaptive changes in the human vestibulo-ocular reflex arc. J Physiol (Lond) 1976; 256;361-79.

7. Gonshor A, Melvill-Jones G. Extreme vestibulo-ocular adaptation induced by prolonged optical reversal of vision. J Physiol (Lond) 1976; 256:381-414.

8. Melvill-Jones G, Davis P. Adaptation of cat vestibulo-ocular reflex to 200 days of optically reversed vision. Brain Res 1976; 103:551-4.

9. Miles FA, Fuller JH. Adaptative plasticity in the vestibulo-ocular responses of the rhesus monkey. Brain Res 1974; 72:512-6.

10. Robinson DA. Adaptation gain control of vestibuloocular reflex by the cerebellum. J Neurophysiol 1976; 39:54-69.

11. Zee DS, Tee RD, Cogan DG, Robinson DA, Engel WK. Ocular motor abnormalities in hereditary cerebellar ataxia. Brain 1976; 99:207-43.

12. Baloh RW, Jenkins HA, Honrubia V, Yee RD, Lau CGY. Visual-vestibular interaction and cerebellar atrophy. Neurology 1979; 29:116-9.

13. Takemori S. Visual suppression test. Ann Otol Rhinol Laryngol 1977; 86:80-5.

≈

CHRONIC EFFECTS OF PHASIC MIDDLE EAR PRESSURE CHANGES

J. M. MILLER, PhD
A. AXELSSON, MD
W. POTTER, BA
SEATTLE, WASHINGTON

In an attempt to better define the mechanisms of barotrauma, middle and inner ear pathology was studied in guinea pigs three weeks following exposure to a brief, sudden middle ear pressure change. Findings included tympanic membrane perforations (particularly dependent upon high negative pressure exposures), vascular hemorrhage (primarily dependent upon high positive pressure exposures), serosanguineous effusions (predominantly dependent upon infection) and serous effusion (dependent upon negative pressure exposure). Round window perforations were common in high pressure animals with infection. Other inner ear membrane changes were infrequent or minimal. Lymphatic hemorrhage was observed as a function of exposure. The clinical implications of these findings and possible mechanisms underlying these changes are discussed in terms of our previously reported study of the immediate effects of such pressure change.

The mechanisms and treatment of barotrauma in man is of long-standing otologic concern. Based upon behavioral and clinical studies in man and histological findings in animals, the mechanisms of barotrauma may be described in terms of middle ear (ME) and inner ear (IE) pathology. Middle ear changes have often been graded. For example, Edmonds and Thomas[1] suggest: grade 0) symptoms without signs; grade 1) injection of the tympanic membrane (TM); grade 2) injection plus slight hemorrhage within the substance of the TM; grade 3) gross hemorrhage within the substance of the TM; grade 4) free blood in the ME evidenced by a bluish, bulging drum and a possible fluid level; and grade 5) free hemorrhage with perforation of the TM. This classification is based upon changes that can be visualized with the otomicroscope. It is also supported by direct observations of ME changes that accompany barotrauma in human and animal models.

Middle ear pathology consists of: 1) effusions: serous, serosanguineous or hemorrhagic;[2-6] 2) mucosal changes;[1,4] 3) vascular distention and hemorrhage;[1-9] 4) ossicular disarticulation and fractures;[1,10-13] and 5) TM perforations.[1-6,8]

Although sensorineural hearing loss following barotrauma in man has been documented, for obvious reasons less is known regarding the underlying pathology. Theories advanced for the explanation of the sensorineural hearing loss have been highly speculative. Since the turn of the century, animal experiments simulating barotraumatic conditions have been performed in an attempt to gain additional information on the histopathological changes of the IE that may underlie hearing loss. Documented and suggested IE pathology has included: 1) membranous labyrinth distortion and rupture;[5,6,14-16] 2) round window (RW) perforation;[17] 3) hemorrhage;[5-7,18-20] and 4) gas bubble formation.[5,6,20]

Recently, tympanotomy has been performed in human cases with clinical symptoms of sensorineural hearing loss, vertigo and nystagmus following barotrauma experiences. A frequently reported finding has been round and oval window fistulas.[1,11,12,21-30] It is somewhat surprising that tympanotomy was not performed before 1971 in these patients, given the long and enthusiastic history of ME surgery. One explanation for this may be that experimental studies suggested a primary etiology of hemorrhage in the IE or membrane breaks, conditions which have not been accessible for surgery. These clinical studies indicate that a difference may exist between experimental animals which primarily show intracochlear pathology and man where the primary, only confirmed pathology has been round and oval window perforations.

Therapeutic suggestions for these patients have been numerous:

1. Bed rest.[1,9,11,12,21,29-33]
2. Avoidance of exercise, coughing, nose blowing, sneezing, straining, etc.[4,21,33]
3. Oral or local decongestants.[1,15]
4. Antibiotics.[1,4]
5. Immediate surgery for tympanic and/or window perforations.[1,11,26]
6. Surgery after delay.[11,12,28-32,34]
7. Low molecular weight Dextran®.[4,28]
8. Heparin®.[20,35]
9. Hyperbaric oxygen therapy.[36]
10. Vasodilators.[1,4,28]

During the past years we have performed a number of studies on animal models with artificially induced ME pressure changes in order to determine its influence on ME and IE function and morphology.[5,6,37-41]

From the Department of Otolaryngology, University of Washington School of Medicine, Seattle.
REPRINTS — Josef M. Miller, PhD, Department of Otolaryngology, RL-30, University of Washington School of Medicine, Seattle, WA 98195.

Our investigations extended our information on pressure induced changes in the ME and confirmed that ME changes, as noted above, were similar for the experimental animal and patients with clinical barotrauma. However, no such similarity was found for the experimental animal and man in regard to cochlear changes. Inner ear membrane distortions and hemorrhage were often demonstrated in our experimental animals while seldom observed in man. Little evidence for RW rupture was found in the experimental animal. A study of RW healing following surgical lesion under aseptic conditions in the guinea pig indicates that the autorepair properties of the RW are impressive in this species.[41] Such data may be interpreted to encourage some delay in surgical treatment of clinical cases with IE barotrauma. However, the healing properties of the RW membrane in the guinea pig and man may differ substantially.

In previous studies no information is provided of the residual and potentially lasting effects of ME pressure changes. It would be of interest to establish the possible histopathological sequelae related to the acutely observed IE membrane distortion and hemorrhage. Also we would like to know if RW membrane healing occurs as readily in the presence of other chronic ME and IE pathology accompanying barotrauma as it does following surgical lesions. In the present study an attempt was made to answer these questions by examining the long-term effects of phasic ME pressure changes in a guinea pig animal model. In this investigation the ME and IE of the experimental subjects were evaluated following a three-week recovery after exposure to a phasic ME pressure.

METHODS

Twenty healthy young guinea pigs (250-300 g) were used in this study. All subjects demonstrated a normal Preyer's reflex. For each subject, randomly one ear was designated as a control and one experimental. Similarly, each animal was assigned to one of four groups, in which the experimental ear was exposed to one of four pressure values, + / − 3000 or 6000 mm H_2O.

Surgical and pressurization procedures were similar to those previously reported.[6] The animals were initially weighed, premedicated with atropine and anesthetized with ketamine. After shaving and preparing the periauricular areas for surgery, a postauricular approach was used to expose the ME bilaterally. The bone defect created in the bulla permitted limited inspection of the ME. The drum and the ME of each subject were examined for infection. Animals with fluid, vessel injection, thickened mucosa or distortion and discoloration of the TM were eliminated.

Following inspection, a Teflon® cannula, 2 mm in diameter, was inserted 1-2 mm into the bulla of the experimental ear, and sealed with bone wax. The cannula was then coupled to a pressurization system and a brief (1-2 seconds) phasic pressure change was applied. The system was controlled by a manually operated valve. Maximum pressure for a given setting and rate of change was approximately constant across animals. Duration of the pressure change varied by up to 25%. Following pressurization of the experimental ear, the cannula was placed in the control ear, sealed and then removed.

In both ears the surgical area was irrigated with a topical antibiotic, the bone defect sealed with bone wax and the soft tissue incision closed with interrupted sutures. Body temperature of each subject was maintained with a heat lamp until recovery from the anesthesia. Animals were placed on chloramphenicol (IM) for ten days following surgery. The subjects were sacrificed three weeks postsurgery. The animals were deeply anesthetized with sodium pentobarbital anesthesia, decapitated and their temporal bones were removed. At the time of removal, the external and ME were inspected with the aid of an operating microscope for soft tissue changes, including vessel distortion and rupture, and the presence of effusions. In the process the ME was widely exposed. Following assessment, the bones were placed in formalin for fixation followed by further histological processing of the inner ear.

The temporal bones were then decalcified in 10% Versene® (dibasic salt of EDTA). The solution was changed daily. The cochleas of three subjects from each group were then assigned for soft-surface preparation.[42,43] Briefly, following decalcification, the soft surface preparation included: apicobasal bisection of the cochlea, staining with buffered 0.5% osmic acid, dehydration in increasing concentrations of alcohol, transfer to glycerin and dissection of the membranous labyrinth for further microscopic studies. The remaining two subjects of each group were processed by celloidin embedding and serial paramodiolar sectioning.[44] Every tenth section was saved. Alternate sections were stained with Harris' hematoxylin and eosin and cresyl violet.

A second assessment of the ME was made with the aid of the operating microscope in the soft-surface preparation material at the time of bisection of the cochlea and staining. In all cases the animals were coded at the time of surgery (for value of the exposure and which ear was exposed). This information was not available at the time of temporal bone removal and initial inspection nor at the time of subsequent ME and IE study. The subsequent examinations were performed by another author with no knowledge of the results of the first examination. Individual observations were kept separate in coded form until completion of the IE study. The initial and second ME evaluation included assessment of TM change, mucosal changes, presence of fluids, and hemorrhage, vessel distention, perivascular hemorrhage and RW perforations. Other IE changes evaluated included pathology of the organ of Corti, endolymphatic and perilymphatic hemorrhage and the occurrence of infection.

RESULTS

One animal, in the + 6000 mm H_2O group, died 20 days following surgery. In all others recovery appeared uneventful.

Middle Ear Effects. Major ME findings are shown in Table 1. The major change of concern in the TM was occurrence of perforations. These were most prevalent in animals exposed to high negative pressures, were found equally often in animals exposed to low negative and high positive pressures and absent in those exposed to low positive pressure. Thickened drum membranes were observed in association with mucosal thickening throughout the ME. Similarly, vessel distention in the TM and hemorrhage were consistent with similar findings elsewhere in the ME mucosa.

A thickened ME mucosa was also found most frequently in animals exposed to high negative pressure. High positive pressure was second in influence, low positive third in effect, and low negative pressure ineffective. The occurrence of serosanguineous fluid in the ME space was related

TABLE 1. MIDDLE EAR PATHOLOGY

Applied Pressure mm H_2O	*Total No. Ears*	*TM[1] Perforation*	*ME & TM Thickened Mucosa*	*Serosanguineous Fluid*	*ME & TM Vessel Distention & Hemorrhage*
+ 6000	4/4*	1/0	3/2	3/2	4/0
+ 3000	5/5	0/0	2/1	2/0	3/0
– 3000	5/5	1/0	0/0	1/0	0/0
– 6000	5/5	3/0	4/2	4/2	3/1

ME - Middle ear; TM - Tympanic membrane.

*Experimental/control.

to magnitude and direction of pressure in the same manner.

Tympanic membrane perforation, mucosal thickening and presence of serosanguineous fluid were more frequently observed following high negative pressure than following high positive pressure. In turn, high positive pressure was more influential than lower pressure values. The greatest vascular changes occurred with high positive pressure. In the case of all pathological findings, except for vessel distention and hemorrhage in the high positive pressure group, some normal cases were found in experimental ears.

Middle ear infection was identified by the presence of purulent secretion. Nine of the 19 experimental ears exhibited infection. In these ears, serosanguineous fluid was a consistent finding. In the 10 animals without infection, 1 exhibited a small amount of serosanguineous fluid and 5 exhibited some serous fluid. These six ears were all exposed to negative pressure. No fluid was found in the remaining four experimental ears which were all exposed to positive pressure. Infections were also observed in 5 of the 19 control ears, in most cases associated with serosanguineous effusion. In no instance was a control ear infection associated with a TM perforation. In one case, however, specific vascular hemorrhage was observed.

Pathology in experimental and control ears independent of direction and magnitude of applied pressure is illustrated in Figure 1. The height of the unshaded bar illustrates the percent occurrence of pathology in the control ears. Figure 2 shows a comparison of the percent occurrence of pathology in animals exposed to ± 6000 mm H_2O versus those exposed to the lower pressure value. Both experimental (unshaded) and control findings (shaded) are illustrated. Note that in all cases there is an increase in percent pathology with the higher pressures. An increase in occurrence of pathology also occurred in the control ears except for TM perforations. No control ear exhibited this pathology.

Inner Ear Effects. Inner ear findings were comparable in the material processed with either of our two histological techniques. Thus the data for each have been combined for the purposes of this report. Five of nine ears exposed to 6000 mm H_2O exhibited RW perforations. Three were exposed to positive pressure, two to negative pressure. One animal exposed to + 3000 mm H_2O also had a perforation. Round window perforations were not found in control ears. In the experimental ears these perforations were always observed in animals with ME infections. In these ears, labyrinthitis was a consistent finding.

Lymphatic hemorrhage was observed in 58% of

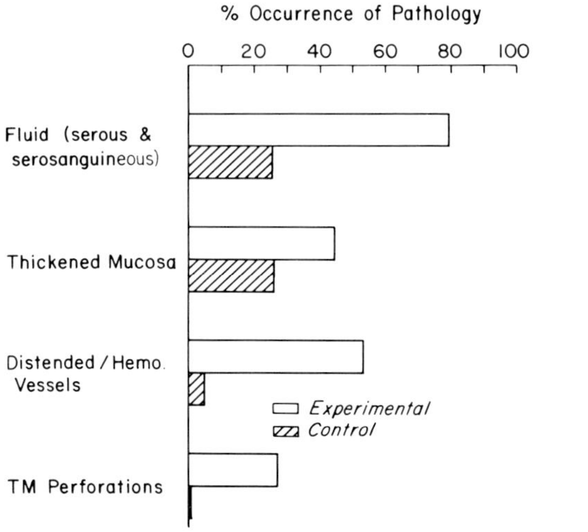

Fig. 1. Frequency of middle ear pathological findings in all experimental and all controlled animals. Hemo -Hemorrhagic; TM - Tympanic membrane.

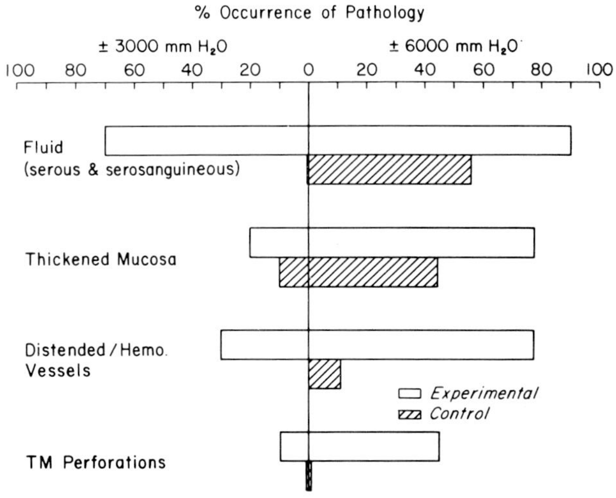

Fig. 2. Frequency of pathological observations in high (+/– 6000 mm H_2O) versus low (+/– 3000 mm H_2O) pressure subjects. Observations in both controlled and experimental ears are shown.

TABLE 2. OCCURRENCE OF PERILYMPHATIC HEMORRHAGE

Applied Pressure mm H_2O	*Total No. Ears*	*Total No. Ears with Hemorrhage*
+ 6000	4	4
+ 3000	5	3
− 3000	5	1
− 6000	5	3

the experimental ears studied. In assessing this pathology, hemorrhage located at the extreme basal end of the scala tympani was excluded.* Lymphatic hemorrhage was related to both magnitude and direction of the applied pressure change (Table 2). Hemorrhage was most frequent with high positive pressure (100%), second in prevalence with high negative and low positive pressures (60%), and least common with low negative pressure (20%). In the control ears, lymphatic hemorrhage (excluding that in the extreme basal end of the scala tympani) was observed in one ear, in the scala vestibuli contralateral to a − 6000 mm H_2O exposed ear.

The presence of endolymphatic hydrops was evaluated in each ear. It was observed in 10 of 19 experimental ears (53%) and 4 of 19 control ears (21%). It was not related in any consistent manner to the magnitude or direction of pressure applied in the experimental ears. In three of the four control ears it was, however, associated with ME infection. In the experimental material endolymphatic hydrops was observed in association with ME infection in three of the ten ears.

DISCUSSION

The principal long-term changes in the ME which appeared directly related to magnitude and direction of applied phasic ME pressure were: 1) TM perforation, 2) vessel distention and hemorrhage, 3) serous effusion, and 4) perhaps mucosal thickening. The interpretation of ME pathology resulting from applied pressure is complicated by the influence of infection. Since serosanguineous effusions occurred frequently in control ears, their occurrence in experimental ears cannot be attributed solely to the applied pressure. The observation that the frequency of this finding was not greatly increased in ears exposed to the higher pressures (6000 mm H_2O) as opposed to the lower values (3000 mm H_2O) is consistent with this interpretation. The finding of mucosal changes more frequently in the high than in the low pressure groups may indicate that pressure changes may be of etiological significance for this pathology. However, the small sample size employed in this study condition the interpretation of this change also. The increase in frequency of effusions and thickened mucosa in control ears of high pressure exposed animals, as compared to low pressure exposures, is in part related to the fortuitous distribution of infection in the control material. However, such differences in control ear pathology of high and low exposed animals was also reported acutely.[6] Thus, infection cannot solely account for this observation. Alternative physiological mechanisms were discussed previously.[6]

The observation of serous effusion only in negative pressure ears and without relation to infection indicates that this effusion is dependent upon pressure. Similarly, the occurrence of perforations, vessel distention and hemorrhage were all related to high pressures. These pathologies were minimal or absent in control ears. This indicates that pressure was the primary causative factor in producing these changes. While the small sample size used in this study restricts interpretation of findings, this may be overcome by the consistency of findings in the present study with those found immediately following phasic pressure.[6] Our interpretation regarding TM perforation, effusions and vessel changes are consistent with the acute findings of the previous study. High negative pressure most frequently caused effusions and TM perforations. Vascular damage was most frequent with high positive pressure changes. The bases for these effects were discussed previously.

In general, the current observations are qualitatively similar to those found in the acute ear. Quantitatively, there are some marked differences. In both cases we have observed that the damage to ME and IE structures appears related to magnitude of applied pressure. Obviously, this is a baseline observation that must be made or reservations should and would be raised regarding the entire approach of these studies. Comparing present findings to those following acute pressure exposure it appears that the ME has remarkable healing abilities. In the absence of infection following three weeks recovery, little hemorrhage is found in the ME and indeed the occurrence of hemorrhage in the IE is much reduced from that observed in the acute preparation. Tympanic membrane rupture was much less commonly found in this material than in the acutely studied material. In part this may reflect healing processes of the drum membrane.

In the previous acute study one instance of RW membrane rupture was observed. In this investigation 25% of the exposed ears exhibited RW rupture. Among the animals exposed to the higher pressures this occurrence was almost 50%. It was consistently found in the presence of ME infection. Given the observation of both the previous acute study and the current chronic study it would appear that ME infection is a necessary but not sufficient condition for RW rupture. The presence of unobserved very small or microscopic RW perforations in some of the previous material cannot be excluded. We suggest that phasic high pressure exposure of the ME of the guinea pig does influence the RW. Moreover, it would appear that ME infection interacts with the

*This finding, basal turn scala tympani hemorrhage, probably reflects the histological procedures employed in removal of the temporal bones.[6]

trauma caused by the pressure change to create a perforation. This study indicates that the rapid healing of the guinea pig RW membrane observed following surgical lesion[41] is inhibited by the presence of infection. The time course of these events would be of interest in defining mechanisms involved.

Generalization of these results to man must of course be done with caution. In the previous acute study of phasic pressure,[6] the absence of RW perforations we interpreted to suggested hesitation in performing ME surgery for RW perforations in man following barotrauma. If ME infection may be associated with barotrauma in man, these current data support the view that the RW may indeed require "sealing." Certainly other IE pathology observed in these animals, particularly the exclusive occurrence of labyrinthitis in RW ruptured ears, reinforce this concern.

ACKNOWLEDGMENT — We wish to acknowledge the excellent histological preparations of serially sectioned material used in this investigation by Mrs. Judith E. Miller.

REFERENCES

1. Edmonds C, Thomas RL. Medical aspects of diving, part 3. Med J Aust 1972; 2:1300-4.

2. Haines HL, Harris JD. Aerotitis media in submariners. Ann Otol Rhinol Laryngol 1946; 55:347-71.

3. Fields JA. Skin diving, its physiological and otolaryngological aspects. Arch Otolaryngol 1958; 68:531-41.

4. Compere WE. Otolaryngologic problems encountered in scuba divers. ORL Digest 1974; 36:21-8.

5. Lamkin R, Axelsson A, McPherson D, Miller J. Experimental aural barotrauma: electrophysiological and morphological findings. Acta Otolaryngol (Stockh) 1975; Suppl 335:1-24.

6. Axelsson A, Miller J, Silverman M. Anatomical effects of sudden middle ear pressure changes. Ann Otol Rhinol Laryngol 1979; 88:368-76.

7. Vail HH. Traumatic conditions of the ear in workers in an atmosphere of compressed air. Arch Otolaryngol 1929; 10:113-26.

8. Bayliss GJA. Aural barotrauma in naval divers. Arch Otolaryngol 1968; 88:49-55.

9. Beasly JW. Inner ear damage due to barotrauma. Wis Med J 1974; 73:143-5.

10. Gregg JB, Ferrell MR. Cochlear and vestibular damage from middle ear pressure change. EENT Month 1967; 46:464-70.

11. Goodhill V. Sudden deafness and round window rupture. Laryngoscope 1971; 8:1462-74.

12. Goodhill V, Brockman SJ, Harris I, Hantz O. Sudden deafness and labyrinthine window ruptures. Ann Otol Rhinol Laryngol 1973; 82:2-12.

13. Azem K, Caldarelli MD. Sudden conductive hearing loss following sneezing. Arch Otolaryngol 1973; 97:413-4.

14. Simmons FB. Theory of membrane breaks in sudden hearing loss. Arch Otolaryngol 1968; 88:41-8.

15. Eichel BS, Landes BS. Sensorineural hearing loss caused by skin diving. Arch Otolaryngol 1970; 92:128-31.

16. Freeman P, Edmonds C. Inner ear barotrauma. Arch Otolaryngol 1972; 95:556-63.

17. Harker LA, Norante JD, Ryu JH. Experimental rupture of the round window membrane. Trans Am Acad Ophthalmol Otolaryngol 1974; 78:ORL 448-52.

18. Heller R, Mager W, Schrotter HV. Luftdruckerkrankungen. Wien: Alfred Holder, 1900.

19. Hill L. Caisson sickness and the physiology of work in compressed air. New York: Longmans Green & Co, 1921:61-85.

20. McCormick JG, Philbrick T, Holland W, Harrill JA. Diving induced sensorineural deafness: prophylactic use of Heparin and preliminary histopathology results. Laryngoscope 1973; 83:1483-501.

21. Pullen FW. Round window membrane rupture: a cause of sudden deafness. Trans Am Acad Ophthalmol Otolaryngol 1972; 76:1444-50.

22. Schuknecht HF, Gacek RR. Surgery on only hearing ears. Trans Am Acad Ophthalmol Otolaryngol 1973; 77:257-66.

23. Freeman P. Inner ear barotrauma. Arch Otolaryngol 1973; 97:429.

24. Edmonds C, Freeman P, Tonkin J. Fistula of the round window in diving. Trans Am Acad Ophthalmol Otolaryngol 1974; 78:444-7.

25. Freeman P, Tonkin J, Edmonds C. Rupture of the round window membrane in inner ear barotrauma. Arch Otolaryngol 1974; 99:437-42.

26. Healy GB, Strong S, Sampogna D. Ataxia, vertigo and hearing loss. Arch Otolaryngol 1974; 100:130-5.

27. Nedzelski NM, Barber HO. Round window fistula. J Otolaryngol 1976; 5:379-85.

28. Grossenbacher R. Pathologie des runden Fensters bei akuter Ertaubung. HNO 1976; 24:227-32.

29. Molvaer OI, Eidsvik S. Dykking og skade av det indre oyret. Tidsskr Nor Laegeforen 1978; 5:263-5.

30. Simmons FB. Fluid dynamics in sudden sensorineural hearing loss. Otolaryngol Clin North Am 1978; 11:55-61.

31. Fraser JG, Garborow PC. Labyrinthine window rupture. J Laryngol Otol 1975; 89:1-7.

32. Goodhill V. Labyrinthine membrane ruptures in sudden sensorineural hearing loss. Proc R Soc Med 1976; 69:565-72.

33. Farmer JC. Diving injuries to the inner ear. Ann Otol Rhinol Laryngol 1977; 86 Suppl 36:1-20.

34. Taylor PH, Bicknell PG. Rupture of the round window membrane. Ann Otol Rhinol Laryngol 1976; 85:105-10.

35. McCormick JG, Holland WB, Brauer RW, Holleman IL. Sudden hearing loss due to diving and its prevention with Heparin. Otolaryngol Clin North Am 1975; 8:417-30.

36. Appaix A, Demard F. Oxygenotherapie hyperbare of swidiles brutales de perception. Rev Laryngol Otol Rhinol (Bord) 1970; 91:951-72.

37. McPherson DL, Miller JM. Effects of middle ear pressure on the auditory periphery. J Acoust Soc Am 1974; 55:62-3.

38. Miller JM, McPherson DL, Axelsson A. Electrophysiological and morphological effects of middle ear pressure changes in the guinea pig. XII International Congress in Audiology, Paris, 1974.

39. McPherson D, Miller J, Axelsson A. Middle ear pressure: effects on the auditory periphery. J Acoust Soc Am 1976; 59:136-42.

40. Miller J, Donaldson J. Primate model for studies of clinical problems of middle ear function. Ann Otol Rhinol Laryngol 1976; 85 Suppl 25:194-201.

41. Axelsson A, Hallen O, Miller J, McPherson DL. Experimentally induced round window membrane lesions. Acta Otolaryngol (Stockh) 1977; 84:1-11.

42. Axelsson A, Vertes D. Methodological aspects of some inner ear vascular techniques. Acta Otolaryngol (Stockh) 1979, in press.

43. Axelsson A, Miller J. Larsson B. A modified "soft-surface-specimen-technique" for examination of the inner ear. Acta Otolaryngol (Stockh) 1975; 80:362-75.

44. Gussen R, Ward PH. Preparation of the temporal bone for histological study. In: Smith C, Vernon J, eds. Handbook of auditory and vestibular research methods. Springfield: Charles C Thomas, 1976:53-71.

≈

OMISSION

In Volume 89, November-December 1980, the following references were inadvertently omitted from page 533 of the article by M. I. Singer, MD, and E. D. Blom, PhD, *An Endoscopic Technique for Restoration of Voice After Laryngectomy*:

15. Griffiths CM, Love JT. Neoglottic reconstruction after total laryngectomy: a preliminary report. Ann Otol Rhinol Laryngol 1978; 87:180-4.

16. Taub S, Bergner LH. Air bypass voice prosthesis for vocal rehabilitation of laryngectomees. Am J Surg 1973; 125:748-56.

17. Singer MI, Blom ED. Tracheoesophageal puncture: a surgical prosthetic method for postlaryngectomy speech restoration. Third International Symposium Plas Reconstr Surg Head Neck, 1979.

18. Blom ED, Singer MI. Surgical prosthetic approaches for postlaryngectomy voice restoration. In: Keith RL, Darley FL, eds. Laryngectomy rehabilitation. Houston: College Hill Press, 1979:251-76.

19. Conley JJ. Vocal rehabilitation by autogenous vein graft. Ann Otol Rhinol Laryngol 1959; 68:990-5.

CUSTOMIZED DILATOR FOR THE TREATMENT OF SUBGLOTTIC STENOSIS IN CHILDREN

NIGEL R. T. PASHLEY, MB, FRCS(C)
ANN ARBOR, MICHIGAN

A new instrument, a customized dilator for use in dilating subglottic stenosis in children, is described. It combines the desirable features of the bougie for use in the laryngeal subglottis and will be useful to any surgeon involved in the treatment of these difficult airway problems in children.

Interest in the treatment of acquired subglottic stenosis in children has increased with recent advances in neonatology. These advances have improved the survival rate of very small preterm infants, many of whom require prolonged ventilatory support. However, there has been a concomitant increase in the incidence of acquired airway damage and the site of injury in these susceptible children is almost invariably the cricoid region.[1]

Treatments include primary dilation or bougienage sometimes combined with topical or injected medications, surgical resection or reconstruction, and simple cricoidotomy.[2] Following surgical reconstruction of the area and prior to a growth phase which may, as recently reported,[1] compensate for the scar contracture and allow for decannulation, it may be desirable to dilate the region. Dilation of the subglottic region is therefore a commonly used surgical adjunct as well as a primary therapy.

The use of a rigid bronchoscope for dilation may not provide the gentle graded sizes required, and so dilators or bougies have been used. The desired properties of such a dilator are suitable cross-sectional shape, graded sizes, a flexible but firm consistency to prevent an inadvertent tear or perforation, and a suitable length and shaft configuration commensurate with performance of the dilation under direct vision.

Dilation of the laryngeal subglottis in children was found to require an instrument of circular cross-sectional shape with a working length of 30 cm. In conjunction with the Pilling Company an instrument was designed with all the desirable features, at a low cost due to the combination of features taken from existing standard instruments (Fig. 1).

A circular cross-sectional shape of firm but flexible material with a flexible narrow shaft was obtained by use of a Jackson esophageal bougie. The shaft was shortened 30 cm from the tip and a handle, angled downward, was added. This allowed direct vision and placement of the bougie during endoscopy.

A full range of sizes was not required because of the anticipated use in children. These dilators are used solely through an anterior commissure laryngoscope which separates the vocal cords and precludes injury or dislocation of the glottic structures.

This type of dilator has been in use ten months and has earned praiseworthy comment from all who previously struggled with the straight-shafted excessively long instrument. We highly recommend such modifications to those engaged in the stressful treatment of these difficult airway problems in children.

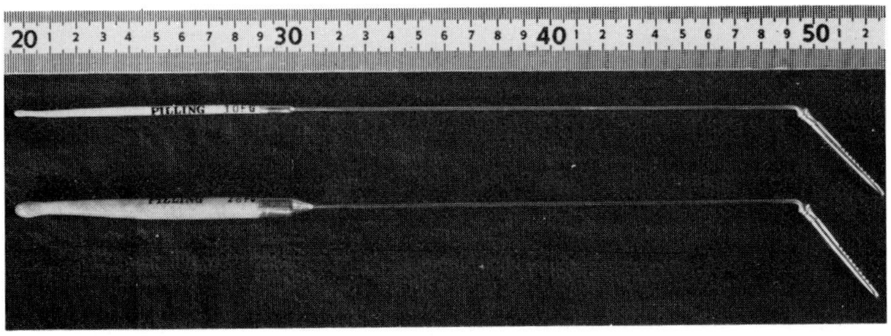

Fig. 1. A customized dilator for the laryngeal subglottis. A shortened shaft has been joined to the gum elastic tip of a Jackson esophageal bougie giving an overall length of 30 cm. The down-angled hand piece from microlaryngoscopy instruments is joined to the shaft and allows an unobscured view while dilation is performed.

REFERENCES

1. Pashley NRT, Papsidero MJ. Acquired stenosis of the upper airway in neonates. An increasing problem. Ann Otol Rhinol Laryngol 1980; 89:512-4.

2. Cotton RT, Seid AB. Management of the extubation problem in the premature child: anterior cricoid split as an alternative to tracheotomy. Ann Otol Rhinol Laryngol 1980; 89:508-11.

From the Department of Otorhinolaryngology, University of Michigan Hospitals, Ann Arbor.

REPRINTS — Nigel R. T. Pashley, MB, Department of Otorhinolaryngology, University of Michigan Hospitals, 1405 East Ann Street, Ann Arbor, MI 48109.

Ann Otol 90:1981

OTOLARYNGIC OSTEOPATHOLOGY IN 14th CENTURY MID-AMERICA
THE CROW CREEK MASSACRE

JOHN B. GREGG, MD
SIOUX FALLS, SOUTH DAKOTA

JAMES P. STEELE, MD
SIOUX FALLS, SOUTH DAKOTA

LARRY ZIMMERMAN, PhD
VERMILLION, SOUTH DAKOTA

HELEN FERWERDA, RTR
YANKTON, SOUTH DAKOTA

PAULINE S. GREGG, RN
SIOUX FALLS, SOUTH DAKOTA

Over 486 people were massacred and buried communally at the Crow Creek Village Site, South Dakota, about 1350 AD. Osseous pathology in the craniofacial area of the victims' skeletons is reviewed and compared to data from other indigenous skeletal populations past and present. The Crow Creek mastoid x-rays are analyzed and compared to four other studies which span over 1000 years of Dakota Territory history. Findings regarding external auditory canal exostoses in the different groups are compared. Unusual findings in the craniofacial area are assessed. Insight into longitudinal epidemiology in one portion of the U.S. is possible through this study.

Two years ago an opportunity was presented to study briefly the remnants of people who died calamitously in a village which existed in South Dakota during the 14th century. Their skeletons were exposed accidentally by erosion into the Missouri River banks at a former village site. Subsequent investigation revealed the magnitude of a horrible massacre (Fig. 1). The investigation of the mass burial included an assessment of the cultural factors, a demographic analysis, and an appraisal of the bones for evidence of pathology.[1]

VIGNETTE OF CROW CREEK HISTORY AND CULTURE

Carbon datings to the years 1325 and 1390 AD indicate that the Crow Creek (CC) villagers were culturally of the initial coalescent variant, ancestral to the Arikara who lived later in the Dakotas along the Missouri River. They descended from groups which were forced out of the Central Plains by drought and had blended with people already living along the river. They were farmers (corn, beans, squash) and hunters, primarily of bison. Villages similar to CC dot the banks of the Missouri River for many miles upstream.

The CC site (39 BF 11), situated on the bluff overlooking the river 13 miles north of Chamberlain, SD, was first excavated during the Missouri River salvage archeology by the Nebraska Historical Society in the mid-1950s. The site, now a National Historical Landmark, was protected on its north boundary by a fortification ditch 4 m wide and 380 m long. A log palisade had been inside the ditch. The true situation had not been found in the late 1950s because the west end of the ditch was not excavated.

Almost every skull of all ages and both sexes bore markings of scalping. Two adult calvaria had evidence of severe periostitis etched into their external surfaces, the patterns strongly suggesting nonlethal scalping long before death of the individuals. Many skulls had recent fractures, most of which could have represented the death blow. The type of skull fracture usually reflected the characteristics of the weapon which had inflicted it. Decapitation pry-marks were present on the basal portion of 33 skulls and 88 upper cervical vertebrae, and cut marks were present on many other bones. Hand bones were almost totally absent and the majority of the foot bones were missing, presumably amputated as trophies or chewed away by carnivores. Although there were over 700 articulations of two or more bones, mostly the skeletons were disrupted. A few bones were burned, suggesting incineration of some bodies. The archeological finding that soil which covered the decedents came from the river bottom quite some distance from the burial site indicated purposeful interment of the massacre victims, possibly by the survivors of the catastrophe.

Although the exact circumstances of this situation are conjectural, it is likely that it was perpetrated by inhabitants of a nearby village, probably of the same culture. Undoubtedly a large force attacked CC. Conceivably the massacre was facilitated by a night-time attack or some communal illness which impaired the villagers' ability to fight or flee. Because many CC skulls had findings suggesting

From the School of Medicine, University of South Dakota, Sioux Falls; the Department of Anthropology, University of South Dakota, Vermillion; and X-Ray Department, Sacred Heart Hospital, Yankton, South Dakota. Financial support was provided by the Grant Review Committee, School of Medicine, University of South Dakota. Crow Creek material was recovered under contract: U. S. Army Corps of Engineers, Omaha District.

REPRINTS — John B. Gregg, MD, 2807 S. Phillips Ave., Sioux Falls, SD 57105.

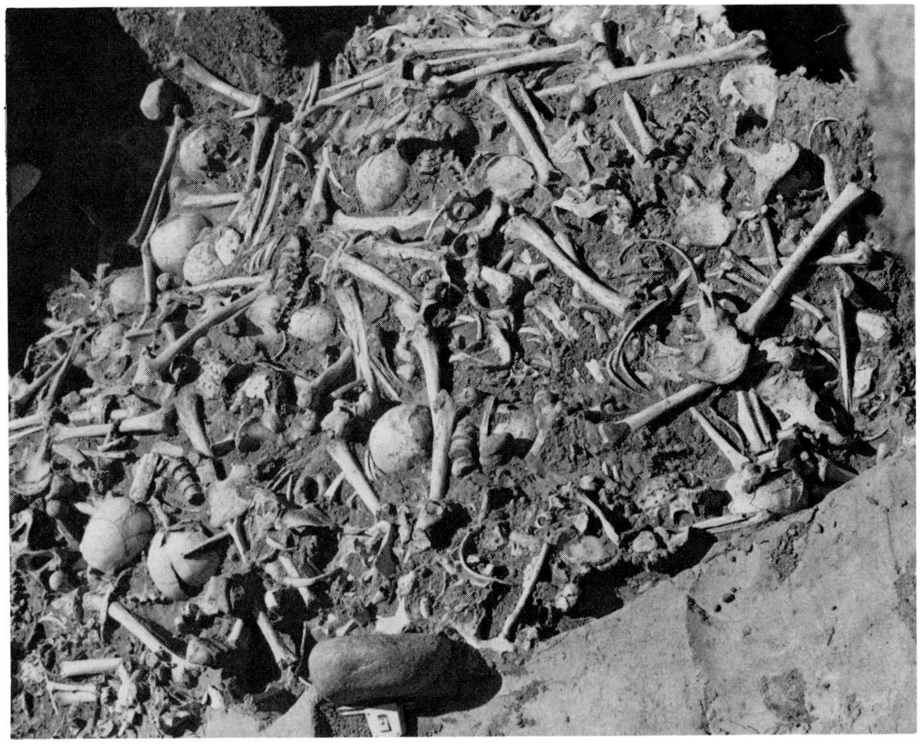

Fig. 1. Overview of the mass burial showing the intermingling of skeletons and the dismembered conditions of remnants.

iron deficiency anemia and many long bones had transverse lines, a viable hypothesis is that warfare followed a disturbance in the food supply.

The temporal bone count of 963 (486 right, 477 left) provided the most accurate estimate of the number of individuals whose skeletons had been exhumed (Table 1). Examination of the CC temporal bones and x-rays of them provided information concerning the frequency and patterns of some otological abnormalities in these people. Through cautious extrapolation between the otological findings and the frequency of other findings in the craniofacial area, estimates concerning other diseases can be made.

OTOLOGICAL FINDINGS

Mastoid Changes Indicating Residua of Otitis Media (Table 2). Law and Stenvers views were taken of 867 temporal bones so as to be comparable with previous skull x-ray studies.[2,3] To promote consistent interpretation, the CC films were evaluated by the same radiologist-otolaryngologist team which had participated in other mastoid projects, and interpreted as *pneumatic, sclerotic, diploic*, or *mixed.* Bilateral mastoid x-rays of 148 of 385 children at the Indian School, Pierre, SD, served as contemporaneous controls for all of the dry bone studies.[4] The fundamental denominator in the total temporal bone project is *a common geographic location.*

Five hundred sixteen (61%) CC mastoids were well pneumatized indicating little effect attributable to upper respiratory infections (URI) or otitis media; 26 (3%) were sclerotic, indicating alteration from otitis media during early life; 242 (29%) showed mixed type air cell patterns suggesting some effect of middle ear disease; and 53 (7%) had diploic or atypical air cells, possibly indicative of otitis media during early life. Two adult mastoids had osteolytic lesions commensurate with cholesteatoma formation (0.2%). Because the frequency of otitis media correlates with the incidence of URI, it is hypothesized that URI during childhood were frequent at CC.

Notably there were fewer CC mastoids with disturbed air cell patterns than in other dry bone mastoid series and a closer statistical relationship of the CC mastoids to the Pierre Indian School children. The smaller amount of mastoid alteration in the Pierre children undoubtedly reflects better socioeconomic conditions. Because the CC people antedated white contact and were not exposed to many of the "herd-type diseases" from Europe, they may have had fewer and less virulent URI than those who lived later. It is interesting that the number of mastoids interpreted as *sclerotic* was *very similar* in all five temporal bone series despite the tremendous

TABLE 1. MINIMUM ELEMENT COUNTS OF MAJOR BONES[1]

Bone	*Left*	*Right*
Temporal, petrous	477	486
Humerus	200	213
Ulna	113	131
Radius	91	115
Femur	367	367
Tibia	262	269
Fibula	143	156

TABLE 2. MASTOID AIR CELL DEVELOPMENT AS SEEN ON X-RAYS OF TEMPORAL BONES

	No. of Bones	Pneumatic No.	%	Sclerotic No.	%	Mixed No.	%	Atypical No.	%
Crow Creek (Proto-Arikara)	837	516	61	26	3	242	29	53	7
W.H. Over Collection* (mixed cultures)	417	220	53	26	6	157	38	14	3
Sully Site (Arikara)	255	116	45.5	12	4.5	92	36	35	14
U.S. National Museum (Sioux)	257	128	50	8	3.1	67	26	54	21
Pierre Indian School (Sioux)†	296	210	71	9	3	35	12	42	14
Total	2,062								

*88 burials (50 temporal bones) were of Middle Plains Woodland origin. Of these 4 were sclerotic, 33 mixed, and 1 was of diploic configuration.
†Children at the Pierre Indian School, located about two miles southeast of Pierre, SD.

differences in time, culture, and socioeconomic conditions represented in this total study. A second significant finding from the x-ray studies is that the frequency of *mixed* mastoid air cell changes has varied during the past 1,000 years, being lowest in today's Indian children. This could indicate that despite the fact that otitis media is *the commonest infection in the upper Midwest today*, second only to the "common cold," it does not affect the air cell development as much now as it did in the past.

Stapes Footplate Fixation. Based upon the demographic data from 332 identifiable CC skeletons (Table 3), 54% of the 486 skeletons, 263 individuals (142 males, 121 females), should have been over 15 years of age at death. If otosclerotic stapes fixation had existed at CC in the same ratio it occurs in U.S. whites today, two instances might have been present. None was found. This agrees with previous studies of ancient Indian temporal bones.[5]

Exostoses and Osteomas (Table 4). Exostoses were found in the external auditory canals of 45 CC temporal bones (4.7%). This is similar to the findings in other upper Missouri River basin (UMRB) skeletons[6] and supports our previous contention that outer ear canal exostoses are *much less frequent* in the Dakotas than was reported in Hrdlicka.[7] Figure 2 shows an unusual exostosis. X-rays of this temporal bone were normal otherwise. Similar, less-marked changes in the tympanic ring bone have been reported in UMRB specimens.[6] One osteoma was found in the squamous portion of a temporal bone.

TABLE 3. SMOOTHED DISTRIBUTION OF CROW CREEK AGES AT DEATH[1]

Age (yr)	Males	Females	Total
0- 1	5	4	9
1- 4	16	16	32
5- 9	36	35	71
10-14	20	20	40
15-19	22	7	29
20-24	21	7	28
25-29	16	7	23
30-34	15	7	22
35-39	4	7	11
40-44	3	8	11
45-49	4	13	17
50-54	7	13	20
55-59	6	13	19
Total	175	157	332

Anomalous Styloid Process. A massive styloid process on the right side and a smaller but larger-than-usual process on the left was found in an adult skull (Fig. 3). X-rays showed no other abnormality.

DENTAL DISEASES

Temporomandibular Joint Alterations. Eight instances of marked temporomandibular joint (TMJ) arthritis were found. Other instances of lesser mandible and mandibular fossa changes were present. The combination of high carbohydrate diet, food processing methods, and ingestion of coarse, tough foods, fostered early deterioration and loss of teeth. This was followed by TMJ changes, similar to those which are seen frequently in other UMRB skeletons.

Tooth Wear and Attrition. In 136 instances involving three or more attached teeth there was moderate to severe attrition of teeth, caries, and frequently tooth pulp exposure. The latter was undeniably a precursor to tooth loss. There were 17 dental abscesses and one abscess apparently of dental origin on the posterior surface of the maxilla. Four antral-oral fistulae and several other tooth abscesses which were forming communications between the maxillary sinus and the mouth were

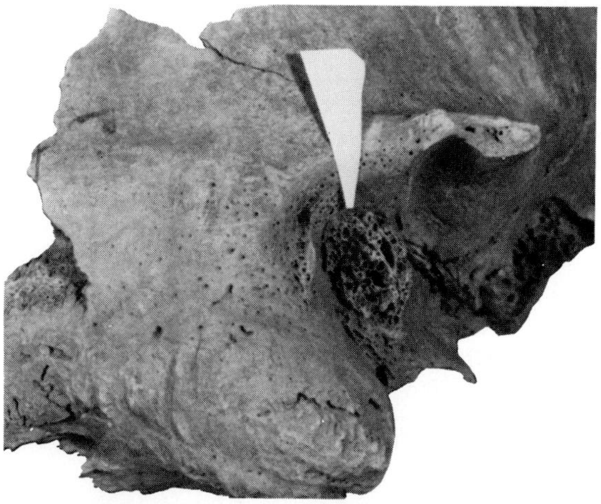

Fig. 2. Spongy bone tumor (arrow) which almost completely occludes an adult right external auditory canal.

TABLE 4. EXOSTOSES IN EXTERNAL AUDITORY CANALS, DAKOTA TERRITORY TEMPORAL BONES

Culture	*Temporal Bones*	*Right Ear*	*Left Ear*	*Bilateral*	*% with Exostoses*
Crow Creek (Proto-Arikara)	963	7	12	26	4.6
Arikara	993	2	5	7	2.1
Arikara-Mandan	50			3	12.2
Mandan	79			2	5.1
Woodland	87	1			1.1
Historic Sioux	301		2	1	1.3
Undetermined	380	1	6	7	5.5
Total	2853	11	25	46	2.9
Pierre Indian School children, Grades K through 12, primarily Sioux	770	None	None	None	None
Overall total	3623	11	25	46	2.25

found. Figure 4 shows an unusual antral-oral fistula. Bone changes within the maxillary sinuses suggesting the effects of long-standing infection were visible in the antral-oral fistula specimens and in one other specimen.

Dental Anomalies. In 11 adult skulls there were anomalies which included anodontia, ectopic, supernumerary, unerupted, and fused teeth, all similar to findings in other UMRB burials.

CRANIOFACIAL ANOMALIES

As they have been in other UMRB skeletons, overt anomalies were conspicuous by their absence. This contradicts today's UMRB findings. Congenital facial clefting was found in 1:220 in a large series of South Dakota native American children[8] and in 1:276 Montana Indian births.[9] Occult palate defects (submucous clefts and bifid uvulas) in South Dakota Indians added to the manifest clefts gave a combined incidence of 1:89.[8] Although it cannot be demonstrated, it is probable that congenital facial clefting did exist in the UMRB in the past. Very likely, children born with disabling congenital anomalies in ancient primitive societies were eliminated by natural means or passive neglect and their bodies did not get into the community cemetery. This hypothesis offers the most plausible explanation for the absence of congenital anomalies which would have been obvious at birth in the CC and other UMRB skeletons.

Two mandibular anomalies were found at CC. Both were isolated specimens from adult males, not articulated or articulable with skulls. In one, the left mandibular head was 2.5 cm higher on the right. The dentition and TMJ surfaces and the remainder of the mandible were normal. On its left side the other mandible showed congenital hypoplasia in the area of the angle and the posterior border of the ascending ramus (Fig. 5). The left mandibular head was poorly developed; the right was normal. Along with a full complement of permanent dentition tooth sockets, the *right* central incisor was smaller and displaced slightly to the right. Wear on the teeth remaining was equal bilaterally, suggesting no interference with mastication. As such, this specimen would be compatible with hemifacial microsomia, grade I variation deformity of Caldarelli et al.[10] If anomalies behaved similarly in the 14th century, this individual had an 86% chance of a deformity of the ossicles (malleus/incus) and a 90.7% chance of a deformed external ear. Al-

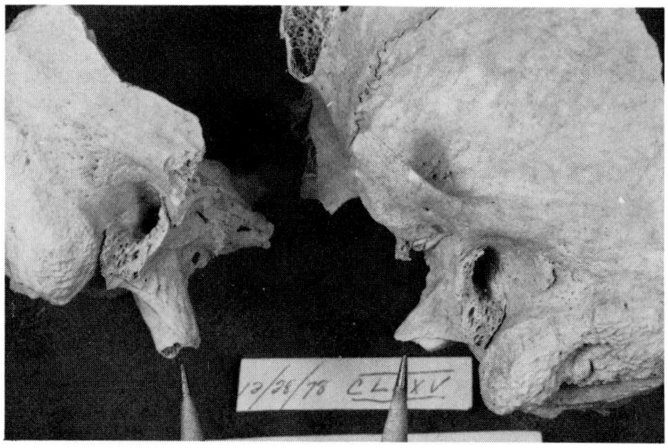

Fig. 3. Right and left temporal bones from the same skull showing an anomalous styloid process on the right side. The styloid on the left is larger in diameter than usual but not as prominent as the right.

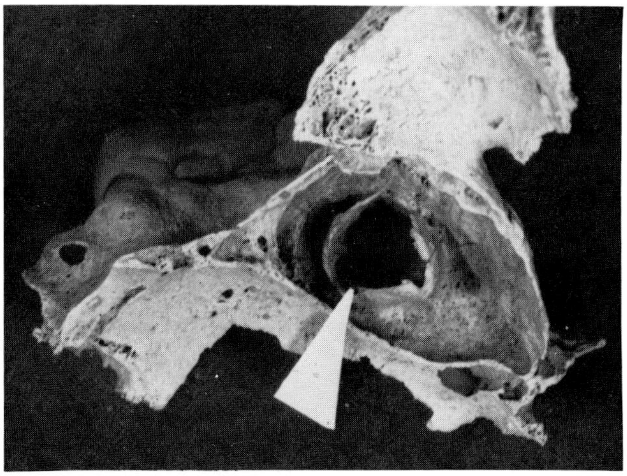

Fig. 4. Right maxilla viewed from above. Note fistula (arrow) extending from the antrum into the oral cavity through the socket of the second molar tooth. A core of metaplastic bone 7 mm deep has built up around the fistula.

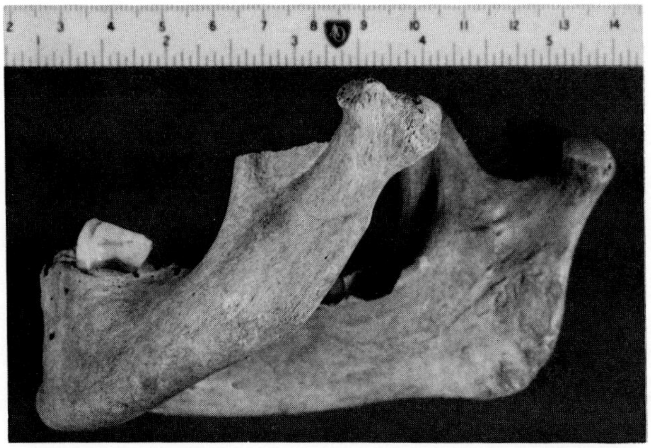

Fig. 5. Isolated adult male mandible with unilateral congenital hypoplasia of the head, angle, and ascending ramus. This bone was not articulable with other portions of a skull.

though this man may have had a unilateral hearing loss and an "Andy Gump" deformity on his left side, he survived into adulthood.

Many occult anomalies were present in the CC skeletons, particularly in the spine, indicating that these people had such abnormalities.[1] The frequency of the occult bone defects is similar to their occurrence in the U.S. today.

NASAL DISEASE

There were five healed nasal pyramid fractures. Four other noses showed paramortem mutilation. Thirteen skulls had septal deformities (8 moderately severe, 5 severe). Septal deformity has been frequent in other UMRB skulls.

OTHER CRANIAL ABNORMALITIES

Sequelae of Severe Old Trauma. These were found in two adult male skulls. In one, an old, well-healed, markedly depressed fracture was in the left frontal region. No other abnormality was apparent. In the other there was a lesion on the lateral surface of the right parietal bone characterized by bone loss and smooth new bone formation. The medial surface of this parietal was intact. The process appeared several months old and stable. It was interpreted as the sequela of head trauma, subperiostial hematoma, avascular necrosis of bone, and cyst formation. Accentuation of the temporal lines indicated stretching of the pericranial structures.

Nutritional Disturbances. Cribra orbitalia and porotic hyperostosis, strongly suggesting iron deficiency anemia, were found in 28 skulls; all but one were children and subadults. X-rays of the postcranial long bones, still being evaluated, show many transverse lines, strongly suggesting community and individual nutritional and metabolic disturbances. Thinning of the cortex and decrease in the medullary trabecular elements was observed in three mandibles and in many other postcranial bones, indicating osteoporosis. Similar changes, possibly less frequent, have been found in other UMRB skeletons.

Notably absent from CC skeletons were evidence of 1) primary or metastatic cancer, although benign bone new-growths were found in various bones, similar to other UMRB findings; and 2) the effects of chronic granulomatous diseases.

Periostial reaction suggesting the effect of treponematosis was found in several CC long bones but not in the skulls.

DISCUSSION

An opportunity to do the final comprehensive "autopsy" upon an entire village whose people lived as a unit and finally perished together at the same moment in time occurred when the CC skeletons washed out of the Missouri River bank in mid-South Dakota in 1978. Because of previous studies upon other skeletal populations recovered from the UMRB, mostly post-white-contact, this situation was a challenge to obtain comparative data regarding diseases, anomalies, and other abnormalities which existed prior to white admixture.

Archeologists know that human temporal bones resist the effects of weathering extremely well. This observation held true at CC. The temporal bone count gave the most accurate indicator of the total human population represented in the enormous pile of bones. Also, the temporal bone assay provided insight into the *incidence* of abnormalities in this portion of the CC skeletons. Despite the incompleteness of data relating to many other bones, by careful extrapolation of information obtained from the temporals with that which *was available* from other segments of the CC skeletons, insight has been gained into the ramifications of disease process elsewhere in the skeletons.

Salient otolaryngic findings in the CC victims' skeletons are presented briefly. The data are compared with information from other peoples of the past and with a control group of South Dakota Indian school children. In the Dakotas today many diseases and abnormalities are very different in the native Americans than in the general population. Through studies such as this, utilizing the approach of longitudinal epidemiology, insight can be gained into the changing patterns of diseases over a millenium, at least in one portion of the North American continent.

ACKNOWLEDGMENTS — Valuable assistance, advice, and support was received from: The William H. Over Museum, University of South Dakota; The Museum of the Historical Society of North Dakota; The Departments of Anthropology at the Universities of Kansas and Tennessee and the Smithsonian Institution; Doctors R. Alex, M.J. Allison, L. Angel, W. Bass, W. Birkby, J. Benitez, W. Hurt, V. Hyams, L. Johnson, R. McGrew, P. Provost, H. Schuknecht, R.E. Stephenson, and T.D. Stewart; Mssrs. G. Galde, C. Miller, M. Swegle and P. Willey; the Anthropology students at the University of South Dakota; the X-Ray Departments at St. Mary's Hospital, Pierre, SD, Sacred Heart Hospital, Yankton, SD, and the Lawrence, Kansas, Hospital. Thanks to Eastman Kodak Company, and Dean W. Hard and the South Dakota Research Council for film.

REFERENCES

1. Zimmerman LJ, Emerson T, Willey P, et al. The Crow Creek site (39 BF 11) massacre: a preliminary report. The University of South Dakota Archeology Laboratory: Vermillion, 1980.

2. Gregg JB, Steele JP, Clifford S. Ear diseases in skulls from the Sully site. Plains Anthropol 1965; 10:233-9.

3. Gregg JB, Steele JP, Holzhueter AM. Roentgenographic evaluation of temporal bones from South Dakota Indian burials. Am J Phys Anthropol 1965; 23:51-62.

4. Gregg JB, Steele JP, Clifford S, Werthman HE. A multidisciplinary study of ear disease in South Dakota Indian children. J So Dak Med Assoc 1970; 23:11-20.

5. Birkby WH, Gregg JB. Otosclerotic stapedial footplate fixation in an 18th century burial. Am J Phys Anthropol 1975; 42:81-4.

6. Gregg JB, Bass WM. Exostoses in the external auditory canals. Ann Otol Rhinol Laryngol 1970; 79:834-9.

7. Hrdlicka A. Ear exostoses. Smithsonian Misc Coll 1934; 93:1-1000.

8. Tupper BJ, Gregg JB, Clifford S. Are cleft palate and cleft lip defects increasing in South Dakota, especially among the Indians? J So Dak Speech Hear Assoc 1967; 7:11-8.

9. Tretsven VE. Incidence of cleft lip and palate in Montana Indians. J Speech Hear Disord 1963; 28:52-7.

10. Caldarelli DD, Hutchinson JG, Pruzansky S, Valvassori GE. A comparison of microtia and temporal bone anomalies in hemifacial microsomia and mandibulofacial dysostosis. Cleft Palate J 1980; 17:103-15.

≈

PAN AMERICAN ASSOCIATION OF OTORHINOLARYNGOLOGY AND BRONCHOESOPHAGOLOGY

The XVIII Congress of the Pan American Association of Otorhinolaryngology and Bronchoesophagology will be held November 2-6, 1982, in San Juan, Puerto Rico. Dr. Hans von Leden has been elected President of the Association.

Ann Otol 90:1981

SURGICAL AND RADIOLOGICAL EFFECTS UPON THE DEVELOPMENT OF SPEECH AFTER TOTAL LARYNGECTOMY

JEAN L. RICHARDSON, DrPH
LOS ANGELES, CALIFORNIA

The data presented examine the relationship between postlaryngectomy communication method, and the extent of total laryngectomy and the use of radiation therapy. The expectations of speech therapy providers were also examined. The author interviewed 60 laryngectomy patients who were six months to 3½ years postsurgery. Surgeries were grouped into four categories and correlated with communication method. The relationship was statistically significant with the most apparent deterrent effect exhibited only for the most extreme surgical excisions. There was no relationship with the use of radiation therapy. In many cases speech therapy providers' expectations were not supported by the data.

INTRODUCTION

Several researchers have attempted to correlate the extent of surgical excision for total laryngectomy (TL) with the ability to learn esophageal speech.[1-9] The production of esophageal voice is generally considered to be dependent upon the trapping of air in the upper esophagus and the vibration of the cricopharyngeus sphincter at the top of the esophagus.[2,10]

Cervical esophagectomy, total pharyngectomy, bilateral radical neck dissection (RND), multiple operations on the neck, and postirradiation fibrosis have been hypothesized to prohibit learning esophageal speech. Research studies, however, have not consistently provided confirmation for a direct correlation between extent of excision and speech. In fact, Smith et al[6] and Sako et al[11] presented findings that were conflicting. Smith et al found that 80% of their subjects who had a TL learned speech and 62% of their subjects who had a TL with RND learned speech.[6] Sako et al found that 50% of their subjects who had a TL learned speech but 61% of their subjects who had a TL with RND learned speech.[11]

Four additional studies failed to confirm a relationship between the extent of surgery and speech.[1,2,5,7] Certain anatomical structures may be critical to the development of esophageal speech while other structures may be removed with little effect. For example, although Diedrich and Youngstrom found that speech skill did not correlate with surgical management, it did correlate with the width of the esophagus, ($r=00.57$, $p=0.01$).[5] Shames et al found a correlation of $r=0.27$ between speech proficiency and intact cricopharyngeus and strap muscles.[3] Vize reported a 90% failure to learn esophageal speech after pharyngolaryngectomy because of the resection of the upper esophagus and cricopharyngeus muscle.[8] Anderson and Thomas demonstrated that rudimentary speech is even possible after a total laryngectomy and glossectomy.[9]

The data presented in this article are part of a larger study of the postsurgical adaptation of laryngectomy patients. Comparisons are made between the communication methods used by patients who experienced different surgical and radiological treatment. In addition the empirical data are compared with provider expectations concerning the effect of treatment modalities on the development of esophageal speech.

METHODS

A five-source cluster sample was used to gain access to 60 TL patients who were six months to 3½ years postsurgery. During a 90-minute home-based interview, the interviewer assessed the subject's primary, secondary, and tertiary methods of communication as well as the intelligibility, volume, and tendency to tire. The interviewer's observational assessment of subject use of communication methods was verified by directly asking the patients to identify their primary and secondary methods of communication. For data analysis purposes, the communication methods were categorized as follows:

1. Esophageal speech (speech created by expelling air from the upper esophagus).

2. Electrolarynx (any type of electrolarynx or Voice Bak® device).

3. Writing, mouthing, and gesturing. Mouthing consists of miming speech, using mouth movements and some buccal sound to communicate. This requires the listener to lip read. Writing is the most prevalent subgroup in this category.

These three categories represent an ordinal scale with esophageal speech considered to be most desirable and writing considered to be least desirable.

Patient exposure to radiation therapy was analyzed using three categories: radiation before surgery (20 subjects), radiation after surgery (10 subjects), and never radiated (30 subjects). None of the subjects received radiation therapy before and after surgery. The extent of radiation therapy was not assessed.

A four-level surgical scale (Table 1) was developed to indicate the extent of surgical excision as a predictor of postsurgical speech. A head and neck cancer surgeon on the UCLA faculty was asked to categorize the subject's operations on the basis of the antici-

From the University of Southern California Comprehensive Cancer Center and School of Pharmacy, Los Angeles. This study was supported by the Administration on Aging Grant No. 90-A-1579(01) and by the American Cancer Society Robert F. Murphy Memorial Graduate Fellowship.

TABLE 1. DISTRIBUTION OF SURGICAL SCALE

Surgical Categories	*Frequency*
Category 1 (N = 27)	
Single surgeries	
TL	22
Radical TL	1
TL with bilateral modified neck dissection	1
TL with functional node dissection on left	1
TL with left or right hemithyroidectomy	2
Category 2 (N = 23)	
Single surgeries	
TL and left RND	11
TL and right RND	4
TL, right RND, and partial thyroidectomy	3
TL and creation of a pharyngocutaneous fistula, later closed	2
TL and creation of a pharyngocutaneous fistula, still used with Voice Bak	1
Multiple surgeries	
TL and further neck exploration	1
TL and further neck exploration and removal of small amount of cancerous tissue	1
Category 3 (N = 8)	
Single surgeries	
TL and bilateral RND	2
TL and left RND, hemithyroidectomy and small partial glossectomy	1
TL, left RND, and cricopharyngeal myotomy	1
Multiple surgeries	
TL and bilateral RND and two operations to close fistula	1
TL, bilateral RND, small partial glossectomy, and one operation to close fistula	1
TL, left RND, and surgical enlargement of the esophagus	1
TL, left RND, and further neck exploration and removal of additional cancerous tissue	1
Category 4 (N = 2)	
Multiple surgeries	
TL, bilateral RND, pharyngectomy, and three reconstructive and two fistula surgeries	1
TL, right RND, and two surgeries to remove part of esophagus	1

TL - Total laryngectomy; RND - Radical neck dissection.

pated effect upon rehabilitation outcome. This proved to be a simple categorization procedure for those patients who had a single operation. For those who had multiple operations the process was slightly more complex. Each patient was categorized individually by comparing the resulting extent of excision with those who had only a single operation. Table 1 shows how surgeries were distributed across the available categories.

During the laryngectomee interview, each subject was asked the names of the professional speech therapists and lay (laryngectomized) instructors with whom they had speech training. Questionnaires were mailed to the 20 providers who were identified; 4 were laryngectomees and 16 were professionals. All four of the lay instructors responded to the interview. Six of the professional speech therapists responded to the interview. Those who did respond had provided the bulk of the speech therapy to the laryngectomee subjects who had been interviewed. Of the 59 people who worked with one or more speech therapists, 49 had worked with at least one of the therapists or lay instructors who responded to the provider questionnaire.

The questionnaire which was mailed to providers elicited data concerning services which they provided and their perceptions of rehabilitation determinants. A comparison of provider expectations and actual experiences is therefore possible.

RESULTS

The four-level scale was cross-tabulated with communication methods. The statistical analysis in-

TABLE 2. RELATIONSHIP BETWEEN SURGERY AND SPEECH METHOD

	Surgical Scale			
Speech Method	*Least Severe 1*	*2*	*3*	*Most Severe 4*
Esophageal speech	70%	44%	50%	0%
Electrolarynx	26%	26%	38%	50%
Writing	4%	30%	12%	50%
Total patients	27	23	8	2

Gamma = 0.42817; Pearson's r = 0.30713; significance = 0.0085.

dicates that there is a significant difference between the communication methods used by subjects in the four surgery categories (Table 2). Category 1 (least severe surgical excisions) clearly had the most favorable communication outcome. Category 4 (most severe surgical excisions) clearly had the least favorable communication outcome. When category 4 is eliminated from the analysis (categories 1, 2, and 3 are compared), the relationship is weakened but remains significant (gamma = 0.37318; Pearson's r = 0.23497, significance = 0.0379). When categories 1 and 4 are eliminated from the analysis (categories 2 and 3 are compared) the relationship is no longer statistically significant (gamma = −0.22689; Pearson's r = −0.13052, significance = 0.2420). Thus categories 2 and 3 are not statistically different from each other in terms of communication outcomes. Categories 1 and 4 are statistically distinct from other categories and from each other.

Further cross-tabular analysis was done between the extent of surgery and the quality of esophageal speech measured by interviewer assessment of intelligibility, volume, and tendency-to-tire during the 90-minute interview. There were no statistically significant relationships between these factors. That is to say, if a person was able to learn esophageal speech, the quality of that speech was not affected by the extent of surgery.

Radiation has been hypothesized to be a factor in the development of speech because radiation decreases the elasticity of the tissues which are utilized to develop esophageal speech. But, the data from this survey do not support the hypothesis that radiation negatively affects speech (Table 3).

The group that never had radiation was expected to have the highest percent of esophageal speakers. Instead, the group that had radiation before surgery achieved the highest percent of esophageal speakers. The group that had radiation after surgery achieved the lowest percent of esophageal speakers as expected. The relationship between the categories of radiation and communication is not statistically significant, therefore it may be concluded that radiation therapy is not a determinant of communication outcome.

Speech therapists and lay instructors were asked in an open-ended question to enumerate which surgical factors they felt would "render a patient un-

TABLE 3. RELATIONSHIP BETWEEN RADIATION AND SPEECH METHOD

Speech Method	Radiation After	Radiation Before	Radiation Never
Esophageal speech	40%	70%	50%
Electrolarynx	50%	15%	30%
Writing	10%	15%	20%
Total patients	10	20	30

Lambda = 0.037; chi square = 4.8; significance = 0.307.

able to learn esophageal speech." The list of opinions offered and the percent of the ten responding speech therapists/lay instructors who listed the surgical factor are presented in Table 4.

It appears from this list that therapists have different opinions about which surgical factors prevent a patient from learning speech. Most speech therapists would agree that the excision of all or most of the tongue, which is a major articulator, is likely to prevent the learning of speech, although in this study a patient who had a small partial glossectomy and a bilateral RND was able to learn speech very intelligibly.

The two patients in category 3 who had surgery to close fistulas were good esophageal speakers. Nonclosing fistulas of themselves do not seem to prevent learning esophageal speech although 20% of the speech therapists/lay instructors felt that they would.

We have cited previous studies that conclude an intact cricopharyngeal muscle is necessary for learning esophageal speech. However, the individual whose record specifically states that he had a cricopharyngeal myotomy (ie, this muscle was cut) *did* use esophageal speech as his primary method of communication.

Many patients who had a TL and one-sided RND learned esophageal speech. Of the four people in category 3 who had a TL and bilateral RND, two learned esophageal speech although 40% of the speech therapists considered RND to be an important deterrent to speech development.

Neither person in category 4 learned speech. One had a pharyngectomy and extensive reconstruction. She inserted a rubber bougie in her throat daily to dilate her esophagus. The other person had multiple operations to remove part of her esophagus. One patient in category 3 who had multiple surgeries to enlarge and dilate his esophagus and inserted a rubber bougie into his throat daily to dilate it at home, also did not learn speech. These three people are

TABLE 4. FACTORS FELT TO RENDER PATIENTS UNABLE TO LEARN ESOPHAGEAL SPEECH

Surgical Factors Cited	Percent of Speech Therapists/Instructors Who Cited Each Factor
Glossectomy or partial glossectomy	50
Negative effects of preoperative or postoperative radiation	30
Tight, narrow, loose, or damaged cricopharyngeal sphincter	40
Nonclosing fistula	20
Extent of tissue removed: particularly RND	40
Excessive pain, immobility, or rigidity	20
Esophageal stenosis	10
Resection of esophagus or pharynx	10
Partial jaw removal	10
Prelaryngectomy stroke	10
Prelaryngectomy colostomy	10

subjects whose medical record or interview indicated surgical excisions on the esophagus.

CONCLUSION

This article examines whether certain postsurgical anatomical changes can be identified as preventing patients from learning esophageal speech. The data presented in this study support the belief that there is a relationship between the extent of surgery and the ability to learn esophageal speech. This deterrent effect is most apparent in the extensive surgeries involving the esophagus and pharynx. Nonclosing fistulas and RNDs were not strong deterrents to learning speech. Radiation was found not to be a deterrent to learning speech although 30% of the therapists/instructors felt it would be.

The beliefs of many speech therapists and lay instructors were not consistent with the findings. Because therapists guide patients into communication methods which they feel are appropriate on the basis of the extent of their surgery, it becomes very important that therapists' and instructors' expectations are accurate. In particular inaccurate responses were concerned with the belief that RND or radiation render a patient unable to learn esophageal speech.

It is clear from this data that though surgery is a factor in learning speech, other factors must account for the failure to learn speech among those people who are not in the more extensive surgical categories. Such factors would include psychological, social support, and speech therapy strategies which could have a larger role in acquiring esophageal speech.

ACKNOWLEDGMENTS — The author wishes to acknowledge the help of Linda B. Bourque, PhD, Dale H. Rice, MD, and Joseph W. Cullen, PhD, in the design of this study and the preparation of this report. Computations and data analysis were carried out at the UCLA Office of Academic Computing.

REFERENCES

1. Robe E, Moore P, Andrews A, Holinger P. A study of the role of certain factors in the development of speech after laryngectomy. Laryngoscope 1956; 66:173-86.

2. Putney FJ. The larynx. In: Nealon T, ed. Management of the patient with cancer. Philadelphia: WB Saunders, 1965: 401-24.

3. Shames F, Font J, Matthews J. Factors related to speech proficiency of the laryngectomized. J Speech Hear Disord 1963; 28:273-87.

4. Bisi RH, Conley JJ. Psychological factors influencing vocal rehabilitation of post-laryngectomy patient. Ann Otol Rhinol Laryngol 1965; 74:1073-8.

5. Diedrich W, Youngstrom K. Alaryngeal speech. Springfield: Charles C Thomas, 1966.

6. Smith J, Rise E, Gralnek D. Speech recovery in laryngectomized patients. Laryngoscope 1966; 76:1540-6.

7. Gilchrist AG. Rehabilitation after laryngectomy. Acta Otolaryngol (Stockh) 1973; 75:511-8.

8. Vize CE. Rehabilitation of the voice after pharyngolaryngectomy and skin repair: I. Cineradiography. Clin Otolaryngol 1976; 1:107-13.

9. Anderson JD, Thomas S. Speech rehabilitation of a laryngectomized glossectomized patient. Laryngoscope 1978; 88: 1666-70.

10. Wepman J, MacGahan J, Rickard J, Shelton N. The objective measurement of progressive esophageal speech development. J Speech Hear Disord 1953; 18:247-51.

11. Sako K, Cardinale S, Marchetta F, Shedd D. Speech and vocational rehabilitation of the laryngectomized patient. J Surg Oncol 1974; 6:197-202.

OBITUARY — SIR ALEXANDER EWING

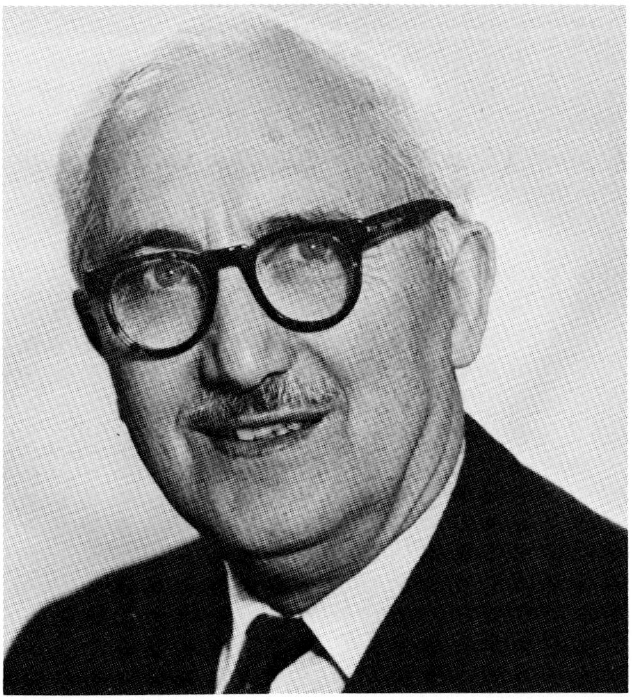

1896-1980

Alexander Ewing, who might rightly be regarded as the founder of British audiology, was born in southeast England in 1896. He received the degree of Master of Arts from the University of Edinburgh, then joined the staff of the Royal Institution for the Deaf in Edinburgh. This was at a crucial point in the history of deaf education in the United Kingdom (UK) since it was at the time when there was a changeover from manual to oral education. Ewing's deep belief that oral methods were paramount in the education of the deaf helped many to be integrated into an essentially normal way of life. At the same time this philosophy attracted not a few critics who believed that visual methods of communication were not given due scope.

In 1922 Ewing joined the staff of the University of Manchester which was then in the forefront of education, having established the first Chair in Education in the UK in 1899. However, the University's choice of a woman, Eileen Goldsack, to head the newly established Deaf Education Department was received with misgivings. Alexander provided a partial solution to this problem by marrying Eileen; their success in making Manchester the country's leading center in deaf education was to be the complete solution. Indeed, references were always to "the Ewings" — never one without the other. This duumvirate not only built up the educational facet of audiology but also spawned the physical and medical facets. The physicist T.S. Littler, who joined the Ewings in the early 1930s, subsequently became the Director of the first Medical Research Council Audiology Research Unit. The physician I.G. Taylor, who joined the team 20 years later, succeeded Ewing, crystallizing the concept of audiology as a medical specialty. It can rightly be claimed that the majority of those in the UK who are now concerned with the care and management of patients with auditory disorders were trained, directly or indirectly, by the Ewings. The recent recognition in the UK of the specialty of Audiological Medicine and the discipline of Audiological Science has been the logical consequence of the efforts of the Ewings' school and a tribute to that team.

Alexander Ewing was also an organizer and, at heart, a scientist. In 1958 he organized a successful International Congress and established the first University course in audiology in the UK. He was always anxious to ensure that whatever he did or taught was based upon sound scientific principles. The bases for this approach were the postgraduate studies that he had undertaken in the late 1920s under the direction of the neuroanatomist, Sir John Stopford. Ewing was probably the first person in the UK to conduct systematic research on hearing-impaired subjects using an electronic audiometer; he collaborated with Littler in studies of auditory adaptation and fatigue. Similarly, he worked with E.D.D. Dickson and Littler in British studies of occupational noise-induced hearing loss.

In 1944 Ewing was designated Director of the Department of Education of the Deaf. He was elected an honorary member of the American Otological Society in 1946. In 1949 he became Ellis Llwyd Jones Professor in the Education of the Deaf in the University of Manchester; 11 years later he was named the first Professor of Audiology in the UK. In the previous year his services to the hearing-impaired were recognized by the conferment of a Knighthood. In 1968 he shared with the late Sir Terence Cawthorne the office of Vice-President of the IX International Congress of Audiology. The British Society of Audiology recognized his contributions to British audiology by electing him one of the first Honorary Life Members. Although his first wife predeceased him, he had, thanks to his second wife, Lady Ethel, a happy and productive retirement. The particular personality characteristics which were often attributed to Alexander Ewing were his kindness and his dedication. Let us hope that his death has not meant the disappearance of the last gentleman-scholar in audiology.

Ronald Hinchcliffe

LETTERS TO THE EDITOR

Dear Editor:

I would like to comment on the use of the term "block nystagmus." Terms denominating various forms of nystagmus characteristics are ever increasing. Adding a new name to a well-known nystagmus pattern is unnecessary and may be confusing.

One of the major controversies in neurotology is the bewildering multiplication of terminology. Terms are used to denominate presence or absence, the plane, direction, intensity, the environmental condition, and the eliciting factor of vestibular nystagmus. In addition to one and the same nystagmic phenomenon, new ad hoc expressions or terms are created by the individual observer or investigator, resulting in a jungle of words and phrases of Latin-Greek-English origin.

In a recent article Olson and Wolfe report on "block nystagmus" recorded in a patient with signs and symptoms of Menière's disease.[1] Eventually computerized tomography and myelography detected a communicating type of hydrocephalus. The authors conclude that certain types of lesions in the brainstem result in "block nystagmus." There is also a figure showing three short sequences of oculographic recordings of what the authors term block or "kip" nystagmus. The first sequence was obtained by positioning the head to the back and right. The second and third records are results of warm and cold irrigations of the left ear. The three records are basically identical and none has the characteristic of a nystagmus.

A criterion of the vestibular nystagmus was formalized close to a century ago as an involuntary rhythmic eye movement composed of a slow and fast component. The illustration in question does not fulfill the basic criterion of a vestibular nystagmus. There is neither a slow nor a fast component recognizable. Instead it is a sequence of back and forth eye movements which are encountered quite frequently in normal individuals as well as in patients. Ever since nystagmus has been recorded, this phenomenon was termed not as a nystagmus but as square waves. It represents a fine, right-left search movement of the eye. It is a very common observation and detectable to various degrees in most people (Fig. 1). Those individuals exhibiting square waves show a marked increase when excited by insecurity or fear, whereas there is considerable decrease at a state of relaxation. Square waves are what Olson and Wolfe call "block nystagmus" although it is not a nystagmus, not of vestibular origin, and certainly not a pathological sign. It is also a common observation that when a square waving subject undergoes thermic or rotatory stimulation, the resulting nystagmus suppresses either partially or totally the underlying square waves. As the stimulatory effect wears out, the square waves gradually return to the prestimulation pattern.

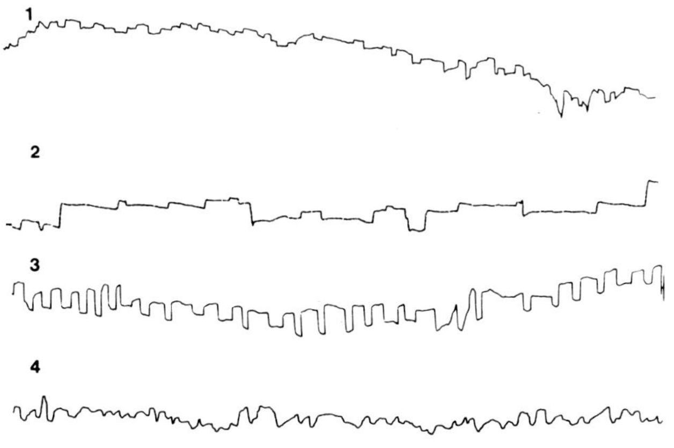

Fig. 1. Four samples of square waves selected from innumerable similar oculographic records of normal individuals and patients. 1) Small amplitude square wave activity. 2) Sequence of square waves with relatively low frequency. 3) High frequency continuous square wave formation. 4) Record of restless eye, or some form of oculomotor incoordination which cannot be considered pathological.

There are further shortcomings in the evaluation of Figure 1. Tracings 2 and 3 represent vestibular stimulations from the left ear. No trace of nystagmus is seen. An absence of vestibular nystagmic response should be interpreted either as left vestibular areflexia or perhaps inadequate stimulation or recording.

It is noteworthy and it was fortunate that this nystagmographic misinterpretation prompted the authors to further investigation including CT scanning and myelography. However, the hydrocephalus so diagnosed would hardly explain the symptoms of recurring attacks of dizziness with a unilateral hearing loss. There is no mention of equal loudness balance testing or SISI score, but with relatively good discrimination and absent tone decay, it can be assumed that it was a cochlear type and not a central hearing loss. Thus, the communicating hydrocephalus may be an unrelated finding concerning the neurotological symptoms.

In conclusion, square waves are not nystagmus, are not a specific sign of central pathology, and occur frequently in normals as well as in patients, particularly when they are in a state of excitement. To use an uncalled-for new term as "block nystagmus" is misleading and can be confusing.

Sincerely yours,
Nicholas Torok, MD

REFERENCES

1. Olson JE, Wolfe JW. Block nystagmus. Ann Otol Rhinol Laryngol 1980; 89:286-7.

REPRINTS — Nicholas Torok, MD
Department of Otolaryngology
University of Illinois Eye and Ear Infirmary
1855 W. Taylor Street
Chicago, IL 60612

Dear Editor:

I enjoyed Dr. Robert Sofferman's "Cranial Arteritis in Otolaryngology" in the May-June 1980 issue of the *Annals of Otology, Rhinology and Laryngology* (89:215-9). I found an otolaryngologist's thoughts about this ophthalmologically important disease very refreshing and informative. However, the author uses the term retinoscopy where he means ophthalmoscopy. Retinoscopy is an objective method of detecting errors of refraction by observing the shadow caused by the margin of the iris upon light reflecting from the retina. Ophthalmoscopy refers to the examination of the fundus of the eye using the ophthalmoscope just as otoscopy means inspection of the ear using an otoscope.

During retinoscopy one can often detect abnormal corneas, lenticular opacities, opacities in the aqueous and vitreous humors and large retinal detachments. However, it would be unlikely retinal pallor or papilledema would be noticed while using this diagnostic method.

I am hesitant to mention some ophthalmologists and optometrists use the term funduscopy in place of ophthalmoscopy for fear it will encourage further correspondence from a comparably nitpicking gynecologist. In any case, the substitution of the term retinoscopy for ophthalmoscopy in this article certainly did not detract in any significant way from this fine review. In fact, there is nothing particularly bright about the small correction, it simply shines a slightly different light upon the problem.

Sincerely,
ALLAN J. FLACH, MD, Pharm D

University of California
San Francisco Medical Center
Veterans Administration Hospital
San Francisco

Dear Dr. Flach:

Doctor Senturia referred your letter to me out of interest and I certainly do appreciate your very kind remarks and constructive criticism. I am a strong believer in semantic accuracy and will certainly plan to use correct terminology in future references to examination of the ocular fundus. The humor in your paragraph three actually brightened my day.

Sincerely,
ROBERT A. SOFFERMAN, MD

University of Vermont
College of Medicine
Section of Otolaryngology
Burlington, Vermont

Dear Editor:

I write with reference to an article entitled "Epiglottitis: Evolution in Management During the Last Decade" by Ralph F. Wetmore, MD, and Steven D. Handler, MD, which appeared in the November-December 1979 issue of *The Annals of Otology, Rhinology and Laryngology* (88:822-6).

I am in the process of updating our review of the management of acute epiglottitis at this hospital from 1964-1976 to 1964-1979. I am therefore somewhat amazed to find in the above article the following statements: "Until the advent of endotracheal intubation for epiglottitis in the early 1970s . . ." and again, ". . . in the early 1970s, several reports appeared recommending endotracheal intubation for epiglottitis" (p. 824).

May I point out that pioneers in the work of prolonged nasotracheal intubation for several conditions including acute epiglottitis in children were Drs. Tom Allen and Ian Steven at the Adelaide Childrens' Hospital about 1963 and Dr. Nerida Dilworth of the Princess Margaret Hospital for Children commenced using the technique in 1964. Their work has been reported in the literature and at meetings since that time as has the work of Dr. Ian McDonald and the late Dr. John Stocks of the Melbourne Children's Hospital, all in Australia.

I cannot understand the failure of this otherwise excellent review to mention this early work, other than perhaps to point out that the people mentioned were, or are, pediatric anesthetists.

Yours sincerely,
PETER BRINE, FFARCS, FFARACS

Princess Margaret Hospital for Children
Perth, Western Australia

Dear Dr. Brine:

I want to thank you very much for taking the time to write the above letter and to bring this matter to our attention. Our statement in the article regarding the advent of endotracheal intubation for epiglottitis in the early 1970s was meant only to indicate the popularity of this technique which appeared at that time. In no way did we mean to minimize or ignore earlier contributions or studies. The omission of the articles that you mentioned was one of oversight and was certainly not intentional.

Yours truly,
STEVEN D. HANDLER, MD

Children's Hospital of Philadelphia
34th Street and Civic Center Boulevard
Philadelphia, Pennsylvania

Dear Editor:

I would like to comment on the manuscript by Drs. Wolfe and Rowe, "Upper Airway Obstruction in Infectious Mononucleosis," presented at the American Broncho-Esophagological Association, April 12-13, 1980, and published in *The Annals of Otology, Rhinology and Laryngology.*[1]

While I agree with the authors' discussion of the management of airway obstruction in mononucleosis, I would like to caution the treating physician when using corticosteroids in patients with infectious mononucleosis. We recently reported the occurrence of peritonsillar abscess in two patients with mononucleosis in whom corticosteroids were used to reduce tonsillar enlargement.[2] At least one other article has reported this complication[3] and I suspect that its occurrence is probably more widespread. Because of the possibility of this complication in a child whose airway is already compromised, I feel that corticosteroids should be used only in selected patients with significant tonsillar enlargement causing airway obstruction *and* who are hospitalized.

REFERENCES

1. Wolfe JA, Rowe LD. Upper airway obstruction in infectious mononucleosis. Ann Otol Rhinol Laryngol 1980; 89:430-3.

2. Handler SD, Warren SW. Peritonsillar abscess as a complication of corticosteroid treatment in infectious mononucleosis. Pediatr Otorhino-laryngol 1979; 1:265-8.

3. Parulekar SS, Rapoport A, Paonessa DF, Kouyoumgian J. Epstein-Barr virus, the ravager. Ann Otol Rhinol Laryngol 1978; 87:729-35.

Yours truly,
STEVEN D. HANDLER, MD

Children's Hospital of Philadelphia
Philadelphia, Pennsylvania

BOOK REVIEWS

Allergy and Clinical Immunology

Edited by *Richard F. Lockey.* Hard cover, black and white illustrations, indexed, 1175 pp, 1979. Medical Examination Publishing Co, Garden City. Price $35.00

The purpose of this text as stated in the introduction is to introduce the rapidly expanding field of clinical immunology and allergy to medical students, interns, residents and practicing physicians. Dr. Samuel Bukantz in an eloquent foreword reminds us that no matter how medicine is specialized and subspecialized, clinical immunology and allergy will be part of all branches and subbranches. This book is divided into two sections. The first deals initially with basic immunology and then relates it to various organs or systems emphasizing clinically relevant areas. The second section deals with allergies.

This book fills its mission in some respects and fails in others. The cost is certainly a plus feature and is within the means, I would think, of most students and physicians. The reader does, however, pay other "prices," in the form of some small type which becomes tiring after a period of prolonged reading, and a relative absence of photographs. This is especially felt in the chapter on allergic dermatoses where the reader has no opportunity to see the lesions of urticaria, atopic dermatitis and contact dermatitis. Perhaps the most bothersome aspect of the book is an exceedingly poor and incomplete index. It is impossible to find such important items in the index as anergy, histamine, slow-reacting substances of anaphylaxis, etc.

This text, through no particular fault of its own, suffers from the problems associated with a field that is virtually exploding with new information. Any text in allergy and clinical immunology is practically outdated by the time it is published. Consider for example, the first chapter on B & T cells. The most recent reference in this chapter is 1976. Therefore, there is a paucity of information on vital areas such as macrophage function and T & B cell interaction. The chapter on insect sensitivity deals only momentarily with pure venom, for this was licensed for skin test and immunotherapy in 1979, only a few months before the book was published.

On the whole, the book is well written and despite the multiple authors, there is some continuity of style. Several chapters are outstanding in the completeness of their coverage. These include immunogenetics, gastrointestinal disorders, malignancies, and asthma. Several other chapters are particularly unique and would be difficult to find elsewhere. I particularly enjoyed chapter 17, "Active and Passive Immunization." Chapter 22, "Immunologic Techniques," provides a reasonable overview of a complex subject. Chapter 43, entitled "Drugs Important in Allergic Diseases" is the result of a survey of 100 allergists and includes tables of the most commonly used antiallergic medications. Chapter 44, written by the editor's father, is the most complete listing available of aspirin- and tartrazine-containing drugs. The final chapter, "Controversies in Allergies" by Thomas Golbert, is an exceedingly comprehensive, well-written, and orderly presentation of various techniques in allergy which are commonly used, but remain totally unproved. It is a highly successful effort to put these procedures in the proper context.

I would not recommend this book to allergists, clinical immunologists and others well versed in the field. The index, as stated earlier, is a significant drawback and I would hope that in the second edition the editor would correct this. The book does, however, provide an inexpensive and reasonably well written and consistent introduction of this fascinating field to the medical student, intern, resident, and practicing physician.

RAYMOND G. SLAVIN, MD
St. Louis, Missouri

Basic Industrial Hearing Conservation

By *David F. Barr* and *Richard K. Miller*. Hard cover, black and white illustrations, glossary, appendix, 125 pages, 1979. Fairmont Press, Atlanta. Price $26.95.

This book is designed as an introductory text for the industrial nurse or audiometric technician. The outline of the book is good; the text is easy to read and accompanied by numerous illustrations. With all of these admirable qualities it is disturbing to find several important omissions. While a discussion of decibel notation is given in Chapter Two, there is no presentation of the meaning of decibel notation with regard to the audiometer in Chapter Four. In Chapter Five, which discusses noise related hearing disorders, the sections dealing with inner ear noise damage and other mechanisms of damage followed by a discussion of both auditory and nonauditory effects of noise on man tend to leave the reader with the impression that nonnoise damage to the inner ear can be easily determined and that the nonauditory effects of noise on man are both measurable and meaningful. In the former category this reviewer wishes that some discussion of hereditary factors and ototoxic drugs had been included and that the review of effects of noise on man had included in its bibliography some of the papers which question the significance of nonauditory effects in typical work-place environments rather than in the laboratory. This reviewer also wishes that the part of Chapter Six which discusses selecting a professional consultant had not equated otolaryngologists with audiologists, and the discussion of disadvantages of outside consultants as compared to the advantages of professional consultants is confusing.

Finally, the chapter on hearing protective devices (Chapter Seven) fails to stress the need for continued monitoring of employees' hearing when protective devices are used.

In summary, this textbook is a useful compilation of material for the industrial nurse, audiometric technician, personnel manager, or safety engineer. Several omissions from the basic considerations have been noted. The reasons and need for continued audiologic surveillance are not stressed sufficiently in the text. The addition of Appendix A which contains a "model industrial audiometric technician course" plus pages for notes implies that this text is to be used as a handbook for such a course. And for that purpose, the text should be satisfactory.

FRANCIS I. CATLIN, MD
Houston, Texas

Clinical Voice Disorders: An Interdisciplinary Approach

By *Arnold E. Aronson*. Soft cover, black and white illustrations, indexed, 254 pp, 1980. Thieme-Stratton, Inc, New York. Price $19.50.

This new clinical text is written by the head of the section of speech pathology at the Mayo Clinic, who is well known in the voice pathology literature for his work on psychogenic voice disorders. It will become a cardinal trainee text in college programs and an important clinical reference periodical for practicing voice pathologists. The new text is clearly Aronson's quintessential statement of his approach to hyperfunctional vocal pathology. Aronson has now formally stated the extrinsic laryngeal muscle relaxation technique that he has developed in the past fifteen years to reduce the musculoskeletal tensions responsible, in large part, for the majority of hyperfunctional voice disorders.

The text begins with an attempt to define abnormal phonation, thereby introducing some basic vocal pathology terminology. Chapter two focuses on anatomy and physiology with an unfortunate omission of respiratory mechanics for phonation. The chapter has, however, an important emphasis on laryngeal suspension via muscular interconnections of the supra- and infrahyoid muscles. There are several original excellent medical illustrations of the extrinsic laryngeal musculature, illustrating the complex but critical suspension phonatory system. The chapter concludes with an interesting discussion of the phylogenetic development of the human larynx. The next chapter deals with normal voice development with an outline of life span changes in pitch from infant cry to the geriatric voice. Chapters four and five discuss organic voice disorders with the addition of several less common voice disorders, (normally found in larger medical centers) such as cri du chat, laryngotracheal cleft, laryngomalacia, and, in adults, cricroarytenoid arthritis, as well as an excellent presentation of the dysphonias found in upper and lower motor neuron disease. Rather than focus on any lengthy comparison of vocal polyps, nodules, or granulomas, Aronson chooses to emphasize the less common and not well documented disorders of vocal pathology. For that reason alone this text is an important addition to the general vocal pathology library. Also included is a much needed presentation of the endocrine-related vocal disorders, such as, hypo- and hyperthyroidism, hyperpituitarism, and amyloidosis. The text also discusses virilization and myxedematous vocal pathology, which is a more common clinical occurrence than previously recorded. Aronson's discussion will alert clinicians to this fact.

Chapter six is one of the best in the text, presenting psychogenic and generalized musculoskeletal tension voice disorders. The emphasis in this chapter is on conversion reaction disorders and their clinical history. Aronson defines many of the common vocal disorders (nodules, ulcer, ventricular dysphonia) as due, primarily, to "musculoskeletal tensions." Utilizing case reports the chapter cleverly outlines the insidious course of major vocal tension pathology and their assessment. Chapter seven deals exclusively with a very popular but less frequently occurring phenomenon: adductor spasmodic dysphonia. It is a thorough and updating report of the management, assessment, and present thinking on etiology of this enigmatic disorder.

The chapter on voice examination is brief but important for college students entering vocal pathology. The chapter on treatment is excellent, presenting for the first time in print Aronson's laryngeal manipulation technique to remediate musculoskeletal tension disorders. The author includes in this chapter, as he does throughout the text, valuable teaching clinical prose between clinician and patient with a strong support for dealing with emotional and environmental stresses that provoke and/or maintain vocal stress. The text ends with a long-awaited chapter on counseling and interviewing techniques. Aronson discusses psychoneurotic personalities and how to deal with them through examples of clinical patient scripts.

This book is an excellent statement of the nature and care of psychogenic voice disorders, neurologic dysphonias, and Aronson's "laryngeal manipulation technique" to relieve common musculoskeletal laryngeal tension. It will serve as both an excellent adjunct to new college trainees in voice pathology, and as a very fine clinical resource for the practicing laryngologist or resident who requires more appreciation of the phonatory consequences of medical disease and their rehabilitation.

RICHARD M. MERSON, PhD
St. Louis, Missouri

The Sounds of Speech Communication: A Primer of Acoustic Phonetics and Speech Perception

By *J.M. Pickett*. Hard cover, black and white illustrations, indexed, referenced, 249 pp, 1980. University Park Press, Baltimore. Price $19.95.

This is the most recent addition to the University Park Press *Perspectives in Audiology* series (Lyle Lloyd, series editor), and provides an important basic science complement to the predominantly clinical discussions of previous volumes.

Pickett cites as his aim "to teach a technical subject, the acoustics of speech and its production, to the nontechnical student;" to this end the book is thoughtfully designed. Sentences and paragraphs are short and constructed for maximum comprehensibility; each chapter is introduced with a preview of its contents and is closed with a short summary; a topical bibliography and a set of laboratory exercises follow the text. The progression of chapter topics is logical and cumulative, an effective structure for a book that hopes to teach. The reader is led gradually from a consideration of basic acoustics to a discussion of vowels as sounds, and thence to other glottis-dependent aspects of speech such as prosody. Later come the consonants and a chapter on the acoustical complexities of the voiced-voiceless distinction among speech sounds.

There are some problems with this book, however, which detract from its effectiveness as an introductory text. The spectogram, an invaluable tool for understanding and studying speech sounds, is often difficult for the beginner. Yet the first spectrogram Pickett uses is a picture of a complete sentence, involving a mix of vowels and consonants and coarticulations that can be confusing for the "nontechnical" student. The author might better have started his discussion of spectrograms with representations of simpler sounds — white noise, tones of tuning forks, etc — to teach the tool before asking for its application.

The author also depends heavily on the spectrogram for displaying speech sounds; as a result, he hides from the reader the rich detail available in the speech waveform, a "picture" of sound that is attracting much attention among current students of acoustic phonetics and speech perception. An oscilloscope would not only complement but also supplement the spectrograph Pickett prescribes for his appended lab exercises: students would have the advantage of seeing the same aspects of sounds rendered in two different ways, and additional exercises focused on the important aspects of fine timing for speech sounds could have been included.

Finally, the prospective student or teacher expecting a "primer of acoustic phonetics and speech perception" will find that the book's subtitle is misleading. Ten of the 12 chapters are on acoustic phonetics; the 11th on "acoustic cues for speech perception" is woefully dependent on experiments using synthetic speech rather than real speech; it is essentially a summary of the work of a single laboratory, though other workers and approaches have been important in this research. The last chapter, purportedly on "models of speech perception" is really a discussion of only one, the "motor theory" of speech perception; all other theorists are demoted to "critics of the motor theory." One might have expected such a bias on the author's part, given his dedication of this book to R.H. Stetson. However, it is very possible that Stetson with his great interest in physiology would be more impressed with recent discoveries about the complex organization of sensory systems than with the continued insistence by some speech scientists that speech depends on physiological arrangements not found in other animals.

The careful teacher might choose to follow closely the first ten chapters of this very good book on acoustic phonetics and use the last two chapters as points of departure for his own presentation on the array of acoustical, psychological, and physiological variables that may be important for the perception of speech.

JUDITH LAUTER, PhD
St. Louis, Missouri

Evoked Potentials

Edited by *Colin Barber*. Hard cover, black and white illustrations, indexed, referenced, 614 pages, 1980. University Park Press, Baltimore. Price $34.50.

An international symposium on evoked potentials was held in Nottingham, England in the spring of 1978. This symposium, attended by investigators from several countries (primarily European) resulted in a large number of papers covering the major areas of evoked potential work. Colin Barber, with the help of Dr. F. Campbell, Professor S. Crews, Mr. W. Gibson, Professor Harding, Dr. A. Starr, Dr. A. Thornton and Professor L. van der Tweel, selected papers from the symposium for publication in this book. Thus, the book does not contain all of the papers presented at the symposium.

The book is divided into two major sections. Part A is a very readable history of evoked potential investigation. It briefly but adequately covers the history of auditory, visual, and somatosensory investigation as well as an overview of the measurement techniques involved in response measurement.

Part B is an assembly of individual current investigations divided into several subsections. The first subsection deals with new developments in stimuli generation and response analysis. Particularly noteworthy is a study which employs laser technology for visual stimulation. The next three subsections cover both basic and clinically applied investigations using visual, auditory, and somatosensory stimuli respectively. I found the separation of basic and applied studies a particularly useful organization. The fifth subsection is concerned with psychological correlates of evoked potentials. The sixth subsection covers drug and metabolic effects of evoked potentials. Finally, the last subsection contains a series of papers that deal with evoked potential work in patients with multiple sclerosis.

The book can serve several purposes. As a reference book, it provides an historical perspective of all major areas of evoked potential work. It provides carefully edited references for both the older classic studies and the more recent studies. This is particularly valuable since individual investigations tend to be published in a wide variety of unrelated and sometimes difficult-to-locate journals, government publications, and various books.

The book also serves as a summary of the current state-of-the-art, but its value depends on a particular outlook. On the one hand, the "current" investigations are already two years old, a fact which poses some problems. Investigators working in a particular area are likely to have already obtained the information and important developments which have occurred since 1978 are not mentioned. On the other hand, a two-year delay for such a large, comprehensive, carefully organized and edited work is certainly reasonable.

A book which contains an historical perspective and an assembly of relatively recent studies in all areas of evoked potentials is beneficial as a means of informing individuals of developments in related areas. Investigators and clinicians will refer to it quite often.

GERALD R. POPELKA, PhD
St. Louis, Mo

TRACHEOMALACIA IN AN INFANT WITH MULTIPLEX CONGENITA (LARSEN'S) SYNDROME

KENNETH M. GRUNDFAST, MD
WASHINGTON, DC
ROBERT KANTER, MD
SYRACUSE, NY
ANWAR MUMTAZ, MD
WASHINGTON, DC
MURRAY POLLACK, MD
WASHINGTON, DC

An infant born with multiplex congenita (Larsen's) syndrome developed respiratory distress 30 days following tracheostomy for relief of upper airway obstruction. The infant had structural and functional abnormalities of the thoracic cage. Tracheobronchoscopy revealed excessive compliance of the trachea with a tendency for collapse of the tracheal rings and obliteration of the tracheal lumen. Continuous positive airway pressure in the range of 20-25 cm H_2O was used to maintain patency of the tracheal lumen and assure adequate ventilation. Hemodynamic and pulmonary barometric complications often observed when high levels of positive airway pressure are utilized in infants were not observed.

The case report demonstrates a relationship between skeletal abnormalities and ineffectual respiratory effort. Although the initial respiratory difficulty evident at birth was from obstruction of the upper airway, the respiratory difficulty occurring subsequent to tracheostomy was caused by an unusual combination of factors. The significance of this report lies in the manner in which the etiology of the respiratory difficulty was determined, and the method utilized for management.

CASE SUMMARY

A male infant weighing 3,572 g at 41 weeks of gestation was delivered vaginally at a local community hospital. The amniotic fluid was meconium-stained; the baby was apneic and flaccid. Orotracheal intubation was accomplished in the delivery room and after ventilation was initiated with a portable manual-assist self-inflating (Ambu®) bag, spontaneous respiration developed. Apgar scores were 6 and 8 at 1 and 5 minutes respectively.

Examination revealed eyes spaced widely apart, prominent forehead, flat nasal bridge, midline cleft of the secondary palate, bilateral dislocations of the knees and elbows, deformities of the hands and feet, and spatulate thumbs. These features were recognized as being characteristic of multiplex congenita (Larsen's) syndrome. The infant breathed spontaneously through the endotracheal tube. Mechanically assisted ventilation was utilized for 48 hours, then the infant was "weaned" from the ventilator. When removal of the endotracheal tube after five days resulted in severe respiratory distress, attempts at reintubation failed and an emergency tracheostomy was necessary to restore adequate ventilation.

At two weeks of age the infant was transferred to the Children's Hospital National Medical Center for further evaluation and management.

The infant developed progressively worsening respiratory difficulty over the next several weeks. Change to a larger diameter tracheostomy tube did *not* improve the infant's condition. Radiographs of the chest revealed no pulmonary parenchymal abnormality, atelectasis, or pneumonia. When tachypnea, retraction, and intermittent cyanosis developed at age 35 days, the infant was taken to the operating room for laryngotracheobronchoscopy in order to determine the cause of the respiratory difficulty. A rigid 3 mm Storz-Hopkins rod lens ventilating bronchoscope was utilized. Although there was some granulation tissue in the tracheal lumen on the cephalad aspect of the tracheostomy site, there was no obstructing lesion within the trachea distal to the tracheostoma. There was excessive compliance of the trachea with a tendency for collapse of the trachea and nearly total obliteration of the lumen whenever positive pressure was not applied via the ventilating bronchoscope. Collapse of the trachea was most accentuated with expiration, but there was not full opening of the tracheal lumen with inspiration unless positive airway pressure was administered. Based on these findings, a diagnosis of severe tracheomalacia was made. As the infant emerged from anesthesia, respiratory difficulty and cyanosis developed. Rapid reinduction of anesthesia with control of respiratory function improved ventilation. These events were interpreted as indicating

From the Departments of Otorhinolaryngology and Anesthesia, Children's Hospital National Medical Center, and the Department of Otolaryngology, Washington Hospital Center, Washington, DC.

Presented at the meeting of the American Broncho-Esophagological Association, Vancouver, British Columbia, May 11-12, 1981.

REPRINTS — Kenneth M. Grundfast, MD, Department of Otorhinolaryngology, Children's Hospital National Medical Center, 111 Michigan Avenue NW, Washington, DC 20010.

that the infant could not maintain adequate respiration without assisted ventilation. Therefore, a decision was made to maintain respiration with administration of paralyzing agents and mechanically controlled ventilation.

When attempts were made to wean the infant from mechanically assisted ventilation, spontaneous respiration would develop whenever the administration of neuromuscular blocking agents was discontinued. However, spontaneous breathing was always associated with labored breathing, abnormal movements of the chest wall, intercostal retractions, agitation, and prolonged expiratory phase of respiration. After several hours without mechanically assisted ventilation, the infant became tired, breath sounds diminished, then cyanosis and bradycardia developed.

Observation of the infant's chest wall movements and analysis of the causes of the respiratory difficulty led to the conclusion that continuous positive airway pressure (CPAP), rather than mechanical control of respiration was the factor most important in maintaining effective respiratory function.

Cinefluoroscopy demonstrated collapse of the trachea with expiration. Increasing levels of CPAP were utilized until it was determined that the infant could maintain adequate ventilation with CPAP in the range of 20-30 cm H_2O. When CPAP lower than 15 cm H_2O was used, the infant developed frequent episodes of cyanosis accompanied by bradycardia.

The fact that CPAP was the key factor in maintaining adequate ventilation was confirmed by two methods. First, transpulmonary pressure, airflow rate, tidal volume and tidal pCO_2 were measured and continuously recorded as the level of CPAP was changed. (This method is described in Kanter R, et al, unpublished report.) Second, tidal breathing of the radionuclide krypton 81-m with scintillation mapping of the thorax showed improved ventilation with increasing levels of CPAP.

A portable apparatus capable of producing CPAP was devised for the infant's use at home. The child was discharged from the hospital at age 14 months requiring CPAP of 15 cm H_2O.

DISCUSSION

The terms "laryngomalacia" and "tracheomalacia" are frequently used to describe disorders in infants characterized by stridor, respiratory difficulty, and partial collapse of portions of the airway. Jackson[1] introduced the term "laryngomalacia" to describe the condition involving passive movements of certain flaccid supraglottic structures associated with stridor in infants. Later Holinger[2] introduced the concept of "tracheomalacia" when he reported the findings of three infants with stridor, dyspnea, signs of airway obstruction and periods of cyanosis. He noted that the tracheal wall was exceptionally flaccid and symptoms disappeared when a bronchoscope was passed through the seemingly collapsed portion of the trachea. The terms "laryngomalacia" and "tracheomalacia" describe disorders with no precise pathologic correlate. Unfortunately, some physicians have a tendency to use the terms interchangeably.

Terminology notwithstanding, it is generally accepted that stridor in infants can be caused by the abnormal movement of anatomic structures that have a normal gross and microscopic appearance. The type of tracheomalacia observed in infants usually is a congenital self-limited condition possibly caused by a delayed maturation of tracheal cartilaginous elements and hypotonia of tracheal myoelastic elements.[3] As a result, the trachea lacks its usual stiffness and the anterior and posterior aspects of the trachea tend to come close together so that the size of the tracheal lumen diminishes. The deformity is most evident during expiration when the normal physiologic tracheal narrowing is markedly accentuated.

Most often, the stridor associated with tracheomalacia in infants is mild and the respiratory difficulty is not life-threatening. Since there is no identifiable lesion and no characteristic pathologic finding, diagnosis of tracheomalacia depends upon endoscopic, radiographic, or other findings that demonstrate abnormal *movement* of tracheal structures. That is, the aberrant process is a dynamic one.

In 1950 Larsen et al[4] described six cases of children with similar congenital deformities. The syndrome that Larsen discovered is characterized by deformities of the joints of the upper and lower extremities, long cylindrical shaped fingers which do not taper normally from base to finger tips, spatulate shaped thumbs, eyes widely spaced apart, prominent forehead, depressed nasal bridge, and a strikingly flattened face. Additional features observed in some cases were cleft palate and failure of spinal segmentation. Biopsy and necropsy have not revealed pathologic changes in muscle as is seen in arthrogryposis multiplex congenita and similar syndromes. At necropsy, one infant with Larsen's syndrome had excessively compliant epiglottis, arytenoid cartilages, trachea and bronchi, with markedly reduced numbers of elastic fibers in the larynx, trachea and bronchi.[5]

Although Larsen did not describe respiratory difficulty or tracheomalacia as characteristic features of the original syndrome, Szabo and Perjes[6] later reported that stridor, tracheomalacia, and respiratory difficulty were observed in infants manifesting the stigmata of Larsen's syndrome. They did not describe the pathophysiology of the respiratory difficulty. Other authors[7,8] also reported laryngomalacia, respiratory difficulty and stridor in infants with Larsen's syndrome.

In 1974 Latta et al reported the case of an infant with Larsen's syndrome who manifested "serious respiratory problems apparently related to laxity of the trachea and rib cage . . . ."[9] Interestingly, Latta et al noted that there had been only a small number of cases reported in the 20 years since the syndrome originally had been described. He postulated that many cases had not been recognized or were categorized as arthrochalasis or arthrogryposis rather than multiplex congenita. Further, he speculated that death from respiratory compromise soon after birth may have hampered the recognition of characteristic features.

DIAGNOSIS AND MANAGEMENT

In the case now being reported, endoscopy, cinefluoroscopy, and radionuclide scanning were utilized to determine that excessive compliance of the trachea was the cause of the respiratory difficulty. Once it was determined that a combination of dynamic factors rather than intraluminal obstruction was the cause of respiratory difficulty, a method was devised for maintaining adequate ventilation. Parameters of pulmonary function were measured as levels of CPAP were varied. It was determined that CPAP in the range of 20-25 cm H_2O was necessary to maintain adequate ventilation.

Ordinarily, use of such high levels of CPAP for an infant would be expected to produce complications. When CPAP greater than 15 cm H_2O is used in infants, risks of pneumothorax and right heart strain are increased. Apparently, the excessive compliance of the trachea and laxity of cartilaginous rib cage structures enabled higher levels of CPAP to be safely used as a means of preventing collapse of the trachea in the presently reported case of an infant with Larsen's syndrome.

Although tracheostomy may sometimes be necessary to bypass an upper airway obstruction in an infant with Larsen's syndrome and tracheomalacia, in some ways the presence of the tracheostomy can have a deleterious effect on ventilation. A review of relevant aspects of pulmonary mechanics shows how the presence of a tracheostomy can adversely affect the infant with tracheomalacia. Normally, the vocal cords partially adduct during the early phase of respiration thereby providing some resistance to the outflow of air as intrathoracic pressure increases. In infants with tracheomalacia, the glottic mechanism may reduce the degree to which the trachea collapses by allowing a brief (0.1 to 0.2 s) increase in intratracheal pressure at the beginning of expiration.[10] A tracheostomy eliminates from the respiratory cycle the transient increase in intratracheal pressure at the beginning of expiration. In a way, CPAP can be conceptualized as an artificial means of providing a pressure similar to the one that occurs during the end of expiration when there is a competent, functioning glottic mechanism. In fact, this case report indicates that high levels of CPAP can exert an intratracheal positive pressure that counteracts the tendency for an excessively compliant trachea to collapse as intrathoracic pressure increases during expiration. Used in such circumstances, the CPAP effectively acts as a stent to keep the airway from collapsing.

SUMMARY AND CONCLUSIONS

The case of an infant with multiplex congenita (Larsen's) syndrome and tracheomalacia is reported. Though this syndrome is relatively rare, it is important for the otolaryngologist-head and neck surgeon to realize that airway obstruction, laryngomalacia, and tracheomalacia can occur in infants with Larsen's syndrome. Management may be difficult, especially if tracheostomy is required. Levels of CPAP higher than ordinarily utilized for infants may be helpful in the management of severe tracheomalacia associated with Larsen's syndrome.

Experience gained in the management of an infant with Larsen's syndrome who required tracheostomy had led to the following conclusions:

Infants with skeletal deformities such as those comprising Larsen's syndrome can develop respiratory difficulty.

Excessive compliance of the trachea (tracheomalacia) can be a major factor contributing to respiratory insufficiency.

Although tracheostomy may be necessary to bypass an obstruction in the upper airway, tracheostomy may accentuate the tendency for an excessively compliant trachea to collapse.

Continuous positive airway pressure can be safely utilized as a means of maintaining adequate ventilation in infants with tracheostomy, tracheomalacia, and certain skeletal abnormalities.

ACKNOWLEDGMENT — The authors wish to thank Mrs. Cynthia Fisher for her assistance in preparation of the manuscript.

Dr. Kanter is presently in the Department of Pediatrics, Upstate Medical Center, Syracuse, N.Y.

REFERENCES

1. Jackson C, Jackson CL. Diseases and injuries of the larynx. New York: MacMillan, 1942.

2. Holinger PH, Johnston KC, Parchet VN, Zimmermann AA. Congenital malformations of the trachea, bronchi, and lung. Ann Otol Rhinol Laryngol 1952; 61:1159-80.

3. Baxter JD, Dunbar JS. Tracheomalacia. Ann Otol Rhinol Laryngol 1963; 72:1013-23.

4. Larsen LJ, Schottstaedt ER, Bost FC. Multiple congenital dislocations associated with characteristic facial abnormality. J Pediatr 1950; 37:574-81.

5. Ronningen H, Bjerkreim I. Larsen's syndrome. Acta Orthop Scand 1978; 49:138-42.

6. Szabo L, Perjes K. Uber die Differenzierung der Ar-

throgryposis Multiplex Congenita und des Larsen-Syndroms. Syndroms Z Orthrop 1974; 112:1275-81.

7. Robertson FW, Koslowski K, Middleton R. Larsen's syndrome. Clin Pediatr 1975; 14:53-60.

8. O'Herlihy C, O'Brien N. Neonatal stridor with Larsen's syndrome. Israel J Med Sci 1977; 13:912-4.

9. Latta RJ, Graham CB, Aase J, Scham SM, Smith DW. Larsen's syndrome: a skeletal dysplasia with multiple joint dislocations and unusual facies. J Pediatr 1971; 14:53-60.

10. Ross BB, Gramosk R, Rahn H. Physical dynamics of the cough mechanism. J Appl Physiol 1955; 8:264-73.

≈

NINCDS NOTES*

TINNITUS GRANTS AWARDED

Two universities have received grants from NINCDS to study tinnitus, a common adult medical problem also known as "ringing in the ears."

At the University of Oregon, Dr. Jack A. Vernon will oversee the development of quantifiable measurements of the condition and its treatments, and the establishment of a tinnitus data registry. The relationship between tinnitus and drugs will also be examined by studying those agents used to relieve the condition and those linked to its possible causes.

On the East Coast, principal investigator Dr. Merrilynn Penner at the University of Maryland will conduct studies of the perceptual and psychophysical characteristics of tinnitus patients. Subjects for this study will be drawn from patients with sensorineural hearing loss resulting from noise exposure or acoustic trauma.

Tinnitus, which is frequently a symptom of more serious disease, affects an estimated 37 million adults, 7.5 million of whom are incapacitated by the problem. The two new NINCDS grants are expected to generate renewed interest in tinnitus research among otologists, neurologists, and audiologists.

TRAINING AWARDS EXPLAINED

Opportunities for participating in NINCDS's grants and awards programs are outlined in a new Institute booklet, *NINCDS Extramural Research and Training Awards*, now available through the Office of Scientific and Health Reports (OSHR).

The publication offers details on 10 categories of research grants, contract awards, and training stipends which assist the Institute in carrying out its programs in neurological and communicative disorders and stroke. The booklet includes information on award application deadlines as well as a brief description of NINCDS's many research interests.

Research grants make up the largest category of support provided by the Institute. Public and private nonprofit organizations which sponsor and conduct biomedical research and development are eligible for grants. Current grantees include universities, medical schools, college hospitals, and research institutes.

Copies of the new guide can be obtained by contacting the Office of Scientific and Health Reports, National Institute of Neurological and Communicative Disorders and Stroke, Bldg. 31, Rm. 8A06, 9000 Rockville Pike, Bethesda, MD 20205; telephone (301) 496-5751.

VOLUNTARY AGENCY PAMPHLET UPDATED

A revised and expanded edition of the NINCDS pamphlet *Voluntary Health Agencies Working to Combat Neurological and Communicative Disorders* is now available.

The pamphlet lists more than 50 voluntary health organizations alphabetically by disease category, and gives addresses, phone numbers, and key personnel for each organization.

Copies can be obtained from the NINCDS Office of Scientific and Health Reports, NINCDS, NIH, Bldg. 31, Rm. 8A06, 9000 Rockville Pike, Bethesda, MD 20205; telephone (301) 496-5751.

BOOKLET SERIES OUTLINES NIH TRAINING OPPORTUNITIES

A new series of pamphlets, *Research and Research-Related Manpower Development Programs Supported by the National Institutes of Health*, outlines postdoctoral and other training opportunities available in the biosciences through NINCDS and its sister organizations.

The four-part series of booklets examines NIH training programs for the following educational levels: postdoctoral, postbaccalaureate, college, and high school. Program summaries are provided in each pamphlet; included is information on eligibility, funding, points of contact, and application deadlines.

For copies of individual booklets or the complete four-part series, contact the Grants Inquiries Office, Division of Research Grants, Rm. 449, Westwood Bldg., 5333 Westbard Ave., Bethesda, MD 20205; telephone (301) 496-7441.

---

*This information is prepared monthly by the Office of Scientific and Health Reports, National Institute of Neurological and Communicative Disorders and Stroke, National Institutes of Health, Bldg. 31, Rm. 8A06, Bethesda, MD 20205, (301) 496.5751.

FLEXIBLE FIBEROPTIC ENDOSCOPY IN DIFFICULT INTUBATIONS

ENJE TH. EDENS, MD ROBERTO L. SIA, MD

GRONINGEN, THE NETHERLANDS

Intubation problems sometimes occur very suddenly and can be divided into two groups. The expected ones include the patients with a short neck and long teeth, cellulitis of the tongue, large oropharyngeal tumors, obstructing laryngeal tumors, congenital and acquired maxillofacial deformities, ankylosis of the temporomandibular joints, fractures or ankylosing spondylitis of the cervical spine, and all patients with a history of previous intubation problems. Unexpected problems can arise in patients who combine large incisors and canines with an inability to open the mouth wide, or when the glottis is invisible because the epiglottis is immobile. The first concern in these cases is to restore consciousness, for the conscious patient shows tonus and this facilitates identification of anatomical landmarks. A 60 cm bronchofiberscope provided with a tube and a freely movable end of 30 cm is suitable. Shorter flexible scopes are not adequate.

Since the days of Asclepiades, the fashionable Greek physician who practiced in the Rome of 100 BC, efforts have been made to find an elegant solution to the problem of difficult respiration. Fabricius, professor of surgery in Padua (1590), stated with reference to surgery of the trachea that "of all the surgical operations performed in man for the preservation of his life by the physician, I have always judged to be the foremost that by which man is recalled from a quick death by a sudden repossession of life, a feat which raises the surgeon nearest to the level of Aesculapius."[1]

Anesthetists, laryngologists and pneumologists sometimes find themselves in an acute situation in which they must quickly decide on a preferably simple method to combat progressive breathing difficulties. Given the aids available today, an emergency tracheotomy is the least elegant solution, even though in some situations a surgical procedure is certainly to be preferred.

Katz and Berci[2] took a step in the right direction when they evolved their rigid optical stylet. According to their principles we developed an intubation telescope (Fig. 1) which is an excellent aid in stridorous patients with obstructing laryngeal tumors, but is by no means in all cases the appropriate instrument to relieve acute dyspnea. The possibilities of an optical stylet or intubation telescope are limited because the introduction is only possible via the oral route.

The following methods have so far been available to anesthetists confronted with difficulties of intubation: a) guided oral intubation,[3] b) blind nasal intubation,[4] and c) cricothyroid puncture with retrograde catheterization.[5] All these methods give rise to more or less marked injuries of the mucosa of the upper air passage. Lesions of the lip, palate or teeth are often seen in these cases. Other patients show bleeding lesions of the nasal and oropharyngeal mucosa. Forced nasal intubation sometimes takes a false route via the posterior pharyngeal wall. Intubation of the esophagus is not uncommon in these cases.

The introduction of the flexible fiberscope paved the way to a more effective solution of the problems in difficult intubation. Without doubt, intubation with a flexible system is far less traumatic than the previously mentioned methods via a rigid McIntosh laryngoscope.[6]

All flexible bronchoscopes with an operative length of about 60 cm, a diameter of about 5.9 mm and a suction device are suitable as an aid in a difficult intubation. The ENT Department of the Groningen University Hospital uses the Olympus BF-B3 R bronchoscope (Fig. 2A). When the instrument is provided with a standard Portex® tube, a free scope length of 30.5 cm remains for manipulation if the endoscopist takes the nasal route. In a comparable situation the 46 cm American Optical

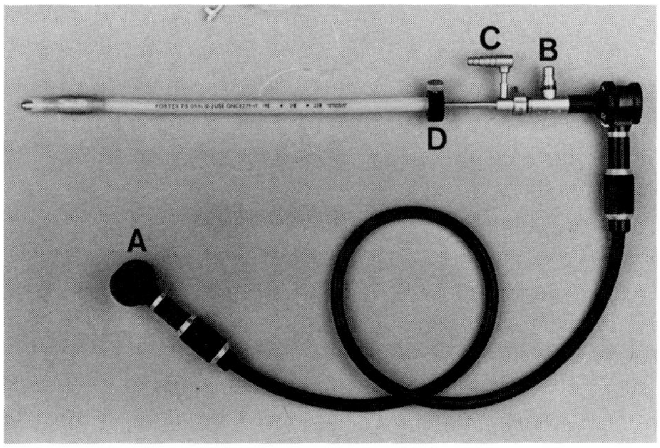

Fig. 1. Intubation telescope (Wolf, Knittlingen, W. Germany). A - Fiberoptic teaching attachment (American Cystoscope Makers, Stamford, Conn.). B - Fiberlight connection; C - Luer connection for washing, suction or oxygen supply; D - Locking device.

From the Ear, Nose and Throat Department and the Department of Anesthesiology, University Medical Center, Groningen, The Netherlands.
Presented at the meeting of the American Broncho-Esophagological Association, Vancouver, British Columbia, May 11-12, 1981.
REPRINTS — Enje Th. Edens, MD, Department of Ear, Nose and Throat, University Medical Center, P. O. Box 30.001, Groningen, The Netherlands.

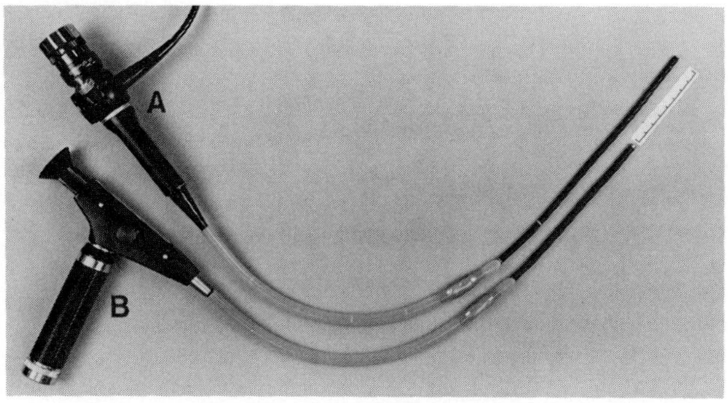

Fig. 2. A - 60 cm bronchofiberscope (Olympus); B - 48 cm flexible laryngoscope (American Optical).

flexible laryngoscope has a free length of only 18 cm for manipulation. In our opinion this is insufficient for effective help in difficult nasal intubation (Fig. 2B).

TECHNIQUE OF INTRODUCTION

The nasal route is the most commonly used. An oral approach is not advisable because, via the base of the tongue, the scope has to be sharply angled in order to reach the glottis. The angle required in the nasal approach is far less acute: the scope makes an almost straight approach to the target. Another advantage of the nasal route is that the expensive instrument cannot be damaged by the patient's teeth. It is advisable to explore the nasal passage in advance so that a proper tube size can be chosen. Blood from the damaged nasal mucosa and secretions often pose problems in that they soil the front lens. Suction of the nose and hypopharynx can prevent many difficulties. Fogging of the lens can be prevented by coating it with a soap solution. In order to minimize frictional resistance, the first 4 cm of the bronchoscope are coated with jelly. While the instrument is being introduced, an assistant should stand by with separated facilities for suction drainage.

In cases in which difficulties are expected, flexible intubation is best done after adequate premedication with diazepam (Valium®) and spraying of the nasal and oral mucosa with a 4% lidocaine (Xylocaine®) solution. The fiberscope with a tube, silicone-coated on the inside, is carefully advanced through the nose to the nasopharynx. Silicone-coating is essential because the fiberscope can be retracted from the tube without any friction. The introduction should be careful because when it is done hastily, the tip can easily disappear into the esophagus behind the larynx. At manipulation with the flexion control, an upward flexion of up to 45° is sufficient to bring the glottis into view. Further flexion of 90° and 130° returns the tip to the base of the tongue or nasopharynx.

In patients already sufficiently anesthetized, the tongue should be pulled out with forceps or with gauze-covered fingers. This maneuver elevates the epiglottis and tenses the piriform sinus, thus faciliating introduction of this instrument. The use of a McIntosh laryngoscope can sometimes surprisingly improve the overall view, provided the mouth can be opened to sufficient width.

When the vocal cords come into view, the tip of the scope is advanced a few centimeters until the tracheal rings can be clearly distinguished. The thumb should continue to fix the flexion control. When the control is released at this critical moment the scopetip flips back from the trachea. At this moment anesthesia is induced, whereupon the free end of the bronchoscope can be passed between the vocal cords. The tube is then retracted from the flexible scope in the trachea.

DISCUSSION

Little is known about the incidence of difficult intubations. Our personal experience indicates a ratio of approximately 1:750 cases. Problem cases

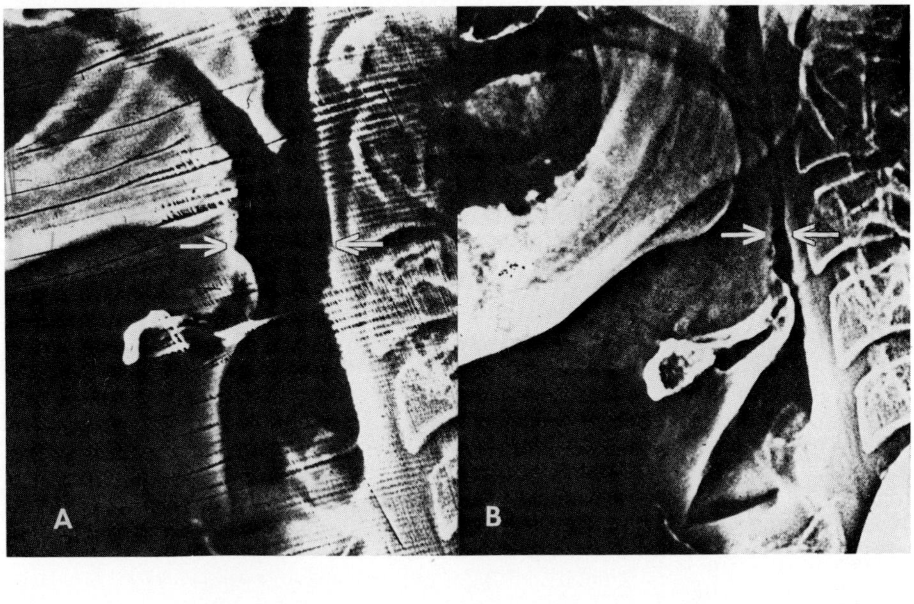

Fig. 3. Radiographic views of oropharynx. A) Conscious patient. Note space between base of tongue and pharyngeal wall. B) Unconscious patient.

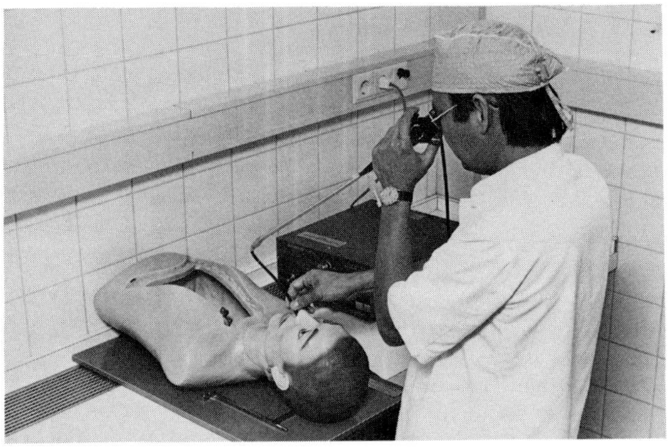

Fig. 4. Nakhosteen bronchoscopy model (C.L.A., Coburg, W. Germany).

can be divided into two groups: expected and unexpected difficult intubations.

The expected difficult intubations comprise some 90% of all cases, the causes of the difficulties being obesity, a short neck, oropharyngeal tumors, cellulitis of the tongue, congenital or acquired maxillofacial deformities, ankylosis of the temporomandibular joint, spondylitis and ankylosis of cervical vertebrae, cervical fractures and a history of previous intubation problems. The unexpected difficult intubations comprise the remaining 10% of cases. The difficulties become apparent soon after injection of barbiturates and muscle relaxants. An overlying epiglottis prevents the vocal cords or even the posterior commissure of the glottis from being brought into view. Another possible cause of unexpected problems lies in the combination of prominent and overly long incisors and canines, and a mouth which cannot be opened to full width.

We have occasionally seen dorsal flexion of the epiglottis due to proliferation of lymphoid tissue of the base of the tongue and pharyngeal mucosa. Touching this region with the laryngoscope quickly caused bleeding and obstruction of the view on the laryngeal inlet.

Unconscious and conscious patients show a distinct difference in oropharyngeal anatomy (Fig. 3). The conscious patient shows tonus of the tongue, epiglottis, piriform sinus and muscles of the floor of the mouth. In the unconscious or paralyzed patient, tonus disappears: the tongue sags back, the epiglottis covers the vocal cords and the piriform sinus shows relaxation. Intubation problems in unconscious or paralyzed patients cannot be adequately solved until tonus is restored. The primary concern is therefore to restore consciousness. When the patient is breathing spontaneously, the nose and pharynx can be cleansed by suction drainage and an attempt can be made to find the laryngeal inlet under local anesthesia.

Fiberoptic intubation requires considerable experience and constant practice. "Flexible experience" can be readily gained during nasal intubations for tonsillectomy or other planned oropharyngeal operations. At the Groningen University Hospital, however, the ENT Department has the benefit of over 600 fiberoptic bronchoscopies carried out annually in collaboration with the pneumologists. Introduction rehearsals on anatomical models (Fig. 4) as proposed by Nakhosteen[7] enable the inexperienced endoscopist to study the possibilities of the flexible bronchoscope at his leisure.

This program provides our department with additional possibilities of instruction in the technique of flexible intubation. We believe that at least 30 successful fiberoptic intubations in both conscious and unconscious patients are required before an endoscopist can be confident of his ability to solve the problems of an unexpected difficult intubation.

REFERENCES

1. Cawthorne T. Two historical tracheostomies. Proc R Soc Med 1968; 61:1169-76.

2. Katz RL, Berci G. The optical stylet. Anesthesiology 1979; 51:251-4.

3. Waters PJ. Guided blind endotracheal intubation. Anaesthesia 1963; 18:130-1.

4. Singh A. Blind nasal intubation. Anaesthesia 1966; 21:400.

5. Powel WF, Ozdil T. A translaryngeal guide for tracheal intubation. Anesth Analg 1967; 46:231-4.

6. Sia RL, Edens ETh. How to avoid problems when using the fibre-optic bronchoscope for difficult intubation. Anaesthesia 1981; 36:74-5.

7. Nakhosteen JR. Fiberbronchoskopie. Stuttgart: Georg Thieme, 1978:27-9.

CARBON DIOXIDE LASER TREATMENT OF METASTATIC MELANOMA OF THE TRACHEA AND BRONCHI

ALBERT H. ANDREWS, JR., MD DAVID D. CALDARELLI, MD

CHICAGO, ILLINOIS

An occasional patient with metastatic or recurrent malignant disease develops intraluminal masses in the trachea and/or the main bronchi. The accuracy of the application, absence of bleeding, slight reaction, and rapid healing make the CO_2 laser applied through the open bronchoscope a valuable palliative treatment for the relief of obstructive dyspnea. This patient is reported because he demonstrated the reduced bleeding which occurred with the bronchoscopic CO_2 lasing as compared to bronchoscopic forceps removal.

It is usually impossible to use two completely different methods of treatment and to make a valid comparison of the two methods in the same patient. The patient reported here had intraluminal, metastatic malignant melanoma of the trachea which necessitated relief of the obstructive dyspnea.

On four occasions bronchoscopic forceps removal was impeded by hemorrhage and on two occasions the CO_2 laser did not cause as much bleeding, and relief of the obstructive dyspnea was comparable with both methods.

CASE REPORT

A 28-year-old male was seen in August 1978 complaining of dyspnea, mild cough and blood-streaked sputum. In February 1976 he underwent a wide excision of right shoulder melanoma with a node dissection. There was no evidence of metastatic disease in the 35 sectioned axillary lymph nodes. Pathologic classification was Clark level V. Chest radiographs and tomography demonstrated two round densities overlying the trachea and three soft tissue masses within the lumen of the trachea and left main bronchus. The trachea was narrowed to 50% of its normal lumen and the left mainstem bronchus was narrowed to 80% of its lumen. A gallium scan showed positive uptake only in the tracheobronchial and lung parenchymal lesions. Bronchoscopically, both tracheal lesions were reddish in color and sessile in nature. They were excised using cup forceps followed by epinephrine pledgets for hemostasis. Postoperatively the patient had minimal hemostasis with less respiratory distress. Three days later the left mainstem bronchial lesion was excised, again with moderate bleeding that was controlled with epinephrine pledgets. The left mainstem bronchus was patent enough to allow a 5 x 40 cm bronchoscope to pass beyond the lesion and to allow visualization of the left bronchial anatomy. No other lesions were visualized. Postoperative course was free of respiratory distress or hemoptysis. Pathologic examination of all lesions revealed metastatic melanoma.

Over the next four months three bronchoscopes were required for the relief of dyspnea and each time bleeding was a problem and required epinephrine pledgets. During this period chemotherapy and palliative x-ray therapy (3900 rads over three weeks) were administered with only mild relief of the respiratory symp-

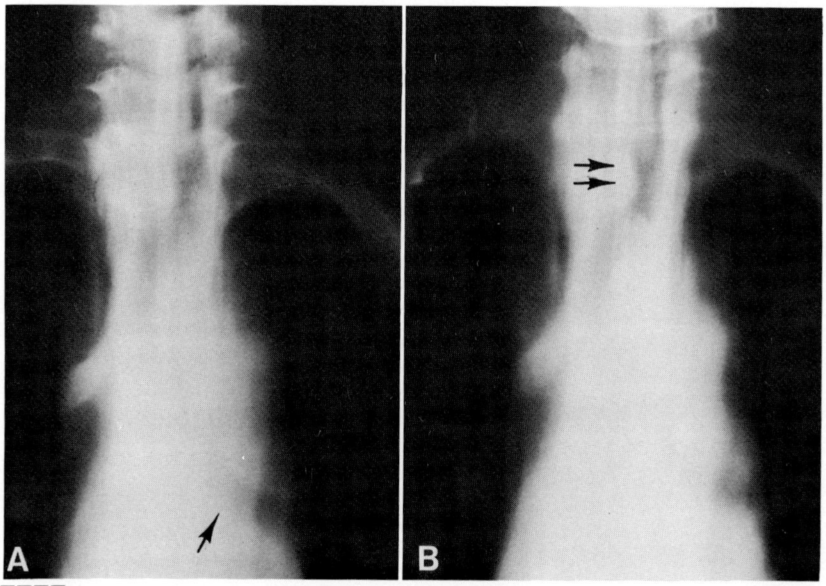

Fig. 1. Tomographic roentgenograms of the chest June 26, 1979. A) Single arrow points to patency of left main bronchus distal to the obstruction. B) Double arrow indicates masses in the right wall of the trachea.

From the Department of Otolaryngology, University of Illinois, and the Department of Otolaryngology and Bronchoesophagology, Rush Medical College, Rush-Presbyterian-St. Luke's Medical Center, Chicago.

Presented at the meeting of the American Broncho-Esophagological Association, Vancouver, British Columbia, May 11-12, 1981.

REPRINTS — Albert H. Andrews, Jr., MD, Department of Otolaryngology, University of Illinois, Eye and Ear Infirmary, 1855 W. Taylor St., Chicago, IL 60612.

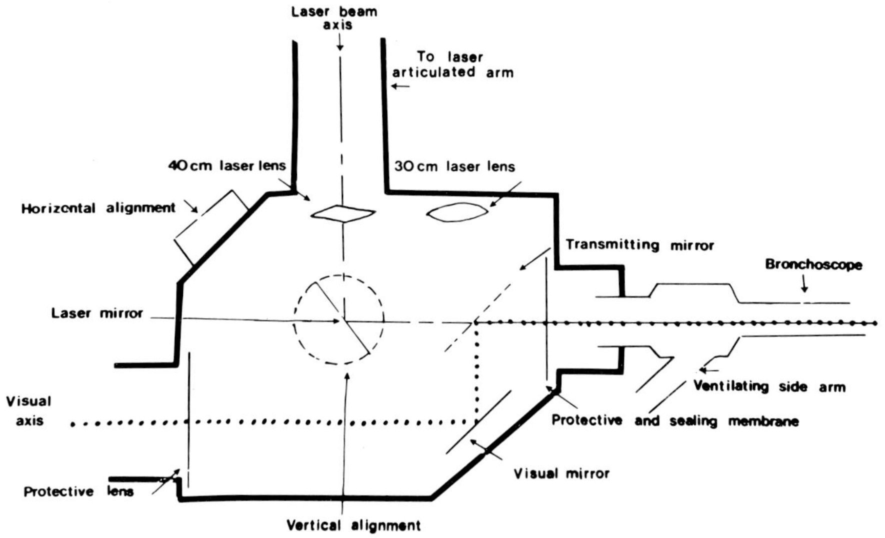

Fig. 2. Diagram of laser bronchoscopic coupler.

toms. Because of the increased bleeding with each bronchoscopy, it was felt that laser excision of the recurrences would provide safer and more complete excision, thus prolonging the interval of palliation.

The patient was admitted to the Eye and Ear Infirmary of the University of Illinois on April 24, 1979, complaining of obstructive intractable dyspnea and hemoptysis. Chest radiographs showed fullness along the right tracheal wall and a density in the carinal area in addition to bilateral multiple rounded densities in the lung fields. Bronchoscopy under general anesthesia showed four masses of 5 to 7 mm in size along the right lateral tracheal wall and a large mass partially obstructing the trachea and almost occluding the left main bronchus. The masses were lased from distally to proximally. At the conclusion the tip of the 8 mm by 40 cm (Wolff International model) bronchoscope could be passed into the left main bronchus. Bleeding was minimal.

The patient had chest pain following the procedure. The chest radiograph showed bilateral pulmonary edema. The patient left the hospital on the third postoperative day with much improved breathing.

Two months later the patient again experienced severe obstructive dyspnea (Fig. 1). Bronchoscopy revealed a mass arising from the right tracheal wall and occluding about 75% of the lumen. Because of difficult ventilation, the bronchoscope was forced past the mass and the obstruction was relieved. A large mass was again found at the carina.

This mass was lased away; however, more bleeding occurred than at the previous lasing. As the bronchoscope was withdrawn the masses were lased away as they appeared at the end of the scope. The patient was discharged on the first postoperative day with much improved breathing.

The patient was readmitted to Presbyterian-St. Luke's Hospital six weeks later because of severe dypsnea. The patient insisted that the shortness of breath was different from that which has been relieved by the CO_2 laser. The patient died on the tenth hospital day of respiratory incompetence due to the pulmonary metastasis.

DISCUSSION

The bronchoscopic coupler (Fig. 2) attaches to the articulated arm of the laser and to the bronchoscope.[1] The coupler directs the infrared beam down the bronchoscope, the vertical and horizontal adjustments allow placing the impact area within the limits of the bronchoscopic field; the coupler contains a membrane which seals the proximal end of the bronchoscope so respiratory support can be given; it contains two lenses for focusing the beam at 30 or 40 cm and allows the endoscopist to see down the bronchoscope without danger to his own eye.

The laser beam is usually adjusted to the center of the field. Bleeding is avoided as much as possible because blood when lased forms an adherent char which can overheat and increase reaction. Care must be exercised to avoid lasing normal tissue beyond the tumor as the tumor is destroyed. Also it is essential to not burn through the tracheal or bronchial wall. At the present time aspiration through the bronchoscope requires separation of the coupler and bronchoscope, a time-consuming process and especially so if it must be done frequently.

Intraluminal obstructing malignant tumors may be lased to supply palliation by relief of obstruction and reduction of cough and bleeding. It is emphasized that lasing of bronchial or tracheal compression is avoided. The advantages to the CO_2 laser include accuracy, precise control of area and depth of burn, minimal reaction, and slight amount of bleeding. The case reported here demonstrated that bleeding was less with the CO_2 laser destruction than with forceps removal. The reduced bleeding permits more adequate removal and therefore improved palliation.[2,3]

REFERENCES

1. Strong MS, Vaughan CW, Polanyi TG, Wallace RW. Bronchoscopic CO_2 laser surgery. Ann Otol Rhinol Laryngol 1974; 83:769-76.

2. Andrews AH, Horowitz SL. Bronchoscopic CO_2 laser surgery. Lasers Surg Med 1980; 1:34-45.

3. Andrews AH, Soltes SF. CO_2 laser for the trachea and bronchi. In: Andrews AH, ed. Endoscopic and microsurgery with the carbon dioxide laser. Littleton, Mass: W-PSG Publishing Company, 1981 (in press).

SPUTUM CYTOLOGIC DIAGNOSIS OF UPPER RESPIRATORY TRACT CANCER

SECOND REPORT

H. BRYAN NEEL III, MD, PhD

DAVID R. SANDERSON, MD ROBERT S. FONTANA, MD

WILLIAM F. TAYLOR, MD LEWIS B. WOOLNER, MD

ROCHESTER, MINNESOTA

Screening for cancer is a popular issue for debate because few, if any, evaluations of the screening process have been conducted on a long-term prospective basis with use of concomitant, unscreened controls. We have found that screening of high-risk persons for presymptomatic lung cancer will identify patients with cancer in the upper and lower respiratory passages. Randomly selected patients enrolled in the Mayo Lung Project have undergone sputum cytologic and chest roentgenographic screening at four-month intervals and were compared with randomly selected matched control subjects who were not intensively screened. The search for upper airway tumors in the head and neck region was instigated by abnormal findings on sputum cytology in 12 screened patients. In the same period, 12 other screened patients with abnormal results of sputum cytology were found to have roentgenographically "occult" lung cancer. This finding emphasizes the importance of the otorhinolaryngologic examination in screening programs for airway cancer. It is also important to emphasize that sputum-negative patients may have obvious, symptomatic tumors of the upper aerodigestive tract that can be easily diagnosed by those who are skilled in examining this area. Contrary to our expectation, there is no definitive evidence that screening has reduced mortality from either upper or lower airway cancer.

Periodic sputum cytology has been incorporated in screening programs designed to detect presymptomatic lung cancer in chronic excessive cigarette smokers.[1-4] This has led to fortuitous identification of cancers of the upper respiratory and alimentary tracts.[5] This observation comes as no surprise because cigarette smoking is an etiologic factor common to both upper and lower respiratory tract cancers.

The present report describes our experience with 54 such cases identified during the course of the Mayo Lung Project for early detection of lung cancer. Thirty-seven of these cases formed the basis of the first report to the American Broncho-Esophagological Association at its annual meeting in 1978.

MATERIALS AND METHODS

During recruitment of subjects for the project, 11,001 patients were interviewed. All patients were men older than 45 years of age who were smoking one pack of cigarettes or more daily or had done so within the previous year. Almost all had smoked heavily for more than 20 years. All patients had a complete medical examination, including a standard 36- by 43-cm chest roentgenogram and cytologic examination of a 3-day "pooled" specimen of sputum.

Those found to have cancer of the respiratory tract on this initial or "prevalence" examination were appropriately treated, but they were excluded from the periodic retesting or "incidence" phase of the project, which is the subject of this report. Also excluded were patients who did not complete the initial screening, patients with limited respiratory reserve who were not candidates for surgical treatment (at least lobectomy), and patients with illnesses considered sufficiently serious to preclude participation in a long-term prospective study.

The remaining 9,211 patients were randomized into a *participant (screened)* group and a *control (comparison)* group. The participant (screened) subjects had roentgenographic and cytologic rescreening at four-month intervals. The patients in the control (comparison) group were advised to have annual rescreening. Intensive efforts were made to secure compliance in the participant (screened) group. Their tests have been paid for by the Mayo Lung Project. The control (comparison) group was merely contacted once a year by a letter-questionnaire that did not mention roentgenography or sputum cytology.

Cytologic Diagnosis. The specimens for sputum cytology in each patient are pooled, three-morning collections of spontaneous deep-cough sputum fixed in 50% alcohol and 2% Carbowax®[5,6] (Doac Pharmacology Company, Inc, Westbury, Long Island, NY).

The cytologic diagnosis of squamous cell cancer is based on conventional cellular criteria for malignancy. The features vary somewhat from case to case but generally include increase in size of the cells and nuclei, variation in size and shape of cells and nuclei, abnormal nuclear-cytoplasmic ratio, nuclear hyperchromasia with coarse chromatin pattern, and a wrinkled or irregular nuclear membrane. Lesser degrees of cellular change are designated squamous cell "atypia" and are generally graded as slight, moderate, or marked in degree. Squamous differentiation in atypical or frankly carcinomatous cells is evidenced by the presence of intracytoplasmic keratin, which imparts a glassy or homogeneous quality to the cytoplasm and is readily detected by a brilliant orange coloration with the Papanicolaou stain.

Generally, a squamous cell carcinoma arising in the upper portion of the respiratory tract cannot be distinguished cytologically from one developing in the lower portion.

Examination. Patients with positive results of sputum cytology and normal chest roentgenograms almost always have squamous

From the Mayo Clinic and Mayo Foundation, Rochester, Minnesota. This investigation was supported in part by Research Grant CB-53886 from the National Institutes of Health, Public Health Service.

Presented at the meeting of the American Broncho-Esophagological Association, Vancouver, British Columbia, May 11-12, 1981.

REPRINTS — H. B. Neel III, MD, PhD, Mayo Clinic, Rochester, MN 55905.

TABLE 1. NUMBER OF MAYO LUNG PROJECT PARTICIPANTS AND CONTROLS WITH CANCER IN THE UPPER AIRWAY OR LUNG THROUGH JULY 1, 1980

Patients	*Participants*	*Controls*
Total entered	4,618	4,593
With upper airway cancer	30	24
Per 1,000 persons/yr	1.2	1.0
With lung cancer	120	83
Per 1,000 persons/yr	4.9	3.5

cancers involving either the upper airway or the first four orders of branching of the tracheobronchial tree.[7,8] Accordingly, one of the first appointments scheduled for these patients is a complete otorhinolaryngologic examination, which is usually conducted in a physician's office. If a tumor of the upper airway is detected, the diagnosis is confirmed by biopsy performed in either the office or the operating room.

Staging. Tumors have been staged according to the recommendations of the American Joint Committee for Cancer Staging and End-Results Reporting (AJC).[9]

RESULTS

Through July 1, 1980, tumors in the upper respiratory and alimentary pathways were detected in 30 patients in the participant (screened) group and 24 patients in the control (comparison) group. Lung cancer was found in 120 participants and 83 control subjects (Table 1). All but one of the tumors in the upper respiratory and alimentary passages were squamous cell carcinomas, as might have been anticipated. The one exception was an oncocytic adenocarcinoma of the larynx that was detected in one of the control (comparison) subjects.

The distribution of cancers by AJC staging was similar in the two groups (Table 2).

In the 30 participant (screened) subjects, the search for cancer in the upper airway was instigated by abnormal sputum cytologic findings in 12 and by symptoms (for example, hoarseness, sore throat, sore in mouth) in 17. In the remaining patient, the tumor was observed during a routine head and neck examination for an inflammatory ear problem (Table 3). One patient in the participant group had a squamous cancer of the anterior tonsillar pillar excised; subsequently, an adenocarcinoma of the lung

TABLE 2. STAGE OF UPPER AIRWAY TUMORS IN MAYO LUNG PROJECT PARTICIPANTS AND CONTROLS

	Participants			*Controls*		
	Detection by		*Total*	*Detection by*		*Total*
Stage	*Cytology*	*Symptoms*	*No.*	*Cytology*	*Symptoms*	*No.*
TIS	1	1	2	0	0	0
I	3	7	10	1	8	9
II	6	6	12	0	5*	5
III	1	0	1	0	3*	3
IV	1	2	3	0	2	2
NS†	0	1	1	1	4	5
Total	12	17	29§	2	22	24§

*One patient had two primary tumors.

†NS - Not staged.

§One participant and one control subject not included — tumors detected on routine head and neck examination.

TABLE 3. DETECTION OF UPPER AIRWAY CANCER IN 30 MAYO LUNG PROJECT PARTICIPANTS

	Method of Detection		
	Cytology	*Symptoms**	*Examination*†
Number of patients	12	17	1
Age (yr)			
Range	50-70	47-73	
Mean	62	61	59
Pack-years			
Range	25-75	23-120	
Mean	52	66	100
Site of cancer			
Larynx	8	9	1
Base of tongue	2	1	—
Soft palate	2	2	—
Floor of mouth	—	3	—
Hypopharynx	—	1	—
Nasopharynx	—	1	—

*All had negative results of sputum cytology before symptoms developed.

†Otorhinolaryngologic examination for ear problem; negative results of sputum cytology.

developed. In the 24 control (comparison) subjects, the search was initiated because of symptoms in 21. Two control subjects had abnormal sputum cytologic findings and concurrent development of symptoms, and one tumor was found on a routine head and neck examination (Table 4).

The time from the collection of positive sputum to the last follow-up of the upper airway tumor was tabulated and related to the status (dead or alive) of the patient. Death rates were calculated from these data. In 7 of these 14 patients, the tumor was localized and treated fairly promptly (from less than 1 month to 5 months); in the other 7, there was a delay in localizing the tumor (from 7 to 46 months) and consequently a delay in treatment. From the time of detection, the subsequent death rate for the early-treated group was 7 per 1,000 months; for the later-treated group it was 12 per 1,000 months. Although these rates do not differ significantly, they are compatible with the theory that effectiveness of screening depends not only on early detection but also on prompt localization, which was not always possible despite intense efforts.

TABLE 4. DETECTION OF UPPER AIRWAY CANCER IN 24 MAYO LUNG PROJECT CONTROLS

	Method of Detection		
	Cytology	*Symptoms*	*Examination**
Number of patients	2	21	1
Age (yr)			
Range		50-73	
Mean	67, 68	64	71
Pack-years			
Range		21-106	
Mean	91	61	106
Site of cancer			
Larynx	2	13	—
Floor of mouth	—	4†	—
Tongue	—	3	1
Hypopharynx	—	1†	—
Hard palate	—	1	—

*Routine otorhinolaryngologic examination; negative results of sputum cytology.

†One patient had two primary tumors.

TABLE 5. SURVIVAL OF MAYO LUNG PROJECT PATIENTS WITH UPPER AIRWAY CANCER

	Participants		Controls	
Total with cancer		30		24
Deaths		12		4
Upper airway cancer	9*		4	
Other cause	3		0	

*Results of sputum cytology negative in five and positive in four.

Survival data are more meaningful now than they were at the time of the first report.[5] Among the 30 participants, 18 are alive and free of tumor and 12 have died; 9 of the 12 died from their upper airway tumors. Among the 24 controls, 20 are alive and free of tumor and 4 have died; all 4 died from their upper airway tumors (Table 5). Of the nine participants who died, four had had positive results and five had had negative results on sputum cytology. For analysis of survival from the time of first detection, the 24 controls were compared with the 30 participants. For controls, the four deaths due to upper airway cancer occurred during an exposure time of 814 person-months, a rate of five deaths per 1,000 months. For participants, the findings were somewhat different; there were nine deaths in 934 person-months, a rate of ten deaths per 1,000 months. Contrary to our expectations, there was no evidence that survival of participant (screened) subjects is better than that of control (comparison) patients. Although there seems to be a difference in Figure 1, these rates are not significantly different.

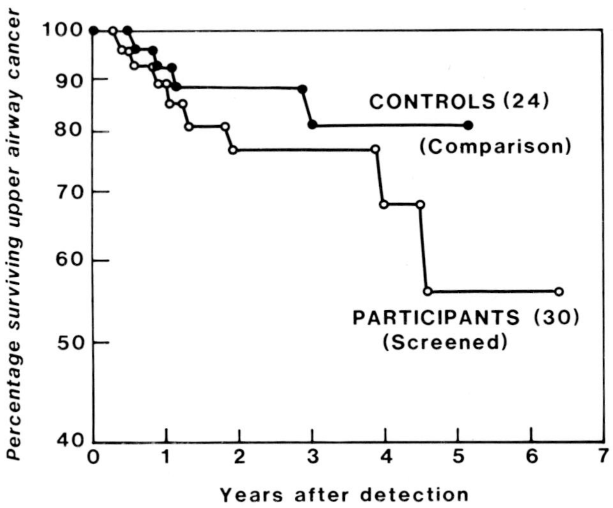

Fig. 1. Actuarial survival curves, showing percentage of patients (screened and comparison subjects) surviving upper airway cancer by years after detection.

DISCUSSION

The Mayo Lung Project was undertaken primarily to evaluate a screening program for lung cancer in high-risk subjects.[1,2] Simply stated, it was designed to answer the question, "Does offering screening for early lung cancer work?"[4] The discovery of several patients with tumors in the *upper* respiratory and alimentary passages in the head and neck region by sputum cytology emphasizes the well-known fact that patients who are at risk for lung cancer are also at risk for squamous cell carcinoma of the head and neck region. This is illustrated by the observation that 54 of the 257 patients (21%) in the project who were found to have cancer through July 1, 1980, had tumors in the head and neck region (excluding the lip).

Cytologic changes may evolve from negative findings or slight atypia to moderate or marked atypia. This transition occurs during the course of months or several years, the time involved being quite variable. Symptoms may develop at approximately the time that sputum cytologic tests become positive.[5]

The search for these tumors in the upper airway of the head and neck region was prompted by abnormal sputum cytologic findings in 12 participant (screened) patients. In the same period, 12 other screened patients with abnormal results of sputum cytology were found to have roentgenographically "occult" lung cancer.[4] Therefore, half of the patients with abnormal findings on sputum cytology had "occult" cancer in the upper airway and half had "occult" cancer in the lower airway (lung). This finding emphasizes the importance of the otorhinolaryngologic examination in screening programs for airway cancer. Those who use sputum cytology as part of a cancer screening program should be aware of the distribution of the cancers in the upper and lower airways.

The 17 participant (screened) patients in whom symptoms developed and the 1 asymptomatic patient who had an otorhinolaryngologic examination for an unrelated problem had negative results of sputum cytology on one or more occasions before the otorhinolaryngologic examination at which their tumors were detected. Thus, sputum cytology may yield negative results at the same time that cancer can be readily detected by a thorough examination of the upper respiratory and alimentary passages; the patient may or may not be symptomatic. Furthermore, the stage of the tumors seemed to be comparable in the participants in whom tumors were detected cytologically and in those in whom they were detected because of symptoms. Similarly, when all participant (screened) and control patients were compared, the various stages of the cancer were about equally represented in the two groups.

Contrary to our expectations, survival in the participant (screened) patients, including those whose examination was instigated by abnormal results of sputum cytology, is no better than that in the control (comparison) patients. Perhaps the similarity of the survival data is related to the fact that the distribution of patients among the various disease stages in the two groups is similar.

The onset of symptoms closely approximated the time that results of sputum cytology become abnormal in many of the patients. Questioning of high-risk patients about symptoms and performing a thorough examination of the upper respiratory and alimentary passages are the usual approaches for early diagnosis. Sputum cytology will help reveal a substantial number of these tumors in high-risk patients, but it does not seem to improve survival over that achieved by localization of the tumor after symptoms develop.

REFERENCES

1. Sanderson DR, Fontana RS. Early lung cancer detection and localization. Ann Otol Rhinol Laryngol 1975; 84:583-8.

2. Taylor WF, Fontana RS. Biometric design of the Mayo Lung Project for early detection and localization of bronchogenic carcinoma. Cancer 1972; 30:1344-7.

3. National Cancer Institute, Cooperative Early Lung Cancer Group. Manual of procedures, Jan 1, 1975.

4. Taylor WF, Fontana RS, Uhlenhopp MA, Davis CS. Some results of screening for early lung cancer. Cancer 1981; 47:1114-20.

5. Neel HB III, Woolner LB, Sanderson DR. Sputum cytologic diagnosis of upper respiratory tract cancer. Ann Otol Rhinol Laryngol 1978; 87:468-73.

6. Saccomanno G, Saunders RP, Ellis H, Archer VE, Wood BG, Beckler PA. Concentration of carcinoma or atypical cells in sputum. Acta Cytol (Baltimore) 1963; 7:305-10.

7. Marsh BR, Frost JK, Erozan YS, Carter D, Proctor DF. Flexible fiberoptic bronchoscopy: its place in the search for lung cancer. Ann Otol Rhinol Laryngol 1973; 82:757-64.

8. Sanderson DR, Fontana RS, Woolner LB, Bernatz PE, Payne WS. Bronchoscopic localization of radiographically occult lung cancer. Chest 1974; 65:608-12.

9. American Joint Committee for Cancer Staging and End-Results Reporting. Manual for staging of cancer. Chicago: American Joint Committee, 1977.

≈

Ann Otol 90:1981

UNUSUAL PRESENTATIONS AND PROBLEMS CREATED BY MISMANAGEMENT OF FOREIGN BODIES IN THE AERODIGESTIVE TRACT OF THE PEDIATRIC PATIENT

SEYMOUR R. COHEN, MD
LOS ANGELES, CALIFORNIA

Nine children who suffered unusual problems because of the mismanagement of ingested or inhaled foreign bodies are reported. The causes of mismanagement are discussed and the details of the histories, examinations and follow-up are given. The serious complications were pulmonary hemorrhage, tracheoesophageal fistulae, mediastinitis resembling a mediastinal tumor, periesophageal infection from perforation, loss of a Fogarty® catheter tip in a segmental bronchus, laryngeal stenosis from a cricothyrotomy in an infant, and the displacing of a foreign body into an almost inaccessible distal bronchus. All of these unusual problems, and the resultant morbidity and financial cost, could have been avoided with proper management and early diagnosis.

This study reports a series of unusual complications and the problems in treatment which were created by the mismanagement of foreign bodies in the aerodigestive tract in children.

The diagnosis and management of foreign bodies in the air and food passages ordinarily poses few, if any, problems for the skillful endoscopist. However, many aspects of mismanagement described in this paper did create problems for the endoscopist, and imposed serious complications which were frequently life-threatening for the child. The unreported morbidity that is created by foreign bodies which are improperly managed has been greatly underestimated, and the resulting excessive financial drain on parents and society is difficult to assess.

In 1936 Jackson[1] reviewed 3,000 cases of foreign bodies and listed carelessness as the primary cause of their ingestion or inhalation in 87% of the patients. Eighty-two percent of the problems occurred in children under 15 years of age. Estimates vary, but the yearly death rate continues to be in the thousands.

The patients presented in this study have been chosen in order to stress the many factors which produced unusual complications and created difficulties in their endoscopic management. The factors which may be responsible for the mismanagement of foreign bodies are listed as follows:

1. Absence of a positive history.
2. Absence of positive roentgenogram findings.
3. Inadequate roentgenographic studies.
4. Omission from the primary diagnosis.
5. Errors created by inexperienced consultants.
6. Inappropriate use of instruments.
7. Inappropriate techniques of removal.
8. Inexperienced endoscopists.
9. Inadequate communication between anesthesiologist and endoscopist.
10. Always expecting the foreign body to be on the right side.[2]
11. Parental ignorance or negligence.

Each patient presented with one of the above problems. Frequently the absence of a positive history seemed to exclude the probability that a foreign body could be the source of the child's problem-symptom complex. When a negative x-ray study was obtained, even though the roentgen studies were inadequate, a foreign body was often ruled out from the differential diagnosis, and in some instances was not even suspected. At times, the x-ray study was merely obtained to "rule out pneumonia." In some of the patients, the respiratory symptoms were not even thought to have arisen from the digestive tract (ie, the hypopharynx or esophagus), and thus the proper diagnosis was completely missed and erroneous therapy was therefore instituted. Inexperienced consultants (in one instance a gastroenterologist and in another an otolaryngologist) misled the pediatrician or primary physician and thus caused serious delay in arriving at the proper diagnosis. In the child reported herein with severe hemoptysis-hematemesis, the consultant's diagnosis of Mallory-Weiss syndrome delayed the diagnosis of a foreign body in the lung which consequently produced life-threatening hemorrhage. In the child with stridor, the ear, nose and throat consultant erroneously made the diagnosis of laryngomalacia, which was then compounded by

From the Department of Surgery, Division of Otolaryngology, Childrens Hospital of Los Angeles and University of Southern California School of Medicine, Los Angeles.
Presented at the meeting of the American Broncho-Esophagological Association, Vancouver, British Columbia, May 11-12, 1981.
REPRINTS — Seymour R. Cohen, MD, 1300 North Vermont Avenue, Los Angeles, CA 90027.

inadequate therapy and misleading and inadequate roentgen studies. The use of the fiberoptic bronchoscope for attempted removal of the foreign body in one instance pushed the foreign body into an almost inaccessible area of the bronchial tree. In another patient the tip of the Fogarty® catheter, lost in a segmental branch of the right upper lobe, fortunately was successfully removed later with the use of the image intensifier. In one child who had a foreign body in the larynx and in the bronchus, attempted removal on three occasions with faulty endoscopic-anesthesia control resulted in repeated unsuccessful endoscopic procedures. This same patient had had a cricothyrotomy because of the severe airway obstruction and then developed a severe laryngeal stenosis. He still wears a tracheotomy tube many months after his original inhalation of the foreign object. Often the parent is not entirely faultless. In the last case reported in this paper, the child's dysphagia was completely ignored until choking became severe to the point of near asphyxiation. This child was found to have a coin in the esophagus which had wandered and had perforated into the trachea, creating mediastinitis. When dysphagia first occurred in this child a single film could have diagnosed her disease and could have prevented this serious complication. This latter foreign body is the only one in the series that was not retrieved by endoscopic means; the child required a thoracotomy.

LITERATURE REVIEW

Cohen et al[2] reported that 62% of the foreign bodies in their series were on the left side of the chest.

Friedberg[3] in 1970, before the American Broncho-Esophagological Association, reported that the journal *Today's Health* published by the AMA contained an article on "The Killer That Came to Dinner."

Friedberg,[4] in his report of the Committee on Prevention of Foreign Body Accidents before the American Broncho-Esophagological Association in 1973 said that stressing the mortality rate caused by foreign bodies was contrary to fact. He stated that while the death rate is more dramatic, creates deeper feelings, and is more provocative, the cost to society of ingested foreign bodies probably exceeds the drama of the death rate in many ways.

LeJeune[5] in his Presidential Address before the American Broncho-Esophagological Association in 1968 reported the case history of a child who had been ailing for four months with cachexia from no identifiable cause. Finally when a film which included the cervical region revealed a foreign body in the postcricoid area, removal was difficult and complications of bilateral vocal cord paralysis made a tracheotomy necessary which was worn for 15 years until an arytenoidectomy was performed.

Yee et al[6] reported on extraluminal foreign bodies, all of which were coins in the food and air passages. They reported four cases of children varying in age from two to eight years in whom external surgery was necessary for removal of a foreign body which had wandered beyond the confines of the esophagus. One had an esophagobronchial fistula which required gastrostomy feedings.

Morioka et al[7] reported on unexpected foreign bodies found on routine preoperative roentgen examinations for other planned surgeries. One patient had been treated for two years for episodes of dysphagia which were attributed to emotional causes. Another patient, who was admitted for routine bilateral myringotomy and ventilating tubes, had a preoperative roentgenogram of the chest which showed a coil spring in the right bronchus. The third patient had been treated for laryngotracheal bronchitis for three days prior to and four days after admission. When no change occurred following therapy the patient was laryngoscoped, revealing a wedge of photographic film in the larynx.

Zavala et al[8] report on the role of the fiberoptic bronchoscope for removal of foreign bodies and indicate that without intensive training in the use of this instrument, the patient will suffer the following:

1. Displacement of the foreign body to an unfavorable position, making its removal difficult.

2. Trauma to the bronchial tree with infection, bleeding or perforation.

3. Airway obstruction secondary to losing the foreign body in the subglottic area.

4. Breaking the foreign body into pieces.

5. Hypoxia and possible cardiac arrest because of failure to utilize supplemental oxygen.

The authors admonish the endoscopist that in children and infants "the rigid tube and not the flexible bronchoscope should be used in pediatric cases because of the small diameter of the trachea and glottis."

Ritter[9] warns against the use of balloons along with radiology to remove foreign bodies in the esophagus because there may be a nonopaque foreign body present or a bone with a sharp point may be within the foreign body. Removal or extraction, he continues, can cause perforation, and if the foreign body is large it may hang up at the cricopharyngeus area, causing obstruction and even death.

CASE REPORTS

Case 1. A 13-year-old male was admitted to the Childrens Hospital of Los Angeles on November 18, 1978. His history was one of being an asthmatic, under treatment with desensitization and medication with prednisone. His present illness started six days prior to admission, when the patient was reported to have swallowed the clip portion of a Lindy® pen. The patient was told to observe his stools for the clip and when it did not pass after six days, a roentgenogram of the abdomen was taken which was reported as normal. Subsequently, a chest roentgenogram was obtained which revealed the metallic foreign body to be in the right mainstem bronchus. He was taken to the operating room by the local otolaryngologist and bronchoscoped with a fiberoptic bronchoscope. The foreign body could not be removed after two hours of surgery. He was transferred to the Childrens Hospital of Los Angeles, where the physical examination on admission was unremarkable except for the inspiratory and expiratory rhonchi and diminished breath sounds in the right base posteriorly. Roentgen studies revealed the metallic foreign body now to be in the right lower lobe bronchus, 7.5 cm from the carina. Laboratory findings were within normal limits. The patient was taken to the operating room following an initial dose of intravenous steroids and antibiotics, and bronchoscopy was performed. Erythema and edema of the larynx and of the right bronchial tree were found. The foreign body could not be seen, and although it could be palpated with a forceps, it could not be removed. Three days later on November 22, after a course of antibiotics and continuation of steroids, bronchoscopy with the aid of the image intensifier made successful surgery of the foreign body possible. The patient was discharged on the day after removal to be followed by his pediatrician. His postoperative roentgenogram of the chest was normal and he was continued on antibiotics for two weeks. The postoperative follow-up indicated that this child had no further problems.

COMMENT. This case illustrates the potential inadequacy and hazards of fiberoptic bronchoscopy in the treatment of foreign bodies in children. It also points to the fact that a report by a child that he has swallowed something does not rule out aspiration. When there is a positive history without a complete examination which includes roentgenograms, waiting for spontaneous extrusion of a foreign body may lead to an incorrect diagnosis and may cause serious complications. It would seem prudent to always adequately examine a patient with roentgenograms on any report of swallowing, choking or aspirating foreign material, and even when findings are negative, to strongly consider endoscopic examination.

Case 2. A male born December 19, 1972, was the product of a normal delivery and pregnancy. The chief complaint was breathing difficulty, and increased difficulty and choking while feeding. Two months prior to his present complaint, this 10-month-old infant began to cry while crawling on the floor, and could not be appeased for a number of hours. Preceding this crying episode, the mother noticed that he had a choking spell. He was taken to his pediatrician that afternoon, after developing fever and swelling in the neck. Roentgenograms of the chest were reported as normal, whereupon he was given penicillin therapy and his temperature soon returned to normal. However, stridor persisted and the child developed increasing difficulties in swallowing. He was referred to an otolaryngologist whose diagnosis was laryngomalacia, and who gave reassurances to the parents that the stridor would disappear with growth and development. However, with an increased difficulty in swallowing, persistence of stridor and loss of weight, the parents requested further consultation. On October 4, 1973, an examination revealed a loud inspiratory fluttering stridor and an expiratory stridor which could be heard at the mouth. There were no neck masses palpable and the pharynx looked perfectly normal. The remainder of the ear, nose and throat examination was within normal limits, except for the presence of a bifid uvula. Roentgenograms of the neck and chest and an esophagram were taken soon after this examination. These roentgenograms revealed a quadrangular discoid opaque foreign body in the soft tissues of the neck in the midprecervical region. There was associated moderate soft tissue swelling into the posterior laryngopharyngeal area with bowing of the cervical tracheal air column. The heart, lungs and mediastinum were perfectly normal. On barium esophagram, only one half of a foreign body appeared to be in the lumen of the cervical esophagus.

The child was admitted to the Childrens Hospital of Los Angeles on October 5, 1973, and on the following morning esophagoscopy and removal of a piece of ceramic porcelain 2 x $1\frac{1}{2}$ cm in size was accomplished. The foreign body had perforated the retropharyngeal and periesophageal tissue. Intravenous penicillin was given and on the following day the child was discharged, but remained on oral antibiotics for a period of two weeks. He was seen periodically and had persistent stridor for approximately three weeks. On October 24, 1973, an esophagoscopy showed the esophagus to be healed and without stricture formation.

COMMENT. This patient's problems were created by the inadequacy of roentgen studies which showed only limited areas on examination. In children, the neck should be included in a chest roentgenogram. If foreign bodies are suspected, the abdominal cavity should also be included in the roentgenological examination. The first x-ray studies of the chest were limited to the level of the clavicle. The original otolaryngologist fell into the trap of assuming that stridor is most often due to laryngomalacia, and therefore made that diagnosis. To and fro stridor is rarely seen in that benign lesion, and feeding difficulties rarely accompany that diagnosis. Ignoring the choking spell that was originally reported by the mother masked this child's problem and created a potentially serious complication.

Case 3. A male child was admitted to the Childrens Hospital of Los Angeles on June 28, 1973, with the diagnosis of a mediastinal tumor mass. This $3\frac{1}{2}$-year-old child lived with his grandmother, who reported that for two months prior to his admission he had developed increasing nocturnal noisy breathing. He had no cough, cyanosis or weight loss. Ten days prior to his admission to the hospital, as part of a routine physical examination, a roentgenogram of the chest was obtained which showed a mediastinal mass. The physical examination revealed a small but active boy with a to and fro stridor associated with suprasternal and intercostal retractions. Prominent lymphadenopathy in the posterior cervical and inguinal regions were found. Hepatosplenomegaly was not found. He was afebrile and had coarse rhonchi in the chest. His admission laboratory studies were within normal limits, except for a 10,400 white blood count. An excisional biopsy of the posterior cervical triangle and inguinal lymph nodes was performed, after a tentative diagnosis was made of Hodgkin's disease, lymphoma or other malignancy. Histopathological examination showed reactive hyperplasia of the lymph nodes. The child was then scheduled for a thoracotomy, but because of the airway obstructive disease, the anesthesiologist requested an otolaryngological consultation for a possible endoscopy to be performed prior to giving the general anesthetic. A foreign body was suspected by the consultant, and an esophagram was advised. The esophagram showed an irregularity and narrowing of the esophageal lumen with marked narrowing of the tracheal airway. Direct laryngoscopy revealed a normal larynx, and tracheal narrowing could be seen when the vocal cords abducted. Esophagoscopy was performed under apneic technique and a foreign body was found imbedded within the folds of the esophagus. A plastic C-shaped package closer was removed. The patient was treated with intravenous antibiotics postoperatively and was fed orally. At the end of one week, esophagoscopy still showed the esophagus to be somewhat narrowed. The bronchoscopy revealed persistent tracheal narrowing in the midportion of the trachea, just above the thoracic inlet. The patient was discharged on antibiotics and was again esophagoscoped two weeks later, at which time the esophagus was healed, although slightly narrowed. On October 1, 1973, esophagoscopy revealed a normal esophagus and he was discharged to continued pediatric care.

COMMENT. This child was misdiagnosed because of a lack of a positive history of foreign body ingestion. The diagnosis of a foreign body was not made because it was not suspected in the primary diagnosis. Tracheal obstruction in children should mandate the exclusion of esophageal disease. The findings on an esophagram spared this child a thoracotomy, and led to accurate diagnosis and management of his problem.

Case 4. This 19-month-old (born August 6, 1978), who was asymptomatic, presented on March 28, 1980, with x-ray evidence of a foreign body in the right upper lobe — a piece of Fogarty catheter which had been broken off during an endoscopic examination performed elsewhere. The past history elicited the information that this child was normal until he choked while eating peanuts and was taken to an outlying hospital. A roentgenogram of the chest on March 19, 1980, with right and left decubitus roentgenograms and fluoroscopy showed marked hyperlucency of the right lung with limited diaphragmatic motion and mediastinal shift to the right during expiration. These findings were compatible with a right-sided bronchial obstruction, for which bronchoscopy was performed. An impacted piece of peanut in the right main bronchus was noted by the surgeon, who used a Fogarty catheter to disimpact the peanut fragment. Subsequently the fragment was removed but it was noticed that a piece of the Fogarty catheter had broken off and had remained in the right upper lobe. A second bronchoscopy was then performed, but the foreign body could not be seen and the child was referred for removal of the foreign body.

The infant was admitted to the Childrens Hospital of Los Angeles on March 28, 1980, when laryngoscopy and bronchoscopy were performed. The foreign body could not be seen since it was in the peripheral area of a segmental bronchus, but was removed with the image intensifier. He was discharged two to three hours after bronchoscopy, to be followed by his pediatrician. A roentgenogram of the chest taken after the foreign body removal showed the chest and lung fields to be normal.

COMMENT. The inappropriate use of an instrument neither designed for nor intended for the removal of foreign bodies created the need for two additional anesthetics and endoscopic procedures when one might have sufficed. The use of a Fogarty catheter to remove a foreign body seems unwarranted in light of this very probable complication.

Case 5. A 17-month-old Laotian female, born in a refugee camp in Thailand, was first seen in a pediatric office ten days prior to her admission to the Childrens Hospital of Los Angeles. The chief complaint was fever 102° F (38.5° C), cough, grunting respirations and increased respiratory rate. A roentgenogram of the chest revealed a left lower lobe infiltrate. Examination showed bilateral basilar rales. On admission to an outside hospital, her temperature was 104° F (40° C) and her laboratory findings showed a hyperchromic microcytic anemia with giardiasis and a urinary culture of 100,000 *Escherichia coli.* She was started on iron and flagyl. A sweat test, SGOT and SGPT were normal. She remained febrile between 99 and 102° F (36.5 to 38.5° C) throughout her hospitalization. Serial roentgenograms showed little change in the left lower lobe infiltrate, but revealed increasing hyperlucency of the left upper lobe with shift of the mediastinum into the right chest. There was no history of a foreign body aspiration. An intermediary PPD was negative, and the parents had normal chest roentgenograms on arriving in this country.

The patient was transferred to the Childrens Hospital of Los Angeles, where examination showed a small Asian female in no distress. Vital signs were within normal limits and the examination was normal, except for the marked reduction in breath sounds over the left chest, with increased resonance to percussion. The heart was normal except for a grade 2/6 systolic ejection murmur. The WBC was 22.8, hemoglobin was 11.3, SMA 12 was normal, blood cultures and stool cultures were negative, *Giardia* was seen in the stools on an ova and parasite stain. The child had a negative PPD and a negative SKSD, but had a positive *Candida* skin test. Gastric aspiration was negative for acid-fast bacillus and tomograms of the chest showed no abnormalities. The patient was treated with antituberculus medication and intravenous cefamandole. Otolaryngology consultation was followed by endoscopic examination. Bronchoscopy on December 14, 1979, showed a large piece of rice in the left lower lobe bronchus, with remarkable reaction around the foreign body. After removal of the foreign body, all chest findings returned to normal, the patient became afebrile, and she was discharged on the second day after bronchoscopic removal of the foreign body. She was readmitted for another endoscopic procedure on January 2, 1980, when purulent secretion was still seen streaming from the left mainstem bronchus, and there was persistent swelling of the mucosa. Because the cultures of the bronchial secretion showed a pneumococcus, the child was discharged on oral antibiotics. Another bronchoscopy was performed on January 21, 1980, at which time there was some inflammation and a roentgenogram of the chest suggested early bronchiectatic changes in the lung.

COMMENT. An absent history, the supposition that refugees most likely have tuberculosis in spite of negative laboratory findings, and the ignoring of the fact that obstructive bronchial lesions may be attributable to foreign bodies led to a delay in diagnosis. This resulted in increased morbidity, expensive hospitalization and the potential for bronchiectasis.

Case 6. A male born June 5, 1977, was first seen on May 30, 1980, with the chief complaints of increasing respiratory difficulty, noisy breathing, difficulty in swallowing and loss of 0.45-0.9 kg (1-2 lb) of weight over a period of two weeks. The following history was obtained. Three and one-half weeks prior to admission the child had a runny nose and low grade fever. He was seen in an emergency room by his pediatrician, was found to have stridor, and had complained of right shoulder pain with violent emesis. He was given an antibiotic. Two weeks prior to admission, he was again seen by his pediatrician with what was described as a croup-like syndrome, for which ampicillin was advised. One and one-half weeks prior to his admission he was again seen, and the child was noted to hold his neck stiffly. The antibiotic was changed to erythromycin. He continued to cough, vomit and have labored breathing and was finally referred for ear, nose and throat examination as a case of unresolved croup. Roentgenograms which were taken originally to determine the status of his airway showed no evidence of disease. There was no history of aspiration or ingestion of a foreign body.

When he was first seen, this 3-year-old male was pale, uncomfortable and munching on a cookie. Soon after attempting to swallow he began to choke, sputter, cough and vomited with severe spasms. Examination of the ear, nose and throat was normal, except that the neck was somewhat stiff and resisted hyperextension. There was tenderness to palpation in the lower portion of the neck and rhonchi were heard in the chest bilaterally. A review of the roentgen studies which had been taken two weeks prior to his being seen showed the chest to be normal but there was fullness in the upper esophagus with a suggestion of air bubble within the esophagus. He was taken to the Radiology Department, where a roentgenogram of the chest revealed a widened mediastinum. A lateral film of the neck and airway showed narrowing of the tracheal airway at the thoracic inlet. The periesophageal area was severely widened. A swallow of barium showed a nonopaque plastic jack in the upper esophagus with a large tracheoesophageal fistula. On the lateral film there was a suggestion that a foreign body projected into the tracheal air column. The child was immediately admitted to Childrens Hospital of Los Angeles and was started on ampicillin and gentamicin. His laboratory findings were within normal limits, except for a WBC of

11,100. The following morning laryngoscopy, bronchoscopy and esophagoscopy were performed. The larynx was normal, but the trachea was found to have a ball prong of the jack projecting into its lumen through a perforation in the party wall. The esophagoscopy showed severe periesophagitis and esophagitis with a perforation through which a portion of the jack extended anteriorly into the trachea. The jack was gently disengaged from the trachea and easily removed. Postoperatively, a nasogastric feeding tube was passed and the child was maintained on his antibiotics with intravenous fluids. Feedings were given only through the nasogastric feeding tube. On the sixth postoperative day, the child being afebrile, oral clear liquids were started and no choking was evident. On June 11, he was taken to the operating room after an esophagram showed no evidence of a persistent tracheoesophageal fistula, and the endoscopy procedures showed the tracheoesophageal fistula to be completely healed with no significant stenosis of the esophagus. He was discharged on the following day on ampicillin and was again seen on June 19 (one week later) at which time he was gaining weight and had completely recovered.

COMMENT. Because the original roentgen studies were reported as negative, a foreign body was no longer suspected. The misinterpretation of the symptoms of stridor and a brassy cough as croup created a life-threatening problem in this child. The persistence of the complaints in spite of adequate antibiotic therapy should have suggested the need for further investigation into the true cause of the symptoms. The prolonged presence of the foreign body caused a tracheoesophageal fistula.

Case 7. A 4-year-old female was admitted to the Childrens Hospital of Los Angeles on September 24, 1980. There was a history of several days of cough and fever prior to admission. The vital signs showed the temperature to be 100.4° F (38.2° C), pulse 170, respirations 60, and the blood pressure to be normal. The ear, nose and throat and heart were normal on examination. The chest examination revealed grunting respirations and coarse breath sounds bilaterally with rhonchi. Her abdomen was soft and bowel sounds were present. The abdomen was distended with air. The WBC was 12.8, and roentgenogram of the chest, which was brought in with the patient, revealed an abnormally tilted coin in the esophagus. On the lateral roentgenogram, the coin could be seen to be partially within the tracheal air column.

Because of her respiratory difficulty, she was immediately taken to the operating room and bronchoscopy was performed. A portion of the coin (a penny which was corroded and black) was seen in the left posterolateral wall of the trachea with a fistula. Esophagoscopy was then performed, but the foreign body could not be seen within the lumen of the esophagus. With each ventilation by the anesthesiologist, an air blast could be heard in the esophagus. Since the foreign body was too large to be removed through the trachea and larynx, a right thoracotomy was performed by the Thoracic Surgery Department. At thoracotomy, a large lymph node mass was seen around the coin, which was blackened from its long presence in the patient. The removal of the coin resulted in a large defect in the trachea, which measured about 1 cm or more in length; the defect was closed.

Postoperatively, the patient was given peripheral hyperalimentation. A barium esophagram two weeks later showed severe aspiration through a large tracheoesophageal fistula, and a gastrostomy was performed. Her postoperative course was complicated by spiking fever, a urinary tract infection, and recurrent pneumonitis. Intravenous cefamandole was given throughout her hospitalization. On November 12, almost six weeks after admission, she was able to take oral feedings without aspiration and she was advanced to a full diet. She was discharged on November 13, 1980, was seen by a thoracic surgeon on December 2, and was found to be doing well, gaining weight, and eating normally. The gastrostomy was completely healed.

COMMENT. This patient represents the difficulties which may develop when the patient or parent does not observe minor symptoms such as dysphagia as this child unquestionably had for a period of time prior to her developing a tracheoesophageal fistula. It was only after severe choking spells occurred that the importance of her symptoms caused the parents to seek medical help. Had the minor symptoms been reported earlier, a roentgenogram of the chest would have shown the coin in the esophagus which could easily have been removed, thus avoiding this life-threatening complication.

Case 8. An 11-month-old male was transferred to the Childrens Hospital of Los Angeles on July 19, 1980. The history documents a choking spell on July 10, 1980, while he was eating a chicken leg. The child became cyanotic and was taken to the local hospital by the paramedics. Because he could not be intubated, a cricothyrotomy was performed.* Laryngoscopy and bronchoscopy showed edema of the vocal cords, but a foreign body was not found. On July 13, 1980, he was again taken to the operating room and direct laryngoscopy and bronchoscopy showed a piece of chicken to be present between the true vocal cords. The tracheotomy tube was removed from the cricothyrotomy incision, following which the child developed severe respiratory obstruction with substernal retractions. Another bronchoscopy was performed, but a foreign body could not be found and a standard tracheotomy was performed to relieve his airway obstruction. Roentgen studies taken postoperatively showed a left upper lobe pneumonia, for which he received treatment with antibiotics. Because of the spiking fevers, he again had laryngoscopy and bronchoscopy, but removal of the foreign body from the left mainstem bronchus was not accomplished. He was therefore transferred to the Childrens Hospital of Los Angeles for further care. On admission, the physical examination revealed a tracheotomized child in no distress. He was taken to the operating room on the day of admission and direct laryngoscopy and bronchoscopy were performed. A foreign body and granuloma were removed from the right mainstem bronchus. A severe laryngeal stenosis was seen on laryngoscopy. Intravenous Keflin® was administered, but he spiked a temperature to 39.7° C and a roentgenogram showed a left perihilar infiltrate consistent with aspiration pneumonitis. A barium esophagram showed aspiration into the trachea and oral feedings were discontinued. He was fed by nasogastric tube and one week later an endoscopic examination showed marked reduction in the sensation of the larynx, consistent with superior laryngeal nerve paralysis. Within two weeks he began to feed normally without aspiration. On July 30, 1980, he became icteric with increased liver enzymes and all laboratory work pointed to his having hepatitis which was most likely halothane-induced. He recovered from this complication and was discharged on August 7, 1980. Numerous laryngoscopies and bronchoscopies and the treatment of his laryngeal stenosis secondary to cricothyrotomy have been performed. He still had a persistent, severe web of the anterior two thirds of the larynx which requires a tracheotomy to support his airway. He feeds well and has a normal tracheobronchial tree.

COMMENT. Inexperienced endoscopy made necessary multiple incomplete and unsuccessful attempts at removal of the foreign bodies. A cricothyrotomy was performed in an infant which created severe complications such as laryngeal stenosis, marked increase in morbidity and costly hospitalizations. If on admission this child had had the laryngeal foreign body removed, or an endotracheal tube had been passed, a cricothyrotomy would not have been necessary.

Case 9. A male born January 11, 1975, was admitted to the Childrens Hospital of Los Angeles on December 8, 1977. The his-

*Although the records state that the surgical procedure was a cricothyrotomy, the scar in the neck, the physical findings, and the clinical course suggest that it was actually a hyothyrotomy.

tory on his admission was that this child had been admitted to an outlying hospital on December 1, 1977, with a two- to three-week history of severe spasmodic cough associated with retching and vomiting. On the night before his admission to that hospital, he had coughed up first 10 cc and then 60 cc of bright red blood. He had been given aspirin intermittently for fever since the onset of his illness. The family history showed that a sibling had died of a ruptured cerebral aneurysm. A roentgenogram of the chest showed a left lower lobe pneumonia. A gastroenterologist was consulted who suggested the diagnosis of Mallory-Weiss syndrome aggravated by aspirin intake. In the past history the child had bronchitis and cough with some wheezing for approximately two months. These symptoms were treated with various antiasthmatic and cough medications. In the outlying hospital he was treated with amoxicillin to control the pneumonia. It was on December 3 and 4, 1977, that he again had emesis of bright red blood. On December 4, he was given erythromycin to cover *Mycoplasma* infection. He continued to spike fevers and there were decreased breath sounds in the left lower lobe. On December 3, his WBC was 11.2 and his hematocrit was 27. On December 4, his hematocrit had dropped to 22 and his WBC was elevated to 15,000. Sputum cultures showed a *Neisseria* species, and a review of the chest roentgenograms showed progressive left lower lobe consolidation.

On December 8, he was transferred to the Childrens Hospital of Los Angeles, where soon after admission he had a hematemesis while coughing. He vomited approximately one-half cup of bright red blood. He required a blood transfusion. Gastroenterology consultation again diagnosed gastrointestinal bleeding, but because of the persistent pneumonia the consulting otolaryngologist suggested that the child might have a foreign body in his left lung.

On December 10 bronchoscopy was performed and revealed a portion of a sunflower seed shell which was imbedded in the left lower lobe. There was a large foreign body granuloma surrounding the shell. After removal of the foreign body, some bleeding occurred which was controlled with the local application of a constricting agent. His postoperative course was uneventful, there was no further bleeding, and he was discharged on December 13.

Because of the roentgen evidence of residual left lower lobe pneumonia, another bronchoscopy was performed on February 1, 1978, and a residual granuloma was removed from the left lower lobe. Narrowing of the left lower lobe bronchus was noted. In March 1980 he again developed fever and cough with x-ray evidence of a left lower lobe infiltrate. Therefore, he was suspected of having bronchiectasis. On April 28, 1978, he was admitted to the Childrens Hospital of Los Angels for endoscopic examination, at which time a bronchogram was performed. There was no evidence of bronchiectasis, but there was narrowing with localized stenosis of the left lower lobe bronchus. Although he had ear, nose and sinus infections, he had not had any recurrent lung disease. He was last seen on January 8, 1981, at which time he was free of pulmonary problems.

COMMENT. Hemorrhage was not considered as being of pulmonary origin and consultation which led to erroneous diagnosis and advice created serious problems for this child. The cough for two months prior to his pneumonia, which was diagnosed as bronchitis, should have indicated the probability of a foreign body in the lung, especially when a pneumonitis followed and failed to clear on appropriate therapy.

CONCLUSIONS

A number of factors were involved in the mismanagement of foreign bodies in the aerodigestive tract in children. Nine children are reported in whom one or more of these factors caused increased morbidity and, at times, serious life-threatening complications. Delayed recognition of the possibility of a foreign body as the cause of the presenting symptoms in these children made repeated hospitalizations necessary, prolonged treatment, and increased the cost of medical care.

The important factors responsible for the mismanagement of foreign bodies were as follows:

1. Failure to think of a foreign body or to ask the older child regarding this possibility.
2. Inadequate roentgenograms, particularly not including the neck in the chest roentgenogram, and failing to use contrast media where necessary.
3. Waiting for spontaneous extrusion of a known swallowed or inhaled foreign object.
4. Assuming a negative history excluded the diagnosis of a foreign body inhalation or ingestion.
5. Not evaluating the esophagus as a cause for persistent and increasing respiratory difficulty.
6. The inappropriate use of a Fogarty catheter and fiberoptic flexible instruments to remove the foreign body.
7. An erroneous diagnosis.
8. Delaying endoscopy in patients with evidence of severe bronchial obstruction.
9. Assuming that negative roentgenograms rule out the possibility of a foreign body diagnosis.
10. The parent ignoring symptoms reported by the child or failing to report a choking spell.

The complications reported in this paper which were created by mismanagement are as follows:

1. The foreign body pushed into an almost inaccessible bronchus by the use of fiberoptic flexible bronchoscopy.
2. Periesophageal perforation with abscess.
3. Mediastinitis misdiagnosed as a tumor of the mediastinum.
4. A lost Fogarty catheter tip in a segmental upper lobe bronchus.
5. Bronchiectasis from delay in removal of a foreign body.
6. Tracheoesophageal fistula in two children with esophageal foreign bodies.
7. Severe laryngeal stenosis from a hyothyrotomy in a child with laryngeal and bronchial foreign bodies.
8. Severe, almost life-threatening pulmonary hemorrhage from an unrecognized foreign body in the bronchus.

When there is a positive history of foreign body ingestion or inhalation, even when the physical findings and roentgen studies are negative, an endoscopic examination is mandatory. When there is a positive history, waiting beyond 24 to 36 hours is not appropriate and may be hazardous to the patient. Expectation that the foreign body will be expelled spontaneously or with the use of bronchodilators and postural drainage is potentially dangerous to the child. The use of fiberoptic flexible endoscopes and Fogarty catheters should be discouraged and has caused complications. Endoscopy, with the high success rate and low morbidity in the hands of skillful endoscopists and anesthesiologists, together with the use of open rigid endoscopes, is the only appropriate form of management of foreign bodies in the aerodigestive tract in children.

There has been serious dilution of patients with foreign bodies in the aerodigestive tract. Thoracic surgeons, pediatric surgeons, pulmonary medical specialists, gastroenterologists and even radiologists are engaging in the removal of foreign bodies. Training programs thus suffer the consequences of a reduced work load which makes difficult adequate training of young endoscopists. The availability and use of the fiberoptic bronchoscope and esophagoscope is a mixed blessing since inadequately trained physicians who use these instruments are potentially dangerous to the pediatric patient.

ACKNOWLEDGMENT — The author gives thanks to his associates Dr. Kenneth Geller and Dr. Jeffrey Birns for their aid in abstracting case reports. To Rose Marie Lapicola gratitude is expressed for the preparation of this manuscript.

REFERENCES

1. Jackson C. Foreign bodies in air and food passages. In: English GM, ed. Otolaryngology. Hagerstown: Harper & Row, 1979:1-94.

2. Cohen SR, Lewis GB, Herbert WI, Geller KA. Foreign bodies in the airway. Five-year retrospective study with special reference to management. Ann Otol Rhinol Laryngol 1980; 89: 437-42.

3. Friedberg SA. Report of the committee on prevention of foreign body accidents. Trans Am Broncho-Esophagol Assn 1970; 116.

4. Friedberg SA. Report of the committee for prevention of foreign body accidents. Trans Am Broncho-Esophagol Assn 1973: 34.

5. Le Jeune FE. Presidential address. Trans Am Broncho-Esophagol Assn 1968:6-13.

6. Yee KF, Schild JA, Holinger PH. Extraluminal foreign bodies (coins) in the food and air passages. Ann Otol Rhinol Laryngol 1975; 84:619-23.

7. Morioka WT, Maisel RH, Smith TW, Cantrell RW. Unexpected radiographic findings related to foreign bodies. Ann Otol Rhinol Laryngol 1975; 84:627-30.

8. Zavala DC, Rhodes ML. Foreign body removal: a new role for fiberoptic bronchoscopy. Ann Otol Rhinol Laryngol 1975; 84:650-6.

9. Ritter FN. Questionable methods for foreign body treatment. Ann Otol Rhinol Laryngol 1974; 83:729-33.

≈

PAN AMERICAN ASSOCIATION OF OTORHINOLARYNGOLOGY AND BRONCHOESOPHAGOLOGY

The XVIII Congress of the Pan American Association of Otorhinolaryngology and Bronchoesophagology will be held November 2-6, 1982, in San Juan, Puerto Rico. Dr. Hans von Leden has been elected President of the Association.

ESOPHAGEAL AND HYPOPHARYNGEAL INJURIES IN PATIENTS WITH CERVICAL SPINE TRAUMA

RICHARD A. POLLOCK, MD
DAVID F. APPLE, JR., MD
JOHN M. PURVIS, MD
H. HERDON MURRAY, MD

ATLANTA, GEORGIA

The authors review their recent experience with four patients referred to the Shepherd Spinal Center, Atlanta, with cervical spine fracture dislocation and quadriplegia. The patients were subsequently found to have tears of the hypopharynx or the esophagus as a complication of their injury. Unexplained fever, swelling of the neck, dysphagia or leukocytosis in the patient with acute cervical spine injury suggest, the authors urge, the possibility of esophageal or hypopharyngeal perforation. The authors review the kinematics and pathophysiology of cervical fractures and provide clues to early detection and management of perforation of the hypopharynx or esophagus, including the use of radiographic study and endoscopy.

INTRODUCTION

The otolaryngologist-head and neck surgeon has been admonished to consider injury to the esophagus or to the hypopharynx in patients with trauma to the larynx and trachea,[1,2] with fractures of the hyoid or facial bones,[3-5] and with penetrating injuries of the neck inflicted by knife or missile.[6,7] Based on recent experience the authors would urge awareness of another dimension: injury to the esophagus or hypopharynx in patients who have sustained fractures of the cervical spine.

CASE REPORTS

Case 1. A 27-year-old male sustained trauma to the neck at a construction site, suffering posterior displacement of C6 into the spinal canal, accompanied by C5 quadriplegia. Atypically, the vertebral bodies of C5 and C7 were not malaligned. At surgery, the sixth vertebral body was removed, and a mushroom-shaped bone graft inserted. The patient was transferred to the Spinal Center in a febrile state. On the fifth postoperative day, swelling, erythema, and tenderness to palpation developed over the anterior cervical wound. A postoperative wound infection was suspected, and the wound incised. After an initial drainage of pus, saliva followed. A diatrizoate meglumine (Gastrografin®) swallow established the presence of a laceration of the cervical esophagus. Despite surgical closure of the rent and appropriate drainage, accompanied by intravenous fluids and antibiotics, the patient had a fulminant course and died. At the time, the laceration was thought to be most likely surgical, ie, iatrogenic.

Case 2. The same year in another part of the city, a 26-year-old male was involved in an automobile accident. The patient sustained a cervical dislocation of C5 on C6, which was promptly reduced by tongs application. A tracheotomy was required four days later because of moderate respiratory distress. On the eighth postoperative day, the patient suddenly became hypotensive and septic. Clinical examination and chest film suggested the presence of pericarditis. Four hundred cubic centimeters of pus were removed by pericardotomy. The patient complained of pain in the left anterolateral neck. Evidence of retropharyngeal abscess on lateral roentgenograms of the neck was overlooked until diatrizoate meglumine swallow, ten days later, revealed a rent in the proximal esophagus. Voluminous pus was encountered in the periesophageal area. Penrose drains were inserted near the site of the posterior esophageal laceration. The patient had a second septic course, but recovered and was transferred to the Spinal Center for further rehabilitation.

Case 3. In 1979 a 24-year-old male was injured in a motorcycle accident sustaining a flexion-compression fracture of C6, associated with complete quadriplegia. The patient, a juvenile-onset, insulin-dependent diabetic, did well for several days, then became febrile. Work-up, including lateral soft tissue of the neck, was unremarkable. A CAT scan clearly delineated a "burst" fracture of C6 but did not show any evidence of abnormality in the esophageal region. On intravenous antibiotics fever progressively resolved. Seven days following the injury, while prone in a Stryker frame, respiratory arrest occurred. An endotracheal tube was inserted, and tracheostomy accomplished. Fiberoptic endoscopy revealed a chronic, macerated and jagged laceration in the posterior wall of the proximal esophagus and the adjacent hypopharynx, immediately overlying the site of fracture. Bone spicules were evident in the laceration at rigid endoscopy. Pus was seen to ooze from the superior apex of the laceration in the hypopharynx, and the presence of a prevertebral abscess was confirmed by repeat lateral soft tissue of the neck. The periesophageal area was approached through the left anterior neck in standard fashion, and drains were inserted. The patient continued a septic course, developed arhythmias, and died 40 days following surgery.

Case 4. A 56-year-old male was injured in an automobile accident in a neighboring state, sustaining dislocation of C5 on C6 and complete quadriplegia. The patient was transferred to the Spinal Center within three days, not having had tracheostomy or any surgical procedure. The patient complained of hoarseness and progressive pain on swallowing, accompanied by tenderness to palpation and swelling of the left lateral neck. Fiberoptic and rigid endoscopy revealed an ecchymotic area, at the center of which was a stellate laceration of the esophagus, anterior to the level of injury. Gastrografin swallow confirmed a limited laceration involving the proximal esophagus. After open discussions with the patient and his family, a nonoperative course was pursued, including the use of nasogastric suction and administration of antibiotics. The patient had an uneventful recovery.

DISCUSSION

Crowe's 1928 description of to-and-fro "whiplash" injury, naval experience with carrier-based catapult aircraft and civilian experience with high-speed automobile collision, ushered in a new era of understanding of cervical injury.[8-12] Although con-

From the Shepherd Spinal Center, Atlanta.

Presented at the meeting of the American Broncho-Esophagological Association, Vancouver, British Columbia, May 11-12, 1981.

REPRINTS — Richard A. Pollock, MD, 105 Collier Road, NW, Suite 4040, Piedmont Professional Building, Atlanta, GA 30309.

TABLE 1. PATHOPHYSIOLOGY OF CERVICAL SPINE INJURY

Mechanism of Injury	*Setting*	*Radiology*	*Autopsy Data*	*Clinical Findings*
Axial	Front-end collision Head and neck unflexed with "on-line" contact	Central compression fracture with "burst" deformity	Intact posterior and anterior ligament complex	Infrequent neurologic deficit Dysphagia
Hyperflexion	Front-end collision Head and neck flexed upon the chest	Flexion-compression Wedge-shaped deformity anterior portion vertebral body	Tears posterior cervical musculature	Posterior neck pain and muscle spasm Dysphagia
Hyperflexion with rotation	Front-end collision Head and neck flexed upon the chest	Fragmentation of the compressed vertebral body with anterior (tear drop) and posterior displacement	Disruption posterior ligamentous complex Avulsion posterior cervical muscles	Frequent neurologic deficits Esophageal laceration Progressive dysphagia and odynophagia
Hyperextension	Rear-end collision Head and neck extended upon posterior upper thorax	Frequently normal	Tears of SCM and longus colli	Tenderness to palpation posterior neck
Hyperextension with rotation	Rear-end collision Head and neck extended upon posterior upper thorax	Fractures of laminae and spinous processes Avulsion (shear and carry) fracture	Avulsion anterior longitudinal ligament and anterior cervical muscles Damage cervical sympathetic chain Hemorrhage into musculature esophagus Development retropharyngeal hematoma	Occasional neurologic deficit Progressive dysphagia and odynophagia Esophageal laceration retropharyngeal hematoma or abscess

troversy still exists, the basic mechanisms by which cervical fractures and related soft tissue injuries occur appear to be vertical compression (axial loading), hyperflexion, and hyperextension, each of which may be combined with rotatory force (Table 1).[13-15]

Vertical compression fractures occur when the head and neck strike "on-line" a firm object. Force is transmitted to the central portion of a vertebral body, creating the typical roentgenographic picture of a "burst" fracture (Fig. 1). Hyperflexion injuries occur when the head and neck are flexed upon the upper chest, a frequent occurrence in front end collisions. The anterior portion of the vertebral body is crushed and compacted to create a wedge-shaped compression deformity of the vertebral body (Fig. 2). By contrast, in hyperextension injuries, common to rear end collision, the head and neck are thrust backward upon the posterior upper thorax, creating in some instances a small "shear and carry" avulsion fracture from the front of one of the vertebral bodies and, less frequently, fractures of the laminae and spinous process (Fig. 3).

The basic mechanism of soft tissue injury appears to be similar to that of fractures,[11] delineated by studies in the experimental animal.[16-18] With vertical compression, unaccompanied by hyperflexion or hyperextension, there is little to no injury to soft tissue. In the experimental animal exposed to hyperflexion, however, soft tissue injury is commonly discovered posteriorly. Tears in the posterior cervical musculature are common and disruption of the posterior ligament complex, though less frequent, may occur, leading to instability of the spine.

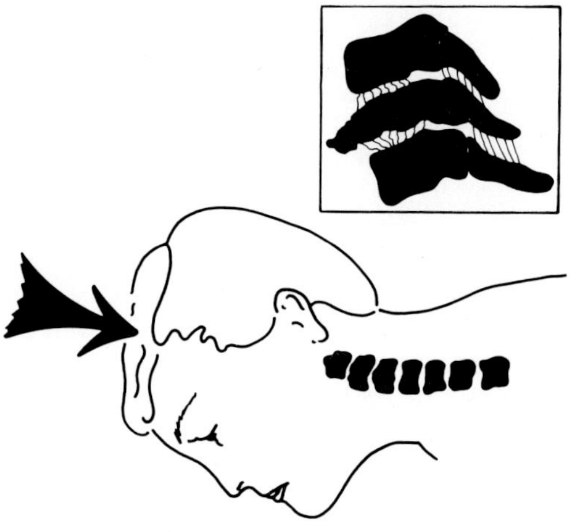

Fig. 1. Vertical compression injury.

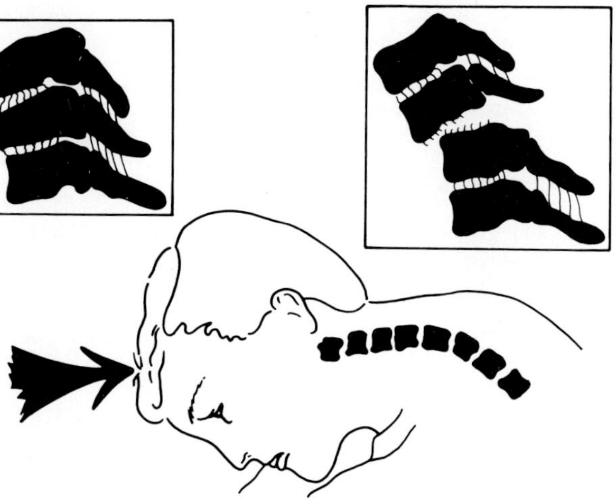

Fig. 2. Hyperflexion injury.

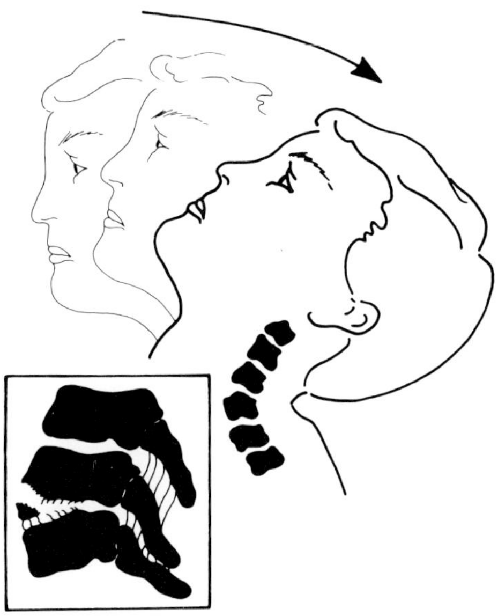

Fig. 3. Hyperextension injury.

Hemorrhagic lesions and edema in the central grey matter and anterior horns of the spinal cord occur within 30 minutes, causing paraplegia or quadriplegia. These lesions become confluent in about four hours, at which time similar changes appear in the peripherally placed white column tracts, associated with reduction in sensory evoked potentials by neurography. Cord necrosis ensues within 24 to 36 hours and neurologic deficit remains essentially unchanged thereafter.[13,19] In the experimental animal exposed to hyperextension, soft tissue injury, by contrast, is usually found anteriorly. Muscle injuries, as documented by McNab,[16] range in severity from minor tears of the sternocleidomastoid to partial avulsion of the longus colli. Such damage in the experimental animal is frequently associated with injury to the cervical sympathetic chain, hemorrhage into the musculature of the esophagus, and development of retropharyngeal hematoma. With hyperextension, hemorrhage and contusion over the upper cervical cord are frequent, but spinal cord injury with paralysis is uncommon in hyperextension injuries.[17,18]

The four case reports of esophageal perforation presented in this publication were associated with hyper*flexion* injuries by routine roentgenographic study, suggesting the danger in assuming that esophageal and other soft tissue injury anterior to the cervical spine must, as is classically the case in the experimental animal and some clinical reports,[9,12,17] occur with hyper*extension* injuries.[20] Obviously, in the patient unrestrained by seatbelt, shoulder strap and head rest, battered about within closed vehicular space or propelled through windshield or open door, injuries may in fact represent a combination of axial, hyperflexion, rotation and hyperextension, leading to combined soft tissue injuries, the radiographs presenting a final summation of all forces brought to bear during the automobile collision.

When damaged during cervical spine injury, the esophagus perforates in the posterior wall in the weak area produced by the sling formation of the cricopharyngeal muscle. The inherent weakness of the posterior musculature, the authors propose, not only renders it susceptible to instrumentation from within the esophagus but renders it susceptible to retrodisplaced bone fragments, thrust anteriorly by the force of automobile collision.

Neck-aching associated with soreness, first of the anterior neck muscles and then 5-7 days later, of the posterior muscles is the most common early symptom of cervical injury.[11] The primary symptoms of hypopharyngeal or esophageal perforation in the cervical area consist of a "sticking sensation" low in the throat which is activated by attempts to swallow. This may be relatively mild when first noted, especially if due to maceration of the lumen wall which allows only slow but progressive contamination of the prevertebral space.[21] With progressive inflammation over the ensuing 24 hours, the pain increases in intensity and becomes constant. Leukocytosis and fever develop. Unlike pain due to midthoracic esophageal rupture, pain associated with cervical perforation is not usually acutely progressive and is not aggravated by respiratory excursion.

When perforation occurs under local anesthesia, subcutaneous emphysema may be noted prior to development of pain. Air dissects easily through the loose tissue of the prevertebral space of the cervical area into the mediastinum, pericardium, and pleural spaces.[21] In approximately 1 in 10 cases of perforation, however, chest and neck radiography remain within normal limits and a large number of cases eventually positive may not be detected for 24 to 36 hours.[22,23]

Primary evidence of esophageal or hypopharyngeal perforation is obtained by endoscopy or by identification of contrast material outside the esophageal lumen. Water-soluble contrast material, such as diatrizoate meglumine, should be used first, with the full understanding that esophagograms are positive in only 50% of patients ultimately found to have esophageal injuries.[6] The value of computerized axial tomography and CAT scan with contrast has not been delineated in a large series of patients. Although such studies of one of our patients were not revealing, the authors suspect that with time, CAT scan with contrast will be proven to be a reasonable second step if routine Gastrografin esophagograms are negative.

If soluble contrast materials have been used and no esophageal injury has been demonstrated, a higher contrast study may be obtained with the use of barium.[24,25] Because barium in the mediastinum has been associated with granulomatous and fibrous tissue reaction, its use probably should be preceded by failure to reveal a perforation at endoscopy.

Esophagoscopy is considered a definitive test in the detection of esophageal perforation, but detection of subsequently proven perforation in some series does not exceed 30%. Defore et al for example, subjected 17 of their 77 patients with penetrating injuries of the esophagus to rigid endoscopy and identified the site of perforation in only 5.[6] The role of the flexible fiberoptic esophagoscope has not been studied in a sufficient number of patients to permit an evaluation of its use. The flexible instrument would appear to be particularly useful, however, in the spinal injury patient in traction for vertebral instability in whom esophageal perforation is suspected.

Prior to the introduction of antibiotics, perforation of the esophagus was nearly always fatal, and treatment limited frequently to incision and drainage of abscess formation. In the antibiotic era, it became fashionable to advocate conservative management, including the use of intravenous fluids, antibiotics, and nasogastric suction,[26-28] a position supported in 1965 by an editorial of JAMA.[29]

Paulson,[30] Mathewson,[31] and Groves[32] took a contrary point of view, suggesting that surgical intervention in some cases was well advised. Youngs and Nicologg, while agreeing that small perforations could be managed conservatively, pointed to the difficulty in delineating the extent of the perforation and the amount of periesophageal contamination. Of 11 patients treated conservatively, 6 subsequently required surgical intervention, 4 of whom died.[33] Although the mortality associated with operative delay led Brewer[34] and Skinner[35] to advocate surgical exploration, reconstruction, and drainage of *all* perforations, Berry,[36] Boyd,[37] and Levine[38] and others advise a selective policy of surgical intervention.

In the presence of an identifiable and small or limited (ie, stellate) cervical laceration and in the absence of leukocytosis or fever, surgery may, in our view, be deferred. Aqueous penicillin would appear to be the first drug of choice, considering the usual flora of the oropharynx and the esophagus,[38] and the bacteria most commonly associated with the gastrointestinal tract. A regimen of 2 million International Units every four hours is preferred (in the presence of normal renal function) because of the abbreviated half-life of aqueous penicillin. Because Gram-negative organisms may be the cause of upper gastrointestinal infection and because Gram-negative colonization of the oropharynx in the elderly is frequent (and in the patient hospitalized over seven days not uncommon), tobramycin or gentamicin may be added to the penicillin regimen. Tobramycin, it should be noted, is less nephrotoxic (and probably less ototoxic) than gentamicin, during the initial three weeks of administration. In the presence of allergy to penicillin, selection of clindamycin, chloramphenicol or cefoxitin seems appropriate. Cefoxitin, a cephalosporin, has the advantage of being effective against several anaerobes, including *Bacteroides fragilis*.[39]

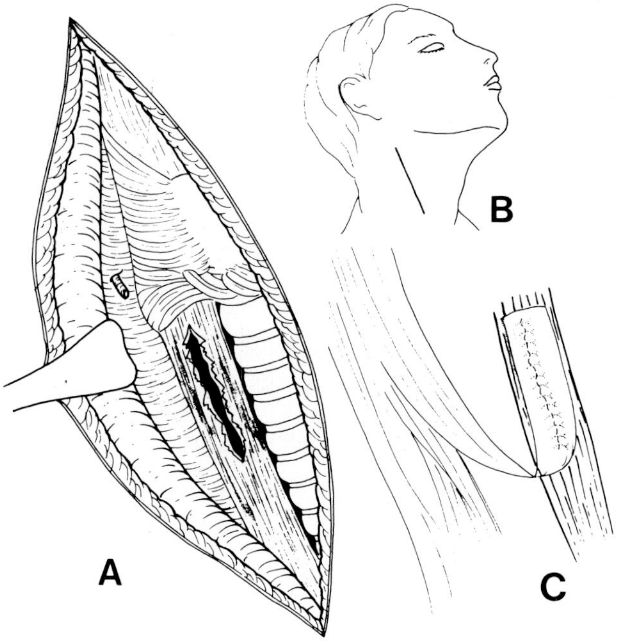

Fig. 4. Surgical closure of esophageal perforation. A) Perforation of the esophagus. B) Neck incision. C) Reinforcing sternocleidomastoid muscle flap.

In the presence of a large perforation, elevated temperature, or increased white-cell count, surgery is immediately advised. An oblique incision is made along the anterior border of the sternocleidomastoid muscle from the upper border of the thyroid cartilage to just above the clavicle. The sternocleidomastoid muscle and the carotid sheath are retracted laterally, and the larynx, trachea, and pharynx retracted medially. The middle thyroid veins and inferior thyroid artery are divided, care being taken to properly protect the recurrent laryngeal nerve. The esophagus is gently lifted forward, the perforation visualized and, if necessary, debrided (Fig. 4). A nasogastric tube is inserted under direct vision. The perforation is closed (with inversion of the mucosa) using 3-0 Dexon® (Davis-Geck) and a two-layer closure. Use of a reinforcing sternocleidomastoid flap may be considered in the presence of compromised tissue. Drains are inserted, and the wound is closed.

CONCLUSION

Esophageal perforation, associated with cervical fractures and/or dislocation, is reported in the English literature, to our knowledge, for the first time. The etiology of esophageal or hypopharyngeal perforation associated with cervical fractures is unknown, but there would appear to be three most probable causes. First, esophageal perforation could occur iatrogenically, during endotracheal intubation or during surgical exploration of the fracture site. In some instances in the past, we suspect that iatrogenic cause has been improperly blamed, a conclusion which may be no longer valid. Second and conceivably, perforation could result from a breakdown of contused esophageal tissue anterior to the fracture site, particularly in the presence of inflammation. Third, a perforation could result from the direct trauma of the cervical fracture, the esophagus in effect being impaled by osteophyte or fracture dislocation. The authors suspect that additional case reports will be forthcoming as an increasing number of patients survive massive vehicular trauma and as awareness of this possible injury-association increases among the orthopedic and otolaryngologic specialties.

REFERENCES

1. Fitzhugh GS, Wallenborn WM, McGovern F. Injuries of the larynx and cervical trauma. Ann Otol Rhinol Laryngol 1962; 7:419-42.

2. Krekorian EA. Laryngopharyngeal injuries. Laryngoscope 1975; 85:2069-86.

3. Forbes SB. Fracture of the greater cornu of the hyoid bone: perforation of the pharynx. J Florida Med Assoc 1931; 17:585-6.

4. Krekorian EA. Perforation of the pharynx with fracture of the hyoid bone. Ann Otol Rhinol Laryngol 1964; 73:583-94.

5. Templer JW. Trauma to the face. In: English GM, ed. Otolaryngology: a textbook. San Francisco: Harper & Row, 1976: 342-64.

6. Defore WW, Mattox KL, Hansen HA, Garcia-Rinaldi R, Beall AC, BeBakey ME. Surgical management of penetrating injuries of the esophagus. Am J Surg 1977; 134:734-8.

7. May M. Civilian neck injuries: a review. Ear Nose Throat J 1980; 59:5-19.

8. Crowe HE. A new diagnostic sign in neck injuries: the continuing revolt against "whiplash." Milwaukee: The Defense Research Institute, 1964.

9. Birsner JW, Leask WH. Retropharyngeal soft tissue swelling due to whiplash injury. Arch Surg 1954; 68:369-73.

10. Severy DM, Mathewson JH, Bechtol CO. Controlled automobile medical phenomena. Can Serv Med J 1955; 11:727-46.

11. Hohl M. Soft tissue injuries of the neck. Clin Orthop 1975; 109:42-9.

12. Howcroft AJ, Jenkins DHR. Potentially fatal asphyxia following a minor injury of the cervical spine. J Bone Joint Surg (Br) 1977; 59B:93-4.

13. Jacobs B. Cervical fractures and dislocations (C3-7). Clin Orthop 1975; 109:18-32.

14. Forsyth HF. Extension injuries of the cervical spine. J Bone Joint Surg (Am) 1964; 46A:1792-7.

15. Heppenstall RB. Fracture treatment and healing. Philadelphia: WB Saunders, 1980.

16. MacNab I. Acceleration injuries to the cervical spine. J Bone Joint Surg (Br) 1964; 46A:1797-9.

17. Ommaya AK, Faas F, Yarnell P. Whiplash injury and brain damage. JAMA 1968; 204:285-9.

18. Wickstrom JK, Rodriquez RP, Martinez JL. Experimental production of acceleration injuries of the head and neck. Highway Safety Research Institute Bull 1967; 181:1-30.

19. Tator CH, Deeks L. Studies of the treatment and pathophysiology of acute spinal cord injury in primates. Paraplegia 1973; 10:344-5.

20. Spenler CW, Benfield JR. Esophageal disruption from blunt and penetrating external trauma. Arch Surg 1976; 111:663-7.

21. Leigh TF, Achord JL. Pharyngeal and esophageal perforations during instrumentation. Am J Roentgenol Radium Ther Nucl Med 1964; 91:757-65.

22. Priviteri CA, Gay BB. Spontaneous rupture of the esophagus. Radiology 1951; 57:48-57.

23. Parkin GJS. The radiology of perforated oesophagus. Clin Radiol 1973; 24:324-32.

24. Vessal K, Montali RJ, Larson SM, Chaffee V, James AE. Evaluation of barium and gastrografin as contrast media for the diagnosis of esophageal rupture or perforations. Am J Roentgenol Radium Ther Nucl Med 1975; 123:307-19.

25. Mattox KL. Evaluation of the esophageal injury patient. Curr Concepts Trauma Care 1980; 11:20-2.

26. Smith CCK, Tanner NC. The complications of gastroscopy and oesophagoscopy. Br J Surg 1956; 43:396-403.

27. Tuttle WM, Barrett RJ. Late esophageal perforations. Arch Surg 1963; 86:695-700.

28. Mengoli LR, Klassen KP. Conservative management of esophagus perforation. Arch Surg 1965; 91:238-40.

29. Editorial: conservative management of esophageal perforation. JAMA 1965; 193:537.

30. Paulson DL, Shaw RR, Kee JL. Recognition and treatment of esophageal perforation. Ann Surg 1960; 152:13-20.

31. Mathewson C, Dozier WE, Hamill JP, Smith M. Clinical experiences with perforation of the esophagus. Am J Surg 1962; 104:257-66.

32. Groves LK. Instrumental perforation of the esophagus: what is conservative management? J Thorac Cardiovasc Surg 1966; 52:1-10.

33. Youngs J, Nicologg D. Management of esophageal perforation. Surgery 1969; 65:264-8.

34. Brewer LA III, in discussion, Mathewson C, Dozier WE, Hamill JP, Smith M. Clinical experiences with perforation of the esophagus. Am J Surg 1962; 104:257-66.

35. Skinner DB, Little AG, Demeester TR. Management of esophageal perforation. Am J Surg 1980; 139:760-4.

36. Berry BE, Ochsner JL. Perforation of the esophagus: a 30 year review. J Thorac Cardiovasc Surg 1973; 65:1-7.

37. Boyd DP, Wittmann CJ. Some principles of treating perforation of the esophagus. Surg Clin North Am 1971; 51:567-74.

38. Levine PA. Hypopharyngeal perforation: an untoward complication of endotracheal intubation. Arch Otolaryngol 1980; 106:578-80.

39. Nair SR, Cherubin CE. Use of cefoxitin, new cephalosporin-like antibiotic, in the treatment of aerobic and anaerobic infections. Antimicrob Agents Chemother 1978; 14:866-75.

Ann Otol 90:1981

INCENDIARY CHARACTERISTICS OF ENDOTRACHEAL TUBES WITH THE CARBON DIOXIDE LASER

AN EXPERIMENTAL STUDY

EDWARD TREYVE, MD

C. THOMAS YARINGTON, JR., MD GALE E. THOMPSON, MD

SEATTLE, WASHINGTON

The ignition characteristics of the American Hospital, Portex®, polyvinyl chloride, and red rubber tracheal tubes commonly available have been evaluated using a standard carbon dioxide laser. The added hazard of the increased combustibility of the impregnated line on endotracheal tubes and the hazard of commonly utilized anesthetic or lubricating materials are discussed. The safety limits which, experimentally, indicate levels of energy and laser burst time which seem to preclude the hazard of ignition are outlined. The potential danger of postburn bronchiolitis is noted, along with appropriate treatment.

At the present time there is a relatively small body of literature with reference to the danger of ignition of endotracheal tubes during use of the carbon dioxide laser in the upper respiratory tract. The majority of articles are anecdotal and refer specifically to the accidental ignition of an endotracheal tube during surgery and the commonly utilized preventive measures which are designed to preclude that complication.[1-3] Specific problems have been addressed: the utilization of muslin-covered tubes to prevent trauma or obstruction from aluminum foil, the utilization of a metal endotracheal tube only now coming onto the market, the use of a moist cotton or gauze pledget below the area of laser targeting, and the utilization of other commonly accepted and self-evident safety precautions attendant to the use of lasers in general. It is the purpose of this presentation to indicate the specific limitations which may be applied with laser surgery to preclude the possible ignition of an endotracheal tube. The parameters include the percent of oxygen utilized, the duration of the laser burst, and the wattage utilized.

MATERIAL AND METHODS

A series of experiments was conducted utilizing a standard Cavitron® carbon dioxide laser and four commonly utilized endotracheal tubes. A flowmeter was attached to the endotracheal tube delivering a flow of air through the tube, or a mixture of air and 30% oxygen. It should be recognized that gas mixtures including greater than 30% oxygen may be expected to support combustion at lower energy and/or time readings. The endotracheal tubes were hit directly with the laser beam in the same spot for five consecutive impulses at the time and power setting indicated, and any evidence of combustion, up to and including ignition, was measured as ignition.

RESULTS

Several potential hazards became immediately apparent. First, the use of common anesthetic ointments, creams, or solutions frequently applied to endotracheal tubes, either for topical anesthesia or lubrication, should be suspect. These agents frequently are made up of vehicles which either are combustible or support combustion. In utilizing

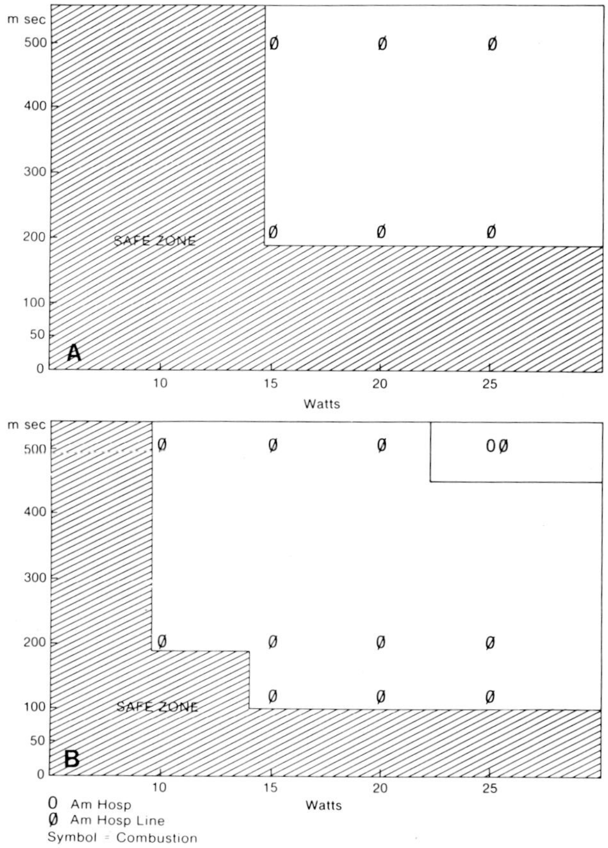

Fig. 1. Combustibility of American Hospital tubes with CO_2 laser in A) air and B) 30% O_2.

From The Mason Clinic, Seattle.

Presented at the meeting of the American Broncho-Esophagological Association, Vancouver, British Columbia, May 11-12, 1981.

REPRINTS — C. Thomas Yarington, Jr., MD, The Mason Clinic, 1100 Ninth Avenue, Seattle, WA 98101.

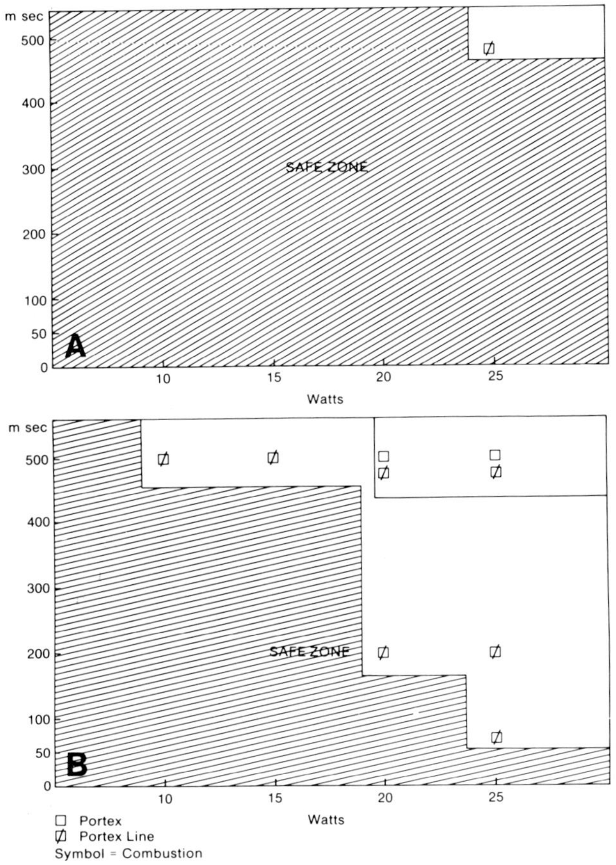

Fig. 2. Combustibility of Portex tubes with CO_2 laser in A) air and B) 30% O_2.

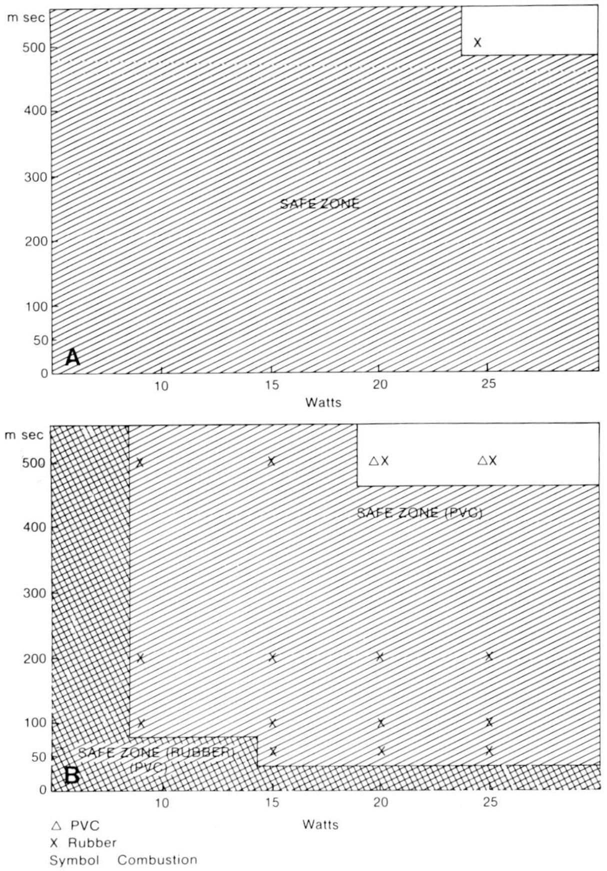

Fig. 3. Combustibility of polyvinyl chloride and red rubber tubes in A) air and B) 30% O_2.

such agents, consideration of the potential hazard should be weighed against their anticipated benefit.

Some commonly utilized endotracheal tubes have a line impregnated upon the tube itself which may or may not be radiopaque. This line, in our experiments, is unusually combustible and at some power settings actually seems to explode. The differences in combustibility of the line itself and the remainder of the tube are indicated in our results and are surprising, significant, and should be considered in tube selection.

Four commonly utilized tubes were evaluated: the standard American Hospital tube and the line impregnated therein, a standard Portex® tube and the line impregnated within it, the standard polyvinyl chloride tube, and the standard red rubber tube.

The American Hospital tube is quite safe, either in air or in 30% oxygen, and is combustible only at energy levels of 20 W at 500 ms and above. Unfortunately, its use is significantly limited by the fact that the impregnated line upon the tube is highly combustible with a safety zone essentially under 10 W at any setting or over 15 W at under 100 ms in oxygen, or under 15 W at any setting or under 200 ms at higher energy levels in air (Fig. 1 A, B).

The Portex tube has similar problems in that the impregnated line upon that tube is more combustible than the tube itself. In air, the tube and line are safe at all but 500 ms above 20 W. In 30% oxygen, however, the safety limit falls, primarily because of the incendiary properties of the impregnated line, to levels of essentially 400 ms, and lower at energy levels above 20 W (Fig. 2).

The red rubber tube is quite safe in air, but has very limited safety in 30% oxygen. In air, below 25 W at 500 ms, the tube is safe, but in a 30% oxygen environment the safety level falls to no setting greater than 5 W at any setting and only below 15 W at 50 ms (Fig. 3).

The polyvinyl chloride tube, without any impregnated line, appears to be the safest tube available. Below 20 W at 500 ms in air or below 15 W at 500 ms in 30% oxygen seem to be very safe areas of operation for the polyvinyl chloride tube (Fig. 3). With conventional protection of the tube with foil wrapping and the prevention of drawing combustible or already ignited material into the tube, as has been reported,[4] a safe procedure should be anticipated.

MANAGEMENT OF COMPLICATIONS

As has been widely reported in the literature, patients who sustain injury through ignition of endotracheal tubes during laser surgery tend to recover without incident. Primarily the treatment is of an acute upper respiratory tract burn, with immediate irrigation of the area, respiratory support, the utilization of anti-inflammatory steroids and antibiotics, and close follow-up during the recovery stage. In our experience with this complication, which has been limited to one case, we performed an elective tracheotomy because of significant concern for upper respiratory or laryngeal edema at the site of the burn and the remote but possible consideration of ventilatory support requirements. The patient was treated with large doses of anti-inflammatory steroids and antibiotics, in much the same manner as has been previously described for the treatment of acute esophageal burns, and followed closely. The anticipated bronchiolitis, as seen following smoke or toxic gas inhalation, was noted in the three to four days following the event and manifested by fine, scattered rales in the chest and a significant drop in the 50-range of partial pressure of oxygen in arterial blood samples. As is usually the case, the bronchiolitis was self-limiting, and the patient made a full recovery, returning to his normal activities. Follow-up bronchoscopy, bronchial biopsies, pulmonary ventilatory studies, and blood gas determinations all returned to and remain at normal levels.

Although several other reports do not indicate a problem with postburn bronchiolitis, it would seem prudent to evaluate the patient for this problem and provide prophylactic therapy which is also therapeutic.

It should be noted that these findings differ considerably from those recently published by Meyers,[5] in which the red rubber tube was found to be safest due to lack of flame production during incineration. Our findings differ considerably in that the red rubber tubes did burn in the same manner in which all of us are familiar with rubber burning. The difference in our recommendations draws attention to the fact that many variables may exist from one laser to another, and even between the incendiary capabilities of similar products. Prudence would dictate that each operator establish safety parameters with his own equipment, and utilize these experimental results merely as a guide.

REFERENCES

1. Birch AA. Anesthetic considerations during laser surgery. Anesth Anal 1973; 52:53-8.

2. Snow JC, Norton ML, Saluja TS, Estanislao AF. Fire hazard during CO_2 laser microsurgery on the larynx and trachea. Anesth Anal 1976; 55:146-7.

3. Burgess GE, LeJeune FE. Endotracheal tube ignition during laser surgery of the larynx. Arch Otolaryngol 1979; 105:561-71.

4. Hirshman CA, Smith J. Indirect ignition of the endotracheal tube during carbon dioxide laser surgery. Arch Otolaryngol 1980; 106:639-41.

5. Meyers A. Complications of CO_2 laser surgery of the larynx. Ann Otol Rhinol Laryngol 1981; 90:132-4.

≈

Ann Otol 90:1981

EFFECT OF TOTAL LARYNGECTOMY ON ESOPHAGEAL MOTILITY

JOHN B. HANKS, MD   SAMUEL R. FISHER, MD   WILLIAM C. MEYERS, MD
KENNETH C. CHRISTIAN, BA   RAYMOND W. POSTLETHWAIT, MD   R. SCOTT JONES, MD
DURHAM, NORTH CAROLINA

Total laryngectomy for cancer can result in dysphagia and altered esophageal motility. Manometric changes in the upper esophageal sphincter (UES), and in proximal and distal esophageal function have been reported. However, most studies have failed to take into account radiation therapy and appropriate controls. We selected ten male patients (54.3 ± 1.9 yr) for longitudinal manometric evaluation prior to laryngectomy then at two weeks and again six months later. No patient received preoperative radiation therapy, had a previous history of esophageal surgery, or developed a postoperative wound infection or fistula. Seven of ten patients had positive nodes and received 6,000-6,600 rads postoperative radiation therapy. Preoperatively 4 of 10 patients complained of dysphagia which did not significantly change following surgery and radiation. Two of three patients who did not complain of dysphagia preoperatively and received radiation postoperatively developed dysphagia. No patient without dysphagia preoperatively who received no radiation therapy developed symptoms. Our studies show that laryngectomy causes alterations in the UES resting and peak pressures but not in the proximal or distal esophagus, or the lower esophageal sphincter. These data also imply radiation therapy may be associated with progressive alterations in motility and symptomatology. Further study regarding the effects of radiation on esophageal motility and function are urged.

INTRODUCTION

Laryngeal carcinoma is a highly curable disease, especially if detected and removed surgically at an early stage. Frequently a total laryngectomy is required. While offering a substantial cure rate for confined lesions, this procedure is associated with a number of postoperative problems. These problems include dysphagia which occurs after laryngectomy as well as other head and neck operations.[1-4] Recently, manometric evaluations of laryngectomy patients have quantitated and characterized motility changes in an attempt to explain postoperative dysphagia.[4-8] Significant alterations in the upper esophageal sphincter (UES) and proximal and distal esophagus have been reported.[4] However, these studies included a mixed surgical population in which the postoperative results were compared to unoperated normal individuals. In addition, many of the patients in these studies had varying amounts of radiation therapy both prior to and after laryngectomy which may have affected esophageal motility independently of laryngectomy. We therefore sought to assess the effect of total laryngectomy on patients in a prospective fashion prior to and two weeks after total laryngectomy in the absence of radiation therapy. All patients were followed and clinical progress monitored for six additional months, after which a third motility study was performed.

METHODS AND MATERIALS

Patients. Ten successive male patients were selected from the Durham VA Hospital prior to total laryngectomy for malignant disease (age 54.3 ± 1.9 yr). All were previous smokers and 6 of the 10 had a history of heavy alcohol consumption. Patients were selected after informed consent was obtained and according to the following criteria: 1) no prior radiation therapy, 2) no prior esophageal or gastrointestinal surgery, and 3) adequate respiratory status.

Patients underwent esophageal motility studies preoperatively and two weeks postoperatively when tolerating a full diet and ready for discharge. No patient had postoperative fistula or wound infection. No esophageal or pharyngeal surgery was done except that done with a standard laryngectomy. All patients were seen in clinic monthly and returned six months after laryngectomy for restudy. Dysphagia was defined as any subjective feeling of difficulty initiating or propulsing a bolus of solid or liquid food. Seven of the ten patients received postoperative radiation therapy, consisting of 6,000 to 6,600 rads at 180-200 rad tissue dose/day using a Varian 4 MV linear accelerator.

Esophageal Manometry Apparatus. Manometric evaluations were performed with the patient in the supine position using a triple lumen polyethylene tube (Arndorfer, Greenfield, Wis.). The lumen openings were 5 cm apart at 120° from each other, each with an internal diameter of 0.2 cm. All three lumens were perfused continuously with water at 1.91 ml/min with a Harvard infusion pump. Pressures from the column of water within the tube were transmitted to external transducers (Gould-Statham, Hato Rey, P.R.) and transcribed by a five-channel recorder (Grass, Model 5-D Polygraph, Quincy, Mass.). Pressures were recorded in millimeters of mercury with the zero reference point being one atmosphere. Restandardization and calibration were performed prior to each study.

Procedure. All patients were fasted overnight and no premedications were administered. Pressure transducers were placed at midchest level with the patient in the supine position. The manometric tube was passed nasally and positioned with all three pressure recording openings in the stomach. The tube was then withdrawn in 1 cm increments at which time the patient swallowed 2 ml of water (wet swallow) and pressure waves were recorded. Graph paper speed was set at 1 cm/s for lower esophageal sphincter (LES), distal and proximal esophagus, and at 5 cm/s for the UES.

Manometric Interpretation. Criteria for evaluation of UES

From the Departments of Surgery, Physiology and Otolaryngology, Duke University Medical Center, and Veterans Administration Center, Durham, North Carolina.

Presented at the meeting of the American Broncho-Esophagological Association, Vancouver, British Columbia, May 11-12, 1981. This paper received First Prize in the Research Essay Contest.

REPRINTS — Samuel R. Fisher, MD, Dept. of Otolaryngology, Head and Neck Surgery, Box 3805, Duke Medical Center, Durham, NC 27710.

TABLE 1. CLINICAL DATA FOR TEN LARYNGECTOMY PATIENTS

Patient No.	Tumor Classification	Site	Operation	Pathology	Nodes
1	$T_3N_2M_0$	PS	TL,LRN	SCCA	+
2	$T_3N_1M_1$	PS	TL	SCCA	+
3	$T_3N_3M_0$	PS	TL, RRN	SCCA	+
4	$T_3N_2M_0$	PS	TL, LRN	SCCA	+
5	$T_2N_0M_0$	Epiglottis	TL, RRN	SCCA	+
6	$T_3N_1M_0$	PS	TL, LRN	SCCA	+
7	$T_3N_2M_0$	Transglottic	TL, RRN	SCCA	+
8	$T_2N_0M_0$	Transglottic	TL	Verrucous	–
9	$T_3N_0M_0$	PS	TL, LRN	SCCA	–
10	$T_3N_1M_0$	PS	TL, RRN	SCCA	–

SCCA - Squamous cell carcinoma; TL - Total laryngectomy; LRN - Left radical neck; RRN - Right radical neck; PS - Pyriform sinus.

body esophagus and LES have been previously described.[4,8] All swallows recorded in the UES and LES were analyzed for resting pressure, postdeglutition ("peak") pressure, degree of relaxation and coordination. A point equidistant between the two sphincters was used to divide the body of the esophagus into proximal and distal segments. Each sphincter was evaluated with 4-6 wet swallows. Each segment of the esophagus was evaluated with 12-14 wet swallows.

TABLE 2. RELATION OF SYMPTOMS TO RADIATION THERAPY

Patient No.	Preoperative Dysphagia	Radiation Therapy	Postoperative Dysphagia
1	+	+	+
2	+	+	+
3	+	+	+
4	+	+	+
5	–	+	+
6	–	+	–
7	–	+	+
8	–	–	–
9	–	–	–
10	–	–	–

The UES and LES were said to be coordinated with the preceding propagative wave (pharyngeal for UES, distal esophageal for LES) when relaxation completely corresponded to the contraction of that wave. Relaxation was complete when intrasphincteric pressures fell to within 5 mm Hg of cervical esophagus (for UES) or intragastric (for LES) pressures. In either distal or proximal esophagus any wave separation between adjacent 5 cm points up to 1.25 s were interpreted as coordinated.

Comparisons between preoperative motility studies and those performed immediately postoperatively and after six months were made using a *t* test for paired values. In addition, comparison between preoperative studies and those for the seven patients receiving radiation therapy were made using *t* test for unpaired values. Probability values less than 0.05 were considered statistically significant.

RESULTS

Clinical Findings. Tables 1 and 2 summarize the clinical experience with these ten patients. All patients had T_3 lesions except for two with a T_2 lesion, and all patients received total laryngectomy. Nine patients had squamous cell carcinoma of which seven had positive nodes. These patients received postoperative radiation therapy as outlined previously.

Table 2 summarizes the incidence of preoperative and postoperative dysphagia. Patients 1-7 received radiation therapy postoperatively. Four of these patients had preoperative dysphagia that did not improve after six months. Two of the other three patients with no preoperative complaints who had radiation therapy had progressive dysphagia at six months. The three patients who had no radiation therapy had minimal or no preoperative dysphagia which did not progress.

Manometric Findings. Table 3 summarizes the manometric evaluation of LES function. Preoperative resting pressures of 11.5 ± 2.1 mm Hg and peak pressures of 29.3 ± 3.9 mm Hg were not statistically altered at either two weeks or six months after laryngectomy. When the seven patients who underwent radiation therapy are compared to the preoperative group, no significant alterations in LES are demonstrated. Likewise, LES coordination of 80.5 ± 8.9% and relaxation of 87.6 ± 7.7% are not altered.

Table 4 summarizes the peak pressures and coordination in the distal and proximal esophagus. Preoperative peak pressures of 25.6 ± 2.7 mm Hg and 18.4 ± 1.3 mm Hg in the distal and proximal esophagus respectively are not statistically altered at two weeks or six months postoperatively. Also, the seven patients receiving postoperative radiation therapy did not demonstrate significant alterations in distal or proximal esophageal function from preoperative values.

TABLE 3. MANOMETRIC ANALYSIS OF LOWER ESOPHAGEAL SPHINCTER

	Resting Pressure (mm Hg)	Peak Pressure (mm Hg)	% Coordination	% Relaxation
Preop (N = 10)	11.5 ± 2.1	29.3 ± 3.9	80.5 ± 8.9	87.6 ± 7
Postop (N = 10)	11.8 ± 1.7	28.2 ± 2.2	67.5 ± 9.2	90.3 ± 5
6 mo (N = 10)	12.1 ± 1.4	26.4 ± 2.4	76.5 ± 9.9	89.2 ± 5
6 mo rad. ther. pts. (N = 7)	12.5 ± 3.0	26.5 ± 3.0	73.6 ± 12.9	95.3 ± 4

TABLE 4. MANOMETRIC ANALYSIS OF DISTAL AND PROXIMAL ESOPHAGUS

	Distal Esophagus		*Proximal Esophagus*	
	Peak Pressure (mm Hg)	*% Coordination*	*Peak Pressure (mm Hg)*	*% Coordination*
Preop (N = 10)	25.6 ± 2.7	89.9 ± 6.2	18.4 ± 1.3	82.6 ± 8.6
Postop (N = 10)	22.7 ± 2.6	83.3 ± 8.6	17.5 ± 2.0	75.5 ± 10.7
6 mo (N = 10)	24.7 ± 7.3	82.8 ± 7.3	17.7 ± 1.9	77.8 ± 6.9
6 mo rad. ther. pts. (N = 7)	25.9 ± 2.7	91.4 ± 4.6	10.0 ± 2.4	83.7 ± 7.4

Table 5 summarizes the manometric findings in the upper esophageal sphincter in the same population of patients. UES resting pressures of 24.5 ± 4 mm Hg significantly decreased to 13.5 ± 2 mm Hg two weeks after laryngectomy. This change persisted unaltered at six months in both the entire population and in the patients who received radiation therapy. In the same manner, peak postdeglutition pressures in the UES significantly decreased from a preoperative value of 37.5 ± 5.9 mm Hg to 21.7 ± 2.7 mm Hg postoperatively. This decrease was maintained at six months in both groups of patients. Coordination and relaxation both showed decreases which attained statistical significance at six months for coordination and postoperatively for relaxation. Again the values obtained for the irradiation patients were not different from those values obtained for the entire group.

Figure 1 illustrates actual motility tracings from one patient at identical anatomic locations, demonstrating the changes which occurred in the upper esophageal sphincter preoperatively and postoperatively.

DISCUSSION

Dysphagia after extensive head and neck surgery is a significant postoperative problem and has been discussed in terms of anatomic and radiologic descriptions.[1,2] In 1957, Schobinger presented radiologic evidence for cricopharyngeal "spasm" after laryngectomy suggesting this was at least partially responsible for postoperative dysphagia.[1]

Most recently, manometric evaluation of the esophagus has allowed a more quantitative analysis of motility in these situations. In 1970, Sandberg analyzed manometric evaluations in postlaryngectomy patients with dysphagia.[3] He reported weaker UES relaxation and contraction pressures after swallowing as well as decreased resting pressures. He specifically stated that he saw no spasm at the level of the cricopharyngeus. Sandberg reported very little data, however, and several of this patients had preoperative radiation therapy.

In a retrospective study, Duranceau reported the comparison of postoperative manometric evaluation in 10 patients (9 total laryngectomies and 1 supraglottic laryngectomy) with 10 "nonsurgical controls." Again, radiation therapy had been administered to some of these patients both preoperatively and postoperatively. He reported significant decreases in resting and peak pressures of the UES as well as significant decreases in coordination and relaxation. However, he also reported significant decreases in peak pressure and coordination in the distal and proximal esophagus. He found no changes in the LES of patients after laryngectomy. He hypothesized that interruption of vagal branches at the level of the UES might be responsible for the changes he saw more distally in the body of the esophagus.

Most recently Welch et al[6] and Gates[7] have used manometric computer modeling to assess UES changes after laryngectomy. In all laryngectomies, the axial and radial asymmetry of the UES disappeared with a mean peak pressure decrease from approximately 120 mm Hg in normal controls to approximately 50 mm Hg in their laryngectomy population. However, he employed intraoperative manometry which did not assess the entire esophagus or LES, nor did it exclude the possible effects of anesthetic agents on the esophageal motion.

We pursued a prospective study of this problem for two reasons. First, using each patient as his own control allows for individual variation in age and pressures, and makes statistical comparison meaningful. Second, the effect of radiation on esophageal motility is unknown. By eliminating patients with

TABLE 5. MANOMETRIC ANALYSIS OF UPPER ESOPHAGEAL SPHINCTER

	Resting Pressure (mm Hg)	*Peak Pressure (mm Hg)*	*% Coordination*	*% Relaxation*
Preop (N = 10)	24.5 ± 4.0	37.5 ± 5.9	100%	96.7 ± 3.3
Postop (N = 10)	13.5 ± 2.0*	21.7 ± 2.7*	73.0 ± 13.2	68.2 ± 11.8*
6 mo (N = 10)	11.1 ± 1.4*	21.4 ± 2.3*	73.0 ± 11.3	76.5 ± 12.6
6 mo rad. ther. pts. (N = 7)	10.0 ± 1.7†	19.8 ± 2.5†	61.4 ± 14.0†	66.4 ± 16.8

*$P < 0.05$ Paired *t* test (Postop or 6 mo to preop).

†$P < 0.05$ Unpaired *t* test (6 mo radiation therapy to preop).

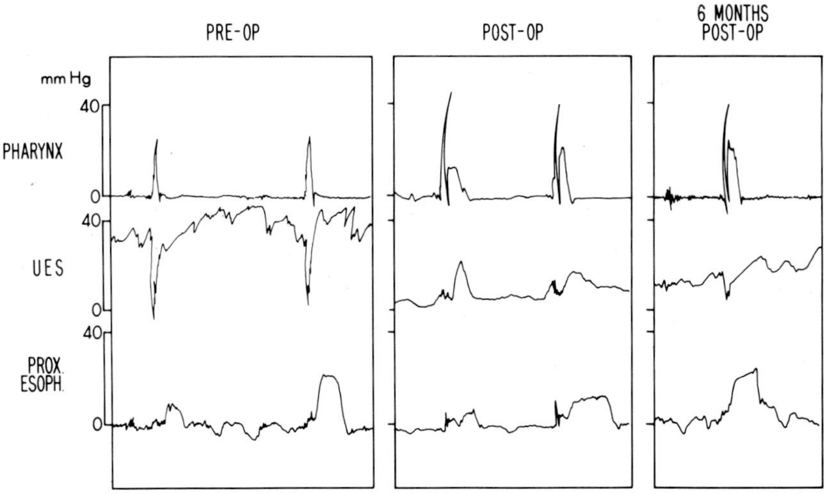

Fig. 1. (Patient 5) Simultaneous pharyngeal, UES and proximal esophageal manometric analysis in preoperative, postoperative and six months postoperative periods. The resting and peak pressures of the UES are significantly affected, while the pharyngeal and proximal esophageal pressures are relatively unaffected.

preoperative radiation, variables are removed which could confuse the results.

Our results agree with Sandberg in that we see no evidence for "spasm" of the cricopharyngeus, but rather we found a consistently weaker UES. Duranceau's findings of alterations in the distal and proximal esophagus were intriguing and perhaps are due to a skewed population and a different control group which included patients who had received radiation therapy. We saw immediate changes only in the UES, which did not progress at six months, regardless of radiation therapy. We did not see changes in the proximal or distal esophagus at any time after laryngectomy.

The effect of radiation therapy on esophageal motility is not clear from our results. Seven patients received postoperative radiation therapy. Four of those seven patients complained of dysphagia preoperatively and continued to complain of this six months later. Two of the other three patients who did not complain of dysphagia became symptomatic following treatment (Table 2). The three patients who did not have radiation therapy had no symptoms of dysphagia either preoperatively or at six months. Surgical technique and reconstruction of the pharyngeal-esophageal mucosa were consistent and do not appear to explain these findings. This seems to imply radiation therapy may alter esophageal motility and function enough to cause symptoms of dysphagia, though this group is not large enough for statistical evaluation.

SUMMARY

Esophageal manometry evaluations of ten laryngectomy patients preoperatively, postoperatively, and at six months reveal significant changes in the UES function which occur immediately after surgery and do not change by six months. No alterations occur in the proximal or distal esophagus. The effect of radiation therapy on esophageal motility is unclear from these studies; however, no dramatic alterations were demonstrated. It is recommended that further study be performed to assess the effect radiation has on esophageal motility and function.

REFERENCES

1. Schobinger R. Spasm of the cricopharyngeal muscle as cause of dysphagia after total laryngectomy. Arch Otolaryngol 1958; 67:271-5.

2. Conley JJ. Swallowing dysfunctions associated with radical surgery of the head and neck. Arch Surg 1960; 80:602-12.

3. Sandberg N. Motility of the pharynx and esophagus after laryngectomy. Acta Otolaryngol (Stockh) 1970; 263:124-7.

4. Duranceau A, Jamieson G, Hurwitz AL, Jones RS, Postlethwait RW. Alteration in esophageal motility after laryngectomy. Am J Surg 1976; 131:30-5.

5. Berlin BP, Fierstein JT, Tedesco F, Ogura JH. Manometric studies of the upper esophageal sphincter. Ann Otol Rhinol Laryngol 1977; 86:598-602.

6. Welch RW, Luckmann K, Rick PM, Draice ST, Gates GA. Manometry of the normal upper esophageal sphincter and its alterations in laryngectomy. J Clin Invest 1979; 63:1036-41.

7. Gates GA. Upper esophageal sphincter: pre- and post-laryngectomy — a normative study. Laryngoscope 1980; 90:454-64.

8. Duranceau A, Fisher SR, Flye MW, Jones RS, Postlethwait RW, Sealy WC. Motor function of the esophagus after repair of esophageal atresia and tracheoesophageal fistula. Surgery 1977; 82:116-23.

Ann Otol 90:1981

HISTOPATHOLOGY OF ACQUIRED SUBGLOTTIC STENOSIS
A DOCUMENTED CASE REPORT

GABRIEL F. TUCKER, JR, MD
CHICAGO, ILLINOIS

LEONARD NEWTON, MD
BRONX, NEW YORK

ROBERT J. RUBEN, MD
BRONX, NEW YORK

The history of a 2,900 g infant who had no stridor at birth and developed subglottic stenosis is presented in detail. The laryngeal lumen, which accepted a 3 mm endotracheal tube at one day of age, diminished to total occlusion at 15 months of age. There was an 8-day intubation and tracheotomy at nine months. At 19 months the patient expired from associated cardiac problems; the larynx was obtained at autopsy and was serially sectioned in the horizontal plane. A series (1mm-Tracer) of 12 sections through the stenotic area is presented. It demonstrates gross distortion of the cricoid cartilage with ossification extending into the right paraglottic larynx.

INTRODUCTION

The whole organ serial section technique originally used to study the spread of carcinoma within the larynx has also been applied to the anatomy and development of the human fetus, embryo, adult human, selected primates, and more recently, larynges of infants and children with congenital and/or acquired laryngeal obstruction. The Laryngeal Development Laboratory welcomes the opportunity to study such postmorten larynges from other institutions. The case presented is the result of such a collaboration which provides clinical documentation of the management and postmortem histological documentation of the laryngeal end result (Fig. 1).

CLINICAL SUMMARY

The patient's mother had one previous, uneventful, pregnancy which was delivered by cesarean section, secondary to cranial pelvic disproportion.

This pregnancy was marked by pre-eclampsia with probable maternal hypertension treated with Apresoline® (20 mg every 6 hours). There was spontaneous rupture of the membranes and the patient was born by cesarean section. After delivery, an attempt at intubation for suctioning was unsuccessful. A nasogastric tube was put in place and gastric irrigation was formed. There was no respiatory distress noted at birth. The patient was transferred immediately to the Hospital of the Albert Einstein College of Medicine for repair of a meningomyelocele found at birth. Other findings revealed IV systolic murmur and a small umbilical hernia. The child also had urinary retention.

On September 2, 1977, the child was taken to the operating room for closure of the meningomyelocele. A No. 3 endotracheal tube was in place for three hours. After the operation severe stridor was noted and the patient was treated with Decadron® and Vaponefrin®. He had a slow recovery of over two days.

On October 12, 1977, the patient was operated for debridement and closure of the sacral wound. Mask anesthesia was noted. No intubation was done that day and postoperative mild retraction was found.

The patient had several subsequent hospitalizations; for diarrhea, dehydration and decreasing cardiac status with respiratory distress. This required a head box; however, he was never intubated.

On June 24, 1978, the patient was admitted to the Bronx Municipal Hospital Center (BMHC) for fever, dehydration, and tachycardia. At that time he had increased respiratory stridor and was intubated on June 27. The respiratory distress ceased and the tachycardia also resolved.

The patient was operated at BMHC on July 5, 1978, where he was extubated and a laryngoscopy was performed by one of our staff. The description at that time was edematous vocal cords with a "ragged" appearance. The patient suffered respiratory distress when the tube was removed and it was immediately replaced.

On July 5, 1978, he had a laryngoscopy at BMHC where edematous vocal cords and a significant subglottic stenosis was noted; a tracheostomy was performed.

On August 28, 1978, an endoscopy revealed a

From the Laryngeal Development Laboratory, Division of Bronchoesophagology/Otolaryngology, Children's Memorial Hospital, Chicago; and the Department of Otorhinolaryngology, Albert Einstein College of Medicine, Bronx, New York. Support of the Edward Shedd Wells Fund is gratefully acknowledged.

Presented at the meeting of the American Broncho-Esophagological Association, Vancouver, British Columbia, May 11-12, 1981.

REPRINTS — Gabriel F. Tucker, MD, Children's Memorial Hospital, 2300 Children's Plaza, Chicago, IL 60614.

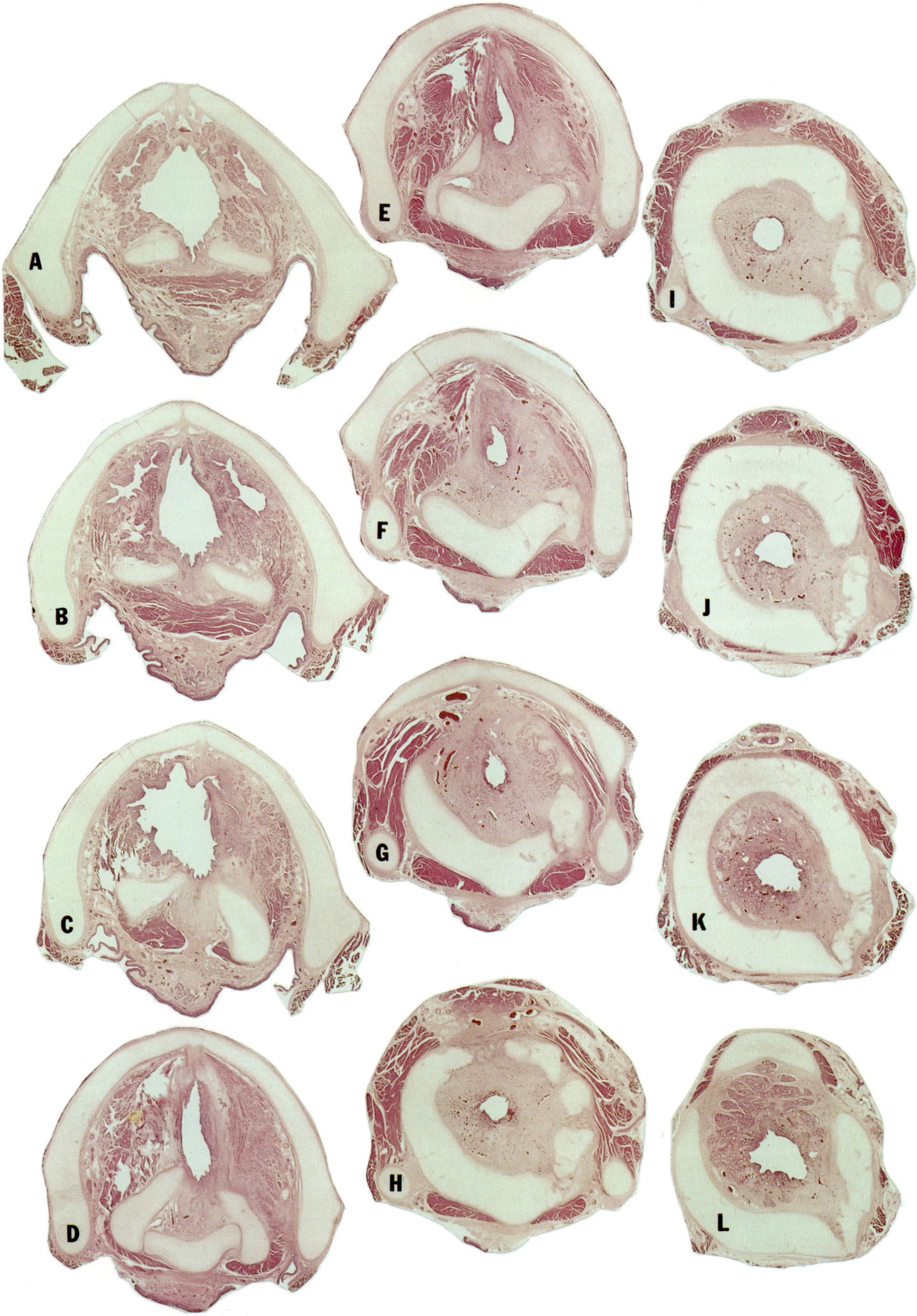

Figure 1.

Fig. 1. The specimen has been serially sectioned in the horizontal plane. Each section is 25 μ thick, thus, in a "tracer" series, every 40th section is approximately 1 mm deeper than its predecessor. The 12 sections selected begin just above the false cord and carry downward in 1 mm steps through the glottis and subglottis to the inferior rim of the cricoid. The larynx is presented as it would be approached by the endoscopist; the uppermost level first, the lowermost last. The posterior larynx is inferior, the anterior is superior. The patient's left is on the observer's left as the section is studied.

Rather than attempting to describe each section in detail, a number of features will be followed through the specimen from one section to the next.

Lumen. Section A shows the lumen just above the false cords; B at the level of the false cords; C shows the lumen of the left ventricle. On the right the floor of the right ventricle was already pushed up into the plane of section and, thus, the right ventricle is not shown. The *posterior commissure* is first seen to be compromised (in section B) by interarytenoid scarring. This becomes more pronounced as one works deeper into the specimen so that space between the arytenoids is replaced by scar tissue all the way down into the subglottic larynx. Similarly, the *anterior commissure* is seen in section D, but as one goes beneath this there is definite scarring which is part of the same subglottic cicatrix. The lumen is at a minimum between sections G and H (the level of the cricothyroid membrane). Also, to be noted in sections A or B are the lumina of the left and right saccules paramedian to the laryngeal lumen itself.

Cartilages. Thyroid — the notch is visible in section A. The thyroid cartilage can be followed relatively undisturbed through the lowermost portions of the inferior cornua (section I). The *cricoid* cartilage is grossly distorted except in its uppermost portion (sections D, E and F). The rim of the cricoid is definitely thick, and in the latter sections it can be seen that there is sequestration of the cricoid cartilage, especially in its right half and in the posterior quadrant. *Arytenoid cartilages* — the left is relatively normal and can be traced through section E (along with this the left cricoarytenoid joint can be seen to be relatively normal). The right arytenoid, however, is foreshortened at the level of the vocal process (section D). The right cricoarytenoid joint is definitely abnormal in sections E and F. In the region just above the superior rim of the right portion of the cricoid and below, the anterior remnant of the right arytenoid is an area of calcification (sections E, F and G). This can be followed from the right glottic soft tissue down into the superior rim of the cricoid where there seems to be very definite *ossification* seen even in section H, both anteriorly and laterally.

Soft Tissues. The supraglottic soft tissues seen in sections A and B are relatively normal. The soft tissues of the left vocal cord are somewhat distorted in sectioning (sections D, E and F), but are relatively normal. The right vocalis muscle is replaced by scarring and the previously mentioned ossification. Other muscles which can be identified are the interarytenoideus (A, B and C), cricoarytenoideus posticus (D-I) and the cricothyroideus (G-L).

The area of scarring, therefore, proceeds from (section B) between the arytenoids posteriorly down into the subglottis and is circumferential around the lumen (sections E onward). It should be also noted that the fibrous structure of the cicatrix changes to a glandular hypertrophy as one leaves the cricoid and approaches the trachea (section L). (H & E, x3.3) subglottic stenosis with a less than 1.5 mm airway in the subglottic space.

On December 13, 1978, laryngoscopy showed the larynx to be normal with normal vocal cord movement. A bronchoscopy was performed and below the vocal cords a greyish-like membrane with a total stenosis of the subglottic space was noted. An opening was created with biopsy forceps and a continuous string was put in place. Bronchoscopy, at that time, revealed a rough and red trachea. The distal trachea and bronchi were normal. The continuous string was left in place through the nose and larynx and out the tracheostomy site, as a guide for future bronchoscopic dilatations.

The pathology report of December 13, 1978, (Path No. S-78-07345) showed fragments of upper respiratory mucosa and fibrous connective tissue. This was the material that was removed in order to open the subglottic space.

On December 22, 1978, the patient was noted to have complete closure of the subglottic space. He was dilated with the No. 3 bronchoscope with great difficulty. On January 3, 1979, he was again dilated with the No. 3 bronchoscope and still had a complete closure.

On January 11, 1979, there was reaction with granulation and edema, on the anterior one third of the vocal cords, from the string. There was less difficulty, however, dilating the child with the No. 3 bronchoscope. Two days later the patient developed increased temperature, and blood cultures were negative. The blood cultures revealed a coagulase negative staff and the patient was treated with Gantrisin®.

He was endoscoped again on January 18, 1979, and the larynx was still normal, there was still significant stenosis, and the child was dilated with the No. 3 bronchoscope. The child was dilated again on January 23. There was still bubbling through the larynx and, again, the child was dilated with the No. 3 bronchoscope (O.D. 16 Fr.).

On February 2, 1979, the patient was endoscoped with a 1-2 mm airway noted. He was dilated again with the No. 3 bronchoscope fairly easily and the No. 3.5 bronchoscope could be passed with some difficulty. On February 4, 1979, the No. 3 bronchoscope was passed easily. On March 7, 1979, the No. 3 bronchoscope was passed with minimal difficulty and stenosis was both fibrous and granular.

The 3 mm bronchoscope was passed easily on March 14, 1979, and a 3.5 bronchoscope was passed with some difficulty. Stenosis was seen to run for approximately 1 cm in length from under the cords to above the tracheostomy, with a 1 mm airway. On March 22, 1979, the stenosis was the same. The patient was dilated again with the No. 3 bronchoscope with difficulty.

On March 23, 1979, an audiogram behavioral response showed responses at 60-70 dB. On April 10, 1979, the patient underwent cardiac arrest. There was no occlusion of the tracheostomy.

An autopsy was done on April 11, 1979, which showed a cyanotic congenital cardiac disease. There was pseudotruncus arteriosus with a variety of tetralogy of Fallot including pulmonary valve atresia with a hypoplastic pulmonary artery and overriding aorta; ventricular septal defect; right ventricular hypertrophy; and bronchial pulmonary artery atresia. The patient also had pulmonary hypertension with tracheostomy in place; subglottic stenosis and chronic passive congestion of the liver.

Additionally, the patient was noted to have multicystic kidneys and surgical repair of sacral meningomyelocele. The cause of death was respiratory insufficiencies secondary to cyanotic congenital cardiovascular disease.

COMMENT

Serial section microscopic examination provides a retrospective look at pathological changes in the larynx invisible to the endoscopist's mucosal perspective. While good correlation is obtained between the difficulty of dilatation and microscopic findings, the origin of such pathological change must remain speculative. Is it congenital? Acquired? Iatrogenic?

This paper is published as a plea for further collaborative studies. This laboratory will welcome the opportunity to study similar documented material from all sources.

ENDOSCOPIC FINDINGS IN SARCOIDOSIS

CHARACTERISTICS AND CORRELATIONS WITH RADIOGRAPHIC STAGING AND BRONCHIAL MUCOSAL BIOPSY YIELD

JOHN R. ARMSTRONG, MD

JAN R. RADKE, MD
PAUL A. KVALE, MD
MICHAEL S. EICHENHORN, MD
JOHN POPOVICH, JR., MD

DETROIT, MICHIGAN

Flexible fiberoptic bronchoscopy was performed in 101 patients with sarcoidosis, and the endoscopic findings were analyzed and correlated with radiographic stages and diagnostic bronchial biopsy. Endoscopic findings included bronchostenosis (26% of patients), mucosal nodularity (64%), hypervascularity (38%), and mucosal edema (55%). The only correlation between these findings and the radiographic stage was the presence of mucosal nodularity observed in 73% of stage I (14/19 patients), decreasing to only 48% in stage III (15/31 patients). Bronchial biopsy yield was 58% for stage I, 62% for stage II, and 46% for stage III, with overall yield of 57%. However, the addition of bronchial biopsies increased the diagnostic yield of the bronchoscopic procedure from 73% for transbronchial biopsies alone to 88% when the two procedures were combined. In the presence of endobronchial stenosis, mucosal nodularity and hypervascularity, bronchial biopsy yield was 91% vs 37% when these were absent. We conclude that the endoscopic characteristics, with the exception of nodularity, do not correlate with radiographic stages. Bronchial biopsy yield is higher in those patients with mucosal nodularity, increased vascularity, and bronchostenosis. Bronchial mucosal biopsy also improved the overall diagnostic yield when it is obtained in conjunction with transbronchial lung biopsy.

INTRODUCTION

The tissue confirmation of sarcoidosis has been greatly facilitated since the introduction and widespread use of the flexible fiberoptic bronchoscope (FFB). Numerous authors have reported their experience with the use of transbronchial lung biopsy with the FFB in the diagnosis of this condition.[1-5] However, the various endobronchial abnormalities that may be visualized with this technique, their frequency with respect to radiographic disease stage, and the potential influence on bronchial biopsy yield has been less well defined.

We have studied 101 patients with sarcoidosis undergoing flexible fiberoptic bronchoscopy. The nature and extent of the gross endobronchial abnormalities in this setting were characterized. In addition, the potential relationships among radiographic disease stage, bronchoscopic mucosal findings, and the bronchial biopsy yields were explored.

METHODS

All patients (101) with sarcoidosis undergoing diagnostic FFB by members of the Division of Pulmonary Medicine between February 1974 and February 1980 are included in this report. Endoscopic findings were described at the time of the procedure and analyzed retrospectively. Particular attention was focused on such endobronchial abnormalities as mucosal nodularity, bronchostenosis, hypervascularity, edema, increased friability, and enlarged bronchial gland openings.

All patients underwent bronchial and/or transbronchial lung biopsy with Olympus BF-2B, BF-3B and BF-2T bronchoscopes utilizing Olympus large cup (FB14-C) or Alligator (FB15-C) forceps in standard fashion.[6] Mucosal biopsies were directed toward areas of greatest visualized abnormality. In the absence of mucosal alterations at least four bronchial biopsy specimens were obtained from several major carini or spurs. A minimum of four transbronchial lung biopsies were taken from the area of greatest radiographic involvement unless excessive bleeding occurred. In individuals without parenchymal infiltrate or with diffuse and homogeneous disease, transbronchial biopsies were taken from either of the lower lobes.

Specimens retrieved at bronchial mucosal and transbronchial biopsy were segregated and processed separately by the Department of Pathology in routine fashion. Typical noncaseating granulomata in the appropriate clinical setting, and in the absence of acid fast organisms or fungal elements, was considered diagnostic.

Each patient was assigned to a radiographic disease stage at the time of bronchoscopy based on the presence of hilar adenopathy alone (stage I), hilar adenopathy and parenchymal infiltrates (stage II) or parenchymal infiltrates without adenopathy (stage III). Correlations between endoscopic findings, radiographic stage, and diagnostic yield on bronchial mucosal biopsy were made. All statistical analyses were performed using x-square contingency tables.

RESULTS

Tissue confirmation of sarcoidosis was obtained at flexible fiberoptic bronchoscopy in 85 of the 101 patients. Twleve of the patients not diagnosed at bronchoscopy had tissue confirmation from other sources; superficial lymph node biopsy (3), mediastinoscopy or mediastinotomy (6), second bronchoscopy (2), and needle biopsy of the lung (1). The four remaining patients were asymptomatic with

From the Division of Pulmonary Medicine, Department of Medicine, Henry Ford Hospital, Detroit.

Presented at the meeting of the American Broncho-Esophagological Association, Vancouver, British Columbia, May 11-12, 1981.

REPRINTS — Jan R. Radke, MD, Division of Pulmonary Medicine, Department of Medicine, Henry Ford Hospital, Detroit, MI 48202.

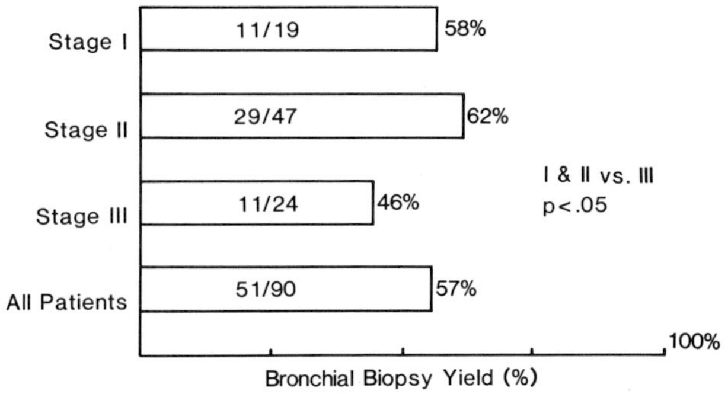

Fig. 1. Bronchial biopsy yield (%) as a function of radiographic disease stage.

symmetrical hilar adenopathy and elevated levels of angiotensin converting enzyme. The adenopathy in this group has remained stable or resolved over an 18-month observation period. There were 57 females and 44 males. Eighty-five patients underwent both mucosal and transbronchial lung biopsy. Eleven had bronchial biopsy alone and five had transbronchial biopsy alone. The overall diagnostic yield for bronchial mucosal biopsy was 57% (51/90). Transbronchial lung biopsy was diagnostic in 73% (70/96) of patients undergoing this procedure.

Among those who had both bronchial and transbronchial biopsies performed, the combined yield rose to 88% (75/85). The correlations between bronchial mucosal biopsy yield and radiographic stages were 58% in stage I disease (11/19), 62% in stage II disease (29/47) and 46% in stage III disease (11/24) (Fig. 1). There was a significantly lower yield from bronchial biopsy among the stage III patients as compared to stage I and II disease ($p < .05$).

The gross morphologic abnormalities described are listed in Table 1. With the exception of mucosal

TABLE 1. COMPARISON OF FREQUENCY OF ENDOSCOPIC FINDINGS AND RADIOGRAPHIC DISEASE STAGE

Gross Finding	*Radiographic Stage %* *I*	*II*	*III*	*Total*
Nodularity	73(14/19)	69(35/51)	48(15/31)	64(64/101)
Stenosis	21(4/19)	27(14/51)	26(8/31)	26(26/101)
Hypervascularity	42(8/19)	39(20/51)	32(10/31)	38(38/101)
Friability	42(8/19)	18(9/51)	29(9/31)	26(26/101)
Edema	58(11/19)	57(29/51)	52(16/31)	55(56/101)
Enlarged Glands	16(3/19)	12(6/51)	6(2/31)	11(11/101)

All differences between stages NS ($p > .05$) except nodularity lower in stage III ($p < .05$).

nodularity, the frequency with which these findings were noted did not vary significantly with radiographic disease stage. The finding of nodularity increased the bronchial mucosal biopsy yield among all patients regardless of radiographic stage, from 52% (14/27) when absent to 68% (43/64) when present. Similarly the diagnostic yield increased from 51% (34/67) in the absence of endobronchial stenosis to 74% (17/23) when this finding was present. Hypervascularity had a similar positive effect increasing bronchial biopsy yield from 51% (29/57) when absent to 63% (23/36) when this finding was present.

As shown in Figure 2, among those patients without either mucosal nodularity, hypervascularity, or bronchostenosis, the total yield at bronchial mucosal biopsy was 37%. In the presence of any two of these endoscopic abnormalities, diagnostic yield rose significantly to 72% ($p < .01$). A further significant increment in diagnostic yield on bronchial mucosal biopsy occurred in the presence of all three abnormalities to 91% ($p < .05$).

Descriptions of other less specific endoscopic abnormalities such as mucosal edema, friability, or enlarged bronchial gland openings were associated

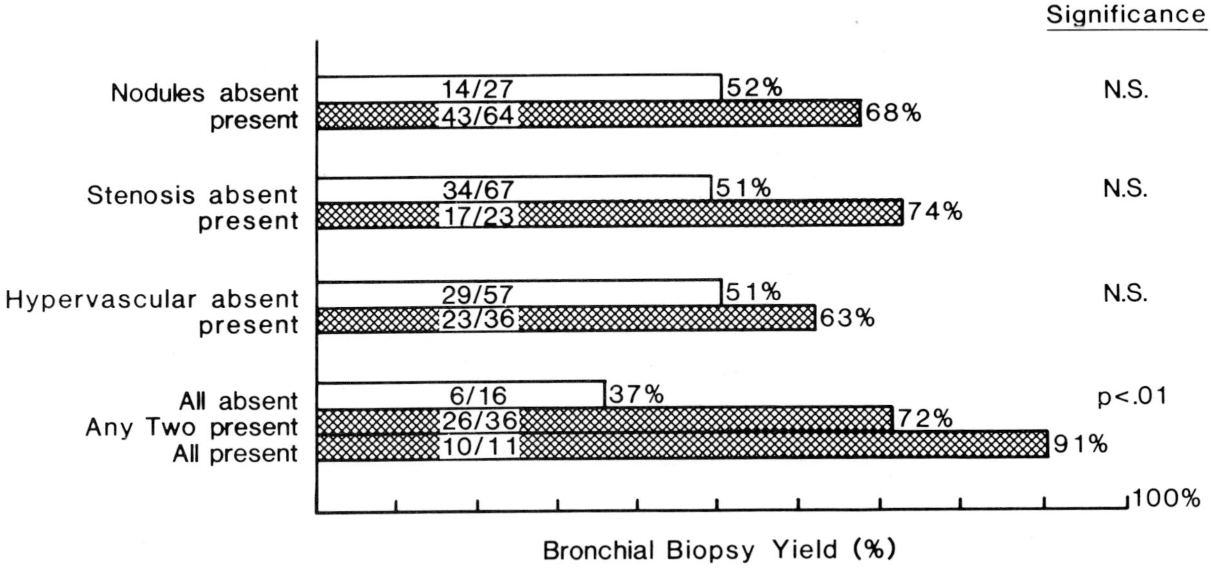

Fig. 2. Bronchial biopsy yield (%) as a function of endoscopic findings.

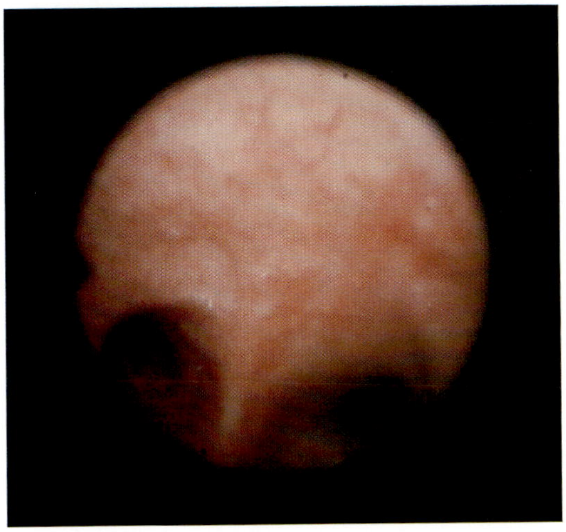

A) Tracheal mucosal hypervascularity. Note vessels running perpendicular to tracheal rings.

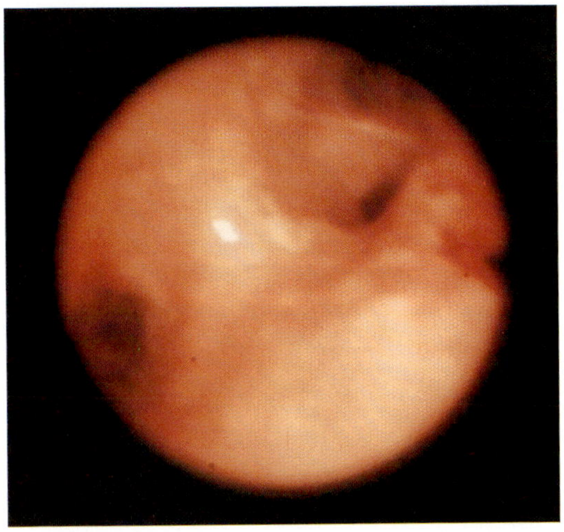

B) Marked mucosal nodularity with irregular bronchial narrowing.

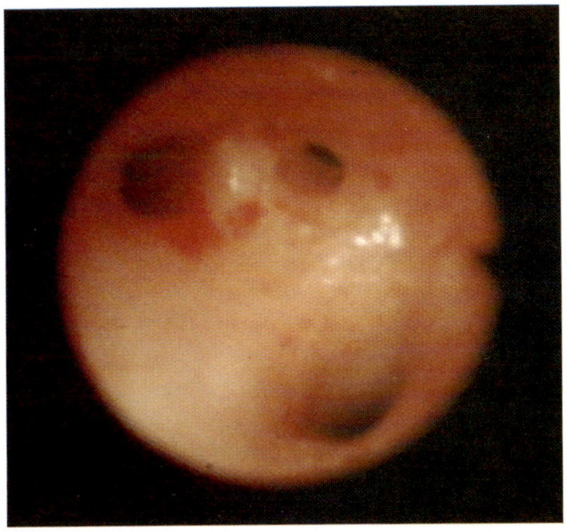

C) Smooth concentric bronchostenosis with widening of the carini. There is suction artifact suggesting increased friability.

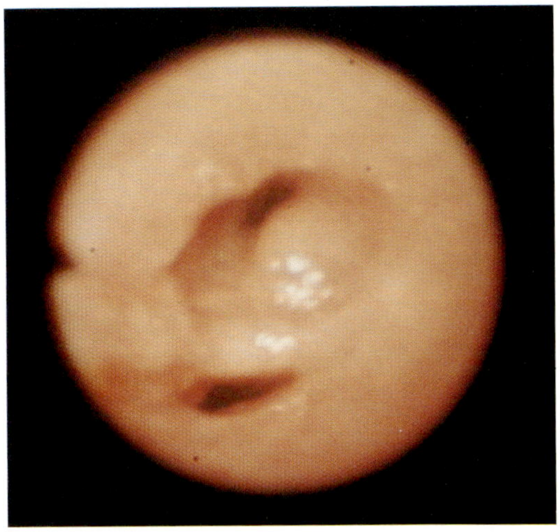

D) Macronodular change nearly obstructing segmental orifice.

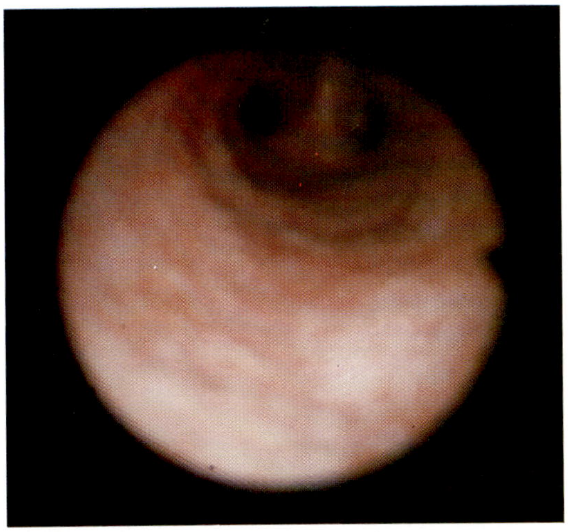

E) Fine nodularity affecting the anterior tracheal wall.

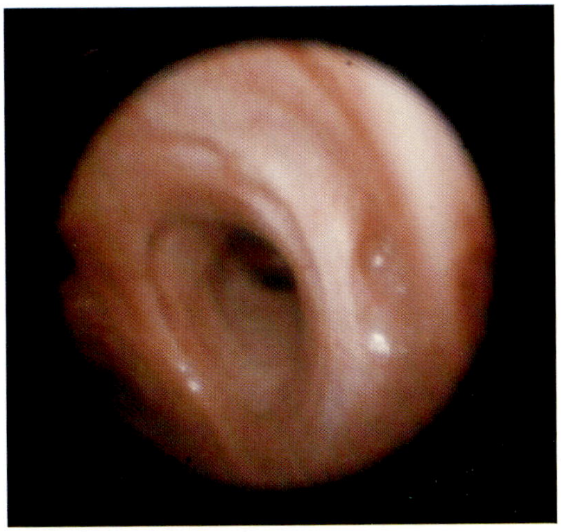

F) Enlarged bronchial gland. The mucosa is atrophic and there is a large vessel circumferentially about the segmental orifice.

Fig. 3. Representative bronchoscopic abnormalities that may be encountered in endobronchial sarcoidosis.

with a slightly higher yield on bronchial mucosal biopsy. However, the relationship between these findings and biopsy yield does not achieve significance when they are considered individually or in combination.

DISCUSSION

In 1941 Benedict and Castleman first reported the diagnosis of sarcoidosis made by means of bronchial mucosal biopsy.[7] It has since been shown that sarcoidosis may frequently involve the bronchial mucosa and submucosa.[8-13] This involvement may range from microscopic granulomatous infiltration in apparently normal appearing mucosa to gross endobronchial distortion of major airways. The utility of mucosal biopsy in these patients has been previously established by other studies utilizing rigid bronchoscopy.[8-13] With the advent of the FFB, attention has shifted towards improving diagnostic yield with transbronchial lung biopsy. While the results from transbronchial lung biopsy depend on the extent of the disease, radiographic staging, and biopsy techniques, yields in excess of 90% have been achieved in some instances.[1,2] Despite this, bronchial biopsy is advocated for all suspected cases of sarcoidosis coming to bronchoscopy.[14] However, the role and efficacy in the context of FFB has not been extensively evaluated. The three major areas considered here are: 1) the relationship between radiographic disease stage and bronchial mucosal biopsy yield, 2) the nature and extent of major endobronchial abnormalities, and 3) the influence these abnormalities may exert on diagnostic yield from bronchial mucosal biopsy.

In our patients the radiographic disease stage affected bronchial mucosal biopsy yields. The yield was significantly lower in stage III disease, although even here it was still 46%. Previous authors, utilizing rigid bronchoscopy, have consistently recorded lowest yields on bronchial biopsy in stage I patients.[8-10,12] Thc reason for this is not entirely clear. However, most of these authors also describe a higher yield in stage II disease.[8,10,12] We also found a higher yield in stage II disease (62%), but maintained a similarly high yield for stage I patients.

Mild changes in the mucosal vascular pattern (eg, parallel clusters of vessels running at right angles to the cartilaginous rings) have been described as an early manifestation of sarcoidosis (Fig. 3).[8] Mucosal nodules 2-4 mm in diameter are frequently described scattered diffusely throughout the major airways.[5,7] These are often associated with mucosal thickening and edema. Progression to plaque-like lesions or even large protuberant nodular excrescences are observed. Frank bronchostenosis and airway obstruction are more advanced pathological changes.[13] The frequency with which the endoscopic abnormalities are distributed among the various disease stages is not well established. Carlens reported no bronchostenosis in 44 patients with radiographic stage I and II disease.[9] However, Stahle described this finding in 6 of 27 (22%) of his patients with radiographic stage I disease,[10] similar to our 26% when all stages were combined. There were no differences among the stages. Mucosal nodularity was our most frequent finding (64%) and was the only abnormality to show a significant variation with stage, decreasing in stage III.

Overall yield on bronchial mucosal biopsy has ranged from 19-63% among the various reported series.[5,8,11,13] Improvement in diagnostic bronchial mucosal yield in the presence of endobronchial abnormalities was reported in the 1960s[8,11,12] and reference to this phenomenon has been made more recently.[3,14] We found that certain abnormalities had a definite influence on yield. The presence of nodules, stenosis and hypervascularity each individually increased the yield. However, all three together were associated with an improvement from 37% if all were absent to 91% if all were present. The association between improved yield and edema, friability, and enlarged bronchial gland openings was less specific. There were 16 patients without mucosal nodules, bronchostenosis or hypervascularity, and 6 had a positive mucosal biopsy (37%). Of these six patients three had negative transbronchial lung biopsies; thus the bronchial biopsy was the only positive tissue obtained during FFB.

We conclude that endobronchial abnormalities do not appear to vary with radiographic disease stage with the exception of mucosal nodularity. This appears to be a significantly less frequent finding in stage III disease. Bronchial mucosal biopsy was also less often diagnostic in stage III disease in our series. The presence of mucosal nodularity, hypervascularity, and bronchostenosis significantly improves bronchial biopsy yield. We recommend that bronchial mucosal biopsies be performed in all suspected cases of sarcoidosis undergoing FFB. If further studies corroborate the high diagnostic yield of bronchial biopsy in the presence of mucosal nodularity, hypervascularity, and bronchostenosis, it may be possible to omit transbronchial lung biopsies in this selected group of patients.

REFERENCES

1. Gilman MJ, Wang KP. Transbronchial lung biopsy in sarcoidosis: an approach to determine the optimal number of biopsies. Am Rev Respir Dis 1980; 122:721-4.

2. Roethe RA, Byrd RB, Hafermann DR. Transbronchoscopic lung biopsy in sarcoidosis: optimal number and sites for diagnosis. Chest 1980; 77:400-2.

3. Koontz CH, Joyner LR, Nelson RA. Transbronchial lung biopsy via the fiberoptic bronchoscope in sarcoidosis. Ann Int Med 1976; 85:64-6.

4. Koerner SK, Sakowitz AJ, Appelman RI, Becker NH, Schoenbaum SW. Transbronchial lung biopsy for the diagnosis of sarcoidosis. N Engl J Med 1975; 293:268-70.

5. Bower GC, Arroyo J, Kvale PA. Bronchial and transbronchial lung biopsy in intrathoracic sarcoidosis, abstract. Am Rev Respir Dis 1977 Suppl 115:90.

6. Zavala DC. Transbronchial biopsy in diffuse lung disease. Chest 1978 Suppl 73:727-33.

7. Benedict EB, Castleman B. Sarcoidosis with bronchial involvement: report of a case with bronchoscopic and pathological observations. N Engl J Med 1941; 224:186-9.

8. Friedman OH, Blaugrund SM, Siltzbach LE. Biopsy of the bronchial wall as an aid in diagnosis of sarcoidosis. JAMA 1963; 183:120-4.

9. Carlens E. Biopsies in connection with bronchoscopy and mediastinoscopy in sarcoidosis; a comparison. Acta Med Scand 1964 Suppl 425:237-8.

10. Stahle I. Bronchial involvement in pulmonary sarcoidosis. Acta Med Scand 1964 Suppl 425:234-6.

11. Turiaf J. Bronchial sarcoidosis. Acta Med Scand 1964 Suppl 425:228-9.

12. Siltzbach LE, Cahn LR. Random biopsy of bronchial and palatal mucosa in the diagnosis of sarcoidosis. Acta Med Scand 1964 Suppl 425:230-3.

13. Olsson T, Bjornstad-Pettersen H, Stjernberg NL. Bronchostenosis due to sarcoidosis. Chest 1979; 75:663-6.

14. Anderson HA. Transbronchoscopic lung biopsy for diffuse pulmonary diseases: results in 939 patients. Chest 1978 Suppl 73:734-6.

≈

GUIDELINES FOR GRANTS

TRUSTEES OF THE RESEARCH FUND OF THE AMERICAN OTOLOGICAL SOCIETY, INC.

The members of the Board of Trustees of the Research Fund of the American Otological Society have determined guidelines for making grants from the Fund. The following is the formulation of policy.

Grants will be given in the area of otosclerosis — its diagnosis and management, the possible causes and underlying conditions, and an understanding of the disorder that may lead eventually to its prevention or cure.

The present lack of understanding of the disorder and the absence of similar conditions in other animals makes research in this field difficult. A direct approach to the disease may or may not be feasible; therefore, a sound strategy would be to use other approaches, such as the investigation of bone development, growth and repair under various conditions, and the study of other diseases that may be similar to otosclerosis. It is possible that investigations which may seem initially remote from otosclerosis may provide information which will eventually lead to a substantive further understanding of the disease process which underlies otosclerosis. The applicant should describe correlations between proposed research with the clinical pathological entity of otosclerosis.

The policy is to aid and encourage research in the immediate field of otosclerosis and also in adjoining fields, if, in the opinion of the Board, there is a substantial promise that results obtained will be of assistance in the ways indicated, and may lead to the attainment of the objective of the further understanding of otosclerosis.

Applications for a research grant from the Research Fund of the American Otological Society may be obtained from the Office of the Secretary-Treasurer of the Research Fund of the American Otological Society. Write to Robert J. Ruben, MD, Secretary-Treasurer, Department of Otolaryngology, Albert Einstein College of Medicine, 1300 Morris Park Avenue, Bronx, NY 10461; telephone (212) 430-3036.

All grant requests must be submitted by January 31, 1982. All grants received after January 31 will not be considered.

A NEW UNIVERSAL BIVALVED SPECULUM DIRECT LARYNGOSCOPE

GEORGE BERCI, MD PAUL H. WARD, MD

LOS ANGELES, CALIFORNIA

A new bivalved slit laryngoscope with an adjustable suspension apparatus is a valuable new instrument for both diagnostic and operative suspension laryngoscopy.

Laryngoscopes can conventionally be divided into two major categories: small diameter scopes designed for diagnostic evaluations, and larger, more cumbersome operating (suspension) instruments. Diagnostic laryngoscopes can be introduced into most patients but have the drawbacks of monocular visualization (with or without the microscope) and limited instrumental and manipulative working space.[1]

Operating laryngoscopes, while overcoming these inadequacies, are sometimes difficult to introduce because of their size. The anatomy of the obese short-necked patient, or of patients with prominent teeth and limited ability to open their mouths further complicate the introduction of the scope. The shape, size and configuration of the tip are important factors that play a role in the safe and easy introduction of the instrument.

This new direct laryngoscope was specifically designed to overcome the deficiencies of both examining and operating scopes (Fig. 1). The straight lower blade is smaller in diameter at the end than other operating laryngoscopes. The upper blade is gently angled to provide a small overall diameter during introduction. After introduction, and upon opening the blades by turning the screw, it acts to lift the anterior commissure (Fig. 1B). This action eliminates the additional wide tip or flange of the Holinger or Dedo type scopes during introduction but provides improved visualization upon opening of the blades.

The fiberoptic bundle for illumination has a flat configuration and contains more fibers for brighter

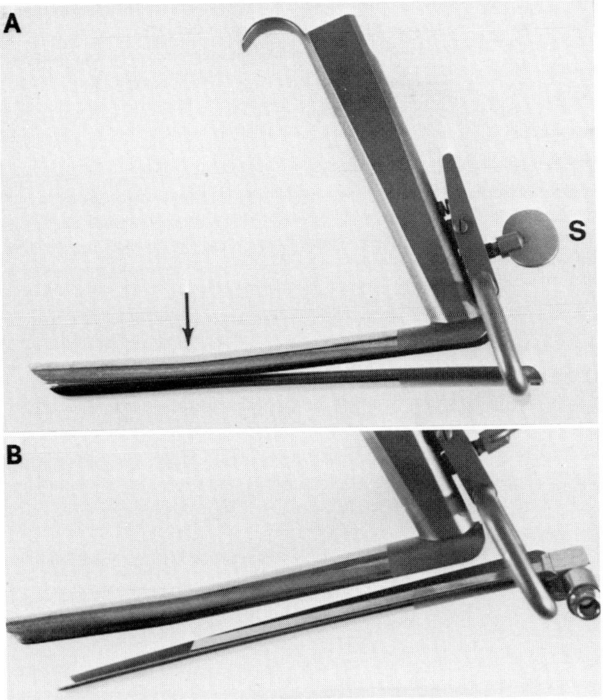

Fig. 1. Slit bivalved laryngoscope. A) In closed position, showing angle of upper blade (arrow) with screw (S) for opening blades. B) In opened position.

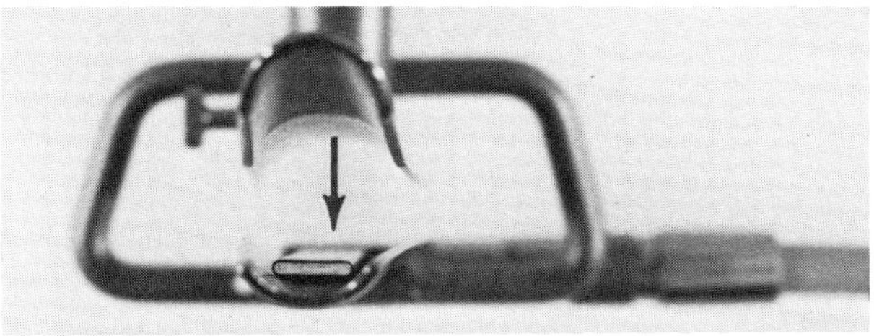

Fig. 2. Laryngoscope (end-on view) showing the flat light carrier positioned at the bottom of the lower blade (arrow). A suction tube or Venturi type injector tube can **be inserted in a slot beside the light carriers.**

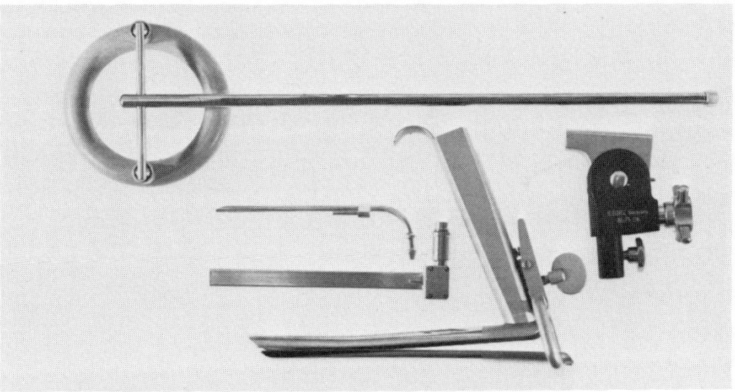

Fig. 3. Complete apparatus including bivalved laryngoscope, light carrier, suction tube and Reicher-Kleinsasser chest support.

From the Division of Head and Neck Surgery, UCLA School of Medicine, Los Angeles.

Presented at the meeting of the American Broncho-Esophagological Association, Vancouver, British Columbia, May 11-12, 1981.

REPRINTS — George Berci, MD, Division of Head and Neck Surgery, UCLA School of Medicine, Los Angeles, CA 90024.

uniform illumination than the conventional small laterally-placed light carriers (Fig. 2). A suction tube for continuous evacuation of smoke, if the laser is being used, can be inserted in a slot next to the light carriers.

The laryngoscope is introduced in a standard fashion and when in position, is attached to a Reicher-Kleinsasser laryngoscope holder and chest support (Fig. 3). The anterior and posterior commissures are seen well and repeated repositioning maneuvers using a standard scope are avoided. The wide bilateral slits allow optimum working space for instruments during microsurgical procedures. Experience thus far suggests this instrument provides a significant advance in laryngoscopy.*

*Manufacturer: Karl Storz Endoscopy-America, Inc., Los Angeles.

REFERENCES

1. Weerda H, Pedersen P, Wehner H, Braune H. A new laryngoscope for endolaryngeal microsurgery. Arch Otorhinolaryngol, Heidelberg: Springer, 1979; 225:103-6. In German.

≈

EXCERPTA MEDICA FOUNDATION TRAVEL GRANTS 1981 AND 1982

Ann Otol 90:1981

VIDEO LARYNGOSCOPY USING A RIGID TELESCOPE AND VIDEO HOME SYSTEM COLOR CAMERA

A USEFUL OFFICE PROCEDURE

EIJI YANAGISAWA, MD
NEW HAVEN, CONNECTICUT

J. RICHARD CASUCCIO, MD
NEW HAVEN, CONNECTICUT

MASAFUMI SUZUKI, MD
TOKYO, JAPAN

A simple but reliable method of videotaping the larynx using the Nagashima rigid laryngoscope (telescope) and a low-cost home video color camera is described. Video laryngoscopy using this technique is a useful office procedure. The video material obtained was of high quality and of great value for teaching, voice analysis, preoperative and postoperative evaluation and documentation of various laryngeal disorders.

Ever since the successful visualization of the larynx via a mirror by Manuel Garcia in 1854, many different methods of laryngeal photography have been tried. They included indirect and direct laryngoscopic photography,[1-4] microscopic photography,[5-11] telescopic photography[12,13] and fiberoptic photography.[14,15] Photographic documentation of the larynx has traditionally been done in still and motion pictures, but more recently videotape recording has gained widespread acceptance.[16-19]

The purpose of this paper is to introduce a simple but reliable method of videotaping of the larynx using a Nagashima rigid telescope (laryngoscope) and a reasonably priced video home system (VHS) color camera.

EQUIPMENT

The equipment used for this technique (Figs. 1 and 2) is as follows:

Nagashima Laryngoscope. This laryngoscope (right-angled SFT-1, Nagashima Medical Instrument Co., Tokyo) is a single integrated unit composed of a telescope and a light transmission system (Fig. 1). It measures 24.5 cm in length and 9 mm in outer diameter. The angle of the prism at the tip of the laryngoscope is 70° providing a right-angled view of the larynx. The rectangular outlets on each side of the lens offer well-balanced illumination of the viewing field. It gives a clear, enlarged view of the larynx which fills the entire screen of the TV monitor when used with the Panasonic® WV3100 camera with a telescopic adaptor. The telescope is connected to the cine-video adaptor and its fiberoptic light cable to a xenon light source (Fig. 3).

Light transmission of the Nagashima laryngoscope was excellent and provided brighter definition of the image than other endoscopes we tried. The reasons for this appeared to be the wide diameter of the telescope, the newer optical lens system it employed, integration of the light cable into the telescope without a connecting joint and a higher number of fibers in the light-transmitting system. This laryngoscope requires no additional light cable nor a special photographic sheath.

Video Camera. There are several excellent color video cameras specially designed for endoscopic documentation. The cost of these cameras is often prohibitive for the practicing otolaryngologist. Because of recent technological advances and wide-

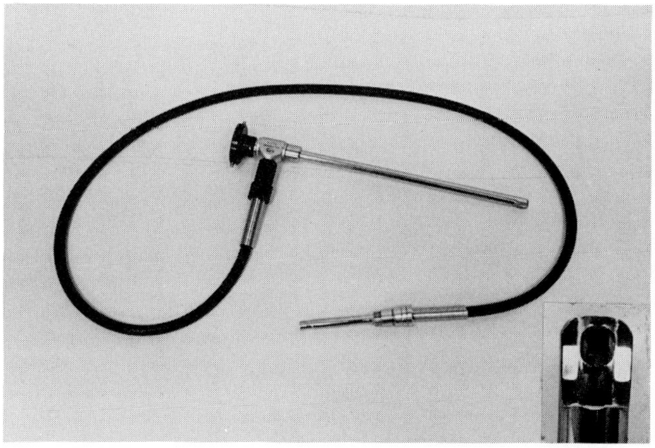

Fig. 1. Nagashima laryngoscope, right-angled SFT-1 composed of a rigid telescope and a fiberoptic light transmission system. Note that the light cable is an integral part of the scope. The inset shows the tip of the laryngoscope with its right-angled viewing prism and two illuminating outlets.

From the Section of Otolaryngology-Head and Neck Surgery, Department of Surgery, Hospital of St. Raphael; the Section of Otolaryngology, Department of Surgery, Yale University School of Medicine; and the Department of Otorhinolaryngology, Keio University School of Medicine, Tokyo.

Presented at the meeting of the American Broncho-Esophagological Association, Vancouver, British Columbia, May 11-12, 1981.

REPRINTS — Eiji Yanagisawa, MD, 98 York Street, New Haven, CT 06511.

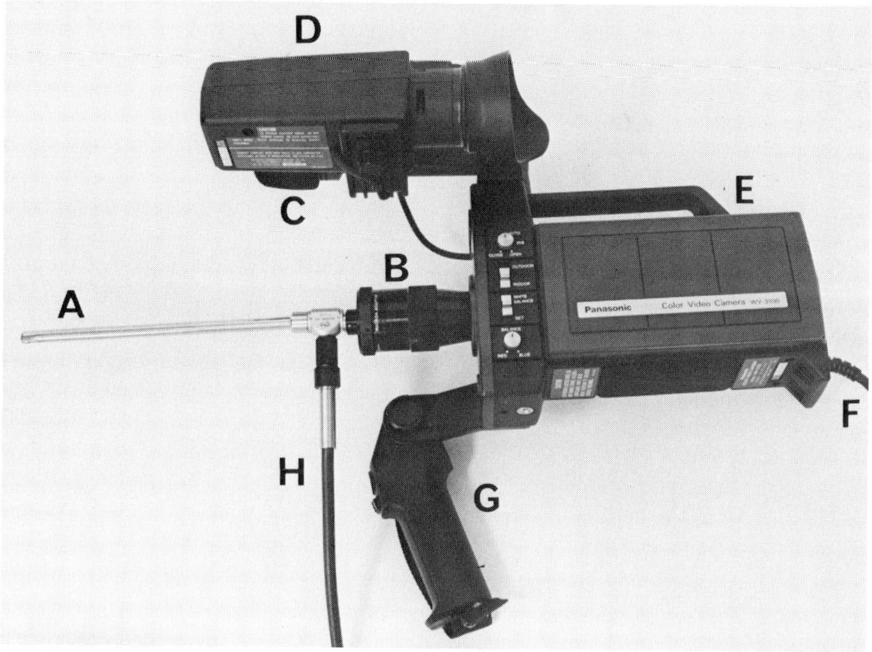

Fig. 2. Equipment for video laryngoscopy. A) Nagashima laryngoscope; B) F-60 mm cine-video adaptor; C) Microphone; D) Viewfinder; E) VHS color camera; F) Camera cable to videocassette recorder; G) Adjustable pistol grip; H) Fiberoptic light cable to xenon light source.

spread use of home video equipment, many compact, low-cost portable color video cameras have now become available. Several of the home video cameras have been tried for video laryngoscopy. Of these, the Panasonic portable color camera WV3100 fulfilled many requirements of laryngeal videotaping.

The Panasonic WV3100 is a fully self-contained, compact and lightweight color camera (Fig. 2). The camera has a $^{2}/_{3}$in (16 mm) integral stripe filter vidicon which receives its power from a Panasonic portable video cassette recorder or an AC adaptor. The $1^{3}/_{8}$ in (35 mm) viewfinder, which is also used for VCR playback, is mounted on the camera head and its position can be easily changed so that the examiner can view the larynx during the procedure (Fig. 2D). The WV3100 comes with telephoto lens (f-60 mm, Nagashima) for routine televising. This lens is detachable and the cine-video adaptor can be connected to the C-mount coupler on the camera body (Fig. 2B). A convenient power switch allows the camera to be turned off when not in use. This will spare the vidicon tube. Another advantage of this camera is that its pistol grip is adjustable which can be turned in such a way that the examiner can hold the pistol grip comfortably in one hand (Figs. 2 and 4).

The price of this camera at the time of this writing is about $900. In view of rapidly advancing video technology and competitive video market, a more compact and sophisticated but reasonably priced video camera may appear in the not-too-distant future. Other lightweight video cameras with a C-mount coupler can also be used for this technique.

Light Source. The standard incandescent light

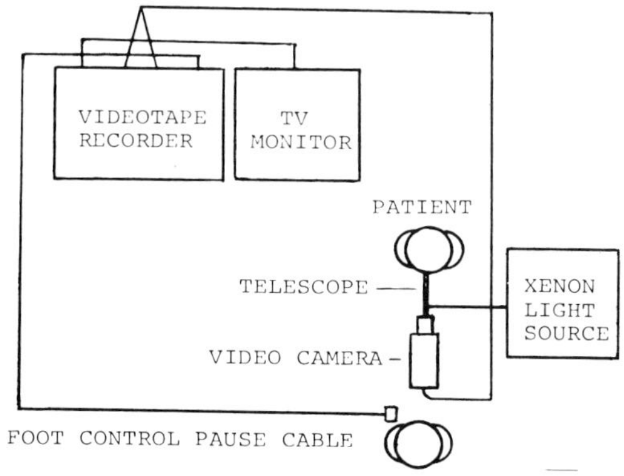

Fig. 3. Schematic diagram of video laryngoscopy system. Note that the videocassette recorder is operated by the examiner using a foot control pause pedal.

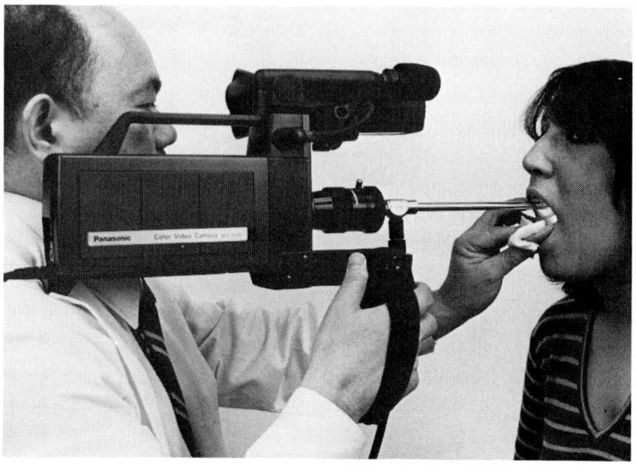

Fig. 4. Technique of video laryngoscopy. The larynx is viewed and centered through the viewfinder of the camera or on the screen of the TV monitor. Note that the camera is balanced with the hand and shoulder.

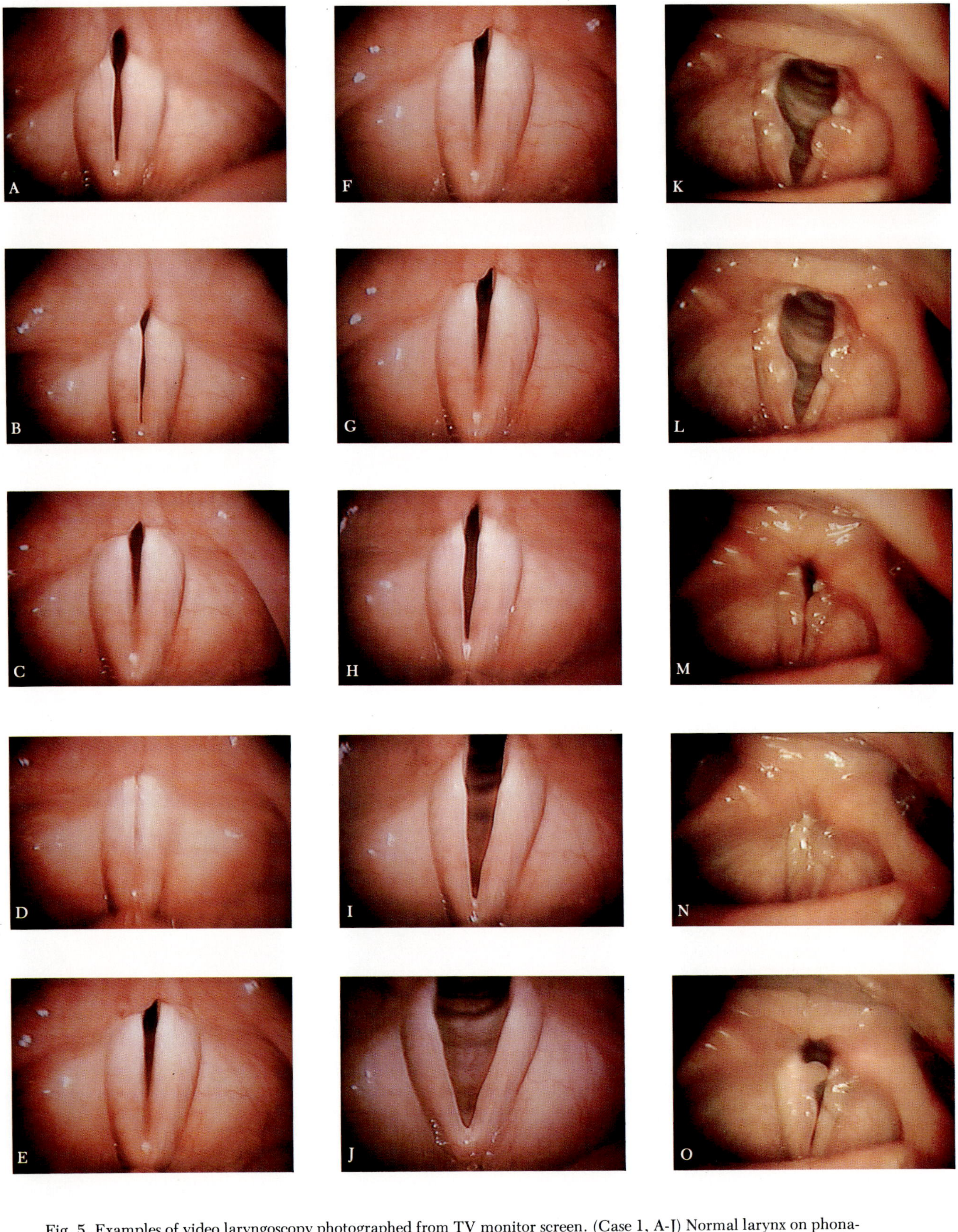

Fig. 5. Examples of video laryngoscopy photographed from TV monitor screen. (Case 1, A-J) Normal larynx on phonation (A-H) and respiration (I-J). (Case 2, K-O) Multiple laryngeal polyps. Note that the polyps move up (K-L) and down (O).

sources did not provide sufficient illumination for video laryngoscopy but the xenon illuminator (Karl Storz 487) designed for cinematography and videotaping provided excellent lighting.

Video Recorder and Monitor. Technically any 3/4 in (18 mm) or 1/2 in (12.5 mm) video recorder can be used. A 3/4in Sony video cassette recorder VO2610 was used in this study. When needed, the 3/4 in videotapes can be transferred to 1/2in format through a series of commercially available coupling devices. A color monitor is ideal for televised laryngoscopy but a more economical portable color television may be substituted.

TECHNIQUE

The patient and examiner sit facing each other (Figs. 3 and 4). The soft palate and the posterior half of the tongue are topically anesthetized with 2% tetracaine hydrochloride (Pontocaine®) solution. The telescope is connected to the video camera via the cine-video adaptor and its fiberoptic light cable to the xenon illuminator (Figs. 2 and 3). The tip of the telescope is dipped in warm water and dried to prevent fogging of the lens during the examination. The video camera and then the illuminator are turned on. The xenon illuminator is set in the high filming mode (15-23 A).

The examiner holds the video camera in one hand and inserts the telescope into the mouth while holding the patient's tongue with the other hand (Fig. 4). When the desired image appears on the monitor screen, video recording is begun. The laryngeal image is centered on the screen by using the viewfinder of the camera or the television monitor. The larynx is videotaped both on phonation and respiration. Every effort should be made to stabilize the camera and the laryngoscope to prevent image movement during videotaping.

RESULTS

Of the 40 consecutive patients studied, video laryngoscopy was successfully performed in all but one patient who could not tolerate the procedure because of anxiety. All patients were adults.

Consistently good results were obtained when the larynx was videotaped using the Nagashima laryngoscope and Panasonic camera WV3100 with the xenon light source in high filming mode. The quality of laryngeal images on the TV monitor screen was much superior to that obtained by a flexible fiberoptic endoscope.

Examples of color pictures photographed from the TV screen of laryngeal conditions in the two patients are shown in Figure 5. The larynx was examined both on phonation and at rest, providing a functional view of the larynx. Not only was vocal cord mobility easily visualized but the vibrations of the vocal folds could be seen in most instances (Fig. 5). The floppy motion of vocal cord polyps passing through the glottis in case 2 was vividly documented by this technique (Fig. 5 K-O). Also the subglottic region, particularly the area under the anterior commissure, could be clearly visualized.

COMMENTS

Video laryngoscopy using a rigid telescope and VHS color camera is a useful office procedure and was found to be of great value for teaching, voice analysis, and preoperative and postoperative evaluation and documentation of various laryngeal disorders.

Video documentation of the larynx by this technique provides many advantages. The technique is simple and as easy as indirect laryngoscopy; yet it gives much useful information difficult to obtain from a brief indirect mirror examination. The entire procedure takes less than ten minutes.

Magnification of the image by both the telescope and the cine-video adaptor provides a view of the larynx which fills the TV monitor screen. The newer optics of the rigid telescope produce a televised picture of high resolution.[5,12,13]

Live viewing by physicians, patients and assisting personnel is possible.[16,17,19] This is an excellent teaching tool for medical students and residents. In many instances, the videotape was shown to the patients and it was extremely helpful for the patient to understand the necessity for treatment.

The taped image can be instantaneously replayed and examined repeatedly. This will eliminate the need for multiple and prolonged examination of the patient. More critical evaluation of the laryngeal image can be done by freezing its motion for a frame by frame examination using a videotape player equipped with a pause capability. This allows the physician to detect a small obscure lesion which may be unrecognized at the time of the initial mirror examination.

One of the most important advantages of video laryngoscopy is the ease of simultaneous voice recording. Voice can be simply recorded by plugging the audio output connector of the camera cable to a cassette recorder. For high fidelity voice recording, the use of a separate external microphone is recommended which is directly connected to the cassette recorder. Simultaneous audio and video documentation is particularly valuable for a preoperative and postoperative voice analysis of the patient. The surgeon can document a progressive improvement or regression of laryngeal disorders of the patient.

One of the disadvantages of this technique is that it is impossible to study an uncooperative patient such as a small child or patients with active gag reflexes. For examination of these patients, a flexible fiberoptic laryngoscope is more useful. Another minor disadvantage is that there is some distortion of the laryngeal image due to the wide angle lens of the telescope.[5] The structures closer to the lens such as the epiglottis and arytenoids appear disappropriately larger than the vocal cords which are farther away from the lens.

It is important to emphasize that not all the home video cameras can be used for this video laryngoscopy with a rigid telescope. Only the cameras equipped with a detachable lens, a C-mount coupler and an adjustable or detachable hand grip can be used for this technique.

SUMMARY

Video laryngoscopy using the Nagashima laryngoscope and VHS color camera is a simple and useful office procedure.

Success of this technique depends upon a) use of a xenon light source, b) adequate topical anesthesia of the pharynx and the base of the tongue, and c) stabilization of the laryngoscope and the camera.

Video material obtained was of high quality and of great value for teaching, voice analysis, permanent records, preoperative and postoperative evaluation and documentation of various laryngeal disorders.

REFERENCES

1. French TR. On a perfected method of photographing the larynx. N Y Med J 1884; 4:655-6.

2. Holinger PA. Photography of the larynx, trachea, bronchi and esophagus. Trans Am Acad Ophthalmol Otolaryngol 1942; 46:153-6.

3. Ferguson GB, Crowder WJ. A simple method of laryngeal and other cavity photography. Arch Otolaryngol 1970; 92:201-3.

4. Rosnagle R, Smith HW. Hand-held fundus camera for endoscopic photography. Trans Am Acad Ophthalmol Otolaryngol 1972; 76:1024-5.

5. Alberti PW. Still photography of the larynx — an overview. Can J Otolaryngol 1975; 4:759-65.

6. Jako GJ, Strong S. Laryngeal photography. Arch Otolaryngol 1972; 96:268-71.

7. Kleinsasser O. Microlaryngoscopy and endolaryngeal microsurgery. Philadelphia: WB Saunders, 1968.

8. Saito S. Phonosurgery — basic study on the mechanism of phonation and endolaryngeal microsurgery. Otologia (Fukuoka) 1977; 23 Suppl 1:171-384.

9. Hirano M. Phonosurgery, basic and clinical investigations. Otologia (Fukuoka) 1975; 21 Suppl 1:239-440.

10. Olofsson J, Ohlsson T. Techniques in microlaryngoscopic photography. Can J Otolaryngol 1975; 4:770-80.

11. Yanagisawa E, Eibling DE, Suzuki M. A simple method of laryngeal photography through the operating microscope: "macrolens technique." Ann Otol Rhinol Laryngol 1980; 89:547-50.

12. Ward PH, Berci G, Calcaterra TC. Advances in endoscopic examination of the respiratory system. Ann Otol Rhinol Laryngol 1974; 83:754-60.

13. Berci G, Calcaterra T, Ward PH. Advances in endoscopic techniques for examination of the larynx and nasopharynx. Can J Otolaryngol 1975; 4:786-92.

14. Sawashima M, Hirose H. New laryngoscopic technique by use of fiber optics. J Acoust Soc Am 1968; 43:168-9.

15. Brewer DW, McCall G. Visible laryngeal changes during voice therapy: fiber-optic study. Ann Otol Rhinol Laryngol 1974; 83:423-7.

16. Tardy ME, Tenta LT. Laryngeal photography and television. Otolaryngol Clin North Am 1970; 3:483-92.

17. Strong MS. Laryngeal photography. Can J Otolaryngol 1975; 4:766-9.

18. Yoshida Y, Hirano M, Nakajima T. A video-tape recording system for laryngo-stroboscopy. J Jpn Bronchoesophagol Soc 1979; 30:1-5.

19. Rayl JE, Rourke D. Application of color television in bronchoesophagology. Ann Otol Rhinol Laryngol 1974; 83:744-9.

FLEXIBLE FIBEROPTIC BRONCHOSCOPY AND PULMONARY CYTOLOGY IN THE EVALUATION OF PATIENTS WITH HEAD AND NECK MALIGNANCIES

TERRY J. GARFINKLE, MD
ROBERT A. WEISMAN, MD JAMES C. DENNENY III, MD
PHILADELPHIA, PENNSYLVANIA

In a study involving 107 patients with new primary tumors of the head and neck and normal chest roentgenograms, the information gained from flexible fiberoptic bronchoscopy and pulmonary cytology was analyzed. A small but significant proportion of the patients (14%) had positive cytologies. Contrary to previous reports, contamination of bronchial washings with tumor cells from head and neck neoplasms did take place. In most patients, the source of contamination appeared to be the passage of the bronchoscope adjacent to the endotracheal tube. Two patients with normal chest radiographs and positive cytologic studies were discovered to have pulmonary metastases within one year of bronchoscopy. It is concluded that malignant involvement of the lungs is unlikely in patients with a normal chest radiograph, normal bronchoscopy, and negative bronchial washings. This informaion appears to be of value in staging patients with head and neck cancer. Positive bronchial washings are always associated with malignancy, either in the head and neck or the lungs, and should be considered an indication for further evaluation. Recommendations are made regarding the technique of bronchoscopy as part of panendoscopy in head and neck cancer patients, and diagnostic strategies are proposed for patients with positive bronchial washings and negative chest radiographs.

INTRODUCTION

In the staging of head and neck malignancies, it has long been recognized that the lungs are a frequent site for neoplastic involvement. The discovery of pulmonary metastases or second primary tumors of the lung in patients with newly diagnosed primary tumors of the head and neck radically alters the therapeutic approach. Malignant involvement of the lung usually portends a grave prognosis. Studies based on postmortem examination demonstrate evidence of pulmonary metastases in as many as 60-80% of patients with squamous cell carcinoma of the head and neck.[1-3] In several reports of multiple primaries associated with head and neck cancers, primary lung carcinoma accounts for 11-25% of second primary tumors,[4,5] with an especially frequent association with oral and laryngeal carcinoma.[6]

The standard approaches to detection of pulmonary malignancies include chest roentgenography, sputum cytology, bronchoscopic biopsy, bronchial brushings, and bronchial washings. In dealing with squamous cell carcinoma of the head and neck, sputum cytologies are not reliable for detection of pulmonary neoplasms, since malignant cells from the head and neck tumor can contaminate sputum. Therefore chest roentgenography and bronchoscopy are the methods of choice in the detection of pulmonary malignancy in these patients. To our knowledge, virtually all the reported experience with these methods has been in patients with primary lung carcinoma.

Chest roentenography may reveal indirect evidence of lung carcinoma, manifested by lobar collapse, consolidation, effusion, mediastinal enlargements or discrete parenchymal nodules. Goldmeier[7] has estimated that a bronchial carcinoma must be at least 1 cm in diameter and contain approximately 1 billion cells before it can be detected on routine chest roentgenography. A neoplasm arising in a main bronchus or within the normal mediastinal and hilar shadows may exceed 2 cm in diameter before it is roentgenographically detectable.[8] Oswald et al[8] observed that 2% of confirmed lung carcinomas could not be detected on routine chest roentgenogram, and most of these arose near the main bronchi. Thus, chest roentgenography is a useful screening procedure, but lesions of significant size may remain undetected.

The development of the flexible fiberoptic bronchoscope by Ikeda et al in 1968[9] has resulted in a dramatic improvement in visualization of the tracheobronchial tree. According to Kovnat et al,[10] 85% of the fifth order subsegmental bronchi and 55% of sixth order bronchi can now be well visualized with this instrument.

With increased visualization has come improvement in the cytologic detection of pulmonary neoplasms. Statistically, cytologic specimens from bronchoscopy are more accurate in the diagnosis of squamous cell carcinoma than adenocarcinoma.[8] Squamous cell carcinoma usually occurs more centrally, while adenocarcinoma tends to arise in the lung periphery. Controversy exists regarding the best method of obtaining cytologic specimens. The data are based on experience in patients with pri-

From the Department of Otorhinolaryngology and Human Communication, Hospital of the University of Pennsylvania, and the Philadelphia Veterans Administration Medical Center.

Presented at the meeting of the American Broncho-Esophagological Association, Vancouver, British Columbia, May 11-12, 1981.

REPRINTS — Robert A. Weisman, MD, 3400 Spruce Street, Philadelphia, PA 19104.

TABLE 1. LOCATIONS OF ORIGINAL AND SECOND PRIMARY MALIGNANCIES (N = 12)

Original Primary	*Second Primary*
Tongue	Larynx
Tongue	Tonsil
Tonsil	Esophagus
Supraglottic larynx	Lymphoma
Supraglottic larynx	Pancreas
Supraglottic larynx	Uterus
Glottic larynx	Pyriform sinus
Glottic larynx	Bladder
Glottic larynx	Prostate
Glottic larynx	Leukemia
Esophagus	Lung
Esophagus	Cecum

mary carcinoma of the lung. Several studies have shown that biopsy and brushings in combination provide the highest yield.[11,12] Others have shown that a combination of biopsy and bronchial washings is superior.[13,14]

Both radiographic and bronchoscopic methods are used frequently for evaluation of the lungs in the staging of head and neck malignancies. Little difficulty exists where there is a roentgenogram strongly suggestive of primary or metastatic carcinoma of the lung. The fact that most patients presenting with head and neck carcinoma are at risk for malignant involvement of the lung but usually have normal chest roentgenograms places importance on bronchoscopic and cytologic assessment in this group. Dellon et al[15] found that direct washings of a series of head and neck tumors resulted in positive cytologies in 72% of cases. The same authors noted that none of these 18 patients had positive pulmonary cytologies and concluded that there is no contamination of bronchial washings from head and neck tumors. This study was limited by its size and the fact that most of the head and neck tumors did not lie in proximity to the path of the bronchoscope. Only one of the patients had carcinoma of the larynx.

It is apparent that the accuracy and effectiveness of bronchoscopically obtained cytologic specimens has not been fully assessed in the setting of concurrent head and neck malignancy. A study was undertaken to address the issue of bronchoscopy in the setting of normal chest roentgenograms for the detection of pulmonary malignancy in patients with head and neck cancer.

METHODS

Patient Selection. The records of patients admitted to the Hospital of the University of Pennsylvania and the Philadelphia Veterans Administration Medical Center from July 1, 1976, to December 31, 1980, with newly diagnosed malignancies of the head and neck were identified. Patients with previous malignancies of the head and neck were excluded. Each patient was systemically evaluated by physical examination, plain chest roentgenograms, barium swallow, complete blood count, electrolytes and enzyme panel. Direct laryngoscopy, bronchoscopy, and esophagoscopy were performed in each case for staging of the tumor. Patients with radiographically demonstrable pulmonary malignancies were excluded from this series.

Technique of Bronchoscopy. Under general anesthesia with endotracheal intubation, flexible fiberoptic bronchoscopy was carried out prior to biopsy of the primary lesion. Bronchoscopy was performed with either a Pentax FB-19A or Olympus BF-5B2 flexible fiberoptic bronchoscope. The bronchoscope was passed through the larynx either adjacent to the endotracheal tube or through the tube while ventilation continued. Careful examination of the entire tracheobronchial tree was carried out in a systematic fashion. Cytologic washings were collected from each main bronchus.

Collection and Analysis of Specimens. Following visual examination of each lung, 10-15 cc of normal saline were instilled into the main bronchus and collected in a Lukens trap. The specimens were carefully labeled, fixed with 95% ethanol, and evaluated by the cytopathologist. Cytologic classification is as follows:

Class I: negative, absence of suspicious cells.
Class II: atypical cytology, no evidence of malignancy.
Class III: suggestion of, but not conclusive of malignancy.
Class IV: strongly suggestive of malignancy.
Class V: conclusive of malignancy.

For the purpose of this study, cytologies of class III, IV, and V were considered significant for malignancy.

RESULTS

All patients in our series had documented squamous cell carcinoma of the upper aerodigestive tract. Of the 107 patients, there were 94 males and 13 females. The average age of our patients was 58.2 years.

Thirteen patients (12%) were found to have either synchronous or metachronous second primary malignancies. The average age of these patients was 60.1 years, slightly older than the average for the entire series. The locations of the second primary malignancies are listed in Table 1.

Fifteen patients (14%) were found to have positive pulmonary cytologies. Two of these patients (2/15) were found to have pulmonary malignancies. One patient had synchronous pulmonary metastases in the hilum; the other developed roentgenographically apparent pulmonary metastases within 12 months. The remaining 13 patients with positive cytologies (13/15) had normal chest roentgenograms and have no detectable pulmonary malignancy to date. Two patients (2/107) with normal chest roentgenograms and negative pulmonary cytologies developed pulmonary metastases within 12 months.

A significant finding was the difference in results associated with the method of passing the bronchoscope through the larynx. In 62 patients (58%) the bronchoscope was passed through the larynx adjacent to a small caliber endotracheal tube. In 45 patients (42%) the bronchoscope was passed through a larger endotracheal tube. There was a significantly greater incidence of false positive cytologies (10/13) when the bronchoscope was passed through the larynx adjacent to the endotracheal tube, as opposed to passage through the tube (3/13) (Table 2). Eight patients (8/13) with false positive cytologies had carcinoma of the larynx (Table 3).

DISCUSSION

The results of this study indicate that bronchoscopy can provide useful information in the staging

TABLE 2. CYTOLOGIC RESULTS ACCORDING TO BRONCHOSCOPIC TECHNIQUE

	Adjacent to Endotracheal Tube	*Through Endotracheal Tube*
True negative	50	40
True positive	1	1
False negative	1	1
False positive	10	3

TABLE 3. LOCATION OF PRIMARY TUMOR IN CASES OF FALSE POSITIVE CYTOLOGIES

Location	*Number*
Lip	1
Floor of mouth	1
Tongue	3
Larynx	8

of head and neck cancer patients. In two patients, a radiologically occult pulmonary metastasis was detected with bronchoscopy and washings. A normal chest roentgenogram, normal bronchoscopy, and normal bronchoscopic cytologies virtually exclude malignant involvement of the lungs. It is also noted that passage of the flexible fiberoptic bronchoscope through the endotracheal tube provides the most reliable cytologic specimens. Contrary to previous reports,[15] contamination of bronchial washings with malignant cells from the head and neck primary can occur. In nearly all such cases, the bronchoscope was passed through the larynx adjacent to a small endotracheal tube. False positive cytologies occurred most commonly in cases of carcinoma of the larynx. This is not surprising, as this phenomenon is probably attributable to the direct contact of the bronchoscope and the tumor.

We also find that consultation with the cytopathologist is helpful in evaluating positive cytologic specimens. Differentiation between adenocarcinoma and squamous cell carcinoma is often possible and histologic comparison of the cytologic specimens with those of the primary tumor may aid in the identification of false positive results.

In the staging of head and neck tumors, it has been our practice to perform panendoscopy under general anesthesia to permit an unhurried and careful examination of all areas with appropriate biopsies. When possible, a large endotracheal tube (8 mm inner diameter or larger) should be used. Prior to biopsy of the primary lesion, bronchoscopy should be performed. Because of its superior diagnostic capabilities, the use of the flexible fiberoptic bronchoscope is preferred. Using an endotracheal tube adapter, the flexible bronchoscope can be passed through the endotracheal tube while ventilation continues. Cytologic specimens are then collected without mechanical contact between the bronchoscope and the primary tumor.

It is concluded that malignant involvement of the lungs is unlikely in patients with a normal chest radiograph, normal bronchoscopy, and negative bronchial washings. Positive bronchial washings should be an indication for further evaluation. All positive cytologies should be reviewed with the cytopathologist and compared with the histology of the primary lesion. Polytomography or computerized axial tomography of the lungs may be indicated in these patients. Repeat bronchoscopy with bronchial washings is recommended in the cases of unexplained positive cytologies. If no explanation is found, or if it felt to be a false positive due to contamination from the head and neck primary, close follow-up with regular chest roentgenograms and physical examination is indicated to detect early pulmonary metastases or the development of a second primary tumor.

REFERENCES

1. Stefani S, Eells RW. Carcinoma of the hypopharynx: a study of distant metastases, treatment failures, and multiple primary cancers in 215 male patients. Laryngoscope 1971; 81:1491-8.

2. Abrahamson AL, Parisier SC, Zamansky M, et al. Distant metastases from carcinoma of the larynx. Laryngoscope 1971; 81:1503-7.

3. Gowen GF, duSuto-Nagy G. The incidence and sites of distant metastases in head and neck carcinoma. Surg Gynecol Obstet 1963; 116:603-7.

4. Marchetta FC, Sako K, Camp F. Multiple malignancies in patients with head and neck cancer. Am J Surg 1965; 110:537-41.

5. Horowitz R, Chemet B. Oral carcinoma and multiplicity of carcinomas. Oral Surg 1968; 26:87-91.

6. Cahan WG. Lung cancer associated with cancer primary in other sites. Am J Surg 1955; 89:494-514.

7. Goldmeier E. Limits of visibility of bronchogenic carcinoma. Am Rev Respir Dis 1965; 91:232.

8. Oswald NC, Hinson KFW, Canti G, Miller AB. The diagnosis of primary lung cancer with special reference to sputum cytology. Thorax 1971; 26:623-31.

9. Ikeda S, Yanai N, Ishikawa S. Flexible bronchofiberscope. Keio J Med 1968; 17:1-16.

10. Kovnat DM, Rath GS, Anderson WM, Snider GL. Maximal extent of visualization of bronchial tree by flexible fiberoptic bronchoscopy. Am Rev Respir Dis 1974; 110:88-90.

11. Chopva SK, Genovesi MG, Simmons DH, Gothe B. Fiberoptic bronchoscopy in the diagnosis of lung cancer. Comparison of pre- and post-bronchoscopy sputa, washings, brushings, and biopsies. Acta Cytologica 1977; 21:524-7.

12. Kvale PA, Bode FR, Kini S. Diagnostic accuracy in lung cancer. Chest 1976; 69:752-7.

13. Saltzstein SL, Harrell JH, Cameron T. Brushings, washings, or biopsy? Chest 1977; 71:630-2.

14. Chaudhary BA, Yoneda K, Burki NK. Fiberoptic bronchoscopy: comparison of procedures used in the diagnosis of lung cancer. J Thoracic Cardiovas Surg 1978; 76:33-7.

15. Dellon AL, Chu EW, Hall CA, Chretien PB. Cytology of bronchial washings. A study of patients with malignant neoplasms of the head and neck. Arch Otolaryngol 1975; 101:465-6.

BRONCHOSCOPIC CRYOTHERAPY

DAVID R. SANDERSON, MD
H. BRYAN NEEL III, MD, PhD ROBERT S. FONTANA, MD
ROCHESTER, MINNESOTA

Bronchoscopic cryotherapy of localized endobronchial tumors can be applied in selected patients who are not candidates for other traditional therapy. Twenty-eight patients were treated on 60 occasions with a closed liquid nitrogen system and a long insulated probe that was specifically designed to be used through an open ventilating bronchoscope. The condition of 15 patients (54%) was improved, as judged by local tumor control, decreased bleeding, or improved airway patency. Fatal complications that could be ascribed to cryotherapy occurred in 2 of the 60 treatments (3%). Two patients have experienced complete control of squamous cell cancers four years and five years nine months after cryotherapy.

Malignant tumors of the tracheobronchial tree constitute a major portion of all neoplasms encountered in clinical practice. Standard therapy consists of surgical resection of those localized lesions in which histologic features suggest that extirpation can be curative. When the disease is limited in extent but resection is not possible, radiation therapy is often used for palliation or occasionally for cure. When the disease has extended outside the thorax, systemic chemotherapy may be selected for palliation.

In some patients in whom disease is confined to the tracheobronchial tree but not amenable to traditional local therapeutic measures, systemic therapy is not recommended. In this selected group of patients, endoscopic cryotherapy can be a useful therapeutic alternative.

BACKGROUND

Experiments with tumors in mice treated by cryotherapy have shown that lower temperatures, repeated freezing and thawing, and larger probe tips produced a higher rate of tumor control[1] (Table 1). An extensive review of the history of cryotherapy for the treatment of cancer and of the experimental and theoretic bases for the application of cryosurgery has been published by one of us.[2] In summary, for consistent control of malignant tumors by cryosurgery, the following factors are important: probe-tip temperatures of −160°C or less, large contact surfaces between the probe tip and the tumor (or use of liquid nitrogen sprays), two or three (repetitive) probe applications, freezing to tumor temperatures of less than −30°C, and rates of freezing greater than 100°C per minute. Heat extraction can be potentiated considerably by inducing ischemia with pharmacologic doses of epinephrine around the tumor. The magnitude of the cold insult and hence the volume of histologic cryonecrosis are not precisely predictable by the size of the ice ball at the time of freezing but are affected by the rate and depth of freezing and the duration of thawing. The combined effects of rapid freezing and slow thawing — generally spontaneous thawing — are maximally lethal to the tumor.

Life-threatening neoplasms that arise primarily in the trachea or bronchi are surgically excised or treated by radiation therapy, or both, whenever possible. We believed that cryosurgery could be used for cure or palliation of certain tracheobronchial neoplasms and that new methods for the treatment of in situ and early invasive bronchogenic tumors, particularly multicentric tumors, would be possible. This impression led to a series of experiments in which the trachea and bronchus were frozen circumferentially by using standardized cryosurgical techniques. We found that this procedure could be done safely. Subsequently, Neel and Sanderson designed a long, insulated probe with interchangeable tips for peroral endoscopic cryosurgery in the trachea and bronchus (Fig. 1). The 55-cm probe, which is now commercially available, is vacuum-insulated except for the interchangeable tips. The interchangeable probe tips allow adaptation for anatomic variations so as to improve contact between the probe tip and the

TABLE 1. TUMOR CONTROL: RELATIONSHIP TO REPETITION OF FREEZING AND TO PROBE TIPS AND TEMPERATURES

Probe Temperature (°C)	*Mice Cured (%)* No. of Freezes 1	2	3	Area of Tip-to-Tumor Contact (Ratio) 1:1	1:4
−180	50	62	83	82	54
−60	7	26	42	44	16

Data from Neel et al.[1]

From the Mayo Clinic and Mayo Foundation, Rochester, Minnesota. This investigation was supported in part by Research Grant CB-53886 from the National Institutes of Health, Public Health Service.

Presented at the meeting of the American Broncho-Esophagological Association, Vancouver, British Columbia, May 11-12, 1981.

REPRINTS — D. R. Sanderson, MD, Mayo Clinic, Rochester, MN 55905.

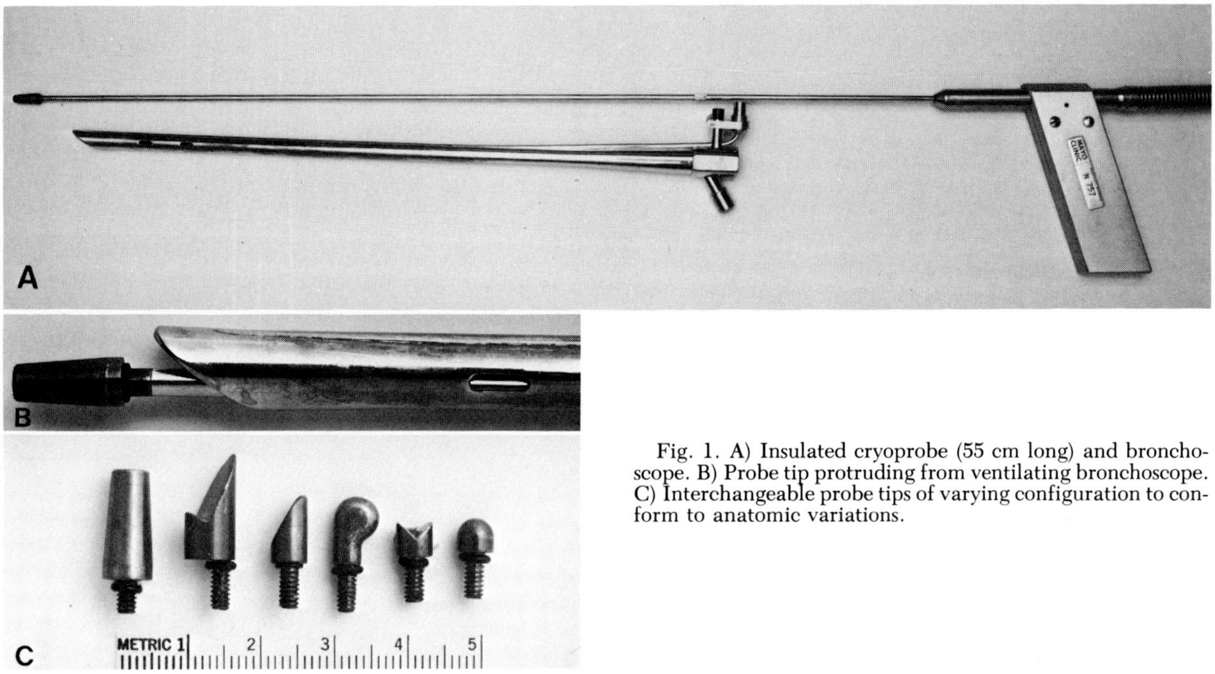

Fig. 1. A) Insulated cryoprobe (55 cm long) and bronchoscope. B) Probe tip protruding from ventilating bronchoscope. C) Interchangeable probe tips of varying configuration to conform to anatomic variations.

tumor. In monkeys and dogs, detailed experimental studies that preceded the clinical experience showed that extensive areas of trachea and bronchi may be safely destroyed by application of a cryoprobe to either the external (serosal) surface or the internal (mucosal) surface. The peroral technique with the long probe was used with the patients who constitute this report.

PATIENTS AND METHODS

Our study group consisted of 23 men and 5 women whose ages ranged from 47 to 77 years (mean age 63 years). Through May 1, 1981, these 28 patients had received cryotherapy on a total of 60 occasions (Table 2). The most frequent diagnosis for which cryotherapy was given was squamous cell bronchogenic carcinoma. Except in one patient with disabling chronic obstructive pulmonary disease and cor pulmonale, all conventional forms of surgical and radiation therapy had been attempted, but disease apparently limited to the thorax still persisted. One patient with a cylindroma and one with tracheopathia osteoplastica had cryotherapy as the primary treatment. One patient had recurrent bronchial carcinoid tumor after left lower lobectomy and numerous prior electrocautery treatments for hemoptysis of varying severity during a 14-year period. One other patient had prior radiation therapy for carcinoma of the esophagus, but an unusually situated mediastinal nodal metastasis invaded the trachea anteriorly and compromised the lumen of the airway.

Patients treated by cryotherapy were selected from those referred for consideration of alternative therapy for endobronchial lesions, after failure of other modalities, or with the clinical impression that none of the conventional modalities offered a high likelihood of success. In most patients, the potential for surgical resection had already been exhausted, and several had received maximal dose radiation therapy. Yet their tracheobronchial lesions were sufficiently limited that systemic chemotherapy was deemed inadvisable. Several patients had localized obstructing lesions that compromised ventilation to major portions of the bronchial tree.

TABLE 2. BRONCHOSCOPIC CRYOTHERAPY: 60 TREATMENTS IN 28 PATIENTS

No. of Patients	*Treatments* *No.*	*Total*
13	1	13
8	2	16
2	3	6
3	4	12
1	5	5
1	8	8
Total 28		60

Only three patients had no prior treatment. One patient had lung cancer and severe obstructive lung disease such that neither resection nor radiation therapy was thought possible. The patient with cylindroma was given cryotherapy as the primary treatment because the size and the extent of the lesion precluded resection and there was doubt about the radiosensitivity of her tumor. (Three years later, radiation therapy was given because of progression of the tumor, and she again experienced remission.) The patient with tracheopathia osteoplastica was reluctantly treated because of concern that some of the nodular projections of osteoid tissue were substantially reducing the lumen of the right main bronchus and there was no effective alternative therapy.

One patient insisted on general anesthesia for bronchoscopy; topical anesthesia was used in all of the other patients. Preparation included nothing by mouth, parenterally administered atropine sulfate and meperidine hydrochloride, and topical anesthesia (200 to 400 mg lidocaine hydrochloride as a 4% solution). An open ventilating bronchoscope (9 mm by 40 cm) was used for inspection, biopsy, and debridement (when necessary) and as the conduit for the 55-cm insulated cryoprobe. Oxygen was delivered continuously via a sidearm connection, and an anesthetist monitored the vital signs and the electrocardiogram.

Initially, the probe tip at room temperature was placed at the desired site in the bronchus, and then liquid nitrogen was circulated. Because this procedure proved exceedingly slow, in later patients we cooled the probe initially before application. Although the probe tip promptly froze to the tumor site, this did not substantially hinder correct positioning. Selection of probe tips was based on which configuration seemed most likely to give maximal tip-to-tumor contact. The long cylinder and the hockeystick ball tip proved most useful.

After the tip temperature was reduced to approximately −160° C, the probe was inserted and applied to the tumor. Transient

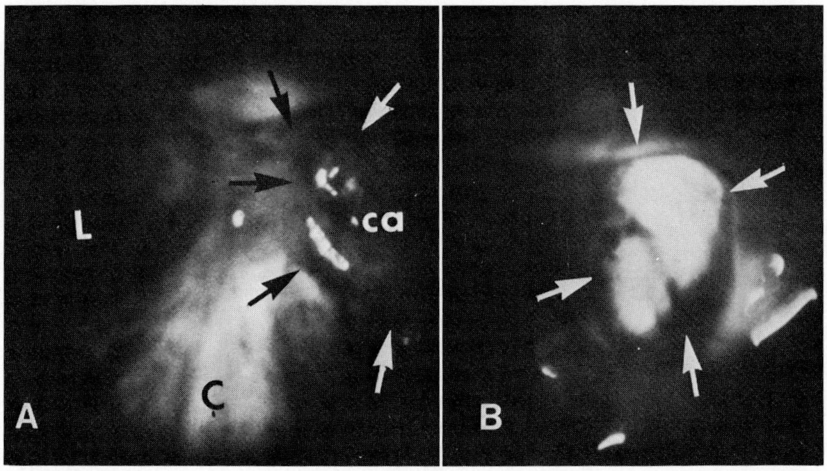

Fig. 2. Squamous cell carcinoma in 51-year-old male. A) Recurrent carcinoma (ca, extent outlined by arrows) in stump of right main bronchus 5 years after pneumonectomy and 1 year after radiation therapy to mediastinum. L - Left main bronchus; C - Carina. (Bright white "flecks" are artifacts.) B) Ice ball (outlined by arrows) in stump during cryotherapy.

warming occurred, but in 1 to 3 minutes, temperatures from −150 to −160° C were again achieved. This level of cooling was maintained for two minutes, and then circulation of nitrogen was discontinued and spontaneous thawing was allowed to occur.

When temperatures increased to between + 5 and + 10° C, the probe tip separated from the tumor spontaneously and the probe could be removed. The ice ball was observed until thawing was complete, and then any secretion or blood was aspirated to again leave a dry field.

The probe was recooled and reapplied for two minutes. Three freezing-thawing cycles were done unless one of the freezes failed to create an ice ball at the desired site, in which case the procedure was repeated.

After the third effective freeze, the bronchoscope was removed and the patient was transferred to the recovery room. After our first half-dozen patients, we used orally administered corticosteroids and antibiotics (prednisone, 10 mg four times daily, and tetracycline hydrochloride, 250 mg four times daily, for three days) routinely, on an empiric basis, in hopes of reducing bronchial edema, which might compromise ventilation in an already narrowed airway.

After cryotherapy, most patients remained hospitalized overnight for observation of any untoward complications and were dismissed the next day. Generally, bronchoscopic examination was repeated 4 to 8 weeks later in order to evaluate the results and often to repeat cryotherapy.

RESULTS

Objective assessment of results from cryotherapy was difficult. Because most patients had malignant tumors that extended beyond the range of the ice ball, control by freezing was not a realistic goal, and palliation was the most favorable outcome that we expected to achieve.

Repeated examinations at 4- to 8-week intervals allowed visual inspection and photographic documentation for comparison before and after response (Table 3). Usually, bronchial biopsy was repeated

TABLE 3. BRONCHOSCOPIC CRYOTHERAPY: RESULTS

Result	*Patients* No.		%
Favorable	15		54
Local tumor control		8	
Decreased bleeding		4	
Improved airway patency		3	
No benefit	13		46

to evaluate the histologic response. Reduction in tumor size or extent after therapy was regarded as local tumor control; this result was noted in eight patients. Of these eight patients, three seemed to have major, sustained local control. One patient with localized verrucous squamous cell cancer of the main carina received cryotherapy on five occasions and exhibited excellent regression of the tumor; however, foci of microscopic tumor cell nests persisted in the biopsy specimen after the fourth freezing treatment. The patient died suddenly of a myocardial infarction while mowing his lawn eight months after the first and five weeks after the fifth freezing procedure. Autopsy disclosed no gross lesion at the carina.[3] Unfortunately, serial sections of the bronchial tree were not done, and thus presence or absence of residual tumor was not determined.

A second patient had right pneumonectomy for squamous cell cancer in 1970. Four years later, recurrent cancer at the stump was confirmed by biopsy and treated with irradiation. One year later, streaking hemoptysis developed and biopsy again confirmed the presence of recurrence (Fig. 2). The stump of the right main bronchus was treated by cryotherapy on three occasions during the next 18 months. The patient was well and free of disease more than five years nine months after initial cryotherapy. Bronchial biopsy specimens from the stump show benign mucous membrane, and results of sputum cytology remain normal.

The third patient had right pneumonectomy for T2 N2 M0 stage III squamous cell cancer in 1973, followed by radiation therapy to the mediastinum. Four years later, he had streaking hemoptysis, bronchoscopy revealed an area (approximately 1 cm^2) of friable mucosa in the midtrachea along the posterolateral wall, and biopsy indicated squamous cell cancer. This area was noncontiguous with the stump and thought to be a second primary focus. Cryotherapy was applied four times during a 1-year period. The most recent biopsy specimen was be-

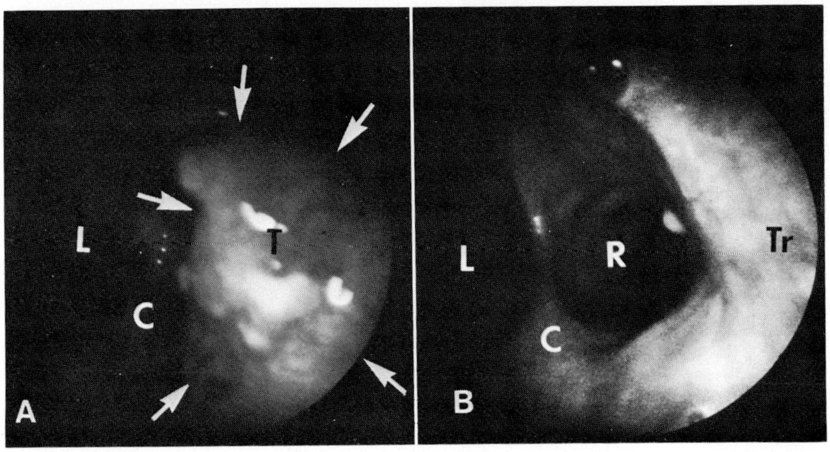

Fig. 3. Adenocystic carcinoma (cylindroma) in 65-year-old female. A) Tumor (T, extent outlined by arrows) filling 50% of lumen of distal trachea. L - Left main bronchus; C - Carina. B) Appearance 3 months after cryotherapy, showing remarkable tumor regression and improved airway patency. L - Left main bronchus; C - Carina; R - Right main bronchus; Tr - Right wall of distal trachea.

nign, and findings on sputum cytology remain normal four years after the first treatment.

The remaining five patients with local tumor control had early regression, only to be followed by more extensive spread of their lesions. Among these patients was the one with cylindroma, who experienced excellent initial shrinkage of tumor (Fig. 3) and relief of symptoms that was sustained for 2½ years. She then had a recurrence and received radiation therapy. Her condition improved, and she is alive with evidence of recurrence five years nine months after initial cryotherapy.

Four patients had major hemoptysis as a prominent symptom before cryotherapy; this symptom decreased in severity after the freezing procedure even though complete local control was not achieved.

In three other patients, wheezing and stridor were severe because of bulky tumors that filled much of the major airway. They experienced dramatic relief of airway obstruction after forceps debridement and cryotherapy of the tumor base. Nevertheless, subsequent progression caused further symptoms and death four weeks to 23 months after initial cryotherapy.

Thus, we found that 15 of the 28 patients (54%) apparently benefitted from cryotherapy. Two patients have had a long-term excellent response and may be cured. A third patient died suddenly of myocardial infarction, and no grossly visible tumor persisted at autopsy examination.

COMPLICATIONS

During cryotherapy, all patients were monitored by electrocardiogram and blood pressure recording. No patient experienced any change in rhythm or any signs of myocardial ischemia during the procedure.

One patient had experienced brisk hemoptysis preoperatively from a large friable polypoid tumor in the left main bronchus. Cryotherapy caused initial shrinkage of tumor tissue and no severe acute bleeding during or immediately after thawing. Five days after cryotherapy, he had another massive hemoptysis and died. Although autopsy was not done, the eschar created by freezing may have sloughed, exposed a major bronchial vessel, and permitted the bleeding. Alternatively, the hemorrhage might have occurred spontaneously in the course of his advanced disease.

The other major complication was in a patient with previous right pneumonectomy and radiation therapy who had recurrent squamous cell cancer at the stump that extended across the carina and into the proximal left main bronchus. Cryotherapy to the carina was given in hope of delaying occlusion of the left bronchus, which seemed imminent. The day after treatment, increased wheezing was noted over the left lung. Despite use of corticosteroids and antibiotics, wheezing and respiratory insufficiency increased during the four days after cryotherapy. Death occurred from respiratory insufficiency, presumably due to edema in the airway (autopsy examination was not done).

DISCUSSION

Cryotherapy in the bronchial tree is capable of inducing coagulation necrosis of tissue and destruction of tumors, but appropriate selection of patients is exceedingly important.

The optimal lesion would be small in surface area, superficial in penetration into the bronchial wall, and situated in the trachea, main bronchi, or accessible lower lobe bronchus. Limitation of probe tip size to the internal diameter of the ventilating bronchoscope restricts the extent of ice ball creation, even with repeated applications. Experimental studies with this closed-probe system have determined the depth of penetration of freezing to be several millimeters; thus, deeply invasive tumors or peribronchial malignant tissue are not likely to be affected.[4] Moreover, the requirement of straight-ahead access via the rigid bronchoscope precludes access to many regions of the bronchial tree, especially the upper lobe branches, with the currently available equipment.

When confronted with a bulky tumor that is crowding the airway, the endoscopist has the alternatives of initial debridement and subsequent freezing of the tumor base or initial application of the cryoprobe to create thrombosis in the tumor vascular supply and subsequent debridement. In some of our patients with a tenuous airway for ventilation, the former sequence was necessary simply to allow for patient comfort and ventilation during the subsequent freezing procedure. Nonetheless, this can produce sufficient endobronchial bleeding to obscure details of the lesion and to hamper later placement of the probe tip. If circumstances permit, it seems preferable to create an ice ball first and then to remove obstructing tumor tissue mechanically with a cup or basket forceps. Bleeding still will occur after thawing, but this generally has not been a major problem. In either situation, direct application of an adrenalin solution (1:20,000) with a long cotton swab is useful for constricting vessels and decreasing bleeding. Throughout this phase of the procedure, suctioning via a velvet eye-tipped aspirator and use of rigid-lens Hopkins telescopes are necessary to achieve optimal visualization and appropriate tip-to-tumor placement. Once the ice ball is formed by the probe-tip contact, bleeding ceases; however, an adequate lumen must remain around the tip and ice ball for ventilation.

After cryotherapy, a necrotic eschar forms in the bronchial tree, which will slough and be expectorated after 2 to 4 weeks. During this early phase, patients may have streaking hemoptysis and an increase in irritative cough. With one exception — the patient who had fatal hemorrhage — bleeding has been minimal in our patients. After expectoration of the eschar, many patients have experienced diminution of the symptom of coughing.

Bronchoscopic cryotherapy does not have wide application. Indeed, most patients with localized endobronchial tumors can more predictably be treated by surgical resection or radiation therapy. There is little point in seeking endobronchial palliation for patients with widespread systemic metastases. Nevertheless, in carefully selected patients with isolated endobronchial tumors in whom the other local therapeutic modalities have been exhausted or in whom further surgical or radiation therapy is not feasible, bronchoscopic cryotherapy does serve as a good alternative for palliation and even long-term tumor control.

REFERENCES

1. Neel HB III, Ketcham AS, Hammond WG. Requisites for successful cryogenic surgery of cancer. Arch Surg 1971; 102:45-8.

2. Neel HB III. Cryosurgery for the treatment of cancer. Laryngoscope 1980; 90 Suppl 23:1-48.

3. Sanderson DR, Neel HB III, Payne WS, Woolner LB. Cryotherapy for bronchogenic carcinoma: report of a case. Mayo Clin Proc 1975; 50:435-7.

4. Carpenter RJ III, Neel HB III, Sanderson DR. Cryosurgery of bronchopulmonary structures: an approach to lesions inaccessible to the rigid bronchoscope. Chest 1977; 72:279-84.

Ann Otol 90:1981

ESOPHAGEAL CANCER RESEARCH IN THE PEOPLE'S REPUBLIC OF CHINA

WU HUAN-HSING, MD, DMR

PEKING, CHINA

Esophageal cancer, which accounts for 21% of all cancer deaths in China, has been the subject of epidemiology studies in the three areas of the country where the disease is most prevalent. In the area of the highest mortality rate, the first field research unit was established to study cancer in high-risk areas. The investigations of this unit for the last 20 years are discussed, including the design and implementation of the studies. The geographic, dietary and cultural factors in the etiology of esophageal cancer are examined. The results of the studies and the clinical applications are explored.

I take great pleasure in conveying to you the greetings of the Chinese Society of Oncology, and wish to express our hopes of increasing contacts and of mutual exchange of visits, to consolidate the friendly ties existing between colleagues of our two countries.

Today I will present some sidelights on the background and significance of cancer work in high-risk areas in China, especially with reference to cancer of the esophagus.

In a large country like China with 9.6 million square kilometers, often one variety of cancer can have high-risk areas thousands of kilometers apart, with completely different climatic and geological conditions. The populations in these areas are all of one ethnic group and are fairly stable, in that for generations, people are born, live, marry, work and die within that same geographic area. As we all know, a stable population provides favorable conditions for long-term epidemiologic studies on the various aspects of a disease.

The present talk is an account of the work carried out in one such county, called Linxian. It is a rural county with a fairly large population (750,000) distributed over an area of 2,000 square kilometers. Statistical figures of prevalence and yearly mortality rates due to cancer of the esophagus for Linxian county and for the whole province show that they top the list compared to the figures for all other provinces and counties of China. (Incidentally, esophageal cancer accounts for over 21% of all cancer deaths in China.)

The field research unit in Linxian was the first one established and has served as a pilot for studies on all other varieties of cancer in their respective high-risk areas. Also, trends in morbidity and mortality rates can be evaluated for Linxian because the county has kept a cancer registry since 1959.

Before commenting on the work done in Linxian county, allow me first to say a few words on the conceptual approach which we have adopted in building our network for cancer investigations, especially the lessons we learned on how to set up a field research team.

Back in the late 1950s, when malignant diseases started to become an important if not one of the major health problems for our government authorities and for the medical profession, new cancer hospitals and cancer research institutes began to be organized in the various large cities of China. The classical concept of organization in such hospitals or institutes is based on the establishment of two main sections, namely the clinical section and the laboratory or experimental section. As it happened in the experience of other countries where cancer work has a much longer history, we very soon also found out the undesirable sharp division in this approach — the gap between the staff of the clinical section and the staff of the experimental laboratory section.

In such a situation, when two parties work separately, isolated from each other, we say in Chinese that there is "no air communication." This means that each section's staff is enclosed in its own airtight space, with no exchange of viewpoints. Such an airtight system of work could create many a misunderstanding between the clinician and the laboratory worker. Once after a scientific discussion, somebody jokingly made the remark that it has been a session of PhDs versus MDs, because the viewpoints were different, each side believing itself to be the wiser. On the one side, the clinician often feels frustrated at being unable to probe deeper into the understanding of the various aspects of the disease such as the mechanism of action of factors involved in carcinogenesis, the evolution of the disease, the search for more reliable or simpler methods of early diagnosis, for means of prevention, etc.

From the Department of Radiation Oncology, Cancer Research Institute, Chinese Academy of Medical Sciences, Peking.

Presented at the meeting of the American Broncho-Esophagological Association, Vancouver, British Columbia, May 11-12, 1981.

REPRINTS — Wu Huan-Hsing, MD, Director, Cancer Research Institute, Chinese Academy of Medical Sciences, Peking, China.

On the other side, the laboratory worker in the midst of his tissue cultures and laboratory animals often gets lost or is led astray in evaluating his experimental results, because there is always that delicate problem of extrapolation of results from the cell in vitro to the experimental animal in vivo and from the animal to the human species itself. Such a situation happened in the work of our own clinical and laboratory sections, for example in their search for the causal factors in esophageal cancer with reference to the role of nitrosamines.

Some years ago, reading an interesting monograph, *Problems of Experimental Oncology* by Graffi and Beilka of Berlin, I was struck by the first lines of the dedication: "To the memory of the millions of experimental animals whose lives were sacrificed to help the cancer patient." Due credit must be given also to the contributions of experimental oncologists, along with the millions of animals, in furthering our understanding of the process of malignant changes in cells or tissues under the influence of carcinogenic or cocarcinogenic agents. At the same time we also have come to realize that however useful are all the species of animals used in experimental oncology, from mice and rats to hamsters, marmosets or monkeys, we always have some reservations in extrapolating the results from animals to man. Pure strain animals living under well-defined environmental conditions and given standard diets are somehow different when compared to even a well-defined ethnic group, living in the same area and with the same occupations in life.

So, a solution had to be found where more direct observations on humans could be carried out. This is where in the last two to three decades, with the advent of the new discipline of cancer epidemiology, the work of both clinical and experimental oncologists was given a new orientation. First, the discovery by the cancer epidemiologists of high-risk areas for some varieties of cancer has provided an opportunity for study. Such high-risk areas look like a vast laboratory provided by nature where clinicians and experimentalists can work together, bringing together these two disciplines and so allowing the "air to communicate" in planning their research projects. This was the beginning of the concept of establishing field research units in high-risk areas. From the descriptive and analytical data provided by the epidemiologists, our clinicians and experimental workers can now plan their research projects with clues related to etiology pathogenesis, diagnosis, treatment and prevention of disease.

After having described the guiding principles underlying our work, allow me now to comment briefly on some of the data acquired from the Linxian field unit.

Numerous statistics for high- and low-risk areas, such as comparative incidence and mortality rates; chemical analysis of samples of soil, water, foodstuffs and cereals; and biochemical investigations in patients and controls, are already reported in many publications. I will try to sum up these figures and give the gist of the investigations with a few comments. These remarks will be in three areas of investigation: 1) geographical features of the high-risk area; 2) etiological factors in relation to external surrounding factors, mode of life and dietary habits; 3) clinical applications of results obtained in the field research unit.

FACTORS RELATED TO CLIMATIC AND GEOLOGICAL FEATURES

Three high-risk areas to be discussed are 1) Linxian county (Henan Province, North China, population 750,000), where during a period of 30 years the mortality rate for esophageal cancer varied from 100 to 150/100,000; 2) Yang Zhong (at the estuary of the large river Yangtze, Central China, population 200,000) with a mortality rate of 99/100,000, a figure close to that of Linxian; and 3) Nan'ao (an island off the coast of Guangdong Province, South China; area about 100 square kilometers; population 50,000, mostly engaged in fishing) with a mortality rate of 87/100,000.

In these three high-risk areas are found the same ethnic population groups but living in completely different climatic and geological conditions and with different modes of life. Linxian is a mountainous area with poor dry arid soil, Yang Zhong a river island on the Yangtze River with damp alluvial soil, and Nan'ao is a small hilly island off the sea coast of Guangdong Province where the population lives mostly on sea products.

When the first epidemiological survey for cancer of the esophagus was started in 1959 in Linxian and surrounding counties, a strong impression given was that a close relationship existed between the high incidence of the disease and the conditions of life in proximity to mountainous areas and areas with arid soil.

By mapping out the mortality rates for Linxian and the surrounding 180 counties, covering a population area of 50 million, the impression was given of "high mortality areas," selectively lying close to the Taihang mountain range, gradually fading off the farther one moves away from the mountains. Such was the initial impression of geological nature and climatic conditions as clues in our search for etiological factors of the disease. A traditional saying in Linxian is three simple Chinese words, "*san pu tung*," literally translated as "three no passages." The first "no passage" means no roads in such mountainous areas, and the second means no irrigation canals or rivers in such a dry area. The third "no passage" describes the tragic fate of so many patients in the late stages of the disease when food or drink cannot pass anymore.

Now the peasants are saying that the first two "no passages" have been solved with the construction of the famous Red Flag Canal, diverting the water of a large river in a neighboring province into Linxian, and the construction of many irrigation canals and roads. The third "no passage" still awaits solution by the medical workers.

ETIOLOGICAL FACTORS IN EXTERNAL ENVIRONMENT, MODE OF LIFE AND DIETARY HABITS

From the above description, it is obvious that we shall have to look further for clues to lead us to the real factors. During the initial stages of investigation, attention was centered on the possible relationship of types of soil on which the crops were grown and of the sources of drinking water from the local wells. Therefore, the chemical composition of samples of soil, crops, foodstuffs, and water from the high- and low-risk areas were analyzed and compared.

The data obtained showed that in high-risk areas the content of one particular trace element, molybdenum, was significantly lower than in samples from the low-incidence areas. Molybdenum has received more attention than other trace elements because it is an important constituent of certain enzymes such as the nitrate reductase. It is known that foodstuffs from Linxian and other areas of high risk contained very low amounts of molybdenum. The molybdenum deficiency in the soil leads to accumulation of nitrates in the cereals and other foodstuffs grown on that soil. In Linxian county itself, by encouraging and advising the farmers to use ammonium molybdate as fertilizer, the nitrite and nitrate levels in vegetables were markedly decreased by 20% on the average, and the vitamin C level increased by 24% on the average.

This is the first clue leading to the formulation of a hypothesis that the excessive amount of nitrites and nitrates in foodstuffs, cereals and water could react in the stomach with secondary amines and form N-nitroso compounds of which some are known as potent carcinogenic agents, and some believed to be organ-specific.

At the same time, our workers in the field unit, by living in the midst of the population investigated, turned their attention to all other factors related to dietary habits, the nature of the food, its nutritional value and even the way the peasants cook and consume food, in other words, their living habits.

Most of the malignancies are now believed to have not only a multifactorial basis for their etiology, but also it is probable that a specific organ malignancy of the same histomorphology may have different spectrum of carcinogenic factors.

One factor that might play a role in initiating or promoting the carcinogenic process in Linxian's cases is the poor oral hygiene of the average peasant, even causing the loss of teeth at an early age. The poorly masticated coarse food, often contaminated by various species of fungi, may be a cause of minute trauma to the delicate esophageal mucosa. Surgical specimens of resected esophageal cancer very often show intracellular inclusions of fungi. According to some authors, the chronic infection of the esophageal mucosa predisposes to the fungal invasion. The fungus itself is experimentally proved to enhance the formation of nitrosamines by reducing nitrates to nitrites, decomposing proteins and increasing the amount of amines.

In one such experiment carried out by our workers, it was noticed that the bad storage of food in the peasant's homes frequently caused contamination of cornbread by fungi of the species belonging to *Fusarium*, *Geotrichum*, *Aspergillus*, etc. The steamed cornbread is prepared by peasants usually once a week or in some families every two or three weeks to save time. Days later, the cornbread would have become moldy inside, and this stale contaminated food was eaten by the peasants. When a small amount of sodium nitrite is added to moldy cornbread and incubated for a week, analysis by gas chromatography and mass spectrometry shows the presence of N-nitroso compounds such as dimethylnitrosamine, diethylnitrosamine, methylbenzylnitrosamine and a recently identified volatile nitrosamine, N-1 methylacetyl-N-3 methylbutyl nitrosamine (MAMBNA). This last compound was found to be mutagenic, according to the Ames test.

Animal experimentation with rats and mice can be summed up as follows. *Fusarium*-contaminated cornbread produces carcinogenic mycotoxins and when $NaNO_2$ is added into the moldy cornbread more papillomas and more carcinomas are produced in experimental animals fed on the cornbread.

Another dietary habit of the area is the heavy consumption of a special variety of pickled vegetables taken together with the cornbread or hot gruel. Sometimes when the peasants are thirsty they take a drink made from the supernatant fluid in the jar containing the pickled vegetables. The taste is very sour and sometimes salty. From the epidemiological data, the mortality rate of esophageal cancer appears to have a close relation to the amount and the duration of consumption of these pickled vegetables.

Two components of the pickled vegetables were analyzed chemically. One is the extract from the vegetables and the other is the fluid from a culture of a fungus most commonly contaminating the pickled vegetables, *Geotrichum candidum, Link.* When mice were fed by gastric intubation with extract fluid from pickled vegetables, papillomas in the forestomach were induced. The chemical substance contained in the pickled vegetables which produces mutagenic effects is probably the Roussin red methyl ester, which curiously enough has not yet been reported as existing in natural products. It was first synthesized by Roussin in 1858. This compound may react with secondary amines to form nitrosamines. It is suggested that the combined action of such chemical carcinogens, eg, nitrosamines formed in vivo from their precursors in food and water and the mycotoxins contaminating the food, and poor nutrition are the chief causative factors of cancer of the esophagus in Linxian county. Dietary deficiencies of vitamins A and C and riboflavin and the poor oral hygiene of the peasants in the high-risk areas are contributing factors.

According to the modern concept of the two-stage carcinogenic process, it would be a great advance in formulating preventive measures if we could classify all the factors studied into one of the two stages, ie, initiating or promoting.

Very often, practical measures of eliminating the promoting factors could well avoid the ultimate malignant degeneration of the esophageal mucosa which had already been acted on by an initiating agent. Also, it would be useful to follow up some of the cases of hyperplasia classified as grade 1 by our cytologists which, due to the action of repair enzymes in the cells, gradually return to mild hyperplasia and ultimately to a normal condition.

One interesting aspect of the epidemiological work in Linxian has been the discovery of the marked prevalence of cancer of the pharyngoesophagus in domestic fowl in the high-risk areas, and then also in a low-risk area where domestic fowl were raised by families who had migrated from the high- to low-risk areas. The domestic fowl of the migrants are fed with the leftovers from household food.

It is worth recalling the beginning of this aspect of the research, which may help to elucidate the etiological factors in human cases. The idea came to M.H. Li in 1970 that animals living in close proximity with human beings under similar environmental factors should be investigated to see if they showed similar lesions of the upper digestive tract. School children of the commune were paid to catch rats for the study. Household rats were first caught and dissected, and the esophageal epithelium of some of them showed hyperplasia or metaplasia. It was presumed that the older the rats the greater the possibilities of finding such lesions, but rats are mostly short-lived owing to infections and parasitic diseases. However, in Linxian, chickens, which run free in the courtyards and are fed remnants of household food, are raised for years, as long as they lay eggs, so it was a fortunate idea to turn from rats to chickens in the search for tumors of the upper digestive tract.

The chickens which were moved from the high-risk areas to low-risk areas but were raised by high-risk area migrant families have provided the clues on the importance of diet in carcinogenesis of esophageal cancer. In the same low-risk area, the hens raised and fed by the local indigenous families showed no sign of the disease.

Various steps have been described which lead to the identification of carcinogenic factors in the environment, in the dietary habits, and in foods contaminated with various fungi and with high contents of nitrates and nitrites, all of which interact in the stomach to form carcinogenic N-nitroso compounds.

I mentioned that the carcinogenesis of one variety of cancer of a specific organ may involve different spectrums or combinations of factors. In relation to esophageal cancer, this assumption can be applied for example to the cases diagnosed at Ille-et-Vilaine in France, where the amount of ethanol consumed in the apple cider is quantitatively related to the prevalence of the disease. However, it has been suggested that the origin of the apples used in making the cider is also suspected of being a factor. It is said that homemade apple cider is more directly related to the carcinogenicity of the drinks, and it is presumed that this is because it is usually made from discarded apples, many of which are more or less rotted. If this is true, then we could advance the same hypothesis for the role of the moldy cornbread or the pickled vegetables of Linxian county. This assumption is backed by our investigators who examined dietary habits in the high risk areas of China. In the three areas studied, nearly all the population consumes some variety of fermented foodstuffs. The fishermen in Nan'ao Island consume fermented fish paste and fish sauce, and in other areas salted vegetables are a major part of the diet. Further detailed investigations are needed to follow up on the clues first provided by the investigators of the Linxian county field unit.

CLINICAL APPLICATIONS OF RESULTS OBTAINED IN THE FIELD RESEARCH UNIT

Three of the many spin-offs from this investigation are the following:

First, the cytosmear examination is an efficient and reliable means of cytologic diagnosis of cancer of the esophagus at a very early stage. Chinese cytologists have now raised the diagnostic accuracy to a very high level, as checked by barium x-ray examination, endoscopic examination and biopsy. The discovery of lesions predisposing to malignant evolution has provided opportunities for experimenting with drugs, eg, retinoid compounds and Chinese herbals, which might restore to normalcy the esophageal epithelium.

Second, there is the understanding of the natural evolution of the disease in time and in space, ie, the various stages from hyperplasia, metaplasia to can-

TABLE 1. TMN CLASSIFICATION OF GROUP 1 PATIENTS (N = 1,644)

Stage	*No. Patients*	%
I	8	0.5
II	304	18.5
III	1,188	72.3
IV	144	8.8

cer in situ and invasive cancer, and the progress of these stages in months and years. Also there is new understanding of the distribution of the lesions, ie, multifocal lesions separated by a stretch of normal mucosa, with early pathological changes of the mucosa (hyperplasia, metaplasia or cancer in situ) at the edge of the actual carcinomatous lesion. The above findings are in accordance with the now generally acknowledged concept of malignant growth in an organ through the process called "surface cancerization."

Third, the mass screening carried out among the population in high-risk areas not only has provided data on the relation of age to incidence and other factors, but also has resulted in the fortunate discovery of many cases at such an early stage (mostly asymptomatic or with very mild symptoms) that the 5-year survival rate of operated cases can reach 85%.

Until the time when effective prophylactic measures result in prevention or marked diminution in the incidence of esophageal cancer, the present approach to reduce the mortality rate of this disease is detection, diagnosis and resection of the lesion at its earliest stages. We have very convincing statistics in relation to postoperative survival rates in two distinct groups of patients treated by our surgical staff under the direction of K. C. Huang. One group are 1,644 patients who were seen in our Peking hospital between 1959 and 1979, with a diagnosis of esophageal cancer, judged operable, and then admitted for treatment (Table 1). The other group were 237 patients who in the course of mass screening (1964-1979) in the high-risk area of Linxian were diagnosed as having esophageal cancer in its very early stages (stage I, $T_1N_0M_0$) and then were treated surgically. The 5-year survival rate for the first group of patients is 30.3% (296/976) while for the second group (early cases) it is 85.9% (110/128).

I hope the account I have given of the significance of working in a high-risk area to search for clues in human carcinogenesis helps us better understand the complexity of the problem. Yet in the complexity of so many pathways leading to the last stage, namely the condition of malignant change, there is maybe that one ultimate path to which all other pathways have to converge. May we hope to find that one last unique path leading to malignancy. The present policy of prophylaxis is to try to block each of the known initial pathways. Efforts could be rewarding if we could also find means of blocking the last path leading to malignancy. Then prevention of cancer in the midst of our modern environment and in our modern habits of lifestyle could be a reality.

≈

Ann Otol 90:1981

CONGENITAL TRACHEAL STENOSIS

BRUCE BENJAMIN, FRACS
JOHN PITKIN, FRACS, FRCS DOUGLAS COHEN, MS, FRACS
SYDNEY, AUSTRALIA

Twenty-one cases of congenital tracheal stenosis seen at the Royal Alexandra Hospital for Children 1971 through 1980 were reviewed with regard to the clinical features, associated anomalies, endoscopic findings and radiological evaluation. Congenital tracheal stenosis was usually a serious problem often associated with other major anomalies of the respiratory tract, esophagus, or skeleton. There was no set pattern of presentation. The presenting features included: persistent wheeze or stridor, atypical "respiratory distress," and atypical "croup" or "bronchiolitis." Documentation of the nature and extent of the stenosis by endoscopy and, if necessary, tracheobronchogram was important for prognosis and to direct treatment. Congenital tracheal stenosis must be considered in infants who present with atypical respiratory tract obstruction, especially where there is an H-type tracheoesophageal fistula, pulmonary hypoplasia or skeletal abnormalities such as hemivertebrae or a thumb abnormality.

INTRODUCTION

Upper airways obstruction due to congenital anomalies has been known for many years. The first reports of congenital tracheal stenosis were of autopsy findings. Later larger series were reviewed, notably that of Holinger et al[1] demonstrating not only the relative incidence of congenital tracheal stenosis but also the clinical features, necessary investigations and available treatment.

In recent years there have been significant advances in evaluation of the pediatric respiratory tract, notably safer, more versatile techniques of anesthesia; closer cooperation between the endoscopist and the pediatrician; miniaturization of endoscopes and high quality fiberoptic systems; improved radiological modalities including arteriography and computerized scanning; use of the Hopkins rigid telescopes and ancillary equipment for routine endoscopic photography.

It is now possible to carefully evaluate, photographically document, and record examples of uncommon or unusual conditions for comparative study.[2]

Congenital stenosis of the trachea has been believed to be very rare. In 1941 Wolman[3] wrote, "The lesion receives meagre comment or no mention at all in well known text books of otolaryngology and pediatrics and the number of cases on record is small." This statement remains true today.

This paper is based on our experience with 21 cases seen over a 10-year period, 1971 through 1980, at the Royal Alexandra Hospital for Children, Sydney, a major pediatric hospital of 350 beds with approximately 7,000 surgical admissions per year.

MATERIALS AND METHODS

All cases of congenital tracheal stenosis recognized clinically or at postmortem between 1971 and 1980 were reviewed from the hospital records, the endoscopic findings, and radiological studies. We have carefully and deliberately excluded cases of acquired tracheal stenosis; congenital subglottic stenosis; bronchial stenosis; tracheomalacia, whether primary or secondary (eg, due to a vascular ring); tracheal compression from external causes and membranous or localized tracheal webs.

All patients except the neonate who died at 21 hours had endoscopic examination, usually with photography. Seventeen of 21 patients also had contrast tracheobronchography. The endoscopic examinations were under carefully controlled conditions of general anesthesia using the Storz equipment with Hopkins telescopes and the Storz endocamera for photographic documentation (Fig. 1). In those cases where contrast tracheobronchography was performed it was always preceded by endoscopy with extreme care and every precaution to ensure against the potential complications. A minimal amount of contrast material was selectively placed in the tracheobronchial tree with radiological control using the image intensifier.

All patients in this study were proven beyond doubt to have congenital tracheal stenosis as judged by one or more of the following criteria: endoscopic evaluation; tracheobronchogram (Fig. 2); exposure of the trachea at thoracotomy in an attempt to surgically correct the deformity, or by postmortem examination. Congenital tracheal stenosis was defined as an intrinsic narrowing of the tracheal lumen, the walls of which are rigid and nondistensible. The malformation may affect part or all of the trachea and often extends into the main bronchi. The tracheal cartilages are smaller than normal, firm and nonpliable and lack the normal structure of the posterior membranous trachea[4] (Fig. 3).

RESULTS

During the 10-year period, 1971 to 1980, there were 21 cases of congenital tracheal stenosis.

Age. The age of presentation was from birth to six years. Four patients presented at birth, another 7 patients by 2 months of age and a further 8 by 12 months of age. Of the remaining two patients, one

From the Royal Alexandra Hospital for Children, Sydney, Australia. This study was assisted by a grant provided by the Royal Alexandra Hospital for Children and the Children's Medical Research Foundation, Sydney.

Presented at the meeting of the American Broncho-Esophagological Association, Vancouver, British Columbia, May 11-12, 1981.

REPRINTS — Bruce Benjamin, FRACS, 231 Macquarie Street, Sydney, N.S.W., 2000 Australia.

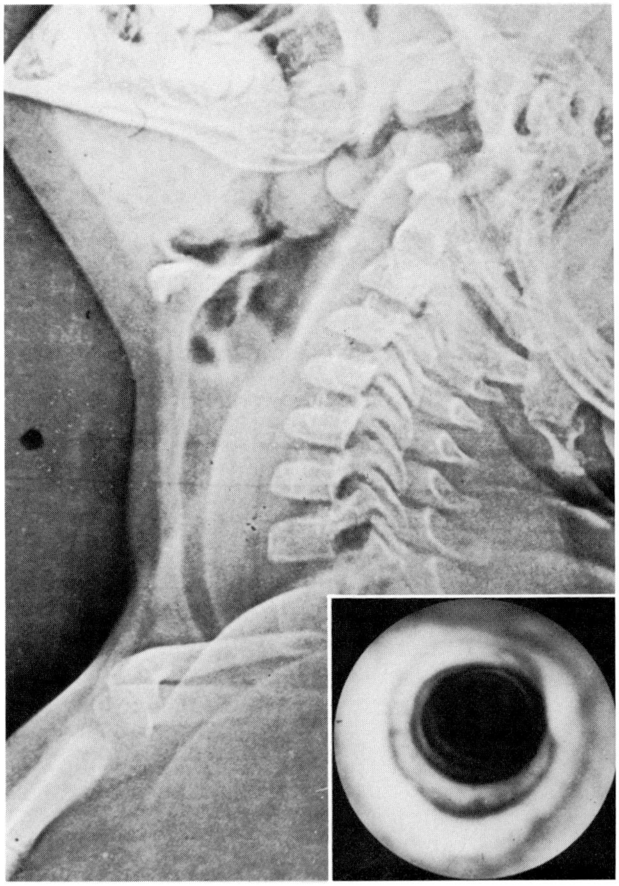

Fig. 1. (Case 6) Xeroradiogram with appearance of "stove-pipe" trachea. Insert) Circular, complete tracheal cartilages seen in the endoscopic view.

presented at $3^{1}/_{2}$ years and the other at six years of age.

Sex. Eleven of the patients were females and ten were males.

Presentation. The mode of presentation is summarized in Table 1 according to the major presenting clinical feature although there were often multiple features. In no case was the correct diagnosis made immediately.

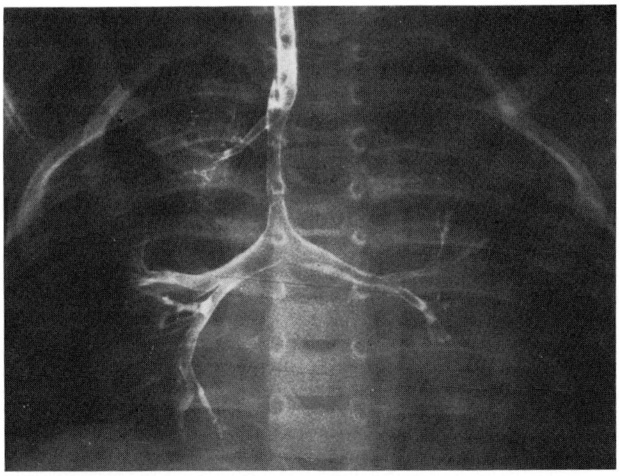

Fig. 2. (Case 17) Tracheal bronchus and lower tracheal stenosis. Note the equal lengths of the right and left main bronchus.

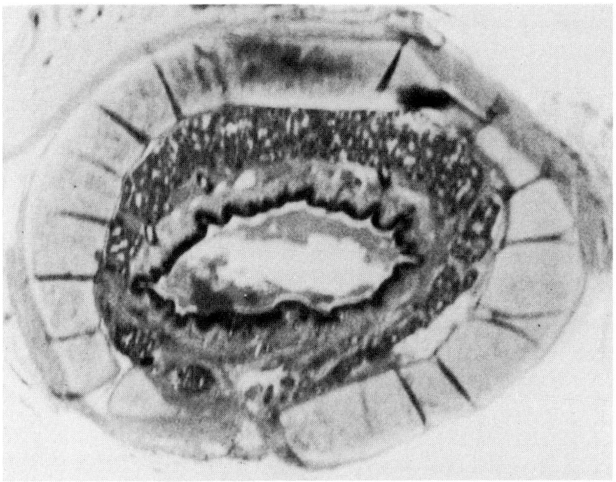

Fig. 3. (Case 15) Cross section of surgically resected segmental stenosis. The tracheal cartilage is virtually complete.

There was often an undue delay in diagnosis because the clinician did not consider the possibility of congenital tracheal stenosis. The period of delay before endoscopic proof varied from two days to nearly five years. The patient diagnosed at six years of age had had symptoms since infancy.

Besides the major presenting clinical features listed in Table 1 other prominent features were bronchiolitis (always atypical and persistent); bronchitis; cough; "near miss" sudden infant death syndrome; respiratory distress, and barking cough.

Four of the patients had repeated croup, often associated with cyanotic attacks. The croup was atypical in that it recurred often, persisted longer than the usual two or three days, failed to respond to the usual treatment, and obviously had some underlying anatomical cause.

Some patients presented with another anomaly often in some other organ system, eg, tracheoesophageal fistula or congenital heart disease.

It is noteworthy that in six patients intubation and ventilation for respiratory failure was required.

TABLE 1. MODE OF PRESENTATION

Clinical Features	*No. Patients*
Total respiratory obstruction at birth	1
Respiratory distress syndrome	3
Respiratory distress	5
Stridor since birth	4
Stridor developing later	2
Wheeze since birth	2
Wheeze developing later	1
Cyanotic attacks	1
Failure to thrive	1
Elective tracheotomy	1

TABLE 2. DETAILS OF EACH CASE (N = 21)

Case	Presenting Age	Sex	Clinical Features	Associated Anomalies	Progress	Tracheo-Bronchial Anatomy
1	2 mo	M	Wheezy since birth, moist cough. Chest x-ray—right upper lobe (CXR-RUL) consolidation.	H-type tracheoesophageal fistula (TEF). Congenital esophageal stenosis. Dextrocardia. Patent ductus anteriosus (PDA).	Initially treated for pneumonia and cardiac failure. Esophageal stenosis dilated, developed repiratory distress. Gastrostomy, H - fistula ligated, discharged well.	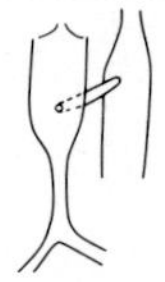
2	2 mo	M	Stridor since birth, failure to thrive, systolic murmur.	Ventricular septal defect (VSD).	Medical treatment for VSD. Thriving, has stridor but no respiratory distress, alive and well.	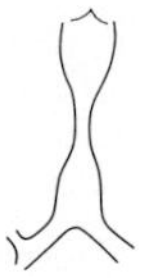
3	3 wk	F	Moist cough, tachypnea. Crepitations. CXR-RUL consolidation.	Vulvalectopic anus. Hypoplastic left thumb. Bilateral proximal radioulnar synostosis. Esophageal reflux.	Pneumonia treated, no further respiratory problems, alive and well.	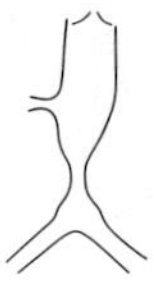
4	2 mo	M	Stridor since birth, developed upper respiratory tract infection (URTI) and cough.	None.	Symptomatic treatment for URTIs, repeated hospital admission for physiotherapy in early childhood. Alive and well; improvement in respiratory symptoms.	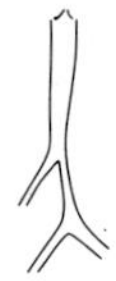
5	Birth	F	Severe respiratory distress, cyanosis, scaphoid abdomen. CXR - right diaphragmatic hernia.	A-V communis. Coarctation of aorta. Rt Bochdalek hernia. Absent left thumb. Hemivertebra L5.	Intubation, ventilation, repair of hernia, continuing deterioration. Died aged 21 hr. No endoscopy. Postmortem (PM) diagnosis.	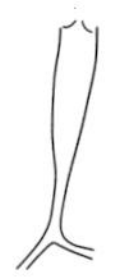
6	1 yr	M	Stridor since birth, recurrent attacks of croup.	Subglottic stenosis.	Symptomatic treatment still has stridor but no respiratory problems. Alive and well.	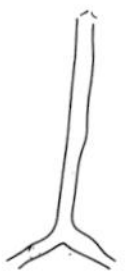
7	Birth	F	Respiratory distress syndrome (RDS) of the newborn with deterioration. CXR—hyperinflated right lung.	Tracheobronchomalacia. Emphysematous unilobar right lung.	Progressive respiratory distress, rapid deterioration following bronchoscopy, no bronchogram. Right pneumonectomy - satisfactory postop, discharged well.	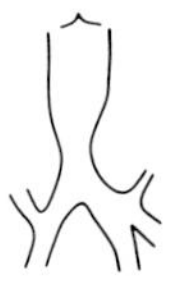
8	Birth	F	RDS of the newborn. CXR-RUL consolidation, left upper lobe (LUL) collapse, ? accessory diaphragm.	Accessory diaphragm and eventration. Hemivertebrae T11-T12. Hypoplastic right lung.	Required intermittent positive pressure ventilation (IPPV) for 4 days. Discharged well.	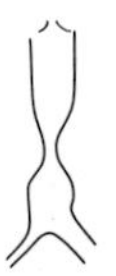
9	10 mo	M	Stridor since birth, repeated cyanotic episodes.	Innominate artery compression.	Tracheopexy at 11 months of age, still has recurrent cough and stridor but no further cyanotic attacks.	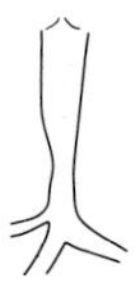
10	Birth	F	Cyanosed at birth, could not be intubated.	Laryngeal hypoplasia. H-type TEF. Hypoplastic right thumb.	Tracheostomy at birth. Tracheal stenosis and H-fistula diagnosed. No bronchogram. Gastrostomy and ligation of fistula, repeated chest infections. Died.	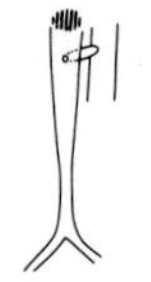
11	7 mo	M	3 episodes of croup, stridor, wheeze, barking cough, respiratory distress.	Hypoplastic lungs.	Investigated following recurrent croup. Narrowed trachea below cords; tracheostomy, rapid deterioration. Died age 7 mo.	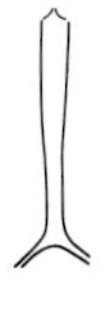

TABLE 2. CONTINUED

Case	*Presenting Age*	*Sex*	*Clinical Features*	*Associated Anomalies*	*Progress*	*Tracheo-Bronchial Anatomy*
12	1 mo	F	Mucusy at birth. Developed cough and tachypnea after primary repair.	TEF with esophageal atresia. Tracheomalacia.	Primary repair of TEF, investigated postop. Respiratory distress and stenosis diagnosed. Alive and well.	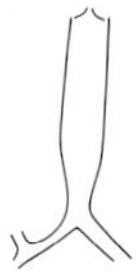
13	5 wk	M	2nd twin. Repeated attacks of cough, stridor, tachypnea, increasing in severity.	Tracheal web.	Treated with antibiotics and oxygen. Deteriorated, required ventilation. Severe stenosis diagnosed, active management stopped. Died age 7 mo.	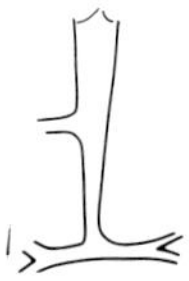
14	2 d	F	Tachypnea and cyanosis requiring ventilation.	H-type TEF. Tracheomalacia. Unilobar lung, emphysema left lung.	H-fistula ligated age 7 days. Postop cyanotic attacks - ventilated, tracheal stenosis "dilated." Tracheal resection age 20 wk. Could not be extubated. Died age 32 wk.	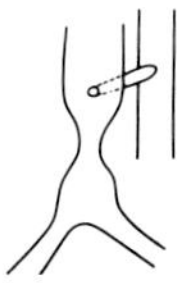
15	4 mo	F	Repeated cyanotic attacks. "Near miss" sudden infant death syndrome, (SIDS), no stridor.	Pulmonary artery sling at PM.	Intubation and ventilation, eventually tracheal stenosis diagnosed. Tracheal resection age 4 mo. Restenosis. Died age 6 mo.	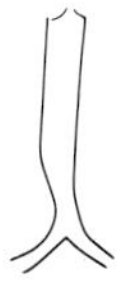
16	3 yr 9 mo	M	Failed intubation for elective orthopedic surgery.	Short left femur. Hypoplastic mandible. Cervical hemivertebrae.	Tracheostomy prior to proposed surgery. Postop respiratory problems, bronchoscopy via stoma - tracheal stenosis. No bronchogram. Thoracotomy; inoperable, deteriorated, died.	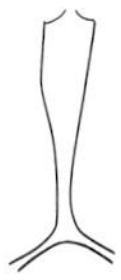
17	9 mo	M	Failure to thrive, stridor since birth, cyanotic episodes. CXR — bilateral patchy opacities.	Laryngomalacia. Subglottic stenosis. Extrahepatic portal hypertension.	Initial chest problems improved with physiotherapy. No major respiratory problems despite repeated anesthetics for mesocaval and splenorenal shunts.	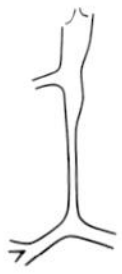
18	6 yr	F	Recurrent wheeze and cough from 18 mo. CXR - hypoplastic right lung.	Hypoplastic right lung.	Recurrent bronchiolitis as a young child treated symptomatically. Improved with age. Alive and well.	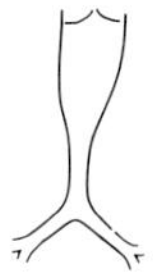
19	10 mo	M	Recurrent croup.	Laryngomalacia.	No major respiratory problems, croup treated with humidification. No bronchogram. Alive and well.	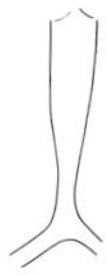
20	5 mo	F	Wheezing since birth, respiratory distress, ? bronchiolitis. Persistent right upper lobe (RUL) collapse.	Hypoplastic right lung.	Diagnosed as bronchiolitis, deteriorated, ventilated. Failure to extubate after 4 wk, bronchoscopy showed stenosis. Died aged 7 mo.	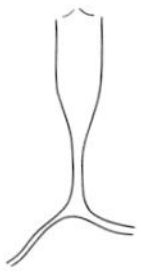
21	3 mo	F	3 wk tachypnea and stridor. CXR — left lung hypoplasia.	Agenesis left lung.	Initial treatment for pneumonia. Tracheal stenosis inoperable. Continued deterioration. Died 4 mo.	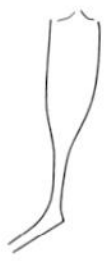

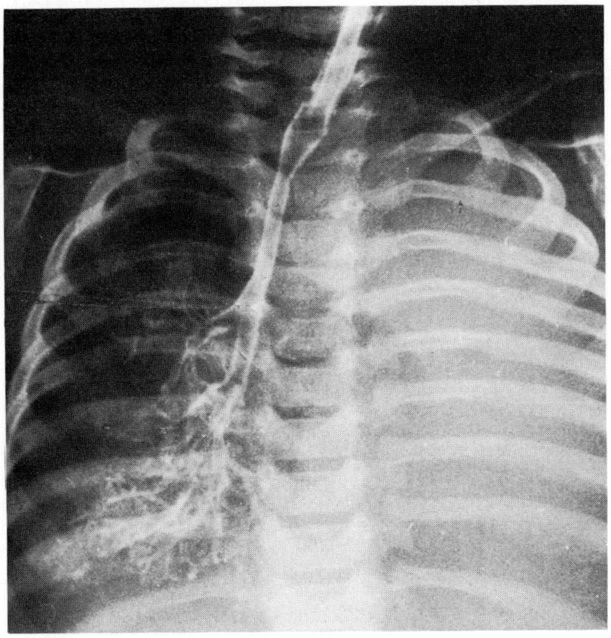

Fig. 4. (Case 21) Congenital stenosis of the trachea with agenesis of the left lung.

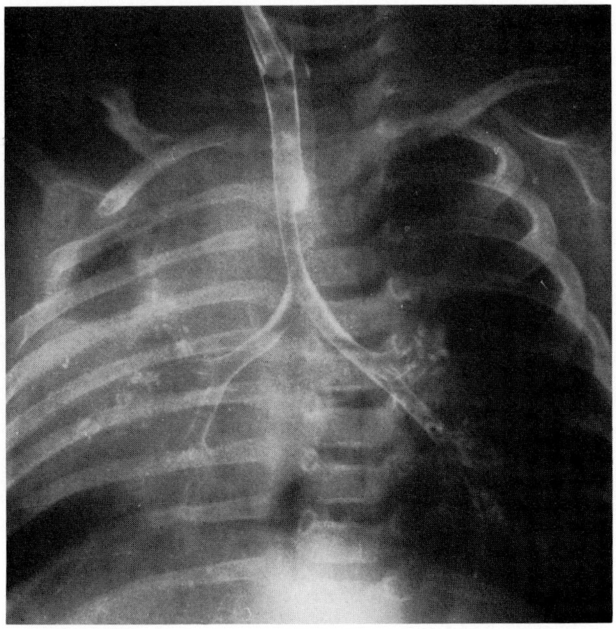

Fig. 5. (Case 1) Congenital stenosis of the lower trachea and main bronchi, the latter being of equal length. Appearance of a pouch at the lower end of the normal upper tracheal segment. There was as associated cervical H-fistula.

Introduction of an endotracheal tube often compounded the problem as the distal tip of the tube formed granulations where it traumatized the upper aspect of the stenosis, leading to further obstruction.

Table 2 summarizes the information about each individual case.

Associated Anomalies. There were only two patients in whom no other congenital anomalies were detected. In the other 19 patients the anomalies can be conveniently divided into a group where the respiratory tract and esophagus were involved and another group where other organ systems were involved.

Associated anomalies of the respiratory tract and esophagus were often found. The commonest association was with bronchial stenosis, only three cases having congenital tracheal stenosis without bronchial stenosis. A tracheal bronchus (Fig. 2) was seen in four cases. Hypoplasia of one or both lungs (Fig. 4) was seen in five cases and unilateral agenesis in one.

There was an association with H-type tracheoesophageal fistula in three cases (Fig. 5), one of whom also had a congenital stenosis of the upper esophagus.

Other anomalies included tracheomalacia, congenital lobar emphysema, accessory diaphragm, diaphragmatic hernia, tracheal web, laryngomalacia, congenital subglottic stenosis, and one patient had laryngeal hypoplasia with complete absence of the glottic and subglottic airway.

Three patients had congenital anomalies of the heart and great vessels, these being atrioventricular communis and coarctation of the aorta, dextrocardia with patent ductus arteriosis and ventricular septal defect.

Congenital anomalies commonly involved the skeleton and included hemivertebrae in either the cervical, thoracic or lumbar regions, hypoplasia or absence of the thumb, proximal radioulnar synostosis, widened pedicles of L2-4 vertebrae and hypoplastic mandible.

Other abnormalities included vulval ectopic anus and extrahepatic portal hypertension.

Outcome. Of the 21 patients 12 are alive, most of them living satisfactorily with their disease except for repeated respiratory infections which usually present as recurrent bronchitis or croup.

One infant with multiple abnormalities, including severe congenital heart disease, died at 21 hours of age (case 5).

Seven patients died before seven months of age, usually due to respiratory failure directly as a result of their congenital tracheal and bronchial stenosis. In two of the five cases (case 14 and case 15) thoracotomy was performed and the localized segment of stenosis resected (Figs. 3 and 6). Although the resection itself was successful both patients died eventually due to the severe nature of the associated bronchial stenosis.

The patient who died at three years and nine months (case 16) was to have planned repeated orthopedic surgery but the inability to extend his cer-

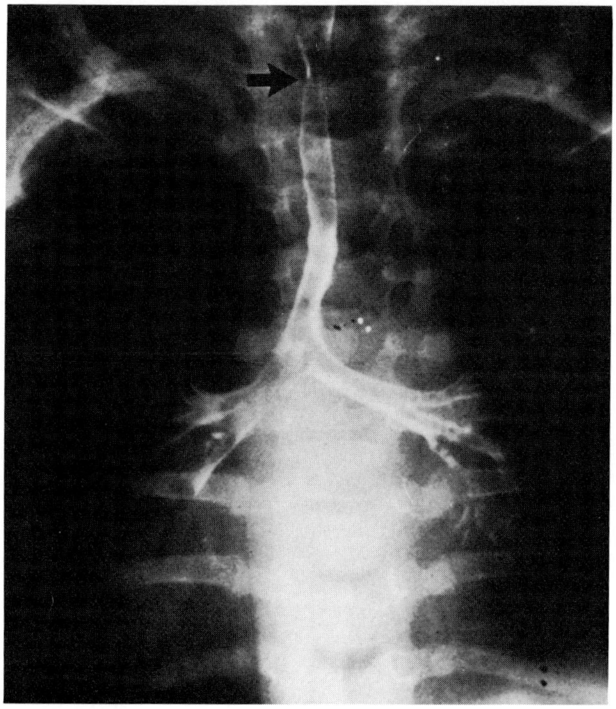

Fig. 6. (Case 15) Diffuse stenosis of trachea and bronchi. The localized "hour-glass" stenosis (arrow) was surgically resected (see Fig. 3) but the patient eventually died due to the associated severe bronchial stenosis.

vical region made endotracheal intubation hazardous. An elective tracheotomy was performed prior to the initial orthopedic operation but no bronchoscopy was performed and the congenital tracheal stenosis was recognized only some days later when the tracheotomy tube began to cause granulations and bleeding from the upper end of the tracheal stenosis. At thoracotomy the trachea was widely exposed and a long, fixed, rigid, congenital tracheal stenosis was found.

DISCUSSION

There are many congenital causes of respiratory tract obstruction but the clinical features are seldom diagnostic in themselves and it may be difficult to distinguish pharyngeal and laryngeal disease from tracheal malformations. In the evaluation of such airway obstruction investigation of the pharynx and larynx without examination of the tracheobronchial tree and, if necessary, of the esophagus, must be regarded as an incomplete examination. This applies not only to radiological but also to endoscopic examination.

In general, infants with congenital tracheal anomalies may present with respiratory obstruction and stridor that may have an inspiratory and/or expiratory component. Although all the patients in this series had some form of respiratory obstruction there was no set pattern to the presentation. Some newborn infants were regarded as having respiratory distress syndrome (Table 1), others had stridor or a persistent wheeze, there were cyanotic attacks, failure to thrive, attacks of atypical bronchiolitis and many were merely labelled respiratory distress. On further analysis, the latter term was found to include bronchiolitis, cyanotic attacks, tachypnea and cough.

It is quite clear then that the neonatologist, pediatrician and laryngologist must be aware of the condition of congenital tracheal stenosis, alert to its clinical manifestations and prepared to entertain the diagnosis in atypical cases.

Endoscopic examination is mandatory to make the diagnosis, to plan treatment, evaluate the presence of other associated anomalies and to assist in the assessment of the prognosis. Endoscopic examination, even by an experienced laryngologist, with expert pediatric anesthesiology, is fraught with danger in these cases. The drying effect of the premedication and the anesthetic gases, the trauma of the passage of the endoscopic instruments and the handling of small newborn babies can easily worsen an already critical situation. In most cases the smallest 2.5 mm Storz bronchoscope (4 mm true external diameter) can be passed only into the upper trachea proximal to the stenosis. Even the smallest Hopkins rigid fiberoptic telescope, which is 2.8 mm in external diameter, is difficult and usually impossible to pass to make a satisfactory evaluation of the lower trachea and bronchi. Contrast tracheobronchography is necessary to evaluate the tracheal stenosis, the main bronchi and the segmental bronchi.

If endoscopic assessment is potentially dangerous then the performance of a contrast tracheobronchogram is even more so and the decision to go ahead with this examination must be critically evaluated in each individual case. Where possible it should be performed when the child is in remission and only in exceptional, life-threatening circumstances should it be performed during an exacerbation. A carefully performed contrast tracheobronchogram with meticulous attention to detail, extreme care with anesthesia and expert postoperative intensive care will clearly demonstrate the nature and extent of the problem. This information is absolutely essential in any patient where surgical correction of the abnormality is being considered.

In most cases conservative management will be indicated, consisting of regular physiotherapy, intensified when there is an intercurrent respiratory infection, humidification of the inspired air, administation of antibiotics when appropriate, and every effort made to avoid the use of an endotracheal tube. The use of corticosteroids in an attempt to minimize mucosal edema and inflammatory swelling remains in dispute. Admission to the hospital for observation and treatment is occasionally necessary.

In general the younger the age at presentation the worse the outcome, but this is by no means always so. Besides the presence of other severe life-threatening anomalies such as untreatable congenital heart disease, children with normal lung tissue have a better prognosis.

Endotracheal intubation to assist ventilation in respiratory failure when the congenital stenosis has neither been recognized nor assessed will almost always make the situation worse. The tip of the endotracheal tube may rest on the upper aspect of the stenosis, create granulation tissue and bleeding, and this situation is further compounded by the trauma of a suction tip during "routine pulmonary suction toilet." In recognized cases it is our practice, where assisted ventilation is absolutely necessary, to carefully position the distal end of the endotracheal tube in what is left of the normal trachea at least 1 cm above the proximal end of the tracheal stenosis. Passage of a suction catheter is kept to an absolute minimum. Every effort is directed toward maintaining optimum humidity of the inspired air and to removing the endotracheal tube as soon as possible.

Although segmental surgical resection must rarely be feasible, the possibility should always be considered. In our series three cases were submitted to thoracotomy. In case 16 a tracheobronchogram had not been performed, and at surgery a rigid "stovepipe" trachea with completely closed rings with thick rigid walls was found occupying the entire lower part of the trachea and no form of surgery was possible. In two other cases with severe manifestations (cases 14 and 15), characterized by life-threatening respiratory infections and recurrent cyanotic attacks, segmental resection of the narrowest part of the tracheal stenosis was successfully performed by one of us (D.H.C.). Previous reports of successful surgery include that of Cantrell and Guild,[5] Mansfield[6] and Harrison et al.[7] Unfortunately each of our latter two patients eventually died of respiratory failure directly due to the very diminished caliber of the right and left main bronchi.

In three of our cases congenital stenosis of the tracheobronchial tree was associated with an H-type tracheoesophageal fistula, among other associated congenital anomalies.[2]

The association with hypoplasia of the lungs is common and is best assessed clinically and by radiological studies.

Cohen and Landing[8] in 1976 reported the association of pulmonary artery sling with tracheostenosis and bronchial abnormalities but we have been able to detect the association only once in our series. We have, of course, seen pulmonary sling in other patients but it is surprising that we have not detected it more often in the patients reported here.

Because of the wide variety of patterns of tracheal and bronchial stenosis seen we have not attempted a classification as we found it more useful to assess each patient's problems separately.

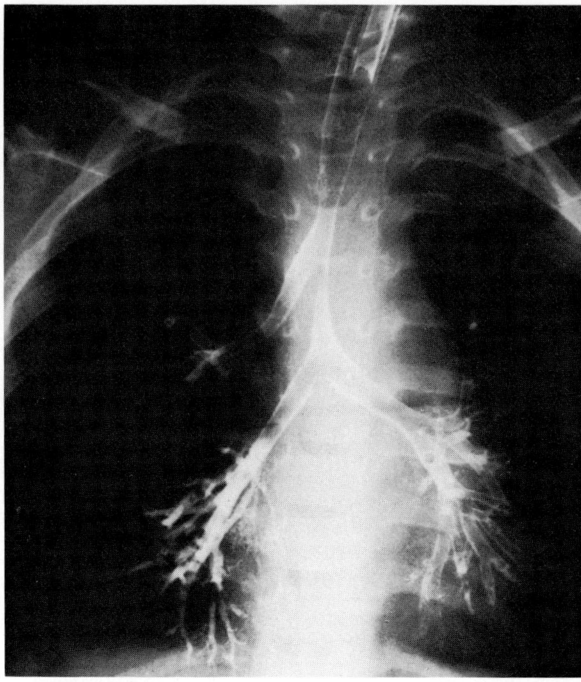

Fig. 7. (Case 4) Congenital stenosis of the trachea and main bronchi with a right tracheal bronchus. Note the short left main bronchus. The narrowest part of the trachea measures less than 2 mm.

We have been surprised that some children seem to live reasonably happily with their disease — the stenosis apparently "growing" with the child — but we cannot substantiate this hypothesis. In those cases where a tracheal bronchus is present it seems possible that respiratory exchange through that bronchus to normal lung may partially account for the child's apparently good respiratory function (Fig. 7).

A final and positive diagnosis can be made only at endoscopic examination, and the association with other abnormalities of the respiratory tract and esophagus must be carefully and thoroughly evaluated. There may be more than one cause of respiratory obstruction, ranging in our series from total absence of the glottic and subglottic airway to commoner conditions such as laryngomalacia.

CONCLUSIONS

Although uncommon, congenital tracheal stenosis can no longer be considered a very rare anomaly. It is a serious major congenital abnormality itself and is very often associated with other major or minor abnormalities. Diagnosis depends upon awareness of the possibility, heightened in the presence of skeletal abnormalities, especially hemivertebrae or an abnormality of the thumb. There is a consistent association with H-type tracheoesophageal fistula.

The diagnosis must be considered and appropriate investigations undertaken for atypical respiratory distress syndrome, unexplained stridor or wheezing, persistent respiratory distress and obstructive cyanotic attacks. The investigations themselves carry certain dangers and should be performed only in a large pediatric hospital where all the necessary items of equipment together with experienced anesthetic personnel and fully staffed postoperative and intensive care wards are available for maximum patient safety.

Conservative treatment is sufficient for most of those who survive infancy. In some cases correction of associated anomalies, eg, an H-type tracheoesophageal fistula, will improve the outlook. There appears to be little place for surgical resection of the stenosis, the limiting factors being the length of the stenosis, the degree of accompanying bronchial stenosis and the associated abnormalities of other major organs.

Documentation of the nature and extent of the stenosis is important for prognosis, for therapy of intercurrent respiratory infections, for consideration for segmental resection and lastly, of vital importance, to allow special precautions to be taken should the child require general anesthesia for some reason in the future.

REFERENCES

1. Holinger PH, Johnson KC, Parchet VN, Zimmerman AA. Congenital malformations of the trachea, bronchi and lungs. Ann Otol Rhinol Laryngol 1952; 61:1159-80.
2. Benjamin B. Endoscopy in congenital tracheal anomalies. J Pediatr Surg 1980; 15:164-71.
3. Wolman IJ. Congenital stenosis of the trachea. Am J Dis Child 1941; 61:1263-71.
4. Greene DA, Congenital complete tracheal rings. Arch Otolaryngol 1976; 102:241-3.
5. Cantrell JR, Guild HG. Congenital stenosis of the trachea. Am J Surg 1964; 108:297-305.
6. Mansfield PB. Tracheal resection in infancy. J Pediatr Surg 1980; 15:79-81.
7. Harrison MR, Heldt GP, Brasch RC, de Lorimier AA, Gregory AA. Resection of distal tracheal stenosis in a baby with agenesis of the lung. J Pediatr Surg 1980; 15:938-43.
8. Cohen SR, Landing BH. Tracheostenosis and bronchial abnormalities associated with pulmonary artery sling. Ann Otol Rhinol Laryngol 1976; 85:582-90.

≈

NINTH CONGRESS OF THE EUROPEAN RHINOLOGIC SOCIETY — THIRD INTERNATIONAL SYMPOSIUM ON INFECTION AND ALLERGY OF THE NOSE AND PARANASAL SINUSES

The Ninth Congress of the European Rhinologic Society and the Third International Symposium on Infection and Allergy of the Nose and Paranasal Sinuses will be held in Stockholm, Sept. 5-8, 1982. For information write: Ninth ERS Congress 1982, c/o Reso Congress Service, S-105 24 Stockholm.

SURGICAL REPAIR IN HYPOPHARYNGEAL AND CERVICAL ESOPHAGEAL CANCER

ANALYSIS OF 162 PATIENTS

D. F. N. HARRISON, MD, MS

LONDON, ENGLAND

Most recent publications dealing with surgical repair following pharyngolaryngectomy or pharyngolaryngoesophagectomy appear to be based upon limited surgical experience of the most differing operations now available. An up to date review of 162 patients, including 68 gastric "pull up" procedures, has the advantage of being a personal series as well as a critical evaluation of each technique based upon personal evaluation.

The anatomical boundaries of the hypopharynx are generally agreed upon as are its divisions into pyriform fossae, posterior pharyngeal wall and postcricoid regions. Although convenient for clinical classification these regions are of course in continuity with each other, probably all being exposed to those factors which make up common denominators in the etiology of most hypopharyngeal cancers. Although the incidence of squamous carcinoma within these three regions varies throughout the world, pyriform fossae remaining the commonest site, survival figures for the whole hypopharynx remain embarrassingly low. This is due to the failure to control local disease and regional and systemic metastases — problems common to many cancers. Despite the enthusiasm and technical advantages of present day radiotherapists and the reemergence of chemotherapy, surgery remains the most effective therapy, although it is frequently associated with other modalities in an attempt to combat what may well be a multifocal disease. This paper is not intended to reexamine in detail the whole problem of hypopharyngeal cancer although the time may well be ripe for such a worthwhile exercise. However, between 1965 and 1980 I have personally operated upon 162 patients with squamous carcinoma of the hypopharynx and although on previous occasions[1,2] various aspects of this condition have been examined in some detail, little has been said regarding the problems in selecting the most appropriate surgical techniques or the causes of failure in relationship to surgical pathology.

DeSanto and Carpenter[3] have most authoritatively reviewed the many varied and often imaginative surgical procedures at present used to rebuild a functional pharynx and esophagus following circumferential resection. In skilled, experienced hands most of these procedures are reasonably safe and effective, but in determining their success in eradicating cancer we meet the same inadequacies encountered with the larynx[4] and the upper jaw:[5] classification.

Difficulties of describing a three-dimensional disease in two-dimensional terms are inherent in all systems and on some occasions may be inconsequential. Within the hypopharynx, spread from region to region is both easy and rapid. Site of origin may be largely guesswork and as Stell et al[6] have emphasized, none of the existing systems of classification takes note of extension into the cervical esophagus or involvement outside the hypopharynx to involve recurrent laryngeal nerves. Invasion of the laryngeal framework may be less important since the larynx is removed in the majority of surgical procedures. Stell has also emphasized the poor prognostic significance of tumors longer than 5 cm although not indicating why this should be so.

The present inadequacies and inherent deficiencies of classification for hypopharyngeal cancer make detailed comparisons between published statistics virtually meaningless unless supported by pathological studies. Most survival rates are so poor that fortunately these undefined errors are relatively unimportant.

INDICATIONS FOR SURGERY

The factors usually considered in determining treatment modality or relative timing of combination therapy are not dissimilar to those met in other sites with the head and neck. Patient fitness, tumor extent including presence of regional metastases and, perhaps less easily defined, the surgeon's personal attitude and experience in reconstructive techniques are all relevant.

The proven extent of on average 10 mm of submucosal extension superiorly in 50 surgical speci-

From the Institute of Laryngology and Otology, London.

Presented at the meeting of the American Broncho-Esophagological Association, Vancouver, British Columbia, May 11-12, 1981.

REPRINTS — D. F. N. Harrison, MD, Institute of Laryngology and Otology, Gray's Inn Road, London, WC1X 8EE, England.

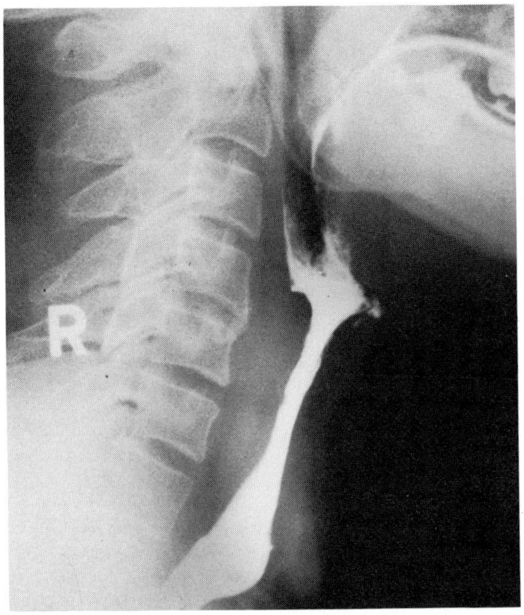

Fig. 1. Radiograph showing narrowing of skin repair secondary to pharyngolaryngectomy.

mens[2] removed by pharyngolaryngectomy and substantiated by examination of a more recent larger group of hypopharyngeal cancers suggests that many "early" neoplasms of pyriform fossae or posterior pharyngeal wall are in fact extensive. Clinical evaluation of regional lymph node metastasis in many individuals is no easier in the upper deep cervical region than in the inaccessible paratracheal chain. A more rewarding and practical philosophy may be to treat all hypopharyngeal neoplasms as advanced irrespective of the erroneous optimism which may be inherent in classification systems. These factors make the determination of those few patients histopathologically suitable for conservation surgery incredibly difficult. As in other sites it may be that these are the only patients who should receive primary radiotherapy. With this exception there remain three excisional procedures: partial pharyngectomy with laryngectomy, total pharyngolaryngectomy and pharyngolaryngoesophagectomy. Site of origin is probably less important than accurate evaluation of tumor extent when planning excisional surgery. My experience with these operations will therefore be discussed in relation to patient selection, technical developments and reasons for failure rather than presentation of possibly quite erroneous "staged" cure rates. Covering a period of 15 years, developments in technical expertise and better understanding of the natural history of this disease has obviously influenced my personal attitude. It is my philosophy for the 1980s which will be discussed.

PARTIAL PHARYNGECTOMY WITH LARYNGECTOMY (42 PATIENTS)

Mucosal abnormalities are common in patients with cancer of the pharyngeal walls, many of whom are heavy smokers and regular users of alcohol. Total removal of all potentially altered mucosa is impossible but resection should be as wide as possible with frozen section check of the margins.[7] If primary pharyngeal repair is to be associated with adequate surgical excision then the primary lesion must invariably be sited within the pyriform fossa. My pathological studies of such tumors has confirmed, as did Kirchner,[8] that invasion of thyroid cartilage and extension superiorly along the lateral wall markedly influences prognosis because of the difficulty of adequate excision. Pyriform apex invasion is of less significance since partial pharyngectomy has always been associated with total laryngectomy in my own cases.

Almost by definition patients treated by this procedure initially had relatively small tumors many of which received curative doses of radiotherapy. Inevitably this reduced the tumor size and since no effective means of tattooing is available in the hypopharynx, delineation of tumor margins is imprecise. Frozen section control is unreliable and inadequate resection occurred in 38% of patients. More radical excision leaves insufficient mucosa for adequate repair and particularly after radiotherapy, fistulization and stricture formation is common (Fig. 1).

Only 62% of patients showing microscopically positive malignant tissue within 5 mm of the margins of resection actually developed local recurrences. However, all had previously received radiotherapy and this figure undoubtedly reflects such factors as difficulty of interpretation, time delay between surgery and preoperative radiotherapy, and the inhibiting effect of postoperative fibrosis on tumor growth. Search of the literature makes it difficult to evaluate the experiences and thoughts of others on the role of partial pharyngectomy and total laryngectomy. Many writers do not clearly separate this operation from the more radical pharyngolaryngectomy.

Donald et al[9] talk of a 3 cm margin of excision which must be difficult to achieve with any pyriform fossa tumor. They continue by commenting that only 2 out of 33 patients with pyriform fossa carcinoma had a margin of 2 mm. Many of their patients were said to be T3/T4 and no figure for local recurrence is given.

In view of the functional problems associated with tight pharyngeal repair and the technical limitations of excision, this operation is now restricted to tumors localized to the pyriform fossa presenting with operable neck metastases or to small tumors recurring after curative radiotherapy.

PHARYNGOLARYNGECTOMY (52 PATIENTS)

Providing that the tumor is confined within the mucosal, muscular or cartilaginous wall of the hypopharynx, and conveniently ignoring the ever-

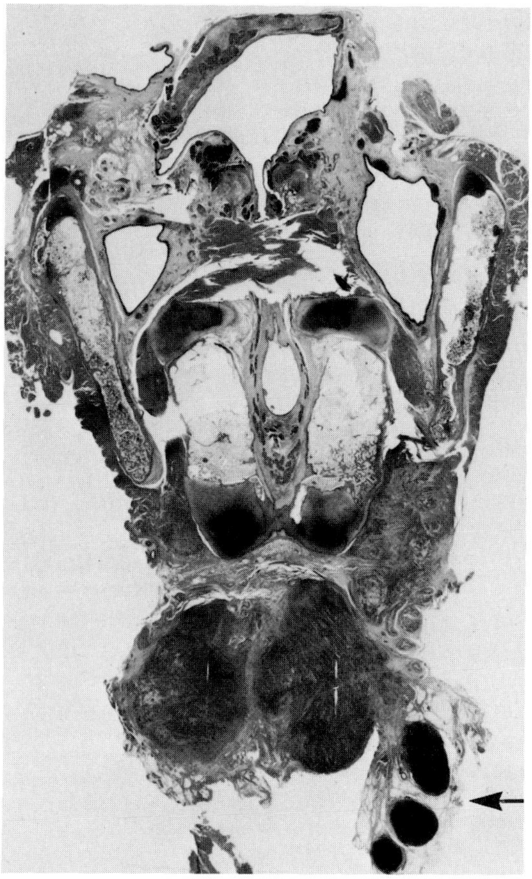

Fig. 2. Whole organ serial section through pharyngolaryngectomy specimen showing inferior limitation of excision and involved paratracheal nodes (arrow).

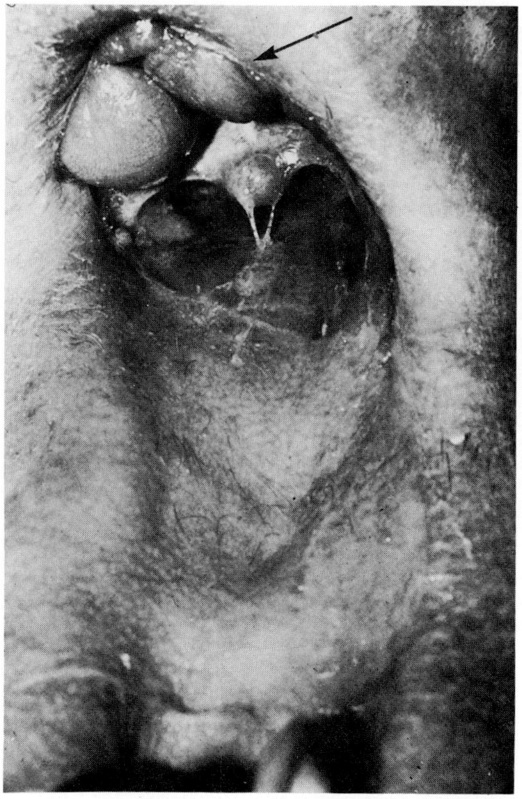

Fig. 3. Pharyngostome with prolapsed tongue after pharyngolaryngectomy and transposition of "trotters" laterally based skin flap (arrow). In cases with doubtful margins of excision repair should be defined.

present problem of regional and systemic metastasis, local control should be obtained by adequate excision above and below the neoplasm. Since excision is limited superiorly and laterally at a level bounded by the lower pole of the tonsil and the soft palate, many tumors are in effect not resectable. Irrespective of the means used to close the pharyngoesophageal defect — and considerable progress has been made to achieve this objective — local recurrence is inevitable in a proportion of all large hypopharyngeal tumors. Inferior resection of the esophagus varies in extent in individual patients. The length of the cervical esophagus is not constant and the lower the resection the more difficult subsequent repair and possibly the greater the risk of leaving local disease or paratracheal node metastasis (Fig. 2).

It is doubtful if preoperative radiotherapy effects sterilization of these margins. Neither is it possible to diagnose extension of the tumor outside these containing walls with certainty. Consequently, potentially curable patients will be found to have nonresectable tumors although removal of prevertebral fascia is feasible.

Development of single-stage repair, even in post-irradiation cases, using a deltopectoral flap and now more effectively musculocutaneous flaps with surface skin grafting, overcomes the intrinsic disadvantages of multistage repair. However, even immediate closure of the operative defect is only sensible if margins are clear — and in many instances they are not.

My experience of 52 patients treated by pharyngolaryngectomy includes not only the pre-"gastric pull-up" era but patients unsuitable or unfit for the more severe visceral interposition procedures. However, some patients have superior extension of disease within pharyngeal musculature or tongue base which makes effective marginal clearance difficult to obtain. In such cases the Wookey operation, leaving the patient with an open pharyngostome and esophagostome, allows a more careful clinical and pathological appraisal of the superior margins. When all is shown to be clear, closure is effected with a split-skin-covered musculocutaneous flap (Fig. 3) with less risk of covering up residual disease.

With tumors extending inferiorly into the cervical esophagus, visceral interposition avoids the anxieties and difficulties of low resection and reconstruction. However, the technique of reconstruction in hypopharyngeal cancer is in itself not related to control of the neoplasm unless limitations in surgical technique prevent adequate resection.

Even in experienced hands, pharyngolaryngec-

TABLE 1. RESULTS OF SURGERY (N = 162)

	Partial Pharyngolaryngectomy No.	%	Pharyngolaryngectomy No.	%	Pharyngolaryngoesophagectomy and Gastric Anastomosis No.	%
Total patients	42		52		68	
Operative mortality	2	(5)	9	(17)	8	(12.0)
Operative morbidity	29	(69)	31	(59)	6	(8.8)
Positive margins	16	(38)	16	(31)	2	(3.0)
Local recurrence	10	(24)	14	(27)	2	(3.0)

tomy with or without primary repair carries a mortality of possibly 20%[6] and in postirradiated patients a morbidity rate which may be as high as 60%. Many of these patients have extensive tumors, and suffer from other more generalized systemic conditions.

The presence of metastatic disease in the neck — a factor which has a markedly detrimental effect on prognosis in all hypopharyngeal cancers — increases morbidity rates by adding the need for radical neck surgery and must be considered when comparing "raw" mortality, morbidity and salvage figures. The high morbidity rate and poor functional results obtained by skin repair, irrespective of the many varied techniques used now, prevents my carrying out pharyngolaryngectomy unless primarily concerned with the upper limits of excision or where there is an early postcricoid carcinoma and a relatively long length of cervical esophagus.

PHARYNGOLARYNGOESOPHAGECTOMY (68 PATIENTS)

The ideal operation for any malignant tumor combines radical resection with restoration of function in a single procedure. It is possible that removal of pharynx, larynx and esophagus with primary anastomosis of stomach to pharynx comes as close to this ideal as is possible. Providing that upper margins are clear and that the tumor is confined within the pharyngoesophageal walls then further local disease can only develop in remaining pharyngeal mucosa — a reality in these high risk cases. Previous radiotherapy does not affect the pharyngogastric repair and only two patients had minor fistulae. Even when accompanied by radical neck dissection, skin necrosis is a rarity and exposed stomach can be skin-grafted. Good case selection should minimize risk of recurrence at the upper margin while manubrial resection[10] allows adequate resection of trachea preventing disease remaining at the tracheoesophageal junction.

However, even with an experienced surgical team — and synchronous surgery reduces operating time to an average of four hours — this is a major procedure. The criteria for case selection can only be determined by those experienced with this technique[1] and the operative mortality of 12% (Table 1) covers any patient not leaving the hospital. It includes the early hazardous period during technique development and a more realistic figure, based on the 23 patients operated upon during the past five years, would be 8.7%. In suitable patients this is a safe, effective, procedure but will not cure the incurable.

DISCUSSION

Despite better understanding of the natural history of hypopharyngeal cancer and the considerable improvements in reconstructive techniques, statistical probability of cure is not likely to improve. Relative high rates of systemic metastases and a propensity for regional metastasis limit prognosis, while late diagnosis and extension of tumor into inaccessible areas reduce likelihood of effective radical excision. There is no real evidence that preoperative radiotherapy realistically improves prognosis although it certainly increases morbidity rates. What improvements there have been are difficult to place in perspective while systems of classification remain obscure and confusing.

During the past 15 years my experience with these problems, both clinically and in the histopathological laboratory, has convinced me of the need for a rational approach based upon careful consideration of each patient. The need for preoperative or postoperative radiotherapy or radical neck dissection combined with radical excision of primary tumor is the primary problem. Reconstructive techniques must be chosen according to the need of each patient and the experience of the surgical team. Only in this way can all patients be given their best chance of survival.

REFERENCES

1. Harrison DFN. Surgical management of hypopharyngeal cancer. Arch Otolaryngol 1979; 105:149-52.

2. Harrison DFN. Pathology of hypopharyngeal cancer in relation to surgical management. J Laryngol Otol 1970; 84:349-67.

3. DeSanto L, Carpenter R. Reconstruction of the pharynx and upper esophagus after resection for cancer. Head Neck Surg 1980; 2:369-79.

4. Harrison DFN. Intrinsic weakness of the TNM system for classification of laryngeal cancer. ORL 1979; 41:241-51.

5. Harrison DFN. Critical look at the classification of maxillary sinus carcinomata. Ann Otol Rhinol Laryngol 1978; 87:3-9.

6. Stell PM, Carden EA, Hibbert J, Dalby JE. Post-cricoid carcinoma. Clin Oncol 1978; 4:215-26.

7. Ballantyne AJ. Principles of surgical management of cancer of the pharyngeal walls. Cancer 1967; 20:663-7.

8. Kirchner JA. Pyriform sinus cancer; a clinical and laboratory study. Ann Otol Rhinol Laryngol 1975; 84:793-803.

9. Donald PJ, Randall Hayes H, Dhaliwal R. Combined therapy for pyriform sinus cancer using postoperative irradiation. Otolaryngol Head Neck Surg 1980; 88:738-44.

10. Harrison DFN. Resection of the manubrium. Br J Surg 1977; 64:374-7.

Ann Otol 90:1981

ENDOSCOPY IN ESOPHAGEAL ATRESIA AND TRACHEOESOPHAGEAL FISTULA

BRUCE BENJAMIN, FRACS

SYDNEY, AUSTRALIA

Between 1970 and 1979 152 infants born with the anomaly of esophageal atresia with or without tracheoesophageal fistula or of congenital tracheoesophageal fistula without atresia were treated at the Royal Alexandra Hospital for Children, Sydney. Recent developments in endoscopic equipment and new techniques of anesthesia allow detailed examination of the respiratory tract and esophagus with minimum trauma and maximum safety. Symptomatology relating to the airway and to the esophagus after surgical repair often occurs in patients who may have tracheomalacia, esophageal anastomotic stricture, esophageal reflux and sometimes recurrent or residual fistula. A definite diagnosis of tracheomalacia can be made by finding the typical triad of anteroposterior narrowing of the tracheal lumen, weakening of the semicircular-shaped cartilages and forward ballooning of the widened posterior membranous tracheal wall. Careful examination of the trachea and esophagus allows identification of an elusive recurrent fistula or an H-type fistula. As the primary results of surgery for esophageal atresia and tracheoesophageal fistula improve, long-term problems are becoming increasingly important. The role of the pediatric endoscopist is vital in the care of these patients.

INTRODUCTION

Previous papers, outstanding among which were those of Fearon[1] and Holinger,[2] have stressed the importance of endoscopy in the overall management of esophageal atresia and tracheoesophageal fistula, and others[3-5] have pointed out the place of endoscopic techniques in the diagnosis of H-fistula or recurrent fistula. The development of sophisticated equipment using fiberoptic illumination together with advances in anesthetic techniques allows greater safety for the patient during endoscopic procedures in the diagnosis and treatment of congenital anomalies. With these refinements in endoscopic techniques the role of endoscopy has become much broader. The purpose of this paper is to outline the place of laryngobronchoesophagology in the overall management of patients with esophageal atresia and/or tracheoesophageal fistula, based on experience at the Royal Alexandra Hospital for Children, Sydney.

MATERIAL AND METHODS

During the ten years 1970 through 1979 we treated 152 cases of esophageal atresia with or without tracheoesophageal fistula and of congenital tracheoesophageal fistula without atresia (Table 1). Analysis of the case histories of these patients forms the basis of this paper.

Approximately one half of the children were submitted to endoscopy, either as a diagnostic procedure before surgical repair or to evaluate or treat postoperative complications. It was sometimes possible to make a preliminary diagnosis from the clinical and radiological features but diagnostic endoscopy was usually necessary to make a complete and accurate assessment. The examination included the pharynx, larynx, tracheobronchial tree and the esophagus.

Preoperative examination for evaluation before definitive repair in the neonatal period was performed only toward the end of the series. In other cases preoperative examination was for investigation of possible H-fistula or recurrent fistula. Endoscopy was performed postoperatively to confirm tracheomalacia with its accompanying features; to ascertain the presence of an associated anomaly of the larynx or tracheobronchial tree; and in the investigation of esophageal stenosis, whether congenital or surgically acquired, and for the evaluation of esophageal reflux. Therapeutic endoscopy was performed for esophageal dilatation and removal of an esophageal foreign body.

The technique of endoscopy was standard. Using a suitable laryngoscope the pharynx, supraglottic larynx and the vocal cords were examined, the latter for both their appearance and movement. Next the Storz rigid bronchoscope was introduced. The tracheobronchial tree was examined and any abnormal secretions were aspirated and collected in a trap bottle for examination and culture. The presence of any abnormal compression, collapse, stenosis, pulsation or altered anatomy of the bronchial segments was noted.

For esophagoscopy we used both the Storz pediatric and the Negus pattern rigid instruments. We generally preferred the latter as they have a wider diameter and are especially useful for open tube manipulation, biopsy removal of foreign bodies and for direct-vision antegrade esophageal dilatation.

The various small diameter Hopkins fiberoptic telescopes whose light may be directed straight ahead or at various angles were used constantly in the larynx and tracheobronchial tree and allowed an excellent view. In the esophagus the telescopes were especially useful for evaluation of the mucosa where gastroesophageal reflux was suspected or for examination of the anterior esophageal wall for the orifice of a tracheoesophageal fistula without atresia. Esophageal examination and telescopic visualization was combined with biopsy in the investigation of gastroesophageal reflux to confirm the diagnosis and to indicate the nature and extent of esophagitis.[6]

TABLE 1. TYPES OF ANOMALY IN TEN-YEAR PERIOD 1970-1979

Atresia, lower fistula	129
Atresia, upper fistula	3
Atresia, double fistula	2
Atresia, no fistula	10
Fistula, no atresia (H-type)	8
	Total 152

From the Royal Alexandra Hospital for Children, Sydney, Australia.

Presented at the meeting of the American Broncho-Esophagological Association, Vancouver, British Columbia, May 11-12, 1981. Recipient of the Seymour R. Cohen Award for Pediatric Laryngology and Bronchoesophagology.

REPRINTS — Bruce Benjamin, 231 Macquarie Street, Sydney N.S.W. 2000 Australia.

The problems confronting the endoscopist and the anesthesiologist varied from patient to patient. Fortunately the majority of patients for diagnostic examination were good risks for anesthesia but some were seriously ill and teamwork between the endoscopic surgeon and the anesthesiologist was essential.

The most common technique of anesthesia for diagnostic examination was spontaneous respiration with nitrous oxide, oxygen and halothane.[7] Topical analgesia, up to 5 mg lidocaine/kg body weight, usually diluted to a 1-2% concentration, was sprayed on the epiglottis, larynx and trachea. Topical analgesia minimized unwanted reflex activity and virtually abolished laryngeal spasm during endoscopy. This spontaneous respiration technique was particularly suitable for diagnostic examination as it allowed the opportunity for careful, unhurried observation and for photography.

Photographs were obtained using the Storz electronic flash-generating equipment with the light-bodied Storz reflex endocamera. Kodak Ektachrome® 35 mm film with a speed of ASA 200 was used.

With complete preoperative assessment by the anesthesiologist and surgeon and with reasonable care, experience and attention to detail, anesthesia and endoscopy caused minimal morbidity and no mortality.

RESULTS

Major and minor congenital anomalies of other organs besides the respiratory tract and esophagus were common and often involved the cardiac, gastrointestinal, genitourinary and skeletal systems. Associated anomalies of the upper respiratory tract and esophagus demonstrated at endoscopy included vocal cord paralysis, congenital subglottic stenosis, stenosis of the tracheobronchial tree, pulmonary hypoplasia, lower esophageal stenosis and gastroesophageal reflux. Problems presenting to the endoscopist were many but tended to occur in a regular, distinct and recognizable pattern. Those anomalies associated with the principal abnormality involving the respiratory tract and esophagus have been analyzed in detail.

Of the 152 patients there were 8 with an H-type tracheoesophageal fistula. An unexpected finding was that five of these had associated anomalies of the upper respiratory tract or of the esophagus (Table 2). It is especially noteworthy that four of the eight had a severe segmental congenital stenosis of the trachea.

There were 43 patients in the series with tracheomalacia confirmed at bronchoscopy. This represents an observed incidence of almost 30%. There were six patients who had bronchoscopy and the trachea showed no signs of tracheomalacia. There was no indication for bronchoscopy in the remainder of the patients but from the clinical features alone it is likely that some of them had a mild degree of tracheomalacia. The 43 patients with proven tracheomalacia were classified as mild (11), moderate (20) or severe (12) on the clinical features. All of these patients had the brassy, barking cough which is one of the characteristic clinical manifestations of tracheomalacia.

Esophagoscopy was not performed in all of the patients who had surgical repair of the esophagus. The esophagus was examined only when indicated by the clinical features and the barium swallow. Of the 144 patients with repaired esophageal atresia there were 40 who required one or more dilatations of an anastomotic stricture. They were classified as mild, needing three or fewer dilatations (18); moderate, needing four or more dilatations (17); and severe, needing a further operation (5).

TABLE 2. ASSOCIATED ABNORMALITIES IN FIVE OF THE EIGHT PATIENTS WITH H-TYPE FISTULA

Case No.	*Tracheal Stenosis*	*Esophageal Stenosis*	*Tracheo-malacia*	*Laryngeal Atresia*
1	+	—	+	—
2	+	—	+	—
3	+	+	—	+
4	+	+	—	—
5	—	+	—	—

There were six recurrent fistulae, a rate of less than 5%. Congenital esophageal stenosis was seen in six cases of which three were in association with H-type fistulae. There were no serious complications of the endoscopic procedures and there was no mortality.

DISCUSSION

Symptoms relating to the airway and to the esophagus after surgical repair of esophageal atresia and tracheoesophageal fistula are often present in the postoperative period and may be due to tracheomalacia, bronchomalacia, tracheal stenosis, esophageal anastomotic stricture, esophageal reflux with or without aspiration and occasionally recurrent or residual fistula. Endoscopy allows evaluation of any associated congenital anomaly, assessment of the degree and extent of the flaccidity and collapse of the trachea in tracheomalacia, dilatation of an esophageal stricture, direct examination and biopsy of esophagitis and identification of a suspected recurrent fistula.

Significant developments in improving and modifying endoscopic equipment to allow better operating conditions include:

1. Adaptation of bronchoscopes to facilitate ventilation.

2. Techniques for positive pressure ventilation during bronchoscopy.

3. Development of the cold light source for use with flexible fiberoptic leads and prisms for proximal lighting of miniature endoscopes.

4. The Hopkins fiberoptic telescopes for use with very small diameter rigid bronchoscopes.

5. Availability of the image intensifier while contrast radiography of the respiratory tract is performed.

These improvements in equipment and fiberop-

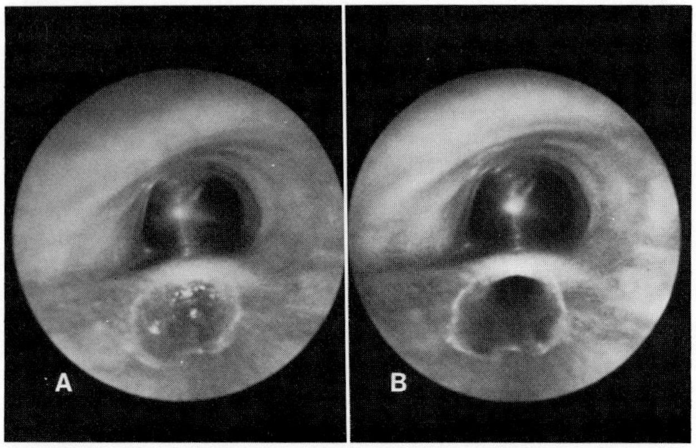

Fig. 1. Endoscopic appearance of the tracheal aspect of an unoperated lower pouch tracheoesophageal fistula; A) closed during expiration and B) open during inspiration. In this patient there is a little reactionary tracheitis around the orifice due to aspiration of gastric juice.

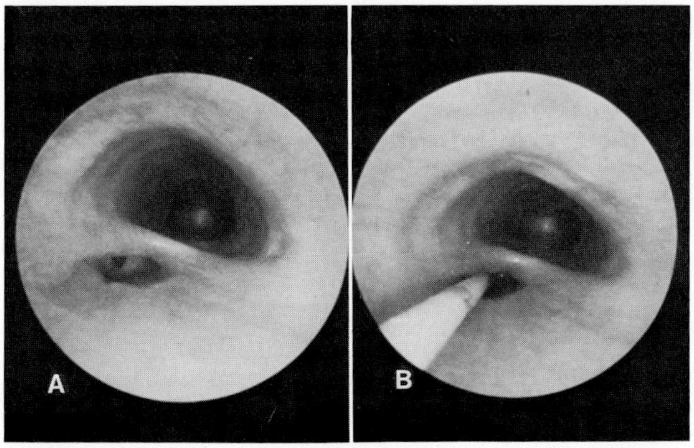

Fig. 2. Tracheal aspect of an unoperated lower pouch tracheoesophageal fistula A) before and B) after passage of a fine catheter through the fistula. In this particular case the orifice of the fistula lies to the left of the midline.

tics allow greater safety for the patient but the varying problems confronting the bronchoesophagologist demand that the operator is absolutely familiar with the complexity of the instruments so that he always has complete control over their passage and manipulation.

Endoscopic examination need not be performed in every child after operation for tracheoesophageal fistula and esophageal atresia. From our experience in this series the indications for endoscopy are as follows.

Diagnostic:

1. Evaluation in a neonate before operative repair.

2. Diagnosis of H-fistula.

3. Assessment of tracheomalacia and associated factors.

4. Identification of recurrent, residual or second fistula.

5. Presence of an associated anomaly, eg, subglottic stenosis or vocal cord paralysis.

6. Evaluation of esophageal stenosis.

7. Evaluation of gastroesophageal reflux.

Therapeutic:

8. Dilatation of esophageal stricture.

9. Removal of esophageal foreign body.

Preoperative Evaluation. A newborn baby with rattling respirations of fine frothy bubbles of mucus and saliva at the lips or nostrils should have the patency of his esophagus tested. The diagnosis of esophageal atresia is established by failure to pass a catheter. Radiological study with contrast material is contraindicated because of the danger of aspiration.

Although the diagnosis of the common anomaly of esophageal atresia with lower pouch fistula is standardized, with the less common varieties of malformation the exact diagnosis may be elusive and may result in delay or even incorrect operative treatment.[3] We have performed diagnostic endoscopy in the neonate with esophageal atresia and tracheoesophageal fistula before definitive surgery on nine occasions and there is valuable information to be obtained for the surgeon prior to repair.

Having examined the larynx, the appearance and movement of the vocal cords and the subglottic region, the bronchoscope is introduced into the trachea. The large opening of the fistula (Fig. 1) is seen on the posterior wall usually in the midline; we have seen several to the left of the midline (Fig. 2) but, as yet, none toward the right. After removal of secretions, the site and size of the fistula and the state of the mucosa, whether it is soiled by gastric juice or whether there are infected secretions, can be accurately judged. If no other associated anomalies in the tracheobronchial tree are found a ureteric catheter is passed via the bronchoscope through the fistula (Fig. 2) and on into the lower esophagus and left in place. The peroral endotracheal tube to continue anesthesia is then passed and lies beside the catheter; the latter enables the surgeon to quickly and confidently identify the fistula at thoracotomy. Finally the blind upper esophageal pouch is inspected.

Endoscopic examination takes about five minutes and immediately precedes the definitive thoracotomy. The exact diagnosis and pathological anatomy is established. It allows assessment of associated malformations which could be important in the operative or postoperative care, eg, subglottic stenosis, tracheomalacia, tracheal or bronchial stenosis, upper esophageal segment fistula, second fistula or an unusual fistula.

We are still evaluating preoperative endoscopy, and whether the final place of this examination is in the atypical or complicated case with known or sus-

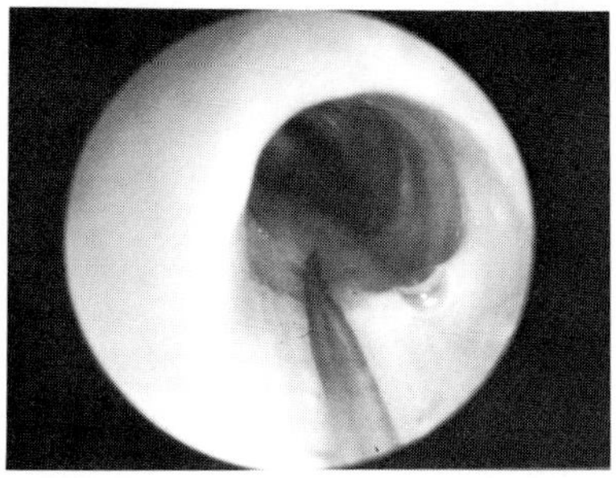

Fig. 3. A fine catheter has been passed through the tracheal orifice of an H-type fistula, seen high on the posterior wall of the trachea.

pected associated anomalies or whether it should be a routine examination remains to be determined. Preoperative endoscopy with telescopes is safe, ensures accurate assessment, gives confidence and comfort to the surgeon and may even modify his approach and surgical technique at the definitive operation. Lastly the endoscopist develops a personal association with the patient and his continuing welfare.

Diagnosis of H-type Fistula. There were eight fistulae without esophageal atresia in the series. The majority of patients developed respiratory symptoms associated with feeding during the first week of life but there was a variable delay until the diagnosis was made.

The key to eventual diagnosis of H-type fistula is awareness of the possibility from the clinical features.[4] Endoscopic identification of an elusive H-type fistula or a recurrent fistula requires meticulous examination of the posterior wall of the trachea and of the anterior wall of the esophagus with angled telescopes.

It is our opinion that diagnostic examination under general anesthesia is not only more reliable but safer than radiological examination of the esophagus.[5] Should inhalation of contrast material occur in the x-ray department, choking, cyanosis and apnea may occur and facilities for resuscitation are not always readily available. It is noteworthy that two of the eight fistulae in this series did not show on barium swallow.

The tracheal orifice of a fistula occurring without esophageal atresia is higher than the orifice of a fistula occurring with esophageal atresia (Fig. 3). It is usually in the cervical region of the trachea and is best seen with an angled telescope. The esophageal aspect of a fistula without esophageal atresia is a characteristic inverted V-shaped slit orifice which may be difficult to identify. Positive pressure ventilation of the trachea through the endotracheal tube after a few milliliters of saline have been instilled into the upper esophagus with an esophagoscope in place has proved to be a useful diagnostic technique in detection of the tracheoesophageal fistula when bubbles of air are seen coming from the fistula itself.[4,5] Endoscopic catheterization of the fistula with a fine catheter facilitates surgical treatment.

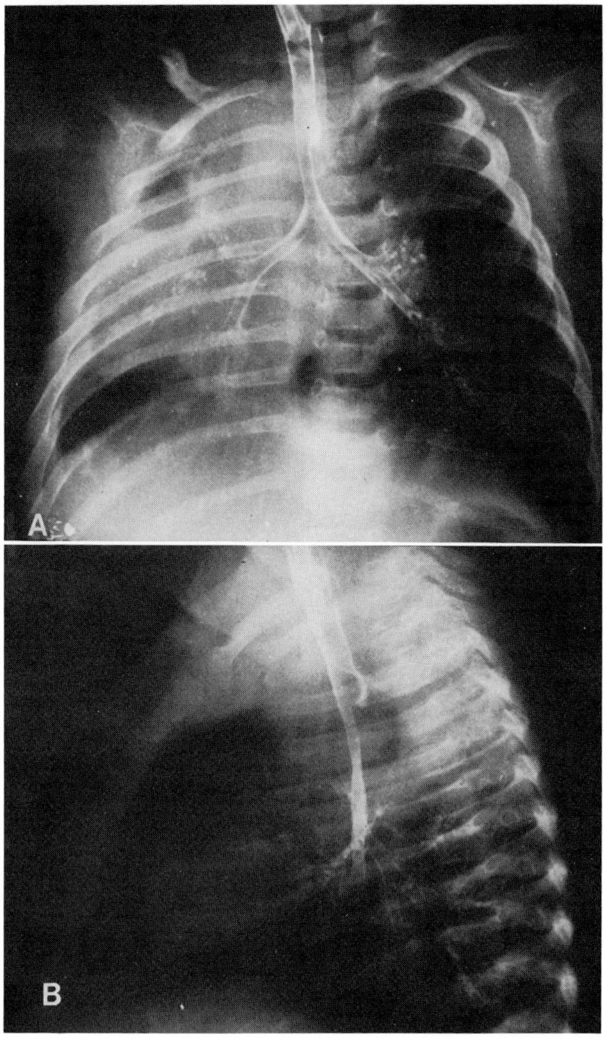

Fig. 4. A, B) Contrast tracheobronchogram of a patient with an H-type fistula showing not only congenital stenosis of the trachea and of both main bronchi but also a blind posterior tracheal pouch. There is right-sided pneumonitis.

An unexpected finding in this series was the high incidence of associated abnormalities of the trachea and/or the esophagus in 5 of the 8 patients (Table 2). Figure 4 illustrates a case with stenosis of the lower trachea and main bronchi, and the blind tracheal pouch can be seen on the posterior tracheal wall.

In our hands endoscopic evaluation has a better success rate in the diagnosis of tracheoesophageal fistula than have contrast x-ray studies and we believe it is safer and gives a more thorough evaluation of associated anomalies of the upper respiratory tract and esophagus.

Tracheomalacia and the Tracheal Pouch. Endoscopy has its most significant and well-established

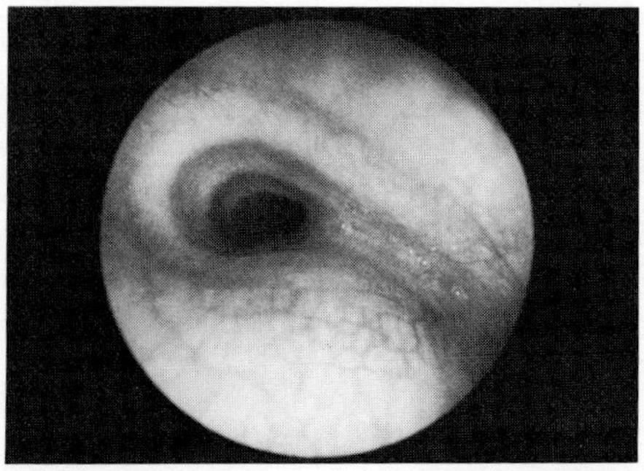

Fig. 5. Tracheomalacia of the lower trachea five weeks after primary repair of tracheoesophageal fistula and esophageal atresia. There is severe anteroposterior collapse more marked on the right side during expiration. Note the wide membranous posterior tracheal wall.

place in the management of patients who have respiratory distress, infection, obstruction, stridor, retention of secretions, barking cough, aspiration, atelectasis, cyanotic attacks or apnea following repair of esophageal atresia.[1,2,5,8,9] In the past these features have been rather loosely considered as "postoperative pulmonary complications." Holinger et al[2] noted that tracheomalacia had been recognized bronchoscopically in the differentiation of the causes of severe stridor in an "appreciable number of cases." We now know that tracheomalacia is the major factor in producing these symptoms.

In our series 43 patients had tracheomalacia confirmed at bronchoscopy but it is likely that many other cases, where bronchoscopy was not indicated, also had some degree of tracheomalacia. All of these patients had the characteristic brassy cough which is a manifestation of tracheomalacia. The anteroposterior narrowing of the soft tracheal segment is accentuated by the raised intrathoracic pressure during coughing.

Patients with tracheomalacia can be divided into mild, moderate or severe on the clinical features.[8] Patients in the mild and moderate groups can be managed conservatively. When the clinical features suggest moderate or severe tracheomalacia, endoscopy is essential to confirm the diagnosis and document the severity. In severe cases there is almost total anteroposterior collapse of the lower trachea (Fig. 5), especially severe during expiration, with a residual lumen which may be only 1-2 mm. Patients classified as severe have upper respiratory obstruction with stridor at rest developing during the first two months of life. All have marked sputum retention, often associated with cyanotic attacks, apneic episodes and sometimes attacks of reflex apnea. These attacks may be aptly referred to as "dying spells" and more than half of those in the severe category have had one or more cardiac arrests. Our experience with operative tracheopexy[8] for patients in the severe group has been encouraging. We now believe that tracheotomy should not be necessary unless there is some unrelated laryngeal or upper respiratory anomaly which itself necessitates tracheotomy.

Because of the collapse, weakness and instability of the tracheal wall in tracheomalacia the changes have been thought for a long time to be due to hypoplasia, dysplasia or absence of the normal framework of the trachea. The detailed work of Wailoo and Emery[10] has been a milestone and has firmly documented the anatomical changes in tracheomalacia. In 40 autopsy specimens with tracheoesophageal fistula, histological analysis for structural deformities showed a deficiency of cartilage in 70%, increased length of transverse muscle in the trachea in 60% and a longer than average internal perimeter of the trachea in 65%. In only six patients was the trachea normal. These changes correlate exactly with our own endoscopic findings where we have observed anteroposterior collapse of the tracheal walls during respiration with wheezing, dyspnea and stridor. The tracheal cartilages have an indented half-circle shape rather than the normal horseshoe shape, and the posterior membranous wall is markedly widened so that during expiration it bulges anteriorly into the residual lumen of the trachea. This typical triad of widened semicircular cartilages, ballooning of the posterior membranous wall and collapse and loss of the tracheal lumen affects several centimeters of the lower trachea. The lumen above is normal but below the changes may affect the caliber of one or other main bronchus for a short segment.

It has now been shown conclusively that this abnormal flaccidity of the trachea, sometimes also involving one or other stem bronchus, is a primary congenital anomaly commonly associated with tracheoesophageal fistula, being part of the whole malformation.

Squamous epithelium has been demonstrated by Emery and Haddadin[11] in the trachea of children with tracheoesophageal fistula who clinically had sputum retention. This may be a congenital malformation or may be due to squamous metaplasia. We believe there are other factors that contribute both to the respiratory obstruction and to the retention of secretions. These include:

1. Tracheal compression by the innominate artery.[12]

2. Food or an impacted foreign body which may fill the dilated upper segment of the esophagus above the esophageal anastomosis particularly where there is an anastomotic stenosis.

3. Approximation of the anterior and posterior walls during coughing which partially obstructs clearing of endobronchial secretions.

4. Aspiration into the trachea as a result of disordered esophageal peristalsis or gastroesophageal reflux.

5. Disordered mucociliary mechanism. The clearing action may be impeded by the wide mouth of the residual pouch of the fistula which crosses the posterior tracheal wall.

The residual pouch of the fistula is invariably seen as a diverticulum varying in length from a few millimeters to 10-15 mm in every case of repaired tracheoesophageal fistula. It is not necessarily related to the surgical technique of the individual surgeon performing the repair. The pouch is usually healthy but occasionally a suture, granulation tissue, discharge, soft tissue reaction or scarring may be seen within it.

It is important to emphasize that the tip of a bronchoscope or an endotracheal tube may enter the fistula pouch. If the distal bevel of an endotracheal tube passes into the residual pouch of a repaired tracheoesophageal fistula the anesthesiologist may be totally unable to ventilate the child. The tube must be withdrawn 1-2 cm and repositioned with the bevel rotated. Normal ventilation is then achieved.

Recurrent Fistula. There were six recurrent fistulae. Only one occurred early after repair; they were diagnosed at the ages of 2, 6, 7, 11, 17 and 18 months respectively. A suspected recurrence of a fistula occurring some time after primary repair may be difficult to prove and is best diagnosed at endoscopy although some will be shown at barium swallow. The recurrent fistula is usually in the pouch of the original fistula. A ureteric catheter passed through the recurrent fistula will be seen at esophagoscopy to enter the esophagus at or just below the anastomotic repair site.

Congenital Esophageal Stenosis. The occurrence of both esophageal atresia and esophageal stenosis in the lower esophagus in the same patient has been considered to be rare.[2,13] Concomitant esophageal atresia and stenosis in the lower segment of the esophagus was seen in three cases in this series. There were also three cases seen in association with H-type fistula (Table 2). These stenoses appeared to have a congenital basis as they were seen in neonates, there were no mucosal changes and there was no association with gastroesophageal reflux.

Gastroesophageal Reflux. The manifestations of gastroesophageal reflux following repair of esophageal atresia are variable. There may be a stricture, failure to thrive, repeated pneumonitis and even apnea from aspiration. Esophagoscopy and biopsy can give useful information.[6] Early recognition and aggressive treatment of gastroesophageal reflux following repair of esophageal atresia may reduce the incidence of acquired stricture formation in the lower esophagus.

Endoscopy does not assist in the evaluation of the additional problem of disordered motility and neuromuscular incoordination of the esophagus.

Esophageal Stricture. When a stricture appears to be forming after surgical anastomosis opinions are divided[2] as to whether dilatation should be performed early or late. We favor early endoscopic inspection and dilatation for best results. Early dilatation may increase the danger of esophageal disruption or even reformation of the fistula unless it is done with great care but it is easier to treat a stricture in the early stages than when it is firm and fibrotic.

Stricture of the esophagus at the site of the end-to-end anastomosis performed for esophageal repair is seen commonly.[1,2] We do not perform esophagoscopy routinely in all patients but of the 144 patients with repaired esophageal atresia in this series 40 required one or more dilatations. Not included in this group are postanastomotic strictures following esophageal replacement using either colon or reversed gastric tube.

It is difficult to know when esophageal dilatation is indicated for postanastomotic stricture. Although there is no acceptable definition of what is an adequate lumen, in our view it is satisfactory to judge on the functional swallowing performance of the child together with the degree of radiographic narrowing on barium swallow. The contrast esophagogram may be unreliable and esophageal evaluation with calibration by dilators may then be the best guide to the capability of the esophagus.

Direct vision bouginage is performed from above through a large diameter Negus rigid esophagoscope using graduated gum elastic bougies. It has not been necessary to leave a string in the lumen of the esophagus except for retrograde dilatation. On occasions in difficult cases retrograde dilatation with Tucker's bougies is preferable and is the method of choice for dilatation of a resistant stenosis. Retrograde bouginage is unlikely to damage the esophagus and is safe for repeated manipulation. We have had few complications from esophagoscopy or dilatation in patients who have had esophageal atresia.

Esophageal Foreign Body. Impaction of an esophageal foreign body occurs more commonly in children with any type of esophageal repair, whether an end-to-end anastomosis, intestinal interposition or gastric tube transplant. Some require repeated removal of foreign bodies from the anastomotic site, usually related to neuromuscular incoordination of the esophagus or more likely to narrowing caused by scar tissue, in which case dilatation may be necessary.

CONCLUSION

The endoscopist should no longer be consulted only in an occasional emergency situation where there is a serious respiratory problem. Correlation of evidence from the history and the findings on physical examination together with the radiological examination generally indicate the necessity for direct endoscopic examination.

As the primary results of surgery for esophageal atresia improve, long-term problems become increasingly important. The dramatic nature of some of these troubles, especially respiratory complications and the overall generally good progress and prognosis of babies using the latest techniques of corrective surgery means that the endoscopist is now a vital member of the team in the care of these patients.

REFERENCES

1. Fearon B. The endoscopic management of congenital atresia of the esophagus. Ann Otol Rhinol Laryngol 1959; 68:1047-69.

2. Holinger PH, Brown WT, Maurizi DG. Endoscopic aspects of post-surgical management of congenital esophageal atresia and tracheo-esophageal fistula. J Thorac Cardiovasc Surg 1965; 49:22-31.

3. Cohen SJ. Unusual types of esophageal atresia and tracheo-esophageal fistulae. Clin Pediatr 1965; 4:271-5.

4. Gans SL, Johnson RO. Diagnosis and surgical management of "H-type" tracheoesophageal fistula in infants and children. J Pediatr Surg 1977; 12:233-6.

5. Benjamin B. Endoscopy in congenital tracheal anomalies. J Pediatr Surg 1980; 15:164-71.

6. Benjamin B, Pohl D. Endoscopy and biopsy in gastro-esophageal reflux in infants and children. Ann Otol Rhinol Laryngol 1980; 89:443-5.

7. Benjamin B, Lines V. Endoscopy and anaesthesia in non-infective airway obstruction in children. Anaesthesia 1972; 283-91.

8. Benjamin B, Cohen D, Glasson M. Tracheomalacia in association with congenital tracheo-esophageal fistula. Surgery 1976; 79:504-8.

9. Editorial, Esophageal troubles after repairs in infancy. Lancet 1978; i:700.

10. Wailoo MP, Emery JL. The trachea in children with tracheo-esophageal fistula. Histopathology 1979; 3:329-38.

11. Emery JL, Haddadin AJ. Squamous epithelium in the respiratory tract of children with tracheo-esophageal fistula. Arch Dis Child 1971; 46:236-42.

12. Fearon B, Shortreed R. Tracheobronchial compression by congenital cardiovascular anomalies in children. Syndrome of apnea. Ann Otol Rhinol Laryngol 1963; 72:949-69.

13. Mortensson W. Congenital esophageal stenosis distal to esophageal atresia. Pediatr Radiol 1975; 3:149-51.

≈

COMPUTER TOMOGRAPHY SCANNING OF THE BRAIN

The National Institute of Neurological and Communicative Disorders and Stroke is the lead sponsor of a National Institutes of Health Consensus Development Conference on "Computer Tomography Scanning of the Brain" to be held at the National Institutes of Health November 4-6, 1981. For information contact: Dr. M. D. Walker, Director, Stroke and Trauma Program, NINCDS, Federal Bldg., Room 8A08, 7550 Wisconsin Ave., Bethesda, MD 20205, (301) 496-2581.

Ann Otol 90:1981

ABNORMAL ESOPHAGEAL MANOMETRY IN GLOBUS HYSTERICUS

TORIBIO C. FLORES, MD

FREDERICK S. CROSS, MD, PhD RICHARD D. JONES, PhD

CLEVELAND, OHIO

Globus hystericus means the "hysterical ball or lump in the throat," and is generally assumed to be of psychic origin. True dysphagia is usually absent. Twelve patients with the globus syndrome were studied at the Esophageal Motility Laboratory of the Saint Luke's Hospital of Cleveland. An organic cause for their symptomatology was ruled out by physical examination, laryngoscopy, esophagoscopy and cine-esophagograms. Ten patients showed significant elevations in esophageal resting pressures and nine had evidence of disordered motor activity in the body of the esophagus. Knowing from previous investigations that a suprasternal discomfort may be elicited from stimulation of the esophagus at different levels, we propose that the globus sensation is a referred one coming from the hypertonic and frequently incoordinated body of the esophagus.

INTRODUCTION

Globus hystericus means the "hysterical ball or lump in the throat."[1] It was first described in the Hippocratic treatises when it was regarded as a disease of menopausal women. The ancients believed that the womb was a floating organ which moved freely around the woman's body cavity and that the "lump in the throat" was caused by this organ rising into the root of the neck.[2]

The term "globus hystericus" implies that because no cause can be found for the sensation of a lump in the throat in most patients, it must have a hysterical or neurotic basis.[3] True dysphagia and weight loss are absent.

In the past, the literature has questioned the assumption that the globus sensation is purely a psychogenic phenomenon. In 1707, John Purcell[4] postulated that the sensation was due to contractions of the strap muscles of the neck pressing on the thyroid cartilage and therefore the globus symptoms were "not vain imaginations and groundless fancies, occasioned by the disturbance of the spirits of the brain, as some physicians are pleased to say, but are real sensations actually felt by the patient." Table 1[1,5,6] lists some other associated factors which have been described.

TABLE 1. OTHER REPORTED ETIOLOGICAL FACTORS ASSOCIATED WITH GLOBUS HYSTERICUS

Maxillary sinusitis
Long uvula
Enlarged lingual tonsils
Chronic pharyngitis
Osteophytes of the cervical spine
"Dry swallow"
Cricopharyngeal sphincter spasm
Goiter — hypothyroidism
Hiatus hernia — acid reflux
Gastroduodenal and biliary lesions
Rectal polyps

Globus hystericus represents approximately 3% of all adult patients seen by an otolaryngologist.[1] This study was interesting because of the frequency with which one sees that patient who does not grossly display a hysterical personality and who seeks treatment for a sensation so vivid and so real, and resents the physician's suggestion that "there is nothing."

It was the objective of this study to attempt a physiological explanation for the globus sensation using esophageal manometry.

PATIENTS AND METHODS

Patients. Twelve patients, ten females and two males, were studied at the Esophageal Motility Laboratory of Saint Luke's Hospital of Cleveland. All patients had been seen by at least one other otolaryngologist in the community, but despite reassurance the globus sensation had persisted. The patients' symptoms had been present from 1 to 14 months. Patient ages ranged from 20 to 73 years. Of the patients 67% were between 40 and 60 years of age (mean of 49 years).

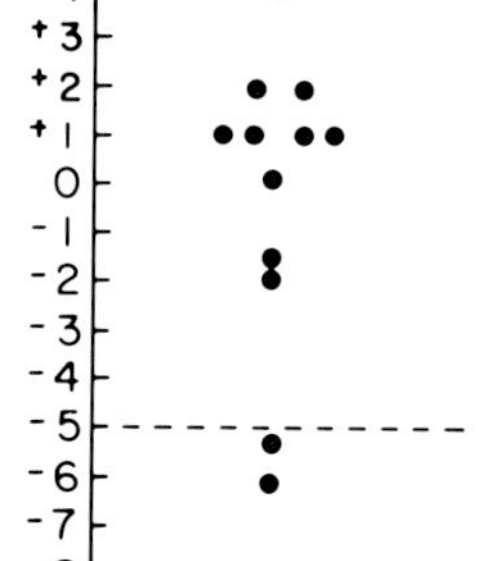

Fig. 1. Average end expiratory resting pressures in mm Hg in body of esophagus for 12 globus patients studied. Dotted line - upper limit of normal.

From the Divisions of Otolaryngology, Thoracic and Cardiovascular Surgery and Surgical Research, Department of Surgery, Saint Luke's Hospital, Cleveland.

Presented at the meeting of the American Broncho-Esophagological Association, Vancouver, British Columbia, May 11-12, 1981.

REPRINTS — Toribio C. Flores, MD, Department of Otolaryngology and Communicative Disorders, Cleveland Clinic Foundation, 9500 Euclid Avenue, Cleveland, OH 44106.

TABLE 2. SUMMARY OF ESOPHAGEAL MOTILITY STUDY

Patient	Age (yr)	Sex	Duration of Symptoms (mo)	Cricopharyngeal Resting Pressures (N:8-50 mm Hg)	Mean Resting Pressures of Body of Esophagus (mm Hg)	Motor Change in Body of Esophagus
1	21	F	2	10	−6.0	Normal*
2	35	F	3	11	+0.1	Normal
3	73	M	12	13	+1.0	DMA, PRv lower 2/3
4	48	F	4	19	+1.0	Normal
5	52	F	1	9	−2.0	DMA, PRv lower 2/3
6	45	F	14	18	+4.0	DMA, PRv entire length
7	53	F	4	15	−5.0	DMA, PRv entire length
8	55	F	3	10	+1.0	DMA, PRv entire length
9	53	F	7	16	+2.0	DMA, PrV entire length
10	55	F	11	16 (Premature contraction)	+0.6	DMA, PRv entire length gastric reflux
11	22	F	3	22	−0.6	DMA, PRv middle 3rd
12	46	M	8	31	+2.0	DMA, PRv lower 2/3 gastric reflux

*Normal - Over 80% of contractions are peristaltic, no spontaneous activity.

DMA - Disordered motor activity (spontaneous, simultaneous, repetitive waves); P - Presence of peristalsis; R - G-e sphincter relaxes, r - Poor or no relaxation; V - Vigorous motor activity, waves over 50 mm Hg; v - Low amplitude waves.

Methods. Physical examinations, laryngoscopies (indirect and/or direct), esophagoscopies and cineesophagograms were performed to exclude an organic lesion.

An assembly of three open-tipped polyethylene catheters spaced 5 cm apart were swallowed. Each catheter had an internal diameter of 0.76 mm, and was continuously perfused at 0.4 ml/minute. Pressure changes were transmitted to external Statham P23Db transducers, and their outputs were amplified and recorded with a Honeywell oscillograph. Resting and deglutitive responses were recorded.

RESULTS

Resting Pressures. Figure 1 is a scatter of the mean resting (end expiratory) pressures in the body of the esophagus. Like intrapleural pressures, normal resting pressures in the body of the esophagus are subatmospheric with a normal upper limit of −5 mm Hg. Ten out of the 12 patients had abnormally high resting pressures ranging from −2 to +4 mm Hg with a mean of +1.1 mm Hg. Resting pressures of the cricopharyngeal sphincter were within normal limits (Table 2). Two patients had evidence of gastroesophageal reflux (Fig. 3).

Deglutition. The act of swallowing normally initiates sequential and coordinated pressure changes in the esophagus (Fig. 2). Nine of the 12 patients showed evidence of neuromuscular incoordination which was seen as spontaneous activity with simul-

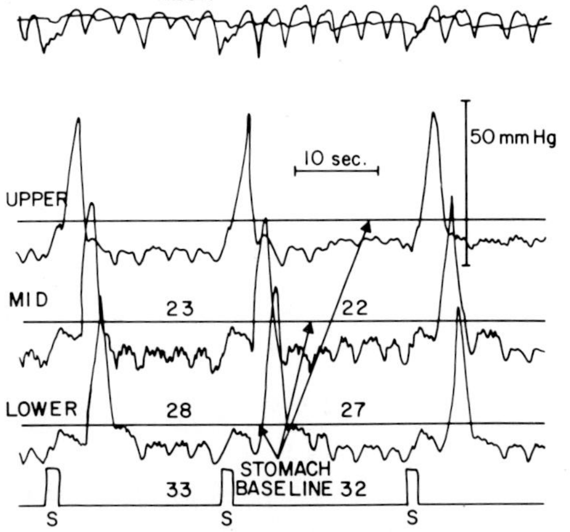

Fig. 2. Normal deglutition study. Numbers represent distance (cm) from incisors. Water swallows (S) initiate a coordinated and sequential passage of peaked peristaltic waves in the midesophagus.

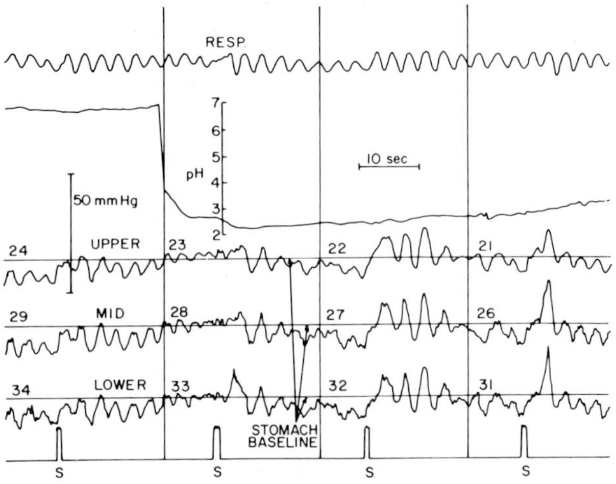

Fig. 3. Several water swallows in the body of the esophagus. Note low amplitude, simultaneous and repetitive activity with deglutition. Note sudden reflux of acid (pH graph) to lower esophagus and poor acid clearing on subsequent swallows.

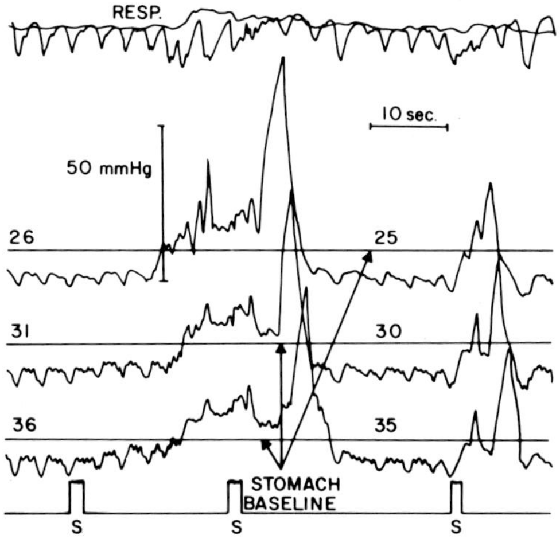

Fig. 4. Disordered motor activity in response to three water swallows in the midesophagus. Note failed peristaltic wave with first swallow and simultaneous and repetitive response with last trial.

taneous and repetitive contractions mostly of low amplitude in the body of the esophagus (Figs. 3-5). This involved the lower two thirds in four patients and the entire length of the esophagus in five.

One of the two patients who had gastric reflux had evidence of dysfunction at the pharyngoesophageal junction seen as premature contraction of the cricopharyngeal sphincter (Fig. 6).

DISCUSSION

Intraluminal pressure studies at the apparent site of the globus sensation, ie, the cricopharyngeal level had been investigated previously but the data presented is contradictory. Caldarelli et al concluded that the globus sensation was not related to cricopharyngeal spasm as he even found cricopharyngeal sphincter pressures even less than his controls.[7] In contrast, Watson and Sullivan said that

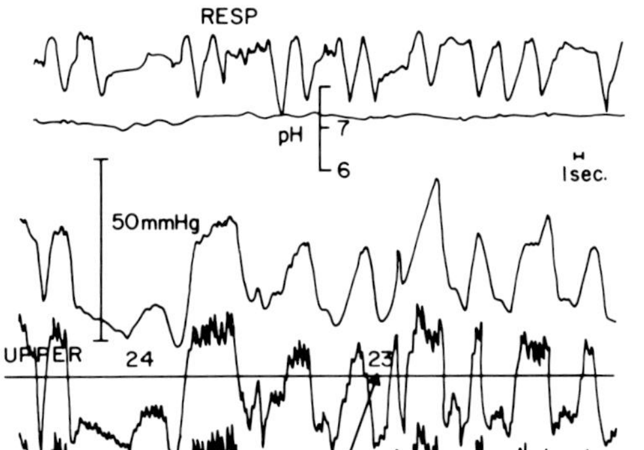

Fig. 5. Disordered motor activity showing simultaneous and repetitive contractions of varying amplitude and duration. Note markedly elevated resting pressures.

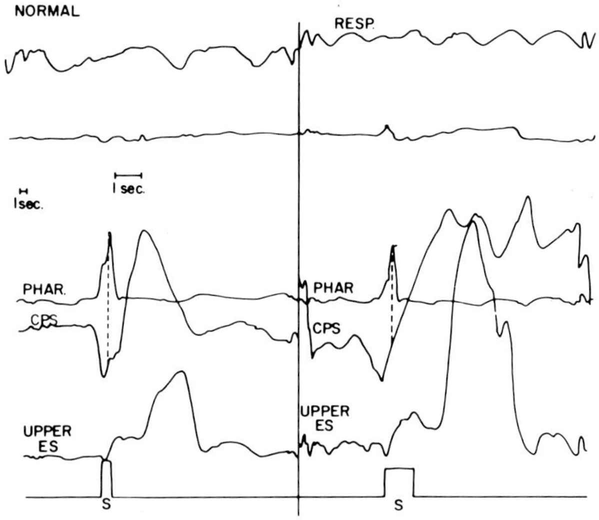

Fig. 6. To the left is a normal response at the pharyngoesophageal junction. The pharyngeal motor wave (PHAR) is coordinated with cricopharyngeal sphincter (CPS) relaxation. Premature cricopharyngeal contraction is seen on the right tracing. PHAR arrives at the CPS as it starts to contract.

"The hypertonicity of the cricopharyngeal sphincter is a cause of the globus sensation."[3] Our data fails to show any elevations in cricopharyngeal pressures (Table 1).

As shown by Nagler and Spiro, intermittent nonperistaltic motor responses in the esophagus may be associated with emotional stress.[8] However, to the best of our knowledge, no one has yet described abnormal motility changes in the body of the esophagus in patients with the sole complaint of a globus sensation.

Our ignorance of the precise mechanism of the swallowing reflex makes it difficult to suggest the pathogenesis in this condition. Some central modification from emotion must cause a derangement in neural control. The absence of abnormal manometric findings in two of our patients may be due to the intermittence of symptoms seen in this disorder.

The distribution of sensory and motor fibers to the upper foregut is very rich and arises from branches of the glossopharyngeal, vagus, sympathetic and phrenic nerves. It is known that the proximal foregut, which includes the pharynx and the cervical esophagus, is most sensitive, and this sensitivity diminishes distally. Clinical experience in other disorders, such as in diffuse esophageal spasm and hiatus hernia, recognizes that symptoms may be referred from lesions situated at more distal sites.[1,9] Experimentally, Jones[10] and Kramer and Hollander[11] showed that a suprasternal choking or pressure discomfort can be elicited by inflating balloons at different levels of the esophagus.

It may thus be assumed that the globus sensation experienced by our patients who showed abnormal esophageal manometric findings was a referred one coming from the hypertonic and incoordinated body of the esophagus.

In summary, esophageal motility studies in 12 patients with globus hystericus showed abnormally high resting pressures in the body of the esophagus in ten (83%). Nine (75%) had evidence of disordered motor activity.

CONCLUSION

Our studies are in agreement with John Purcell's statement 270 years ago that the globus symptoms are "not vain imaginations and groundless fancies . . . but are real sensations actually felt by the patient,"[1] a thought which should come to the mind of the reassuring clinician.

The sensation of a lump in the throat may be a referred one coming from a hypertonic and frequently incoordinated body of the esophagus. The etiology remains uncertain, possibly psychogenic, but appears to result in a physiologic derangement.

ACKNOWLEDGMENT — We would like to thank James Bayer and Mrs. Sylvia Kaminski for their help in the preparation of the manuscript.

REFERENCES

1. Malcomson KG. Globus hystericus vel pharyngis. J Laryngol Otol 1968; 82:219-30.

2. Pratt LW, Tobin WA, Gallagher RA. Globus hystericus-office evaluation by psychological testing with the MMPI. Laryngoscope 1976; 86:1540-51.

3. Watson WC, Sullivan SN. Hypertonicity of the cricopharyngeal sphincter: a cause of globus sensation. Lancet 1974; 2:1417-9.

4. Purcell J. A treatise of vapours or hysteric fits. 2nd ed. London, 1707.

5. Mair IWS, Schroder KE, Modalshi B, Maurer HJ. Aetiology of the globus symptom. J Laryngol Otol 1974; 88:1033-40.

6. Rigby RG. The present status of globus hystericus. Laryngoscope 1952; 62:401-5.

7. Caldarelli DD, Andrews A, Derbyshire AJ. Esophageal motility studies in globus sensation. Ann Otol Rhinol Laryngol 1970; 79:1098-100.

8. Nagler R, Spiro HM. Serial esophageal motility studies in asymptomatic young subjects. Gastroenterology 1961; 41:371-9.

9. Henderson RD, Ho CS, Davidson JW. Primary disordered motor activity of the esophagus (diffuse spasm). Ann Thorac Surg 1974; 18:327-36.

10. Jones CM. Digestive tract pain. New York: Macmillan Co, 1938.

11. Kramer P, Hollander W. Comparison of experimental esophageal pain with clinical pain of angina pectoris and esophageal disease. Gastroenterology 1955; 719-43.

≈

CASSELBERRY AWARD

The American Laryngological Association announces that it will receive essays or theses relating to the art and science of laryngology and rhinology for consideration of the Casselberry Award for 1981-82. The Award is open to physicians, interns, residents and graduate students in laryngology and rhinology in the Americas and scientists in the field in laryngology and rhinology. For information write to: William M. Trible, MD, Secretary, American Laryngological Association, 1234 19th Street, NW, Washington, DC 20036.

Ann Otol 90:1981

ESOPHAGEAL HIATAL HERNIA IN INFANTS AND CHILDREN

BLAIR FEARON, MD — ISRAEL BRAMA, MD

TORONTO, ONTARIO, CANADA

Although prior to 1950 esophageal hiatal hernia (EHH) in children was a seldom recognized entity, it has since then become well known. The symptoms in children are considerably different from those in adults. The cause of EHH is still somewhat in doubt. The term gastroesophageal reflux (GER) is often applied as a diagnosis where the diagnosis is uncertain. The authors have reviewed case histories of 56 patients admitted to the Hospital for Sick Children, Toronto, from 1972 to 1980. A comparison is made with 101 cases admitted between 1952 and 1960. It is our firm belief that all patients with symptoms of GER should be esophagoscoped for definitive diagnosis as well as for assessment of the esophagus. Because there is a high rate of respiratory complications in infants and children with GER, bronchoscopy should be carried out concurrently with the esophagoscopy. Infants with GER are at risk from the possibility of aspiration and it is possible that an unknown number of sudden infant death syndrome is due to this factor. The majority of patients with EHH can be managed by a medical regime. Those with esophageal strictures are treated by dilatation but many require surgical correction.

It is not our contention or expectation in this presentation to settle the controversy regarding the causes of esophageal hiatal hernia (EHH), and/or gastroesophageal reflux (GER), and their complications. Rather we wish to emphasize the importance of open tube esophagoscopy in the assessment and the diagnosis in infants and children with symptoms and signs secondary to GER.

Esophageal hiatal hernia is a condition in which there is a displacement of the distal esophagus and part of the stomach into the thorax through the hiatus of the diaphragm. There are three types (Fig. 1): hiatus or sliding hernia (A-C); paraesophageal or rolling hernia (D, E); congenitally short esophagus with thoracic stomach or brachyesophagus (F, G). Harrington[1] described a similar condition as dilated esophagus, but this is radiologically and clinically like a hiatal hernia. The distal esophagus is dilated and the hiatus itself is open or patulous (Fig. 2). However, the esophagogastric junction (EGJ) is in its normal position. This is now known more commonly as achalasia. In the majority of patients the cause of EHH is uncertain, but in a small proportion of patients it may be due to surgery of the esophagus or an esophageal abnormality such as congenital atresia of the esophagus, corrosive stricture, abdominal injury and following spinal surgery for scoliosis.

It was not really until the 1950s that EHH was described extensively. Indeed, in our institution prior to 1952, the condition of EHH was rarely recognized despite the fact that in a review of the records of esophageal strictures, many were considered congenital, but were obviously secondary to EHH. In fact, the first patient with this problem who came to our attention was in 1952. This was a 9-year-old boy who had been chronically ill since infancy and an earlier esophagoscopy in another center described a midthoracic stricture with multiple papillomata beyond the stricture. What were thought to be papillomata were gastric rugae. In the next eight years 101 cases of EHH were esophagoscoped and reported by the senior author.[2]

ANATOMY

The esophagus is a two-layered muscular tube extending from the pharyngeal musculature (cricopharyngeus) to the esophagogastric junction (EGJ). The proximal end is at the cricoid cartilage and the

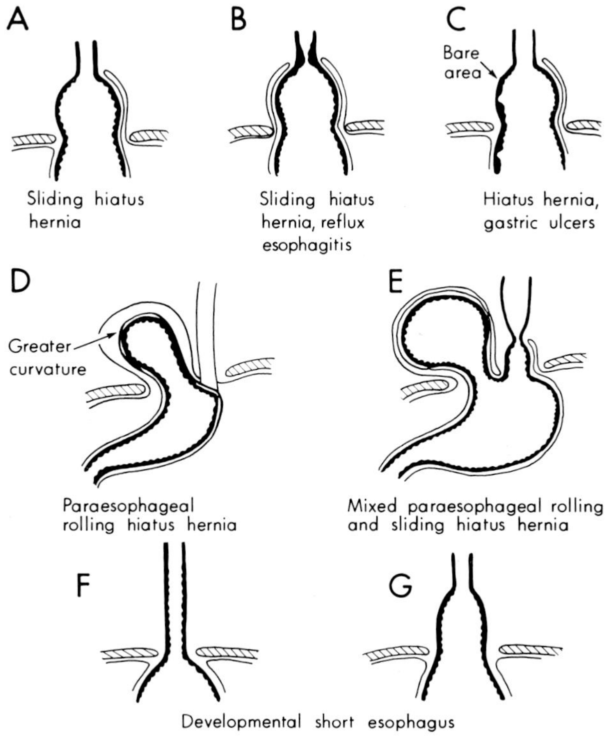

Fig. 1. Types of esophageal hiatal hernia.

From the Department of Otolaryngology, Hospital for Sick Children and the University of Toronto.

Presented at the meeting of the American Broncho-Esophagological Association, Vancouver, British Columbia, May 11-12, 1981.

REPRINTS — Blair Fearon, MD, Medical Arts Building, Suite 308, 170 St. George Street, Toronto, Ontario, Canada M5R 2M8.

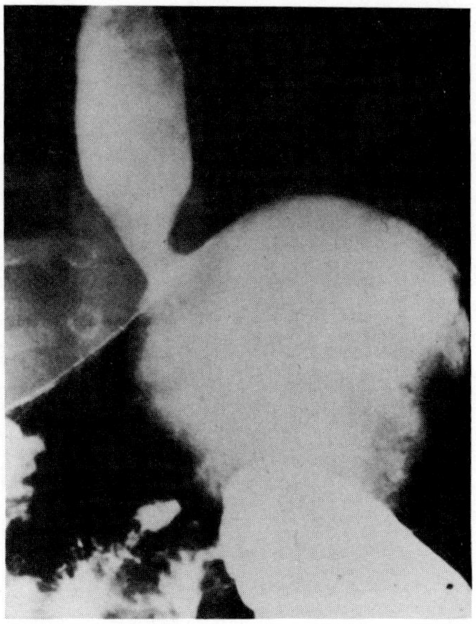

Fig. 2. Achalasia.

distal end is demarcated by a reflexion of peritoneum from the stomach to the inferior surface of the diaphragm. Hayward[3] has described it as a tube lined mainly by stratified squamous epithelium with glands in the mucosa and variable small islands near the upper end and around the whole circumference of the lower 1-2 cm. He has described the epithelium between the squamous epithelium of the esophagus and gastric epithelium as being columnar and this area being very mobile, resulting in changes in appearance with the esophageal and gastric movement. This Hayward describes as "junctional epithelium." Hayward also defines cardia as "the sphincteric lower part of the esophagus between the phreno-esophageal ligament and the gastro-esophageal junction."

PATHOLOGY

The pathology of an EHH has been described by many authors, but in particular by Harrington,[1] Allison,[4] Belsey,[5] Swyer,[6] Putney,[7] and most recently in an excellent text on the esophagus by Henderson.[8] Even so there is yet no unanimity of opinion as to what really constitutes an EHH. Recently there seems to be a tendency, in particular by internists, to employ the phrase gastroesophageal reflux in patients who have symptoms and signs of reflux of gastric contents into the esophagus without bothering to determine the cause of the GER. To the authors, GER is a symptom complex and not a diagnosis.

According to Allison,[4] there is no intrinsic stricture at the lower end of the esophagus, but rather an extrinsic stricture mechanism which in the normal person allows the passage of the food bolus in the esophagus into the stomach, but effectively prevents a reflux of gastric contents in the opposite direction by the pinchcock action of the fibers of the right crus forming the margins of the esophageal hiatus, the sharp backward angulation of the lower end of the esophagus caused by the contractions of the crura, and the acute angle of entry of the esophagus into the stomach. The efficiency of this mechanism depends on the normal arrangements of the fibers of the crus, especially posteriorly, where the muscular ring of the hiatus is weakest; the muscular tone and activity of these fibers; and the normal relationship of the cardia to the hiatus, with the EGJ lying wholly below the diaphragm. Henderson[8] describes a high pressure zone in the intra-abdominal segment of the normal esophagus preventing reflux. On the other hand, Botha[9] states that a hiatal hernia is always present when there is reflux. In contrast to a congenitally short esophagus, which is relatively rare, a hernial sac is always there when a recessed peritoneal cavity projects upwards through the hiatus in front of the stomach. Cohen and Snape[10] regard the lower esophageal incompetence as always the cause of GER. Regardless of the cause of EHH or GER, there is a failure in the mechanism that prevents GER, which results in reflux of acid-gastric-peptic secretion into the esophagus, which is ill-equipped to withstand the corrosive action, or allows stomach contents to pass up the esophagus into the airway. The occurrence of hiatal herniation in early infancy supports the view that the EHH was considered congenital in origin due to a developmental abnormality of the diaphragm. Whether the primary failure of the pinchcock is due to a congenital deficiency of the right crus at the posterior margin of the hiatus, or to a defect of the phrenoesophageal ligament, is uncertain. On the other hand, Terracol and Sweet[11] consider that many cases that are thought to be due to an EHH are, in fact, congenitally shortened esophagus with thoracic stomach. They use the term brachyesophagus for this condition.

In children we feel that there are two distinct types of problems as seen by esophagoscopy. In the majority of cases of EHH, the EGJ is relatively high above its normal position, but the hiatus itself is open, permitting the esophagoscope to pass into the abdominal stomach with little, if any, resistance (Fig. 3). In this type the reflux seems to have relatively minor effect on the esophageal mucosa. In a small number of patients, we find that the EGJ is high with the proximal stomach entrapped by the hiatus (Fig. 4). In these there is pronounced resistance in passing the esophagoscope into the stomach. It would seem that in the latter type, gastric secretions are entrapped by the hiatus and the proximal stomach, creating a much more severe effect on the esophagus and especially on the EGJ, the most vulnerable part of the esophagus.[12]

SYMPTOMS AND SIGNS

Although Henderson[8] states that the commonest symptom in adults is pain, we have found that

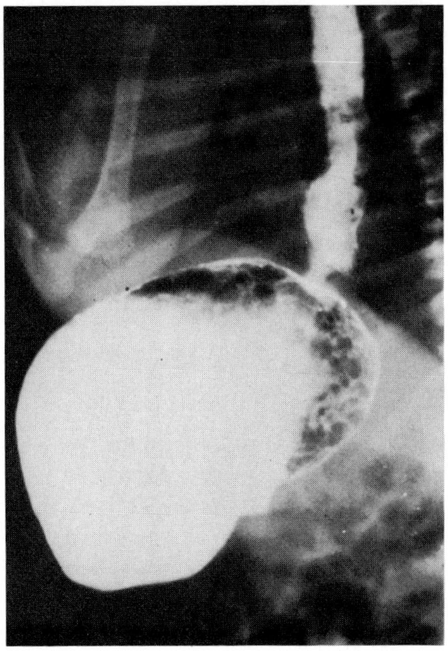

Fig. 3. High esophagogastric junction where esophagoscope passes readily into stomach.

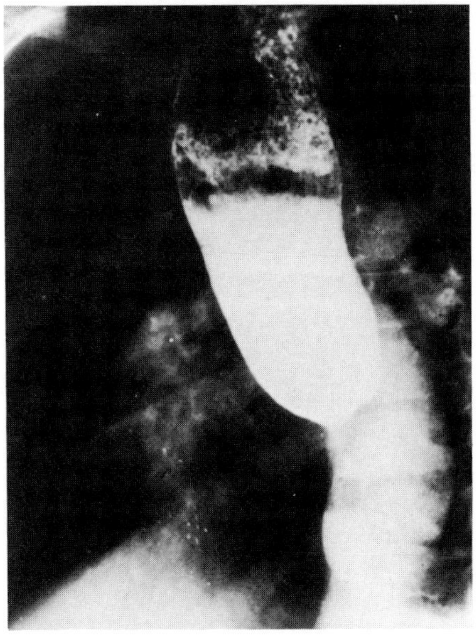

Fig. 4. Entrapment of proximal stomach by hiatus and a second fluid level caused by stricture at the EGJ.

vomiting and regurgitation are the commonest symptoms in children. Next in frequency are respiratory symptoms including severe respiratory distress and perhaps death, repeated pneumonia, continual bronchitis, and persistent asthmatoid breathing. Other findings are dysphagia, dystrophy, melena and severe anemia. The authors feel strongly that an unknown number of sudden infant death syndrome (SIDS) cases are secondary to the effects of an unrecognized EHH, either from massive aspiration of gastric contents, or from laryngospasm initiated by the effect of gastric secretion on the larynx. Even a small amount of concentrated acid in the larynx may cause fatal laryngospasm and this might not be recognized at postmortem. Indeed, in our first series reference, two patients being treated in hospital for a diagnosed EHH died suddenly from the effects of GER.

In children, the symptoms date from birth in half the patients. As recently as 1952, Thorek[13] stated that in the majority of cases of EHH in adults, symptoms begin after the age of 40. Had it been possible in many of these patients to obtain a history of their early childhood, it might have been found that they had a problem then. We have known adults with EHH to have had "feeding problems" or even strictures treated in early childhood and to have been free of symptoms until they were in their 30s or 40s.

DIAGNOSIS OF ESOPHAGEAL HIATAL HERNIA

The diagnosis of EHH is a most controversial one and the solution is far from settled. Henderson[8] states that EHH is a radiological diagnosis only, despite the fact that in 428 patients he treated surgically for reflux, the diagnosis was made radiologically in 69.4% and reflux was diagnosed only in 12.6%. Since these patients were all adults, it seems only reasonable to conclude that the radiological diagnosis in infants and children is likely to be more inexact. Whether or not reflux is always due to EHH, reflux is certainly responsible for most of the symptoms encountered.

Because this presentation is primarily on the endoscopic findings in patients with GER or EHH, it is not concerned with other adjunctive investigations. We know that there can be severe reflux determined by endoscopy in the absence of radiological findings. But needless to say, radiography is mandatory in the investigation of GER. Unfortunately, however, clinicians often accept the normal x-ray report as final, regardless of the fact that the patient has obvious evidence of reflux.

Since many patients have undiagnosed tracheobronchial symptoms that might be due to GER, it is our firm belief that all such patients should have bronchoscopy concurrent with esophagoscopy. Where the symptoms are primarily from the airway, we examine the tracheobronchial tree first and then the esophagus. When the problem is primarily esophageal, we follow the esophagoscopy by bronchoscopy.

Our endoscopic procedures are carried out under general anesthesia in an operating room which has a permanently placed image intensifier with facilities for taking radiographs. Continuous breathing endotracheal anesthesia is employed for esophagoscopy and inhalation anesthesia via bronchoscope for bronchoscopy.[14] For esophagoscopy we prefer to use the Holinger-Jackson full-lumen aspirating esophagoscope of a size suitable to the age of the pa-

TABLE 1. SIGNS AND SYMPTOMS IN THE 56 PATIENTS

Regurgitation or vomiting	38	67.8%
Respiratory complications	21	35.5%
Dysphagia	17	30.35%
Hematemesis	10	17.8%
Epigastric or retrosternal pain	9	16.0%
Failure to thrive	5	8.9%
Melena	4	7.1%
Anemia	3	5.3%
Dystrophy	3	5.3%

tient, ranging from a 4 x 30 cm for the average newborn to a 7 x 53 cm in the older teenager. The purpose of the esophagoscopy is several fold: to determine whether or not there are abnormalities in the esophageal lumen; whether or not there is GER and the degree and character of same; the status of the esophageal mucosa; and in particular, the position of the EGJ relative to the hiatus. Moreover it is important to know whether or not the hiatus itself is closed tightly, entrapping a part of the stomach above the diaphragm, or whether it is widely open allowing free and constant reflux from the stomach. Although not essential, magnification with either the proximally placed telescope or with the Hopkins telescope is most valuable especially in the recognition of the EGJ. The EGJ can be identified where there is the change from the smooth folds of the esophagus to the typical gastric rugae. Biopsy, using center-action angled cup forceps, can be carried out to supplement and verify the visual diagnosis. Biopsy also serves to identify changes in the esophagus secondary to reflux as described by Benjamin et al.[15] Once the EGJ is identified, the tip of the esophagoscope is placed at the junction and the position of this tip can be determined by fluoroscopy or by radiograph. It must be remembered that where there has been a longstanding GER, the lower esophageal mucosa may be altered to a columnar epithelium as described by Hayward.[3]

Where secondary strictures have developed, they must be treated by dilatation and the authors prefer to do the dilatation with graduated sizes of scopes.[16] Palmer has stated that in instances of severe esophagitis causing stricture and shortening of the esophagus, dilatation has proven to be not only remarkable for the relief of symptoms, but also the esophagus may lengthen to its original position.[17] We certainly can confirm that this is true in several of our patients where dilatation alone was so effective that surgical correction of the EHH was considered unnecessary. Although we have not established that the esophagus in these patients has lengthened, nonetheless we do know that they have been free from significant symptoms 25 years later.

Laryngobronchoscopy is important first of all to determine whether or not there are abnormalities of the tracheobronchial tree that are unrelated to GER. The senior author has been guilty of missing an H-tracheoesophageal fistula in a proven EHH, because he concluded that all symptoms were due to the EHH. Furthermore, it is important to establish whether or not aspiration of GER may be affecting the tracheobronchial mucosa and to what degree. Secretions are always collected for bacteriological study as well as for pathological study where indicated. The size of bronchoscopes used for various ages as well as the technique have been documented elsewhere.[14]

CASE STUDIES

To compare the current status of EHH with that reported in the 1952-1960 series, case reports on patients admitted between 1972 and 1980 were reviewed. We were greatly surprised to find that only 56 patients with EHH were admitted in this latter period, whereas approximately 300 cases were diagnosed in eight years of the earlier series. This difference can be explained in part by the fact that in the 1950s, most major problems in children throughout Ontario were referred for management to the Hospital for Sick Children. There are now many pediatric units, not only throughout the province of Ontario but even in the Toronto area itself, equipped to handle such cases. We have not included patients seen by us in other hospitals.

In the 56 patients there were 33 males and 23 females. In 27 (48%) symptoms and signs dated from birth and in 8 (14.2%) under a year. Ten (17.8%) of the patients developed esophageal strictures before the diagnosis of EHH was made. Two other patients had congenital esophageal atresia with tracheoesophageal fistula repair; two others had a repair of a congenital tracheoesophageal fistula. Two patients had surgery previously for presumed pyloric stenosis, although pyloric stenosis was not found at laparotomy. In one teenaged patient, the symptoms followed corrective surgery for a severe scoliosis.

Esophagoscopy was performed in only 33 (59%) including some that had EHH surgery. In 15 (26.7%) where the esophagus was considered normal on radiograph, the diagnosis was arrived at by esophagoscopy. The ten patients with esophageal stricture were treated by either prograde or retrograde dilatation. It has been our experience that patients with strictures prior to EHH correction require very little stricture treatment subsequent to the surgery.

In Table 1 is a list of the signs and symptoms in the 56 patients. Although the number of cases reported in this series is smaller than in our first report, the symptomatology and the complications in percentages are remarkably similar (Table 2).

A diagnostic tool, the use of radionucleotides, was used on one of our patients and this type of test may be vitally important in establishing the correct diagnosis of GER or EHH. The following is the case history of the patient in brief.

TABLE 2. SYMPTOMATOLOGY AND COMPLICATIONS OF EHH

Vomiting or regurgitation	90%
Respiratory symptoms including severe respiratory distress, repeated pneumonia, bronchitis, cough, expiratory wheeze	39%
Hematemesis	25%
Dysphagia	24%
Dystrophy	12%
Melena	12%
Severe anemia	10%
Excessive mucus	5%

A 9-year-old boy was admitted to our service with a history of recurrent stridor, choking spells, and shortness of breath, occurring mainly at night after going to bed. The complaint started several months earlier and three months prior to this admission, he was bronchoscoped at another hospital with negative findings. Examination showed a normal, well developed boy for his age. A barium esophagogram was described as being normal. Laryngobronchoscopy showed no abnormalities. Esophagoscopy, however, revealed the EGJ to be 3-4 cm above its normal position and there was a mild esophagitis. Our conclusion was that the patient had an episodic laryngospasm secondary to EHH reflux. He was discharged on an appropriate dose of Maxaran® (metoclopramide monohydrochloride). The patient's symptoms improved remarkably, but because he was making "unusual gurgling sounds" during his sleep he was admitted to the surgical service for another evaluation. Barium examination of the upper gastrointestinal tract was again reported as being normal. Pressure studies showed both the upper and lower esophageal sphincters to be normal. Neurological examination and radiological examination of the chest indicated no abnormalities. The patient then was fed technetium sulfur colloid and delayed films were taken. This test confirmed the original esophagoscopic diagnosis of GER from an EHH. Surgical correction was not deemed necessary and the patient has continued to do well on therapy.

MANAGEMENT OF ESOPHAGEAL HIATUS HERNIA

The primary role of the endoscopist in the management of EHH is to determine the diagnosis and to assess the status of the esophagus and, additionally, the laryngotracheobronchial complex. However, we should take the responsibility of directing the type of treatment.

Where there is pathology in the esophagus and/or tracheobronchial tree, follow-up endoscopy must not be neglected. Where there is severe secondary airway obstruction, tracheotomy should be performed and maintained until the problem is controlled. This does not necessarily mean surgical correction. Infants with GER, either from EHH or other causes, are potentially at risk from the possibility of massive aspiration or from chemical laryngospasm. Undoubtedly an unknown number of SIDS cases is due to aspiration.

The majority of patients with EHH respond to conservative measures. In time many of the infants "grow out of their symptoms," especially when they begin to stand and walk.

Medical management includes positioning, thickened feedings, antacid and other drug therapy. We have had particularly good results with the use of metoclopramide monohydrochloride. A few patients with severe strictures and brachyesophagus do remarkably well with dilatations alone. As soon as possible, we have them proceed with self-bouginage. Patients who have esophageal strictures prior to surgical correction of the EHH require very little further dilatation. Recurrence of a stricture suggests recurrence of the EHH.

In recent years in our institution, the division of general surgery has preferred the Dor-Nissen repair of EHH. The success rate has been high and seems to avoid the "gas bloat syndrome" of the Nissen fundoplication.[18]

REFERENCES

1. Harrington S. Esophageal diaphragmatic hernia. Surg Gynecol Obstet 1955; 100:277-92.

2. Fearon R, Briant D, Comet V. Esophageal hiatal hernia in children. Paper presented at Seventh Panamerican Congress of Oto-Rhino-Laryngology and Bronchoesophagology, Miami Beach, 1960:201-15.

3. Hayward J. The phreno-esophageal ligament in hiatal hernia repair. Thorax 1961; 16:41-5.

4. Allison P. Reflux esophagitis, sliding hiatal hernia and the anatomy of repair. Surg Gynecol Obstet 1951; 92:419-31.

5. Belsey R. Diaphragmatic hernia. In: Jones FA, ed. Modern trends in gastroenterology. London: Butterworths: 1952:128-78.

6. Swyer P. Partial thoracic stomach and esophageal hiatus hernia in infancy and childhood. Am J Dis Child 1955; 90:421-51.

7. Putney F. Esophagogastric incompetency. Laryngoscope 1959; 69:297-305.

8. Henderson R. The esophagus: reflux and primary motor disorders. Baltimore: Williams & Wilkins, 1980:53.

9. Botha G. The gastroesophageal junction. London: J & A Churchill, 1962.

10. Cohen S, Snape W. The pathophysiology and treatment of gastroesophageal reflux disease. Arch Intern Med 1978; 138:1399-1401.

11. Terracol F, Sweet R. Diseases of the esophagus. Philadelphia: WB Saunders, 1958:145.

12. Fearon B. Lower esophageal disease in infants and children. Ann Otol Rhinol Laryngol 1961; 70:1124-39.

13. Thorek P. Diseases of the esophagus. Philadelphia: JP Lippincott, 1952:611.

14. Fearon B. Pediatric endoscopy. Vol 3. Hagerstown: Harper Row, 1979:1-17.

15. Benjamin B, Pohl E. Bale P. Endoscopy and biopsy in gastroesophageal reflux in children. Ann Otol Rhinol Laryngol 1980; 89:443-5.

16. Cotton R, Fearon B. Esophageal strictures in infants and children. Can J Otolaryngol 1972; 1:224-29.

17. Palmer E. The hiatus hernia-esophagitis-esophageal stricture complex. Am J Med 1968; 44:566-79.

18. Ein S, Shandling B, Stephens C, Simpson J. Partial gastric wrap-around as an alternative procedure for the treatment of hiatus hernia. J Pediatr Surg 1979; 14:343-5.

Ann Otol 90:1981

DUPLICATION OF THE ESOPHAGUS

DIRAN O. MIKAELIAN, MD

JOHN J. O'KEEFE, MD SIMON SIMONIAN, MD

PHILADELPHIA, PENNSYLVANIA

Two patients with tubular esophageal duplications and the embryologic development of the esophagus are presented. The several theories in the formation of the esophageal duplications have been reviewed. As of yet, no definite explanation can be advanced for this developmental anomaly.

INTRODUCTION

Duplications of the alimentary tract are rare congenital malformations.[1-5] Even rarer are duplications of the esophagus, especially in the region of the cervical esophagus.[6] This paper presents the clinical manifestations of such patients with signs and symptoms, their diagnosis, pathology and management. Two cases are reported. Several theories as to the pathogenesis of these anomalies are discussed.

CLINICAL MANIFESTATIONS

Signs and Symptoms. There are two types of esophageal duplications: cystic and tubular.

Most patients with cystic duplications present in early childhood; however, they may remain asymptomatic and show only when complications occur. The presenting symptoms in early life may be an expanding mediastinal mass with symptoms referable to structures in the mediastinum being compressed.[2-5]

1. Vascular compression. Cyanosis and engorgement of head and neck vessels.

2. Digestive. Difficulty in swallowing, regurgitation and vomiting.

3. Respiratory. Dyspnea, obstructive emphysema and recurrent respiratory infections.

4. Mediastinitis due to rupture of duplication.

On the other hand, in tubular duplications patients complain of recurrent dysphagia, distress on swallowing and occasional chest pain. When complications occur, such as rupture, they present with all signs and symptoms of acute mediastinitis.

Radiologic studies reveal a cystic mass in the posterior mediastinum in cystic duplication. Barium swallow may show either a tubular duplication with connection to the esophageal lumen or cystic duplications with no communication. In fact, they may show cystic compression with obstruction of the esophageal lumen. Careful endoscopy may reveal the opening in tubular duplications, while cystic duplications may show esophageal obstruction.

Such patients may also have other associated congenital malformations.[2,4,7] Most of these occur in the vertebral bodies in the form of scoliosis, fusion, spina bifida anterior and hemivertebrae. Esophageal atresia distal to the duplication and various combinations of tracheoesophageal fistulas have also been reported.[7,8]

Histologically, tubular duplications have a stratified squamous epithelium similar to that of the esophagus and a submucosa containing glandular structures. There is a distinct muscular layer which often mingles with the muscular layer of the true esophagus as most tubular duplications occur in the wall of the esophagus. There is no serosa.

In cystic duplications the mucosa varies between a stratified squamous epithelium to gastric mucosa with gastric glandular elements in the submucosa. The fluid may contain gastric secretions. There is again a definite muscular layer.[4,5]

Surgery is the treatment for these anomalies. Most of the literature on this subject is found in thoracic surgery publications. However, when duplications occur in the cervical esophagus, patients may present themselves to the head and neck surgeon.

CASE REPORTS

Case 1. This is a 54-year-old male whose present illness started with fever and cough and was diagnosed as having acute pharyngitis. He was treated with Ancef®, and the fever subsided.

Three weeks following this episode, he again developed fever and chest pain with some difficulty in swallowing and was admitted to the hospital. Chest radiograph showed a widened mediastinum. A bronchoscopy was performed which revealed the tra-

From the Department of Otolaryngology, Jefferson Medical College, Philadelphia.

Presented at the meeting of the American Broncho-Esophagological Association, Vancouver, British Columbia, May 11-12, 1981.

REPRINTS — Diran O. Mikaelian, MD, Jefferson Medical College, Department of Otolaryngology, 1025 Walnut Street, Philadelphia, PA 19107.

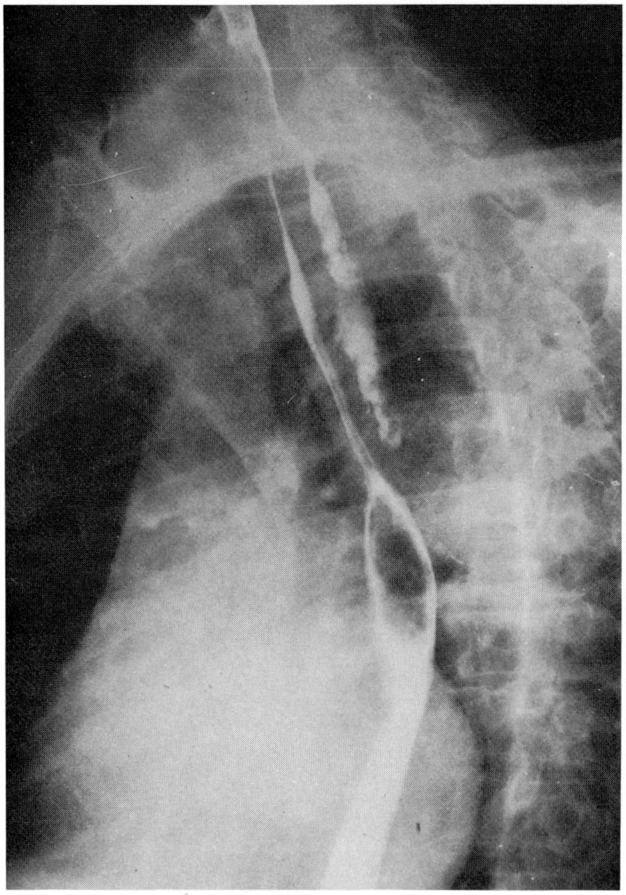

Fig. 1. Perforated esophagus with barium in mediastinum.

chea pushed forward by a retrotracheal mass. A barium swallow revealed a perforated esophagus with barium going into the posterior mediastinum (Fig. 1). Soon after, he was taken to the operating room and the mediastinal abscess was drained through a left supraclavicular approach. He was started on intravenous antibiotics and the fever subsided. He was placed on nasogastric (NG) tube feeding which was removed in three weeks because the patient started losing weight. The left supraclavicular drain was gradually withdrawn and came out subsequently by itself.

A repeat barium swallow revealed the fistula to be patent still, but there was no collection. He was observed for a period of one month when symptoms of mediastinitis recurred, and this was drained through the previous drain site. During these two hospitalizations, the patient had repeated direct laryngoscopies and esophagoscopies, and no abnormalities were noted. He was discharged from the hospital and was being followed on an outpatient basis. During this time, the patient decided to have a second opinion.

On physical examination, the drain tube in the left supraclavicular area was the only positive finding, with some fullness in the left lower part of the neck. Mirror laryngoscopy was normal.

His previously done radiographs were obtained which revealed a conical outpouching from the cervical esophagus on the left side. This reached the upper mediastinum (Fig. 2).

Under general intubation anesthesia, the patient underwent an esophagoscopy using the Jesberg esophagoscope. No abnormalities were noted. With the use of the Dedo microlaryngoscope, the upper part of the cervical esophagus was entered just beyond the cricopharyngeus. At this time, a second lumen was seen in the wall of the cervical esophagus on the left side next to its normal lumen (Fig. 3). The opening of this tract was almost as wide as the normal esophagus, and the mucous membrane cover-

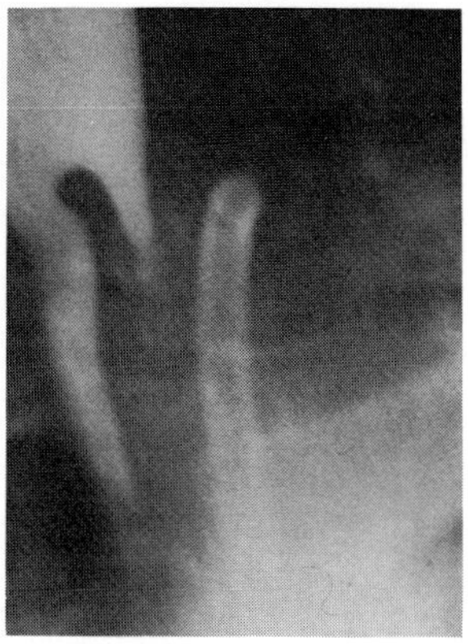

Fig. 2. Tubular duplication, partial, of cervical esophagus.

ing it appeared the same as that of the esophagus. The tract came to a tapered end and was 5 cm long as measured with a filiform catheter. Subsequent radiologic studies failed to demonstrate a second opening in the distal segment of the esophagus.

Under general anesthesia, a left neck exploration was performed. During the dissection, a lot of fibrosis was encountered around the cervical esophagus. An assistant introduced a short, wide Jesberg scope and the fistulous tract was visualized. A No. 12 Jackson bougie was inserted gently in the lumen of the double esophagus and palpated in the neck wound. Dissection was then incorporated in the wall of the esophagus. The tract extended to the superior mediastinum and came to a blind end. It was completely removed. This left dehiscence in the esophageal wall 6.5 cm long which was closed in two layers using 3.0 chromic catgut sutures. The esophagoscope was withdrawn. The patient was maintained on NG tube feeding for ten days. After a negative fistula test, he was started on oral feedings. Barium swallow done three months later failed to show any more tracts, and the patient has remained asymptomatic since.

Light microscope study of the removed specimen revealed a tract covered with stratified squamous epithelium with subepithelial fibrosis and chronic inflammatory changes. Esophageal glandular elements and a muscular wall could be identified (Fig. 4).

Case 2. A 55-year-old male presented himself with difficulty on swallowing of three months' duration. He had enjoyed a healthy life. Head and neck examination was normal, and chest radiograph was normal. He was advised to stop drinking all types of alcoholic beverages and placed on a bland diet. However, his symptoms persisted and subsequently he underwent a barium

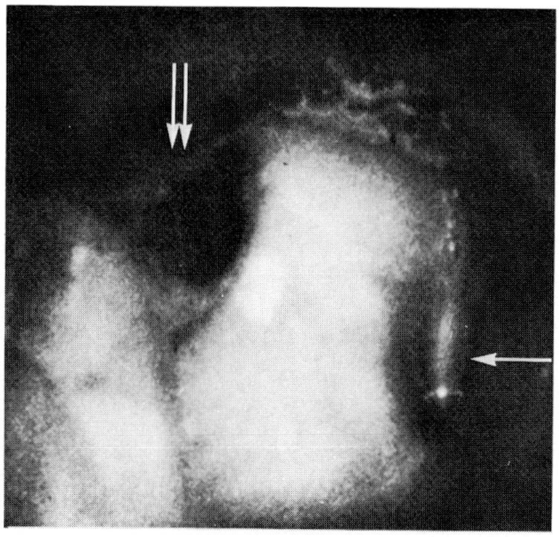

Fig. 3. Two openings in the lumen of the cervical esophagus. Bougie on right in main lumen (arrow). Opening on left is duplicated esophagus (double arrow).

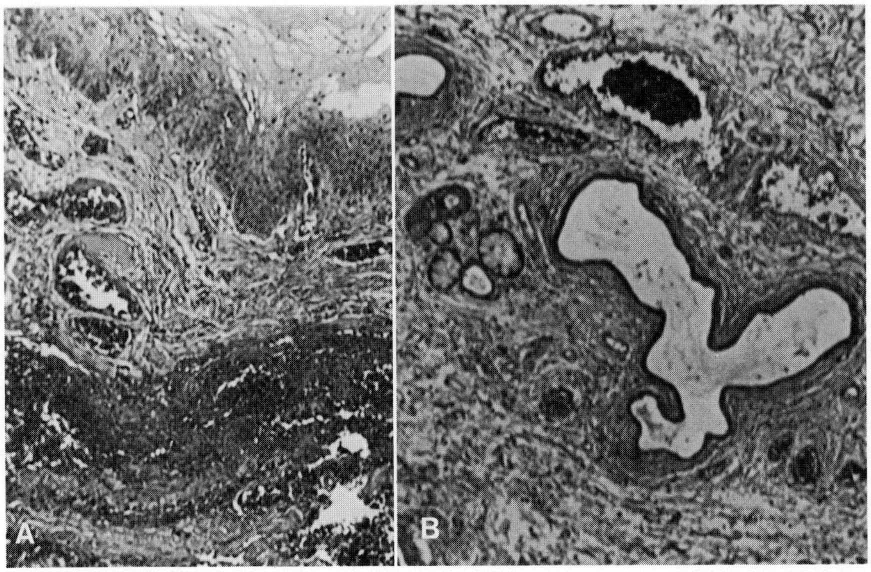

Fig. 4. A) Light microscopy reveals stratified squamous epithelium with submucosa and muscular layer in duplicated esophagus (H & E, x25). B) Glandular structures in submucosa (H & E, x40).

swallow which revealed a double esophagus in the thoracic segment with narrowing of the proximal esophagus (Fig. 5).

At esophagoscopy a moderate stenosis was seen in the proximal esophagus; however, a No. 7 Jackson scope could be introduced. Passing through the narrow segment, a larger lumen was seen and two openings in the lumen of the esophagus were identified. No attempts were made to pass the scope into the secondary openings.

Postoperatively the patient did well. He was advised as to the nature of the disease and managed only by dietary advice and chewing habits. He has done very well since and is minimally symptomatic with occasional difficulty on swallowing. No surgical correction was advised.

DISCUSSION

The terminology of alimentary tract duplications is indeed confusing.[9] They have been commonly called enterogenous cysts, enteric cysts, gastroenteric cysts, etc. In most of the alimentary mediastinal cysts, no communication exists with the lumen of the esophagus.

In contrast to cystic anomalies, most tubular reduplications have been found to communicate with the esophageal lumen and are intimately related to the wall of the true esophagus. These can occur in different combinations (Fig. 6).

To understand this anomaly, a brief summary of the embryology of the esophagus is in order.[10,11] At around the age of 2 weeks, the entodermal epithelium has started to form the primordial buds for the future formation of the esophagus and tracheobronchial tree. At the age of 4 weeks, a definite groove appears separating the trachea from the esophagus. There is no actual lumen at this time. By five weeks, the esophagus elongates and the epithelial cells become two-layered. By the seventh week, vacuolization sets in and starts the formation of the primitive lumen. With the gradual development of the embryo, these vacuoles coalesce and form the definitive lumen of the esophagus on the human fetus.

Several theories have been advanced to explain the origin of the esophageal duplications:

1. Errors of revacuolization. This theory was advanced originally by Keith[12] and later supported and elaborated upon by Bremer.[13] During the embryonic development of the esophageal lumen, errors or malfusions occur in the esophageal vacuoles with persistence of the latter resulting in cystic malformations. However, this theory fails to explain tubular duplications.

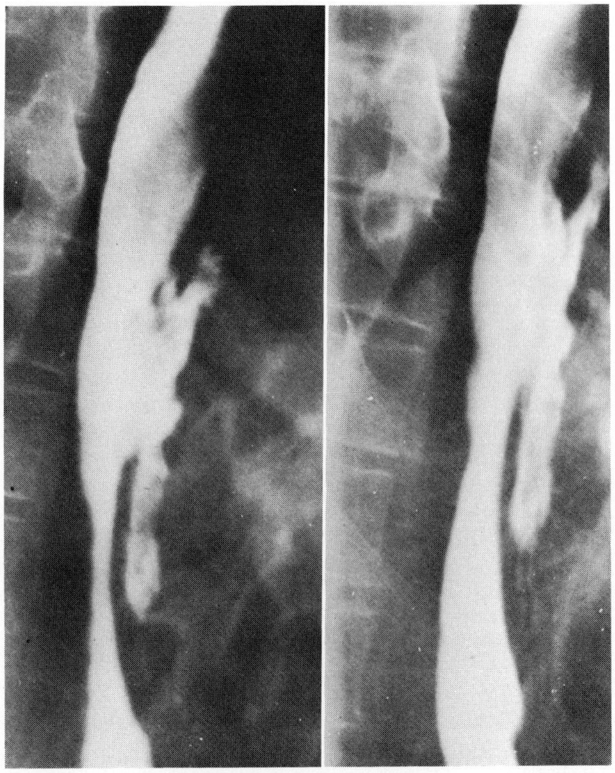

Fig. 5. Tubular duplication of thoracic esophagus. Left oblique view.

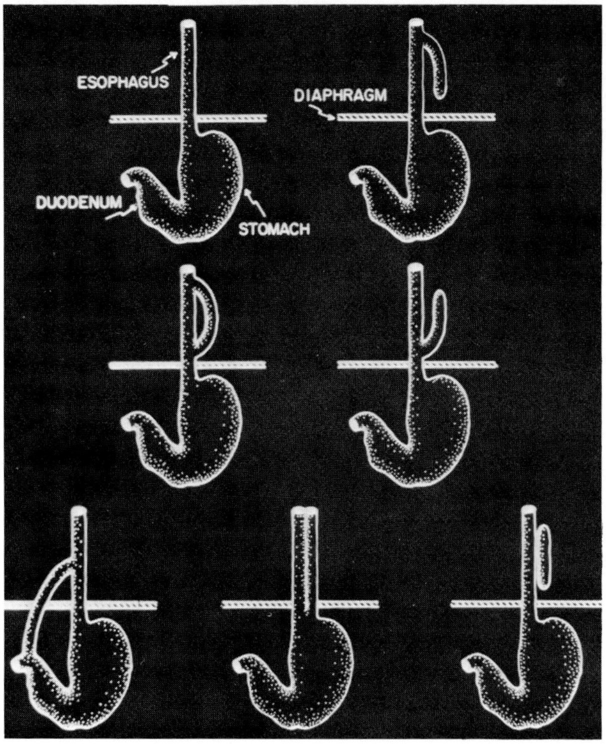

Fig. 6. Types of tubular esophageal duplications reported in the literature.

2. Attempts of twinning. This theory, advanced by Ravitch,[14] does not hold well because duplication of other structures in and around the esophagus has not been encountered.

3. Alimentary diverticulae. Lewis and Thyng[15] advanced the theory that most duplications arose from alimentary tract diverticulae. Such diverticulae are commonly found in animals, eg, pigs, rabbits, etc, but have been rarely described in human fetuses. They are even rarer in the region of the esophagus. This theory also does not explain cystic duplications.

4. Notochordal theory of Veeneklass.[16] In 1952, Veeneklass advanced the theory that during embryonic life, the notochord is adjacent to the primordium of the esophagus and that during normal growth the notochord separates from the esophagus. In errors of development, the notochord does not separate from the primitive esophagus and with further growth, that portion of the esophagus separates from the rest of the developing esophagus and thus forms a cyst between the vertebral bodies and the normal esophagus. As mentioned earlier, such patients have abnormalities of the vertebral bodies.

As of yet, there is no clear cut explanation for duplications of the esophagus. A review of the literature failed to disclose an experimental animal model.

The present authors believe that the two types of duplications, ie, cystic and tubular, have separate origins in their development. None of the above theories satisfactorily explains the pathogenesis of these errors of development. The authors themselves have no theories of their own to offer.

REFERENCES

1. Frank CR, Paul LW. Congenital reduplication of the esophagus. Radiology 1949; 53:417-9.

2. Basu R, Forshall I, Rickham PP. Duplication of the alimentary tract. Br J Surg 1960; 47:477-84.

3. Borrie J. Duplication of the esophagus. Br J Surg 1961; 48:611-9.

4. Ladd WE, Scott HW Jr. Esophageal duplications or mediastinal cysts of enteric origin. Surgery 1944; 16:815-35.

5. Langston HT, Tuttle WM, Patton TB. Esophageal duplications. Arch Surg 1950; 61:949-56.

6. Gans SL, Lackey AD, Zuckerbraun L. Duplications of the cervical esophagus in infants and children. Surgery 1968; 63: 849-52.

7. Hemalatha V, Batcup G, Brereton RJ, Spitz L. Intrathoracic foregut cyst (foregut duplication) associated with esophageal atresia. J Pediatr Surg 1980; 15:178-80.

8. O'Connell DJ, Kelleher J. Congenital intrathoracic bronchopulmonay foregut malformations in childhood. J Can Assoc Radiol 1979; 30:103-8.

9. Sieber WK. Alimentary tract duplications. Arch Surg 1956; 73:383-92.

10. Arey LB. Developmental anatomy. 7th ed, rev. Philadelphia: WB Saunders, 1974:245-7.

11. Payne SW, Olson MA. The esophagus. Philadelphia: Lea and Febiger, 1974:1-3.

12. Keith A. Human embryology and morphology. Baltimore: William Wood, 1933.

13. Bremer JL. Diverticula and duplications of the intestinal tract. Arch Pathol 1944; 38:132-40.

14. Ravitch MM. Hind-gut duplication — doubling of colon and genital urinary tracts. Ann Surg 1953; 137:588-601.

15. Lewis FT, Thyng FW. Regular occurrence of intestinal diverticula in embryos of the pig, rabbit and man. Am J Anat 1907; 7:505-19.

16. Veeneklass GMH. Pathogenesis of intrathoracic gastrogenic cysts. Am J Dis Child 1952; 83:500-7.

Ann Otol 90:1981

HORSERADISH PEROXIDASE STUDIES IN ANIMALS WITH NEUROMUSCULAR TRANSPOSITIONS

G. DAVID NEAL, MD
DWIGHT SUTTON, PhD
GREGORY DUNCAN, BS
CHARLES W. CUMMINGS, MD
SEATTLE, WASHINGTON

Horseradish peroxidase (HRP) is used to trace axonal connections from the motor end-plate to the driving neuron. This technique has confirmed that the neurons activating the sternothyroid muscle are located in the cervical spinal cord, while those controlling the posterior cricoarytenoid (PCA) are found in the nucleus ambiguus ipsilaterally. Eight rabbits underwent a sternothyroid ansa pedicle implantation to the PCA at the time of sectioning the recurrent laryngeal nerve ipsilaterally. After two months, four of these animals received HRP injections into the previously implanted PCA. Brainstem staining HRP did not reveal any retrograde transport to the motor neurons that were known to control the sternothyroid. Possible reasons for the failure of retrograde transport are discussed.

INTRODUCTION

One of the more vexing problems in otolaryngology remains vocal cord paralysis. This is frequently idiopathic, but may result from surgical, traumatic or neoplastic causes. Following axonotmesis of a recurrent laryngeal nerve, the crossed regeneration of fibers to abductors and adductors will leave the patient with a functionally paralyzed vocal cord in the paramedian position. If both recurrent nerves are severed, an inadequate airway results, since there is no muscle functioning to abduct the cords in inspiration. It is this situation that has inspired many to attempt to develop procedures to reinnervate the posterior cricoarytenoid (PCA) muscle.

The surgical attempts at selective reinnervation of the PCA have either involved direct implantation of the proximal end of the recurrent nerve or transposing another nerve and suturing it to the muscle fibers of the PCA.[1-3] Varying degrees of success have been reported in nearly all series and the reasons for success or failure were not clear. The best clinical results have been achieved by Tucker[4] using a neuromuscular pedicle based on a branch of the ansa cervicalis to a strap muscle. Electromyographic (EMG) work has confirmed that the omohyoid or sternothyroid muscles fire at the onset if inspiration during labored respirations induced by hypercapnea or increased airway resistance. This muscle has the added advantage that its subsequent paralysis is not noticed by the patient.

The purpose of this study was to elucidate further the mechanism of the clinical improvement after the ansa pedicle reinnervation. Our previous work in dogs had led us to believe that there were other possible reasons for abduction postsurgery than just reinnervation. Some chronic animals had apparent abduction with stressed ventilation, but were found to have the PCA replaced with fibrous tissue at autopsy. Another possibility we felt was that the scarification of the inferior constrictor muscle at the time of implantation led to tethering or neural ingrowth sufficient to provide the noted abduction.[5] We had noticed that delay between the time of denervation and implantation of pedicle was inversely related to the likelihood of success. Accordingly, we chose a model for reinnervation where all known factors would be favorable for success, ie, the method of sternothyroid implantation was performed during the same operation as the severing of the recurrent laryngeal nerve (RLN).

METHODS

All work was carried out in New Zealand white rabbits. The initial reinnervation surgery was performed at 1.5-2 kg. Animals were then maintained for eight weeks prior to evaluation.

Type 4 horseradish peroxidase (HRP) (Sigma) was used as a neuroanatomic tracer. A 0.05 ml aliquot of 30% HRP in normal saline was injected into the muscle to be studied. An amount sufficient to produce a definite brown discoloration of the muscle was used. If we wished to trace from the nerve itself, a Gelfoam® pledget soaked with 30% HRP was wrapped about the cut nerve end.

The injection of the aliquot was done transorally via a 25.4 cm long hypodermic needle fashioned from 22 gauge steel tubing, after elevation of the larynx using a pediatric Jackson laryngoscope.

Seventy-two hours following the HRP injection, the rabbits were perfused with 500 ml Ringer's lactate at 37°C to wash out as

TABLE 1. RESULTS OF HRP INJECTIONS INTO STRAP MUSCLES

Rabbit No.	*Site Injection*	*Spinal No. Cells*	*Nucleus Ambiguus*
1	Steroid thyroid	34	0
2	Steroid thyroid	19	0
3	Ansa pedicle	32	0
4	Ansa pedicle	22	0

From the Department of Otolaryngology, University of Washington, Seattle.

Presented at the meeting of the American Broncho-Esophagological Association, Vancouver, British Columbia, May 11-12, 1981.

REPRINTS — G. David Neal, MD, Department of Otolaryngology RL-30, University of Washington, Seattle, WA 98195.

TABLE 2. LABELING OF NEURONS FOLLOWING INJECTION OF PCA OF UNOPERATED ANIMALS

	Labeled Cells	
Rabbit No.	*Spinal Cord*	*Nucleus Ambiguus*
5	15	17
6	15	18
7	18	21

much blood from the brain as possible. Immediately following, they were perfused with 2% glutaraldehyde to fix the tissue in situ. The brainstem and cervical spinal cord were then removed and transferred to 20% sucrose in phosphate buffer. They were subsequently cut into 40 μ horizontal sections and reacted with H_2O_2 and trimethyl benzidine and counterstained with neutral red.

Data retrieval consisted of viewing every fifth section under phase contrast microscopy and counting the cells containing the reaction product.

RESULTS

Four rabbits were used to map the projections of the ansa cervicalis into the spinal cord. The motor neurons labeling with the HRP were found to be strongly labeled and entirely contained within the periaqueductal grey region of the anterior horn. The rostral-caudal extent of this tract was entirely confined to cervical levels 1 and 2 and did not extend into the medulla where confusion with the nuclei of the vagus was possible. There were essentially no contralateral projections. The results are summarized in Table 1. The specific mapping of each strap muscle is the topic of another article now in submission.

Four animals were used for EMG and histologic studies of their larynges after innervation. Six to eight weeks following their ansa pedicle implantation the ability to abduct the vocal cord under hypercapnic drive was again assessed. In each case, the visual appearance was that of a unilateral vocal cord paralysis. Histologically, however, the ansa pedicle was in place without muscle atrophy. There was little fibrous tissue bridging from the pharyngeal constrictor fibers to the PCA, and the muscle appeared well vascularized. The EMG potentials recorded from PCA at the time of inspiration were of low amplitude and impossible to differentiate from the transmitted firing of surrounding muscles.

The final study consisted of retrograde tracing from the left posterior cricoarytenoid to its innervating neuron. In the control (unoperated) animals, there was heavy labeling of the nucleus ambiguus ipsilaterally (Table 2). The four animals with recurrent laryngeal nerves and ipsilateral ansa pedicle implants did not show any label in either the nucleus ambiguus or the anterior horn cells of the upper spinal cord. In fact, they showed no labeled cells at all.

Conclusion. It is clear from this data that we cannot document a neural connection to the PCA eight weeks following pedicle implantation and section of the RLN. We did not expect that reinneravtion via sprouting from the RLN would be likely since the centimeter segment was removed far from the larynx. However, we did anticipate innervation either from other nearby vagal efferents or from the implanted ansa cervicalis fibers.

DISCUSSION

One cannot conclude from this data that reinnervation is not the method by which eventual return of abduction is achieved. We do not know of any studies where the time course of an axon's ability to transport HRP has been studied following transpositions such as the ansa pedicle implant. It has been possible to transport HRP across a neurorrhaphy of the peroneal nerve in rats at three months, but many of the cells did not label.[6] It is possible that we did not wait long enough for reinnervation to sufficiently establish itself for HRP transport. It is also possible that the dynamics of HRP transport are different postreinnervation such that longer than 72 hours is necessary to achieve labeling of cells in the brainstem. Finally, the experimental sample is small and random chance may have caused us to fail to find labeled cells in the implanted animals.

REFERENCES

1. Hengeres AS, Tucker HM. Restoration of the abduction in the paralyzed canine vocal cord. Arch Otolaryngol 1973; 97:247-50.

2. Sato F, Ogura JH. Functional restoration for recurrent laryngeal paralysis: an experimental study. Laryngoscope 1978; 88:855-70.

3. Iwamura S. Functioning remobilization of the paralyzed vocal cord in dogs. Arch Otolaryngol 1974; 100:122-9.

4. Tucker HM. Human laryngeal reinnervation — long term experience with the nerve muscle pedicle technique. Laryngoscope 178; 88:598-604.

5. Neal GD, Sutton D, Cummings CW. Delayed reinnervation of the unilateral vocal cord paralysis in dogs. Otolaryngol Head and Neck Surg (in press).

6. Brushart TM, Mesulam MM. Alterations in connections between muscles and anterior horn motorneurons after peripheral nerve repair. Science 1980; 208;603-5.

Ann Otol 90:1981

USE OF VIDEOTAPE IN DIAGNOSIS AND TREATMENT OF CANCER OF LARYNX

HORST R. KONRAD, MD
JOHN BUSSEN
DAN M. HOPLA, MD
FREDERICK C. GRISWOLD

SPRINGFIELD, ILLINOIS

Sophisticated endoscopic techniques coupled with new developments in medical videotaping have made this combination a clinically useful technique in the diagnosis and management of laryngeal cancer. Preoperative tapings in the physician's office and taping at laryngoscopy and biopsy allow for better assessment and permanent record of size and location of lesion, location of biopsies, and physiologic impairment of laryngeal function. All personnel participating in treatment including radiotherapists, surgeons, pathologists, radiologists, chemotherapists, and speech therapists can clearly see the lesion and contribute more usefully to decisions regarding treatment. Videotaping during and after radiotherapy and chemotherapy and after partial laryngectomy can aid in assessing response to treatment, provide a permanent record for comparison, and aid in detecting treatment failure or recurrence. Finally, these techniques aid our educational process for future physicians by permanently and objectively recording the appearance of lesions, treatment, and outcome. (The presentation included actual videotape material used in the processes described.)

The combination of modern endoscopes and videotaping techniques has given us a new tool in the objective evaluation of laryngeal lesions and their resultant effect on the airway, vocal cord, and voice function. Information obtained in this way may alter our understanding of laryngeal cancer, the natural history of disease, and the effect of treatment.

Just as CT scanning has extended our ability to evaluate cartilaginous invasion,[1,2] extension to pre-epiglottic space, and nodal metastases, videotaping gives us the best assessment of mucosal extent, airway, vocal cord motion, and proximity to nearby important anatomic structures.

From May 1979 to March 1981, we recorded 123 patients with laryngeal lesions, 97 preoperatively/postoperatively in the clinic, and 26 during direct laryngoscopy in the operating room. The technique and selected cases are presented to demonstrate the usefulness of these methods in the clinic and the operating room.

Size of airway, vocal cord mobility, and voice quality can best be evaluated in the outpatient clinic with the 90° Ward-Berci laryngoscope with concomitant voice and videorecording. No anesthesia is required in most patients. Topical anesthetic spray is useful in some patients and the rare patient who has a hyperactive gag reflex can be recorded with 5-10 mg of IV diazepam. The telescope is inserted similar to a mirror and the examiner can either view through the telescope if one uses an articulating arm, or on the television monitor.

Storz Hopkins rod telescopes (90°, 0°, and 70°) (Fig. 1) were coupled to a videocamera directly or through the Storz articulating arm. Although we used a Hitachi FP-1020 three-tube broadcast camera, recent lightweight one-tube cameras such as the Sanyo-Syn Optics, Hitachi GP-5 medical camera, or the Circon MV9270 can also be used for the purposes discussed here although with some decrease in image quality. We used a sophisticated editing system with one inch (25 mm) type C Ampex VTRs which permits complete control over film speed including still framing, but standard ¾ in (18.75 mm) videoplayers such as are used for home videorecording permit repeated evaluations of the findings and permanent recording of the data. Recordings can be done via indirect laryngoscopy in the clinic or directly in the operating room (Fig. 2).

With direct laryngoscopy, under general or topical anesthesia, extension along mucosal surfaces can be assessed and recorded. The 0° telescope gives the best view of the overall airway and the size of the lesion. By placing a calibrated marker on the lesion, size in millimeters can be directly measured. Although the 70° telescope has more angular distortion, tumor extent relative to structures such as anterior commissure, ventricles, false cord, and subglottic larynx can be measured indirectly. Biopsy sites can be recorded interoperatively using either the 0° or 70° telescope.

The recordings made serve several purposes. A permanent record of voice, size of lesion, airway, and vocal cord mobility is recorded in the clinic. Size, extent of lesion, proximity to important anatomic structures and biopsy location are recorded and measured in the operating room.

From the Division of Otolaryngology, Department of Surgery, and the Biomedical Communications Department, Southern Illinois University School of Medicine, Springfield.

Presented at the meeting of the American Broncho-Esophagological Association, Vancouver, British Columbia, May 11-12, 1980.

REPRINTS — Horst R. Konrad, MD, Department of Surgery, SIU School of Medicine, P.O. Box 3926, Springfield, IL 62708.

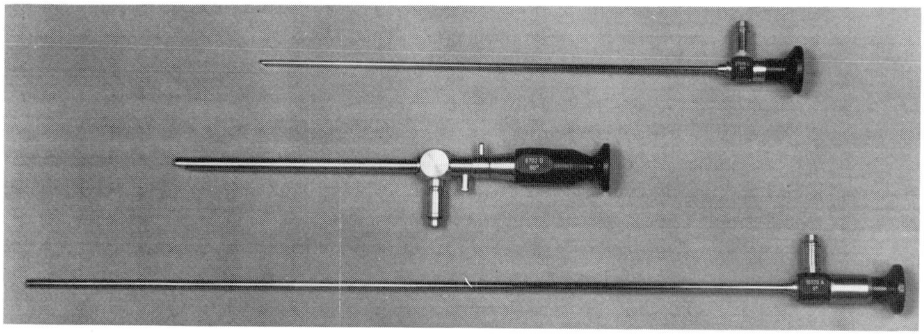

Fig. 1. Hopkins rod telescopes. Upper: 70° telescope. Middle: 90° Ward-Berci laryngoscope. Lower: 0° telescope.

This information is used in several ways.

Type and Extent of Operation. Mucosal margins of tumor can be easily evaluated and proximity to anterior commissure, vocal cord, and subglottic extension observed and measured with the use of a calibrated marker. To date, decisions regarding extent of lesion have been accurate as confirmed during definitive resection.

Adequacy of the Airway. Although adequacy of the airway can be judged without recording in most cases, a patient with borderline airway can be videotaped and the videotape replayed several times to assess the airway at leisure rather than repeating examination of the patient.

Size of Lesion for Accurate Staging. Once a permanent record which includes vocal cord motion is obtained, staging of lesion can be accomplished easily and if a question regarding stage comes up at a later date, the tape can be replayed to check the accuracy of the original decision.

Voice Quality. Voice quality is permanently recorded for reference or comparison of posttreatment voice. Such questions as comparison of voice quality for the T2 lesion treated by different methods (radiation vs partial laryngectomy) can be answered by having an impartial trained listener decide on voice quality without knowing how each patient was treated simply by listening to the voice on the audio channel of each pretreatment and posttreatment recording. We have not yet performed this study but are recording each patient's voice for this purpose.

Vocal Cord Mobility. Assessment of vocal cord mobility is easier when one can replay the record and is simplified when one can use an editor with slow motion and stop-frame capability. We have two cases where our visual observation regarding vocal cord paralysis was shown to be incorrect on subsequent examination of the videotape.

Consultation. Interdisciplinary head and neck tumor conferences with clinical radiologist, pathologist, speech pathologist, radiation therapist, and chemotherapist are vastly improved by the use of videotape. In the past, the head and neck surgeon used indirect laryngoscopy to view the lesion and then describe it to his colleagues. Now each consulting clinician can personally see the lesion. This serves to improve our colleagues' understanding of cancer of the larynx and improves the relevance of their consultation. In questionable cases, the videotape of the larynx can be sent with histological material to another institution for consultation.

Assessment of Response to Radiation Therapy or Chemotherapy. All participating physicians, including radiation therapists and chemotherapists,

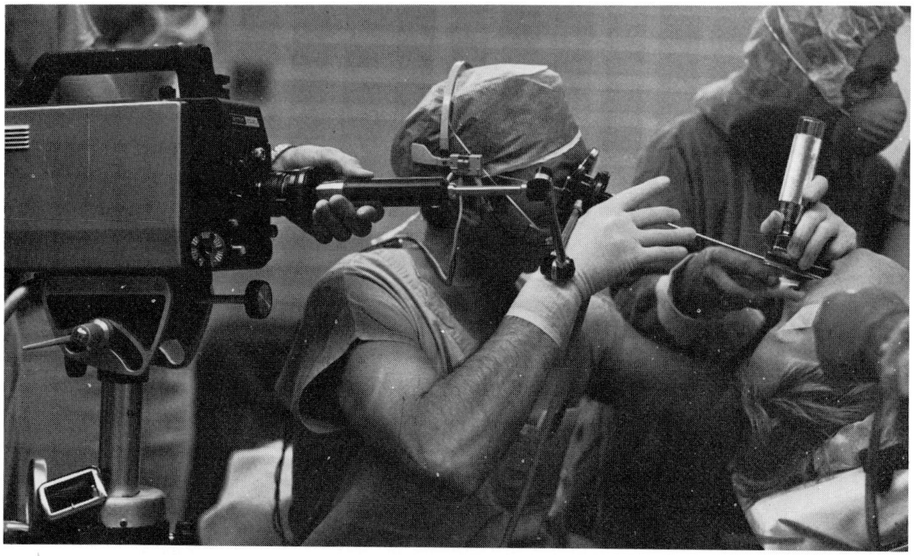

Fig. 2. The 70° telescope is used through a laryngoscope connected to a television camera via a Storz articulating arm.

can view the lesion and evaluate response to treatment. In these days of chemotherapy protocols, such evaluations can be made by a third party who does not know which arm of the study the patient is in, therefore giving a more objective assessment of response.

Patient Education. Patients with laryngeal cancer frequently have poor understanding about the anatomy, physiology, and pathology of the larynx. By showing them the recording of their own lesion, better explanation of the disease and its treatment is possible. We can also show them post-treatment results of other patients with similar lesions to obtain better informed consent.

Education of Medical Students. By videotaping many patients with laryngeal cancer, we can vastly improve the exposure to pathology for these students. In the past, their experience was limited to the patients on the service during their head and neck surgical rotation.

Education of Primary Care Physicians. Primary care physicians rotating through otolaryngology need to learn about laryngeal cancer. The graphic impact of these lesions on videotape makes a much stronger impression than a verbal description.

Education of Head and Neck Residents. Our own residents can be given a rich experience in carcinoma of the larynx early in their training program. In addition, we use videotape to observe a resident's technical skills during biopsy or endoscopic procedures. By playing back the recording, we can point out good and bad technique to the resident. The instant replay features permit much quicker feedback than recording on movie film.

By having an objective record of the lesion and simultaneous voice recordings, we can use this data to accomplish all of the above goals.

The pioneering work of Holinger[3] in cinephotography of the larynx and recent work by Ward and Berci[4] led to the use of videotape for the objective documentation of laryngeal lesions. The development of a high output light source and high quality optics permit the recording of laryngeal lesions on videotape. The flexibility to edit tape and the lower production costs (approximately one half of movies) and the instant replay features make video an attractive method for recording laryngeal lesions. Recently lightweight cameras have been adapted to endoscopes of all kinds including arthroscopes, gastrointestinal endoscopes, and laparoscopes. Videorecording and playback equipment is also becoming more available in medical centers, general hospitals, physicians' offices, and even in the home.

Although the initial cost is high ($4,000 for three endoscopes, $4,000 for the light source, and $3,000 to $60,000 for recording and editing equipment), once the recordings are made they can be used in several ways: first, for clinical decisions regarding the patient's care; later for the education of patients and primary care physicians and specialists in head and neck surgery.

REFERENCES

1. Gregor RT, Lloyd GAS, Michaels L. Computed tomography of the larynx: a clinical and pathologic study. Head Neck Surg 1981; 3:284-96.

2. Ward PH, Hanafee W, Mancuso A, Shallit J, Berci G. Evaluation of computerized tomography, cinelaryngoscopy, and laryngography in determining the extent of laryngeal disease. Ann Otol Rhinol Laryngol 1979; 88:454-6.

3. Holinger PH, Johnston KC. Bronchoscopy and endoscopic photography. Surg Clin North Am 1957; 37:1311-25.

4. Ward PH, Berci G, Calcaterra TC. Indirect endoscopic examination of the larynx and nasopharynx. In: Berci G, ed. Endoscopy. New York: Appleton-Century-Crofts, 1976: 587.

MANAGEMENT OF LARYNGOTRACHEOESOPHAGEAL CLEFT

ROBIN T. COTTON, MD J. TRACY SCHREIBER, MD

CINCINNATI, OHIO

Laryngotracheoesophageal cleft (LTE) is a rare disorder that is still associated with a high mortality. Often the mortality is associated with other coexisting severe congenital anomalies, but even in those infants in whom the LTE cleft is the only anomaly, the mortality rate is still unacceptably high. This paper explores two avenues aimed at reducing the mortality. There are two main factors responsible for the high mortality. First, the diagnosis may be difficult and hence delayed; and second, once the diagnosis is made, management reported to date does not adequately prevent aspiration of stomach contents, which is the main mechanism of the infant's death. With respect to early diagnosis, the key symptom is respiratory distress exacerbated by attempts at feeding. The key diagnostic radiological procedure is a cine-esophagram which shows a high spillover of contrast into the trachea on swallowing. The definitive diagnosis is made by endoscopy. Endoscopic evaluation can be confusing but if the anomaly is considered by the surgeon, an important maneuver at endoscopy, under general anesthesia, is to pass an endotracheal tube into the larynx. The tube stents open the edges of the cleft, which can clearly be seen while performing esophagoscopy, thus confirming the diagnosis. With respect to early management, the commonest cleft is a partial LTE cleft. Initially the airway should be maintained either by placement of an endotracheal tube or a tracheotomy. The more entensive the cleft, the more easily does the indwelling tube slip over the edge of the defect into the esophagus. In all but the mildest of clefts, gastric decompression and alimentation are required. This still allows for considerable reflux of gastric contents into the lungs, and we advocate a high total gastric section with a double gastrostomy to minimize the possibility of aspiration of stomach contents. After the infant's general condition is stabilized, definitive early surgical repair is undertaken. This paper includes a detailed case report of one patient, illustrating the above points of early diagnosis, total gastric division and early repair.

INTRODUCTION

The purpose of this report is to add a further case of laryngotracheoesophageal (LTE) cleft to the 59 cases documented in the English literature[1] and to stress that early diagnosis and management is the key factor in reducing the high mortality rate of this disorder. Total gastric division rather than gastrostomy is advocated to prevent aspiration of stomach contents.

LTE is a rare congenital anomaly that is associated with a high mortality. This reflects not only the severity of the anomaly itself, but the consequences of delayed diagnosis and treatment, and other coexistent major congenital anomalies.

The cleft involves the absence of fusion of the posterior cricoid lamina, thus creating an abnormal communication between the larynx and hypopharynx. The defect in partition may be confined to the larynx, or extend down the tracheoesophageal septum to the carina (Fig. 1). Various terms have been used to describe this defect, including LTE cleft and persistent esophagotrachea. The relative incidence of these clefts is not known, except to note that they are rare. In 1975 Cohen[2] reported on 7 cleft cases, 4 of which were confined to the larynx, and stated that his review of the literature to date revealed only 2 or possibly 3 of approximately 30 reported LTE clefts limited to the larynx. However, he pointed out that while the more extensive cleft is incompatible with life unless surgically repaired, posterior cleft limited to the larynx is an anomaly compatible with life and its occurrence, therefore, cannot be truly evaluated since with careful medical management and with growth and development of the child, symptoms of this anomaly usually subside. Thus Montgomery and Smith[3] reported a case of posterior cleft limited to the larynx diagnosed at the age of 48. There was no reported history of neonatal respiratory or feeding difficulties, though three episodes of pneumonia occurred between 1 and 15 years.

CASE REPORT

A male was born on September 15, 1977, to a 28-year-old mother after 36 weeks of pregnancy complicated only by marked polyhydramnios. Birth weight was 2,608 g and Apgar rating was 8. Because of an imperforate anus the child was transferred to a children's hospital for further care. Only mild respiratory distress was noted. Feedings were withheld because of the anticipated repair of the imperforate anus. At the time of intubation for this surgery (the day of birth) some difficulty was encountered, and laryngoscopy, bronchoscopy and esophagoscopy performed. A preliminary diagnosis of LTE cleft was made, confirmed by cinebarium swallow and a nasogastric tube inserted under direct vision. Several episodes of cyanosis occurred in the first few days of life due to both the displacement of the tracheotomy tube over the inferior margin of the cleft into the esophagus and to aspiration. Bilateral chest tubes were inserted on the fourth day of life.

On the eighth day of life the baby was transferred to Children's Hospital Medical Center, Cincinnati, for further management. Upon arrival the child's condition was stable with two chest tubes present and tracheotomy and nasogastric tubes in place.

On that day, laryngoscopy, bronchoscopy and esophagoscopy were performed. With an endotracheal tube in place, stenting

From the Department of Otolaryngology and Maxillofacial Surgery and the Division of Thoracic Cardiovascular Surgery, University of Cincinnati College of Medicine.

Presented at the meeting of the American Broncho-Esophagological Association, Vancouver, British Columbia, May 11-12, 1981.

REPRINTS — Robin T. Cotton, MD, Dept. of Otolaryngology, Children's Hospital Medical Center, Elland Avenue, Cincinnati, OH 45229.

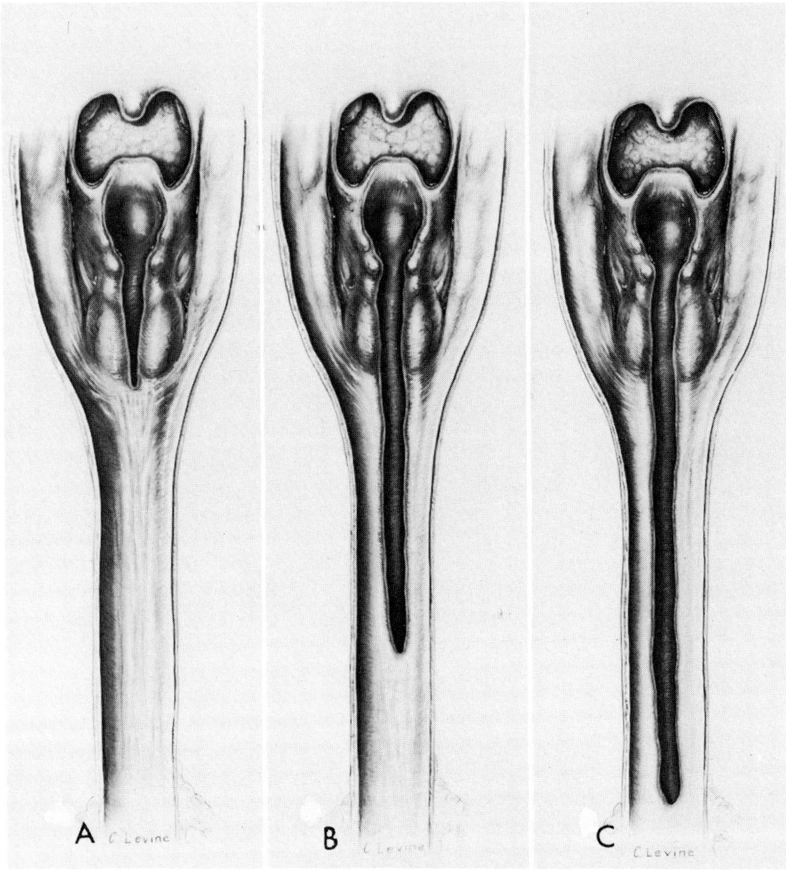

Fig. 1. A) Cleft larynx. B) LTE cleft (partial). C) LTE cleft (complete).

open the margins of the cleft, the diagnosis of LTE cleft was readily confirmed. Without the endotracheal tube in place the margins of the cleft readily came together, and it was easy to appreciate how easily the diagnosis could be missed. Using the measuring technique described by Fearon and Whalen[4] the cleft extended 3 cm below the level of the vocal cords. Above the carina there were 2.25 cm of intact wall between trachea and esophagus (Fig. 1B). The total length of the trachea was 5.25 cm and the tracheotomy entered the trachea a few millimeters below the inferior margin of the cleft. With the diagnosis confirmed, a high gastric division with double gastrostomy was performed (Fig. 2) preserving the innervation and vascular supply to the two segments of stomach. The stomach segments were closed with surgical staples. The upper gastrostomy tube was solely for drainage purposes, while the lower was for feedings. Following this maneuver, the danger of aspiration was much reduced over the conventional gastrostomy. The chest tubes were removed the following day, and on September 26, 1977, the AP chest radiograph was reported as normal, apart from the presence of a tracheotomy tube.

At this point, it was felt the baby was out of any immediate life-threatening situation and that some weight gain would be appropriate prior to definitive repair of the cleft. Stabilization of the tracheotomy tube, however, was a problem, and the baby had several episodes of respiratory distress and cyanosis caused by the tracheotomy tube slipping through the cleft into the esophagus. A variety of tracheotomy tubes of various lengths and different consistencies were tried, but the problem recurred. Definitive repair was then performed on October 19, 1977.

General anesthesia was induced through the tracheotomy tube and continued via a 3.5 mm Portex® endotracheal tube. The neck and chest area was prepped in the event a thoracotomy might be necessary, but the intention was to repair the cleft through a cervical approach. Via an incision along the anterior border of sternocleidomastoid muscle (Fig. 3A), the major vessels of the neck were dissected and retracted laterally. A posterolateral hypopharyngotomy and upper esophagotomy were performed (Fig. 3B) exposing the cleft (Figs. 3C and 4C). With some upward traction the inferior margins of the cleft could be elevated from the mediastinum into the surgical area. The arytenoid prominences could be seen.

Two flaps of mucosa were elevated from the esophagus (Figs. 3D and 4D) to create a two-layer closure (Figs. 3E, F and 4E). No attempt was made at interarytenoid closure for fear of creating a supraglottic stenosis. The hypopharyngotomy and esophagotomy were closed in two layers (Fig. 4F), followed by the neck wound, and a drain left in place.

Postoperatively the child progressed well. A barium swallow performed on November 1, 1977, identified some pharyngonasal reflux, no tracheoesophageal fistula, and a minimal amount of contrast material aspirated into the trachea. Endoscopy was performed on December 10, 1977, at which time the pertinent findings were right vocal cord paresis, normal left cord mobility; tracheomalacia; intact tracheoesophageal septum, and normal esophagus.

We felt in no hurry at this point to perform any further restoration surgery and the patient was discharged home on tracheotomy and gastrostomy care and sham feedings. Three episodes of pneumonia occurred from 2 to 14 months of age, since which time there have been no pulmonary problems.

The tracheotomy was removed on November 8, 1978; reanastomosis of the stomach was performed on October 1, 1979; barium swallow on May 29, 1980, was normal, and the gastrostomy removed. The patient's present weight is 13.5 kg (25th percentile) and height is 95 cm (50th percentile). He is taking all feeding by mouth without difficulty.

DISCUSSION

Richter[5] is credited with the first diagnosis of this anomaly in 1792 though, as no autopsy was per-

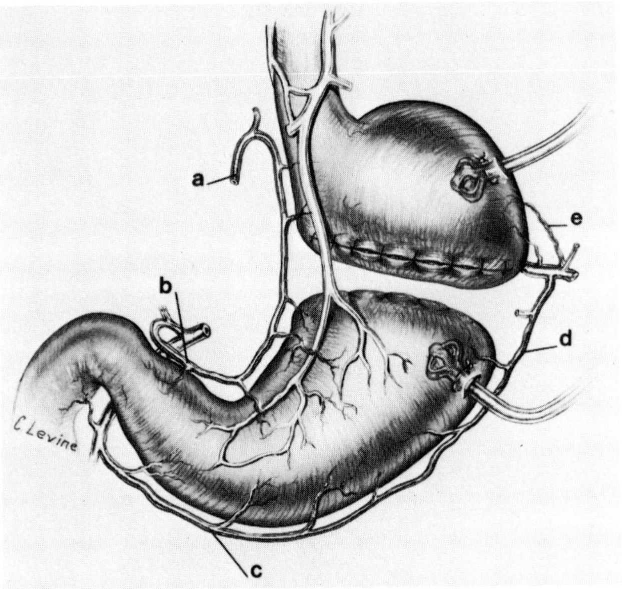

Fig. 2. Total gastric division with preservation of neurovascular supply and double gastrostomy. Arteries: a - left gastric artery; b - right gastric artery; c - right gastroepiploic artery; d - left gastroepiploic artery; e - short gastric artery.

formed, the case is not verified. Finlay[6] described the second case in 1949, and the first successful surgical repair was reported in 1955.[7] In all, 59 cases have been documented in the English literature at last review.[1] There is an extensive European literature on this subject however. The mortality remains high, in part due to coexistent major anomalies such as tracheoesophageal fistulas and/or esophageal atresia or cardiovascular and pulmonary defects. The embryology and histopathology has been extensively reviewed in the literature.[1,2]

The clinical presentation is that of *respiratory distress*, *feeding problems*, and *repeated aspiration*. It is important to note that in this case report the first feeding was withheld because of the imperforate anus, and the diagnosis was made prior to any feeding. The symptomatic severity is likely to be proportionate to the extent of the cleft, and small clefts may remain asymptomatic for a long period of time.[3] The diagnosis is made by careful consideration of the history, an awareness of the anomaly, radiographic studies and endoscopy.

In the maternal history, polyhydramnios is commonly mentioned in the literature. Symptoms of respiratory and feeding problems in the neonate (Table 1) will lead the astute physician to consider the anomaly and proceed with radiographic and endoscopic evaluation.

A cine-esophagram will show spillover of contrast medium into the trachea, but may be negative unless carefully performed.[2] The radiologist should be alerted to the possibility of multiple tracheoesopha-

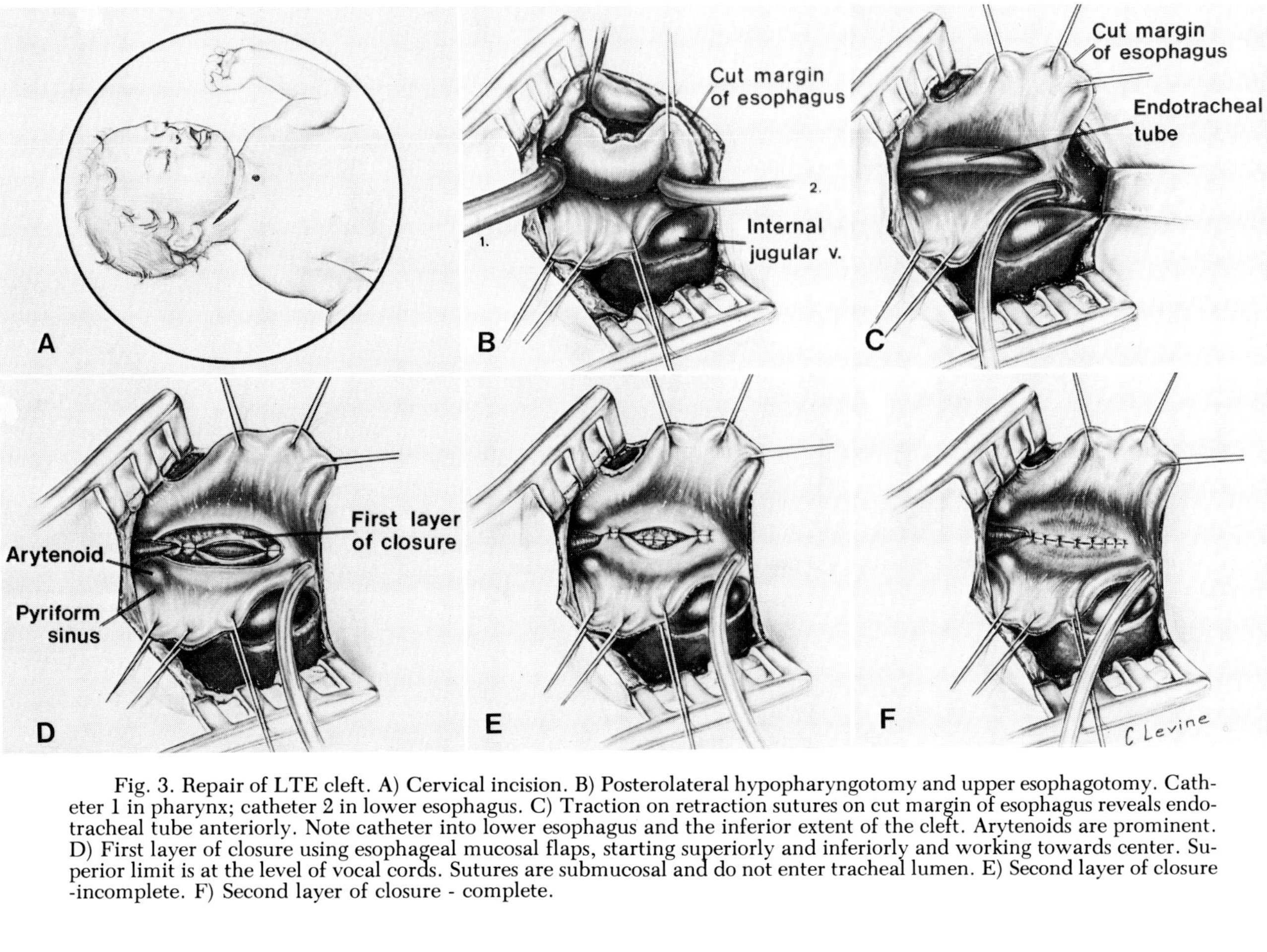

Fig. 3. Repair of LTE cleft. A) Cervical incision. B) Posterolateral hypopharyngotomy and upper esophagotomy. Catheter 1 in pharynx; catheter 2 in lower esophagus. C) Traction on retraction sutures on cut margin of esophagus reveals endotracheal tube anteriorly. Note catheter into lower esophagus and the inferior extent of the cleft. Arytenoids are prominent. D) First layer of closure using esophageal mucosal flaps, starting superiorly and inferiorly and working towards center. Superior limit is at the level of vocal cords. Sutures are submucosal and do not enter tracheal lumen. E) Second layer of closure -incomplete. F) Second layer of closure - complete.

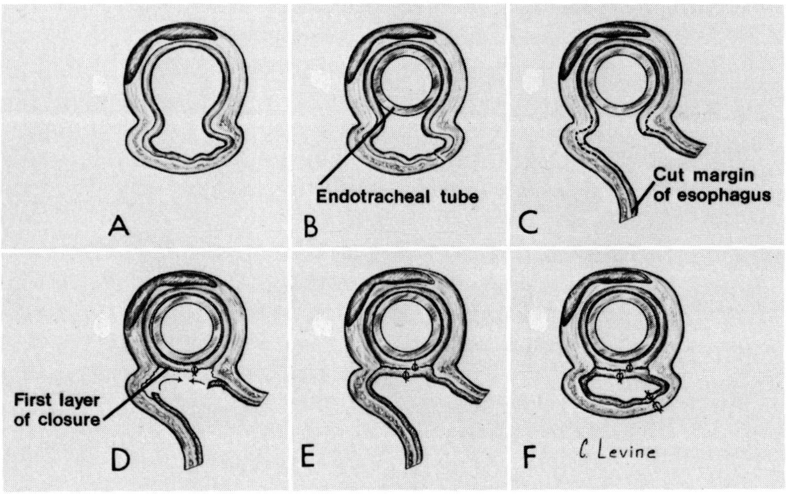

Fig. 4. Repair of LTE cleft (transverse section). A) Diagram of cleft between trachea and esophagus. Notice some deficiency in tracheal rings. B) Endotracheal tube used as a guide to sizing the trachea to be created at repair. Note the site of hypopharyngotomy and upper esophagotomy. C) Esophageal mucosal flaps elevated, borrowing tissue from esophagus to create trachea. D) First layer of closure, showing submucosal placement of sutures and knots away from tracheal lumen. E) Second layer of closure not directly overlying first layer. F) Repair completed.

geal fistulas and/or esophageal atresia existing in conjunction with a LTE cleft.

The endoscopic examination is crucial to making the definitive diagnosis. Unless the lesion is considered by the endoscopist, however, the lesion may not be diagnosed. The literature has many reports indicating difficulty and delay in the diagnosis of these clefts.[2,8-11] If the lesion is considered, and endoscopy performed with an endotracheal tube in place, the edges of the cleft are separated by the stenting action of the tube, and the cleft becomes obvious. If this step is omitted, then the edges of the cleft tend to approximate, and the diagnosis is missed. This maneuver does not appear to be stressed in the previous literature.

The differential diagnosis has been carefully considered by Cohen[2] and includes other anatomical defects, central nervous system lesions, esophageal disorders, and a variety of neuromuscular disorders. In the management of a LTE cleft, it is important to provide respiratory support, prevent aspiration and perform appropriate surgical repair.

Respiratory support may be provided by an endotracheal tube initially, but a tracheotomy will soon be required. Burroughs and Leape[12] reviewed the literature in 1974 and found that all patients who were operated on required tracheotomy for prolonged periods of time (1-4 years) and the situation has not improved since that time. The more extensive the cleft, however, the less secure is the airway because the tube has a constant tendency to slip over the inferior edge of the defect and into the esophagus.

TABLE 1. SYMPTOMS OF RESPIRATORY AND FEEDING PROBLEMS IN THE NEONATE

Respiratory distress
Cyanosis
Weak or absent cry
Stridor
Intermittent apnea
Feeding problems
Excessive secretions
Aspiration pneumonia

Once the airway is secure, it is imperative to prevent aspiration. Gastric decompression and alimentation by tube are essential, as the most critical problem of an infant with a LTE cleft is that of repeated aspiration leading to pneumonia and death. A nasogastric tube may be sufficient initially, but has two dangers. First the presence of a nasogastric tube may contribute to reflux and aspiration, and secondly the tube may dislodge forward through the cleft to obstruct the airway.[13] For these reasons a gastrostomy has been the recommended procedure in the past. However this does not eliminate the danger of aspiration, as evidenced by the fact that the literature quotes many examples of serious aspiration problems even though gastrostomy has been performed, both before[14,15] surgical repair of the cleft and after repair.[16,17] For this reason, it is important to minimize the possibility of reflux of gastric contents into the esophagus until after both successful surgical repair of the cleft and restoration of adequate esophageal physiology. This may take several months. For this reason we would recommend a high gastric division and double gastrostomy as early as possible in the management of this condition, before the child either succumbs to massive aspiration or the lungs are irreversibly damaged. Although this has been alluded to briefly in the anesthetic literature,[18] the authors have not found a case report in the surgical literature.

For extensive clefts, the surgical procedure of choice is the posterolateral pharyngoesophagotomy approach. This appears to be the most widely used procedure. The anterior approach through a laryngofissure technique has been used for short clefts[10,11] but there is no reported long-term survivor when this approach has been used for the long partial cleft or complete cleft.[19]

CONCLUSIONS

Laryngotracheoesophageal cleft is a rare disorder that is still associated with a high mortality.

In attempting to diagnose a child who is aspirating the endoscopist should look specifically for the cleft with an endotracheal tube in place. This stents open the margins of the cleft.

Aspiration is the major cause of death. Gastrostomy alone is insufficient to prevent recurrent aspiration before or after surgical repair. High gastric division with double gastrostomy is recommended as early initial management, with later reanastomosis once adequate physiology has been restored following repair of the cleft.

REFERENCES

1. Lim TA, Spanier SS, Kohut RI. Laryngeal clefts: a histopathologic study and review. Ann Otol Rhinol Laryngol 1979; 88:837-45.
2. Cohen SR. Cleft larynx. Ann Otol Rhinol Laryngol 1975; 84:747-56.
3. Montgomery WW, Smith SA. Congenital laryngeal defects in the adult. Ann Otol Rhinol Laryngol 1976; 85:491-7.
4. Fearon B, Whalen JS. Tracheal dimensions in the living infant. Ann Otol Rhinol Laryngol 1967; 76:964-74.
5. Richter CF. Dissertation medico de infanticido in artis obstetriciae, thesis, Leipzig, 1792.
6. Finlay HVL. Familial congenital stridor. Arch Dis Child 1949; 24:219-33.
7. Pettersson G. Inhibited separation of the larynx and the upper part of the trachea from the esophagus in a newborn: report of a case successfully operated upon. Acta Chir Scand 1955; 10:250-5.
8. Pracy R, Stell PM. Laryngeal cleft: diagnosis and management. J Laryngol Otol 1974; 88:483-6.
9. Pillsbury HC, Fischer ND. Laryngotracheoesophageal cleft. Arch Otolaryngol 1977; 103:735-7.
10. Jahrsdoerfer RA, Kirchner JA, Tahler SU. Cleft larynx. Arch Otolaryngol 1967; 86:108-13.
11. Bell DW, Christiansen TA, Smith TE, Stucker FJ. Laryngotracheoesophageal cleft: the anterior approach. Ann Otol Rhinol Laryngol 1977; 86:616-22.
12. Burroughs N, Leape LL. Laryngotracheoesophageal cleft; report of a case successfully treated and review of the literature. Pediatrics 1974; 53:516-22.
13. Beazer R, De Sa DS, Freeland AP, Robertson NRC. Laryngoesophageal cleft. Arch Dis Child 1973; 48:912-5.
14. Delahunty JE, Cherry J. Congenital laryngeal cleft. Ann Otol Rhinol Laryngol 1969; 78:96-106.
15. Imbrie JD, Doyle PJ. Laryngotracheoesophageal cleft; report of a case and review of the literature. Laryngoscope 1969; 79:1252-74.
16. Donahoe PK, Hendren WH. The surgical management of laryngotracheoesophageal cleft with tracheoesophageal fistula and esophageal atresia. Surgery 1972; 73:363-8.
17. Zachary RB, Emery JL. Failure of separation of larynx and trachea from the esophagus; persistent esophagotrachea. Surgery 1961; 49:525-9.
18. Ruder CB, Glaser LC. Anesthetic management of laryngotracheoesophageal cleft. Anesthesiology 1977; 47:65-7.
19. Pettit RN, Butcher RB, Bethea CM, King TD. Surgical correction of complete tracheoesophageal cleft. Laryngoscope 1979; 89:804-11.

Ann Otol 90:1981

GRASSHEADS IN THE TRACHEOBRONCHIAL TREE: TWO DIFFERENT OUTCOMES

MARY J. SPENCER, MD
VICTORIA E. MILLET, MD
JESSIE L. SHERROD, MD
JAMES P. DUDLEY, MD
YVONNE J. BRYSON, MD

LOS ANGELES, CALIFORNIA

Many vegetable foreign bodies can produce serious pulmonary complications because of chemical irritation to the airway. Barley grass, a type of grasshead, does not induce such a reaction because of its resistance to organic decay. Complications which may occur are illustrated by the clinical course of two patients with aspiration of this foreign body. In the first patient the grasshead entered the trachea with the flowering unit first and the stem following. In the second patient the stem entered the trachea first. Recurrent pneumonias were noted in the first patient. Despite its presence in the right stem bronchus for three years, no further episodes of pneumonia followed its removal. In the second patient the grassheads could not be removed endoscopically. They migrated into the right lower lobe producing pneumonia and ultimately resulting in a brain abscess. The difference of entry of the same foreign body into the trachea, stem first versus flowering unit first, is an essential factor in altering the clinical outcome.

A variety of foreign bodies can find their way into the tracheobronchial tree of children.[1] Many of these in the vegetable family can produce serious damage because of chemical irritation to the airway. Despite their failure to induce a similar kind of reaction because of their resistance to organic decay, grassheads consisting of a stem and a flowering unit can be responsible for serious pulmonary complications. An example of two of the clinical syndromes which may be produced by the different presentations of the grasshead to the tracheobronchial tree is demonstrated by the following two cases involving inhalation of barley grass, a type of grasshead. Despite the similarity of the inhaled foreign bodies, the clinical course of these two patients is strikingly different. Although foreign body aspiration was initially considered in each case, both children were asymptomatic when seen in the emergency room and initial chest roentgenograms were normal. Bronchoscopy was not performed on either patient until complications occurred.

CASE REPORTS

Case 1. A 4-year-old girl was referred to the UCLA Hospital and Clinics for evaluation of a nonproductive cough of three weeks duration and a persistent right lower lobe infiltrate which had failed to resolve after a prolonged course of oral antibiotics. When the parents were specifically questioned about possible aspiration of a foreign body they recalled that three years prior to admission, when the child was 9 months of age, a sudden episode of choking, coughing, and cyanosis had occurred when she was crawling on the lawn. At that time her symptoms cleared rapidly, and a chest roentgenogram was normal. However, within 24 hours the child developed high fever and a cough. A chest roentgenogram six days after the episode demonstrated a right lower lobe infiltrate. Symptoms resolved after one month of oral antibiotic therapy, but the pulmonary infiltrate did not resolve. During the ensuing 3-year period the child had frequent febrile episodes associated with a nonproductive cough which were considered to be recurrent upper respiratory infections. Each episode rapidly responded to oral antibiotic therapy, and no chest roentgenograms were obtained.

Physical examination showed a thin child with height in the 40th percentile and weight in the 10th percentile. Auscultation of the chest revealed dullness to percussion and rales and rhonchi at the right posterior lung base.

Laboratory data included a hemoglobin of 12 g/dl, a white blood count of 22,000/mm^3 with 55% neutrophils, 1% bands, 1% eosinophils, 40% lymphocytes, and 3% monocytes, and an erythrocyte sedimentation rate of 52 mm at one hour. A right lower lobe infiltrate was demonstrated on chest roentgenogram.

Because of the chronic problem and the history of apparent aspiration, bronchoscopy was performed. A grasshead, subsequently identified as barley grass, surrounded by purulent exudate was found intact in the right main stem bronchus (Fig. 1). Minimal mucosal erythema and edema were noted. *Escherichia coli*, *Hemophilus influenzae*, *Staphylococcus aureus*, viridans streptococci, and *Neisseria* species were recovered. Intraoperative bronchography revealed the presence of bronchiectasis in the right lower lobe. The child responded rapidly to

From the Departments of Pediatrics and Surgery, Division of Head and Neck Surgery, UCLA School of Medicine, Los Angeles.
Presented at the meeting of the American Broncho-Esophagological Association, Vancouver, British Columbia, May 11-12, 1981.
REPRINTS — James P. Dudley, MD, Department of Surgery, Division of Head and Neck Surgery, UCLA School of Medicine, Los Angeles, CA 90024.

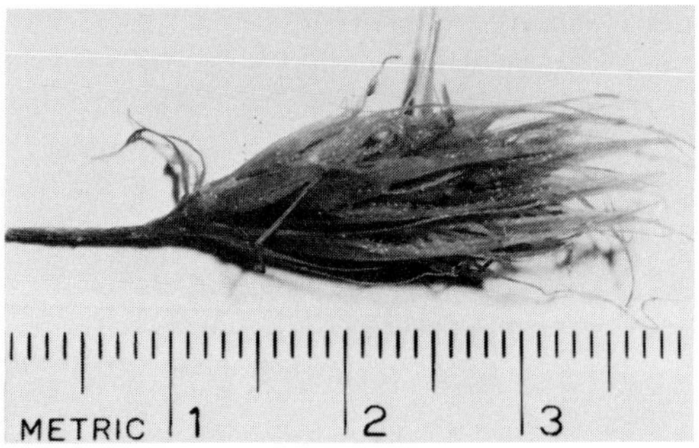

Fig. 1. Grasshead (barley grass) removed three years after entering the right main stem bronchus.

intravenous antibiotics, was discharged, and lost to follow-up care.

Case 2. A 19-month-old boy was referred to UCLA Hospital and Clinics because of fever, vomiting, and lethargy for ten days. One day before admission amoxicillin therapy was begun. On admission, physical examination revealed a pale, irritable, somnolent child who refused to walk. He had marked nuchal rigidity, hypotonia, and a rectal temperature of 38.6° C. Laboratory data included a peripheral white blood cell count of 22,800/mm^3 with 75% neutrophils, 20% lymphocytes, 5% monocytes, and an erythrocyte sedimentation rate of 44 mm at one hour. Lumbar puncture revealed a CSF which contained 2,075 leukocytes/mm^3 with 93% being neutrophils, protein 215 mg/dl, and glucose 5 mg/dl; no bacteria were seen on Gram stain. A right lower lobe infiltrate was observed on chest roentgenogram.

The child was treated with antibiotics intravenously for presumed bacterial meningitis. Bacterial cultures of the CSF, blood, and urine revealed no growth, and counterimmunoelectrophoresis of the CSF failed to reveal any evidence of infection. The child's symptoms improved, but because of persistent fever, an EMI scan of the brain was performed on the eighth hospital day. A right parietal lobe abscess adjacent to and communicating with an enlarged right lateral ventricle was observed. Surgery was performed, and viridans streptococci were cultured from the abscess cavity.

One week after admission because of persistent right lower lobe infiltrate on chest roentgenogram, the parents were carefully questioned regarding possible aspiration of a foreign body. It was then revealed that the child had had a severe coughing spell while playing in a freshly cut grass field three months prior to admission. A chest roentgenogram at that time revealed no abnormality. Several days following the coughing episode the child was treated for pneumonia although a repeat chest roentgenogram was not done. For three weeks prior to this admission, the child had a history of foul-smelling breath.

Bronchoscopy was performed on the eighth hospital day and again seven days later. Both studies revealed purulent exudate in the right main stem bronchus. Two weeks later the right lower lobe was removed because of increasing mucopurulent sputum and persistence of the right lower lobe infiltrate. Two heads of barley grass were recovered from the removed lung. *Escherichia coli, Eikenella corrodans*, and viridans streptococci were cultured from lung tissue. Recovery has been complicated by hydrocephalus for which permanent ventriculoperitoneal shunts were inserted.

DISCUSSION

Although our two patients both inhaled barley grass, an extrusive type of grasshead, uncommon complications occurred. One patient developed a brain abscess, a previously unreported complication of grasshead inhalation. The grasshead reached the distal portion of the right lower lobe producing bronchial obstruction, pneumonia, and brain abscess. In the other case the grasshead entered the bronchus, with the spikelet leading and the stem trailing. This prevented the usual migration of the grasshead through the lung parenchyma. The grasshead thus remained lodged in the bronchus as an inert nonopaque object for three years and resulted in bronchiectasis of the right lower lobe.

The clinical features of grasshead aspiration are determined by the physical characteristics of the specific grass and their resistance to decay. Their silicious coat provides a protection against organic decay.[1-5] Grassheads are composed of flowering units called spikelets which consist of a group of one to five flowers on a short stem.[5,6] A grasshead once inhaled usually descends to the right bronchus with the stem leading into the lung and the spikelet or flowering unit trailing.[6] Since its irregular shape does not produce a ball-valve phenomenon,[4-6] expiratory wheezing may be absent in subjects who have aspirated this grass.

There are two basic types of grasshead, the nonextrusive and the extrusive type. The spikelets of the nonextrusive type of grass, represented by timothy or rye grass, are close together and soft and tend to lodge and remain in one place in the tracheobronchial tree. They are removed by bronchoscopy or by lung resection. The spikelets of the extrusive type (barley grass), in contrast, are firm and sharp and are set at an acute angle to the rigid stem. With this arrangement, the to-and-fro movement of the tracheobronchial tree can propel the grasshead distally into the lung if the stem goes into the trachea first and spikelets follow. The grasshead can be propelled into the more distal and ever smaller bronchioles where it obstructs the lumen. It may even go on to perforate the chest wall within weeks to months after the episode of inhalation.[4,5,7] Serious complications such as pulmonary hemorrhage and rarely death have been reported.[8]

The inhalation of grassheads, if unrecognized, can be responsible for serious complications. Bronchoscopists should be aware that they can present themselves to the trachea in two different ways. In the first they enter the airway with the flowering units leading the way and the stem trailing. In this instance the foreign body can remain as an inert object for years in the bronchus. In the second manner of aspiration the stem enters first with the flowering units trailing. This presentation permits the flowering unit to be propelled into the lung requiring resection of the lung.

REFERENCES

1. Pyeman C. Inhaled foreign bodies in childhood: a review of 230 cases. Med J Aust 171; 1:62-8.

2. Clery A, Ellis F, Schmidt H, et al. Problems associated with aspiration of grass heads (inflorescences). JAMA 1959; 171:1478-84.

3. Jackson C. Foreign bodies in the air and food passages. In: English GM, ed. Otolaryngology. Vol. 5. Hagerstown: Harper and Row, 1977: 1-33.

4. Woolley P. Grass inflorescence as foreign bodies in the respiratory tract. J Pediatr 1955; 46:704-5.

5. Godrey RC. The behavior of inhaled grass inflorescences. Lancet 1957; 2:273-4.

6. Windsor HM. Massive hemopysis from intrabronchial foreign body. Med J Aust 1951; 1:694.

7. Choremis C, Theodorow S, Athanasiades TH, et al. Spontaneous elimination of inhaled grass florescences through the lung and chest wall. Arch Dis Child 1964; 39:406-8.

8. William HE, Phelan PD. The "missed" inhaled foreign body in children. Med J Aust 1969; 1:625-8.

Ann Otol 90:1981

EPIGLOTTIC LARYNGOPLASTY FOR COMPLICATED LARYNGEAL STENOSIS

STEVEN M. SOBOL, MD
BENJAMIN WOOD, MD
HOWARD LEVINE, MD
HARVEY M. TUCKER, MD

CLEVELAND, OHIO

The technique of epiglottic laryngoplasty, previously described for reconstruction following near total laryngectomy for glottic carcinoma, has been used in selected patients with severe glottic and subglottic stenosis. Our experience in four patients suggests that it is useful for 1) laryngeal stenosis in which there is loss or collapse of the external cartilaginous framework, and 2) laryngeal stenosis which is refractory to the usual forms of therapy. The technique is a technically simple, one-stage procedure which provides its own endolaryngeal mucosal lining, as well as autogenous cartilaginous support. It has been successful in restoring adequate airway and preserving voice without interfering with deglutition or laryngeal competence in most patients.

INTRODUCTION

While most cases of glottic and subglottic stenosis can be managed successfully by either conservative endoscopic techniques or one of several conventional open laryngoplasty and stenting procedures, there remain certain ones that are refractory to such management. It is often difficult to achieve a satisfactory airway in patients with extensive combined glottic and subglottic stenosis and in those who have sustained loss or collapse of the cartilaginous skeleton. The purpose of this report is to describe our experience with the use of epiglottic laryngoplasty, previously reported for management of carcinoma of the larynx,[1] in appropriately selected cases of laryngeal stenosis.

CASE REPORTS

Case 1. This 56-year-old female was treated with full course radiation therapy for a T_1B epidermoid carcinoma of the anterior right and left true vocal cords in 1978. She underwent a frontolateral partial vertical laryngectomy for local recurrence several months later at another institution. Decannulation was not possible because of postoperative laryngeal stenosis and she was referred to our clinic for evaluation and therapy. Laryngoscopy revealed a dense anterior glottic-subglottic stenosis with normal left arytenoid mobility and a fixed right arytenoid. There was no evidence of recurrent disease on either gross or microscopic examination.

Laryngotomy and epiglottic laryngoplasty, combined with cricoid split and hyoid interposition were performed. An endolaryngeal stent was placed and anchored to the tracheotomy tube. Postoperatively the patient developed a local wound infection which resulted in subsequent slough of the hyoid bone graft. Local wound care and antimicrobial therapy resulted in complete healing and an airway adequate for day-to-day activity. She was decannulated successfully four months after surgery.

Case 2. This 27-year-old female was referred for treatment of severe glottic stenosis sustained at age 25 following prolonged intubation for barbiturate overdose. Right arytenoidectomy and laser excision of the stenosis with placement of an endolaryngeal stent had been unsuccessful. Several subsequent attempts at microlaryngoscopic scar excision and stenting were similarly inadequate to permit decannulation.

A thyrotomy with epiglottic reconstruction was performed. Healing was satisfactory, with the formation of an airway which should have been sufficient for decannulation. However, severe psychiatric problems precluded decannulation; the patient continues to wear a tracheotomy tube which is corked almost continuously.

Case 3. This 50-year-old female was treated with full course radiation therapy for carcinoma of the glottis in 1976. Several months following radiation therapy she developed increasing airway obstruction. Several laryngoscopic examinations with biopsy revealed severe glottic and arytenoid edema and granulation tissue without evidence of recurrent carcinoma.

Partial laryngectomy with epiglottic reconstruction was performed for what was suspected to be possible recurrent carcinoma. Final pathologic diagnosis was "chronic radiation-induced laryngeal stenosis with cartilage destruction." The patient was successfully decannulated five months after surgery. She has suffered mild bouts of aspiration of liquids since surgery, but none sufficiently severe to warrant further surgical intervention.

Case 4. This 30-year-old male was referred because of laryngeal stenosis. He had sustained laryngotracheal trauma resulting in bilateral vocal cord paralysis and subglottic stenosis secondary to cricoid crush injury in a motorcycle accident. He had under-

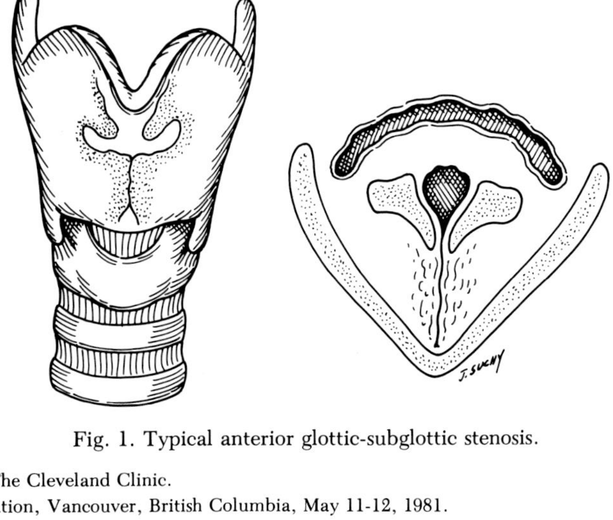

Fig. 1. Typical anterior glottic-subglottic stenosis.

From the Department of Otolaryngology and Communicative Disorders, The Cleveland Clinic.

Presented at the meeting of the American Broncho-Esophagological Association, Vancouver, British Columbia, May 11-12, 1981.

REPRINTS — Harvey M. Tucker, MD, 9500 Euclid Avenue, Cleveland Clinic, Cleveland, OH 44106.

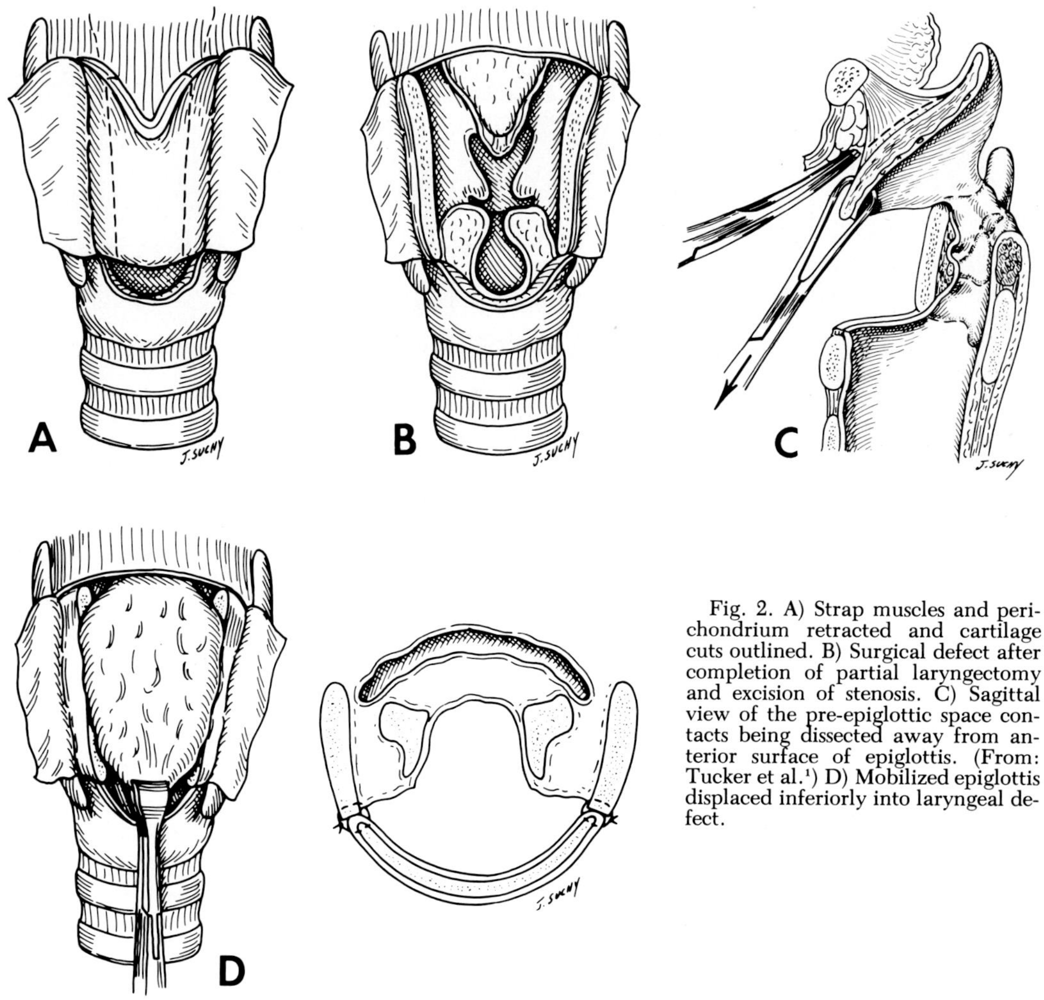

Fig. 2. A) Strap muscles and perichondrium retracted and cartilage cuts outlined. B) Surgical defect after completion of partial laryngectomy and excision of stenosis. C) Sagittal view of the pre-epiglottic space contacts being dissected away from anterior surface of epiglottis. (From: Tucker et al.[1]) D) Mobilized epiglottis displaced inferiorly into laryngeal defect.

gone bilateral Woodman arytenoidectomies prior to his referral. His airway was inadequate without a tracheotomy in place. Laryngoscopy confirmed total glottic and anterior subglottic stenosis. Thyrotomy, anterior cricoidectomy with excision of the stenosis and epiglottic laryngoplasty was performed. The patient was decannulated successfully within one month.

He did well for several months until he began to develop progressive airway obstruction. Repeat laryngoscopic examination revealed recurrent subglottic-tracheal stenosis which required laser dilatations and stenting. He is now breathing well without the need for a tracheotomy tube.

TECHNIQUE

Patients with complicated glottic and subglottic stenosis are evaluated by both indirect and direct laryngoscopy and bronchoscopy in order to assess the thickness and length of stenosis and the status of vocal cord and arytenoid mobility. Laryngographic, tomographic and CAT scan examinations may be used in selected cases to help ascertain the conditions of the cartilaginous framework and degree of stenosis.

The technique of near total laryngectomy with epiglottic reconstruction has been reported in a previous publication.[1] A modification of the technique for laryngeal stenosis is used (Fig. 1). A low collar or neck crease incision is made at the level of the cricoid and a subplatysmal flap is elevated to the level of the hyoid bone. The strap muscles are separated in the midline and retracted to expose the underlying thyroid cartilage. The perichondrium of the thyroid cartilage is incised in the midline, elevated off the thyroid alae bilaterally and retracted laterally. The perichondrial incisions are extended along the superior and inferior borders of the thyroid alae. Midline thyrotomy or appropriate vertical parallel cartilaginous cuts are outlined with brilliant green and completed with a Stryker saw (Fig. 2A). The position of these cuts is determined by the extent of glottic and subglottic scarring which must be resected. The larynx is entered and the stenosis is excised under direct vision (Fig. 2B). The arytenoids should be preserved whenever possible. The cricothyroid membrane and a portion of the anterior cricoid arch may also be removed if the stenosis warrants it. As opposed to surgery for malignancy, this resection need not be performed en bloc, and may be tailored to the individual case. The base of the epiglottis is then grasped and the pre-epiglottic contents are dissected away, deep to lingual epiglottic mucosa, staying in the plane immediately anterior to the underlying epiglottic cartilage (Fig. 2C). The hyoepiglottic and glossoepiglottic ligaments are transected for better mobilization. Superior mucosal attachments must be preserved since they represent the remaining blood supply to the mobilized epiglottis. The epiglottis is displaced inferiorly into the defect and sutured with nonabsorbable material to the cut edges of the thyroid alae laterally and the cricoid or first two tracheal rings inferiorly (Fig. 2D). A mucosa-to-mucosa closure is neither necessary nor possible. Since these tissues are usually redundant they will lie in sufficiently close proximity to each other. The overlying perichondrial flaps and strap muscles are then approximated. The flap is replaced and a suction catheter apparatus is placed.

If a portion of the cricoid arch must be removed, an endolaryngeal stent may be left in place for three to six weeks. We prefer the Kotton Silastic® stent.[2]

Broad spectrum antibiotics which are begun preoperatively are maintaind for several days after surgery. A cuff tracheotomy tube is used but the cuff may be deflated by the second postoperative day. Tube feedings are maintained via a nasogastric tube for approximately one week postoperatively. Decannulation is undertaken as soon as the patient is able to tolerate corking of the tracheotomy tube. Patients may not be allowed to eat until decannulation is complete and the tracheotomy site healed. In patients who require a stent, however, perioral feeding may be started prior to tracheal decannulation.

DISCUSSION

Because laryngeal and subglottic stenosis can be of varying degrees of severity, no single procedure can be appropriate for all cases. The ultimate goal of any such procedure is to 1) establish adequate airway without the need for tracheotomy, and 2) maintain phonatory capability. Most uncomplicated cases of glottic or subglottic stenosis will respond to one of the more conventional techniques. Those cases not amenable to conservative management such as dilatation or endoscopic laser excision with stenting are generally considered for an open transcervical procedure. The choice of technique depends on the degree of stenosis and anatomic location.

Near total laryngectomy with epiglottic reconstruction has been used successfully in the management of selected cases of glottic carcinoma, even when recurrent after radiation therapy.[1] This technique is attractive because it is a one-stage procedure which can provide an adequate airway without tracheotomy, maintain satisfactory phonatory function and allow satisfactory deglutition without significant aspiration despite the removal of as much as both vocal cords and one arytenoid cartilage. The modification of this technique described in this paper may be applicable in cases of complicated glottic and sublottic stenosis.[3]

Laryngeal stenosis may be complicated by the loss or collapse of the cartilaginous framework and in such cases is often difficult to manage. This situation is most often seen following blunt laryngeal trauma with fragmentation or devitalization of the cartilaginous framework. Previous partial laryngeal surgery may be complicated by similar stenosis. When there is concomitant infection, radiation therapy may cause laryngeal chondritis with distortion and collapse of the laryngeal cartilaginous skeleton. Because it restores cartilaginous support, the technique of partial laryngectomy with epiglottic reconstruction may have particular advantage over other techniques in these circumstances.

CONCLUSIONS

Epiglottic laryngoplasty for glottic carcinoma has been a successful reconstructive technique. It has provided 1) reliable restoration of airway, 2) maintenance of acceptable phonatory function, and 3) satisfactory deglutition. This technique should offer similar advantages in appropriately selected cases of severe laryngeal stenosis. Experience in four patients, although far from definitive, has supported this expectation.

REFERENCES

1. Tucker H, Wood B, Levine H, Katz R. Glottic reconstruction after total laryngectomy. Laryngoscope 1979; 89:609-17.

2. Kotton B. Treatment of subglottic stenosis in children by prolonged dilatation. Laryngoscope 1979; 89:1983-90.

3. Kennedy T. Epiglottic reconstruction of laryngeal stenosis secondary to cricothyroidostomy. Laryngoscope 1980; 90:1130-6.

SURGICAL APPROACH TO THE MEDIAL ORBITAL WALL

DONALD F. N. HARRISON, MD
LONDON, ENGLAND

There is a need for the head and neck surgeon to be familiar with the anatomy of the orbit, for the practice of his specialty may require deliberate entry into this region, either for access or to carry out specific procedures. A review of 561 occasions in which entry into the orbit was desirable revealed that 478 (85%) were primarily for exposure of the medial orbital wall. A variety of operative techniques were required together with knowledge of the relevant anatomy and possible hazards.

It is not always appreciated that management of paranasal sinus disease may necessitate deliberate entry into the orbit, either for access or to carry out specific procedures. With increasing experience and confidence this route may also be used as a formal approach to the sphenoidal sinus or orbital floor. My training in ophthalmology, together with access to clinical material from a large ophthalmic hospital, has provided an opportunity to gain such expertise. Recent analysis of 527 specific occasions of deliberate orbital exploration[1] and analysis of 35 additional patients showed that 85% of these procedures were primarily for exposure of the medial orbital wall (Table 1). As with most sinus surgery, safety and success are largely related to sound anatomical knowledge, and orbital exploration is no more hazardous than other surgical procedures in this region.

SURGICAL ANATOMY OF THE MEDIAL ORBITAL WALL

This is the only wall which is not obviously triangular; being roughly oblong it consists of four bones united by vertical sutures: a) frontal process of maxilla, b) lacrimal bone, c) orbital plate of ethmoid (lamina papyracea), and d) small part of the body of the sphenoid. Most of the bony wall is occupied by the thin, almost transparent lamina papyracea, with the hard compact lacrimal bone and sphenoid anteriorly and posteriorly. This is of considerable importance since the floor of the lacrimal fossa is frequently absent and the lacrimal sac then becomes intimately related to anterior ethmoidal cells. The optic foramen lies within part of the sphenoid bone and overenthusiastic removal of the posterior part of the lamina papyracea may produce a "fissure fracture" into the canal (Fig. 1).

Although importance is attached to such constant features as the lacrimal crest and the anterior-posterior ethmoidal arteries, it is essential to appreciate that they are not constant in position or appearance. Rontal et al[2] measured the distance of the foraminae for anterior-posterior ethmoidal arteries and the optic foramen from the lacrimal crest. I have examined 40 orbits during exenteration and 54 dissected cadavers. Taking the anterior lacrimal crest as the focal point, average measurements of 22 mm to the anterior ethmoidal foramen, 37 mm to the posterior foramen, and 40 mm to the optic canal were obtained. However, variations were considerable, particularly the distance from posterior ethmoidal foramen to optic canal (range 2-9 mm).

Absence of the anterior ethmoid foramen is found in 16% of orbits, and over 30% show multiple foramina for the posterior ethmoidal artery. The only safe conclusion from these measurements is that undue reliance should not be placed on these landmarks, nor on "average" measurements of position. Increasing use of coronal tomography has confirmed the variable level of the cribriform plate. This is substantiated by findings during external ethmoidectomy and craniofacial surgery where this bone is found to vary in size, thickness, and level as related to the anterior ethmoidal foramen (Fig. 2). Of considerable surgical importance is the orbital periosteum which not only protects globe and periorbital tissues but acts as an effective barrier to penetration by neoplasms, infection, and surgical instruments! Although fixed to the orbital margin, sutures, fissures, foramina, and lacrimal fossa, it passes through the superior orbital fissure, optic foramen, and ethmoidal canals to join the periosteal layer of the dura. Most orbital surgery will therefore be intraorbital but extraperiosteal.

INTRANASAL ETHMOIDECTOMY

Although generally employed as a standard procedure in the management of recurrent nasal polyps and other specific pathology, this operation carries with it a constant fear of damage to orbital contents or cribriform plate. Access is frequently limited and surgical tuition inadequate. Although this cannot be seriously considered as an effective surgical approach to the medial orbital wall, the most commonly reported complication is to the orbit and its contents. Eichel,[3] speaking at the American Trio-

From the Professorial Unit, Royal National Throat, Nose and Ear Hospital, London.

Presented at the meeting of the American Laryngological Association, Vancouver, British Columbia, May 10-11, 1981.

REPRINTS — Donald F. N. Harrison, MD, Institute of Laryngology and Otology, Royal National Throat, Nose & Ear Hospital, 330/332 Gray's Inn Road, London, WC1X 8EE.

TABLE 1. SURGICAL APPROACHES TO THE MEDIAL ORBITAL WALL

Approach	*No. of Occasions*
Transorbital ethmoidectomy (Patterson's)	188
External ethmoidectomy	
Orbital infections	22
Ligation ethmoidal arteries	4
Frontoethmoidectomy	75
Lateral rhinotomy	161
Craniofacial approach	28
Total	478

logical Society in 1978, said he accepted a 25% incidence of orbital ecchymosis, and hemorrhage was the most common complication in the 1,000 operations reported by Freedman and Kern.[4] Damage to the orbital surface of the lamina papyracea as a result of intranasal surgery carries a constant risk of intraorbital but extraperiosteal bleeding. Anterior tracking of blood produces a periorbital hematoma, erroneously considered by some as the hallmark of a successful operation. Posterior bleeding can cause proptosis and visual loss necessitating removal of nasal packing or exploration.[5] The true morbidity of this procedure, particularly in unskilled hands, is unknown, nor is its effectiveness known in the treatment of ethmoidal disease. However, in no way can it be seriously considered as a realistic approach to the medial orbital wall.

With the exception of the surgical management of ethmoidal neoplasms, most surgery to this region of the orbit is exenteration of ethmoidal cells for recurrent nasal polyposis. Complete removal of the ethmoidal labyrinth is only feasible via a craniofacial approach and the varying relationship of posterior cells to optic foramen, as shown by axial tomography, illustrates the hazards of any indirect approach to this region.

PATTERSON'S EXTERNAL ETHMOIDECTOMY

The value of the transorbital approach to the ethmoid described by Patterson in 1939[6] lies in the almost invisible scar and more direct access, although it is possibly more difficult technically than traditional procedures. The skin incision is confined to the nasojugal fold and the orbital margin reached by separation of the fibers of orbicularis oculi. Careful freeing of orbital periosteum from the bony rim reveals the origin of the inferior oblique muscle (except in 9% of patients where this muscle is entirely intraperiosteal) and, medially, the nasolacrimal sac (Fig. 3). As dissection advances this gap opens to reveal orbital floor and medial wall as far posteriorly as the posterior ethmoidal foraminae. Mobilization of the lacrimal sac provides access to the anterior ethmoidal cells and removal of the lamina papyracea is performed under direct vision. This is continued until the compact bone of the sphenoid surrounding the optic canal is seen, when further removal of ethmoid cells is carried out transnasally. Although controlled hypotension simplifies this operation, the ethmoidal arteries present no problem in the normotensive state since removal of bone around the foraminae allows contraction and hemostasis. Apart from transient epiphora, probably from edema of the sac or orbicularis fibers, complications in 188 operations on 121 patients were minimal.

Since removal of the orbital floor is possible as far laterally as the infraorbital nerve, this procedure has been combined with lateral orbitotomy for orbital decompression, providing direct, safe, and quick access with the sure knowledge that all bone has been removed. Visualization of the sphenoidal sinus is excellent and this operation is useful in providing access for transethmoidal transsphenoidal hypophysectomy.

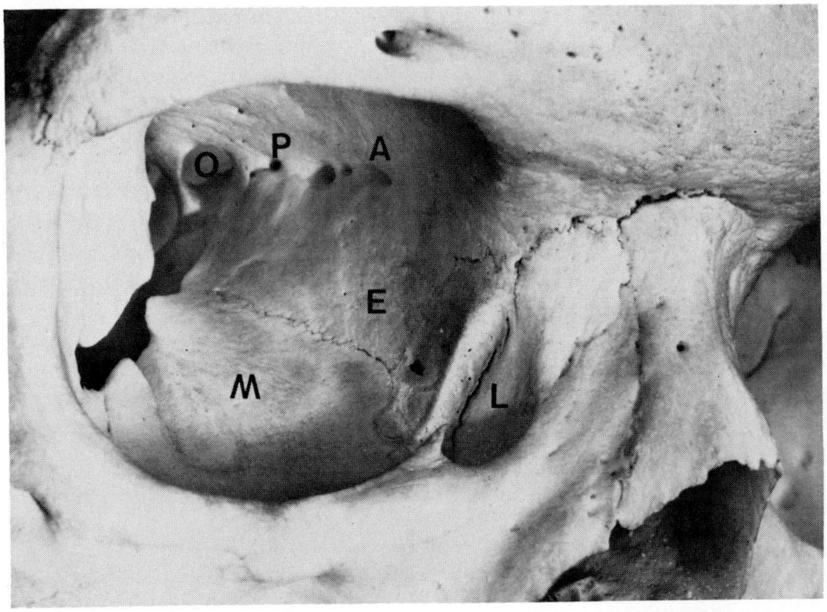

Fig. 1. Medial bony wall of orbit. L - Lacrimal fossa; M - Orbital plate of maxilla; E - Lamina papyracea; O - Optic foramen; A-P - Anterior and posterior ethmoidal foraminae.

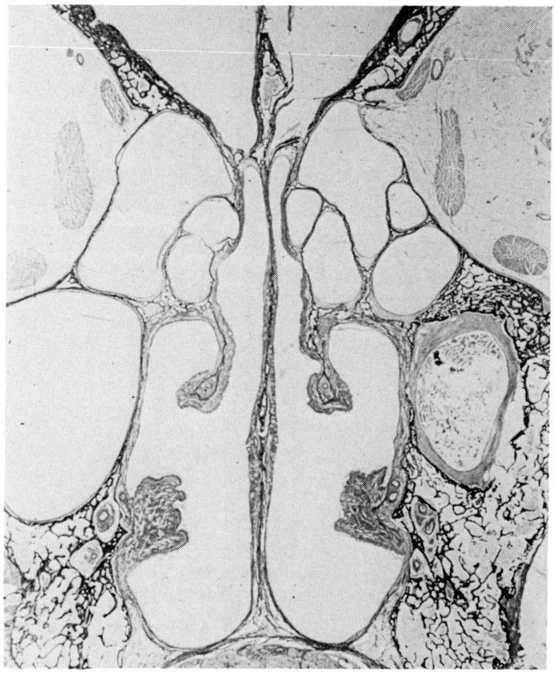

Fig. 2. Coronal section through nasofrontal region showing relationship of cribriform plate to medial orbital wall.

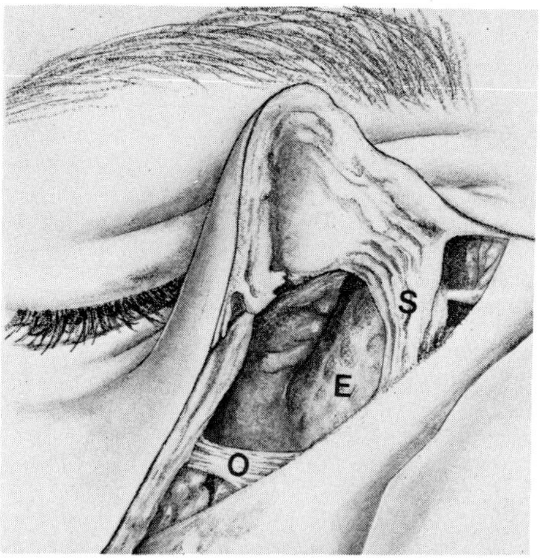

Fig. 3. Tendon of inferior oblique muscle and lacrimal sac revealed via Patterson's approach. Lamina papyracea is seen deep to these structures. E - Lamina papyracea; S - Lacrimal sac; O - Tendon of inferior oblique.

FRONTOETHMOIDECTOMY

Exposure of the frontal sinus or frontonasal duct is not possible by transorbital ethmoidectomy alone, and although chronic suppuration is no longer a major reason for frontoethmoidectomy, 75 operations were performed primarily for mucocele, osteoma, and a variety of benign lesions affecting this region. Although the skin incision is relatively standardized, the actual procedure relates more to the condition being treated rather than the eponymous title of its originator. Forty-nine patients were operated upon for frontoethmoidal mucoceles (38% proved to be pyoceles), and details of most of these have been reviewed by Evans.[7] All had a palpable swelling either at the medial canthus or below the superior orbital rim. Over 80% presented with proptosis and almost half gave a history of previous nasal surgery. Since it is rarely possible to be certain of the real extent of these mucoceles, a standard Killian incision is used and the orbital periosteum elevated widely to provide complete exposure of both the medial orbital wall and frontoethmoidal region. Retraction of orbital contents is best performed with copper retractors to avoid undue pressure on the globe (important in the myopic eye when retinal detachment is possible). In the established frontal mucocele (pure ethmoidal mucoceles are uncommon), the frontonasal duct is assumed to be abnormal. Indeed, most are associated with recurrent polyposis or damage from previous surgery. Consequently, partial ethmoidectomy preserving the middle turbinate, if possible, is usually performed and no attempt is made to reconstruct the frontonasal region. A silicone tube is left in situ, being removed when it no longer fits tightly. Twelve of the 49 patients had a pure ethmoidal mucocele being treated by removal of the lamina papyracea alone.

Invariably, the supraorbital nerve and vessels must be coagulated and the trochlea detached from its origin. Preservation of orbital periosteum requires careful dissection with pyoceles, although it may be impossible to avoid rupture of the thin sac wall. Despite extensive proptosis, less than half of these patients complained of preoperative diplopia, possibly because of habituation, for there is often a long history of diplopia. However, return of the eye to a normal position and restoration of binocular vision frequently leads to a temporary complaint of diplopia.

The natural history and pathology of most paranasal sinus osteomas included in this series have been described by Atallah and Jay.[8] There is considerable difficulty in determining the site of origin of large frontoethmoidal osteomas, and a frontoethmoidal approach is essential even for those apparently localized to the orbital plate of the ethmoid, if only to provide access for removal (Fig. 4). Two patients had osteomas attached by narrow pedicles from the lamina papyracea, producing severe proptosis. Fracture of the pedicle by a localized blow with dissection of attached orbital periosteum allowed removal after considerable manipulation. The base was then removed by limited ethmoidectomy. Osteomas filling the whole ethmoidal labyrinth are too big and convoluted for this approach, and require lateral rhinotomy. Piecemeal removal with cutting burr risks damage to the cribriform plate and is less satisfactory than wide exposure with direct removal of the whole mass.

EXTERNAL ETHMOIDECTOMY

Apart from the occasional deliberate occlusion of

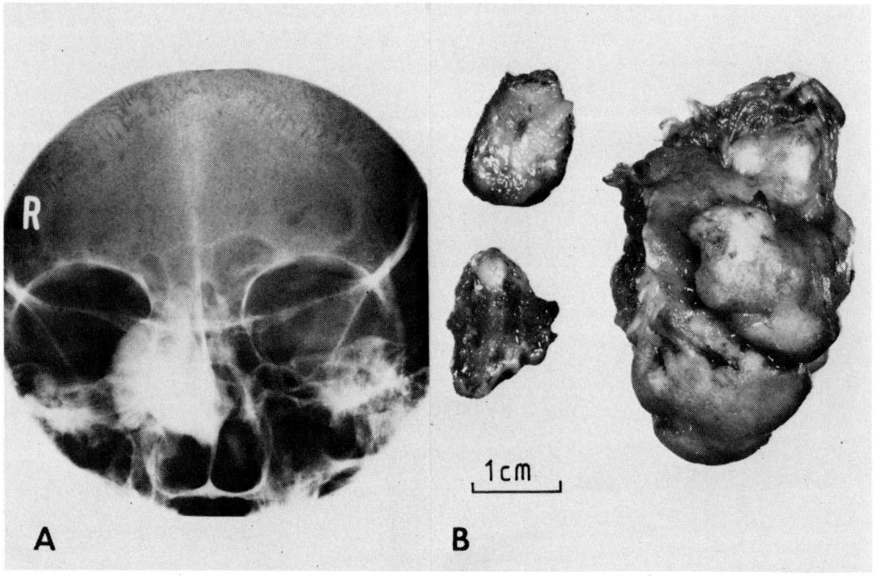

Fig. 4. A) Ethmoidal osteoma with B) specimen removed by lateral rhinotomy. R - Right.

the anterior or posterior ethmoidal arteries for intractable hemorrhage, my experience with limited external ethmoidectomy has been for drainage of orbital infections. Although the use of antibiotics has radically changed the management of sinus infections and incidence of orbital involvement, complications still occur. Organisms are usually *Staphylococcus aureus* or *Hemophilus influenzae*, and orbital invasion, probably by septic thrombophlebitis, may occur within 48 hours. Increasing proptosis with limitation of eye movement suggests abscess formation, and in children a subperiosteal abscess usually discharges close to the medial canthus.

Elevation of orbital periosteum must be carried as far as the posterior extent of the lamina papyracea. Twenty-two of the 42 patients with orbital cellulitis required external drainage and in 10, pus was present extraperiosteally, either with evidence of osteitis or a dehisence in the underlying bone. Removal of the orbital plate is recommended to ensure free drainage into the nose. If pus is not found the skin incision may be extended to allow further periosteal elevation, although clinical judgment will determine the limitations of this exploration.

LATERAL RHINOTOMY

The original purpose of this approach was to provide access for removal of ethmoidal neoplasms, and it is only in recent years that the considerable potential of the operation has been appreciated.[9] In most instances the skin incision need reach no higher than the medial palpebral ligament, allowing almost complete exposure of the lacrimal sac and medial orbital wall. Why "medial maxillectomy" should be added to operative descriptions is hard to understand since any lateral rhinotomy encompasses partial maxillectomy, partial ethmoidectomy, etc.[10]

Some ethmoidal carcinomas are treated with radiotherapy followed by lateral rhinotomy in the hope that residual, undetectable tumor might be removed as early as possible. Benign lesions, such as angiofibromas, hamartomas, or transitional cell papillomas, can be removed by this approach with minimal cosmetic disability. However, the cribriform plate remains and the resection is limited superiorly, particularly with neoplasms arising primarily in ethmoid or olfactory epithelium.

Increasing experience with the craniofacial approach combined with lateral rhinotomy (a midline forehead incision is joined to the lateral rhinotomy — external ethmoidectomy incision inferiorly) has convinced me of the low morbidity and excellent visualization of this technique. Wide resection of the floor of the anterior cranial fossa is carried out under direct vision using the operating microscope and drill without the need for neurosurgical assistance. The orbit is always entered from above as well as medially, allowing posterior removal of the medial wall as far as the optic canal. If uninvolved orbital periosteum is available posteriorly, then localized excision with closure of the orbital defect utilizing fascia lata allows preservation of the eye. In three patients this has been possible with subsequent normal movement and vision. We have now reached the stage when potentially curable or even benign tumors of the ethmoid reaching the cribriform plate area can be offered a truly oncological operation, and less may well be considered unethical.

The frequency with which surgeons enter the orbit, deliberately or occasionally accidently, is undoubtedly underestimated. A sound knowledge of the relevant surgical anatomy will reduce the risk of producing damage to orbital contents or surrounding structures. Without the confidence and expertise that such knowledge brings, surgery to the medial wall of the orbit may be inadequate or accompanied by an unacceptable morbidity.

REFERENCES

1. Harrison DFN. The ENT surgeon looks at the orbit. J Laryngol Otol 1980; Suppl 33:1-43.

2. Rontal E, Rontal M, Guilford FT. Surgical anatomy of the orbit. Ann Otol Rhinol Laryngol 1979; 88:382-6.

3. Eichel BS. The intranasal ethmoidectomy procedure: historical, technical and clinical considerations. Laryngoscope 1972; 82:1806-21.

4. Freedman HM, Kern EB. Complications of intranasal ethmoidectomy: a review of 1000 consecutive operations. Laryngoscope 1979; 89:421-32.

5. Leopold DA, Kellman RM, Gould LV. Retro-orbital hematoma and proptosis associated with chronic sinus disease. Arch Otolaryngol 1980; 106:442-3.

6. Patterson N. External operations on the frontal and ethmoidal sinuses. J Laryngol Otol 1939; 54:235-44.

7. Evans C. Aetiology and treatment of fronto-ethmoidal mucocoele. J Laryngol Otol 1981; 95:361-75.

8. Atallah N, Jay MM. Osteomas of the paranasal sinuses. J Laryngol Otol 1981; 95:291-304.

9. Harrison DFN. Lateral rhinotomy: a neglected operation. Ann Otol Rhinol Laryngol 1977; 86:1-7.

10. Schramm VL, Myers EN. Lateral rhinotomy. Laryngoscope 1978; 88:1042-5.

≈

NINCDS NOTES*

HEARING-SPEECH-LANGUAGE RESEARCH REPORT AVAILABLE

The NINCDS Research Program: Hearing, Speech, and Language, a new research report published by the Institute's Office of Scientific and Health Reports, is now available in limited quantities.

The report contains information for investigators and health practitioners involved with the communicative disorders. Included in the report are brief summaries of research on auditory and speech prostheses, taste and smell, otitis media, and aphasia.

Copies of the publication can be obtained by contacting the Office of Scientific and Health Reports, NINCDS, Bldg. 31, Rm. 8A06, Bethesda, MD 20205; (301) 496-5751.

REVISED GUIDELINES SET FOR PROGRAM PROJECT AND CENTER GRANTS

The NINCDS has issued revised guidelines for program project and center grant proposals, restating and clarifying that subprojects be directed toward a unified research goal and suggesting guidelines for dollar limitations on annual direct costs.

The guidelines also recommend that applicants submit a letter of their intent to seek support before applying for new grants or for renewal of currently active grants.

The new guidelines were published in the July 31, 1981, issue of *NIH Guide to Grants and Contracts.* Copies have been sent to program directors and principal investigators of current NINCDS program projects and research centers. Detailed guidelines are also available from Director, Extramural Activities Program, NINCDS, Federal Bldg., Rm. 1016, Bethesda, MD 20205; (301) 496-9248.

MAJOR CHEMOSENSORY CENTER RECEIVES NINCDS FUNDING

A three-year grant by NINCDS has provided funds for a major new center for basic and clinical research in taste and smell. The Connecticut Chemosensory Clinical Research Center, directed by Dr. Frank A. Catalanotto of the University of Connecticut at Farmington, encompasses a multidisciplinary program conducted by scientists at the Center and at Yale University, the John B. Pierce Foundation Laboratory, and the Worcester Foundation for Experimental Biology. Clinical studies focus on chemosensory functions in aging, multiple sclerosis, neurological deficits, obesity, and diabetes. Laboratory investigations will explore the basic anatomy and physiology of taste and smell, animal models of disorders, the effects of chronic exposure to odor, regeneration in the olfactory system, and the development of sound and practical measurements of the chemosensory abilities of people.

DEMENTIA BOOKLET AVAILABLE

NINCDS'S Office of Scientific and Health Reports has produced a new pamphlet, *The Dementias: Hope Through Research,* for patients' families and others interested in the problems and prospects of dementia patients.

The pamphlet delves into the misconceptions about the dementias, and the causes, symptoms, diagnosis, and treatment of this group of neurological disorders.

Single copies of *The Dementias* can be obtained from the Office of Scientific and Health Reports, NINCDS, Bldg. 31, Rm. 8A06, Bethesda, MD 20205; (301) 496-5751.

*This information is prepared monthly by the Office of Scientific and Health Reports, National Institute of Neurological and Communicative Disorders and Stroke, National Institutes of Health, Bldg. 31, Rm. 8A06, Bethesda, MD 20205; (301) 496-5751.

Ann Otol 90:1981

JUVENILE NASOPHARYNGEAL FIBROMA

RICARDO TAPIA ACUÑA, MD
MEXICO CITY, MEXICO

The large number of cases of nasopharyngeal fibroma seen in Mexico gives Mexican otolaryngologists considerable experience with this disease. This report includes studies on 322 patients seen by the author. It is important to recognize that nasopharyngeal fibroma is not just a tumor, but a disease with particular characteristics, such as prevalence among young males. Clinically it is quite different from other tumors of the pharynx, nose or accessory sinuses.

In nasopharyngeal fibroma, the history includes occasional or frequent epistaxis that sometimes requires blood transfusion.[1-4] The tumor is located in the nasopharynx; it is of a hard consistency and can invade the sphenoid sinus in maybe 90% of the cases, and one or both choanae, with consequent nasal obstruction. It also may invade other nasal cavities, such as a fossa, the ethmoidal or maxillary sinus, the orbit, the pterygomaxillary space or even inside the cranium.

The tumor appears as a compact mass, generally smooth, grey or reddish, that bleeds at slightest contact. If a biopsy is performed, control of the subsequent hemorrhage becomes difficult. Packing for several hours or days might be indispensable to avoid deterioration of the general condition of the young patient.

ETIOLOGY

It is well-known that race, age and sex are the most important factors in the development of nasopharyngeal fibroma. In this series, 80% of the patients were Mexican natives, 18% were of mixed race, and only 2% white. Geographic variables, such as altitude and climate, are not significant factors, since these patients came from all parts of Mexico. All were male. Their karyotypes demonstrated no pathologic features.

Follow-up on some patients who were treated more than 20 years before showed that they are married and have normal children, and that the development of primary and secondary sexual characteristics and the endocrine glands was normal. Flora of the nose and pharynx are usually normal. Heredity is not a factor in this disease; none of the relatives of the patients have had similar tumors. There was no history of syphilis, tuberculosis or other specific infections. Blood tests were normal or showed some anemia or a slight increase in white cells. The age of the patients ranged from 10 to 25 years. The only exception was one patient 35 years old who had suffered the disease since adolescence.

PATHOLOGY

The tumor is constituted by fibrous tissue with stellar cells supported by immature fibroblasts. Multiple vessels can be seen in a stroma of myxomatous tissue. The most important characteristic of such vessels is that they are devoid of elastic or muscular fibers and are filled with blood. This explains the presence of severe hemorrhage when the tumor is touched. It is nourished by the ophthalmic artery and secondarily by the internal maxillary artery. It is very important to remember this when planning treatment. Though nasopharyngeal fibroma is considered a benign tumor, the consequence of its growth can be fatal.

DIAGNOSIS

Clinically, diagnosis is based on the patient's sex, age at onset, characteristics and location of the tumor and the experience of the examiner in previous cases. Biopsy might be unnecessary or even dangerous. Unfortunately the specialist is consulted only when the disease is advanced enough to cause obstruction of the nose or when the patient is in bad condition due to repeated hemorrhages. Deformity of the soft palate is common. One can visualize the tumor by retracting the palate or even by depressing the tongue of the patient. Deformity of the nasal pyramid, exophthalmus, deviation of one of the eyes and troubled vision are common. Complete blindness with no hope of recovery occurred in one case. Conventional radiography of the nose and pharynx is helpful. In the past arteriography was performed to search the cranium for the presence of part of the tumor. At the present time computerized axial tomography (CAT scan), which gives excellent images, is preferred. Sometimes a deformity of the face is the only symptom. This happens when the tumor has destroyed the pterygoid process and has gone out through the lateral wall of the mouth. This was seen in two patients.

TREATMENT

At the beginning, it is important to improve the

Presented at the meeting of the American Laryngological Association, Vancouver, British Columbia, May 10-11, 1981.
REPRINTS — Ricardo Tapia Acuña, MD, Av. Insurgentes Sur No. 300, México 7, D.F.

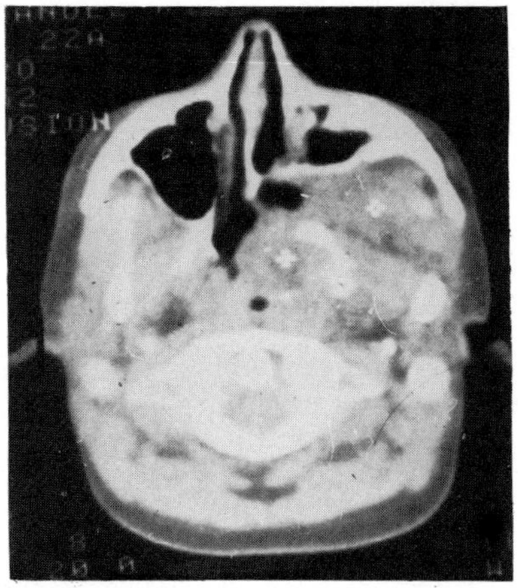

Fig. 1. (Case 1) CAT scan showing the destruction of the wall of the cranium.

general condition of the young patient. Blood transfusions are indicated if repeated hemorrhages have caused anemia. It is better to give small amounts of blood every 48 hours than to give a large amount that might provoke a new hemorrhage. Radiotherapy is useless and might complicate the surgical procedure. Diethylstilbestrol, which has been recommended by some colleagues, is not only useless but also produces disagreeable side effects, such as increased breast size, which might last for a long time. In some patients in this series electrocoagulation was used with some success to reduce the size of small residual tumors; in these particular cases cryotherapy was tried without any good result.

Surgery, with complete removal of the tumor, is the only way to obtain radical cure. The technique differs according to the size of the fibroma, organs which are invaded and, most important, any prior surgical intervention. If a previous operation has failed, the tumor creates adherences that make the second attempt at removal more difficult. A conservative procedure is that in which the retropalatine approach is used, the tumor grasped with a good forceps, the index finger of the right hand introduced through a horizontal incision in the soft palate to guide a dissector or a curette into a nasal fossa with the purpose of isolating the tumor. This procedure has to be done rapidly to avoid unnecessary loss of blood. Meanwhile, an assistant surgeon must be pulling down the tumor by the forceps that holds it. The wound of the palate is sutured and the nose and pharynx are packed. In cases in which the size of the tumor makes it difficult to introduce the tracheal tube for anesthesia, it is preferable to tracheotomize the patient for this purpose and close the opening when the operation is finished.

Unfortunately there are many cases in which surgical treatment is not so simple. When the fibroma has destroyed the ethmoid and invaded the orbit and the maxillary sinus, it might be necessary to

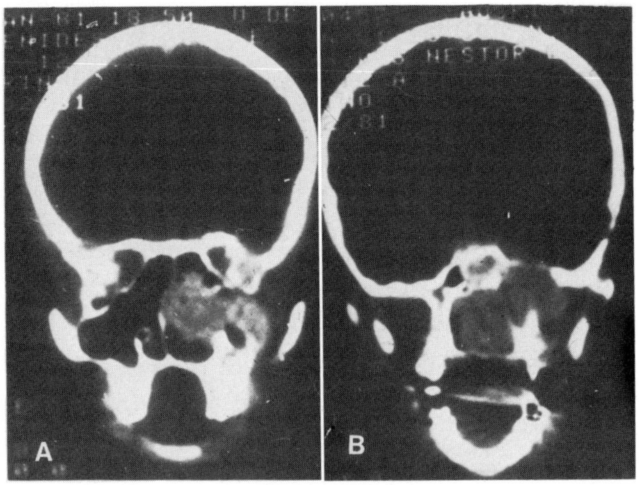

Fig. 2. (Case 2) CAT scans showing various degrees of invasion of tumor into cranium.

open the latter and combine this approach with the retropalatine one. In a few cases (discussed below) it has been necessary to request the assistance of a neurosurgeon.

A blood transfusion is necessary during the operation in every case. Usually 500 cc are enough. In the case of craniotomy not less than 2000 cc of blood was transfused. An appropriate administration of liquids is very important, as in any major surgery.

RESULTS OF TREATMENT

Before discussing the results of the treatment, it is important to distinguish between a residual tumor and a relapse. Either may occur. A residual tumor gives symptoms shortly after removal. A relapse generally comes more than one year after the operation, and in the interim the patient has been free of symptoms. A second operation was required for one of every ten of the patients in this series, and at least half shortly following the first surgery. No mortality has occurred in this series. Two of the cases are especially interesting.

Case 1. A 22-year-old male, married, father of a child, was operated on ten years ago and had some relapse after being free of symptoms for seven years. Recently he began to suffer headaches and epileptic attacks. A neurologist gave him some drugs that did not improve his condition and he returned to this office for advice. Because of his history of nasopharyngeal fibroma, a CAT scan was done, which showed a tumor invading the temporal fossa inside the cranium (Fig. 1). A neurosurgeon performed a craniotomy and at the same time a Denker operation was performed. This revealed a small tumor outside the meninges which was isolated and removed totally through the maxillary sinus. Bleeding was very slight. The opening of the cranium was closed and the sinus packed for 72 hours. Postoperative treatment consisted of the administration of antibiotics and diphenylhydantoin combined with phenobarbital. Soon neurologic symptoms disappeared and the patient was able to resume normal activities.

Case 2. A boy, 11 years old, had been operated twice for nasopharyngeal fibroma a few months before consulting this office. Clinically and radiologically there was a large tumor occupying the facial sinuses and part of the orbit of the right side with destruction of the bone at the level of the temporal cranial fossa (Fig. 2). A Caldwell-Luc operation was performed, and when the tumor was touched, a major hemorrhage resulted, undoubtedly from the sphenopalatine artery. A tied packing was necessary and later a ligation of the external carotid artery, which controlled bleeding. Again, the assistance of the neurosurgeon was necessary and the problem was solved in a similar way.

CONCLUSION

As a result of long-term observation of 322 patients with juvenile nasopharyngeal fibroma, the following conclusions are drawn:

1. This is a benign tumor that may cause important damage, even death.

2. It is prevalent in young males. Similar tumors seen in female or older patients are not this particular disease.

3. The only important etiologic factor identified is race.

4. CAT scan is very important for diagnosis.

5. Surgery is the elective procedure for treatment. The removal of the tumor is not difficult if it is located exclusively in the nasopharynx and has not been touched before with surgical instruments.

6. A joint effort between the otolaryngologist, the ophthalmologist and the neurosurgeon is very important in some cases.

7. It can be estimated that in 5% of cases there will be residual tumors left, even if surgical procedure has been done adequately.

8. Relapse may occur in approximately 10% of all cases. Patients must be seen periodically after the operation.

9. To control the hemorrhages in cases in which the pterygomaxillary space has been invaded by the tumor, ligation of the external carotid artery is preferable to any other similar procedure.

REFERENCES

1. Rodriguez H. A new surgical approach to nasopharyngeal angiofibroma. Cancer 1966; 19:458-60.

2. Tapia Acuña R. The nasopharyngeal fibroma and its treatment. Arch Otolaryngol 1956; 64:451-5.

3. Tapia Acuña R. Nasopharyngeal fibroma. Acta Otolaryngol (Stockh) 1973; 75:119-26.

4. Wilson CP. Observations on the surgery of the nasopharynx. Ann Otol Rhinol Laryngol 1957; 66:5-35.

≈

PAN AMERICAN ASSOCIATION OF OTORHINOLARYNGOLOGY AND BRONCHOESOPHAGOLOGY

The XVIII Congress of the Pan American Association of Otorhinolaryngology and Bronchoesophagology will be held November 2-6, 1982, in San Juan, Puerto Rico. Dr. Hans von Leden has been elected President of the Association.

HISTOCHEMICAL CHARACTERISTICS OF MUSCLE FIBER TYPES IN THE POSTERIOR CRICOARYTENOID MUSCLE

LESLIE T. MALMGREN, PhD RICHARD R. GACEK, MD

SYRACUSE, NEW YORK

The muscle fiber type composition of the human posterior cricoarytenoid muscle (PCA) was examined using a large battery of histochemical techniques. Staining for myosin ATPase (pH 9.9) indicated that the muscles were composed of 52% ± 11.8 SD type 1 (slowly contracting) fibers and 48% ± 11.9 SD type 2 (rapidly contracting) fibers. In order to obtain information concerning the probable fatigue resistance of the type 2 fibers, serial sections were processed to determine the relative extent of ATPase inactivation at various pH levels in the acid range and to obtain data concerning the relative activities of oxidative and glycolytic enzymes and their substrates. The great majority of the type 2 fibers were of the 2A (fatigue resistant) fiber type. This indication of a capacity for prolonged activity was substantiated by the presence of high activities of succinic dehydrogenase, a mitochondrial enzyme which is involved in oxidative metabolism. Type 2C fibers (generally considered to be an undifferentiated fiber type) were also present but relatively rare. The overall enzyme profiles of many of the muscle fibers in the human PCA differed from those typical of fibers having the same alkaline ATPase and acid ATPase characteristics in most other mammalian muscles. Since muscle fiber biochemistry reflects the activity pattern of the motor unit, these unusual enzyme profiles may be the result of activity patterns that are associated with the inspiratory cycle and/or patterns of activity that are relatively specific to the PCA. Four of the ten muscles examined had unequivocal evidence of muscle fiber type grouping, a manifestation of partial denervation followed by reinnervation. This is interesting since most of the cases were in the fifth decade. Muscle fiber type grouping has been shown to occur selectively in certain other human muscles and to increase with age, eventually resulting in muscle atrophy. This suggests the possibility that the human PCA is for some reason selectively vulnerable to partial denervation and indicates the need for more extensive data concerning the relationship of muscle fiber type grouping in the PCA and other laryngeal muscles to age.

INTRODUCTION

Although the posterior cricoarytenoid muscle has an important role as an inspiratory muscle,[1-5] very little is known about the biochemical basis for the physiological characteristics of the various types of motor units in this muscle.

It has been observed in other mammalian muscles that the physiological characteristics of various motor units are correlated with the histochemical enzyme profiles of the muscle fibers in the motor unit.[6,7] Furthermore, there is considerable evidence indicating that both the physiological characteristics of the motor unit and the enzyme profiles of the included muscle fibers reflect the pattern of activity of the motor unit.[8-10]

The activity patterns of many of the motor units in the posterior cricoarytenoid (PCA) muscles differ from those in most other muscles in that they are active during each inspiratory cycle.[4] In addition, there is a considerable diversity in the activities of individual motor units of this muscle in response to certain stimuli and in the duration of their activity during each period of inspiration.[4] Consequently it would be expected that, if the activity of each muscle fiber determines its specific biochemical characteristics, the biochemical differentiation of the PCA would be seen as a complex mosaic of muscle fiber types reflecting the diverse activities of the individual motor units. Data available for the cat PCA indicate that the physiological characteristics and enzyme profiles of many of the muscle fibers differ from those observed in most other mammalian muscle fiber types.[11] Although Teig and coworkers[12] have determined the percentage composition of type 1 (low alkaline stable ATPase) and type 2 (high alkaline stable ATPase) muscle fibers in the human PCA, there is as yet no information available concerning the relative activities of glycolytic and oxidative enzymes and their substrates in the muscle fiber types in this muscle. Since these data are essential to an understanding of the differentiation, physiology, and pathology of the motor units in the human PCA, we have examined the enzyme profiles of the muscle fiber types in this muscle using a large battery of histochemical techniques.

METHODS

The muscles were obtained from six male volunteers of various ages (43, 51, 52, 57, 59, and 64 years) who were undergoing laryngectomy for malignancy. All of these cases except one had not received radiation treatment. The muscles were removed at the time of surgery and immediately frozen by rapid immersion in 2-methylbutane cooled to its freezing point with liquid nitrogen. Before freezing, the muscles were tied on splints to maintain a slightly stretched length.[13] They were then stored in a liquid nitrogen refrigerator (-196°C) until they were processed in order to stabilize enzyme activities.

Transverse sections (10μ thick) of the muscles were cut in a cryostat, mounted on coverslips, and allowed to dry at room temperature. Each muscle section of the series was processed using a different histochemical technique. The stains used included alkali stable and acid stable ATPase,[14] succinic dehydrogenase,[13] NADH tetrazolium reductase,[13] phosphorylase,[15] menadione-

From the Department of Otolaryngology and Communication Sciences, Upstate Medical Center, Syracuse, New York.

Presented at the meeting of the American Laryngological Association, Vancouver, British Columbia, May 10-11, 1981.

REPRINTS — Leslie T. Malmgren, PhD, Department of Otolaryngology and Communication Sciences, Upstate Medical Center, Syracuse, NY 13210.

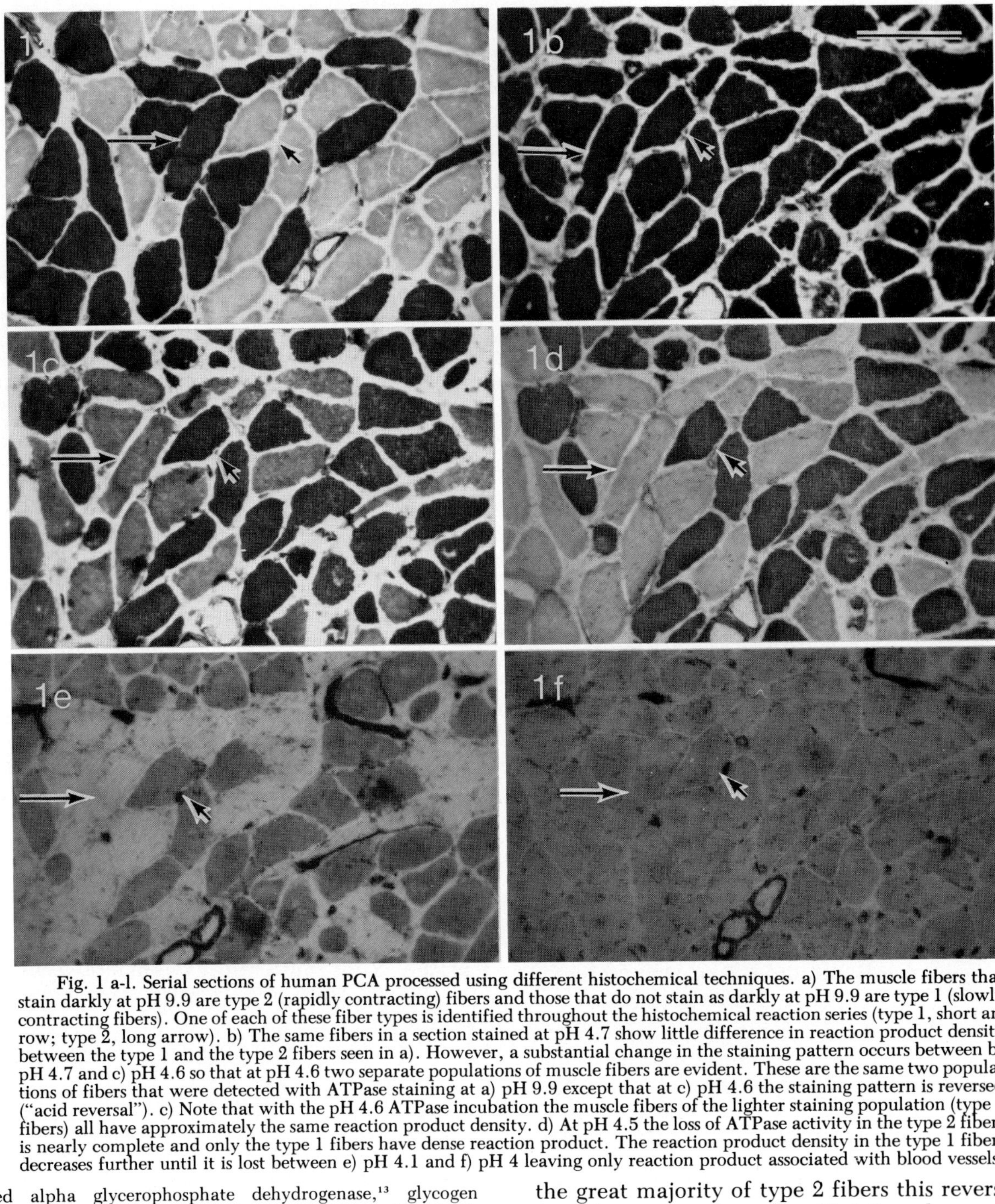

Fig. 1 a-l. Serial sections of human PCA processed using different histochemical techniques. a) The muscle fibers that stain darkly at pH 9.9 are type 2 (rapidly contracting) fibers and those that do not stain as darkly at pH 9.9 are type 1 (slowly contracting fibers). One of each of these fiber types is identified throughout the histochemical reaction series (type 1, short arrow; type 2, long arrow). b) The same fibers in a section stained at pH 4.7 show little difference in reaction product density between the type 1 and the type 2 fibers seen in a). However, a substantial change in the staining pattern occurs between b) pH 4.7 and c) pH 4.6 so that at pH 4.6 two separate populations of muscle fibers are evident. These are the same two populations of fibers that were detected with ATPase staining at a) pH 9.9 except that at c) pH 4.6 the staining pattern is reversed ("acid reversal"). c) Note that with the pH 4.6 ATPase incubation the muscle fibers of the lighter staining population (type 2 fibers) all have approximately the same reaction product density. d) At pH 4.5 the loss of ATPase activity in the type 2 fibers is nearly complete and only the type 1 fibers have dense reaction product. The reaction product density in the type 1 fibers decreases further until it is lost between e) pH 4.1 and f) pH 4 leaving only reaction product associated with blood vessels.

linked alpha glycerophosphate dehydrogenase,[13] glycogen (PAS),[13] Sudan black B (lipid),[13] acid phosphatase[16] and trichrome.[17] Equivalent fields in each of the serial sections were photographed, and an enzyme profile for each muscle fiber examined was compiled from the respective reaction product densities obtained with each of the histochemical techniques.

RESULTS

In the human PCA muscles examined ($n = 10$) 52% ± 11.8 SD were type 1 muscle fibers and 48% ± 11.9 SD type 2 muscle fibers.

The relative reaction product densities of type 1 (low ATPase at pH 9.9) and the type 2 (high ATPase at pH 9.9) reversed in the acid pH range (Fig. 1). In the great majority of type 2 fibers this reversal occurred at approximately pH 4.6 and was nearly complete by pH 4.5. This group of type 2 fibers behaved as a homogeneous population, and there was little evidence for diversity within this group with regard to the extent of inactivation of ATPase at different points in the acid reversal sequence. There were, however, infrequent type 2 fibers that retained an intermediate ATPase reaction product density (less than type 1 fibers) at pH 4.3. The type 1 fibers showed a loss of ATPase activity between pH 4.1 and 4 with essentially no difference among the various type 1 fibers in the extent of ATPase inactivation.

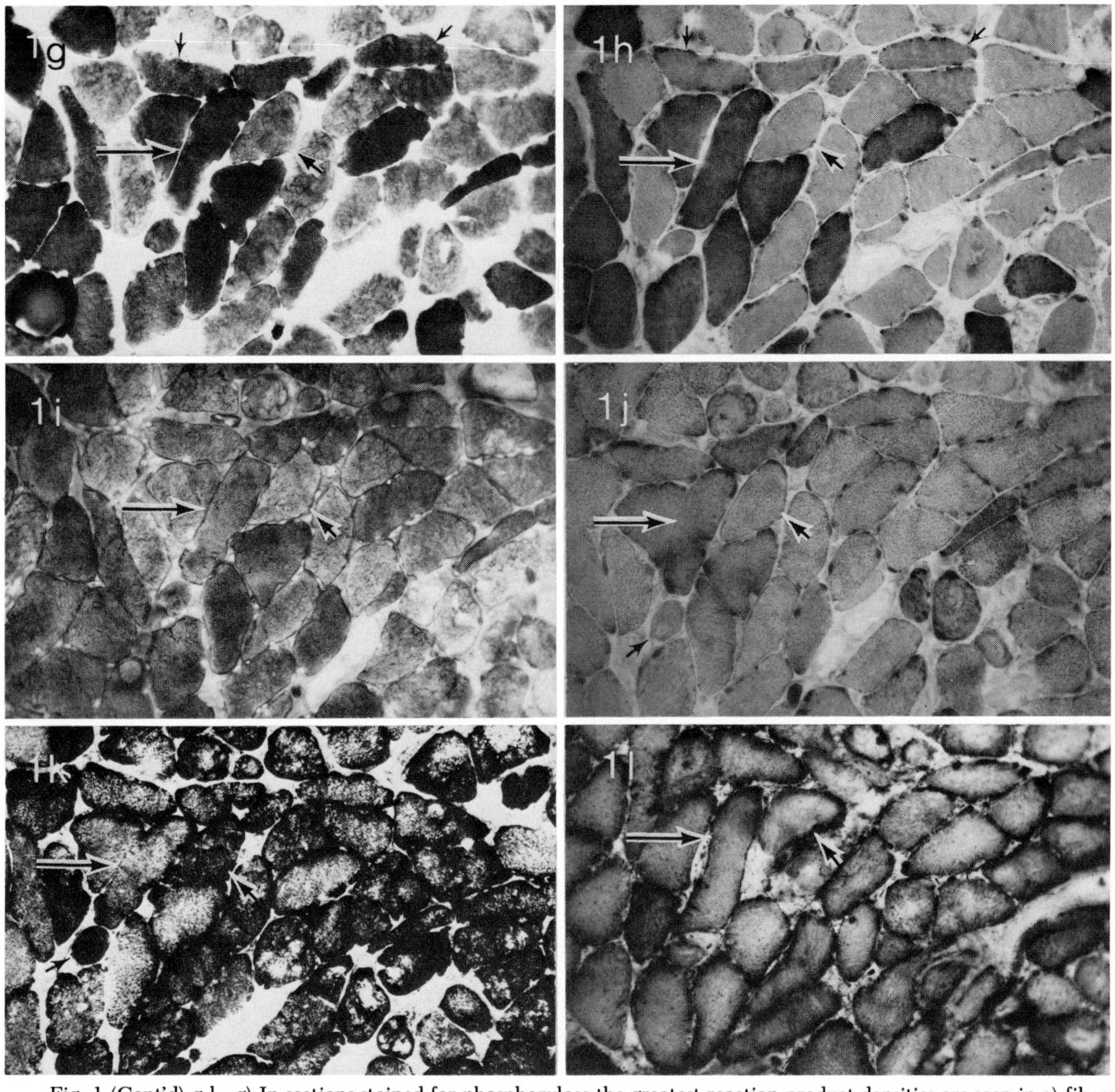

Fig. 1 (Cont'd) g-l. g) In sections stained for phosphorylase the greatest reaction product densities are seen in a) fibers that stain darkly for alkaline ATPase (type 2 fibers). However some of the type 2 fibers stain less darkly for phosphorylase than others (small arrows). The type 2 fibers also stain more densely than the type 1 fibers for menadione-linked αGPD. Some of the type 2 fibers that had less phosphorylase reaction product than other type 2 fibers (small arrows) also have h) much lower menadione-linked αGPD reaction product densities (small arrows) than other type 2 fibers. i) PAS (glycogen) staining is also generally somewhat less dense in the type 1 fibers than in type 2 fibers. j) Staining for succinic dehydrogenase shows variation in reaction product density among the fibers, but no obvious relationship is evident between staining intensity and fiber type. Some of the fibers show j) relatively low reaction product density for succinic dehydrogenase (small arrow) and k) relatively high reaction product density for NADH tetrazolium reductase (small arrow). In general NADH tetrazolium reductase reaction product is most dense in k) type 1 muscle fibers (short arrow). l) There is little difference in the staining intensity of Sudan black B (lipid) among the fiber types. Bar: 100μ.

In general the reaction product densities for the "glycolytic marker" enzymes, phosphorylase, and menadione-linked alpha glycerophosphate dehydrogenase (αGPD) were higher in the type 2A fibers than in the type 1 fibers (Fig. 1 g-i). However, there was a very wide range of phosphorylase and αGPD reaction product densities in the 2A fiber group (Fig. 1 g, h). Almost all of the muscle fibers in the PCA had high succinic dehydrogenase (SDH) activities (Figs. 1 j and 2). Although there were differences among fibers in relative SDH reaction product densities, there was no consistent difference between the type 1 and type 2A fibers in reaction product density. However some of the type 1 fibers differed from the other type 1 fibers and from the 2A fibers in that they had little staining for SDH. In contrast to the results obtained for SDH activities, staining for NADH tetrazolium reductase (NADH-TR) indicated fairly consistent differences in reaction product densities between type 1 and type 2A fibers. The reaction product densities in the type 1 fibers were typically higher than those in type 2A fibers. Staining with Sudan black B did not reveal any difference in lipid content between the type 1 and the type 2A fibers.

As indicated, in addition to type 1 and type 2A fibers, the human PCA included some infrequent

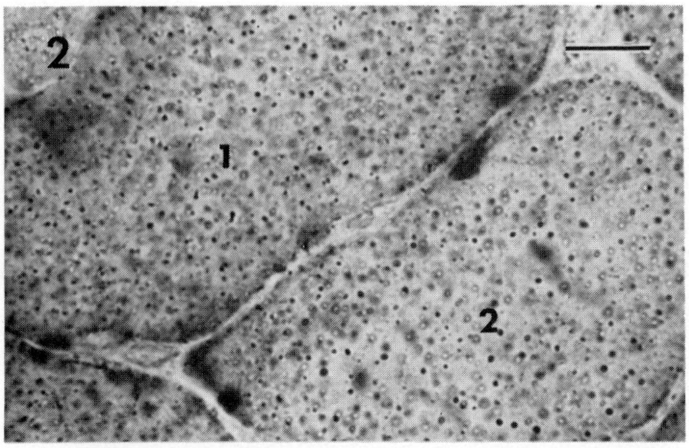

Fig. 2. High magnification of a type 1 (1) and a type 2 (2) muscle fiber in the same field as in Fig. 1j processed for the localization of succinic dehydrogenase activity. Numerous punctate sites of succinic dehydrogenase reaction product (a mitochondrial enzyme) are found in both the type 1 and the type 2 muscle fiber (some of the sites of staining are out of the focal plane and appear less distinct). Bar: 10μ.

type 2C fibers. The reaction product densities for this fiber group were generally intermediate to high for phosphorylase, low to intermediate for αGPD, low to intermediate for PAS (glycogen) staining, high for NADH-TR, low to high for SDH and intermediate for Sudan black B (lipid).

The distributions of type 1 and type 2 muscle fibers were examined in a total of ten PCA muscles (6 cases with both right and left PCA on 4 of the 6 cases). Muscle fiber type grouping (Fig. 3b) was clearly present in 4 of 10 muscles (4 of 6 cases examined). In the 4 cases where both the left and the right PCA muscles were taken, 2 had clear type grouping in the left PCA but not in the right PCA and 1 had type grouping in the right PCA and not in the left PCA.

DISCUSSION

General Characteristics of Muscle Fiber Types. In this study we have classified the muscle fiber types in the human PCA according to Brooke and Kaiser[18,19] since this system has been used most frequently in investigations dealing with human muscle fiber types. In this system muscle fibers are classified into 1 of 4 categories (types 1 and 2 A, B, or C) on the basis of the characteristics of their myosin ATPase. An initial classification of the fibers into two major groups (system of Engel, 1962)[17] is made on the basis of their ATPase reaction product density in sections that are preincubated in a solution having a pH in the alkaline range (we use pH 9.9). The fibers that have relatively little staining after this alkaline preincubation are categorized as type 1 fibers and those that stain darkly under these conditions are classified as type 2 fibers.[17] The type 2 fibers are then classified into subgroups on the basis of the extent of ATPase inactivation present when serial sections are preincubated at pH 4.6 or at pH 4.3.[18,19] Type 2 fibers that have marked inactivation of ATPase activity at pH 4.6 are classified as 2A fibers. Those that retain substantial activity at pH 4.6, but show almost complete inactivation at pH 4.3, are categorized as type 2B fibers. The 2C fiber is relatively rare in human muscle and is distinguished from 2A or 2B fibers by its retention of substantial ATPase activity after preincubation at pH 4.3.

Using glycogen depletion techniques, Burke et al[6,7] examined the relationship between the histochemical and the physiological characteristics of single motor units in the cat. They found that the type 1 fibers had the slowest contraction times, developed the smallest tensions, and were the most resistant to fatigue. The type 2B fibers had the fastest contraction times, developed the greatest tensions, and were the least resistant to fatigue. Finally, the type 2A fibers were found to have contraction times nearly as rapid as the 2B fibers, intermediate tensions and an intermediate fatigue resistance. The activities of the enzymes of energy metabolism as well as the concentrations of the related substrates were consistent with the physiological characteristics of each of these fiber types. The enzyme profiles of type 2 fibers indicated a high

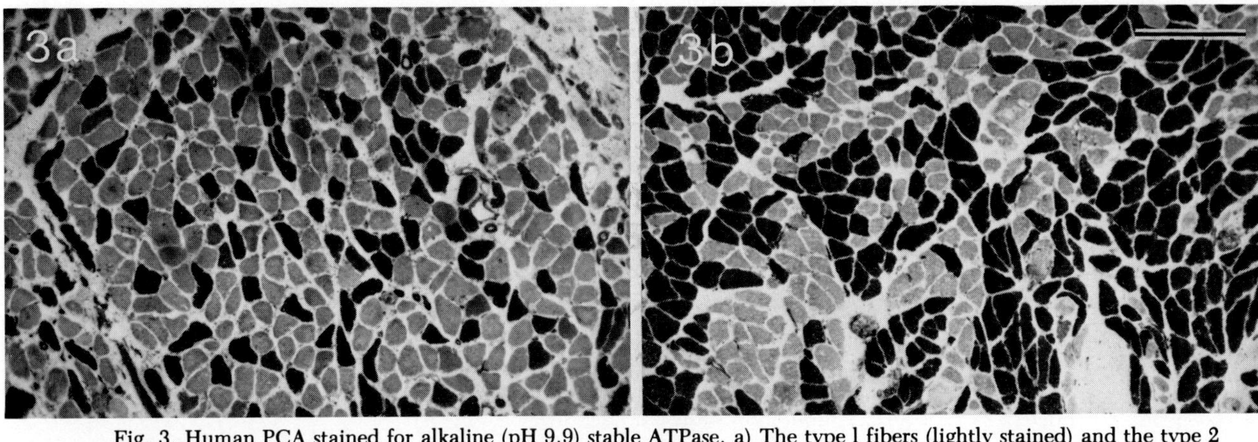

Fig. 3. Human PCA stained for alkaline (pH 9.9) stable ATPase. a) The type 1 fibers (lightly stained) and the type 2 fibers (darkly stained) are randomly distributed, which is generally considered to be normal. b) The distribution of type 1 and type 2 muscle fibers in a number of the human PCA muscles differed from the random distribution in that fibers of the same type are grouped together ("muscle fiber type grouping"). Bar: 200μ.

capacity for oxidative metabolism which correlated with their extreme resistance to fatigue while the type 2B fibers were found to be adapted primarily for short-term activity based on anaerobic glycolysis. As with the physiological parameters, the enzyme profiles of the type 2A fibers represented an intermediate form in that they indicated a high capacity for either anaerobic glycolysis or oxidative metabolism. Similar combined physiological and histochemical studies have been recently carried out on single motor units in the human medial gastrocnemius muscle and the results indicate that there are the same correlations between the physiological characteristics of motor units and the enzyme profiles of each of the muscle fibers included with them.[20]

Type 2C fibers are relatively rare in adult human muscles and they are considered to be an undifferentiated or precursor fiber.[19,21,22]

Muscle Fiber Types in the Human PCA. Our results concerning the type 1 and type 2 muscle fiber percentage composition in the human PCA (n = 10; 52% ± 11.8 SD type 1 and 48% ± 11.9 SD type 2) are in good agreement with those of Teig and coworkers[12] (n = 7; 67% ± 8.6 SD type 1 and 33% ± 8.6 SD type 2). They reported a gradual inactivation of type 2 fiber ATPase activity in the range 4.6-4.2. On the basis of these findings they concluded that it was not possible to be certain which muscle fibers corresponded to the different subgroups of type 2 fibers. Although we have also noted that the inactivation of the ATPase activity in the type 2 fiber is to some extent gradual within the 4.6-4.2 pH range, the major inactivation of type 2 fiber ATPase occurs at approximately pH 4.6. This pH value is close to that which would be expected for type 2A muscle fibers.[18,19] In addition to this population of type 2 fibers there is another group of type 2 fibers which have distinctly different acid reversal characteristics and are relatively rare in the human PCA. These fibers retain substantially more ATPase activity at pH 4.3, which would place them in the 2C fiber type category.[18,19]

As indicated, in the human PCA, the pH range at which acid reversal occurs in type 2 fibers suggests that most of the type 2 fibers are 2A fibers and that the remaining type 2 fibers are 2C fibers. However, our results for the "glycolytic" marker enzymes, phosphorylase and αGPD, suggest that there may be two additional populations of fiber subtypes within the 2A category. Another possibility would be that there is a single population having a wide range of values for these glycolytic enzymes.

In general, there is a tendency in both human and animal muscles for the relative activities of the various oxidative enzymes to show parallel relative reaction product densities in an individual fiber type as compared to reaction product densities in other fiber types.[13] The results that we have obtained for the muscle fiber types in the human PCA indicate a departure from this general tendency for parallel oxidative reaction product densities in that most of the type 1 fibers have higher NADH-TR activities than the type 2 fibers while staining for SDH activity shows variation in reaction product density among the fibers, but no obvious relationship between staining intensity and fiber type. It has been reported [23] that, in the cat PCA, certain muscle fibers differ from other mammalian muscle fibers in that the relative reaction product densities for SDH and NADH-TR show a nonparallel relationship in certain fibers. However, in the cat, the fibers that have nonparallel staining for these oxidative enzymes show a consistent total enzyme profile. They found that the type 1 fibers that had nonparallel staining for these oxidative enzymes were characterized by a low SDH activity but a high NADH-TR activity and a low staining for phosphorylase and glycogen. In the type 2 fibers that had nonparallel staining for the oxidative enzymes, the order of the oxidative enzyme levels was reversed with a high SDH activity and a low activity for NADH-TR. It was indicated that, in the PCA, the nonparallel type 1 fiber was the most common type 1 fiber while type 2 fibers in this muscle more commonly had parallel staining for SDH and NADH-TR. Although we have noted some type 1 fibers of the variety indicated by Edström and coworkers[23] (low SDH, high NADH-TR) in the human PCA, they do not appear to be common as they are in the cat. The human PCA differs from that of the cat in that most of the fibers, regardless of fiber type, have fairly high densities of SDH.

Muscle fibers having nonparallel staining for different oxidative enzymes have also been found to occur in other mammalian muscles. Type 1 fibers in the cat stapedius muscle have high NADH-TR activities but low SDH activities (Lyon MJ, Malmgren LT, unpublished data). Quantitative histochemical studies in the rabbit have also indicated a similar incomplete correlation between SDH values and NADH-TR values when data from the soleus, extensor digitorum longus, psoas and diaphragm are pooled.[10] It was suggested that one possible explanation for this finding might lie in the existence of diaphorases that are not part of the electron transport chain and that variations in the activities of these other diaphorases might account for the observed incomplete correlation between SDH values and NADH-TR values.

Physiological Implications of PCA Enzyme Profiles. In general, it can be concluded that the muscle fibers in the human PCA can be divided into three types on the basis of their ATPase characteristics alone, type 1, type 2A and type 2C. However, it is important to note that the combinations of relative reaction product densities that we have observed for glycolytic and oxidative enzymes and their substrates are not consistent with the enzyme profiles that are classically expected[13] for these fiber types. Since there is a close correlation between the enzyme profiles of muscle fibers and their activity patterns [8,9,24] it seems likely that the unusual enzyme profiles observed in the muscle fibers in the human PCA reflect the duration of activity of the individual motor units involved in the inspiratory cycle and/or other patterns of motor unit activity specific to the PCA. The diversity of motor unit activity patterns reported for individual motor units in the PCA[4] could well account for the diversity that we have observed in the enzyme profiles in these muscle fibers.

Although the contraction time of the cat PCA (20-25 ms) is fast in comparison with other mammalian muscles, the PCA is extremely fatigue resistant (equal to soleus).[23,25] The quantitative results available from biochemical investigations indicate that there is generally a correspondence between metabolic fluxes and the enzyme activities of the respective pathways.[26] Since the enzyme profiles that we have observed in the human PCA as well as those in the cat PCA[23] differ from those of classical muscle fiber types,[13] it is likely that metabolic fluxes in many of the muscle fiber types in the PCA would also differ from those of fiber types in most other mammalian muscles. Such a difference in energy metabolism might reflect an adaptation for the combination of rapid contraction times and fatigue resistance characteristic of the PCA.[25]

We found that the human PCA lacked type 2B (fatigue susceptible) muscle fibers. Half of the fibers present were of the extremely fatigue resistant[20] type 1 variety and the remaining half was composed almost entirely (rare type 2C fibers also present) of type 2A fibers which are also fatigue resistant.[20] In addition, almost all of the fibers, regardless of type, had high activities of succinic dehydrogenase (Fig. 2), a mitochondrial enzyme involved in oxidative metabolism. This indicates that the great majority of muscle fibers in the human PCA are equipped metabolically for fatigue resistance during prolonged activity.

"Fiber Type Grouping": Partial Denervation of PCA. When a muscle is partially denervated the remaining axons in the regions containing denervated muscle fibers receive a stimulus to sprout and reinnervate the denervated fibers.[27,28] Since the motor neuron determines the enzyme profiles of the muscle fibers that it innervates, the fiber types of the reinnervated muscle fibers shift to that characteristic of the new motor unit. As a result, the normally random mosaic of different muscle fiber types is interrupted by groups of muscle fibers with similar histochemical characteristics ("muscle fiber type grouping").

Unequivocal evidence of muscle fiber type grouping was present in 4 of the 10 human PCA muscles examined. In a previous study Teig and coworkers[12] reported muscle fiber type grouping in the PCA of 1 of 7 laryngectomy cases as well as a PCA muscle obtained at autopsy from a person without a history of laryngeal disease. One obvious implication of the presence of muscle fiber type grouping in this muscle is that the motor unit sizes would have been increased, in some cases greatly, in the PCA muscles where type grouping was evident. This would mean that the control of these muscles would be more coarse than in the normal PCA.

In a study of 36 human muscles in male subjects between 17 and 30 years, Johnson and coworkers[29] noted there was no muscle fiber type grouping in the great majority of the muscles examined. However muscle fiber type grouping was regularly present in the extensor digitorium brevis.[29,30] The extent of type grouping in this muscle was found to increase with age, and it was concluded that the etiology involved a slow process of denervation and reinnervation, probably as a result of intermittent compression of the nerve branch to this muscle. In middle-aged and elderly subjects, groups of atrophic fibers were present in the extensor digitorum brevis indicating that the rate of partial denervation was exceeding that of the reinnervation.[30] A more extensive study will be necessary to adequately examine the relationship between age (our cases were 43, 51, 52, 57, 59 and 64 years) and the extent of type grouping in the human PCA and to determine if type grouping occurs selectively in the PCA or if it is commonly found in other laryngeal muscles as well. It will also be of interest to examine the balance between partial denervation and reinnervation with advancing age to determine if this partial denervation eventually advances to muscle atrophy.

The cause of muscle fiber type grouping in the human PCA remains to be determined. Since the nerve fibers supplying the PCA have a scattered distribution within the recurrent laryngeal nerve[31,32] a selective compression of the abductor fibers at this level seems unlikely. Teig et al[12] have called attention to the possibility that terminal nerve branches in the PCA might be selectively prone to damage during endoscopy or when large lumps of food are swallowed. Another possibility would be that the specific activity patterns of certain motor units in the PCA lead to an early neuronal cell death.

Type grouping also occurs in the PCA muscle of apparently normal horses.[33] Laryngeal paresis with impaired abductor function ("roaring horses") is a well recognized problem in the horse, and it has been suggested that the muscle fiber type grouping observed in "normal" horses might, with time, advance to become a clinical problem. It has also been suggested that the muscle fiber type grouping observed in the PCA muscles of normal horses might result in a slight interference with normal breathing which, although not detectable clinically, would increase the animal's work of breathing and thereby decrease its athletic ability. Similar considerations might be applied to man as well, and this may be of particular importance in societies where the mean age of the population is increasing. Muscle fiber type grouping has been shown to increase with age in other human muscle.[29,30]

ACKNOWLEDGMENTS — We wish to thank Ms. Carol Horzempa for her excellent technical assistance. We are grateful to Dr. Precha Emko for his cooperation in providing tissue. We also thank Mrs. Pat Kane for her very helpful secretarial assistance.

REFERENCES

1. Green JH, Neil E. The respiratory function of the laryngeal muscles. J Physiol 1955; 129:132-41.

2. Faaborg-Andersen K. Electromyographic investigation of intrinsic laryngeal muscles in humans. Acta Physiol Scand 1957; 41: Suppl 140.

3. Hast MH. The respiratory muscle of the larynx. Ann Otol Rhinol Laryngol 1967; 234:489-97.

4. Suzuki M, Kirchner JA. The posterior cricoarytenoid as an inspiratory muscle. Ann Otol Rhinol Laryngol 1969; 78:849-64.

5. Wyke B. Respiratory activity of intrinsic laryngeal muscles: an experimental study. In: Wyke B, ed. Ventilatory and phonatory control systems. New York: Oxford University Press, 1974.

6. Burke RE, Levine DN, Zajac FE, Tsairis P, Engel WK. Mammalian motor units: physiological-histochemical correlation in three types of the cat gastrocnemius. Science 1971;174:709-12.

7. Burke RE, Levine DN, Tsairis P, Zajac FE. Physiological types and histochemical profiles in motor units of the cat gastrocnemius. J Physiol 1973; 234:723-48.

8. Pette D, Ramirez BU, Müller W, Simon R, Exner GV, Hildebrand R. Influence of intermittent long-term stimulation on contractile histochemical and metabolic properties of fibre populations in fast and slow rabbit muscles. Pfluegers Arch 1975; 361:1-7.

9. Salmons S. The response of skeletal muscle to different patterns of use — some new developments and concepts. In: Pette D, ed. Plasticity of muscle. Berlin: de Gruyter, 1980:387-99.

10. Spurway NC. Histochemical typing of muscle fibres by microphotometry. In: Pette D, ed. Plasticity of muscle. Berlin: de Gruyter, 1980:31-44.

11. Engel WK, Cunningham GG. Rapid examination of muscle tissue: an improved trichrome method for fresh-frozen biopsy sections. Neurology(NY) 1963; 13:919-23.

12. Teig E, Dahl HA, Thorkelsen H. Actomyosin ATPase activity of human laryngeal muscles. Acta Otolaryngol (Stockh) 1978; 85:272-81.

13. Dubowitz V, Brooke MH. Muscle biopsy: a modern approach. London: WB Saunders, 1973.

14. Guth L, Samaha FJ. Procedure for the histochemical demonstration of actomyosin ATPase. Exp Neurol 1970; 28:365-7.

15. Meijer, AE. Improved histochemical methods for demonstration of the activity of alpha-glucan phosphorylase. I. The use of glucosyl acceptor dextran. Histochemie 1968; 12:144-51.

16. Barka T, Anderson PJ. Histochemical methods for acid phosphatase using hexazonium pararosanilin as coupler. J Histochem Cytochem 1962; 10:741-53.

17. Engel WK. The essentiality of histo- and cytochemical studies of skeletal muscle in the investigation of neuromuscular disease. Neurology 1962; 12:778-94.

18. Brooke MH, Kaiser KK. Some comments on the histochemical characterization of muscle adenosine triphosphatase. J Histochem Cytochem 1969; 17:431-2.

19. Brooke MH, Kaiser KK. Muscle fiber types: how many and what kind? Arch Neurol 1970; 23:369-79.

20. Garnett RA, O'Donovan MJ, Stephans JA, Taylor A. Motor unit organization of human medial gastrocnemius. J Physiol 1979; 287:33-43.

21. Brooke MH, Kaiser, KK. The use and abuse of muscle histochemistry. Ann NY Acad Sci 1974; 228:121-44.

22. Brooke MH, Williamson E, Kaiser KK. The behavior of four fiber types in developing and reinnervated muscle. Arch Neurol 1971; 25:360-6.

23. Edström L, Lindquist C, Mortensson A. Histochemical properties of intrinsic laryngeal muscle. In: Wyke B, ed. Ventilatory and phonatory control systems. London: Oxford University Press, 1974:392-407.

24. Streter FA, Mabuchi K, Köver A, Gesztelyi I, Nagy Z, Furka I. Effect of chronic stimulation on cation distribution and membrane potential in fast-twitch muscles of rabbit. In: Pette D, ed. Plasticity of muscle. Berlin: deGruyter, 1980:441-51.

25. Mortensson A, Skoglund CR. Contraction properties of intrinsic laryngeal muscle. Acta Physiol Scand 1964; 60:318-36.

26. Pette D, Hofer HW. The constant proportion enzyme group concept in the selection of reference enzymes in metabolism: trends in enzyme histochemistry and cytochemistry. CIBA Foundation Symposium 73, 1980: 231-44.

27. Karpati G, Engel WK. "Type grouping" in skeletal muscles after experimental reinnervation. Neurology 1968; 18:447-55.

28. Kugelberg E, Edström L, Abbruzzse M. Mapping of motor units in experimentally reinnervated rat muscle: interpretation of histochemical and atrophic fibre patterns in neurogenic lesions. J Neurol Neurosurg Psychiatry 1970; 33:319-29.

29. Johnson MA, Polgar J, Weightman D, Appleton D. Data on the distribution of fibre types in thirty-six human muscles: an autopsy study. J Neurol Sci 1973; 18:111-29.

30. Jennekens FG, Tomlinson BE, Walton JN. The extensor digitorium brevis: histological and histochemical aspects. J Neurol Neurosurg Psychiatry 1972; 35:124-32.

31. Malmgren LT, Lyon MJ, Gacek RR. Localization of abductor and adductor fibers in the kitten recurrent laryngeal nerve: use of a variation of the horseradish peroxidase tracer technique. Exp Neurol 1977; 55:187-98.

32. Malmgren LT, Gacek RR. Acetylcholinesterase staining of fiber components of the cat and the human recurrent laryngeal nerve: topography of laryngeal motor regions. Acta Otolaryngol (Stockh) 1981; 91:337-52.

33. Gunn HM. Histochemical observations of laryngeal skeletal muscle fibers in "normal" horses. Equine Vet J 1972; 4:144-8.

Ann Otol 90:1981

OBSERVATIONS ON CENTRAL NEUROLOGIC ETIOLOGY FOR LARYNGEAL DYSFUNCTION

PAUL H. WARD, MD

DAVID G. HANSON, MD　　GEORGE BERCI, MD

LOS ANGELES, CALIFORNIA

Observations of patterns of laryngeal dysfunction in patients with known as well as unrecognized neurological disease have provided the basis for a new classification. Representative patients are used to describe typical patterns of laryngeal dysfunction which occur with afferent and efferent (upper motor neuron, extrapyramidal, cerebellar and nuclear pathways) neurological disorders. The value of cinephotography in documenting and avoiding the pitfalls of brief indirect laryngoscopy is emphasized as a factor in achieving a correct diagnosis in patients with laryngeal diseases of central origin.

The laryngologic literature detailing the functional results of peripheral injury to the nerve supply to the laryngeal musculature is voluminous. However, it is relatively recently that the abnormalities of function have been visually documented for detailed analysis.[1,2] Studies of cinephotographic documentation of these disorders now allow comparisons between patients and lesions that will continue to refine our understanding of the functional results of individual peripheral neural lesions in a manner not possible with undocumented examinations.

This kind of description has not been applied, to any substantial degree, to laryngeal dysfunction that originates from central neurologic lesions. This communication describes the authors' experience in direct telescopic observation of laryngeal function, with photographic documentation, in clinically documented central neurologic disorders. This type of study offers new insights into the normal control of laryngeal function as well as improving our ability to define the functional abnormalities in patients with recognized and unrecognized central neurological disorders.

The vocal and speech processes are erroneously conceived by most observers as simplistic and automatic since in the normal adult they are carried out with spontaneity and lack of conscious effort. Only brief reflection is needed to recognize that the physiology of the entire language and speech process is indeed complex. This involves encoding sensory inputs, organizing and conceptualizing them into linguistic form, selecting appropriate words and sentences and converting these words and concepts into a program of sequential neural impulses. All this is translated into neuromuscular action by the respiratory system, laryngeal and pharyngeal musculature, and articulatory structures, eventuating in speech. The complexity of the system is further increased by the acoustical output of speech which is almost simultaneously monitored by the auditory, visual, and proprioceptive systems. This feedback is coordinated in the central nervous system where modification of the entire linguistic process recurs. The central compensatory mechanisms may obscure the original pathological changes.

The process of vocalization is largely unconscious for most individuals. It is only when there is a functional abnormality that the patient usually becomes aware of speech and vocal patterns. When dysfunction occurs it is quickly apparent to patient and physician alike that the coordination of respiratory, alimentary, postural, and speech functions of the glottis are controlled by a finely balanced, very complex physiology. It is perhaps useful to think of laryngeal function in terms of a phylogenic hierarchy of priorities. It appears that the primal function of the glottis was sphincteric protection of the airway. Closure of the airway in the act of swallowing or stimulation of the pharynx is an automatic reflex that takes precedence over voluntarily controlled function. The cough reflex can be, to some degree, suppressed but may override even swallow and gag reflexes. These functions are controlled centrally and depend on normal integration of sensory and proprioceptive afferent input from the upper respiratory tract. The primitive gag reflex involves more than simple closure of the vocal folds. The larynx is observed to close with tight sphincteric approximation of the false vocal folds, the petiol of the epiglottis, and the interarytenoid fold. Loss of the control of this reflex in relation to sensory input may be expected to affect laryngeal function in a spectrum of pathology depending on the location and severity of the lesion.

From the Department of Surgery, Division of Head and Neck Surgery (Otolaryngology), UCLA School of Medicine, and the Department of Surgery, Cedars-Sinai Medical Center, Los Angeles. This work was supported in part by the Brian W. Lawrence Fund of the Blalock Foundation.

Presented at the meeting of the American Laryngological Association, Vancouver, British Columbia, May 10-11, 1981.

REPRINTS — Paul H. Ward, MD, Division of Head and Neck Surgery, UCLA School of Medicine, Los Angeles, CA 90024.

In higher forms, the larynx becomes increasingly important in posture, ie, in support of the upper body for lifting and straining and functions unconsciously to regulate intrapulmonary pressures. Finally the importance of the glottis in phonatory function becomes increasingly apparent in organisms that communicate by vocalization. Cortical control over the larynx becomes increasingly conscious in the production of speech and is distinctly voluntary in the highly trained and controlled vocal apparatus of the professional singer.

Injury to the peripheral pathways of neural control to the larynx results in the predictable dysfunctions of well-recognized paralytic dysphonias.[3] Functionally these disorders result in loss of movement of the affected laryngeal muscles and dysphonia which will vary according to the degree of compensatory changes in function that the patient may employ. There is considerable compensation that can occur which may complicate assessment of the original pathology. Prolonged observation is often the only way that an accurate functional description can be made.

Disorder of the central laryngeal pathways both afferent and efferent by a variety of pathologies manifests in patterns that may be typical for the specific neurologic disease. It is this observation of characteristic functional abnormalities in given neurologic disorders that has prompted this report. The authors have had the opportunity to examine and photograph the larynges and record the voices of a significant number of patients with known neurological disorders, undiagnosed dysphonia, or dysfunction and incoordinated breathing disorders. A typical history has included examination by several physicians, psychiatrists, laryngologists, and neurologists. The same patient may have been told by different examiners that he or she had vocal cord paralysis and at other times that the larynx was normal. These patients have often been referred to psychiatrists or speech pathologists for nonorganic speech problems. Others have had their intermittent problems diagnosed as due to central sleep apnea or asthma. It is clear that the standard mirror examination of the larynx is totally inadequate for the definition of problems due to central neurologic disease. A fleeting glance with the mirror is unlikely to reveal subtle abnormalities in control, and results in an inadequate report of an anatomically normal larynx with good (or paralyzed) vocal cord motion. The abnormal signs and symptoms produced in other body structures containing voluntary muscles are well-recognized. It is clearly reasonable that the larynx, a structure whose functions are largely controlled by voluntary striated muscle, should also exhibit recognizable deviations from normal when there is damage to its central neural pathways.

The following classification is proposed for correlation of observed patterns of laryngeal dysfunction with the site of lesion in the central nervous system.[4]

Central Neuronal Network

A. Afferent sensory, autonomic
B. Efferent motor
    1. Upper motor neuron (cortex and pyramidal tracts)
    2. Extrapyramidal (recticular substance)
    3. Cerebellar
    4. Nuclear (lower motor neuron)

Representative cases are presented that illustrate the functional laryngeal deficits that result in lesions at various levels in the central neuronal network.

AFFERENT SYSTEM DISEASE

Relatively little is known and minimal reference is made in the literature concerning the afferent pathways except that they are known to exhibit and pass centrally through the superior laryngeal and vagus nerves.[5] Several patients were observed whose laryngeal dysfunction appears to be primarily one of override of more primitive reflexes due to faulty coordination of sensory input with functional needs.

Case 1. This 39-year-old male was examined because of his severe difficulty with speech. A schoolteacher, his problem had manifest initially by changes in personality and ataxia. As his symptoms progressed, a diagnosis of progressive suprabulbar palsy was made. His speech difficulty was initially characterized by difficulty in initiating phonation. His voice when first examined sounded like spastic dysphonia. He had extreme difficulty initiating phonation and the quality was forced. Examination of the head and neck was unremarkable except for a very active gag reflex, which could be initiated by simply touching the nasal mucosa, and lead to sometimes prolonged laryngospasm. It was possible to examine the larynx with a fiberoptic telescope only after topical anesthesia of the entire nose and pharynx. There was full range of motion of the arytenoids and a marked tendency to spasm. Bilateral superior laryngeal nerve blocks resulted in reversal of the dysphonia to a normal phonatory pattern. Single superior nerve block had little effect on the very spastic quality of his voice. Unilateral recurrent laryngeal nerve block resulted in some improvement but there was still significant difficulty initiating phonation as the nonparalyzed cord continued to spasm.

The patient's disease progressed to the point where he was unable to initiate any phonation. Swallowing also caused laryngeal spasm. Trunkal apraxia affected his ability to walk, write, and care for himself. There was progressive involvement of the disease, producing impairment of voluntary eye movement, dysphonia, and dementia.

COMMENT. The laryngeal dysfunction in this patient appeared to be related to progressive loss of control over or inhibition of the primitive protective glottic reflexes. When there was stimulation of almost any area of the upper airway mucosa there was a marked gag reflex and laryngeal spasm. Superior laryngeal nerve block and topical anesthesia (ie, interruption of afferent sensory input) resulted in essentially normal phonatory movements and normal speech.

Case 2. This 72-year-old female has been followed for 2½ years. She presented with articulatory problems, initially slurring of words and marked difficulty in tongue control. Her voice subsequently became very spastic in quality. She had difficulty initiating phonation and her voice was strained. Initiation of phonation was accompanied by facial grimaces similar to those seen in advanced spastic dysphonia. There was a markedly increased gag reflex. Examination of the larynx could be accomplished only with topical anesthesia of the pharynx with bilateral topical superior laryngeal nerve blocks. There was full range of motion of the left vocal cord. The right vocal cord was in an intermediate position and did not move voluntarily but showed involuntary abduction and adduction. Though involuntary movement persists, the patient has progressively lost essentially all voluntary control of tongue movements. She has progressed to complete aphonia because of often prolonged laryngeal spasm which occurs with attempts at phonation and with swallowing. It has been necessary to place a cervical esophagostomy for feeding. The patient has learned to manipulate the esophagostomy tube very carefully in order to avoid prolonged laryngeal spasm from the stimulation of the esophageal mucosa. There are no apparent abnormalities in other cranial nerves in this patient. She has normal motor function other than the 12th cranial nerve, she walks and writes well, drives her own car, and lives by herself. CT scan shows pontine atrophy and she was initially diagnosed as having pontocerebellar atrophy type II. However, she had few cerebellar signs.

COMMENT. This patient's primary problem appears to be failure to successfully integrate sensory and proprioceptive input for control of the tongue and larynx. This results in completely ineffective tongue movements and in the override of laryngeal closure reflexes with normal stimulation of the upper airway mucosa. As in the prior case the laryngeal spasm can be relieved by blocks of the superior laryngeal nerves.

It is believed that these cases represent suprabulbar sites of lesions that result in loss of normal control over laryngeal protective reflexes. The overbalance of the primitive gag reflex results in major disruption in deglutition and speech. The spastic component of laryngeal dysfunction can be alleviated by interruption of the superior laryngeal fiber transmission.

Another function of the larynx is its role in respiration. Glottic closure is important in the stabilization of the chest for lifting, and has a role in the regulation of intrathoracic pressures. There is some question about the precise nature of relative roles of active muscular abduction versus a biomechanical "spring action" in opening the larynx in deep rapid respiration but there is no question that deep inspiration results in the normal patient in hyperabduction of the vocal folds.[6] There is good evidence in animals of neural reflexes in respiratory sensors.[7] At least two patients in our study clearly provide evidence that central neuromuscular function plays an important role in the opening of the glottis with respiration. Brainstem and higher lesions can cause isolated abduction spasm and other disorders of position in relationship to normal respiratory control.

EFFERENT MOTOR SYSTEM DISEASE

UPPER MOTOR NEURONS (CORTEX AND PYRAMIDAL)

The experimental studies by Furstenberg and

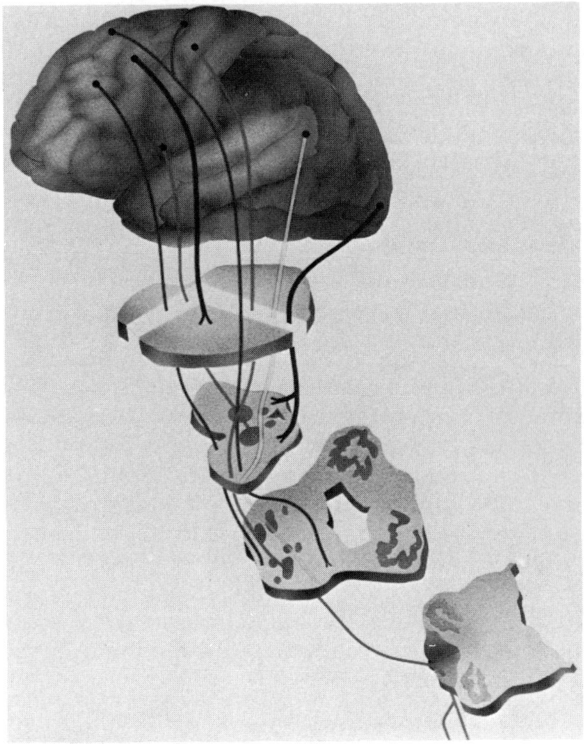

Fig. 1. Drawing of the cerebral cortex showing upper motor neurons. Fibers from the precentral gyrus (Broca's area) pass through the internal capsule making up the pyramidal tracts to eventually synapse in the nucleus ambiguus and other brainstem nuclei.

Magielski[8] and by Kirikae and coworkers[9] demonstrated that stimulation of the frontal motor area as well as many other cortical areas in monkeys and cats produces activity in the electromyographically monitored laryngeal muscles.[8,9] In man, Broca's area 4 of the precentral gyrus of the dominant hemisphere is important in initiation of vocalization and speech (Fig. 1). Stimulation of the cortex during craniotomy (under local anesthesia) has revealed that vocalization can be elicited. Sounds were produced by stimulation of the frontal, parietal, and occipital lobes as well as Broca's area.[10]

Neurons from the speech cortex join the cortical bulbar tracts and pass through the internal capsule and cerebral peduncle to form the pyramidal tracts. A partial decussation takes place in the medulla prior to synapse in the nucleus ambiguus. Diseases that involve the upper motor neurons will have variable effects on the function of the larynx depending on the location of the lesion. The changes may be subtle or incapacitating, but do not cause complete paralysis of laryngeal musculature. Rather, these lesions result in loss of normal coordination of respiratory and phonatory movements of the laryngeal muscles. There may be aggravating involvement of the articulators as well. These patients may also experience variable degrees of difficulty in understanding written and spoken words and in formulating and expressing meaningful speech. Dysarthria, aphonia and dysphonia are the clinical manifestations. Strokes or vascular accidents involve these areas secondary to thrombosis, embolism, or hemorrhage of the middle cerebral artery. Because the upper motor neurons responsible for articulation, phonation, and respiration come from both hemispheres, and their fiber tracts have undergone partial decussation, only bilateral lesions have a severe effect on the muscles of the larynx. Because the changes in the larynx are subtle, in unilateral lesions they have often gone unnoticed. Even the minor abnormalities caused by a unilateral hemispherical lesion, however, can be recognized if motion pictures of the larynx are carefully studied. Bilateral damage to Broca's area results in first a flaccid and then spastic paresis of the laryngeal muscles. Because other motor pathways take over control of the lower motor neurons, there is limited wasting or atrophy of the laryngeal muscles. The striking appearance of the larynx in patients with bilateral vascular accidents, widespread cerebral atherosclerosis (causing suprabulbar or pseudobulbar palsy), and cerebral palsy (secondary to anoxia, kernicterus toxic drugs or viral infections) is manifested by variable patterns of incoordination of the laryngeal musculature. The incoordination of respiration and laryngeal function results in production of sounds that are sometimes harsh and excessively loud or may be breathy, weak, and fading. Concomitant involvement of the articulators causes slow slurred speech with distorted sounds and defective resonance. The following case exemplifies this type of upper neuron lesion.

Case 3. A 28-year-old female was referred for severe airway obstruction. She had a history of "asthma," rheumatic valvular heart disease, and ten mild strokes. She had sustained a right hemiparesis, but had made remarkable progress in rehabilitation and was ambulatory with crutches. The embolizations were attributed both to ingestion of birth control pills and to valvular heart disease, which was complicated on one hospitalization by subacute bacterial endocarditis.

Her first stroke, causing a right hemiparesis, occurred three years prior to being seen at UCLA. It was accompanied by severe respiratory distress requiring intubation on two occasions. A year later "respiratory infection" again resulted in obstruction and two additional intubations. Two years after the onset of hemiparesis a "respiratory infection" and severe airway obstruction necessitated a tracheostomy. This was closed subsequently but had to be reopened two weeks prior to her referral to UCLA.

During the previous three years the patient sustained at least ten minor strokes accompanied by severe respiratory obstruction and varying degrees of dysphonia. The "asthma" was nonresponsive to steroids and she was under the care of a psychiatrist for "functional voice and breathing problems." A number of competent laryngologists had seen her and had reported on several occasions the presence of a normal larynx. Several other examiners described a swollen epiglottis and supraglottis, and she was told at a large well-known midwestern clinic and by several other laryngologists that she had a "bilateral abductor paralysis."

Upon initial examination this pleasant, cheerful, well-developed female was breathing through a bivalved tracheostomy tube and walked with the assistance of crutches. She was determined to overcome her illness and wanted to get rid of her tracheostomy. She was stridorus on inspiration and her voice was a bit raspy and breathy. Examination and photography of the larynx showed the cords remaining near the midline in a slightly bowed position most of the time. There were quivering motions of the arytenoids

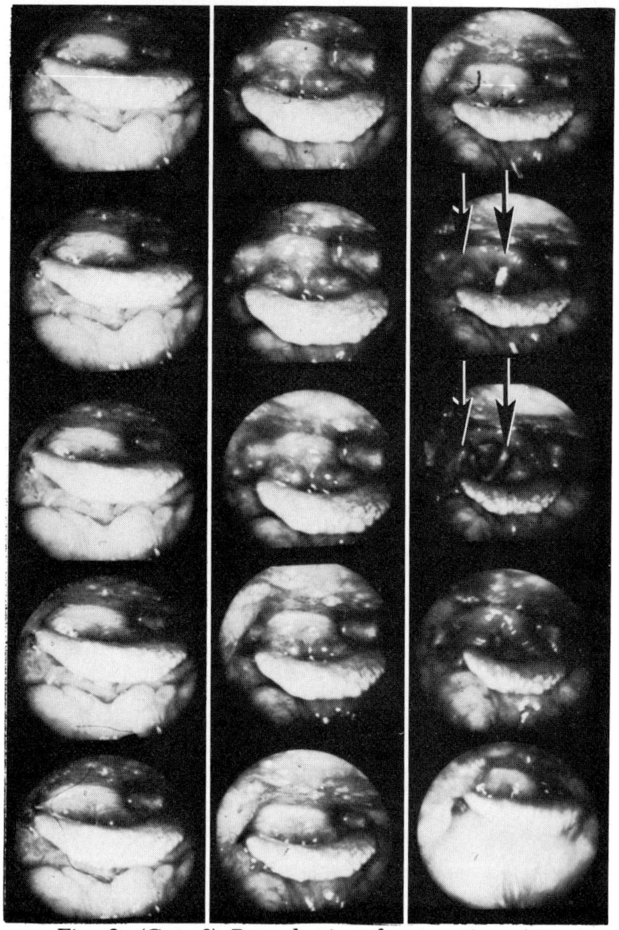

Fig. 2. (Case 3) Reproductions from motion picture telescopic views of the larynx. There was a "spastic" closure of the aryepiglottic folds, epiglottis, and vocal cords. The first two vertical rows were the characteristic appearance. Only rarely was there involuntary wide abduction of the cords as seen in the third row (arrows). Note the lag of the right cord producing the laryngeal asymmetry.

and, after long periods of observation, spontaneous, involuntary wide abduction of the cords. During the next few months, improvement of the control and voluntary abduction of her cords (documented on film) paralleled the improvement in the hemiparesis.

Four months later she sustained another "small stroke" and had to leave her tracheostomy tube open because of shortness of breath. The larynx was filmed two weeks after her hospitalization and at that time there was marked spasticity of the entire larynx with tne epiglottis, aryepiglottic folds, and cords squeezed together. On two occasions during several minutes of filming the larynx opened as the cords involuntarily abducted widely (Fig. 2).

During the next $2\frac{1}{2}$ years, motion pictures were taken of her larynx during different phases of recovery after two additional small strokes. Because she was hospitalized elsewhere following her strokes, the immediate poststroke, upper motor neuron, flaccid, paralytic phase was not observed. The spastic supraglottic and glottic paresis of the larynx that we observed several weeks after the strokes gradually resolved into what has been commonly called "bilateral abductor paralysis." This was in actuality a paresis, because at other times she voluntarily and involuntarily abducted both vocal cords. There was some asymmetry of the larynx with a lagging paretic motion of the right cord. The patient's larynx was filmed before and after hypnosis (by her psychiatrist) which showed no effect upon the voluntary or involuntary motions of her laryngeal muscles.

COMMENT. This is a rather typical history of patients with central laryngeal paresis or paralysis. Unless the stroke is massive with many other neurological signs and symptoms the patients may be seen only by laryngologists for airway obstruction and a hoarse voice. The brief mirror or even telescopic views of the larynx may suggest a swollen larynx if it is in the spastic phase. As resolution takes place, the laryngeal appearance of a superior and recurrent bilateral "abductor paralysis" may be the interpretation unless prolonged, careful examination reveals the presence of rare voluntary and involuntary abductions of the cords. The dysphonic episodes and the shortness of breath accompanied by stridor are often interpreted and treated as asthma. Failure to respond to steroids is characteristic of these patients.

This patient's strokes were caused by emboli, primarily to the middle cerebral artery or its branches. The patient's other neurological signs suggest confinement to the left hemisphere although there may have been bilateral diffuse embolization. The laryngeal response involved the entire larynx, although during recovery there was a more marked paresis of the right side of the larynx (the side of her hemiparesis). This patient is still under observation and by repeated filmings of her larynx it is hoped that additional knowledge will be obtained about upper motor neuron (pyramidal tract) paresis of the larynx.

Case 4. This 79-year-old female developed deterioration of her speech over a period of seven days. This occurred about seven years ago and the speech pattern has been stable since that time. She had no other symptom, at that time or since, other than a mild unsteadiness of her hands. She is bright, fully oriented, and lives alone and cares for herself.

The voice is characterized by ataxic short choppy phrases. Words and sentences are stopped short and breathing is similarly interrupted. On laryngeal examination there is constant motion of the arytenoids and involuntary abduction and adduction of the glottis during respiration and speech.

Neurological examination shows no other abnormalities of the cranial nerves. Muscle strength is normal and symmetrical as are deep tendon reflexes. There are no pathological reflexes. There are no abnormal cerebellar signs. There is a mild constructional apraxia in copying objects but mental status is otherwise normal. CT scan with and without contrast is normal. The neurologic diagnosis was that this patient had a small isolated cortical infarct, and that the disability was unlikely to improve.

COMMENT. The patient's lesion, which is not well identified as to precise location, has interrupted the normal control of vocal cord positioning with respiration. The glottis involuntarily abducts widely during phonation and will also adduct completely during deep inspiration. This constant motion is superimposed on voluntary actions, and is suggestive of the kind of abnormality that would be expected with extrapyramidal disease. However it is difficult to imagine an extrapyramidal lesion specific enough to involve only laryngeal muscular control. It is postulated that the lesion may involve important cortical input to the extrapyramidal system.

Case 5. A 65-year-old business man, in prior good health, collapsed in coma with a left hemiparesis. On CT scan the site of lesion appeared to be a small hemorrhage confined to the thalamus. The patient made a fair recovery but remained hemiparetic on the left. The patient's constant aspiration of all fluids remained a serious problem after his stroke. On laryngeal examination there was marked hyperabduction of the left vocal cord at rest, with the right cord in normal position. On attempts at phonation the left cord lagged in its movements toward the midline in relation to the right, and complete closure was effected only with forced cough. As the patient's hemiparesis became less spastic his aspiration improved as well.

COMMENT. This patient appears to represent an example of isolated unilateral abductor spasm associated with a thalmic hemorrhage.

EXTRAPYRAMIDAL LESIONS

The corpus striatum with caudate and lenticular nuclei and the basal ganglia, the globus palidus, and substantia nigra, are included with the reticular substance in the extrapyramidal system. These areas of the brain are thought to be important to coordination of synergistic control of the laryngeal muscles in both respiration and speech. Athetoid and choreatoid movements are characteristic of patients with extrapyramidal lesions and these functional changes may be seen in the larynx of affected patients. This dysfunction manifests in poorly controlled phonatory efforts. Several cases of Parkinson's disease as a cause of vocal cord paralysis are reported in the literature.[11-13] Unless these were caused by lesions extending beyond the extrapyramidal system it is likely that more lengthy examination would reveal these patients had only paresis rather than paralysis.

Degeneration of the basal ganglia and reticular substance is responsible for the tremor and rigidity that is characteristic of Parkinson's disease. Several forms of parkinsonism can now be differentiated, including postencephalitic, arteriosclerotic, and idiopathic (Fig. 3). Parkinsonian symptoms may accompany other syndromes, such as Shy Drager syndrome, where there are lesions extending beyond the extrapyramidal system. Laryngeal photographic examination of patients with Parkinson's disease shows an apparently characteristic functional appearance. Patients with postencephalitic Parkinson's disease tend to have a greater degree of tremor in the laryngeal muscles. On examination, quivering involuntary movements of the interarytenoid muscles and false vocal folds may be particularly apparent. This tremor results in a quivering quality to the voice. There is a full range of adductor and abductor motion in these patients.

Patients with idiopathic hypokinetic parkinsonism characteristically have weak breathy voices. Phrasing is limited due to rapid loss of air. Photographic examination of the larynx of these patients reveals a consistent appearance. There is normal range of motion of the arytenoids but inability to tense the vocal cords. This is manifested sometimes by marked bowing of the cords and difficulty with

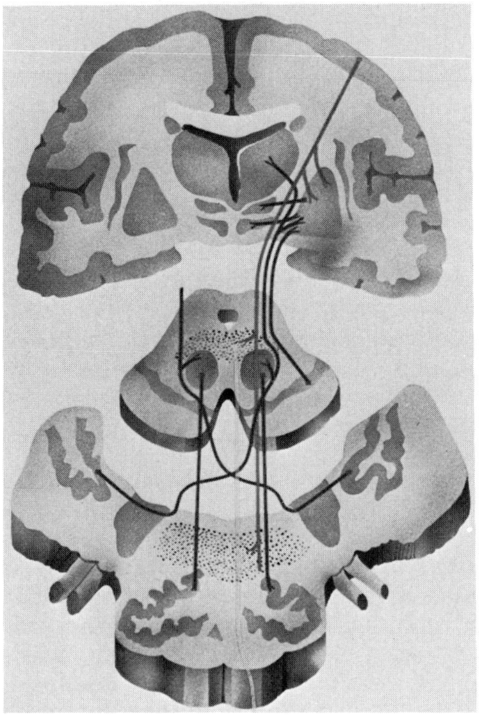

Fig. 3. Diagram of the extrapyramidal system which includes the caudate and lenticular nuclei, the basal ganglia, the globus palidus and substantia nigra as well as the reticular substance (stippled areas).

pitch changes. Tremor is usually not a significant component of the laryngeal function pattern.

The following cases are examples of extrapyramidal disease causing parkinsonism and atypical parkinsonism which exhibited altered laryngeal function.

Case 6. This 65-year-old female was diagnosed as having Parkinson's disease 15 years previously. During the ensuing years she had a gradual progression in the severity of her pill-rolling tremor, forward-leaning gait, cog-wheel rigidity, and loss of facial expression. Her voice was noted to be fairly normal although her speech was slow and had a quivering sound. Examination of the larynx showed quivering tonicity, pseudomyoclonic motions of the aryepiglottic folds with irregular involuntary adduction or abduction of the cords. There was voluntary adduction during phonation; however, the quivering and involuntary motions tended to produce incompetence of the glottic chink, resulting in a comparable quivering characteristic to the voice.

COMMENT. This pattern has been observed and photographed in several other patients with well-documented postencephalitic parkinsonism. Shy Drager syndrome is a rare disorder that is characterized by progressive autonomic failure. These patients subsequently develop bulbar and cerebellar signs in addition to parkinsonian symptoms. The pathology described in the few cases available shows degenerative lesions in the pigmented basal nuclei in addition to the dorsal motor nucleus of the vagus.[14,15] Involvement of the dorsal motor nucleus of the vagus should result in a progressive paralysis of the laryngeal muscles as this is a lower motor nuclear lesion. This would be in contradistinction to the preserved, though poorly controlled, movement that is characteristic of higher neurological lesions. Photographic examination clearly demonstrates that such is the case. Shy Drager syndrome patients are, in our experience, characterized by a progressive abductor paresis of the larynx. While the degree of paresis may fluctuate the overall course is toward complete abductor paralysis and respiratory failure.[16] It is of interest that Shy Drager syndrome patients can also be differentiated from parkinsonian patients by acoustic and perceptual analysis of voice recordings (Hanson DG et al and Ludlow C et al, unpublished data).

Case 7. This 70-year-old male was admitted in coma with severe respiratory distress which required tracheostomy. The patient had noted progressive difficulty in breathing over a period of a month. The patient's wife noted progressive stridor during this time. The patient had been previously well. The only neurologic symptom that he had noted was the onset of a mild resting tremor in the right arm approximately two months prior to hospitalization. Examination after tracheostomy revealed marked prominence of the neck and mediastinal vasculature.

The larynx was described, on direct and indirect examination, to be very edematous but otherwise normal. After tracheostomy there was rapid resolution of the venous distention and mediastinal widening. The larynx was reported as returning to normal, but was difficult to examine well. The patient's hospital course was complicated by the onset of urinary retention which required catheterization. After discharge the patient developed difficulty with lightheadedness and fainting when he was in an upright position, and was confined to a wheelchair. At this point the patient was accepted in referral.

Laryngeal examination showed the vocal cords to be in a paramedian position with no abduction beyond this position over prolonged observation. In phonation the cords were abducted to the midline with inward rotation of the arytenoids. There was impaired ability to tense the vocal cords, manifest by bowing of the cords during phonation. On the basis of abductor paresis of the vocal folds, along with evidence of progressive failure of the autonomic nervous system and early evidence of basal ganglia disease, a diagnosis of Shy Drager syndrome was suggested which was subsequently confirmed by further neurological consultation.

Case 8. A 58-year-old male was referred to UCLA with an unusual group of symptoms. The patient gave a history of progressive weakening of his voice, slowing of his speech with slurring, shortness of breath, deterioration of penmanship, general weakness, unsteadiness, and loss of potency over the previous $1^1/_2$ to 2 years. He had been seen by several physicians, laryngologists, neurologists, and a psychiatrist. Several laryngologists informed him that his vocal cords were paralyzed. The urologist diagnosed a neurogenic bladder. The neurologist's clinical diagnosis was Shy Drager syndrome.

On examination the patient appeared his stated age. His speech was mildly dysarythric and slowed. The incoordination of his breathing resulted at times in his voice becoming weaker and trailing off as he ran out of air. He exhibited mild decrease in his ability to perform the finger-to-nose test and would fall to the right on tandem walking. Study of the motion pictures of his larynx failed to confirm the previously diagnosed vocal cord paralysis. At rest his vocal cords were positioned in an almost medial position with only 1-2 mm of glottic chink. There were fine quivering, tremorous motions of both arytenoids and aryepiglottic folds. The patient's larynx was repeatedly observed and photographed during the following $1^1/_2$ years as he showed the neurological signs of progressive olivopontocerebellar degeneration. The cerebellar and brainstem atrophy was confirmed by CT scan. The laryngeal motions were a progressive increase in the irregular tremor of the arytenoids and aryepiglottic folds with periodic involuntary adductions or abductions of the bowed medially positioned vocal cords.

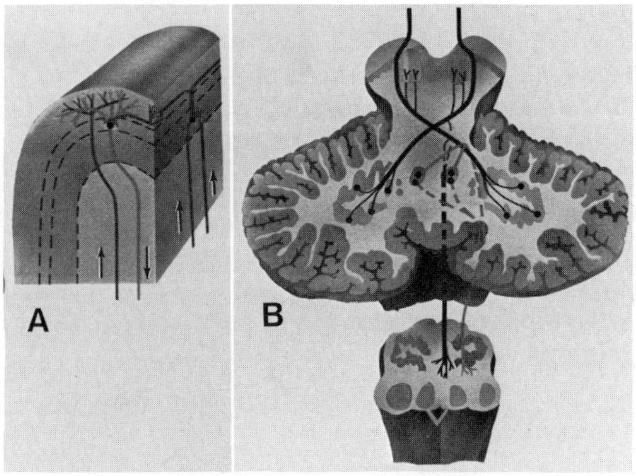

Fig. 4. Drawing of A) cerebellar cortex supplying neural fibers that impinge upon the deep nuclei of B) cerebellum. Messages are then relayed to the extrapyramidal system as well as to the brainstem nuclei including the nucleus ambiguus.

COMMENT. The typical course of laryngeal abnormality in the Shy Drager syndrome is a progressive loss of voluntary and respiratory abductor function and loss of voicing control. In addition to extrapyramidal disease, this probably represents a progressive involvement of the dorsal motor nucleus of the vagus that may eventually produce a paralysis of the vocal cords rather than a paresis.

Progressive airway obstruction is not characteristic of Parkinson's disease. The difference between patients with Parkinson's symptoms and patients with panautonomic failure in addition to Parkinson's can be explained by the additional pathology in the dorsal motor nuclei in the latter. The laryngeal abnormalities in the Shy Drager patients probably represent a combination of extrapyramidal and nuclear pathologies. They may have cerebellar findings as well, as occurred in case 8.

In these cases of extrapyramidal and combined extrapyramidal and cerebellar and nuclear degeneration, the characteristic laryngeal abnormalities were tremor and incoordination of laryngeal motions with involuntary abduction and adduction of the cords progressing towards actual paralysis. The tendency of the cords to stay in a somewhat adducted position for significant periods of time had led to an original diagnosis of vocal cord paralysis. The voice changes, breathiness, and shortness of breath were due to incoordination of laryngeal musculature during vocalization and breathing.

CEREBELLAR

As with the higher central nervous system centers, the cerebellum supplies neural fibers that impinge upon the nucleus ambiguus and other brainstem nuclei (Fig. 4). The general signs and symptoms of cerebellar disease are ataxia, nystagmus, adiadochokinesis and bradyteleokinesis. Myoclonus of the palate, pharyngeal, and laryngeal musculature contributes to the changes in speech and voice. The larynx of patients with disruption of the cerebellar pathways shows frequent involuntary contractions of the vocal cords. The jerky irregular abductions and adductions of the vocal cords produce a variety of spasmodic, explosive-to-weak, and breathy sounds. Acute lesions of the cerebellum may result in extreme hyperkinesia of all respiratory muscles and phonatory movements.[17] There can be enormous tension, resulting in a spasmodic, extremely low grunting phonation. The aryepiglottic folds may be squeezed together during phonation producing a cerebellar form of ventricular dysphonia. With recovery there is some compensation and the voice and the airway may improve.

Patients with Arnold-Chiari malformation (ACM) may have cerebellar and/or brainstem damage when there is herniation through the abnormally enlarged foramen magnum. Many patients with ACM have stridor as a presenting symptom. In most of the reported cases this was attributed to a bilateral vocal cord paralysis.[18-22] The incidence of stridor and abnormal vocal cord function is probably much more common than has been reported. Concern about the frequently present meningocele and accompanying hydrocephalus overshadows, at least to some degree, the airway symptoms. Many of these patients die secondary to their increased intracranial pressure and perhaps also from the airway obstruction. The appearance of the larynx in ACM had been called "bilateral abductor paralysis" by Holinger and coworkers.[22] This probably represents inadequate length of the period of observation of the larynx. These patients may appear to have a paralysis but in actuality, if observed for sufficient time, would very likely have involuntary abduction of the cords. Snow and Rogers recognized, after repeated direct laryngoscopy under light general anesthesia, a return in vocal cord function in one of their two cases.[20] Smith reported two cases of laryngeal paralysis associated with meningomyelocele in which there was some "return" of vocal cord function.[23] In one of the cases vocal cord function reportedly returned to "normal" four months before death.

The pathology of ACM is characterized by a herniation or protrusion of cerebellar tissue and medulla oblongata through the foramen magnum. These tissues overlap in the spinal canal resulting in compression of the cerebellum and cervical spinal cord. The degrees of malformation were divided by Chiari into three categories of herniation:[20] 1) the lower cerebellum alone into the upper vertebral canal, 2) the lower cerebellum and lower part of the medulla into the upper portion of the vertebral canal, and 3) the whole cerebellum into a cervical spina bifida and meningocele.

The following case was seen by the senior author 13 years prior to the diagnosis of ACM. The abnormal laryngeal function is illustrative of patients with ACM and serves to clarify the reasons for the probable misinterpretation of the appearance of the larynx in previously reported cases.

Case 9. The patient was originally referred to the senior author at Vanderbilt School of Medicine in 1967. The patient was $1\frac{1}{2}$ years of age when first seen. He had required a tracheostomy 30 minutes after birth for severe respiratory distress. The tracheostomy tube was still in place and all efforts to remove it were unsuccessful. The parents were told by several previous examiners that he had a bilateral vocal cord paralysis. A meningomyelocele present at birth was repaired at ten weeks of age.

Upon examination the infant was well developed but small for his age. The tracheostomy tube could be occluded as long as the infant was unaware that a plug was being inserted.

Direct laryngoscopic examination was performed with the patient wrapped and without anesthesia. The laryngoscope was placed in the valluculae, elevating the tongue, hyoid, and epiglottis, thereby allowing prolonged observation of the larynx. During quiet breathing the cords were in a paramedial position with a 1-2 mm glottic chink providing an adequate but marginal airway. The larynx was observed for 7-10 minutes and periodically there were spontaneous involuntary wide abductions of the vocal cords. The tracheostomy tube could again be plugged as long as the child did not feel any movements around the tube. Removal of the tube and manual occlusion of the stoma caused the cords to go into a midline adducted position. The infant would begin to get cyanotic, requiring release of the tracheostome obstruction and reinsertion of his tube. He was hospitalized and the direct laryngoscopic examination repeated several times without anesthesia. Heavy sedation was tried on one occasion during laryngoscopy to see if possible "supratentorial influence" could be responsible for the phenomena observed upon occluding the stoma. The laryngeal findings remained unchanged. The parents were informed that the infant possibly had a paresis but that he definitely had the ability to adduct and abduct the vocal cords involuntarily if not voluntarily. The patient was subsequently cared for by other physicians and laryngologists, having his tracheostomy closed at $3\frac{1}{2}$ years of age. In ensuing years he had several "respiratory infections" with severe respiratory distress. At age 13 he had one of these episodes and required a repeat tracheostomy. He and the parents were again told by several different laryngologists that he had bilateral vocal cord paralysis. Around this time in the course of his problems he began to experience some unsteadiness of gait and incoordination during participation in sports.

One year after his most recent tracheostomy, at age 14, the parents brought the patient to Los Angeles for follow-up examination. Since the patient had again been told that he had a bilateral vocal cord paralysis, the parents were interested in reinnervation or other surgical procedures that might allow closure of his tracheostoma.

The examination of the patient at this time revealed a well-developed 14-year-old male who was somewhat small for his age. He wore a tracheostomy tube that was plugged but had to be opened at night because he developed severe stridor when sleeping. He appeared to have a normal gait and the Romberg sign was absent. Nevertheless, he still complained of feeling unsteady.

Motion pictures of the larynx were obtained which showed the vocal cords in a bowed "abductor paralysis" position for long periods of time. The airway was marginally adequate but there was no shortness of breath except after strenuous exercise. Both cords would adduct during phonation with some visible lag or paresis of the right side. Periodically there were spontaneous involuntary wide abductions of the vocal cords. At times there were incoordinated quivering or flopping motions of the cords and aryepiglottic folds. During his evaluation axial views of the skull revealed the typical enlarged foramen magnum resulting in the recognition and diagnosis of Arnold-Chiari malformation. His tracheostomy tube was left in place and it was recommended that it be converted into a permanent stoma by the technique described previously.[24] The stoma can be plugged with a skin-colored obturator prosthesis that can be worn or removed as needed.

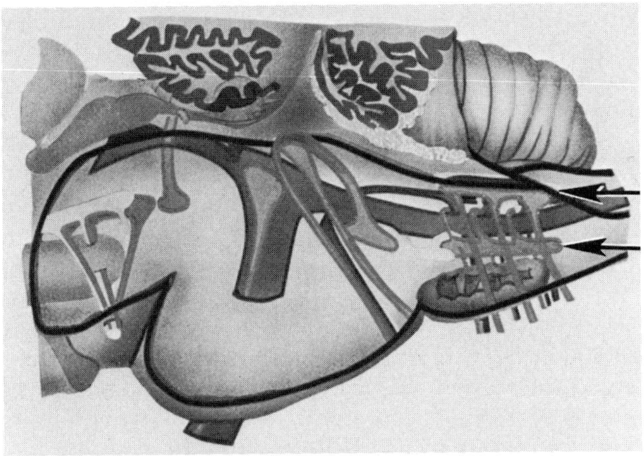

Fig. 5. Schematic drawing of the intramedullary course of some of the cranial nerve nuclei. The dorsal and ventral tenth nerve (nucleus ambiguus) are indicated by arrows.

COMMENT. This patient's problem stimulated our interest in central laryngeal paresis 14 years ago. After the initial examination of the patient's larynx it was obvious that there was abnormal involuntary behavior of the laryngeal musculature but there was certainly not a bilateral vocal cord paralysis as was reported to the patient's parents by other laryngologists. It was postulated at that time that there was abnormality of the central pathways supplying his laryngeal muscles. This was believed to be either a problem associated with his meningomyelocele or a learned reflex-type breathing and laryngeal reaction pattern secondary to the breathing through his tracheostomy since birth. Further observations of other patients with central nervous system disease and abnormal laryngeal physiology provided better insight into this patient's problem. The fortuitous opportunity to get a 13-year follow-up examination and motion picture studies of this patient added to our knowledge of central laryngeal paresis.

Roentgenograms of the base of the skull provided the belated diagnosis of ACM and helped localize the area of the neural involvement. It appears likely that his lesion is herniation of a portion of the cerebellum in view of his incoordination and the involuntary motions of the larynx. The paresis of the right cord and recent unsteadiness could, however, represent compression of the vestibular nuclei and the nucleus ambiguus or a combination of both cerebellar and brainstem involvement.

NUCLEAR (LOWER MOTOR NEURON)

Lesions in the brainstem and medulla oblongata that involve the tenth nerve nucleus (dorsal and ventral nucleus ambiguus) are often associated with paresis and paralysis of other cranial nerve nuclei (Fig. 5). Deglutition, phonation, articulation and facial expression may all be affected to varying degrees. Unilateral paresis and/or paralysis or the nucleus ambiguus produces a classic appearance of the ipsilateral vocal cord similar to that caused by high division of the vagus nerve resulting in paralysis of the superior laryngeal and recurrent laryngeal nerves. There is total paralysis of the cricothyroid and the other intrinsic laryngeal muscles supplied by the superior and recurrent laryngeal nerves. The vocal cord is flaccid, nonmobile and positioned in a paramedian to cadaveric position depending upon the degree of postinjury atrophy and scarring that has taken place. There is a classic shift of the posterior position of the larynx away from the intact contracting cricothyroid muscle of the nonparalyzed side. The paralyzed cord is at a different level and is often more hyperemic than the opposite normal functioning cord. The dysphonia is characterized by a breathy, weak whisper voice. Compensatory movement by the opposite cord may produce some voice improvement but is rarely complete because of the extreme lateral position of the flaccid cord. Due to dysphagia and loss of the afferent sensory input from the larynx and trachea, aspiration may become severe. Pooled secretions contribute to the gurgling component of the voice. Clinicians experienced in dealing with bulbar poliomyelitis cases were familiar with this problem. Dysphonia with what appears to be an idiopathic peripheral vagal paralysis may be one of the early presenting symptoms of bulbar lesions.[17] Bilateral disease caused by lesions such as syringomyelia and amyotrophic lateral sclerosis can result in a dysphonia with a marginally adequate airway (since both cords are held in an intermediate to cadaveric position). In the author's experience, a marginally adequate airway, complicated by inability to manage secretions and severe aspiration, necessitated a tracheostomy in one amyotrophic lateral sclerosis patient with bulbar involvement.

The following case is illustrative of findings in the larynx in a patient with unilateral lower motor neuron (nuclear) paralysis.

Case 10. A 32-year-old male awoke on November 24, 1979, with a feeling of unsteadiness and numbness of his left arm and face. He had double vision, was hoarse, and had difficulty clearing his throat and swallowing. He vomited dark material and was admitted to a hospital. He signed out of the hospital six days later and presented in the UCLA Emergency Room. He had several complicated medical problems that included pneumonitis, plural effusion, and pulmonary embolism which were evaluated and treated prior to clarification of his neurological problem. A neurological examination revealed slight head tilt to the right. Spontaneous, direction-fixed rotatory nystagmus with the fast phase to the right was noted upon admission. The diplopia appeared due to a sixth nerve paresis. There was a Horner's sign, decreased left gag reflex, sternocleidomastoid and hypoglossal muscle strength. Finger to nose testing revealed poor coordination. Electronystagmography was performed with electrodes applied medial and lateral to each eye and above and below the left eye to record bilateral horizontal monocular and unilateral vertical monocular eye movements respectively. With eyes open fixating in the midposition the patient had a persistent right-beating spontaneous nystagmus that increased in amplitude with gaze to the right and changed to a left-beating horizontal nystagmus with gaze to the left. Vertical gaze both up and down slightly increased the horizontal nystagmus but did not induce any vertical nystagmus. With eyes open in darkness, the spontaneous right beating nystagmus increased in amplitude and the eyes tonically deviated to the left. Horizontal saccadic eye movements showed marked asymmetry with hypometria to the right and hypermetria to the left. The patient frequently required 5-10 small saccades to make a 20° refixation to the right. Peak velocity of horizontal saccades was within normal limits. Horizontal smooth pursuit was symmetrically impaired at all target velocities. Horizontal optokinetic responses were also symmetrically impaired but counterclockwise responses were significantly greater than clockwise responses. The vestibulo-ocular reflex was within normal limits when the patient was rotated in darkness but the patient had impaired fixation suppression of vestibular nystagmus.

The larynx was examined and photographed two weeks after the onset of his illness. There was a typical lower motor neuron paralysis of the left vocal cord in the paramedial position. There was no motion of the cricothyroid or any of the intrinsic muscles of the left vocal cord. Phonation produced a shifting of the posterior larynx toward the normal right side. The paralyzed cord was more hyperemic and at a different level than the intact right cord.

These multiple neurological findings were compatible with Wallenburg's medullary infarction syndrome. The final diagnosis was a vascular accident, probably embolization of the posterior inferior cerebellar artery. The patient has been followed for six months with marked improvement in his signs and symptoms. His voice has remained hoarse and breathy and he has been offered Teflon injection to fill out his paralyzed cord in an effort to improve his speech.

COMMENT. Lower motor neuron lesions of the nucleus ambiguus are easily recognized because of the usually multiple surrounding brain lesions. The peripheral manifestations of involvement of other cranial nerve nuclei are similar to actual damage to the main trunk of the peripheral portion of the nerves as they leave the skull. The total paralysis of the abductors and adductors of the left vocal cord produced the same appearance in the larynx that is seen with combined superior and recurrent laryngeal paralysis. The same appearance and behavior of the larynx is produced by a high vagus nerve section. The destruction of lower motor neurons leads to atrophy of the muscles involved and, therefore, the more lateral displacement of the vocal cord diminishes the degree of compensation of glottic closure.

UNKNOWN CENTRAL PARESIS

Since developing an interest in central laryngeal paresis and paralysis, a number of patients have been examined, photographed, and studied who have laryngeal symptoms and signs but no recognized neurological disease. The variety of signs and symptoms has included intractable cough, shortness of breath, hoarseness, asthma, and vocal cord paresis and paralysis. The laryngeal dysfunction in these patients appears similar to that seen with the previously described cases of known involvement of the central laryngeal pathways.

The following recent case is so typical that the diagnosis of probable central laryngeal paralysis or paresis was suggested to the perplexed referring physician after hearing the history over the telephone.

Case 11. This 20-year-old well-developed, well-nourished female college student was transferred to UCLA following an emergency tracheostomy the previous evening for severe respiratory obstruction and vocal cord paralysis. The patient was the product of a difficult labor and delivery. At three months of age she developed "severe stridorous respirations" which were evaluated by her pediatrician and attributed to a "severe respiratory infection." Throughout childhood and in her teens she had recurrent episodes of "respiratory distress" resulting in hospitalization. Her mother recalls that these were always accompanied by stridorous breathing. She was diagnosed and treated for asthma by a number of different physicians. Indirect and direct examinations of the larynx by several otolaryngologists were always reported to show a normal larynx. One particularly severe attack of respiratory distress and stridor occurred following a spinal anesthesia and knee surgery. Again, indirect and direct laryngoscopy and bronchoscopy were normal.

The patient's most recent hospitalization followed the administration of an allergy injection. She developed severe air hunger, airway obstruction and stridor. This was interpreted initially as laryngeal edema secondary to anaphylaxis. She was treated immediately with bronchodilators, antihistamines, and epinephrine without significant benefit. Examination by a competent otolaryngologist upon her arrival at the intensive care unit revealed a normal larynx. She received extensive medical, cardiologic, neurologic and psychological workups which were essentially within normal limits. Included in the evaluation were a normal skull series and CT scan. While in the radiology department getting tomograms she again developed respiratory distress and stridor. The radiologist was unable to get abduction of the cords during inspiration. The same laryngologist was called and performed indirect laryngoscopy. This time the cords were noted to be in an adducted position and could not be made to abduct. He noted once "when the patient was distracted the cords abducted normally." The senior author was called by telephone and after hearing this history suggested the likelihood that she had a central laryngeal paresis. It was agreed to accept her in transfer in order to evaluate her problem further. The evening prior to transferring hospitals she developed another episode of severe respiratory obstruction with stridor that was unresponsive to intermittent positive pressure breathing and epinephrine. Examination of the larynx again revealed a "bilateral vocal cord paralysis or adductor spasm." The obstructive symptoms became worse, requiring an emergency tracheostomy.

Immediately after transfer the patient's larynx was examined and photographed. It has subsequently been rephotographed both from above and indirectly and retrograde through a 90° telescope inserted into her tracheostome. During periods of acute respiratory distress, when she has difficulty in talking and cannot tolerate plugging of her tracheostomy tube, the cords are maintained almost approximated in the midline and only rarely is there a spontaneous abduction. When not having an adductor spasm or abductor paresis, the cords are maintained in a partially adducted position with a "marginal" 2-3 mm airway. There are periodic spontaneous wide abductions of the cords accompanied by an irregular flapping or tremulous motion of the aryepiglottic folds.

The tracheostomy was converted into a permanent tracheostoma and the patient fitted with a skin-colored stomal button. It was interesting that the rather traumatic, time-consuming process of making and fitting the stomal button caused her to go into acute respiratory distress that required unplugging the stoma.

COMMENT. This patient was the product of a difficult labor and a traumatic birth. It seems likely that she sustained some central nervous system trauma that could be responsible for interruption of some of her central laryngeal pathways that have resulted in her laryngeal dysfunction. Historically, her laryngeal and breathing problem began at age three months with a respiratory infection accompanied by "severe respiratory difficulty and stridor." Infection involving the central pathways is a possible but less likely etiological factor.

Like some of our other patients with recognized or unrecognized neurological disease, she was diagnosed and treated for 20 years for "asthma." The lack of response to drugs, including epinephrine and steroids, and the acute bouts of severe respiratory obstruction and stridor, raise doubt about the diagnosis of asthma, although she may have both diseases.

The variable appearance of the larynx described by different observers as normal or at other times as paralyzed or spastic is the typical experience of patients with central laryngeal dysfunction.

The behavior of this patient's larynx is somewhat similar to that of the patient with the upper motor neuron paresis (case 3). This patient, however, had no other known localizing neurological abnormalities.

A permanent tracheostome with a skin-colored obturator has been created for this young, athletic college student. This provides a safety mechanism enabling her to remove the obturator in periods of respiratory distress. It is cosmetically acceptable, the voice is normal, and essentially normal activities are possible. Should a diagnosis and successful treatment for her problem be found, the stoma can be surgically closed.

DISCUSSION

Little attention has been previously given to paralysis and paresis of central laryngeal origin. The careful examination of the larynx and documentation, by motion picture filming and stop frame analysis, has provided some new insights. The study of the larynges of patients with known localizing neurological diseases has provided the basis for classification. The speech chain of input (afferent) and output (efferent) neural impulses is very complex but it is now possible to recognize lesions affecting these pathways. Diseases and lesions of the efferent laryngeal pathways can be further subclassified as upper motor neuron, extrapyramidal, cerebellar, and nuclear.

Throughout this study the observation was made that movements of the larynx are abnormal whenever the various central pathways responsible for laryngeal motions and voice production are involved. Common to all central nervous system lesions affecting the larynx is a lack of coordination and control. Although the speech may not be significantly affected, careful observation and assessment of laryngeal motion reveals variable findings. These include paresis, paralysis, involuntary abduction and adduction, tremor, and incoordinated quivering motions.

The general tonicity of the muscles can vary from

flaccid to spastic depending upon the acuteness and location of the lesion. The lower motor neuron (nuclear) lesions produce a motor paralysis similar to that produced by section of the peripheral nerves.

Due to bilateral cortical upper motor neuron representation with crossing of neural pathways and alternate, phylogenetically older, neural pathways, transmission of neural impulses to the laryngeal musculature is rarely completely blocked except when the lesion is extensive.

A number of cases without recognized central nervous system disease but with laryngeal dysfunction and with behavior of the musculature similar to that seen in patients with known CNS lesions have been studied. In all 18 documented cases of idiopathic paralysis of the vocal cords there was a total unilateral paralysis similar to the patient with a nuclear lesion (case 1). There was not a single case of isolated idiopathic recurrent laryngeal nerve paralysis. Many patients presenting with signs and symptoms of intractable cough, laryngospasm, shortness of breath, "asthma," and dysphonia with vocal cord paresis and paralysis have been examined, photographed and studied. In some of these the laryngeal pathophysiological behavior is similar to that seen in cases with known disruption of central laryngeal pathways. The spastic, quivering motions of the larynges of patients with spastic dysphonia, while not identical, certainly have similarity to the motions of the larynx observed particularly in patients with degenerative diseases of the extrapyramidal areas. There are reports of peripheral nerve degeneration in specimens taken during sectioning of the recurrent laryngeal nerves. The loss of nerve fibers has not been confirmed in our small series studies by light and electron microscopes. The almost symmetrical bilateral spasticity and tremor of the cords perhaps should call for a reconsideration of the likely site or sites of the lesions responsible for spastic dysphonia.

Several of the patients were diagnosed and treated for asthma because of the episodes of acute respiratory distress and wheezing. Different, competent laryngologists examined the larynges of the same patients and reported "bilateral abductor paralysis," bowed cords, and a completely normal larynx. In many cases psychiatrists were consulted because the patient's problems were considered functional. In case 3, filming of the larynx before and after hypnosis was required to prove to her physicians and psychiatrist that her intermittent "abductor paralysis" was not psychogenic in origin. With or without hypnosis the vocal cords were positioned in the midline for lengthy periods but periodically would abduct. In similar cases there appears to be impaired ability to voluntarily abduct the cords (as normally produced by deep inspiration). Perhaps this is due to the approximately 3 to 1 adductor to abductor muscle mass. It is also possible that the protective swallowing reflex may contribute to maintaining lengthy glottic closure. In all of the cases studied to date only bilateral peripheral recurrent laryngeal lesions produced a true "bilateral abductor paralysis." If the lesion involves the central neural system (except bilateral nuclear) there results a paresis and not a paralysis. Meticulous observation will demonstrate occasional involuntary abductions of the cords demonstrating intact neural pathways with deranged central programming or recircuiting of the neural message by older pathways.

ACKNOWLEDGMENTS — The authors are indebted to Ms. Maureen DeBoise for preparation of the illustrations and to Mrs. Margaret Partlow and Mr. Eric Partlow for their assistance in preparation of the motion picture accompanying the presentation of this paper.

REFERENCES

1. Ward PH, Berci G, Calcaterra TC. Advances in endoscopic examination of the respiratory system. Ann Otol Rhinol Laryngol 1974; 83:754-69.

2. Ward P, Berci G, Calcaterra TC. Superior laryngeal nerve paralysis: an often overlooked entity. Trans Am Acad Opthalmol Otolaryngol 1977; 84:78-89.

3. Arnold GE. Vocal rehabilitation of paralytic dysphonia: III. Present concepts of laryngeal paralysis. Arch Otolaryngol 1957; 65:317-36.

4. Ward PH, Hanson DG, Berci G. Photographic studies of the larynx in central laryngeal paresis and paralysis. Acta Otolaryngol (Stockh) (in press).

5. Kirchner JA. Intrathoracic injury to the motor nerve supply to the larynx. Acta Otolaryngol (Stockh) 1977; 83:163-9.

6. Fink RB, Demarest RJ. Laryngeal biomechanics. Cambridge: Harvard Press, 1978.

7. McCaffrey TV, Kern EB. Laryngeal regulation of airway resistance. II. Pulmonary receptor reflexes. Trans Am Broncho-Esophagol Assoc 1980; 92-6.

8. Furstenberg AC, Magielski JE. A motor pattern in the nucleus ambiguus: its clinical significance. Ann Otol Rhinol Laryngol 1955; 64:788-93.

9. Kirikae I, Hirose H, Kawamura S, Sawashima M, Kobayashi T. An experimental study of central motor innervation of the laryngeal muscles in the cat. Ann Otol Rhinol Laryngol 1967; 71:222-39.

10. Penfield W, Roberts L. Speech and brain-mechanism. Princeton: Princeton University Press, 1959.

11. Montgomery WW. Surgical laryngeal closure to eliminate chronic aspiration. N Engl J Med 1975; 292:1390-1.

12. Holinger LD, Holinger PC, Holinger PH. The etiology of bilateral abductor vocal cord paralysis. Ann Otol Rhinol Laryngol 1976; 85:428-36.

13. Plasse H, Lieberman A. Bilateral vocal cord paralysis in Parkinson's disease. Arch Otolaryngol 1981; 107:252-3.

14. Roessmann U, Van den Noort S, McFarland DE. Idiopathic orthostatic hypertension. Arch Neurol 1971; 24:503-10.

15. Bannister R, Oppenheimer ER. Degenerative diseases of the nervous system associated with autonomic failure. Brain 1972; 95:457-74.

16. Williams A, Hanson D, Calne D. Vocal cord paralysis in Shy-Drager syndrome. J Neurol Neurosurg Psychiatry 1979; 42:151-3.

17. Arnold G. Disorders of laryngeal function. In: Paparella

MM, Shumrick DA. Otolaryngology. Philadelphia: W.B. Saunders, 1980; 2470-88.

18. Cavanaugh F. Vocal palsies in children. J Laryngol Otol 1955; 69:399-419.

19. Graham MD. Bilateral vocal cord paralysis associated with meningomyelocele and the Arnold-Chiari malformation. Laryngoscope 1963; 73:85-92.

20. Snow JB, Rogers KA Jr. Bilateral abductor paralysis of the vocal cords secondary to the Arnold-Chiari malformation and its management. Laryngoscope 1965; 75:316-21.

21. Bluestone CD, Delerme AN, Samuelson GH. Airway obstruction due to vocal cord paralysis in infants with hydrocephalus and meningomyelocele. Ann Otol Rhinol Laryngol 1972; 81:778-83.

22. Holinger PC, Holinger LD, Reichert TJ, Holinger PH. Respiratory obstruction and apnea in infants with bilateral abductor vocal cord paralysis, meningomyelocele, hydrocephalus, and Arnold-Chiari malformation. J Pediatr 1978; 99:368-73.

23. Smith MEN. The association of laryngeal studor with meningomyelocele. J Laryngol Otol 1959; 73:188-96.

24. Fee WF, Ward PH. Permanent tracheostomy: a new surgical technique. Ann Otol Rhinol Laryngol 1977; 86:635-8.

≈

GUIDELINES FOR GRANTS

TRUSTEES OF THE RESEARCH FUND OF THE AMERICAN OTOLOGICAL SOCIETY, INC.

The members of the Board of Trustees of the Research Fund of the American Otological Society have determined guidelines for making grants from the Fund. The following is the formulation of policy.

Grants will be given in the area of otosclerosis — its diagnosis and management, the possible causes and underlying conditions, and an understanding of the disorder that may lead eventually to its prevention or cure.

The present lack of understanding of the disorder and the absence of similar conditions in other animals makes research in this field difficult. A direct approach to the disease may or may not be feasible; therefore, a sound strategy would be to use other approaches, such as the investigation of bone development, growth and repair under various conditions, and the study of other diseases that may be similar to otosclerosis. It is possible that investigations which may seem initially remote from otosclerosis may provide information which will eventually lead to a substantive further understanding of the disease process which underlies otosclerosis. The applicant should describe correlations between proposed research with the clinical pathological entity of otosclerosis.

The policy is to aid and encourage research in the immediate field of otosclerosis and also in adjoining fields, if, in the opinion of the Board, there is a substantial promise that results obtained will be of assistance in the ways indicated, and may lead to the attainment of the objective of the further understanding of otosclerosis.

Applications for a research grant from the Research Fund of the American Otological Society may be obtained from the Office of the Secretary-Treasurer of the Research Fund of the American Otological Society. Write to Robert J. Ruben, MD, Secretary-Treasurer, Department of Otolaryngology, Albert Einstein College of Medicine, 1300 Morris Park Avenue, Bronx, NY 10461; telephone (212) 430-3036.

All grant requests must be submitted by January 31, 1982. All grants received after January 31 will not be considered.

Ann Otol 90:1981

TREATMENT OF CARCINOMA OF THE EPIGLOTTIS

JOSEPH B. NADOL, JR., MD
BOSTON, MASSACHUSETTS

One hundred five cases of primary squamous cell carcinoma of the epiglottis were reviewed and the results of treatment compared. The cure rate by radiation therapy for epiglottic carcinomas, both suprahyoid and infrahyoid, was poorer than previously reported cure rates for all supraglottic carcinomas ($p < 0.01$). This may be due to unsuspected anterior extension of infrahyoid tumors into the preepiglottic space and thyroid cartilage. The cure rate (five years with no evidence of disease) for suprahyoid lesions was superior to that of infrahyoid lesions for all stages of primary size and nodal metastases and for all treatments. It is suggested that initial staging of primary epiglottic carcinomas should include the designation of suprahyoid or infrahyoid. The role of xeroradiography as an adjunct to staging and the implications for treatment are discussed.

INTRODUCTION

A variety of treatment regimens have been proposed for supraglottic carcinoma. These include radiotherapy,[1,2] surgical excision, either total or supraglottic partial laryngectomy,[3-7] and a planned combination of radiation therapy and surgical excision.[1,5,6,8-10] Although these reports include cases in which the tumor is limited to or originated in the epiglottis, little attempt has been made to separately analyze the treatment of epiglottic carcinoma. Because it was the author's clinical impression that carcinoma of the epiglottis, particularly that arising from the infrahyoid portion, constitutes a unique group as judged by its biological behavior, a retrospective study was undertaken to evaluate the treatment of squamous cell carcinoma of this site.

MATERIALS AND METHODS

Case histories of 1,476 patients with carcinoma of the larynx diagnosed between 1962 and 1975, as cataloged by the Head and Neck Tumor Registry of the Massachusetts Eye and Ear Infirmary and Massachusetts General Hospital (Cox Cancer Center), were reviewed. This produced 115 cases in which the clinical description was sufficient to allow the designation of the epiglottis as the primary site. Follow-up of at least five years was available in 105 cases. Patients who died of other diseases before five years were excluded from the study.

Tumor classification was performed according to the protocol of the American Joint Committee for Cancer Staging.[11] Assessment of the primary tumor was accomplished by indirect mirror examination, direct laryngoscopy, plain films, tomography, and contrast studies of the pharynx and larynx.

The distribution of the 105 patients with primary squamous cell carcinoma of the epiglottis by TNM classification is shown in Table 1. Tumors were divided into two groups, based on their location with reference to the hyoid bone. Suprahyoid tumors were defined as limited to the lingual surface and rim of the epiglottis. Tumors extending to the infrahyoid portion were defined by involvement of the laryngeal surface of the epiglottis inferior to the level of the hyoid bone. By clinical examination, this would correspond to a level on the epiglottis inferior to the floor of the valleculae. Of the 105 tumors, 82% were infrahyoid in location, whereas 18% were suprahyoid in location. Of the 19 suprahyoid lesions, 3 (16%) had clinical evidence of nodal metastases (N_1 to N_3) at the time of first examination. Of the 86 cases of infrahyoid carcinoma, 28 (33%) had evidence of neck metastases at the time of presentation.

Treatment regimens were divided into five types (Table 2).

1. Radiation therapy: 6,000 to 7,000 rads by external beam ^{60}Co to the primary tumor and both necks.

2. Combined radiation and surgery: preoperative radiotherapy of 4,000 to 4,500 rads to the primary and both necks followed by either total laryngectomy or supraglottic laryngectomy, with or without radical neck dissection.

3. Surgical treatment: either supraglottic laryngectomy or total laryngectomy, with or without radical neck dissection.

4. Radiation failure with attempted surgical salvage: treated with radiation for cure as in regimen 1 and subsequent surgical treatment because of residual primary carcinoma or metastatic disease in the neck.

5. Surgical failure with radiation salvage: primary surgery for cure and postoperative radiation therapy because surgical margins were positive for carcinoma.

The cure rates for each of these five treatment regimens are tabulated in Table 2. The overall cure rate for radiation therapy was determined by combining patients in regimens 1 and 4, thereby including both patients in whom only radiation was given and also patients in whom failure of radiation occurred requiring surgical salvage. This composite evaluation of cure rate by primary radiation therapy is tabulated in Table 3. Analysis of statistical significance was performed by the chi square test.

RESULTS

Lesions Without Palpable Nodal Metastases. For all T_1 lesions of the epiglottis the overall cure rate by radiation therapy alone is 9/13 (69%). Recurrence at the primary site was the cause of radiation failure in three of four cases, and salvage by surgery was achieved in one of three patients. For T_2 lesions the cure rate for radiation treatment alone was 8 of 19 (42%). Six died of distant metastases, and surgical salvage was attempted in five, four of whom had recurrence at the primary site. This compares to a cure rate of 78% ($p < .10$) for surgery alone for T_2 lesions.

From the Department of Otolaryngology, Harvard Medical School and the Massachusetts Eye and Ear Infirmary, Boston. This work was supported by the National Institutes of Health, Teacher-Investigator Award No. 5 K07 NS00174-04.

Presented at the meeting of the American Laryngological Association, Vancouver, British Columbia, May 10-11, 1981.

REPRINTS — Joseph B. Nadol, Jr., MD, Massachusetts Eye and Ear Infirmary, 243 Charles Street, Boston, MA 02114.

TABLE 1. DISTRIBUTION OF EPIGLOTTIC CARCINOMA PATIENTS BY TNM CLASSIFICATION (N = 105)

	N_0	N_1	N_2	N_3	Total (N_0-N_3)
T_1					
S	3	0	0	0	
I	15	3	0	1	
Total	18	3	0	1	
T_2					
S	4	0	0	1	
I	31	9	2	0	
Total	35	9	2	1	
T_3					
S	0	0	0	0	
I	5	4	0	0	
Total	5	4	0	0	
T_4					
S	9	1	0	1	
I	7	2	3	4	
Total	16	3	3	5	
Totals, (T_1-T_4)					
S	16	1	0	2	19
I	58	18	5	5	86
Total	74	19	5	7	105

S - Suprahyoid; I - Infrahyoid.

For T_3 lesions there were insufficient data to warrant any comparison between treatments. For T_4 lesions the cure rate for radiation treatment alone was 5 of 10 (50%).

Lesions with Palpable Nodal Metastases. If metastases were palpable at the time of presentation, radiation therapy alone was infrequently sufficient for cure, and either planned combined radiation and surgery or surgery alone indicated. The influence of nodal metastases on cure rates is also presented in Table 4. The combined 5-year cure rate for all treatments was 68% for N_0 cases, 42% for N_1 cases, 60% for N_2 cases, and 17% for N_3 cases.

Comparison of Suprahyoid and Infrahyoid Primary Disease. From Tables 1 through 3 it is clear that tumors arising from the infrahyoid portion of the epiglottis have a poorer prognosis than those located exclusively in the suprahyoid portion. Thus, for T_1N_0 and T_2N_0 lesions of the suprahyoid portion of the epiglottis the cure rate by radiotherapy was 3 of 4 (75%) compared to 14 of 28 (50%) for lesions arising in the infrahyoid portion. For advanced lesions (T_3N_0 and T_4N_0) the comparative success rate for radiation therapy was 4 of 6 (67%) for suprahyoid lesions, and 3 of 7 (43%) for lesions arising in the infrahyoid portion of the epiglottis. Likewise, in cases with nodal metastases, the overall 5-year cure rate is consistently better for lesions arising in the suprahyoid portion of the epiglottis. Thus, for lesions in all stages the cure rate by radiation treatment is 62% for suprahyoid and 40% for infrahyoid

TABLE 3. CURE RATES OF RADIATION FOR PRIMARY EPIGLOTTIC CARCINOMA*

TNM	Radiation Therapy Cure Rates	Cure Rates for Surgical Salvage of Primary Recurrence	Cure Rates for Surgical Salvage of Neck Metastases
T_1			
S	3/3 (100%)	—	—
I	7/13 (54%)	1/4	—
Total	10/16 (63%)	1/4	—
T_2			
S	1/2 (50%)	—	—
I	9/20 (45%)	1/4	0/1
Total	10/22 (45%)	1/4	0/1
T_3			
S	—	—	—
I	2/5 (40%)	1/2	—
Total	2/5 (40%)	1/2	—
T_4			
S	4/8 (50%)	2/2	1/2
I	1/10 (10%)	1/1	4/4
Total	5/18 (28%)	1/3	5/6
Totals, T_1-T_4			
S	8/13 (62%)	2/2 (100%)	1/2
I	19/48 (40%)	4/11 (36%)	4/7
Total	27/61 (44%)	6/13 (46%)	5/9

*No evidence of disease for five years.

S - Suprahyoid; I - Infrahyoid.

TABLE 2. RESULTS OF TREATMENT OF EPIGLOTTIC CARCINOMA*

TNM	Radiation Only	Planned Combined Radiation & Surgery	Surgery Only	Radiation Failure & Surgical Salvage	Surgical Failure & Radiation Salvage	All Treatments
T_1						
S	3/3 (100%)	—	—	—	—	3/3 (100%)
I	7/9 (78%)	2/2	2/2	1/5	1/1	13/19 (68%)
Total	10/12 (83%)	2/2 (100%)	2/2 (100%)	1/5 (20%)	1/1	16/22 (73%)
T_2						
S	1/2 (50%)	2/3	—	—	—	3/5 (60%)
I	9/16 (56%)	5/10	9/12	1/4	—	24/42 (57%)
Total	10/18 (56%)	7/13 (54%)	9/12 (75%)	1/4	—	27/47 (57%)
T_3						
S	—	—	—	—	—	—
I	2/3	1/4	—	1/2	—	4/9
Total	2/3	1/4	—	1/2	—	4/9 (44%)
T_4						
S	4/6 (67%)	1/1	1/1	2/2	1/1	9/11 (82%)
I	1/9 (11%)	3/4	—	3/3	—	7/16 (44%)
Total	5/15 (33%)	4/5 (80%)	1/1	5/5	1/1	16/27 (59%)
Totals, T_1-T_4						
S	8/11	3/4 (75%)	1/1	2/2	1/1	15/19 (79%)
I	19/37	11/20 (55%)	11/14	6/14	1/1	48/86 (56%)
Total	27/48	14/24	12/15	8/16	2/2	63/105 (60%)

*No evidence of disease for five years.

S - Suprahyoid; I - Infrahyoid.

TABLE 4. CURE RATES BY TNM CLASSIFICATION (ALL TREATMENTS)*

	N_0	N_1	N_2	N_3	*Totals* (N_0-N_3)
T_1					
S	3/3	—	—	—	
I	11/15	2/3	—	0/1	
T_2					
S	2/4	—	—	1/1	
I	18/31	5/9	1/2	—	
T_3					
S	—	—	—	—	
I	3/5	1/4	—	—	
T_4					
S	9/9	0/1	—	0/1	
I	4/7	0/2	2/3	1/4	
Totals					
T_1-T_4					
S	14/16 (88%)	0/1	—	1/2	15/19 (79%)
I	36/58 (62%)	8/18 (44%)	3/5 (60%)	1/5 (20%)	48/86 (56%)
Combined	50/74 (68%)	8/19 (42%)	3/5 (60%)	2/7 (17%)	63/105 (60%)

*No evidence of disease for five years.

S - Suprahyoid; I - Infrahyoid.

lesions respectively (Table 3). For combined radiation and surgery the cure rate was 3 of 4 (75%) for suprahyoid lesions compared to 11 of 20 (55%) for infrahyoid lesions (Table 2). For all treatments combined the 5-year cure rate for suprahyoid lesions was 15 of 19 (79%) compared to 48 of 86 (56%) for infrahyoid lesions ($p<0.10$, Table 2).

DISCUSSION

Relative Cure Rates for Supraglottic and Primary Epiglottic Carcinoma. Comparison of the results of the present study with the results of megavoltage radiation therapy for all supraglottic carcinomas[2] suggests that primary epiglottic carcinomas, particularly of the infrahyoid portion, are considerably less radiosensitive than supraglottic carcinomas in general. For T_1N_0 and T_2N_0 lesions of the supraglottis, Wang[2] reported a cure rate of 30/36 (83%), compared to a cure rate by radiation therapy in this series of 17/32 (53%, $p<0.01$) for all T_1N_0 and T_2N_0 lesions, and 14/28 (50%, $p<0.01$) for infrahyoid

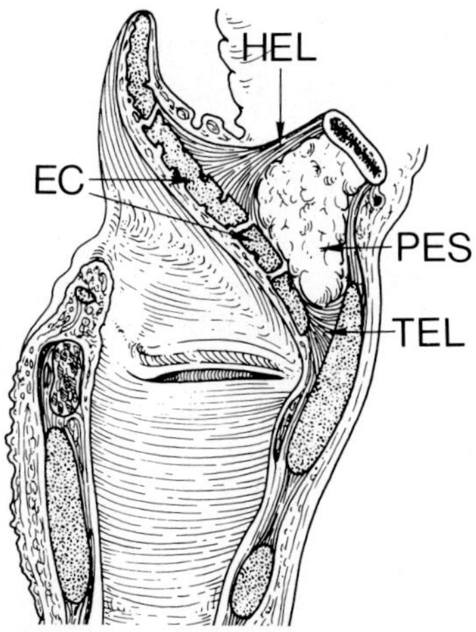

Fig. 1. Drawing of sagittal section of larynx. The epiglottic cartilage (EC) is cribrose providing a natural pathway of extension to the preepiglottic space (PES). Only the hyoepiglottic ligament (HEL) and thyroepiglottic ligament (TEL) separate the preepiglottic space from the base of tongue and the thyroid cartilage, respectively.

T_1N_0 and T_2N_0 lesions. Fletcher et al[1] have also shown a poorer cure rate by radiation therapy for infrahyoid compared to suprahyoid epiglottic carcinoma. Similarly, when compared to conservation surgery with or without radiation therapy for supraglottic carcinoma,[6] the 5-year cure rates demonstrated in this study for all treatments (Table 1) are somewhat poorer, and the group of infrahyoid primary tumors considerably poorer, than for the general class of supraglottic carcinoma.

These facts suggest that epiglottic carcinoma, particularly that arising from the infrahyoid portion of the epiglottis, carries a poorer prognosis regardless of the treatment protocol than the general class of supraglottic carcinomas. Analysis of the relative rates of regional metastases and of the special anatomic characteristics of the epiglottis provide possible explanations for this difference.

The incidence of nodal metastases from supraglottic squamous cell carcinoma has been reported as 23% by Ogura et al,[6] and 33% by Coates et al.[7] Wang[2] found incidence of nodal metastases of 22% for T_1 and T_2 lesions, 45% for T_3 lesions, and 63% for T_4 lesions of the supraglottic larynx. In the present series the incidence of nodal metastases from suprahyoid and infrahyoid lesions combined was 31/105 (30%). However, for suprahyoid lesions the incidence was 3/19 (16%) compared to 28/86 (33%) for infrahyoid lesions. When the various stages of primary disease are analyzed, the differences between suprahyoid and infrahyoid lesions persist. Thus, for suprahyoid lesions the incidence of nodal metastases was 1/8 (13%) for T_1 and T_2 lesions combined and 2/11 (18%) for T_3 and T_4 lesions combined, compared to 15/61 (25%) for T_1 and T_2 lesions and 13/25 (52%) for T_3 and T_4 lesions of the infrahyoid region ($p<0.10$). The greater incidence of regional metastases for infrahyoid lesions would be expected to adversely affect the prognosis for cure of these lesions.

The anatomic characteristics of the epiglottis

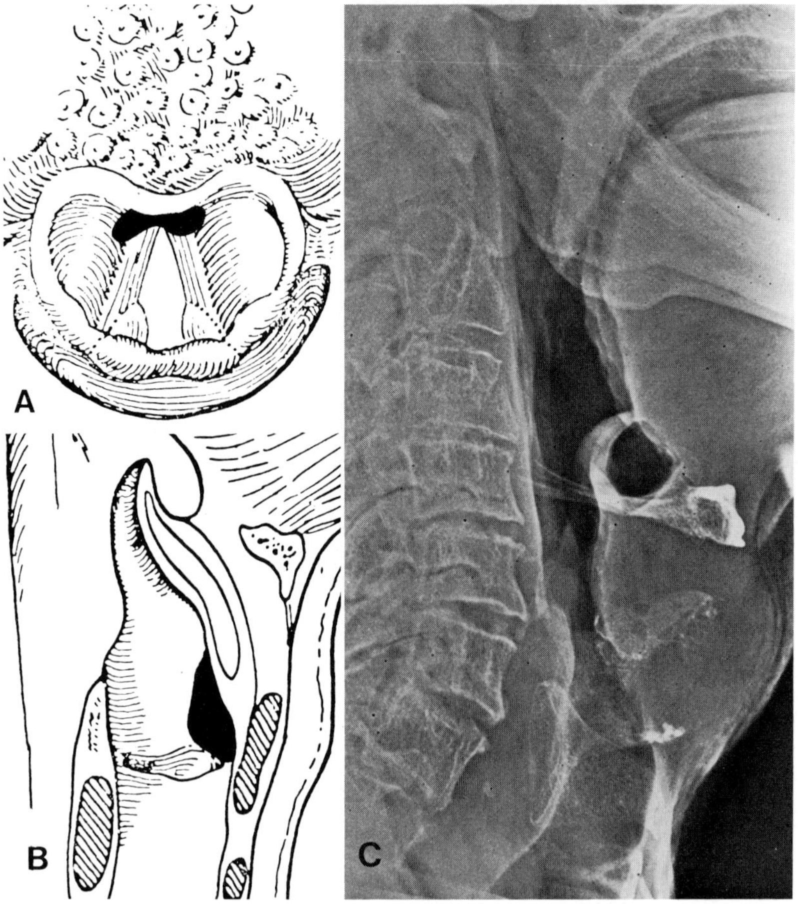

Fig. 2. A, B) The primary tumor was limited to the laryngeal surface of the epiglottis and the anterior portion of both false cords in this 74-year-old male. The tumor extended to the level of the true cords, but there was no subglottic extension. Initial classification was $T_2N_0M_0$. C) A lateral xerogram of the neck demonstrated a mass measuring 4 x 5 cm in the preepiglottic space. The thyroid cartilage was partially destroyed.

may also influence the relative prognosis for suprahyoid and infrahyoid lesions. As can be seen in Figure 1, the cartilage of the epiglottis is perforated resulting in natural channels from the laryngeal surface of the epiglottis through the cartilage of the epiglottis into the preepiglottic space. Likewise, other than the hyoepiglottic ligament, there is no anatomical barrier between the laryngeal surface of the epiglottis and the base of the tongue. Theoretically, this would allow earlier escape of tumor from the mucosal confines of the larynx and access to the rich lymphatic and vascular supply of the tongue base.

Clinically, anterior extent of tumor may be suspected by fullness or a mass in the suprahyoid area or beneath the thyrohyoid ligament. In addition, xeroradiography may be of considerable assistance in evaluating the anterior extent of the tumor. Figures 2 and 3 demonstrate the usefulness of this technique. In both cases the tumors were classified as T_2 infrahyoid lesions by clinical and radiographic evaluation. However, xeroradiography demonstrated marked tumor invasion of the preepiglottic space, which raised the stage to T_3. Thus, the poorer prognosis for infrahyoid epiglottic carcinoma may be due to unassessed or unexpected extension into the preepiglottic space and escape from the anatomical boundaries of the larynx. Kirchner and Som[4] found that microscopic invasion of the thyroid cartilage was rare unless the inferior mucosal extent of tumor was below the anterior commissure, suggesting a "tight barrier" at the level of the anterior commissure preventing downward extension of tumor of the epiglottis. However, that deep extension anteriorly and inferiorly can occur is illustrated in Figures 3 and 4.

Another difficulty in the management of epiglottic carcinoma, particularly of the infrahyoid portion, is the limited value of mirror examination of the primary tumor site after treatment, particularly radiation therapy. This is demonstrated in Figure 4. This patient was classified as having a $T_2N_0M_0$ squamous cell carcinoma of the infrahyoid portion of the epiglottis and received 6,500 rads of radiation therapy. Total laryngectomy became necessary for recurrent tumor eight months later. Figure 4 B demonstrates the surgical specimen from the perspective of an indirect laryngoscopy showing little if any evidence of tumor, and no tumor was visible by mirror examination. When viewed from the opened posterior aspect of the larynx (Fig. 4 C), the tumor is more obvious. However, the actual extent of tumor into the preepiglottic space, base of tongue, and to the thyroid cartilage as shown in Figure 4 D could not be anticipated from the surface appearance.

Implications for Tumor Staging. The present TNM system for supraglottic tumors is not ideally

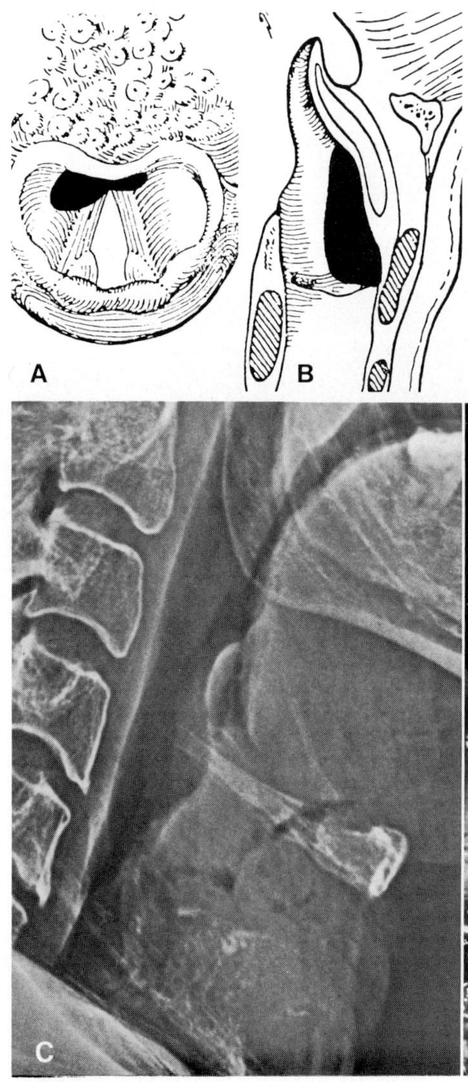

Fig. 3. A, B) The primary tumor was limited to laryngeal surface of epiglottis and anterior aspects of both false cords in this 42-year-old male. It extended to the anterior commissure but not into the subglottic space. Initial classification was $T_2N_{3b}M_0$. C) A lateral xerogram demonstrated marked infiltration of soft tissue anterior to the epiglottis. Gas present in this mass suggested central necrosis. D) Photograph of sagittal section of laryngectomy specimen demonstrates deep anterior infiltration and invasion of preepiglottic space and thyroid cartilage. Central necrosis with an air pocket was present in the preepiglottic space.

suited to classification of epiglottic carcinoma. The T staging bears no relation to actual tumor size. Thus, a small lesion of the lingual surface of the epiglottis may be staged as T_4 by extension to the mucosa of the tongue base whereas a much larger lesion involving the laryngeal surface of the epiglottis and extending to both false cords would be staged as a T_2 lesion. As a result, the cure rates by radiation therapy (Table 3) bear little relation to the T classification. For example, the cure rate by radiation was 9/13 (69%) for T_1N_0 lesions, 8/19 (42%) for T_2N_0 lesions, and 5/10 (50%) for T_4N_0 lesions, which are not statistically different ($p > 0.10$). Furthermore, the anatomical location of the tumor in relation to the hyoid bone, which seems to affect prognosis, is not considered in the present TNM classification.

Treatment Protocol for Epiglottic Carcinoma. Based on the results of this study, the author's present protocol for treatment of epiglottic carcinoma is as follows:

For T_1 and T_2 lesions, as confirmed by xeroradiography in infrahyoid lesions, a trial course of 4,500 rads of radiation therapy to the primary and both necks is given. Direct laryngoscopy and biopsy of the original primary site may be necessary, particularly with infrahyoid tumors, to assess the response to radiotherapy. If there is still residual carcinoma, the radiation treatment is considered to be preoperative, and a resection is performed as indicated by the original limits of the lesion. If the primary lesion has disappeared, radiation therapy to the primary is completed to 6,500 rads. The alternate therapy of supraglottic laryngectomy with or without preoperative radiation therapy is supported by the reported cure rates.[4-6] For N_0 disease, a full course of radiation therapy is given to both necks as well. With palpable nodal disease (N_1 to N_3) radical neck dissection is performed after 4,500 rads.

For T_3 and T_4 disease, a combined approach of preoperative radiotherapy followed by surgery as indicated by the location and size of the primary lesion and presence of nodal metastases is performed. This is in conformance with the improved survival rate seen with combined therapy for advanced T_3 and T_4 carcinomas of the supraglottis.[10] Although primary radiation therapy may convert palpable

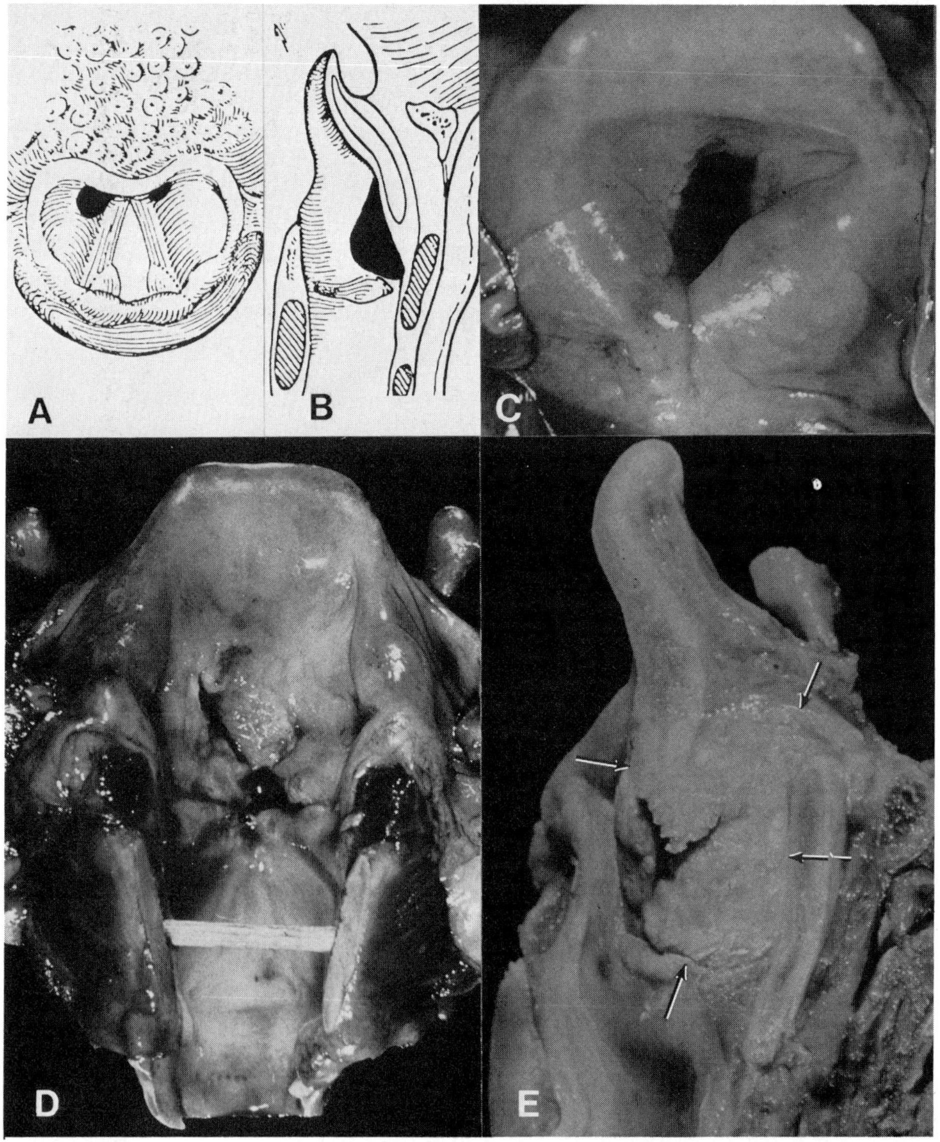

Fig. 4. A, B) Pretreatment extent of primary epiglottic carcinoma, classified as $T_2N_0M_0$ in a 74-year-old female. The patient then underwent 6,500 rads of radiotherapy to the larynx and both necks. Eight months later, although no tumor was visible by indirect laryngoscopy, direct laryngoscopy was performed because of referred otalgia, and a recurrent tumor was found. C) Laryngectomy specimen as seen from the perspective of indirect laryngoscopy. D) Laryngectomy specimen opened in posterior midline. Residual tumor and ulceration are limited to laryngeal surface of epiglottis. E) Sagittal section of laryngectomy specimen demonstrated deep anterior infiltration into the preepiglottic space and to the thyroid cartilage.

nodal metastases to N_0 disease, as determined histologically, this occurs in a minority of cases,[10] and neck dissection is performed in all cases where nodes were palpable prior to radiotherapy. Furthermore, there is some evidence to suggest that preoperative radiation followed by radical neck dissection is superior to surgery alone for palpable nodal metastases from the supraglottic larynx.[6]

REFERENCES

1. Fletcher GH, Jesse RH, Lindberg RD. The place of radiotherapy in the management of the squamous cell carcinoma of the supraglottic larynx. Am J Roentgenol 1970; 108:19-26.

2. Wang CC. Megavoltage radiation therapy for supraglottic carcinoma: results of treatment. Radiology 1973; 109:183-6.

3. Som ML. Conservation surgery for carcinoma of the supraglottis. J Laryngol Otol 1970; 84:655-78.

4. Kirchner JA, Som ML. Clinical and histological observations on supraglottic cancer. Ann Otol Rhinol Laryngol 1971; 80:638-45.

5. Rowley NJ, Boles R. Symposium on malignancy: I. Supraglottic carcinoma: a 10-year review at the university hospital. Laryngoscope 1972; 82:1264-72.

6. Ogura JH, Sessions DG, Spector GJ. Conservation surgery and radiotherapy for epidermoid carcinoma of the supraglottic larynx. Laryngoscope 1975; 85:1808-15.

7. Coates HL, Devine KD. Carcinoma of the supraglottic larynx: a review of 221 cases. Arch Otolaryngol 1976; 102:686-9.

8. Vermund H. Role of radiotherapy in cancer of the larynx as related to the TNM system of staging: a review. Cancer 1970; 25:485-504.

9. Flynn MB, Jesse RH, Lindberg RD. Surgery and irradiation in the treatment of squamous cell cancer of the supraglottic larynx. Am J Surg 1972; 124:477-81.

10. Wang CC, Schulz MD, Miller D. Combined radiation therapy and surgery for carcinoma of the supraglottic and pyriform sinus. Laryngoscope 1972; 82:1883-90.

11. Manual for staging of cancer 1978. Chicago: American Joint Committee for Cancer Staging and End-Results Reporting, 1978:40-1.

≈

NINTH CONGRESS OF THE EUROPEAN RHINOLOGIC SOCIETY — THIRD INTERNATIONAL SYMPOSIUM ON INFECTION AND ALLERGY OF THE NOSE AND PARANASAL SINUSES

The Ninth Congress of the European Rhinologic Society and the Third International Symposium on Infection and Allergy of the Nose and Paranasal Sinuses will be held in Stockholm, Sept. 5-8, 1982. For information write: Ninth ERS Congress 1982, c/o Reso Congress Service, S-105 24 Stockholm.

HYPOTHYROIDISM FOLLOWING TREATMENT FOR HEAD AND NECK CANCER

DONALD P. VRABEC, MD　　TIMOTHY J. HEFFRON, MD

DANVILLE, PENNSYLVANIA

One hundred ninety-six head and neck patients were studied to determine the effects of radiation therapy and surgery on thyroid function. Serum thyroid-stimulating hormone (TSH) levels were obtained as a screening test for primary hypothyroidism. Elevated TSH levels were found in 57 of the 196 patients (29.1%). The highest incidence of abnormal TSH values (66%) occurred in the group treated with combination radiation therapy and surgery, including partial thyroidectomy. TSH levels rose early in the posttreatment period with 60% of the abnormal values occurring within the first three posttreatment years. Posttreatment thyroid dysfunction was twice as common in women (48.6%) as in men (25.4%). When serum thyroxine levels by radioimmunoassay (T_4RIA) were correlated with the elevated serum TSH levels, a similar pattern was seen with 65% of the patients in Group 3 having a decreased T_4RIA level indicating overt hypothyroidism. Pretreatment levels of thyroid function including thyroid antibody studies should be established for all patients. Serial TSH levels should be done every three months during the first three posttreatment years and semiannually thereafter as long as the patient will return for follow-up care. All patients treated with combination radiation therapy and surgery who develop elevated TSH levels should be treated with thyroid replacement therapy. Patients receiving radiation therapy alone should receive replacement thyroid therapy if they develop a depressed T_4RIA value or a pattern of gradually increasing TSH levels.

INTRODUCTION

Thyroid dysfunction is not ordinarily considered to be a major complication of the therapy for head and neck cancer. It is our clinical impression that this complication is common and more serious than is generally recognized. Although the normal thyroid gland is traditionally considered to be resistant to external radiation, at one time external radiation was the standard treatment for thyrotoxicosis. Today, another form of ionizing radiation, iodine 131, is the more commonly employed treatment modality for thyrotoxicosis while surgical excision of a portion of the thyroid gland is employed in a lesser number of cases. Myxedema has been reported as a complication of each of these modalities, being more commonly seen following the use of ^{131}I.[1-4]

Currently, radiation therapy, either alone or in combination with surgery, has an important role in the therapy for head and neck cancer. External radiation therapy is administered using bilateral cervical and anterior supraclavicular portals. These portals usually include the thyroid gland within the field of radiation. Additionally, it is standard clinical practice when doing a laryngectomy for cancer to remove the isthmus and the ipsilateral lobe of the thyroid gland. This is especially true with transglottic and subglottic laryngeal cancer. It logically follows that if these same two modalities can be used to ablate the hyperactive thyroid, they may have a similar though untoward effect when the normal thyroid is incidentally encompassed in a treatment regimen for a head and neck malignancy. The reports of several clinical investigators verify this contention. Bartels and Kusakcioglu[5] and Bird and Bryce[6] report hypothyroidism as a sequela to external radiation administered to the neck. In a study of 41 patients who had received high-dose external radiation therapy for laryngeal or hypopharyngeal cancer more than ten years earlier, Einhorn and Wikholm[7] found clinical hypothyroidism in 7.3% of the patients while biochemical evidence of decreased thyroid reserve was present in all 41 patients. Ballantyne[8] reported hypothyroidism as a common finding in patients who had undergone radiation to the neck at the M.D. Anderson Hospital and Tumor Institute. Several authors[9-12] report a substantial increase in hypothyroidism when external radiation is combined with laryngectomy and hemithyroidectomy.

Along similar lines, the incidence of hypothyroidism following radiation therapy in patients with lymphoma has been well documented.[13,14] This finding was more frequent in patients who had undergone prior lymphangiography, suggesting that an expanded extrathyroidal iodide pool may increase the susceptibility to hypothyroidism in the irradiated subject. The common clinical use of iodide-containing expectorants in this patient population suggests the possibility of inducing overt clinical hypothyroidism in the marginally compensated hypothyroid patient.

It is the purpose of this paper 1) to determine the effect of various combinations of radiation therapy and surgery on the thyroid function of the head and neck cancer patient, 2) to explore the time relationships between completion of therapy and the onset of clinical or subclinical hypothyroidism, 3) to recommend preoperative and postoperative screening procedures that will alert the clinician to impend-

From the Department of Otolaryngology, Geisinger Medical Center, Danville, Pennsylvania.

Presented at the meeting of the American Laryngological Association, Vancouver, British Columbia, May 10-11, 1981.

REPRINTS — Donald P. Vrabec, MD, Geisinger Medical Center, Danville, PA 17822.

TABLE 1. RESULTS OF THYROID-STIMULATING HORMONE IN POSTTREATMENT HEAD AND NECK CANCER PATIENTS (N = 196)

	Patients with Elevated TSH	*Patients with Normal TSH*	*Total Number*	*% with Elevated TSH*
Group 1	14	86	100	14
Group 2	10	36	46	21.7
Group 3	33	17	50	66
Total	57	139	196	29.1

TSH - Thyroid-stimulating hormone.

ing hypothyroidism in its earliest stages, and 4) to discuss management alternatives when clinical or biochemical signs of hypothyroidism are identified.

METHODS AND MATERIALS

The medical records of the patients undergoing treatment for head and neck malignancies at the Geisinger Medical Center during the 12-year period from 1969 to 1980 were reviewed. Included in the study were all patients who received therapeutic levels of radiation therapy to the region of the thyroid gland as well as those patients receiving combined radiation therapy and surgery. During this period, it was our standard clinical practice to treat stage I carcinoma using radiation therapy as the principal treatment modality. Selected stage II cancers were also treated with radiation therapy while more extensive lesions were treated with combined surgery and radiation therapy. During the earlier years of this study, preoperative radiation therapy was more frequently employed, while during the latter years of this study postoperative radiation therapy was the treatment of choice. As a general rule, clinically palpable metastatic disease in the neck was treated with an en bloc radical neck dissection and 5,000 rads of radiation therapy. N_0 neck disease was treated by resecting the primary area and administering 5,000 rads of radiation therapy through bilateral cervical and supraclavicular ports.

This study included all patients receiving therapeutic levels of radiation therapy to the head and neck area in whom the thyroid gland was included within the radiation portals. Also included were the patients receiving radiation therapy to the thyroid area in whom surgery was done in the thyroid area, whether or not thyroid tissue had been removed. Patients with stage I laryngeal cancer were included in the study since their treatment portals included at least half of the thyroid gland and there was sufficient scatter radiation to warrant concern. Patients excluded from this study were those 1) with a prior history of thyroid disease, 2) with prior thyroid surgery, 3) with abnormal preoperative thyroid function studies, 4) with tumor invasion into the thyroid gland, 5) in whom the operative specimen contained microscopic evidence of abnormal thyroid tissue, 6) in whom the entire thyroid gland was included in the operative specimen, 7) with recurrent carcinoma, 8) not living at the time of the study, 9) lost to follow-up, and 10) who, for any other reason, did not fall within the defined limits of the study. No attempt was made to differentiate those patients receiving preoperative radiation therapy from those receiving postoperative radiation therapy.

Three hundred fifty-one patients fell within the defined limits of the study and were contacted to cooperate in the study. One hundred ninety-six patients agreed to cooperate. Thyroid-stimulating hormone (TSH) levels determined by the radioimmunoassay method were used as the principal screening parameter for primary hypothyroidism. In most patients, a serum thyroxine level by radioimmunoassay (T_4RIA) was also obtained in order to correlate these two values.

The patient population was subdivided into three groups: group 1, patients receiving radiation therapy alone; group 2, patients receiving radiation therapy and neck surgery in the thyroid area but without removal of thyroid disease; group 3, patients receiving radiation therpay and surgery, including partial thyroidectomy.

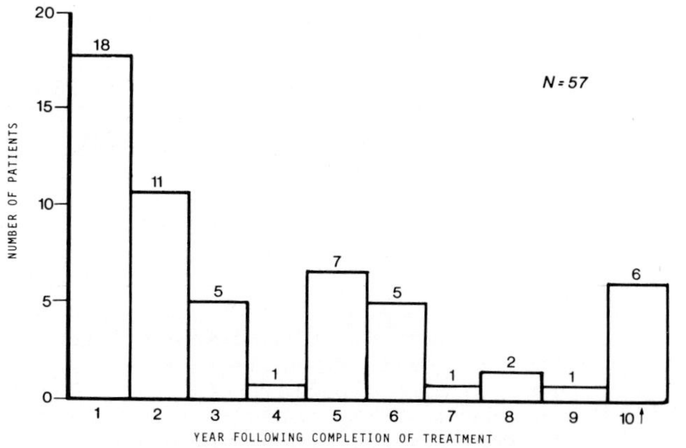

Fig. 1. Graph showing year following completion of treatment in which elevated TSH was first discovered for all patients with elevated TSH.

The medical records of these 196 patients were reviewed and correlated with thyroid function studies to determine the incidence of clinical or subclinical hypothyroidism. The time relationships between the completion of therapy and the onset of clinical hypothyroidism were noted.

RESULTS

Fifty-seven of the 196 patients (29.1%) had elevated TSH levels (Table 1). Group 1, receiving radiation therapy as their sole treatment modality, was comprised of 100 patients. Fourteen patients (14%) had elevated TSH levels. Group 2 was comprised of 46 patients who received radiation therapy and surgery without removal of thyroid tissue. The incidence of elevated TSH levels in this group was 21.7%. There were 50 patients in group 3, all of whom were treated using combined radiation therapy and surgery, including partial thyroidectomy. Thirty-three of the 50 patients (66%) exhibited elevated TSH levels.

Sixty-six percent of the patients in group 3, 40% of the patients in group 2, and 64% of the patients in group 1 developed TSH elevations during the first three years following completion of therapy. Figure 1 is a composite of the three groups showing the year following completion of treatment in which an elevated TSH level was first appreciated. The overall incidence of abnormal TSH values during the first three years following completion of treatment was 59.7%.

The correlation between the sex of the patient and the TSH level is given in Table 2. Thirty-five (17.9%) of the 196 patients were female. Seventeen (48.6%) of the 35 female patients developed abnormally high TSH levels while only 41 (25.4%) of the 161 male patients developed abnormally high TSH values. This female preponderance was found in each of the three groups with 44.4% (8 of 18) in group 1, 22.2% (2 of 9) female patients in group 2, and 87.5% (7 of 8) female patients in group 3 displaying abnormally high TSH values. The corresponding values for the male patients were 8.5% (7 of 82) in group 1, 21.6% (8 of 37) in group 2, and 61.9% (26 of 42) male patients in group 3.

TABLE 2. COMPOSITE CHART OF ALL SUBJECTS CORRELATING SEX OF PATIENT WITH TSH VALUES

	Male	*Female*	*Total*
Normal TSH	120	18	138
Elevated TSH	41 (25.4%)	17 (48.6%)	58
Total	161	35	196

To evaluate the reliability of serum TSH as a screening test for primary hypothyroidism, serum T_4RIA were measured on all but a few of the 196 patients. In no instance was the T_4RIA found to be depressed in the absence of an abnormally elevated TSH. T_4 by RIA testing was done on 54 of the 57 patients with elevated TSH levels. Two of the remaining three patients had been placed on thyroid supplement therapy by their family physician on the basis of serum TSH elevation and the clinical picture. The third patient was unable to return for additional thyroid function testing.

Table 3 displays the incidence of depressed T_4 levels in those patients with an elevated TSH for each of the three patient groupings. In group 1, 30.8% of the patients with elevated TSH had a concomitant depression in the serum T_4RIA. In group 2, 50% of the ten patients with elevated TSH levels had a concomitant decrease in the T_4RIA level. In group 3 (patients receiving combined radiation and surgery, including partial thyroidectomy), 64.5% of the 31 patients with an elevated TSH level also had a depressed serum T_4RIA level. Of further interest is that 5 of the 11 remaining patients with elevated TSH levels in group 3 were found to have borderline low T_4RIA levels ranging between 5.6-6 μg/dl (normal range 5.5-11.5 μg/dl).

DISCUSSION

The finding that external radiation therapy to the thyroid gland, alone or in combination with a surgical procedure, will depress thyroid function is not new. The important feature is that the similarities between early hypothyroidism and the emotionally exhausted and depressed state of the head and neck cancer victim may be striking. There has been a relative lack of emphasis placed on the likelihood of concurrent thyroid injury during the course of treatment for head and neck malignancy. As a consequence, the busy practitioner may not be alert to this possibility until overt hypothyroidism develops. The results of this study emphasize the significant incidence of thyroid dysfunction in the head and neck cancer victim. Thyroid hypofunction may develop from any combination of the commonly employed treatment modalities. It is most frequently seen when portions of the thyroid gland have been resected in patients receiving combination radiation and surgical treatment for their malignancy. The portion of the thyroid gland remaining is not capable of assuming the function of the entire gland. Lindsay et al[15] described acute epithelial injury associated with necrotizing vasculitis and thrombosis resulting from high-dose radiation. Concomitant surgery interferes with the arterial blood supply and venous drainage to the remaining thyroid lobe, and as a result it lacks sufficient reserve to increase its function and produce an adequate supply of thyroid hormone. The result is a hypothyroid state.

TABLE 3. INCIDENCE OF HYPOTHYROIDISM IN PATIENTS WITH ELEVATED THYROID-STIMULATING HORMONE LEVELS

	Patients with Elevated TSH Levels	*Patients with Depressed T_4 Levels*	*% Hypothyroid*
Group 1	13	4	30.8%
Group 2	10	5	50.0%
Group 3	31	20	64.5%

One of the purposes of this study is to alert the clinician to hypothyroidism as a major complication of the treatment for head and neck cancer. This awareness combined with a simple and reliable screening procedure should result in more frequent recognition of hypothyroidism in this patient population. The TSH by RIA is a reliable yet simple method to determine early thyroid dysfunction. TSH values rise relatively soon after withdrawal of thyroid hormone in the hypothyroid patient and fall soon after replacement therapy is reinstituted. Serum TSH levels would, therefore, seem to be especially useful in assessing mild or developing hypothyroidism. Utigar[16] found that TSH levels are almost invariably elevated in patients with primary hypothyroidism and that "this finding must now be considered virtually a sine qua non for this diagnosis." In hypothyroidism secondary to pituitary dysfunction, the TSH level is virtually undetectable.

If hypothyroidism is defined as a lack of availability of thyroid hormone to meet normal tissue requirements, then an elevated TSH must reflect thyroid deficiency. In our study of 196 patients, the TSH was elevated in 29.1% (Table 1). When the group was subdivided according to treatment modalities, the lowest incidence (14%) was reported in the group treated with radiation therapy alone, while the highest incidence (66%) was seen in that group treated with combination radiation and surgery including partial thyroidectomy. These results clearly indicate that external radiation through the thyroid gland in dose ranges customarily used to treat malignancy will impair thyroid function in a significant number of patients. When external radiation therapy is combined with surgery, the incidence of thyroid dysfunction rises, being highest when portions of the thyroid gland are included in the resected specimen.

The importance of making the diagnosis of hypothyroidism in these patients lies in the fact that treatment with thyroid hormone replacement is simple, inexpensive, effective, and usually without major side effects.

A depressed serum T_4RIA level accompanying an elevated TSH level is traditionally recognized as diagnostic of primary hypothyroidism. Patients with normal T_4RIA levels and elevated TSH levels are considered to be in a "latent" or "compensated" hypothyroid state. In order to determine the relative incidence of overt and compensated hypothyroidism in our study group, the T_4RIA levels are correlated with TSH levels (Table 3). A similar pattern evolved with the highest incidence of overt hypothyroidism seen in group 3 (combination radiation and surgical therapy including partial thyroidectomy). Of further interest is the finding in group 3 of borderline low T_4RIA levels in 5 of the 11 patients in the "compensated hypothyroid" category.

Although plasma TSH and T_4RIA levels change inversely, it is recognized that there is not good correlation between the degree of reduction in serum T_4RIA and the degree of elevation of TSH.[16] It is, however, unequivocal that in primary hypothyroidism the TSH is always elevated before the development of T_4RIA depression. During this period of compensated hypothyroidism the T_4RIA levels are maintained by the elevated TSH levels.

Although there is no question as to the propriety of replacement thyroid therapy in the patient with overt clinical hypothyroidism, the question of replacement therapy in the patient with compensated hypothyroidism raises a controversy. Some clinicians feel that the T_4RIA levels should be followed serially and that replacement thyroid therapy should be withheld until depressed T_4RIA levels are demonstrated. Others contend that even in patients with elevation of TSH alone, it is appropriate to begin replacement therapy. Their rationale is based on the following facts: 1) to lessen production of TSH will prevent possible pituitary hyperplasia and sella turcica enlargement, 2) elevated TSH in the presence of radiation-damaged thyroid tissue is known to be carcinogenic, and 3) replacement therapy will reduce the incidence and severity of true hypothyroidism.

Based on the incidence of abnormal and borderline T_4RIA values in the current study we recommend replacement thyroid therapy for all patients in groups 2 and 3 (combination radiation and surgical treatment with or without partial thyroidectomy) who develop an elevated TSH level. Patients in group 1 (radiation therapy alone) should be followed closely with serial TSH and T_4RIA studies and all who develop a depressed T_4RIA value or display a pattern of gradually rising TSH levels should receive thyroid replacement therapy.

The time relationships between completion of therapy for the malignancy and the discovery of an elevated TSH level were explored. However, in a retrospective study such as this, the results cannot be completely accurate. To be accurate, preoperative and serial postoperative TSH levels should be obtained. In some of our patients many months had passed between the completion of therapy for the malignancy and the initial determination of the TSH level. Commonly it was the onset of overt clinical manifestations of hypothyroidism that prompted the investigation.

Despite the shortcomings in this study, the highest incidence of TSH elevation was found during the first posttreatment year while 60% of the abnormal TSH values were obtained during the first three posttreatment years (Fig. 1).

The unusually high incidence of hypothyroidism in the posttreatment female cancer patient has not been previously reported. The explanation for this finding is elusive but may be somehow related to estrogen levels, especially with patients taking supplemental estrogen therapy. This information could not be reliably correlated using data extracted from the medical records in this study group. Another possible explanation for female susceptibility may be subclinical Hashimoto's thyroiditis. This entity is three to four times more common in the female. Here again a prospective study might be designed to clarify these possibilities using pretreatment and serial posttreatment thyroid antibody studies and controlled administration of estrogens.

One final item of interest relates to the use of iodide in the posttreatment cancer patient. As early as 1948 the Wolff-Chiakoff effect was described[17] in which it was demonstrated that large doses of iodide induced an inhibition of thyroid hormone synthesis in the rat. In 1973 it was demonstrated[18] that daily administration of a saturated solution of potassium iodide (SSKI) causes a notable decrease in serum T_4 and an increase in serum TSH levels. Braverman et al[19] demonstrated that euthyroid patients who had undergone ^{131}I treatment for toxic goiter developed myxedema with elevated TSH and decreased T_4 levels after small pharmacologic doses of iodide. These biochemical changes induced by the iodide were accompanied by severe clinical symptoms of hypothyroidism.

As it is not an uncommon clinical procedure to administer saturated solution of potassium iodide (SSKI) as an expectorant in the posttreatment head and neck cancer patient, the medical records of the patients in groups 1, 2, and 3 were reviewed to determine iodide exposure. Nineteen of the 57 patients with elevated TSH levels had received iodide sometime during their posttreatment clinical course. However, because the exposure was sporadic and unrelated to timely TSH determinations no reliable correlation could be established. Here again an interesting prospective study might be designed to clarify the efficacy of iodide therapy in the posttreatment cancer victim.

SUMMARY

The medical records of 196 patients were reviewed in order to evaluate the effects of radiation therapy and surgery on thyroid function in the head and neck cancer patient. The following conclusions were reached.

1. Hypothyroidism is a major complication of the surgical treatment of head and neck cancer.

2. Measurement of TSH levels by the radioimmunoassay method is a reliable screening procedure to detect early primary hypothyroidism.

3. Abnormally elevated TSH levels were found in 29.1% of the group, with the highest incidence (66%) developing in the group treated with combination radiation therapy and surgery, including partial thyroidectomy.

4. The highest incidence of abnormal TSH values occurred during the first posttreatment year. Overall, 60% of the abnormal TSH levels developed within the first three years following completion of therapy.

5. There was a disproportionately higher incidence of abnormal values in the female patients.

6. Pretreatment levels of thyroid function including thyroid antibody studies should be done for all patients. Posttreatment TSH levels should be obtained at least every three months during the first three years and semiannually thereafter.

7. Thyroid replacement therapy should be administered to all patients who have undergone combination radiation and surgical treatment whenever abnormally elevated TSH levels develop.

8. Patients receiving radiation therapy as a sole treatment modality should be followed in a similar manner and replacement thyroid therapy administered if T_4RIA levels fall below normal or if a rising pattern of TSH levels can be demonstrated.

REFERENCES

1. Groover TA, Christie AC, Merritt EA, Coe FO, McPeak EM. Roentgen irradiation in treatment of hyperthyroidism: statistical evaluation based on 305 cases. JAMA 1929; 92:1730-4.

2. Markson JL, Flatman GE. Myxoedema after deep x-ray therapy to the neck. Br Med J 1965; 1:1228-30.

3. Green M, Wilson GM. Thyrotoxicosis treated by surgery or iodine-131: with special reference to development of hypothyroidism. Br Med J 1964; 1:1005-10.

4. Adler RA, Corrigan DF, Wartofsky L. Hypothyroidism after X irradiation to the neck: three case reports and a brief review of the literature. Johns Hopkins Med J 1976; 138:180-4.

5. Bartels EC, Kusakcioglu O. Hypothyroidism subsequent to x-ray therapy. Lahey Clin Found Bull 1965; 14:64-71.

6. Bird RJ, Bryce DP. Longterm effects of heavy irradiation to the neck. J Otolaryngol 1980; 9:18-23.

7. Einhorn J, Wikholm G. Hypothyroidism after external irradiation to the thyroid region. Radiology 1967; 88:326-8.

8. Ballantyne AJ. Late sequelae of the radiation therapy in cancer of the head and neck with particular reference to the nasopharynx. Am J Surg 1975; 130:433-6.

9. Schimpff SC, Diggs CH, Wiswell JG, Salvatore PC, Wiernik PH. Radiation-related thyroid dysfunction: implications for the treatment of Hodgkin's disease. Ann Intern Med 1980; 92:91-8.

10. Murken RE, Duvall III AJ. Hypothyroidism following combined therapy in carcinoma of the laryngopharynx. Laryngoscope 1972; 82:1306-14.

11. Fuks Z, Glatstein E, Marsa GW, Bagshaw MA, Kaplan HS. Long-term effects of external radiation on the pituitary and thyroid glands. Cancer 1976; 37:1152-61.

12. Lavelle RJ. Thyroid function after radiotherapy and total laryngectomy in the treatment of carcinoma of the larynx. Ann Otol Rhinol Laryngol 1971; 80:593-8.

13. Glatstein E, McHardy-Young S, Brast N, Eltringham JR, Kriss JP. Alterations in serum thyrotropin (TSH) and thyroid function following radiotherapy in patients with malignant lymphoma. J Clin Endocrinol Metab 1971; 32:833-41.

14. Smith RE, Adler RA, Clark P, Brinck-Johnsen T, Tulloh ME, Colton T. Thyroid function after mantle irradiation in Hodgkin's disease. JAMA 1981; 245:46-9.

15. Lindsay S, Dailey ME, Jones MD. Histologic effects of various types of ionizing radiation on normal and hyperplastic human thyroid glands. Trans Am Goiter Assoc 1954; 11: 1179-1218.

16. Utiger RD. Thyrotropin radioimmunoassay: another test of thyroid function. Ann Intern Med 1971; 74:627-9.

17. Wolff J, Chiakoff IL. Plasma inorganic iodide as homeostatic regulator of thyroid function. J Biol Chem 1948; 174:555-64.

18. Vagenakis AG, Downs P, Braverman LE, Burger A, Ingbar SH. Control of thyroid hormone secretion in normal subjects receiving iodides. J Clin Invest 1973; 52:528-32.

19. Braverman LE, Woeber KA, Ingbar SH. Induction of myxedema by iodide in patients euthyroid after radioiodine or surgical treatment of diffuse toxic goiter. N Engl J Med 1969; 281:816-21.

Ann Otol 90:1981

SIGNIFICANCE OF POSITIVE BRONCHIAL CYTOLOGY IN PRESENCE OF SQUAMOUS CELL CARCINOMA OF UPPER AERODIGESTIVE TRACT

JONAS T. JOHNSON, MD
ANDREW DEKKER, MD
JOSEPH TURNER, MD
EUGENE N. MYERS, MD, FACS

PITTSBURGH, PENNSYLVANIA

The otolaryngologic literature reflects the high incidence of second primary neoplasms found in patients with a squamous cell carcinoma of the upper aerodigestive tract. Most commonly the second tumor is bronchogenic in origin. Routine panendoscopy (direct laryngoscopy, bronchoscopy, esophagoscopy) has been recommended in patients presenting with a squamous cell carcinoma primary in the upper aerodigestive tract. We have questioned the usefulness of obtaining bronchial washings during bronchoscopy in a patient who has an established primary in the upper aerodigestive tract. Perhaps false-positives would occur due to desquamation of tumor cells into the tracheobronchial tree. The authors address the incidence of false-positive washings encountered in a prospective evaluation of bronchial cytology encountered in 100 consecutive patients with primary squamous cell carcinoma of the upper aerodigestive tract who do not have primary bronchogenic carcinoma. A single false-positive (1%) was encountered. It is concluded that epithelial carcinoma of the larynx and upper aerodigestive tract rarely shed identifiable tumor cells into the tracheobronchial tree. When malignant cells are found with bronchial washings, every effort should be made to localize a second primary tumor in the lung.

The high incidence of second primary neoplasms of the aerodigestive tract in patients with a known squamous carcinoma of the upper aerodigestive tract is well recognized. Fifteen percent to 30% of patients may at some time during their lives develop a second primary carcinoma.[1-3] One third of these may be synchronous with the discovery of the initial squamous cell carcinoma.

The alarming rate of synchronous primaries has led many authors to advocate routine panendoscopy (direct laryngoscopy, bronchoscopy, esophagoscopy) of the upper aerodigestive tract in an attempt to avoid overlooking a second primary tumor.

The most commonly encountered second primary tumor is bronchogenic carcinoma. An accepted method to detect bronchogenic carcinoma is through cytodiagnosis of bronchial washing. This observation suggests that routine collection of bronchial washings during panendoscopy of patients with a known squamous cell carcinoma primary in the upper aerodigestive tract would improve our ability to diagnose occult carcinomas of the lung.

The theoretic reservation for the use of bronchial washings to diagnosis coexistent primary carcinoma of the lung in the presence of a known primary in the upper aerodigestive tract must be raised. Would tumor cells desquamated by the primary cancer in the upper aerodigestive tract be recovered in the tracheobronchial tree? If so, the interpretation of the cytologic specimen would not be useful.

Clearly, the examination of sputum collected by expectoration would have limited value since contamination cannot be eliminated. Exfoliative cytology has been successfully employed to diagnose lesions of the larynx,[4] esophagus,[5] pharynx,[6] and oral cavity.[7-9]

The objective of the present study was to determine the incidence of false-positive cytologic findings obtained with bronchial washings in patients with a primary squamous cell carcinoma of the upper aerodigestive tract.

METHODS

One hundred patients evaluated at the Eye and Ear Hospital of Pittsburgh were studied consecutively and prospectively. When panendoscopy was done bronchial washings were obtained. Patients with radiographic findings compatible with the diagnosis of bronchogenic carcinoma of pulmonary metastasis were excluded because the intent of this study was to document the incidence of false-positive bronchial cytology. Other authors have previously discussed the value of bronchial cytology in the evaluation of a pulmonary lesion.[10-12]

A rigid Jackson bronchoscope was used in all cases. No attempt was made to "wash" the instrument after passing through the upper airway prior to obtaining washings. Each mainstem bronchus was then irrigated with 10 cc normal saline and aspirated for cytology in separate containers.

The specimens were individually labeled and forwarded to the cytology laboratory. Four slides were prepared from each specimen by pipetting particulate sediment onto an albumen-coated, frosted slide. The slide were then fixed in 95% alcohol. Subsequently, the slides were stained with the Papanicolaou stain. The cytologic findings were reported as normal, atypical, suspicious, or positive, in which case the cell type in usually given (Table 1). During the course of this study the cytologist was not aware that the study was in progress. At the termination of the study all specimens were reviewed retrospectively by one of us. No change in initially reported results was necessary.

From the Departments of Otolaryngology and Pathology, University of Pittsburgh School of Medicine.
Presented at the meeting of the American Laryngological Association, Vancouver, British Columbia, May 10-11, 1981.
REPRINTS — Jonas T. Johnson, MD, Eye and Ear Hospital of Pittsburgh, 230 Lothrop Street, Pittsburgh, PA 15213.

TABLE 1. CYTOLOGIC INTERPRETATION

Normal	Epithelial cells, no evidence of malignancy
Atypical (benign)	Abnormal cells due to circumstances other than a neoplastic process (ie, infection)
Suspicious	Process may be neoplastic but sufficient criteria to make diagnosis of malignancy not present. Clinical correlation needed
Positive	Malignant cells present. Attempt to predict histologic cell type usually possible

All patients were then followed for a minimum of six months in order to determine whether a bronchogenic carcinoma had been present which was not detected by the bronchial washings.

RESULTS

The study was terminated when 100 patients with untreated squamous cell carcinoma of the upper aerodigestive tract and a normal chest radiograph had undergone panendoscopy and bronchial washing. Half of the patients had laryngeal tumors and half a variety of other head and neck lesions (Table 2). All stages of laryngeal disease were represented in approximately equal numbers (Table 3).

None of the 50 patients with laryngeal cancer had positive cytology. In four cases atypical cells were reported. This was interpreted as evidence of possible inflammation and was not considered evidence of malignancy. In one case suspicious cells were reported. A primary bronchogenic tumor could not absolutely be ruled out, but is unlikely from the clinical point of view. This patient has shown no evidence of bronchogenic carcinoma during one year of follow-up. Perhaps these suspicious cells may have been from the laryngeal tumor. However, suspicious cells are considered nondiagnostic by our laboratory.

Examination of the data from the other 50 patients demonstrates a broad representation of mucosal head and neck sites (Table 4). One patient with squamous cell carcinoma of the tonsil was found to have positive bronchial cytology. The remaining 49 patients had uniformly negative cytology.

This one exception deserves special note. The patient is a 61-year-old male who had been treated first in 1969 for a squamous cell carcinoma of the mobile tongue. He continued to use alcohol and smoke heavily. In 1979 he was found to have two separate primary lesions. A 2 cm lesion was noted on the tonsillar pillar and a 1 cm lesion on the posterior pharyngeal wall. Bronchial washings obtained at the time of panendoscopy showed cells consistent with squamous cell carcinoma; however, full chest tomography was normal. The patient subsequently underwent excision of the pharyngeal lesions. Repeat bronchoscopy and washings done in November 1980 were negative. Follow-up in this patient to date has not demonstrated the development of a clinically evident carcinoma. The patient represents the only case in 100 (1%) in which it is likely that malignant cells from an upper aerodigestive primary tumor may have been aspirated and recovered by bronchial washings.

TABLE 2. TUMOR SITES IN PATIENT POPULATION STUDIED

Site	*No. of Patients*
Larynx	50
Other upper aerodigestive tract sites	50
	100

TABLE 3. BRONCHIAL CYTOLOGY IN PATIENTS WITH LARYNGEAL TUMORS

Stage	*No. of Pts.*	*Negative*	*Atypical*	*Suspicious*	*Positive*
T_1	9	9	0	0	0
T_2	16	16	0	0	0
T_3	13	10	2	1	0
T_4	12	10	2	0	0
Total	50	45	4	1	0

It should be stressed that a number of obvious second primary pulmonary carcinomas were encountered during the course of this study. In almost all cases the pulmonary carcinoma was evident on routine chest radiograph and positive bronchial cytology was usually obtained. These patients were excluded from our data.

An illustrative case is that of a 76-year-old male who presented with a transglottic carcinoma. The preoperative chest radiograph demonstrated a lesion of the right lower lobe. Panendoscopy confirmed the squamous cell carcinoma of the larynx. Bronchoscopy demonstrated only erythema at the orifice of the right lower lobe bronchus. However, bronchial washings were positive for squamous cell carcinoma. It is unclear if this represented a second primary or metastatic disease; however, the patient's overall condition precluded surgical treatment of his pulmonary disease. Subsequently, therapy was undertaken with a palliative intent.

The objective of this study is to investigate the significance of positive cytology in the presence of a primary squamous cell carcinoma of the upper aerodigestive tract. The study does show that positive cytology is important because head and neck lesions do not commonly shed detectable tumor cells into the tracheobronchial tree. Perhaps malignant cells are in fact desquamated and cleaned by mucociliary action or alveolar phagocytosis. Desquamated malignant cells from

TABLE 4. BRONCHIAL CYTOLOGY IN PATIENTS WITH NONLARYNGEAL HEAD AND NECK TUMORS (N = 50)

	No. of. Pts.	*Negative*	*Atypical*	*Suspicious*	*Positive*
Oral cavity	14	14	0	0	0
Tonsil	14	13	0	0	1
Base of Tongue	10	10	0	0	0
Pharynx	10	10	0	0	0
Cervical esophagus	2	2	0	0	0
Total	50	49	0	0	1

an upper aerodigestive primary tumor are not detectable by commonly practiced cytology techniques. Therefore, obtaining a specimen for bronchial cytology plays an important part in the diagnosis of an unsuspected bronchogenic carcinoma.

Bronchial cytology played an important role in another patient encountered during the course of the study. The patient is a 49-year-old male admitted for evaluation of a T_4 pharyngeal lesion. Preoperative chest radiograph was within normal limits. Routine panendoscopy was performed. Histologically the pharyngeal lesion was squamous cell carcinoma. Bronchial washings were interpreted as positive for tumor consistent with oat cell carcinoma. The patient subsequently underwent a pulmonary CT scan which demonstrated nodules not noted on routine chest radiograph. The patient was subsequently treated for disseminated oat cell carcinoma and surgery on his pharynx was avoided. In this case, the information gained from the bronchial washing clearly helped us avoid what would have been inappropriate surgery in this unfortunate man.

DISCUSSION

Our findings substantiate the results of Dellon et al.[13] In a series of 18 patients with head and neck lesions, positive washings were not encountered in any patient in spite of the fact that 72% of these patients have positive cytology when the lesion was specifically washed and aspirated.

This study provides evidence to support the statement that the shedding of malignant cells into the proximal tracheobronchial tree and their subsequent recovery on bronchial washings is unusual. In our series of 100 patients, only one patient (1%) had evidence of probable shedding from an upper aerodigestive source. In fact, in the 50 patients with laryngeal lesions who would seem to be at highest risk, no false-positive cases were countered.

A corollary of this statement is that bronchial washings should be routinely obtained as a part of the panendoscopic evaluation of the patient with a head and neck primary. In our experience, a false-positive is a very unusual occurrence and positive washings deserve full and careful search for a subclinical primary carcinoma of the lung.

REFERENCES

1. Marchetta FC, Soho K, Camp F. Multiple malignancies in patients with head and neck cancer. Am J Surg 1965; 110:537-41.
2. Horowitz R, Chomet B. Oral carcinoma and multiplicity of carcinomas. Oral Surg 1968; 26:87-91.
3. Gluckman JL, Crissman JD, Donegan JO. Multicentric squamous-cell carcinoma of the upper aerodigestive tract. Head Neck Surg 1980; 3:90-6.
4. Glennie HRR, Gilbert JG, Melcher DH, Linehan J, Wadsworth PV. The place of cytology in laryngeal diagnosis. Clin Otolaryngol 1976; 1:131-6.
5. Prolla JC. Histopathology and cytology in detection. JAMA 1973; 223:1554-6.
6. Hopp ES. Cytologic diagnosis and prognosis in carcinoma of the mouth, pharynx and nasopharynx. Laryngoscope 1958; 68:1281-7.
7. Sandler HC. The cytologic diagnosis of tumors of the oral cavity. Acta Cytol 1964; 8:114-20.
8. Molinari R, Pilotti S, Rilke F. Clinical evaluation of cytological diagnosis of nasopharyngeal malignancies. In: de-The G, Ito Y, eds. Nasopharyngeal carcinoma: etiology and control: proceedings of an international symposium. Lyon: International Agency for Research on Cancer, 1978.
9. Friedmann I. Exfoliative cytology as an aid in the diagnosis of tumours of the throat, nose and ear. J Laryngol Otol 1951; 65:1-9.
10. Burke MD, Melamed MR. Exfoliative cytology of metastatic cancer in lung. Acta Cytol 1968; 12:61-74.
11. Russell WO, Heinrich WN, Mountain CF, Griffith KM, Chang JP. Cytodiagnosis of lung cancer. Acta Cytol 1963; 7:1-15.
12. Koss LG, Melamed MR, Goodner JT. Pulmonary cytology — a brief survey of diagnostic results from July 1, 1952 until Dec. 31, 1960. Acta Cytol 1964; 8:104-13.
13. Dellon AL, Chu EW, Hall CA, Chretien PB. Cytology of bronchial washings. Arch Otolaryngol 1975; 101:465-6.

Ann Otol 90:1981

LARYNGEAL REINNERVATION FOR UNILATERAL VOCAL CORD PARALYSIS: LONG-TERM RESULTS

HARVEY M. TUCKER, MD

MELINDA RUSNOV, MA

CLEVELAND, OHIO

Since 1976 modified nerve-muscle pedicle reinnervation for restoration of adductor function in unilaterally paralyzed vocal cords has been performed at the Cleveland Clinic. This technique has been reserved for patients with "valuable" voices such as clergymen, public speakers, professional singers and actors. It was felt that this technique should offer potential for restoration of quality of voice and in particular of pitch control, superior to that usually obtained by Teflon® injection, because of restoration of the ability to tense the vocal cord. In this regard nerve-muscle pedicle reinnervation is potentially superior to any of the other techniques available for medialization of the unilaterally paralyzed cord. At the present time 27 patients have undergone this surgery and have been followed long enough (at least one year) to determine if the procedure was successful or not. All of these have been subjected to preoperative and postoperative voice recordings on high quality tape equipment. Some of them have been subjected to voice printing for vocal analysis. There have been no complications in the group and all but two of the patients have achieved significant voice improvement as a result of the surgery. The details of current technique and demographic data and follow-up will be presented.

Unilateral vocal cord paralysis may be managed in three general ways. These include Teflon® or Gelfoam® injection, surgical medialization of the vocal cord, and/or nerve-muscle pedicle reinnervation for restoration of phonation.[1,2] Of these the procedure of choice is Teflon injection because it is rapid, inexpensive, and offers good results in most cases. In the occasional patient who has an unusually large posterior glottic chink or where the arytenoid is ankylosed or limited in motion as well as paralyzed, Gelfoam or Teflon alone will usually not be adequate and some means of surgical medialization must be undertaken. In the past these patients have been managed by any of several techniques designed to interpose autogenous cartilage to force the arytenoid to the midline and with it the vocal cord. Such an approach yields satisfactory results in most cases and in the occasional patient in whom this does not produce an acceptable improvement in voice, a minimal Teflon injection can be superimposed on the partially medialized vocal cord, usually yielding good results. Both of these techniques, however, suffer from the failure to restore tensing capability in the vocal cord and with this the ability to regain good pitch control. For this reason, a modified nerve-muscle pedicle technique for reinnervation of adductor function has been employed at the Cleveland Clinic Foundation since 1976 in carefully selected patients with unilaterally paralyzed vocal cords.[2] The technique has been reserved for patients with so-called "valuable" voices. This group includes clergymen, public speakers, professional singers and actors. Because nerve-muscle pedicle reinnervation of the adductor division not only can produce active medialization of the vocal cord, but also has the potential to restore the ability to tense the vocal cord, it was anticipated that superior quality of voice could be achieved by this technique. Of necessity, the original report dealt mostly with the technical aspects of the operation and with a small initial group of patients. Since that time 31 patients have undergone the procedure and all of these have been followed long enough to determine whether or not the procedure was successful. This report includes our long-term experience in this larger group of patients subjected to reinnervation for unilateral vocal cord paralysis.

METHODS

Patient Selection. As noted in the introduction, only certain patients have been offered the opportunity to select vocal cord reinnervation for unilateral cord paralysis. Review of several series[3] shows that most cases of unilateral vocal cord paralysis not due to direct trauma to the recurrent nerve will spontaneously recover or will compensate within six months to one year to a sufficient degree that no other intervention is needed. Moreover, Teflon injection offers at least adequate results for the vast majority of those patients who require some type of intervention for restoration of voice. It is only the occasional patient who needs to consider some more extensive procedure in hopes of achieving an *excellent* voice including restoration of pitch control. Of necessity, however, this group of patients must be chosen in subjective rather than objective fashion. To limit the procedure only to certain professions seemed to be a reasonable approach but as experience has accumulated it is apparent that certain patients who do not fall into these categories also are willing and, indeed, insist upon undergoing the more extensive surgical procedure in hopes of achieving the best possible voice. In presenting the surgical alternatives to patients with unilateral vocal cord paralysis, the point is always made that Teflon injection is the procedure of choice because of its reliability, simplicity, and limited expense. Most of them have agreed that this was the approach that they preferred. Those patients who have indicated interest in nerve-muscle pedicle reinnervation were counseled by the surgeon and the speech pathologist preoperatively and in many cases were given the opportunity to converse with patients who had already undergone the procedure to hear what sort of results had been achieved.

Technique. The surgical technique has not changed appreciably since it was first reported in 1977.[2] Through a neck

From the Department of Otolaryngology and Communicative Disorders, The Cleveland Clinic Foundation.

Presented at the meeting of the American Laryngological Association, Vancouver, British Columbia, March 10-11, 1981.

REPRINTS — Harvey M. Tucker, MD, The Cleveland Clinic Foundation, Department of Otolaryngology, 9500 Euclid Avenue, Cleveland, OH 44106.

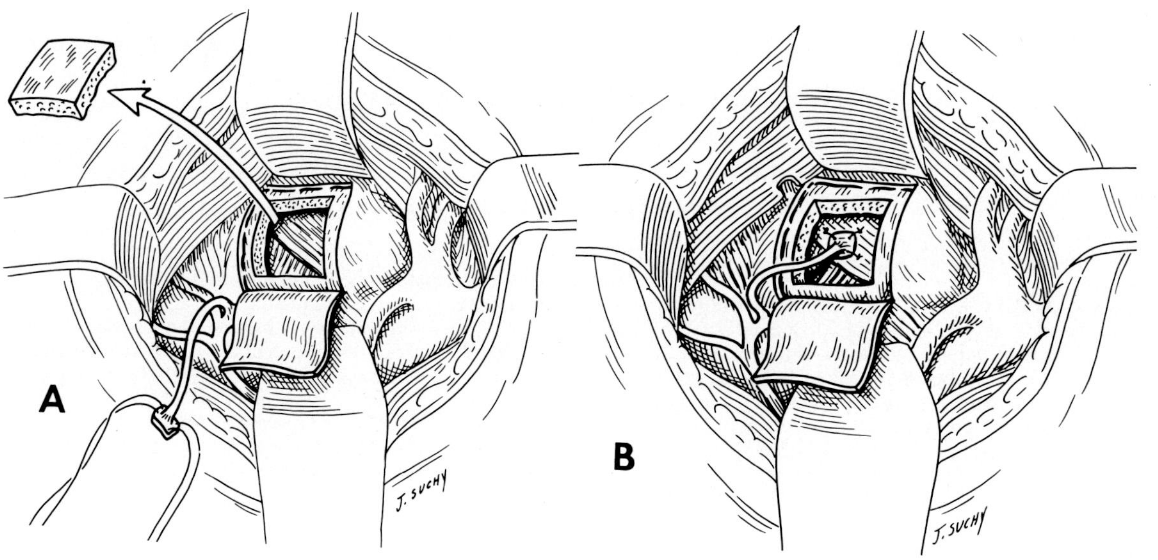

Fig. 1. A) Nerve-muscle pedicle prepared, cartilage "window" removed, revealing underlying laryngeal adductor muscles. B) Nerve-muscle pedicle sutured into place.

crease incision to one side of the midline at about the level of the lower border of the thyroid cartilage, a nerve-muscle pedicle is obtained, usually from the anterior belly of the omohyoid muscle. When necessary, any of the branches to the other strap muscles can be used instead (Fig. 1A). A window is made in the lower half of the thyroid ala on the same side using an oscillating saw and through this the fibers of the lateral thyroarytenoideus muscle (a major adductor of the larynx) are exposed. The nerve-muscle pedicle is transposed to this recipient bed (Fig. 1B). Postoperatively, patients are permitted to eat as soon as they have recovered from anesthesia and no attempt is made to prevent them from talking. Up to 12 mg of dexamethasone (Decadron®) has been given intravenously as a supramaximal dose in order to limit postoperative edema which might follow since these patients have unilateral cord paralysis, must be intubated, and laryngeal surgery is being performed. There have been no postoperative problems with the airway in any of these patients.

RESULTS

There have been no complications as a result of the surgical procedure to date. All patients have healed promptly and have been able to leave the hospital three to five days after surgery. There was an immediate, although generally minimal, improvement in voice following the surgical procedure. This was felt to be due to a combination of postoperative edema coupled with the detachment of some of the lateral fibers of the thyroarytenoideus from the inner surface of the thyroid cartilage, thus producing some mechanical medialization of the cord. In most cases this initial improvement deteriorated postoperatively so that by two weeks after surgery the patient's voice was roughly equivalent to what it had been before the operation. Patients were followed at 2-week intervals when possible, but because several of them came from great distances some were not followed more often than once every two months. In all cases, however, they were encouraged to send either tapes or to call on the telephone at roughly 2-week intervals to apprise us of their progress. The referring physician was contacted in every case so that the patients were seen in follow-up at roughly 2-week intervals. The earliest voice improvement thought to be due to active restoration of tonus or movement in the reinnervated cord was noted at approximately $3^1/_2$ weeks after surgery. In no case was there significant improvement in voice that did not begin within four months after the surgery. Therefore, if there was no improvement after four months the procedure was considered a failure and, if the patient so desired, some other means of restoration of voice was undertaken (Table 1). Postoperative voice recordings were obtained at intervals in most of the patients. On several of these, voice spectograms were obtained in an attempt to arrive at some reliable assessment of the quality of voice that had been achieved. It was our conclusion that such analysis is not sufficiently precise to provide an objective measurement of voice quality and, therefore, could not be used to assess the results obtained. Therefore, the voice results obtained were graded subjectively by the surgeon, the patient and/or a speech pathologist as normal, greatly improved, somewhat improved, or no improvement. The results of these assessments are tabulated in Table 2. All patients in

TABLE 1. TIME OF ONSET OF VOCAL CORD MEDIALIZATION POSTREINNERVATION

	<6 wk	*6-12 wk*	*13-18 wk*	*Failures*
Tonic medialization	1	9	5	4
Active adduction	3	7	2	

TABLE 2. RESULTS OF NERVE-MUSCLE PEDICLE REINNERVATION FOR UNILATERAL VOCAL CORD PARALYSIS

Total Pts	*Normal Voice*	*Greatly Improved*	*Somewhat Improved*	*No Improvement*
31	10	16	1	4

the series have been followed at least six months since surgery and all but four of them have been followed for a period longer than one year. There have been two cases in which there was an initial good result within a 4-month period, but whose voice quality subsequently deteriorated back to the breathiness that existed before the surgery. In both of these cases the patient reported an upper respiratory infection shortly before the diminution in voice quality. Both of these patients regained the previous vocal improvement in a period of one to three months without further intervention other than speech therapy. All of the remaining patients who were improved after reinnervation have maintained it without regression to previous poor voice quality.

DISCUSSION

If nerve-muscle pedicle reinnervation can achieve successful active or tonic medialization of the paralyzed vocal cord in a majority of patients, it should offer the possibility of better voice results than can be expected after Teflon injection because of restoration of tensing capability in the cord. It is not possible to compare the results achieved with reinnervation to those achieved by either Teflon injection or surgical medialization since adequate controls cannot be established. Therefore, one is reduced to making subjective assessments of vocal quality. On the basis of these it appears that reinnervation can produce normal or near-normal voice results in properly selected patients. Whether or not a surgical procedure of this magnitude is justified by the possibility of better voice result is unresolved and will have to be subject to individual preference of the operating surgeon and the patient. If the alternatives are fairly presented with the relative advantages and disadvantages made clear, it would seem that in most cases the patient can make a valid decision as to how he or she wishes to proceed.

Nerve-muscle pedicle reinnervation offers both advantages and disadvantages when compared to other techniques. The *advantages* include the potential for better voice quality and pitch control and the fact that this procedure does not preclude the successful use of either of the other two general approaches. The *disadvantages* include the need for an open surgical procedure under general anesthesia and the time that must elapse between the operation and eventual improvement in the voice.

Passive mobility of the arytenoid is critical to success or failure of both Teflon injection and nerve-muscle pedicle reinnervation. It is important to assess this móbility under general anesthesia with use of paralytic agents before a decision is made how best to treat the patient. In reviewing some 200 patients with unilateral vocal cord paralysis[3] it was noted that fixation was uncommon as compared to bilateral vocal cord paralysis in which one third of all patients who had had paralysis for longer than six months also developed ankylosis of the cricoarytenoid joint. It appears that the remaining mobile parts of the larynx produce enough passive movement of the paralyzed cricoarytenoid joint to maintain its mobility. As a result, ankylosis or limitation of motion is an uncommon occurrence in unilateral paralysis when it is not due to inflammatory or traumatic problems involving the cricoarytenoid joint itself. Patients who sustain unilateral paralysis after trauma that may have produced a temporary dislocation of the arytenoid should be assessed very carefully before a decision is made how to proceed. If the joint is fixed, the surgeon should give serious consideration to surgical medialization by cartilage interposition since this is really the only procedure that will successfully medialize a fixed cricoarytenoid joint.[1]

CONCLUSIONS

Teflon injection remains the procedure of choice for the management of most patients with unilateral vocal cord paralysis who do not either recover spontaneously or compensate to satisfactory voice levels. Nerve-muscle pedicle reinnervation may be employed as a means of reanimation of unilaterally paralyzed vocal cords with good-to-excellent voice results within four months of surgery in carefully selected cases. It is not possible to objectively assess the quality of voice obtained by this technique as compared to other alternatives since controls cannot be realistically established. The procedure may offer a good alternative to Teflon injection or surgical medialization in patients who desire voice restoration of best possible quality.

REFERENCES

1. Tucker HM. Management of the patient with an incompetent larynx: a review. Am J Otolaryngol 1979; 1:47-56.

2. Tucker HM. Reinnervation of the unilaterally paralyzed larynx. Ann Otol Rhinol Laryngol 1977; 86:789-94.

3. Tucker HM. Vocal cord paralysis — 1979: etiology and management. Laryngoscope 1980; 90:585-90.

PANENDOSCOPY FOR SECOND PRIMARIES IN HEAD AND NECK CANCER

ROBERT H. MAISEL, MD HUBERT VERMEERSCH, MD

MINNEAPOLIS, MINNESOTA

Four hundred patients with biopsy-proven squamous cell carcinoma of the upper aerodigestive tract were studied for evidence of a synchronous second primary tumor. The protocol of study included in most cases direct laryngoscopy, metal tube bronchoscopy, and esophagoscopy. Chest x-ray studies were performed on all patients and many had barium swallow x-ray studies. Asymptomatic second head and neck primary tumors were found only in the vallecula and esophagus among this series of patients. Metachronous second primary tumors were presented as early as one month after the original endoscopy and were located in areas which had been carefully examined by endoscopy and appeared asymptomatic to the examining physician at the time of the original evaluation. Based on this series of patients, we recommend careful indirect laryngoscopy and oral examination, direct laryngoscopy and esophagoscopy as well as a barium swallow for patients with clinically suspicious mucosal lesion of the upper aerodigestive tract. In view of our failure to discover a single lung carcinoma which was not evident from chest x-ray studies, we recommend bronchoscopy, which adds some morbidity to the endoscopic procedure, not be included unless a specific clinical suspicion is entertained. However, because of the important treatment implications which follow the diagnosis of a new squamous cell carcinoma of the upper aerodigestive tract, we feel it is imperative that the entire esophagus be evaluated in the course of the pretreatment exploration of the patient. Although few esophageal tumors were discovered, their implications in terms of surgical resection and debilitation without much likelihood of long-term patient survival has encouraged us to continue the above described procedure.

The concept of multiple separate tumors of the head and neck has long caught the attention of interested medical researchers. Billroth appears to be the first to describe a patient in the literature with multiple primary cancers.[1] In 1932 Warren and Gates[1] described a large series of patients with multiple tumors, and Moertel[2] felt this explosion of multiple cancer cases coincided with the increased survival from the initial cancer which began to occur due to the improvements in medical and surgical treatment in the 1920s and 1930s.

Patients with epidermoid carcinoma of the upper aerodigestive tract usually smoke and drink.[3] This presumed carcinogenic environment also suggests the concept of field cancerization first described for the oral cavity by Slaughter.[4] In the otolaryngology literature, the range of multiple tumors has been described in those studies which paid particular attention to it to be between 1 and 20%.[5-11]

Moertel[2] classified multiple primary tumors functionally in three categories. Category 1, multicentric cancers, includes two or more cancers of the same tissue and organ. Moertel also grouped multiple cancers of the same tissue shared by contiguous organs (pharynx and larynx) and cancers in each of bilateral paired organs in this category. Category 2 includes tumors of different organs or tissues and category 3 includes those patients with multiple tumors in category 1 and another tumor from a different organ.

Multiple tumors can also be defined by time of discovery. Simultaneous tumors are discovered during the evaluation of the first tumor and include those second tumors discovered by physical examination and by the usual radiographic and endoscopic evaluation, as well as any further workup dictated by the symptoms described to the attending physician. Synchronous tumors are considered those second tumors not discovered by the above workup, either because the tumors were not present, not recognized, or the appropriate tests were not done, but which were uncovered less than six months after the completion of this evaluation. Metachronous tumors are those which are detected more than six months after the first tumor. Again, the completeness of the initial workup will determine the frequency of metachronous tumors, since failure to inquire about respiratory symptoms as well as neglecting to obtain a chest x-ray study would almost by definition make a second simultaneous primary tumor in the lung a metachronous tumor since its symptoms may not show for many months.

The contribution of otolaryngologists and other head and neck surgeons has been to highlight the possibility of discovering a second primary tumor. It has been felt by many writers that the presence of one head and neck tumor suggests a second primary tumor, usually from among category 1.[2] Various authors[5,6,8,9] have recommended that the workup for head and neck cancer include upper aerodigestive panendoscopy with biopsy of any suspicious lesion. Shapshay et al[10] reviewed their experience with 150 patients over two years and found nine (6%) simultaneous esophageal cancers concurrent with the index cancer of the head and neck. They

From the Department of Otolaryngology, University of Minnesota, and Hennepin County Medical Center, Minneapolis.

Presented at the meeting of the American Laryngological Association, Vancouver, British Columbia, May 10-11, 1981.

REPRINTS — Robert H. Maisel, MD, Department of Otolaryngology, University of Minnesota Hospitals, Minneapolis, MN 55455.

TABLE 1. ENDOSCOPIC EVALUATION OF PATIENTS WITH HEAD AND NECK TUMORS (N = 449)

	No Direct Laryngoscopy	*Direct Laryngoscopy*	*Bronchoscopy*	*Esophagoscopy*	*Panendoscopy*	*Total*
Oral	93	21	1	3	17	135
Oropharynx	27	28	10	—	15	80
Hypopharynx	—	28	—	4	17	49
Larynx	2	138	10	10	25	185
Total	122	215	21	17	74	449

concluded that esophagoscopy was indicated in all new head and neck cancer patients.

Our interest in this problem was heightened by a familiarity with the above literature. Even when examination is carefully and easily accomplished, we have seen experienced physicians not recognize asymptomatic tumors of the head and neck on office examination. We made a retrospective study of our patients at the University Hospital and Hennepin County Medical Center.

METHODS

Patients with squamous cell cancers of the mucosa of the superior aerodigestive tract (except lip, sinus, and nasopharynx) seen in clinic or hospital from January 1, 1971, through December 31, 1980, were included and categorized as to location of the index primary. The categories included oral cavity (tongue, floor of mouth, palate, and cheek), oropharynx (tongue base, tonsil, and pharynx), hypopharynx (pyriform sinus and postcricoid lesions, as well as posterior pharyngeal lesions) and intrinsic laryngeal lesions. Chest x-ray and barium swallow studies when done were described as normal or suggesting neoplasm and the results of indirect laryngoscopy and direct laryngoscopy were compared. Bronchoscopy and esophagoscopy when performed were either normal or biopsy-positive for a second tumor.

We used the criteria of Warren and Gates[1] to recognize multiple tumors. These criteria specify that the tumors must be clearly histologically malignant and geographically distinct. The possibility that the two tumors represent metastasis from a single site had to be ruled out. Lung cancer presented a particularly difficult problem; we used the clinical criteria of multiple pulmonary nodules to define a metastatic lesion and endobronchial lesions to define a separate pulmonary primary. In questionable cases the clinician's judgment was accepted..

RESULTS

In a review of 494 charts, 20 were excluded because of incomplete information and 25 were rejected because the tissue type or tumor location did not fit our protocol. In 449 patients with squamous cell carcinoma of the head and neck, 185 had a primary tumor in the larynx, 49 in the hypopharynx, 135 in the oral cavity, and 80 in the oropharynx (Table 1). Seventy-four patients had triple endoscopy and 38 patients had double endoscopy. All patients, except two with laryngeal/hypopharyngeal lesions, had a direct laryngoscopy for diagnosis. Forty-four percent of patients with oral and oropharyngeal lesions had endoscopy while 56% had examination and biopsy only. Among the 449 patients in the study, 36 simultaneous double tumors were found (Table 2). Seventeen of the 36 tumors were in the lung. Chest x-ray studies were abnormal for all 17 patients and bronchoscopic biopsies or washings were positive in 5 of these patients. The four esophageal tumors occurred in patients who had oral cavity or oropharyngeal lesions. Two esophageal cancers were biopsied and a subsequent barium swallow x-ray study was normal. Two other patients had abnormal barium swallow x-ray studies preceding the biopsies. In all patients with double symptomatic tumors the tumor closest to the anterior incisor was considered the index primary and the more distal tumor considered secondary. Asymptomatic tumors were always second primaries. Twenty-one patients with oral cavity and oropharyngeal lesions had subsequent tumors. Four of the 49 patients with hypopharyngeal tumors had secondary tumors and 19 among the 185 laryngeal tumor patients had secondary tumors (Table 3).

DISCUSSION

Our study leads us to agree with Vrabec's concept of a multicentric zone which involves all the squamous epithelial-lined aerodigestive tract including the lower tracts of esophagus and lung.[8] It is this target area that is the likely site for any secondary primary tumors. Our finding of 36 patients with simultaneous second primaries among 449 patients studied is consistent with the literature. Gluckman[6] was able to show a 9.2% incidence of simultaneous primaries while Cohn and Peppard[9] reported 8%, and Shapshay et al[10] 14%. Gluckman[6] found 7.4% of simultaneous second primaries were discovered in the head and neck, while Cohn and Peppard[9] noted less than 4% in their series of patients; Shapshay et al[10] reported 6% and Vrabec[8] 7.5%. These series are not strictly comparable with respect to metachronous primaries since there is no uniform follow-up period.

Our data (Table 4) show an 8% incidence of

TABLE 2. PATIENTS WITH SIMULTANEOUS PRIMARY TUMORS (N = 36)

	Oral Cavity/ Oropharynx	*Hypopharynx*	*Larynx*	*Lung*	*Esophagus*	*Other*
Oral cavity/oropharynx	3	3	2	4	4	1
Hypopharynx	—	—	1	—	—	1
Larynx	—	3	—	13	—	1
Total		12		17	4	

TABLE 3. PATIENTS WITH METACHRONOUS PRIMARY TUMORS (N = 44)

	Oral Cavity/ Oropharynx	*Hypopharynx*	*Larynx*	*Lung*	*Esophagus*	*Other*
Oral cavity/oropharynx	7	2	4	8	—	—
Hypopharynx	2	—	—	1	1	—
Larynx	6	2	—	8	—	3

simultaneous second primaries. We therefore conclude that second primaries coincidental to head and neck tumors occur rather frequently and that most are in the head and neck (3%) or the lung (4%). Most second primaries in the lung are discovered by x-ray studies.

It is noteworthy that the upper aerodigestive tract second primaries which accounted for 12 cases were recognized on the admission history and physical examination by the otolaryngologist in only seven instances. Many of the index primaries were completely evaluable without a direct laryngoscopy and general anesthetic. Two of the soft palate tumors were completely definable through bimanual palpation and it was only because of the full panendoscopy, insisted upon by the staff physician, that there were discovered a vallecular primary in one patient and an esophageal primary in the other. Similarly, one patient with a very large and painful tongue tumor whose extent was defined completely by office examination had a vocal cord carcinoma discovered by laryngoscopy. Laryngoscopy was done only for completeness of examination since the vocal cord tumor was not suspected, the poor voice quality of the patient having been considered secondary to lingual fixation by the tongue tumor.

Based on these cases we recommend general anesthesia and direct laryngoscopy if the patient's medical condition will permit and if treatment is planned for the primary tumor.

All 17 of the simultaneous second primaries in the lung were discovered by x-ray studies. Bronchoscopy confirmed five and the rest required thoracotomy, mediastinoscopy or autopsy for tissue diagnosis. No patients who had bronchoscopy with a normal chest x-ray study had a bronchogenic carcinoma. Weaver et al recognize early diagnosis of lung cancer to be difficult, with less than 30% of proven lung cancers identified by bronchoscopy.[5]

Vrabec[8] reported that 10-15% of laryngeal carcinoma patients are likely to develop lung carcinoma. He further stated that 6% of lung carcinoma patients have a laryngeal carcinoma at diagnosis.

TABLE 4. REPORTED SIMULTANEOUS PRIMARY TUMORS

Authors	*All SP Tumors*	*Second Primary in Head and Neck*
Gluckman[6]	9.2%	7.4%
Cohn and Peppard[9]	8.0%	<4.0%
Shapshay et al[10]	14.0%	6.0%
Maisel and Vermeersch	8.0%	3.0%

SP — Simultaneous primary.

Our data were not designed to agree with or refute this last statement, as we did not evaluate patients admitted with a diagnosis of pulmonary carcinoma. However, 13 of 183 patients with laryngeal carcinoma in our study had a simultaneous lung cancer and 17 other patients did develop what the attending physicians regarded as a second primary tumor in the lung some time after their initial diagnosis.

Support for considering a solitary pulmonary nodule as a new primary lesion is offered by Cahan, who reports a $3^1/_2$ to 1 chance that a solitary pulmonary shadow is a separate tumor and not metastatic.[12] It is felt that a second tumor in the lung is not due to x-ray therapy to the primary since it is beyond the port of radiation and probably reflects a result of the same carcinogenic bathing that precipitated the first tumor, possibly in the presence of a reduced immune surveillance. Since no bronchoscopies revealed a lung cancer in this high-risk population unless the chest radiograph is abnormal, we suggest that bronchoscopy not be mandatory in the workup of the head and neck cancer patient. Particularly in large and bulky base of tongue and laryngeal carcinomas, the technique of bronchoscopy where the bronchoscope is used for intubation puts the patient's airway at significant risk with the necessity for an emergency tracheostomy and the possibility of a period of hypoxia. Therefore without indications we do not perform bronchoscopy on head and neck tumor patients.

Goldstein and Zornoza[13] reviewed a 30-year experience comprising approximately 10,000 patients with head and neck carcinoma. Their study showed that less than 1% of the patients with head and neck cancer had developed an esophageal cancer. Eighty-nine of 850 patients with esophageal cancer had a head and neck cancer. For esophageal cancer, the incidence of subsequent stomach or colon carcinoma approximated the population statistics for these patients with esophageal carcinoma. Cahan et

TABLE 5. REPORTED HEAD AND NECK CANCER PATIENTS WITH ESOPHAGEAL CANCER

Authors	*%*	*Ratio*
Goldstein and Zornoza[13] (n = 10,000)	<1	Of 10,000 tumors
Cahan et al[14] (n = 7,000)	<1	60/7000
Thompson et al[15] (n = 3,000)	1	35/3000
Shapshay et al[10] (n = 150)	6	9/150
Maisel and Vermeersch (n = 449)	1	5/449

TABLE 6. PERCENTAGE OF SECOND PRIMARY TUMORS

	Simultaneous	*Metachronous*
Oral Cavity/Oropharynx	7.5%	10.0%
Hypopharynx	4.0%	8.5%
Larynx	9.0%	10.0%

al[14] similarly reviewed a large series of patients and found less than 1% of the head and neck cancer patients had a double primary in the esophagus, either simultaneously or subsequently. Thompson et al[15] reviewed more than 3,000 head and neck cancer patients and found 35 double primaries with the esophagus (Table 5).

In the study of Odette et al,[16] 10 of the 42 patients with double primaries had an esophageal tumor simultaneous or metachronous to a head and neck lesion. The recent article of Shapshay et al[10] suggests that 6% of their head and neck cancer patients when carefully studied showed a simultaneous esophageal carcinoma.

Vrabec[8] reports 7 of 11 simultaneous esophageal cancers had a normal contrast x-ray study of the esophagus. Gluckman[6] and Gluckman et al[7] also noted the same phenomenon and Shapshay's group had four negative x-ray studies among nine tumors.[10]

Our results show four cases of simultaneous esophageal carcinoma which were discovered on direct esophagoscopy with biopsy. Two of these patients had a normal barium swallow x-ray study. Only one patient developed an esophageal carcinoma metachronous to his index tumor. Although esophagoscopy will discover the rare tumor (4 of 449), this expensive, somewhat risky, and time-consuming procedure may not be cost effective in head and neck cancer. If, however, the frequency of seond tumors described by Shapshay is confirmed in other studies, esophagoscopy must be part of the routine pretreatment evaluation for all squamous cell carcinomas of the mucosa of the head and neck. Therefore, although our results do not conform to those of Shapshay[10] but are more in keeping with Gluckman et al,[7] who discovered four tumors among 259 endoscopies, we continue to evaluate whether esophagoscopy should be part of the routine examination in all patients with a mucosal head and neck carcinoma, to avoid failing to discover a small esophageal tumor whose symptoms are not clear or not present.

We are concerned that the early discovery of this second tumor may still not improve survival. Presently esophageal carcinoma when less than 3 cm in size at discovery has a 3-10% two-year survival.[17] A surgeon's philosophy on what to do for the primary tumor in the presence of a second tumor that has a very low opportunity for cure will determine his recommended treatment protocol. (It is not yet known what the two- and five-year survival will be for esophageal tumors which present without symptoms and are discovered only through routine endoscopy because of upper aerodigestive carcinoma.) Obviously, the results in these esophageal carcinomas can never improve beyond the cure rate of the original index primaries.

Table 3 shows the metachronous primaries discovered in our series and reveals 19 second primaries among the 185 laryngeal cancers, an incidence of 10%, which is similar to the incidence of simultaneous second primaries from among patients with laryngeal tumors. Oral cavity and oropharynx cases showed 21 metachronous primaries among 215 cases, an incidence of 10% compared to 16 simultaneous primaries. Kogelnik et al[18] felt the soft palate was the source of the highest incidence of multiple primaries in the head and neck, while Wagenfeld et al[19] noted supraglottic laryngeal patients to have a crude risk rate for simultaneous primary of 4% with a metachronous risk of 8%. For our series the hypopharynx showed a lower incidence of simultaneous tumors than other sites, but all three categorized sites had a similar risk of metachronous disease (Table 6). The results of our study suggest that the risk of a second cancer either in the head and neck, the lung, and less frequently in the esophagus in patients with head and neck carcinoma (in the relatively low-risk tumors), is almost equal to the risk of metastatic disease from the initial primary neoplasm.[20]

In general, if two or more simultaneous tumors are discovered, the order of treatment is established which is most expedient for the patient. If both tumors are potentially curable they should be treated individually, as though each were the sole lesion, although obviously physiologic effects of treatment to the first on the organ containing the second tumor must be considered in the overall treatment plan.[11] Our present protocol for evaluation of new patients with head and neck carcinoma therefore includes a direct laryngoscopy with palpation of the nasopharynx and base of tongue, as well as direct examination of the base of the tongue, vallecula, pyriform sinuses, and endolarynx. Esophagoscopy to the point of the gastric junction is done in all patients if possible. Any suspicious lesions are biopsied. Bronchoscopy is not done unless the chest x-ray study is abnormal or symptoms and signs of inflammatory disease or neoplasm suggest the need for bronchoscopy.

We are not yet prepared from our results to change our posttreatment examination protocol. Cohn and Peppard felt routine chest x-ray studies should be carried out every three months, barium esophagogram every six months and routine endoscopy performed annually for the first three years after treatment.[9] We feel that close surveillance in the office with every 6-month chest x-ray study remains all that is necessary. We are not yet prepared to recommend follow-up barium swallows or esophageal endoscopy on a routine basis to our postoperative patients.

SUMMARY

We evaluated the charts of 449 patients with head and neck cancer. Thirty-six simultaneous second primary tumors were found. Four second head and neck tumors were first noticed on direct laryngoscopy. No lung cancer was discovered unless the x-ray study was abnormal. Two asymptomatic esophageal tumors were seen. Forty-four metachronous tumors were noted. We conclude direct laryngoscopy and possibly esophagoscopy are necessary in the pretreatment evaluation of head and neck cancer. Bronchoscopy has not been of value in this series unless a firm clinical suspicion is present. Periodic re-endoscopy is not warranted from our data.

REFERENCES

1. Warren S, Gates O. Multiple primary malignant tumors: a survey of the literature and a statistical study. Am J Cancer 1932; 16:1358-414.

2. Moertel CG. Multiple primary malignant neoplasms. Cancer 1977; 40:1786-92.

3. Wynder EL, Mushinski MH, Spivak JC. Tobacco and alcohol consumption in relation to the development of multiple primary cancers. Cancer 1977;40:1872-9.

4. Slaughter DT. Multicentric origin of intra-oral carcinoma. Surgery 1946; 20:133-46.

5. Weaver A, Fleming SM, Knechtges TC, Smith D. Triple endoscopy: a neglected essential in head and neck cancer. Surgery 1979; 86:493-6.

6. Gluckman JL. Synchronous multiple primary lesions of the upper aerodigestive system. Arch Otolaryngol 1979; 105:597-8.

7. Gluckman JL, Crissman JD, Donegan JO. Multicentric squamous-cell carcinoma of the upper aerodigestive system. Head Neck Surg 1980; 3:90-6.

8. Vrabec DP. Multiple primary malignancies of the upper aerodigestive system. Ann Otol Rhinol Laryngol 1979; 88:846-54.

9. Cohn AM, Peppard SB. Multiple primary malignant tumors of the head and neck. Am J Otolaryngol 1980; 1:411-7.

10. Shapshay SM, Hong WK, Fried WP, Sismanis A, Vaughan CW, Strong MS. Simultaneous carcinomas of the esophagus and upper aerodigestive tract. Otolaryngol Head Neck Surg 1980; 88:373-7.

11. Brownson RJ, Sessions DG, Porubsky ES, Ogura JH. Simultaneous malignant tumors in patients with head and neck cancer. Arch Otolaryngol 1973; 97:347-9.

12. Cahan WG. Lung cancer associated with cancer primary in other sites. Am J Surg 1955; 89:494-514.

13. Goldstein HM, Zornoza J. Association of squamous cell carcinoma of the head and neck with cancer of the esophagus. Am J Roentgenol 1978; 131:791-4.

14. Cahan WG, Castro EB, Rosen PP, Strong EW. Separate primary carcinomas of the esophagus and head and neck region in the same patient. Cancer 1976; 37:85-9.

15. Thompson WM, Oddson TA, Kelvin F, Daffner R, Postlethwait RW, Rice RP. Synchronous and metachronous squamous cell carcinomas of the head, neck and esophagus. Gastrointest Radiol 1978; 3:123-7.

16. Odette J, Szymanowski T, Nichols RD. Multiple head and neck malignancies. Trans Am Acad Ophthalmol Otolaryngol 1977; 84:805-13.

17. Cederqvist C, Nielsen J, Berthelsen A, Hansen HS. Cancer of the esophagus. Acta Chir Scand 1978; 144:233-40.

18. Kogelnik HD, Fletcher GH, Jesse RH. Clinical course of patients with squamous cell carcinoma of the upper respiratory and digestive tract with no evidence of disease five years after initial treatment. Radiology 1975; 115:423-7.

19. Wagenfeld DJH, Harwood AR, Bryce DP, vanNostrand AWF, deBoer G. Second primary respiratory tract malignant neoplasms in supraglottic carcinoma. Arch Otolaryngol 1981; 107:135-7.

20. Sugarbaker EV, Jesse RH. Second primary carcinoma of the "foregut:" high risk of head and neck patients. Presented to Society of Surgical Oncology, Hilton Head, SC, May 3, 1977.

LARYNGEAL COMPLICATIONS OF NASOGASTRIC TUBES

ROBERT A. SOFFERMAN, MD RICHARD N. HUBBELL, MD

BURLINGTON, VERMONT

The association of bilateral vocal cord paralysis with relatively short-term nasogastric tube use is represented in four case histories. A prospective study of the effects of nasogastric tubes on the normal human larynx discovered arytenoid edema in approximately one third of patients. A literature review, possible pathophysiologic mechanisms to explain the condition, and basic medical management are described.

In 1934, Paine[1] presented a comprehensive review of the evolution and uses of the nasogastric tube. The most pertinent writings are extracted from him in the following historical sketches. A 1790 publication by John Hunter described the use of a fresh eel skin stretched over a whalebone and introduced into the stomach for feeding a patient with paralysis of deglutition. This represented the first written documentation of the use of a stomach tube. In 1813, Physick, a Philadelphia surgeon, described gastric lavage via an urethral catheter in a case of accidental morphine poisoning. Kussmaul popularized the use of tubes in the treatment of gastric disease and his papers are said to have been responsible for Billroth's interest in gastric surgery. Since those beginnings, nasogastric tubes have found further uses in the monitoring and treatment of gastrointestinal hemorrhage and decompression of the distended upper gastrointestinal tract.

Although the initial nasogastric tubes were manufactured of red rubber, current preferences are for less irritating polyethylene and silicone materials. Regardless of physical composition, all of the tubes produce local tissue problems over time. Some of the more commonly mentioned irritative complications are nasal alar necrosis, epistaxis, nasopharyngitis and eustachitis, and arytenoid edema. The progression of arytenoid edema to bilateral paralysis of the vocal cords in adduction is a rare occurrence. Nevertheless, three cases of bilateral vocal cord paralysis associated with the use of nasogastric tubes have occurred at the University of Vermont from July 1978 to the present. An additional case contributed by a recently graduated resident alert to the process permits an analysis of four patients with this clinical syndrome. Prior to an in depth literature survey, this association seemed to be unique and set the foundation for a prospective analysis of the effects of the nasogastric tube on the normal human larynx.

CASE REPORTS

Case 1. A 60-year-old female was admitted to the surgical service of the Medical Center Hospital of Vermont (MCHV) with a 12.5 kg weight loss and right lower quadrant mass of three months' duration. Barium enema confirmed a carcinoma of the cecum and terminal ileum and a right hemicolectomy was subsequently accomplished. A nasogastric tube was inserted by the anesthesiologist at the beginning of the procedure and maintained for the next four days. For each of the first three postoperative days, she complained of pharyngodynia and then developed respiratory distress and hoarseness on the fourth day. The otolaryngology service was consulted and panendoscopy and tracheostomy were accomplished. Endoscopic findings included bilateral arytenoid and postcricoid edema, bilateral vocal cord paralysis in adduction, and a small left postcricoid abscess which was evacuated (Fig. 1). Treatment consisted of removal of the nasogastric tube, institution of steroids, and parenteral antibiotics. Three days later, indirect laryngoscopy revealed return of normal right cord mobility and arytenoid appearance. By the following day, both cords were found to be mobile and decannulation of the tracheotomy tube was accomplished seven days after drainage of the abscess. Laryngeal recovery was complete and rapid.

Case 2. A 74-year-old male was admitted to MCHV with a right CVA and dense left hemiplegia. A nasogastric tube was inserted for nutritional support and maintained for nine days. On day 8, he complained of a sore throat and developed progressive acute stridor the next day. The nasogastric tube was removed; the patient would not cooperate for mirror laryngoscopy. Direct laryngoscopy under anesthesia demonstrated bilateral abductor paralysis and arytenoid edema. Esophagoscopy revealed a linear ulceration of the posterior lamina of the cricoid with exposed cartilage (Fig. 2). A tracheotomy was performed, and the patient begun on parenteral hyperalimentation. Three days after tracheotomy the patient was examined with a fiberoptic bronchoscope under topical anesthesia. There was little resolution in the edema, and both cords remained immobile. By the end of the second week following the onset of the cord paralysis, repeat laryngoscopy with the flexible fiberscope indicated return of bilateral cord motion and resolution in edema. Tracheal decannulation was performed without incident.

Case 3. This 34-year-old male sustained a head injury in a snowmobile accident. A linear temporal fracture with midbrain contusion was diagnosed and nasotracheal intubation utilized for respiratory support. He was placed in barbiturate coma for two weeks after insertion of a cranial pressure monitor. Nutrition was maintained via a nasogastric tube from the outset. The nasotracheal tube was converted to a tracheotomy tube 12 days postinjury. One month after injury, he was unable to tolerate occlusion of the tracheotomy tube and although his neurologic improvement was theoretically sufficient to allow him to handle oral feedings, the nursing staff consistently reported his reluctance to swallow because of apparent throat discomfort. Subsequent to his having been removed from the barbiturate protocol, he frequently removed his own nasogastric tube. At least 12 nasogastric

From the Section of Otolaryngology, Department of Surgery, University of Vermont Medical School, Burlington.

Presented at the meeting of the American Laryngological Association, Vancouver, British Columbia, May 10-11, 1981.

REPRINTS — Robert A. Sofferman, MD, 1 South Prospect St., Burlington, VT 05401.

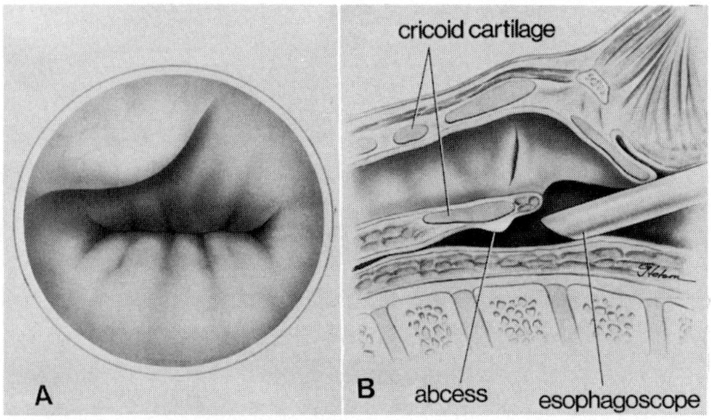

Fig. 1. (Case 1) Postcricoid abscess identified at esophagoscopy. A) Endoscopic view. B) Diagrammatic lateral view.

tube reinsertions were required during the two weeks preceding otolaryngologic consultation. Again, fiberoptic laryngoscopy with topical anesthesia allowed an accurate assessment of the larynx and esophageal introitus. This method of laryngoscopy was required because of the patient's inability to cooperate with conventional indirect mirror examination. Both vocal cords were paralyzed in adduction and the postcricoid tissues were markedly edematous, especially on the right side. Direct laryngoscopy with biopsy revealed proliferative interarytenoid granulation tissue but no evidence of a postcricoid abscess (Fig. 3). A gastrostomy was later accomplished to provide improved nutrition and resting of the cervical esophagus. The vocal cords remain immobile now three months after injury and he still requires the gastrostomy for hyperalimentation. It is possible that the indwelling endotracheal tube for 12 days contributed to the laryngeal insult, but the repeated nasogastric tube reinsertions and amount of postcricoid pathology would seem to place most of the blame on the esophageal tube.

Case 4. A 75-year-old female with Osler-Weber-Rendu disease was admitted to Theda Clark Regional Medical Center, Menasha, Wisconsin, for evaluation of anemia and gastrointestinal bleeding. Gastroscopy, duodenoscopy, and exploratory laparotomy were performed and a nasogastric tube placed. Nine

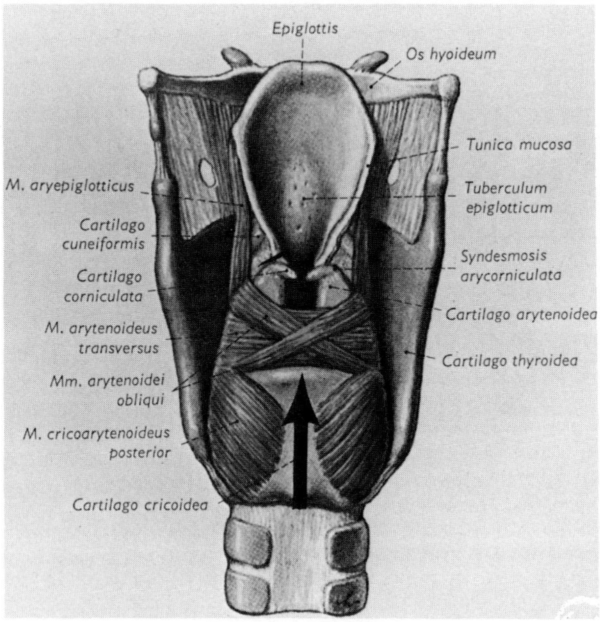

Fig. 2. (Case 2) Black arrow shows location of postcricoid ulceration and proximity to posterior cricoarytenoid muscles. (From Pernkopf E. Atlas of Topographical and Applied Human Anatomy. Baltimore: Urban & Schwarzenberg, Inc., 1980. Published with permission.)

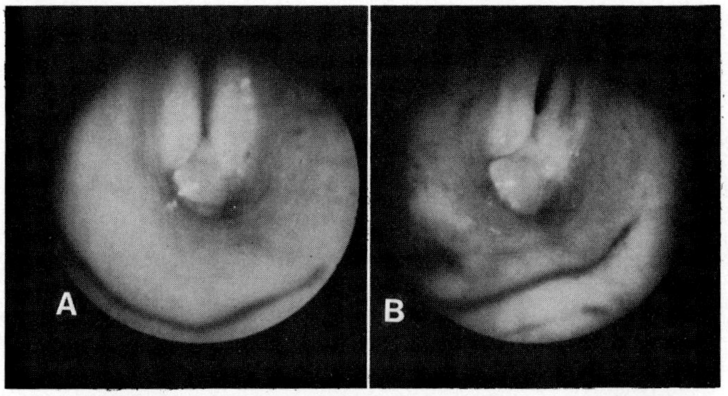

Fig. 3. (Case 3) Interarytenoid granuloma as visualized retrograde with the Hopkins laryngoscope through the tracheotomy site. A) Appearance of cords during phonation. B) Limitation of abduction during attempted inspiration.

days later she experienced stridor and subsequent mirror laryngoscopy identified bilateral vocal cord paralysis and arytenoid edema. A tracheotomy was accomplished and the patient followed closely. On the fifth posttracheotomy day, some vocal cord movement returned bilaterally with progressive and complete laryngeal recovery by 15 days subsequent to initial symptoms and removal of the nasogastric tube.

METHODS

Fifty-seven patients (28 males, 29 females) admitted to the surgical and gynecologic services at the MCHV and Fanny Allen Hospital from Feb. 12 to April 18, 1980, received nasogastric tubes and were included in the study. One of the authors (R.H.) examined each patient preoperatively with indirect laryngoscopy and then daily thereafter until the tube was discontinued and the examination returned to baseline.

Patients were questioned about previous neck injury, neck trauma, thyroid surgery, and stroke to eliminate preexisting neurogenic causes of vocal cord paralysis. Inquiries concerning gout and rheumatoid arthritis were initiated to exclude cricoarytenoid arthritis as an alternate cause of arytenoid edema. Recent hoarseness, pharyngodynia, and otalgia were investigated as background symptoms prior to nasogastric intubation and daily thereafter until removal of the nasogastric tube. Patients with any of these preexisting entities or symptoms were eliminated from the study. The following data were recorded from each patient's chart: age, sex, primary surgical diagnosis, and smoking history. The nasogastric tube size, type, and nostril employed were noted. Duration of the surgical procedure, position of the patient on the operating table, and difficulty of endotracheal intubation were recorded. The anesthesiology staff cooperated in the analysis in examining the larynx prior to extubation to determine the presence or absence of arytenoid edema. A normal terminal direct view of the larynx or normal postoperative indirect laryngoscopy on the ward was felt to essentially eliminate the likelihood of adverse effects of the endotracheal tube on the larynx. A schema for quantification of endolaryngeal edema and cord mobility was established before each patient was studied.

RESULTS

The mean age of patients was 53.8 years (range 17 - 83 years). The mean duration of nasogastric intubation was 3.6 days (range 1 - 11 days). Eighty-nine percent of patients experienced intubation for six days or less. Arytenoid edema was the only pathologic change identified and no patients demonstrated vocal cord paresis. Thirty-two percent of patients developed arytenoid edema and nearly half of these had at least one day when the edema was of "moderate" severity. The onset of edema averaged 2.6 days postintubation (range 1 - 5 days) and resolved by a mean of 1.5 days (one half - 3 days) after tube removal. No patients showed edema at the end of surgery. Pharyngodynia was noted by 77% of the patients. Hoarseness was reported in 42% of the cases. Otalgia was evident in 14% of the patients at some time during the intubation.

Most patients had polyethylene Salem sumps ranging from No. 14 - 18 French, with 75% of the tubes being No. 16 French. Two tubes were adult cantors. There was no correlation between the size of the tube and laryngeal pathology. Furthermore, there was no uniform correlation between laryngeal findings and any of the variables considered above prior to nasogastric intubation. Arytenoid edema seemed to occur as a random event.

DISCUSSION

Wolff and Kessler[2] lay unique claim to the association of postcricoid ulceration and vocal cord paralysis with the use of nasogastric tubes. Similarly, the rarity[3] and severity of this complication stimulated our interest in reporting this as a new entity. A careful review of the literature proved conclusively that we of the modern era of otolaryngology are simply rediscovering a previously well-described pathologic process. In 1939, Iglauer and Molt[4] presented a series of ten cases implicating the nasogastric tube as the direct cause of postcricoid ulceration and bilateral cord paralysis. Holinger and Loeb[5] added another four similar cases in 1946. For unknown reasons, the literature remained dormant regarding this entity with resurgent, sporadic reports in the 1970s.[6,7] In fact, many case reports place emphasis on the endotracheal tube and do not mention or recognize the nasogastric tube as the true source of the problem.[8-10] Holinger et al,[11] in an excellent 1976 review of 389 cases of bilateral abductor paralysis, do not implicate the nasogastric tube in any aspect of their retrospective analysis.

The cases presented by Iglauer and Molt[4] are very graphic and give the strongest clue that the nasogastric tube is the specific culprit. The series was reported in 1939 before the routine use of endotracheal intubation for delivery of general anesthesia, limiting the endotracheal tube as a culpable agent when laryngeal complications evolve from the surgical setting. Furthermore, many patients in this series developed stenosis of the posterior endolarynx suggesting that postcricoid chondritis spreads forward to involve the inner surface of the cricoid. Although the endotracheal tube is often designated as the offending agent because of the endolaryngeal locus of the fibroinflammatory process, Iglauer and Molt demonstrate that the pathology begins outside the larynx. Endotracheal tubes can produce the same syndrome,[12,13] but evidence seems to skew the pathophysiologic insult to the postcricoid area. Interestingly, duration of esophageal intubation does not necessarily correlate directly with the severity of symptoms; one case of bilateral cord paralysis evolved after only 24 hours with a nasogastric tube, with rapid recovery after removal and steroid-antibiotic therapy.[14]

A pathophysiologic mechanism must be proposed and there is likely to be more than one cause. Since paralysis has developed with both rubber and polyethylene tubes, it is unlikely that one can implicate a structural variable. The larynx is a very dynamic structure, moving vertically with swallowing and coughing against this foreign body. The cricopharyngeus muscle is in a tonic state of contraction, pulling the tube against the postcricoid lamina with its thin mucosal cover. Finally, the cricoid and larynx rest against the cervical spine when the patient is supine, with the nasogastric tube compressed precariously between the two rigid structures. Subsequent to ulceration of the posterior cricoid plate, a diffuse inflammatory process develops and can even lead to abscess formation (case 1). If the inflammatory process develops into perichondritis and anterior cricoid infection, a posterior subglottic stenosis can evolve and tether the vocal cords, impairing abduction. Since in many instances the bilateral vocal cord paralysis is of short duration, some form of myopraxia or neuropraxia is likely. The posterior cricoarytenoid muscles arise from the postcricoid lamina and, if temporarily malfunctioning, would present the appearance of bilateral vocal cord paralysis. Perhaps a posterior recurrent laryngeal neuropraxia is the true physiologic deficit. One could also imagine an inflammatory spasm of the interarytenoid muscle as a cause for the temporarily adducted position of the true cords.

Our study indicates that localized laryngeal inflammation develops early in the course of nasogastric intubation and that discomfort symptoms are very common. Just as Holinger pointed out in 1946,[5] it is crucial to recognize the importance of hoarseness, otalgia, and pharyngodynia as harbingers of laryngeal complications. An autopsy series[2] addressing hypopharyngeal and cervical esophageal instrumentation identified a 60% injury rate, but remarkably only 2% of the complications were identified antemortem. Fifteen percent of the injured series demonstrated ulceration into and often through the posterior cricoid cartilage. Often patients with indwelling nasogastric tubes are either unwilling or mentally incapable of cooperating for mirror laryngoscopy. We have found the flexible bronchoscope and especially the thinner fiberoptic laryngonasopharyngoscope to be an excellent tool in the evaluation and follow-up of these patients (cases 2 and 3).

Eade et al[15] have questioned the routine use of nasogastric tubes in gastrointestinal surgery and illustrate the safety in withholding them in 130 of 143 consecutive major abdominal surgical procedures. Among principal reasons for deferring nasogastric tubes were patient discomfort and a very real concern for laryngeal complications. Perhaps either more judicious use of gastric tubes or the employment of soft polymer silicone (Silastic) tubes will reduce the incidence of laryngeal pathology. The importance of recognizing the aforementioned clues to impending laryngeal edema and paralysis cannot be overemphasized. The nasogastric tube should be removed and the larynx followed closely, either with indirect laryngoscopy or the fiberoptic laryngoscope. Antibiotics and steroids have been associated with recovery in two of our patients and probably should be considered in the overall management of the patient with bilateral cord paralysis secondary to nasogastric tubes. Seven of eight patients in the Iglauer and Molt series[4] who survived required chronic tracheotomy due to permanent laryngeal stenosis. Since these patients were managed during the 1930s before the availability of appropriate antibiotics, perhaps the high incidence of permanent laryngeal pathology was related to poor control of the established inflammatory process.

In summary, this combined clinical report and prospective study is designed to realert the medical and surgical community to this serious complication of nasogastric tubes. The study illustrates that laryngeal changes occur in nearly one third of patients, and that the process can develop after only a few days of esophageal intubation.

ACKNOWLEDGMENT — David Ostrowski, MD, participated in the study of this entity while in recent otolaryngology training at the University of Vermont. The authors wish to express their gratitude for his contribution of case 4 to the report.

REFERENCES

1. Paine JR. The history of the invention and development of the stomach and duodenal tubes. Ann Intern Med 1934; 8:752-63.

2. Wolff AP, Kessler S. Iatrogenic injury to the hypopharynx and cervical esophagus. Ann Otol Rhinol Laryngol 1973; 82:778-83.

3. Foster CA, Meyerhoff WL. Cricoid chondritis. Ear Nose Throat J 1980; 59:28-31.

4. Iglauer S, Molt WF. Severe injury to the larynx resulting from the indwelling duodenal tube. Ann Otol Rhinol Laryngol 1939; 48:886-904.

5. Holinger PH, Loeb WJ. Feeding tube stenosis of the larynx. Surg Gynecol Obstet 1946; 83:253-8.

6. Canalis RF, Jenkins HA, Osguthorpe JD. Acute laryngeal abscesses. Ann Otol Rhinol Laryngol 1979; 88:275-9.

7. Clemons JE, Portella W. Laryngeal abscess. Otolaryngol Head Neck Surg 1971; 87:339-41.

8. Hahn FW, Martin JT, Lillie JC. Vocal cord paralysis with endotracheal intubation. Arch Otolaryngol 1970; 92:226-9.

9. Holley HS, Gildea JE. Vocal cord paralysis after tracheal intubation. JAMA 1971; 215:281-4.

10. Nuutinen J, Kärjä J. Bilateral vocal cord paralysis following general anesthesia. Laryngoscope 1981; 91:83-6.

11. Holinger LD, Holinger PC, Holinger PH. Etiology of bilateral abductor vocal cord paralysis. Ann Otol Rhinol Laryngol 1976; 85:428-36.

12. Ellis PD, Pollister WK. Recurrent laryngeal nerve palsy and endotracheal intubation. J Laryngol Otol 1975; 89:823-6.

13. Minuck M. Unilateral vocal cord paralysis following endotracheal intubation. Anesthesiology 1976; 45:448-9.

14. Bland JB, Emerson CW, Wilson RS. Acute laryngeal edema 24 hours after passage of a nasogastric tube. Anesthesiology 1976; 45:555-7.

15. Eade GG, Metheny D, Lundmark VO. An evaluation of the practice of routine postoperative nasogastric suction. Surg Gynecol Obstet 1955; 101:275-9.

Ann Otol 90:1981

LARYNGEAL INJURIES SECONDARY TO NASOGASTRIC TUBES

MICHAEL FRIEDMAN, MD

HOWARD BAIM, MD
MAREK STOBNICKI, MD
THOMAS FERRARA, MD

VICKI SHELTON, MD
THOMAS CHILIS, MD
EMANUEL SKOLNIK, MD

CHICAGO, ILLINOIS

Laryngeal complications secondary to nasogastric intubation have been reported rarely in recent literature. Recent experience with three patients who developed laryngeal injuries related to nasogastric tubes prompted retrospective, experimental, and prospective studies to determine the mechanism of laryngeal injury. A review of the literature, as well as the clinical findings in our three patients, point to midline tube placement and the subsequent development of cricoid chondritis as the underlying etiology. An experimental study using anesthetized dogs was designed to compare histologically the effect on the larynx with nasogastric tubes placed in the midline, as opposed to nasogastric tubes in the lateral position. Results of the histologic study confirmed that midline tubes generate severe inflammation in the postcricoid region. One hundred patients were then evaluated roentgenographically to determine the incidence of midline tube placement in a random sample. Six percent of the patients had nasogastric tubes in the midline. Patients who have nasogastric tubes in place for more than three days or have a severe amount of discomfort should have an x-ray film to determine position of the tube. Midline tubes should be removed or replaced.

Nasogastric tubes have been used widely in medicine, particularly in the surgical field, since their development. With the advent of the duodenal tube and suction techniques, postoperative mortality and morbidity related to gastric distention and perforation occurred rarely by the mid-1930s. Initially, nasogastric tubes were made of soft rubber, but with the development of polyethylene and Silastic compounds, nasogastric tubes composed of these synthetic materials have been demonstrated to elicit less inflammation and tissue reaction than soft rubber tubes.

Today, nasogastric tubes not only are used in the preoperative and postoperative management of abdominal surgical conditions, but also have gained widespread popularity in use for enteral alimentation. In spite of their commonplace usage, complications secondary to nasogastric intubation have been reported rarely. After treating several patients recently with cricoid chondritis thought to be secondary to nasogastric intubation, we undertook this retrospective, prospective, and experimental study of laryngeal injuries occurring as a result of nasogastric intubation.

INTRODUCTION

Early reports of cricoid chondritis after nasogastric intubation appeared in 1939 when Wangensteen[1] mentioned two cases that he and his coworkers encountered. Iglauer and Molt[2] in 1939 provided the first extensive discussion of injury to the larynx resulting from an indwelling duodenal tube. They presented ten cases from their own experience and reported two others. Of their own 10 patients, 8 developed laryngeal stenosis that required tracheostomy. The average period of intubation was $8^1/_2$ days, and in all but one instance, symptoms developed while the tube was in place. Early symptoms included pain, dysphagia, blood-streaked sputum, hoarseness, and dyspnea, which increased in severity over days and weeks, necessitating tracheostomy in all but 2 of the 10. Their examination in the acute stage revealed inflammation and edema of the larynx and subglottic area which progressed in varying degrees of laryngeal fixation and stenosis over a prolonged period. The pathologic features of the early manifestations of the disease are well illustrated in two patients in whom autopsy findings were included. Both patients died shortly after removal of their nasogastric tubes (present six days in one patient, nine days in the other). Ulcerations of the anterior esophageal wall at the level of the cricoid cartilage with exposure of perichondrium as well as intense inflammation were noted.

Holinger and Loeb,[3] in 1946, described four cases of laryngeal injury secondary to nasogastric tube trauma. Three of the patients developed laryngeal stenosis weeks after the initial injury which required tracheostomy. In the fourth patient, who succumbed to the primary disease process (during which time she had a tube in place less than a week), postmortem findings revealed a deep ulcer in the mucosa covering the posterior aspect of the cricoid cartilage, extending through the esophageal walls to expose an area of cricoid.

Foster and Meyerhoff[4] in 1980 reported a case of cricoid chondritis secondary to nasogastric intubation, which was successfully treated with in-

From the Department of Otolaryngology, University of Illinois Hospital and Eye and Ear Infirmary, and the Departments of Otolaryngology, Surgery, Pathology, and Radiology, Illinois Masonic Medical Center, Chicago.

Presented at the meeting of the American Laryngological Association, Vancouver, British Columbia, May 10-11, 1981.

REPRINTS — Michael Friedman, MD, 30 North Michigan Avenue, Chicago, IL 60602.

travenously administered antibiotics, hyperbaric oxygen, and tracheostomy. By direct laryngoscopy, they noted a midline cleft in the postcricoid area with exposed cartilage. Cultures grew *Pseudomonas*, which was sensitive to a carbenicillin-gentamicin regimen.

Holinger and Loeb agreed with the etiologic theory of Iglauer and Molt. They all noted mucosal erosion with ulceration in the postcricoid region, intense inflammation, and exposure of underlying cartilage, progressing to chondritis, necrosis, loss of cartilaginous laryngeal support, and severe chronic laryngeal stenosis. The relative absence of submucosa in the postcricoid region, as well as the rigidity imposed by cervical vertebrae and cricoid cartilage, contributed to the development of the ulceration.

Questions currently remain concerning the identification of patients at risk for the development of laryngeal injuries after nasogastric intubation, recognition of early symptoms, and appropriate treatment to avoid long-term severe laryngeal stenosis. Is there evidence that midline nasogastric tubes cause more inflammation than laterally placed tubes? In what percentage of cases does midline placement of the tubes occur? What is the early course of the disease and how should it be treated to avoid long-term complications?

Three patients from our experience are described, followed by an experimental study and a prospective study of 100 intubated patients designed to provide answers to the lingering questions.

CASE REPORTS

Case 1. A 67-year-old female was admitted to the hospital with the diagnosis of carcinoma of the colon. She had been an insulin-dependent diabetic for approximately five years. With her diabetes under good control, she underwent an abdominal-perineal resection. At surgery, a No. 18 Salem sump nasogastric tube was passed without difficulty. She had an uneventful operative course with endotracheal extubation in the recovery room approximately one hour after the end of the procedure. She had pain in the operative site noted by the medical staff on the third postoperative day with odynophagia recorded in the nurses' notes. On the fourth postoperative day, she complained of a severe sore throat. At the end of the fourth day she also had mild stridor. On the fifth postoperative day she had increased odynophagia and progressive stridor which required emergency tracheostomy.

Direct laryngoscopy at that time revealed an exact midline position of the nasogastric tube at the level of the postcricoid area. The arytenoids were markedly inflamed and edematous. Both vocal cords were immobile. One cord was in the median position and the other was in the paramedian position. The nasogastric tube was removed, and a deep ulcer in the postcricoid area with exposed cartilage was noted. Cultures of the ulcerated area grew *Enterobacter aerogenes* sensitive to gentamicin.

The patient was treated with intravenously administered gentamicin and penicillin. Indirect laryngoscopy was performed regularly until the 14th day of antibiotic therapy when direct laryngoscopy showed healing of the ulcer and markedly decreased arytenoid edema. The left cord at that time was judged to have fair mobility, while the right cord was still immobile.

Over the next 14 days she received a tapering course of corticosteroids. At that time indirect laryngoscopy revealed mobility of both cords with a mild decrease in abduction. Her airway was adequate, however, and the tracheotomy tube was removed. She had no further airway problems. Her voice was normal.

Case 2. A 62-year-old male was admitted to the hospital with the diagnosis of carcinoma of the stomach. The patient underwent an esophagogastrectomy with insertion of a No. 18 Salem sump nasogastric tube at surgery.

He complained occasionally of a mild sore throat in the first several postoperative days. He did develop a wound infection and abdominal abscess, necessitating prolonged nasogastric intubation. By the 12th postoperative day, he complained of sore throat. He had a breathy voice as well as increased pulmonary congestion. During postoperative days 12 through 24, oral feeding was attempted. The patient could not swallow, however, because of severe odynophagia, which was complicated further by aspiration when he attempted to swallow liquids. Because of the patient's inability to swallow, the general surgery service left the nasogastric tube in place.

On the 24th postoperative day, an otolaryngologic consultation was requested to evaluate the odynophagia. Direct laryngoscopy on the 25th postoperative day showed a midline position of the nasogastric tube in the postcricoid area. There was marked inflammation of the arytenoids and the left cord was immobile. The tube was removed and a midline ulcer with exposed cartilage was noted. Under direct visualization the tube was replaced to a lateral position. Cultures from the ulcerated area grew *Staphylococcus aureus* (coagulase positive) and *Enterobacter colititia*. The patient was treated with methicillin and gentamicin. The patient had a progressive downhill course with severe aspiration, pneumonia, and respiratory failure. He eventually had a respiratory arrest and died.

Case 3. A 77-year-old male was admitted to the hospital with a diagnosis of small bowel obstruction. He had a previous history of abdominal aortic aneurysm, which had been repaired approximately six months prior to this admission. The patient underwent a small bowel resection with lysis of adhesions. A No. 18 Salem sump nasogastric tube was placed without difficulty in the operating room. He was extubated at the end of the procedure.

On the fifth postoperative day the patient complained of hoarseness and sore throat, and the general surgery service removed the nasogastric tube. On the seventh postoperative day the nasogastric tube was reinserted for gastrointestinal decompression. Over the next several days the patient had severe aspiration and a very weak, ineffective cough. Respiratory failure developed, and he was transferred to the intensive care unit. Direct laryngoscopy performed without anesthesia showed a midline position of the nasogastric tube. There was no mobility of the left cord and decreased mobility of the right cord. The nasogastric tube was removed and a midline ulcer was found. A therapeutic bronchoscopy was also performed at that time. Cultures of the necrotic postcricoid tissue grew *Escherichia coli* sensitive to gentamicin. On a regimen of intravenously administered gentamicin the patient had gradual improvement in his pulmonary status and an improved cough. On the 21st postoperative day, indirect laryngoscopy showed healing of the ulcer and improved mobility of both cords. On phonation, less than a 1 mm glottic chink remained.

The patient was discharged from the hospital and was lost to follow-up.

COMMENT

Our conclusion based on endoscopic findings in these three patients, as well as the findings previously reported, is that patients with midline tube placement are at high risk to develop laryngeal complications. Based on this supposition, we undertook an experimental study using anesthetized dogs.

TABLE 1. LARYNGEAL INFLAMMATION IN EXPERIMENTAL DOGS

Group/Dog	Inflammation Midline	Left Lateral	Right Lateral
Midline			
1	2+ to 3+	2+ to 3+	2+ to 3+
2	2+ to 3+	2+ to 3+	1+ to 2+
3	2+ to 3+	0	0
4	2+ to 3+	+/−	1+
Lateral			
5	0 to 1+	+/1 to 1+	+/− to 1+
6	+/− to 1+	+/− to 1+	+/− to 1+
7	0 to +/−	+/−	1+
8	1+ to 2+	+/−	+/−
9*	+/−	+/−	+/−

*Tube was in place for six weeks.

0 - No inflammation; +/− - Minimal inflammation; 1+ - Mild inflammation.

2+ - Moderate inflammation; 3+ - Marked inflammation.

EXPERIMENTAL STUDY

The animal model was designed to study the effects of nasogastric tubes placed in the postcricoid area and compare them with the effects of tubes placed laterally. Mongrel dogs weighing 20 to 30 kg were used.

To determine the relative size of the postcricoid area in dogs, a series of polyethylene tubes was used. Tubes beginning with No. 12 French and ending with No. 36 French were passed into the postcricoid area and repositioned from one pyriform sinus to the other. Even the largest tube passed easily from one side to the other and was not compressed while in the midline position. We believed that the No. 28 French tube in the dog was comparable in size to a No. 12 French tube in the human.

Originally, the experiment was designed to mimic nasogastric intubation in hospitalized patients. It was not possible in the dogs, however, to maintain the nasogastric tubes in the midline position following placement. Because of the relatively large size of the hypopharynx and larynx in the dog, tubes initially placed in the midline migrate laterally following anesthesia. Therefore, dogs were maintained under anesthesia for 24 hours to ensure immobility of the tubes.

Eight dogs of the same size were anesthetized, endotracheal tubes inserted, and the dogs placed on respirators. In four dogs a No. 28 French Argyle chest tube was inserted through the mouth and into the postcricoid area. Gauze sponges in each pyriform sinus held the tube in position. In four other dogs, the tubes were placed in the pyriform sinus and gauze sponges placed in the postcricoid area. At the end of 24 hours, the dogs were killed. The larynx and pharynx were removed immediately, placed in formalin, and submitted to the pathologist.

One dog was used to determine the effect of length of intubation on laterally placed tubes. A No. 14 French Levin tube was passed through the nose and attached to a No. 28 French tube in the pharynx (No. 28 French tube would not pass through the nose). The combined tubes were placed

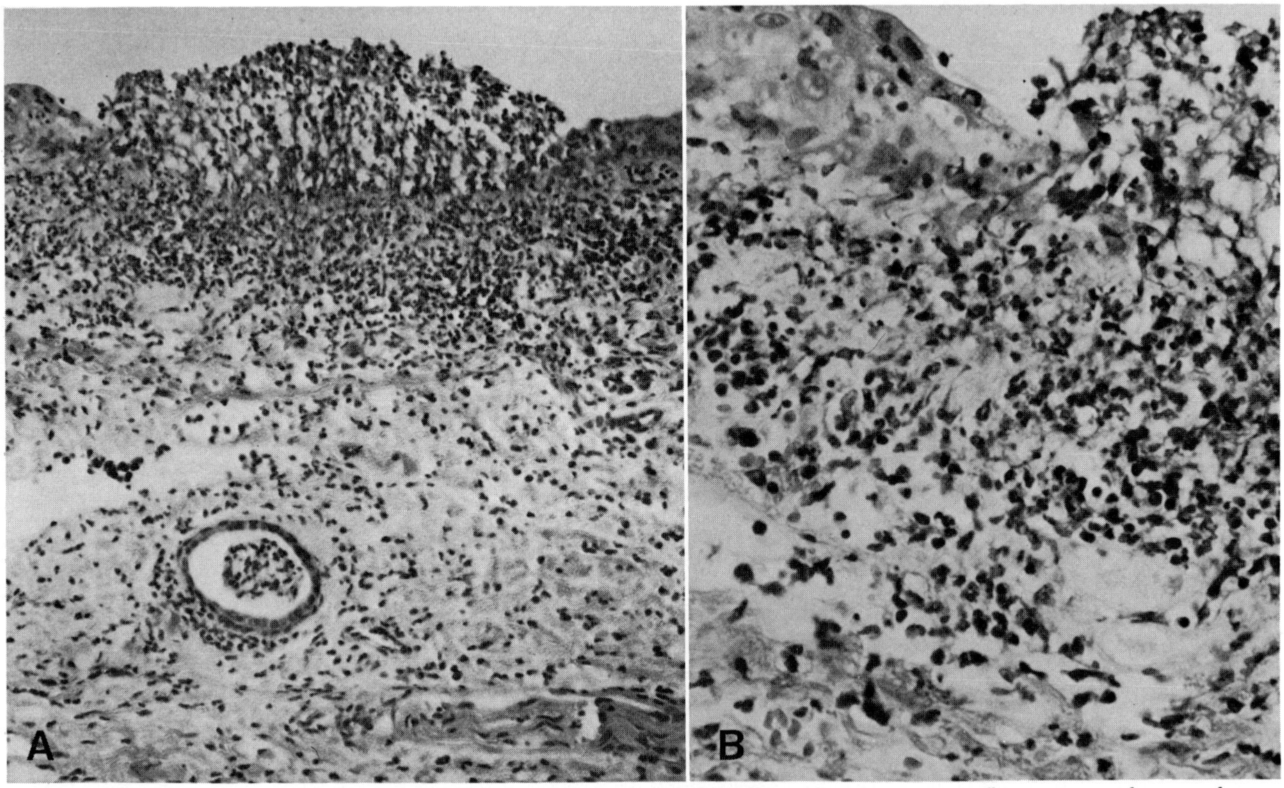

Fig. 1. A) Low-power view of postcricoid mucosa of dog with midline tube. Note severe inflammation with mucosal ulceration. B) High-power view of postcricoid mucosa after midline tube placement.

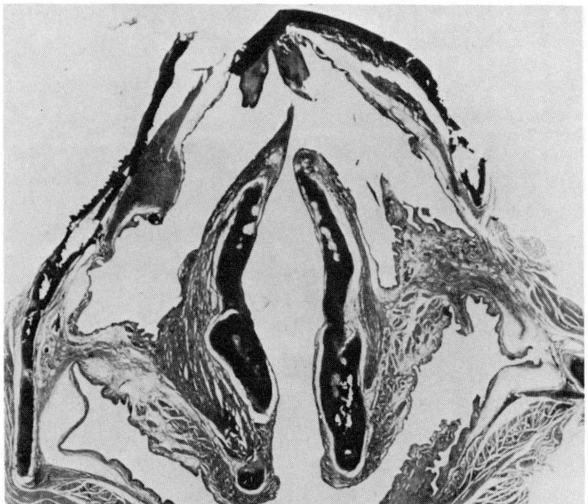

Fig. 2. A) Whole mount of larynx of dog with laterally placed tube. B) High-power view of mucosa surrounding laterally placed tube. Note complete absence of inflammation.

laterally in the pyriform sinus under direct visualization. A large plastic protective collar was then placed, and the dog allowed to awaken. At various intervals thereafter, the tube position was evaluated to ensure maintenance in the lateral position. At six weeks, the dog was killed.

From each larynx, several blocks were taken from both the postcricoid area and the pyriform sinus area. After routine paraffin embedding, sections were stained by hematoxylin and eosin. Histological examination of the mucosa was performed by the pathologist without knowledge of the tube position. The degree of inflammatory reaction in the mucosa was recorded for each area of each specimen, using the following scale: 0, no inflammation; +/−, minimal inflammation; 1+, mild inflammation (5 polymorphonuclear leukocytes [PMN]/high power field); 2+, moderate inflammation; 3+, marked inflammation (focally 100 PMN/high power field) with or without erosive changes. Results of histologic studies are shown in Table 1.

Larynges with tubes in the midline demonstrated moderate to marked inflammation in the postcricoid area with variable inflammation in the lateral hypopharynx (Fig. 1). Three of four larynges with tubes in the pyriform sinus showed minimal inflammation in both the postcricoid area and lateral hypopharynx (Fig. 2). One dog (No. 8) with a laterally placed tube had mild-moderate inflammation in the postcricoid region, possibly attributed to the dog's awakening during anesthesia and struggling to extract both the endotracheal and nasogastric tubes. The larynx of the dog with the tube in the laterally placed position for six weeks (No. 9) showed only minimal inflammation of both postcricoid region and the lateral hypopharynx. Histologic findings were comparable to the findings in the dogs with laterally placed tubes examined after 24 hours.

PROSPECTIVE CLINICAL STUDY

The clinical finding in the patients presented and results of the experimental study point to midline tube placement as the precipitating factor in laryngeal injuries occurring as a result of nasogastric intubation. We next undertook a study to determine the incidence of midline placement of nasogastric tubes. One hundred consecutive patients with nasogastric tubes were evaluated roentenographically, excluding patients with head and neck tumors. Five positions of tube placement were identified by x-ray film.

Tube position was called midline only when the x-ray film showed its location to be exactly in the center of subglottic air shadow and overlying the midline of the glottis. Intermediate positions L1 (for left) and R1 (for right) were defined as tubes just lateral to the midline. The far lateral positions were

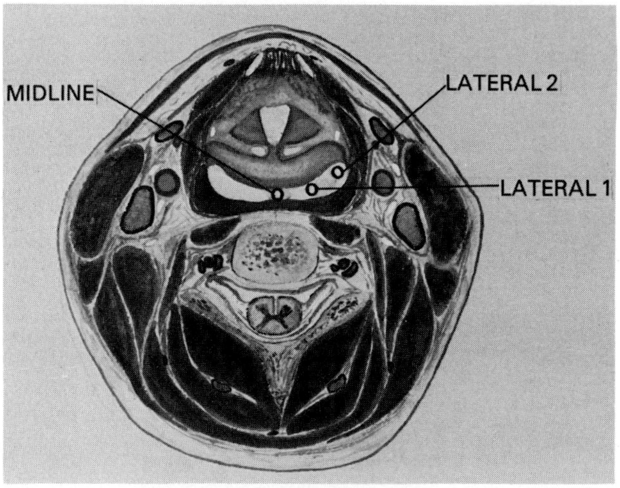

Fig. 3. Cross section of neck at level of cricoid cartilage demonstrating tube position anatomically.

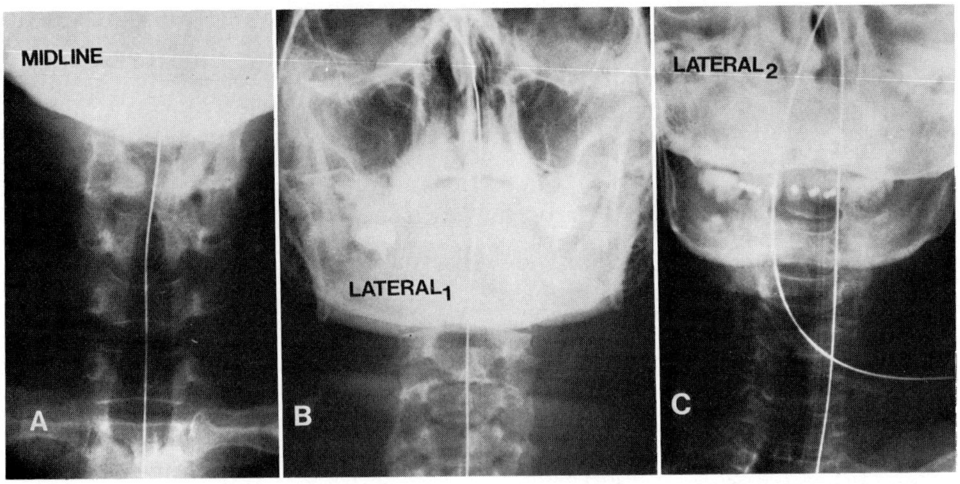

Fig. 4. X-ray films showing placement of nasogastric tube. A) Midline. B) Intermediate position. C) Lateral position.

denoted as L2 (left) and R2 (right). Tube positions are diagrammed in Figure 3, and Figure 4 shows x-ray films denoting tube positions. Distribution of tube positions is illustrated in Figure 5.

From these statistics, it is seen that the vast majority of nasogastric tubes are laterally placed, with only 6% present in the midline, to be in position to cause erosion of postcricoid mucosa. Patients with midline tubes were reevaluated by follow-up x-ray films in 24 hours and found to have the tube in the same position. All patients in our series had midline tubes removed or replaced to a lateral position in less than three days.

DISCUSSION

In spite of widespread use of nasogastric tubes in both the medical and surgical disciplines, laryngeal complications are rare. One of the primary reasons is that midline tube placement is uncommon, occurring in only 6% of cases in a random sample. All three patients with laryngeal injuries described in this report had midline tubes placed. The microscopic findings of severe laryngeal inflammation with atraumatically placed midline tubes in the dogs, as opposed to mild inflammation in the laterally placed tubes, offer further evidence to support this conclusion (Table 1).

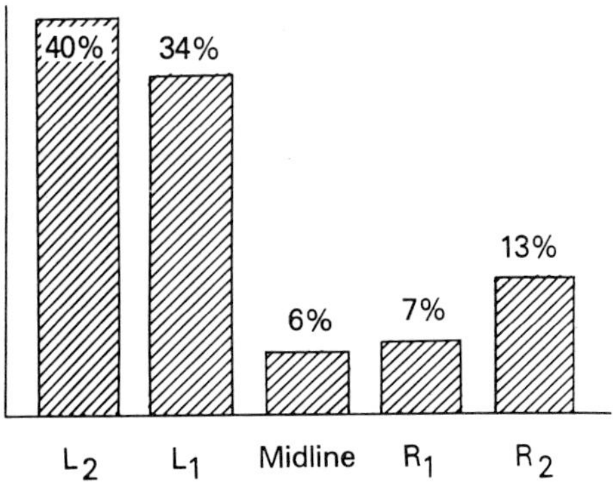

Fig. 5. Distribution of nasogastric tube positions in random sample of patients.

These data substantiate the thoughts of Holinger and Loeb[3] and Iglauer and Molt,[2] as well as provide more insight into the mechanism of the laryngeal injury. The midline-placed nasogastric tube, impinged between the cricoid cartilage and cervical vertebrae, facilitates erosion of the postcricoid mucosa. With exposure of the cartilage, contaminated by saliva, chondritis of the cricoid ensues. If the disease process is not reversed, laryngeal edema and inflammation progress to cartilage necrosis, laryngeal mobility, and subglottic stenosis.

Fortunately, with the availability of antibiotics, long-term severe laryngeal stenosis can be prevented in many cases. In the discussions from 1939 and 1946,[1-3] when antibiotics were not available, the effects of untreated chondritis were seen. Today, with aggressive management through the use of appropriate antibiotics, the delayed sequelae of chondritis can be avoided.

CONCLUSIONS AND RECOMMENDATIONS

To prevent laryngeal injury after nasogastric tube insertion, the following points are emphasized.

Anteroposterior neck x-ray films are easy to obtain and should be considered after nasogastric intubation for three days or the development of symptoms. No patient in this series who developed chondritis had a tube in place for less than three days. The majority of patients who developed chondritis, however, had tubes in place for only one to two weeks, certainly not a prolonged time. Obtaining antero-posterior x-ray films definitely should be undertaken in unconscious patients expected to require nasogastric intubation for an extended time period. Patients with midline tube placement should have the tube replaced to a lateral position. Indirect laryngoscopy should be done in all cases of midline tube placement where possible.

Pain is an important early symptom, both severe localized odynophagia and radiation of pain to the ears. The overwhelming majority of patients in these studies experienced pain prior to removal of the nasogastric tube. Other early symptoms included blood-tinged sputum, dysphagia, and mild hoarseness. Recognition of pain as an early warning signal should alert the clinician to the possibility of the development of mucosal ulcerations. At this point, an anteroposterior neck x-ray film should be obtained. If the tube is midline, it should be repositioned immediately. If the tube is in a lateral position and the pain increases or persists, the tube should be moved to a contralateral position.

Patients with persistent symptoms after replacement of the nasogastric tube should be evaluated endoscopically. Additionally, in patients with evidence of respiratory obstruction or decreased cord mobility, direct laryngoscopy is imperative. At this time, mucosal erosions can more easily be identified and appropriate cultures taken.

Although not specifically evaluated, we observed that the tubes placed atraumatically in the midline of dogs were more mobile than standard nasogastric tubes used in patients. A question remains as to the amount of inflammation caused by small Silastic tubes specifically designed only for enteral alimentation.

Early chondritis should be managed aggressively with parenteral antibiotics. Reported cultures have produced Gram-negative rods responding to various regimens of gentamicin and carbenicillin. Tracheostomy may be required for airway protection.

Although laryngeal injuries secondary to nasogastric intubation are relatively rare, it is of paramount importance to identify high-risk patients, recognize early symptoms, and aggressively manage the onset of cricoid chondritis to prevent long-term sequelae.

REFERENCES

1. Wangensteen OH. Experiences with employment of suction in the treatment of acute intestinal obstruction. Surg Gynecol Obstet 1939;68:851-68.

2. Iglauer S, Molt WF. Severe injury to the larynx resulting from the indwelling duodenal tube. Ann Otol Rhinol Laryngol 1939; 48:886-904.

3. Holinger PH, Loeb WJ. Feeding tube stenosis of the larynx. Surg Gynecol Obstet 1946;83:253-8.

4. Foster CA, Meyerhoff WL. Cricoid chondritis. Ear Nose Throat J 1980;59:106-9.

≈

Ann Otol 90:1981

ANESTHESIA FOR LARYNGEAL LASER SURGERY IN THE INFANT AND CHILD

W. M. BRUMMITT, MD
TORONTO, CANADA

BLAIR FEARON, MD
TORONTO, CANADA

I. BRAMA, MD
JERUSALEM, ISRAEL

Currently available anesthetic techniques for laryngoscopy and bronchoscopy are briefly evaluated. Recently reported complications from the literature are reviewed. Satisfactory anesthetic techniques are shown to be limited by the physical dimensions of the instruments as well as the extreme limitations of the flow capacity of the small airway itself. The technique used at the Hospital for Sick Children for the past ten years is described. It is based upon spontaneous respiration with inhalation anesthesia, supplemented by topical lidocaine (Xylocaine). Size and age of the patient are not limiting factors. The safety and effectiveness of this technique are supported by representative blood gas studies as well as the clinical records of over 400 cases.

This paper describes the management of anesthesia and ventilation appropriate for almost all kinds of endoscopic procedures in children. The technique is safe, uncomplicated, and minimally stressful for both surgeon and anesthetist.

The Department of Otolaryngology at the Hospital for Sick Children, Toronto, performs over 250 endoscopic procedures each year. A large series of bronchoscopies has been reported[1] and a description of our earliest anesthetic experiences with laser surgery is in press.[2] Up to December 1980, 149 laser treatments were performed on 37 patients (Table 1). Their ages ranged from 3 weeks to 31 years (mean age is 8 years). The smallest patient weighed 2 kg; the single adult was anesthetized nine times. Most children were of school age with papillomata or vocal nodules. Symptoms of dyspnea and respiratory distress (Table 2) were not accompanied by cyanosis.

Fifteen anesthetists on our staff administered the anesthetics and their techniques varied in only minor detail. Age did not alter the technique which, in all cases but one, provided moderately deep anesthesia with spontaneous respiration, no paralysis, and no catheter or other anesthetic equipment in the airway. During the operation anesthesia was maintained by insufflation of anesthetic vapor in oxygen, above the larynx, assuring a high level of oxygen at all times. Suppression of reflexes was assured by thoroughly spraying the airway from carina to pharynx with lidocaine (Xylocaine). The local lidocaine dose was strictly limited so as not to exceed 4 mg/kg.[3] The average dose was 2.2 mg/kg.

None of the children were premedicated on the ward. Although it is not unusual for older children to benefit from generous doses of diazepam, in the younger children we depend greatly on personal communication with the child by all members of the hospital staff. Narcotic premedication is contraindicated if anesthesia is dependent on spontaneous respiration.

TABLE 1. PATIENTS WITH LARYNGOTRACHEAL LESIONS TREATED BY LASER

Diagnosis	*No. Patients*	*No. Procedures*
Laryngeal papillomatosis	11	84
Vocal cord nodules	10	10
Subglottic hemangioma	3	13
Vocal cord palsy (granuloma postintubation)	3	3
Acquired stenosis		
Traumatic laryngeal stenosis and granuloma	2	5
Postintubation laryngeal and tracheal granuloma	3	23
Congenital laryngeal web	2	4
Granuloma	2	4
Laryngeal cyst	1	3
Total	37	149

Eleven of the children chose to have a gas (N_2O) induction. Regardless of age, the anesthetists' choice for induction in the remainder was thiopentone and atropine followed by N_2O and halothane and then methoxyflurane (Penthrane) by face mask. Once the anesthetized patient was stable, the N_2O was turned off and halothane turned well down (0.5%). Thus methoxyflurane insufflation with a high concentration of oxygen became the principal means of providing a well-relaxed, areflexic but adequately breathing patient in 80% of the cases. Halothane oxygen was used in the remainder (Table 3). Arterial oxygen levels were always higher than normal and $PaCO_2$ levels ranged from 37-59 torr.

Mean operating room time was 58 minutes, and mean exposure time to methoxyflurane was 43 minutes. Recovery room time for methoxyflurane was

From the Departments of Anaesthesiology and Otolaryngology, Hospital for Sick Children, Toronto.
Presented at the meeting of the American Laryngological Association, Vancouver, British Columbia, May 10-11, 1981.
REPRINTS - W. M. Brummitt, MD, Department of Anaesthesia, Hospital for Sick Children, 555 University Avenue, Toronto, Ont. M5G 1X8, Canada.

TABLE 2. SYMPTOMS OF PATIENTS RECEIVING LASER TREATMENTS

	No. of Patients
Hoarseness	24
Stridor	9
Dyspnea	18
Respiratory distress	13
Croupy cough	6
Feeding problems	3
Low voice	1
High pitch cry, nasal regurgitation	1

93 minutes compared with 87 minutes in the five cases which had halothane alone. The notoriously slow recovery time of methoxyflurane did not delay discharge from the recovery room significantly.

Although there was severe airway obstruction in several of the cases, there were no airway or significant anesthetic complications. One 10-year-old had a reflex bradycardia of 56 requiring atropine, and one seriously ill patient had a drop in blood pressure under 90 mm/kg.

Methoxyflurane has unique properties. It is potent at very low concentrations (Minimal Alveolar Concentration of 0.17%) so that oxygen concentrations above 95% can be used at all times. It provides excellent analgesia and relaxation without depressing respiration or risking explosion. Exposure time in adults at least is limited by its renal toxicity which is dose related and therefore controllable. Our attempts to substitute less toxic alternatives such as halothane, enflurane, or isoflurane not only reduce the quality of our technique but the latter two consistently produce hypoventilation. All three have the added risk of partially anesthetizing the endoscopist during times of open insufflation.

If serious exposure to personnel, especially the surgeon, is to be avoided then scavenging of anesthetic vapors must be performed whenever possible. Complete scavenging is easily attained until the laryngoscope is used. However, during insufflation at the time of inspecting and operating on the larynx, the surgeon and anesthetist should wear either a compressed air mask or charcoal absorbent mask for maximum protection.[4]

The unique characteristics of the small airway have defeated our efforts to substitute any technique which would completely eliminate the noxious vapor problem from the operating room. The physical characteristics of the infant's airway tend to create problems for the anesthetist accustomed to adult patients. The tongue is relatively large, the larynx is high, anterior and obscured by a floppy epiglottis. Because of the high position of the larynx and large tongue, the small pharyngeal airway is readily obstructed. The infant has a high metabolic demand for oxygen, and high alveolar ventilation requirements for CO_2 removal. Despite this, the thorax is mechanically inefficient and the alveolar system is incompletely developed.

TABLE 3. ANESTHESIA IN PEDIATRIC ENDOSCOPY

Anesthetic Agents	% of Cases	Mean Recovery Room Time (min)
Methoxyflurane with halothane	80%	93
Halothane alone	18%	87

The physical limitation of gas flowing through a small tube is of critical importance in management of the small airway. This is compensated for in the lower bronchial airways because the total cross-sectional area of all bronchi increase greatly as ventilatory gases flow distally. It is the cricoid orifice, the narrowest portion of the upper airway, which is critical to flow. Poiseuille's law states that flow through a tube is inversely proportional to the fourth power of the radius, thus:

normal cricoid internal diameter: $r = 2$ mm, $r^4 = 16$
with 1 mm of edema: $r = 1$ mm, $r^4 = 1$.

Maximum flow at the cricoid is reduced 16 times by 1 mm of edema in an infant, compared to only a 50% reduction in the adult. Similarly, flow is disproportionally reduced by an endotracheal tube or bronchoscope which may have a wall thicker than 1 mm. Furthermore, limitations of space available for expiratory escapement would limit the use of the Cardin tube to children whose upper trachea could accommodate a 6½ mm tube or larger.

The introduction by Sanders[5,6] of the jet-venturi technique for ventilatory patients undergoing surgery of the upper airway has been an effective alternative to less desirable techniques of anesthetic management. Unfortunately when the jet becomes a significant portion of a small air passage, then small variations in pressure or even minor alterations in the direction of the jet produce variations of up to 300% in flow and in intrathoracic pressure.[7] The possibility of hypoventilation or hyperventilation and the risk of airway rupture[8,9] increase as the size of the airway diminishes. A single inspiratory jet inflation has produced massive emphysema.[10] Furthermore, the equipment reduces the surgeon's vision and the high flows can cause seeding of papillomata, displacement of tumor, fragmentation of foreign bodies, and venturi entrainment of blood and debris. If the patient is paralyzed his functional anatomy is altered. If a cannula or endotracheal tube is in place during laser surgery, there is also a fire hazard.[11] We feel categorically that jet ventilation by cannula in the infant trachea is very dangerous "and should be abandoned forthwith."[12]

When respiratory failure is present one may be forced to use the "skateboard" anesthetic technique by either paralyzing the patient or pumping him with anesthetic to a point of apnea, and alternately allowing the surgeon a short peek, then re-establishing gas exchange by gentle, hand-controlled, relatively low-flow artificial respiration. This is a time-consuming and unsatisfactory but at times necessary compromise for both surgeon and anesthetist.

For anatomic, pathologic, and especially for physical reasons, we do not yet have a safe and effective alternative to insufflation anesthesia and spontaneous respiration if the patient is small and able to breathe on his own. This technique is readily teachable, applicable to all endoscopy in infants as well as older patients, and clinically safe. The airway is uncluttered and, provided the surgeon will take precautions to avoid inhaling anesthetic vapor, his work is not interrupted by the anesthesiologist, and their mutual concern to support artificially the patient's ventilation is served.

REFERENCES

1. Kim IG, Brummitt WM, Humphry A, Siomra SW, Wallace WB. Foreign body in the airway: a review of 202 cases. Laryngoscope 1973; 83: 347-54.

2. Chinyanga HM, Kennedy MG, Steward DJ. Anaesthetic experience using a standard technique for laryngeal surgery in infants and children. Can Anaesth Soc J (in press).

3. Pelton DA, Daly M, Cooper PD, Conn AW. Plasma lidocaine concentrations following topical aerosol application to the trachea and bronchi. Can Anaesth Soc J 1970; 17: 250-5.

4. Gange MA. Protection for theatre staff against halothane pollution. Nurs Times 1978; 75: 1600.

5. Carden E. Positive pressure ventilation during anaesthesia and bronchoscopy: a laboratory evaluation of two recent advances. Anaesth Analg 1973; 52: 402-6.

6. Sanders RD. Two ventilating attachments for bronchoscopes. Del Med J 1967; 391: 170-5.

7. Miyasaka K, Sloan IA, Froese AB. An evaluation of the jet injector (Sanders) for bronchoscopy in paediatric patients. Can Anaesth Soc J 1980; 27:117-24.

8. Oliverio R, Ruder CB, Fermon C, Cura A. Pneumothorax due to ball valve obstruction during jet ventilation. Anesthesiology 1979; 51: 255-6.

9. Tate N. Excessive airway pressure during anaesthesia, letter. Anaesthesia 1979; 34: 212.

10. Vivori E. Anaesthesia for laryngoscopy. Br J Anaesth 1980; 52: 638.

11. Devries P. CO_2 laser: a fire hazard when used in upper airway. The Medical Post, November 18, 1980: 2.

12. Steward DJ, Fearon B. Anaesthesia for laryngoscopy. Br J Anaesth 1981; 53: 320.

≈

CASSELBERRY AWARD

DOCUMENTATION IN PEDIATRIC LARYNGOLOGY

BRUCE BENJAMIN, FRACS
SYDNEY, AUSTRALIA

Endoscopy in pediatric laryngology continues to develop and broaden its horizons. The need for documentation of the various pathological conditions has become more apparent. The upper lateral airways radiological study together with endoscopic photography allows permanent objective documentation of the changes occurring in any part of the upper respiratory tract from the nose and nasopharynx to the bronchi and segmental openings. This combination of radiological study and single frame color photography is the most convenient means of studying the pathology, natural history, and results of treatment as well as for clinical research and teaching in training programs.

In 1854 Manuel Garcia, a Spanish singing teacher, first saw his own larynx in the act of vocalizing.[1] Since that time it has been a problem for an assistant, an observer, or for students to view the larynx and respiratory tract for comparative study. With the advent of microsurgery and fiberoptic endoscopy, provision of an observer eyepiece has become standard but the various observer systems have become more complicated and expensive. Attempts to overcome this problem of suitable documentation of disease include detailed written descriptions of the pathological findings at operation supplemented by diagrams; carefully drawn colored diagrams for teaching (notably those of Netter);[2] clinical photographs; x-ray studies and endoscopic photographs both still and cine.

Endoscopy in pediatric laryngology and bronchoesophagology continues to develop and broaden its horizons. New and challenging problems demand a multidisciplinary approach involving pediatric specialists in many fields. Advances in anesthesia and endoscopic techniques now allow safer, more comprehensive and more detailed examination. The otolaryngologist has the overall expertise and training in monocular endoscopic evaluation and microsurgical techniques that are essential in the management of the respiratory and esophageal problems encountered, and the need for a simple means of permanent documentation of the changes seen in various pathological conditions has become apparent.

At the Royal Alexandra Hospital for Children, Sydney, we have found that a combination of the lateral airways radiograph or xeroradiogram together with endoscopic photography gives useful objective information for reference, comparison and teaching, and to observe progress or change.

RADIOLOGICAL DOCUMENTATION

It is well known that the lateral airways radiograph or, more recently, the xeroradiogram, can demonstrate pathological changes in the pediatric airway and larynx. It seems reasonable, except in extreme emergencies, to have both a chest radiograph and lateral airways study before undertaking diagnostic endoscopic evaluation of the pediatric patient with obstruction of the upper airways.

Xeroradiography has been used for some years in the evaluation of the upper respiratory tract[3,4] and has a useful application in the larynx. Its unique properties of enhancing the air and soft tissue edge and having a wide recording latitude are distinct advantages over conventional radiological techniques. In many patients the airway can be seen from the nasal cavities above to the bifurcation of the trachea below (Fig. 1) showing details of the oropharynx and larynx which are more difficult to delineate with standard radiographic technique. The higher radiation dosage associated with xeroradiography must be carefully considered and balanced against the clinical needs for the particular patient and the possibility of added useful information.

There are many variations in the appearance seen in a normal lateral airways radiograph in infants and children and experience in interpretation will distinguish the normal from the abnormal.[5] The most reliable landmark in the larynx is the laryngeal ventricle which is normally distended with air, depending on the phase of respiration in which the film is taken. Common artifacts sometimes open to misinterpretation include a forward buckle of the posterior wall of the trachea below the larynx; "bunching" of the true vocal cord giving the appearance of a soft tissue mass; blurring of the vocal cord and laryngeal ventricle to make the features in the area difficult to distinguish; air in the piriform fossa giving the appearance of an air-containing cyst in the arytenoid region; a ridge in the posterior pharyngeal wall due to contraction of part of the

From the Royal Alexandra Hospital for Children, Sydney, Australia.
Presented at the meeting of the American Laryngological Association, Vancouver, British Columbia, May 10-11, 1981.
REPRINTS — Bruce Benjamin, FRACS, 231 Macquarie Street, Sydney, Australia 2000.

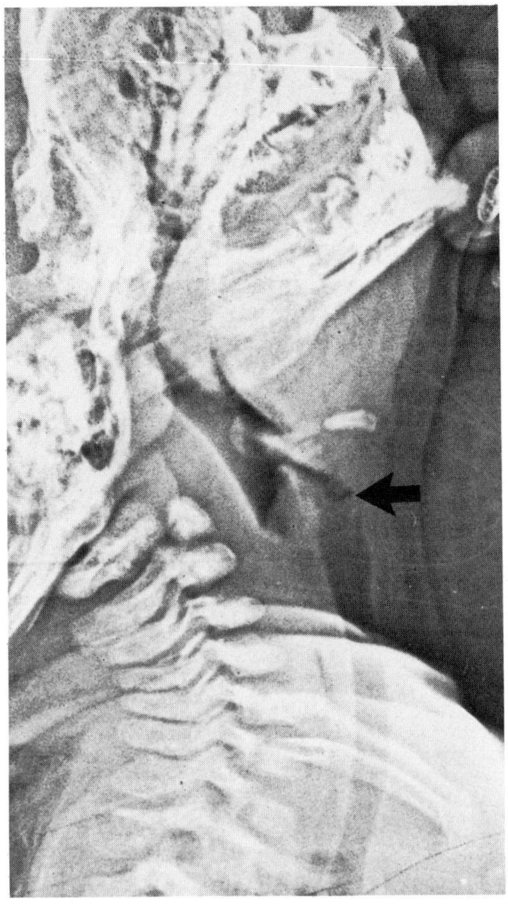

Fig. 1. Lateral airway xerogram in a normal infant. The intrathoracic trachea shows clearly. The ventricle of the larynx (arrow) is seen with the true cords below it and the false cords above. The supraglottic structures (including the arytenoids and epiglottis); the posterior pharyngeal wall; the base of the tongue; the soft palate and the nasal airways are all well seen.

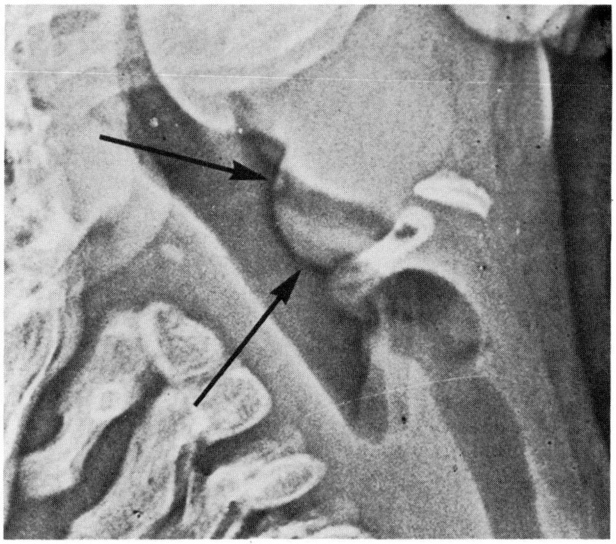

Fig. 2. Thyroglossal duct cyst (arrows) at the base of the tongue above and in front of the epiglottis.

constrictor muscle; elevation of the soft palate so that the nasopharyngeal airway appears narrow; and a number of other variations from normal.

It must be emphasized that correct positioning and exposure technique is the most important factor in avoiding many of these variations from the normal appearance. The film must be taken with the cervical spine in extension (Fig. 1) and the head of the child as far back as it can be comfortably placed, so long as this does not aggravate any preexisting airway problem.

The lateral radiograph of the pharynx shows the adenoid mass to good advantage and this is a common clinical indication for the study. Evaluation of the posterior pharyngeal wall and prevertebral soft tissues is of vital importance where a retropharyngeal abscess is suspected from the clinical features. Less common conditions such as encephalocele, teratoma, chordoma, dermoid cyst, angiofibroma, rhabdomyosarcoma and others may be documented.

Induction of anesthesia or commencement of instrumentation in the presence of a large lesion in the laryngopharynx such as a mass of papillomata or a cyst may precipitate a critical situation. The surgeon and anesthetist will be fully prepared, for example, to decompress a cyst in the larynx or pharynx when the radiograph has revealed it preoperatively (Fig. 2). Other causes of obstruction seen in this region include ectopic thyroid tissue, enlargement of chronically infected lingual tonsils, cystic hygroma, hemangioma, and so on. The radiological appearances in croup and acute epiglottitis are well known.

A clear example of the value of radiology is the demonstration of the altered anatomy allowing hypermobility of the tongue to cause pharyngeal obstruction in the Pierre Robin syndrome (Fig. 3). Congenital subglottic stenosis and some cases of congenital laryngeal web (Fig. 4) or subglottic hemangioma can be suspected as the cause of airway obstruction from the radiographs alone.

We have, as yet, found no place for the contrast laryngogram in the investigation or documentation of laryngeal problems in infants and we have no experience with computerized scanning in this field in pediatrics.

The lateral airways radiograph does not replace endoscopy in the assessment of the upper respiratory tract but it may give useful information prior to endoscopic examination.

PHOTOGRAPHIC DOCUMENTATION

Holinger[6] used the Holinger-Brubaker endoscopic camera to reproduce, in a manner that had never been done before, the findings of the endoscopist and by any standard the photography was superb. Unfortunately, however, the camera was expensive and heavy. It was large and cumbersome and could not be satisfactorily applied routinely to the infant and child.

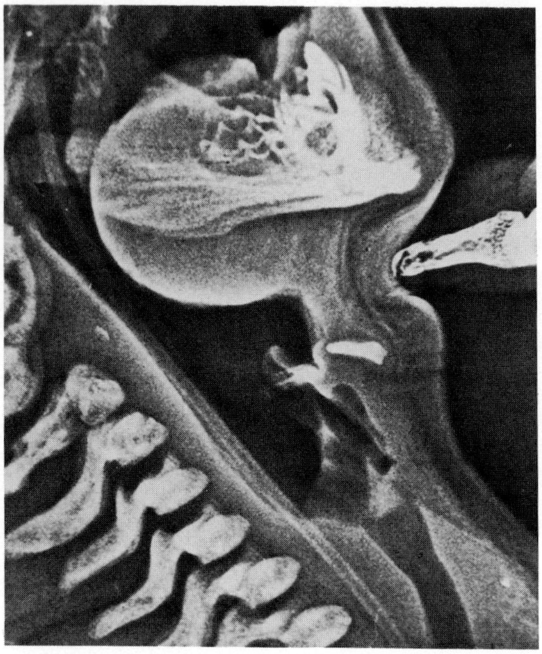

Fig. 3. Pierre Robin syndrome showing micrognathia and glossoptosis. Intermittent upper airway obstruction is caused by a hypermobile tongue with a narrow and unstable origin.

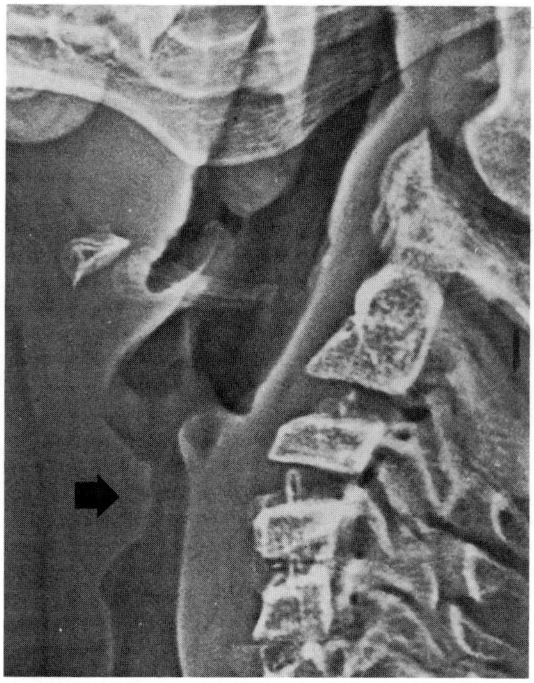

Fig. 4. Large congenital laryngeal web associated with severe congenital subglottic stenosis (arrow). It is remarkable that the child, aged 3, survives with such a narrow airway.

Many different methods of laryngeal photography have been described and these were reviewed by Yanagisawa[7] who himself described a simple method of laryngeal photography through the eyepiece of the operating microscope.

Endoscopic photographs of the glottis can be obtained using the Zeiss operating microscope,[8] the usual method being with the camera attached to a beam-splitter but the depth of field is very small and focusing is critical. In fact the field becomes almost two-dimensional and the technique can be applied in the larynx in only a few instances in infants and children. It is of course, not suitable for the nasopharynx, oropharynx, tracheobronchial tree or esophagus.

With the development of fiberoptic lighting, application of the Hopkins rod telescopes and miniaturization of endoscopic instruments, photographic documentation has become a practical reality.[9] The Storz instrumentation lends itself to photography of diseases previously described but never pictorially documented. The equipment for flash photography can be used with a variety of small diameter telescopes whose light may be directed straight ahead or at various angles. We use these telescopes constantly in the nose, nasal cavity, larynx, tracheobronchial tree and esophagus. The Hopkins rod telescope has light transmitted to it through a flexible fiberoptic cable. The telescope has a wide angle of view and for photography the focus is from about 5 mm to infinity. The flexible fiberoptic cable not only transmits light from an external light fountain but also incorporates flash illumination for color or black and white still photography.

Using general anesthesia, supplemented by local anesthesia, direct laryngoscopy is performed first with the naked eye and then a more detailed evaluation is made using the Hopkins telescopes, straight ahead and angled 30, 70 or 120° (for retrograde visualization of the nasopharynx). For routine 35 mm color photography we use the Storz lightweight miniature motor-drive endocamera. However, an adaptor is available to couple any 35 mm single lens reflex camera to the Hopkins telescope. Normally 200 ASA Kodak Ektachrome® 35 mm film is used but 400 ASA Ektachrome is used for photography of the nasopharynx because there is some loss of light transmission through the 120° retrograde telescope (Fig. 5).

Initially some practice is required to be sure that the field of view is exactly central in the telescope and in the desired plane as this is most important for orientation by the viewer and to compare the left and right sides. There is a very wide latitude in the depth of focus (Fig. 6) so that focusing does not usually present any problem. Photographs can be readily taken even in the small airways of the tracheobronchial tree in premature and newborn babies (Fig. 7) using the smallest telescope which is merely 2.8 mm in external diameter.

Photographic documentation offers positive proof of what the laryngologist sees. For instance laryngeal trauma due to prolonged intubation can be shown to our colleagues in anesthesia when we meet to discuss these problems. For teaching purposes photographs showing croup and other causes of

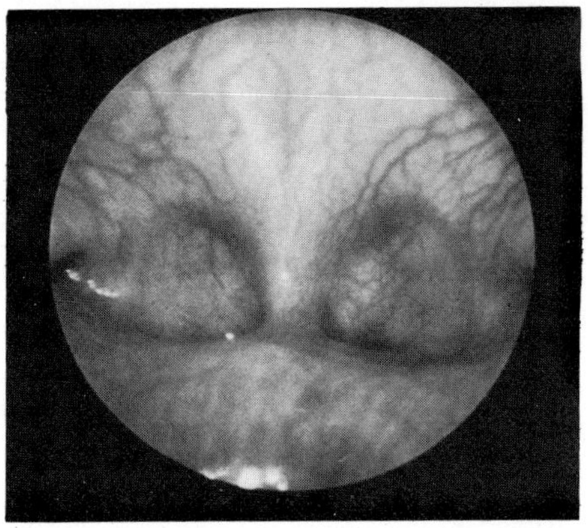

Fig. 5. Bilateral posterior congenital choanal atresia in a newborn baby. The eustachian tube opening is visible on the left.

acute inflammatory airway obstruction such as acute epiglottitis, are dramatic reminders to students who might otherwise be unfamiliar with these conditions.

Composite photography also allows comparison say, of vocal nodules (Fig. 8) which vary in their site, size and disposition. Laryngomalacia is the commonest cause of congenital laryngeal stridor and serial, composite still photographs will show the changes in the supraglottic tissues and arytenoids during inspiration. However, where dynamic changes in the larynx need to be demonstrated, video cassette television recording and cinephotography are the best modalities. We have recorded pathology in the larynx, tracheobronchial tree and esophagus on cinefilm or video cassette using the Storz equipment, the Hopkins telescopes, the xenon light source and the Wittmoser articulated optical arm. This system gives superb image quality with natural color reproduction in the documentation of many conditions such as laryngomalacia, vocal cord paralysis or tracheal compression with changes of the lumen during inspiration and expiration.

CONCLUSIONS

While a careful written description of the pathological findings remains the cheapest and most convenient routine form of documentation, especially when supplemented by suitable diagrams, various

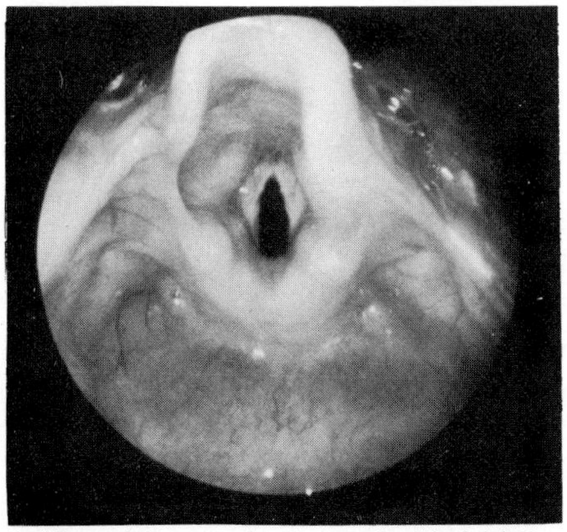

Fig. 6. Normal larynx of a 6-month-old child showing the vocal cords, supraglottic structures and piriform fossae.

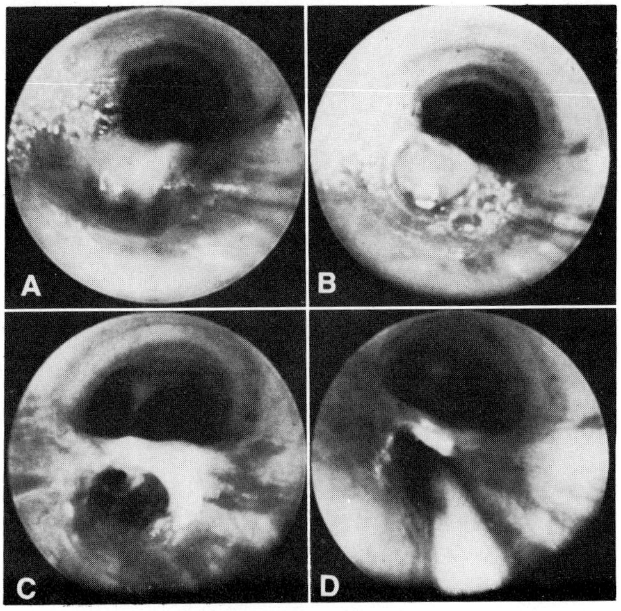

Fig. 7. A neonate with tracheoesophageal fistula and esophageal atresia showing the appearance of the trachea before definitive repair. A-C) Gastric juice bubbles up the fistula and contaminates the tracheobronchial tree. D) A catheter is placed through the fistula for easier identification at thoracotomy.

forms of permanent objective documentation serve better for comparative study, teaching, clinical research and for the improvement and expansion of training programs.

The upper lateral airways radiological study consistently gives valuable information and the application of radiological studies, together with unrestricted endoscopic photography allows permanent documentation of the changes occurring in any part of the anatomical areas being studied — from the nose and nasopharynx to the bronchi and segmental bronchial openings.

The combination of radiological study and single

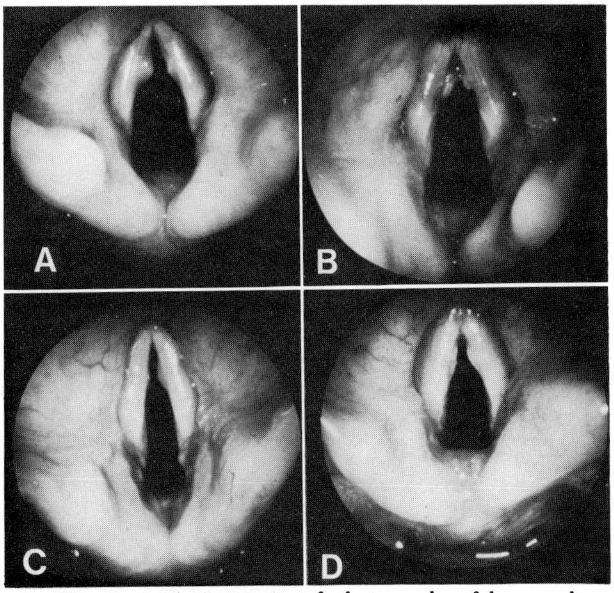

Fig. 8. A-D) Composite of photographs of laryngeal nodules in four children.

frame endoscopic color photography affords the best means of studying the pathology, natural history and results of treatment and is especially valuable in consultation with colleagues in other branches of pediatric medicine and surgery and in the widespread dissemination of information regarding the diagnosis and management of diseases seen by the pediatric otolaryngologist.

REFERENCES

1. Versatile valve. MD Aust 1973; Dec:39-43.

2. Saunders WH. The larynx-CIBA clinical symposia. Netter FH, illus. 1966;6.

3. Doust DD, Ting YN. Xeroradiography of the larynx. Radiology 1974; 110:727-30.

4. Zizmor J, Noyek AM. An atlas of otolaryngologic radiology. Philadelphia: WB Saunders Co, 1978.

5. Benjamin B. Xeroradiography of the upper airways in pediatrics. Aust Radiol 1979; 23:214-24.

6. Holinger PA, Brubaker JD, Brubaker JE. Open tube, proximal illumination mirror and direct laryngeal photography. Can J Otolaryngol 1975; 4:781-5.

7. Yanagisawa E, Eibling DE, Suzuki M. A simple method of laryngeal photography through the operating microscope. Ann Otol Rhinol Laryngol 1980; 89:547-50.

8. Strong MS. Laryngeal photography. Can J Otolaryngol 1965; 4:766-9.

9. Ward PH, Berci G, Calcaterra TC. Advances in endoscopic examination of the respiratory system. Ann Otol Rhinol Laryngol 1974; 83:754-60.

≈

PLASTIC SURGERY OF THE AGING FACE

"Plastic Surgery of the Aging Face," the biannual symposium of the American Academy of Facial Plastic and Reconstructive Surgery, will be held Jan. 30-Feb. 2, 1982, in Birmingham, Alabama. For registration details write: E. Gaylon McCollough, MD, Director, Aging Face Symposium, 1516 South 20th St., Birmingham, AL 35202.

Ann Otol 90:1981

PSEUDOLARYNGEAL PARALYSIS: A POSTINTUBATION COMPLICATION

SEYMOUR R. COHEN, MD

LOS ANGELES, CALIFORNIA

Seven patients in the pediatric age group who had severe posterior glottic stenosis are reported. All of these patients had been misdiagnosed as having bilateral vocal cord paralysis because of errors in observing the actual findings in the larynx. On cursory examination of the larynx, the findings resembled vocal cord paralysis, thus the name "pseudolaryngeal paralysis" was given to this disease entity. This paper describes in some detail the case histories, the endolaryngeal findings, and the therapy which was instituted and followed. The difficulties in managing this problem are also reviewed. Three of the seven patients were decannulated, two with persistent stress stridor and reduced exercise tolerance. Four other patients have improved, but are still in the process of being treated. The success of the therapy appears to be dependent on the severity of the scarring, whether there was fibrosis of the interarytenoideus muscle, and whether the cricoarytenoid joints were involved. It is hoped that by reporting this difficult problem, a more rapid and successful form of management will be developed.

This study reports a group of six patients who developed isolated posterior glottic stenosis following intubation and were misdiagnosed as having bilateral abductor vocal cord paralysis. Because the clinical picture of these children and the examination of the larynx so closely resembled vocal cord paralysis, the lesion has been named "pseudolaryngeal paralysis." Because this lesion when coexisting with other laryngeal damage prolongs the need for a tracheotomy, another patient with a more complex laryngeal stenosis and associated severe posterior glottic stenosis is also included in this report.

This paper presents another serious postintubation laryngeal problem that is very difficult to treat and which apparently has not received adequate attention by members of the profession who treat these children. In the patients reported in this study, the error in diagnosis appeared to be a failure to observe the esoteric changes in the larynx. All of these patients were referred to the author with the diagnosis of bilateral vocal cord paralysis. Usually more than one examiner had seen the patient. At times the opinions of the examining physicians varied as to the true cause of the obstruction within the larynx.

Posterior glottic scarring frequently occurs in the severely damaged postintubated larynx and is associated with subglottic and laryngotracheal involvement. Any form of trauma to the larynx (and especially endotracheal intubation) may create severe anatomic defects with consequent physiological dysfunction.

The literature is replete with papers that describe the effect of intubation but which have stressed subglottic stenosis and the difficulties in treating that complication. It would appear from reviewing the literature that too little concentrated attention has been given to this important lesion of the intubated larynx, ie, posterior glottic stenosis. The obstruction caused by this lesion, even when isolated, may create the prolonged need for airway support by a tracheotomy.

PATHOPHYSIOLOGY

Pressure by endotracheal intubation with ischemia and infection within the posterior glottis results in scarring of varying severity within one of three areas. These are the interarytenoid area, posterior commissure, and vocal process area of the larynx. The changes may be present in only one part or may involve a combination of these areas of the larynx. The patients who are reported had isolated lesions in the posterior glottic region without other damage to the larynx. In some of the children, lesser involvement made management easier and improvement in the airway was seen earlier. Because the lesion may be so hidden from view, incomplete or careless visualization of the larynx may cause an erroneous diagnosis of bilateral abductor paralysis. This may be particularly true when examinations do not include passive motion tests for cricoarytenoid fixation.

The scarring of the posterior glottic area of the larynx in all of the patients was of such a magnitude that the vocal cords failed to abduct and the arytenoid mobility was defective or impaired. It is probable that there is a varying degree of cricoarytenoid fixation or ankylosis in some patients. It is possible that some of the cases of laryngeal paralysis

From the Department of Surgery, Division of Otolaryngology, Childrens Hospital of Los Angeles and University of Southern California School of Medicine.

Presented at the meeting of the American Laryngological Association, Vancouver, British Columbia, May 10-11, 1981.

REPRINTS — Seymour R. Cohen, MD, 1300 North Vermont Avenue, Los Angeles CA 90027.

following intubation which have been reported may indeed have been due to this posterior glottic scarring.

The most commonly reported iatrogenic postintubation laryngeal problem is subglottic stenosis. The effects of intubation trauma vary from minor lesions such as granulomata in the larynx (particularly on the vocal cords), to complete disruption of the normal laryngeal anatomic pattern.

The otolaryngologist tends to accentuate the effects of prolonged intubation. However, duration of intubation is only one factor in the creation of laryngeal disease. More important factors are the age of the patient, the size of the endotracheal tube, the presence of infection, trauma during intubation, hypotension, hypoxemia, motion of the tube and head from improper fixation of the endotracheal tube, nasotracheal versus orotracheal intubation, the piston action of the ventilator, inadequate hydration, and inadequate moisture content of the inspired air.

The mucosa covering the arytenoids and interarytenoid areas overlies a very thin mucoperichondrium with very little submucosa. When the posterior-lying endotracheal tube (Fig. 1A) presses against this area, ischemia is produced and ulceration, with the exposure of perichondrium, may result. Infection then occurs with resultant perichondritis, following which healing is by fibrosis of the ulcerated, infected area (Fig. 1B). The interarytenoideus muscles and interarytenoid area may become fibrosed, and contraction of the scar then pulls the arytenoid cartilages together. Ulceration and fibrosis of the vocal process areas result in the fusion of the posterior ends of the true vocal cords, and the posterior commissure may be replaced by scar. In some cases it may be assumed that cricoarytenoid inflammation and joint fixation could occur, or that at least some limitation of joint motion may result. Where the intervocal process scar is very thin but restricts abduction, the examiner may only see the failure of abduction, and thus may erroneously diagnose the problem as bilateral abductor paralysis of the larynx. Where the entire posterior glottic area is fibrosed, the skillful endoscopist should have no problem in making a proper diagnosis.

LITERATURE REVIEW

In 1973 Jaffe[1] described three unusual laryngeal problems in children. One of these children who was intubated for only four days after open heart surgery and who required a tracheotomy, was incorrectly diagnosed as having bilateral vocal cord paralysis. The patient had repeated laryngeal examinations over a period of two years (1970 and 1971) and was said each time to have had bilateral vocal cord paralysis. Suspension microlaryngoscopy showed dense adhesions at the posterior margins of the vocal cords. Incision of this scar released the arytenoids and allowed for motion of the vocal cords, but the patient still wore the tracheotomy tube eight months later.

Holinger and Schild[2] reported on injuries to the pharynx, larynx, and trachea. One of their cases showed postintubation synechia between the arytenoids. However, the child had no airway problems. These authors listed edema, ulceration, granulations with late development of the glottic and subglottic stenosis, synechia formation, fixation of the cricoarytenoid joints and complications of exuberant granuloma in the subglottic areas, as being responsible for the prolonged need for a tracheotomy following endotracheal intubation. Dwyer et al[3] wrote that the points of greatest pressure from endotracheal intubation were the posterior commissure of the glottis, the medial surface of the arytenoids, the vocal processes, and anterior subglottic and tracheal areas.

Hawkins,[4] in reporting on the effects of prolonged intubation for hyaline membrane disease in the neonate, showed autopsy findings of the larynx. Ulcerations were found in the area beneath the arytenoid and in the anterior subglottic area. He stated that the posterior commissure at the glottic level did not seem to be the point of excessive pressure. There were some ulcerations of the arytenoids, but ulcerations were more severe below the vocal process. He attributed this to the higher position and posterior tilt of the funnel-shaped neonatal larynx which allowed the malleable endotracheal tube to assume a position which exerted less pressure on the surrounding laryngeal tissue, particularly within the interarytenoid area. Benjamin (personal communication) referred to this problem of posterior glottic stenosis as one of the most difficult management problems of lesions of the pediatric larynx.

Woodman and Pennington[5] in 1976 cautioned against the use of arytenoidectomy in patients with localized fibrosis or ankylosis of the arytenoids because successful lateralization is thereafter difficult or impossible.

CASE REPORTS

Case 1. A 1-year-old female was first seen Oct. 2, 1975. She was the product of a 37-week gestation, normal pregnancy, and uncomplicated delivery. Her birth weight was 2,464 g, and she was noted to have stridor and airway obstruction of sufficient magnitude to require intubation. The vocal cords were reported normal following extubation, but stridor recurred and reintubation was necessary. The second procedure was extremely difficult and was associated with shock and cardiac arrest. She was resuscitated and ventilated with the endotracheal tube and was transferred to a children's hospital in London on Oct. 18, 1974. The cause of her airway problem was not found, and she was extubated two days later. Although hoarseness was noted initially, her airway appeared adequate and she was discharged on Oct. 30, 1974. She was again seen on Nov. 28, 1974, with moderately severe stridor and retractions which had become progressively worse over a period of one week. Examination then showed a very stridorous infant with sternal, infracostal, and diaphragmatic retractions. Intubation was again required, at which time supraglottic and

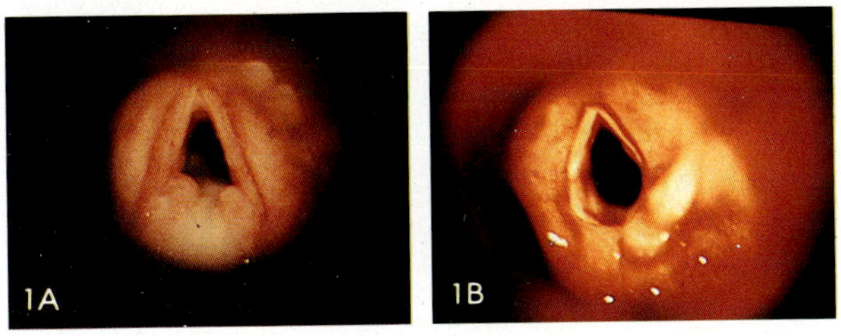

Fig. 1. A) Endotracheal tube lies posteriorly placed with large granulomata at the vocal process. The anterior portions of the larynx and glottis are free of disease. B) Endotracheal tube has been removed and the posterior glottic ulceration and exposure of cartilage can be seen. The trauma is limited to the posterior portion of the larynx.

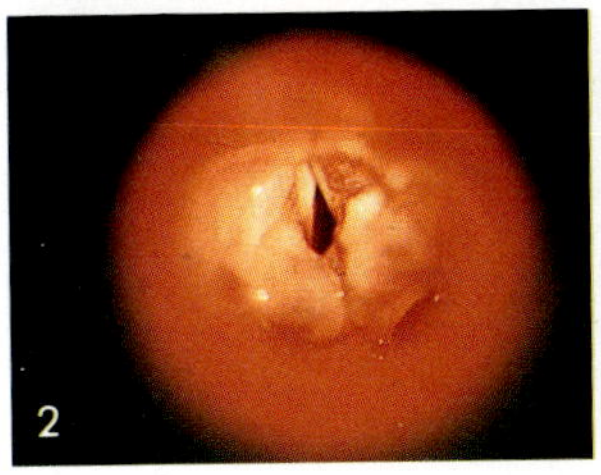

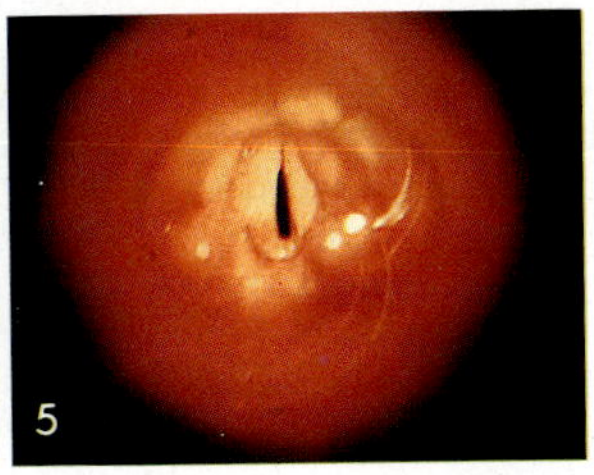

Fig. 2. (Case 1) Persistent interarytenoid web. The vocal cords abduct to the paramedian position posteriorly, but remain adducted anteriorly.

Fig. 5. (Case 4) Child who was involved in an automobile accident was intubated and had tracheotomy. Vocal cords are minimally abducted. Intervocal process scar is seen and limits abduction. Interarytenoid space is free of disease.

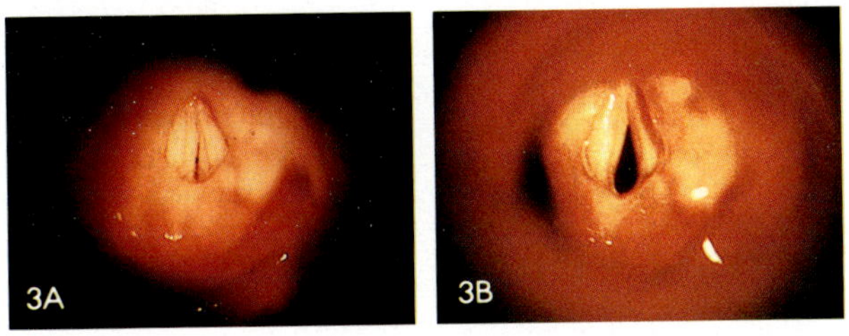

Fig. 3. (Case 2) Child intubated for 3 weeks for treatment of respiratory distress syndrome. A) Vocal cords appear duplicated, are in the midline, and cannot be passively abducted. Interarytenoid, intervocal process, and posterior commissure scarring are seen. B) After 11 laser surgical treatments the airway is seen to be adequate. Duplication of the vocal cords is still apparent, abduction is satisfactory, but persistence of the interarytenoid scar is noted.

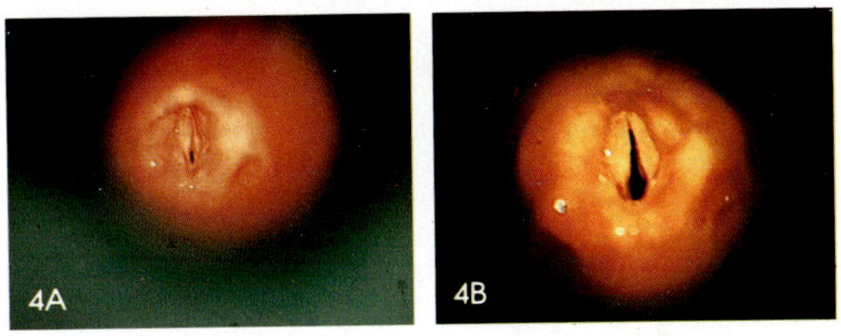

Fig. 4. (Case 3) Larynx of a premature infant who required nasotracheal intubation for one week. A) Vocal cords are adducted. Glottic chink is minimal from scarring in the posterior commissure and intervocal process area. B) Vocal cords abduct more posteriorly, but less anteriorly and the posterior glottis is patent. Intervocal process scar is now absent.

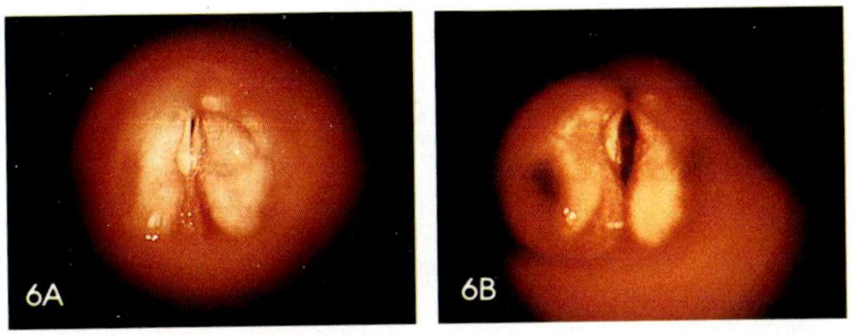

Fig. 6. (Case 5) Child who swallowed a caustic substance and had multiple esophageal strictures and a colon esophagus interposition. A) Vocal cords are in adduction. The interarytenoid and intervocal process areas are scarred, and the posterior commissure is obliterated. The arytenoids are posteriorly displaced. B) Larynx as seen after three laser surgeries. The interarytenoid scar has been disrupted, and the posterior commissure is now deeply V-shaped. The vocal cords abduct to the paramedian position.

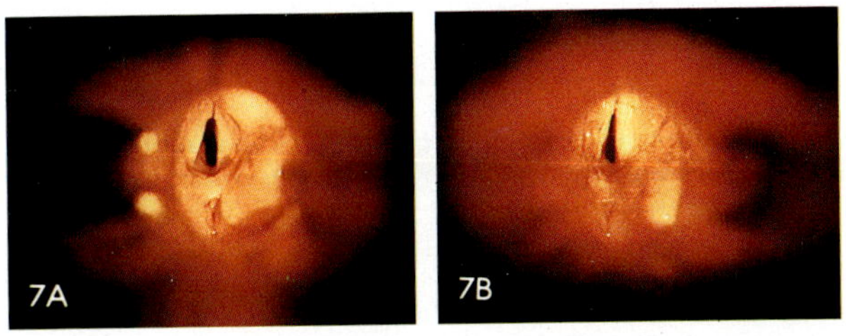

Fig. 7. (Case 6) Child with history of ingesting a quantity of medication and required intubation, resuscitation, and dilatations. A) Vocal cords appear almost in the midline. Scarring of the interarytenoid area and fixation of the arytenoids are noted. The posterior commissure is obliterated. There appears to be an anterior web. B) Some abduction of the vocal cords is noted after laser surgery. Scarring in the posterior glottic area is noted, there is still some anterior webbing of the vocal cords, and the airway has improved.

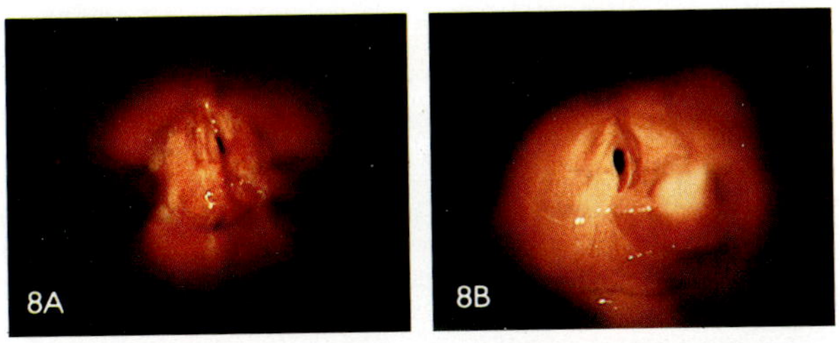

Fig. 8. (Case 7) Child involved in an automobile accident who required tracheotomy, stenting, and dilatations. A) Anterior portion of the vocal cords appears normal. Vocal cords have been artificially separated to expose the severe intervocal process, interarytenoid and posterior commissure scarring. Airway is poor; subglottic area is free of disease. B) Vocal cords abduct to the paramedian position. There is persistence of the interarytenoid scarring. Posterior commissure has not returned to normal.

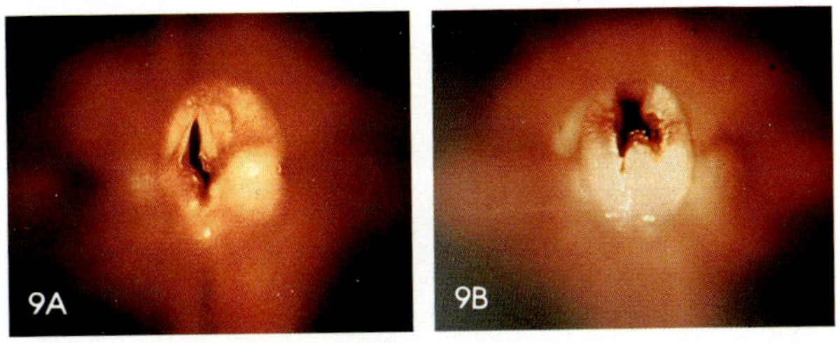

Fig. 9. A) Example of a larynx following laser surgery with a linear cut into the scar posteriorly and through the interarytenoid area on the right side. B) Example in which a double linear cut was made with the laser on each side of the exposed scar of the posterior glottis. This leaves a tongue of scar and tissue in the midportion of the posterior glottis.

vocal cord edema, without significant subglottic stenosis, was seen. A chest roentgenogram, barium esophagogram, and serum calcium were normal. She was subsequently extubated and discharged on Dec. 23, 1974. At the time of her discharge minimal stridor was present, but two days later she was readmitted with vomiting and airway obstruction and required a short period of intubation. In late January 1975, her weight deteriorated and she appeared more distressed; therefore an elective tracheotomy was performed on Feb. 4, 1975, when she was four months of age. Direct laryngoscopy at the time of her tracheotomy showed a bilateral recurrent laryngeal paralysis. Following her tracheotomy she thrived, but remained hospitalized for a prolonged period of time. Another laryngoscopy performed on July 1, 1975, revealed "bilateral vocal cord recurrent paralysis." The child was discharged on Sept. 1, 1975, to return to the United States with her parents.

She was first seen on Oct. 2, 1975, and was admitted to the Childrens Hospital of Los Angeles on Oct. 28, 1975. Direct laryngoscopy and bronchoscopy revealed a small larynx for a 1-year-old, with cricoarytenoid fixation, posterior commissure web, and a large fibroma proximal to the tracheotomy site within the tracheal lumen. The diagnosis of posterior glottic stenosis or pseudolaryngeal paralysis of the larynx was made on the basis of these findings. She was followed at infrequent intervals, and on March 31, 1976, endoscopic examination again revealed the severe posterior glottic problem. In May 1976, incision of the web with triamcinolone acetonide (Kenalog) injection was performed. Multiple procedures followed with incisions of the web-like stenotic lesion and application of triamcinolone acetonide. Because airway obstruction still persisted, on Oct. 10, 1977, a large fibroma was removed from the trachea by external neck incision. On Feb. 8, 1978, she was decannulated, and a tracheocutaneous fistula which still persisted was not closed. Following extubation she developed two episodes of pneumonia, one of which required hospitalization. Exercise tolerance was reduced so that running caused shortness of breath, and any stress by exercise produced inspiratory stridor. In late May 1978, the tracheotomy tube was replaced in order to further treat the posterior glottic stenosis. Her response to incisions was unsatisfactory so that in March 1979, laser surgery to the posterior glottic scar was started on a monthly basis. On Aug. 29, 1978, she again was decannulated. Since then, her voice has been breathy and high pitched and there has been inspiratory stridor with stress and reduced exercise tolerance. During 1980 a direct laryngoscopy and bronchoscopy were performed, which showed the larynx to have remained smaller than usual for a child of her age. The vocal cords moved to the paramedian position, but an interarytenoid web was still present. The subglottic area and trachea were perfectly normal (Fig. 2).

In March 1981, she was again seen in the office and examination revealed the inspiratory stridor with stress and exercise. The parents reported that she could not keep up with her friends and had limited exercise tolerance. The tracheocutaneous fistula was still patent. Further treatment will be necessary to improve the airway.

Case 2. A male child born prematurely on Aug. 4, 1974, was the product of a normal pregnancy. His birth weight was 2,240 g. He was intubated for three weeks for treatment of respiratory distress syndrome. Following extubation he was discharged, but required a number of hospitalizations for what was diagnosed as recurrent bronchitis. Each episode required treatment with oxygen tent and humidification. The parents were told that he had suffered "tracheal scarring." On Dec. 2, 1975, after a respiratory infection, he developed progressive respiratory difficulty and was hospitalized because of cyanosis and breathing difficulties. He was intubated with considerable difficulty and was placed on a respirator for a few days, but extubated himself during a seizure and was reintubated. He was then transferred to another medical center on Dec. 6, 1975. On examination he was alert and active with an endotracheal tube in place and with spontaneous respirations but with flaring of his nasal alae. On Dec. 9, 1975, he was taken to the operating room with a preoperative diagnosis of possible subglottic stenosis. When the endotracheal tube was removed, an exophytic growth was seen on the left vocal cord and this was thought to be papillomatosis of the larynx. A biopsy, however, showed fibrinous exudate. Subglottic stenosis was diagnosed and a tracheotomy was performed. On Jan. 12, 1976, direct laryngoscopy revealed the supraglottic structures to be normal but the arytenoids and false cords were moderately edematous. The subglottic space and trachea were normal. When the patient was awakened from the anesthetic, vocal cord abduction was found defective and a diagnosis of bilateral vocal cord paralysis was made. The patient was subsequently transferred to another physician's care. On March 14, 1977, direct laryngoscopy and bronchoscopy again showed "typical bilateral vocal cord abductor paralysis of the larynx." Extubation was impossible and he was referred for evaluation and treatment of the paralyzed larynx.

This patient was seen in consultation on March 29, 1977, and was admitted to the hospital for endoscopic examination. Direct laryngoscopy revealed severe glottic laryngeal stenosis with webbing of the interarytenoid area and a small anterior vocal cord web (Fig. 3 A). The subglottic area and trachea were normal. Periodically for the next 24 months, incisions of the posterior glottic stenosis were made with knife and scissors and triamcinolone acetonide was applied or injected. His airway improved and he tolerated plugging of the tracheotomy tube. His voice was fairly good, but high pitched. By Feb. 7, 1979, the airway had improved so that he tolerated plugging of the tracheotomy tube for long periods of time. However, exercise tolerance was reduced. From November 1977 until May 1979, he was followed in the office, and because of exercise intolerance with the tracheotomy tube plugged, he was admitted for laser surgery. On May 7, 1979, the posterior glottic stenotic lesion was treated with the laser. After 11 laser surgical treatments, direct laryngoscopy on Sept. 3, 1980 (Fig. 3 B) revealed the airway to be adequate and the patient was decannulated. On Feb. 20, 1981, the tracheocutaneous fistula was closed and the larynx was intubated for this procedure. His first postoperative visit on Feb. 26, 1981, showed the neck to be healing nicely and his airway and voice were excellent.

Case 3. A female born prematurely on April 5, 1972, had respiratory distress syndrome of the neonate. Her birth weight was 1,512 g and she required nasotracheal intubation for about one week. She was the product of a normal pregnancy and normal delivery.

The patient was first seen Sept. 15, 1972, with the chief complaint of noisy breathing. Examination showed a small infant with inspiratory stridor and a normal cry. She had xiphoid retractions and rhonchi in the chest, but the remainder of the physical examination was within normal limits. Endoscopic examination was advised but was rejected by the parents, and she was not seen again until Jan. 15, 1973. At that time, the complaint was that of increasing stridor and difficulty in feeding. The examination showed inspiratory crowing type of stridor with evidence of airway obstruction. Stress or crying caused xiphoid retractions. A lateral x-ray film of her airway showed no abnormality of the laryngeal subglottic or tracheal airway. Because of the increase in airway obstruction, she was admitted to the hospital on March 12, 1973, for direct laryngoscopy. The examination revealed a severe laryngeal stenosis (Fig. 4 A). The preliminary diagnosis was probable paralysis or fixation of the vocal cords. The left vocal cord was fixed in the midline and the right vocal cord moved approximately 2 mm from the midline. The subglottic area was not examined and the larynx was not manipulated because of the possibility of increasing the airway obstruction. The parents had imposed limitations on the examination and also refused any suggestions of a tracheotomy or artificial airway. It was felt that her airway was very tenuous and that a tracheotomy was necessary. She was not examined again until May 1975, when while on vacation in Hawaii, severe respiratory distress and obstruction occurred and an emergency tracheotomy was performed. The patient was transferred to the hospital on May 13, 1975, in excellent condition with a normally functioning tracheostomy. Her condition was stable and on May 14, 1975, direct laryngoscopy revealed bilateral vocal cord fixation in the midline due to posterior glottic stenosis. Cricoarytenoid fixation was evident by passive motion testing. She was discharged from the hospital on May 15, 1975. On June 16, 1975, she was readmitted for evaluation of her airway and a granuloma of the trachea was removed. Dilatation of the larynx was attempted, and triamcinolone acetonide was injected into the posterior commissure area, but no improvement occurred. For the next two years, periodic laryngoscopies with incisions of the posterior glottic scar with a knife or scissors were accomplished. The incisions were made down to the perichondrium. On Feb. 7, 1977, she was decannulated (Fig. 4 B). The tracheocutaneous fistula was closed on June 14, 1978, at which time the larynx tolerated intubation quite well. Since decannulation, the patient's voice has been excellent with very good tonal qualities. Stress, however, produces stridor. She is normally active, dances and runs, but becomes stridorous. A recent report from her pediatrician indicates she is well, but that inspiratory stridor with stress exercise persists. The parents do not want any further treatment or examinations.

Case 4. A 6-year-old male born June 14, 1972, was first seen in consultation July 11, 1978. The history was one of having been hospitalized for three to four weeks because of injuries sustained in an automobile accident. Originally having been intubated, he required a tracheotomy to support his airway and for tracheobronchial toilet. He recovered from his multiple injuries but following removal of the tracheotomy tube, stridor and moderately severe airway obstruction were noted. He was referred with the diagnosis of possible vocal cord paralysis or subglottic stenosis. Examination revealed a comfortable child with a normal examination of the head and neck. His voice was husky and both inspiratory and expiratory stridor were noted. A tracheotomy scar was present in the neck, which was completely healed. There were numerous scars on the right chest wall. The patient was admitted to the hospital on July 12, 1978, for endoscopic examination. Direct laryngoscopy (Fig. 5) revealed postintubation scarring of the posterior glottic area. The interarytenoid and intervocal process areas were bound together, and the subglottic space and tracheal lumen were normal. Five direct laryngoscopies with incisions of the posterior web were done, with improvement of the status of his airway. He was seen on March 27, 1979, after an injury to his face. Indirect laryngoscopy showed excellent mobility of both vocal cords and his voice was remarkably improved. Unfortunately, he has not been examined since April 1979, and a follow-up report is not available.

Case 5. A female seven years of age, born Aug. 22, 1972, was first seen in consultation Aug. 26, 1980. The patient was referred by her pediatric surgeon in Arizona for evaluation of her airway problem. She had been endoscoped many times and diagnosed as having either bilateral vocal cord paralysis and/or subglottic and upper tracheal stenosis. This patient had swallowed a caustic substance at about $1\frac{1}{2}$ years of age and suffered severe damage to the esophagus with multiple strictures. She had required a colon-esophagus interposition. Following surgery, she developed frequent episodes of stridor with respiratory obstruction. On April 7, 1977, soon after closure of an esophagocutaneous fistula, she was admitted to an Arizona hospital because of increasing respiratory difficulties. Endotracheal intubation was required to relieve the severe obstructive airway problem. She was then extubated and was transferred to the Arizona Children's Hospital. However, because of the inability to deal with her airway problem at that hospital, she was transferred to the Good Samaritan Hospital on April 20, 1975. A tracheotomy was performed, at which time laryngeal examination showed "supraglottic airway obstruction" which was said to be due to the original caustic ingestion. She was then transferred back to the children's hospital, where numerous tracheal dilatations were performed which were reported to have resulted in a normal tracheal diameter. On July 31, 1975, the tracheotomy tube was removed, but required replacement because of severe airway obstruction. She was discharged on Oct. 27, 1975, with a Shiley tube in place with the diagnosis of tracheal stenosis. On June 20, 1976, laryngoscopy revealed bilateral abductor paralysis of the larynx and the examiner felt that prior to this date, vocal cord paralysis had been obscured by the succinylcholine chloride (Anectine) used during anesthesia for examination of the larynx. In July 1978 she was admitted to the Sacred Heart Medical Center in Spokane, where the laryngeal diagnosis was subglottic stenosis. The stricture of the esophagus-colon anastomosis required dilatation every two weeks to maintain its patency. She was referred for management of her airway problems on Aug. 27, 1980, when she was admitted to the Children's Hospital of Los Angeles. Direct laryngoscopy and bronchoscopy revealed pseudolaryngeal paralysis (Fig. 6 A) with interarytenoid and posterior glottic scarring and dislocation of the arytenoids. The immediate subglottic area and trachea were perfectly normal. A stricture of the colon-esophagus anastomosis was dilated at that time and the patient was changed to a Holinger tracheotomy tube. On Nov. 24, 1980, and each month until Feb. 3, 1981 (a total of four treatments), suspension microlaryngoscopy and laser surgery were performed. She was treated with long-term antibiotics and it was noted that her larynx had improved considerably within the very short period of treatment (Fig. 6 B). She tolerates plugging of her tracheotomy tube all through the day and will probably be decannulated in the very near future. Her response to laser surgery is most encouraging.

Case 6. A 4-year 9-month male living in a foster home was transferred to the hospital for endoscopic evaluation Feb. 13, 1978. Little is known about his past history. A few of the important historical facts are that two years prior to his having been referred for treatment, he apparently ingested an unknown quantity of medication and required intubation and resuscitation. Because of severe airway obstruction following extubation, a tracheotomy was performed. A diagnosis of laryngeal paralysis or subglottic stenosis was made and treatment with dilatations followed. Because he could not be decannulated, he was referred for further management. On admission to the hospital his vital signs and x-ray film of the chest were normal. The physical examination was normal, except for the presence of a tracheotomy tube which functioned normally. Direct laryngoscopy (Fig. 7 A) revealed the vocal cords to be fixed in the midline with little or no abduction. There was interarytenoid scarring at the vocal process and the posterior commissure was completely obliterated. An anterior tracheal granuloma was found and was removed. The diagnosis was posterior glottic stenosis or pseudolaryngeal paralysis.

Dilatations of the stenosis proved fruitless; therefore on Aug. 14, 1978, incisions with laryngeal knife and scissors were done. The larynx was dilated each time with a bronchoscope, and triamcinolone acetonide was applied locally or was injected. Antibiotics were given intermittently. Some improvement occurred, but was inadequate to warrant decannulating the patient. Since Feb. 19, 1978, suspension microlaryngoscopy and laser surgery have been used periodically. Local applications and injections of triamcinolone acetonide were used together with antibiotics. By the end of 1980, he tolerated plugging of the tracheotomy tube for prolonged periods of time. During the past three months, his voice has been excellent and he functions normally even with stress when the tracheotomy tube is plugged (Fig. 7B). He is almost ready for decannulation.

Case 7. A 17-year-old female was referred for laser surgery of a laryngeal stenosis. She was first seen on Oct. 21, 1980. The history revealed that one year before consultation she had been in an automobile accident, at which time she suffered a fracture of the larynx and required a tracheotomy for airway support. Multiple procedures had been performed with stenting and dilatations of the larynx. However, on each occasion, soon after removal of the stent, closure of the larynx occurred. Examination on her first visit revealed a healthy-appearing adolescent in no distress, but totally dependent upon her tracheotomy tube. Closure of the tracheotomy tube created severe airway obstruction. Her voice was somewhat husky and hoarse. Indirect laryngoscopy revealed a severe glottic stenosis with a pinpoint opening. She was admitted to the hospital on Nov. 19, 1980, for suspension microlaryngoscopy and laser surgery. The direct laryngoscopy showed webbing of the entire larynx at the level of the vocal cords (Fig. 8 A). The interarytenoid, intervocal process, and posterior commissure areas were fused, and a small anterior web was also seen. An anterior subglottic stenosis was also present. Laser surgery was applied to the posterior glottic scar and triamcinolone acetonide was applied locally. Antibiotics were ordered and she was discharged on the day of surgery. She has had four treatments since then, with laser surgery used on the area of scarring, resulting in marked improvement each time. Her voice has now improved tremendously, although it is still slightly husky. She tolerates plugging of the tracheotomy tube for long periods of time. Further treatment will be necessary before decannulation is possible (Fig. 8 B).

DISCUSSION

The prognosis of posterior glottic stenosis (pseudolaryngeal paralysis) is dependent on the severity of the lesion and the degree and depth of involvement of the larynx.

When minor changes such as intervocal process scarring are present, simple incisions of the scar band may be curative. When, however, the posterior glottic stenosis involves the interarytenoid area and posterior commissure region, increased difficulties will be encountered in correcting the airway obstruction. If the interarytenoideus muscle or cricoarytenoid joints are involved, any method of treatment may be disappointing.

Dilatations of this laryngeal lesion have proven useless, and injections of steroids to soften the scar have not proven beneficial. Stenting after disruption of the scar, whether by knife, scissors or laser surgery, has not been used. This form of treatment was not used in order to avoid any potential further damage to the larynx.

Open laryngeal surgery, whether to excise scar, introduce mucosal grafts, or for incising of the lamina of the cricoid and widening of the postcricoid region with cartilage implant, has not been used. While the rationale for these procedures may exist, the inability to assess the pathology of the cricoarytenoid joint rules against this type of corrective surgery. Arytenoidectomy was not employed since the usual contraindications existed in these patients.

Incision with laser surgery, knife, or scissors seems to be a slow but effective method of dealing with this difficult problem. Either linear cuts parallel to the vocal cord extending posteriorly from the vocal process through the interarytenoid area, or notching of the scar at the vocal process, have been used (Fig. 9 A). Whenever possible, a linear cut is made on each side parallel to the vocal cord which leaves a tongue of tissue between the laterally placed cuts (Fig. 9 B). As suggested by B. Benjamin (personal communication) the cuts must be made deeply and down to the cricoid mucoperichondrium. Plugging the tracheotomy tube soon after treatment may facilitate movement of the vocal cords and can limit refixation.

The effect of steroid therapy cannot be assessed, but the use of antibiotics is felt to be most beneficial.

It is probable that no single modality of therapy can be used because of differences in the severity of the lesion. Whether cricoarytenoid joint activity returns to complete normalcy is unknown, particularly after inactivity of the joints over long periods of time.

Hopefully, this report will increase the awareness of this not uncommon postintubation complication, stimulate newer techniques of therapy in children with pseudolaryngeal paralysis of the larynx, and lessen the morbidity of this lesion.

ACKNOWLEDGMENT — The author gives thanks to his associates Drs. Kenneth Geller and Jeffrey Birns for their aid in abstracting case reports. To Rose Marie Lapicola gratitude is expressed for the preparation of this manuscript.

REFERENCES

1. Jaffe BF. Unusual laryngeal problems in children. Ann Otol Rhinol Laryngol 1973; 82:637-42.

2. Holinger PH, Schild JA. Pharyngeal, laryngeal and tracheal injuries in the pediatric age group. Ann Otol Rhinol Laryngol 1972; 81:538-45.

3. Dwyer CS, Kronenberg S, Saklad M. The endotracheal tube: a consideration of its traumatic effects. Anesthesiology 1949; 10:714-28.

4. Hawkins DB. Hyaline membrane disease of the neonate: prolonged intubation in management: effects on the larynx. Laryngoscope 1978; 88:201-24.

5. Woodman D, Pennington CL. Bilateral abductor paralysis. Ann Otol Rhinol Laryngol 1976; 85:437-9.

Ann Otol 90:1981

BILATERAL VERTICAL PARTIAL LARYNGECTOMY FOR BILATERAL VOCAL CORD CARCINOMA

HUGH F. BILLER, MD WILLIAM LAWSON, DDS, MD

NEW YORK, NEW YORK

This paper presents a technique of partial laryngectomy for tumors involving both vocal cords. The resection includes both vocal cords, adjacent cartilage and one arytenoid. Staged reconstruction consists of rotating the remaining posterior border of the thyroid cartilage 90° in order to obtain adequate anteroposterior length. A temporary laryngostome is formed. The results in four patients, followed for a minimum of three years, are presented.

Tumors which involve the anterior commissure and both vocal cords with normal mobility can be resected by a frontolateral approach with preservation of a significant portion of one thyroid ala on the side of lesser involvement. The cord adjacent to the preserved thyroid ala is resected subperichondrally. This subperichondral resection is oncologically satisfactory provided the vocal cord does not exhibit fixation or diminished mobility which infers vocalis muscle invasion. Preservation of the thyroid ala when the adjacent cord exhibits vocalis muscle invasion leads to an increased incidence of local recurrence.[1] Therefore, in larynges in which both vocal cords are involved with tumor, and decreased mobility or fixation of the cord is present, the oncologic procedure indicated requires resection of both adjacent thyroid alae. Reconstruction following bilateral thyroid ala resection usually results in a significant incidence of laryngeal stenosis.

The purpose of this paper is to present a technique of resection and reconstruction of the larynx following bilateral vocal cord and adjacent thyroid cartilage resection which provides rehabilitation of the airway with preservation of its protective function and the voice. The results of this procedure performed on five patients are presented.

METHODS

Patient Selection. This procedure is indicated in a very select group of patients with glottic carcinoma (Table 1). The criteria for case selection include tumor involving the anterior commissure and both vocal cords; mobility of the cord diminished bilaterally or one cord fixed and the other with diminished motion; subglottic involvement of less than 1 cm anteriorly and laterally, with no subglottic involvement posteriorly; involvement of the arytenoid should be limited to the vocal process and the anterior surface of the arytenoid; one arytenoid including vocal process must be free of tumor, with no fixation on the side of arytenoid preservation. This procedure is not indicated after radiation failure. Cartilage invasion anteriorly or anterolaterally may be present.

Accurate delineation of the extent of the tumor is determined by indirect and direct laryngoscopy and computerized tomographic scanning.

Procedure. The technique of reconstruction utilized in these cases is similar to that presented in 1974.[2] General anesthesia is maintained through the tracheotomy side. The incision and outline of the skin flaps is the same as described by Conley[3] (Fig. 1). If hair-bearing tissue is present, the flaps are de-epithelized. The strap muscles are separated in the midline and the thyroid cartilage and cricoid cartilage are completely exposed following transsection of the sternothyroid muscles at their insertions. Methylene blue is used to mark the thyroid cartilage cuts. The perichondrium is not elevated. The bilateral thyroid cartilage cuts are made vertically, approximately 1 cm anterior to the posterior border of the thyroid alae (Fig. 2A). An oscillating saw is utilized to section the cartilage. A transverse incision is made in the cricothyroid membrane at the upper border of the cricoid cartilage. This incision is extended laterally along the superior border of the cricoid on the side of arytenoid preservation. Direct visualization of the mucosa is required before it is incised. The patient is paralyzed, the undersurface of the vocal cord is inspected, and the extent of tumor involvement is visualized. The subglottic cut continues posteriorly until the level of the vocal process is encountered. The vocal process of the arytenoid to be preserved is visualized and the cord is sectioned at the level of the vocal process. This incision is continued superiorly to transsect the posterior aspect of the false cord and aryepiglottic fold. The thyrohyoid membrane is then incised at the upper border of the thyroid cartilage. Following this, retraction of the thyroid ala towards the

TABLE 1. CHARACTERISTICS OF PATIENTS WITH BILATERAL VERTICAL PARTIAL LARYNGECTOMY (N = 5)

Patient	*Tumor Margin*	*Vocalis Muscle Invasion*	*Decannulation*	*Aspiration*	*Recurrent Tumor*	*Survival (yrs.)*
1	Neg.	Pos.	Yes	No	No	7
2*	Neg.	Pos.	Yes	No	No	6
3	Neg.	Pos.	Yes	No	No	6
4	Neg.	Pos.	Yes	No	No	3
5†	Neg.	Pos.	—	—	—	—

*Cervical metastases, neck dissection, two years.

†Patient died following first stage.

From the Department of Otolaryngology, The Mount Sinai Hospital Medical Center, New York.

Presented at the meeting of the American Laryngological Association, Vancouver, British Columbia, May 10-11, 1981.

REPRINTS — H. F. Biller, MD, Department of Otolaryngology, The Mount Sinai Hospital, 100th Street and Fifth Avenue, New York, NY 10029.

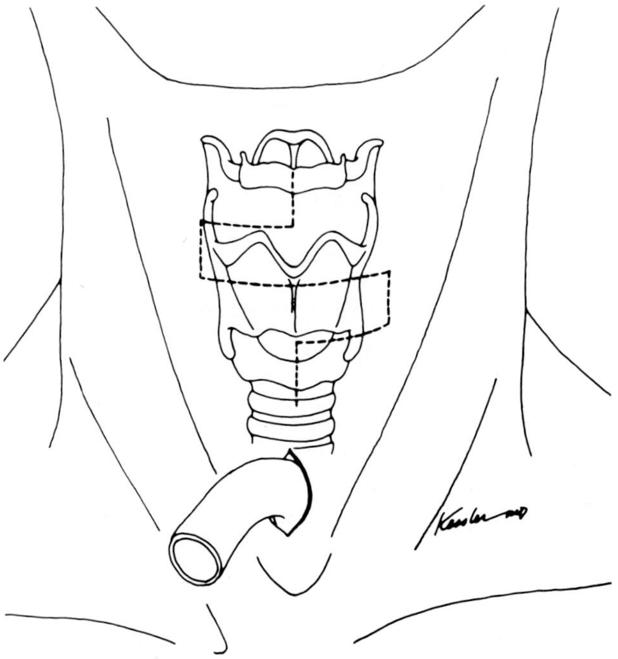

Fig. 1. Skin incision allows formation of two pedicle flaps which are utilized to resurface the resected area.

opposite side exposes the contralateral cord. The subglottis is now incised on the opposite side. The thyrohyoid membrane is divided and the posterior cut is made either through the vocal process, body of the arytenoid, or the cricoarytenoid joint depending upon tumor extent. Reconstruction is initiated by suturing the petiole of the epiglottis anteriorly to the infrahyoid tissues. The posterior remnants of thyroid cartilage are mobilized by severing the cricothyroid articulation and separating the pyriform sinus mucosa from the medial aspect. The inferior constrictor muscle is left attached to the cartilage. The posterior thyroid ala (Fig. 2B) is then rotated forward 90° (Fig. 2C). In order to perform this rotation, the inferior constrictor muscle is separated from the superior aspect of the thyroid ala. Following rotation of the alae anteriorly it becomes evident that they project excessively and must be shortened so as to extend only slightly anterior to the cricoid arch. A wire suture passed from the cricoid to the thyroid ala stabilizes the cartilage in its new position. A small piece of cartilage is also wired to the cricoid to replace the arytenoid if it has been resected. The skin flaps are now advanced into the operative defect and are sutured to the cut margin of the vocal process on one side and the mucosa over the neoarytenoid on the opposite side (Fig. 3). The remaining skin incisions are closed in layers. A nasogastric tube is inserted and a tracheotomy tube replaces the endotracheal tube. Healing of the laryngostome is usually complete in 3-6 weeks. During this time, one is able to observe when an adequate airway is present. During this period granulations may require cauterization. The patient is fed on the seventh postoperative day. Aspiration into the trough is generally noted during the first few days. The time of closure of the laryngostome is determined by 1) complete healing of the suture lines, 2) absence of aspiration, 3) adequate airway patency when the laryngostome is closed by Vaseline® gauze. Closure of the laryngostome is performed under general anesthesia. A circumferential incision is made around the laryngostome and the skin is undermined medially and turned in forming the first layer of the closure. The external defect is closed by rotating an adjacent cervical flap. The donor defect of this flap is either closed primarily or skin grafted. The tracheotomy tube is removed seven days later.

RESULTS

This type of resection and reconstruction has been performed in five patients for whom sufficient time has elapsed to assess tumor control. These patients had a prior biopsy of invasive squamous cell carcinoma. There was bilateral vocal cord involvement with both cords demonstrating either diminished mobility, or with one cord fixed and the contralateral cord having diminished mobility. The arytenoid cartilage was removed in four cases. The margins of resection were free of tumor in all cases. The vocalis muscle was invaded bilaterally in all cases. In the four patients who underwent the second stage, all developed good airways, adequate glottic closure, and satisfactory voice. One patient died of a pulmonary embolism prior to the second stage.

DISCUSSION

The technique of utilizing the remaining thyroid cartilage pedicled on the inferior constrictor muscle has enhanced laryngeal reconstruction following extended partial laryngeal resection. Modifications of this technique have been used successfully for arytenoid and cricoid replacement.[4] The present technique similarly allows successful reconstruction in patients who ordinarily would undergo total laryngectomy for such lesions. Tucker,[5] following similar resections, reconstructed the larynx by utilizing the epiglottis. Subsequent to this presentation, we interrupted the use of our staged reconstructive procedure and utilized the epiglottic laryngoplasty in six patients. Our results were unsatisfactory in those patients in whom the entire thyroid ala was resected bilaterally to the level of the vocal process. In these cases the larynx was foreshortened in the anteroposterior axis resulting in marginal airways. Although these patients could be decannulated, the airway

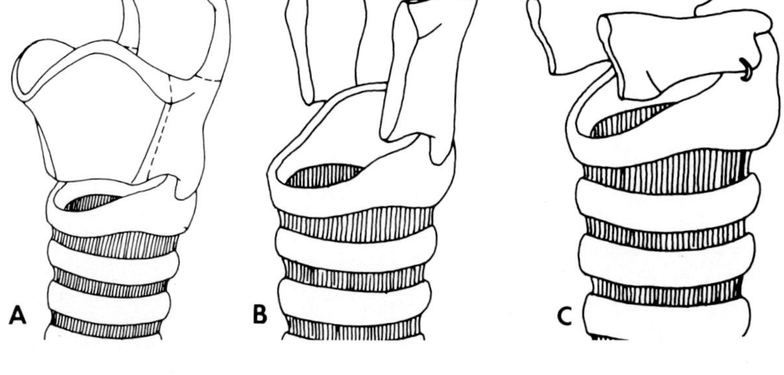

Fig. 2. A) Outline for posterior thyroid cut, which is vertical and approximately 1-1.5 cm anterior to posterior border. B) Position of posterior thyroid ala following resection and prior to rotation. C) Position of posterior thyroid ala following rotation and stabilization.

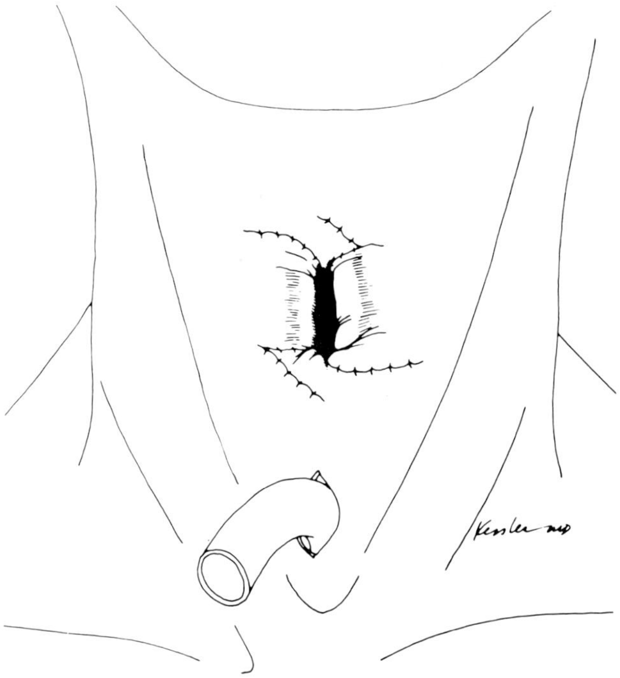

Fig. 3. Creation of laryngostome after flap advancement.

was sufficient to allow only minimal physical exertion and became compromised with respiratory infections. The airway was acceptable in those patients in whom the thyroid cartilage was not completely resected on one side. In these patients the vocal cord was removed subperichondrally with preservation of the overlying cartilage.

It became apparent that the epiglottic laryngoplasty was an adequate method of reconstruction when sufficient cartilage is maintained on one side in order to preserve the anteroposterior diameter of the larynx. In those cases where the thyroid alae are resected to the level of the vocal process bilaterally an inadequate airway will result.

The present series demonstrates that the reconstructive technique employed results in adequate laryngeal function. Although the patients aspirated saliva for the first few days postoperatively, this was no longer present at seven days. The resultant airway is excellent and the voice is good but husky.

The adequacy of tumor control is dependent upon case selection. Decreased or absent cord mobility is usually related to tumor invading the vocalis muscle. The patient who exhibits decreased cord mobility or fixation secondary to posterior subglottic extension or infiltration of the cricoarytenoid joint is not a candidate for this procedure.

The follow-up period in this small series is sufficient to conclude that in selected cases of bilateral glottic carcinoma partial laryngeal resection yields adequate survival in patients who would otherwise be treated by total laryngectomy.

REFERENCES

1. McGavran MH, Spjut HJ, Ogura JH. Laryngofissure in the treatment of laryngeal carcinoma: a critical analysis of success and failure. Laryngoscope 1959; 69:44-53.

2. Biller HF, Blaugrund SM, Som ML. Decreasing limitations of partial laryngectomy for vocal cord cancer. Can J Otolaryngol 1975; 4:432-3.

3. Conley J. Regional skin flaps in partial laryngectomy. Laryngoscope 1975; 85:942-9.

4. Biller HF, Som ML. Vertical partial laryngectomy for glottic carcinoma with posterior subglottic extension. Ann Otol Rhinol Laryngol 1977; 86:715-8.

5. Tucker HM, Wood BG, Levine H, Katz R. Glottic reconstruction after near total laryngectomy. Laryngoscope 1979; 89:609-17.

≈

TRACHEOESOPHAGEAL PUNCTURE FOR ALARYNGEAL VOICE RESTORATION

BENJAMIN G. WOOD, MD
HARVEY M. TUCKER, MD
MELINDA G. RUSNOV, MA
HOWARD L. LEVINE, MD

CLEVELAND, OHIO

Thirty-two tracheoesophageal punctures (TEP) were performed on 30 patients by The Cleveland Clinic Foundation Department of Otolaryngology and Communicative Disorders. In all cases, the Blom-Singer duckbill prosthesis was utilized for alaryngeal voice restoration. Ninety-three percent of patients were able to produce significantly better voice following TEP when compared to their preoperative mode of communication. The preoperative orientation/evaluation format, surgical technique, success-failure ratios, and possible factors affecting successful TEP voice restoration are examined.

INTRODUCTION

From February 1, 1980, to April 30, 1981, 32 tracheoesophageal punctures (TEP) were performed on 30 total laryngectomy patients by The Cleveland Clinic Foundation Department of Otolaryngology and Communicative Disorders. In all cases, the Blom-Singer duckbill prosthesis was utilized for alaryngeal voice restoration. All 30 surgical procedures were accomplished by the senior author, with the preoperative and postoperative speech pathology support being provided by a single individual (MGR).

If the total laryngectomy was accomplished by one of the members of The Cleveland Clinic Foundation Department of Otolaryngology, the abovementioned speech pathologist reviewed in detail the various modalities of alaryngeal voice communication available to the patient. Total laryngectomees specifically seeking or referred for surgical voice restoration underwent an intensive preoperative orientation to the surgical procedure with the same speech pathologist (Table 1). Patients desiring further consideration for surgical candidacy were next *jointly* evaluated in the outpatient clinic by the surgeon and the speech pathologist. This preoperative evaluation included a complete otolaryngological-head and neck examination, an air insufflation test, a detailed explanation of the TEP and postoperative regimen, and, finally, patient selection. We continue to utilize the air insufflation test for prognostic purposes despite a significant number of false-negative results. In Table 2 the patient criteria, which we feel largely determine the success or failure of this particular surgical procedure, are listed in descending order of importance.

TABLE 1. PREOPERATIVE ORIENTATION OF TRACHEOESOPHAGEAL PUNCTURE PATIENTS

Alaryngeal voice restoration: various alternatives (historical development of Singer-Blom technique)
Review of pertinent anatomic and physiologic principles
Representative postop results (live, videotaped)

TABLE 2. CRITERIA FOR SELECTION OF TRACHEOESOPHAGEAL PUNCTURE PATIENTS

Supratentorial factors
Motivation
Learning capability
Patient expectations
Adequate manual dexterity and vision
Stomal factors
Anatomy
Size
Maturity
General physical status, especially the cardiopulmonary system
Results of air-insufflation test

SURGICAL TECHNIQUE

The senior author adopted Singer and Blom's technique with minor modifications.[1] Under general anesthesia and complete neuromuscular relaxation, pharyngoscopy and esophagoscopy is carried out with the largest conventional esophagoscope available. The base of the tongue is palpated for suspicious areas of induration and the lumen of the stoma digitally examined for peritracheal extrinsic masses.

A specially adapted Robert's esophagoscope (0.9 x 1.3 x 30 cm) is then introduced and rotated 180° so that the dorsal "window" can be palpated directly beneath the posterior tracheal wall. A No. 14 gauge angiocather needle (No. 16 gauge angiocatheter x 61 cm) is fashioned in a "gentle-C" and introduced through the tracheoesophageal wall into the lumen of the esophagoscope via the dorsal "window" (Fig. 1). The puncture is made at the 12-o'clock position approximately 1-1.5 cm inferior to the mucocutaneous junction on the posterior tracheal wall. The No. 16 gauge angiocatheter is

From The Cleveland Clinic Foundation.

Presented at the meeting of the American Laryngological Association, Vancouver, British Columbia, May 10-11, 1981.

REPRINTS — Benjamin G. Wood, MD, The Cleveland Clinic Foundation, 9500 Euclid Avenue, Cleveland, OH 44106.

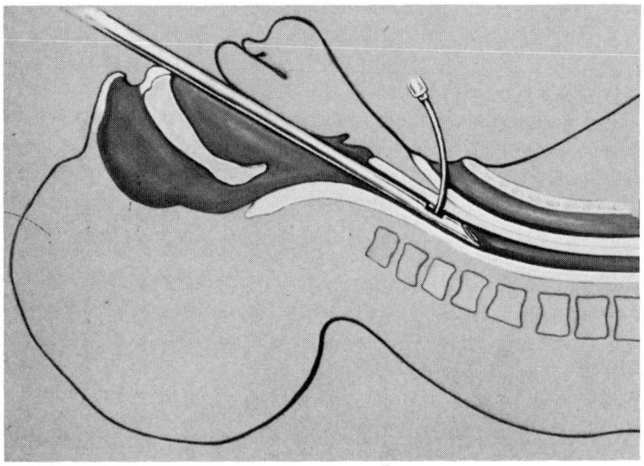

Fig. 1. No. 14 gauge angiocatheter needle being introduced through the tracheoesophageal wall and into the dorsal "window" of the specially adapted esophagoscope.

then threaded out of the oral cavity and the distal end secured to a No. 12 French Argyle catheter. With the puncture site being dilated with a fine, curved hemostat, the Argyle catheter is pulled through the esophageal lumen and into the oral cavity. Stenting of the tracheoesophageal fistula tract is accomplished in either a circumferential or distal esophageal manner (Fig. 2A, B). The Argyle catheter(s) are left in place for 48-72 hours. Thereafter, the patient is referred to the speech pathologist for instruction relative to the "dynamics" of the Blom-Singer prosthesis (ie, fitting, digital stomal occlusion, placement, and retention). Most patients are discharged from the hospital within two or three days and followed on a regular outpatient basis by both the surgeon and speech pathologist for a minimum of one year.

RESULTS

Thirty patients underwent 32 tracheoesophageal punctures for alaryngeal voice restoration utilizing

TABLE 3. CHARACTERISTICS OF TRACHEOESOPHAGEAL PUNCTURE PATIENTS (N = 30)

Male: female	19:11
Age range	44 - 77 yrs
Follow-up time	1 - 15 mo
Preop communication (No. of patients)	
Writing/nonvocal speech	10
Artificial device	15
Artificial device and esophageal speech	2
Esophageal speech	3

the Blom-Singer duckbill prosthesis between February 1, 1980, and April 30, 1981. Two patients required repeat TEP for complete stenosis of the fistula tract following displacement of the prosthesis due to incorrect taping. This series consisted of 19 males and 11 females ranging in age from 44 to 77 years. Follow-up ranged from 1 to 15 months; analysis of pre-TEP modes of communication is presented in Table 3. All ten patients who utilized writing and/or nonvocal speech had refused the use of an artificial device, and as one might expect, opted against conventional esophageal speech training. The 15 individuals who relied solely on artificial devices either did not attempt to develop conventional esophageal speech skills or quickly withdrew from available speech pathology programs.

A patient was deemed a success if the post-TEP voice was judged better than the pre-TEP mode of communication by the patient, one or more family members, and the speech pathologist. Twenty-eight patients were classified as successes while two were felt to be failures (Table 4). One of these two subsequently obtained good voice following a partial pharyngeal myectomy and superior esophageal myotomy. The other patient developed a cervical cellulitis when the TEP was mistakenly placed too superior in the tracheal stoma. This readily responded to systemic antibiotic therapy and removal

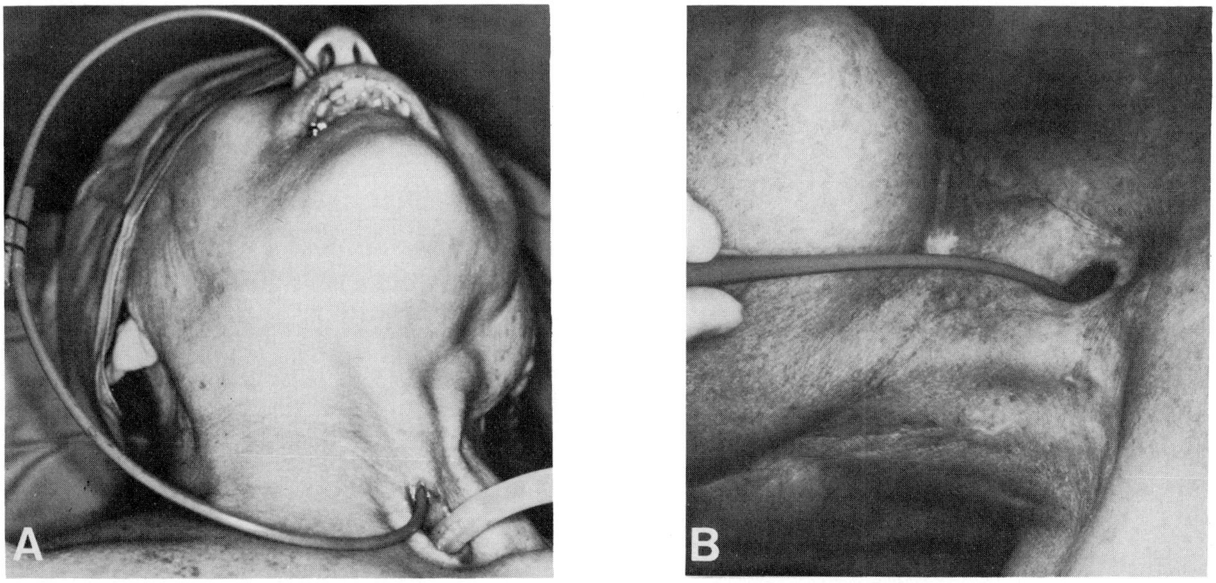

Fig. 2. A) Circumferential stenting using two No. 12 Argyle catheters. B) Distal esophageal stenting using one No. 12 Argyle catheter.

TABLE 4. EVALUATION OF TRACHEOESOPHAGEAL PUNCTURE PROCEDURE (N = 30)

		No. of Patients
Successes		28
Failures		2
Salvaged with partial pharyngeal myectomy/superior esophageal myotomy	1	
Technical error (patient refused repeat TEP)	1	
"Adjusted" successes		25
Failures		3
Required repeat TEP (incorrect taping)	2	
Prosthesis removed at patient's request (unrealistic expectations)	1	

TABLE 5. MORTALITY AND MORBIDITY OF TRACHEOESOPHAGEAL PUNCTURE PATIENTS (N = 2)

Deaths	0
Mediastinitis	0
Chronic aspiration	0
Persistent tracheoesophageal fistula following removal of prosthesis	0
Significant crusting/increased tracheobronchial secretions	0
Cervical cellulitis	1
Acute post-TEP "leak"	1

of the Argyle catheter stent, but the patient subsequently refused a repeat procedure. It is obvious that the above results are skewed in that approximately 80% of our patients had not developed any esophageal speech capability. Any functional alaryngeal speech obtained from the TEP would therefore, in most cases, be superior to their preoperative mode of communication. The authors feel, however, that the resultant alaryngeal voice is more than just functional when compared to conventional esophageal speech (see below). Also, these patients were willing to undergo a secondary surgical procedure and assume long-term care of the Blom-Singer prosthesis, but not to pursue esophageal speech training for the optimal length of time.

"Adjusted" successes are not based on alaryngeal voice restoration criteria but on the design of this particular surgical procedure and the biomechanical properties of the Blom-Singer prosthesis. Since this technique does not provide for the creation of a permanent fistula and the duckbill prosthesis is not self-retaining, prolonged displacement of the prosthesis will usually result in reasonably rapid stenosis of the tract, thus requiring a repeat TEP. One patient expected unrealistic voice production from the procedure and after four months demanded that the operation be reversed. The prosthesis was removed and the fistula tract healed spontaneously within 72 hours without sequelae. The author includes this as a failure since he strongly suspected during the preoperative evaluation that this might occur, but encouraged the patient to proceed with surgery anyway.

No deaths occurred as a result of surgery (Table 5). No cases of mediastinitis, chronic aspiration, or persistent patency of the tracheoesophageal fistula were noted in this series. Significant stomal crusting and/or increased tracheobronchial secretions due to the presence of the prosthesis was not observed. One case of cervical cellulitis occurred which has been alluded to previously. One patient developed an acute post-TEP salivary "leak" with symptomatic aspiration. This readily resolved following aggressive silver nitrate ($AgNO_3$) cautery of the fistula tract and reduction in the size of the stent.

The speech pathologist subjectively compared the post-TEP voices with conventional esophageal speech. The patients were rated in terms of intelligibility, fluency, pitch and volume variability, phrasing, and external noise factors. The majority of these patients were felt eventually to have achieved voice equal to or better than superior conventional esophageal voice. In the future, the authors intend to address this aspect of post-TEP voice restoration with a study utilizing objective criteria.

DISCUSSION

Twenty-eight (93%) of the 30 patients comprising this series were able to produce voice following TEP with the Blom-Singer prosthesis. All of the 28 patients found this method significantly better than their pre-TEP mode of communication. The authors feel that these results are possibly due to the following factors:

1. The otolaryngological-head and neck oncologic patient population seen at the Cleveland Clinic Foundation.
2. The preoperative orientation and evaluation format, which may result in improved patient selection.
3. The concept of a single "surgeon - speech pathologist team" approach.
4. Finally, and probably most importantly, excellent speech pathology support.

ACKNOWLEDGMENT — The authors are extremely grateful for the assistance of Ms. Kathy Jung (Department of Medical Illustrations) and Mrs. Elaine Mead (Department of Otolaryngology) of the Cleveland Clinic Foundation in the preparation of this manuscript for publication.

REFERENCES

1. Singer MI, Blom ED. An endoscopic technique for restoration of voice after laryngectomy. Ann Otol Rhinol Laryngol 1980; 529-33.

Ann Otol 90:1981

LIMITATIONS OF THE BLOM-SINGER TECHNIQUE FOR VOICE RESTORATION

J. OLIVER DONEGAN, MD

JACK L. GLUCKMAN, MD

JAGDEV SINGH, MD

CINCINNATI, OHIO

The loss of voice following total laryngectomy is a severe blow to a patient's functional and psychological well-being. Since the first laryngectomy numerous attempts at voice restoration have been attempted with only limited success. The tracheoesophageal puncture with insertion of the Blom-Singer valve is a major development in neoglottic reconstruction. Initial reports on the use of this technique have been very encouraging. Our initial experience has not been entirely satisfactory. The difficulties encountered include: 1) inability to manage the prosthesis in the home setting; 2) anatomical problems; 3) inability to produce fluent speech. While it is our impression that this new technique is the simplest and most effective method of voice restoration, it is not appropriate for all laryngectomees. Great care should be exercised in patient selection, and this may eliminate many of the difficulties encountered.

INTRODUCTION

The loss of speech following total laryngectomy constitutes a severe blow to the patient's functional and psychological well-being. The restoration of speech, therefore, is a major priority in the rehabilitation of these patients. Esophageal speech remains the best and preferred method for vocal rehabilitation. However, a certain percentage of patients (approximately 50%) are unable to learn this method of phonation. These patients are compelled to resort to electronic devices in order to communicate. Over the years a wide variety of innovative procedures have been devised to help these patients, but with no single procedure offering reliable reproducible results.[1-4]

In recent years Singer and Blom have developed a technique which overcomes many of the difficulties encountered with other procedures.[5] This simple techinque has now been adopted as the procedure of choice by many surgeons with apparently good results, and obviously represents a major breakthrough in neoglottic reconstruction. The advantages cited for this new technique are: 1) simplicity; 2) minimal morbidity; and 3) high rate of success. For these reasons approximately 18 months ago this technique was adopted as the primary method of voice restoration at the University of Cincinnati Medical Center in those patients who had failed to develop esophageal speech. Our results to date have been somewhat disappointing with a significant number of problems being encountered, particularly among our VA patients, and our experience with these problems is the basis of this report.

METHODS

Twenty-three patients treated between February 1980 and February 1981 at the University of Cincinnati Medical Center underwent duckbill neoglottic reconstruction. There were 17 males and 6 females in the series. Their ages ranged from 51 to 77 years. Fourteen patients of the 23 had undergone radical neck dissection associated with the laryngectomy. Either preoperative or postoperative radiation therapy was used in 50% of the patients. All patients had failed to develop esophageal speech after a minimum of six months therapy.

The patients were assessed preoperatively by the surgeon and the speech therapist. The air insufflation test was used in all patients in an attempt to predict the outcome of the procedure, but was found to be of limited value in predicting success or failure of the tracheoesophageal puncture.

The operative procedure was performed as described by Singer and Blom.[5] A midline tracheoseophageal fistula was created and stented open for 48 hours by a No. 14 Foley catheter. On removal of this catheter the duckbill prosthesis was inserted and the speech therapist instructed the patient in the use and care of the tube. The average hospital stay was five days.

RESULTS

A successful outcome was considered achieved if the patient attained fluent and intelligible speech and was willing and able to maintain the prosthesis unaided. Inability to achieve these goals was regarded as a failure. Unlike Singer and Blom we have included willingness and ability to maintain the prosthesis in the criteria for success.[5] We feel this is necessary in reporting results as fluency of speech only is not a true indication of how well these patients achieve vocal rehabilitation. Of the 23 patients in this series, 13 were deemed successful (56%), and there were 10 failures. Seven of the failures were due to the patients' inability to care for the prosthesis in a home setting despite having

From the Department of Otolaryngology and Maxillofacial Surgery, University of Cincinnati Medical Center.

Presented at the meeting of the American Laryngological Association, Vancouver, British Columbia, May 10-11, 1981.

REPRINTS — J. Oliver Donegan, MD, Dept. of Otolaryngology and Maxillofacial Surgery, University of Cincinnati Medical Center, Cincinnati, OH 45267.

achieved fluent speech. The problems encountered included difficulty manipulating the prosthesis into position after cleaning and difficulty maintaining the prosthesis in position, and a few simply left the prosthesis out for prolonged periods allowing the fistula to close. One stated he noted blood and purulent secretions in the fistula tract on cleaning and he allowed it to close in spite of having developed fluent speech. Another patient developed a stricture in the fistula tract, and it too was allowed to close before adequate dilatation could be performed. This patient also had developed fluent speech. Three others in the failure group had nonfluent speech. One patient had pharyngeal reconstruction performed with a free jejunal graft. Her speech was of unacceptable quality, probably due to the voluminous nature of the jejunal lumen. This was partially corrected by the simultaneous compression of the jejunum while speaking, which increased the volume and quality of the speech somewhat. However, she became discouraged and eventually decided that she did not want to continue with it. The other two nonfluent speakers had problems with pharyngeal spasm and redundant pharyngeal mucosa.

DISCUSSION

The Blom-Singer technique is a dramatic advance in neoglottic reconstructive surgery. The operative procedure itself is technically simple with few complications, and satisfactory results may be expected. There are limitations to this procedure, however, and they may be divided into three groups.

Inability to Manage the Prosthesis. This accounted for the largest number of failures (7) in spite of careful screening preoperatively. Most of this group of patients were from the VA Hospital series. This group was less willing and able to cope with the use and care of the prosthesis than others. We feel that perhaps more careful counselling preoperatively and postoperatively and more careful selection of patients in the future will remedy this particular reason for failure. The clinical psychologist may be of help in screening these patients.

Anatomical Problems. Ideally the tracheal stoma must be located above the sternum and must be of adequate dimensions. If stomal stenosis exists this should be revised prior to performing the tracheoesophageal fistula. A recessed stoma may make taping and care of the tube more difficult but can usually be overcome with assistance from the speech therapist. If pharyngeal stenosis exists then it is less likely that this procedure will be successful. If stenosis is suspected preoperatively a barium swallow should be performed to assess the pharyngeal and esophageal lumen. Pharyngeal and esophageal dilatation may remedy a moderate stenosis. A stenosis secondary to the use of a deltopectoral flap for reconstruction is more difficult to deal with and it is unlikely that a successful outcome will be achieved in these patients.

Inability to Produce Fluent Speech. Only three of our failures were due to inability to produce fluent speech. One of these patients had apparent difficulty with pharyngeal muscular spasm and a great amount of effort was necessary on his part to produce any speech at all. The speech that was produced was nonfluent and the patient became dissatisfied with this and allowed the fistula to close. Another of the failures had fluent speech which, however, was very intermittent. He too became dissatisfied and allowed the fistula to close. It was noted in this patient at the time of the procedure that he had quite an amount of redundant mucosa in the pharynx and this may have contributed to the patient's difficulties in producing speech. The possibility that an inferior constrictor myotomy may correct the problem of pharyngeal spasm should be considered.[6]

CONCLUSION

To date we have used the Blom-Singer method of voice restoration on 23 patients. Our success rate is somewhat disappointing and below that reported by Blom and Singer. Our experience so far is in conflict with their statement that this is an effective procedure for voice restoration in a majority of patients who have undergone removal of the larynx.

While relatively safe and easy to perform it is not a method that will work for all patients. In particular, the patients must be well motivated and demonstrate a clear understanding of the difficulties in the use and care of the stoma and the prosthesis.

Esophageal and pharyngeal stenosis and tracheal stomal stenosis are also relative contraindications to this procedure. These should be corrected and the neoglottic reconstruction performed at a later date. In our series the major reason for failure was patient dissatisfaction with this method of voice production, either because they rejected the quality and manner of voice production or because they did not have the energy and persistence that is necessary for a successful outcome. We do not wish to condemn this excellent technique, but to advise regarding its limitations as its use becomes more widespread. We feel that the technique will not be successful in all laryngectomees, particularly those who are poorly motivated, physically unwell or alcoholic, and a significant number of head and neck patients fall into this group. Despite our relatively poor results, it is our impression that this technique is the simplest and most effective method of voice restoration available. We feel that with more careful patient selection some of the difficulties encountered by us will be overcome.

REFERENCES

1. Asai R. Laryngoplasty after total laryngectomy. Arch Otolaryngol 1972; 95:114-9.

2. Komorn RM. Vocal rehabilitation in the laryngectomized patient with a tracheo-esophageal shunt. Ann Otol Rhinol Laryngol 1974; 83:445-51.

3. Conley JS, DeAmesti F, Pierce M. A new surgical technique for the vocal rehabilitation of the laryngectomized patient. Ann Otol Rhinol Laryngol 1958; 67:655-64.

4. Staffieri M, Serafini I. La riabilitazione chirurgica della voce e della respirazione dopo laryngectomia totale. 29th National Congress of the Associazione Otologi Ospedalieri Italiana Bologna: Associazione Otologi Ospedalieri Italiana 1976; 57-111.

5. Singer MI, Blom ED. An endoscopic technique for restoration of voice after laryngectomy. Ann Otol Rhinol Laryngol 1980; 89:529-33.

6. Singer MI, Blom ED. A selective myotomy for voice rehabilitation after total laryngectomy. Presented at the Joint Meeting of the Society of Head and Neck Surgeons and The American Society for Head and Neck Surgery, Phoenix, Arizona, March 8-11, 1981.

≈

WINTER MEETING — MONT TREMBLANT

The University of Toronto and the Cleveland Clinic are the cosponsors of the fourth Winter Meeting - Mont Tremblant Feb. 7-13, 1982, at Mont Tremblant Lodge, Quebec. AMA Category 1 credit of 17 hours. For further information contact: W. S. Crysdale, MD, Meeting Director, 555 University Ave., Suite 6118, Toronto, Ontario, Canada M5G IX8.

FURTHER EXPERIENCE WITH VOICE RESTORATION AFTER TOTAL LARYNGECTOMY

MARK I. SINGER, MD

ERIC D. BLOM, PhD

RONALD C. HAMAKER, MD

INDIANAPOLIS, INDIANA

The current report describes a 40-month experience with 129 patients undergoing voice restoration by endoscopic tracheoesophageal puncture and use of a removable silicone valve. Successful acquisition of voice was achieved in 88% of patients with minimal complications. Observations of this group of laryngectomy patients suggest that esophageal voice is profoundly affected by the residual function of the pharyngeal constrictor musculature. Selective division of these muscles will enhance voice acquisition in a large number of failed esophageal speakers.

INTRODUCTION

In 1979 we reported an endoscopic technique for voice restoration after total laryngectomy.[1] A 60-case experience over a 28-month period was presented the following year.[2] It was remarkably free of failure or complications. The current report describes an additional year of experience with a total of 129 patients.

The endoscopic procedure and use of a removable valve (duckbill voice prosthesis) have not been modified. The results continue the trends described in the initial reports with negligible deterioration of success over 40 months. In addition, Johns and Wetmore subsequently reported their experience with this technique and achieved comparable results.[3,4] The problems of tracheal reflux and stenosis of the tracheoesophageal puncture are controlled by the valved prosthesis.

REVIEW OF RESULTS

Successful acquisition of voice occurred in 113 of 129 patients (88%), based on fluency and intelligibility. Acoustic, aerodynamic, and intelligibility features of tracheoesophageal speech have been analyzed in other publications.[5-7] The overall assessments often equal or exceed superior esophageal speech.

Nine patients were unable to maintain the voice prosthesis in spite of speech acquisition (Fig. 1). Routine maintenance involves daily stoma hygiene, cleaning the prosthesis, and replacement with prescribed skin adhesives. Patients previously unable or unwilling to care for their tracheostomas were limited in their ability to handle the voice prosthesis. Visual problems, generalized infirmity, or disinterest precluded satisfactory adaptation to this method of vocal rehabilitation. Three patients with exceptionally low tracheostomas failed to use the prosthesis over time. In this group of failures, the prosthesis was removed and the puncture spontaneously closed in 12 to 24 hours.

An individualized vocal prosthesis may have solved the mechanical problem for a number of these patients; however, the risk of aspiration of saliva or the prosthesis itself would have been increased. Approximately 20% of the patients will experience occasional extrusion of the voice prosthesis, requiring replacement after dilatation of the tracheoesophageal puncture, and additional supervision of their stoma care regimen. Two of the patients accidently aspirated the voice prosthesis without consequence. The prostheses were retrieved with a flexible fiberoptic bronchoscope.

Problems relating to the tracheoesophageal puncture procedure have remained minimal. One patient developed cervical subcutaneous emphysema after he inadvertently removed the stent. There have been four marked inflammatory reactions around the stoma in irradiated patients. This problem required the use of a silicone tracheal vent tube or laryngectomy tube until the reaction resolved.

The most important group of problems is related to tracheal reflux (Fig. 2). Although salivary contamination of the trachea can be a serious problem, no patients experienced aspiration pneumonia. Two patients had intractable leakage around the voice prosthesis and required a second procedure to close the puncture. Intermittent aspiration was reported by three patients three months to one year postoperative. They are treated by repeated applications of electrocautery to the tracheoesophageal puncture to enhance stenosis. Nine others experienced minimal leakage which has been eliminated by a single application of electrocautery.

In spite of a patent tracheoesophageal puncture and functional voice prosthesis, 16 patients failed to

Presented at the meeting of the American Laryngological Association, Vancouver, British Columbia, May 10-11, 1981.

REPRINTS — Mark I. Singer, MD, 1633 N. Capitol Avenue, Medical Tower Inn, Suite 780, Indianapolis, IN 46202.

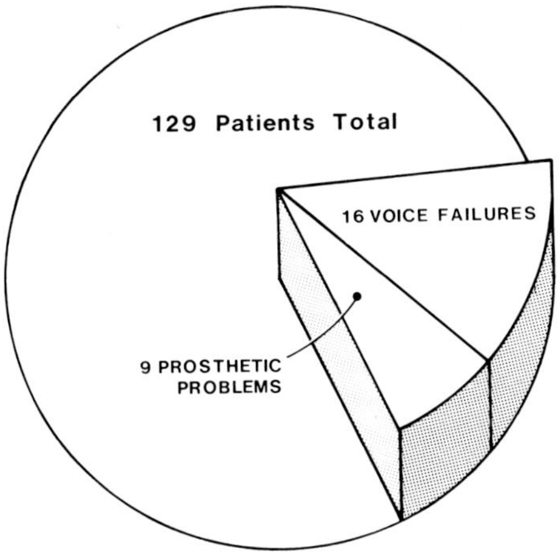

Fig. 1. Numbers of patients with phonatory or prosthetic difficulties.

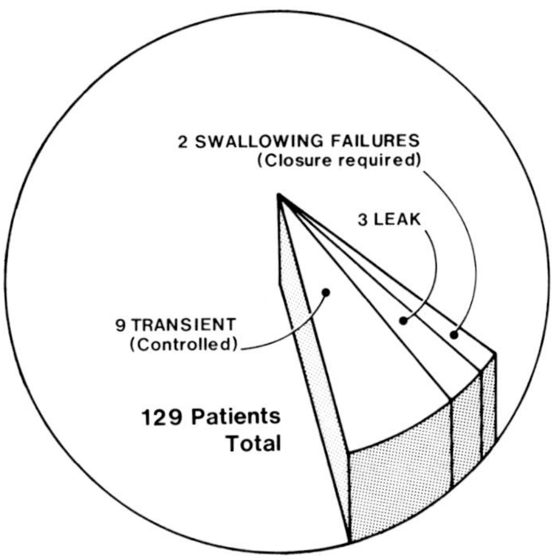

Fig. 2. Patients with leakage into trachea (reflux).

develop satisfactory speech (Fig. 1). All were assessed by preoperative insufflation of the esophagus with voice failure correlating with complete cessation of airflow during speech or brisk esophageal distention. The 16 patients were predicted by insufflation, while 13 additional patients demonstrated some limitation to airflow or lack of fluency, but eventually acquired satisfactory speech after tracheoesophageal puncture.

It became apparent that a subpopulation of esophageal speech failures could not achieve airflow across the pharyngoesophagus. This group had developed negligible esophageal speech before evaluation. During esophageal insufflation, little or no air entered the pharynx to produce sound. It appeared that the pharyngoesophageal transition zone failed to relax or was in spasm. The esophageal air distention test remains useful for preoperative assessment of spasm and should be used in all patients.

HISTORICAL REVIEW

Seeman is credited in 1922 with the earliest descriptions of the physiology of esophageal speech stressing the importance of preservation of anatomic structures for "substitute" phonation.[8] He devised a method of transnasal esophageal insufflation to measure the tension in the upper esophageal sphincter, and noted that high tensions, 40-80 mm/Hg, were associated with especially difficult speech rehabilitation. This region of the pharyngoesophagus has been called the vicarious glottis, pseudoglottis, neoglottis, or pharyngoesophageal segment.

Negus attributed the origin of sound to the cricopharyngeus muscle in the esophageal speaker.[9] With the development of improved radiographic techniques, Templeton and Kredel were able to demonstrate the cricopharyngeus.[10] During the Valsalva maneuver, a posterior pharyngeal mass was observed protruding into the lumen at the level of the cricopharyngeus. It represented a "heavy, soft tissue shadow, measuring about 1 cm in depth and 1 cm in width." Air was not observed to cross the sphincter, and with increasing pressure the mass appeared progressively more prominent.

Lindsay et al employed this method of the Valsalva test in laryngectomized patients and demonstrated the cricopharyngeus in contraction when intrathoracic pressure was increased by occlusion of the tracheostomy tube.[11] They described the participation of the muscle in esophageal voice production and suggested that "proficiency of the esophageal voice is related to the degree of control over the cricopharyngeus muscle."

The spastic contraction of the cricopharyngeal muscle forms a "cross-roll" at the posterior hypopharyngeal wall according to Brunner.[12] He felt that this was analogous to Passavant's bar in the epipharynx which is formed by contraction of the superior pharyngeal constrictor, and labelled the described x-ray findings the "hypopharyngeal bar." Brunner suggested that the bar was caused by increased air pressure in the hypopharynx, consistent with Negus's proposal that the function of the cricopharyngeus muscle is to prevent esophageal inhalation.

It had been held that conservation of structures at laryngectomy would maximize esophageal voice production. In 1934 Kallen wrote, "The surgeon should be interested in preparing the patient as favorably as possible for the phonetician. He should save as much tissue as is safely possible. Every fold of mucous membrane, every favorably placed cicatricial band, every muscle, or muscle remnant may serve as the basis of the development of a pseudoglottis. Many a striking case of pseudovoice owes its development to the hand of the watchful surgeon."[13]

DeCroix et al described the innervation of the cricopharyngeus muscle with particular emphasis on the fibers originating from the recurrent laryngeal

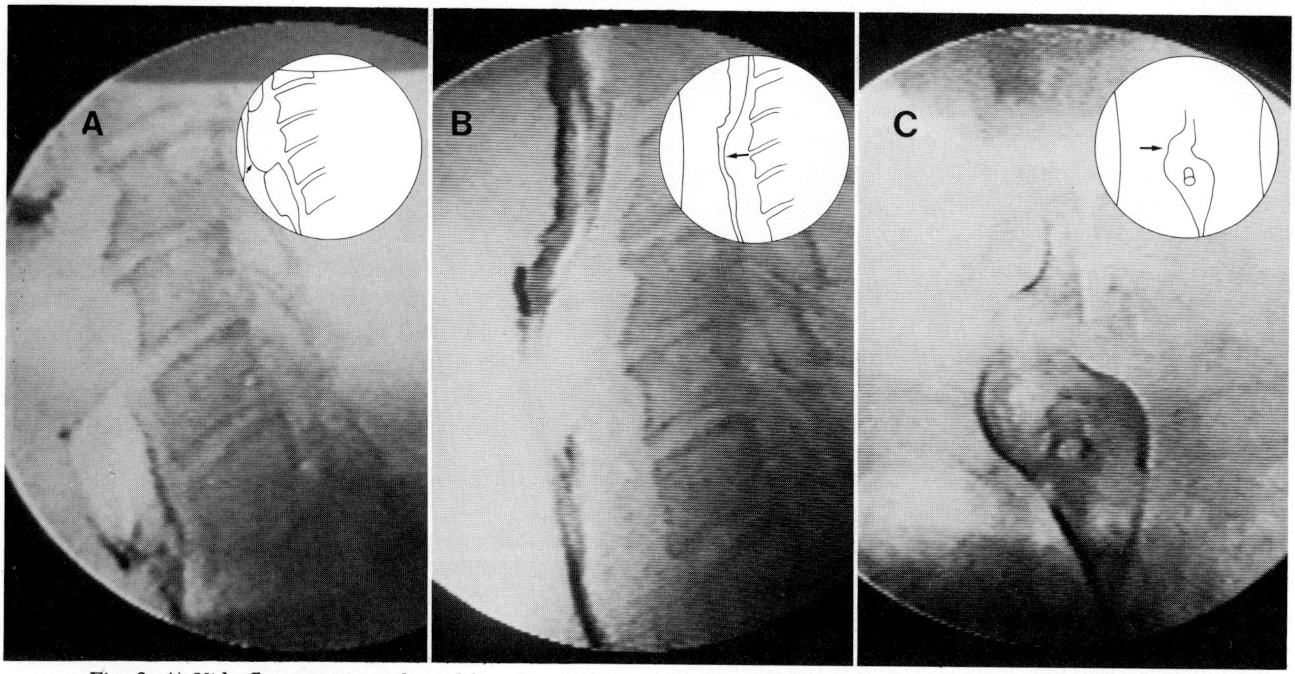

Fig. 3. A) Videofluoroscopic study and line drawing (inset) of pharyngeal muscle mass (arrow) during phonation. B) Reduction of pharyngeal muscle mass (arrow) after anesthetic infiltration. C) Pharyngoesophageal insufflation (arrow) after myotomy with voice prosthesis in place.

nerve.[14] They reasoned, "Under the influence of education the neo-glottis adapts itself progressively to a neuromuscular function which is identical with that of the larynx and thereby becomes the seat of a new and improved vibratory movement. We conclude by stating that it is theoretically possible to reeducate all laryngectomees provided the necessary anatomical conditions have been observed."

Storchi and Micheli-Pellegrini challenged this attractive theory.[15] They confirmed the neuroanatomy of the pharyngoesophageal sphincter with regard to the recurrent nerve, but went on to state, "For the purposes of phonation, the cricopharyngeus muscle [must] have the ability to relax . . . to allow air to pass from the esophagus to the hypopharynx . . . it is the air itself which, at the moment . . . it passes through the stricture of the sphincter becomes sonorous, rather than being the latter which produces the basic sounds, vibrating under a refined voluntary control."

Kirchner and coworkers assessed the pharynx after laryngectomy and noted the posterior pharyngeal wall muscle masses previously described, and attributed them to surgical detachment of the cricopharyngeus and inferior and middle constrictor muscles from their insertions into the larynx and hyoid bone.[16] Intraluminal manometry after laryngectomy revealed the presence of reduced tone in the pharyngoesophageal segment, and failure to relax in a normal manner.[17]

The pharyngoesophageal "high pressure zone" in a *resting state* was recently measured by a force-summing manometric probe in successful and failed esophageal speakers.[18] Identical pressures for speakers 70 ± 18 mm/Hg and nonspeakers 59 ± 18 mm/Hg were observed, and it was concluded that this was not a critical determinant for the acquisition of esophageal speech. Furthermore, there was wide variation in the duration of sphincter relaxation among patients. Based on these observations, it was concluded that a myotomy would not be useful for the rehabilitation of the failed esophageal speakers.

RESULTS

From our group of 16 tracheoesophageal voice failures, 14 agreed to further assessment and revision myotomy of the pharyngeal constrictor muscles. Eight underwent transtracheal esophageal insufflation with simultaneous videofluoroscopy. A consistent finding in all of the patients was the presence of a retropharyngeal mass, corresponding radiographically with the pharyngeal constrictors (Fig. 3A). The axial length of this mass ranged from 1 to 4 cm, and was increasingly prominent with increasing esophageal distention. The mass effectively occluded the pharynx preventing airflow for voice. With relaxation the muscle mass was not observed, and no patients reported dysphagia.

A parapharyngeal nerve block was used to relax the sphincter in all patients and to demonstrate the capacity for airflow and fluent voice (Fig. 3B, C). The details of this technique and subsequent myotomy are described in a companion paper.[19] The results of this revision technique are encouraging. All 14 patients eventually acquired tracheoesophageal voice (Fig. 4). Three of the patients required a com-

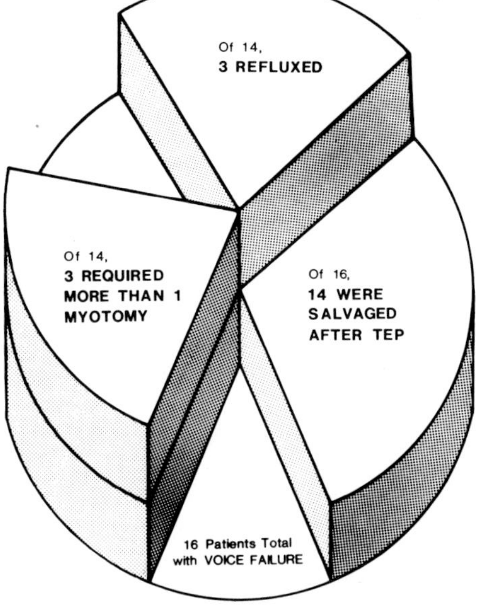

Fig. 4. Results of pharyngeal constrictor myotomy after tracheoesophageal puncture.

pletion myotomy for residual spasm. This was found to be secondary to preservation of the middle pharyngeal constrictor muscle, which is now sectioned in all cases when it is present. There have been three cases of transient esophageal reflux, two minor wound infections, and one postoperative hematoma.

There have been no postoperative fistulae although the lumen of the pharynx was entered in two cases, and was repaired primarily. Also, none of the patients have become late failures with resumption of spasm. Of particular interest, two patients developed conventional esophageal voice following myotomy, and one poor esophageal speaker has improved after constrictor myotomy. Three pharyngeal speakers developed successful tracheoesophageal voice, but no change was detected in their pharyngeal speech habit.

Eight additional patients underwent constrictor myotomy in conjunction with tracheoesophageal puncture. They were selected on the basis of inadequate airflows during transnasal esophageal insufflation. All were successful tracheoesophageal speakers following the combined procedure.

CONCLUSION

The method of speech rehabilitation by tracheoesophageal puncture and silicone voice prosthesis continues to offer a majority of patients a safe and effective rehabilitation. Its midline placement superior in the tracheostoma makes it accessible for most patients. The uncomplicated endoscopic technique demands no new skills for the surgeon. Voice sustained by exhaled pulmonary air of varying pressure assumes many of the characteristics of natural speech, and is eagerly accepted by the patients. It appears to be a satisfactory alternative speech for the alaryngeal patient.

The tracheoesophageal puncture offers a minimally invasive vantage point for observing the laryngectomized pharynx. From the initial reports of esophageal speech to the contemporary interest in laryngeal restorative techniques, a certain mystery existed regarding the mechanism of sound production. The radiographic and manometric procedures reviewed have been limited by either the transient appearances of the muscles constituting the pharyngoesophageal segment, or by artifactual distortion of the region by manometric probes preventing accurate measurement of the speech function. Transtracheal esophageal insufflation with a speaking patient provides a reproducible method for radiographic assessment of the pharyngeal constrictor muscles. The muscle tone can be readily altered by pharyngeal nerve plexus block or myotomy and the resultant speech function immediately assessed.

The long-held view that the cricopharyngeus is the principal structure for esophageal speech production must be reconsidered in light of the observed contributions from the inferior and middle pharyngeal constrictors. In addition, changing the architecture of this region by selective pharyngeal constrictor myotomy has consistently enhanced voice production in 22 patients. The musculature of the upper esophageal segment provides tone for apposition of mucosal surfaces thereby regulating airflow and voice source production. Alteration of the tonic segment of myotomy does not eliminate the generation of sound as may have been feared from the concepts in the literature.

The observation that three patients developed esophageal speech after pharyngeal constrictor myotomy has significant implications. It has been widely felt that esophageal speech failure has no anatomic basis, but the fault is with the patient.[20] The devastation of laryngectomy has profound psychologic effects; with the loss of human voice, the patient loses a portion of his humanity as well. It is the rare patient who lacks the motivation to regain speech.

Using the transtracheal esophageal puncture to study the mechanism of esophageal speech as well as for vocal rehabilitation, it is concluded that anatomic factors may profoundly affect the acquisition of esophageal speech. Alaryngeal speech is more complex than the cricopharyngeus muscle or the variable morphology of the postlaryngectomy pharynx, but it is also simpler than the exquisite neuromuscular activity of the larynx.

The pharyngoesophageal transition zone is complexly innervated and is capable of variable adjustments of tone with differing air pressures, swallowing, and reflux. The partial denervation of this region after laryngectomy has great importance for the ability to tolerate pharyngoesophageal airflow for alaryngeal speech. The air-distended esophagus will stimulate pharyngeal constrictor contraction and in the laryngectomized condition, inability to relax may occur in as many as 15 to 20% of failed esophageal speakers. Selective division of the pharyngeal constrictor muscles will permit relaxation and voice acquisition will be possible for a larger number of laryngectomy patients.

REFERENCES

1. Singer MI, Blom ED. Tracheoesophageal puncture: a surgical prosthetic method for post laryngectomy speech restoration. Read before the Third International Symposium on Plastic and Reconstructive Surgery of the Head and Neck, 1979.

2. Singer MI, Blom ED. An endoscopic technique for restoration of voice after laryngectomy. Ann Otol Rhinol Laryngol 1980; 89:529-33.

3. Johns ME, Cantrell RW. Voice restoration of the total laryngectomy patient: the Singer-Blom technique. Otolaryngol Head Neck Surg 1981; 89:82-6.

4. Wetmore SJ, Krueger K, Wesson K. The Singer-Blom rehabilitation procedure. Laryngoscope (in press).

5. Robbins J, Dudley BL, Singer MI, Blom ED, Fisher HB. An acoustic study of voice after tracheoesophageal puncture. Read before the Annual Convention of the American Speech-Language-Hearing Association, Detroit, 1980.

6. Weinberg B, Horii Y, Blom ED, Singer MI. Airway resistance during esophageal phonation. J Speech Hear Res (in press).

7. Dudley BL, Robbins J, Singer MI, Blom ED, Fisher HB. An intelligibility study of tracheoesophageal speech. Read before the Annual Convention of the American Speech-Language-Hearing Association, Detroit, 1980.

8. Seeman M. Speech and voice without larynx. Cas Lek Cesk 1922; 41:369-72.

9. Negus VB. The mechanism of the larynx. St. Louis: CV Mosby, 1929.

10. Templeton FE, Kredel RA. The cricopharyngeal sphincter — a roentgenologic study. Laryngoscope 1943; 53:1-12.

11. Lindsay JR, Morgan RH, Wepman JM. The cricopharyngeus muscle in esophageal speech. Laryngoscope 1944; 54:55-65.

12. Brunner H. X-ray examination of the cricopharyngeal sphincter "hypopharyngeal bar." J Laryngol Otol 1952; 66:276-82.

13. Kallen L. Vicarious vocal mechanisms. Arch Otolaryngol 1934; 20:360-503.

14. DeCroix G, Libersa C, Lattard R. The anatomical and physiological foundations of voice re-education in laryngectomees. J Franc d'Otolaryngol 1958; 7:549-73.

15. Storchi OF, Micheli-Pellegrini V. A proposito dell' innervazione ricorrenziale del musculo cricofaringeo e della sue importanze nelle fonazione dei laringectomizzati. Bolletino del malettie dell' orechio delle gole del naso 1959; 77:3-14.

16. Kirchner JA, Scatliff JH, Dey FL, Shedd DP. The pharynx after laryngectomy. Laryngoscope 1963; 73:18-33.

17. Dey FL, Kirchner JA. The upper esophageal sphincter after laryngectomy. Laryngoscope 1961; 71:99-115.

18. Welch RW, Luckmann K, Ricks PM, Drake ST, Gates GA. Manometry of the normal upper esophageal sphincter and its alterations in laryngectomy. J Clin Invest 1979; 63:1036-41.

19. Singer MI, Blom ED. A selective myotomy for voice restoration after total laryngectomy. Arch Otolaryngol (in press).

20. Diedrich WM, Youngstrom KA. Alaryngeal speech. Springfield: Charles C. Thomas, 1966: 129-48.

≈

Ann Otol 90:1981

VOICE BUTTON PROSTHESIS REHABILITATION OF THE LARYNGECTOMEE

ADDITIONAL NOTES

WILLIAM R. PANJE, MD

DUANE VANDEMARK, PhD

BRIAN F. MCCABE, MD

IOWA CITY, IOWA

Forty laryngectomy patients in Iowa have received a tracheoesophageal fistula and voice button prosthesis. The fistula was successfully completed in all patients using local anesthesia. Delayed insertion of the voice prosthesis, approximately a month after the fistula is created, appears to be helpful in establishing the respiratory muscle control needed to achieve tracheoesophageal speech. In addition, delayed insertion allows for longer fistula maturation, recognition by the patient that speech is formed by vibrations within the pharyngoesophageal segment, and improved ability to manage the fistula site by proper insertion of the stent. The tracheoesophageal fistula-voice button prosthesis technique has proved to be a relatively simple, uncomplicated, reproducible and inexpensive method of achieving effective speech in a majority of laryngectomy patients.

The voice button (Panje Voice Button Prosthesis, Xomed, Inc.) is a biflanged silicone device which when inserted into a preformed tracheoesophageal (TE) fistula allows the laryngectomy patient to produce esophageal speech by expressing air from the trachea into the esophagus. The passage of air through the upper esophagus and pharynx causes these structures to vibrate, producing a low-pitched sound similar to esophageal speech. A one-way flutter valve located at the esophageal end of the prosthesis prevents aspiration of liquids and foods.

A previous report indicated the voice button could be successfully used in approximately 80% of an unselected group of 24 laryngectomees.[1] Most of this group had had irradiation in addition to a wide-field laryngectomy. Further observations of these plus an additional 16 patients with the voice button prosthesis are reported.

Forty patients have received tracheoesophageal fistulas for restoration of speech following laryngectomy. They comprised an unselected group of wide-field laryngectomy patients requesting a better form of communication and meeting specified criteria (Table 1). Initial analysis of these patients revealed that 80% were failures in esophageal speech or electrolarynx use. Most of the patients used buccal speech or writing to communicate.

CONTRAINDICATIONS

A narrow stoma (< 1.5 cm diameter) was a contraindication to utilization of the voice button technique. This problem is corrected by placing 6-8 radial incisions approximately 3 cm long in the stomal verge and expanding it to accept a No. 12 laryngectomy tube. The "stab" TE fistula previously described[1] is also accomplished at this time. After the fistula site has matured and the radial stomal incisions have healed, a Pilling tracheostomal stent (No. 8 or 9) can be placed to prevent restenosis of the stoma. A small U-shaped aperture is cut in the upper part of the stent to accommodate placement of the voice button or continued use of the TE fistula stent (No. 14 French Coude red rubber catheter). The tracheostomal stent does not interfere with the development of prosthetic esophageal speech and in some cases has provided for better finger-thumb stomal occlusion during phonation.

Chronic obstructive lung disease and dexterity problems are also contraindications. To do the procedure in marginal patients with these kinds of problems may contribute to very limited success with the voice button and dissatisfaction of both patient and surgeon. Marginal patients may require a disproportionate amount of help from the surgeon and speech pathologist in learning to use the voice button. In some instances they are unable to use it correctly, the prosthesis is removed, and the fistula allowed to close. Lack of motivation and the patient's inability to use the prosthesis due to physical and psychological factors have been the major reasons for discontinuing its use.

Three patients had esophageal speech previous to placement of the voice button. The principal reasons they gave for requesting the voice button were inability to produce voice of adequate volume and to sustain speech without tiring, the longer time required to communicate with esophageal speech, and lack of intelligibility. All of these patients have indicated their preference for the voice button over

From the Department of Otolaryngology and Maxillofacial Surgery, Division of Head and Neck Surgical Oncology, University of Iowa Hospitals, Iowa City.

Presented at the meeting of the American Laryngological Association, Vancouver, British Columbia, May 10-11, 1981.

REPRINTS — William R. Panje, MD, Department of Otolaryngology and Maxillofacial Surgery, University of Iowa Hospitals, Iowa City, IA 52242.

TABLE 1. INDICATIONS FOR VOICE BUTTON-TRACHEOESOPHAGEAL FISTULA SPEECH

Patients with total laryngectomy
Tracheostoma >1.5 cm diameter
Good pulmonary status (avoid patients with asthma, severe COPD, recurrent pneumonia)
Good dexterity (avoid amputees and patients with arthritis or parkinsonism)
Unacceptable communication skills
Three to six months postradiation therapy

COPD - Chronic obstructive pulmonary disease.

esophageal speech. Additionally, they have been able to maintain their original form of esophageal speech, and are encouraged to use it, especially when both hands are being utilized in some other capacity (work situations, weather protection).

The voice prosthesis does not appear to fail faster in esophageal than in nonesophageal speakers. For optimal rehabilitation, we recommend that the laryngectomee learn both esophageal and tracheoesophageal (voice button) speech, esophageal for short conversations and voice button for prolonged conversation.

MANAGEMENT OF PROBLEM AREAS

Several limiting factors may be encountered with the voice button. One potential problem is a thick tracheoesophageal party wall. The stab technique of creating the TE fistula as previously outlined is crucial in avoiding subsequent thick wall problems. The maximal intralumenal diameter of the esophagus must be demonstrated before performing the stab fistulization. This is achieved by using an esophageal dilator (Hurst, Maloney) that has been previously emptied of its mercury. The dilator is used as a locator and is easily passed into the esophageal lumen. No. 30 and No. 40 French dilators are adequate for this task. The locator will trace the location of the esophagus in relation to the trachea. Once the locator is passed and the point of maximal bulge of the tracheoesophageal wall is noted, additional anesthesia is given (1% lidocaine [Xylocaine] with 1:100,000 epinephrine delivered via a 3.8 cm No. 25 gauge needle). Then a needle is inserted at the point of maximal forward bulge of the tracheoesophageal party wall, approximately 1-1.5 cm below the superior verge of the tracheal stoma. The needle should be inserted perpendicular to the posterior tracheal wall and passed until the locator is contacted. This will indicate the thickness of the tracheoesophageal parting wall. If more than 1 cm of needle is needed to reach the locator, the needle should be withdrawn and reinserted at a point 5 mm inferior to the previous insertion. This locates the point of minimal party wall thickness. The area is usually found 1-1.5 cm from the superior tracheal stoma verge.

A second difficulty in achieving total success with the voice button prosthesis has been pharyngoesophageal spasm. In our earlier report, 2 of 24 patients exhibited aphonia, with and without a prosthesis, despite having a sufficiently patulous TE fistula. One of these patients developed TE speech only after heavy diazepam (Valium®) sedation and topical anesthesia of the pharynx and trachea. Spontaneous closure of the fistula site was allowed in both cases. Four other patients in this earlier series demonstrated difficulty in achieving sustained speech. These patients usually produced 3-5 syllables before becoming aphonic. Of particular interest in these latter patients was the intense amount of straining involved in their effort to speak. Straining appeared to be intensified with inconsistent stoma closure and anxiety of the patient. Two of these patients have subsequently allowed closure of the fistula site and returned to their original form of communication.

Recently Singer and Blom have noted the problem of pharyngoesophageal spasm in a minority of their tracheoesophageal duckbill prosthesis patients.[2] They noted a dramatic reversal of poor esophageal phonation in patients following pharyngoesophageal segment anesthesia. They have also demonstrated that a complete pharyngomyotomy can restore TE speech. Interestingly some of these selected patients were able to attain intelligible esophageal speech and requested removal of the duckbill prosthesis.

Examination of our last 16 patients revealed only one case of pharyngospasm. Based on our previous experience we expected this problem in at least four patients. Although our results are very preliminary, introducing speech in the tracheosesophageal patient prior to placement of the voice prosthesis appears to be of significance in avoiding the spasm problem.

With early training the patient is taught the mechanics of TE fistula speech when minimal air resistance is encountered; he learns how to manage stenting of the fistula site, and he realizes from concrete experience that the speech is produced in the pharyngoesophageal segment (upper esophageal sphincter) and not by the voice prosthesis per se. (The voice prosthesis allows air to enter the pharynx, prevents closure of the fistula site, and inhibits aspiration.) Resistance to air flow through the TE fistula is at its least for one hour after removal of the No. 14 French catheter stent. The fistula site begins constricting after one hour and airflow resistance increases concomitantly. Reinsertion may be difficult or even impossible if the stent or prosthesis is left out longer than an hour. The patient is instructed in stomal capping and simple muscle relaxation techniques, and is encouraged to practice TE speech by removing the stent three or four times a day for up to one hour. The patient is cautioned never to take fluids or foods when the stent is out during these speech practice periods.

When intelligible sustained speech without

straining is achieved, the voice prosthesis can be inserted. This period may vary from 2 to 6 weeks following establishment of the TE fistula. (Note that this is at variance with our original recommendation of placing the voice button 10 to 14 days following establishment of the fistula.) Insertion of the voice prosthesis is not indicated if the patient cannot develop TE fistula speech, since the prosthesis will increase the pulmonary effort needed to generate esophageal speech, and thus interfere with establishment of the muscular coordination needed for sound production.

REFERENCES

1. Panje WR. Prosthetic vocal rehabilitation following laryngectomy — the Voice Button. Ann Otol Rhinol Laryngol 1981; 90:116-20.

2. Singer MI, Blom ED. A selective myotomy for voice rehabilitation after total laryngectomy. Read before the joint meeting of the Society of Head and Neck Surgeons and the American Society for Head and Neck Surgery, Phoenix, 1981.

≈

Ann Otol 90:1981

ROLE OF CHEMOTHERAPY IN THE MULTIDISCIPLINARY APPROACH TO ADVANCED HEAD AND NECK CANCER: POTENTIALS AND PROBLEMS

THOMAS J. ERVIN, MD
RALPH R. WEICHSELBAUM, MD
RICHARD L. FABIAN, MD
DANIEL D. KARP, MD
MARSHALL R. POSNER, MD
DANIEL MILLER, MD

BOSTON, MASSACHUSETTS

Chemotherapy as initial treatment for advanced squamous carcinoma has received much recent attention. Despite sparse experimental data supporting its usefulness, such chemotherapy is now used for a variety of advanced malignancies. This experience is conceptually reviewed, with special emphasis on squamous carcinoma of the head and neck. Factors which influence treatment results, such as drug dosage, radiation treatment planning, and surgical resection, will require careful analysis in the evolution of the multidisciplinary approach to advanced head and neck cancer.

INTRODUCTION

Traditionally, chemotherapy is used in situations where systemic disease is manifest or strongly suspected. Chemotherapy for local disease has been reserved for palliation after other local control measures such as surgery or radiation have failed. Within the past five years there has been a proliferation of new protocols employing preoperative or preradiation chemotherapy. At the forefront of such efforts has been the treatment of advanced squamous carcinoma of the head and neck; other tumors such as ovarian cancer, lymphoma arising in extranodal sites, lung cancer, testicular cancer, esophageal cancer, and osteogenic sarcoma, have been treated in similar fashion. The purpose of this article is to examine such effort, focusing particularly on our experience with squamous carcinoma of the head and neck, and attempting to summarize the experience to date as well as to post some explanation for the rationale and results of this chemotherapeutic approach. In this paper, preoperative or preradiation chemotherapy is called "induction chemotherapy."

EXPERIMENTAL DATA

There is little experimental evidence supporting the usefulness of chemotherapy prior to, rather than after, local treatment. Animal models demonstrate presurgical adjuvant chemotherapy to be as effective as postoperative adjuvant chemotherapy in prolonging survival and preventing distant metastases (Skipper HE, personal communication, 1977). These data would suggest that short-course but effective chemotherapy prior to local treatment does not select for clones which will be refractory to further treatment by radiation therapy or adjuvant chemotherapy. In an experimental murine model, Looney et al[1] reported similar antitumor effects from preoperative and postoperative chemotherapy. However, local toxicity was enhanced with preoperative chemotherapy in their study. Further information on the inducibility of resistance to radiotherapy in solid tumors by prior exposure to chemotherapy is needed.

In tumor model systems where early dissemination of tumor is common, long-term cure is dependent upon systemic treatment as well as adequate local control. In such studies it is apparent that the dose of chemotherapy as well as the total tumor cell burden is critical to successful systemic treatment.[2] As most human antitumor regimens (like animal models) are designed at doses which may be the steep portion of the dose-response curve, small increases in drug doses (like small increases in radiation doses) can have a logarithmic relationship to tumor cell kill.[3,4] Chemotherapy delivered prior to local treatment is better tolerated generally with less host toxicity.[5] The use of induction chemotherapy may allow for increased doses of highly effective chemotherapy to be given, thus increasing overall tumor cell kill.

In model systems, effective chemotherapy cannot be expected to eradicate all tumor cells in most large solid tumors.[6] Therefore, induction chemotherapy prior to local treatment cannot compromise local treatment measures. For example, enhancement of radiation toxicity by previous administration of chemotherapy is well documented, and care must

From the Divisions of Medicine and Surgical Oncology, Sidney Farber Cancer Institute, and the Joint Center for Radiation Therapy, Harvard Medical School, Boston.

Presented at the meeting of the American Laryngological Association, Vancouver, British Columbia, May 10-11, 1981.

REPRINTS — Thomas J. Ervin, MD, Sidney Farber Cancer Institute, 44 Binney Street, Boston, MA 02115.

TABLE 1. CHEMOTHERAPY AS INITIAL TREATMENT FOR ADVANCED MALIGNANCY

Tumor	*Findings*	*References*
Oat cell carcinoma	No survival advantage to initial RT Pre-RT and post-RT chemotherapy equal	10, 11
Non-small-cell lung cancer	↑Response rate, ↑survival ↑Drug-radiation toxicity	12
Ovarian cancer	↑DFS ↑Removal of all gross disease at "second look"	13
Esophageal cancer	↑Resectability rate ↑3-year survival No increase in local toxicity	14
Squamous carcinoma of the head and neck	↑Surgical resection rate ↑Survival No ↑ survival	15, 16
Osteogenic sarcoma	↑DFS for patients responding to chemotherapy vs. patients not responding to chemotherapy prior to surgery	8
Breast cancer	↑DFS in inflammatory breast cancer vs. historical controls treated with irradiation alone	17

RT — Radiotherapy; DFS — Disease-free survival; ↑—increase.

be used to choose drugs with acceptable cross-toxicity. The use of high-dose chemotherapy may increase the chance for cure when chemotherapy does not significantly compromise local treatment; it allows for more effective combinations of surgery and radiation to be delivered to the primary tumor sites(s).

In most cases the combination of chemotherapy and local treatment has at least additive cytotoxic properties. A question to be answered is whether or not the therapeutic ratio is altered. With chemotherapy plus radiation alone, the question remains unanswered for most human tumors. However, an additional treatment measure, such as surgery without additive toxicity, can be exceedingly important. The fact that surgery *can be performed* on some primary tumors may make a contribution to overall local control. This issue is particularly important in head and neck cancer because 70% of patients who die from this disease do so with only local tumor.

In vitro culturing of tumor cells has become commonplace, yet certain solid tumors are refractory to such techniques. For easily cultured tumors, in vitro exposure to chemotherapeutic agents is predictive for antitumor effect in vivo.[7] For the majority of commonly treated solid tumors, the clonogenic assay is not routinely available. Some tumors, including lung cancer, colon cancer, and head and neck cancer, also need systemic treatment in addition to local therapy. Induction chemotherapy provides a clonogenic assay of sorts, providing measurable evidence of antitumor activity which can be used as justification for the design of adjuvant chemotherapy protocols. Specifically, evidence for rapid tumor cell kill suggests that such treatment may provide an excellent systemic effect while avoiding the development of a resistant cell line within the primary tumor which might metastasize distantly. Such effective chemotherapy seems to be essential for successful adjuvant treatment.[8] As a clinical correlate in humans, there is evidence from the osteogenic sarcoma experience that a significant response to induction high-dose methotrexate with leucovorin rescue prior to surgical resection of the primary lesion is predictive for long-term disease-free survival following discontinuation of all treatment.[9]

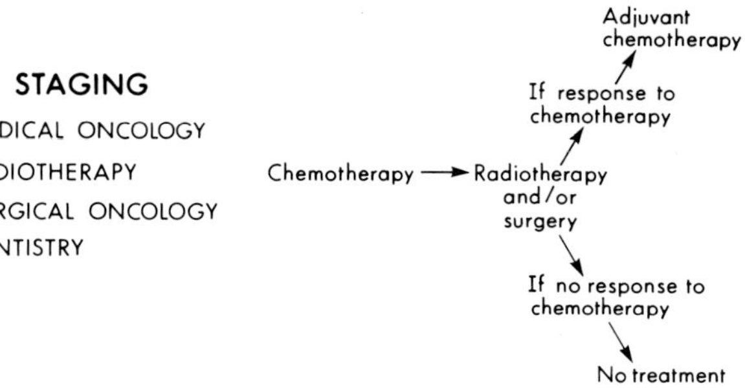

Fig. 1. Multidisciplinary approach to advanced squamous carcinoma of the head and neck.

INDUCTION CHEMOTHERAPY IN HUMANS

Despite the paucity of supportive animal data, induction chemotherapy is used in a variety of human neoplasms. In some cases, the objective of such treatment is systemic control, whereas in other instances the goal is both to increase local control and eradicate distant metastases. A summary of the findings reported in a representative group of such tumors is shown in Table 1. In general, chemotherapy response rates were equal or superior to those seen with the same chemotherapeutic agents administered after local treatment. Toxicity was manageable and did not significantly compromise local treatment, ie, surgical staging or resection, or radiation. Survival appeared to be improved in studies in which, by virtue of a response to chemotherapy, patients received combined systemic and local therapy. Despite these positive findings, controlled trials showing an advantage for induction chemotherapy are lacking.

SQUAMOUS CARCINOMA OF HEAD AND NECK

The problem facing the clinical treating advanced squamous carcinoma of the head and neck is usually one of increasing local control. Of patients who fail local therapy, 70% recur with only local disease.[18] Despite an increasing incidence of distant metastases, systemic disease alone is not a major problem. At the Sidney Farber Cancer Institute and many other centers, in an attempt to increase local control and decrease systemic spread of disease, induction chemotherapy for advanced unresectable or marginally resectable squamous carcinoma of the

TABLE 2. INDUCTION AND ADJUVANT CHEMOTHERAPY (HD-MTX-LDV) IN ADVANCED HEAD AND NECK CANCER PATIENTS (N = 21)

		No. of Patients
Response		11 (52%)
No response		10 (48%)
	Survival	
Responders		>48 mo median
Nonresponders		15 mo median
	p = 0.02	

head and neck was initiated. The general treatment program is outlined in Figure 1.

Induction and adjuvant treatment consisted of high-dose methotrexate at a dose of 3 - 7 g/m² with leucovorin (MTX-LCV) given weekly for four consecutive weeks. The full details of the treatment are reported elsewhere.[15,19] Responders to induction (HD-MTX-LCV) then received adjuvant chemotherapy following completion of radiation therapy or surgery. Significant response was considered *greater than 50%* reduction of all measurable tumor. The survival difference between responding and nonresponding groups is statistically significant ($p = 0.02$, two-sided exact test, Table 2). All patients still surviving are disease-free. Response to MTX-LCV was not related to T or N stage. However, base of tongue lesions proved refractory to HD-MTX-LCV chemotherapy. The initial response to HD-MTX-LCV influenced subsequent treatment planning. Responding patients more often received combination local therapy, the essential difference being the addition of surgical resection. Despite increased local control rates seen in responding patients, the incidence of distant metastases was the same in both groups.[12]

A number of investigators have reported positive results using induction chemotherapy prior to, and in some cases after, surgery and/or radiation. A summary of these studies is reported in Table 3. From this experience a few generalizations and qualifications should be made. First, induction chemotherapy has not been shown in a randomized, prospective trial to improve disease-free survival or overall survival in patients with advanced head and neck cancer. This question is being partially addressed in a national study; however, results are incomplete and the treatment regimen used may not be optimal. Second, combination chemotherapy protocols employing high-dose chemotherapy provide the best regression rate, suggesting a steep-dose response curve for head and neck cancer. Third, most uncontrolled clinical trials suggest an improvement over earlier treatments involving radiation and/or surgery without chemotherapy, a finding, which while encouraging, must be muted by the fact that staging criteria, surgical and radiotherapeutic techniques, and supportive care for head and neck cancer patients have all improved or changed during the past ten years. Finally, it appears that the use of induction chemotherapy is practical and does not materially impair local treatment measures. In fact, the major impact of induction therapy for head and neck cancer may be that its use allows for the addition of more non-cross-toxic treatment, ie, surgery, to be added to the treatment regimen.

DISCUSSION

The potential role of induction chemotherapy as initiation of the multidisciplinary approach to advanced malignancy remains to be defined. Our experience with advanced squamous carcinoma suggests that induction chemotherapy may "upstage" advanced lesions so that combined local therapy, specifically the addition of complete surgical resection, can be performed. The usefulness of combined

TABLE 3. STUDIES USING INDUCTION CHEMOTHERAPY IN HEAD AND NECK CANCER

Chemotherapy	*No. of Patients*	*Findings*	*Reference*
HD-MTX-LCV	21	↑DFS $p = 0.02$ in responders ↑Resectability rate in responders	15
CDDP-BLEO	43	↑DFS compared to historical controls Continued relapses > 2 yrs	19
CDDP-VIN-BLEO	77	↑DFS compared to historical controls Continued relapses > 2 yrs No added toxicity Best results in stage III patients	20
MTX	312	No difference in survival overall ↑DFS oropharynx, hypopharynx, supraglottic larynx ↑RT induced mucositis (18%)	21
CDDP-VINBL-BLEO	23	No difference in DFS compared to historical control	22
MTX (with RT)	15	↑Resectability rate in oral lesions	23
CDDP-BLEO-HD-MTX-LCV	8	↑Resectability rate	24
CDDP-BLEO-MTX-VIN	25	↑Disease free status ↑Resectability rate Slight ↑ in RT - induced mucositis	25
MTX-LCV	30	↑DFS compared to historical controls	26
VIN-BLEO-MTX-5 Fu-H-CORT	101	↑DFS compared to historical controls	27
MTX-LCV	30	↑DFS compared to historical controls	28
CDDP-BLEO-VIN	34	↑DFS at 1 yr	29

HD-MTX-LCV — High dose methotrexate with leucovorin rescue; MTX-LCV — Methotrexate with leucovorin rescue; MTX — Methotrexate; CDDP — Cis-platinum; BLEO — Bleomycin; Fu — Fluorouracil; VIN — Vincristine; VINBL — Vinblastine; H-CORT — Hydrocortisone; DFS — Disease-free survival; RT — Radiotherapy; ↑—increase.

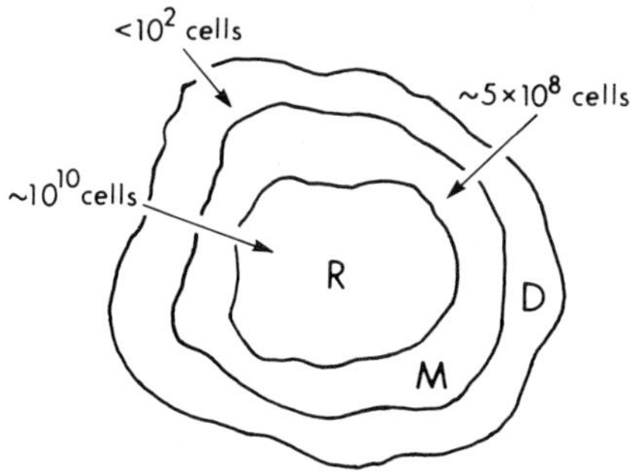

Fig. 2. Idealized compartmentalized model for advanced carcinoma of the head and neck. R — Resectable tumor comprising >90% of total tumor volume; M — Marginal tumor incompletely resectable by conventional surgery; D — Disseminated micrometastases outside standard radiation and surgical treatment fields.

surgical-radiation treatment for squamous carcinoma of the head and neck has been noted previously.[30,31] The mechanism by which chemotherapy might contribute to the success of combined treatment is unclear. Taylor et al noted an increased two-year disease-free survival rate in patients with advanced squamous carcinoma of the head and neck treated with induction and adjuvant low-dose methotrexate. However, a documented antitumor response to induction low-dose methotrexate did not, in their study, correlate with long-term survival or local control. This would suggest that tumor regression did not alter local treatment in their study.[27]

Differences between previous reports[27,28] and our experience could be explained by chemotherapy dose differences. For chemotherapy-sensitive tumors such as squamous carcinoma of the head and neck, the dose response curve may be very steep, that is, a small variation in dose may produce a large difference (10 to 10^2 cells) in tumor cell kill. While this suggestion is extrapolated from cytokinetically homogeneous tumors models, there is evidence in humans to suggest that dosage may be a critical variable in the success of cancer chemotherapy.[32] It is reasonable to postulate that a response to high-dose chemotherapy in our study was more effective due to increased tumor cell killing. This may reflect the increased resectability rate in our series, as well as the correlation between response and overall survival. It is also reasonable to suspect that combination chemotherapy, if used at full dosage, might exploit this principle further. Drugs such as cis-platinum and bleomycin have shown remarkable efficacy in squamous carcinoma of the head and neck.[5,33-36] Certainly these drugs, in addition to methotrexate, should be exploited at full dosage both as induction and adjuvant chemotherapy for this neoplasm.

Careful coordination between the surgeon, radiotherapist, and medical oncologist is essential in the administration of multidisciplinary therapy. Surgical resection fields must be planned prior to treatment to encompass the initial volume of tumor. Review of pathologic specimens[37] after chemotherapy does indicate tumor regression toward a hypoxic or resistant core of tumor; however, in our experience, tumor deposits are often demonstrable at a distance from such resistant core tumor in carefully sectioned resection specimens removed after chemotherapy. The surgeon must remove the entire area initially encompassed by tumor to achieve maximal tumor cell removal. This can only be done by careful prechemotherapy tumor mapping and operative planning. Additionally, radiotherapy must be planned to include the initial tumor volume so that additional radiation can be directed to areas at high risk of harboring tumor cells. Such careful coordination is necessary to avoid compromising local treatment which follows the chemotherapy.

It is possible to construct a theoretical model for head and neck cancer which might predict whether or not this "up-front" chemotherapy will be of help. The design of such a model must reflect experimental tumor systems,[6] as well as the small amount of cytokinetic data available for squamous carcinoma of the head and neck.[38] The chemotherapy data are taken from our own experience.[5] The model is not meant to be definitive (it certainly has inconsistencies), but rather to stimulate discussion.

Figure 2 represents a compartmentalized view of head and neck cancer of approximately 10^{10} cell size. Ninety percent of the tumor (10^9 cells) is resectable, 1 to 10% of the tumor is at the margin of resectability, and a very small percentage (between 0 and 100 cells) is distant from the regional tumor.

For simplicity, it is assumed that doubling time, cell cycle time, cell loss fraction, and percent of cells in cycle are constant throughout the tumor. This is not representative of a "wild-type" cancer, but since these factors would be expected to shift at the margins and in the distant sites in favor of susceptability to drug-induced killing, it is not unreasonable.

In this kind of tumor two cycles of combination chemotherapy produce a response, for 6 months in large tumors and 12 months in small tumors. Extrapolating from animal systems, the cell kill produced by these responses can be estimated. Using response durations of 6 and 12 months, and assuming a doubling time of 20 days, two courses of chemotherapy would be predicted to kill 10^3 cells at the primary site (analogous to the advanced tumor situation) and approximately 10^5 cells at the margin and distant sites (areas analogous to a small tumor).

Based on the tumor model, this amount of cell kill would suggest the following conclusions.

1. Regarding the resectable volume of tumor, the tumor reaches the limits of detectability at 10^7, but enough cells remain that there is a significant

probability of drug-resistant or radiation-resistant cells (10^{-6} mutation rate) among them. For the primary tumor, then, further aggressive surgery and/or radiation therapy would be needed for total cell destruction.

2. At the margin, the tumor burden decreased from 10^8 to approximately 10^3 cells. With this number of cells, given a 10^{-6} mutation rate to drug-resistant strains initially, some residual drug-resistant tumor would be expected. This area might be eradicated by further chemotherapy (adjuvant) or radiotherapy at greater than adjuvant doses. It is in this area that a finite number of recurrences can be expected, despite optimizing current therapy. The area at the margins will require further investigation; possibly hypoxic sensitizers, hyperthermia, or new agents might be useful.

3. Distant micrometastasis should be uncommon in advanced head and neck cancer. Assuming that drug and radioresistant cells are not selectively metastasizing distantly, it would be expected that a 10^5 cell kill would effectively reduce this population of cells to near zero. A decrease in distant metastases as the only site of recurrence would be expected in these patients.

In summary, there has been significant progress in the area of chemotherapeutic treatment of head and neck cancer. Currently protocols appear effective enough to both increase the resectability rate of these tumors and decrease the failure rate at both primary and distant sites. Further studies, both randomized and phase II, will be required to develop the optimal role for chemotherapy in the multidisciplinary treatment of advanced head and neck cancer.

REFERENCES

1. Looney WB, Ritenour ER, Hopkins HA. Solid tumor models for the assessment of different treatment modalities. Cancer 1981; 47:860-9.

2. Schabel FM. Animal models as predictive systems. In: Cancer chemotherapy - fundamental concepts and recent advances. 19th Annual Clinical Conference on Cancer, Houston, 1974. Chicago: Year Book Medical Publishers, 1975:323-55.

3. Bruce WB, Meeker BE, Valeriote FA. Comparison of the sensitivity of normal hematopoietic and transplanted lymphoma colony forming cells to chemotherapeutic agents administered in vivo. J Natl Cancer Inst 1966; 36:233.

4. Steel GG. Growth kinetics of tumours. Oxford: Clarendon Press, 1977: 244-67.

5. Ervin TJ, Weichselbaum RR, Miller D, Meshad MW, Posner M, Fabian RL. Platinum, bleomycin, methotrexate (P-B-M): a treatment for patients with advanced squamous carcinoma of the head and neck. Cancer Treat Rep (in press).

6. Laster WR, Mayo JG, Simpson-Herren L, et al. Success and failure in the treatment of solid tumors. II. Kinetic parameters and "cell cure" of moderately advanced carcinoma 755. Cancer Chemother Rep 1969; 53:169-88.

7. Salmon SE, Humberger AW, Soehnler B, Durie BGM, Alberts DS, Moon TE. Quantitation of differential sensitivity of human tumor stem cells to anticancer drugs. N Engl J Med 1978; 298:1321-7.

8. Piro AJ, Hellman S. Effect of primary treatment modality on the metastatic pattern of mammary carcinoma. Cancer Treat Rep 1978; 62:1275-80.

9. Rosen G, Murphy ML, Huvos AG, Gutierrez M, Marcove RC. Chemotherapy, en bloc resection, and prosthetic bone replacement in the treatment of osteogenic sarcoma. Cancer 1976; 37:1-11.

10. Fox RM, Woods RL, Brodie GN, Tattersall HN. A randomized study: small cell anaplastic lung cancer treated by combination chemotherapy and adjuvant radiotherapy. Int J Radiat Oncol Biol Phys 1980; 6:1083-5.

11. Salazar OM, Creech RH. "The State of the Art" toward defining the role of radiation therapy in the management of small cell bronchogenic carcinoma. Int J Radiat Oncol Biol Phys 1980; 6:1103-17.

12. Eagan RT, Fleming TR, Lee RE, Ingle JN, Frytak S, Creagam ET. Chemotherapy response as a prognosticator for survival in patients with limited squamous cell lung cancer treated with combined chemotherapy and radiotherapy. Int J Radiat Oncol Biol Phys 1980; 6:879-83.

13. Smith JP, Delgado G, Rutledge F. Second-look operation in ovarian carcinoma. Cancer 1976; 38:1438-42.

14. Marcial VA, Valez-Garcia E, Cintron J, Yarach AA. Radiotherapy preceded by multidrug chemotherapy in carcinoma of the esophagus. Cancer Clin Trials 1980; 3:127-30.

15. Ervin TJ, Weichselbaum RR, Miller D, Frei E III. Improved survival in patients with advanced squamous carcinoma of the head and neck responding to preoperative high-dose methotrexate-leucovorin (HD-MTX), abstracted. Proceedings of the Meeting of the American Association for Cancer Research 1980. Baltimore: Waverly Press, 1980: 562.

16. Shaw HJ, Dalley VM, Hill BT, Price LA. Prospects for improved survival in head and neck cancer using a kinetically based adjuvant chemotherapy protocol, abstracted. Report of the International Head and Neck Oncology Research Conference, Rosslyn, Va, 1980. US Department of Health and Human Services, Public Health Service.

17. Buzdan AU, Montague ED, Hortobaggi GN, Blumenchein GR. Management of inflammatory carcinoma of breast with combined modality approach. Paper presented at the International Conference on the Adjuvant Therapy of Cancer, Tucson, Ariz, 1981.

18. Probert JC, Thompson RW, Bagshaw MA. Patterns of spread of distant metastases in head and neck cancer. Cancer 1974; 33:127-33.

19. Weichselbaum RR, Miller D, Pitman SW, Kirkwood J. Initial adjuvant weekly high dose methotrexate with leucovorin rescue in advanced squamous carcinoma of the head and neck. Int J Radiat Oncol Biol Phys 1978; 4:671-4.

20. Hong WK, Shapshay SM, Bhutani R, et al. Induction chemotherapy in advanced squamous head and neck carcinoma with high-dose cis-platinum and bleomycin infusion. Cancer 1979; 44:19-25.

21. Muhyi AS, Drelichman A, Jacobs J, et al. Adjuvant chemotherapy with cis-platinum, oncovin and bleomycin followed by surgery and/or radiotherapy in patients with advanced previously untreated head and neck cancer — final report. Paper presented at the Third International Conference on the Adjuvant Therapy of Cancer, Tucson, Ariz, March, 1981.

22. Fazekas JT, Sommer C, Kramer S. Adjuvant intravenous methotrexate or definitive radiotherapy alone for advanced squamous cancers of the oral cavity, oropharynx, supraglottic larynx or hypopharynx. Int J Radiat Oncol Biol Phys 1980; 6:533-41.

23. Brown AW, Blom J, Butler WM, Garcia-Guerrero G, Richardson MF, Henderson RL. Combination chemotherapy with vinblastine, bleomycin and cis-diamminedichloroplatinum (II) in

squamous cell carcinoma of the head and neck. Cancer 1980; 45:2830-5.

24. Weitz J. Multi-disciplinary approach to the treatment of advanced squamous cell carcinoma of the oral cavity. Paper presented at the meeting of the New York Head and Neck Society, 1981.

25. Leone LA, Ohnuma T. Combined high-dose MTX rescue, bleomycin and cis-platinum for untreated stage III and localized stage IV for advanced squamous carcinoma of the head and neck, abstracted. Proceedings of the Meeting of the American Society of Clinical Oncology 1979. Baltimore: Waverly Press, 1979.

26. Schuller DE, King GW, Smith RE, Wilson HE, James AD, Batley F. Combination therapy protocol for stage III or IV carcinoma of the oral cavity, oropharynx and hypopharynx. Laryngoscope 1980; 90:1263-72.

27. Taylor SG IV, Bytell DE, Sisson GA, et al. Methotrexate-leucovorin with immunotherapy as adjuvant to surgery and radiotherapy in stage III-IV head and neck squamous cancer patients. In: Salmon SE, Jones SE, eds. Adjuvant therapy of cancer. Amsterdam: Elsevier/North Holland Biomedical Press, 1977.

28. Price LA, Hill BT. Safe and effective combination chemotherapy for squamous cell carcinoma of the head and neck. J Laryngol Otol 1980; 94:89-90.

29. Tarpley JL, Chretien PB, Alexander JC Jr, Hoye RC, Block JB, Ketcham AS. High dose methotrexate as a preoperative adjuvant in the treatment of epidermoid carcinoma of the head and neck. Am J Surg 1975; 130:481-6.

30. Spaulding MB, Klotch D, Early A, et al. Clinical and histologic evaluation of the response of advanced cancer of the head and neck to adjuvant chemotherapy. Report of the International Head and Neck Oncology Research Conference, Rosslyn, Va, 1980. US Department of Health and Human Services, Public Health Service.

31. Wang LC, Schulz MD, Miller D. Combined radiation therapy and surgery for carcinoma of the supraglottis and pyriform sinus. Laryngoscope 1972; 82:1883-90.

32. Frei E III, Canellos GP. Dose: a critical factor in cancer chemotherapy. Am J Med 1980; 69:585-94.

33. Elias EG, Chretien PB, Monnard E, et al. Chemotherapy prior to local therapy in advanced squamous cell carcinoma of the head and neck: preliminary assessment of an intensive drug regimen. Cancer 1979; 43:1025-31.

34. Holoye PY, Byers RM, Gard DA, Goepfert H, Guillmondegui OM, Jesse RH. Combination chemotherapy of head and neck cancer. Cancer 1978; 42:1661-9.

35. Caradonna R, Paladine R, Ruchdeschel JC, et al. Methotrexate, bleomycin and high dose dichlorodiammine platinum (II) in the treatment of advanced epidermoid carcinoma of the head and neck. Cancer Treat Rep 1979; 63:489-91.

36. Vogl SE, Kaplan BH. Chemotherapy of advanced head and neck cancer with methotrexate, bleomycin and cis-diamminedichloroplatinum II as an efective outpatient schedule. Cancer 1979; 44:26-31.

37. Shapshay SM, Hong WK, Incze JS, et al. Histopathologic findings after cis-platinum bleomycin therapy in advanced previously untreated head and neck carcinoma. Am J Surg 1978; 36:534-8.

38. Nervi C, Archangeli G, Badaranco G, et al. The relevance of tumor size and cell kinetics as predictors of radiation response in head and neck cancer. Cancer 1978; 41:900-6.

TREATMENT OF LARYNGEAL STENOSIS

A CONSERVATIVE NEW APPROACH

SIDNEY A. PEERLESS, MD
CINCINNATI, OHIO

HAROLD R. PILLSBURY III, MD
NEW HAVEN, CONNECTICUT

ALTER G. PEERLESS, MD
CINCINNATI, OHIO

One of the most perplexing problems in laryngology is the treatment of laryngeal scar tissue. This can be supraglottic, glottic, or infraglottic. Two acceptable methods of treatment have been surgical and endoscopic. Endoscopic treatment consists of dilatation, excision of scar tissue with a laser, removal of scar tissue with insertion of a stent, and removal of scar tissue with injection of intralesional cortisone. Twelve cases are reported, treated with microscopic removal of scar tissue followed by voice rest and beclomethasone dipropionate (Vanceril) inhalations, a topical steroid. All twelve cases showed marked improvement measured by improved glottic opening and improvement of voice quality. Further evaluation of this method of treatment should be done as an auxiliary treatment to our present accepted regime of treatments in this troublesome condition.

Laryngeal stenosis with its abnormal voice and restricted airway can interfere with normal living, physically and psychologically. The multitude of procedures used in the treatment of this condition indicates that no one procedure gives successful results in all cases. In this report we are recommending a new conservative approach of excision of the obstructing scar tissue under microlaryngoscopy followed by voice rest, beclomethasone dipropionate (Vanceril) inhalations, and antibiotics. Our results in 12 selected cases have been excellent in improving the quality of voice and respiratory exchange.

Etiology. Holinger and Johnson[1] have stated that chronic laryngeal stenosis may be congenital, inflammatory, traumatic, neoplastic, or neurogenic. Inflammatory, traumatic, postoperative, and, possibly, congenital lesions in their final forms present as firm cicatricial tissue stenosing in the airway. Whether the lesions in the inflammatory or traumatic categories are due to acute laryngeal infections, prolonged or traumatic intubations, or laryngeal trauma from automobile accidents, missile wounds, burns, caustic burns, or high tracheotomy, the development and pathological findings are probably similar. First, disruption of the different layers of the larynx in varying degrees is associated with an acute inflammatory response. This is followed by secondary infection of the area, possibly involving the perichondrium and cartilage. A varying amount of necrosis and ulceration then occurs followed by proliferation of granulation tissue with the formation of firm contracted cicatrix. Each of these conditions, of course, is best treated early, whatever the cause. Inevitably, however, the later, severe stage of stenosis occurs in many cases. The similarity of the granulation and cicatricial stages of this disease process to other scar-forming processes in the body brought us to try procedures developed for the latter on the patient with laryngeal stenosis.

Steroids in the Treatment of Scar Tissue. Baker and Whitaker[2] demonstrated in 1950 that direct application of corticosteroids over a long period of time produced thinning of the dermis limited to the area of treatment. He further showed that corticosteroids administered during wound healing stopped fibroplasia and the growth of granulation completely. The cutaneous atrophy seen following local injection of steroids was substantiated later by Schetman et al.[3] The first treatment of hypertropied scars dates back to 1951 when Conway and Stark[4] reported on decreased itching and pain in keloids after they injected corticotropin and cortisone parenterally. Though they did get some response, their results failed to indicate that this was the answer for decreasing scar tissue formation. In 1954, Griswold[5] injected hypertrophic scars with hydrocortisone, and, although he could not successfully produce regression, he could arrest progression of the lesion. It was not until the late 1950s when new biochemical changes of the basic hydrocortisone molecule occurred, enhancing its antiinflammatory properties, that researchers were able to improve their results. Murray,[6] in 1963, successfully used triamcinolone in the treatment of keloids. He reported good results in whites and fair results in blacks from excision followed by injection of the wound margins. Maguire[7] later had similar good experience with just the intralesional injection of triamcinolone acetonide. By 1966, Griffith[8] was able to report success on 56 keloids treated with triamcinolone acetonide, with or without excision,

From the Department of Otolaryngology, University of Cincinnati College of Medicine, and Yale University College of Medicine, New Haven, Connecticut.

Presented at the meeting of the American Laryngological Association, Vancouver, British Columbia, May 10-11, 1981.

REPRINTS — Sidney A. Peerless, MD, 315 Goodman Street, Cincinnati, OH 45219.

and in the same year, Ketchum et al[9] presented a clinical series of 195 kinds of abnormal scar tissue of which approximately 90% regressed with intralesional triamcinolone acetonide. The latter authors were also able to show that the amount of atrophy following steroid therapy was both greater and more rapidly attained when treating a hypertrophic scar than when treating a true keloid, and when treating a young scar rather than one present for years. In 1970, Griffith et al[10] were able to report a follow-up study of 163 keloids and hypertrophic scars in over 90% of which the steroid injection was effective in reducing the size of the lesions.

Ashcraft and Holder,[11] in 1969, reported their results with the use of intralesional steroid in the treatment of short esophageal strictures. Improvement was shown in 15 dogs with experimental lesions and in a small group of patients. A report later that year by Holder et al[12] presented ten children with short to moderately short esophageal strictures. Five obtained excellent results and five poor to questionable response. One failure was felt to have too long a stricture. In three, a series of strictures were found after resolution of a short upper stricture. The fifth developed a localized paraesophageal abscess.

The mechanism of action of corticosteroids on connective tissue is still not clear. It has been assumed that changes in protein synthesis by diversion of amino acids to carbohydrate formation induced by the steroid interfere with the proliferation of fibroblasts and, in turn, with the production of colloid. If this assumption is correct, then the "dissolution" of a scar can be explained, at least in early stages; it is a dynamic rather than static lesion, with destruction of old fibroblasts and collagen and replacement with new going on continuously and simultaneously. By blocking fibroplasia, then, the body would continue to resorb the lesion. To help substantiate this hypothesis of blockage of collagen synthesis, Castor[13] demonstrated interference with formation of the mucopolysaccharide chondroitin necessary in collagen synthesis by adrenocorticosteroids in human connective tissue cell cultures.

Another possible mechanism is the enhancement of collagen breakdown by steroids. Ketchum et al[14] in 1967 showed an increase in the saline-extractable collagen fraction of formed collagen in vitro and in vivo when triamcinolone was used with bacterial collagenase. This might suggest that steroids increase the action of a human collagenase on collagen. Although collagenase in the human has not been isolated, inferential evidence of its existence comes from the changes in treated scars and from such phenomena as the involuting postpartum uterus and the cirrhotic liver. Thus, at least two possible mechanisms of action of intralesional steroids can be postulated, inhibition of collagen synthesis and enhancement of collagen breakdown.

Injectable Steroids in the Treatment of Laryngeal Stenosis. Bonchek[15] reported using steroid injections and dilatation in a patient with subglottic stenosis and felt that this method is worthy of consideration. Waggoner et al[16] reported good results in treating four children with subglottic stenosis with injections of triamcinolone acetonide suspension combined with hyaluronidase and gentle dilatations.

Rosen and Vered[17] reported three cases of acquired laryngeal stenosis treated with pericutaneous interstitial injections of triamcinolone acetonide using mirror laryngoscopy. The laryngeal airway and the phonation have been satisfying for a period of 2 to 6 years of close follow-up.

Lyons et al[18] reported six patients with acquired laryngeal stenosis treated microlaryngoscopically with carbon dioxide laser excision of the obstructing lesions and injected with interstitial steroids. All of these patients now have adequate airways and improved voices.

In the present study it was decided that inhalations of steroids might be useful in the treatment of laryngeal stenosis.

The Vanceril Inhaler is a metered-dose aerosol unit containing a microcrystalline suspension of 10 mg beclomethasone dipropionate,[19] an antiinflammatory steroid, in propellants (trichlorofluoromethane and dichlorodifluoromethane) with oleic acid as a dispersing agent. Each actuation releases approximately 50 μg of the active component.

Beclomethasone 17, 21-dipropionate (chemical name 9-chloro-ll, 17-21-trihydroxy-16 β-methylpregna-1, 4-diene-3, 20 dione 17, 21 dipropionate) is a diester of beclomethasone, a synthetic corticosteroid which is chemically related to prednisolone. It differs from prednisolone only in having a chlorine at the 9-alpha and a methyl group at the 16-beta position in place of hydrogen. Animal studies showed that a beclomethasone dipropionate has potent and antiinflammatory activity. When administered systemically to mice, the antiinflammatory activity was accompanied by other typical features of glucocorticoid action including thymic involution, liver glycogen deposition, and pituitary-adrenal suppression. However, after systemic administration to rats, the antiinflammatory action was associated with little or no effect on other tests of glucocorticoid activity.

Beclomethasone dipropionate is sparingly soluble and is poorly mobilized from subcutaneous or intramuscular injection sites. However, systemic absorption occurs after all routes of administration. When given to animals in the form of an aerosolized suspension, the drug is deposited in the mouth and nasal passages, the trachea and principal bronchi, and in the lung; a considerable portion of the drug is also swallowed. Absorption occurs rapidly from all respiratory and gastrointestinal tissues, as indicated by the rapid clearance of radioactively labeled drug from local tissues and appearance of tracer in the circulation. There is no evidence of tissue storage of beclomethasone dipropionate or its metabolites. Lung slices can metabolize beclomethasone dipropionate rapidly to beclomethasone 17-monopropionate and more slowly to free beclomethasone (which has very weak antiinflammatory activity). However, irrespective of the route of administration (injection, oral or aerosol), the principal route of excretion of the drug and its metabolites is the feces. Less than 10% of the drug and its metabolites is excreted in the urine. In humans, 12 to 15% of an orally administered dose of beclomethasone dipropionate was excreted in the urine as both conjugated and free metabolites of the drug.

The mechanisms responsible for the antiinflammatory action of beclomethasone dipropionate are unknown. The precise mechanism of the aerosolized drug's action in the lung is also unknown.

The long-term effects of beclomethasone dipropionate in human subjects are still unknown. In particular, the local effects of the agent on developmental or immunologic processes in the mouth, pharynx, trachea and lung are unknown. There is also no information about the possible long-term systemic effects of the agent.

It was also decided to use antibiotics to reduce possible infection because of the influence of infection in increasing scar tissue. Sasaki[20] has shown that, in general, wounds uncomplicated by infection stabilize and heal with minimal scarring. This analog is applicable to endolaryngeal wounds as well.

METHODS

Following is an outline of the analytic framework within which the 12 patients with glottic stenosis are reviewed.

CLASSIFICATION

Our cases were classified as to the area of stenosis, glottic, supraglottic or subglottic, as suggested by Montgomery[21].

METHOD OF TREATMENT

1. Patients were classified as to the location of stenosis.

2. All patients were anesthesized with thiopental sodium, nitrous oxide, oxygen, and succinylcholine chloride.

3. Microlaryngoscopic removal of scar tissue was done with biting forceps and scalpel.

4. Voice rest for two weeks was instituted.

5. Inhalations of beclomethasone dipropionate were performed four times daily for one month. In infants, aerosol therapy was used.

6. Antibiotics were used.

7. Endoscopic follow-up was done at varying intervals.

RESULTS

All patients showed marked improvement in voice quality and respiratory exchange. The advantages of this approach are that 1) it is a noncomplicated method of application of steroids to the entire surgical area with the least amount of trauma, 2) there is minimal trauma to the larynx, and 3) intralaryngeal splints are unnecessary. Infections of localized *Candida albicans* were the only complications seen. There were treated with oral nystatin (Mycostatin).

CASE STUDIES

The 12 patients presented below had beclomethasone dipropionate inhalation treatment after removal of stenotic scar tissue. Five had had previous surgery with unsatisfactory results.

Case 1. A 2-day-old female presented with absent cry. Laryngoscopy revealed a 60% glottic and subglottic web. When this was removed the airway improved and the cry returned but became high-pitched. One year later laryngoscopy revealed a 35% glottic web, which was removed. The patient developed croup postoperatively and was given IV dexamethasone (Decadron) and racemic epinephrine and humidity. Beclomethasone dipropionate was given by mask and voice returned to normal. Twelve months later laryngoscopy revealed the web to be resolved.

Case 2. A 7-year-old male presented with high-pitched voice since birth. Direct laryngoscopy revealed a 30% anterior glottic web which was removed by forceps. Beclomethasone dipropionate inhalation therapy was given. Direct laryngoscopy three months later revealed the web to be resolved.

Case 3. A 54-year-old male presented with carcinoma of the right vocal cord, without paralysis. A hemilaryngectomy was done. A biopsy one year postoperatively was negative for carcinoma, but a 60% glottic and subglottic stenosis was present. Scar tissue was removed by microlaryngoscopy, followed by beclomethasone dipropionate therapy. Voice and airway were excellent one year postoperatively.

Case 4. A 52-year-old male presented with carcinoma of the right vocal cord. A hemilaryngectomy was done. A biopsy one year postoperatively was negative for carcinoma but 50% glottic stenosis was present. Removal by microlaryngoscopy was followed by beclomethasone dipropionate therapy. Marked improvement in voice quality and respiratory exchange occurred. Direct laryngoscopy three months later revealed a good glottic opening.

Case 5. A 60-year-old female presented with carcinoma of the right cord. A hemilaryngectomy was done, with a resultant postoperative 60% glottic and subglottic stenosis. One year later, microlaryngoscopic removal of scar tissue was followed by beclomethasone dipropionate therapy. Good postoperative results were maintained through the 2-year follow-up.

Case 6. A 48-year-old female developed 50% glottic and supraglottic anterior stenosis secondary to removal of papillomata. One year later, microlaryngoscopic removal of stenosis was followed by beclomethasone dipropionate therapy. She made a good recovery with satisfactory results.

Case 7. A 50-year-old male schoolteacher developed papillomata of the larynx requiring eight surgical procedures. Laser removal was followed six weeks later by the development of a fungating carcinoma of the right cord which was treated with

6,500 rads of cobalt therapy. He developed a 50% anterior glottic and subglottic stenosis with voice loss. A biopsy one year later was negative, and scar tissue was removed by microlaryngoscopy, followed by beclomethasone dipropionate therapy. His voice was of good quality, and respiratory exchange was excellent. These results were maintained through the 2-year follow-up.

Case 8. A 20-year-old male presented with a history of papillomatosis since infancy and over 20 operations. A tracheotomy done at age 5 remained to age 16. After removal of the tracheotomy tube a 60% stenosis of the glottic, subglottic and supraglottic areas was found. Tissue was removed by microlaryngoscopy on two occasions, followed by beclomethasone dipropionate inhalations. Excellent results were obtained, and the patient went on to become a football player.

Case 9. A 30-year-old male presented with a history of neck injury at ten years of age with destruction of the larynx and severance of the trachea. Treatment involved 16 surgical procedures and a tracheotomy tube until age 24, when laryngeal reconstruction was followed by laryngotracheal anastomosis and removal of the tracheotomy tube. He developed a 60% stenosis of the glottic, subglottic and supraglottic areas. Tissue was removed six months later by microlaryngoscopy followed by beclomethasone dipropionate therapy. Excellent results were achieved and the patient returned to college.

Case 10. A 30-year-old female had a crushed larynx from an automobile accident. Three previous operative procedures had been done. She presented with loss of voice, shortness of breath, and supraglottic, glottic and subglottic stenosis with absence of the epiglottis. Microlaryngoscopic removal of scar tissue was followed with beclomethasone dipropionate therapy. Excellent results were maintained through the 2-year follow-up.

Case 11. A 50-year-old male developed voice change after endotracheal intubation for herniorrhaphy. Laryngoscopy three months later revealed a 30% anterior glottic stenosis. Removal by microlaryngoscopy was followed with beclomethasone dipropionate therapy. Good results with voice and airway were maintained through the 1-year follow-up.

Case 12. A 54-year-old female developed hoarseness after endotracheal intubation for hysterectomy. Examination four months later revealed a 30% anterior glottic stenosis which was removed by microlaryngoscopy followed by beclomethasone dipropionate. Excellent results were maintained through the 2-year follow-up.

CONCLUSION

Inhalant of beclomethasone dipropionate is an excellent adjunct therapy for the treatment of laryngeal stenosis. Further studies of the effects of steroids on scar tissue should be undertaken.

REFERENCES

1. Holinger PM, Johnson KC. The management of chronic laryngeal stenosis. Ann Otol Rhinol Laryngol 1958; 67:496-515.

2. Baker BL, Whitaker WL. Interference with wound healing by the local action of adrenocortical steroids. Endocrinology 1950; 46:544-51.

3. Schetman D, Hambrick GW, Wilson CE. Cutaneous changes following local injections of triamcinolone. Arch Dermatol 1963; 88:820-8.

4. Conway H, Stark RB. ACTH in plastic surgery. Plast Reconstr Surg 1951; 8:354-77.

5. Griswold ML Jr. Effects of adrenal cortical preparations on scar hypertrophy. Plast Reconstr Surg 1954; 13:454-61.

6. Murray RD. Kenalog and the treatment of hypertrophied scars and keloids in Negroes and whites. Plast Reconstr Surg 1963; 31:275-80.

7. Maguire HC Jr. Treatment of keloids with triamcinolone acetonide injected intralesionally. JAMA 1965; 192:325-6.

8. Griffith BH. The treatment of keloids with triamcinolone acetonide. Plast Reconstr Surg 1966; 38:202-8.

9. Ketchum LD, Smith I, Robinson DW, et al. The treatment of hypertrophic scar, keloid and scar contracture by triamcinolone acetonide. Plast Reconstr Surg 1966; 38:209-18.

10. Griffith BH, Monroe CW, McKinney P. A follow-up study on the treatment of keloids with triamcinolone acetonide. Plast Reconstr Surg 1970; 46:145-50.

11. Ashcraft KW, Holder TM. The experimental treatment of esophageal strictures by intralesional steroid injections. J Thorac Cardiovasc Surg 1969; 58:685.

12. Holder TM, Ashcraft KW, Leape L. The treatment of patients with esophageal strictures by local steroid injections. J Pediatr Surg 1969; 4:646-53.

13. Castor CW. Adrenocorticoid suppressions of mucopolysaccharide formation in human connective tissue cell cultures. J Lab Clin Med 1962; 60:788-98.

14. Ketchum LD, Robinson DW, Masters FW. The degradation of mature collagen: a laboratory study. Plast Reconstr Surg 1967; 40:89-91.

15. Bonchek LI. Successful treatment of postintubation subglottic stenosis with intralesional steroid injections. Ann Thorac Surg 1973; 15:84-7.

16. Waggoner LG, Belenky WM, Clark, CE. Ann Otol Rhinol Laryngol 1973; 82:822-6.

17. Rosen G, Vered IF. Triamcinolone acetonide injection for laryngeal stenosis. J Laryngol Otol 1975; 89:1043-6.

18. Lyons GD, Owens R, Lousteau R, Trail M. Carbon dioxide laser treatment of laryngeal stenosis. Arch Otolaryngol 1980; 106:255-6.

19. Physician's desk reference, 35th ed. Oradell: Medical Economics Co, 1980:1632-4.

20. Sasaki C. Tracheostomy-related subglottic stenosis: bacteriologic pathogenesis. Laryngoscope 1979; 89:857-65.

21. Montgomery WW. Management of glottic stenosis. Otolaryngol Clin North Am 1979;16:841-7.

Ann Otol 90:1981

LARYNGOTRACHEAL RECONSTRUCTION IN CHILDREN
FIVE-YEAR FOLLOW-UP

ROBIN T. COTTON, FRCS(C), FACS
CINCINNATI, OHIO

JOHN N. G. EVANS, FRCS
LONDON, ENGLAND

Congenital and acquired subglottic stenosis is a commonly encountered problem in the pediatric population. In acquired cases endotracheal intubation is responsible for its development in the great majority of cases, but high tracheotomy, laryngeal burns, external neck trauma, and tumors, both intrinsic and extrinsic, are occasionally seen. The management of mature subglottic stenosis in children remains a controversial issue. The prevailing attitude of otolaryngologists is to perform a tracheotomy and hope for decannulation after one or two years, due to the expected growth of the larynx. Unfortunately, some of the acquired lesions are so severe that often no lumen is demonstrable. In such cases no amount of growth will allow extubation. A variety of endoscopic methods, such as dilation with or without resection using diathermy or laser, are certainly helpful in the early phases of wound healing while the scar tissue is soft and pliable. To deal with the mature, hard, fibrous, unresponsive scar various authors have proposed differing laryngotracheal reconstructive techniques. The authors discuss a unique experience of laryngotracheal reconstruction in 103 children. They define their indications for the three procedures that are most widely used, and address the issue raised by opponents of laryngotracheal reconstruction in children, namely the consideration that laryngeal growth potential may be adversely affected by such external operations. The authors have evidence that this has not occurred in 35 cases followed for a minimum of five years.

This study was undertaken to evaluate the results of laryngotracheal reconstruction (LTR) in children, with particular emphasis on the 5-year follow-up. The incidence of subglottic and upper tracheal stenosis in children has increased over the past decade and a half. This has occurred following the reintroduction of long-term endotracheal intubation as a means of respiratory support in 1965.[1] Since that time this method of respiratory support has been widely practiced in many countries of the world. Laryngotracheal complications of this procedure are well described.[2,3]

The authors have analyzed their operative cases of LTR for subglottic stenosis in children from January 1972 to December 1980. Both authors have been interested in developing methods to correct subglottic and upper tracheal stenosis in children and have published results individually.[4,5] They have also been close friends for many years and have had frequent discussions of the problems of pediatric laryngotracheal stenosis.

This study reviews 103 consecutive children who have had LTR by the authors, 55 at the Hospital for Sick Children, London (UK), and 48 at Children's Hospital Medical Center, Cincinnati (USA) (Table 1); 35 of the cases were available for follow-up of five years or more. This study does not review all cases of subglottic stenosis seen during this time period, but only those severe enough to require LTR. Previous studies[5] indicate about 60% of children with subglottic stenosis requiring a tracheotomy for six weeks or longer eventually require LTR. This figure should not be extrapolated to other institutions; our figures are biased because these cases are referred from widely scattered sources, and only a small proportion of the cases originate in our institutions. The two series are closely matched for age and sex (Tables 2 and 3). The etiology of the stenoses is outlined in Table 4. The majority of cases developed stenosis subsequent to prolonged endotracheal intubation.

TABLE 1. LARYNGOTRACHEAL RECONSTRUCTION IN CHILDREN, 1972-1980 (N = 103)

Series	*No. of Patients*
UK	55
USA	48

METHODS

Methods of surgical reconstruction used in the 103 children are detailed in Table 5. The methods used for reconstruction in the subgroup of 35 available for five years are outlined in Table 6.

The surgical details of the laryngotracheoplasty (LTP) have been described previously.[4] Briefly, a castellated incision is created in the larynx and upper trachea (Fig. 1A), the subglottis is entered and scar tissue removed (Fig. 1B). A rolled Silastic stent is placed in the glottis, subglottis, and upper trachea to guide the mucosa in its healing process, and segments of cartilage are sewn together in a distracted position (Fig. 1C). The stent is removed endoscopically at six weeks.

The surgical details of the costal cartilage graft (CCG) have been described.[5] A midline cartilaginous incision is made from

TABLE 2. AGE AT OPERATION (N = 103)

Age (Years)	*No. of Patients* UK	USA	*Total*
0-2	30	23	53
3-5	14	16	30
6-15	11	9	20
	55	48	103

From the Department of Otolaryngology and Maxillofacial Surgery, University of Cincinnati, and the Hospital for Sick Children, London.
Presented at the meeting of the American Laryngological Association, Vancouver, British Columbia, May 10-11, 1981.
REPRINTS — Robin T. Cotton, MD, Department of Otolaryngology, Children's Hospital Medical Center, Elland and Bethesda Avenue, Cincinnati, OH 45229.

TABLE 3. SEX INCIDENCE IN LARYNGOTRACHEAL RECONSTRUCTION (N = 103)

	No. of Patients UK	USA	Total
Males	32	29	61
Females	23	19	42
	55	48	103

immediately below the vocal cords to the tracheotomy site (Fig. 2A), the lumen is entered by dividing the mucosa, but the scar tissue is left untouched (Fig. 2B). The lumen is now widened by placing a CCG, perichondrial lining towards the lumen, between the cut edges of the cartilage (Fig. 2C). No stent is used.

For severe combined glottic, subglottic, and upper tracheal stenosis, a modification of the Rethi operation[6-8] is recommended. This involves use of the castellated incision anteriorly in the larynx and upper trachea, removal of scar tissue and division of the posterior cricoid plate (Fig. 3A). Stenting is necessary either with a Montgomery Silastic laryngeal stent (Fig. 3B) or a Teflon Aboulker prosthesis (Fig. 3C). The stent remains in place three or four months and is removed endoscopically.

RESULTS

The results in this series of children are tabulated in Table 7. Of the 9 not extubated, 5 have been operated on within the last six months and extubation is expected; only 4 are long-term failures. There has been one surgical mortality which occurred in the early postoperative period with accidental extubation of the patient and failure to reinsert the tracheotomy tube. Seven of the 103 patients required a second attempt at reconstruction prior to extubation. In the subgroup of 35 patients available for 5-year follow-up there was no mortality. Two remain with tracheotomies in place.

Following removal of the stent in the LTP, there is an average time lapse of 3½ months before extubation (range of 3 weeks to 20 months). For the CCG procedure, extubation occurs on average at 2½ months from the time of operation (range of 2 weeks to 12 months). In the modified Rethi operation, there is a marked difference between the two methods of stenting; using the Montgomery Silastic laryngeal stent there is an average of 7½ months prior to extubation of the patient following stent removal, while using the Teflon Aboulker prosthesis, extubation is usually possible within two weeks.

After successful extubation, no patient has developed or been treated for upper airway obstruction. Several have undergone subsequent endotracheal anesthesia uneventfully for unrelated conditions, and several are now old enough to be in competitive sports, doing well with an unrestricted airway.

TABLE 4. ETIOLOGY OF STENOSIS (N = 103)

Type of Stenosis	No. of Patients UK	USA	Total
Congenital	28	1	29
Acquired			
Intubation	24	38	62
External trauma	1	1	2
High tracheotomy	2	2	4
Burn			
Thermal	0	4	4
Chemical	0	1	1
Dystrophic cartilage	0	1	1
	55	48	103

TABLE 5. METHODS OF LARYNGOTRACHEAL RECONSTRUCTION (N = 103)

	No. of Patients UK		USA		
Laryngotracheoplasty	52		8		
Costal cartilage graft	3		21		
Modified Rethi principle	0		18		
Resection	0		1		
	55	+	48	=	103

DISCUSSION

The arguments for and against surgical reconstruction of the pediatric larynx and trachea have been discussed in a previous publication.[5] Two arguments are proposed against operative intervention. First, it is stated that as the laryngotracheal complex increases in size, the problem eventually will be outgrown. While this may be true of congenital subglottic stenosis, neither clinical observation nor published data support this conclusion in stenosis secondary to intubation, external injury, or burns.

Second, it has been felt that extensive surgery on the growing larynx may interfere with normal growth, though experimental work[9] suggests that this is not the case. Among the patients in this study, none has any evidence of failure or retardation of laryngeal growth. Many of the patients in the 5-year follow-up group are competing in athletic events without unusual dyspnea. Physiologic studies are presently being performed on those older patients and on matched controls, and the results of these studies are expected to show that normal laryngeal growth patterns occur in operated patients.

Prior to surgical reconstruction, all conservative efforts to establish a satisfactory airway must be considered. In the initial phases of injury when active infection with mucosal ulceration and subglottic granulation tissue is present, careful endoscopic bouginage, removal of granulation tissue, local and systemic steroid therapy, and culture and appropriate antibiotic therapy, together with time, may often allow satisfactory resolution and decannulation. In some instances, use of the laser or endoscopic diathermy is advocated for the management of early subglottic stenosis. While this may be appropriate under controlled situations, a word of

TABLE 6. METHODS OF LARYNGOTRACHEAL RECONSTRUCTION IN CASES WITH 5-YEAR FOLLOW-UP (N = 35)

	No. of Patients UK		USA		
Laryngotracheoplasty	21		1		
Costal cartilage graft	0		9		
Modified Rethi principle	0		4		
	21	+	14	=	35

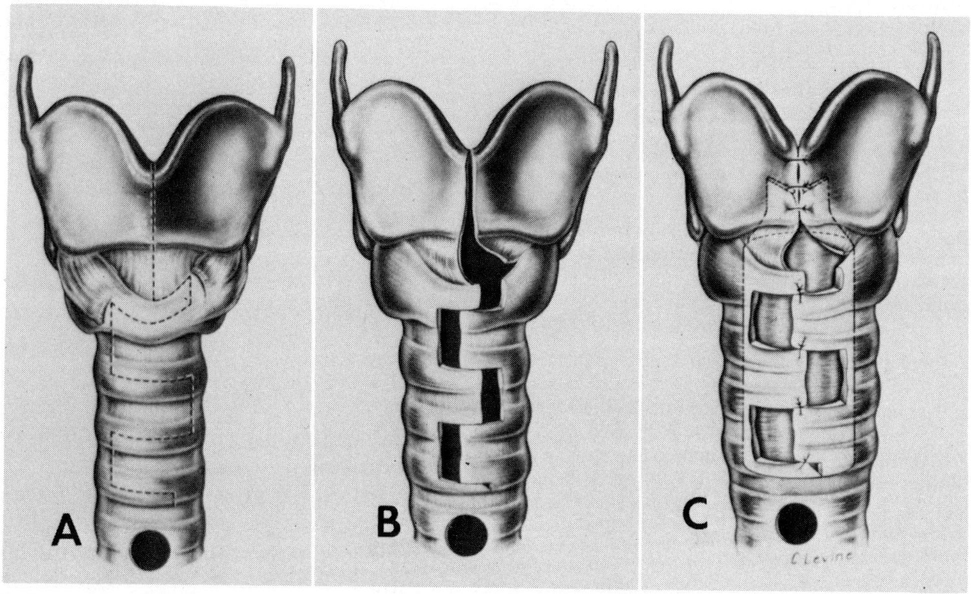

Fig. 1. Laryngotracheoplasty. A) Thyrotomy with stepped incision in cricoid and upper tracheal cartilages. B) Distraction of cartilaginous segments allowing access to lumen for resection of scar. C) Rolled Silastic stent in lumen, and cartilaginous segments sewn in distracted position.

caution is necessary, since some of the most severe stenoses that the authors have had to manage have occurred in failures from these modalities of therapy. In such circumstances it is impossible to separate the injurious nature of the original insult from the possible iatrogenic effect of the laser or endoscopic diathermy.

Surgical reconstruction should only be performed in those stenoses in which tracheotomy has been required. The stenosis should be mature and the lumen either nonexistent or so small that decannulation in the foreseeable future would be impossible. Vocal cord movement must be carefully assessed to identify either paralysis or tethering due to scar.

With regard to choice of operation, the CCG and LTP operations are largely but not completely interchangeable. In both operations, a preoperative lumen must be present. For isolated, mainly anterior subglottic stenosis the costal cartilage graft procedure is ideal. It is one surgical procedure, with no

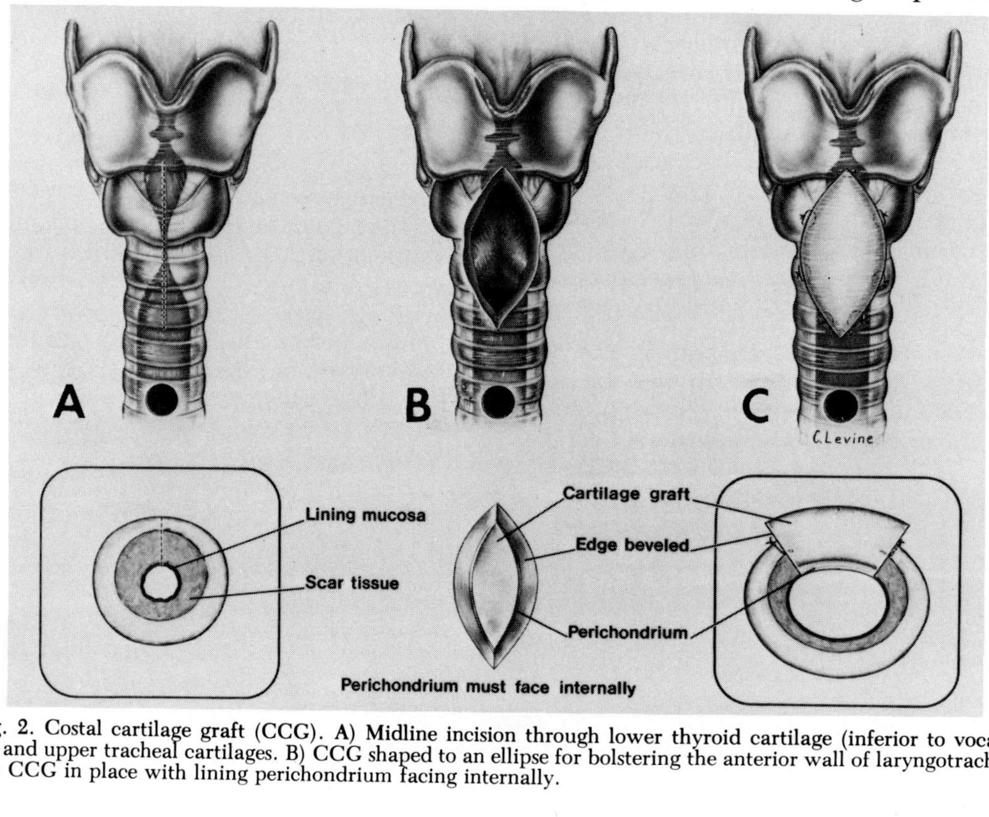

Fig. 2. Costal cartilage graft (CCG). A) Midline incision through lower thyroid cartilage (inferior to vocal cords), cricoid, and upper tracheal cartilages. B) CCG shaped to an ellipse for bolstering the anterior wall of laryngotracheal complex. C) CCG in place with lining perichondrium facing internally.

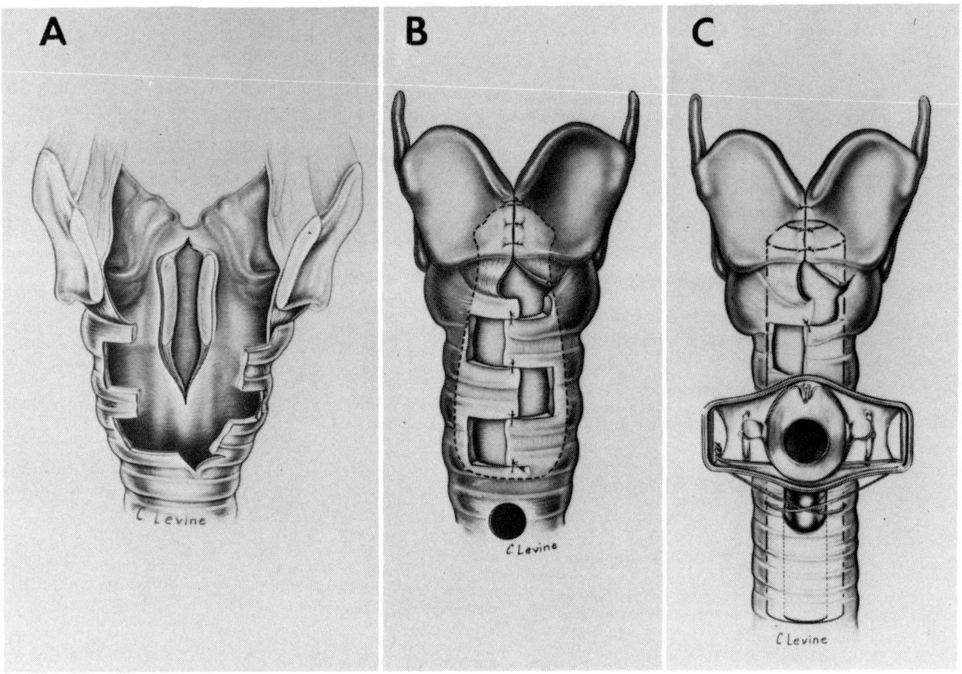

Fig. 3. Modified Rethi procedure. A) Stepped incision with exposure of posterior cricoid lamina. B) Stenting with the Montgomery Silastic stent. C) Stenting with the Aboulker Teflon stent.

stent, and extubation generally occurs about eight weeks postoperatively. Also, in those patients in whom little or no cartilage is present anteriorly, and in whom the castellated incision is not then possible, costal cartilage is preferred. Lengthy segments of cartilage may be grafted into the trachea.[10]

If there is mainly posterior subglottic scarring or if there is an anterior glottic web coexisting with the subglottic stenosis, the LTP is the operation of choice. The disadvantages of the LTP relative to the CCG include the necessity for stenting and its attendant necessity for endoscopic removal. Further, the presence of the stent itself induces granulation tissue formation, especially at the anterior commissure, which necessitates a variable number of endoscopic procedures for its removal after the stent is out. This accounts for the average extubation time of 3½ months after stent removal.

If there is combined posterior glottic and subglottic stenosis, the Rethi principle of splitting the posterior lamina of the cricoid followed by three or four months' stenting is a reliable procedure. The reliability may be increased by using the Aboulker Teflon prosthesis rather than the Montgomery Silastic prosthesis. The former induces very little granulation tissue formation, and since the stent is long (Fig. 3C) it eliminates the problem of suprastomal collapse that occurs immediately above the tracheotomy stoma in younger patients.

The increased incidence of congenital subglottic stenosis in the Evans series (UK) compared with the Cotton series (USA) is puzzling. The high incidence of congenital subglottic stenosis in the UK series is supported by the review of subglottic stenosis of the larynx in the infant and child by Fearon et al[11] who reported that 80% of their cases were clearly congenital. The fact that congenital subglottic stenosis is not a single entity but represents a variety of histopathologic conditions has been reviewed recently by Tucker et al.[12] It is also evident from the review of Holinger et al[13] that acquired stenosis is generally more severe and difficult to treat than is congenital stenosis. Isolated congenital subglottic stenosis requiring airway support is a rare lesion at Children's Hospital Medical Center, Cincinnati. Those few cases seen that have required airway support have been managed, prior to 1977, by tracheotomy and a wait-and-see period for natural growth. Only one (Table 4) required LTR. Since 1978, congenital subglottic stenosis requiring airway support has been managed by the anterior cricoid split procedure.[14]

CONCLUSIONS

Not all cases of subglottic stenosis requiring a tracheotomy in children require a laryngotracheal reconstruction (LTR).

Severe laryngotracheal stenosis in children that has failed to respond to conservative management should be considered for LTR.

In 103 cases of LTR, there is no clinical, radio-

TABLE 7. RESULTS OF LARYNGOTRACHEAL RECONSTRUCTION IN CHILDREN

Patient Series	*Extubated*	*Not Extubated*	*Mortality*
Total UK and USA (N = 103)	93	9	1
5-year follow-up (N = 35)	33	2	0

logical, endoscopic or functional evidence of change in laryngeal growth patterns.

The costal cartilage graft (CCG) and laryngotracheoplasty (LTP) techniques are largely interchangeable. However, isolated anterior subglottic stenosis is preferentially treated by the CCG procedure. Isolated posterior subglottic stenosis or any subglottic stenosis with an anterior glottic web is preferably treated by the LTP technique. The modified Rethi operation is reserved for combined subglottic and posterior glottic stenosis and for those cases that do not have any lumen.

REFERENCES

1. McDonald IH, Stocks J. Prolonged nasotracheal intubation. Br J Anaesth 1965; 37:161-5.

2. Hawkins DB. Hyaline membrane disease of the neonate; prolonged intubation in the management: effects on the larynx. Laryngoscope 1978; 88:201-24.

3. Lindholm CD. Prolonged endotracheal intubation. Acta Anaesthesiol Scand 1969; Suppl 33.

4. Evans JNG, Todd GB. Laryngotracheoplasty. J Laryngol Otol 1974; 88:589-97.

5. Cotton R. Management of subglottic stenosis in infancy and childhood. Ann Otol Rhinol Laryngol 1978; 87:649-57.

6. Rethi A. An operation for cicatricial stenosis of the larynx. J Laryngol Otol 1956; 70:283-93.

7. Cotton R, Richardson MA, Seid AB. Management of combined advanced glottic and subglottic stenosis in infancy and childhood. Laryngoscope 1981; 91:221-5.

8. Grahne B. Operative treatment of severe chronic traumatic laryngeal stenosis in infants up to three years old. Acta Otolaryngol (Stockh) 1971; 72:134-7.

9. Calcaterra TC, McClure R, Ward PH. Effect of laryngofissure on the developing canine larynx. Ann Otol Rhinol Laryngol 1974; 83:810-3.

10. Majeski JA, Schreiber JT, Cotton R, MacMillan BG. Surgical correction of tracheal stenosis in the pediatric burn patient. J Trauma 1980; 20:81-6.

11. Fearon B, Crysdale WS, Bird R. Subglottic stenosis of the larynx in the infant and child: methods of management. Ann Otol Rhinol Laryngol 1978; 87:645-8.

12. Tucker GF, Ossoff RH, Newman AN, Holinger LD. Histopathology of congenital subglottic stenosis. Laryngoscope 1979; 89:866-77.

13. Holinger PH, Kutnick SL, Schild JA, Holinger LD. Subglottic stenosis in infants and children. Ann Otol Rhinol Laryngol 1976; 85:591-9.

14. Cotton R, Seid AB. Management of the extubation problem in the premature child: anterior cricoid split as an alternative to tracheotomy. Ann Otol Rhinol Laryngol 1980; 89:508-11.

BOOKS RECEIVED

Pernkopf Atlas of Topographical and Applied Human Anatomy. Volume 1 — Head and Neck

Second revised edition. Edited by Helmut Ferner, MD. 231 color illustrations and 108 black and white illustrations, indexed, hard cover, 308 pages, 1980. Urban & Schwarzenberg, Inc., Baltimore, $98.

Structure-Activity Relationships in Clonidine-like Imidazolidines and Related Compounds

By P. B. M. W. M. Timmermans, W. Hoefke, H. Stahle, and P. A. van Zwieten. Series: Progress in Pharmacology, volume III, No. 1. Black and white illustrations, indexed, soft cover, 104 pages, 1980. Gustav Fischer Verlag, Stuttgart, $42.50.

Reeducation de l'Aphasique Adulte

By Anne Tissot. Black and white illustrations, indexed, soft cover, 110 pages, 1980. Masson, Paris.

Disorders of Auditory Function III

Edited by Ian G. Taylor and Andreas Markides. Black and white illustrations, indexed, hard cover, 334 pages, 1980. Academic Press, London, $38.

Tympanoplasty and Stapedectomy. A Manual of Techniques

By Ugo Fisch. Black and white illustrations, indexed, soft cover, 79 pages, 1980. Thieme-Stratton, New York, $24.

Acoustical Factors Affecting Hearing and Performance

Edited by Gerald A. Studebaker, PhD, and Irving Hochberg, PhD. Black and white illustrations, indexed, hard cover, 430 pages, 1980. University Park Press, Baltimore, $34.50.

Readings in Speech Following Total Laryngectomy

Edited by Bernd Weinberg, PhD. Black and white illustrations, soft cover, 588 pages, 1980. University Park Press, Baltimore, $24.95.

Surgical and Prosthetic Approaches to Speech Rehabilitation

Edited by Donald P. Shedd, MD, and Bernd Weinberg, PhD. Black and white illustrations, indexed, hard cover, 310 pages, 1980. G. K. Hall, Boston, $32.50.

Ear, Nose and Throat Radiology. Advanced Exercises in Diagnostic Radiology

By June B. Unger, MD, and Katherine A. Shaffer, MD. Black and white illustrations, indexed, soft cover, 171 pages, 1980. W. B. Saunders, Philadelphia, $13.95.

Long Term Treatment in Cleft Lip and Palate. Proceedings of the First International Symposium, August 23rd/24th, 1979, Department of Pediatric Surgery, University of Bern, Switzerland

Edited by Beat Kehrer, Theddy Slongo, Brigitte Graf, and Marcel Bettex. Black and white illustrations, indexed, 338 pages, 1981. Hans Huber Publishers, Berne.

Antimicrobial Prescribing™

By Harold C. Neu, MD. Soft cover, 111 pages, Antimicrobial Prescribing, Inc., Princeton.

Manual of Otolaryngology

By Raymond P. Wood II, MD, and Jerry L. Northern, PhD. Index, black and white illustrations, soft cover, 235 pages, The Williams & Wilkins Company, Baltimore. $15.95.

Changing the Body. Psychological Effects of Plastic Surgery

By John M. Goin, MD, and Marcia Kraft Goin, MD. Indexed, hard cover, 225 pages, 1981. Williams & Wilkins, Baltimore, $30.

Anatomy and Physiology of Speech

By Harold M. Kaplan, PhD. Indexed, soft cover, 180 pages, 1981. Graceway Publishing Co., Flushing, NY.

Diseases of the Ear, Nose and Throat. A Guide to Diagnosis and Management

By D. Thane R. Cody, MD, CM, PhD, Eugene B. Kern, MD, MS, and Bruce W. Pearson, MD, FRCS(C). Black and white illustrations, indexed, hard cover, 476 pages, 1981. Yearbook Medical Publishers, Chicago.

Craniofacial and Upper Cervical Arteries. Functional, Clinical and Angiographic Aspects

By Pierre L. Lasjaunias, MD, with the collaboration of Alex Berenstein, MD. Color and black and white illustrations, indexed, hard cover, 195 pages, 1981. Williams & Wilkins, Baltimore, $57.

The Primary Acoustic Nuclei

By Rafael Lorente de No, MD. Black and white illustrations, indexed, hard cover, 171 pages, 1981. Raven Press, New York, $32.

The History of Central Institute

By Helen S. Lane. Black and white illustrations, indexed, soft cover, 293 pages, 1981. Central Institute for the Deaf, St. Louis.

Hearing Assessment with the Acoustic Reflex

Edited by Gerald R. Popelka, PhD. Indexed, hard cover, 168 pages, 1981. Grune & Stratton, New York, $17.50.

The Oral Speech Mechanism Screening Examination

By Kenneth O. St. Louis and Dennis M. Ruscello. Black and white illustrations, soft cover, 33 pages, 1981. University Park Press, Baltimore, $13.95.

X-RAY STUDY OF THE MONTH

LARYNGEAL CYST

NELSON C. GOLDMAN, MD
JACKSONVILLE, FLORIDA

PATIENT

A 12-year-old male with a two-week history of increasing voice changes was seen to be in slight respiratory distress. Indirect laryngoscopy revealed the presence of a large cystic mass of the left supraglottic larynx. The vocal cords were not visible.

RADIOGRAPHS

Lateral and frontal xeroradiographs (Fig. 1A, B) without contrast media demonstrated a 4 x 3 cm rounded mass on the left side of the larynx extending into the midline. Significant distortion of the anatomy is present, particularly on the left side, with compression of the ventricles. The mass appeared to have a fluid density.

DIAGNOSIS

At the time of surgery a tracheotomy was first performed under local anesthesia. The laryngeal cyst was then removed by way of a submucosal resection through an external cervical approach. The cyst did not communicate with the laryngeal lumen and on pathological examination was found to be lined with ciliated respiratory columnar epithelium.

DISCUSSION

Cystic lesions of the larynx filled with mucus that are non-air-containing and do not communicate with the laryngeal lumen are described as being saccular cysts.[1] They are to be differentiated from laryngoceles which do communicate with the lumen of the larynx and are filled with air. Saccular

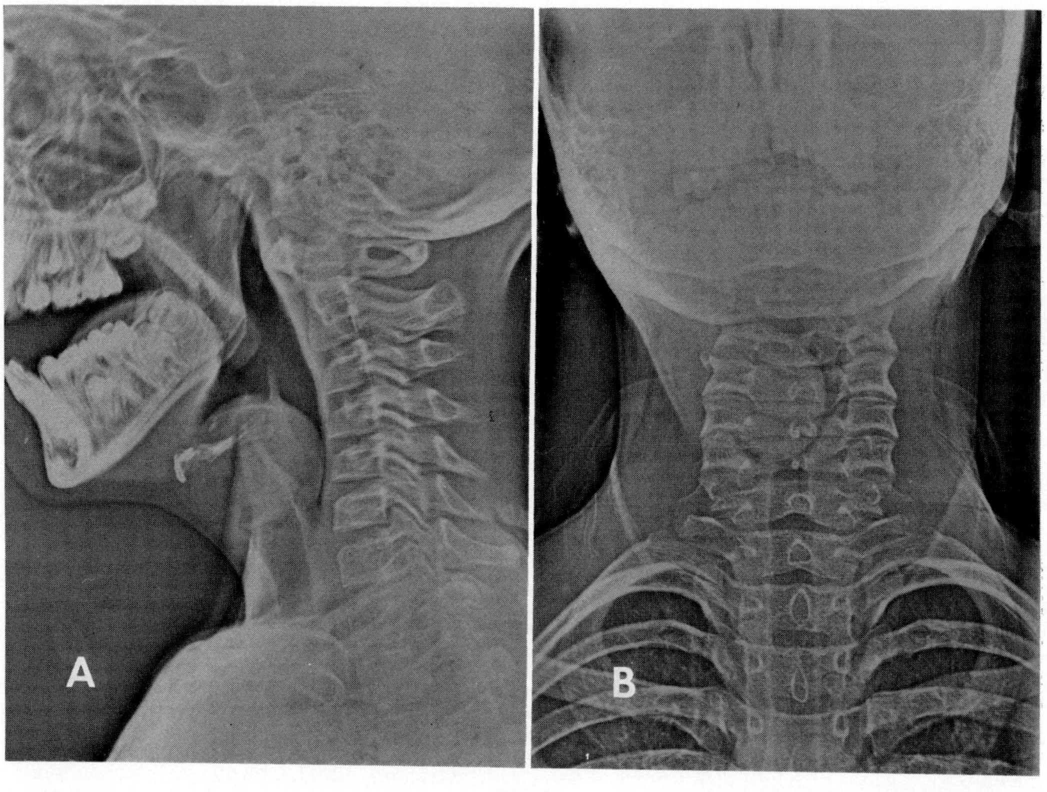

Fig. 1.

REPRINTS — Nelson C. Goldman, MD, Samuel Wells Medical Complex, 3599 University Boulevard, South, Jacksonville, FL 32216.

cysts in infants and children are usually treated with aspiration; large cysts and recurrent cysts are treated by the external approach after appropriate evaluation.

Radiological examination of the larynx may produce a multidirectional orientation of benign or malignant disease to the normal laryngeal structures. Indirect laryngoscopy permits evaluation of the larynx only from above. Radiographically the greatest information may be obtained by contrast radiography; however, its use is complicated by the need for local anesthesia and patient cooperation. This may not be possible to perform in the pediatric patient. Xeroradiography has been shown to produce excellent detail of the laryngeal structures and, as in this case, is superior to conventional soft tissue radiography.

ACKNOWLEDGMENT — The author wishes to express his thanks to the offices of Drs. Mori, Bean and Brooks for their fine x-rays.

REFERENCES

1. Holinger LD, Barnes DR, Smid LJ, Holinger PH. Laryngocele and saccular cysts. Ann Otol Rhinol Laryngol 1978; 87:675-85.

ENG OF THE MONTH

PERIODIC ALTERNATING NYSTAGMUS

RICHARD W. BABIN, MD
IOWA CITY, IOWA

CASE REPORT

A 46-year-old male presented with a chief complaint of headaches of one year duration increasing in frequency to one to two times daily. The patient was born with a thoracic myelomeningocele and secondary paralysis of the lower extremities. This had not been repaired and he had been functioning on self-care, wheelchair bound, in a nursing home. On presentation, the patient was noted to have a direction-changing gaze nystagmus with the eyes open. This nystagmus would beat to the right with gaze far right, and to the left with gaze far left. In neutral gaze, the patient was described by various observers as having either left- or right-beating nystagmus. Cranial nerve examination was otherwise noted to be unremarkable and cerebellar function was described as intact. Skull roentgenograms revealed platybasia and computerized tomography demonstrated moderate hydrocephalus, secondary to Arnold-Chiari deformity. He underwent a ventriculojugular shunt with resolution of his headaches.

Following an uneventful postoperative recovery, he was referred to Otolaryngology for evaluation of a fluctuating hearing loss associated with head fullness present for three to four years. The patient had never experienced tinnitus or vertigo. Tympanic membranes were noted to be normal in appearance and mobility, bilaterally (AU). Weber was midline and Rinne test showed air conduction greater than bone conduction with the 128, 256, and 512 Hz forks, AU. Examination of the eyes showed a brisk right-beating nystagmus on right gaze which promptly changed direction on left gaze. On neutral gaze, he demonstrated periodic alternating nystagmus. There was no vertical component to his nystagmus, even on upward or downward gaze. The remainder of the head and neck examination was unremarkable. An initial audiogram showed normal hearing and discrimination on the right (AD). There was a moderate low frequency neurosensory hearing loss on the left (AS), with 30 dB at 250 Hz, 50 dB at 500 Hz, and 10 dB at 1000 Hz. Discrimination was excellent, AS.

A repeat audiogram, two weeks later, showed complete resolution of the hearing loss AS with 10 dB levels at 250, 500, and 1000 Hz. No tone decay could be elicited, AU. Polytomography of his temporal bones revealed bilaterally symmetric internal auditory canals. Cochlear and vestibular aqueducts were of normal dimensions.

An electronystagmogram (ENG) was performed using our usual routine. During calibration, a fine left-beating spontaneous nystagmus was evident in both gaze positions (20° lateral to neutral gaze). The direction-changing characteristics of the patient's nystagmus became evident on pendulum tracking where lateral gaze was farther from neutral position (Fig. 1). Here there was a right-beating nystagmus on far right gaze and a left-beating nystagmus on far left gaze. Both these tasks were, of course, done with eyes open. With eyes open at the neutral position, an initial left spontaneous nystagmus of 10°/sec was noted (Fig. 2A). This was suppressed in part by closing the eyes (Fig. 2B). Positional testing was then undertaken with eyes closed. It soon became evident that there was a direction-alternating nystagmus of two minutes duration with about 10 seconds without nystagmus between direction changes. This periodic alternating nystagmus was in no way influenced by position, positioning, or positive or negative fistula test.

Five milliliters of ice water AS, begun during left-beating nystagmus alternans (eyes closed), resulted in premature right-beating nystagmus of 5°/sec (Fig. 3A). Visual fixation did not diminish the magnitude of this nystagmus (Fig. 3B). Five milliliters of ice water AD during a period of right-beating nystagmus alternans resulted in the premature production of a left-beating nystagmus (Fig. 3C). Again, visual fixation did not diminish this nystagmus (Fig. 3D).

DISCUSSION

Periodic alternating nystagmus is an uncommon pattern of horizontal or horizontal-rotatory nystagmus in which periods of right-beating nystagmus alternate with equal periods of left-beating nystagmus. There is characteristically 5 to 20 seconds of inactivity between direction changes. An entire

From the Department of Otolaryngology and Maxillofacial Surgery, University of Iowa, Iowa City.
REPRINTS — Richard W. Babin, MD, Department of Otolaryngology and Maxillofacial Surgery, University of Iowa, Iowa City, IA 52242.

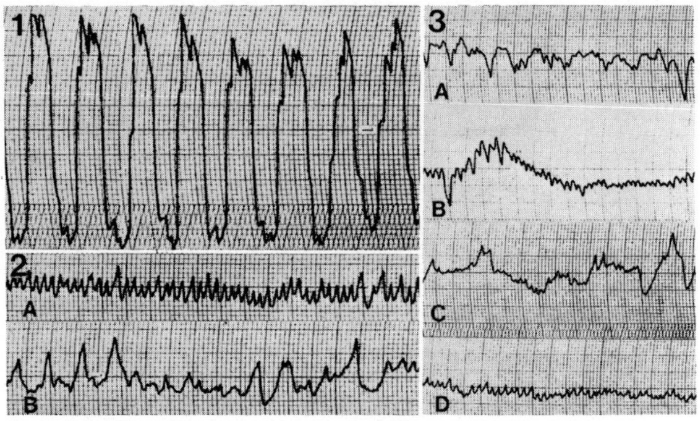

Fig. 1. Pendulum tracking (eyes open) showing right-beating nystagmus at far right gaze and a left-beating nystagmus at far left gaze.

Fig. 2. A) Left-beating spontaneous nystagmus in neutral gaze present at onset of ENG. B) Partially suppressed by closing eyes. This nystagmus decreased in magnitude and subsequently reversed directions 57 seconds beyond segment B).

Fig. 3. A) Right-beating nystagmus induced by a 5 ml ice-water irrigation AS initiated during left-beating nystagmus alternans with eyes closed. B) Same nystagmus as A showing no suppression with eyes open. C) Left-beating nystagmus induced by a 5 ml ice-water irrigation AD initiated during right-beating nystagmus alternans with eyes closed. D) Same nystagmus as C showing lack of visual suppression.

cycle may have a periodicity of 2 to 12 minutes. During peaks of maximum velocity, the patient may be unable to maintain gaze fixation and experience oscillopsia. At least one case has been reported, however, where the alternating nystagmus was only apparent with the eyes closed.[1] Patients have been described in whom opening or closing the eyes interrupted the rhythm or reversed the direction of the nystagmus.

Davis and Smith reviewed 40 cases in the literature prior to 1971, only 3 of which were in English.[2] They added eight additional cases. Table 1 includes the conditions associated with periodic alternating nystagmus in the cases reviewed by Davis and Smith, their reported cases, and the present case. It is generally agreed that periodic alternating nystagmus is generated at a site more central in the nervous system than the end-organ or primary afferent nerves. It has been noted that barbiturates will block periodic alternating nystagmus at dosages that do not eliminate brisk caloric response.[3] This has been taken as evidence that alternating nystagmus is generated at a site outside of the vestibulo-ocular reflex arc, per se. The only two cases having undergone neural autopsy had posterior fossa lesions. One had the Arnold-Chiari deformity and the other had arachnoid cyst caudal to the cerebellum.[2,4] Certainly, the preservation of appropriate caloric responses in this and other reported cases despite opposite-beating spontaneous nystagmus argues against a peripheral disorder. A central etiology is also suggested by the direction-changing gaze nystagmus and lack of ocular fixation suppression of caloric nystagmus.[5,6]

TABLE 1. ETIOLOGIC CONSIDERATIONS IN PERIODIC ALTERNATING NYSTAGMUS

Chronic otitis media with fistula
Cerebral trauma
Vertebrobasilar artery insufficiency
Encephalitis
Syphilis
Demyelinating diseases
Cerebellar lesions
Friedreich's ataxia
Tumors of corpus callosum
Arnold-Chiari deformity
Congenital nystagmus with or without albinism
Total amaurosis

This case presentation emphasizes the importance of prolonged observation of spontaneous or latent nystagmus. The patient described was seen initially by four different physicians and the alternating nature of his midgaze nystagmus was not appreciated until the direction discrepancy became apparent in the record. Even during an electronystagmogram, the independence of nystagmus changes from head positioning may not be readily apparent. This is especially true since a normal caloric response overrides the alternating nystagmus. While periodic alternating nystagmus is not specific for any single disease process, the differential posed in Table 1 suggests a starting point and general course of a work-up of a patient with this sign. The posterior fossa pathology present in this patient correlates well with three ENG findings considered strong indicators of central nervous system pathology: direction-changing gaze nystagmus, loss of eye fixation, suppression of caloric response, and periodic alternating nystagmus.

REFERENCES

1. Toglia JU. Periodic alternating nystagmus. Arch Otolaryngol 1968; 88:148-51.

2. Davis DG, Smith JL. Periodic alternating nystagmus. Am J Ophthalmol 1971; 72:757-62.

3. Bodo G. Approach to the generation centre of nystagmus alternans by means of drug tests. Acta Otolaryngol (Stockh) 1961; 53:328-32.

4. Towle PA, Romanul F. Periodic alternating nystagmus: first pathologically studied case. Neurology 1970; 20:408.

5. McCabe BF, Ryu JH. Vestibular physiology in understanding the dizzy patient. Rochester: American Academy of Ophthalmology and Otolaryngology, Inc, 1979: 54.

6. Barber HO, Stockwell CW. Manual of electronystagmography. St. Louis: CV Mosby, 1976: 99.

OTOLOGY IN TODAY'S MEDICAL SETTING

HAROLD F. SCHUKNECHT, MD
BOSTON, MASSACHUSETTS

I feel highly privileged to be the Guest of Honor of the American Otological Society. The honor is enhanced by the fact that this Society is one of the oldest and most dignified of the specialty societies in America. While the American Otological Society is primarily a scientific organization and, by law, cannot and does not engage in political activities, it probably should play a more active role in shaping the destiny of otology in American medicine. Enormous changes are occurring in the organization, technology and delivery of medical care, and nowhere is this more evident than in otolaryngology. Otology, as a scientific art in medicine, was born in the great medical centers of the European continent and Great Britain in the last century. Otology came of age in America at about the turn of the century but, for the most part, it was encompassed in the domain of the eye, ear, nose and throat physician. With the growth of medical sophistication, the two specialties of ophthalmology and otolaryngology diverged and the certification boards were established. The logic of separation of these two disciplines eventuated in the recent division of the joint American Academy into separate academies.

Otolaryngology itself has undergone some very significant changes in the past two decades. With the surge of otologic surgery in the 1940s and 1950s came a progressive and effective involvement of otolaryngologists in the subspecialties of major head and neck surgery, plastic surgery and allergy. As otologic surgery moved from treating the prevalence of disease to treating the incidence of disease, the volume of surgery decreased. Meanwhile, the role of the otolaryngologist as head and neck surgeon, plastic surgeon, and allergist gained strength and, in fact, has rather shaken the medical profession, especially those specialty groups which viewed this development as an encroachment upon their domains, artificial as they were.

This neomorphogenesis in otolaryngology has quite naturally generated some internal difficulties in our training programs. Speaking as an otologist and department chairman, I would like to share with you some of my thoughts concerning these problems.

It is quite clear that most otolarynology programs cannot adequately train residents to be proficient in all aspects of otolaryngology because sufficient time and clinical resources are simply not available. Increasing the time requirement for residency training from four to five years as mandated by our American Board of Otolaryngology, will be helpful but will not totally solve the problem. The difficulty is perceived quite clearly by the residents themselves as evidenced by the increasing demand for additional training following their residencies. For example, of the six residents who are completing their otolaryngology training at the Massachusetts Eye and Ear Infirmary this year, three are entering accredited 2-year residencies in plastic surgery; one, who is also a board certified pediatrician, has accepted an academic position; another is entering private practice; and one has been appointed to a clinical and research fellowship in otology.

Those of us who are responsible for training programs have the responsibility for maximizing the educational effectiveness of the available clinical material, teaching faculty, and financial resources. At the Massachusetts Eye and Ear Infirmary this goal is not being achieved. We have trained residents as best we could in the broad field of otolaryngology; some are pursuing further education in plastic surgery and almost certainly will never practice otology; others are pursuing further education in otology and probably will never perform major head and neck surgery. Quite obviously, we have not made the best use of our teaching efforts and clinical materials. This is a national problem which deserves the thoughtful consideration of the members of the American Otological Society.

Now that we have a 5-year residency training program, an immediate expedient might be the establishment of concentrated fifth year subspecialty electives. This plan would certainly be feasible in the larger training programs. It would allow for better use of clinical material and better training for the resident in his chosen field of subspecialization. This plan could also include a pathway for the training of otolaryngology generalists. Such a plan would have to be endorsed by the American Board of Otolaryngology and require some flexibility in the requirements for surgical experience. Further

From the Department of Otolaryngology, Massachusetts Eye and Ear Infirmary, Boston.
Address of the Guest of Honor at the meeting of the American Otological Society, Inc., Vancouver, British Columbia, May 9-10, 1981.

down the road, of course, the Board will have to grapple with the issue of subspecialty certification, a very logical formulation, but an immensely sensitive issue with major implications for reimbursement of professional fees by third party payers.

Otolaryngology, which was literally "hanging on the ropes" 30 years ago, has made a remarkable resurgence into the ranks of respectable specialties of medicine. We can credit this development to the confidence, capability and vision of many great American otolaryngologists. If we are to maintain the present high level of professional competence in otology, we will soon have to make some further changes in the structure of our training programs and the requirements for certification.

PANEL ON EXPERIENCES WITH MIDDLE EAR VENTILATING TUBES

TYMPANOSTOMY TUBES: THE CONSERVATIVE APPROACH

R. F. NAUNTON, MD
WASHINGTON, DC

The clear advantage accruing from the use of tympanostomy tubes in the treatment of otitis media with effusion is immediate improvement in hearing; there are also disadvantages entailed, such as scarring of the drum, risk of continuing otorrhea and interference with the patient's normal physical activities. All possible forms of medical treatment should be exhausted (antihistamine decongestants, politzerization) before resorting to tympanostomy tubes. There is a small group of children with severe chronic nasal obstruction and otitis media with effusion for whom adenoidectomy is likely to be required.

INTRODUCTION

My attitude towards the use of tympanostomy or ventilation tubes in the treatment of otitis media with effusion (OME) has always tended to be one of cautious procrastination, cautious because there are situations where procrastination can be the thief of something, if not of time. This may be described as conservatism; but from the Oxford dictionary definition of conservatism, "Keeping from change, decay or destruction," we have to conclude that each one of us is or should be a conservative. As with so many things, those who treat OME are all somewhere on the continuum between too much and too little. Nevertheless, it has been clear to me, as children have been brought for a second opinion, that some of our colleagues are far too anxious to use tubes.

I believe that all physicians are under an obligation to provide medical care based on sound scientific principles; but in the area of OME there is as yet a dearth of scientifically based information, depending somewhat upon the acceptable definition of "scientifically based." There remain many uncertainties about the correct mode of treatment of this common problem, let alone its etiology. I can bring you no new answers or dictums, only impressions and more questions.

IMPORTANT POINTS IN THE NATURAL HISTORY OF OME

Clearly there are very many important points to be made concerning the natural history of OME; the literature on the subject is voluminous. However, a number of points of practical importance can be identified as bearing significantly on the question of conservatism in the treatment of the problem, whether supporting or denying the conservative approach to the use of tubes.

OME is principally a disorder of children. It occurs frequently in association with upper respiratory infections (URI) and commonly it is self-limiting, resolving with or without treatment, leaving no indication of permanent residua.[1] This observation supports the concept that at least some delay is appropriate before resorting to the use of tubes, in order to allow time for spontaneous resolution; it may also explain the striking findings of Grote and Kuijpers[2] that OME was frequently associated with infection elsewhere in the upper respiratory tract, particularly the paranasal sinuses, and that sinus lavage led to resolution of the OME in about 85% of their cases with sinusitis and OME.

There is evidence that allergy and the use of antibiotics are rarely associated with OME[3,4] and that disorders of eustachian tube function commonly but not invariably play a primary role.[4] In all probability there is no single causative factor for OME although some of these factors or mechanisms may be implicated more commonly than others.

It seems self-evident that swallowing while the nose is obstructed causes a reduction in middle ear pressure and that repeated swallows further decrease the pressure; this is the classical Toynbee maneuver. The maneuver is most simply reproduced by pinching the nose shut and then swallowing; the resulting abnormal middle ear pressure can be corrected by opening the nose and swallowing once or twice. Incidentally Toynbee thought that the change in middle ear pressure he observed was toward the positive; it remained for Politzer to demonstrate that the pressure change was actually

From the Communicative Disorders Program, National Institute of Neurological and Communicative Disorders and Stroke, National Institutes of Health, Washington, DC.

Presented at the meeting of the American Otological Society, Inc., Vancouver, British Columbia, May 9-10, 1981.

REPRINTS — R. F. Naunton, MD, Director, Communicative Disorders Program, NINCDS, NIH, Washington, DC 20205.

negative. The child with a chronic severe nasal obstruction reproduces the Toynbee maneuver each time he swallows but he cannot correct the problem by opening the nose; every time he swallows the problem grows worse. Elverland et al[1] suggested that a similar problem develops in children who sniff vigorously and repeatedly; this possibility is less compelling than the Toynbee maneuver. Pursuing the relationship further it would appear that in the rather rare case with severe irreversible nasal obstruction due to adenoid hypertrophy, surgical conservatism has no place, and an adenoidectomy is indicated. This proves to be the case, and in examples of this type the results of adenoid surgery are often dramatic. It may also explain the findings of others, including Grote and Kuijpers,[2] that removal of large adenoids not necessarily producing total nasal obstruction is only of minor value in resolving OME.

The hearing impairment resulting from OME varies between individuals and from day to day between zero and about 40 dB. It is not unusual for hearing to be normal in an ear that is apparently completely fluid-filled, a clinical observation that can be confirmed by tympanometry and audiometry; so in any discussion of the advisability of screening children by audiometry or tympanometry, it may be important to distinguish between screening for hearing impairment and screening for middle ear pathology; the child in trouble may have either one or both of these problems.

Much has been written about the devastating effects on language development of a profound hearing impairment present in infancy or early childhood (Whetnall and Fry,[5] Northern and Downs[6]). We know far less about the effect of moderate chronic or recurrent hearing impairment although it seems self-evident that linguistic, social and cognitive development may be impeded to a significant extent.[7] The otologist who discounts the educational significance of a minor or moderate hearing impairment is probably an otologist who himself has never suffered a transient mild hearing impairment.

The etiology of cholesteatoma continues to puzzle clinicians; children commonly suffer from OME, and they also suffer from middle ear cholesteatoma. There is, however, no irrefutable evidence that the former will lead to the latter, with or without uncomplicated treatment.

PROBLEMS ASSOCIATED WITH THE USE OF TUBES

The most important problem or question related to the use of tubes is that the underlying disease may be unaffected by this mode of treatment. Here again the evidence is unclear; if, as has commonly been assumed in the past, OME is the result of tubal inadequacy, then it would seem likely that ventilation will not influence the basic problem; if, on the other hand (and the evidence on this point is growing), OME is the result of an immune response, then adequate ventilation and removal of fluid may well lead to permanent resolution. In this regard it should be remembered that even a poorly pneumatized ear has far more space to become fluid-filled than just the mesotympanum; all of the contained fluid must be drained off or encouraged to drain before the ear can be said to have returned to normal.

The child with a ventilation tube in place must be cautious, as must his parents, to keep water out of the ear against the risk of middle ear contamination and purulent infection. The need for this precaution is a nuisance to all concerned and constantly reminds the child that he is "different": he may not swim — or if he swims he must not get water in the ear(s) — and he must shower or tub with great care. Some of our colleagues deny the need for the caution to keep water out of the ear but this might well still present some medicolegal hazards.

Scarring of the drum is a familiar sequel to the use of tubes (or is its scarring attributable wholly or partially to the chronic problem itself for which the tube is "treatment"?) The scars run the gamut from a circular atrophic and weakened area in the drum, the size of the tube previously inserted but later extruded or removed, to a massive tympanosclerotic plaque occupying a substantial part of the pars tensa. The former is the place where the drum will give way the first time there is a significant pressure differential between the middle and external ears (too vigorous nose blowing, diving, recurrence of a eustachian tube problem); the latter is the bête noire of the middle ear surgeon who is attempting a myringoplasty to repair a chronic perforation where little remains of the drum but plaque. Morgan[9] found tympanosclerosis in a relatively small percentage of cases in connection with the use of ventilation tubes, while Møller reported a considerably higher incidence. Møller[10] and Tos and Poulsen[11] agree that tympanosclerosis of the drum commonly has little effect on hearing; nevertheless, there is a positive correlation between the magnitude of scarring or tympanosclerosis and the amount of hearing impairment.

Otorrhea may occur after tube insertion in between 5%[12] and 68%[13] of cases; Barfoed and Rosborg[8] report a 34% incidence despite a ban on swimming.

When the ventilation tube is removed or extruded, the hole it leaves behind may not always close spontaneously; estimates of the frequency of this complication vary but it is probably less than 5%.[12,14]

It is common experience that tubes tend to be extruded sooner or later; and more often than not, whether they are extruded or deliberately removed, the associated drum defect will close. The original problem may then recur and, depending again on the individual surgeon's preference for conservatism, tube(s) may be required again. McLelland[14] reports a 14% incidence of this problem while in Barfoed and Rosborg's cases[8] 61% required repeat tube insertions. In children this requires another anesthetic together with the attendant risks of anesthesia. Every time a tube or anesthetic is required, there is question of cost, whether to family or to third party payer.

Other complications of tube insertion are reported (cholesteatoma, ossicular disruption, sensorineural impairment) but these, even if they are genuine complications of skillful tube insertion, merit no more than mention.

BENEFITS OF TUBES

The clear advantage of tubes, and on this point there is little or no controversy, is that skillful placement accompanied by careful aspiration of fluid or glue from the mesotympanum leads to immediate resolution of the hearing problem, an improvement that will usually continue as long as the tube stays in place and remains patent. This single but impressive fact has led to the popularity of the procedure despite the disadvantages associated with tubes.

Tubes may have no direct influence on the underlying disease; but this remains uncertain and the possibility remains that the use of tubes, in some circumstances, encourages the resolution of the basic problem. The figures of Kokko and Palva[12] appear to lend credence to this possibility.

CONSERVATIVE APPROACH TO THE USE OF TUBES IN OME

Patient Evaluation. This should be thorough and appropriate, rather than done by rote; it should not be unnecessarily exhaustive, exhausting, or expensive. If there is reason to believe that the problem has developed recently in association with URI, treatment should be directed towards the URI and time allowed for spontaneous resolution (2-4 months); if there is a respiratory allergy, it should be treated; if there is severe chronic nasal obstruction from adenoids, adenoidectomy will probably be required. In those cases not of recent onset, allergy or severe adenoidal obstruction requiring surgery will not commonly be encountered. The majority of long-standing cases will therefore call for nonsurgical treatment.

Nonsurgical Treatment. There are several reasons for using oral decongestants or oral decongestant-antihistamine preparations despite the common perception, like my own, that they are of little value. It is abundantly clear that these preparations do not produce spectacular results (if they did, there would be no argument about their efficacy); but there is some evidence that they may have some beneficial effect;[15] they are largely free from the risk of untoward side effects; and parents, indoctrinated by the advertising media, have confidence in this type of medication and in the physician who prescribes them as a first approach to treatment.

Early in his care of the child with OME the physician should introduce the idea of politzerization. The procedure may not be completed on the first visit, nor should it be forced on a reluctant child; but a gradual introduction to a procedure that may prove later to be of great importance will avoid unhappiness on all sides and, in the right hands, practically guarantee success later.

While nonsurgical treatment continues, any hearing impairment may be expected to persist. Parents and teachers should be alerted to this and preferential seating provided in class in the sense that the child should be close to the teacher but have other children directly in front of him (eg, seated at one end of a semicircle of desks; or seated next to the front in a conventional classroom setting). This should be done without encouraging the child to look upon himself as physically handicapped, any more than the child who wears glasses need be or is usually regarded in this light.

The last paragraph refers indirectly to parent counselling, a matter of great importance but one which is unfortunately often the first to suffer in a busy office practice.

Assuming that despite antihistamine decongestants the OME persists, the next step is closer attention to politzerization, introduced earlier. The change in the appearance of the drum(s) is the indication of success, and a single session of politzerization may temporarily resolve the problem. Parents can be taught to use a mini-Politzer inflator but unfortunately they will be largely dependent on the child to report whether the correct end-point has been reached.

If this were the best of possible worlds, we would prescribe a low-powered hearing aid at this point, to be used until the problem has resolved. I have prescribed hearing aids in this situation with a final outcome satisfactory to all parties; but the majority of parents and children still see a hearing aid as a major social stigma, outweighing the seriousness of a hearing problem; and the cost of a hearing aid is often an absolute bar to its prescription.

Nitrous Oxide (N_2O). Reference is appropriate at this point to the potential value of N_2O as a means of ventilating a fluid-filled middle ear, only to dismiss it. There has been a low background level of interest in this question for a considerable time, based upon the well-recognized phenomenon of rapid diffusion of an inhaled gas which is highly soluble in the blood (eg, N_2O or acetylene) into the middle ear spaces. The result is a rapid elevation of middle ear pressure which can lead to eustachian tube opening, discharge of middle ear fluid and pressure equalization. Might this offer a convenient noninvasive method of treating OME? Bluestone et al[16] and Johnson et al[17] have concluded that only fluids of low viscosity could be cleared in this manner from the middle ear.

There are two overriding considerations as this possible treatment method is considered: first, no middle ear pressure changes will result from gas inhalation alone unless air is present in the middle ear, and air will be present only if the OME has been of brief duration or if the eustachian tube is continuing to ventilate the middle ear to some extent; and second, if the procedure does work (because there was air present in the middle ear from the start) the middle ear will remain relatively free of fluid *but filled with nitrous oxide*; as gas-administration stops, the gas transfer will then reverse with equal rapidity and the net result will be a rapidly developing severe negative pressure in the middle ear that will be equalized by transudation of fluid into the middle ear again.

Surgery. In those few cases where there is severe chronic nasal obstruction from adenoids and adenoidectomy is recommended, the question of simultaneous tonsillectomy should be decided on its own merit, rather than because the two procedures are so conveniently carried out together, or in an effort to avoid the later necessity of a second anesthetic. The morbidity and risks of a tonsillectomy are greater than those of a second general anesthetic. It is wise, however, to carry out a simultaneous myringotomy and middle ear aspiration in order to further increase the chances that the adenoidectomy will resolve the OME. My preference is not to use tympanostomy tubes at this point because the chances of OME resolution without the use of tubes is very high; and if tubes are used, an additional anesthetic will be required later to remove them; (there is a law that states that the tubes you want to extrude themselves will stay in place, and vice versa).

Failing all other measures, the final steps in my hands have been tympanostomy and insertion of tubes.

REFERENCES

1. Elverland HH, Hagueto OK, Mair IWS, Schrøder KE. Influence of adenoid hypertrophy on secretory otitis media. Ann Otol Rhinol Laryngol 1981; 90:7-11.

2. Grote JJ, Kuijpers W. Middle ear effusion and sinusitis. J Laryngol Otol 1980; 94:177-83.

3. Juhn SK, Paparella MM, Kim CS, Goycoolea MV, Giebink S. Pathogenesis of otitis media. Ann Otol Rhinol Laryngol 1977; 86:481-92.

4. Tos M, Poulsen G, Borch F. Etiological factors in secretory otitis. Arch Otolaryngol 1979; 105:582-8.

5. Whetnall E, Fry DB. The deaf child. Springfield: CC Thomas, 1964.

6. Northern JL, Downs MP. Hearing in children. Baltimore: Williams and Wilkins, 1978.

7. Ruben RJ, Hanson DG. Summary of discussion and recommendations made during the workshop on otitis media and development. Ann Otol Rhinol Laryngol 1979; 88 Suppl 60: 107-11.

8. Barfoed C, Rosborg J. Secretory otitis media: long-term observations after treatment with grommets. Arch Otolaryngol 1980; 106:553-6.

9. Morgan WC. Tympanosclerosis. Laryngoscope 1977; 87: 1821-5.

10. Møller P. Tympanosclerosis of the eardrum in cleft palate patients. Acta Otolarngol 1981; 91:91-4.

11. Tos M, Poulsen G. Secretory otitis media. Arch Otolaryngol 1976; 102:672-5.

12. Kokko E, Palva T. Clinical results and complications of tympanostomy. Ann Otol Rhinol Laryngol 1976; 85 Suppl 25: 277-9.

13. Herzon FS. Tympanostomy tubes: infectious complications. Arch Otolaryngol 1980; 106:645-7.

14. McLelland CA. Incidence of complications from use of tympanostomy tubes. Arch Otolaryngol 1980; 106:97-9.

15. Cantekin EI, Rockette HE, Bluestone CD, Beery QC. Effect of decongestant with or without antihistamine on eustachian tube function. Ann Otol Rhinol Laryngol 1980; 89 Suppl 68: 290-5.

16. Bluestone CD, Beery QC, Paradise JL. Audiometry and tympanometry in relation to middle ear effusions in children. Laryngoscope 1973; 83:594-604.

17. Johnson LP, Parkin JL, Stevens MH, Otto WC, McCandless BA. Action of general anesthesia on middle ear effusions. Arch Otolaryngol 1980; 106:100-2.

CHRONIC NONSUPPURATIVE OTITIS MEDIA

COMPARISON OF TYMPANOSTOMY TUBES AND MEDICATION VERSUS VENTILATION

BEVERLY W. ARMSTRONG, MD
CHARLOTTE, NORTH CAROLINA

ROBERT B. ARMSTRONG, MD
NEW YORK, NEW YORK

Experiences with tympanostomy tubes extending over a period of 29 years are compared with the computer-assisted analysis of a questionnaire that was submitted to 500 otolaryngologists. Ventilating tubes are being used by 99.4% of the respondents in the group and are estimated to achieve good to excellent results in 90% of patients treated. Appropriate use of tympanostomy tubes has significantly reduced the incidence of chronic ear disease. A comparison of prophylactic antibiotics and prophylactic ventilating tubes for the prevention of acute otitis media showed that 91% of the participants in the survey found ventilating tubes to be more effective than antibiotics. Benefits from ventilating tubes far outweigh the small number of tube-induced complications.

INTRODUCTION

We are aware of those who endorse medical treatment for nonsuppurative otitis media, and we are equally aware that medical treatment has been implicated as a cause of the disease as well as a factor contributing to its chronicity. From a few dissenting voices, and they are few indeed, we have heard that ventilating tubes are without value and may even do more harm than good. We disagree. With a desire to avoid bias, we undertook to survey 500 prominent, well-qualified otolaryngologists practicing throughout the world, and we employed the same selection criteria that were used in a similar survey conducted in 1968.[1] Responses (325) were received in time for computer-assisted analysis. The results of the survey and some comparisons with our own experience are offered for information. In some instances percentages have been rounded off.

MEDICAL TREATMENT AND RESULTS

At the outset we inquired about the modalities used as medical treatment of nonsuppurative otitis media. Decongestants and antihistamines, singly or in combination, were used most commonly. Inflation performed in the office and/or by the patient at home was also used as an adjunct by the majority of physicians. A smaller percentage of respondents used antibiotics, allergy treatment, intranasal medication, corticosteroids or other modalities. L. W. Welsh commented: "I am not convinced that medical care plays any part in the successful treatment of this problem. I can cite one of our local large pediatric hospitals where the pediatricians have given up use of antihistamines and decongestants."*

Next, physicians were asked to estimate the response to medical treatment alone. In general, those respondents who had referral practices had less success with medical management, reflecting a skew in their patient population which included a disproportionate number of patients who had already failed with nonsurgical management. H. G. Birck wrote: "My practice is a total referral practice and therefore I do not know how many patients have already received decongestants, steroids, antibiotics, etc. I very rarely resort to medical treatment as practically all of my patients have been through that mill already. I personally do not believe that any of these are of value." T. Palva stated: "I only see cases of long-standing disease, and use no medical treatment."

We have found medical treatment to be up to 80% effective in the first few weeks after onset, but the respondents in our survey estimate it at only 50%. Most otolaryngologists abandon medical treatment after one to two months (average 1.8 months) in favor of tympanostomy tubes. We agree, if the patient has fluid in both ears, but might extend the period of observation to 3, 4, or even 6 months when only one ear is involved. Of those participating in our survey, 32% insert tubes in one month or less. This hardly gives medical treatment a fair chance and gives rise to the criticism that tubes are overutilized. Tubes should not be used indiscriminately because most of the patients with serous otitis media get well, treated or not.

SURGICAL TREATMENT

Tympanostomy tubes were intended for chronic nonsuppurative otitis media[1,2] and should be used after failure of medical therapy or initially when untreated patients have had fluid for years. While a few respondents to our survey have found myringotomy to be effective for some patients, the overwhelming majority (99.4%) use tubes when appropriate. G. O. Proud, one of the two respondents

*All quoted material taken from questionnaires.

From the Charlotte Eye, Ear and Throat Hospital, Charlotte, North Carolina.
Presented at the meeting of the American Otological Society, Inc., Vancouver, British Columbia, May 9-10, 1981.
REPRINTS — Beverly W. Armstrong, MD, 1600 East Third Street, Charlotte, NC 28204.

who has stopped using tubes, elects to have his patients wear a hearing aid "indefinitely" in preference to intubation, presumably because tubes are "only temporary. Didn't cure. Complications." Other less common indications for ventilating tubes will not be dealt with here.

From the wide variety of tubes available only two are necessary. A Teflon tube 1 cm in length with a relatively small flange will suffice for short-term (two to three months) ventilation, and a Teflon tube of the same length with a broader flange at a 45° angle to the shaft will afford long-term ventilation. Both tubes are 0.113 cm in diameter.

We do not like grommets. Grommets admittedly are less apt to become plugged with dried blood or secretion, but their disadvantages far outweigh their virtues. The exterior flange is a barrier to migrating epithelium that collects debris and encourages crusting, granuloma formation and extrusion. We have seen accumulation of epithelial debris around long tubes but never a granuloma. Grommets are short, so short that they can get lost in the middle ear, and they do not protect the middle ear from water nearly as well as long tubes. G. D. L. Smyth found that "the Armstrong tube stays in very much longer than the Sheppard and Paparella" (personal communication).

The location of the tube is extremely important if long-term ventilation is to be achieved. The migration pattern of epithelium on the drumhead is well known and led to the conclusion that tubes should be placed in the anterosuperior quadrant. We advocate a radial incision that extends into the fibrous annulus and placement of the tube snugly against the annular fibers. The angled flange permits alignment so the shaft of the tube is not in contact with the canal wall.

Result. Having inquired about how the otolaryngologists used tubes, they were asked to assess the results of this treatment in the management of nonsuppurative otitis media. On the average, the group surveyed estimated that 90% of patients achieved a good to excellent result, 8% a fair result and 2% a poor response. As another indicator of the efficacy of tubes, physicians were asked to compare hearing in ears treated with tubes with the contralateral ear, if uninvolved, or other control. On the average, 90% of the tubed ears were estimated to have hearing as good or better than the control group. Five percent of treated ears were estimated to be equal to the control group and 5% worse.

Excellent results without known recurrence have been obtained in 87% of our patients after initial tube insertion, and another 12% remained free of fluid after being reintubated for one to six recurrences. We have several patients with eustachian malfunction or occlusion who will be reintubated periodically until they develop a permanent perforation. We believe that patients should be observed carefully after intubation and that the period of observation should be continued after extrusion or removal of the tube.

One of the benefits claimed for tubes is their effect on the incidence of chronic ear disease. Of the participants in this survey 83% believed tubes have reduced the frequency of chronic ear disease, 15% stated they had little or no effect, while 2% thought they had increased chronic ear disease. The bare statistics can be animated by some of the comments offered. W. M. Wallenborn indicated he had "done one mastoidectomy in three years (and) formerly did 20 to 40 a year." A. Weisskopf has found "practice with children much more pleasant" with tubes. A. J. Scalco's feeling that "tubes have more emphatically reduced chronic ear problems and drainage than any other single entity" is similar to D. B. Kamerer's contention that "tubes are certainly far ahead of whatever is in second place." As J. D. Clemis summarized the situation with a touch of poetic exaggeration: "(Tubes) damn near put us out of business."

Prophylactic Tubes Versus Antibiotics. Ventilating tubes originally proposed as an adjunct in the treatment of chronic nonsuppurative otitis media are also being used to prevent recurrent attacks of acute otitis media. The otolaryngologists in our survey were asked to assess use of antibiotics and tympanostomy tubes prophylactically to prevent recurrent acute otitis media. Of the respondents 35% advocated prophylactic antibiotics, and they estimated that 50% of their patients benefited from such treatment. In comparison, 64% of the respondents indicated that they use tubes prophylactically to reduce the frequency or prevent recurrent attacks of otitis media. The relative merits of these two modalities can be inferred because 91% of all respondents expressed the opinion that prophylactic tubes are more effective than prophylactic antibiotics. W. S. Gibson, Jr. volunteered: "I recently studied a large group of children with recurrent otitis media under two years (the so-called 'otitis-prone child') and placed tubes in their ears. There were practically no more infections in children with tubes who had previously had more than six acute episodes." Gebhart in his award-winning Triological thesis this year reported that "the presence of tympanostomy tubes significantly prevented multiple episodes of acute otitis media."

Complications. No surgical treatment is without its complications. Analysis of the survey indicated that drainage following tube insertion occurred in 10%, persistent perforation in less than 1% and cholesteatoma in less than 1%. Buckingham[4] concluded the incidence of cholesteatomas caused by or following intubation to be 0.5%. He went on to emphasize, however, that this is outweighed by the benefits of intubation in preventing atelectasis and cholesteatoma.

In our patients drainage has occurred in 7%, and the tube had to be removed in less than 1%. Two permanent perforations have been observed in 29 years. Both patients had a long history of chronic serous otitis media, and the perforation was viewed as a fortunate event, not as a complication. Granuloma formation has never been observed in patients in whom we had inserted the ventilating tube, nor have we seen a cholesteatoma that we could relate to tube insertion. We are of the opinion that cholesteatomas related to tube insertion are probably initiated by forcefully inserting a blunt or broad-flanged tube that is not only traumatic but causes inversion of keratinizing epithelium into the middle ear. This danger is minimized with a beveled flanged tube.

Comments. We asked the question whether or not tubes are being used too frequently. We learned that 50% of the respondents thought that tubes were used appropriately. However, many of them added "appropriately in my own hands." It seems that the response to the question depended on whether or not the physician chose to answer for his own practice or that of others. We join the 40% who expressed their opinion that tubes were used too frequently. We believe that overutilization is common because many tubes are inserted without an adequate period of observation with or without medical treatment. We also find ourselves in agreement with the 10% of our respondents who thought tubes were being used too infrequently. We are confident that some patients who need ventilating tubes are not getting them. Attic cholesteatomas are still much too common, and adequate ventilation should practically eliminate this serious problem.

CONCLUSIONS

Enthusiastic acceptance of ventilating tubes has been expressed, and their value in treating nonsuppurative otitis media demonstrated. The prophylactic use of ventilating tubes in the "otitis media prone child" significantly prevents multiple episodes of acute otitis media.

Our convictions about ventilating tubes are perhaps better expressed in the words of others: Wallenborn: "I firmly believe that the ventilation tubes have had the most beneficial effect in controlling and preventing recurrent ear infections, secretory otitis media, hearing loss, and speech defects of all modalities." R. W. Cantrell: "I believe the tympanostomy tube is the greatest single contribution to otology in the past 50 years." V. F. Mersol: "It is my personal feeling that tubes have done as much for the ear disease-prone child as the Salk vaccine did for polio." L. L. Pratt: "By the use of tubes, we have raised a generation free of ear disease, when tubes were used properly."

ACKNOWLEDGMENT — We express our appreciation to the contributors who shared their experiences with us and without whose help this material could not have been obtained.

REFERENCES

1. Armstrong BW. What your colleagues think of tympanostomy tubes. Laryngoscope 1968; 78:1303-13.

2. Armstrong BW. A new treatment for chronic secretory otitis media. Arch Otolaryngol 1954; 59:653-4.

3. Gebhart DE. Tympanostomy tubes in the otitis media prone child. Laryngoscope 1981 (in press).

4. Buckingham RA. Cholesteatoma and chronic otitis media following middle ear intubation. Laryngoscope 1981 (in press).

COMMENT

RALPH J. CAPAROSA, MD

PITTSBURGH, PENNSYLVANIA

Doctors Armstrong and Naunton have presented their true feelings as to whether or not tympanostomy should be performed. Armstrong has covered completely the history of his own initial survey (ten years following the introduction of the tube) and the most recent survey. In his first survey only two respondents of more than 350 were opposed to tubal insertion. In the most recent survey, there is only one otolaryngologist who prefers the use of a hearing aid to the insertion of tubes. That otologist is entitled to his opinion; I discuss this option not to dignify it, but to state that it is cruel, insensitive, and shameful. Armstrong suggests his indications for this surgery and states that sometimes it is overutilized, but in some patients it is underutilized. Having had the opportunity to review his

From the Pittsburgh Otolaryngological Clinic.

Presented at the meeting of the American Otological Society, Inc., Vancouver, British Columbia, May 9-10, 1981.

written manuscript, I submit that his presentation today and his written paper are very sound.

Naunton's experience must have been learned in a pediatric setting. Of what value antibiotics, antihistaminics, or judicious neglect are, needs a bit more elaboration than suggesting that in the majority of patients these methods of management will suffice. The explanation as to the validity of these three approaches plus the fourth, the hearing aid, is not well defended by Naunton.

In reality, the question is not, "Is the tympanostomy a good operation?" but rather, "When is it indicated?" Several factors influence when the procedure should be performed. One of these is, at what stage of the disease the patient is seen. In some practices, the patient may be seen very early. In others, such as those of us who practice in a center city area, the patients are usually not seen until they have had an abundance of medical therapy 6-10 months following the onset of the problem. In most of these youngsters, the parents become a little disenchanted with the doctrine, "Let's wait and see." They also are concerned about the overabundance of antibio tics, the decibel level of television, the report card, and the irritability of both patient and parents. Of equal importance with the history is the physical examination. The examination, of course, should include an evaluation of the nose, nasopharynx and oropharynx. Any obstruction to the physiological nasal breathing portends more severe problems than in the patient who does not have obstruction. Examination of the ears should be performed under the microscope. The appearance of the eardrum is the single most significant part of the examination and determines whether or not a tympanostomy should be performed. I have categorized the appearance of the eardrum as follows:

1. The middle ear contains fluid with air bubbles or there is a fluid level.

2. There is a very light-colored fluid with excellent mobility.

3. The color of the eardrum is a deep reddish-blue with increased vascularity of the surface and poor mobility.

4. The tympanic membrane is black.

In any of the above, retraction is of added significance. Changes suggesting early or beginning atrophy, along with retraction, should encourage early use of the tympanostomy tube.

In the first and second categories, it is my feeling that judicious neglect is an acceptable approach. If there is some specific indication for antibiotics, they should be used. It is my feeling that the latter will do nothing to clear the fluid and the use of antihistaminics or decongestants has been ineffectual. Most likely in these two categories fluid will clear itself in a very short period. The deep reddish-blue discolored eardrum will not respond to antibiotics, judicious neglect, or any other medical therapy. In my office, these patients are most frequently seen after long, overtreated antibiotic trials or in the long judiciously neglected patients. In the case of the black eardrum, there will be no spontaneous clearing in response to any type of medical therapy.

As far as the adult is concerned, in those with a very short history, usually a myringotomy will suffice without the use of a tube. If there is a prolonged history, or repeated attacks, I feel that a tube should be inserted. This is performed under phenol anesthesia. The examination of the nasopharynx is essential in all of these patients.

In summary, I believe that Armstrong has solid evidence for the continued use of tympanostomy tubes if the indications are present.

USE OF TYMPANOSTOMY TUBES IN OTITIS MEDIA

WILLIAM L. MEYERHOFF, MD, PhD

MINNEAPOLIS, MINNESOTA

Tympanostomy tubes (TT) are frequently employed as treatment for otitis media (OM) although there is little clinical or experimental evidence of their efficacy. Potential detriments of TT include cost, risk of inhalation anesthesia, intraoperative complications, and tympanic membrane (TM) damage. Potential benefits include elimination of the conductive hearing loss (CHL), reduction in the occurrence of acute purulent OM, and avoidance of sequelae. The cost/benefit ratio of TT has never been accurately determined and morbid complications of inhalation anesthesia and the surgical procedure appear to be rare. There is evidence that TT significantly reduce the CHL of OM as well as reduce the incidence of recurrent acute purulent OM and help avoid sequelae. It is therefore determined that the risk of TT insertion for middle ear effusion (occasional TM changes) can be justified, in properly selected patients, by the benefits (immediate improvement in hearing and reduction in the incidence of recurrent acute purulent OM).

INTRODUCTION

Tympanic membrane (TM) intubation as a form of therapy for otitis media (OM) has been known for over 100 years but was not well accepted until 1954 when reintroduced by Armstrong.[1] Tympanostomy tubes (TT) were to serve two primary functions: middle ear (ME) ventilation and pressure equalization. It was hoped that, through these functions, TT would prevent the accumulation of middle ear effusion (MEE) and thereby eliminate its associated conductive hearing loss, recurrent infections, and sequelae. Subsequent to Armstrong's 1954 publication, controversy has arisen regarding the use of TT, not only between professional disciplines but within the discipline of otology itself.

Unfortunately, much of the information on TT is anecdotal or retrospective. As beneficial as TT appear to some observers, to others they appear unnecessary and hazardous. In spite of the controversy and paucity of scientific study, Paradise[2] estimated that 2 million TT are inserted annually in the United States for the treatment of persistent MEE and for the prevention of recurrent acute purulent OM. He warned that TT insertion was not without hazard and should be utilized only when the condition being treated was troublesome enough to warrant a surgical procedure and only when equally effective but less risky alternatives were not available.

Obviously, when considering any therapeutic modality, potential benefits must be weighed against potential detriments. In the case of TT for the treatment of OM the potential benefits are elimination of conductive hearing loss (CHL), reduction in the occurrence of acute purulent OM, and avoidance of sequelae. The potential detriments include cost, inhalation anesthesia, surgical complications, and damage to the TM, ME, and inner ear as the result of postoperative infection.

POTENTIAL DETRIMENTS

Cost. Although cost is a definite consideration in the delivery of health care no one has been able to determine the cost effectiveness of TT in the treatment of OM. Armstrong[3] observed that it is difficult to compare the immediate surgical costs of TT insertion to the long-term costs of the otitis prone patient. He also noted that the value of hearing, preserved or restored, is incalculable and, therefore, impossible to include in any computation of a cost-benefit ratio.

Anesthesia. In a review of the literature and in personal communications with several active otologists the author was unable to document a single morbid complication or death from inhalation anesthesia during TT insertion. In addition, a review of tonsillectomy and adenoidectomy by Pratt and Gallagher[4] described over 1,300,000 surgical procedures with no mention of anesthetic complication. Therefore, although it is conceivable that complications of inhalation anesthesia have occurred with the placement of TT, they must be rare.

Surgical Complications. Case reports of aberrant jugular bulb, aberrant carotid artery, and persistent stapedial arteries being injured during ME surgery exist. Similarly, unusual instances of incudostapedial joint disarticulation with TT insertion have also been reported. The exact incidence, however, of such complications are not known and thought to be extremely rare.[5]

Effect of Tympanostomy Tubes on the Tympanic Membrane. Harell and Shea[6] warned that long-term use of TT resulted in frequent and serious complications and described occurrences of post-operative tympanosclerosis and atrophic changes in the drumhead. Similar warnings have been issued

From the Departments of Otolaryngology, University of Minnesota and Hennepin County Medical Center, Minneapolis. This research has been supported in part by "Pathogenesis of Otitis Media," NIH-NINCDS Grant No. NS14538.

Presented at the meeting of the American Otological Society, Inc., Vancouver, British Columbia, May 9-10, 1981.

REPRINTS — William L. Meyerhoff, MD, PhD, Hennepin County Medical Center, 701 Park Avenue South, Minneapolis, MN 55415.

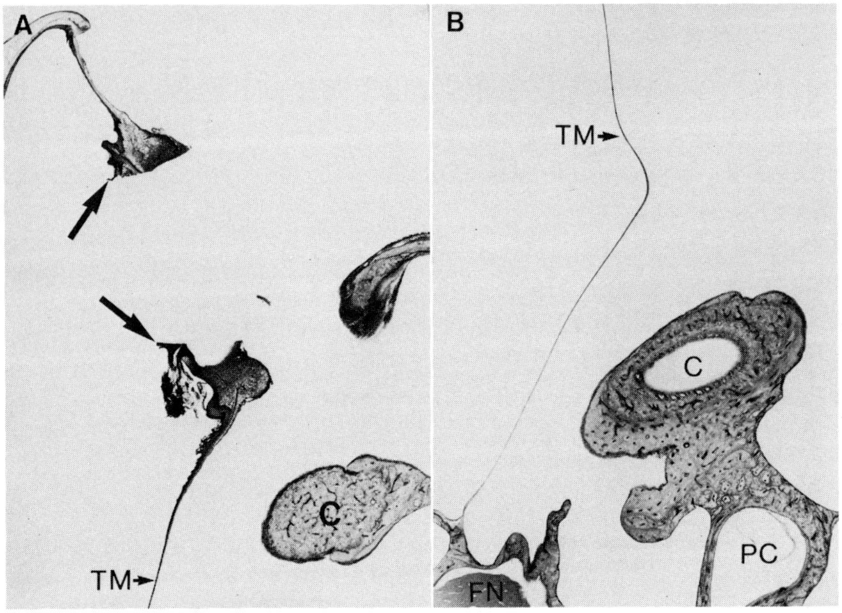

Fig. 1. A) Tympanic membrane (TM) of a chinchilla with a tympanostomy tube in place. The reaction to the tympanostomy tube (arrows) can be identified as well as the basal turn of the cochlea (C). B) The tympanic membrane (TM) of a chinchilla following extrusion of the TT appears perfectly normal. The facial nerve (FN), posterior semicircular canal (PC), and basal turn of the cochlea (C) can be identified. (x20)

by others who, in retrospective studies, have identified tympanosclerosis and TM perforation, atrophy, and retraction in patients previously treated with TT.[7-11] No attempt is made in these publications to eliminate the disease process itself as a predisposing factor in the development of these TM changes nor is any attempt made to subdivide patients on the basis of underlying disease (maxillary sinusitis, allergy, cleft palate, or nasopharyngeal infection or neoplasm).

Buckingham,[12] using serial Kodachrome studies, documented TM changes that occurred subsequent to TT insertion. He recorded TM perforation, granuloma, cholesteatoma, and TM atrophy and atelectasis. It was convincing from the photographs that many of these conditions occurred at or near the previous site of the TT. Whether these changes were a result of the tube or sequelae of the disease process itself is speculative, however, since similar TM changes are seen in otitis prone patients who have never had TT inserted.

Brown et al[13] did attempt to separate TM changes due to TT from those that occur as a result of the otitis process by placing TT in only one ear of 60 patients with bilateral persistent MEE. They reported an immediate 16 dB improvement in hearing in the intubated ear but, at the end of five years, the intubated TM demonstrated a higher incidence of scarring and tympanosclerosis. This scarring and tympanosclerosis did not appear to significantly affect the hearing and no case of cholesteatoma or TM perforation was identified.

Stenfors and Winblad[14] inserted solid, biflanged polyethylene rods through the TM of healthy adult rats. These rats were sacrificed at intervals and their ears were studied morphologically with the light microscope and scanning electron microscope. At three days following insertion of the polyethylene rod inflammatory cells, granulocytes, and fibrin accumulated around the circumference of the rod and evidence of mild ME inflammation was present. By three weeks, these changes had totally resolved. Also, at three days, hyperplastic epithelium began to appear around the circumference of the rods and this remained as long as the rods were in place. Following extrusion, however, this hyperplastic epithelium disappeared and no atrophy or scarring could be identified at the insertion site.

Similar findings were observed in a pilot study by Meyerhoff and D. A. Shea (unpublished data, 1981). The authors placed Paparella type I TT through both TM of 25 healthy adult chinchillas following 90-second sterilization of one external auditory canal (EAC) with 70% alcohol. A mild local inflammatory reaction could be seen bilaterally around all tubes early in the postoperative course. This was replaced by a mild fibrous reaction and epithelial hyperplasia (Fig. 1A). With extrusion of the TT this fibrous band was similarly extruded, the TM healed, and no permanent changes could be observed (Fig. 1B). The results of these studies provide evidence that TT insertion does not cause frequent irreversible changes in the TM in the absence of OM and its predisposing factors.

Effect of Tympanostomy Tubes on the Middle Ear. Herzon[15] noted that 7.9% of his patients developed otorrhea within ten days of TT insertion. He admitted that these early infections may be a continuation of an active infection present at the time of surgery and that the TT might be serving as a drain. In the same study, an additional 14% of patients developed otorrhea beyond the first ten days postoperatively and the author speculated that this was either a result of water contamination or the development of a new episode of purulent OM. Others have reported postoperative otorrhea and chronic OM as a complication of TT insertion but,

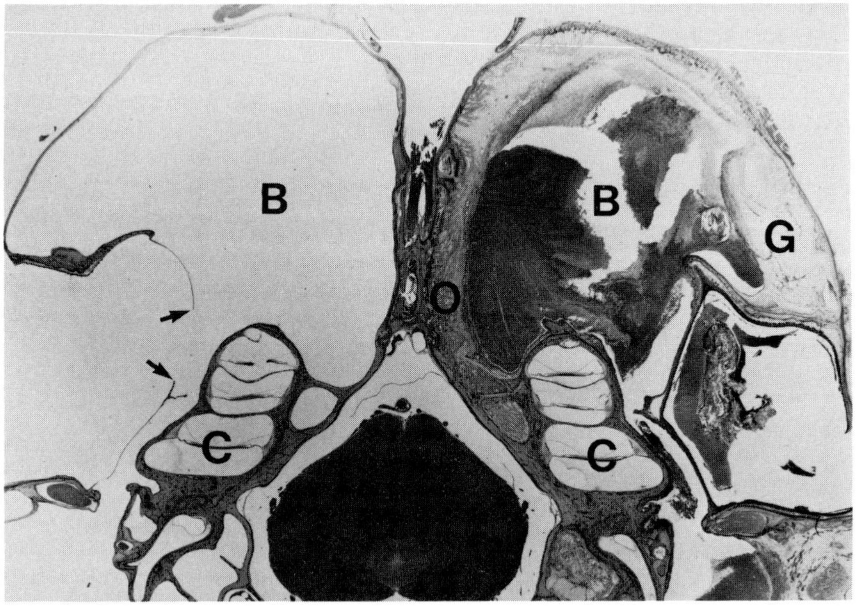

Fig. 2. Bullae (B) of a chinchilla that underwent palatal clefting 14 days previously. Exudate can be seen in the ear without the TT with osteoneogenesis (O) and granulation tissue (G). The cochleae can be identified (C) as can the hole in the TM (arrows) where the TT was placed. (x5)

like Herzon, they did not attempt to separate these cases of OM on the basis of etiology, and no preoperative patient history was available. Further, if attempts to preoperatively sterilize the EAC existed, they were not reported.[7,10,11]

When Stenfors and Winblad[14] inserted their solid, biflanged, polyethylene rods through the TM of healthy rats they observed the presence of thin serous fluid at the myringotomy site for several days postoperatively but no animals developed purulent otorrhea. In the 1981 pilot study of Meyerhoff and Shea 12% of the ears without preoperative sterilization with 70% alcohol developed purulent otorrhea around the Paparella type I TT. In the ears with preoperative sterilization, however, there was no case of postoperative otorrhea. This finding suggests that surgical contamination might be one factor in the development of postoperative otorrhea.

Meyerhoff et al[16] also inserted TT in the right TM of 25 chinchillas followed by mechanical clefting of the soft palate. Within 24 hours of clefting all animals developed sterile MEE in the nonintubated ear which became purulent by day 10 (Fig. 2). Although three intubated ears developed postoperative otorrhea, no other evidence of sterile or purulent MEE in the intubated ears could be identified.

In a later experiment, Meyerhoff et al[17] sterilized the EAC of 45 chinchillas with alcohol and inserted TT in the right TM. Subsequently, they inoculated the chinchillas' nasopharynges with *Streptococcus pneumoniae* and influenza A virus, a combination known to result in OM in about 70% of animals.[18] Unlike the cleft palate model, OME developed with equal frequency in the intubated and nonintubated ears. In the intubated ears this OM manifested as otorrhea. These experiments suggest that not only does preoperative sterilization of the EAC affect the incidence of postoperative OM and otorrhea but that the varied underlying precipitating factors of the otitic process may also play a role.

Karlan et al[19] also recognized the pathophysiologic status of the ME and EAC contamination as factors influencing the development of postoperative otorrhea although they did not address these problems in their experiment. They did, however, demonstrate a difference between the susceptibility of Teflon and Silastic to infection when placed through the TM making the composition of TT a third variable in the occurrence of postoperative otorrhea and ME inflammation.

POTENTIAL BENEFITS

Conductive Hearing Loss. It was determined by Cooper et al[20] following study of 1,133 ears that those with TM demonstrating no compliance reversal (Jerger's type B tympanogram) had an average associated conductive hearing loss of 22 dB in the speech frequencies. It was further concluded by Lewis et al[21] that type B tympanograms were quite stable with less than 10% reverting to normal over a two-month observation period. While E. Harford (unpublished data, 1981) demonstrated that surgical removal of MEE and placement of TT immediately reduced the average conductive hearing loss by 21 dB in 41 consecutive patients, Lildholdt et al[22] reported no long-term (12 months) differences in auditory thresholds between ears with MEE that had been treated with TT insertion and those that had not been so treated. In the latter study, however, no interim thresholds nor psychosocial or educational effects of temporary hearing loss were measured.

Although the significance of temporary hearing loss is not totally agreed upon, Needleman[23] identified linguistic problems and strained relationships between parents and children when the children suffered OM and its associated hearing loss. These linguistic problems and strained relationships eventually resulted in detriment to the child's social development and academic success. The Communicative Disorders Program of the National Institute of Neurological Disorders and Stroke similarly concluded that recurrent and persistent MEE does significantly affect long-term auditory function, speech, language, cognition, and socialization of the developing child.[24]

Incidence of Acute Purulent Otitis Media. Samuel et al[25] studied 30 young children with intractable recurrent purulent OM in whom ME ventilating tubes were used as a treatment and they concluded that 82% of their patients were definitely improved following insertion of the tube. With the addition of associated adenoidectomy they were able to achieve total remission from recurrent purulent OM in 93% of their cases.

Gebhart[26] prospectively studied 95 children 36 months of age and younger with refractory recurrent, acute, purulent OM. These patients were randomly placed in two groups: one receiving TT and the other, aggressive medical treatment. The patients were followed at monthly intervals for six months during which time acute purulent OM occurred statistically less frequently in those children with the TT.

Middle Ear Sequelae. Sequelae including ossicular erosion, osteoneogenesis, fibrosis of the subepithelial space and scarring have all been described following OM in humans.[27] These changes have also been identified in experimental animals with OM. Tympanostomy tubes appear, in some models, to reduce the incidence and severity of these sequelae. In the 25 chinchillas with mechanical clefting of the soft palate and unilateral TT that were described by Meyerhoff et al[16] not only did purulent OM develop statistically more often in the nonintubated ears than in those with TT but, with time, the nonintubated ears also developed irreversible sequelae (Fig. 2). The animals were sacrificed at intervals following palate clefting and the temporal bones studied morphologically with the light microscope. Although mild inflammation could be identified in nine intubated ears, the inflammation in the nonintubated ears was more severe, more frequent, and associated with the irreversible changes of ossicular erosion, osteoneogenesis, and fibrosis of the subepithelial space.

The 45 chinchillas in which Meyerhoff et al[17] inoculated the nasopharynges with *S pneumoniae* and influenza A virus developed MEE with equal frequency in the intubated and nonintubated ears. The animals were sacrificed at intervals following nasopharyngeal inoculation and histologic study of the temporal bones confirmed the equal frequencies of MEE in the intubated and nonintubated ears.

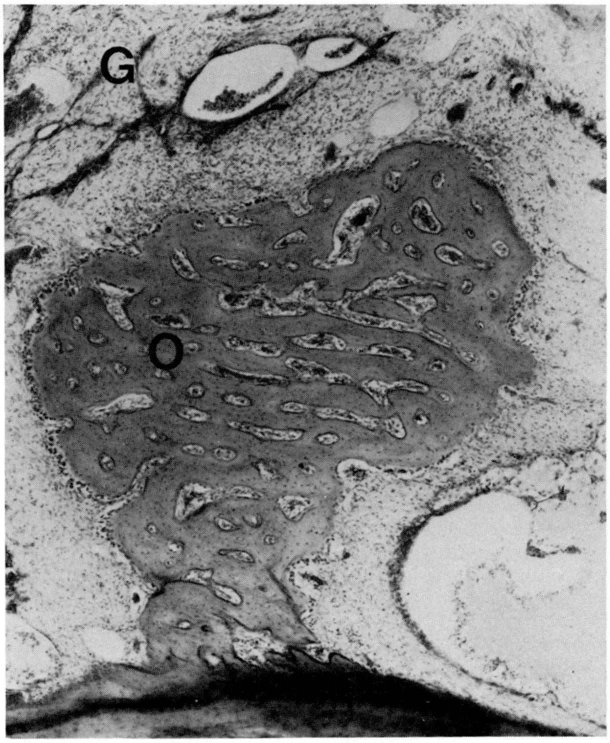

Fig. 3. New bone formation (O) and granulation tissue (G) can be identified in the subepithelial space of a chinchilla. This chinchilla had its nasopharynx inoculated 14 days previously with influenza A virus and *S pneumoniae*. A TT was placed in the contralateral ear and no chronic irreversible changes could be identified. No TT was placed in the ear from which this section was taken. (x65)

The severity of the process in the intubated ears was subjectively less, however, and there were more irreversible pathologic changes in the subepithelial space of the nonintubated ears (Fig. 3).

Inner Ear. Aside from the catastrophic condition of suppurative labyrinthitis other, more subtle, complications of OM such as sensorineural hearing loss and endolymphatic hydrops are known to occur. Hulka[28] described changes in bone conduction thresholds in patients with acute purulent OM and Paparella et al[29] noted that the mean bone conduction audiograms from patients with chronic OM were significantly worse than normative data. Further, Paparella et al[30] demonstrated both clinical and histologic evidence of endolymphatic hydrops in patients with otherwise asymptomatic OM.

It is postulated that the round window membrane is the site of communication between the ME and the inner ear. Round window membrane permeability to different substances and localized perilymphatic labyrinthitis with sensorineural hearing loss in cases of OM has been well documented.[31,32] There is no available evidence, however, that the presence of a TT and its serving as a drain would alter the pathophysiology or frequency of these processes.

CONCLUSIONS

As discussed in the introduction, the efficacy of

any treatment regimen depends on the benefit/risk ratio.

The cost effectiveness of TT as a treatment for OM is difficult to determine. Surgical and anesthestic fees are substantial as are operating room costs. Nonsurgical outpatient care of the otitis prone patient is also expensive, however, and the value of hearing restoration and preservation is, at present, impossible to assess. For this reason it is felt that cost should not be a deterrent to the placement of TT. Further, although the incidence and severity of anesthestic and surgical complications associated with TT insertion are not precisely known, they do not appear to be significant enough to warrant these potential problems as deterrent factors for this procedure.

There is good evidence that TM changes occasionally occur following TT insertion but there is little evidence that separates those TM changes that are due to the TT from those that are secondary to the process of OM itself. The results of animal experiments suggest that, in the absence of ME disease, TT cause little or no permanent TM damage.

The cause and effect of postoperative otorrhea and ME inflammation is not well understood although otorrhea and ME inflammation do occasionally occur following TT insertion. Whether this otorrhea is stimulated by the TT or whether the TT merely serves as an escape for effusion resulting from other local and regional factors is speculative. Animal experiments show that otorrhea rarely occurs postoperatively if the ME is free of disease, the EAC is properly sterilized, and the least reactive material is used. Middle ear inflammation does occur following TT insertion in certain animal models for OM but no more frequently than inflammation in the nonintubated ears. Whether TT increase or decrease the incidence of inner ear disease in OM is not known.

There is no doubt that TT usually correct the conductive hearing imposed by the MEE and presumably the educational and psychological ramifications. The incidence of recurrent acute OM appears clinically to be reduced by the insertion of TT and the results of animal experiments suggest that TT reduce also the incidence and severity of ME sequelae in OM.

For these reasons it is concluded that, in the hands of capable surgeons and competent anesthetists and anesthesiologists, TT insertion as a treatment for OM is almost free of intraoperative and postoperative complications while eliminating the CHL and reducing the incidence of recurrent acute OM and its sequelae. With proper patient selection (intractable MEE), appropriate treatment of associated conditions (maxillary sinusitis, allergy, nasopharyngeal infections), sterilization of the EAC and the use of least easily infected materials, TT insertion is an efficacious procedure.

REFERENCES

1. Armstrong BW. A new treatment for chronic secretory otitis media. Arch Otolaryngol 1954; 59:653.
2. Paradise J. On tympanostomy tubes: rationale, results, reservations, and recommendations. Pediatrics 1977; 60:86-90.
3. Armstrong BW, Armstrong RB. Tympanostomy tubes, their use, abuse, and cost-benefit ratio. Laryngoscope 1979; 89:443-9.
4. Pratt LW, Gallagher RA. Tonsillectomy and adenoidectomy: incidence and mortality, 1968-1972. Otolaryngol Head Neck Surg 1979; 87:159-66.
5. Goodman RS, Cohen NL. Aberrant internal carotid artery in the middle ear. Ann Otol Rhinol Laryngol 1981; 90:67-9.
6. Harell M, Shea J. Hazards of ventilation tubes. Adv Otorhinolaryngol 1978; 23:22-8.
7. Barfoed C, Rosborg J. Secretory otitis media: long term observations after treatment with grommets. Arch Otolaryngol 1980; 106:553-6.
8. Donaldson JA. Surgical management of eustachian tube dysfunction and its importance in middle ear effusion. Pediatrics 1978; 61:774-7.
9. Gundersen T, Tonning F. Ventilating tubes in the middle ear. Arch Otolaryngol 1976; 102:198-9.
10. Pappas JJ. Middle ear ventilation tubes. Laryngoscope 1974; 84:1098-117.
11. McLelland CA. Incidence of complications from use of tympanostomy tubes. Arch Otolaryngol 1980; 106:97-9.
12. Buckingham RA. Cholesteatoma and chronic otitis media following middle ear intubation. Presented at the meeting of the middle section of the American Laryngological, Rhinological, and Otological Society, Inc, Oklahoma City, January 23, 1981.
13. Brown MJ, Richards SH, Ambegaokar AG. Grommets and glue ear: a five-year follow up of a controlled trial. R Soc Med J 1978; 71:353-6.
14. Stenfors L, Winblad B. Tympanic membrane changes after installation of polyethylene grommets. Acta Otolaryngol (Stockh) 1980; 90:16-24.
15. Herzon F. Tympanostomy tubes: infectious complications. Arch Otolaryngol 1980; 106:645-7.
16. Meyerhoff WL, Shea DA, Foster CA. Otitis media, cleft palate and middle ear ventilation. Otolaryngol Head Neck Surg 1981 (in press).
17. Meyerhoff WL, Giebink GS, Shea DA, Le CT. Effect of tympanostomy tubes on the pathogenesis of acute otitis media. Am J Otolaryngol 1981 (in press).
18. Giebink GS, Berzins IK, Marker SC, Shiffman G. Experimental otitis media after nasal inoculation of *Streptococcus pneumoniae* and influenza A virus in chinchillas. Infect Immunol 1980; 30:445-50.
19. Karlan M, Skobel B, Grizzard M, et al. Myringotomy tube materials: bacterial adhesion and infection. Otolaryngol Head Neck Surg 1980; 88:783-95.
20. Cooper JC, Langley LR, Meyerhoff WL, Gates GA. The significance of negative middle ear pressure. Laryngoscope 1977; 87:92-7.
21. Lewis N, Dugdale A, Canty A, Jerger J. Open-ended tympanometric screening: a new concept. Arch Otolaryngol 1975; 101:722-5.

22. Lildholdt T, Courtois J, Kortholm B, Schou JW, Warrer H. The diagnosis of negative middle ear pressure in children. Acta Otolaryngol (Stockh) 1980; 89:459-64.

23. Needleman H. Effects of hearing loss from early recurrent otitis media on speech and language development. In: Jaffe BF, ed. Hearing loss in children. Baltimore: University Park Press, 1977.

24. Hanson DG, Ulvestad RF. Otitis media and child development. Ann Otol Rhinol Laryngol 1979; 88 Suppl 60.

25. Samuel J, Rosen G, Vered Y. Use of middle ear ventilation tubes in recurrent acute otitis media. J Laryngol Otol 1979; 93:979-81.

26. Gebhart D. Tympanostomy tubes in the otitis media prone child. Presented at the 84th annual meeting of the American Laryngology, Rhinology, and Otological Society, Vancouver, Canada, May 14, 1981.

27. Meyerhoff WL, Kim CS, Paparella MM. Pathology of chronic otitis media. Ann Otol Rhinol Laryngol 1978; 87:749-60.

28. Hulka JH. Bone conduction changes in acute otitis media. Arch Otolaryngol 1941; 33:333-50.

29. Paparella MM, Brady D, Hoel R. Sensorineural hearing loss in chronic otitis media and mastoiditis. Trans Am Acad Ophthalmol Otolaryngol 1970; 74:108-15.

30. Paparella MM, Goycoolea MV, Meyerhoff WL, Shea DA. Endolymphatic hydrops and otitis media. Laryngoscope 1979; 89:43-54.

31. Schachern PA. The round window membrane following application of staphylococcal exotoxin: an electron microscopic study. Presented at the eastern section of the American Triological Society, Philadelphia, 1981.

32. Goycoolea MV, Paparella MM, Goldberg B, Carpenter AM. Permeability of the round window membrane in otitis media. Arch Otolaryngol 1980; 106:430-3.

≈

NINCDS NOTES*

INSTITUTE REPORTS ON FY 81 TRAINING AWARDS

Training and development awards granted by NINCDS totaled over $16.5 million in FY 81, a figure that includes funding for both competitive awards and continuation payments for previously awarded multiple-year grants. New and competitive renewal awards were funded in four categories: individual and institutional National Research Service Awards (research fellowships), Research Career Development Awards (RCDAs), and Teacher Investigator Development Awards (TIDAs). Over $1.9 million was awarded to 104 individual NSRA grantees, and $274,000 was awarded to support four institutional National Research Service Awards (training grants). Twenty-four TIDAs claimed approximately $1 million in Institute funds, while $339,000 went to nine RCDA recipients. Applications for NINCDS training and development awards must be received by October 1, February 1, and June 1 of each year. Approximately ten months are required to review the applications and notify applicants of the results. Additional information on these programs may be obtained by contacting Dr. John W. Diggs, Deputy Director, Extramural Activities Program, NINCDS-NIH, Bethesda, MD 20205; (301) 496-4188.

INSTITUTE CREATES INTRAMURAL COMMUNICATIVE DISORDERS BRANCH

A new Communicative Disorders Branch has been established in the NINCDS Intramural Research Program to focus on research problems involving speech, language, and hearing. The new branch will enable the Institute to develop and support an integrated clinical program devoted to the sensory-motor mechanisms of the ear, nose and throat and other aspects of communicate disorders. Staff scientists will investigate speech and language dysfunctions, and design and evaluate treatment procedures as well as prosthetic devices. Branch resources will include NIH Clinical Center facilities for patients undergoing surgical and diagnostic or treatment procedures. A branch chief has not yet been named.

NINCDS PUBLISHES STUTTERING PAMPHLET

The perplexing nature of stuttering and recently developed techniques to overcome this disorder are explained in a new NINCDS pamphlet, *Stuttering: Hope Through Research.* The 20-page booklet describes NINCDS-supported efforts to identify the cause of stuttering, and explains therapeutic techniques such as biofeedback and larynx control. Warning signs of stuttering in children, such as a rise in pitch as the child draws out a syllable, are also described. In addition, the publication lists seven health organizations concerned with the speech disorder. Single copies of the new pamphlet can be obtained by contacting the Office of Scientific and Health Reports, NINCDS, Building 31, Room 8A06, 9000 Rockville Pike, Bethesda, MD 20205; (301) 496-5752.

*This information is prepared monthly by the Office of Scientific and Health Reports, National Institute of Neurological and Communicative Disorders and Stroke, National Institutes of Health, Building 31, Room 8A06, Bethesda, MD 20205; (301) 496-5751.

AUDITORY PROCESSING ABILITIES IN CHILDREN WITH PREVIOUS MIDDLE EAR EFFUSION

KIMBERLY HOFFMAN-LAWLESS, MA
ROBERT W. KEITH, PhD ROBIN T. COTTON, MD
CINCINNATI, OHIO

The present study was designed to determine whether auditory processing disorders are present in children with documented middle ear effusion (MEE) that required surgical treatment. Children with previous MEE and control subjects, in two age groups, were studied using five tests of auditory processing abilities: low-pass filtered speech, staggered spondaic word test, speech in noise, auditory sequential memory, and sound blending. Results found differences in groups at mean age 7 on the filtered speech test, but no statistical differences were found on any other test at age 7 or on any test at mean age 9. The results indicate that well-managed MEE appears to have no long-term effects on children acquiring this disease.

INTRODUCTION

The recent otolaryngologic literature indicates an increasing interest in the complications and sequelae of otitis media (OM). Results of two international symposia on otitis media with effusion (OME) finds an impressive amount of data on all aspects of this subject.[1,2] However, very little information was presented during these meetings on effects of middle ear effusion (MEE) on speech, language, and cognitive development and on auditory processing abilities. In fact, there is less scientific data available on these subjects than on the epidemiology, physiology, microbiology, immunology, and other topics related to MEE. Studies that are available have found positive correlations among all types of speech, language, auditory processing, behavioral and learning disorders, and the presence of chronic OME.[3-9]

While there may be a clear link between histories of recurrent MEE and delays in the development of verbal communication skills, the cause and effect relationship is not known. In fact, the suggestion has been made that "predisposition to language-learning disabilities may be responsible for the occurrence of chronic OM as well."[10] Criticism of research implicating conductive hearing impairment as a causal agent in learning disability, language dysfunction, and central auditory problems has been voiced by Ventry[11] who calls for more rigorous research on these subjects. That recommendation was made also in the guidelines for the use of acoustic impedance measurement in screening for middle ear (ME) disease in children.[12] The task force making those recommendations concluded that "evidence for early treatment of otitis media with effusion to avoid unfavorable long-term developmental consequences in children is not conclusive and more studies are necessary to confirm this possibility."

In a workshop on OM and child development,[13] a suggestion was made that the kinds of auditory processing problems identified in children with chronic ME disease are more likely to be delays and not permanent. These conclusions run contrary to the results of animal model studies that indicate reduction of sound stimulation in the developing auditory nervous system leads to mainly irreversible anatomical defects.[14]

The present study was designed to investigate two interrelated hypotheses: 1) whether auditory processing abilities of children with medically confirmed early MEE are different from children with no history of MEE, and 2) whether these differences, if they exist, persist as children grow older.

METHODS

Four groups of ten subjects each were chosen for study. They were selected without regard to socioeconomic status. There were eight males and two females in each of the groups. The two experimental groups were comprised of children having documented histories of OME. All experimental subjects had persistent MEE lasting nine months or longer indicated by tympanometric findings and verified by otoscopic examination. Tympanometric findings indicating possible MEE included peaked or rounded tympanograms with negative pressures exceeding -200 mm H_2O and flat tympanograms. Otoscopy was always performed by the same examiner. Experimental group 1 had a mean age of 7 years with an age range from 6 years 2 months to 7 years 9 months. Experimental group 2 had a mean age of 9 years with an age range from 8 years 2 months to 9 years 8 months. The experimental subjects acquired MEE during their first four years of life, although most subjects acquired their disease between their second and fourth years. All had been under the care of the same otologist and had surgical placement of ventilation tubes before their fifth birthday. In order to be included as subjects, the children were required to be free of ME disease with normal ME function at the time of the study. No child who had failed to respond to treat-

From the Department of Otolaryngology and Maxillofacial Surgery, University of Cincinnati Medical Center.
Presented at the meeting of the American Otological Society, Inc., Vancouver, British Columbia, May 9-10, 1981.
REPRINTS — Kimberly Hoffman-Lawless, MA, Div. of Audiology and Speech Pathology, Univ. of Cincinnati, Cincinnati, OH 45267.

ment or had continuing ME problems was included in this study. Confirmation of medical histories was accomplished through review of each child's medical record. According to their parents, these children were all functioning well in a normal classroom at the time of the study.

Two groups of children with ages similar to the experimental population served as a control population. The mean age of control group 1 was 6 years 9 months with an age range from 6 years 4 months to 7 years 8 months. Control group 2 had a mean age of 8 years 9 months and an age range from 8 years 2 months to 9 years 10 months. The control subjects had no known history of OM with MEE. According to their parents, they were functioning well in a normal classroom and exhibited apparently normal articulation and language skills.

Subjects in all groups were required to have hearing thresholds between 0 and 15 dB in the speech frequencies with speech discrimination scores better than 88% at 30 dB SL. Normal impedance measurements were required of all subjects with ME pressure between 0 and −200 mm H_2O, static compliance between 0.3 and 1.5 cc of equivalent volume of air, and acoustic reflex thresholds less than 95 dB HL at 500, 1000 and 2000 Hz. These findings indicated the presence of normal ME function in all children at the time studied.

Procedures. Prior to the experimental procedures the following hearing tests were performed: pure tone thresholds at 500, 1000, 2000 and 4000 Hz; speech reception thresholds; speech discrimination scores in quiet using half lists of PBK words; and impedance measurements. Results of these tests were used to determine the child's eligibility to participate in the study. Audiometric testing was done with a Maico MA-17 audiometer, and a Grason-Stadler model 162 speech audiometer with input from an Akai 400-PS MK-11 reel-to-reel tape recorder at 19.05 cm (7½ in)/s. The earphones used were TDH-39 10 Ω with MX-41/AR cushions.

Five tests of auditory processing ability were administered to each subject. These tests were selected on the basis of their suitability for the age groups tested and their purported ability to identify auditory processing problems, as indicated by our review of the literature. All of the tests were prerecorded on low-noise magnetic audio tape. The tests include the following:

1. A filtered speech test consisting of kindergarten PB-50 lists 1B and 1C, low pass filtered at 1000 Hz with an 18 dB/octave rejection rate.[15] Test items were presented monaurally at 50 dB HL.

2. The staggered spondaic word test (SSW) consisting of all 40 items of list E presented at 50 dB HL.[16] The four test conditions of the SSW were right noncompeting (RNC), right competing (RC), left competing (LC), and left noncompeting (LNC).

3. A speech-in-noise test consisting of kindergarten PB-50 lists 4A and 4B presented monaurally at 50 dB HL in the presence of speech babble noise at +8 dB S/N. The speech babble noise was recorded with two males and two females reading aloud material from different sources (Palanker S, unpublished master's thesis). No single speaker is predominant, nor is any speaker consistently intelligible on the speech babble recording.

4. The auditory sequential memory test from the *Illinois Test of Psycholinguistic Abilities.*[17] Sequences of numbers increasing in length from two to eight digits were presented binaurally at 50 dB HL.

5. The sound blending test of the *Goldman-Fristoe-Woodcock Auditory Skills Test Battery.*[18] Sounds of words spoken singly were presented binaurally at 50 dB HL.

Instructions to subjects were given before each test presentation. The bias of order and sequence effect was minimized by randomizing the order of test presentation. Ear effects were minimized by alternating the ear presented first on the filtered speech, staggered spondaic word, and speech-in-noise tests.

RESULTS

Results of the filtered speech test are shown in Figure 1, where mean percentage of words correct is plotted for experimental and control groups at each age level. An analysis of variance found significant differences between groups (F = 4.09, df = 1/36, p ≤ .01). There was no significant difference between ears (F = 1.24, df = 1/36, p ≥ .05). Inspection of mean data shown in Figure 1 indicates that significant differences were due to differences in performance of experimental and control groups at age 7. The difference between group means at that age was 6.5%. There is no longer a difference between groups at age 9 where the difference between group means was 1.9%.

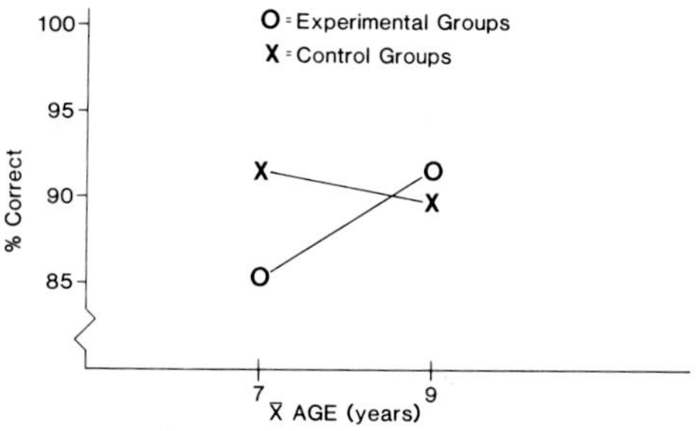

Fig. 1. Mean scores obtained by groups on the 1000 Hz low pass filtered PBK word test.

The SSW test results are shown on Figure 2. On this figure the mean percentage of errors for both groups is plotted for each of the four test conditions. Results of younger age groups is shown on the left, of older groups on the right. There was no significant difference between groups on this test (F = .08, df = 1/36, p ≥ .05), although there was an expected improvement of mean scores with age. In addition, the right ear competing scores were better than left ear competing scores, as normally expected.

The speech-in-noise test results are shown on Figure 3, where mean percentage of scores correct are plotted by group and age. The analysis of variance failed to show any difference between groups

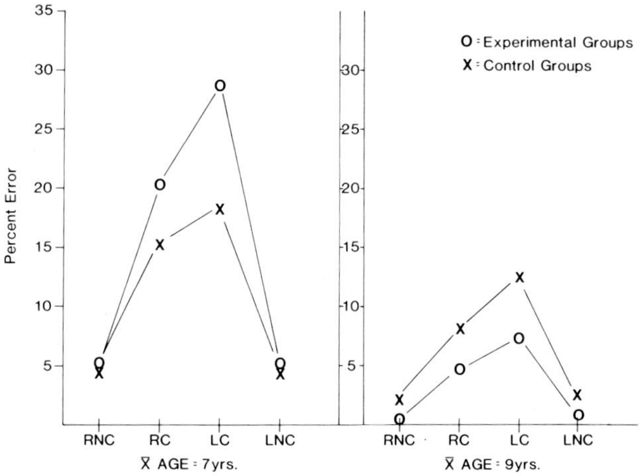

Fig. 2. Mean error scores obtained by groups on the Staggered Spondaic Word test. Left - Younger age groups; Right - Older age groups. The four test conditions were right noncompeting (RNC), right competing (RC), left competing (LC), left noncompeting (LNC).

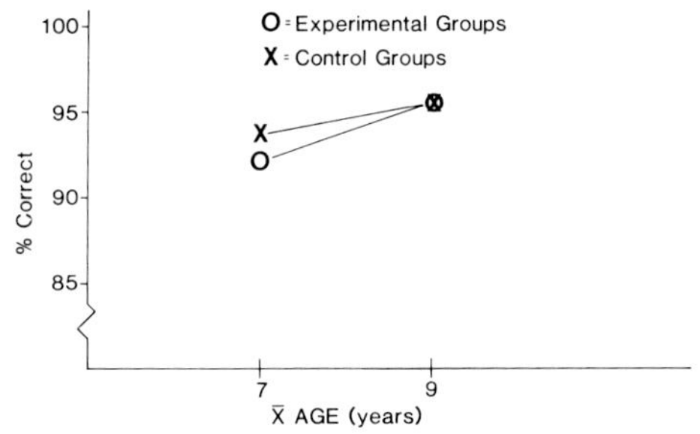

Fig. 3. Mean scores obtained by groups on the PBK words in the presence of speech babble noise at + 8 dB S/N ratio.

($F = 0.76$, $df = 1/36$, $p > .05$). In addition, neither the sequential memory test nor the sound blending test yielded significant differences between groups. The difference of mean raw scores for treatment and control groups was 0.3 or less on the sequential memory test for both age groups. Similarly, the difference of mean raw scores for treatment and control groups on the sound blending test was 1.3 or less.

DISCUSSION

The results of this study fail to identify a clear link between a history of MEE exceeding nine months in children 4 years or less who were adequately treated and the presence of disordered auditory processing abilities. The findings of a difference between the younger age experimental and control groups on the low pass filtered speech test was statistically significant at the 0.01 level of confidence; however, the 6.5% difference between group means was not clinically meaningful and would not be considered as having implications for auditory language learning. Nevertheless, the finding of statistical differences that were present in group means of children 7 years old and absent in the 9-year-olds tends to confirm the hypothesis of temporary delays rather than permanent differences in auditory abilities of children with MEE who are adequately treated.

The lack of differences between groups on all other measures presents several possibilities. The auditory processing tests may not have been sufficiently sensitive to subtle differences among groups, although they have shown differences in studies conducted on auditory learning-disabled subjects. In addition, children who receive effective medical or surgical care of their persistent MEE may be less apt to acquire disorders of central auditory abilities, since their conductive hearing loss is minimized.

Finally, central auditory defects may be more inclined to occur in otitis-prone children who acquire MEE in the first few months of life when the auditory nervous system is still developing. Children who continue to have fluctuating hearing loss over the period of time when the auditory nervous system is immature and when they are acquiring speech, language and auditory perceptual skills would undoubtedly be at higher risk for central auditory disorders.

In fact, each of the several possibilities listed here represents a research question that should be investigated. From the results reported here, we would especially encourage prospective longitudinal study of otitis-prone children from the age of identification until speech and language skills are well established. Future investigators should heed the recommendations on experimental design reported in the proceedings edited by Hanson and Ulvestad.[13]

REFERENCES

1. Lim DJ, Bluestone CD, Saunders WH, Senturia BH. Recent advances in middle ear effusions. Ann Otol Rhinol Laryngol 1976; 85 Suppl 25.

2. Senturia BH, Bluestone CD, Lim DJ, Saunders WH. Recent advances in otitis media with effusion. Ann Otol Rhinol Laryngol 1980; 89 Suppl 68.

3. Holm V, Kunze L. Effect of chronic otitis media on language and speech development. J Pediatr 1969; 43:833-9.

4. Kaplan G, Fleshman J, Binder T, Baum C, Clark P. Long-term effects of otitis media: a 10-year cohort study of Alaskan Eskimo children. J Speech Hear Disord 1969; 33:132-46.

5. Howie V, Ploussard J, Sloyer J. Natural history of otitis media. Ann Otol Rhinol Laryngol 1976; 85 Suppl 25:18-30.

6. Paradise J. Management of middle-ear effusion in infants with cleft palate. Ann Otol Rhinol Laryngol 1966; 85 Suppl 25:285-8.

7. Lewis N. Otitis media and linguistic incompetence. Arch Otolaryngol 1976; 102:387-90.

8. Needleman H. Effects of hearing loss from early recurrent otitis media on speech and language development. In: Jaffe B, ed. Hearing loss in children. Baltimore: University Park Press, 1977.

9. Zinkus P, Gottlieb M, Shapiro M. Developmental and psychoeducational sequelae of chronic otitis media. Am J Dis Child 1979; 132:1100-4.

10. Hersher L. Letter to the editor. Am J Dis Child 1980; 134:94.

11. Ventry IM. Effects of conductive hearing loss: fact or fiction. J Speech Hear Disord 1980; 45:143-56.

12. Harford ER, Bess FH, Bluestone CD, Klein JO. Impedance screening for middle ear disease in children. New York: Grune & Stratton, 1978:3-7.

13. Hanson DG, Ulvestad RF. Otitis media and child development, speech, language and education. Ann Otol Rhinol Laryngol 1979; 88 Suppl 60:108.

14. Ruben RJ. A review of transneuronal changes of the auditory central nervous system as a consequence of auditory defects. Int J Pediatr Otorhinolaryngol 1980; 1:269-77.

15. Farrer S, Keith RW. Filtered word testing in the assessment of children's central auditory abilities. Ear and Hearing (in press).

16. Katz J. The staggered spondaic word test. In: Keith RW, ed. Central auditory dysfunction. New York: Grune and Stratton, 1977, chap 4.

17. Kirk S, McCarthy J, Kirk W. Illinois test of psycholinguistic abilities. Urbana: University of Illinois Press, 1968.

18. Goldman R, Fristoe M, Woodcock R. Goldman-Fristoe-Woodcock auditory skills test battery. Circle Pines, Minn.: American Guidance Service, 1974.

RECURRENT MIDDLE EAR EFFUSION IN CHILDHOOD: IMPLICATIONS OF TEMPORARY AUDITORY DEPRIVATION FOR LANGUAGE AND LEARNING

ROBERT J. SAK, MA

ROBERT J. RUBEN, MD

BRONX, NEW YORK

Eighteen healthy, normal hearing (PTA ≤ 15dB, better ear), neurologically intact, 8 to 11-year-old children who had documented histories of middle ear effusion (MEE) before the age of five years were evaluated by a battery of audiological, psychological, language and achievement tests. Each was compared to his/her non-MEE sibling who was tested at the same age. All the children (n = 36) tested in the bright normal range of verbal ability (WISC-R) and none had been diagnosed previously as learning disabled. Paired comparison of sibling data revealed that the effusion subjects had deficits in verbal ability, auditory decoding and spelling skills when compared with their control siblings. Significant strength in visual sequential memory in the MEE subjects suggests the availability of compensatory strategies for auditory deficits. Data analysis on the basis of sex and/or birth order differences could not explain the differences between siblings.

Fluctuating conductive hearing loss associated with middle ear effusion (MEE) creates a condition of temporary partial auditory deprivation. During episodes of effusion, normal auditory input is attenuated and distorted. Recurrent episodes of MEE in early childhood — a critical period for language development — have been associated with cognitive, language and learning deficits in the school-age child.[1-4]

Howie[1] reported significant differences in the IQs of school-age children with three or more episodes of acute otitis media in the first year of life as compared with the IQs of children with no such history. However, that study did not control for hearing levels, achievement levels, or socioeconomic factors. Studies by Kaplan et al[3] and Ling[4] reported depressed achievement levels associated with a history of recurrent MEE. However, included in these studies were children with significant hearing loss at the time of testing, a condition which would in itself contribute directly to poor test performance on an achievement test battery. Holm and Kunze's[2] evaluation of the speech and language abilities of 5- to 9-year-old children with histories of recurrent MEE before 2 years of age revealed significant delay in language skills, involving the reception and processing of auditory information or the production of verbal responses. This study lacked controls for levels of intellectual functioning and hearing at the time of the evaluation. In general, studies of an association between the early history of recurrent MEE and subsequent deficits have been open to criticism on the grounds that the design of these studies did not control for other significant variables.[5,6]

The present study assessed the association of recurrent MEE which occurred in the preschool period with subsequent cognitive, linguistic and academic performance while evaluating hearing level and middle ear status. A sibling control paradigm was used in which one child had a documented history of recurrent MEE in the preschool period (below five years of age) and the other child did not. The advantage of this model over all previous studies lies in the statistical expectation of greater homogeneity in genetic and environmental factors in the pairs of siblings.

METHODS

Experimental Design. A review of medical records of the Hospital of the Albert Einstein College of Medicine and Montefiore Hospital and Medical Center identified all children who had documented diagnoses of recurrent MEE dating from before their fifth birthday. Children who would be between the ages of 8 and 11 years during the time period of the study were considered potential candidates for inclusion. Parents of these children were contacted by mail to determine if they would be interested in participating in the investigation. If the parent was interested, additional criteria had to be met. The child with the history of recurrent MEE (effusion sibling - ES) had to have a sibling without a history of recurrent MEE (control sibling - CS) who would also be between the ages of 8 and 11 during the period of the study. Children had to be free of neurological and neuromuscular diseases, craniofacial malformations, and severe emotional difficulties. No subject could have been diagnosed as being learning disabled prior to the study. Excluded from the study were children with Wechsler Intelligence Scale for Children - Revised (WISC-R) full scale IQs below 85 (1 SD below the mean). Each child had to have a pure tone audiometric average of equal to or less than 15dB in the better ear. Eighteen sibling pairs met the criteria for inclusion in the study.

Evaluation Procedure. Although the age range of all children in the study was 8 to 11 years of age, sibling pairs were evaluated at the same chronological age (see Table 1).

Audiometric evaluation consisted of air conduction, bone conduction, speech reception thresholds, discrimination tests, middle ear pressure, acoustic reflex evaluation, tympanometry, and mea-

From the Department of Otorhinolaryngology, Albert Einstein College of Medicine of Yeshiva University and Montefiore Hospital and Medical Center, Bronx, New York. This work was supported by grants from the William T. Grant Foundation and the New York State Health Research Council.

Presented at the meeting of the American Otological Society, Inc., Vancouver, British Columbia, May 9-10, 1981.

REPRINTS — Robert J. Sak, MA, Albert Einstein College of Medicine of Yeshiva University, 1300 Morris Park Avenue, Bronx, NY 10461.

TABLE 1. AGE, SCHOOL GRADE LEVEL, SEX AND BIRTH ORDER CHARACTERISTICS OF SUBJECTS (N = 36)

	Effusion Sibling N = 18	*Control Sibling* N = 18
Age*	9 yr 7 mo	9 yr 7 mo
School grade*	4.6	4.7
Sex		
Males	13	8
Females	5	10
Birth order		
Older	8	10
Younger	10	8

*At time of evaluation.

surement of compliance. An otorhinolaryngological examination was performed and a complete medical history was obtained at the time of evaluation. The battery of psychological tests included the following:

1. Wechsler Intelligence Scale for Children - Revised (WISC-R).[7] The WISC-R provides separate direct measures of verbal and performance skills. The full scale intelligence quotient (IQ) is derived from verbal and performance quotients.

2. Raven's Coloured Progressive Matrices (RCPM).[8] The RCPM is a nonverbal measure of mental ability involving the linguistic mediation of problem solving strategies.

3. Illinois Test of Psycholinguistic Abilities (ITPA).[9] A test in psycholinguistic skills involved in the communicative process as conceptualized by the authors, Kirk, McCarthy and Kirk. Eleven subtests assess auditory and visual efficiency in receptive (decoding), organizing and expressive (encoding) abilities. Data on the 13 sibling pairs whose age range did not exceed the ceiling level for the ITPA (ten years three months) is reported.

4. Wide Range Achievement Test (WRAT).[10] A widely used diagnostic test of reading skills (word attack and word recognition), spelling and arithmetic computation.

5. Durrell Analysis of Reading Difficulty (DARD).[11] Graded reading paragraphs providing measures of oral reading and comprehension, and silent reading and oral recall.

Characteristics of the Population. Age, grade, sex and birth order of all subjects are given in Table 1. The mean age of ES and CS subjects at the time of evaluation were the same: nine years, seven months of age. The mean educational grade levels for ESs and CSs were 4.6 and 4.7 respectively. The distribution of males and females in both groups differed. In the ES group there were 13 males and 5 females and in the CS group there were 8 males and 10 females. Eight of the ESs were the older and ten were the younger of their sibling pair.

Table 2 details the history of recurrent MEE in the ES cases. Fifty percent (n = 9) of the ES subjects had their first episode of MEE in the first 24 months of life and the other 50% (n = 9) between their 25th and 48th month. The number of episodes of

TABLE 2. HISTORY OF RECURRENT MIDDLE EAR EFFUSION IN EFFUSION SIBLING SUBJECTS (N = 18)

Age at first episode		
Month		Subjects
Birth - 24		9
25-48		9
Total number of episodes		
Episodes		Subjects
3-6		7
>6		11
Age at first bilateral myringotomy		
Month		Subjects
13-24		1
25-48		17
Total number of myringotomies		
N	Range	Average
43	1-8 bilateral	2.5

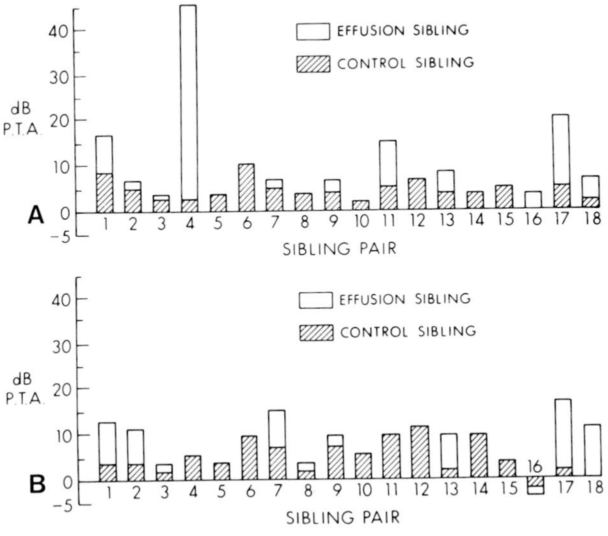

Fig. 1. Comparison of ES and CS pairs on dB pure tone average (PTA) 500 Hz - 2kHz at time of evaluation. A) Right ear; B) Left ear.

MEE as obtained from the history revealed that 61% of the ESs (n = 11) had more than six episodes. Parents estimated the number of episodes of MEE in ES subjects to range from three to "almost continuously" during the preschool period. One of the ESs had a myringotomy with insertion of tympanotomy tubes performed before the 24th month of life. The other 17 subjects had the initial procedure between the 25th and 48th month. ESs had from one to eight bilateral myringotomies with insertion of tympanotomy tubes.

Audiometric findings are given in Figure 1. The audiological evaluations were done at the time of the psychological and otological assessments. All of the 18 CSs had bilateral pure tone averages in the speech frequencies 500, 1000, 2000 Hz equal to or less than 10dB (ANSI 1969). Thirteen of the ESs had bilateral pure tone averages equal to or less than 10dB PTA. Four of the ESs had a unilateral hearing loss equal to or less than 10dB in the better ear and one had a unilateral hearing loss of 15dB in the better ear. All of the ESs and CSs had speech reception thresholds (SRT) equal to or less than 10dB bilaterally or unilaterally. Normal speech discrimination ability (92-100%) was obtained when measured with phonetically balanced monosyllables presented at 30dB sensation level (SL) relative to the SRT.

Abnormal impedance as defined by a middle ear pressure of greater than − 100mm of water and/or static compliance of less than 0.4 - 1.6cc and/or the presence of a tympanotomy tube was found in 50% (9) of the ES cases and only 22% (4) of the CS subjects.[12] Retracted and restricted tympanic membranes were the most common abnormalities.

The CS medical histories, obtained from the parents, revealed that nine of the CSs had at least one episode of MEE in the preschool period. None of the CSs had myringotomies.

RESULTS

Statistical analysis of the psychological and educational test data was based upon comparison of sibling data using paired *t* tests of significance.

Intelligence. WISC-R scores for the two groups are shown in Table 3. Both ESs and CSs attained mean verbal quotients in the above average range of ability. The sibling pairs are not statistically distinguished from one another on the basis of performance quotient or full scale IQ. The two groups did not differ significantly on the nonverbal measure of

TABLE 3. WECHSLER INTELLIGENCE SCALE FOR CHILDREN — REVISED (WISC-R): VERBAL, PERFORMANCE AND FULL SCALE IQs

WISC-R	*Effusion Sibling Mean ± SD*	*Control Sibling Mean ± SD*	*Paired t Test*
Verbal quotient	111.00 ± 12.11	116.11 ± 13.52	p< .05
Performance quotient	103.33 ± 12.95	104.00 ± 13.17	NS*
Full scale IQ	108.16 ± 12.72	111.50 ± 13.63	NS

*Nonsignificant.

mental ability (RCPM). However, the ESs had significantly depressed verbal quotients when compared to their CSs (p< .05). This would suggest that deficits were in the area of verbal language, and not due to overall nonverbal reasoning deficiencies.

Analysis of intelligence test ratings on the basis of sex and birth order of the siblings revealed no significant differences between male and female subjects or between younger and older siblings.

Psycholinguistic Abilities. Eleven subtests of the ITPA were given to 13 sibling pairs whose ages did not exceed the ten-year, three-month limit for the test. These included 16 males and 10 females. Raw scores were converted to scale scores for analysis. Statistically significant differences between the siblings were found on two of the subtests: auditory reception and visual sequential memory. Table 4 provides mean and standard deviation data for both ES and CS subjects on the ITPA subtests. ESs were deficient in auditory reception relative to the CSs (p< .05). They were more proficient than their control siblings on the visual sequential memory subtest (p< .01), the only psycholinguistic measure in which the ESs demonstrated superiority over their CSs. All other subtest ratings were in the direction of greater proficiency for the CSs although not at statistically significant levels. Analysis of the subtest scores on the ITPA by sex revealed differences favoring females on both the visual sequential memory and visual association subtests, both at p< .05. The greater representation of females in the control group notwithstanding, the ESs performed better than their CSs on the same subtest representing a reversal in significance. Female superiority on the visual association subtest of the ITPA was not maintained when the data was analyzed on the basis of condition rather than by sex.

Sex and Birth Order. Differences found in the comparison of ES and CS subjects could not be explained by sex and/or birth order differences. This finding is of particular interest as data analysis by sex indicated females performed better than males on the visual sequential memory test (ITPA). Male subjects were more highly represented in the ES than in the CS group by a ratio of 2:1. The implication of the ESs strength in the visual sequential memory task becomes all the more significant as the finding runs contrary to what would be expected on the basis of the sex distribution of the subjects in the study. Previous retrospective studies have noted a preponderance of males in their MEE samples but have not reported on the possible contribution of sex to their findings.[2,13]

Achievement. All subjects were rated on both a) the discrepancy between current grade placement and achievement level; and b) standard scores for the three achievement tests; reading, spelling and arithmetic. Table 5 provides the mean and standard deviations for the two groups in the three achievement areas. In spelling achievement level, a significant negative discrepancy from actual grade placement was found in the ESs (p< .05). Standard scores for the two groups did not differ significantly for any of the three achievement tests. However, the data in Table 5 points in the direction of greater academic proficiency of the sibling controls.

Reading Comprehension. The two groups were not significantly different in their performance on either the oral reading or silent reading paragraphs of the Durrell Analysis of Reading Difficulty. Table 6 provides oral and silent reading grade level attainments for both the ES and CS subjects as well as the reading level discrepancy from actual grade placement. As might be expected on the basis of intelli-

TABLE 4. ILLINOIS TEST OF PSYCHOLINGUISTIC ABILITIES SUBTEST SCALE SCORE MEANS

	Effusion Sibling Mean ± SD	*Control Sibling Mean ± SD*	*Paired t Test*
Auditory reception	31.92 ± 5.49	37.53 ± 7.63	p< .05
Visual reception	36.30 ± 7.89	37.00 ± 4.58	NS
Visual memory	39.30 ± 7.22	34.84 ± 7.16	p< .01
Auditory association	34.46 ± 8.15	37.92 ± 5.54	NS
Auditory memory	35.07 ± 5.10	36.53 ± 4.61	NS
Visual association	35.46 ± 7.55	38.76 ± 6.40	NS
Visual closure	30.92 ± 6.89	32.30 ± 5.02	NS
Verbal expression	32.07 ± 2.56	32.69 ± 3.56	NS
Grammatic closure	37.53 ± 7.94	39.15 ± 7.19	NS
Manual expression	34.46 ± 5.28	36.69 ± 5.58	NS
Auditory closure	37.84 ± 4.05	38.69 ± 6.65	NS
Sum of scale scores*	347.53 ± 38.84	361.61 ± 30.31	NS

*Sum of ten subjects (excluding auditory closure).

TABLE 5. WIDE RANGE ACHIEVEMENT TEST STANDARD SCORES AND ACHIEVEMENT LEVEL ± GRADE LEVEL DISCREPANCY

	Effusion Sibling Mean ± SD	*Control Sibling Mean ± SD*	*Paired t Test*
Reading (word recognition & decoding)			
Standard score	111.61 ± 9.59	117.00 ± 16.18	NS
Achievement level ± grade level	1.35 ± 1.42	2.24 ± 2.05	NS
Spelling			
Standard score	110.11 ± 10.68	117.55 ± 16.45	NS
Achievement level ± grade level	0.82 ± 1.24	2.02 ± 2.19	p<.05
Arithmetic computation			
Standard score	103.27 ± 37.00	110.22 ± 18.82	NS
Achievement level ± grade level	−0.38 ± 0.78	0.77 ± 2.19	NS

gence test performance, the mean reading grade levels are consistent with current grade placement. Virtually all children showed greater proficiency on the oral reading and comprehension task than on silent reading with oral recall.

DISCUSSION

The results of the present investigation demonstrate a pattern of depressed verbal ability, auditory decoding and spelling skills in the absence of current hearing loss in the ESs. These findings differentiate the paired siblings, one of whom has had a history of recurrent MEE before five years of age and the other who had not. Although sibling data in the retrospective study of psychoeducational sequelae of recurrent MEE has not been previously reported in the literature, other studies[6] have suggested a similar pattern: depressed language and auditory processing skills and impaired academic achievement as a result of recurrent MEE in early life.[2,3]

The differences between the ESs and the CSs in the present report, while significant, are not so great as to result in a major functional deficit, eg, specific learning disability. This lack of a major functional deficit is due to the design of the study in that any children who would have had a significant functional educational deficit were excluded.[14] The results in this study show what are probably the most minimal deficits secondary to recurrent MEE in the preschool years.

The ESs in this study — intellectually bright youngsters with specific auditory decoding deficit — do not show pervasive psycholinguistic or achievement problems. Spelling is affected but other areas of achievement (as measured by the WRAT) are not. No deficits are found in other auditory-verbal or visual-motor functions related to psycholinguistic development. The more pervasive deficits reported in other studies[2-4,6] may have been due in part to the presence of a number of other factors excluded from this study. In addition to auditory decoding deficits resulting from recurrent MEE in the preschool period, hearing loss, socioeconomic disadvantage, and low average mental ability have been characteristic of the populations previously studied.[2-4]

In contrast to the present study, Zinkus and Gottlieb[13] and Bennett et al[15] have approached the problem from the point of view of the learning disabled child. Zinkus and Gottlieb[13] found that among learning disabled children described as having auditory processing deficits, those with a history of chronic MEE in early childhood could be differentiated from those without such a history; the former group showed more pervasive language and cognitive deficits than the latter. Bennett et al[15] found a higher incidence of chronic MEE, middle ear pathology and hearing loss among learning disabled children than among a control group without learning problems. The children in these studies would not have met the criteria for inclusion in the present investigation. It can be hypothesized that the children with MEE in the Zinkus and Gottlieb[13] and Bennett et al[15] studies were more cognitive- and/or sensory-impaired and may have been unable to effectively compensate for an auditory processing deficit.

The subjects in the present study represent a relatively homogeneous group of children: bright, achieving, middle class youngsters whose deficits, though statistically significant, were not of sufficient magnitude to be considered functionally significant. The possibility of a compensatory shift in the cognitive strategy of these subjects who had endured periods of temporary partial auditory deprivation in early childhood was suggested by the findings of a significant deficit in auditory decoding skills with a concurrent strength in the area of visual sequential memory. Holm and Kunze[2] speculated that young children of a lower socioeconomic background (as were the subjects in their retrospec-

TABLE 6. DURRELL ANALYSIS OF READING DIFFICULTY — ORAL AND SILENT READING GRADE LEVELS AND DISCREPANCY RATINGS BETWEEN READING LEVEL AND GRADE PLACEMENT

	Effusion Sibling Mean ± SD	*Control Sibling Mean ± SD*	*Paired t Test*
Oral reading grade level	4.70 ± 1.04	4.74 ± 1.36	NS
Oral reading grade level ± current grade level	−0.02 ± 0.83	0.10 ± 1.15	NS
Silent reading grade level	4.07 ± 0.93	4.12 ± 1.36	NS
Silent reading grade level ± current grade level	−0.63 ± 0.87	−0.52 ± 1.12	NS

tive study) might be disadvantaged in attempting to compensate for depressed language functioning associated with conductive hearing loss. The present findings would support their view.

The present report specifically excluded children with a functionally significant hearing loss and/or learning disability. Yet the pattern of statistically significant findings which emerged is consistent with those reported by previous investigators[1-4,13,15] who studied more heterogeneous and impaired populations. It is hypothesized that a basic pattern of depressed verbal ability, auditory decoding deficit and achievement discrepancy from expected levels may be associated with the early history of recurrent MEE. This basic pattern may then take on functional significance under less optimal conditions than those reported in the present investigation. Recurrent MEE in the child who has a persistent hearing loss and/or is less cognitively competent and/or is socioeconomically disadvantaged may contribute to the greater functional deficit. The ability of the ESs in the present study to compensate for a basic deficit in auditory decoding via another channel, visual sequential memory, may reflect their otherwise intact neuroperceptual functioning and a lack of other disabling conditions. The presence of at least high average intelligence may be a necessary prerequisite for the development of compensatory skills. The ability to effect significant compensatory modes may not be available to all children affected by recurrent MEE.

The evidence of the effect of early auditory deprivation on auditory behavior is consistent with many anatomical and physiological studies.[16] For example, electrophysiological data on the full-term human infant suggest that middle and inner ears are virtually mature at birth and that the maturation of the auditory system occurs over the next 18 months.[17] The first year and a half of life appears to be a highly critical period for the effects of auditory deprivation.[16]

As a retrospective study, the present investigation is open to the problems inherent in such an investigation. The deficits which have been described may reflect a variety of characteristics for which we have little objective information: age at onset of the recurrent MEE, severity and duration of the individual episodes, range of hearing impairment throughout the course of the episode, and treatment. The early history of MEE, age at onset and the number of episodes were obtained from parents at the time of the evaluation. Half of the ESs in the present study were noted by history to have their first episode of effusion at less than 24 months of age. However, recent data would suggest that most of the group may have had MEE during the first year of life.[18]

The limitations of a retrospective study notwithstanding, the present sibling control paradigm offers a number of advantages which make it a useful instrument for this type of investigation. The siblings are 50% genetically identical. There is a minimal variation in expected cognitive functioning with sibling pairs.[19] The socioeconomic, psychological and pedagogical factors for sibling pairs are similar. Recurrent episodes of MEE with attendant temporary partial auditory deprivation during the preschool years appear to be related to compromised auditory function and a pattern of vulnerability in auditory processing and achievement in the school-aged child even after auditory acuity has been restored. Other factors such as hearing level, socioeconomic background and intelligence may determine, at least in part, the degree to which the "risk" becomes manifest as a real functioning impairment. Since recurrent MEE in the preschool child is a risk factor for future language and learning disability these children should be monitored audiometrically and otologically in order to maintain hearing levels at the lowest threshold.

SUMMARY

1. A sibling paradigm was used to study the effects of recurrent ME in early childhood on subsequent cognitive, language and achievement skills.

2. Audiological, otological and psychological evaluations were performed on 18 sibling pairs tested at the same age with an age range from 8 to 11 years.

3. The ES subjects were significantly depressed in verbal functioning, auditory decoding, and spelling skills when compared to their sibling controls. The differences did not imply functional significance.

4. The ES subjects were significantly better than their CSs in visual sequential memory, despite the breakdown by sex of the ES and CS subjects which would have predicted the reverse.

ACKNOWLEDGMENTS — The authors wish to express appreciation to Laurence Rotkin, PhD, for the statistical analysis of the data.

REFERENCES

1. Howie VM. Acute and recurrent acute otitis media. In: Jaffe BF, ed. Hearing loss in children. Baltimore: University Park Press, 1977; 421-30.

2. Holm VA, Kunze LH. Effect of chronic otitis media on language and speech development. Pediatrics 1969; 43:833-9.

3. Kaplan GJ, Fleshman JK, Bender TR, Baum C, Clark PS. Long-term effects of otitis media — a ten-year cohort study of Alaskan Eskimo children. Pediatrics 1973; 52:577-85.

4. Ling D. Rehabilitation of cases with deafness secondary to otitis media. In: Glorig A, Gerwin KS, eds. Otitis media: proceedings of the national conference. Springfield, Ill: Charles C. Thomas, 1972; 249-53.

5. Ventry IV. Effects of conductive hearing loss: fact or fiction. J Speech Hear Dis 1980; 45:143-56.

6. Rapin I. Conductive hearing loss: effects on children's language and scholastic skills. A review of the literature. Ann Otol Rhinol Laryngol 1980; 88:3-11.

7. Wechsler D. Wechsler intelligence scale for children — revised. New York: Psychological Corporation, 1974.

8. Raven JC. Coloured progressive matrices. London: H. K. Lewis, 1956.

9. Kirk S, McCarthy J, Kirk W. Illinois test of psycholinguistic abilities. Urbana: University of Illinois Press, 1964.

10. Jastak J, Jastak S. Wide range achievement test. Wilmington: Guidance Associates, 1965.

11. Durrell D. Durrell analysis of reading difficulty. New York: Harcourt, Brace and World, 1955.

12. Feldman A, Wilber L. Acoustic impedance and admittance — the measurement of middle ear function. Baltimore: Williams and Wilkins, 1976.

13. Zinkus PW, Gottlieb MI. Patterns of perceptual and academic deficits related to early chronic otitis media. Pediatrics 1980; 66:246-53.

14. Horowitz FD. Design factors in the assessment of intelligence issues and implications in otitis media research. Ann Otol Rhinol Laryngol 1979; 88:64-74.

15. Bennett FC, Ruuska SH, Sherman R. Middle ear function in learning-disabled children. Pediatrics 1980; 66:254-60.

16. Ruben RJ, Rapin I. Plasticity of the developing auditory system. Ann Otol Rhinol Laryngol 1980; 89:303-11.

17. Keith RW. Middle ear function in neonates. Arch Otolaryngol 1975; 101:376-9.

18. Shurin PA, Pelton SI, Donner A, et al. Persistence of middle ear effusion after acute otitis media in children. N Engl J Med 1979; 300:1121-3.

19. Paul SM. Sibling resemblance in mental ability: a review. Behav Genet 1980; 10:277-90.

≈

Ann Otol 90:1981

PANEL ON EXPERIENCES WITH TESTING EUSTACHIAN TUBE FUNCTION

CURRENT CLINICAL METHODS, INDICATIONS AND INTERPRETATION OF EUSTACHIAN TUBE FUNCTION TESTS

CHARLES D. BLUESTONE, MD — ERDEM I. CANTEKIN, PhD

PITTSBURGH, PENNSYLVANIA

Eustachian tube (ET) dysfunction is the most important factor in the pathogenesis of otitis media and related conditions. The importance of the function of the ET in relation to the middle ear-mastoid air cell system is compared to the critical role that laryngeal function has in its relation to the tracheobronchial-pulmonary system. However, because of its obscure location, the ET is not as easily assessed by clinical or laboratory methods as is the larynx, and therefore, its function is not as well understood. Most clinicians do not include ET function testing as part of their evaluation of patients with middle ear (ME) disease. Pneumatic otoscopy, the Toynbee test, tympanometry, the 9-step inflation-deflation tympanometric test, and the patulous tube test can be performed when the tympanic membrane is intact. The modified inflation-deflation test employing the pump-manometer of the electroacoustic impedance bridge can assess the function of the ET when the tympanic membrane is not intact. These tests are helpful in the diagnosis of the presence or absence of abnormal ET function; if a dysfunction is present, these tests help to determine whether or not the tube is obstructed (mechanically or functionally) or abnormally patent, and in some instances, the degree of the malfunction. Even though testing of the function of the ET in the clinical setting has severe limitations at present, and further research is needed, information can be gained which is useful in the diagnosis and management of ME disease. Failing to recognize and assess the function of the ET in relation to the ME and mastoid in selected patients is as irrational as ignoring the function of the larynx in patients with disease of the lower respiratory tract.

INTRODUCTION

Abnormal function of the ET appears to be the most important factor in the pathogenesis of middle ear (ME) disease. This hypothesis was first suggested more than 100 years ago by Politzer.[1] However, later studies[2-5] suggested that otitis media (OM) was a disease primarily of the ME mucous membrane, ie, due to infection or allergic reactions in this tissue, rather than related to dysfunction of the ET. Figure 1 is an attempt to incorporate these hypotheses and thus, to resolve the controversy.

The vast majority of patients with OM and related conditions have (or have had in the past) abnormal function of the ET that may cause secondary mucosal disease of the ME, ie, inflammation.[6] Infection is secondary to reflux, aspiration, or insufflation of nasopharyngeal bacteria up the ET and into the ME.[7] Inflammation (infection or possibly allergy) may also cause intrinsic mechanical obstruction of the ET.[8] Unrelated to the function of the ET, hematogenous spread of bacteria into the ME may also result in OM; the commonly postulated example of this mechanism is meningitis associated with OM in infants. A much smaller number of patients may have primary mucosal disease of the ME as a result of allergy (although this has not been proven), or, more rarely, an abnormality of the cilia, eg, Kartagener syndrome.[9]

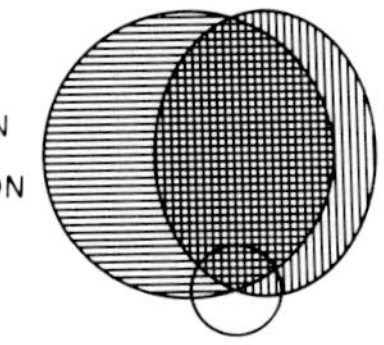

Fig. 1. Etiology and pathogenesis of otitis media.

Since abnormalities of ET function may result in ME disease, we need to review our current knowledge of the physiology and pathophysiology of the ET with regard to the pathogenesis of OM before selecting methods to test tubal function and interpreting the results of these tests for the purpose of selecting among management options. The function of the ET will be compared with the function of the larynx to put into perspective for the modern otorhinolaryngologist the importance of the ET.

COMPARISON OF THE FUNCTIONS OF THE EUSTACHIAN TUBE AND LARYNX

The physiologic functions of the ET cannot be isolated from the other components of the ME system: the nose, nasopharynx, and palate at the proximal end, and the ME and mastoid air cells at the distal end (Fig. 2). Likewise, the larynx is within a system made up of the pharynx at the proximal

From the Department of Otolaryngology, University of Pittsburgh School of Medicine, and Children's Hospital of Pittsburgh. Supported in part by a grant from the National Institute of Neurological and Communicative Disorders and Stroke, 1P01-NS-16337.

Presented at the meeting of the American Otological Society, Inc., Vancouver, British Columbia, May 9-10, 1981.

REPRINTS — Charles D. Bluestone, MD, Department of Otolaryngology, Children's Hospital of Pittsburgh, 125 DeSoto Street, Pittsburgh, PA 15213.

	EUSTACHIAN TUBE		LARYNX
PHYSIOLOGY	HEARING —	VENTILATION — PROTECTION	PHONATION
	PUMP —	DRAINAGE —	COUGH
PATHOPHYSIOLOGY		OBSTRUCTION MECHANICAL FUNCTIONAL ABNORMAL PATENCY	
PATHOLOGY	RETRACTION POCKET	ATELECTASIS	SEGMENTAL ATELECTASIS
	MIDDLE EAR EFFUSION	EFFUSION	PULMONARY EDEMA
	REFLUX OTITIS MEDIA	INFECTION	ASPIRATION PNEUMONIA
	SUPPURATIVE OTITIS MEDIA		BACTERIAL PNEUMONIA

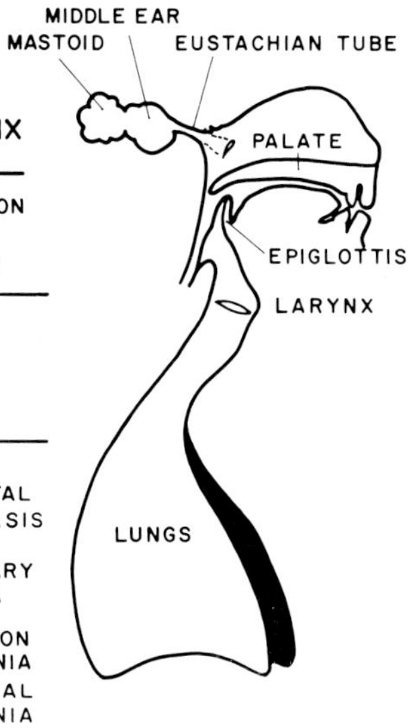

Fig. 2. Nose-nasopharynx-eustachian tube-middle ear-mastoid system compared to the pharynx-larynx-tracheobronchial-pulmonary system.

end, and the tracheobronchial-pulmonary system distally. Within their respective systems, the ET and the larynx play critical roles in the functions of the ME and lungs, respectively, in their connections to the aerodigestive tract. The tympanic membrane (TM) and malleus (which may be compared to a rib) and tensor tympani muscle (which may play a role similar to that of the intercostal muscles) could even be compared to the rib cage and diaphragm of the pulmonary system. The mastoid air cell system, in its role as a reservoir for gas for the ME, can also be compared to the reserve volumes of the lungs. Physiologically, both the ET and the larynx have ventilatory, protective, and drainage functions. The ET *ventilates* the ME to regulate ME pressure, which maintains optimum *hearing*. The larynx ventilates the lungs to provide respiration which, in man, has also evolved phylogenetically into *phonation*. In order to perform these critical physiologic functions, the ET and larynx must *protect* the ME-mastoid and the tracheobronchial-pulmonary systems from unwanted secretions. In the absence of swallowing, the ME and mastoid are protected (also from nasopharyngeal sound pressures) by the functional collapse of the normal ET; however, during swallowing, the normal ET actively opens due to contraction of one muscle, the tensor veli palatini,[10-12] and the palate seals off the nasopharynx from the contents of, and extreme pressure developed in, the oropharyngeal cavity. The larynx, on the other hand, is open (by the activity of one paired muscle) when swallowing is not occurring but closes during swallowing activity. The epiglottis, although less important in humans, protects the glottis during swallowing much like palatal closure protects the nasopharyngeal end of the ET.

Both systems have *clearance* (or drainage) functions primarily provided by the mucociliary activity of their mucosal linings, but the larynx is integrally involved in coughing, acting to clear (and therefore to protect) the lungs. Likewise, the ET is now thought to have a pump-like activity that actually "milks" secretions out of the ME and mastoid.[13]

The pathophysiology of the ET can also be compared to that of the larynx. Both can be obstructed mechanically (anatomically) or functionally. Clearly, both structures can have intrinsic (due to inflammation) or extrinsic (as from a tumor) mechanical obstructions. However, *functional* obstruction of the ET is much less easy to visualize conceptually than this type of obstruction of the larynx and tracheobronchial tree. Functional obstruction of the larynx caused by bilateral vocal cord paralysis (in the median or paramedian position), or laryngomalacia, or, more distally, tracheobronchial malacia, is well known and understood. However, an abnormally compliant (floppy) ET or an abnormal tubal opening mechanism, even though it may have similarities to the pathophysiology of laryngeal dysfunction, is not as easily understood. This is because the larynx, trachea, and bronchi are more readily available for examination, and have been studied much more than the ET. Other instances in which laryngeal abnormalities may lead to disease include 1) *aspiration* pneumonia caused by an abnormally patent or incompetent glottis (eg, paralysis of the vocal cords in the lateral position); 2) reflux esophagitis, which can also cause aspiration pneumonia, resulting from incompetence of the esophagogastric junction; and 3) cricopharyngeal achalasia resulting in a similar condition. The analogies in the ME system include 1) "reflux otitis media" caused by the reflux of nasopharyngeal secretions through an abnormally patent (patulous or semipatulous) ET; and 2) the *aspiration* through the ET of secretions into a ME that has high negative pressure. Nasal obstruction may have an effect on both ET (Toynbee phenomenon)[7] and pulmonary function.

Some of the pathologic conditions found at the distal ends of the two systems are also comparable.

Atelectasis of the TM, which is analogous to pulmonary atelectasis, is the result of hypoaeration of the ME. A retraction pocket of the posterosuperior or pars flaccida areas of the TM could be likened to segmental pulmonary atelectasis, for instance, atelectasis of the right middle lobe; both of these conditions may result from the unique anatomies of the parts involved. A middle ear effusion (MEE) which is sterile may develop in a way similar to that in which pulmonary edema develops, and suppurative OM could be compared to bacterial pneumonia in their pathogenesis.

In conclusion, then, the larynx plays a well-recognized and critical role in the functioning of the pulmonary system, but while the ET plays a similar role in the ME system, this latter role is poorly understood. This is due to the obscure location of the ET and the limited methods available to assess its function. The larynx and tracheobronchial-pulmonary system have been extensively studied by many different methods, some of which are quite simple. For instance, laryngeal function can readily be assessed by indirect laryngoscopy, one of the simplest assessment techniques, although more sophisticated laryngeal and pulmonary function tests are available and used frequently in clinical practice as well as in the laboratory. Unfortunately, since the ET is not as accessible to the clinician or investigator, and therefore has not been studied as extensively as its counterpart, it is thus not as well understood. However, in spite of these disadvantages, it is as important to assess the function of the ET of a patient with tympanic membrane-middle ear-mastoid disease as it is to assess the function of the larynx of a patient who has tracheobronchial or pulmonary disease. The various instruments available to the clinician and investigator, as well as the methods of assessment of ET function, have been described in detail elsewhere.[14] In the following discussion only the instruments and assessment techniques available to the clinician will be reviewed.

INSTRUMENTATION NEEDED TO ASSESS EUSTACHIAN TUBE FUNCTION IN THE CLINICAL SETTING

Prior to the examination of the patient, the presence of certain signs and symptoms may be helpful in determining if ET dysfunction is present. However, as in the assessment of laryngeal and pulmonary function, the presence or absence of these signs and symptoms, eg, airway obstruction, stridor, hoarseness, dyspnea, cough, may only help in determining if dysfunction is present and, when present, may not determine the type, location, or severity. Likewise, conductive hearing loss, otalgia, otorrhea, tinnitus, or vertigo may or may not be present with ET dysfunction.

Otoscopy. Visual inspection of the TM is one of the simplest (and oldest) ways to assess the functioning of the ET; however, like auscultation of the chest to diagnose pulmonary disease, it has severe limitations. The appearance of a MEE or the presence of high negative ME pressure, or both, as determined by the *pneumatic* otoscope,[15] is presumptive evidence of ET dysfunction, but the type, ie, obstruction (functional vs mechanical), as well as the degree of abnormality, cannot be determined by this method. Moreover, a normal-appearing TM cannot be considered to be evidence of normal functioning of the ET: for instance, a patulous or semipatulous ET may be present when the TM appears to be normal. In addition, the presence of one or more of the complications or sequelae of OM (such as a perforation or atelectasis, as observed through the otoscope) may not correlate with dysfunction of the ET at the time of the examination, since ET function may improve with growth and development.

Many otolaryngologists use the otomicroscope to improve the accuracy with which OM and related conditions are diagnosed. For assessment of TM mobility, the otomicroscope, when used with the Bruening pneumatic otoscope and a nonmagnifying lens, is superior to the conventional otoscopes.

Nasopharyngoscopy. Indirect mirror examination of the nasopharyngeal end of the ET is also an old but still important part of the clinical assessment of a patient with ME disease. For instance, a neoplasm in the fossa of Rosenmüller may be diagnosed by this simple technique. The development of endoscopic instruments has greatly improved the accuracy of this type of examination but, unlike indirect and direct laryngoscopy (and bronchoscopy), the function of the ET cannot be determined with the aid of currently available instruments.

Tympanometry. The use of an electroacoustic impedance instrument to obtain a tympanogram is an excellent way of determining the status of the TM-ME system, and can be helpful in the assessment of ET function.[16] The presence of a MEE or high negative ME pressure as determined by this method usually indicates impaired ET function; however, unlike the otoscopic evaluation, the tympanogram is an objective way of determining the degree of negative pressure present in the ME. Unfortunately, assessing the abnormality of values of negative pressure is not so simple: high negative pressure may be present in some patients, especially children, who are asymptomatic and who have relatively good hearing, while in others, symptoms such as hearing loss, otalgia, vertigo, and tinnitus may be associated with modest degrees of negative pressure or even with normal ME pressures. Alberti and Kristensen[17] have suggested that the limits of normal ME pressure for adults are between +50 and −50 mm H_20, while Brooks[18] feels that the normal ME pressure in children may be as low as −175 to −200 mm H_20. However, these values depend upon the time of day, season of the year, or the con-

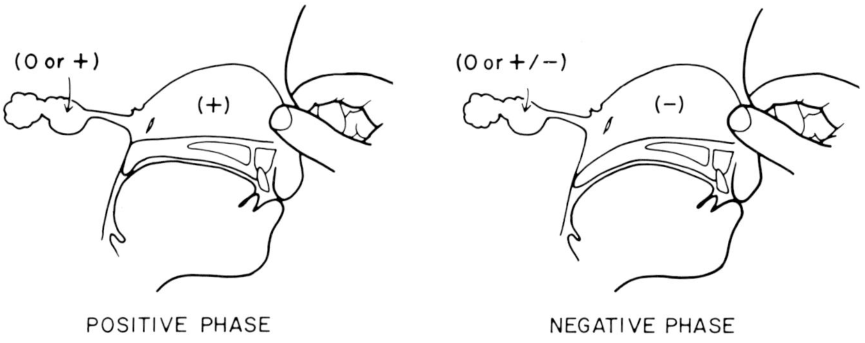

Fig. 3. Toynbee test of ET function. During closed-nose swallowing a positive pressure develops within the nasopharynx, followed by a negative pressure phase. If the ET opens during the test, the ME pressure will change depending upon the timing of the tubal opening and pressure gradient.

dition of the other parts of the system, such as the presence of an upper respiratory tract infection. For instance, a young child with a common cold may have transitory high negative pressure within the ME while he has the cold, but be otherwise otologically normal. The decision as to whether or not high negative pressure is abnormal or is only a physiologic variation should be made taking into consideration the presence or absence of signs and symptoms of ME disease. If severe atelectasis or adhesive otitis of the TM-ME system is present, the tympanogram may not be a reliable indicator of the actual pressure within the ME.

Therefore, a resting pressure that is high negative is associated with some degree of ET obstruction, but the presence of normal ME pressure does not necessarily indicate normal ET function. An analogy can be made to the evaluation of pulmonary function employing chest x-ray films. Abnormal pulmonary function is most likely associated with radiographic evidence of severe disease of the lung, but the finding of a normal-appearing roentgenograph of the chest does not necessarily indicate normal pulmonary function.

Manometry. The pump-manometer system of the electroacoustic impedance bridge is usually adequate to assess ET function clinically when the TM is not intact. However, due to the limitations of the manometric systems of all of the commercially available instruments, a controlled syringe and manometer (a water manometer will suffice) should be available when these limitations are exceeded, eg, when ET opening pressure is in excess of +400 to +600 mm H_2O.

METHODS OF ASSESSING EUSTACHIAN TUBE FUNCTION

Classical Tests of Tubal Patency. Valsalva and Politzer have developed methods to assess patency of the ET; ET catheterization achieves the same results. When the TM is intact and the ME inflates following one of these tests, then the tube is not totally mechanically obstructed. Likewise, if the TM is not intact, passage of air into the ME would indicate patency of the tube. The success of these tests can be determined subjectively by the use of the otoscope, a Toynbee tube, or a stethoscope at the ME end of the system. The assessment is more objective when a tympanogram is obtained when the TM is intact, or when the manometer on the impedance instrument is observed when the TM is not intact. However, inflation of the ET-ME from the nasopharynx end of the system by one of these classical methods only is an assessment of tubal patency and not function, and failure to inflate the ME does not necessarily indicate a lack of patency of the ET. Elner et al[19] reported that 86% of 100 otologically normal adults could perform the Valsalva test. In young children, the Valsalva test is usually more difficult to perform than the Politzer test. However, in a recent study by Bluestone and coworkers,[20] 6 of 7 children who had a traumatic perforation but who were otherwise otologically "normal" could perform the Valsava test as compared to only 11 of 28 children who had a retraction pocket or a cholesteatoma. The Valsalva and Politzer maneuvers are more beneficial as management options in selected patients than they are as methods to assess tubal function.

Toynbee Test. One of the oldest and still one of the best tests of ET function is the Toynbee test (Fig. 3). The test is usually considered positive when an alteration in ME pressure results. More specifically, if negative pressure (even transitory in the absence of a patulous tube) develops in the ME during closed-nose swallowing, the ET function can be considered most likely to be normal. When the TM is intact, the presence of negative ME pressure must be determined by pneumatic otoscopy or, more accurately, by obtaining a tympanogram before and immediately following the test (Fig. 4). When the TM is not intact, the manometer of the impedance bridge can be observed to determine ME pressure. In the Elner et al study,[19] the Toynbee test was positive in 79% of normal adults. Cantekin et al[21] reported that only 7 of 106 ears (6.6%) of subjects (mostly children) who had had tympanostomy tubes inserted for OM could perform a modification of the Toynbee test (closed-nose equilibration attempt with applied negative ME pressure of 100 or 200 mm H_2O). Likewise, in a series of patients, most of whom were older children and adults with chronic perforations of the TM, only 3 of 21 (14.3%) passed the test. However, in children with a traumatic perforation of the TM but who other-

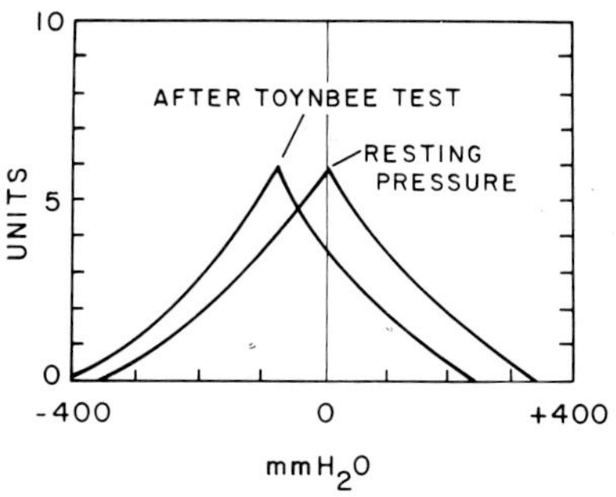

Fig. 4. Tympanogram obtained before and after Toynbee test. Negative ME pressure is objectively demonstrated in the ME, which is considered to be associated with good ET function.

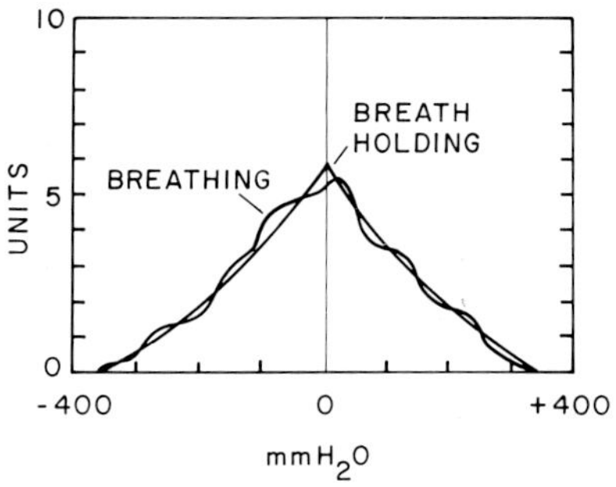

Fig. 5. Diagnosis of a patulous ET employing the tympanogram.

wise had a negative otologic history, three of ten (30%) could pass the test. In the Bluestone et al study[20] of "normal" children with traumatic perforations, six of seven children could change the ME pressure as compared to *none* of the 21 ears of children who had a retraction pocket or a cholesteatoma. The test is of greater value in determining normal versus abnormal ET function in adults than in children. The test is still of considerable value since, regardless of age, if negative pressure develops in the ME during or following the test, the ET function is most likely normal, since the ET actively opens and is sufficiently stiff to withstand nasopharyngeal negative pressure, ie, it does not "lock." If positive pressure is noted or no change in pressure occurs, the function of the ET still may be normal and other tests of ET function should be performed.

Patulous Eustachian Tube Test. If a patulous ET is suspected, the diagnosis can be confirmed by otoscopy or objectively by tympanometry when the TM is intact.[16] One tympanogram is obtained while the patient is breathing normally, and a second is obtained while the patient holds his breath. Fluctuation of the tympanometric trace which coincides with breathing confirms the diagnosis of a patulous tube (Fig. 5). Fluctuation can be exaggerated by asking the patient to occlude one nostril with the mouth closed during forced inspiration and expiration or by performing the Toynbee maneuver. When the TM is not intact, a patulous ET can be identified by the free flow of air into and out of the ET using the pump-manometer portion of the electroacoustic impedance bridge. These tests should not be performed while the patient is in a reclining position since the patulous ET will close.

Nine-Step Inflation-Deflation Tympanometric Test. Another method of assessing the function of the ET when the TM is intact, developed by Bluestone,[22] is called the 9-step inflation-deflation tympanometric test, although the applied ME pressures are very limited in magnitude. The ME must be free of effusion. The 9-step tympanometry procedure may be summarized as follows (Fig. 6):

1. The tympanogram records resting ME pressure.

2. Ear canal pressure is increased to + 200 mm H_2O, with medial deflection of the TM and a corresponding increase in ME pressure. The subject swallows to equilibrate ME overpressure.

3. While the subject refrains from swallowing, ear canal pressure is returned to normal, thus establishing a slight negative ME pressure (as the TM moves outward). The tympanogram documents the established ME underpressure.

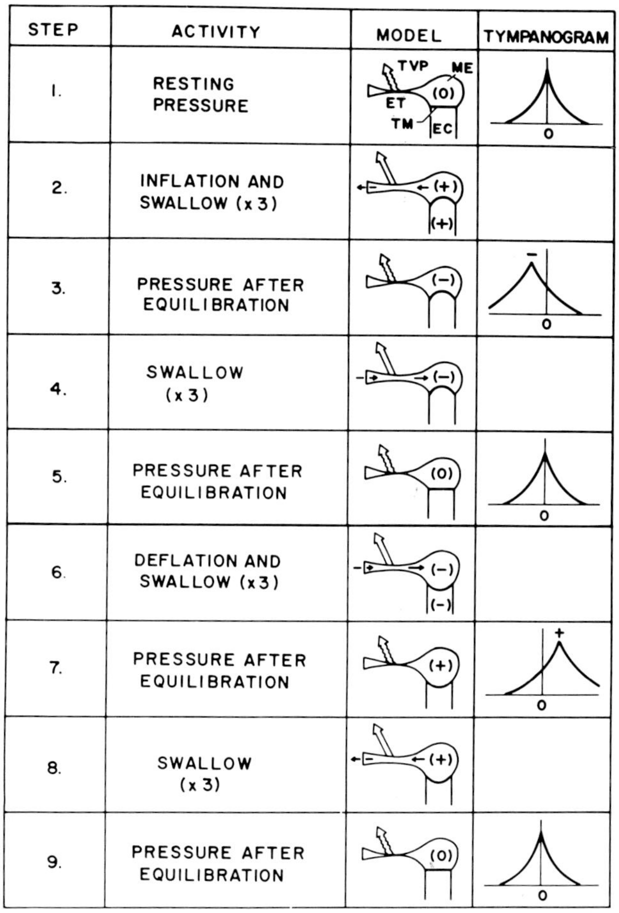

Fig. 6. Nine-step inflation-deflation tympanometric test. TVP - Tensor veli palatini muscle, ET - Eustachian tube, ME - Middle ear, TM - Tympanic membrane, EC - Ear canal.

NINE-STEP INFLATION-DEFLATION TYMPANOMETRIC TEST FINDINGS

	Function Test Findings (Ears)				
Groups of subjects	*All Positive*	*Some Positive*	*None Positive*	*Total Ears*	*% All or Some Positive*
Normal adults (N = 27)	39	10	5	54	90.7
Abnormal adults (N = 42)	18	26	36	80	55.0
Normal children (N = 44)	11	19	58	88	34.1
Abnormal children (N = 18)	7	8	61	76	19.7

4. The subject swallows in an attempt to equilibrate negative ME pressure. If equilibration is successful, airflow is from nasopharynx to ME.

5. The tympanogram records the extent of equilibration.

6. Ear canal pressure is decreased to − 200 mm H_2O, causing a lateral deflection of the TM and a corresponding decrease in ME pressure. The subject swallows to equilibrate negative ME pressure; airflow is from the nasopharynx to the ME.

7. The subject refrains from swallowing while external ear canal pressure is returned to normal, thus establishing a slight positive pressure in the ME as the TM moves medially. The tympanogram records the overpressure established.

8. The subject swallows to reduce overpressure. If equilibration is successful, airflow is from the ME to the nasopharynx.

9. The final tympanogram documents the extent of equilibration.

In an attempt to determine the usefulness of this method of testing ET function, four groups of subjects, all of whom had intact TM and no otoscopic or tympanometric evidence of MEE, were evaluated:

1. Normal adults — 27 adults without a prior history of otologic disease.

2. Abnormal adults — 42 adults with a prior history of otologic disease.

3. Normal children — 44 children between 2 and 15 years of age without a prior history of otologic disease.

4. Abnormal children — 48 children between 2 and 15 years of age, all of whom had otoscopic and tympanometric evidence of a MEE in the recent past.

The table shows the findings in these four groups of subjects. The ability to perform all or any one of the steps progressively increased with advancing age and the absence of a past history of otologic disease. Conversely, the percentage of ears in which *no* function was present progressively increased from the normal adult group (9.3%) to the abnormal children group (80.3%). Of the 46 ears in these children, regardless of past history, in whom a ME pressure of − 50 mm H_2O or less was found, only 3 (7%) could perform any of the tests. Likewise, of 13 ears with high negative pressure in the abnormal adult group, only two (15.3%) could pass any of the tests. These findings verify the presence of ET obstruction when high negative ME pressure is identified.

The test is simple to perform and can give useful information regarding ET function and should be part of the clinical evaluation of patients with suspected ET dysfunction. In general, most normal adults can perform all or some parts of this test, but even normal children have difficulty in performing this test.

Modified Inflation-Deflation Test (Nonintact Tympanic Membrane). When the TM is not intact, the pump-manometer system of the electroacoustic impedance bridge can be used to perform the modified inflation-deflation ET function test, which assesses passive as well as active functioning of the ET.[21,23] The ME should be free of any drainage for an accurate assessment of ET function using this test. Figure 7 illustrates the procedures employed during the test. The ME is inflated, ie, positive pressure is applied, until the ET spontaneously opens. At this time, the pump is manually stopped and air is discharged through the ET until the tube closes passively. The pressure at which the ET is passively forced open is called the opening pressure, and the pressure at which it closes passively is called the closing pressure. The patient is then instructed to equilibrate the ME pressure actively by swallowing. The residual pressure remaining in the ME after swallowing is recorded. The active function is also recorded by applying over- and underpressure to the ME, which the patient then attempts to equilibrate by swallowing. The residual pressure in the ME following equilibration of + 200 mm H_2O or half of the passive opening pressure is recorded. The residual negative pressure which remains in the ME after the attempt to equilibrate applied negative pressure of − 200 mm H_2O is also noted. This procedure is not performed in patients who cannot equilibrate applied overpressure. If the ET does not open following application of positive pressure using the electroacoustic impedance bridge, and no reduction in positive pressure occurs during swallowing, then the ET must be assessed using a manometric system other than the electroacoustic impedance bridge manometric system. The opening pressure may be higher than 400 to 600 mm H_2O pressure, or not present at all (severe mechanical

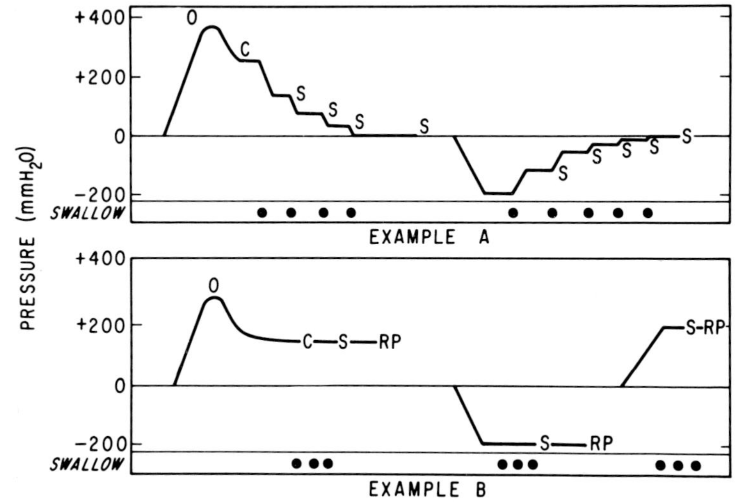

Fig. 7. Procedure and symbols used in describing the modified inflation-deflation test employing the pump-manometer system of an electroacoustic bridge. The figure shows strip-chart recordings, but the results of the test can be read directly from the equipment readout and noted manually. RP - Residual pressure, O - Opening pressure, C - Closing pressure, ● - Mark for swallow, S - Pressure after swallow.

obstruction). Example A in Figure 7 shows that following passive opening and closing of the ET during the inflation phase of the study, the patient was able completely to equilibrate the remaining positive pressure. Active swallowing also completely equilibrated applied negative pressure (deflation). This is considered to be characteristic of normal ET function. Example B shows the ET passively opened and closed following inflation, but subsequent swallowing failed to equilibrate the residual positive pressure. In the deflation phase of the study, the patient was unable to equilibrate negative pressure. Inflation to a pressure below the opening pressure but above the closing pressure could not be equilibrated by active swallowing. This type of result is considered to be abnormal but may be found in a few subjects who do not have any obvious otologic disease.

Failure to equilibrate the applied negative pressure may indicate locking of the ET during the test. This type of tube is considered to have increased compliance or to be "floppy" in comparison to a tube with perfect function. The tensor veli palatini muscle is unable to open (dilate) the tube. The speed of application of the positive and negative pressures is an important variable in testing ET function with the inflation-deflation test. The faster the positive pressure is applied, the higher the opening pressure. During the deflation phase of the study, the faster the negative pressure is applied, the more likely it is that the locking phenomenon will occur.

Even though the inflation-deflation test of ET function does not strictly duplicate physiologic functions of the tube, the results are helpful in differentiating normal from abnormal function. The mean opening pressure for apparently normal subjects with a traumatic perforation and negative otologic history reported by Cantekin and coworkers[24] was 330 mm H_2O ($\pm$ 70 mm H_2O). If the test results reveal passive opening and closing within the normal range, residual positive pressure can be equilibrated by swallowing and applied negative pressure can also be equilibrated completely, then the ET can be considered to have normal function. However, if the tube does not open to a pressure of 1000 mm H_2O, one can assume that total mechanical obstruction is present. This pressure is not hazardous to the ME or inner ear windows if the pressure is applied slowly. An extremely high opening pressure (eg, greater than 500 to 600 mm H_2O) may indicate partial obstruction, whereas a very low opening pressure (eg, less than 100 mm H_2O) would indicate a semipatulous ET. Inability to maintain even a modest positive pressure within the ME would be consistent with a patulous tube, ie, one which is open at rest. Complete equilibration by swallowing of applied negative pressure is usually associated with normal function, but partial equilibration, or even failure to reduce any applied negative pressure may or may not be considered abnormal since even a normal ET will lock when negative pressure is rapidly applied. Therefore, inability to equilibrate applied negative pressure may not indicate poor ET function, especially when it is the only abnormal parameter.

Elner et al[19] studied 102 adults with intact TM and a negative otologic history. They used the microflow technique and pressure chamber to evaluate ET function, but the results of this type of testing are comparable to the results of the inflation-deflation test when the TM is not intact. They reported that only 5% could not equilibrate to some degree an applied pressure of + 100 and 7% could not equilibrate − 100 mm H_2O. Bylander[25] compared the ET functioning in 53 children with that in 55 adults, all of whom had intact TM and who were apparently otologically healthy. Employing a pressure chamber, she reported that 53% of the children could not equilibrate applied negative intratympanic pressure (− 100 mm H_2O) by swallowing, whereas only 9% of the adults were unable to perform this function. Children between 3 and 6 years of age had worse function than those in the

7-to-12-year age group. In addition, she also found that even normal children who had tympanometric evidence of high negative pressure within the ME had poor ET function. From these two studies, it can be concluded that even in apparently otologically normal children, ET function is not as good as in adults, which would contribute to the higher incidence of ME disease in children compared to adults. In the Cantekin et al study,[21] only 8 of 108 ears (7%) of subjects (primarily children) with tympanostomy tubes could equilibrate an applied pressure of -200 mm H_2O to any degree and none of 67 ears could equilibrate -100 mm H_2O. In subjects with chronic dry perforations, 4 of 30 ears (13%) could equilibrate -100 mm H_2O, and none of 17 ears could equilibrate -200 mm H_2O. These results were compared to those obtained from a group of subjects with traumatic perforations of the TM; in this latter group 12 of the 27 (44%) ears equilibrated a pressure of -200 mm H_2O.

Other Methods Available for Laboratory Use. There are other methods available to test the functioning of the ET, but they are limited to use in the laboratory for investigational purposes at present. When the TM is intact the microflow technique[26] or an impedance method,[25] both of which require a pressure chamber, or sonometry[27,28] may be used. When the tympanic membrane is not intact the forced-response test[29] may be used. Sonometry and the forced-response test show great promise for future use in the clinical setting.

CLINICAL INDICATIONS FOR TESTING EUSTACHIAN TUBE FUNCTION

Diagnosis. One of the most important reasons for assessing ET function is the need to make a differential diagnosis in a patient who has an intact TM without evidence of OM but has symptoms that might be related to ET dysfunction (such as otalgia, snapping or popping in the ear, fluctuating hearing loss, tinnitus, or vertigo). An example of such a case would be a patient who has a complaint of fullness in the ear without hearing loss at the time of the examination, a symptom which could be related to abnormal functioning of the ET or could be due to inner ear pathology. A tympanogram that reveals a high negative pressure (-50 mm H_2O or less) is presumptive evidence of tubal obstruction, whereas normal resting ME pressure is not diagnostically significant. However, when the resting intratympanic pressure is within normal limits and the patient can develop negative ME pressure following Toynbee's test or can perform all or some of the functions in the 9-step inflation-deflation tympanometric test, the ET is probably functioning normally. Unfortunately, failure to develop negative ME pressure during the Toynbee test or inability to pass the 9-step test does not necessarily indicate poor ET function. Tympanometry is not only of value in determining if ET obstruction is present: it can also identify abnormality at the other end of the spectrum of ET dysfunction; the presence of an abnormally patent ET can be confirmed by the results of the tympanometric patulous tube test.

Screening for the presence of high negative pressure in certain high-risk populations (ie, children with known sensorineural hearing losses, developmentally delayed and mentally impaired children, children with cleft palates or other craniofacial anomalies, American Indian and Eskimo children, and children with Down syndrome) appears to be helpful in identifying those individuals who may need to be monitored closely for the occurrence of OM.[30]

Tympanometry appears to be a reliable method for detecting the presence of high negative pressure as well as of otitis media with effusion (OME) in children.[31-33] The identification of high negative pressure without effusion in children is indicative of some degree of ET obstruction. These children as well as those with MEE should have follow-up serial tympanograms since they may be at risk of developing OME.

However, the most direct method available to the clinician today for testing ET function is the inflation-deflation test. A perforation of the TM or a tympanostomy tube must be present in order to perform this test. The test uses the simple apparatus described earlier, with or without the electroacoustic impedance bridge pump-manometer system. This test will aid in determining the presence or absence of a dysfunction, and the type of dysfunction (obstruction vs abnormal patency) and severity of dysfunction when one is present. No other test procedures may be needed if the patient has either functional obstruction of the ET tube or an abnormally patent tube. However, if there is a mechanical obstruction, especially if the tube appears to be totally blocked anatomically, then further testing may be indicated. In such instances, retrograde-prograde radiographic contrast studies of the ET-ME, which are used primarily for research purposes, can be performed to determine the site and cause of the blockage.[6] In most cases in which mechanical obstruction of the tube is found inflammation is present at the ME end of the ET (protympanic or bony portion), which usually resolves with medical management or ME surgery. Serial inflation-deflation studies show resolution of the mechanical obstruction. However, if no ME cause is obvious, other studies should be performed to rule out the possibility of neoplasm in the nasopharynx.

Management. Patients with recurrent acute or chronic OME should have ET function studies as part of their otolaryngologic workup. The management of such patients may depend on the results of these studies, as mechanical obstruction of the ET may indicate treatment different from that for functional obstruction. For instance, adenoidectomy may not be indicated in a child with a small adenoid mass and tubal function test results that indicate functional obstruction; however, the operation may benefit the child with marked mechanical obstruction of the ET.[34,35]

Patients in whom tympanostomy tubes have been inserted may benefit from serial ET function studies. Improvement in function as indicated by inflation-deflation tests might aid the clinician in determining the proper time to remove the tubes. Cleft palate repair,[36,37] adenoidectomy,[34,35] elimination of nasal and nasopharyngeal inflammation,[8] treatment of a nasopharyngeal tumor, or growth and development of a child[38] may be associated with improvement in ET function.

Studies of the ET function of the patient with a chronic perforation of the TM may be helpful in determining preoperatively the potential results of tympanoplasty surgery. Holmquist[39] studied ET function in adults before and after tympanoplasty and reported that the operation had a high rate of success in patients with good ET function (ie, those who could equilibrate applied negative pressure) but that in patients without good tubal function surgery frequently failed to close the perforation. Miller and Bilodeau[40] and Siedentop[41] reported similar findings but Ekvall,[42] Lee and Schuknecht,[43] Andreasson and Harris,[44] Cohn et al,[45] and Virtanen et al[46] found no correlation between the results of the inflation-deflation tests and success or failure of tympanoplasty. Most of these studies failed to define the criteria for "success" and the postoperative follow-up period was too short. Bluestone et al[47] assessed children prior to tympanoplasty and found that of 51 ears of 45 children, 8 ears could equilibrate an applied negative pressure (-200 mm H_2O) to some degree, and in 7 of these ears, the graft took, no MEE occurred, and no recurrence of the perforation developed during a follow-up period of between one and two years. However, like the studies in adults, failure to equilibrate an applied negative pressure did not predict failure of the tympanoplasty.

The conclusion to be drawn from these studies is that if the patient is able to equilibrate an applied negative pressure, regardless of age, the success of tympanoplasty is likely, but failure to perform this difficult test will not help the clinician in deciding not to operate. However, the value of testing a person's ability to equilibrate negative pressure lies in the possibility of determining from the test results if a young child is a candidate for tympanoplasty when one might decide on the basis of other findings alone to withhold surgery until the child is older. These tests are also of value in the diagnosis of severe or total mechanical obstruction, conditions which contraindicate the performing of a myringoplasty; further evaluation and medical or surgical management of such patients may be indicated depending upon the condition of the ear. When a tympanoplasty is performed and the function of the ET is thought to be poor, a tympanostomy tube should be inserted.

In children and adults, tympanoplasty frequently fails when performed on ears in which an acquired cholesteatoma is present. This has been attributed to poor ET function in these ears.[47] Bluestone et al[20,48] reported that, using the modified inflation-deflation and forced-response ET function tests, they have found that in almost all subjects the ET constricts during swallowing instead of dilating, as it does normally. This abnormality is one involving functional obstruction of the ET. However, preoperative testing of a patient with a cholesteatoma can be helpful in deciding whether a tympanoplasty should be performed and, if it is done, whether a tympanostomy tube should be inserted at the time of surgery. Eustachian tube function may be normal if the cholesteatoma is congenital,[20] secondary to trauma (implantation), or present in an adult in whom tubal function has improved following the development of an acquired cholesteatoma in childhood.

Failure to obstruct the ME end of the ET surgically at the time of radical mastoidectomy for the eradication of cholesteatoma may result in troublesome postoperative otorrhea secondary to reflux of nasopharyngeal bacteria.[49] Assessment of ET function by the inflation-deflation manometric technique or by performing a Valsalva or Politzer test (observing the manometer) is helpful in determining if the ET is still patent following a radical mastoidectomy from which otorrhea is a postoperative complication.

Failure to consider the function of the ET as a critical variable may be the reason why it is so difficult to interpret the results of clinical studies of various techniques advocated for surgical reconstruction of the ME and mastoid. Prospective clinical trials that include, among other important factors, controlling for ET function, are urgently needed.

CONCLUSION

Even though the testing of ET function is not an exact science and more research on such testing is needed, the methods presently available to the clinician provide useful information related to the diagnosis and management of ME disease. Not to include ET function testing as part of the modern otorhinolaryngologist's diagnostic assessment of selected patients is as irrational as failing to perform laryngeal and pulmonary function tests in the diagnosis and management of patients with disease of the lower respiratory tract.

ACKNOWLEDGMENTS — The authors would like to thank Sandi Arjona and Diana Mathis for assistance in preparation of the manuscript; Margaretha Casselbrant, MD, PhD, for assistance in analysis of portions of the data; Jon Coulter for preparation of the artwork; and Vera Spector for technical assistance.

REFERENCES

1. Politzer A. Ueber die Willkurlichen Bewegungen des Trommelfells. Weiner Med Halle Nr 1862; 18:103.

2. Zollner R. Anatomie, Physiologie und Klinik der Ohrtrompete. Berlin: Springer Verlag, 1942.

3. Suehs OW. Secretory otitis media. Laryngoscope 1952; 62:998-1027.

4. Senturia BH, Gessert DF, Carr CD, Caumann HS. Studies concerned with tubotympanitis. Ann Otol Rhinol Laryngol 1958; 67:440-7.

5. Sadé J. Pathology and pathogenesis of serous otitis media. Arch Otolaryngol 1966; 84:297-305.

6. Bluestone CD, Paradise JL, Beery QC. Physiology of the eustachian tube in the pathogenesis and management of middle ear effusions. Laryngoscope 1972; 82:1654-70.

7. Bluestone CD, Beery QC. Concepts on the pathogenesis of middle ear effusions. Ann Otol Rhinol Laryngol 1976; 85 Suppl 25:182-6.

8. Bluestone CD, Cantekin EI, Beery QC: Effect of inflammation on the ventilatory function of the eustachian tube. Laryngoscope 1977; 87:493-507.

9. Fisher R, McManus J, Entis G, Cotton R, Ghory J, Avsden-Moore R. Middle ear ciliary defect in Kartagener's syndrome. Pediatrics 1978; 62:443-5.

10. Rich A. Physiological study of eustachian tube and its related muscles. Bull Johns Hopkins Hosp 1920; 31:206-14.

11. Cantekin EI, Doyle WJ, Reichert TJ, Phillips DC, Bluestone CD. Dilation of the eustachian tube by electrical stimulation of the mandibular nerve. Ann Otol Rhinol Laryngol 1979; 88:40-51.

12. Honjo I, Okazaki N, Kumazawa T. Experimental study of the eustachian tube function with regard to its related muscles. Acta Otolaryngol (Stockh) 1979; 87:84-9.

13. Honjo I, Okazaki N, Nozoe T, Ushiro K, Kumazawa T. Experimental study of the pumping function of the eustachian tube. Acta Otolaryngol (Stockh) 1981; 91:85-9.

14. Bluestone CD, Cantekin EI. Eustachian tube dysfunction. In: English GM, ed. Otolaryngology. Hagerstown: Harper and Row, 1980.

15. Bluestone CD, Shurin P. Middle ear diseases in children: pathogenesis, diagnosis, and management. Ped Clin North Am 1974; 21:379-400.

16. Bluestone CD. Assessment of eustachian tube function. In: Jerger J, Northern J, eds. Clinical impedance audiometry. New York: American Electromedics Corp, 1980:83-108.

17. Alberti R, Kristensen R. The clinical application of impedance audiometry. Laryngoscope 1970; 80:735-46.

18. Brooks D. Electroacoustic impedance bridge studies on normal ears of children. J Speech Hear Res 1971; 14:247.

19. Elner A, Ingelstedt S, Ivarsson A. The normal function of the eustachian tube. Acta Otolaryngol (Stockh) 1971; 72:320-8.

20. Bluestone CD, Casselbrant ML, Cantekin EI. Functional eustachian tube obstruction in the pathogenesis of acquired cholesteatoma in children. The Netherlands: Kugler Publications BV, 1981 (in press).

21. Cantekin EI, Bluestone CD, Parkin LP. Eustachian tube ventilatory function in children. Ann Otol Rhinol Laryngol 1976; 85 Suppl 25:171-7.

22. Bluestone CD. Assessment of eustachian tube function. In Jerger J, ed. Handbook of clinical impedance audiometry. New York: American Electromedics Corp, 1975.

23. Ingelstedt S, Ortegren U. Qualitative testing of the eustachian tube function. Acta Otolaryngol (Stockh) 1963; Suppl 182:7-23.

24. Cantekin EI, Bluestone CD, Saez C, Doyle WJ, Philips D. Normal and abnormal middle ear ventilation. Ann Otol Rhinol Laryngol 1977; 86 Suppl 41:1-15.

25. Bylander A. Comparison of eustachian tube function in children and adults with normal ears. Ann Otol Rhinol Laryngol 1980; 89 Suppl 68:20-4.

26. Ingelstedt S, Ivarsson A, Jonson A. Mechanics of the human middle ear: pressure regulation in aviation and diving, a nontraumatic method. Acta Otolaryngol (Stockh) 1967; Suppl 228:1-57.

27. Virtanen H. Sonotubometry: an acoustical method for objective measurement of auditory tubal opening. Acta Otolaryngol (Stockh) 1978; 86:93-103.

28. Murti K, Stern R, Cantekin EI, Bluestone CD. Sonometric evaluation of eustachian tube function using broadband stimuli. Ann Otol Rhinol Laryngol 1980, 89 Suppl 68:178-84.

29. Cantekin EI, Saez CA, Bluestone CD, Bern SA. Airflow through the eustachian tube. Ann Otol Rhinol Laryngol 1979; 88:603-12.

30. Harford E, Bess R, Bluestone CD, Klein J. Impedance screening for middle ear disease in children. New York: Grune and Stratton, 1978.

31. Beery QC, Bluestone CD, Cantekin EI. Otologic history, audiometry and tympanometry as a case finding procedure for school screening. Laryngoscope 1975; 85:1976-85.

32. Brooks D. An objective method of detecting fluid in the middle ear. J Int Audiol 1968; 7:280-6.

33. Brooks D. Electroacoustic impedance bridge studies on normal ears of children. J Speech Hear Res 1971; 14:247-53.

34. Bluestone CD, Wittel R, Paradise JL, Felder H. Eustachian tube function as related to adenoidectomy for otitis media. Trans Am Acad Ophthalmol Otolaryngol 1972; 76:1325-39.

35. Bluestone CD, Cantekin EI, Beery QC. Certain effects of adenoidectomy on eustachian tube ventilatory function. Laryngoscope 1975; 85:113-27.

36. Bluestone CD, Paradise JL, Beery QC, Wittel R. Certain effects of cleft palate repair on eustachian tube function. Cleft Palate J 1972; 9:183-93.

37. Paradise JL, Bluestone CD. Early treatment of universal otitis media of infants with cleft palate. Pediatrics 1974; 53:48-54.

38. Holborow C. Eustachian tube function. Arch Otolaryngol 1970; 92:624-6.

39. Holmquist J. The role of the eustachian tube in myringoplasty. Acta Otolaryngol (Stockh) 1968; 66:289-95.

40. Miller GF, Bilodeau R. Preoperative evaluation of eustachian tubal function in tympanoplasty. South Med J 1967; 60:868.

41. Siedentop KH. Eustachian tube dynamics, size of the mastoid air cell system, and results with tympanoplasty. Otolaryngol Clin North Am 1972; 5:33-44.

42. Ekvall L. Eustachian tube function in tympanoplasty. Acta Otolaryngol (Stockh) 1970; Suppl 263:33-42.

43. Lee K, Schuknecht HF. Results of tympanoplasty and mastoidectomy at the Massachusetts Eye and Ear Infirmary. Laryngoscope 1971; 81:529-43.

44. Andreasson L, Harris S. Middle ear mechanics and eusta-

chian tube function in tympanoplasty. Acta Otolaryngol (Stockh) 1979; Suppl 360:141-7.

45. Cohn AM, Schwaber MK, Anthony LS, Jerger JF. Eustachian tube function and tympanoplasty. Ann Otol Rhinol Laryngol 1979; 88:339-47.

46. Virtanen H, Palva T, Jauhiainen T. The prognostic value of eustachian tube function measurements in tympanoplastic surgery. Acta Otolaryngol (Stockh) 1980; 90:317-23.

47. Bluestone CD, Cantekin EI, Douglas GS. Eustachian tube function related to the outcome of tympanoplasty in children. Laryngoscope 1979; 89:450-8.

48. Bluestone CD, Cantekin EI, Beery QC, Douglas GS, Stool SE, Doyle WJ. Functional eustachian tube obstruction in acquired cholesteatoma and related conditions. In McCabe BF, Sadé J, Abramson M, eds. Cholesteatoma, first international congress. Birmingham: Aesculapius, 1977.

49. Bluestone CD, Cantekin EI, Beery QC, Stool SE: Function of the eustachian tube related to surgical management of acquired aural cholesteatoma in children. Laryngoscope 1978; 87:1155-63.

TESTING EUSTACHIAN TUBE FUNCTION

JAMES L. SHEEHY, MD

LOS ANGELES, CALIFORNIA

This paper reviews the concepts, attitudes and experience at the Otologic Medical Group (OMG) in regard to testing eustachian tube function. At OMG eustachian tube function tests are not performed prior to reconstructive surgery in cases of chronic otitis media and the reasons for this are reviewed. The lack of significant incidence of serous otitis media in postoperative patients substantiates the conclusion that there is no rationale for preoperative eustachian tube function tests in patients who are to undergo reconstructive surgery for chronic otitis media.

At the Otologic Medical Group (OMG) eustachian tube function tests are rarely performed prior to surgery for correction of chronic otitis media. Our concepts of the role of the eustachian tube and the lack of importance of preoperative tubal function testing have evolved over a number of years. These concepts are intimately related to, and have modified, our philosophy of surgery for chronic otitis media. The OMG publications on this subject will be reviewed to demonstrate how and why these concepts have evolved.

EARLY EXPERIENCES

In 1958, Compere,[1] when he was closely associated with OMG, worked with W. House on tympanic clearance studies using water-soluble radiopaque media. Compere commented that a "tubal ear" may very well be a tubotympanic problem rather than a nasal or nasopharyngeal problem, that obstruction of the tube may be due to mucous membrane edema, granulations or inspissated mucus in the tubotympanum. Despite the now obvious conclusion from this, House stated that if it could be determined preoperatively that fluid would not drain through the eustachian tube, then the middle ear should not be closed by grafting procedures.

In 1960 W. House[2] commented on the need for elimination of mucous membrane edema and granulations preoperatively and the use of polyethylene tubing in the eustachian tube at the time of surgery. He concluded that closure of the eustachian tube seriously limited the possibility of success in tympanoplasty.

By 1963 eustachian tube function tests were not being performed in most cases. The approach at OMG was to operate, if indicated, regardless of possible tubal malfunction. It was felt that if the function of the eustachian tube could not be reestablished the tympanoplasty would not be successful.[3] The possibility of a two-stage procedure for gain in hearing was mentioned indicating that we had begun to think of the apparent eustachian tube problem more in terms of adequacy of the mucous membrane. But it was some time before this concept was crystallized.

The important word in the above paragraph is *reestablished.* We had learned that most of our patients whose eustachian tube function was nil using the Compere test, but who nonetheless required surgery for elimination of disease, did well following tympanoplasty. This confirmed the concept stated in Compere's paper. As a result of this experience we began in the early 1960s to perform surgery electively on patients generally thought to be poor risks in regard to eustachian tube function: adults with a cleft palate repair or with a chronic sinusitis-bronchitis syndrome.

One of these cases demonstrated that our evolv-

From the Otologic Medical Group, Inc., Los Angeles. Supported by funds from the House Ear Institute, Los Angeles.

Presented at the meeting of the American Otological Society, Inc., Vancouver, British Columbia, May 9-10, 1981.

REPRINTS — James L. Sheehy, MD, 2122 West Third Street, Los Angeles, CA 90057.

ing concept was probably correct. This was a 42-year-old female with situs inversus, bronchiectasis, chronic sinusitis and large bilateral central perforations with constant mucoid drainage. The hearing levels were 40 and 45 dB. She had become adjusted to her lifelong otorrhea. Her main problem was that she could not wear an air conduction aid because of the discharge and was unhappy with her bone conduction aid. The referring otolaryngologist was understandably hesitant to close the perforations.

Surgery was offered to obtain dry ears but with the understanding that middle ear effusion probably would develop and that further loss of hearing or graft failure could develop. The ossicular chains were intact, the mucous membrane was edematous but not hypertrophic, and the outer surface fascia graft technique was used on both sides at separate operations. Both operations resulted in a thick but mobile tympanic membrane without middle ear effusion. The hearing was restored to the point where an aid was not necessary.

This and subsequent similar cases made us realize that the lateral surface fascia grafting technique had an important advantage over techniques we had used prior to 1963: in patients who had infection at the time of surgery, or who had a major mucous membrane problem, the grafted membrane was often thicker than a normal membrane. This increased rigidity resulted in a better bellows effect, so to speak, to help ventilate the middle ear in the patient whose eustachian tube function might be marginal. And if tubal malfunction persisted postoperatively the tympanic membrane was less likely to become thin and atelectatic. If transtympanic ventilation was necessary this thicker-than-normal membrane accepted the ventilation tube better.

As a result of this experience we began to appreciate more fully the role of the tympanic membrane in middle ear ventilation. Previously a nonfixed atelectasis was thought to be due to persistent eustachian tube malfunction; transtympanic ventilation was the only solution. We now began to realize that some cases of this type, should there be a significant hearing problem, might well be best served by tympanic membrane reconstruction to reestablish the bellows effect, to allow the middle ear to develop the negative pressure it normally does, a negative pressure which then serves to aspirate air from the nasopharynx when the eustachian tube opens.

LATER DEVELOPMENTS

Although tubal malfunction is not a contraindication to tympanoplasty, in order for tympanoplasty to be successful, tubal function must be reestablished.[4] By 1965 eustachian tube function testing, as part of the preoperative evaluation of patients with chronic otitis media, had been abandoned at OMG.

In 1967 we began systematically performing operations in two stages.[5] This concept of staging had been reported by Rambo[6] and by Tabb,[7] but had not been generally accepted. Although we initially staged some of our operations in the early and mid-1960s because of mucous membrane problems it was in fact the residual cholesteatoma problem which spurred us on. With more staging of surgery in cholesteatoma cases it became apparent that we could obtain a ventilated middle ear space even in some cases with little or no remaining mucous membrane in the middle ear. This led to better hearing results and, incidentally, a decrease in the incidence of recurrence of cholesteatoma (retraction pockets).

In 1969 House, Glasscock and Miles reported on the technique of eustachian tuboplasty through a middle fossa approach.[8] Seven patients who had bilateral closure of the eustachian tube had surgery on one ear. The usual finding was fibrous closure of the isthmus. Following removal of this obstruction Silastic sheeting was inserted. Brackmann[9] reported that four of seven patients had long-term success. Eustachian tuboplasty, however, has not been pursued at OMG because of the magnitude of the surgical procedure, the difficulty in case selection and the ease and effectiveness of transtympanic ventilation. Glasscock has performed only one tuboplasty in ten years (Glasscock ME, personal communication).

As we reconstructed, in two stages, the more badly diseased ears, we began to encounter patients who had persistent tubal insufficiency or no tubal function at all postoperatively. The recognition and treatment of this problem was commented on in 1970.[10]

By 1973 we reported on the systematic use of plastic sheeting in tympanoplasty, usually as part of a two-stage procedure.[11] Our experience over the preceding seven years had led us to two conclusions: 1) persistent tubal malfunction need not result in failure in tympanoplasty; 2) permanent transtympanic ventilation is necessary in some cases to maintain hearing and prevent retraction pockets. One could often operate on the chronically draining ear with cholesteatoma and little or no tubal function, eliminate the infection, graft the tympanic membrane, restore the sound pressure transfer mechanism, and then ventilate the middle ear space transtympanically to maintain hearing.

RESULTS

The results of three recent studies have confirmed that our concepts are correct. In 1977 we reported on 1,024 primary cases of cholesteatoma requiring mastoid surgery. Postoperative serous otitis media was detected in only 7%.[12] In half of these the problem was transient. In half, however, long-term transtympanic ventilation was required. The incidence of persistent serous otitis media in the 6-and-under age group was only slightly higher: 2/33 cases. This confirmed that even in the badly diseased ear, not preselected for surgery on a basis of tubal function tests, the incidence of tubal malfunction was low, even in young children.

In 1980 we reported results in 472 myringoplasty operations.[13] Serous otitis media was detected postoperatively in only one case. A recent review of 1,026 revision tympanoplasty procedures revealed transient serous otitis media in 4%; persistent serous otitis media, requiring a ventilation tube in 3%; and postoperative atelectasis as a cause of failure in 1%.[14]

DISCUSSION

All would agree that eustachian tube malfunction plays a major role in the development of chronic otitis media. And all would agree that one of the prerequisites for hearing improvement in reconstructive middle ear surgery is an air-containing, mucous membrane-lined middle ear space.

In the early days of tympanoplasty it was often said that surgery should not be performed unless the eustachian tube had normal function. As more experience was gained this concept was modified: a tympanoplasty would not be successful unless eustachian tube function was reestablished.

With the advent of staged procedures and the use of plastic sheeting, it became apparent that although it was desirable to have normal tubal function the operation could be successful without this. If a mucosal lined space could be established the middle ear space could be ventilated transtympanically if necessary, as it was in 4% of our cholesteatoma cases.

CONCLUSION

At OMG we do not test eustachian tube function prior to reconstructive middle ear surgery and see no rationale for doing so.

REFERENCES

1. Compere WE. Tympanic clearance studies. Trans Am Acad Ophthalmol Otolaryngol 1958; 62:444-54.

2. House WF. The function of the eustachian tube. Arch Otolaryngol 1960; 71:405-7.

3. House WF, Sheehy JL. Functional restoration in tympanoplasty. Arch Otolaryngol 1963; 78:304-9.

4. Sheehy JL. Surgery of chronic otitis media. In: English GM, Maloney W, eds. Vol 1. New York: Harper & Row, 1965: 24.

5. Sheehy JL, Paterson ME. Intact canal wall tympanoplasty with mastoidectomy: 8 years experience. Laryngoscope 1967; 77:1502-42.

6. Rambo JHT. The use of paraffin to create a middle ear space in musculoplasty. Laryngoscope 1961; 71:612-9.

7. Tabb HG. The surgical management of chronic ear disease with special reference to staged surgery. Laryngoscope 1963; 73:363-83.

8. House WF, Glasscock ME, Miles J. Eustachian tuboplasty. Laryngoscope 1969; 79:1765-82.

9. Brackmann DE. Middle ear eustachian tuboplasty. Presented to the Pacific Coast Oto-Ophthalmologic Society, Portland, Ore., May, 1973.

10. Sheehy JL. Tympanoplasty with mastoidectomy: a reevaluation. Laryngoscope 1970; 80:1212-30.

11. Sheehy JL, Crabtree JA. Tympanoplasty: staging the operation. Laryngoscope 1973; 83:1594-1621.

12. Sheehy JL, Brackmann DE, Graham MD. Complications of cholesteatoma: a report on 1,024 cases. In: McCabe BF, Sadé J, Abramson AA, eds. First International Conference on Cholesteatoma. Birmingham: Aesculapius, 1977: 420-9.

13. Sheehy JL, Anderson RE. Myringoplasty: a review of 472 cases. Ann Otol Rhinol Laryngol 1980; 89:331-3.

14. Sheehy JL, Robinson JV. Revision tympanoplasty: recurrent and residual cholesteatoma. Presented at the Second International Conference on Cholesteatoma and Mastoid Surgery, Tel Aviv, March, 1981.

COMMENT

JAMES JERGER, PhD

HOUSTON, TEXAS

Drs. Sheehy and Bluestone have succeeded in highlighting key issues with clarity and insight. Both gentlemen are in agreement on two basic points: first, they both acknowledge that eustachian tube malfunction plays a major role in the development of chronic otitis media; second, they both agree that past and present tests of eustachian tube function are not reliable predictors of the results of

From the Department of Otorhinolaryngology and Commmunication Sciences, Baylor College of Medicine, Texas Medical Center, Houston.

Presented at the meeting of the American Otological Society, Inc., Vancouver, British Columbia, May 9-10, 1981.

REPRINTS — James Jerger, PhD, Dept. of Otorhinolaryngology and Communication Sciences, Baylor College of Medicine, Texas Medical Center, Houston, TX 77030.

tympanoplasty in children. Our own experience has certainly been in concurrence with these conclusions.

Beyond these points of basic agreement, however, Sheehy and Bluestone take seemingly divergent paths. Sheehy says that, with respect to reconstructive middle ear surgery, he does not test eustachian tube function and sees no rationale for doing so. Bluestone, on the other hand, argues that in spite of imperfect knowledge of eustachian tube physiology, and in spite of acknowledged limitations of existing tests, eustachian tube function should be evaluated in patients with middle ear disease.

Are these views contradictory, or do they represent the same edifice viewed from different perspectives? I suggest that Sheehy's conclusion is reasonable from the viewpoint of the practicing clinician while Bluestone's position is sound from the viewpoint of the teacher-investigator. I can agree with each. Sheehy reasserts the findings of a number of respected investigators — Ekvall, Palva and Karÿa; Holmquist and Hallen; Siedentop et al; MacKinnon; and Cohn — that existing eustachian tube function tests show relatively poor capacity to predict success of tympanoplasty. Based on these results there can be little quarrel with Sheehy's intensely practical conclusion that, from the viewpoint of the middle ear surgeon, the results of eustachian tube function tests have little immediate relevance. He and his associates have, therefore, elected to dispense with them.

Bluestone would not, I am sure, quarrel with the rationale for this decision. But he makes the important additional point that we are unlikely to develop better tests without a more comprehensive understanding of eustachian tube function, and there is no better laboratory for such investigation than the patient with middle ear disorder.

Bluestone views the problem from a different perspective than Sheehy. While agreeing on the negative predictive value of existing tests he sees a very good reason for continuing to think about and to develop new ways of measuring eustachian tube function. For Bluestone this research route is the only possible route to a more rational and effective clinical management of patients with middle ear disease. He feels, and I agree with him, that eustachian tube function is an essential key to the effective resolution of middle ear disease and that the ultimate answer to better surgical prognosis lies in more sensitive, yet more physiologic, evaluation of the eustachian tube. For these compelling reasons he urges us to expand, not contract, our research horizons, a sentiment with which I am sure Sheehy would concur.

In addition to the very important issue of prognosis for reconstructive surgery, there is a growing concern for the possibly deleterious deprivation effects of chronic middle ear disease during early childhood. This is a potential problem of incredible scope with long-term ramifications affecting a very large number of children. At present serial tympanometry is perhaps our most effective mass screening technique. But we are all aware of the many problems associated with the tympanogram as an index of eustachian tube function. There can be no question of the need for better tests of eustachian tube function, and there can be no question of the need for further research in this important area. Viewed from this perspective, I can do no less than urge full support for Bluestone's viewpoint.

In the year 2000 we will celebrate the 500th anniversary of the birth of Bartolommeo Eustachio. Perhaps by then the pooled knowledge of clinicians and researchers working together will have brought us to a truly complete understanding of Eustachio's remarkable tube.

NEURAL CONNECTIONS BETWEEN THE MIDDLE EAR, EUSTACHIAN TUBE AND BRAIN

IMPLICATIONS FOR THE REFLEX CONTROL OF MIDDLE EAR AERATION

AVRIM R. EDEN, MD

GALVESTON, TEXAS

This study was designed to investigate the neuroanatomic connections between the middle ear (ME), eustachian tube, and brain. The neural tracer, horseradish peroxidase (HRP), was injected into the promontory mucosa of the ME in six adult rabbits. Following a 24-48 hour survival, the brain was perfused with fixative and the HRP reacted by the tetramethylbenzidine (TMB) blue reaction process. Two groups of HRP-labeled neurons were noted in the ipsilateral brainstem: 1) a well-defined cluster of HRP-labeled neurons in the nucleus of the solitary tract, and 2) a more widely scattered group of labeled neurons in the inferior salivary nucleus. The labeled neurons in the solitary tract may represent the direct central sensory projections of the glomus tympanicum. In a second set of animals HRP was injected into both the tubal and palatal muscles to identify the motor innervation of the eustachian tube musculature; HRP-labeled motoneurons were noted in the trigeminal motor nucleus and nucleus ambiguus, respectively. Assuming that the glomus tympanicum cells can sense changes such as oxygen concentration in their immediate environment in the ME like the related glomus cells in the carotid and aortic bodies which also project to the solitary tract, then the neuroanatomic relationships of the HRP-labeled neurons in this study to other respiratory neurons in the medulla suggest the possibility of a polysynaptic ME aeration reflex. The relevance of these results to the pathogenesis of otitis media with effusion is discussed.

INTRODUCTION

The precise control of middle ear (ME) aeration is unknown. Periodic opening of the eustachian tube (ET) is said to maintain air in the ME and mastoid at atmospheric pressure. Although changes in the anatomical configuration of the ET from birth to adulthood have been clearly described, mechanical factors alone cannot account fully for the widespread phenomenon of ME hypoventilation manifesting clinically, for example, as otitis media with effusion (OME) in 5-10% of otherwise healthy elementary school age children.[1]

This study was designed to investigate the neuroanatomic connections between the ME, ET, and brain to determine their relationship to other brainstem respiratory neurons, and to investigate the possibility of reflex neural control of ME aeration.

MATERIALS AND METHODS

Group 1. Under Innovar anesthesia (1 ml/kg) one ME of each of six adult New Zealand white rabbits was entered by a lateral approach through the bulla to expose the oval and round windows and promontory of the ME. The neural tracer horseradish peroxidase (10 μl of 50% HRP in saline) was slowly injected into the component nerves of the tympanic plexus and submucosa of the promontory using a Hamilton microsyringe and micromanipulator. Care was taken to avoid spread of the tracer to the oval and round windows and the horizontal portion of the facial nerve. The postauricular incision was sutured and the animal allowed to survive 24-48 hours.

The brain was fixed at the end of the allotted survival period by transcardiac perfusion under deep anesthesia. An initial 50 ml normal saline flush at 37°C was immediately followed by 1000 ml of quarter strength Karnovsky's fixative (1.25% glutaraldehyde and 1% paraformaldehyde) in 0.1M phosphate buffer (pH 7.4) at 4°C. The fixative was in turn followed by 1000 ml of 20% sucrose-phosphate buffer. The brain was dissected, cryosectioned at 40 μ intervals, and reacted by the tetramethylbenzidine (TMB) blue reaction process.[2] The mounted brain sections were counterstained with neutral red.

Group 2. In a second set of five anesthetized adult rabbits, horseradish peroxidase (10μl of 50% HRP in saline) was slowly injected under direct vision into both the tubal and palatal muscles. The animals were allowed to survive 24-48 hours. The brain was fixed, dissected, sectioned, and reacted for HRP as described above.

RESULTS

Group 1. Following the tympanic plexus injections two groups of HRP-labeled neurons were noted in the ipsilateral brainstem. A well-defined cluster of intensely labeled multipolar neurons was observed in the nucleus of the ipsilateral solitary tract[3,4] (Figs. 1 and 2). The tympanic plexus injections also yielded a group of HRP-labeled neurons in the salivary nucleus (Fig. 3), ventrolateral to the solitary tract and dorsal to the facial nucleus (Figs. 1 and 2). There were no labeled cells in the facial nucleus, trigeminal motor nucleus, or contralateral brainstem.

Group 2. The combined tubopalatal muscle injections also yielded two groups of labeled neurons. A compact cluster of intensely labeled multipolar motoneurons was noted in nucleus ambiguus (Figs. 1 and 2). A second group of heavily labeled motoneurons was noted in the ventral most part of the

From the Department of Otolaryngology, University of Texas Medical Branch, Galveston. Supported in part by grants from the National Institutes of Health (NINCDS NS 16082) and the Deafness Research Foundation.

Presented at the meeting of the American Otological Society, Inc., Vancouver, British Columbia, May 9-10, 1981.

REPRINTS — Avrim R. Eden, MD, Department of Otolaryngology, University of Texas Medical Branch, Galveston, TX 77550.

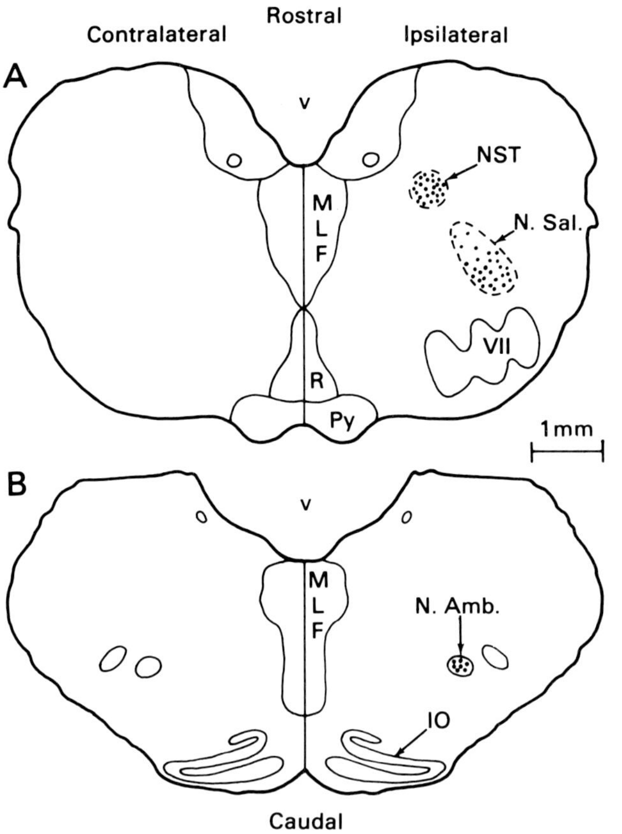

Fig. 1. Coronal diagrams of the rabbit brain to show the location of HRP-labeled neurons (dots) A) in the nucleus of the solitary tract (NST) and salivary nucleus (N. Sal.) following tympanic plexus injections, and B) in nucleus ambiguus (N. Amb.) following palatal muscle injection. The number of dots does not reflect the exact number of labeled cells but rather the relative distribution within the different nuclei. MLF — Median longitudinal fasciculus; R — Raphe nucleus; Py — Pyramid; V — Ventricle; VII — Facial nucleus; IO — Inferior olive.

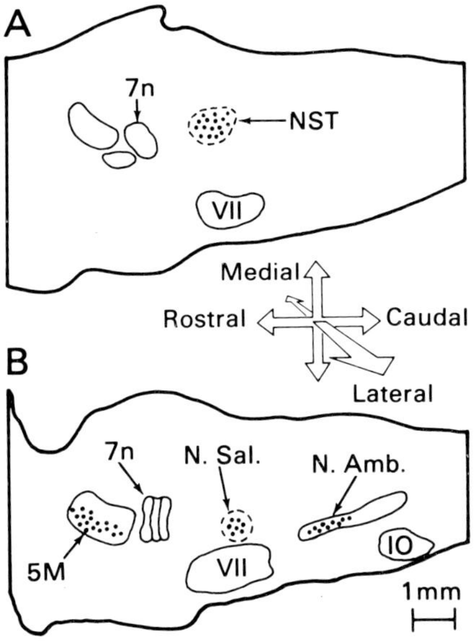

Fig. 2. Sagittal diagrams of the rabbit brain to show the location of HRP-labeled neurons (dots) following ipsilateral tympanic plexus injections in A) the nucleus of the solitary tract (NST), and B) salivary nucleus (N. Sal.), and, following tubopalatal muscle injections, in the trigeminal motor nucleus (5M), and nucleus ambiguus (N. Amb.). The number of dots does not reflect the exact number of labeled cells but rather the relative distribution within the different nuclei. VII — Facial nucleus; 7n — Facial nerve tract; IO — Inferior olive.

trigeminal motor nucleus (Fig. 2). Since the palatal and tubal muscles were injected in combination and bilaterally, possible crossed and/or separate innervation of these two muscle groups could not be defined.

There were no other labeled cells in the brainstem. Specifically noteworthy was the absence of labeling in the trigeminal mesencephalic nucleus. The extracranial ganglia of the vagus and glossopharyngeal nerves were not examined.

DISCUSSION

The neuroanatomic relationships of the HRP-labeled neurons described above to other central respiratory neurons suggest the existence of a mechanism whereby the degree of ME aeration may be monitored and regulated (Fig. 4).

Respiratory neurons in the medulla have been divided into two groups.[5] The nucleus of the solitary tract (NST) together with part of the dorsal motor nucleus of the vagus (DmnX) form the dorsal respiratory group (DRG). Motoneurons in nucleus ambiguus, nucleus retroambiguus, the facial and retrofacial nuclei, the trigeminal motor nucleus (5M), and the hypoglossal nucleus form the ventral respiratory group (VRG) (Table 1). The DRG is the primary respiratory oscillator initiating the rhythm of the inspiratory-expiratory cycle. Projections from the DRG to the motoneuron pool of the VRG[6] control the cyclic action of the respiratory tract musculature (nasal alae, soft palate, tongue, larynx, trachea, and bronchi). Projections from the DRG and VRG to spinal cord motoneurons (phrenic and intercostal nerves) and the pontine pneumotaxic center complete the complex central control of respiration.

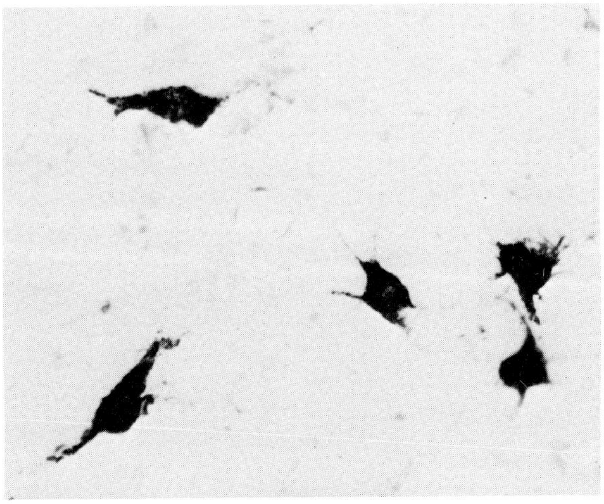

Fig. 3. Lightfield photomicrograph of HRP-labeled neurons (black) in the salivary nucleus following ipsilateral tympanic plexus injection.

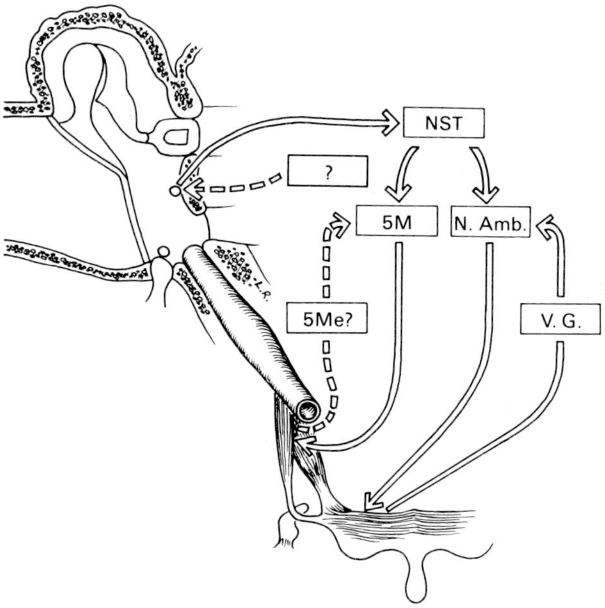

Fig. 4. Diagram to illustrate the neural connections between the ME, ET, and brain as described in the text. HRP-labeled neurons in the nucleus of the solitary tract (NST) following tympanic plexus injection may represent the sensory projections from the ME. HRP-labeled tubopalatal muscle motoneurons are located in the trigeminal motor nucleus (5M) and nucleus ambiguus (N. Amb.). Cell bodies subserving tubopalatal muscle proprioception are generally thought (hence the ?) to be located in the trigeminal mesencephalic nucleus (5Me?) and extracranial vagal ganglia (V.G.), respectively. The absence of HRP-labeled neurons in 5Me in our studies suggests an alternative location in the semilunar ganglion. The boxed ? indicates the possibility of efferent projections from regulatory neurons in the medulla to the ME (see text).

We have demonstrated HRP-labeled neurons in the DRG following tympanic plexus injections and in nuclei of the VRG following tubopalatal muscle injections in the rabbit. It is our contention that these neurons are part of a mechanism for 1) monitoring the degree of ME aeration through sensory projections to the DRG, and 2) reflexly controlling ET function by higher order projections from the DRG to the tubopalatal motoneurons in the VRG.

The exact location of the sensory cell bodies subserving tubopalatal muscle proprioception (and thereby modulating muscle tonus) is controversial, since it is widely held that trigeminal motor nucleus innervated muscle proprioceptive neurons, eg, jaw muscles, are located within the brain in the trigeminal mesencephalic nucleus (5Me) rather than in the trigeminal semilunar ganglion.[7] Indeed, Wild and Zeigler[8] have demonstrated pigeon jaw closing muscle proprioception in this brainstem nucleus. Even though we noted many intensely labeled motoneurons in 5M from the tubal muscle injections, we did not observe labeled cells in 5Me. We suggest, therefore, that in the rabbit, tubopalatal muscle proprioceptive neurons are more probably located in extra CNS sites such as the semilunar and petrosal ganglia (Fig. 4).

TABLE 1. RESPIRATORY NEURONS IN THE MEDULLA

Dorsal Group	*Ventral Group*
Solitary tract nucleus	N ambiguus
Dorsal motor nucleus of X	N retroambiguus Facial nucleus Retrofacial nucleus Trigeminal motor nucleus Hypoglossal nucleus?*

*Inclusion of the hypoglossal nucleus in the ventral respiratory group is not without controversy.[5]

The specificity of HRP-labeled neurons is directly related to the precision of the neural tracer application. HRP injected into the tympanic plexus will be taken up by all components of that plexus (Table 2) and transported retrogradely in the axoplasm to the parent cell bodies.[2] HRP does not appear to cross synapses to second order neurons. Cell bodies of all tympanic plexus nerves (even those whose existence is the subject of neuroanatomic controversy) are located in peripheral ganglia. Thus HRP taken up by these axons will not result in labeling of neurons in the brain, the exception being those of the preganglionic secretomotor fibers from the salivary nuclei (Figs. 1-3) to the parotid gland.[9]

We were surprised to note heavily labeled neurons in the nucleus of the solitary tract (NST) since it was expected that the cell bodies subserving the innervation of the tympanic glomus body (TGB) would be located in the petrosal ganglion; only their central axons should project to terminal fields within the NST. Some caution, therefore, is indicated in interpreting this data. These NST labeled cells may be part of the the adjacent dorsal motor nucleus of the vagus (DmnX) which is, however, included in the dorsal respiratory group. It is also possible that the labeled NST neurons are efferent to, rather than sensory afferent projections from, the ME.

The exact function of the TGB is unknown, but its similarity to other glomi has been noted by several investigators.[9] For example, the carotid body glomus cells are small modified neurons with few dendritic processes and no axons. They are connected to one another and to the axonal terminals of the glossopharyngeal (Hering's) nerve by reciprocal synapses. The synaptic arrangements and ultra-

TABLE 2. TYMPANIC PLEXUS

Nerve	*Cell Bodies*
Sensory IX (Jacobson)	Petrosal ganglion
Sensory X (Arnold)	Jugular ganglion
Caroticotympanic	Sup. cervical ganglion
Pregangl. secretomotor	Inf. salivary nucleus Sup. salivary nucleus?
Sensory (taste) VII?*	Geniculate ganglion
Sensory V?*	Semilunar ganglion
Glomus tympanicum	Solitary tract nucleus?** Dorsal motor nucleus of X?**

*Inclusion of these nerves in the tympanic plexus is not without controversy.

**Preliminary evidence presented in this paper suggests strongly but not yet conclusively that axons from these neurons project to the middle ear.

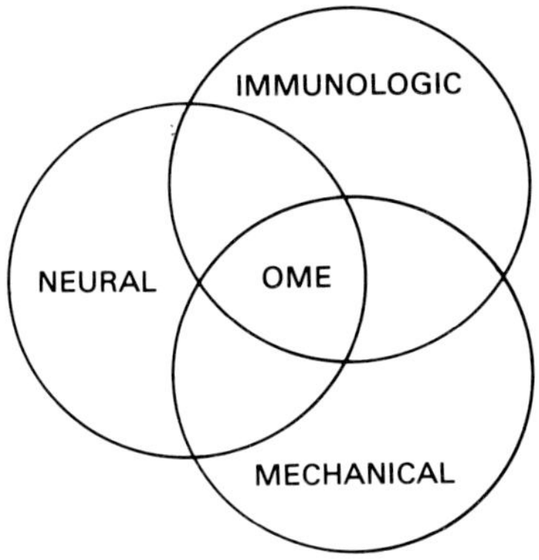

Fig. 5. Diagrammatic representation of the interaction between anatomic, immunologic, and neural factors in the pathogenesis of OME.

structural characteristics, eg, large dense-core vesicles, of the glomus cells suggest that they have multifunctional capabilities.[10] Sensory afferents from the carotid and aortic arch bodies project to the NST to form the afferent limbs of the complex and parallel respiratory-cardiovascular reflex arcs.[11,12]

We suggest that the tympanic glomus cells may have similar capabilities to those in the carotid body in that they may be able to act as a ME chemosensory organ responsive to changes such as oxygen concentration in the ME and that projections to the NST may form the afferent limb of a polysynaptic ME aeration reflex (Fig. 4). Also, since oxygen concentration in the ME space appears to be determined mainly by diffusion from capillaries,[13] efferent projections from DmnX (a respiratory-vascular reflex center) to the ME may regulate the ME oxygen concentration by their influence on the ME vasculature.

Unpublished observations (Eden AR) on developmental aspects such as the ratio of unmyelinated to myelinated nerve fibers in the tympanic plexus lead to speculation that the higher incidence of, for example, OME in children may be due partly to immaturity of the neural elements.

In conclusion, we suggest that the traditional view of the pathogenesis of OME be broadened to include a more dynamic interaction between mechanical factors occasioned by anatomic changes during growth, local ME immunologic mechanisms (perhaps even modulated by efferent projections from DmnX to the ME), and modulation of the ME environment by the neural interconnections between the tympanic plexus, ET, and brain (Fig. 5).

ACKNOWLEDGMENTS — I thank Joseph Torey Nalbone and Elisa Jo Castro for their expert technical assistance. Beryl Eden typed the manuscript.

REFERENCES

1. Sadé J. Secretory otitis media and its sequelae. New York: Churchill Livingstone, 1979.

2. Mesulam MM. Tetramethyl benzidine for horseradish peroxidase neurohistochemistry: a non-carcinogenic blue reaction-product with superior sensitivity for visualizing neural afferents and efferents. J Histochem Cytochem 1978; 26:106-17.

3. McBride RL, Klemm WR. Stereotaxic atlas of rabbit brain, based on the rapid method of photography of frozen, unstained sections. Commun Behav Bio 1968A; 2:179-215.

4. Meessen H, Olszewski J. A cytoarchitectonic atlas of the rhombencephalon of the rabbit. New York: S. Karger, 1949.

5. Kalia MP. Anatomical organization of central respiratory neurons. Ann Rev Physiol 1981; 43:105-20.

6. Beckstead RM, Morse JR, Norgren R. The nucleus of the solitary tract in the monkey: projections to the thalamus and brain stem nuclei. J Comp Neurol 1980; 190:259-82.

7. Brodal A. Neurological anatomy. 2nd ed. New York: Oxford University Press, 1969.

8. Wild JM, Zeigler HP. Central representation and somatotopic organization of the jaw muscles within the facial and trigeminal nuclei of the pigeon *(Columba livia)*. J Comp Neurol 1980; 192:175-201.

9. Schuknecht HF. Pathology of the ear. Cambridge: Harvard University Press, 1974.

10. Shepherd GM. The synaptic organization of the brain. 2nd ed. New York: Oxford University Press, 1979.

11. Wallach JH, Loewy AD. Projections of the aortic nerve to the nucleus tractus solitarius in the rabbit. Brain Res 1980; 188:247-51.

12. Chalmers JP, Korner PI, White SW. The relative roles of the aortic and carotid sinus nerves in the rabbit in the control of respiration and circulation during arterial hypoxia and hypercapnia. J Physiol (Lond) 1967; 188:435-50.

13. Ostfeld E, Blonder J, Crispin M, Szeinberg A. The middle ear gas composition in air-ventilated dogs. Acta Otolaryngol (Stockh) 1980; 89:105-8.

Ann Otol 90:1981

PANEL ON TREATMENT OF BELL'S PALSY

EARLY DECOMPRESSION OF THE FACIAL NERVE IN BELL'S PALSY

JACK L. PULEC, MD

LOS ANGELES, CALIFORNIA

Decompression of the facial nerve for 200 patients with Bell's palsy has been performed by the author during the past 17 years. These procedures were accomplished without injury to the facial nerve or inner ear. In no case was the incus removed nor the tympanic membrane or posterior bony canal wall disturbed with the exception of two translabyrinthine procedures in which the incus and inner ear were removed. Of 34 patients with normal nerve excitability preoperatively all had 100% recovery of facial motion. In 147 others followed for one year or more and whose nerve excitability was absent preoperatively, there was obtained an average of 80% recovery of motion and usually some degree of synkinesis. One patient who had a missing segment of nerve and a nerve graft performed failed to obtain any facial motion. Biopsy of facial nerve fibers during surgery has been found to be a feasible and useful technique. There is still no way to establish a prognosis when one still has a chance to avoid a bad result. The best one can do is to carefully follow serial electrical tests and perform surgery at the time when electrical studies begin to deteriorate. It is hoped that deterioration will develop slowly enough that a third degree injury will not have developed by the time that surgery is performed. Considering the results of this series of cases it would seem that the best results can be obtained by early surgical decompression for Bell's palsy. The patient must be informed of the possibility and the decision regarding the nature and timing of treatment should be a subjective one made after a careful analysis of the available facts and each patient's own circumstances. The availability of a promptly accomplished and precisely performed facial nerve decompression allows every patient to have a minimal risk of disabling permanent facial deformity.

The disfigurement of a facial paralysis can cause a patient to have a lifetime of agony and disappointment. A discussion of the treatment of no other disease stimulates more controversy than that for Bell's palsy. Surgical techniques are now available to reach every portion of the facial nerve without the production of additional injury to the nerve or to hearing. The purpose of this paper is to report on 200 patients with Bell's palsy treated surgically by the author during the past 17 years. This demonstrates that decompression of the nerve can be accomplished with minimal morbidity, and that the best results can be obtained when surgery is accomplished early in the course of the disease.

EXAMINATION

Without exception every patient with facial palsy should have a complete examination to establish the diagnosis and topognosis. Many lesions associated with the facial nerve in the brainstem, cerebellopontine angle, temporal bone, and soft tissue of the face can produce facial paralysis which appears the same as Bell's palsy. The diagnosis is, therefore, one of exclusion. Every patient who develops a facial paralysis whether complete or incomplete should have a careful otologic and neurologic evaluation[1] including audiogram for pure tone and speech, electronystagmogram, and roentgenograms of the temporal bone. Should these tests be abnormal, if the paralysis has been of gradual onset, or should spasms or twitching of the face be present, a Pantopaque myelogram of the posterior fossa and internal auditory canals and computerized tomography with enhancement should be made.

Topognosis is determined by testing the function of the branches of the facial nerve. The edema which is associated with Bell's palsy almost always starts at the stylomastoid foramen and extends proximally in the more severe cases for varying distances. The chorda tympani nerve can be most conveniently examined with the electric taste tester. Function of the stapedius nerve is determined by eliciting a stapedius reflex using impedance audiometry. The most important topognostic test is the tear test. This qualitative test is performed by placing strips of filter paper behind each lower eyelid. Irritation of the cornea normally produces saturation of the paper for a length of 2-3 cm within one minute. The absence of tearing signifies that there is involvement of the geniculate ganglion or medial to it.

PROGNOSIS

There is still no clear way to determine prognosis at the time of onset of the paralysis. The fact that it is impossible to predict for certain which patient will and which will not have a good and prompt recovery is the major problem which prevents physicians from being able to select patients for surgery who would otherwise have a poor result. Nevertheless, certain findings do provide some indication of the status of the nerve and should be considered in the decision to do surgery.

From the Pulec Ear Clinic, Los Angeles. Sponsored by Ear International, Los Angeles.

Presented at the meeting of the American Otological Society, Inc., Vancouver, British Columbia, May 9-10, 1981.

REPRINTS — Jack L. Pulec, MD, Pulec Ear Clinic, 1245 Wilshire Blvd., Los Angeles, CA 90017.

Patients who have an incomplete paralysis can for practical purposes be expected to make a full and complete recovery and should not be included in most discussions about medical or surgical treatment. The presence of severe pain of the mastoid tends to indicate a more severe edema of the nerve and a poor prognosis. Persons with cardiovascular disease, the elderly, those with diabetes mellitus, and pregnant women near term have a less favorable outlook for complete recovery. Patients who sustain a second or recurrent facial paralysis tend to have a constricted fallopian canal which leads easily to entrapment of the nerve by any edema which it might develop. Recurrent episodes ultimately result in poor facial function. The topognostic tests also have some limited value in suggesting prognosis. Patients who have involvement of a greater length of the facial nerve within the temporal bone and especially those who have reduced tearing can be expected to generally have a poorer prognosis.

Most patients with complete idiopathic facial palsies that recover begin to do so within five days of onset. Although an occasional patient may have complete paralysis for months without ever developing measurable nerve degeneration, prolonged paralysis usually results in a poor recovery.

The nerve excitability test is the most commonly used electrical examination. Electromyography and electroneurography are now commonly in use, and provide more detailed and graphic demonstration of facial function. Evoked electromyography[2] has been utilized in this series during the past four years. From a practical standpoint it has added nothing to our ability to determine prognosis over the simpler nerve excitability test. Both methods detect the development of nerve degeneration or demyelination. The tests have limited value in indicating a bad prognosis after the fact. They are misleading in cases where the nerve becomes demyelinated since those cases mistakenly appear to have a bad prognosis when, in fact, they usually make a complete spontaneous recovery despite any type of therapy.

PROBLEM

Since there is no way to definitely determine prognosis at the onset of a complete facial paralysis the physician is faced with the dilemma of which patient should have surgery and when it should be offered. Sunderland[3] has described the three fundamental types of nerve fiber injury, and in relation to the endoneurium, perineurium and epineurium, provides the basis for his classification of nerve trunk injuries. Five degrees of injury of increasing severity are described which involve successively and in progression 1) conduction in the axons, 2) loss of continuity of the axons without breaching the endoeurium, 3) loss of continuity of nerve fibers, 4) the perineurium and funiculi, and 5) loss of continuity of the nerve trunk. It would be desirable to be able to determine before hand which patient will develop loss of axons and loss of continuity of nerve fibers. So long as only a conduction block is present, complete and prompt perfect recovery is possible. If injury could be limited to the second degree without progression to loss of continuity of nerve fibers, even though recovery is delayed for several months, the result should ultimately be excellent. If the degree of injury progresses to the third and fourth degree with scarring, loss of continuity of nerve fibers, and loss of perineurium and funiculi, complete recovery is not possible. Synkinesis invariably results from this type of injury. The fifth degree of injury with complete loss of continuity of the nerve trunk will result in no recovery at all and requires a nerve graft.

TABLE 1. BELL'S PALSY RECOVERY IN 156 CASES*

Recovery	*% of Total Cases*
Complete	48
Incomplete	
No disability	5
Trivial disability	22
Poor result	20
Not traced	5
Herpes oticus	
Poor result	66

*From Matthews.[4]

The problem that exists in the practical management of Bell's palsy is that the separation between the development of a first and second degree injury is extremely small and all parts of the facial nerve do not have uniform severity of injury. The progression from a first to a second or third degree injury can occur so rapidly that even in a very carefully followed patient permanent changes cannot always be avoided.

The patient and the surgeon have a choice of proceeding with surgical decompression early in the course of Bell's palsy before any degeneration develops, or delaying surgery until signs of degeneration occur. The problem with the first option is that some patients will undergo surgery who would have made a complete spontaneous recovery. The problem with the second option is that the patient accepts a significant risk of incomplete recovery and the development of synkinesis.

It is generally accepted that patients with incomplete facial paralysis require no surgical treatment and will make a spontaneous recovery. Patients with complete facial palsy who make spontaneous recovery will generally do so within five days of the onset of the paralysis. Without surgical treatment approximately 50% will undergo some degeneration and delayed recovery and up to 35% will ultimately have a poor result with incomplete recovery and synkinesis (Table 1).[4-6] As shown in a previous report[7] the only sure way to avoid risk of permanent disability is to offer surgical decompression of the nerve early before any degeneration occurs.

TREATMENT

MEDICAL

Medical treatment of Bell's palsy offers limited and unreliable results. Efforts are directed to the reduction of edema and the increase of circulation to the nerve. These include administration of nicotinic acid orally in doses of several hundred milligrams daily and the administration of histamine intravenously daily. Prednisone in doses of 40 to 60 mg daily often produces disturbing side effects. The use of medical treatment at the onset of Bell's palsy of both the complete and incomplete types seems to be indicated during the time required to complete the examination. Medical treatment would seem to have some value in the management of Bell's palsy but its use should not affect the decision to recommend surgery.

SURGICAL

Techniques for the total exposure and decompression of the facial nerve,[1,8,9] grafting techniques,[10] and the management of tumors[11,12] have been perfected, and our ability to work around and on the nerve without producing injury has become standard practice over the past 17 years. Three approaches are used to reach the nerve in the temporal bone. For the majority of cases who have good hearing with nerve involvement distal to the geniculate ganglion the approach is through the mastoid and facial recess.

Two approaches are available for the patient with absence of tearing, indicating that the lesion is extending medial to the geniculate ganglion. Total facial nerve decompression by the translabyrinthine approach is used for the rare patient with Bell's palsy who has had a preexisting useless labyrinth. Total decompression of the entire nerve without disturbing the middle or inner ear is accomplished by combining the mastoid and tympanic approaches with the middle cranial fossa approach. Accurate placement of the temporary craniectomy is critical to obtain adequate exposure of the facial nerve through the middle cranial fossa. Details of the surgical technique have been thoroughly described.[1,7,8] In addition to an adequate knowledge of the temporal bone, modern training in surgical technique and experience, it is extremely important that the surgeon use and maintain the appropriate instruments to accomplish the surgery. The most important and most frequently neglected instrument is a delicate, light, and easy-to-direct drill with an angled handpiece. The handpiece is held by the surgeon with his thumb and fingers like a pencil and he must have a light touch if accurate surgery is to be performed. Use of the heavy air-powered drills commonly available in operating theaters is difficult to control even by the most experienced surgeon and provides an additional hazard to the facial nerve and its surrounding structures. Decompression of the facial nerve without removal of the incus, tympanic membrane, or posterior canal wall should be routine if appropriate equipment is used.

Of the circumference of bone surrounding the facial nerve sheath 180° should be removed, and decompression involves the longitudinal incision of thick constricting facial nerve sheath. The nerve in acute Bell's palsy will usually swell when the sheath is incised. It is convenient to assess edema as 1+ when the facial nerve diameter increases by 25%; 2+ to represent a 50% increase in facial nerve diameter; 3+ when the diameter increases by 75% and 4+ when the nerve diameter is 100% or more of its normal diameter. If one expects to cause no injury to the facial nerve it must never be bumped or bruised or touched with the suction tip. Curettes should not be used within the fallopian canal to remove bone. Should a tumor be found or the nerve be absent or fibrotic, the area can be excised and grafted. After the sheath has been incised and the nerve adequately inspected blood is allowed to accumulate over the nerve with no cover of any sort. The external wound is closed. Nothing is placed upon the nerve fibers or within the middle ear or mastoid cavity.

Facial Nerve Biopsy. Histopathologic examination of the facial nerve fibers in the human have been studied for the first time (Pulec JL and Kurokawa M, unpublished data). The ability to decompress a normally functioning nerve without reducing function in surgery for chronic otitis media and idiopathic hemifacial spasm has contributed to the development of the facial nerve biopsy without the addition of any noticeable disability. Experience in 21 cases of geniculate neuralgia demonstrated that up to 30% of the cross-sectional area of the motor trunk of the facial nerve could be excised; if done without producing injury to the remaining fibers, it will produce no facial weakness.[13] A technique has been developed to excise a very small fascicle from the facial nerve as a biopsy without the production of any deficit or harm to the patient. This information has been correlated with the preoperative history, electrical testing of the nerve, and postoperative recovery (Pulec JL and Kurakawa M, unpublished data). Correlation with electrical testing, the extent of surgical edema at the time of surgery, and postoperative results have been excellent, and objectively demonstrate the actual edema and extent of nerve injury. Specimens taken from the normal part of the nerve proximal to the edematous portion can show the area of involvement. Clear differences can be seen between the chorda tympani (Fig. 1A) and the edematous motor portion of the nerve within the fallopian canal (Fig. 1B). These histopathologic changes support the need and rationale for surgical decompression in Bell's palsy.

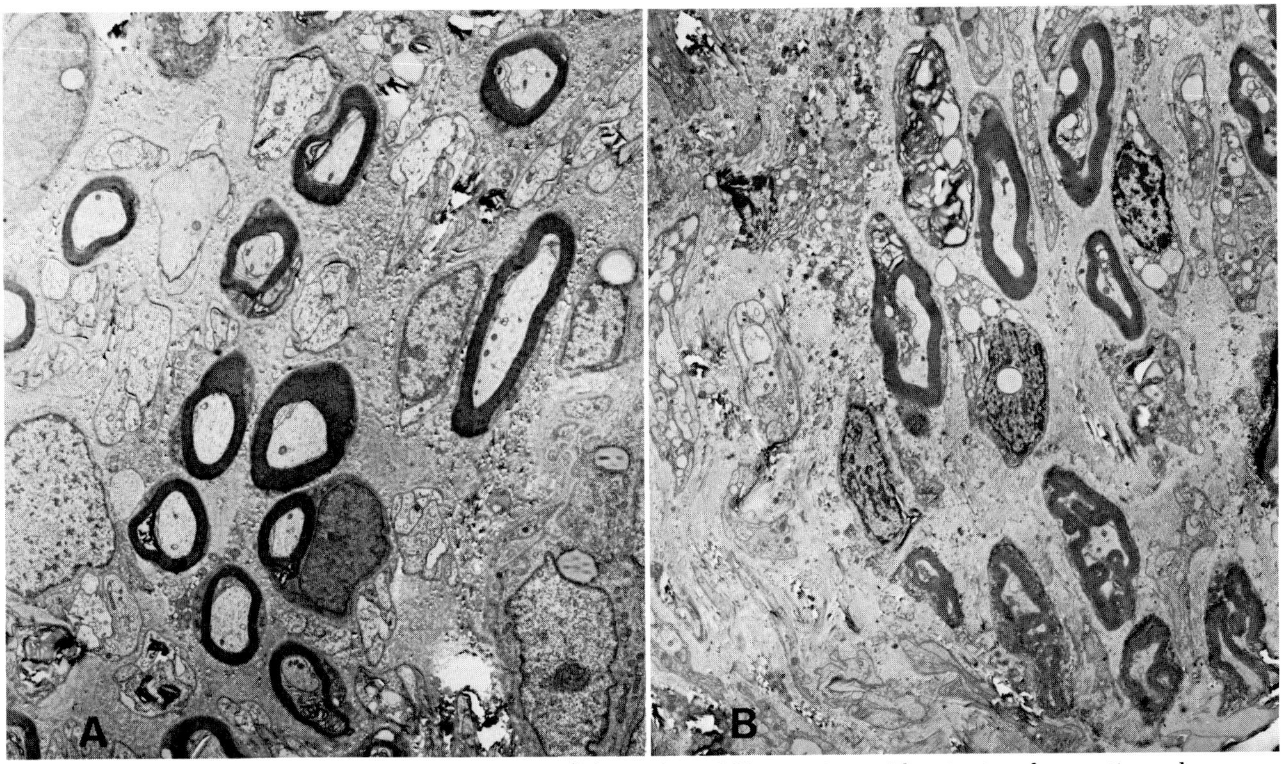

Fig. 1. (Case 2) A) Chorda tympani nerve. Most of the myelinated fibers are intact. There is minor degeneration and unraveling of the innermost layer of the myelin sheath. Perineurium collagen fibers are normal. Schwann cell nuclei and vacuoles within the Schwann cell cytoplasm are seen. B) Facial nerve. There is a moderate degree of degeneration of the myelin sheath and much greater than that within the chorda tympani nerve. Schwann cell cytoplasms contain many vacuoles. There is a minimal increase of the collagen fibers. (x6000)

RESULTS

During a 17-year-period from 1964 to 1981 the author has decompressed the facial nerves of 200 patients with Bell's palsy utilizing the techniques already described. The first 100 patients were reported previously[7] and are included in this report to which an additional 100 patients have been added. Each patient had a complete neurootologic examination including audiometric, electronystagmographic, topognostic, and radiographic examinations to substantiate the preoperative diagnosis of Bell's palsy. Patients who had a dry eye determined by the tear test underwent total decompression of the facial nerve. The remaining group underwent decompression from the stylomastoid foramen to the cochleariform process by working through the facial recess. The nerve sheath was then opened, and if edema extended to the end of the incision, the portion between the cochleariform process and the geniculate ganglion was subsequently exposed and decompressed. The extent of the edema correlated in almost every case with the topognostic determination.

Total decompression was accomplished in 35 patients by the mastoid and middle cranial fossa approaches and in 2 patients by the translabyrinthine approach for patients who had a preexisting inner ear hearing loss. The remaining 163 patients had decompression of the mastoid and tympanic segments only (Table 2).

Two patients included in this series had small neuromas involving the stapedius nerve and concomitant edema of the facial nerve probably from pressure of the neuroma. These neuromas were undetected preoperatively and diagnosis was Bell's palsy. Both had complete recovery following surgery. During the period involved in the study in this report the author has surgically removed 19 additional facial nerve neuromas for a total of 21, or an incidence of 10% compared to the number of cases operated on for Bell's palsy. An additional three facial nerve angiomas were surgically removed. In addition to the 200 patients in this series of Bell's palsy, the author has performed 44 facial nerve grafts and six facial anastomoses exclusive of hypoglossal facial anastomosis.

One year or more follow-up was available for 181 of the 200 patients. Postoperative facial recovery was 100% in all 34 patients who had surgery performed while their preoperative nerve excitability tests were normal. Recovery averaged 80% for 147 patients whose nerve excitability was absent preop-

TABLE 2. FACIAL NERVE DECOMPRESSION FOR BELL'S PALSY

Surgical Procedure	*No. Pts.*
Mastoid tympanic	163
Total decompression	
Approach	
Middle fossa	35
Translabyrinthine	2

TABLE 3. FACIAL NERVE DECOMPRESSION FOR BELL'S PALSY*

Nerve Excitability	*No. of Pts.*	*% Recovery*
Normal	34	100
Absent	147	80

*One-year follow-up for 181 of 200 patients.

eratively in one or more branches (Table 3). The facial nerve was missing for several millimeters in each of two cases, both of whom obtained facial nerve grafts. One patient had an excellent result and the other patient had complete failure with no recovery at all presumably due to technical failure of the graft procedure. Patients with normal nerve excitability preoperatively obtained their surgery between five days and eight months after the onset of their palsy. All had recovered facial function within three weeks of the procedure. Of the 181 patients with one year follow-up, 147 patients with absent nerve excitability preoperatively had surgery between eight days and five years after the onset of their paralysis. Although most patients who had nerve degeneration developed some synkinesis, their results were generally good or satisfactory. Eleven patients with absent nerve excitability preoperatively had complete recovery with no synkinesis whatever. Adequate functional result has been obtained in all but one whose graft failed, and a reasonably good cosmetic result was obtained in most cases (Table 4).

In no case was there injury to the inner ear. Four cases had a 10 dB or less conductive hearing loss and one had a 29 dB conductive hearing loss postoperatively. None had symptoms of vertigo or changes in the electronystagmogram postoperatively.

CASE REPORTS

Case 1. This 28-year-old professional trombone player noticed a slight problem changing registers when playing his trombone two weeks before he was seen on August 13, 1975. Three days before he had started losing air around his mouthpiece, and on the following day he had total right facial paralysis and the onset of constant pain in the mastoid, numbness of the right side of the tongue, and tinnitus.

Physical examination revealed a complete right facial paralysis with normal tearing, normal excitability bilaterally, and absent taste to the electric taste test on the right side. Audiogram was normal for pure tones and speech. Electronystagmogram was normal for caloric and positional tests. Impedance audiometry was normal bilaterally and petrous pyramid x-ray studies were normal.

On August 15, 1975, under a general anesthetic the facial nerve decompression was performed from the stylomastoid foramen to the cochleariform process. There was 2+ edema from the stapes to the pyramid and 1+ edema in the mastoid segment. Facial motion had cosmetically returned to normal on February 10, 1976, but he was unable to properly play his trombone.

COMMENT. This case with normal preoperative nerve excitability of a dial setting of 2.2 on the Hilger stimulator represents a case in which significant nerve injury apparently occurred before surgery even though the procedure was performed five days after the onset of palsy. His recovery was cosmetically complete; however, he was unable to continue as a professional trombone player. The severe economic implications of this problem demonstrate how even a subtle change and a result acceptable to everyone else can still be unsatisfactory for a patient who has had Bell's palsy.

TABLE 4. FACIAL NERVE DECOMPRESSION RESULTS

	% Motion	*% Synkinesis*	*No. of Pts.*
Normal	100	0	45
Good	80	10	91
Satisfactory	70	20	17
Fair	50	50	27
None	0	0	1
Total			181

Case 2. This 27-year-old male was seen on June 18, 1980, with a history of having had a right complete facial paralysis for four weeks which had been preceded for three days with severe mastoid pressure and headaches. He had had tinnitus for three days at the onset.

Physical examination revealed a complete right facial paralysis. Tear test was normal, taste test had no reaction, and there was absent nerve excitability on the right side. Impedance audiometry revealed absent stapes reflex on the right. Audiogram was normal for pure tones and speech. Electronystagmogram was normal for caloric testing but had a 2° left beating spontaneous nystagmus. Evoked electromyelogram revealed reduced amplitude with normal distal latency with relatively elevated stimulation. Petrous pyramid x-ray studies were normal.

On June 24, 1980, under general anesthesia, a right facial nerve decompression was performed from the stylomastoid foramen to the geniculate ganglion. There was 3+ edema of the nerve from the geniculate ganglion to the pyramid and 2+ edema of the entire mastoid segment. The chorda tympani was removed along with a biopsy from the posterior edge of the external genu for light and electron microscopic studies (Fig. 1A, B). Within nine months he obtained complete recovery.

COMMENT. This case represents the first to be reported of electron microscopic examination of a biopsy of the motor portion of the facial nerve in a patient with Bell's palsy. The chorda tympani nerve appears to be normal with no injection, hemorrhage, or edema, and there are minor degenerative changes showing unraveling of the myelin sheath and degeneration of axon cytoplasm. There is no marked increase in the numbers of unmyelinated fibers and no evidence of axon regrowth. The motor trunk specimen shows moderate degeneration of the myelinated fibers. The fibers are decreased and most of them fall into the vacuolar degeneration. There is, however, only a mild extent of proliferation of collagen fibers. There are no signs of regenerating axons and this suggests that axon regrowth is disturbed by nerve edema. Nerve injury in this case seems confined to the first and second degree. This is also supported by the patient's good recovery. This case represents second degree injury.

Case 3. This 13-year-old female was seen on August 17, 1976, with a history of right facial paralysis of 2½ weeks' duration. Two days following the onset of the palsy she was placed on 60 mg prednisone daily and took it until the time of my examination.

Physical examination of ears, nose, and throat was entirely normal with the exception of a complete right facial paralysis. Audiogram was normal for pure tones and speech. Electronystagmogram was normal for caloric and positional testing. Petrous pyramid x-ray studies showed no abnormality. The electric taste test showed a threshold greater than 400 μA on the right side compared to 190 μA on the left side. Tear testing revealed 2.5 cm saturation of the Schimer test papers on each side. Nerve excitability revealed no reaction to maximal stimulation on the right side. Impedance audiometry showed no stapedius reflex on the right side.

On August 20, 1976, three weeks after the onset of palsy a right facial nerve decompression was performed and the nerve was exposed from the stylomastoid foramen to the geniculate ganglion by working through the facial recess. The nerve had 1+ edema beginning at 1 mm distal to the geniculate ganglion and extending to the cochleariform process. From the cochleariform process to the stapedius nerve there was 4+ edema and the remaining mastoid portion had 2+ edema. She was discharged from the hospital the following day and obtained maximum recovery within eight months. When last seen on March 27, 1979, she had 100% overall motion with 2% synkinesis. She had only an occasional twitch of the right eye and both the patient and the author felt that the result was excellent.

COMMENT. Bell's palsy in an attractive little girl carries great implications for a lifetime of disability and heartbreak. The three-week delay of surgery during the futile use of prednisone contributed to the loss of nerve excitability and nerve degeneration and subsequent prolonged delay in recovery. The mild synkinesis in this case has not been disabling or troublesome, but indicates that a portion of the nerve sustained a third degree injury and the major portion of the nerve a second degree injury.

Case 4. A 9-year-old female was seen on May 14, 1975, with a history of having had a right otitis media which had been treated with antibiotics one month before. There had been no otorrhea and only a low grade fever. Recovery was prompt but 1½ weeks before examination the patient developed a complete right facial paralysis. She was placed on steroids. At the time of examination, there was a total right facial paralysis and right serous otitis media. Audiogram for pure tones and speech was completely normal. Electronystagmogram showed no abnormality. Petrous pyramid x-ray studies were within normal limits. A reliable taste test could not be obtained. Tear testing revealed 3 cm saturation of paper on each side. Hilger nerve excitability testing showed a reading of 2 on the left and 7 on the right side. Stapedius reflexes were normal bilaterally. A diagnosis of right Bell's palsy and right serous otitis media was made.

On May 19, 1975, under general anesthesia, a right facial nerve decompression was performed. The nerve was exposed from the stylomastoid foramen to the geniculate ganglion by working through the facial recess. There was 2+ edema from the stylomastoid foramen to the cochleariform process. The middle ear was filled with mucus. Within three months recovery was almost complete and within seven months there was 98% recovery with 10% synkinesis evident primarily when she attempted to whistle. The overall result was excellent.

COMMENT. This case is similar to case 3 in that surgery was delayed for four weeks and use of steroids was ineffective to prevent nerve degeneration. Fortunately, decompression was performed early enough to minimize the progression into a third degree injury. Recovery although not perfect was quite satisfactory.

Case 5. This 51-year-old female was examined on March 25, 1977, with a history of having flown to Honolulu and having taken the Pearl Harbor Cruise during which she was exposed to cool sea air. Three days later she awoke with a complete right facial paralysis, instability but no nausea, and right hearing loss. She had pain in the right ear the first two weeks. She was given betamethasone sodium phosphate (Celestone) 6 mg twice daily. She gave a history of having had a mastectomy for carcinoma one year before. Her husband had had Bell's palsy which lasted for two weeks and had made a full recovery two years before.

Physical examination of the ears, nose, and throat was normal with the exception of the presence of right serous otitis media, a right 18dB conductive hearing loss, and a total right facial paralysis. Vestibular testing with electronystagmography showed a 50% reduced vestibular response on the right side. Petrous pyramid x-ray studies showed no abnormality. Electric taste test was not performed. The tear test produced 1.5 cm saturation on each side. Nerve excitability was completely absent on the right side with the Hilger stimulator. The prognosis was explained to the patient and facial nerve decompression was recommended. The patient was reluctant to have surgery and did not return to the office until May 16, 1977. The right serous otitis media persisted and the tear test remained normal. Electromyography showed severe nerve involvement. CT scan of the temporal bones with enhancement showed no abnormality and no evidence of metastatic carcinoma. Because of a strong possibility of metastatic breast carcinoma within the temporal bone a total facial nerve decompression was performed using the mastoid and middle cranial fossa approaches on June 1, 1977. No tumor was found at surgery. There was 2+ edema of the nerve from the stylomastoid foramen to a point 2 mm medial to the cochleariform process. Her postoperative course was uneventful and after six months there was 80% recovery with 75% synkinesis. Two years after surgery despite intensive self-physical therapy her appearance was significantly improved but she still had major complaints of right nasal obstruction and drooping eyebrow.

COMMENT. This case represents a common situation in that surgery is delayed in the hope that spontaneous recovery will occur. Patients tend to accept the curbside advice from friends and neighbors who have had or have known someone who has had an incomplete or mild facial paralysis which recovered promptly without treatment. Physicians who do not see large numbers of patients with facial paralysis also tend to take a casual approach and do not recommend early surgery. This patient delayed surgery for three months and subsequently developed a major third degree nerve injury. Despite the reasonably good amount of recovery she was disappointed because of the synkinesis.

DISCUSSION

Surgical decompression of the facial nerve is now generally available to patients in most parts of the country. With this availability of the procedure, acceptance of its use is growing. Although no operative procedure is perfect and 100% free from risk and complication, 200 cases of facial nerve decompression performed by the author have been associated with no mortality and no significant morbidity. In none was the inner ear function made worse. Four patients sustained conductive hearing losses no greater than 10 dB and one who has maintained a postoperative serous otitis media has a 29 dB loss. In all other cases hearing and vestibular function remain at the preoperative level. Attention to precise and careful surgical technique with the utilization of good instruments and a smooth running angled electric drill with a light touch will yield good results. The facial nerve sheath can be exposed and incised and the facial fibers manipulated and biopsied without the production of facial paralysis if proper procedures are followed. These methods can and have been taught to a large number of otologic surgeons who have taken fellowships or who have attended the Advanced Temporal Bone Surgical Dissection Course at Ear International or other such training areas.

Despite the development and general usage of evoked electromyography there is still no way to learn the prognosis of a facial palsy at the present time. When third degree injuries occur to the nerve, the damage is permanent and irreparable. Some reduced function and synkinesis will inevitably follow. In our present society facial deformity represents a major serious disability. Based on this series of 200 cases it seems that surgical decompression can be done with minimal morbidity, and when performed before the nerve dies, will result in completely normal recovery. If decompression is accomplished often an excellent result is obtained although it is not a certainty, and recovery is delayed if decompression is performed in the early stages of a second degree injury. Should the patient wish to take this risk for permanent morbidity surgery is not performed unless there is evidence of reduced nerve excitability or electromyographic changes. Decompression of the nerve even in the late stages is of great value. The amount of recovery and reduction of synkinesis is better with decompression than without. In addition to the improvement in regeneration allowed by decompression, other lesions can be identified such as areas of missing nerve or facial nerve tumor which can be excised and repaired by a graft. The author has surgically removed 21 facial nerve neuromas and three angiomas of the facial nerve during the same time period of the 200 decompression cases for Bell's palsy reported in this communication. This is an incidence of over 10%. Two of these tumors were unsuspected and the patients were felt to have Bell's palsy.

Biopsy of small fascicles of human facial nerves during surgical decompression has been shown to be useful to predict results after surgery. The presence of normal nerve as demonstrated by electron microscopy at the proximal end of the decompression gives reassurance that an adequate procedure has been performed. Biopsy of the edematous portion of the nerve provides information about the actual degree of injury and therefore provides reassuring information concerning expected recovery.

Distinctly better results have been obtained in patients who have had early decompression of the facial nerve for Bell's palsy compared with those who have surgery performed at a later time. It would seem that "early" is a relative term and the actual time can vary greatly. For practical purposes the term "early" might best be confined to surgery performed within seven days of the onset of paralysis. Decompression performed on an emergency basis within hours might yield superior results but is probably impractical and unwise since greater benefits are derived when a deliberate thorough examination and adequate preparation of the patient and the surgical team can be accomplished.

CONCLUSION

Decompression of the facial nerve for 200 patients with Bell's palsy has been performed by the author in the past 17 years. These procedures were accomplished without injury to the facial nerve or inner ear. In no case was the incus removed nor the tympanic membrane or posterior bony canal wall disturbed with the exception of two translabyrinthine procedures in which the incus and inner ear were removed. Of 34 patients with normal nerve excitability preoperatively all had 100% recovery of facial motion. In 147 others followed for one year or more and whose nerve excitability was absent preoperatively, an average of 80% recovery of motion and usually some degree of synkinesis was obtained. Only one patient who had a missing segment of nerve and a nerve graft performed failed to obtain any facial motion. Biopsy of facial nerve fibers during surgery has been found to be a feasible and useful technique. There is still no way to establish a prognosis when one still has a chance to avoid a bad result. The best that one can do is to follow carefully serial electrical testing and perform surgery at the time when electrical studies begin to deteriorate with the hope that deterioration has developed slowly enough that a third degree injury will not have developed by the time surgery has been performed. Considering this series of cases it would seem that the best results can be obtained by early surgical decompression for Bell's palsy. The patient must be informed of the possibilities, and the decision regarding the nature and timing of treatment should be a subjective one made after a careful analysis of the available facts and each patient's own circumstance. The availability of a promptly accomplished and precisely performed facial nerve decompression allows every patient to have a minimal risk of disabling permanent facial deformity.

REFERENCES

1. Pulec JL. Total decompression of the facial nerve. Laryngoscope 1966; 76:1015-28.

2. Esslen E. The acute facial palsies. Investigations on the localisation and pathogenesis of meato-labyrinthine facial palsies. New York: Springer Verlag, 1977.

3. Sunderland S. A classification of peripheral nerve injuries

producing loss of function. Brain 1951; 74:491-516.

4. Mathews WB. Prognosis in Bell's palsy. Br Med J July 22, 1961; 215-7.

5. Taverner D. Medical management of idiopathic facial (Bell's) palsy. Proc R Soc Med 1973; 66:554-6.

6. Adour KK, Swanson PJ Jr. Facial paralysis in 403 consecutive patients: emphasis on treatment response in patients with Bell's palsy. Trans Am Acad Ophthalmol Otolaryngol 1971; 75:1284-2301.

7. Pulec JL. Bell's palsy: diagnosis, management and results of treatment. Laryngoscope 1974; 84:2119-40.

8. Pulec JL. Total facial nerve exposure. Arch Otolaryngol 1969; 89:179-83.

9. Pulec JL. Idiopathic hemifacial spasm: pathogenesis and surgical treatment. Ann Otol Rhinol Laryngol 1972; 81:664-76.

10. Pulec JL. Facial nerve grafting. Laryngoscope 1969; 79:1562-83.

11. Pulec JL. Facial nerve tumors. Ann Otol Rhinol Laryngol 1969; 78:962-83.

12. Pulec JL. Symposium of ear surgery. II. Facial nerve neuroma. Laryngoscope 1972; 82:1160-76.

13. Pulec JL. Geniculate neuralgia: Diagnosis and surgical management. Laryngoscope 1976; 86:955-64.

PATHOMECHANISMS IN CELL METABOLISM: A KEY TO TREATMENT OF BELL'S PALSY

EBERHARD STENNERT, MD

GÖTTINGEN, FEDERAL REPUBLIC OF GERMANY

In light of current research the classic theory on the vicious circle of Bell's palsy has to be reconsidered. New findings through electron microscopy and biochemistry concerning the structure and metabolism of cells have presented aspects which have consequences for treatment of the disease. These aspects deal mainly with the pathomechanisms of cell metabolism whose interactions also cause a vicious circle, leading to a breakdown of microcirculation and ultimately to the death of the cells due to hypoxia and acidosis. It is therefore suggested that the aim of an effective therapy must be the early normalization of cell metabolism by improving microcirculation. A fitting treatment protocol is presented and the extraordinarily good results are discussed.

INTRODUCTION

It was more than 30 years ago that Kettel[1] and Hilger[2] advanced a theory of a combined primary and secondary ischemia as the cause of Bell's palsy. "According to Hilger, the primary feature of the pathogenesis is an arteriolar constriction, the impetus being derived from autonomic nervous impulses to the vessel concerned."[3] It is the author's personal conviction that, in light of the present state, such views concerning the etiology of Bell's palsy can no longer be maintained.

There is growing evidence gained through clinical observation, neurophysiological and laboratory findings and also postmortem examinations that Bell's palsy is 1) either an isolated disease of the peripheral nerve due to various etiological factors, or 2) often the only clinical symptom of a number of other diseases. Present research suggests that exposure to cold, stress, hypertension, hypercholesterolemia, diabetes, or other vascular diseases, pregnancy, familial disposition, intoxication, and numerous immunological processes all have to be regarded as factors causing or coacting in the development of this disease. Furthermore, it can be assumed that the number of influencing factors is even larger than hitherto recognized.[4-10]

In addition there is no longer any doubt that viruses also play an important role in acute facial pareses. Thus far there has been positive proof that the following cause the disease: herpes simplex, varicella zoster, cytomegalovirus, Epstein-Barr, influenza A and B, mumps, and adenoviruses.[11-16]

It is the aim of this contribution not simply to point out that the present knowledge about the etiology of Bell's palsy is going to change, since diagnostic procedures are becoming more sophisticated, but rather to question whether the ideas about the pathophysiology of Bell's palsy can still be explained by this classic theory, which has, after all, been with us for 35 years. What do we know today about the pathomechanisms in cases of acute peripheral nerve paralysis and what consequences does this have for therapy? Before discussing these questions, the therapeutic method which has been

From the ENT Department, University of Göttingen, Federal Republic of Germany. This investigation was supported by research grants of the Deutsche Forschungsgemeinschaft.

Presented at the meeting of the American Otological Society, Inc., Vancouver, British Columbia, May 9-10, 1981.

REPRINTS — Eberhard Stennert, MD, ENT Department, University of Göttingen, Geiststrasse 5-10, 3400 Göttingen, Federal Republic of Germany.

TABLE 1. TREATMENT PROTOCOL FOR BELL'S PALSY

Days of Treatment	*Dextran 40[a] with Sorbitol or Mannitol (10%) ml/day*	*Pentoxifylline[b] ml/day*		*Cortisone[c] (Prednisolone-equivalent dose [mg/day]) < 70 kg*	*> 70 kg*	*Replacement*
Inpatient						
1	2 x 500/16 hr*	10		200	250	
2	2 x 500/16 hr	10		200	250	Potassium[e]
3	2 x 500/16 hr	15		150		
4	500/ 8 hr	15		150		
5	500/ 8 hr	15		100		
6	500/ 8 hr	15	by infusion	100		Fluid[f]
7	500/ 8 hr	15		75		oral or iv (ca. 1000
8	500/ 8 hr	15		50		ml/day) control of
9	500/ 8 hr	15	oral[d]	40		hematocrit: 35-38
10	500/ 8 hr	15		20		
Outpatient						
11				15		
12				12.5		
13				10		
14				7.5		
15				5		
16				2.5		
17				2.5		
18				2.5		

[a]Onkovertin N® with sorbitol 10%, [b]Trental®, [c]Solu-Decortin H®, [d]Ultralan®, [e]Kalinor® Brause-Tbl., [f]Sterofundin®.
*Therapy with infusions twice per day should last for 3 x 24 hrs. Cortisone — as well as pentoxifylline — dose divided into both infusions.

used with considerable success in the ENT Department of Göttingen University will be described.

METHODS

Patients for whom initial diagnosis is Bell's palsy are admitted at once as inpatients. After taking 10 ml of blood to determine basic laboratory values, infusion therapy (Table 1) is started immediately. If there are no contraindications of fluid load, 1000 ml dextran are given on each of the first three days over a 16-hour period. Thereafter the infusion is reduced to 500 ml and is given daily over an 8-hour period; these 8-hour infusions may sometimes be given on an outpatient basis. Cortisone, up to an amount of 50 mg prednisolone-equivalent, as well as pentoxifylline are added directly to the dextran solution thus simplifying therapy.

After cortisone has been decreased to 40 mg per day, the remaining treatment is then performed orally and in a circadian fashion (6-8 am) to avoid an irreversible atrophy of the adrenal cortex. Dextran solution is supplemented with 10% sorbitol or mannitol. The glomerular filtration rate can thus be considerably increased and thereby possible damage to the kidney caused by crystalline deposits in the tubuli avoided. Since hyperosmolarity of dextran leads to elimination, particularly of potassium during diureses, one should ensure a sufficient replacement of fluid and potassium.

The following factors should be regarded as contraindications: left heart failure, renal insufficiency, recent history of peptic ulcer, pregnancy, bacterial infections, and coagulation defects. Diabetes is by no means a contraindication, since an increase of blood sugar can be easily compensated for, and values return to normal when treatment is completed. During the course of infusion, patients should be monitored as to blood pressure and heart rate daily and blood glucose, electrolytes, creatinine and hematocrit every other day.

For follow-up all patients were investigated upon admission, at the end of infusion therapy, and then four weeks as well as four to six months thereafter. Both clinical and neurophysiological methods were used. Since, however, mimic function and the patient's own subjective judgment are of the greatest importance for the patient, this discussion restricts itself to the clinical methods of investigation with the exception of the electromyogram (EMG) analysis. Clinical examination included: 1) careful anamnesis; 2) assessment of the paralytic degree by means of our Paralysis and Secondary Defect Score; 3) careful evaluation of mimic innervation when frowning, closing eyes, wrinkling nose, exposing teeth and whistling. For statistical analysis the activity patterns in the EMG were divided into five stages given the identification numbers 0 to 4. These data were recorded routinely from the following muscles: m. frontalis, m. orbicularis oculi, m. levator labii, m. zygomaticus, m. orbicularis oris.

RESULTS

Of 150 consecutive patients 132 were actually available for follow-up; 63 were male and 69 female. The mean age was 41.6 years; the range from 16 to 75 years. The mean duration of paresis from its onset until the beginning of treatment was 5½ days with a range from 1 to 20 days.

Table 2 illustrates the development of Bell's palsy during the 10-day infusion therapy. Upon admission 70 patients (53%) suffered from a clinically complete paralysis; an additional 36 (27%) of the whole group also had a complete paralysis as established by the EMG. After termination of the 10-day treatment only 32 patients (24%) still suffered from a clinically complete paresis. This means that during therapy there was a change from clinically complete to incomplete paresis in 54% of our patients.

TABLE 2. DEVELOPMENT OF BELL'S PALSY DURING TEN-DAY INFUSION THERAPY (N = 132)

Degree of Paralysis	*Initially Pt.*	*%*	*After 10 Days Infusion Pt.*	*%*	*Change (%)*
Clinically complete	70	53	32	24	54
EMG complete	36	27	8	6	78
Paralysis index	6.0		3.0		
EMG index	1.3		2.6		

The direct influence of therapy becomes even more evident through the use of the particularly sensitive EMG. After ten days we were able to demonstrate a silent EMG in only eight remaining cases (6%); thus electromyographically 78% had changed from complete to incomplete. The mean paralysis index of the whole group was 6 at the beginning and had decreased to 3 after ten days of treatment. The average EMG activity pattern consisted of only single oscillations. After termination of the treatment protocol it corresponded closely to a transitory pattern.

The final outcome, according to careful investigation of the mimic function, showed a complete recovery rate of 94%. Moreover, seven of the remaining eight patients with incomplete recovery had to be classified as "good," according to the various evaluation systems.[17-21] The only patient with "fair" results did not start therapy until the 18th day postonset. In addition, one patient of the remaining incomplete cases suffered from a severe paresis due to a chronic alcoholic intoxication and another patient developed a complete paralysis on both sides.

DISCUSSION

What is the rational basis of our treatment protocol? Electron microscopy and biochemistry have given us completely new insights into the secrets of the structure and metabolism of cells. The main pathophysiological reactions responsible for morphological damage can be briefly summarized as follows.

The blood, actually functioning as a large organ 1) supplies the cells with life-supporting substances whose absence makes survival even for a short period of time impossible, eg, most importantly oxygen and glucose, and 2) eliminates cellular poisons, such as carbon dioxide and ammonia. In order to fulfill their function, the erythrocytes have to be extremely specialized; this, however, also means that their function can be easily disturbed. One of their main characteristics is their flexibility; however, in an acid plasma their membrane quickly becomes rigid, thus leading to an increased disturbance of microcirculation.

With the exception of a few diseases which directly effect the axon or myelin sheath, the vast majority of damaging factors affect primarily the vascular connective tissue. The endothelium of the capillaris becomes edematous and increasingly permeable; capillary leaks can even develop, so that plasma escapes. This has two consequences. 1) Passage of the capillaries becomes impossible because of the swelling of the endothelium on the one hand and of the growing rigidity of the erythrocytes on the other. 2) Due to the edema of the interstice and the flowing of the plasma into the intercellular spaces, the transit necessary for oxygenation of the cells becomes impossible.

This breakdown of microcirculation leads to hypoxia and acidosis. The unavoidable consequence of such hypoxic-acidotic metabolism is the death of the cells. This cell destruction also includes a rupturing of the nucleus and of lysosomes with releases of proteolytic enzymes, formation of toxic peptides and activation of kinin and kallikrein. At this point the vicious circle is complete: the destruction of the tissue has escalated to such an extent that a metabolic catastrophe is imminent. Consequently, the aim of an effective therapy must therefore be the early normalization of cell metabolism, which, above all, means the improvement of microcirculation. The drugs used in our treatment protocol are capable of positively influencing this pathomechanism as follows.

Cortisone. Its strong antiphlogistic and antiedematous effect is clinically and experimentally well established. Its involvement in all phases of the inflammatory tissue reactions is based on three main cooperative efficiencies: an antiexudative, an antitoxic and an antiproliferative. It is therefore suggested that in all cases of Bell's palsy cortisone acts by elimination of the edema, avoidance of immunological reactions, and reduction of proliferative formations.

Low Molecular Dextran. The strong rheological effect, especially in the terminal blood vessels, has also been demonstrated in many studies and is mainly due to an extensive hemodilution. It thereby decreases local concentration of hematocrit, blood viscosity, blood flow resistance and sludge-phenomenon of the erythrocytes, but increases the microcirculatory pressure gradient and oxygen perfusion. In cases of Bell's palsy this drug is therefore regarded as helpful by its improvement of blood fluidity in the terminal vessels and resorption of extravasal plasm due to its hyperosmolarity.

Pentoxifylline. The key role of the erythrocytes for the regulation of cell metabolism was already pointed out. Pathophysiological changes due to low flow conditions and acidosis quickly lead to aggregation and rigidity of the red cells and also to an increased secretion of platelet factor 3. Numerous experimental and clinical studies during recent years could verify the following main actions of the xanthine derivate: improvement of red cell deformability, inhibition of platelet aggregation and decrease of blood viscosity, which is caused by an increase in ATP-level and an enhancement of cAMP formation.[22,23]

The advantages of our therapy are threefold.

1. It can be rendered anywhere at any time; it does not require the skills of extremely specialized surgeons.

2. It can be started immediately without waiting until such a degree of irreversible damage has occurred that the prospects of recovery become very limited.

TABLE 3. SCHEME OF NERVE IMPAIRMENT ACCORDING TO MORPHOLOGICAL CRITERIA

Degree	*Morphological Criteria*	*Characteristics of Repair*
Neurodyspraxia (metabolic dysfunction)*	? Disturbance of membranes with inability for polarization	?
Neurapraxia	Demyelination	Remyelination
Axonotmesis	Wallerian degeneration	
	With preservation of perineurium plus endoneural tubes	Intrafascicular "isomorphic" neurotization[26]
	With preservation of perineurium but with damage of endoneural tubes	Intrafascicular "heteromorphic" neurotization[26]
Neurotmesis	Partial or complete deterioration of different numbers of fascicles with continuity of epineurium	Extrafascicular neurotization (always "heteromorphic" or even "neuromatous")[27]
	Complete section	

*Classification of nerve injuries according to Seddon[25] should be extended by a fourth degree, for which the term "neurodyspraxia" is proposed, and which is characterized by only functional disturbances of the neurites mainly due to a metabolic disturbance of the Schwann cells. This stage shows a quick reversibility if improvement of microcirculation is performed at once. As soon as the endoneural tubes and, moreover, the perineurium is damaged, thus leading to a heteromorphic reneurotization, complete recovery can no longer be expected regardless of therapy applied.

3. It confronts the disease at its roots; the drugs actually affect the pathomechanisms involved in the disease, restoring the ability of the organism to function normally.

Decompression on the other hand is based on a mechanistic conception of nerve functioning and remains in the truest sense of the word superficial. The mechanical compression of the neurites most probably plays a secondary role since the decisive disturbing factors are hypoxia and acidosis of the various types of cells of the nerve tissues.

At present the considerable success of our therapeutic concept can only be estimated by comparing our results with the percentage of spontaneous recovery. As it was stressed previously[24] complete recovery must be assumed with a rate of 50-60%, if reinvestigation is performed carefully.

The effectiveness of our treatment protocol is also demonstrated by its direct influence during the 10-day infusion period. This can only be explained as follows: nerve fibers still suffering from a "neurodyspraxia," which is the first degree of impairment according to our classification of nerve injuries (Table 3) and which is characterized by a disturbance of the metabolism of the Schwann cells with inability for depolarization and repolarization, are actually normalized within a short time.

In consequence, it is of great importance to begin treatment immediately on those patients with clinically complete or progressively incomplete paralysis. Our investigations have shown that the percentage of secondary defects increases rapidly if such patients are not treated within ten days postonset at the latest. A similar prognosis is however also to be expected as soon as the EMG is silent or registers only single oscillations. By starting infusion therapy as soon as possible one has the time to perform all clinical tests necessary to finalize the diagnosis of Bell's palsy without endangering the patient's chances of complete recovery.

ACKNOWLEDGMENTS — I thank Drs. C. H. Limberg and W. Ostner, members of the Department of Otorhinolaryngology, University of Göttingen, for their help. I am grateful to Mr. David Starr, MA, Lecturer in English, University of Göttingen.

REFERENCES

1. Kettel K. Bell's palsy. Pathology and surgery. Arch Otolaryngol 1947; 46:427-72.

2. Hilger JA. The nature of Bell's palsy. Laryngoscope 1949; 59:228-35.

3. Kettel K. Nerve grafting and nerve suture in postoperative facial palsies. Proceedings of the Fourth International Congress of Otolaryngology 1949; 1:355.

4. Abraham-Inpijn L, Devriese PP. Hypertension and diabetes mellitus in Bell's palsy. Paper presented at the IV International Symposium of Facial Nerve Surgery, Los Angeles, Sept 2-5, 1980.

5. Adour KK, Byl FM, Hilsinger RL Jr, Kahn ZM, Sheldon MI. The true nature of Bell's palsy: analysis of 1,000 consecutive patients. Laryngoscope 1978; 88:787-811.

6. Devriese PP. On etiology and pathogenesis of Bell's palsy. Paper presented at the IV International Symposium of Facial Nerve Surgery, Los Angeles, Sept 2-5, 1980.

7. Gomez JG. Incidence and management of Bell's palsy according to geographic distribution. In: Fisch U, ed. Facial nerve surgery. Amstelveen: Kugler, 1977:319-36.

8. Hilsinger RL, Adour KK, Doty HE. Idiopathic facial paralysis, pregnancy, and the menstrual cycle. Ann Otol Rhinol Laryngol 1975; 84:433-42.

9. Lundgren A, Ödkvist LM, Hendriksson K-G, Larsson LE, Karlberg BE, Jerlvall L. Facial palsy in diabetes mellitus — not only a mononeuropathy? Adv Otorhinolaryngol 1977; 22:915-7.

10. McGovern FH, Konigsmark BW, Sydnor JB. An immunological concept for Bell's palsy. Laryngoscope 1972; 82:1594-601.

11. Blatt I, Freeman J. Bell's palsy III: further observations on the pathogenesis of Bell's palsy and the results of chorda tympani neurectomy. Trans Am Acad Ophthalmol Otolaryngol 1969; 73:420-38.

12. Djupesland G, Berdal P, Degré M, Stein R, Skrede S. Acute peripheral facial palsy and viral infection. In: Fisch U, ed. Facial nerve surgery. Amstelveen: Kugler, 1977:397-402.

13. McCormick DP. Herpes simplex virus as cause of Bell's palsy. Lancet 1972; 29:937-9.

14. Peitersen E, Caunt AE. The incidence of herpes zoster antibodies in patients with peripheral facial palsy. J Laryngol Otol 1970; 84:65-70.

15. Proctor G, Corgill DA, Proud G. The pathology of Bell's

palsy. Trans Am Acad Ophthalmol Otolaryngol 1976; 82:70-80.

16. Tomita H. Viral etiology of Bell's palsy. In: Fisch U, ed. Facial nerve surgery. Amstelveen: Kugler, 1977:356-63.

17. Adour KK, Swanson PJ. Facial paralysis in 403 consecutive patients. Trans Am Acad Ophthalmol Otolaryngol 1971; 75:1284-1301.

18. Botman JWM, Jongkees LBW. The result of intratemporal treatment of facial palsy. Pract Otorhinolaryngol (Basel) 1955; 17:80-100.

19. Janssen FP. Proefschrift Univ. Amsterdam: Jacob von Campen, 1963.

20. May M. Facial paralysis, peripheral type: a proposed method of reporting. Laryngoscope 1970; 80:331-90.

21. Stennert E, Limberg CH, Frentrup KP. New aspects in facial nerve surgery; paralysis and secondary defect score. In: Baker DC, ed. Clin Plast Surg 1979; 458-65.

22. Ambrus HL, ed. Pentoxifylline, pharmacological and clinical research. Symposium on Pentoxifylline, Athens, March 22, 1978. J Med 1979; 10.

23. Müller R. Pentoxifylline — a biomedical profile. In: Ambrus JL, ed. Pentoxifylline, pharmacological and clinical research. Symposium on Pentoxifylline, Athens, March 22, 1978. J Med 1979; 10.

24. Stennert E. New concepts in treatment of Bell's palsy. Paper presented at the IV International Symposium of Facial Nerve Surgery, Los Angeles, Sept 2-5, 1980.

25. Seddon HJ. Three types of nerve injury. Brain 1943; 66:238-88.

26. Hiller F. Die Bedeutung des mesodermalen Gewebes bei der Nervenregeneration. Experimentelle Untersuchungen an Nervenverletzungen und Transplantaten. Dtsch Z Nervenheilkd 1949; 160:176-95.

27. Hiller F. Nerve regeneration in grafts. J Neuropath Clin Neurol 1951; 1:5-25.

COMMENT

RICHARD R. GACEK, MD

SYRACUSE, NEW YORK

The controversy regarding the treatment of Bell's palsy is well demonstrated by the presentations regarding use of steroids and surgical decompression of the fallopian canal. The controversy comes from the fact that the etiology of Bell's palsy, or idiopathic facial palsy, is unknown. Of the various theories put forth to explain Bell's palsy, the one implicating viral neuritis has gained the most support. A mechanism of paralysis based on ischemia secondary to microvascular occlusion has not been supported scientifically. In fact, experimental studies on other peripheral nerves have demonstrated that it is virtually impossible to deprive the intraneural compartment of its blood supply by occluding the vessels in the epineurium.[1] On the other hand several studies have demonstrated a probable association between the herpes simplex virus (HSV) and Bell's palsy based on indirect evidence in the form of elevated viral antibodies.[2-7] 1) Significantly higher levels of HSV antibodies have been observed in patients with Bell's palsy compared to comparable controls. However, direct evidence of the virus infection in such cases of facial palsy has not been found. 2) The only available temporal bone report describing the changes in the early stages of Bell's palsy is that of Proctor et al[8] where acute inflammatory changes and demyelination throughout the entire course of the facial nerve was observed. Edema of the nerve was also present in their specimen. 3) Demyelination in the central portion of the trigeminal nerve has been observed following inoculation of the HSV peripherally (nose) in laboratory animals (mice and rabbits).[9,10] It is thought that the virus may have a direct cytopathic effect on cells that are responsible for maintaining myelin or may bring about an antigen-antibody response which results in demyelination. These clinical, histopathological and experimental observations support the thesis that Bell's palsy may be the result of a viral neuropathy or neuritis with inflammation, edema and demyelination of the nerve responsible for the palsy. It has, in fact, been suggested that the viral infection caused a polyneuropathy involving nearby cranial nerves such as IX, X, and XI.

Only the inflammatory changes and edema are amenable to presently available forms of treatment. The anti-inflammatory properties of steroids support its use in the treatment of Bell's palsy. Although previous reports have not been unanimous in demonstrating a beneficial effect on the outcome in this disorder,[11-13] it is possible that high-dose steroids administered in a manner described by Stennert may be effective. His results showing a 96% complete recovery rate are superior to those achieved in other similar series. The conclusion will be strengthened by similar results obtained using a comparable treatment program in a well-controlled series of patients with Bell's palsy. The addition of

From the Department of Otolaryngology, SUNY-Upstate Medical Center, Syracuse.

Presented at the meeting of the American Otologic Society, Vancouver, British Columbia, May 9-10, 1981.

REPRINTS — Richard R. Gacek, MD, Department of Otolaryngology, SUNY-Upstate Medical Center, 750 E. Adams St., Syracuse, NY 13210.

other components in the medical treatment of this disorder as used by Stennert seem unnecessary and possibly associated with risk involving renal function, electrolyte imbalance and cardiac arrhythmia. There is no scientific basis for the use of dextran in idiopathic facial paralysis.

Edema of the facial nerve has also been the target of surgical treatment for Bell's palsy. If surgical decompression of the facial nerve is used, then exposure of the entire course of the facial nerve canal from internal auditory canal to the stylomastoid foramen is required. However, several basic observations mitigate against the effectiveness of such surgical treatment.

1. It has not been clearly established that significant swelling of the facial nerve is present in Bell's palsy. In addition to observations at surgery that reflect no swelling of the nerve, it should be remembered that normal nerves expand when the perineurium is incised.[14] This herniation of nerve fibers through the incised perineurium reflects the intraneural pressure found in normal nerve and is associated with a focal demyelination. Therefore, incision of the perineurium can be expected to produce a traumatic effect upon axons.

2. Since the perineurium is the effective barrier between the intraneural and extraneural environments, it must be incised the total length of the nerve if effective decompression is to be achieved. However, the multifascicular arrangement of the facial nerve and its perineurium in the labyrinthine and tympanic segments prevents complete and safe incision by surgical means.

3. Compression of axons by increased intraneural fluid pressure as proposed in Bell's palsy has not been demonstrated by clinical or experimental means. It is not analogous to other compression syndromes (carpal tunnel) which are effectively relieved by surgical decompression. In these syndromes direct compression of axons is manifested by a narrowing of the nerve trunk diameter. The proposed indirect compression of axons by increased intraneural pressure in Bell's palsy is associated with an unchanged or increased nerve trunk diameter.

4. Other nerves which travel along a bony canalicular course and may be involved by a virus, such as the inferior alveolar nerve, do not show a propensity for loss of function when edematous.

In addition to these doubts regarding the safety and effectiveness of total facial nerve surgical decompression, there are associated risks which must be justified by significant beneficial results. These risks include 1) almost certain risk of variable degree of conductive hearing loss due to ossicular manipulation and/or repositioning required to expose the epitympanic segment of the facial nerve; 2) possible risk of sensorineural hearing loss either from transmitted acoustic trauma through the ossicular chain or direct injury to the basal turn of cochlea near the labyrinthine segment of facial nerve; and 3) possible intracranial complications of middle cranial fossa surgery. Furthermore, the use of biopsy of the facial nerve as proposed by Pulec is unwarranted and dangerous. It is unwarranted because 1) the artifact in nerve tissue incurred by even careful surgical removal precludes accurate interpretation and 2) the variation in pathological changes along the nerve associated with an inflammatory process renders the biopsy specimen undependable. It is dangerous to intentionally remove any portion of the nerve because of the unknown degree of trauma to the remaining axons of the facial nerve.

The use of medical or surgical treatment in idiopathic facial palsy must be justified by end results superior to those obtained when Bell's palsy is allowed to run its natural course. Peitersen[15] has reported on a series of 1,011 patients with Bell's palsy seen over a 15-year period in which no treatment was given. The significant results in this group of patients were that all the patients had some return of facial function. Of these patients 84% had either normal function (71%) or insignificant sequelae (13%). An additional 12% of the patients had moderate sequelae but an acceptable result. Only 4% had severe sequelae with facial asymmetry and synkinesis. The patients with the worst prognosis, as indicated by diminished nasolacrimal reflex, developed the severe sequelae in about 1 out of 3, a result which is similar to that achieved by surgery.

The results of medical or surgical treatment previously reported do not surpass the outcome seen when *no treatment* is administered for Bell's palsy. Nevertheless, it seems reasonable to administer steroids since they carry the least risk and do have a logical basis for use because of their anti-inflammatory properties. Surgery, on the other hand, carrying risk of either conductive or sensorineural hearing loss, the significant morbidity and possible mortality of middle cranial fossa surgery, and trauma to axons from incision of the perineurium cannot be justified because of its ineffectiveness compared with the natural course of the disorder. Perhaps the only indication for surgical exploration of the facial nerve in idiopathic facial nerve paralysis is in those cases where no return of function is observed 1½ to 2 years following the onset of paralysis. Surgical exploration may then be justified in order to determine whether the cause of the facial paralysis is other than idiopathic such as a facial nerve tumor. Correction of such a neoplasm by resection of the facial nerve with grafting may be carried out to improve facial function.

REFERENCES

1. Olsson Y. Vascular permeability in the peripheral nervous system. In: Dych PJ, Thomas PK, Lambert EH, eds. Peripheral neuropathy. Vol 1. Philadelphia: WB Saunders, 1975:190-200.

2. Adour KK, Bell DN, Hilsinger RL. Herpes simplex virus in idiopathic facial paralysis (Bell's palsy). JAMA 1975; 233:527-30.

3. Brodie SW. Virology studies and Belll's palsy. J Laryngol Otol 1979; 93:563-8.

4. Grose C, Feorino PM, Dye LA. Bell's palsy and infectious mononucleosis. Lancet 1973; 2:231-2.

5. Leeming RD. Varicella-zoster virus and facial palsy. J Laryngol Otol 1976; 90:365-71.

6. McCormick DP. Herpes simplex virus as a cause of Bell's palsy. Lancet 1972; 1:937-9.

7. Vahlne A, Edstrom S, Arstila P, et al. Bell's palsy and herpes simplex virus. Arch Otolaryngol 1981; 107:79-81.

8. Proctor B, Corgill DA, Proud G. The pathology of Bell's palsy. Trans Am Acad Ophthalmol Otolaryngol 1976; 82:70-80.

9. Kristensson K, Svennerholm B, Persson L. Latent herpes simplex virus trigeminal ganglionic infection in mice and demyelination in the central nervous system. J Neurol Sci 1979; 43:253-64.

10. Townsend JJ, Baringer JR. Comparative vulnerability of peripheral and central nervous tissue to herpes simplex virus. J Neuropathol Exp Neurol 1976; 35:100.

11. Adour KK, Winger BJ, Bell DM, Manning J. Prednisone treatment for idiopathic Bell's paralysis. N Engl J Med 1972; 287:1284.

12. May M, Welte R, Hardin WB, Sullivan J. The use of steroids in Bell's palsy: a prospective controlled study. Laryngoscope 1976; 86:111.

13. Taverner S. Medical management of idiopathic (Bell's) palsy. Proc R Soc Med 1973; 66:554.

14. Sunderland S. The effect of rupture of the perineurium on the contained nerve fibers. Brain 1946; 69:149.

15. Peitersen E. Natural history of Bell's palsy. Acta Otolaryngol (Stockh) 1981 (in press).

≈

ASSOCIATION FOR RESEARCH IN OTOLARYNGOLOGY

The annual Midwinter Meeting of the Association for Research on Otolaryngology will take place January 18-21, 1982, at the Dolphin Beach Resort, St. Petersburg Beach, Florida. People wishing to register should contact Donald W. Nielsen, PhD, Secretary-Treasurer, Otological Research Laboratories, 7036 Education and Research Building, Henry Ford Hospital, 2799 West Grand Blvd., Detroit, MI 48202.

Ann Otol 90:1981

TOTAL ENERGY AND CRITICAL INTENSITY CONCEPTS IN NOISE DAMAGE

W. DIXON WARD, PhD
ARNDT J. DUVALL III, MD
PETER A. SANTI, PhD
CHRISTOPHER W. TURNER, MS
MINNEAPOLIS, MINNESOTA

Groups of chinchillas were given a series of noise exposures of approximately equal energy ranging from 22 minutes at 120 dB SPL to 150 days at 82 dB. For all exposures involving levels of 112 dB or less, the same average permanent hearing losses (15-20 dB) and degree of outer hair cell destruction (8-10%) resulted, thus confirming the validity of the total energy principle for assessing the hazard associated with single continuous exposures at moderate levels. The 22-minute, 120-dB exposure, however, produced a 60-dB hearing loss and massive hair cell destruction (70-80%), indicating that some critical level had been exceeded, thus producing acoustic trauma. Further histological study suggests that the massive destruction is a result of breaks in the organ of Corti, produced by severe mechanical stress, that permit the mixture of endolymph with perilymph, thus creating a hostile environment for the hair cells.

Traditionally, damage to the auditory system caused by sound has been divided into two classes: acoustic trauma (AT), caused by a single short exposure to a sound of very high intensity, and noise-induced hearing loss (NIHL), the product of repeated exposures at moderate intensities. Considerably more is known about AT than NIHL, largely because short exposures are easier to control, and because the results are generally spectacular, in a physiological sense. Yet more slowly developing NIHL is equally important in our modern noisy world.

Indeed, if one particular theory is correct, the hearing of everyone is being affected by noise. This theory, sometimes called the "equal energy" theory, although "total energy" is more accurate, postulates that cumulative damage to the auditory system is a function only of the total acoustic energy that has reached the cochlea during the lifetime of the individual, except for the effect of individual differences in susceptibility that may be ascribed to variability in cochlear structure from person to person. If this were correct, then every sound would exact its toll on the auditory system and we should all be doomed to eventual deafness, if from nothing more than the sound of our own voice.

Obviously, this is quite unlikely. Although most people do lose hearing sensitivity as time passes, and part of this is no doubt due to noise, it is hard to believe that the pattern of noise exposure makes absolutely no difference in the amount of damage, that rest periods that interrupt a noise exposure never reduce its effect, and that there are no durations of ordinary levels that are completely safe. Yet this extreme position is seriously held by influential persons in the field of international standards. The practical importance of this controversy is so great that our laboratories have been testing the total-energy theory in depth, giving chinchillas a series of exposures that include some of equal energy but with levels and durations that range from AT to NIHL, and then assessing both the changes in auditory sensitivity and structural damage to the cochlea. By so doing we hope not only to determine the degree to which the total-energy theory is approximately correct but also perhaps to shed light on the question of the difference in processes involved in AT and in NIHL.

Earlier research has established that the total-energy hypothesis seemed to hold, at least qualitatively, for AT in the chinchilla. An exposure of 30 minutes at 123 dB produced approximately the same hearing loss (50 to 60 dB) as two hours at 117 dB.[1] However, the cochlear destruction in these animals was so extensive that its quantification was difficult. It seemed desirable, therefore, to adopt some method for assessing in a consistent manner at least one type of structural damage to the auditory system, and to study the total-energy theory using noise exposures that give substantially less damage, so that the method can provide an unequivocal indication of an increase or decrease in total damage from one exposure to another.

EXPERIMENT 1

The general procedure is as follows: monauralized chinchillas are exposed to a 700- to 2800-Hz band of noise of approximately constant spectrum in a reverberant room that is designed to minimize standing waves and hence provide a uniform field. Behavior thresholds at octave frequencies are assessed by means of standard conditioned avoidance tech-

From the Department of Otolaryngology, University of Minnesota, Minneapolis. This research was supported by NINCDS grants NS 12125 and NS 04615.

Presented at the meeting of the American Otological Society, Inc., Vancouver, British Columbia, May 9-10, 1981.

REPRINTS — W. Dixon Ward, PhD, 2630 University Ave SE, Minneapolis, MN 55414.

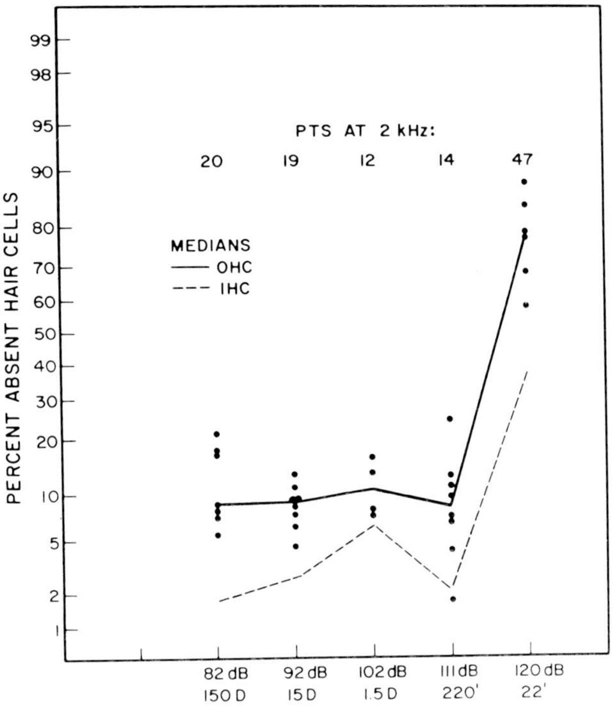

Fig. 1. Percent absent inner (AIHC) and outer (AOHC) hair cells in chinchillas, 30 days or more after exposure to 700-2800-Hz noise at the levels and durations indicated on the abscissa. Points represent AOHC counts in individual ears, and the solid line connects group medians. Median AIHC counts are shown by the dashed line. The numbers at the top denote the mean permanent threshold shift (PTS) at 2 kHz resulting from the various exposures.

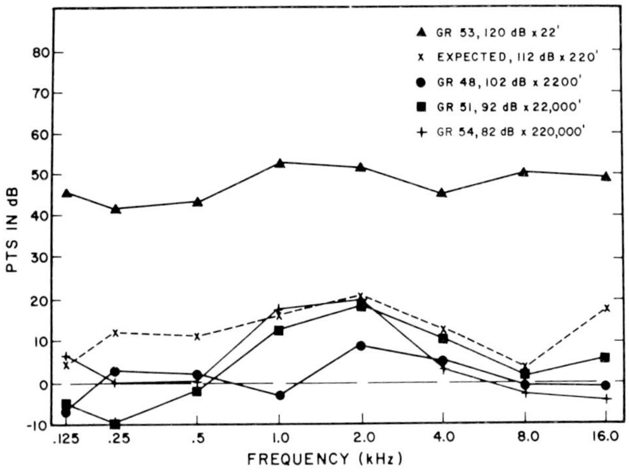

Fig. 2. Permanent threshold shifts (PTS) produced in monauralized chinchillas by various exposures of equal total energy. Average of four animals per group.

niques[2] before exposure, during exposure (when exposures are longer than one day), and for at least 30 days after exposure, in order to assess temporary and permanent hearing losses. The four animals that constitute a typical exposure group, plus two exposed nonbehaviorally-tested animals and one or two nonexposed controls, are then sacrificed and a complete census of the hair cells is taken. Cochlear hair cells are serially assessed from soft surface preparations in which the hair cell stereocilia have been stained with alcian blue and their nuclei with ruthenium red.[3] A hair cell is classified as "absent" if it is missing or has no stereocilia; the number of present and absent hair cells are plotted to produce a cytocochleogram.

Preliminary studies had shown that a loss of about 10% of the outer hair cells (OHC) would be produced by an exposure of 220 minutes at 112 dB. This dose was therefore taken as the standard, since either increases or decreases from the value of 10% destruction could be reliably assessed, indicating how the damage changed as the noise levels were made lower or higher, with durations correspondingly longer or shorter. Groups of animals were exposed at 102 dB for 2200 minutes or 1.5 days (ten times longer but at one tenth the intensity of the 220 minute 112 dB exposure), at 92 dB for 15 days, and at 82 dB for 150 days. Only one exposure at a higher level was included in this particular series: 22 minutes at 120 dB, a dose known from other pilot studies to produce more than 10% damage, even though the total energy was somewhat less than for the other exposures. Since one group of animals had been run at 111 dB for 220 minutes, we did not actually give a 220-minute exposure at 112 dB, but assumed that the 111 dB group would have given about the same results.

Results and Discussion. The damage produced by these exposures is shown in Figure 1, expressed in percent hair cell loss over the entire cochlea, using probability coordinates. The points represent absent outer hair cell (AOHC) counts for individual ears, and the solid line connects group medians of the AOHC counts. The median inner hair cell (IHC) loss is shown by the dashed line. The differing number of ears for the various conditions results from the death of a few animals before the end of the experiment. It is clear that single, essentially uninterrupted exposures of this particular energy do in fact cause equal total cochlear damage as long as the SPL involved is 111 dB or less.

All exposures cause less damage to the IHC than to the OHC; only two of the 32 animals whose cochleas are represented in Figure 1 showed a greater IHC loss than OHC loss. Approximately the same permanent threshold shift (PTS) at 2 kHz was also produced by these lower-intensity exposures. Figure 2 shows the PTS for all groups; the only consistent difference is that the PTSs are somewhat greater at high frequencies for the exposures involving higher intensities, consistent with the spread of excitation to remote frequencies as intensity increases.

A corresponding spread of results was observed in the spatial distribution of damage. Although damage is distributed widely throughout the cochlea even when the level is only 82 dB, apical damage was relatively more severe for the higher-intensity exposures. For example, the mean percent AOHC in the four behaviorally-tested animals in group 54

(150 days at 82 dB SPL) in the first, second, and third turns was 10.3%, 10.9%, and 4.5%, respectively, while in group 45 (220 minutes at 111 dB SPL), the corresponding values were 6.6%, 7.4% and 8.6%. There was a slight but significant tendency for the third row of OHC (those farthest from the IHC) to display more damage than the first and second rows; in the 111 dB 220 minute group, for example, the average AOHC values were 8.6%, 8.7% and 11.7% for the first, second and third rows, respectively.

An attempt was made to correlate individual PTS with individual AOHC counts and distributions, with a marked lack of success. We find, as do other laboratories studying the chinchilla,[4-7] moderately large gaps in the OHC population yet normal hearing at what we believe to be the appropriate frequency, and conversely, significant hearing loss accompanied by a normal appearing complement of hair cells. Noise exposure causes both OHC destruction and hearing loss, but it is clearly incorrect to say that OHC destruction causes hearing loss (in the sense of a loss of auditory sensitivity). The role of the OHC in the hearing process remains a mystery.

However, considering only averages, the total-energy theory holds, for both hair cell destruction and hearing loss, down to levels as low as 82 dB for the chinchilla. An extrapolation of this trend to even lower levels implies that if a chinchilla spent its entire life of 16 years or so in a 66 dB environment, it would have this same 10% AOHC loss due to noise exposure.

However, if one asks how far the total-energy principle extends upward, the exposure at 120 dB makes it obvious that 111 dB may, on the average, be the limit for this particular dose of energy. The exposure of 22 minutes at 120 dB, which should have produced an AOHC loss of perhaps 8%, instead nearly wiped out the organ of Corti in all four animals, causing AOHC losses of over 50% in each of them. Apparently we have made the transition from NIHL to AT with this upward step in level, even though it was a downward step in energy. That is, the "critical" level for this particular noise dose has been exceeded.

The idea that there exists a critical intensity for a particular dose of total energy, below which the effects of noise are perhaps biochemical in nature but above which the effects may be primarily structural, has become fairly well accepted. The structural anomalies have been studied extensively, and include phenomena such as detachment of the tectorial membrane from the hair cells, disconnection of the organ of Corti from the basilar membrane, and rupture of Reissner's membrane.[8] However, secondary effects from such structural changes could well ensue, eg, damage induced by the intermixture of perilymph and endolymph which creates an environment hostile to the welfare of hair cells.[9-11] The structural damage induced by exceeding the critical level, that is, may act in a synergistic fashion: by allowing mixture of cochlear fluids, it may multiply manyfold the biochemical effects that would have existed in moderation even if the tissues had remained intact.

Our earlier studies on the effect of a 15-minute exposure at 123 dB SPL,[12,13] well above the critical intensity for this duration according to the present results, showed that the stria vascularis displayed a marked edema six hours after exposure, although not immediately afterwards, that lasted several days. As yet it is not clear just what role this edema plays in the development of hair cell destruction. However, one possibility is that stria edema is associated with the mixture of endolymph and perilymph, either reflecting an adverse reaction to a higher concentration of sodium ions than normal in the immediate vicinity, or indicating "overwork" as the stria attempts to restore the normal ionic balance,[14] if that is its function.

In either case, it seemed worthwhile to study simultaneously the condition of the stria vascularis and that of the organ of Corti, in order to test the hypothesis that above a critical intensity, for a particular time of exposure, mechanical breaks occur in cells that seal the endolymphatic from the perilymphatic spaces, and that the combination of mechanical disruption and fluid exchange through these breaks results in greater hair cell loss than is observed at lower intensities but the same total energy.

EXPERIMENT 2

Ten chinchillas were exposed to 111 dB for 220 minutes and ten more to 120 dB for 22 minutes for investigation of mechanical breaks in the organ of Corti and stria edema, as the 111 dB exposure was below the critical point for all eight cochleas in that group (Fig. 1), while the 120 dB exposure was clearly above it, again for all six of the animals. Following exposure, the animals were sacrificed, three or four at a time, either immediately, 24 hours, or three days after exposure.

For anatomical examination the animals were decapitated, and one cochlea from each animal was fixed by perilymphatic perfusion of 2% osmium tetroxide in phosphate buffer. After fixation, the cochleae were dehydrated with ethanol and embedded whole in Epon. Radial sections (2μ thick) of the scala media were sectioned from each of the three cochlear turns and stained with toludine blue. To obtain objective though only semiquantitative data, all slides were evaluated dichotomously in two respects. If the anatomical integrity of the organ of Corti was disrupted, thus indicating a break in the seal between the endolymphatic and perilymphatic spaces, the organ of Corti was given a positive rating. If the stria vascularis was edematous, the stria was rated as positive. Coexistence of stria

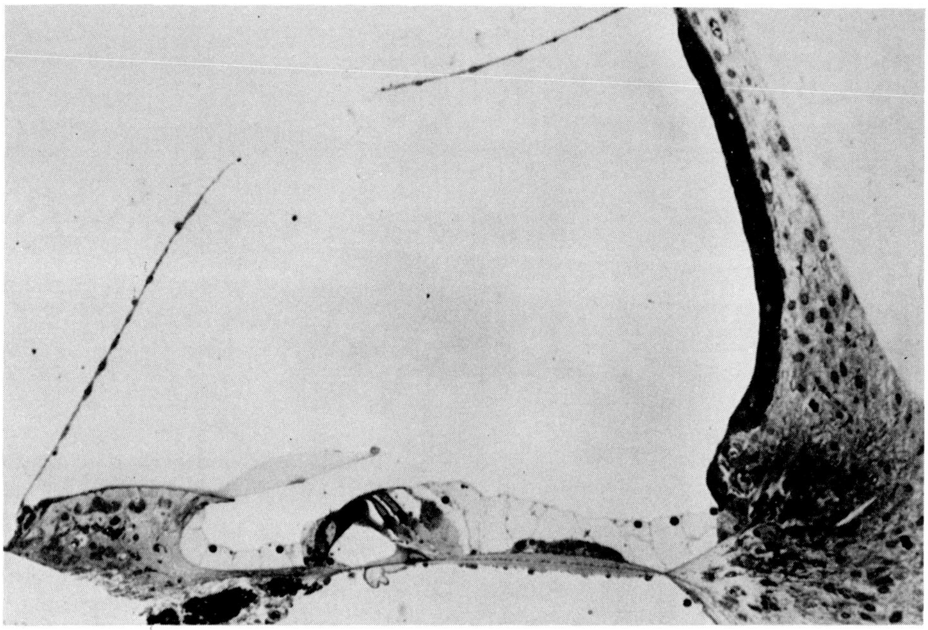

Fig. 3. Photomicrograph of a 2-μm radial section of the scala media in turn 1 of an animal exposed to 111 dB SPL noise for 220 minutes and sacrificed immediately. Note the absence of organ of Corti disruption and the lack of stria edema. (Approximately x390)

edema and organ of Corti disruption could thus be compared in the two groups.

The results are shown in Table 1. After the 111-dB-sound exposure no breaks were observed between the cells that seal the organ of Corti, and stria edema was observed in only one animal (Fig. 3). However, immediately after the 120-dB exposure, there was substantial tearing of the organ of Corti off the basilar membrane (Fig. 4A) and stria edema was almost universal 24 hours after the exposure (Fig. 4B). It appears that hair cell loss is greater after the more intense, shorter duration exposure due to intermixing of endolymphatic and perilymphatic fluids through the permeable basilar membrane.[15,16] This fluid imbalance is reflected in the subsequent development of stria edema.

These data provide supporting evidence for Bohne's theory[11] on one of the mechanisms of noise damage in the cochlea, at least after intense sound exposure. Goldstein and Mizukoshi[17] observed swelling and rupture of hair cells (similar to that observed after intense sound exposure) that has been suspended in artificial endolymph. Bohne[11] demonstrated similar hair cell destruction after

TABLE 1. PERCENTAGE* OF 2 μm SECTIONS THAT SHOWED ORGAN OF CORTI BREAKS (OCB) AND STRIA EDEMA (SE)

Exposure	Morphology	Sacrifice Times Immediate	24 hr	3 days
111 dB SPL 220 min	OCB	0 (0/16)	0 (0/13)	0 (0/16)
111 dB SPL 220 min	SE	0 (0/16)	31 (4/13)†	0 (0/16)
120 dB SPL 22 min	OCB	33 (4/12)	20 (3/15)	10 (2/21)
120 dB SPL 22 min	SE	0 (0/12)	93 (14/15)	86 (18/21)

*No. damaged/no. of sections.

†Edema in one animal.

artificial endolymph had been perfused through the scala tympani. Tasaki and Fernandez[18] had earlier demonstrated decreased cochlear microphonics and action potentials following similar perfusion of the scala tympani with endolymph. Thus, for intense sound exposures during which the organ of Corti is torn from the basilar membrane, fluid intermixing appears to be a significant factor in hair cell degeneration. That intermixing of fluid is the mechanism involved is supported by the development of stria edema following disruption of scala media integrity after intense sound exposures[9] or as the result of surgical tears in Reissner's membrane.[19]

DISCUSSION

For a single uninterrupted exposure whose energy is that corresponding to an exposure of 220 minutes at 112 dB SPL, the total-energy theory holds until the SPL involved exceeds 112 dB, perhaps in the neighborhood of 115 or 116 dB SPL. It does not necessarily follow, however, that 115 dB would also be the average critical intensity for less severe exposures, say those with one tenth as much energy. That is, if a reference exposure of 22 minutes at 112 dB were subjected to a procedure like the one used here, it might well turn out that 2.2 minutes at 122 dB gave no more damage, and that only when the exposure was to 0.22 minutes at 132 dB would the damage suddenly soar. Further research must test the generality of 115 dB as a critical intensity for the chinchilla, one that divides AT from NIHL.

The present results also do not bear on the applicability of the total-energy theory to interrupted exposures nor to the question of the "threshold of damage" exposure. A quantitative analysis of how much reduction in effectiveness is afforded by the ordinary quiet intervals between daily noise exposures is still to be performed.

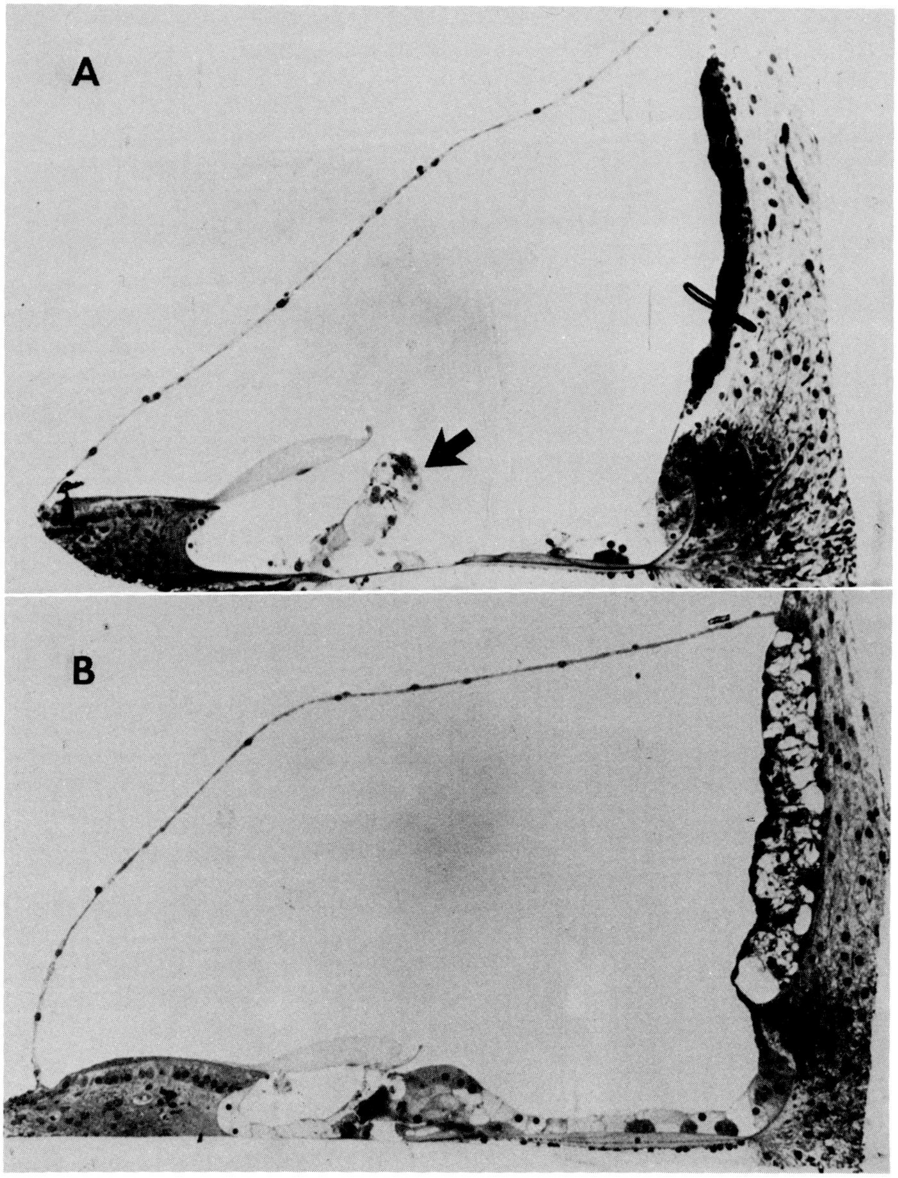

Fig. 4. A) Photomicrograph of a radial section of the scala media turn 1 of an animal exposed to 120 dB SPL noise for 22 minutes and sacrificed immediately. Note that sensory and supporting cells of the organ of Corti have been mechanically torn (arrow) from the basilar membrane while the stria appears normal. (Approximately x380) B) Photomicrograph of an animal that received the 120 dB 22-minute sound exposure and was sacrificed 24 hours after the exposure. There is evidence of cellular repair in the organ of Corti while the stria vascularis is edematous. (Approximately x390)

The present results are at least in line with earlier chinchilla studies, although few researchers have employed a noise similar to the two-octave-wide band (700-2800 Hz) employed in all our recent experiments. Dolan et al[20] exposed one animal to 114 dB for a 600- to 2400-Hz noise for eight hours, and this one animal showed the massive destruction characteristic of AT. Lipscomb et al,[7] on the other hand, used 8-hour exposures to a pinkish noise at 110 dB overall, with about 106 dB in the 700- to 2800-Hz region; a loss in hair cells of only 4% was found, consistent with the thesis that the critical intensity (for this dose) had not been reached.

Two experiments have, however, used exactly the same noise spectrum we employ, in attempts to duplicate some results we presented earlier.[21] We found that some chinchillas exposed for 15 minutes at 123 dB SPL, although showing the extensive hair cell destruction that is characteristic of AT, had apparently completely recovered behaviorally, so that no PTS was produced. Indeed, in a subsequent group of animals given the same exposure in an attempt to confirm those results, an animal with "complete wipeout" (no hair cells at all) in the first turn nevertheless showed a complete gradual recovery to pre-exposure thresholds even at 8 and 16 kHz. Fortunately, these bizarre results were never published, because we now are confident that some elusive artifact was operating for all those animals, even though its nature has never been deduced. It was at least not a vibration artifact, because insertion of an earplug raised the animal's apparent threshold by the expected 20 to 30 dB. Coincident with the move of our laboratories to a new building, the artifact completely disappeared, in that the 123-dB 15-minute exposure now produces not only the severe hair cell destruction of AT but also a 60-dB PTS over most of the auditory range, just as Clark et al[22] found using a testing technique with positive reinforcement instead of shock avoidance. On the other hand, Hunter-Duvar and Bredberg[5] report that of four exposed chinchillas, only one showed wipeout over a large area of the basilar membrane. The other three had negligible HC losses (1-3%) and only 15-20 dB of PTS; it appears that the critical intensity for these three chinchillas was a bit higher than average.

The implications of the present results for human exposure standards are not clear-cut, except for use in limiting unusually extended exposures that may occur under some circumstances in the military area, as in submarines. Even then, caution must be used. The chinchilla is known to be considerably more sensitive to noise damage than the guinea pig, by 15 to 25 dB,[23] quite apart from considerations of the differential conduction of sound to the cochlea.[24] Is the human ear more like that of the guinea pig or the chinchilla? One bit of evidence suggests that the answer is the guinea pig. In an unreported study performed several years ago, ten human subjects were exposed to this noise for 10 and 100 minutes at 100 dB SPL. The average temporary threshold shift at 2, 2.8 and 4 kHz, measured two minutes after exposure, was 9 and 25 dB, respectively. If one can assume that an asymptote of threshold shift is reached after about 12 hours of exposure, the figures cited predict that the value of this asymptotic threshold shift would be about 38 dB. This is very near the value of 39 dB observed in our chinchillas exposed to 82 dB SPL, which implies a difference in susceptibility to temporary threshold shift of some 18 dB.

If this relation can be generalized, then the critical intensity of 700- to 2800-Hz noise for guinea pig and man for a 220-minute exposure should be somewhere around 130 to 135 dB SPL. This is not to say, of course, that 220 minutes at 130 dB of *any* sound would be safe. For example, Erlandsson et al[25] find that the critical intensity of a 3850-Hz pure tone for six hours is just under 120 dB for the guinea pig, and Spoendlin and Brun[26] find values of about 125 dB for a 1-hour exposure to broadband noise, 135 dB for a 3-minute exposure.

We have demonstrated mechanical breaks in the cells that seal the endolymphatic and perilymphatic spaces following exposures which exceed the critical level for the chinchilla. The formation of stria edema indicates that intermixing of fluids occurred through these breaks. Thus, a mechanism for hair cell loss is the presence of endolymph beneath the reticular lamina. Voldrich[27] has recently shown a fourfold increase in hair cell damage in the guinea pig when an intense sound exposure (145 dB of 1000-Hz third octave band noise for five minutes) is immediately followed by a continuous, ordinarily subtraumatic, exposure to the same noise at 90 dB for 30 minutes. He demonstrated that the first sound exposure produced mechanical breaks in the cells of the organ of Corti and suggested that the ensuing intermixing of fluids is enhanced by the mechanical vibrations of the second subtraumatic sound exposure. Hamernik and Henderson[28] found a potentiation of the effects of impulse and continuous noise in the chinchilla which might also be explained by this mechanism.

Obviously, the surface of the critical exposure problem has been scarcely scratched.

ACKNOWLEDGMENTS — We thank Beth Prieve for her assiduous cochlear dissection and hair cell counting, and Tom Kiester, Sherry Gregg, Cheryl Holmgren, Chris Dietrich, Blake Iserman, Lenore Holte, and Janet Harvey for threshold measurements. Thanks are also due Marnie Cushing, Susan Rolle, and Margaret Hukee for technical assistance.

REFERENCES

1. Ward WD, Nelson DA. On the equal-energy hypothesis relative to damage-risk criteria in the chinchilla. In: Robinson DW, ed. Occupational hearing loss. London: Academic Press, 1971: 225-31.

2. Nelson DA, Kiester TE, Turner CW, Ward WD. Automated conditioned-avoidance audiometry in the chinchilla. J Aud Res 1976; 16:209-37.

3. Santi PA, Muchow DC. Morphometry of the chinchilla organ of Corti and stria vascularis. J Histochem Cytochem 1979; 27:1539-42.

4. Eldredge DH, Miller JD. Acceptable noise exposures — damage risk criteria. In: Ward WD, Fricke JE, eds. Noise as a public health hazard. ASHA Reports No. 4, 1969; 110-20.

5. Hunter-Duvar IM, Bredberg G. Effects of intense auditory stimulation: hearing losses and inner ear changes in the chinchilla. J Acoust Soc Am 1974; 55:795-801.

6. Ades HW, Trahiotis C, Kokko-Cunningham A, Averbuch A. Comparison of hearing thresholds and morphological changes in the chinchilla after exposure to 4 kHz tones. Acta Otolaryngol (Stockh) 1974; 78:192-206.

7. Lipscomb DM, Axelsson A, Vertes D, Roettger R, Carroll J. The effect of high level sound on hearing sensitivity, cochlear sensorineuroepithelium and vasculature of the chinchilla. Acta Otolaryngol (Stockh) 1977; 84:44-56.

8. Lim DJ, Dunn DE. Anatomic correlates of noise induced hearing loss. In: Cantrell R, ed. Noise — its effects and control. Otolaryngol Clin North Am 1979; 12:493-513.

9. Lawrence M, Yantis PA. Individual differences in functional recovery and structural repair following overstimulation of the guinea pig ear. Ann Otol Rhinol Laryngol 1957; 66:595-621.

10. Duvall AJ, Sutherland CR, Rhodes VT. Ultrastructural changes in the cochlear duct following mechanical disruption of the organ of Corti. Ann Otol Rhinol Laryngol 1969; 78:342-57.

11. Bohne BA. Mechanisms of noise damage in the inner ear. In: Henderson D, Hamernik RP, Dosanjh DS, Mills JH, eds. Effects of noise on hearing. New York: Raven Press, 1976.

12. Duvall AJ, Ward WD, Lauhala K. Stria ultrastructure and vessel transport in acoustic trauma. Ann Otol Rhinol Laryngol 1974; 83:498-514.

13. Santi PA, Duvall AJ. Stria vascularis pathology and recovery following noise exposure. Otolaryngology 1978; 86:354-61.

14. Duvall AJ, Santi PA, Hukee M. Cochlear fluid balance: a clinical/research overview. Ann Otol Rhinol Laryngol 1980; 89:335-41.

15. Ilberg CV. Elektronenmikroskopische Untersuchungen uber Diffusion und Resorption von Thoriumdioxyd an der Meerschweinchenschnecke: 4. Mitteilung Basilarmembran und Cortisches Organ. Arch Otorhinolaryngol 1968; 192:384-400.

16. Duvall AJ, Sutherland CR. Cochlear transport of horseradish peroxidase. Ann Otol Rhinol Laryngol 1972; 81:795-815.

17. Goldstein AJ, Mizukoshi O. Separation of the organ of Corti into its component cells. Ann Otol Rhinol Laryngol 1967; 76:414-26.

18. Tasaki I, Fernandez C. Modifications of cochlear microphonics and action potentials by KCl solution and by direct currents. J Neurophysiol 1952; 15:497-512.

19. Duvall AJ, Rhodes VT. Ultrastructure of the organ of Corti following intermixing of cochlear fluids. Ann Otol Rhinol Laryngol 1967; 76:688-708.

20. Dolan TR, Murphy RJ, Ades HW. A comparison of the permanent deleterious effects of intense noise on the chinchilla resulting from either continuous or intermittent exposure. In: Henderson D, Hamernik RP, Dosanjh DS, Mills JH, eds. Effects of noise on hearing. New York: Raven Press, 1976.

21. Ward WD, Duvall AJ III. Behavioral and ultrastructural correlates of acoustic trauma. Ann Otol Rhinol Laryngol 1971; 80:881-96.

22. Clark WW, Clark CS, Moody DB, Stebbins WC. Noise-induced hearing loss in the chinchilla, as determined by a positive-reinforcement technique. J Acoust Soc Am 1974; 56:1202-9.

23. Drescher DG, Eldredge DH. Species differences in cochlear fatigue related to acoustics of outer and middle ears of guinea pig and chinchilla. J Acoust Soc Am 1974; 56:929-34.

24. Mitchell C. Susceptibility to auditory fatigue: comparison of changes in cochlear nerve potentials in the guinea pig and chinchilla. J Acoust Soc Am 1976; 60:418-22.

25. Erlandsson B, Hakanson H, Ivarsson A, Nilsson P, Wersall J. Hair cell damage in the guinea pig due to different kinds of noise. Acta Otolaryngol (Stockh) 1980; Suppl 367.

26. Spoendlin H, Brun JP. Relationship of structural damage to exposure time and intensity in acoustic trauma. Acta Otolaryngol (Stockh) 1973; 75:220-6.

27. Voldrich L. Noise-noise effect upon the spreading of the posttraumatic progressive necrosis in the organ of Corti. Arch Otorhinolaryngol 1979; 222:169-73.

28. Hamernik RP, Henderson D. The potentiation of noise by other ototraumatic agents. In: Henderson D, Hamernik RP, Dosanjh DS, Mills JH, eds. Effects of noise on hearing. New York: Raven Press, 1976.

≈

PAN AMERICAN ASSOCIATION OF OTORHINOLARYNGOLOGY AND BRONCHOESOPHAGOLOGY

The XVIII Congress of the Pan American Association of Otorhinolaryngology and Bronchoesophagology will be held November 2-6, 1982, in San Juan, Puerto Rico. Dr. Hans von Leden has been elected President of the Association.

NEURAL GENERATORS OF BRAINSTEM EVOKED POTENTIALS
RESULTS FROM HUMAN INTRACRANIAL RECORDINGS

AAGE R. MØLLER, PhD
PETER J. JANNETTA, MD
MARGARETA B. MØLLER, MD, PhD
PITTSBURGH, PENNSYLVANIA

Recordings were made from the auditory nerve near its entrance into the brainstem during neurosurgical operations for cranial nerve disorders. The recorded compound action potentials in response to 2000 Hz tonebursts at 90 dB were characterized by a negative peak with a latency of 3.0 to 3.7 ms. When these compound action potentials were compared with the brainstem evoked potentials (BSEP) recorded from the scalp during the operation or before the operation, it was found that the latency of the main peak of the compound action potential matched the latency of the vertex negative wave located between waves II and III (P_2) and the potentials recorded from the nerve were found to match the $N_2P_2N_3$ complex of the scalp-recorded BSEP. The results indicate that the auditory nerve is the neural generator of the two first peaks in the human BSEP, in contrast to the results of experiments in animals which show that the second peak originates in the cochlear nucleus.

INTRODUCTION

Auditory brainstem evoked potentials (BSEP) are widely used in the diagnosis of disorders affecting the auditory nervous system as well as of more general nervous system disorders such as multiple sclerosis.[1-4] The BSEP that can be recorded on the scalp, usually by placing electrodes on the vertex and the mastoid, are characterized by a series of peaks and valleys. Usually five peaks are identified during the first 10 ms after the onset of a transient stimulus such as a click or a toneburst, but as many as seven or eight peaks can often be seen.[5,6] The neural generators of these peaks are believed to be the various nuclei of the ascending auditory pathway.[6-9]

Earlier it was assumed that each peak could be associated with the activity in a particular nucleus of the ascending auditory pathway. Substantial evidence has been provided regarding the origin of the first peak in the BSEP. Studies by Portman et al[10] show that this peak probably originates in the auditory nerve since its latency matches closely that of the compound action potential (N_1) that can be recorded from the round window. The neural generators for the subsequent peaks are less well known but they have been assumed to be the various nuclei of the ascending auditory pathway. The most simplistic hypothesis assigns the origin of the second peak to the cochlear nucleus, of the third to the superior olive, of the fourth to the lateral lemniscus, and the origin of the fifth peak to the inferior colliculus.

The exact locations of the neural generators of the BSEP have been established in animals either by recording from specific nuclei and comparing the latencies of the recording potentials with those of the scalp-recorded potentials, or by removing certain neural structures or severing nerve tracts and noting the effects of these lesions.[9,11-15] The effects of verified lesions on the BSEP recorded in man have been similarly studied.[1-4,8,13,16,17] Both types of studies have in some cases supported the above hypothesis of the location of the neural generators for the scalp-recorded BSEP, and in other cases the results of such studies have indicated a different and more complex pattern for the origin of these potentials. In particular, later studies[4,11,12,16] seem to show that the previous hypothesis regarding localization of the neural generators of the BSEP was an oversimplification and that, in fact, the electrical activity in more than one nucleus may contribute to a particular peak of the scalp-recorded BSEP, and the activity in a particular nucleus may contribute to more than one peak as well. The results of studying the latency of the response of single nerve cells in particular nuclei of the ascending auditory pathway have shown that groups of neurons with different latencies can be identified. That indicates that there are a different number of neurons between the sensory cells and the various neurons in a particular auditory nucleus. This is contrary to the hypothesis that the cochlear nucleus is composed of only second-order neurons, the superior olive of third order neurons, etc. The results of single unit recordings thus lend support to the hypothesis that each nucleus of the ascending auditory pathway is likely to contribute to more than one peak in the BSEP.

It has been suggested by others[18] that the first five waves of the BSEP in man originate from structures that are peripheral to the lateral lemniscus, and

From the Divisions of Physiological Acoustics, Audiology and Speech Pathology, Departments of Otolaryngology and Neurological Surgery, University of Pittsburgh School of Medicine. This study was supported by the Deafness Research Foundation and the National Institutes of Health (Division of Research Resources) Grant No. 2507RR05779-05.

Presented at the meeting of the American Otological Society, Inc., Vancouver, British Columbia, May 9-10, 1981.

REPRINTS — Dr. A. R. Møller, Division of Physiological Acoustics, Department of Otolaryngology, Eye and Ear Hospital, 230 Lothrop Street, Pittsburgh, PA 15213.

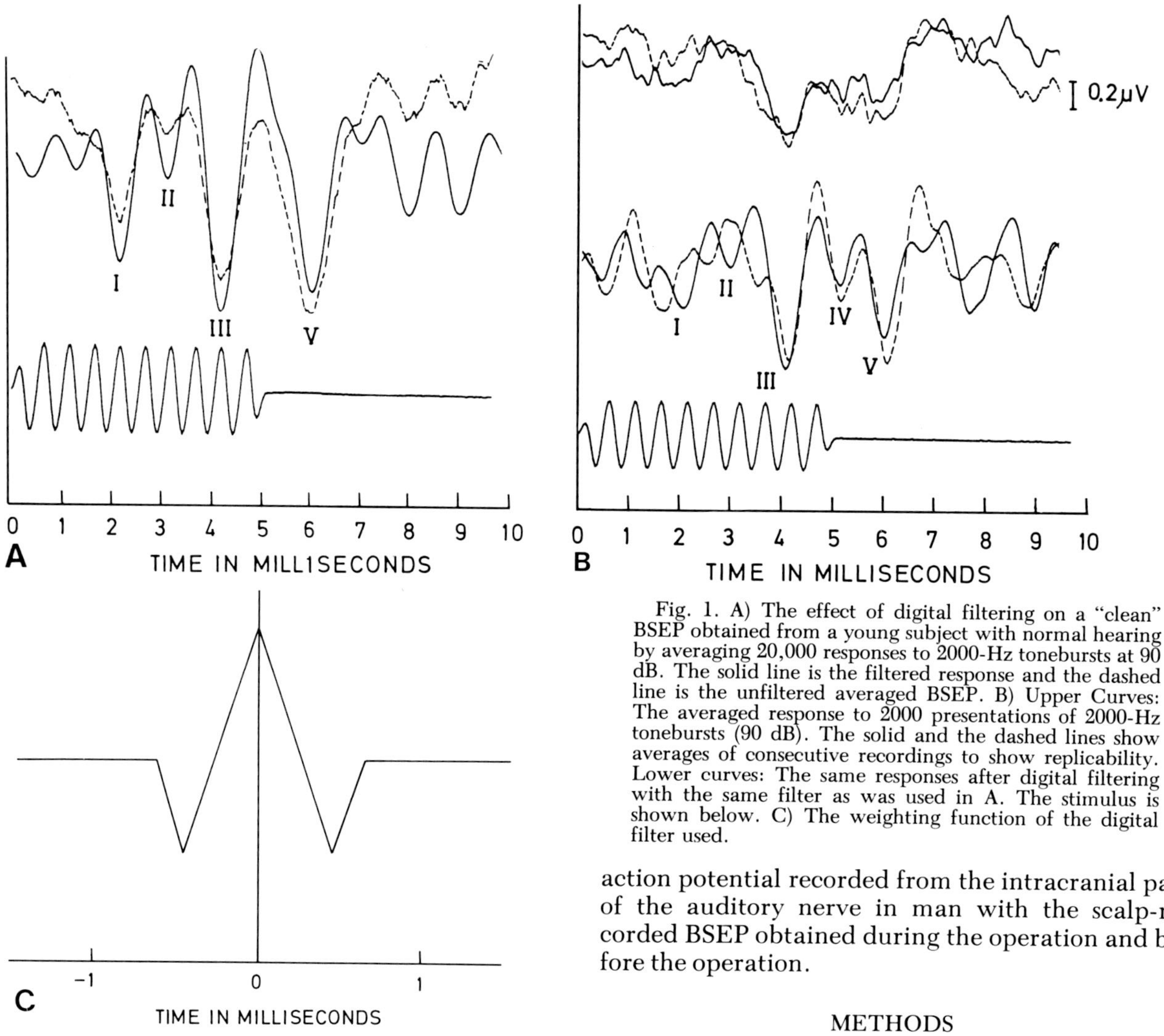

Fig. 1. A) The effect of digital filtering on a "clean" BSEP obtained from a young subject with normal hearing by averaging 20,000 responses to 2000-Hz tonebursts at 90 dB. The solid line is the filtered response and the dashed line is the unfiltered averaged BSEP. B) Upper Curves: The averaged response to 2000 presentations of 2000-Hz tonebursts (90 dB). The solid and the dashed lines show averages of consecutive recordings to show replicability. Lower curves: The same responses after digital filtering with the same filter as was used in A. The stimulus is shown below. C) The weighting function of the digital filter used.

that thus the commonly used BSEP does not include responses from the inferior colliculus.

There are obvious difficulties in interpreting the results of studies designed to determine the locations of the neural generators of the BSEP. Several factors such as the difference in size between the heads of the different animals used in animals studies and that of man makes it difficult to transfer the results of animal studies to man. In studies using human subjects with different pathologies it is impossible to determine exactly the extent and location of the lesions. Not until recently have the results of recording directly from the ascending auditory pathway in man been published. It was shown that the response from the intracranial part of the auditory nerve in man has a much longer latency that that of the first peak in BSEP.[19] The results of such studies support the hypothesis that the contributions from the various nuclei of the ascending auditory pathway are complex and that there are characteristic differences between the results obtained in man and those obtained in experimental animals such as cats.

In the present study we compare the compound action potential recorded from the intracranial part of the auditory nerve in man with the scalp-recorded BSEP obtained during the operation and before the operation.

METHODS

The studies were performed in patients with cranial nerve disorders (hemifacial spasm and trigeminal neuralgia) in whom the intracranial nerve was exposed during microvascular surgery.*

The BSEP was recorded before and after the operation using silver silver-chloride surface electrodes placed on the forehead and the ipsilateral mastoid. A ground electrode was placed on the contralateral earlobe. The sound stimulus was 2000 Hz, 5 ms long tonebursts with a rise and fall time of 0.5 ms (to 90 and 10% of the maximal amplitude, respectively). The tonebursts were presented with an interstimulus time interval of 150 ms. The sounds were presented through earphones (Sennheiser HX414) and the patients were seated in a reclining chair in a sound-insulated room.

The intensities of the sound stimuli used in studies of the BSEP are often given in the literature in terms of a certain hearing level. However, since it required a much shorter time for the part of the nervous system involved in generation of the BSEP to integrate sound (on the order of a few milliseconds) than it does for the subjective loudness of a sound to be determined (on the order of 100 ms), it is not meaningful to describe the intensity of the stimuli used in BSEP studies in terms of the hearing level. The intensity of the tonebursts can be described by the hearing level of a toneburst of the same physical amplitude, but with a duration longer than 100 ms. The sounds used in the present study are characterized in that way. Thus 90 dB means that the toneburst has an amplitude that

*The protocol for recording was reviewed by the hospital human experimentation committee and all patients were fully informed about the recording procedure.

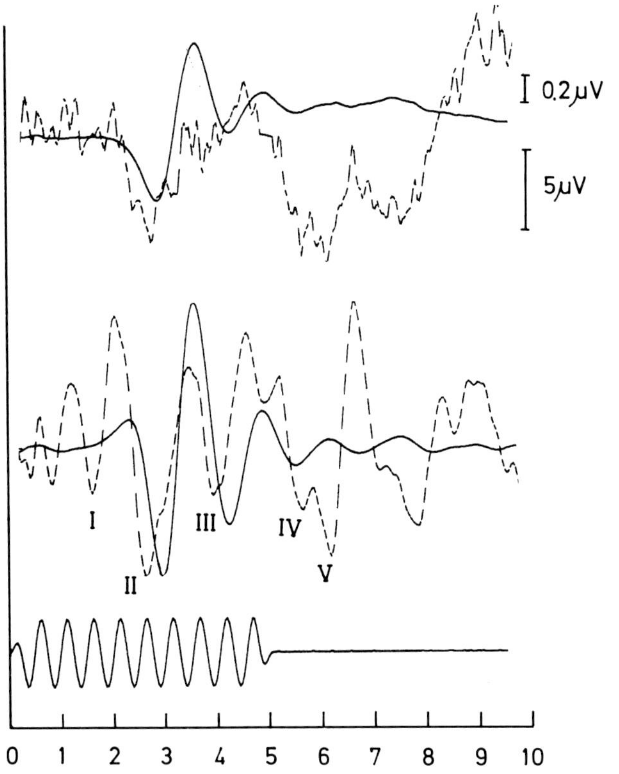

Fig. 2. Upper curves: Typical compound action potential of the auditory nerve recorded intracranially (solid line) compared with the scalp-recorded BSEP (dashed line). No digital filtering. Lower curves: The same recording after digital filtering. The stimulus is shown below.

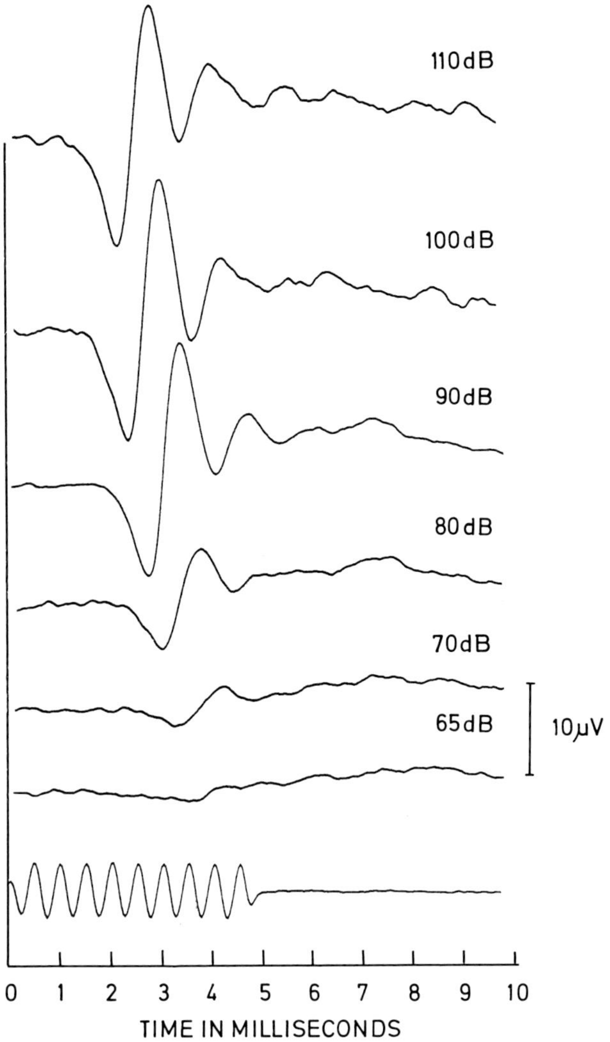

Fig. 3. The compound action potential of the auditory nerve at different stimulus intensities. Recording passband was 3 Hz to 5 kHz. No digital filtering.

is the same as that of a 100 ms or longer toneburst with a hearing level of 90 dB. The hearing level of the 5 ms tonebursts with an amplitude that corresponds to 90 dB HL is about 75 dB, but they are as efficient in eliciting a response from the peripheral auditory system as is a toneburst of longer duration. Thus, if the tonebursts are prolonged to about 100 ms, they will have a hearing level of 90 dB but be as efficient in eliciting the BSEP response as the 5 ms tonebursts.

The recorded potentials were amplified and filtered (highpass 23 Hz and lowpass 3.4 kHz) and averaged (Nicolet 1170). The averaged signal was transferred to disk storage in a PDP 11/60 computer.[20] The averaged BSEP were filtered using a digital filter.[21] The digital filtering used in the present study suppressed background noise without shifting the peaks in the recorded response as is the case when conventional (analog) filters are used. Also the digital filters used in the present study enhanced the peaks in the recorded BSEP, making it easier to identify the individual peaks. The distortion of the BSEP waveform by the digital filtering can be seen in Figure 1A, which shows a "clean" BSEP, obtained by averaging the response to a very large number of stimuli (20,000) before and after filtering. It is seen that filtering does not displace the peaks in time but enhances the peaks slightly. When the BSEP recordings are more noisy, as is the case in practice where many fewer responses are averaged, the distortion of the BSEP by filtering is no greater than that shown in Figure 1 for the "clean" BSEP. The efficiency of the digital filter in suppressing the background noise when the responses to fewer stimuli are averaged has been shown earlier,[21] and is illustrated in Figure 1B which shows the BSEP averaged from many fewer responses. Figure 1C shows the weighting function that characterizes the filter used.

The intracranial recordings were performed during microvascular decompression operations to alleviate either hemifacial spasms or trigeminal neuralgia. The patients were operated upon in the contralateral lateral decubitus position under general endotracheal anesthesia. Following retromastoid craniectomy, a vertical incision one fingerbreadth long was made to the mastoid eminence.[22-24] In these procedures the cerebellum falls away with little or no retraction after the dura mater has been opened and the cerebrospinal fluid has been released from the subarachnoid space. The auditory nerve was exposed during the operation and the recording electrodes were placed on the nerve with the reference electrode placed on the adjacent cerebellum. The electrodes used for recording the compound action potentials from the nerve were Teflon-coated silver wires. The uninsulated tip of each electrode was chlorated and a cotton wick was sutured to it. Before the electrode was placed on the nerve, the wick was soaked in saline.

During the operation, BSEP were also recorded from the scalp. This was done using a technique slightly different from that used for the preoperative and postoperative recordings of BSEP. In the operating room, needle electrodes were placed on the vertex and the ipsilateral earlobe or just above the mastoid. The sound stimuli were the same as used preoperatively and postoperatively but presented through insert earphones. The scalp-recorded potentials and intracranially recorded potentials were amplified using identical (Grass P511H) amplifiers and recorded on magnetic tape using a four-track FM tape recorder (Tandberg Type T1R 115). The filters of the amplifiers were set at 3 Hz highpass and 10 kHz lowpass. The upper cut-off frequency of the tape recorder was 10 kHz at the tape speed used (15 ips). Trigger pulses and the

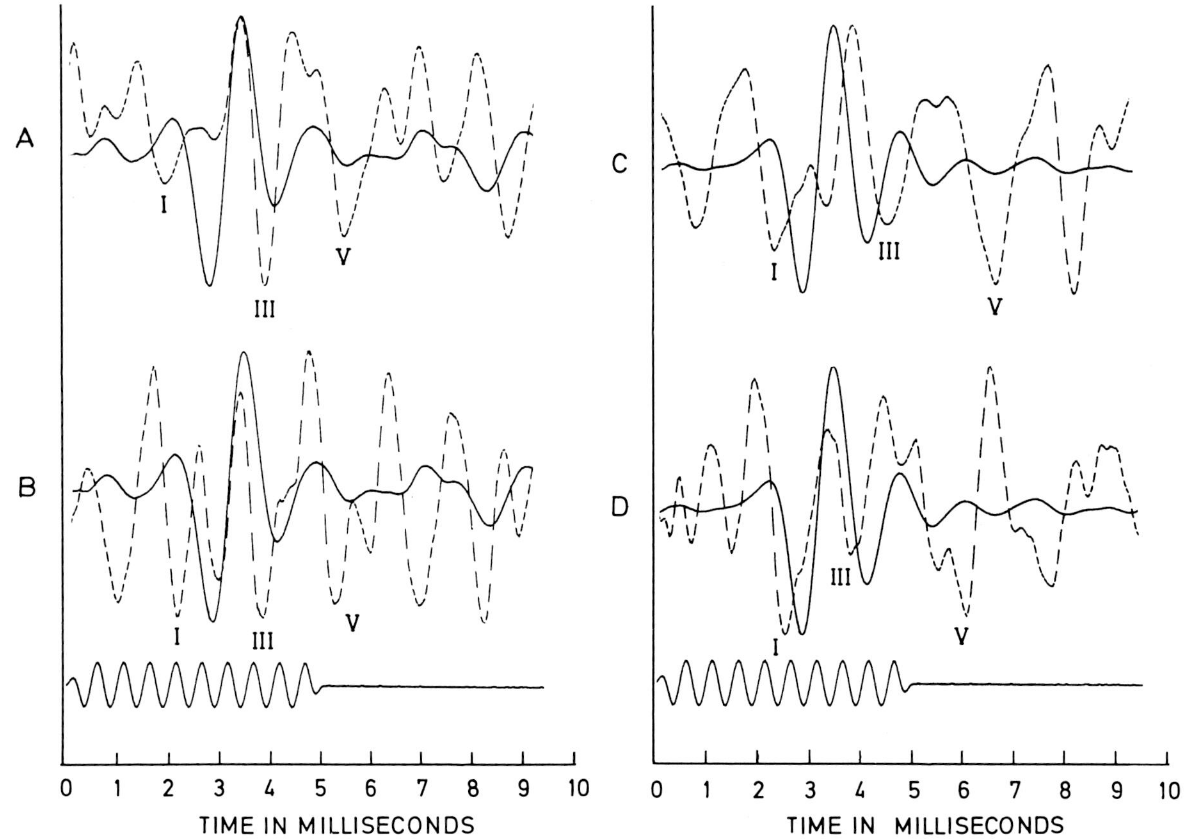

Fig. 4. Intracranially recorded compound action potentials (solid lines) superimposed on the BSEP recorded before the operation (A,C) and during the operation (B,D) for two subjects. All curves were digitally filtered.

sound were recorded on the two remaining tracks of the tape. The potentials recorded in the operating room were averaged and filtered using the same equipment and methods as used for processing the potentials recorded preoperatively and postoperatively.

The literature does not offer a uniform standard with regard to the way to display the BSEP and how to mark (name) the peaks. In the graphs shown in the present paper, an upward deflection indicates vertex (or forehead) negativity and negativity of the nerve recording. That convention was adopted because electrical activity of the nervous system is commonly displayed with negativity upwards and because the vertex (or forehead) is the more active of the two electrodes. The vertex positive (mastoid negative) peaks of the scalp recordings are marked with Roman numerals I, II, III, IV, V or named N_1, N_2, . . .N_5, while the vertex negative peaks are named P_1, P_2, . . .P_5. This notion originates from the time when it was assumed that the vertex electrode was regarded as the reference electrode and the mastoid electrode was regarded as the active electrode. (For further discussion regarding recording conventions see Jewett and Willison[6] and Terkildsen et al.[25])

RESULTS

Figure 2A shows a typical response from the intracranial part of the auditory nerve together with the scalp-recorded BSEP as it appears without digital filtering. It is seen that the compound action potential of the auditory nerve is dominated by a large negative deflection, the latency of which is about 3.2 ms. The main peak is usually preceded by a small positive peak and it is followed by a smaller positive and then a second small negative deflection. That triphasic shape of the compound action potential is what can be expected since the field potentials of a long bundle of axons is the second derivative of the action potential.[26] The comparison between the latency of the various peaks of the BSEP and the nerve response is best made after the recordings have been subjected to digital filtering. Thus Figure 2B shows the same recording as in Figure 2A, after the response was filtered digitally using the filters that are shown in Figure 1. When the various peaks of the BSEP are enhanced by the filtering, they appear much more distinctly and it is seen that the main negative peak in the compound action potential recorded from the nerve appears at the same time as the P_2 peak of the BSEP. Generally it is seen that the compound action potential recorded from the nerve matches the $N_2P_2N_3$ complex of the BSER.

The latency of the negative peak in the compound action potential of the nerve varies from subject to subject, between 3 and 3.7 ms, when the stimulus is a 2000 Hz tone at 90 dB. The latency increases when the stimulus intensity is decreased, as can be seen from Figure 3 which shows the response from another subject obtained at different sound intensities. In this subject, as is usually the case, a small positive deflection is seen immediately before the main negative peak. It is seen that the waveform also changes with decreasing sound intensity and the negative peak becomes broader.

Figure 4 shows a comparison between the potentials recorded from the nerve and those recorded from the scalp (BSEP) in two of the patients. The upper graph compares the intracranial response with the scalp-recorded BSEP done before the operation when the patient was seated in a sound-insulated room. The lower graph compares the same intracranial response with the BSEP recorded from the scalp during the operation. It is seen that in both cases the negative peak of the compound action potential recorded from the nerve matches the latency of the vertex negative peak that is located between the second and the third vertex positive peaks (II, III) of the scalp-recorded BSEP. The curves in Figure 4 were all subjected to digital filtering. The BSEP recorded from the scalp during the operation is not of the same quality as the ones recorded in a sound-insulated room, but the different peaks can be identified easily and they appear with approximately the same latencies as those of the BSEP recorded preoperatively and postoperatively.

DISCUSSION

The results of the present study indicate that the neural generator of the second (vertex negative) peak in the BSEP is the intracranial portion of the auditory nerve. That means that it is not only the first wave in the scalp-recorded BSEP which originates in the auditory nerve, but most likely both of the two first waves. The difference in latency between the two first waves can be accounted for by the travel time in the auditory nerve to its entrance into the brainstem.

Although exact data on the length of the human auditory nerve are not available in the literature, to the best of the knowledge of the authors, the length of the human auditory nerve can be estimated to be between 1 and 1.5 cm. Most of the fibers of the auditory nerve have diameters between 2 and 4μ as reported by Engstrom and Rexed[27] and Lazorthes et al.[28] The conduction velocity of the auditory nerve in man can be estimated to be 10 to 20 m/s on the basis of the fiber diameters. This makes the travel time from the peripheral part of the auditory nerve to its entrance into the brainstem 1 to 1.5 ms, which is in good agreement with the difference in latency of peaks I and II in the ordinary BSEP, assuming that the second peak originates in the auditory nerve close to its entrance into the brainstem. In contrast, the results of experiments on cats indicate that the first peak of the scalp-recorded BSEP originates in the auditory nerve and the second peak originates in the cochlear nucleus in these animals.

The results of the present study are supported by the findings of Stockard et al[2] who found, in a patient with brain death affecting the brainstem and presumably the entire ascending auditory pathway including the cochlear nucleus, that two waves could be discerned in the BSEP. They concluded from these results that the auditory nerve itself may be the neural generator of not only the first but also the second wave in the scalp-recorded BSEP in humans.

The fact that the compound action potential of the nerve in some cases appears slightly earlier than the P_2 component of the BSEP may be a result of the electrode being placed slightly peripheral to the exact part of the nerve that is the major generator of the scalp-recorded potentials. It may be speculated that it is the region of the nerve near the entrance of the nerve into the brainstem that is the main generator of the scalp-recorded potentials.

The question then naturally arises as to why the entire nerve does not give off electrical activity that can be recorded on the scalp. There may be several reasons for this. One may be related to the fact that the nerve travels for most of its length in the bony canal of the internal auditory meatus which is likely to have a much lower electrical conductivity than the brain tissue and cerebrospinal fluid, thus electrically insulating this part of the nerve. Another reason may be that the wave of activity traveling along the nerve contributes only slightly to the volume-conducted potential recorded at a point which is relatively far away and along a path subtended by a small solid angle from the direction of travel of the wave.[26]

The results of the present study thus show that there may be fundamental differences between the neural generators of the BSEP in man and those of the experimental animals (mostly cats) used in earlier studies of neural generators.

REFERENCES

1. Stockard JJ, Stockard JE, Sharbrough FW. Detection and localization of occult lesions with brain stem auditory responses. Mayo Clin Proc 1977; 52:761-9.

2. Stockard JJ, Stockard JE, Sharbrough FW. Brain stem auditory evoked responses in clinical neurology — methodology, interpretation, clinical application. In: Aminoff MJ, ed. Electrodiagnosis in clinical neurology. New York: Churchill Livingstone, 1980; 370-413.

3. Stockard JJ, Rossiter VS. Clinical and pathological correlates of brain stem auditory response abnormalities. Neurology (NY) 1977; 27:316-25.

4. Starr A, Achor LJ. Auditory brain stem responses in neurological diseases. Arch Neurol 1975; 32:761-8.

5. Sohmer H, Feinmesser M. Cochlear action potentials recorded from the external ear in man. Ann Otol Rhinol Laryngol 1967; 76:427-8.

6. Jewett DL, Williston JS. Auditory evoked far fields averaged from the scalp of humans. Brain 1971; 94:681-96.

7. Sohmer H, Feinmesser M, Szabo G. Sources of electrocochleographic responses as studied in patients with brain damage. Electroencephalogr Clin Neurophysiol 1974; 36:663-9.

8. Thornton ARD. Interpretation of cochlear nerve and brain stem evoked responses. In: Naunton RF, Fernandez C, eds. Evoked electrical activity in the auditory nervous system. New York: Academic Press, 1978: 429-42.

9. Buchwald JS, Huang CM. Farfield acoustic responses: origins in the cat. Science 1975; 189:382-4.

10. Portman M, Cazals Y, Negrevergme M, Aran JM. Transtympanic and surface recordings in the diagnosis of retrocochlear disorders. Acta Otolaryngol (Stockh) 1980; 89:362-9.

11. Britt RH, Rossi GT. Neural generators of brain stem auditory evoked responses. I. Lesion studies. Neurosci Abstr 1980; 6:594.

12. Rossi GT, Britt RH. Neural generators of brain stem evoked responses. II. Electrode recording studies. Neurosci Abstr 1980; 6:595.

13. Starr A, Achor LJ. The generators of the auditory brainstem potentials as revealed by brainstem lesions in both man and cat. In: Naunton RF, Fernandez C, eds. Evoked activity in the auditory nervous system. New York: Academic Press, 1978; 443-52.

14. Achor LJ, Starr A. Auditory brain stem responses in the cat. I. Intracranial and extracranial recordings. Electroencephalogr Clin Neurophysiol 1980a; 48:154-73.

15. Achor LJ, Starr A. Auditory brain stem responses in the cat. II. Effects of lesions. Electroencephalogr Clin Neurophysiol 1980b; 48:174-90.

16. Starr A, Hamilton A. Correlation between confirmed sites of neurological lesions and abnormalities of far field auditory brain stem responses. Electroencephalogr Clin Neurophysiol 1976; 41:595-608.

17. Stockard JJ, Sharbrough FW, Tinker JA. Effect of hypothermia on the human brain stem auditory response. Ann Neurol 1978; 3:368-70.

18. Kevanishvili ZS. Sources of the human brainstem auditory evoked potential. Scand Audiol 1980; 9:75-82.

19. Møller AR, Jannetta PJ, Bennett M, Møller MB. Intracranially recorded responses from the human auditory nerve: new insights into the origin of brain stem evoked responses (BSEP). Electroencephalogr Clin Neurophysiol 1981a; 52:18-27.

20. Møller AR, Møller MB, Millner D. A computer system for auditory evoked responses. Proc HICSS-14 Symposium 1981b; 2:430-8.

21. Møller AR. A digital filter for brain stem evoked responses (BSER). Am J Otolaryngol 1980; 1:372-7.

22. Jannetta PJ. Treatment of trigeminal neuralgia by suboccipital and transtentorial cranial operations. Clin Neurosurg 1977; 24:538-49.

23. Jannetta PJ. Neurovascular compression in cranial nerve and systemic disease. Ann Surg 1980; 192:518-24.

24. Jannetta PJ, Abbasy M, Maroon JC, Ramos FM, Albin MS. Etiology and definitive microsurgical treatment of hemifacial spasm: operative techniques and results in 47 patients. J Neurosurg 1977; 47:321-8.

25. Terkildsen K, Osterhammel PO, Huis in't Veid F. Far field electrocochleography, electrode positions. Scand Audiol 1974; 3:123-9.

26. Lorente de No R. Analysis of the distribution of the action currents of nerve in volume conductors. Study Rockefeller Inst Med Res 1947; 132:384-482.

27. Engstrom H, Rexed B. Uber die Kaliber Verhaltnisse der nerven Fasern im N. Stato-acusticus des Menschen. Z Mikrosk Anat Forsch 1940; 47:448-55.

28. Lazorthes G, Lacomme Y, Gaubert J, Planel H. La constitution du nerf auditif. Presse Med 1961; 69:1067-8.

≈

NINTH CONGRESS OF THE EUROPEAN RHINOLOGIC SOCIETY — THIRD INTERNATIONAL SYMPOSIUM ON INFECTION AND ALLERGY OF THE NOSE AND PARANASAL SINUSES

The Ninth Congress of the European Rhinologic Society and the Third International Symposium on Infection and Allergy of the Nose and Paranasal Sinuses will be held in Stockholm, Sept. 5-8, 1982. For information write: Ninth ERS Congress 1982, c/o Reso Congress Service, S-105 24 Stockholm.

PANEL ON TINNITUS CONTROL

MANAGEMENT OF THE TINNITUS PATIENT

JOHN W. HOUSE, MD
LOS ANGELES, CALIFORNIA

At the Otologic Medical Group, we see many patients complaining of tinnitus. Because tinnitus is a symptom the underlying cause and disease process must be identified and evaluated. Most patients complaining of tinnitus will not require special treatment. In this paper we discuss the treatment of patients who are severely disturbed by their tinnitus. We also discuss the effects of surgery on tinnitus. This surgical treatment includes stapedectomies, translabyrinthine eighth nerve sections and translabyrinthine removal of acoustic neuromas. In patients with tinnitus as a primary complaint, stapedectomy can be expected to improve the tinnitus in 50%. In patients undergoing translabyrinthine section of the vestibular nerve, 45% reported improvement and 55% reported the tinnitus to be the same or worse. Following translabyrinthine removal of acoustic tumors, 40% felt that their tinnitus was better, 50% said it was worse and only 10% felt it was the same preoperatively. When the patients' symptoms are severe, we have recommended biofeedback training, tinnitus maskers, and, when appropriate, hearing aids. Of 132 patients undergoing biofeedback training, 77% of the patients reported some degree of relief. No patients were worse. Our acceptance and utilization of the tinnitus maskers has not been as successful. Of 42 patients undergoing tinnitus masker evaluations, only 17% eventually purchased the maskers. We have found that patients with some degree of hearing loss benefit greatly from the use of hearing amplification.

"Any management which is based upon a single panacea for the treatment of a symptom and not a disease will result in failure."

The preceding statement is the conclusion of an excellent article written 31 years ago by Goodhill, discussing tinnitus management.[1] In discussing tinnitus it is important to keep in mind the fact that it is a symptom not a disease. Objective tinnitus refers to a sound in or around the ear which can be heard by an observer. This type is most commonly associated with a vascular lesion or anomaly. It may be caused by muscle spasm, such as palatal myoclonus. On the other hand subjective tinnitus can be heard only by the patient. It is usually associated with a sensorineural hearing loss, but may occur in patients with a conductive hearing loss or normal hearing.

The incidence of tinnitus in the general population is unknown. Most people will say that they have experienced occasional, brief ringing in the ears, frequently associated with exposure to loud noise. Fowler[2] pointed out that 86% of patients with ear disease have tinnitus. Over the years our experience has been in agreement with this figure.

EVALUATION

The patient complaining of the symptom of tinnitus requires an otologic and, if necessary, a neurootologic evaluation. When such a patient is seen at the Otologic Medical Group (OMG), we obtain an audiogram including pure tone air and bone conduction and speech testing (speech reception thresholds and phonetically balanced word discrimination). The audiometric testing is performed routinely, even though the patient may not be aware of a hearing loss. It is common to find patients with tinnitus who are not aware of a hearing loss and are experiencing no difficulty with their hearing. These patients seek medical attention only because of their tinnitus.

After the hearing tests the patient is seen by the otologist who takes a history and performs an ear, nose and throat examination. A neurological examination will be performed if there is indication of possible neurologic or central disorder. Following this initial evaluation, further tests may be ordered. Commonly, these are not necessary because it is apparent from the screening audiometry, history and examination that the problem is due to past noise exposure, aging or other benign processes.

When does one suspect more serious pathology and order further tests? If the tinnitus is associated with a progressive or fluctuating hearing loss, or if the symptom or findings are unilateral or asymmetrical. A high index of suspicion is important for further evaluation. Tests include radiographs of the internal auditory canals, ENG, auditory brainstem response (ABR), impedance audiometry with reflex decay test and blood tests (FTA, glucose tolerance, lipids and thyroid). If any of these tests suggests a retrocochlear lesion then a CAT scan with infusion of iodine is obtained. If this shows a tumor then further CAT scans are not performed. If the CAT scan is negative then 4 cc of oxygen are instilled into the

From the Otologic Medical Group, Inc., and the Department of Otolaryngology, University of Southern California, Los Angeles. Supported by funds from the House Ear Institute.
Presented at the meeting of the American Otological Society, Inc., Vancouver, British Columbia, May 9-10, 1981.
REPRINTS — John W. House, MD, 2122 West Third Street, Los Angeles, CA 90057.

subarachnoid space in order to provide contrast in the internal auditory canals. This technique provides the ability to find intracanicular tumors. When the patient's tinnitus is of the objective type, with an audible bruit, then anterior-posterior and lateral polytomography is obtained in order to examine the vascular structures of the temporal bone (carotid artery and jugular vein). Angiography and jugular venogram may be indicated. Other factors, such as history of trauma or positive neurologic findings may indicate further neurological or neurosurgical evaluation.

MANAGEMENT

Because tinnitus is a symptom, treatment is usually directed at the underlying disease process. The most common causes of tinnitus are sensorineural hearing loss due to aging, vascular changes, or past noise exposure. If the hearing is impaired then amplification with the appropriate hearing aids will usually help to lessen the patient's awareness of the tinnitus. In most cases, if the hearing is not impaired, then a thorough explanation of the problem and reassurance will suffice.

A small percentage (5%) of our patients are severely disturbed by the symptom of tinnitus. It is difficult to say why this small group of patients is so disturbed by their symptoms. In the past we have performed psychological evaluations finding that they tended to have depressive or anxiety neuroses and psychosomatic tendencies.[3,4] It is difficult to say if the tinnitus causes these problems or whether the basic personality makeups of the patients cause them to have difficulty coping with the tinnitus. We have measured the loudness of tinnitus in patients who are disturbed by the tinnitus and in those who are not particularly concerned about it. The relative loudness of the tinnitus was the same in both groups.

Patients who are severely disturbed by the tinnitus will seek any help that is available to eliminate the noise in their ears or head. It is to these patients that we recommend an avenue of treatment in order to provide some degree of relief, such as biofeedback, tinnitus maskers or appropriate hearing aids. Because of the variable results with surgical procedures we do not advise a destructive operation. We have reviewed a large number of patients who have undergone these procedures for reasons other than tinnitus to ascertain what happens to tinnitus with these procedures.

Surgical Treatment of Tinnitus. In 1941, Dandy[5] described his experience with tinnitus in 401 patients in whom he sectioned the auditory nerve for Menière's disease. He felt that 50% of the patients have improvement in their tinnitus. He stated that "tinnitus may or may not disappear after nerve section, and if it persists, it may or may not be improved . . . No promise can be made concerning tinnitus, which a sensible person learns to disregard."

TABLE 1. TINNITUS FOLLOWING TRANSLABYRINTHINE NERVE SECTION

Tinnitus	*Postoperative Condition* No.	%
Absent	1	2
Improved	43	43
Unchanged	16	27
Worse	17	28

Objective tinnitus tends to respond to surgical management better than subjective tinnitus. Ward et al[6] review the evaluation, diagnosis and surgical treatment of lesions causing objective tinnitus. Among the situations presented are cases of venous hum causing objective tinnitus. By ligating the internal jugular vein, relief of the tinnitus was accomplished. Similar results are obtained with A-V malformations and glomus tumors.

A common complaint of patients with otosclerosis is tinnitus. Successful stapedectomy can now be anticipated over 90% of the time. But what about relief of the tinnitus? In our experience and that of other authors, tinnitus does not always disappear or improve even with successful surgery. Glasgold and Altmann[7] studied 190 operated ears in patients with otosclerosis. Tinnitus was present in 78.9%. Following surgery the 103 ears with successful results were reviewed. Of this group 40% had disappearance of tinnitus; 34% had decrease; 20% no change, and 3% were worse. Sheehy has reviewed a large number of patients who underwent stapedectomy surgery and found similar results (personal communication).

Translabyrinthine Eighth Nerve Section. In patients with intractable vertigo or chronic disequilibrium and who have nonserviceable hearing in the affected ear, we will perform a translabyrinthine section of the superior and inferior vestibular nerves. Sixty-eight patients who underwent a translabyrinthine section of the vestibular and, at times, the cochlear nerves, were asked about their tinnitus both before and after surgery. Preoperatively, 60 patients (88%) had tinnitus. Following surgery, 45% said that the tinnitus was either gone or better while 55% reported that it is the same or worse (Table 1).

Because of my interest in tinnitus, careful note has been made of patients' tinnitus responses to various forms of treatment including translabyrinthine section of the eighth nerve. The patients have been questioned preoperatively and postoperatively. In addition, many of them have undergone a tinnitus matching test before and after surgery. If the patients have tinnitus preoperatively then the cochlear nerve as well as the vestibular nerve is sectioned. Surprisingly the tinnitus will usually be matched identically after surgery for both frequency and relative loudness. Subjectively, most of the patients report that the tinnitus is the same.

There were 17 patients in this smaller group. Like the larger series, the majority of the patients (11) had the surgery because of vertigo due to Menière's disease. Two patients each were diagnosed as having dizziness due to trauma and neuronitis. Of the 17, 12 (71%) reported having tinnitus before surgery. The cochlear nerve as well as the vestibular nerves were sectioned in ten cases. Following surgery, 3 patients (all cochlear and vestibular nerve sections) reported an improvement in the tinnitus while 10 said it was the same and 3 felt the tinnitus was worse (no follow-up on one patient). This represents less than a 20% chance of improving tinnitus by sectioning the vestibular nerve. These results suggest that by cutting both the vestibular and cochlear nerve the tinnitus may be improved. However, one of the three patients who say that their tinnitus was made worse had undergone a cochlear nerve section.

Acoustic Neuroma Surgery. Like the translabyrinthine nerve section, removal of acoustic neuromas involves removal of the bony labyrinth of the entire eighth nerve. This allows study of the efficacy of such surgery in helping relieve tinnitus. A few years ago a series of 500 consecutive acoustic neuromas were reviewed.[8] As part of this study questionnaires were sent to the patients inquiring about their postoperative condition including items regarding their tinnitus. Of the 500 patients, 414 (83%) had tinnitus prior to surgery. Only 55 (11%) said that it was their first symptom.

Postoperatively, 40% of the patients felt that their tinnitus was better. Half of them said that it was worse and only 10% found it to be the same as preoperatively. With increasing interest in tinnitus, several recent acoustic neuroma patients have been questioned closely in the office on routine follow-up visits regarding the present status of the tinnitus. Of the 11 postoperative acoustic neuroma patients, only 1 (9%) said that it was better, 6 (55%) said it was the same, and 4 (36%) reported that the symptom was worse than prior to surgical removal of the tumor. These figures vary from those reported in the larger series of patients. The difference may have to do with the timing and manner of questioning. The patients were asked to rate their tinnitus during many months of the postoperative period. This follow-up could have made them more aware of the tinnitus than most patients who have undergone such surgery.

Biofeedback. Since 1975 we have been using biofeedback as a treatment modality for our patients with severe tinnitus[3,9] and have continued to be happy with the results. Biofeedback is not a new form of therapy. It has been used for approximately 25 years for the control of pain and other stress-related disorders. It is a method of teaching the patient to exert conscious control over areas of the body which were thought previously to be outside the control of the conscious mind. Instruments are used which will sense and amplify impulses coming from parts of the body which one wishes to alter. This information can then be used by the patient to modify and alter the specific physiologic processes. For our purpose, we used biofeedback information from the frontalis muscle and skin temperature from the fingers. The patients are to relax the muscles and at the same time to increase peripheral circulation. When the patient is able to do this and achieve a significant degree of relaxation, perception of their tinnitus is lessened greatly. In some cases where stress is a major cause of the tinnitis (muscle spasm, neck pain, temporomandibular joint symptoms, etc), we see the tinnitus disappear as the patient is able to relax and become more aware of bodily tensions. There seems to be a reflex arc where muscle tension in the face and neck causes an increase in tinnitus.

TABLE 2. RESULTS OF BIOFEEDBACK TRAINING (N = 132)

	No.	*%*
Total relief	20	15
Greatly improved	38	29
Improved to tolerance level	44	33
No change	30	23
Worse	0	0

In order for this form of treatment to be successful, the patient must be willing to cooperate. It is an active form of treatment requiring hourly sessions each week and daily exercises at home. Some of the patients are unable or unwilling to devote this much time and effort. For those who do complete the biofeedback training, about 3 out of 4 will have some degree of improvement with none of the patients being worse (Table 2).

The percentage of patients who show improvement in their tinnitus using biofeedback training has improved since we first began the program six years ago. As our experience has grown we have learned to be more selective in the patients we refer for treatment. The patients who do the best are those who do not show severe psychologic disorders and the ones who are well motivated to help themselves. We have been using psychologists to do the training. The therapists stay in the room with the patient during the training sessions and help the process by teaching relaxation exercises. We continue to be happy with biofeedback as a viable form of treatment to help the patients achieve relief from their symptoms.

Tinnitus Maskers and Hearing Aids. Since 1977 we have been performing tinnitus masker evaluations and recommending maskers when appropriate. In 1979 we reported our results in the first 45 patients to undergo a tinnitus masker evaluation.[10] Since then we have continued to offer the masker to patients with severe tinnitus and continue to have similar results as reported in 1979.

Vernon first described his use of the tinnitus masker in 1977.[11] In 1978 Vernon and Schleoning reported results in 158 patients using hearing aids, tinnitus maskers and "FM-masking."[12] An important facet of tinnitus relief is the use of hearing aids. As he points out Saltzman[13] first proposed this in 1949, but with effective middle ear surgery, conductive deficits could be corrected. Vernon stresses the effectiveness of a properly fitted and prescribed hearing aid for patients with either a conductive or sensorineural hearing loss.

In Vernon's initial series, 72% of the overall group experienced effective relief of their tinnitus. More recently Schleoning et al[14] reported their results with a group of 72 patients who underwent testing and fitting at the tinnitus clinic in Oregon during 1979. In this more recent series, 36 patients were advised to try maskers, 24 purchased them, and 21 continue to wear them. Five patients reported complete relief of their tinnitus and 14 reported partial relief. Success records were better for patients who were advised to try hearing aids. Seventeen patients were advised to try aids, 14 purchased them, and 12 are still wearing them. In this group one patient has reported complete relief from tinnitus while eight had partial relief. They report similar results with the tinnitus instrument (a combination masker and hearing aid). Of the 78 patients who were evaluated 8 (10%) reported completed relief with the masker, hearing aids, or tinnitus instrument. An additional 36 (46%) obtained some degree of relief with these modalities.

Pulec et al[15] reported an 82% success rate with tinnitus masking in his office. However, he is reporting 23 of 28 patients who were able to have tinnitus masked in the office during the evaluation. He did not say how many of these patients purchased or could be considered successful users of the masker.

We reviewed charts of the first 45 patients to undergo the masker evaluation. The follow-up period was 6 to 15 months. Patients were sent questionnaires regarding their tinnitus, experience with the tinnitus masker or hearing aids. Forty-two patients returned the questionnaire. The group of 45 patients consisted of 31 males and 14 females from age 17 to 73. Half of the patients had had tinnitus less than two years and 13 had the symptom over five years. The most common diagnosis was presbycusis. Five patients had normal hearing and one patient had a conductive hearing loss.

A total of 27 patients were advised to try the masker (Table 3), and were given a prescription and referral to a hearing aid dealer. Fourteen patients followed this recommendation. Seven patients chose to purchase the masker after a rental trial period. At the time of the initial study, six patients were wearing the masker daily and one occasionally. Since then three patients continue to use their maskers, and one patient wears it almost 24 hours per day.

TABLE 3. EXPERIENCE WITH TINNITUS MASKER (N = 42)

	No.	%
Advised to try	27	64
Trial rental	14	33
Masker purchased	7	17

Instead of the tinnitus masker, 15 patients were advised to obtain hearing aids. Fourteen patients tried aids and nine continue to wear them. Seven patients report that the aids help their tinnitus. The use of aids continues to be dramatic in the treatment of tinnitus. We have found that many times the patient may not be aware of the hearing loss or may only complain of difficulty in some situations. This is particularly true in patients with moderate or severe high frequency sensorineural hearing loss. In these patients binaural hearing aids with high frequency emphasis and open molds will improve their ability to hear and understand speech in many situations while helping their tinnitus. Because of our good results in tinnitus patients with the use of hearing aids we will usually recommend hearing aids instead of tinnitus maskers.

CONCLUSIONS

Because tinnitus is a symptom there is no universal cure. All patients who are complaining of tinnitus deserve a complete evaluation. The underlying cause of the tinnitus symptom should be treated. In most cases the cause is not treatable as such and, therefore, a thorough explanation of the problem will, in most cases, satisfy the patient. If the tinnitus remains a problem for the patient many courses of treatment may be offered. We have found that if a hearing loss exists then hearing aids can be very effective in reducing the severity of the tinnitus. With the increased hearing ability many patients find the tinnitus no longer to be a problem.

At times the patient is literally driven to distraction by the tinnitus. With these patients a careful history will help to better ascertain the extent of the problem. The ability of the patient to sleep and to concentrate during the day helps to determine the severity of the tinnitus. If the patient tends to awaken in the middle of the might and finds it difficult to get back to sleep "because of the tinnitus," he is probably suffering from some degree of depression. In these cases biofeedback is our next choice because 3 out of 4 patients who undergo biofeedback training will gain some degree of relief. More important, most patients become aware of how their bodily tensions affect their tinnitus. This greater awareness helps the patients to understand the various factors which affect the tinnitus. Most of our biofeedback patients find that they no longer require medications to sleep, are taking less tranquilizers, and are generally better able to function in everyday situations. We have found a correlation between the overall mental health of the patient and his ability to perform in biofeedback. The more psychopathic the person is the more likely the tinnitus will fail to improve with biofeedback. The "healthy neurotics" do well with biofeedback. They are able to reduce their tinnitus and become more aware of some of the dynamics involved with it.

A small group of our patients have benefitted from the use of the tinnitus masker and are grateful for the relief the masker provides. Certainly it is not a panacea, but it does offer some relief and should be offered as a possible treatment to these patients.

The best results of treatment of tinnitus occur after complete evaluation, examination, and thorough explanation to the patient.

REFERENCES

1. Goodhill V. The management of tinnitus. Laryngoscope 1950; 60:422-50.
2. Fowler EP. Head noises in normal and disordered ears. Arch Otolaryngol 1944; 39:498-503.
3. House JW, Miller L, House PR. Severe tinnitus: treatment with biofeedback training (results in 41 cases). Trans Am Acad Ophthalmol Otolaryngol 1976; 84:697-703.
4. House PR. Personality of the tinnitus patient. CIBS Symposium 1981; 85 (in press).
5. Dandy WE. Surgical treatment of Meniere's disease. Surg Gynecol Obstet 1941; 72:421-5.
6. Ward PH, Babin R, Calcaterra TC, Konrad HR. Operative treatment of surgical lesions with objective tinnitus. Ann Otol Rhinol Laryngol 1975; 84:473-81.
7. Glassgold A, Altmann F. The effects of stapes surgery on tinnitus. Laryngoscope 1966; 76:1524-31.
8. House WF, Luetje CM, eds. A history of acoustic tumor surgery: 1800-1900, early history. Vol. 1. Baltimore: University Park Press, 1979.
9. House JW. Treatment of severe tinnitus with biofeedback training. Laryngoscope 1978; 78:406-12.
10. House JW, Johnson EW. Tinnitus: tinnitus masker and biofeedback training. Trans Pac Coast Otoophthalmol Soc Annu Meet 1979; 60:115-20.
11. Vernon J. Attempts to relieve tinnitus. J Am Audiol Soc 1977; 2:124-31.
12. Vernon J, Schleoning A. Tinnitus: a new management. Laryngoscope 1978; 88:413-9.
13. Saltzman M, Ersner MJ. A hearing aid for the relief of tinnitus aurium. Laryngoscope 1947; 51:358-66.
14. Schleoning A, Johnson R, Vernon J. Evaluation of a tinnitus masking program: a followup study of 598 patients. Vol. I. Baltimore: Williams & Wilkins, 1980.
15. Pulec J, Hodell S, Anthony P. Tinnitus: diagnosis and treatment. Ann Otol Rhinol Laryngol 1978; 87:821-33.

MEDICAL TREATMENT OF TINNITUS

JOHN J. SHEA, MD

JOHN R. EMMETT, MD
KIT MAYS, MD

DANIEL J. ORCHIK, PhD
WILLIAM WEBB, MD

MEMPHIS, TENNESSEE

Medical treatment is presented as the best hope of the various treatment methods available for the management of tinnitus. A test dose of 100 mg lidocaine given rapidly intravenously will give good or partial temporary relief to approximately 80% of patients with tinnitus. More permanent relief can then be achieved by the oral anticonvulsants carbamazepine or primidone but the side effects of these drugs are occasionally too severe to justify their use. Three preliminary clinical studies of the oral amide of lidocaine, tocainide hydrochloride, were conducted and results with 600 mg four times daily are very promising. Further long-term clinical trials with tocainide will be started soon. It would appear that local anesthetics when given intravenously block the multisynaptic slow pathways in tinnitus as well as in chronic pain, with which there are many other similarities. The delay in wave V in the BSER and the sudden sleep induced in patients with a good response to intravenous lidocaine further confirm the site of action of these drugs in the brainstem and reticular formation. Until tocainide is available for general use it is possible to control tinnitus with large doses of intravenous lidocaine, 100 mg given rapidly and 400 mg slowly with EKG monitoring each day for several days, and then at weekly intervals, as in the treatment of clausalgia. Because patients with disabling tinnitus, as with chronic intractable pain, are rigid, insecure, chronically depressed and fatigued, a mood-elevating tranquilizer drug combination such as perphenazine-amitriptyline is of great value in maintaining these patients. While medical treatment is not the final answer it is the best treatment available and it offers a promising direction for further study.

From the Departments of Otolaryngology and Maxillofacial Surgery, Anesthesia and Psychiatry, University of Tennessee Center for the Health Sciences, the Shea Clinic, Memphis.

Presented at the meeting of the American Otological Society, Inc., Vancouver, British Columbia, May 9-10, 1981.

REPRINTS — John J. Shea, MD, Shea Clinic, 1060 Madison Avenue, Memphis, TN 38104.

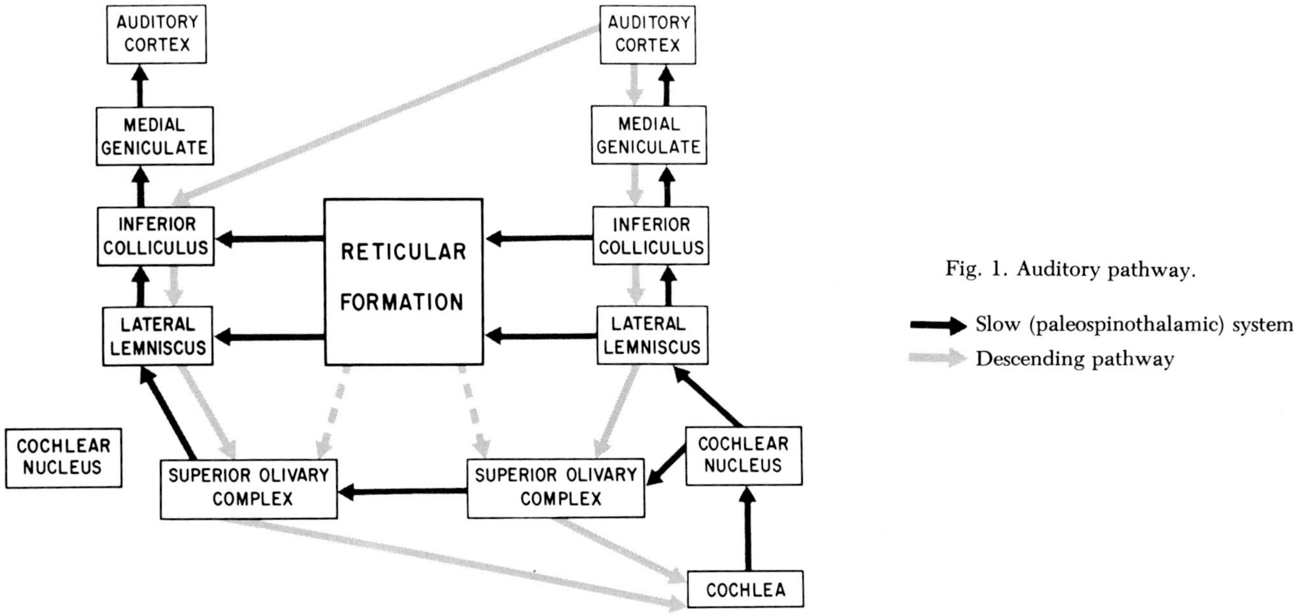

Fig. 1. Auditory pathway.

Medical treatment offers the best hope, we believe, of the various treatment methods available for the management of tinnitus. This is a preliminary report of the progress to date of a combined investigation and tinnitus treatment program.

One finds mention of the treatment of tinnitus as early as 400 BC in the writings of Hippocrates, and it is hard to find a remedy for the relief of tinnitus that has not been tried. Neither masking[1] nor psychotherapy nor intravenous local anesthetics are new in the battle against tinnitus. Barany[2] in 1935 was apparently the first to observe relief from tinnitus from procaine injected into the nasal turbinates. When so injected procaine is so rapidly absorbed into the circulation as to be equivalent to intravenous injection. Lewy[3] in 1937 reported on the beneficial effects of intravenous procaine and nupercaine. Gejrot[4,5] in 1963 and 1976 and Englesson et al[6] in 1976 reported on the beneficial effect of intravenous lidocaine on tinnitus in Menière's disease and other causes of tinnitus.

Tinnitus is so widespread nearly every adult who listens for it in quiet has some from time to time. Goodhill[7] found as many as 20 conditions with which tinnitus occurred. Bothersome tinnitus however is almost always associated with a hearing loss or other sensory defect.[8,9]

Patients vary tremendously in their reaction to tinnitus. Even though it is present constantly most patients learn to live with it, while others suffer enormously from it, and become obsessed with it to the exclusion of all else. Sleeplessness, chronic fatigue, personality changes, and in extreme cases, the threat of suicide increase the problems of management.

There is within the auditory pathway a well-established reflex arc with afferent and efferent fibers conducting a steady discharge in both directions from the hair cells through the brainstem, with abundant connections to the reticular formation, to the thalamus, cortex and back (Fig. 1). When damage occurs to the hair cells or the neural pathways that transmit their output, this reflex arc is altered in such a way that the perception of sound is increased, usually for the very frequencies for which the damaged hair cells or neural pathways are to receive or transmit sound. This observation about the matching of tinnitus to the area of hair cell damage has been well documented. What is not clear is where and how the perception of sound is increased when the reflex arc is disturbed.

Tinnitus usually begins when the hearing loss occurs, but it may be delayed for many months or years. It usually starts and stops suddenly, but it may be gradual in onset. It may fluctuate in intensity and pitch, and it may disappear completely. Nervous tension and increased awareness aggravate it, while relaxation and diminished awareness make it less disturbing. The exact cause for the onset may be obvious, such as exposure to noise, drug intoxication, head injury, etc, or it may begin without apparent cause.

These characteristics of tinnitus make it similar to certain other disorders of sensory perception and motor function, most notably clausalgia, phantom limb pain, trigeminal, facial and glossopharyngeal neuralgia, myopalatal clonus and hemifacial spasm. The pain and/or clonic muscular contractions of these disorders are thought to be due to a central pool of abnormal rhythmic neuronal hyperactivity that becomes facilitated by an alteration in the usual pattern of neural discharge[10] (Fig. 2). Lidocaine, procaine, chlorprocaine, and other local anesthetic agents when given intravenously have a blocking action on each synapse of approximately

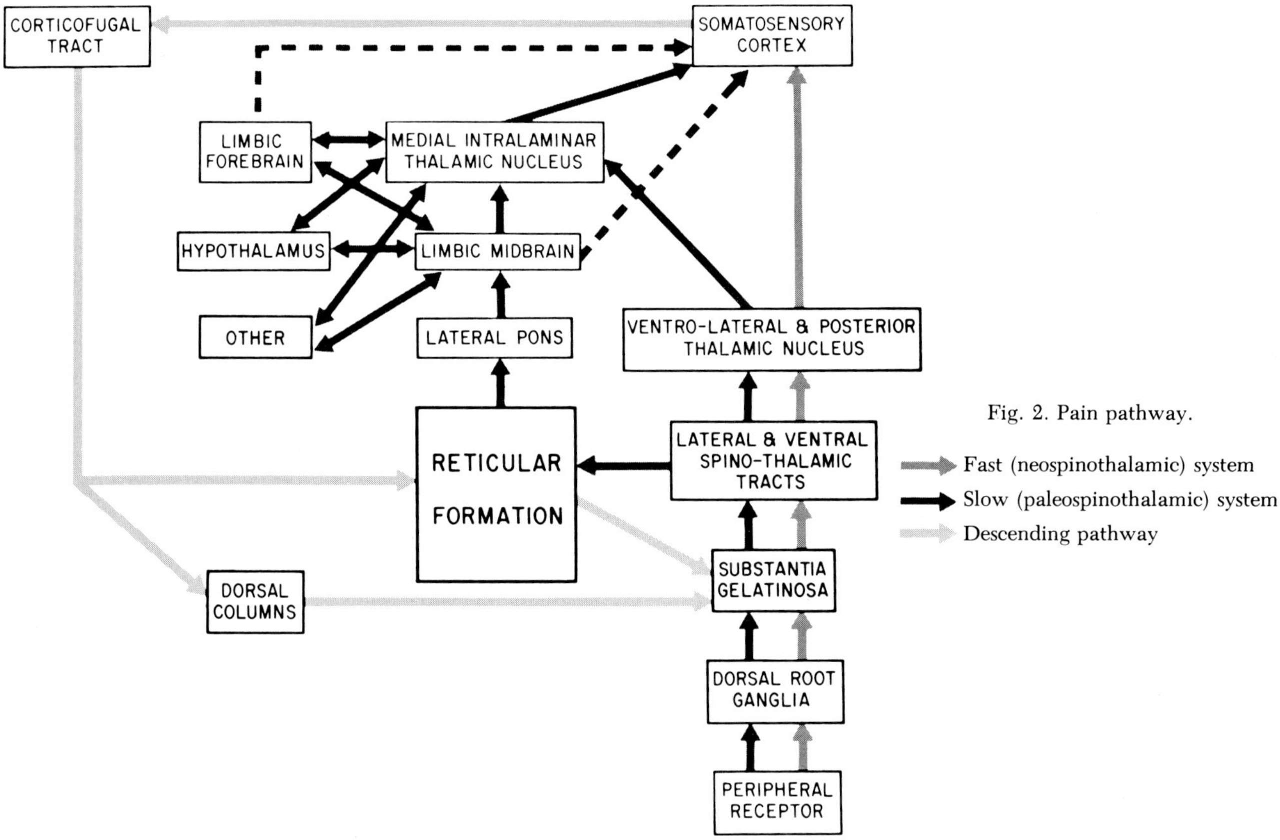

Fig. 2. Pain pathway.

10% but their maximum effect is on the multisynaptic "slow" systems rather than the direct "fast" systems. This effect is well seen in the action of these drugs on chronic visceral pain transmitted through the multisynaptic "slow" paleospinothalamic pathway as opposed to sudden sharp pain or other sensations transmitted through the direct "fast" neospinothalamic pathway.

The similarity of action of these same drugs on tinnitus is very striking: good relief of the low frequency roaring, buzzing white noise as in Menière's disease but less benefit on the high frequency intense ringing. In fact, in many patients with both types of tinnitus the low frequency generalized noise is relieved but the high-pitched intense ringing is made relatively louder, especially at first.

With neural pathways for tinnitus and pain so similar, and with a similar reaction to local anesthetic drugs given intravenously, other similarities are also present. The patients with chronic intractable pain are psychologically similar to the patient with chronic intractable tinnitus — rigid, obsessive, neurotic, insecure, chronically fatigued and depressed — and they respond to local anesthetic drug therapy better if maintained on a combination long-acting anticonvulsant analgesic (perphenazine) and a mood elevator (amitriptyline) such as Etrafon.

The effect of masking on tinnitus would appear to pass through the direct "fast" pathway to block it in the thalamus and cortex, similar to the action of percutaneous and direct neural stimulation of the fast pathway to block the "gate" for pain in the thalamus and cortex. The refractory period for tinnitus and pain occasionally seen after stimulation would also fit into this theory very well.[11]

Bernhard and Bohm[12] described the effect of intravenous lidocaine on epileptic seizures in both experimental animals and human patients. Intravenous lidocaine is known to cause convulsions when given in doses in excess of 10 mg/kg because it selectively blocks the "segmental inhibitory synaptic influences" within the CNS.[13] Intravenous procaine and lidocaine and their oral amides are already widely used to suppress ventricular and other cardiac arrhythmias, which are another form of spontaneous hyperactivity in the conductive neural pathways of the heart. Hatangdi et al[14] extended this concept further and used intravenous lidocaine as a diagnostic test in postherpetic neuralgia.

Intravenous lidocaine has been similarly used in the diagnosis and treatment of intractable central pain in the Pain Clinic of the Auckland General Hospital by Melding et al.[15,16] They observed that some pain patients with coincidental tinnitus reported temporary relief from tinnitus following intravenous lidocaine injection. The duration of temporary relief was quite variable, from three to five minutes to as long as several days, far outlasting the lidocaine effect.

The suppressive effect of lidocaine on tinnitus fits

into this concept very well, since intravenous lidocaine is a potent short-term anticonvulsant as well as a local anesthetic.[12] This concept is strengthened by the observation that in analogous central pain states oral anticonvulsants have caused long-term remissions of pain.[14] Just how oral anticonvulsants work in the central nervous system is not known for sure but they would appear to reduce increased irritability wherever it is present. The next logical step was to give a long-acting oral anticonvulsant to the patients whose tinnitus reacted favorably to the short-acting intravenous lidocaine.[15,16]

Accordingly, 100 mg of lidocaine given rapidly intravenously was used as a test to select patients to be given the oral anticonvulsant treatment. Melding et al[16] found that patients with little or no response to intravenous lidocaine never responded to oral anticonvulsants.

Very often the relief from 100 mg intravenous lidocaine is only temporary, a few minutes, but in some the relief is more prolonged, like the refractory period from a masker, and in a small percentage (about 2%) the relief is permanent. This is not surprising because of the tendency of tinnitus to start suddenly, without apparent cause, even long after the hearing loss begins, and in some patients to stop just as suddenly.

In their series of 125 patients, 56% had excellent or good relief, 24% had only partial relief, and 20% had no relief from tinnitus when given up to 1,000 mg of carbamazepine (Tegretol) daily. They found that lidocaine and carbamazepine are most helpful in patients with hair cell damage, and least helpful to those with conductive hearing loss and other forms of sensorineural hearing loss. Guided by their experience, in 1977 we decided to begin a clinical trial of intravenous lidocaine and smaller doses of oral carbamazepine than had been used by the New Zealand group.

TREATMENT PROGRAM

The patients selected for this study had long-standing intractable tinnitus, and could no longer cope with the problem. Most of them had been seen and treated by several otologists with no relief, and were ready to try anything. All the necessary general and otologic examinations were performed to make the diagnosis, and the tinnitus was matched for pitch and intensity. With the patient supine 100 mg of lidocaine in 5 cc of water was injected intravenously rapidly in 10 to 30 seconds depending on the response of the patient. The patient was asked to report any change in the tinnitus and other sensations in the ear, and the hearing was tested at once. Those patients who had a favorable response to intravenous lidocaine, about 80%, were started on 200 mg of carbamazepine twice a day, the dose being increased weekly by increments of 200 mg to a maximum of 800 mg per day.

Results with carbamazepine were good[17] — 4% complete and 78% partial relief, and 18% no relief (generally the same as reported by Melding et al[16]) — but too many patients experienced serious side effects of the drug, such as depression of the white blood count, liver dysfunction, and diplopia. Because of the serious side effects from carbamazepine, we began a similar study with another short-acting oral anticonvulsant primidone (Mysoline). Our results with primidone were much the same as with carbamazepine, except for less serious side effects, and for that reason it was generally more satisfactory. The usual dose given was 250 mg daily for the first week, 250 mg twice a day the second week, 250 mg three times daily the third week, and finally 250 mg four times daily the fourth, until a good response had been obtained. Fortunately blood dyscrasia and liver damage with primidone are very rare and so the blood count and liver function tests do not need to be monitored with primidone as with carbamazepine.

Because the first pass of primidone through the liver breaks it down into its two component anticonvulsant parts, phenylethylmalonamide and phenobarbital, and phenylethylmalonamide enhances the anticonvulsant action of phenobarbital in animals, we also tried 60 mg of phenobarbital three times a day in patients with a positive response to lidocaine with some benefit. The results were not as good as with primidone or carbamazepine, but interestingly enough, in many patients having benefit from phenobarbital the tinnitus was not only less intense but shifted in frequency from low to higher tone, with very real benefit to the patient. Except for occasional drowsiness phenobarbital was almost without side effects, but unfortunately was of less benefit than primidone, carbamazepine or the original intravenous lidocaine.

It was at this time we learned about a primary amine analog of lidocaine, tocainide hydrochloride, that could be taken by mouth, that was undergoing Phase III clinical trials in patients with cardiac arrhythmias. Tocainide has similar pharmacodynamics to lidocaine, except it can be taken by mouth because it lacks lidocaine's first-pass hepatic degradation. Its half-life is long (11 hours versus 100 minutes for lidocaine) and it is well tolerated by the patient. The most common adverse effects at high doses are central nervous system tremor, dizziness, paresthesia, gastrointestinal anorexia, nausea, and vomiting, and are rapidly reversible upon stopping the drug. No major or permanent side effects have been reported. Cardiac patients have been maintained on daily oral tocainide for periods of up to four years without serious adverse effects, and without regular monitoring of blood chemistries.

A double-blind study involving 31 patients in which one group received 200 mg tocainide four times a day and one group received a placebo re-

TABLE 1. DOUBLE-BLIND DOSE-RANGING STUDY WITH 200 MG TOCAINIDE

No. Patients	*Dose*	*Results*
10	200 mg 4x daily	No statistical difference
10	200 mg 2x daily alternating with matching placebo	
11	Matching placebo 4x daily	

vealed no significant differences in tinnitus relief between the two groups (Table 1). A single-blind study in which 600 mg tocainide four times a day was administered to 12 patients showed 80-98% relief from tinnitus in 10 of the 12 patients who tolerated the drug (Table 2). A double-blind dose-ranging study involving 56 patients who had previously been shown to have a temporary reduction in their level of tinnitus with intravenous lidocaine was begun. Nineteen patients received the active drug (tocainide 600 mg four times daily) throughout the study. Seventeen patients received a matching placebo. Twenty patients received the active drug (tocainide 600 mg twice daily) alternating with a placebo. The tocainide was given every six hours for a total of ten doses[18] (Table 3).

The study was discontinued because of nausea in 6 patients (32%) in the tocainide 600 mg four times daily group, 3 patients (15%) in the tocainide 600 mg twice daily group, and in 2 patients (12%) in the placebo group. Six (46%) of the 13 patients remaining in the tocainide 600 mg four times daily group had 40-100% tinnitus relief. Seven (41%) of the 17 patients remaining in the tocainide 600 mg twice daily group had 40-100% relief. One (7%) of the 15 patients remaining in the placebo group had 40-100% relief.

Not surprisingly these same drugs, intravenous lidocaine, carbamazepine, primidone, and tocainide, are of value in the control of objective tinnitus from palatal myoclonus.

We have observed that in approximately 60% of patients in whom intravenous lidocaine reduces the tinnitus there is a sudden change in the BSER, a shift in the latency of wave V, for as long as the lidocaine effect remains, usually from 10-30 minutes (Fig. 3). Only a shift in latency of 0.3 ms or greater is accepted as that value exceeds typical intrasubject variability, and the prolongation in wave V latency has ranged from 0.3 ms to more than 1 ms. Strangely enough, a significant latency shift in the BSER has never been observed in any patient who reported the tinnitus was unchanged or increased following intravenous lidocaine.

In addition to this effect on the BSER, it would appear that lidocaine acts on the reticular formation where wakefulness is located, because most patients with a good response to intravenous lidocaine will first report numbness of the lips, face and tongue, and then close their eyes and fall asleep as the lidocaine effect on the tinnitus is perceived.

TABLE 2. SINGLE-BLIND STUDY WITH 600 MG TOCAINIDE (N = 12)

No. Patients	*Dose*	*Results*
12	4x daily	80-98% relief

TABLE 3. DOUBLE-BLIND DOSE-RANGING STUDY WITH 600 MG TOCAINIDE (N = 56)

No. Patients	*Dose*	*Pts Experiencing 40-100% Relief*
19	600 mg 4x daily	46%
20	600 mg twice daily alternating with matching placebo	41%
17	Matching placebo four times daily	7%

We began to study the personality of patients with disturbing intractable tinnitus because such a study was already underway in the Pain Clinic of the University of Tennessee in patients receiving the same treatment for chronic intractable pain. As House[19] and others have reported previously, patients with disturbing intractable pain and tinnitus tend to be anxious, inflexible, depressed and obsessive personalities, unable to ignore the pain or tinnitus. While our results are very preliminary we too have verified that patients with disabling intractable tinnitus are similarly desperate, rigid, inflexible, and obsessive, which adds greatly to the problems of management.

Because some of these patients are so fatigued by their battle with tinnitus they are disturbed psychologically and often depressed. We found psychiatric counseling reinforced with one of the mood-elevating tranquilizer combinations such as perphenazine-amitriptyline (Etrafon, Triptafen DA, or Triavil) to be of great value in managing the most disturbed patients.

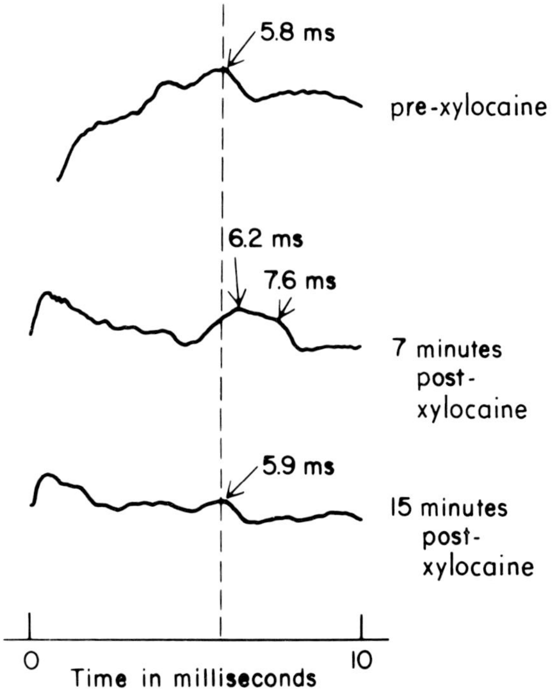

Fig. 3. BSER before and after administration of intravenous lidocaine in patients in whom tinnitus is reduced by the drug.

The widely used and abused drug diazepam (Valium) generally makes patients with chronic pain and intractable tinnitus depressed without relieving the problem and makes them worse.

While awaiting sufficient tocainide to conduct extensive clinical trials we have found that some patients with the most disturbing tinnitus can be managed in much the same way as patients with clausalgia. We give large doses of intravenous lidocaine daily for four or five days to bring the tinnitus under control and then at regular intervals afterwards, usually weekly, to maintain control. We give the first 100 mg rapidly to get an effective blood level and then 400 mg more given slowly with a calibrated intravenous drip, with an EKG monitor running to be sure there is no delay in conduction in the myocardium, which is the only serious hazard of such a large dose of intravenous lidocaine. After such a large and prolonged intravenous dose of lidocaine most patients will have relief from tinnitus from several hours to several days, which is a great help in assuring the patient that something can be done for the tinnitus, so as to learn to cope with it.

It is interesting that intravenous procaine, procainamide, and chlorprocaine, which are more effective than intravenous lidocaine in the control of chronic pain, are less effective than intravenous lidocaine in the relief of tinnitus, which implies that lidocaine exerts a specific effect at one or more places in the ear and/or CNS to control tinnitus. It is interesting that those patients helped by intravenous procaine or procainamide are also helped by procainamide by mouth, but we have refrained from giving procainamide by mouth because of its tendency when given by mouth for long periods of time to sensitize the patient to it and cause a positive test for disseminated lupus erythematosus and in some patients actually cause the disease itself.

Mexilitine, the oral form of the local anesthesia mexitil, was reported by McCormick and Thomas to be ineffective in controlling tinnitus.[20]

Another advantage of medical treatment of tinnitus is that it is of value in patients with little or no hearing with whom maskers and/or hearing aids would be of no value and biofeedback hard to teach.

SUMMARY AND CONCLUSIONS

We believe that the medical management of tinnitus, using intravenous lidocaine, tocainide, and other such new local anesthetic drugs as they are found in the future, supplemented with tranquilizer-mood elevator drugs and psychotherapy, offer real insight into the nature of tinnitus and hope for patients suffering from it. We have found a hearing aid to be of some value in patients with disabling tinnitus associated with a hearing loss, but we have not found a masker to be accepted by the patient if the alternative of drug treatment is available. We have had no experience with biofeedback in the treatment of tinnitus, but it is reasonable to expect it could alter the multisynaptic transmission in the brain and be of value in tinnitus treatment.

Like the patient with chronic disabling pain who refuses to be relieved by whatever is done, the patient with chronic disabling tinnitus is skeptical and resistant to any form of treatment. When the test dose of intravenous lidocaine is given and the tinnitus at least relieved, hope is restored, and the patient for the first time begins to believe that something can be done.

The delay in the wave V that occurs in the BSER and the somnolent state that the intravenous lidocaine induces in those patients who get a reduction in tinnitus from intravenous lidocaine suggests that the drug is acting to block multisynaptic systems within the brainstem and especially in the reticular formation. More detailed work needs to be done to locate and identify the site and mode of action of lidocaine and other local anesthetics and anticonvulsants within the CNS.

The results of our three preliminary studies of tocainide are very promising for affording most patients with disabling tinnitus a method of easily managing their tinnitus and continuing to live productive lives. Several patients in our studies, having experienced the benefits of tocainide by mouth, have traveled to England or Canada to obtain the drug and are very content with sustained reduction of the tinnitus from 60-80%.

As with chronic pain so with disabling tinnitus, some patients with a positive test response to intravenous lidocaine will not get relief from oral anticonvulsants or oral amides of local anesthetics (tocainide) until given the large dose treatment with intravenous lidocaine for one or more days to block the irritable pathway in the brain completely. Having gotten such good relief patients can be maintained on tocainide supplemented with relatively small doses of amitriptyline and perphenazine as compared to the large doses required of the similar drug carbamazepine. Strangely enough, the benefit derived from this drug combination in tinnitus and chronic pain is at a lower dose level than that required to achieve a true psychiatric effect and would appear to be a more direct action on the tinnitus and pain pathway.

While we do not claim to have the final answer in the treatment of tinnitus, we do believe it is the best treatment available and our experience with intravenous lidocaine, carbamazepine, primidone, perphenazine-amitriptyline, and oral tocainide has given us new insights into the nature of tinnitus and offers a promising direction for study.

REFERENCES

1. Saltzman M, Ersner MS. A hearing aid for the relief of tinnitus aurium. Laryngoscope 1947; 57:358-66.

2. Barany R. Die Beeinflussung des Ohrensausens durch intravvenos Injizierte lokalanaesthetica. Acta Otolaryngol (Stockh) 1935; 23:201-3.

3. Lewy RB. Treatment of tinnitus aurium by the intravenous use of local anesthetic agents. Arch Otolaryngol 1937; 25:178-83.

4. Gejrot T. Intravenous xylocaine in the treatment of attacks of Meniere's disease. Acta Otolaryngol (Stockh) 1963; Suppl 188:190-5.

5. Gejrot T. Intravenous xylocaine in the treatment of attacks of Meniere's disease. Acta Otolaryngol (Stockh) 1976; 82:301-2.

6. Englesson S, Larsson B, Lindquist NG, Lyttkens L, Stahle J. Accumulation of ^{14}C-lidocaine in the inner ear. Acta Otolaryngol (Stockh) 1976; 82:297-300.

7. Goodhill V. A tinnitus identification test. Ann Otol Rhinol Laryngol 1952; 61:778-88.

8. Venters RS. Discussion on tinnitus: subjective tinnitus or tinnitus aurium. Proc R Soc Med 1953; 46:825-9.

9. Reed GF. An audiometric study of two hundred cases of subjective tinnitus. Arch Otolaryngol 1960; 71:84-94.

10. Anderson LS, Black RG, Abraham J, Ward AA. Neuronal hyperactivity in experimental trigeminal deafferentiation. J. Neurosurg 1971; 355:444-52.

11. Vernon J. Attempts to relieve tinnitus. J Am Audiol Soc 1977; 2:124-31.

12. Bernhard CG, Bohm E. On the central effects of xylocaine with special reference to its influence on epileptic phenomena. Acta Physiol Scand 1954; 31: Suppl: 114: 5-6.

13. De Jong RH, Robles R, Corbin RW. Central actions of lidocaine — synaptic transmission. Anesthesiology 1969; 30:19-23.

14. Hatangdi VS, Boas RA, Richards EG. In: Bonica JJ, ed. Advances in pain research and therapy. New York: Raven Press, 1976:583-7.

15. Melding PS, Goodey RJ, Thorne PR. The use of intravenous lidocaine in the diagnosis and treatment of tinnitus. J Laryngol Otol 1978; 92:115-21.

16. Melding PS, Goodey RJ, Thorne PR. The treatment of tinnitus with oral anticonvulsants. J Laryngol Otol 1979; 93:111-2.

17. Shea JJ, Harell M. Management of tinnitus aurium with lidocaine and carbamazepine. Laryngoscope 1978; 88:1477-84.

18. Emmett JR, Shea JJ. Treatment of tinnitus with tocainide hydrochloride. Otolaryngol Head Neck Surg 1980; 88:442-6.

19. House JW, Miller L, House PR. Severe tinnitus treatment with biofeedback training. Trans Am Acad Ophthalmol Otolaryngol 1977; 84:697-703.

20. McCormick MS, Thomas JN. A sequential double-blind controlled trial of mexilitine in the relief of tinnitus. Clin Otolaryngol 1980; 5: 79-80.

COMMENT

VICTOR GOODHILL, MD, FACS

LOS ANGELES, CALIFORNIA

Attempts to help patients with tinnitus have challenged physicians for centuries.

What is tinnitus? Is it always abnormal? A healthy person with no ear disease who sits quietly in an audiometric "soundproof" booth or in an anechoic chamber may "hear" internal body sounds. This "visceral tinnitus" is normal and represents an awareness of one's body "at work," of sounds produced by breathing, heart action, blood circulation, middle ear muscle contractions — by normal living.

Fortunately we subconsciously ignore such sounds. If we deliberately try to hear such body sounds we rarely succeed because of the masking effects of environmental sounds. Even in a quiet bedroom at night there is a constant ambient noise level of 20-30 dB sufficient to mask out the ability to hear one's own physiological sounds.

Tinnitus, a troubling human symptom, occurs when such internal signs are of higher intensity levels than the level of masking environmental sounds. It may or may not be of ear origin and is neither a disease nor a syndrome. It must be considered a symptom resulting from any one of a number of lesions.

The otologist can "cure" tinnitus due to cerumen or foreign body impaction in the anterior canal. The tinnitus accompanying otosclerosis is frequently relieved following a successful stapes operation. The tinnitus accompanying secretory otitis media may disappear the moment the fluid is aspirated from the middle ear. The tinnitus of Menière's disease may decrease or disappear following such medical treatments as a low-sodium diet, the use of diuretics or control of allergy, or following certain surgical procedures. Tinnitus due to cochlear drug ototoxicity (such as that caused by salicylates,

From the Department of Surgery (Otology), UCLA Medical School, Los Angeles.

Presented at the meeting of the American Otological Society, Inc., Vancouver, British Columbia, May 9-10, 1981.

REPRINTS — Victor Goodhill, MD, Otosurgical Group Medical Clinic, 469 N. Roxbury Drive, Beverly Hills, CA 90210.

quinine, ototoxic antibiotics, etc) may be relieved by withdrawing the offending drug. Tinnitus due to noise-induced hearing loss or acoustic trauma may be partially relieved by the removal of the offending noise source. The pulsating tinnitus due to a tympanic glomus tumor may be completely relieved following surgery, even if the hearing level is unchanged.

However, there are patients with specific otologic lesions in whom specific otologic therapy is not effective insofar as the tinnitus is concerned. The patient with coexistent cochlear and stapedial otosclerosis may regain considerable hearing following stapedectomy, but the tinnitus may persist because of the cochlear lesion. The patient with tinnitus accompanying Menière's disease may be relieved of vertigo following medical or surgical therapy, but the tinnitus may persist. The patient whose acoustic neurinoma has been successfully removed may still have persistent tinnitus, even if the entire eighth nerve has been resected.

The problem cases are those with decompensated tinnitus. The conversion of decompensated to compensated tinnitus may be accomplished by the otologist. Regardless of the underlying lesion and its therapy, the patient whose tinnitus is a major symptom requires special management which should be carried out by the responsible otologist, rather than by a surrogate therapist.

For many patients the symptom of tinnitus is very frightening. Anxieties regarding the tinnitus may not be volunteered by the patient. Some patients may think that tinnitus is the prelude to total deafness. To others tinnitus implies a sign of a brain tumor. To still others tinnitus means a prelude to a stroke. For some patients tinnitus may be mistakenly interpreted as the beginning of serious mental disease. Although there are remote realities to some of these concerns, for most patients these worries are inappropriate. Such anxieties may even be concealed by the patient.

Simple reassurance as to the real cause and significance of the tinnitus as a component of an ear condition will go far in helping alleviate such anxieties. Inappropriate concerns should be discussed frankly. Reassurance by the physician who carried out the original otologic diagnostic studies and therapy is infinitely more effective than reassurances by another physician or by a psychotherapist.

It is necessary to explain to the patient what ear tinnitus usually represents — that it is real and not imagined, that it is *not* an illusion or a hallucination or a delusion. It is an auditory paresthesia. In this regard it is frequently valuable to give the patient the example of a phantom limb with neuron memory. The amputee with no leg may have "pain" in his absent little toe. The high-pitched tinnitus in a patient with 4 kHz noise-induced hearing loss and a cochlear basal turn lesion may have a "phantom" neuron memory tinnitus comparable to the phantom limb of the amputee.

In the vast majority of patients, the tinnitus accompanying a nonprogressive conductive or sensorineural lesion will become less of a problem with the passage of time. In most patients, such tinnitus may disappear completely as a symptom, but may return temporarily at times of fatigue, stress, or upper respiratory infections. It is thus appropriate and imperative than an optimistic prognosis be given. Such reassurance per se is necessary and will convert decompensated tinnitus in many patients to compensated tinnitus.

J. House has ably delineated the complexity of tinnitus and has outlined the kinds of examinations necessary to localize etiology. He has clarified differences between subjective and objective tinnitus. He has devoted attention to personality factors which might contribute to decompensated tinnitus and he has shared his experiences with biofeedback, tinnitus maskers, and hearing aids in order to accomplish compensated tinnitus in his patients. (I was interested in his report of attempts at tinnitus matching which I tried to accomplish a number of years ago.[1])

He eloquently describes the patients who are "driven to distraction by their tinnitus." It is encouraging to note that in his experience 3 out of 4 patients will obtain "some degree of relief" with biofeedback training. Only a "small group" of his patients have benefitted from the use of tinnitus maskers. I have not used either biofeedback or tinnitus maskers.

Shea and his associates report that "the medical treatment of tinnitus offers the best hope" for management and share their experiences with intravenous lidocaine, tocainamide and other drugs accompanied by psychotherapy. They report favorable responses to these various medical management techniques. I have not used such drugs.

Both House and Shea and his colleagues have alluded to the subjectivity factors in tinnitus and have wisely stressed the need for the high index of suspicion necessary in the examination of the patient with tinnitus in order to avoid missing a serious lesion, emphasizing radiography, electronystagmography, BSER studies, and the entire gamut of contemporary neuro-otologic diagnostic techniques necessary to rule out possible intratemporal and extratemporal lesions.

In both papers there are wise emphases on otologic diagnostic thoroughness and on the avoidance of simplistic mechanistic approaches to the management of the tinnitus patient.

At this point in otologic history there are some disturbing trends which must be faced with reference to the tinnitus problem. Frequently the management of tinnitus patients is nonmedical. For example, Borton et al, in a study on electromyographic feedback treatment for tinnitus aurium,[2] report a detailed study of a single patient in which the relationships between behavioral severity ratings of tinnitus and electromyographic (EMG) activity recorded at the frontalis muscle were investigated. A careful within-subject, double reversal experimental design was utilized. Auditory biofeedback procedures and EMG responses were measured and judged. Psychological strategies were developed by the subject that apparently were associated with increases as well as decreases in EMG activity. However, in this study there is no reported diagnosis of the lesion. The subject in the investigation is described as a 60-year-old female with moderate to severe unilateral sensorineural hearing loss of sudden onset accompanied by severe ringing tinnitus. An audiogram is reproduced. In this very carefully designed and carried out scientific study there is no information regarding otologic examination, radiographic findings, and potential medical diagnostic aspects. We do not know whether this patient had a tumor, a perilymph fistula, labyrinthine hydrops, or any of the many other otologic lesions which can produce a sudden unilateral sensorineural hearing loss.

It is rather difficult to attempt to evaluate the efficacy of electromyographic feedback therapy in a patient whose disease is not even mentioned. The treatment in great detail of the symptom called tinnitus without reference to specific diagnosis is not unusual in contemporary literature.

Another problem which requires serious consideration by the otologic profession is the question of safety and effectiveness of masking devices. In a recent study on tinnitus masking devices,[3] Loavenbruck concludes that "a most serious concern is the question of potential risk to residual hearing and overall health from the continuous noise levels emitted by tinnitus masker devices." The author recommends that until there is sufficient data to indicate safety efficacy of such devices that the use and the presentation of these devices as a form of treatment for tinnitus should be restricted by federal regulatory authorities.

In a recent hearing aid company advertisement, directed primarily to audiologists and hearing aid dispensers, a tinnitus masking hearing aid adapter was advanced as an excellent accessory to help hearing aid users who have tinnitus. How many patients with clear-cut or obscure organic temporal bone lesions or intracranial lesions will now be buying tinnitus maskers from hearing aid dispensers without adequate otologic studies is difficult to assess. Undoubtedly this will occur frequently.

Tinnitus is always a medical problem. It may be due to subjective or objective causes and may not always be associated with a hearing loss. The patient with tinnitus is a medical-otologic responsibility.

Tinnitus is a serious human complaint.[4] I know of no more tragic description of tinnitus than that of Ludwig van Beethoven when he discussed his hearing loss in a letter to his friend Wegeler and had these words to say about his tinnitus: " . . . my ears whistle and buzz continually day and night. I can say I am living a wretched life."

In summary, both House's and Shea's contributions are informative. The management of tinnitus, however, remains a major challenge.

Neither biofeedback, nor complex drug regimens, nor tinnitus maskers are substitutes for that kind of strong and repeated reassurance and support that only the otologist can give to the patient to convert decompensated to compensated tinnitus.

The otologist can be the most effective "stress reducer" and "tinnitus masking force."

REFERENCES

1. Goodhill V. Tinnitus identification test. Ann Otol Rhinol Laryngol 1952; 61:778-86.

2. Borton TE, Moore WH, Clark SR. Electromyographic feedback treatment for tinnitus aurium. J Speech Hear Disord 1981; 46:39-45.

3. Loavenbruck A. Tinnitus masking devices: safe and effective? ASHA 1980; 22:857-61.

4. Goodhill V. Ear diseases, deafness and dizziness. Hagerstown, MD: Harper & Row, 1979; 731-9.

Ann Otol 90:1981

PANEL ON MENIÈRE'S DISEASE

ENDOLYMPHATIC SAC ENHANCEMENT SURGERY FOR MENIÈRE'S DISEASE

AN EXTENSION OF CONSERVATIVE THERAPY

MICHAEL M. PAPARELLA, MD MARCOS GOYCOOLEA, PhD, MD

MINNEAPOLIS, MINNESOTA

It is our hypothesis that the primary goal of endolymphatic sac surgery in cases of intractable Menière's disease or syndrome is for the purpose of enhancing absorption of endolymph. Our experience includes 251 cases over a period of 15 years. In this report we discuss rationale, current methods, and results in a series of 176 cases since 1974.

Whenever a patient consults an otologist for disturbing or incapacitating vertiginous spells usually associated with progressive fluctuant hearing loss due to Menière's disease or syndrome over a long period of time in spite of prolonged medical therapy, in general three choices exist: 1) continue medical therapy, 2) destructive surgery, and 3) conservative surgery.

Continued empirical medical therapy is largely symptomatic and does not alter the progressive course of the disease. The destruction of the vestibular labyrinth or entire labyrinth (labyrinthectomy) or vestibular nerve (vestibular neurectomy) results in total or partial loss of function without any reason to expect preservation or improvement of function. One of several conservative procedures designed to decompress or absorb endolymph can be used with a theoretical opportunity to preserve or improve function. The purpose of this report is to discuss our experience and rationale of utilizing the third approach.

In patients with Menière's disease and Menière's syndrome, the primary intent is to eliminate or reduce vertigo in addition to preserving and, if possible, improving auditory function. Recognizing our inability to definitively treat idiopathic hydrops or Menière's disease, we will discuss our experience and surgical results in attempting to promote endolymphatic sac enhancement since our last series which ended in 1974. We will also discuss the method employed since that time. Our primary indication for surgery was intractable vertigo.

Pathophysiological Considerations. Whether one accepts the longitudinal or radial flow theory of endolymph, or both, or other theories, it is generally understood that endolymphatic hydrops is likely due to an excess of endolymph production or a deficiency of endolymph absorption. The stria vascularis is considered the prime site for endolymph production while the endolymphatic sac is believed to be the most important site for endolymph absorption. Assuming endolymphatic hydrops to be a significant pathological correlate for Menière's disease, any procedure which enhances or improves endolymph absorption should lead to a long-term lessening of hydrops and improvement of symptoms or findings whether due to excessive production or deficient absorption or both.

A group of scientists met at Dusseldorf, Germany, to discuss the current status of research for Menière's disease.[1] In discussing pathogenesis, they considered morphological factors, biochemical interaction, and membrane transport among other things. There was general agreement that our knowledge is scanty and much relevant research is needed. Enzyme systems were discussed, especially sodium-postassium ATPase which is highly concentrated in the stria. The stria is considered to be primarily responsible for the maintenance of the unique ionic composition of the endolymph and for generation of the endocochlear potential. The stria has received more attention than the endolymphatic sac to date. The endolymphatic sac in Menière's disease has been found by some to have perisaccular fibrosis which means increased fibroblastic activity in the subepithelial space. Important investigations of the electrical potentials and ionic profiles of the sac have been initiated by the Dusseldorf team. These investigators found no significant resting potential and potassium approximately nine times lower than that in the cochlear duct. The same team demonstrated for the first time the sac is involved in active transport. Ions were thought to be secreted or ab-

From the Department of Otolaryngology, University of Minnesota, Minneapolis.

Presented at the meeting of the American Otological Society, Inc., Vancouver, British Columbia, May 9-10, 1981.

REPRINTS — Michael M. Paparella, MD, Department of Otolaryngology, University of Minnesota, Minneapolis, MN 55455.

TABLE 1. SYMPTOMS ON WHICH DIAGNOSIS OF MENIÈRE'S DISEASE MADE IN DECREASING ORDER OF IMPORTANCE

90+ % of Diagnosis = History
Vertigo
Hearing loss
Pressure
Tinnitus
Loudness intolerance
Diplacusis
Family history
Stress
Previous treatment

sorbed with little concomitant water flow. They felt it certain, however, that we are dealing with some bulk flow from the cochlear duct towards the sac on a slow time scale. "Leaky" interepithial cell junctions are found in the duct and sac as contrasted to the "tight" junctions in the stria. The epithelial cells of duct and sac produced a mucoprotein substance which might assist endolymph attraction. A cell type occurs in the human duct that is different from any of those found in animals. The experiments of Kimura[1] in which endolymphatic hydrops resulted subsequent to obstruction of the vestibular aqueduct in animals were discussed. The utriculoendolymphatic valve, probably an important mechanism in Menière's disease, was not discussed.

Medical Diagnostic Considerations. In discussing treatment of Menière's disease or Menière's syndrome, it is important to define the disease through diagnosis so that we are discussing the same thing. The diagnosis of Menière's disease is largely (90%) made from the history. History is based on the symptoms in Table 1 with vertigo, hearing loss, and pressure being most important. Patients are strongly advised to answer the questions briefly and succinctly as it is well known such patients have a high anxiety apprehension titer. Ancillary tests, but especially audiometry and ENG, are essential. The early low tone loss leading to a flat audiometric lesion in Menière's disease is well known. In many patients we noted a peak audiometric pattern with comparatively good hearing at 2,000 Hz with poorer hearing below and above that point to be a common configuration (Fig. 1). The patient is treated conservatively for a long period of time using all the various empirical methods of management. In our opinion, the most important aspect of conservative treatment is psychological assurance whether used preoperatively or postoperatively. Other diagnoses are ruled out, and although glycerol tests are done routinely, they have not demonstrated predictive significance in these cases.

Surgical Rationale. It is generally axiomatic in medicine that given equal outcomes preservation or improvement of function in the treatment of disease is preferable to destruction of function. In Menière's disease, many currently advocate vestibular neurectomy as the preferable surgical approach after failure of medical therapy for vertigo.[2] This procedure

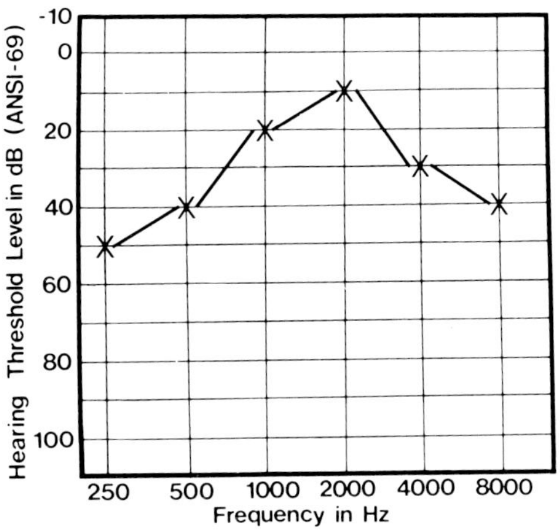

Fig. 1. Characteristic peak audiogram with better hearing at 2000 Hz.

which is intracranial instead of otological can have grave risks, including loss of hearing. Moreover, as we have seen, many patients with Menière's disease (D. Austin estimates 40%; personal communication) develop the disease in the second ear which might occur many years after initial disease in the first ear. As we shall see, the risk of carefully done endolymphatic sac surgery (cochlear deafness) is 2% or the same as carefully done stapedectomy surgery for otosclerosis. Recognizing the disease leads to often fluctuant but progressive sensorineural hearing loss over time, this risk factor seems reasonable. For these and other reasons, we practice an extension of conservative therapy which is endolymphatic sac enhancement. If the second ear becomes involved subsequently, we are grateful for making every attempt to preserve and improve function in the first ear.

SURGICAL METHOD

The salient stepwise features of the method currently employed are as follows:

1. A complete simple mastoidectomy using a postauricular approach, thinning the posterior bony canal wall, enlarging the aditus and identification of the incus.

2. Drilling of the solid angle to but *never* below the level of the dome of the horizonal semicircular canal.

3. Thinning of bone over Trautmann's triangle and lateral sinus.

4. Using a fenestrometer 10 mm is measured from the tip of the short process of the incus or fossa incudis along the axis of the horizontal semicircular canal (30° from the tegmen) and a point is mentally marked; then 12 mm is measured from the fossa incudis at an angle of 45° from the tegmen and another point mentally marked. This demarcation zone is never invaded as it includes the posterior inferior semicircular canal which must be avoided.

5. The dura is uncovered by removing bone around the zone and in an exaggerated way in the infralabyrinthine cell tract or region as the sac is commonly found inferior and anterior to the inferior tip of the posterior semicircular canal.

6. If there is no Trautmann's triangle, the lateral sinus is decompressed and retracted downward to gain access below the posterior semicircular canal.

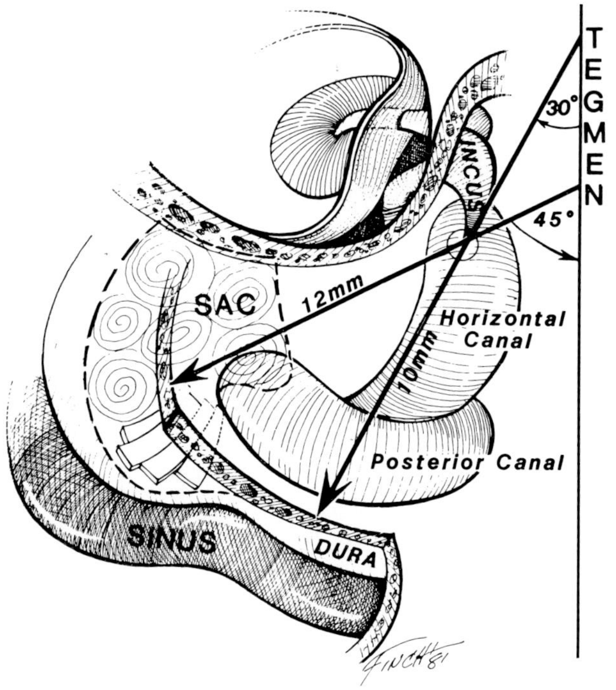

Fig. 2. Surgeon's view inside of mastoid. The posterior canal wall is thinned. Depth of drilling is carried to but *never* below the dome of the horizontal semicircular canal. 10 mm are measured from the fossa incudis (circle) along the axis of the horizontal canal and 12 mm are measured about 45° from the tegmen using a fenestrometer. Removal of bone exposes dura of posterior cranial fossa and if need be the lateral sinus around the demarcated bony zone. The endolymphatic sac is seen in the infralabyrinthine region containing T-shaped coiled Silastic with extensions and spacers seen posteriorly.

7. The sac is entered beneath the solid bony shelf by depressing dura, opening the sac with sickle knife and bluntly probing the sac lumen to see the shiny epithelial lining. An inserted Whirlybird can usually be twirled gently within the sac.

8. Silastic sheeting (0.01 cm) is cut in T-shaped struts (usually two) and several spacers of Silastic are cut. The Silastic T struts are coiled within the sac with a stem entering into the mastoid. Spacers are used to separate the dura from the bone of the posterior canal (Fig. 2).

9. Gelfoam moistened with an antibiotic steroid solution is placed on top.

10. Gold foil is then applied over the Gelfoam to prevent postoperative fibroblastic invasion of the sac. A fascial graft is placed on top and held with additional Gelfoam. A myringotomy tube is usually placed in the tympanic membrane to assist postoperative healing unless the subarachnoid space is uncovered (a rare occurrence).

11. Meticulous attention must be paid to removing bone dust, debris, etc, from the wound to avoid postoperative wound infection which can quickly spread to labyrinthitis.

The primary goal is to enhance endolymph absorption function. The steps which are designed to help achieve this include: 1) enlargement of the sac, 2) releasing bony pressure on the sac, 3) providing intralumenal surfaces of Silastic along which nanoliters of endolymph can diffuse, 4) providing collateral blood supply, and 5) use of gold foil to prevent fibroblastic postoperative sac invasion.

Of the various surgical pitfalls, the most important is nonentry of the sac lumen. The lumen must be bluntly probed and the shiny epithelium seen. It is easy to create a false lumen in the fibrous dura. Another pitfall to be avoided is inadvertently entering the posterior semicircular canal. Exposure of the sac in the infralabyrinthine cell tract which leads to the jugular bulb region and our method of measurement help avoid the above two pitfalls. Other pitfalls include bleeding from the lateral sinus (treated by pressure and Gelfoam), exposure of spinal fluid, and postoperative wound infection, all of which should be controllable.

TABLE 2. MENIÈRE'S SYNDROME CASES (N = 21)

Chronic or recurrent otitis media and Menière's syndrome	6
Delayed hydrops	4
Otosclerosis and Menière's syndrome	3
Posttraumatic hydrops	3
Lues and Menière's syndrome	5

RESULTS

Results from sac surgery must be considered soft, not hard data, as contrasted with destructive procedures such as labyrinthectomy or vesticular neurectomy where results could be considered more definitive. This is because with sac surgery the underlying disease continues although symptoms and findings may improve because of presumed enhancement of endolymph absorption. Several patients with frequent daily or weekly episodes of vertigo have been observed over a period of years in whom vertigo was eliminated only to recur with less frequency, for example, three years after surgery. Moreover, the indications for surgery and the many variables of Menière's disease and Menière's syndrome will profoundly influence any reported results.

In a previous report, 75 cases of endolymphatic sac surgery were discussed.[3] Since that series ended in 1974, 176 patients have received surgery for a total personal series of 251 cases over a period of 15 years. In the present study, 21 patients had Menière's syndrome in which a known causative factor was identified while 155 cases had idiopathic vertigo and/or hearing loss (presumed hydrops) or Menière's disease.

We use and agree with the variations of Menière's described in the AAOO committee report which includes vestibular Menière's and cochlear Menière's disease.[4] Of the 176 cases discussed here, 155 were considered to have Meniére's disease while 21 had Menière's syndrome with known causes (Table 2).

Results occurring in the Menière's disease group are seen in Table 3. Duration of Menière's disease in this group prior to surgery ranged from 1 to 26 years with an average duration of 6.8 years. Patients' ages were from 9 to 80 years of age, the average being 46 years. Ten patients who developed Menière's disease in childhood are included in the classical Menière's disease group. Follow-up varied from a minimum of 6 months, as of this writing, to 72 months, with an average of 30.5 months. Because of the small numbers, the percentages listed for groups other than classical Menière's disease are of little relevance.

TABLE 3. RESULTS IN 155 CASES CORRELATING SYMPTOMS AND MENIÈRE'S DISEASE DIAGNOSIS

Category	*Number*	*Vertigo*	*Hearing*	*Pressure*	*Tinnitus*	
Classical Menière's disease	132	11 (8%)	71 (55%)	20 (15%)	28 (21%)	Same
		22 (17%)	58 (44%)	78 (59%)	67 (51%)	Better
		1 (1%)	2 (1.7%)	3 (2%)	0	Worse
		98 (74%)	1 (1%)	31 (24%)	37 (28%)	Eliminated
Vestibular Menière's disease	12	0		1 (8%)		Same
		1 (8%)		6 (50%)		Better
		0		0		Worse
		11 (92%)		5 (42%)		Eliminated
Cochlear Menière's disease	7		5 (72%)	5 (72%)	4 (57%)	Same
			2 (28%)	2 (28%)	3 (43%)	Better
			0	0	0	Worse
			0	0	0	Eliminated
Previous surgery (tack)	4	0	3 (75%)	0	0	Same
		1 (25%)	1 (25%)	3 (75%)	3 (75%)	Better
		0	0	0	0	Worse
		3 (75%)	0	1 (25%)	1 (25%)	Eliminated

Often the second ear showed some form of sensorineural hearing loss in unilateral Menière's. On occasion, although the characteristic peak audiometric configuration was seen, the patient might not have any symptoms referable to the second ear. It seems likely in many patients considered to have unilateral disease that the opposite side is involved but has not become clinically manifest. The relative frequency of bilaterality, of course, influences the results. In many instances, the second ear became involved years following initial disease in the first ear.

Revision sac surgery was done in only four ears in this series, in which the primary procedure was done by the authors in two cases and by others in two cases. In each instance, the lumen had not been adequately identified and created, mostly because of lack of dural exposure along the infralabyrinthine cell tract or space especially since the cell tract did not exist in these patients.

Four patients in the classical Menière's disease category had Menière's disease in an only hearing ear. In each case, the opposite labyrinth was functionless due to another disease process earlier in the patient's lifetime. In each instance, surgery was reluctantly considered only when the hearing dropped to moderate or severe levels with prolonged incapacitating vertigo. These cases are of special interest in assessing the procedure because of the elimination of influence from the opposite ear. In each of these cases, vertigo was eliminated and hearing improved. These cases, as was true of vestibular Menière's, turned out to have the best results in that vertigo was eliminated while hearing, pressure and tinnitus were dramatically improved (Fig. 3).

Based on personal experience, the patient is advised of the pros and cons of sac enhancement surgery in the following way. There is approximately a 90% or greater chance of improvement of vertigo (less frequent and/or less intense episodes) and approximately a 70% or greater chance of elimination of vertigo. Although some of the patients in the 8th percentile were judged to have similar vertigo postoperatively as compared to preoperatively, with careful questioning most in this group showed some slight improvement. To date, not a patient in this series (according to our records) has required a labyrinthectomy or vestibular neurectomy. The patient is advised of approximately a 40% or so chance that the hearing will improve, a 98% chance hearing will be preserved with a major risk factor consisting of approximately 2% severe cochlear deafness postoperatively. Psychological reassurance, and if need be, medical treatment are applied postoperatively the same way they are used preoperatively.

DISCUSSION

Since the initial description of endolymphatic sac surgery by Portmann[5] and the reintroduction of the procedure by House,[6] a number of others have described the efficacy of this approach. In our opinion, it is an established method for managing Menière's disease and/or syndrome. It is our hypothesis that the procedure, when successful, enhances absorption of endolymph thus decreasing endolymphatic hydrops and associated symptoms. The fact that function is retained or restored with little risk renders this procedure a natural extension of conservative therapy.

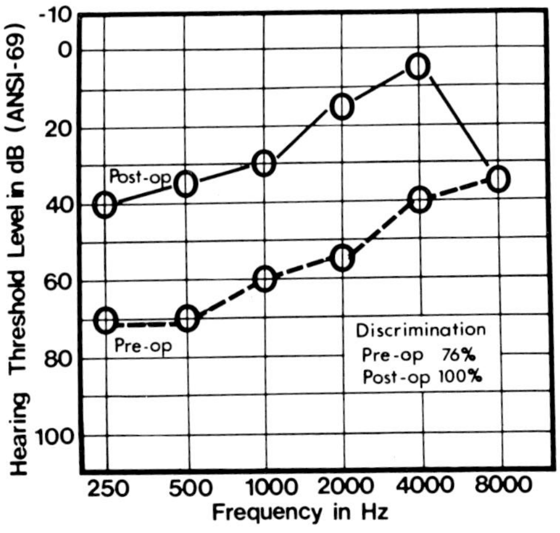

Fig. 3. Preoperative and postoperative audiograms in a patient with classical Menière's disease in an only hearing ear.

The method described is intended to enhance absorption of endolymph in the sac. There are approximately 4 to 6 μl of endolymph in a normal human temporal bone (Juhn SK, personal observations). With idiopathic endolymphatic hydrops, perhaps that number could be doubled. When endolymph reaches the sac, minute volume amounts of endolymph are involved, probably measured in nanoliters (1000th of 1 μl). The shunt[6] and valve method[7] probably work for the same reasons described here. Endolymph during sac surgery is never seen in any abundance, the characteristic feature being shiny epithelium lining the lumen of the sac. Moreover, it is hard to conceive of nanoliters of endolymph reaching, let alone moving, a valve enormous in comparison.

It appears feasible that by enlarging the sac lumen, providing surfaces (Silastic sheeting) along which endolymph can pass by surface pressure, improving collateral blood supply and removing bony pressure, endolymphatic absorption will be improved. Indeed, these results are an improvement over our last reported results and it is believed this is so because of better accomplishing the surgical objectives. There are many variables, too numerous to discuss here, wherein pathological manifestations of disease interact with the surgical approach.

It is our belief that the utriculoendolymphatic valve plays an important role in the pathogenesis of vestibular Menière's as compared to cochlear Menière's and in classical Menière's in which on the one hand vertigo is the dominant symptom whereas on the other hand cochlear loss is the dominant symptom in many patients. Schuknecht[8] previously described the importance of utriculoendolymphatic valve in separating the pars superior from the pars inferior in explaining episodic attacks of Menière's. We believe the function of the valve is important in explaining patients' symptomatology and the results achieved from sac enhancement surgery as well. For example, patients with vestibular Menière's did very well in terms of elimination of vertigo as did classical Menière's patients in whom vertigo was a severe symptom up until time of surgery.

Vertigo is the primary indication for surgery in this series although hearing gain subsequent to surgery defined by the AAOO guidelines seemed better than our last report. In addition to the role of the utriculoendolymphatic valve, as mentioned above, it is likely that patients with recent fluctuant hearing loss or temporary threshold shift due to Menière's have a better chance of hearing gain from surgery than those with permanent threshold shift.

It is fortuitous that the endolymphatic sac is located at a remote site from the rest of the labyrinth. This location allows for a transmastoid exposure and probably a built-in safety factor so the effects of surgical or medical treatment of the sac should cause no direct harm to the labyrinthine endorgans. This feature may some day prove useful for treating other diseases of the endolymphatic system.

Although there is a paucity of research on the sac, morphological studies appear with greater frequency in the literature which influence our understanding of the disease. Some authors have described nonvisualization of the vestibular aqueduct using polytomography.[9] Temporal bone studies have not confirmed closure of the aqueduct in Menière's patients.[10] It is probable that obstruction of the vestibular aqueduct occurs rarely, if at all, in Menière's disease. On the other hand, as we observed in these cases, many patients have apparently abnormal structures within the mastoid, especially including the position of the lateral sinus and definition of Trautmann's triangle. These structural abnormalities which will be the subject of another study are especially notable in patients with Menière's syndrome following previous chronic otitis media and mastoiditis. Such changes could influence endolymphatic sac and duct development and ultimate function. If there are structural deformities, perhaps a promotion of collateral blood supply might assist endolymph absorption.

The method of measurement to avoid the posterior inferior semicircular canal derives from our previous study in which gross anatomical characteristics of the sac were measured in patients and in dry temporal bone specimens.[11] These studies also confirm the presence of the sac in a more anterior and inferior location relative to the inferior tip of the posterior canal as we originally thought. This observation is confirmed by Arenberg[7] and D. Plester (personal communication). Exposure of this region (infralabyrinthine) has consistently led to visualization and treatment of the sac lumen, which is from our observation critical to optimizing the success of the procedure.

REFERENCES

1. Report of Post Symposium Conference, International Symposium on Pathogenesis, Diagnosis and Treatment of Meniere's Disease, Dusseldorf, Germany, May 12-14, 1980.

2. Fisch U, Sterkers JM, Garcia-Ibanez E. First International Symposium on Recent Advances in Ear Surgery. Alexandria, Egypt, March 30, 1981.

3. Paparella MM, Hanson D. Endolymphatic sac drainage for intractable vertigo (method and experiences). Laryngoscope 1976; 86:697-703.

4. Alford BR. Meniere's: criteria for diagnosis and evaluation of therapy for report. Committee on hearing and equilibrium. Trans Acad Ophthamol Otolaryngol 1979; 1462-4.

5. Portmann G. Surgical treatment by opening of the saccus endolymphaticus. Arch Otolaryngol 1927; 6:309-19.

6. House WF. Subarachnoid shunt for drainage of endolymphatic hydrops. Laryngoscope 1962; 72:713-29.

7. Arenberg IK. Endolymphatic sac valve implant surgery. Laryngoscope 1979; 89:Suppl 17 26-39.

8. Schuknecht HF. Further observations on the pathology of Meniere's disease, Ann Otol Rhinol Laryngol 1962; 71:1039-53.

9. Clemis J, Valvassori G. Recent radiographic and clinical observations on the vestibular aqueduct. A preliminary report. Otolaryngol Clin North Am 1968; 339-46.

10. Yuen S, Schuknecht HF. The vestibular aqueduct and endolymphatic duct in Meniere's disease. Arch Otolaryngol 1972; 96:553-5.

11. Shea D, Chole R, Paparella MM. The endolymphatic sac: anatomical considerations. Laryngoscope 1979; 89:88-94.

METABOLIC MANAGEMENT IN MENIÈRE'S DISEASE

BRUCE PROCTOR, MD
DETROIT, MICHIGAN

CONRAD PROCTOR, MD
ROYAL OAK, MICHIGAN

Pollution in the bloodstream by abnormal amounts of metabolites (sugar, insulin, triglycerides and cholesterol) over an extended period of time will have an adverse effect upon the small blood vessels: the arterioles, capillaries and venules. If the microcirculation of the inner ear becomes afflicted, it may produce endolymphatic hydrops. Control of blood pollution can usually be achieved by intelligent dietary management; and, in the case of Menière's disease, the clinical relief is gratifying. Carbohydrate and lipid metabolism is complicated. If the new insulin-glucose tolerance test is used, it will detect many more cases of glucose intolerance. Fifty consecutive cases of Menière's disease were studied for abnormal levels of metabolites. Thirty-eight (76%) of these cases had either an abnormal glucose tolerance test (using the Wilkerson point system) or at least borderline insulin levels: a) abnormal insulin levels, 35 cases; b) borderline insulin values, 3 cases; c) abnormal glucose tolerance with normal insulin values, no cases; d) both normal glucose tolerance and normal insulin production, 12 cases.

INTRODUCTION

Menière's disease, with its characteristic fluctuating sensorineural hearing loss, episodic vertigo, tinnitus and fullness in the affected ear, is inconstant, both in its behavior and in its response to treatment. Its puzzling remissions and exacerbations with periodicity make evaluation of treatment methods difficult. Remissions may be frequent or at long intervals. Most remissions last from six months to six years in 80% of cases. In a long-term study of 200 cases reported by McNally et al,[1] the interval of remissions averaged four years in length. Results of any form of treatment must, therefore, be assessed in the light of unpredictable remissions.

Because attacks of Menière's may occur at varying intervals, with or without treatment, whether medical or surgical, great care and extended time are essential in establishing effectiveness of procedures. Symptomatic relief refers to the immediate relief following the use of medications. Temporary relief would indicate freedom from dizziness for at least six months. Cures should not be assessed until five years have elapsed. Clinical documentation of studies of results of procedures must be carefully made over a period of several years, perhaps as many as ten, before valid conclusions can be drawn.

Clinically satisfactory results have been obtained in approximately 90% of all Menière's cases, in relieving bouts of vertigo with medical treatments. In view of this fact, medical treatment, with surgery as a last effort, is the preferred way to go. Intractable vertigo which has incapacitated an individual is the only basis for the more radical surgical method, when everything else has failed.

The preservation of hearing is an important consideration in the decision for surgery. It remains to be proven that there is sustained preservation or improvement of hearing to warrant an attempt to preserve hearing in surgery for Menière's disease. This is true particularly at an early stage, when hearing may be fluctuating.

There are two phases of medical treatment of Menière's. First, to obtain symptomatic relief from acute vestibular symptoms. Second, to plan a course of treatment with the objective of palliating and even curing the disease. The latter may take one of several directions, depending upon what the etiology is thought to be. These may be metabolic disorders, vasomotor disturbances, allergies, endocrine diseases, syphilis, avitaminosis, toxic factors and psychogenic disorders.

We will, therefore, present the possible effects of disorders of glucose metabolism and/or unsaturated fatty acid metabolism upon inner ear disturbance, with particular reference to Menière's disease.

From Wayne State University, School of Medicine, Detroit, and William Beaumont Hospital Research Institute, Royal Oak, Michigan.
Presented at the meeting of the American Otological Society, Inc., Vancouver, British Columbia, May 9-10, 1981.
REPRINTS — Bruce Proctor, MD, 3535 West 13 Mile Road, Royal Oak, MI 48072.

TABLE 1. WILKERSON POINT SYSTEM

Time	*Plasma Glucose (mg/100 ml)*	*Wilkerson Points**
Fasting	130 or more	1.0
1 hr	195 or more	0.5
2 hr	140 or more	0.5
3 hr	130 or more	1.0

*Two points or more are judged diagnostic of diabetes.

METHOD

Fifty cases (consecutive) of Menière's were studied as outpatient cases. Twenty-seven patients were females, whereas 23 were males. The average age was 45, with a range from 18 to 71. A metabolic workup on all 50 patients included a 5-hour insulin-glucose tolerance test. This was preceded by a 3-day, 300 g daily carbohydrate diet. In order to more easily detect low sugar levels, after 100 g of glucose, blood sugar levels were obtained at 2½ and 3½ hours, as well as at the standard fasting, 30-minute, 1-, 2-, 3-, 4- and 5-hour times. Insulin levels were determined at fasting, 30-minute, 1-, 2-, 3-, and 4-hour times. Serum cholesterol and triglycerides were obtained after a 14-hour fast and prior to the 3-day prep diet. Other studies included a CBC (to rule out anemia, blood dyscrasia, etc), FTI (complete thyroid workup when FTI was abnormal, to rule out hyothyroidism, etc), VDRL and/or FTA-ABS, and fasting serum cortisol (to rule out adrenal disorders). The total cost of metabolic studies was approximately $500.

The glucose tolerance test was evaluated according to the Wilkerson Point System (Table 1), as recommended by the American Diabetes Association.[2] If the fasting glucose was 130 or more mg %, the patient was given 1 Wilkerson point; if the 1-hour glucose was 195 or more, 0.5 Wilkerson point; if the 2-hour glucose was 140 or more, 0.5 Wilkerson point; and if the 3-hour glucose was 130 or more, 1 Wilkerson point. The glucose tolerance test was considered abnormal (and the patient was judged a diabetic) when the total number of Wilkerson points was two or more. If the patient had 0.5 to 1½ Wilkerson points, the glucose tolerance test was considered equivocal, or borderline.

Following Kraft's criteria,[3] insulin levels were considered abnormal if 1) the 2-hour level was 50 or more microunits, 2) the sum of the 2-hour and 3-hour values exceeded 100 μU, 3) the fasting insulin was above 50μU, 4) all insulin values were below 30μU, 5) the peak insulin value occurred after one hour. Insulin levels were borderline if the total of the 2-hour and 3-hour levels was greater than 60 but less than 100μU. Kraft's criteria were based on 3,650 patients randomly referred for glucose tolerance testing. These patients serve as the controls for this study. The average age of Kraft's patients was 46, with 64% being female, 36% male.

Fasting cholesterol and triglycerides were age-adjusted, according to Fredrickson and Levy.[4] Up to age 19, cholesterol over 230 mg% and triglycerides over 150 mg% were considered clearly abnormal. At age 20 and over, triglycerides of over 200 were abnormal. Cholesterol was abnormal ages 20-29 if over 240, ages 30-39 if over 270, ages 40-49 if over 310, and age 50 or more if over 330. Patients were considered to have borderline hyperlipidemia when either cholesterol exceeded 220 or triglycerides exceeded 150 below the age of 55.

RESULTS

The results of these studies were noteworthy. Thirty-eight of the 50 Menière's patients (76%) were found to have either an abnormal glucose tolerance test or at least borderline insulin levels. Thirty-five patients (70%) had clearly abnormal insulin levels, with another three (6%) having borderline insulin values. There were no patients having abnormal glucose tolerance with normal insulin values. Twelve patients had both normal glucose tolerance and normal insulin production. One (2%) of the Menière's patients had abnormal glucose tolerance according to Wilkerson's criteria (2 points or more), with eight patients having borderline glucose tolerance (0.5 to 1½ Wilkerson points). Ten patients had glucose levels which fell below 50 during the glucose tolerance test.

Nine patients (18%) demonstrated definite hyperlipidemia with elevated triglycerides (Type IV), none having type IIA (elevated cholesterol), none having type IIB (elevated cholesterol and triglycerides) hyperlipidemia. Another 11 patients had borderline hyperlipidemia, according to Fredrickson's criteria. Only thirty patients (60%) had completely normal age-adjusted serum cholesterol and triglycerides after the 14-hour fast. Four patients (8%) had abnormal fasting serum cortisol determinations.

Patients with abnormal glucose or insulin values were instructed to follow a low-carbohydrate high-protein diet with interval feedings. Cholesterol and/or triglyceride intake was limited when indicated according to the lipoprotein phenotype.

The response to treatment in the 38 patients with abnormal glucose and/or insulin values was gratifying. Applying the criteria of the Committee on Hearing and Equilibrium[5] (vertigo control means absence of definitive vertigo spells for ten times the average interval between spells before treatment), 35 of the 38 Menière's patients (92%) with abnormal insulin levels achieved control of their vertigo. Three patients of the 38 (8%) improved hearing to normal levels. Four patients of the 38 (10%) reported absence of tinnitus.

DISCUSSION

We are concerned in this study with abnormal glucose metabolism and its possible effects on microcirculation in the inner ear. Newer laboratory tests and their interpretation by internists researching in this field may help in the medical management of some cases of Menière's disease.

In 1980,[6] the AMA "estimated" there are 6.5 million diabetics in the United States (1.9 million receiving insulin injections), with another 1.8 million undiagnosed. Kraft[3] believes that the best means of diagnosing diabetes mellitus "in situ" is with the insulin-glucose tolerance test. Updegraft[7] states that the most common cause of vertigo is impaired carbohydrate and insulin metabolism. He also noted that when diabetes is manifest and insulin-dependent, vertigo occurs much less frequently.

The role of insulin in the formation of hypertriglyceridemia must also be evaluated in these patients. Not only did 76% of the 50 Menière's disease patients in this study exhibit some degree of abnormality in insulin levels, but 9 patients (18%) also showed a triglyceride abnormality. Olefsky et al[8] have proposed a scheme that states: insulin resistance → hyperinsulinemia → increased triglyceride production rate → increased plasma triglyceride levels. In other words, he believes that insulin plays an important role in the genesis of hypertriglyceridemia through its influence on triglyceride production. Olefsky[9] has also shown more recently that insulin deficiency is the cause of blood-sugar rises in the insulin-dependent type I "juvenile" diabetic patient, but that insulin resistance is commonly at work in the noninsulin-dependent type II diabetic patient. The main cause of insulin resistance appears to involve target-tissue defects, either at the receptor or postreceptor site.

Abnormal metabolites circulating in the blood may be considered as a form of pollution. They may well have a profound effect on the microcirculation of the inner ear. Hawkins[10] has demonstrated pathological findings in the organ of Corti of patients with diabetes, aging, ototoxic drugs, and even noise exposure. These changes were loss of outer hair cells and their replacement by extensions of the phalangeal plates that form scars. He felt that the common factor in injury to the inner ear in these patients involved gradual devascularization. Even though outer hair cells were considerably hardier in the face of anoxia than the stria vascularis, they ultimately depended upon the blood flow through the inner and less constant outer spiral vessels.[11] Vasoconstriction appeared to be the dominant pathological finding of Hawkins in diabetes, aging, ototoxic drugs, and noise-induced hearing loss.

In 1977, Stout[12] reported that exposure of arterial tissue to insulin results in proliferation of smooth muscle cells, inhibition of lipolysis, and synthesis of cholesterol, phospholipid, and triglyceride. He reasoned that chronic exposure to elevated insulin levels would result in the development of lipid-filled lesions which would promote changes in the arteries and eventually progress to atherosclerosis.

Schuknecht,[13] in examining 11 temporal bones of diabetics, found changes in small blood vessels that appeared specific for diabetes mellitus, namely, greater intimal thickening and PAS deposits in the capillaries and arterioles.

CONCLUSION

Fifty patients with Menière's disease were studied with regard to their glucose metabolism. Metabolic testing consisted of a 5-hour glucose tolerance test with insulin levels and a lipid profile. Thirty-five patients (70%) had clearly abnormal insulin levels. Nine patients (18%) had definite hyperlipidemia, eleven (22%) had borderline hyperlipidemia, and 30 (60%) had completely normal cholesterol and triglycerides. (The incidence of hyperlipidemia in the world's population is only 5%.[14]) Seventy-six percent of the patients were noted to have either abnormal glucose tolerance or at least slightly abnormal insulin levels.

Patients with abnormal glucose tolerance or abnormal insulin levels were treated with a multiple-feeding, low-carbohydrate high-protein diet, with restriction of cholesterol and/or triglycerides in appropriate cases. Ninety-two percent of the appropriate patients treated with this diet achieved control of their vertigo on a temporary relief basis.

As a result of these findings, it becomes apparent that the earliest identification of carbohydrate imbalance with an insulin-glucose tolerance test is extremely important in the management of Menière's disease. Hyperlipidemia is often associated with inner ear dysfunction; but impaired circulation, possibly resulting from abnormal glucose and insulin levels, may be the primary cause of Menière's disease. The standard glucose tolerance test is of little value in diagnosing abnormal carbohydrate metabolism unless it is done concurrently with insulin levels.

REFERENCES

1. McNally WJ, Stuart EA, McKercher DD, Lockhart HB. A review of two hundred cases of vertigo. Proc Fourth Intern Congress Otolaryngol London 1949; 195-239.

2. Standardization of the oral glucose tolerance test. Report of Committee on Statistics Am Diab Assoc June 14, 1968. Diabetes 1969; 18:299-307.

3. Kraft JR. Detection of diabetes mellitus in situ (occult diabetes). Lab Med 1975; 6:10-22.

4. Fredrickson DS, Levy RI. The dietary management of hyperlipoproteinemia: a handbook for physicians and dieticians. Natl Heart Lung Inst, Natl Inst Health Bethesda, 1973.

5. Alford BR. Committee on hearing and equilibrium. Meniere's disease: criteria for diagnosis and evaluation of therapy for reporting. Trans Am Acad Opthalmol Otolaryngol 1972; 76:1462-4.

6. AMA News July 18, 1980; 23:1.

7. Updegraff WR. Impaired carbohydrate metabolism and idiopathic Meniere's disease. Ear Nose Throat J 1977; 56:160-3.

8. Olefsky JM, Farquhar JW, Reaven GM. Reappraisal of the role of insulin in hypertriglyceridemia. Am J Med 1974; 57:551-60.

9. Olefsky JM. Beyond the beta cell. Diabetes Forcast 1980; 53:26-8.

10. Hawkins JE Jr. Comparative otopathology: aging, noise and ototoxic drugs. Adv Otorhinolaryngol Basel: Karger 1973; 20:125-41.

11. Lawrence M, Wever EG. Effects of oxygen deprivation upon the structure of the organ of corti. Arch Otolaryngol 1952; 55:31-7.

12. Stout RW. The relationship of abnormal circulating insulin levels to atherosclerosis. Atherosclerosis 1977; 27:1-13.

13. Schuknecht H. Pathology of the ear. Cambridge: Harvard Univ Press, 1974.

14. Proctor C. Diagnosis, prevention and treatment of hereditary sensorineural hearing loss. Laryngoscope 1977; 87 Suppl 7:1-60.

COMMENT

HAROLD F. SCHUKNECHT, MD
BOSTON, MASSACHUSETTS

Paparella is of the opinion that the endolymphatic saccotomy procedure enhances the resorption of endolymph, thus decreasing endolymphatic hydrops and its associated symptoms. He feels that by enlarging the sac lumen, providing Silastic surfaces along which endolymph can pass by surface pressure, improving collateral blood supply and removing bony pressure, endolymph resorption will be improved. There is no evidence, of course, that this actually happens. It would seem more probable to me that opening the sac, manipulating instruments within it, and then introducing a foreign body would have the opposite effect. The endolymphatic sac consists of a series of interconnected small cystic spaces and ducts with a special epithelial lining. Certainly much of this epithelium, whatever its function, is destroyed by the operation. Fibrous tissue proliferation is a consequence of any surgical procedure and might further compromise any remaining sac function. The tissue injury associated with the surgery would quite naturally produce an inflammatory exudate which should cause a retrograde flow in the endolymphatic duct for a few days. Why then doesn't the patient have an aggravation of the symptoms in the immediate postoperative period? Also, I would expect the Silastic implant to become totally ensheathed in fibrous tissue. It seems unreasonable that any continuity would be maintained with the endolymphatic duct. Additionally, there is the problem of endolymph flow in ears with Menière's disease. Many ears, and possibly most ears with advanced endolymphatic hydrops, have such severe membrane distortions that the outflow of endolymph can be blocked at the ductus reuniens, saccule, saccular duct, utricular duct and sinus of the endolymphatic duct (Fig. 1). These are some of the reasons that sac surgery seems irrational to me.

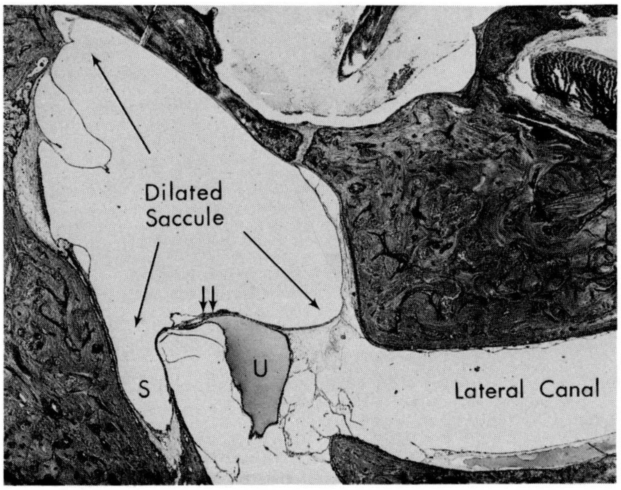

Fig. 1. Severe endolymphatic hydrops in patient with classical Menière's disease. The saccule has herniated into the sinus (S) of the endolymphatic duct, and has blocked the utriculoendolymphatic valve (double arrows). There is a proteinaceous precipitate in the endolymph of the pars superior (utricle and canals). U—Utricle.

The results which he reports are impressive but unfortunately there is no way of developing a meaningful control population. I have personally not been able to reproduce his results and have given up trying.

Proctor studied 50 patients by performing 5-hour glucose tolerance tests with insulin levels and lipid profiles. He found that 96% of the patients had either abnormal glucose tolerance or abnormal insulin levels and he concludes that impaired circulation, possibly resulting from abnormal glucose and insulin levels, may be the primary cause of Menière's disease. I am told by specialists in diabetes that the Danowski method for interpretation of glucose tolerance is prone to overdiagnose diabetes and is not a satisfactory method for diagnosing diabetes. I have also been informed that the measurement of insulin levels is of little use in diagnosing diabetes because of the great variability of the levels.

There are other problems with the metabolic hypothesis. For example, insulin-dependent diabetics do not have an increased incidence of Menière's disease. If there is a metabolic cause for Menière's disease, why are 70% unilateral with the opposite ear showing no evidence of the disease? Even if there is so-called metabolic pollution of the inner ear or vascular changes, how does that cause hydrops?

The sac operation has haunted us for more than 50 years and metabolic therapy for longer than I can remember. It is doubtful that these approaches will endure. While it may be impossible to control any study on Menière's disease, therapies should at least be logical. Today's presentations fall short of satisfying that criterion.

From the Department of Otolaryngology, Massachusetts Eye and Ear Infirmary, Boston.
Presented at the meeting of the American Otological Society, Inc., Vancouver, British Columbia, May 9-10, 1981.

ENDOLYMPHATIC DUCT OBSTRUCTION FROM A JUGULAR BULB DIVERTICULUM

ROBERT A. JAHRSDOERFER, MD
WAYNE S. CAIL, MD ROBERT W. CANTRELL, MD
CHARLOTTESVILLE, VIRGINIA

Herniation of the jugular bulb into the middle ear is uncommon. Extension of a jugular bulb diverticulum into the petrous pyramid is rare. In ten previously reported cases in the literature, only the radiographic appearance of the lesion was stressed. Of interest to otolaryngologists is the fact that in seven of the cases there was an ipsilateral sensorineural hearing loss. Other symptoms included tinnitus and vertigo. One patient had been diagnosed as having Menière's disease. We document an additional case (a patient who had "classical Menière's disease") and report the first known surgical exploration of this venous anomaly. The diverticulum extended high into the petrous bone and was found to obliterate the distal segment of the endolymphatic duct. To our knowledge, this is the first time that a cause and effect relationship has been recognized between endolymphatic hydrops and a jugular bulb diverticulum. We propose that the diverticulum, by obstructing the endolymphatic duct, was directly responsible for the Menière's-like symptoms.

INTRODUCTION

Endolymphatic hydrops is known to occur in two forms, a primary form of unknown etiology in which are recognized the classical symptoms of Menière's disease, and a secondary form linked to known diseases or trauma that directly affects the ear. In this secondary category are found congenital lues, otosclerosis, poststapedectomy complications, acoustic trauma, temporal bone fractures, and bony obliteration of the endolymphatic duct.[1-3]

Endolymph is believed to be secreted by the stria vascularis and to flow longitudinally through the endolymphatic system to be absorbed in an area of the endolymphatic sac called the pars rugosa. Deficient absorption in the sac, or obstruction to the endolymphatic duct, may lead to increased fluid pressure, or hydrops, in the endolymphatic system. The endolymphatic duct arises from the confluence of the saccular duct and the utricular duct and is enclosed within a bony channel called the vestibular aqueduct. The vestibular aqueduct originates from the medial wall of the vestibule, and in its proximal course through the otic capsule runs parallel to the crus commune. It then turns at an angle of 90° to pursue a downward course ending on the back wall of the petrous bone.[4] There is a gradual flat widening of the vestibular aqueduct in its peripheral extent that blends into a shallow foviate impression in the bone facing the posterior fossa. This area houses the endolymphatic sac.

Jugular Bulb. The jugular bulb is the uppermost part of the internal jugular vein that projects through the jugular fossa into the tympanum where it becomes continuous with the sigmoid sinus.[5] In the normal temporal bone, the jugular bulb is covered by a variable thickness of bone in the hypotympanum and is not readily seen in the middle ear on otoscopy. On occasion, the jugular bulb may be high; that is to say, it may be located above the level of the bony annulus. In this position, its bony covering may be thinned or completely lacking.

In three separate studies,[6-8] the jugular bulb was found to be high in 7, 6, and 3.5% of temporal bones examined histologically. A high jugular bulb bears some relation to the degree of pneumatization of the mastoid air cell system. In a poorly pneumatized mastoid the sigmoid sinus is more anterior, the jugular fossa tends to be deep, and the jugular bulb has a correspondingly high dome[4] (Fig. 1).

The degree of pneumatization also affects the morphology of the vestibular aqueduct. Wilbrand et al[4] have shown that in sparsely pneumatized mastoids the peripheral part of the vestibular aqueduct is shorter, the triangular area narrower, and the external aperture smaller. It was noted that this type of vestibular aqueduct can be found in conjunction with a high jugular fossa.

A high jugular bulb has enormous clinical relevance. To be ignorant of this anomaly is to invite a surgical misadventure. The high jugular bulb is particularly vulnerable to injury from a myringotomy or paracentesis, or when turning a tympanomeatal flap.

REVIEW OF LITERATURE

Jugular bulb diverticula until recently have been reported largely as a radiographic curiosity.[9-11] However, in 1978, Dilenge[12] published an account of two patients with a jugular diverticulum each of

From the Departments of Otolaryngology and Maxillofacial Surgery and Radiology, University of Virginia School of Medicine, Charlottesville.
Presented at the meeting of the American Otological Society, Inc., Vancouver, British Columbia, May 9-10, 1981.
REPRINTS — Robert A. Jahrsdoerfer, MD, University of Virginia Medical Center, Charlottesville, VA 22908.

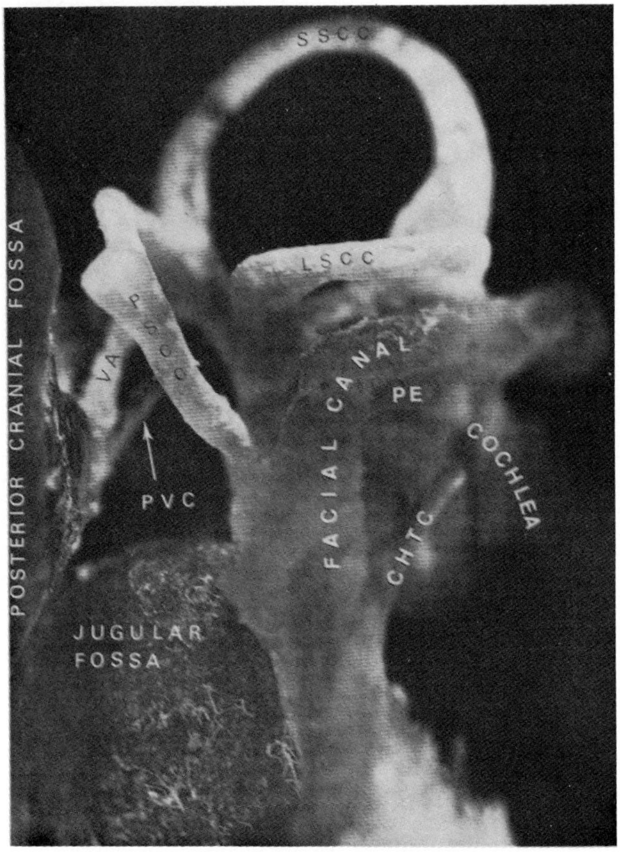

Fig. 1. Plastic mold of right inner ear from petrous bone lacking pneumatization. Note extremely high jugular fossa and its relation to the vestibular aqueduct (VA). PVC — Paravestibular canaliculus; CHTC — Chorda tympani canal; SSCC — Superior semicircular canal; LSCC — Lateral semicircular canal; PSCC — Posterior semicircular canal. From Wilbrand et al.[4] Reprinted with permission.

whom suffered from a diminution in hearing with tinnitus and vertigo. In 1980, Stern and Goldenberg[13] reported three patients who had a jugular bulb diverticulum and observed that all had a sensorineural hearing loss. They postulated that the diverticulum by encroaching on the internal auditory canal may have contributed to the sensorineural hearing deficit. Graham,[5] in an excellent thesis on the jugular bulb, documented one case of a diverticulum. F. T. Shaia related one additional case (personal communication).

Of these ten reported cases, six were in females who ranged in age from 48 to 74 with a mean age of 60. There were two males both described as being "in their 30s." In two cases, neither the age nor the sex was mentioned. The diverticulum was located on the left side in 5 patients, on the right side in 2 patients, and in 3 patients the side of involvement was not mentioned.

Of special interest is the fact that seven patients had a sensorineural hearing loss on the same side as the diverticulum. One patient had a normal pure tone audiogram but the auditory brainstem responses were abnormal. In two patients the hearing was not mentioned. Tinnitus was noted in 5 patients, vertigo or dizziness in 2 patients, otalgia in 2 patients, and facial twitching in 1 patient. It should be stated that some of these reports were for the purpose of radiographic illustration only and the history was either terse or omitted completely. When necessary, an attempt was made to contact the authors of these published cases to solicit the history. Nonetheless, in six cases there was no mention of either dizziness or vertigo as a presenting or related symptom.

REPORT OF A CASE

A 51-year-old female had her first attack of vertigo, tinnitus, and fullness in the left ear in March 1976. A second attack one month later prompted her to seek medical attention. An audiogram showed a low frequency 50 dB sensorineural hearing loss with a positive slope, dropping off to 85 dB at 8 kHz. The discrimination score was 92%. One week later she was free of her tinnitus and dizziness, and her hearing in the low frequencies had returned to normal. A vestibular function test and routine IAC radiographs were normal.

She was admitted to the University of Virginia Hospital in October 1976 for recurring attacks of vertigo, tinnitus, and fullness in her left ear. An

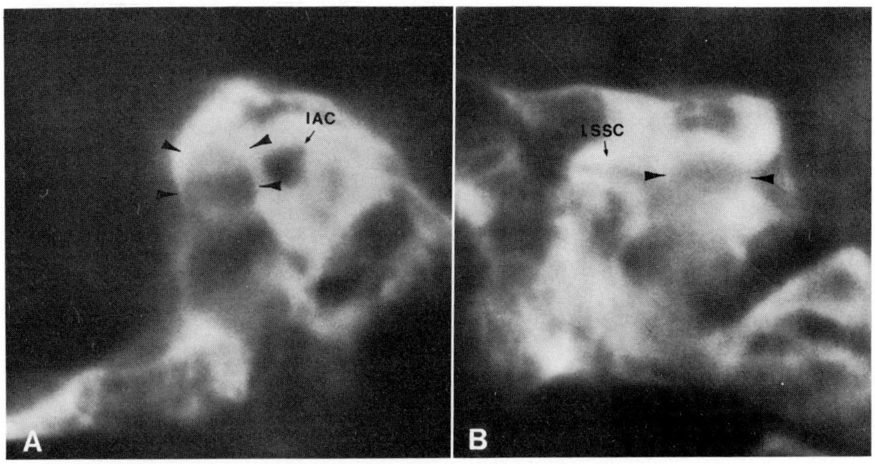

Fig. 2. A) Left lateral tomogram showing jugular diverticulum (arrows) extending high into posterior petrous bone. Note position of internal auditory canal (IAC). B) Left PA tomogram at 11.8 cm. Note jugular diverticulum (arrows) extending into petrous apex. LSSC — Lateral semicircular canal.

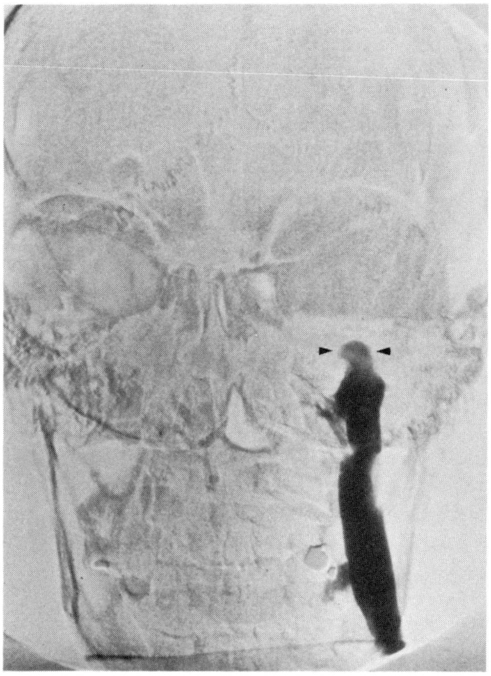

Fig. 3. Left jugular venogram showing diverticulum arising from jugular bulb and extending into petrous apex (arrows).

audiogram showed a flat sensorineural hearing loss of 60-65 dB. Multidirectional polytomography of her temporal bones was reported as within normal limits. Site of lesion testing suggested cochlear pathology. A diagnosis of Menière's disease was made for which she was treated medically.

She returned on November 30, 1977, having had five acute episodes of vertigo with nausea and vomiting, tinnitus, hearing loss, and a sensation of falling to the left. The attacks had occurred over a one-month time period. Audiometric testing again showed a flat 60 dB sensorineural hearing loss in the left ear and the discrimination score had fallen to

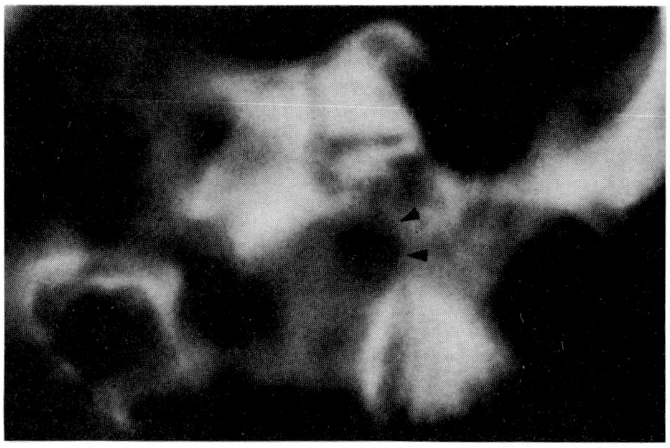

Fig. 5. PA tomogram of left temporal bone showing a high jugular bulb (arrows) presenting in middle ear. Note smooth contour of jugular bulb.

50%. By November 1979 she was averaging four acute vertiginous attacks a week. A vestibular function test showed decreased function of the left labyrinth and the discrimination score had fallen to 38%.

In May 1980 she was admitted for an endolymphatic shunt procedure. Preoperative tomography revealed a diverticulum of the left jugular bulb extending high into the posterior and medial aspect of the left petrous bone (Fig. 2A, B). Venous phase films from a carotid arteriogram showed a normal sigmoid sinus bilaterally, and a jugular diverticulum on the left. The diverticulum was more clearly delineated by retrograde jugular venography (Fig. 3). A review of her tomographs from four years earlier also showed the diverticulum but it appeared slightly smaller and was less clearly seen.

One week later she was readmitted for a translabyrinthine eighth nerve section. At operation, the diverticulum was identified arising from a broad base on the jugular bulb and ascending in the pet-

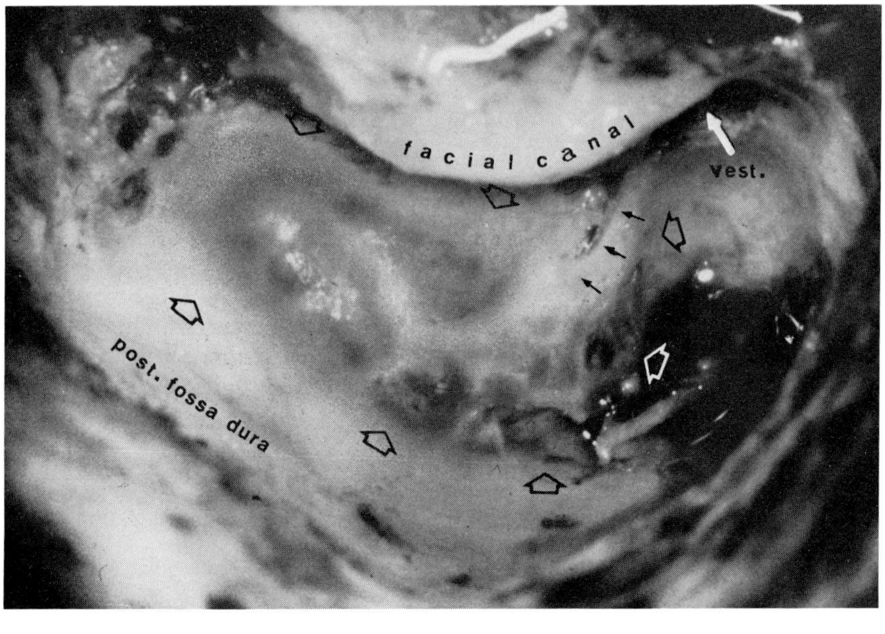

Fig. 4. Photograph taken at operation. Surgeon's position, left ear. The semicircular canals have been drilled away. Note jugular diverticulum (open arrows) extending high into petrous bone and obliterating the endolymphatic duct (small arrows). Solid white arrow points to vestibule.

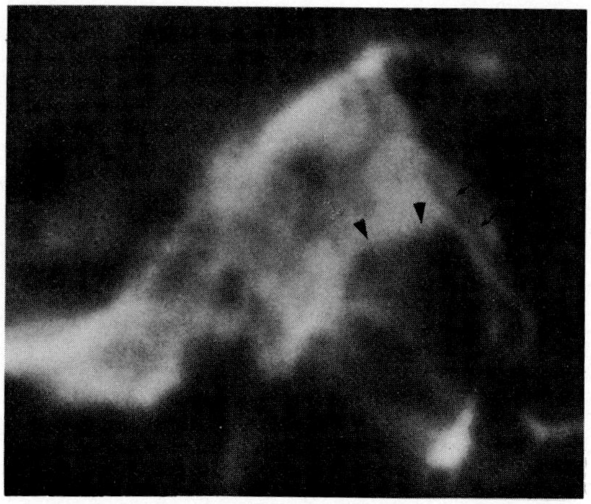

Fig. 6. Lateral tomogram in a patient with congenital atresia and poor mastoid pneumatization. Note smooth contour of elevated jugular bulb (large arrows) and its relation to the vestibular aqueduct (small arrows).

rous bone to the level of the internal auditory canal. The endolymphatic duct was seen to splay over the surface of the diverticulum and to be obliterated by it (Fig. 4). The vestibular nerves and the cochlear nerve were sectioned. There has been no vertigo or tinnitus in one year's time.

DISCUSSION

The jugular bulb may be elevated in the hypotympanum and present as a bluish mass in the middle ear. As previously mentioned, there is a greater likelihood of this occurring in poorly pneumatized mastoid bones. However, the contour of the high jugular bulb is usually smooth and curvilinear (Figs. 5 and 6). A jugular diverticulum, on the other hand, may be considered a true venous anomaly. It is an irregular outpouching of the jugular bulb that may rise to the very top of the petrous bone. It may erode into the internal auditory canal as noted by Graham[5] or obliterate the endolymphatic duct as seen in this case.

There are characteristic differences between a jugular diverticulum and a high jugular bulb. A jugular diverticulum presents more medial and posterior in the petrous bone than does a high jugular bulb. A jugular diverticulum does not invade the middle ear, is not visible on inspection, and is not exposed to surgical trauma from a myringotomy or tympanotomy. The diagnosis of a jugular diverticulum is made radiographically; a high jugular bulb is diagnosed by otoscopic examination.

The hearing loss from a jugular diverticulum is sensorineural from encroachment on the endolymphatic duct or sac, or possibly on the internal auditory canal. The hearing loss from a high jugular bulb is usually conductive from dampening of the ossicular chain movement or blockage of the round window.[14] Tinnitus, if present, is continuous or intermittent in patients with a jugular diverticulum; tinnitus is uncommon in patients with a high jugular bulb. Patients with a jugular diverticulum may be dizzy or vertiginous, symptoms that are most unlikely from a high jugular bulb. Finally, a jugular diverticulum may cause signs and symptoms that mimic classic Menière's disease.

This last point warrants further analysis One of two patients with a jugular diverticulum reported by Dilenge[12] had been followed for attacks of Menière's disease for seven years. Our case report, described herein, fulfilled all the criteria for a diagnosis of Menière's disease. Graham[5] related a case in which a 35-year-old male with Menière's disorder underwent surgery for a subarachnoid endolymphatic shunt. He stated that "the sigmoid sinus and jugular bulb were identified as was a structure presumed to be the endolymphatic sac. Upon incising this, it was obvious that this was a very high jugular bulb and this structure completely obscured the area of the normal endolymphatic sac." In our opinion, this "very high jugular bulb" probably represented a jugular diverticulum which, by its location, may have precipitated the patient's Menière's symptoms.

Many questions need to be asked about this venous anomaly. How common is it? What causes it? Does it increase in size? Is it dangerous? In 239 temporal bone polytomographic examinations done at the University of Virginia over the past year, two patients were noted to have a jugular diverticulum. One case was that of Shaia's, mentioned earlier; the other was an elderly female with sudden onset of facial paralysis on the ipsilateral side. As the diverticulum was of moderate size we believe its existence in relation to the facial paralysis is probably coincidental.

We don't know what causes a jugular diverticulum. Does it increase in size? There is some evidence to suggest that a jugular bulb has the ability to slowly expand and cause thinning of the overlying bone. Graham documented two cases in which a slow growth of the jugular bulb was apparent.[5] In our patient, there appeared to be some slight increase in size over a four-year time span.

Is it dangerous? While there are no published reports of spontaneous rupture of a high jugular bulb or diverticulum, the diverticulum is at risk of being injured during mastoidectomy by the unwary surgeon. Profuse hemorrhage, not unlike that from a torn sigmoid sinus, would be the consequence. Aside from this, the diverticulum is dangerous only insofar as it impinges on the endolymphatic duct or sac, or possibly the internal auditory canal.

In conclusion, we have presented evidence to suggest a cause and effect relationship between endolymphatic hydrops and a jugular diverticulum. We propose that the jugular diverticulum obstructed the endolymphatic duct or sac and was directly responsible for the Menière's-like symptoms in these patients.

REFERENCES

1. Clark SK, Rees TS. Posttraumatic endolymphatic hydrops. Arch Otolaryngol 1977; 103:725-6.

2. Pulec J. Meniere's disease: results of a two and one-half year study of etiology, natural history and results of treatment. Laryngoscope 1972; 82:1703-14.

3. Clemis JD, Valvassori GE. Recent radiographic and clinical observations on the vestibular aqueduct. Otolaryngol Clin North Am 1968; 1:339-46.

4. Wilbrand HF, Stahle J, Rask-Andersen H. Tomography in Meniere's disease — why and how. Adv Oto-Rhino-Laryngol 1978; 24:71-93.

5. Graham MD. The jugular bulb: its anatomic and clinical considerations in contemporary otology. Laryngoscope 1977; 87:105-25.

6. Korner O. Die Otitiscen Erkrankungen des Hirns, der Hirhaute und der Blutleiter. Frankfurt: J. Alt, 1894.

7. Overton SB, Ritter FN. A high placed jugular bulb in the middle ear: a clinical and temporal bone study. Laryngoscope 1973; 83:1986-91.

8. Subotic R. The high position of the jugular bulb. Acta Otolaryngol (Stockh) 1979; 87:340-4.

9. Britton BH. Glomus tympanicum and glomus jugulare tumors. Radiol Clin North Am 1974; 12:543-51.

10. Noyek AM, Holgate RC, Wortzman G, et al. Sophisticated radiology in otolaryngology. J Otolaryngol 1977; 6 Suppl 3:73-94.

11. Unger JD, Shaffer KA. Advanced exercises in diagnostic radiology. Ear, nose and throat radiology. Philadelphia: W. B. Saunders, 1980:29.

12. Dilenge D. The jugular "notch." J Can Assoc Radiol 1977; 28:274-7.

13. Stern J, Goldenberg M. Jugular bulb diverticula in medial petrous bone. AJR 1980; 134:959-61.

14. Glasscock ME, Dickins JRE, Jackson CG, Wiet RJ. Vascular anomalies of the middle ear. Laryngoscope 1980; 90:77-88.

≈

GUIDELINES FOR GRANTS

TRUSTEES OF THE RESEARCH FUND OF THE AMERICAN OTOLOGICAL SOCIETY, INC.

The members of the Board of Trustees of the Research Fund of the American Otological Society have determined guidelines for making grants from the Fund. The following is the formulation of policy.

Grants will be given in the area of otosclerosis — its diagnosis and management, the possible causes and underlying conditions, and an understanding of the disorder that may lead eventually to its prevention or cure.

The present lack of understanding of the disorder and the absence of similar conditions in other animals makes research in this field difficult. A direct approach to the disease may or may not be feasible; therefore, a sound strategy would be to use other approaches, such as the investigation of bone development, growth and repair under various conditions, and the study of other diseases that may be similar to otosclerosis. It is possible that investigations which may seem initially remote from otosclerosis may provide information which will eventually lead to a substantive further understanding of the disease process which underlies otosclerosis. The applicant should describe correlations between proposed research with the clinical pathological entity of otosclerosis.

The policy is to aid and encourage research in the immediate field of otosclerosis and also in adjoining fields, if, in the opinion of the Board, there is a substantial promise that results obtained will be of assistance in the ways indicated, and may lead to the attainment of the objective of the further understanding of otosclerosis.

Applications for a research grant from the Research Fund of the American Otological Society may be obtained from the Office of the Secretary-Treasurer of the Research Fund of the American Otological Society. Write to Robert J. Ruben, MD, Secretary-Treasurer, Department of Otolaryngology, Albert Einstein College of Medicine, 1300 Morris Park Avenue, Bronx, NY 10461; telephone (212) 430-3036.

All grant requests must be submitted by January 31, 1982. All grants received after January 31 will not be considered.

Ann Otol 90:1981

CENTRAL VESTIBULAR SIGNS, POSTERIOR FOSSA PATHOLOGY AND COMPUTERIZED TOMOGRAPHY-REGIONAL BLOOD BRAIN CIRCULATION

ARVIND KUMAR, MD, FRCS

NICHOLAS TOROK, MD GALDINO VALVASSORI, MD

CHICAGO, ILLINOIS

Central vestibular signs are sensitive indicators of lesions in the posterior fossa. With the availability of computerized tomography and computerized tomography-regional blood brain circulation, the identification of suspected retrolabyrinthine lesions has improved considerably. This is a report about the reliability of central vestibular signs in predicting posterior fossa lesions.

INTRODUCTION

The objective of a neurotological examination is to establish the presence and location of a lesion, whether it is labyrinthine or intracranial. This can be determined with significant accuracy by a vestibular evaluation which includes the Torok monothermal differential caloric test.[1]

Before the advent of computerized axial tomography (CT scan) confirmation of neurotologically suspected posterior fossa lesions was limited. The scope of diagnostic capabilities widened considerably with the availability of the CT scan. But in spite of this advancement, no abnormality could be detected in a large number of patients with persistent symptoms and reconfirmed central vestibular signs. A presumptive diagnosis of vertebrobasilar insufficiency was often made though no objective proof of such a circulatory abnormality could be established.

A new form of radiographic assessment based on the hemodynamic evaluation of regional blood flow within the brain objectively demonstrates disorders of brain perfusion.[2] It is thus possible to localize and document abnormalities of circulation in suspected cases of vertebrobasilar insufficiency.

The purpose of this paper is twofold: 1) it reports about the accuracy and reliability of central vestibular signs in predicting intracranial lesions of diverse pathological nature, and 2) it shows the value of CT-regional blood brain circulation (CT-rBBC) in identifying hitherto unproved lesions which were strongly suspected by persistent central vestibular signs.

METHODS

Our neurotological test protocol includes 1) calibration, 2) sinusoidal eye tracking, 3) optokinetic response recording, 4) detection of spontaneous nystagmus, 5) caloric test series, 6) postural test, and 7) vestibulospinal and equilibrium function tests.

Eye movements are recorded by the photoelectric method described by Torok et al,[3] using the Beckman R611 amplification and recording unit. The vestibular examination is performed with the patient sitting comfortably in a semidarkened room. The recording and nystagmogram analysis is done in an adjacent room, separated by a one-way glass partition thus preventing the patient from distraction by students and observers.

Test procedures 1) through 3) are performed in the conventional manner. Spontaneous nystagmus is recorded with the eyes first in the midposition (II°) and then deviated 30° to the right and left (I°R and I°L). In each of these positions the recording is made with a near fixation of about 35 cm and also without fixation, the eye being open but in complete darkness. A search for vertical nystagmus is executed in a similar manner.

For the caloric test, the Torok monothermal differential method is utilized. The technique of this test has been described.[1,4]

In the postural test, the patient is instructed to hold the gaze at midposition, fixating on the face of the physician, who observes the eyes for nystagmus through a series of nine positions: seated, lying on the back with head and neck extending beyond the edge of the examining table, head (supported in physician's hands) turned 90° to the right, returned to center, left, center, head hanging, center, and finally back to sitting posture. Each position is held for a minimum of 30 seconds. Eye movements are recorded throughout the test. The patient is instructed to report any sensation of dizziness. If either dizziness or nystagmus is induced in any position, the critical positioning is repeated to verify reproducibility or fatigability.

The vestibulospinal function test commonly used is the arm tonus reaction[5] for possible past-pointing. When unidirectional spontaneous horizontal nystagmus is recorded, the past-pointing test determines whether the most likely origin of the nystagmus is labyrinthine or central. The tests of equilibrium function are the Romberg (both normal and tandem) and gait (with eyes open and closed).

Detection of one or more central vestibular signs is the crucial element in the neurotologic test procedure. Table 1 summarizes the vestibular signs which indicate a retrolabyrinthine posterior fossa lesion.

In patients showing one or more central vestibular signs further diagnostic studies are carried out depending on the nature of the presumed lesion. If a cerebellopontine angle tumor is suspected, detailed auditory site of lesion tests, brainstem evoked responses

From the Department of Otolaryngology, Abraham Lincoln School of Medicine, University of Illinois, Chicago.

Presented at the meeting of the American Otological Society, Inc., Vancouver, British Columbia, May 9-10, 1981.

REPRINTS — Arvind Kumar, MD, Room B.45, 1855 W. Taylor Street, Chicago, IL 60612.

TABLE 1. SUMMARY OF VESTIBULAR SIGNS INDICATING RETROLABYRINTHINE POSTERIOR FOSSA LESIONS

Test	*Central Vestibular Sign*
Calibration	Calibration overshoot or undershoot
Sinusoidal eye tracking	Saccadic eye tracking
Optokinetic responses	Optokinetic asymmetry Optokinetic fatigue
Spontaneous nystagmus and arm tonus reaction	Horizontal unidirectional nystagmus without past pointing Gaze nystagmus Vertical nystagmus
Caloric responses	Vestibular decruitment Hyperactive responses
Postural study	Nystagmus unaccompanied by dizziness Nystagmus with dizziness, both persisting for as long as critical position is maintained and both being reproducible Vomiting unaccompanied by vertigo

(BSER) and tomography of the petrous bone are obtained. If the tomograms show an asymmetry of the internal canals or evidence of erosion, a CT scan is the next diagnostic procedure. In those instances where the scan is negative and clinical evidence strong, patients undergo posterior fossa myelography. With the development of CT-pneumocisternography the visualization of the cerebellopontine angle and the interior of the internal auditory canal is possible. Thus even small intracanalicular lesions can be demonstrated with accuracy.[6] This technique has therefore now replaced posterior fossa myelography.

In those instances where an infarct or a vertebrobasilar insufficiency is the presumptive diagnosis, patients are referred directly for CT scan and CT-rBBC studies, both of which can be performed consecutively in one sitting. When vertebrobasilar insufficiency is documented by CT-rBBC studies, additional cerebral hemodynamic evaluation[7] provides a physiologic assessment of the direct and indirect carotid and vertebral arterial blood flow. The final step in the evaluation is cerebral vascular angiography. When an area of inadequate regional blood flow is identified and an accessible vascular obstruction localized, vascular reconstruction is recommended.[8]

RESULTS

The neurotological examination revealed one or more central vestibular signs in 229 patients seen between January 1979 and December 1980. Fully comprehensive studies including CT-rBBC, where indicated, were possible in 116 patients. Attrition was due to several factors, not the least of which was a reluctance on the part of the patient and the referring physician to have CT-rBBC studies when recent CT scans had been reported normal. Out of the 116 patients who could be comprehensively investigated, a retrolabyrinthine lesion was identified in 108. The central vestibular signs could thus be confirmed in 93% of the patients. The most frequent central vestibular signs were spontaneous nystagmus and vestibular decruitment (Table 2). The age of these patients varied from 14 to 81 years

TABLE 2. CENTRAL VESTIBULAR SIGNS (N = 108)

Spontaneous nystagmus	74
Vestibular decruitment	56
Postural nystagmus sine vertigo	32
Vestibular hyperactivity	24
Oculomotor dysfunction	13
Vestibular areflexia	3

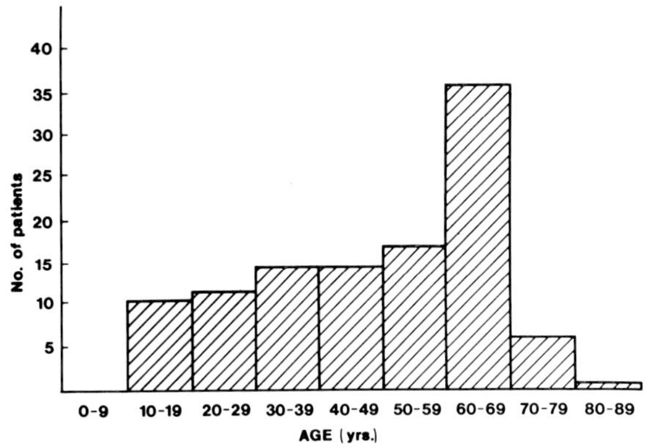

Fig. 1. Age distribution of patients with central vestibular signs.

(Fig. 1). The different pathologic entities diagnosed are shown in Table 3. The most frequent abnormality was a disorder of cerebral circulation. The age distribution of patients with cerebral flow abnormalities is shown in Figure 2.

There were seven patients in whom the central vestibular signs could not be confirmed by any of the currently available diagnostic techniques. In addition there was one patient in whom the neurotological examination was normal but the CT scan showed a small tumor at the skull base. This was the only false negative.

DISCUSSION

Dizziness or disequilibrium is a frequent complaint of patients seen by otolaryngologists, neurologists, internists, cardiologists and family practitioners. The evaluation of these patients often includes CT scanning in the expectation that intracranial lesions missed by other diagnostic procedures could be detected. This is not always the case because if only a few and thick tomographic sections are obtained, a small tumor or infarct can be missed between two consecutive sections or masked by the computer averaging of multiple point measurements within the section. Therefore, if a posterior fossa lesion is strongly suspected, thin section computerized tomography is necessary with cuts made in both the axial and direct coronal planes. As the availability of specific radiological procedures such as CT-rBBC and CT-pneumocisternography

TABLE 3. VARIETY OF PATHOLOGIC CHANGES DETECTED BY CENTRAL VESTIBULAR SIGNS

Circulatory defect	61	S/P subdural hematoma	1
Brainstem/cerebellar atrophy	26	Aqueduct stenosis	1
Tumor	14	Basilar artery aneurysm	1
Neuronitis, encephalitis(?)	7	Hemiplegia	1
Brainstem/cerebellar infarct	6	Ramsay-Hunt syndrome	1
Multiple sclerosis	6	Cysticercosis	1
Lues	5	Normal pressure hydrocephalus	1
CNS malformation	2	Megacisterna magna	1
Brainstem cyst	2	Neurofibromatosis	1
Toxicosis (drugs)	2	Septum pellucidum cyst	1
Epilepsy	2		

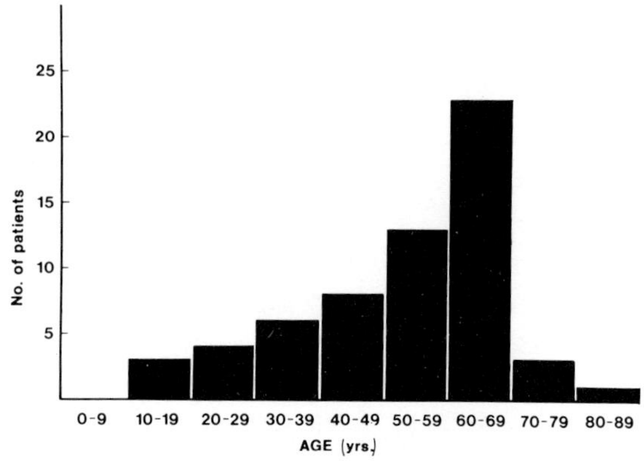

Fig. 2. Age distribution of patients with central vestibular signs and proven cerebral hemodynamic abnormalities.

becomes widespread, the selection of the test most likely to provide diagnostic confirmation will become an important consideration, both from the point of view of radiation exposure and cost.

A screening test which differentiates labyrinthine from retrolabyrinthine lesions would assist greatly in selection of the confirmatory test likely to substantiate the diagnosis. Brainstem evoked response testing (BSER) is being increasingly utilized for this purpose. The test, however, has several disadvantages and limitations: 1) it can only detect lesions confined to or affecting the auditory pathway; 2) in the presence of a significant hearing loss, the characteristic waveforms are not obtainable thus making it difficult to evaluate amplitude or latency; and 3) even if the limited scope of the test is accepted, a further disadvantage is the high rate of false positive results obtained in a search for cerebellopontine angle lesions. Kinney and Nodar[9] have reported 34% false positives in their series. Our own experience with a diverse group of patients complaining of dizziness is similar.

In contrast, the vestibular examination is sensitive, reliable, and capable of indicating lesions of diverse nature anywhere in the posterior cranial fossa. In the present study the central vestibular signs were confirmed in 93% of the patients. This high degree of vestibular test reliability may be explained by two factors.

Use of Photoelectric Nystagmography (PENG). The principle of this method of recording eye movements has been described.[3,10] PENG is far more sensitive in recording eye movements since it directly senses actual excursions of the eye whereas the widely used electronystagmography (ENG) depends on the small and variable corneoretinal potential to detect eye movements. With ENG small amplitude nystagmus often cannot be deciphered because of limited sensitivity to the signal and contamination of the record by competing signals such as EKG, EEG, and muscle potentials. Some of the other difficulties and inaccuracies of electro-oculography have been reviewed recently by Carpenter.[11] In an effort to evaluate objectively the accuracy of both systems, simultaneous records of PENG and ENG were made following cold caloric stimulation of the labyrinth. The records are shown in Figure 3. Although the calibration with both was equal, and filter settings identical, the ENG tracing is hardly legible and does not lend itself to any analysis. Thus a low amplitude spontaneous nystagmus can easily be missed on an ENG recording and an important clinical sign lost. In the present study, spontaneous nystagmus was the most frequently recorded pathological sign.

Use of the Torok Monothermal Differential Caloric Test. This technique provides a very valuable sign of posterior fossa lesions, namely vestibular decruitment. The reliability of this sign has been demonstrated in earlier reports by Torok[12,13] and Kumar.[1] The Fitzgerald-Hallpike bithermal caloric test,[14] though widely used, does not provide an accurate differentiation between labyrinthine and retrolabyrinthine lesions. This was shown by clinical and experimental studies of McCabe and Ryu[15] who felt that "directional preponderance is worthless as a localizing or even a general test of vestibular disease." Perhaps it is because of this dissatisfaction that rotatory testing is again being investigated as a diagnostic modality. Rubin[16] recently reported on the value of the sinusoidal harmonic acceleration test (SHA) in vestibular diagnosis but he concedes that the SHA test cannot be used to the exclusion of other ENG recorded vestibular function tests.

Between 1968 and 1978 the technique of vestibular evaluation was the same as described here. Patients with central vestibular signs were fully investigated by the then available neuroradiologic techniques. Space-occupying lesions, particularly in the cerebellopontine angle, could be diagnosed even when these masses were small. With the availability of the CT scan, the scope of diagnostic capability advanced considerably. Thus it became possible to

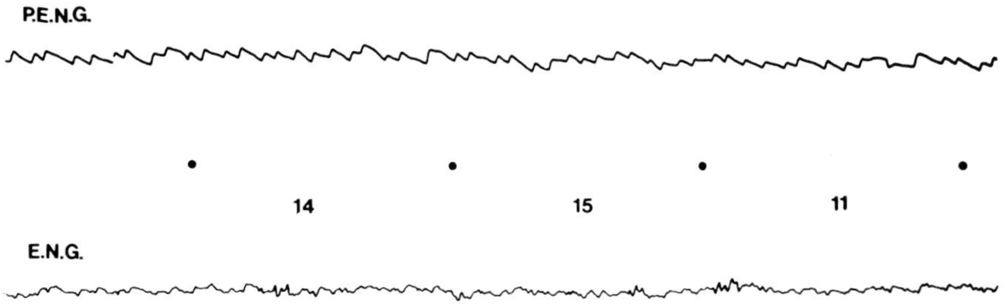

Fig. 3. Simultaneous recording of thermally induced nystagmus with photoelectric nystagmography (PENG) and electronystagmography (ENG). The calibration on both systems was equal.

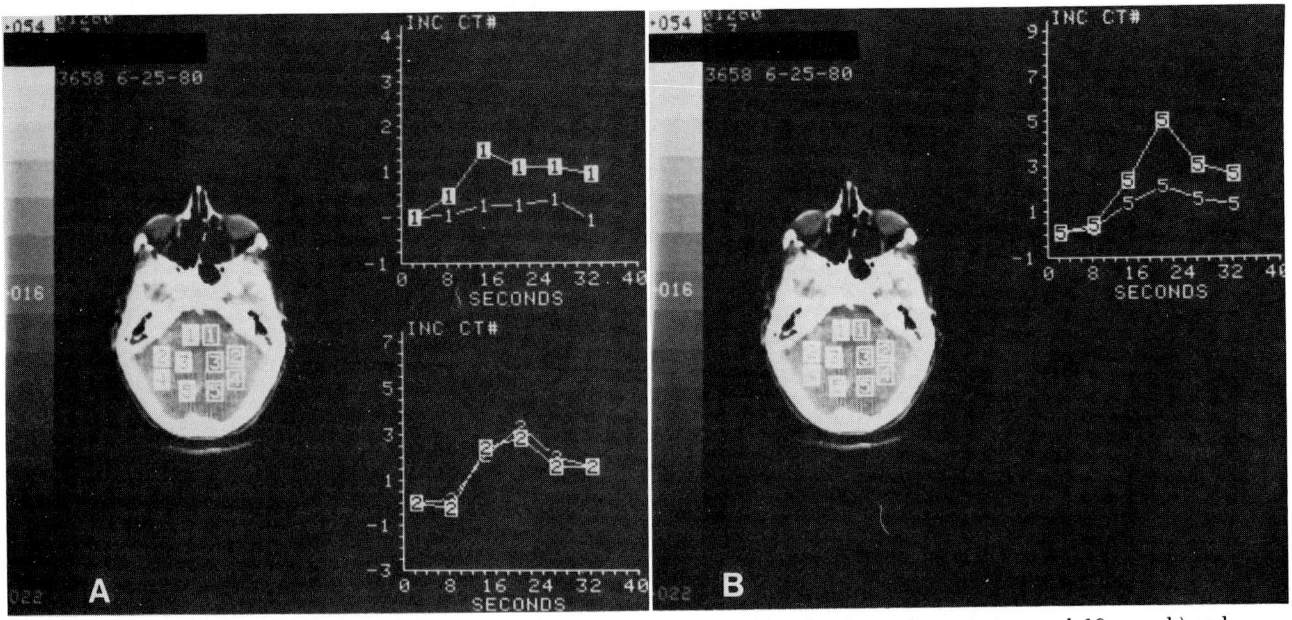

Fig. 4. A, B) CT regional blood brain circulation curves showing both delay (normal transit time peak 16 seconds) and diminished (normal amplitude 3-7 CT #) cerebellar and brainstem perfusion (unboxed 1 and unboxed 5; boxed and unboxed 2 show delay).

identify a variety of aberrations of structure, hemorrhage, infarction, atrophy and tumors located outside the cerebellopontine angle with one noninvasive study. Still, there remained a large number of patients with complaints of dizziness where all the tests were normal except for the central vestibular signs. A presumptive diagnosis of vertebrobasilar insufficiency was usually made in these instances though there was no objective proof of such a circulatory disorder. Angiography proved to be of limited value as it could demonstrate neither small vessel disease nor abnormalities of cerebrovascular hemodynamics. The latter can occur without lesions of any of the major neck or intracranial vessels in patients with reduced cardiac output, hypotension or hypovolemia. The development of CT-rBBC was a significant advance since for the first time an abnormality of cerebral perfusion could be objectively demonstrated and thus central vestibular signs confirmed.

The history and test results of a 65-year-old female exemplify the reliability of the vestibular examination in predicting an intracranial lesion and the CT-rBBC in demonstrating the cause. The patient complained of frequent momentary spells of imbalance for the preceding one year. Six weeks prior to being examined she experienced two severe spells of imbalance and spinning, accompanied by nausea. There was no history of loss of consciousness, visual disturbances or neurological symptoms. The hearing on the right side had been slightly decreased for the previous 11 years. Otoscopy revealed normal external canals and tympanic membranes. The audiogram showed a pure tone average of 43 dB on the right and 26 dB on the left with discrimination scores of 96% bilaterally. The vestibular test results were a clearly recorded gaze nystagmus and a right type II vestibular decruitment.[13] The culmination frequencies were:

	10ml	100ml		Ratio
Right	29	28	=	0.9
Left	29	35	=	1.2

Since these two findings were suggestive of a retrolabyrinthine lesion, the patient underwent a CT scan and CT-rBBC studies. The scan demonstrated moderate cerebellar brainstem and occipital lobe atrophy but no evidence of a space-occupying lesion in the posterior fossa. The dynamic infratentorial study showed markedly delayed circulation in both cerebellar hemispheres (Fig. 4).

Does the demonstration of blood flow abnormality necessarily imply that it is in fact the cause of vertiginous symptoms? The following case report answers the question. A 67-year-old female complained of a "floating" sensation of 5 weeks' duration whenever she stood up from a sitting or supine position. The frequency and severity of these symptoms progressively increased, and eventually she found walking without support almost impossible. There was no history of visual symptoms or loss of consciousness, and there were no hearing complaints. Past medical history was unremarkable. Examination of both ears was normal. Pure tone audiogram showed symmetrical, high-frequency sensorineural hearing loss of mild to moderate severity. The speech discrimination scores on both sides were normal. The vestibular test results indicated normal eye tracking and optokinetic responses. There was no spontaneous nystagmus and the postural study was normal. With the caloric test

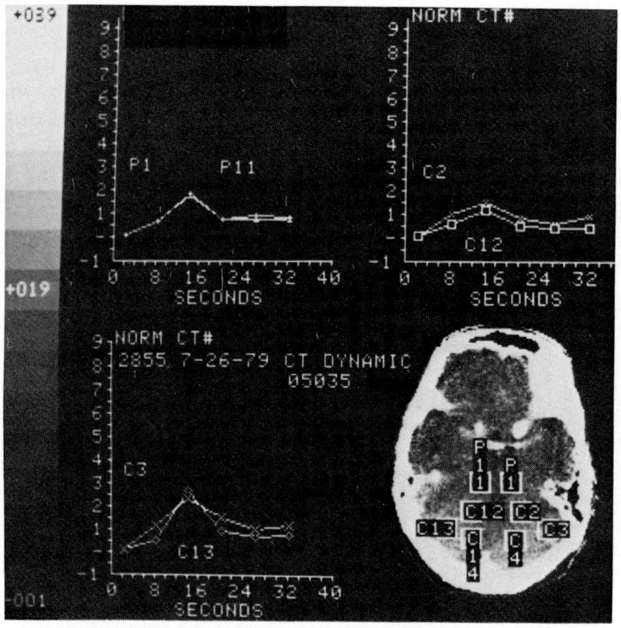

Fig. 5. CT regional blood brain circulation curves showing low amplitude of the curves indicative of diminished perfusion in brainstem and cerebellum (normal amplitude 3-7 CT #).

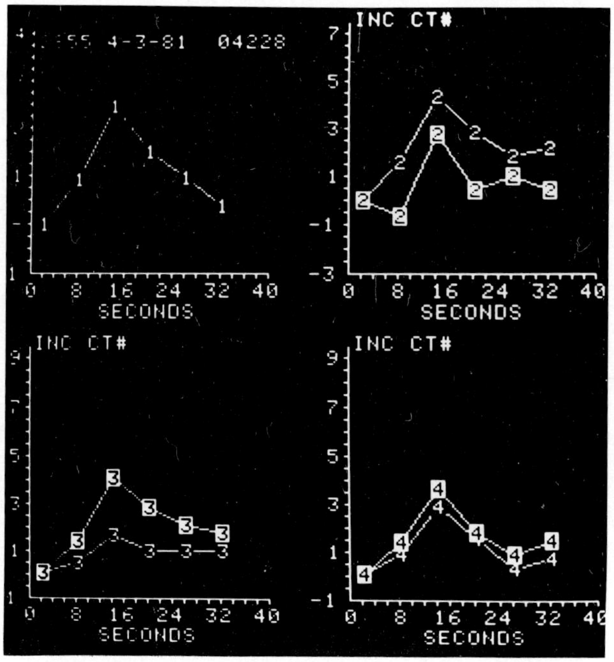

Fig. 6. CT-rBBC 18 months after surgical correction of obstruction in major neck vessels. There is definite increase in amplitude of curves indicating improved perfusion. The measurements were made in the same areas as in Fig. 5.

a bilateral type II decruitment was obtained. The culmination frequencies were:

	10ml	100ml		Ratio
Right	23	19	=	0.8
Left	28	27	=	0.9

The Romberg test was positive and walking without support was not possible. In view of the bilateral type II vestibular decruitment, intracranial pathology was suspected, on the basis of which CT scan with dynamic flow studies was obtained. The scan was normal but the flow studies indicated vertebrobasilar insufficiency (Fig. 5). Detailed hemodynamic evaluation including angiography showed an obstruction of the right internal carotid, the left vertebral, and the left subclavian arteries. A reconstruction of the right internal carotid artery and the left vertebral artery was carried out and the left subclavian artery was decompressed. Two months after surgery the patient was completely asymptomatic. Eighteen months later the neurotological examination was repeated. The culmination frequencies for the caloric test were:

	10ml	100ml		Ratio
Right	28	36	=	1.2
Left	28	35	=	1.2

The CT-rBBC examination was also repeated, and marked improvement in the total cerebral circulation was noted. The flow curves of the posterior fossa are shown in Figure 6. The validity and reliability of both vestibular decruitment and CT-rBBC were thus established.

SUMMARY

Central vestibular signs such as vestibular decruitment are accurate indicators of retrolabyrinthine posterior fossa lesions. The rate of confirmation of abnormalities suspected by vestibular testing improved considerably with the availability of the CT scan. Despite this advance many patients frequently remained undiagnosed while their symptoms of dizziness continued. A presumptive diagnosis of vertebrobasilar insufficiency was often made without objective evidence of such an abnormality. A new form of radiographic assessment based on the hemodynamic evaluation of regional blood flow within the brain served to demonstrate objectively these circulatory defects. CT-rBBC studies thus served to confirm the validity of persistent central vestibular signs in these patients. In this series of patients posterior fossa lesions were suspected in 116 patients by the vestibular tests. In 108 an abnormality could be confirmed, thus giving an identification rate of 93%.

ACKNOWLEDGMENT — The authors wish to express their sincere appreciation to Glenn Krol, BS, for his valuable assistance in testing subjects and collecting data.

REFERENCES

1. Kumar A. The diagnostic advantages of the Torok monothermal differential caloric test. Laryngoscope 1981; 91:1679-94.

2. Valvassori GE, Dobben GD. Vertebrobasilar insufficiency. Ann Otol Rhinol Laryngol 1979; 88:689-92.

3. Torok N, Guillemin V, Barnothy JM. Photoelectric nystagmography. Ann Otol Rhinol Laryngol 1951; 60:917-26.

4. Torok N. Differential caloric stimulations in vestibular diagnosis. Arch Otolaryngol 1969; 90:52-7.

5. Wodak E, Fischer MH. Eine neue Vestibularisreaction. Munchn Med Wchnschr 1922; 6:193.

6. Mafee M, Valvassori GE, Dobben GD, Kumar A, Carney AL. Diagnostic and scientific validity of CT and dynamic CT regional brain circulation (rBC) in patients with abnormal audiometric and vestibular testing. Radiology (in press).

7. Carney AL, Anderson EM, Burns E. Cerebral hemodynamic evaluation. In: Carney AL, Anderson EM, eds. Advances in neurology; diagnosis and treatment of brain ischemia, Vol. 30. New York: Raven Press, 1981: 335-59.

8. Carney AL, Anderson EM. Carotid and distal vertebral bypass for carotid occlusion: case report and technique. Clin Electroencephalog 1978; 9:105-9.

9. Kinney SE, Nodar RH. Brainstem auditory evoked potentials for detection of retrocochlear pathology. Ann Otol Rhinol Laryngol 1980; 89:291-5.

10. Nykiel F, Torok N. A simplified nystagmograph. Ann Otol Rhinol Laryngol 1963; 72:647-54.

11. Carpenter RHS. Movements of the eyes. London: Pion Ltd, 1977: 320-2.

12. Torok N. A new parameter of vestibular sensitivity. Ann Otol Rhinol Laryngol 1970; 79:808-17.

13. Torok N. Vestibular decruitment in central nervous system disease. Ann Otol Rhinol Laryngol 1976; 85:131-5.

14. Fitzgerald G, Hallpike CE. Studies in human vestibular function. I. Observations on the directional preponderance ("Nystagmusbereitschaft") of caloric nystagmus resulting from central lesions. Brain 1942; 65:115-37.

15. McCabe B, Ryu J. Vestibular physiology in understanding the dizzy patient. Am Acad Otolaryngol: Rochester, Minn, 1979: 42.

16. Rubin W. SHA as a modality for monitoring patient progress. Laryngoscope 1981; 91:1282-5.

≈

CASSELBERRY AWARD

The American Laryngological Association announces that it will receive essays or theses relating to the art and science of laryngology and rhinology for consideration of the Casselberry Award for 1981-82. The Award is open to physicians, interns, residents and graduate students in laryngology and rhinology in the Americas and scientists in the field in laryngology and rhinology. For information write to: William M. Trible, MD, Secretary, American Laryngological Association, 1234 19th Street, NW, Washington, DC 20036.

PANEL ON STAPES SURGERY

TOTAL FOOTPLATE EXTRACTION IN STAPEDECTOMY

MENDELL ROBINSON, MD

PROVIDENCE, RHODE ISLAND

The concept of total footplate removal in stapedectomy surgery is recommended as the preferred technique providing that the surgery is atraumatic. Only that part of the footplate which can be removed easily should be removed; in 4,761 consecutive stapedectomies a total footplate removal could be accomplished in 74%. Total and partial footplate removal necessitates a connective tissue graft to seal the oval window and must be coordinated with a suitable prosthesis which is efficient, functional and self-centering. The successful results between total and partial footplate removal are not statistically significant when employing the criteria of air-bone gap closure to within 10 dB, but when comparing the complete air-bone gap closure rate there is a statistically significant difference with total footplate removal providing a more favorable hearing result.

INTRODUCTION

In 1958 Shea advocated total stapes footplate removal as mandatory for a successful result in using the polyethylene tube prosthesis and a vein graft.[1] Stapedectomy techniques using a wire prosthesis also necessitated a total footplate removal for the most successful result. In 1965, Robinson[2] recommended a total stapes footplate removal providing that only that part that could be removed easily should be removed. This principle was established to minimize cochlear trauma during the footplate removal. However, partial or total footplate removal necessitates a tissue graft to seal the oval window and a prosthesis to fit the created fenestra whether it be total removal, partial removal or a "drillout." In 1968 Moon in his series with the author's prosthesis and Gelfoam (the small fenestra technique) reported a fistula rate of 2.5% with the piston technique and he subsequently returned to a connective tissue graft with partial removal of the footplate.[3] His results were comparable with Robinson's results using the same prosthesis.

Austin reported in 1980 a comparison of results of total stapedectomy vs partial stapedectomy, tissue seal and no tissue seal, and the small fenestra stapedectomy of Smyth's.[4] His statistical analysis using Chi-square tables for success or failure, sensorineural loss, fistula, and complete closure were computed. He concluded that a tissue seal provides a better success rate, a significantly lower risk of fistula and a better hearing result in terms of complete closure or overclosure of the air-bone gap. He also noted that in addition to the increased risk of sensorineural complications and fistulae the small diameter pistons did not provide as good a hearing result.

It is not possible to separate the type of footplate removal and the type of prosthesis used. Footplate surgical principles must be coordinated with the type of oval window seal and the prosthesis employed. The purpose of stapedectomy surgery is to create a functional sound-conducting mechanism in a most efficient and safe manner.

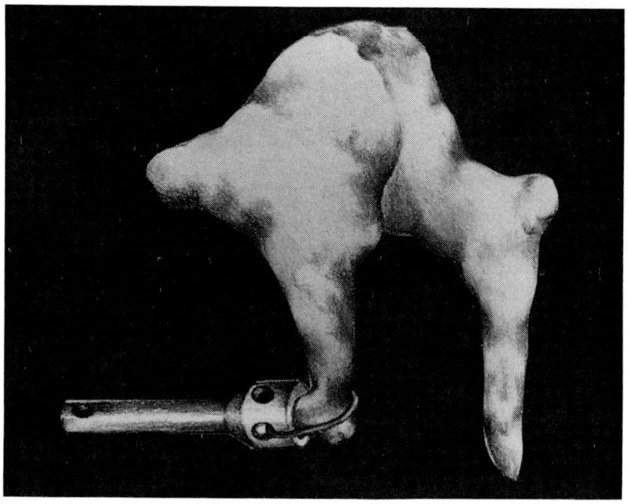

Fig. 1. Physiological attachment of the Robinson stainless steel stapes prosthesis to the lenticular process of the incus.

METHOD

Total footplate removal in every case is an impossibility because of the variable degrees of otosclerotic involvement of the footplate and the annular ligament. The principles followed are:

1. Remove all of the footplate that comes out easily.

2. Thick infiltrated footplates require drilling to create a thin blue area, which is then removed, resulting in a partial footplate removal of 0.8 mm or larger.

3. A thin vein graft is placed over the entire oval window. Edges of the graft must overlap the margins of the fenestra to avoid fistulization. The graft is slightly indented into the opening.

4. The prosthesis, a self-centering design in use for 20 years, is inserted into the graft indentation and then attached to the lentic-

Presented at the meeting of the American Otological Society, Inc., Vancouver, British Columbia, May 9-10, 1981.

REPRINTS — Mendell Robinson, MD, 130 Waterman St., Providence, RI 02906.

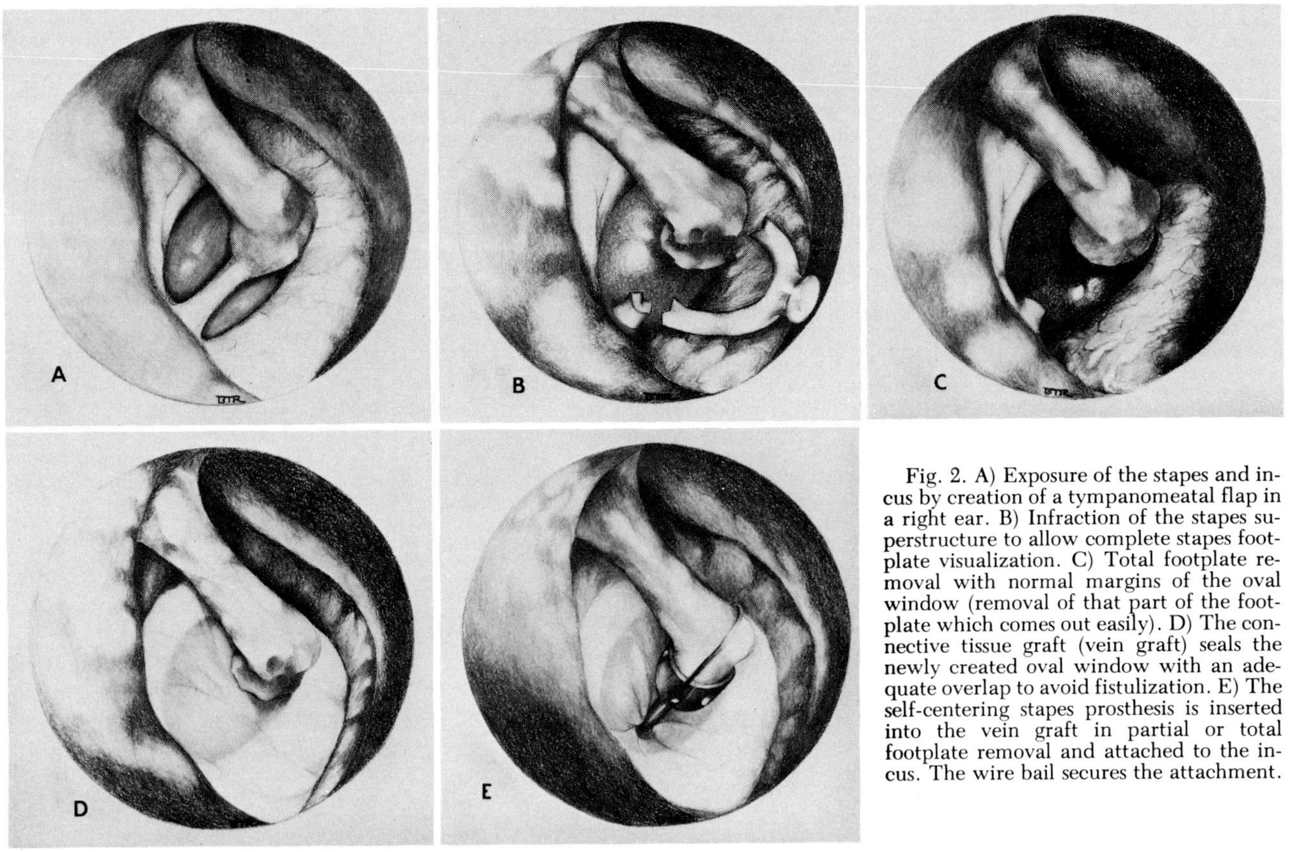

Fig. 2. A) Exposure of the stapes and incus by creation of a tympanomeatal flap in a right ear. B) Infraction of the stapes superstructure to allow complete stapes footplate visualization. C) Total footplate removal with normal margins of the oval window (removal of that part of the footplate which comes out easily). D) The connective tissue graft (vein graft) seals the newly created oval window with an adequate overlap to avoid fistulization. E) The self-centering stapes prosthesis is inserted into the vein graft in partial or total footplate removal and attached to the incus. The wire bail secures the attachment.

ular process of the incus, the most natural physiological point of attachment. As long as an opening 0.8 mm or larger is created the graft and prosthesis will function efficiently (Figs. 1 and 2).

RESULTS

By following the previously enumerated principles and techniques the initial and late results have been consistently the same in studies conducted in 1962, 1964, 1966 and 1975 (Table 1).[5-7] In each study the ratio of total footplate removals to partial footplate removals has been similar (Table 2).

In 4,761 consecutive cases from 1961-1981 the air-bone gap closure to 10 dB is essentially the same in total and partial footplate removal, and the difference is not statistically significant (97 vs 96%). However, using Chi-square tables, and using complete air-bone gap closure as the criteria for success, there is a significant difference between those cases in which the footplate was totally removed and those cases in which the footplate was partially removed (83 vs 78%). Obliterative otosclerosis (drill-out) has a lower success rate of 90% closures to within 10 dB and a lower complete closure rate (64%), which also is statistically significant. However, the obliterative cases comprise only 3% of the overall group (Table 3).

TABLE 1. POSTOPERATIVE AUDIOMETRIC RESULTS (AIR-BONE GAP CLOSURE TO 10 dB)

Cumulative No. Cases	*Year of Study*	*% Total Cases Successful Closure to 10 dB (6 mo Postop)*	*% Delayed Loss >10 dB (1-20 Yr Postop)*
76	1962	90.1	0.0
762	1964	96.0	1.0
1336	1966	96.4	1.4
3277	1975	95.5	2.8
4761	1981	96.5	3.1

COMPLICATIONS

As previously reported by Robinson in 1978 at the AAOO Annual Meeting, the immediate and delayed complication rate has been extremely low and has remained constant throughout the serial studies from 1962-1981. Air-bone gap closures to within 20 dB have varied from 1.5 to 2.9%. Failure to close to within 20 dB has been approximately 1.5%. Immediate severe or total cochlear losses are rare and have occurred in 0.2% (1 out of 50). Delayed conductive losses have been 1.8% and delayed cochlear losses 1.3%. The latter consists of bone conduction loss of more than 10 dB and speech discrimination loss of more than 10% from the best postoperative level.

With the use of the vein graft the occurrence of perilymphatic fistula has been rare; its incidence is 0.1% (6 cases), all of whom were noted to have an inadequate size vein at the time of the original surgery. There is only one known case of a granuloma occurring during the immediate postoperative period as this entity is extremely rare using the vein graft connective tissue technique.

TABLE 2. COMPARISON OF TOTAL AND PARTIAL REMOVAL OF FOOTPLATE

	TOTAL REMOVAL		PARTIAL REMOVAL		DRILLOUT
	HOOK	DRILL	HOOK	DRILL	
TOTAL NO. OPERATIONS: 4761	2999	524	524	571	143
PERCENTAGE	63%	11%	11%	12%	3%

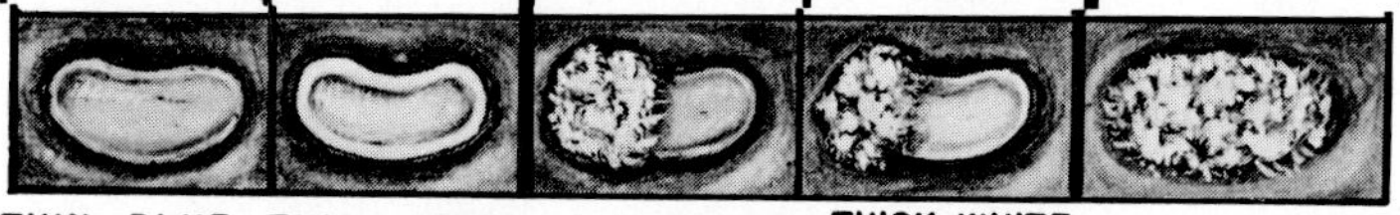

THIN BLUE FOOTPLATE — THICK WHITE MARGINS — THIN BLUE ISLAND — THICK WHITE PARTIALLY OBLITERATIVE — OBLITERATIVE

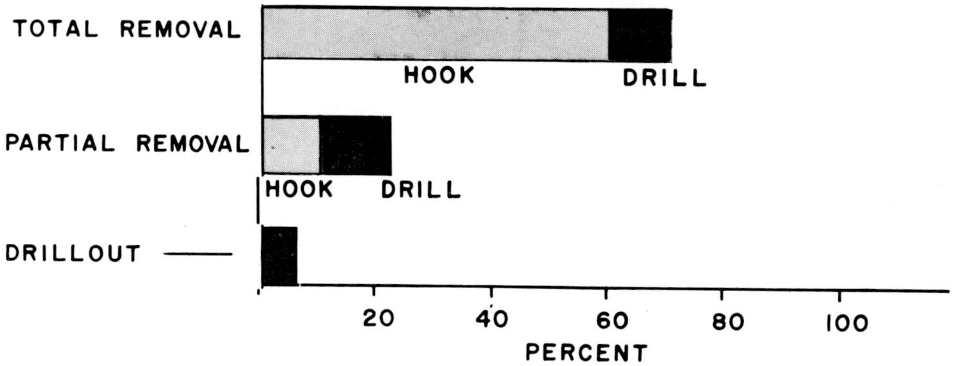

DISCUSSION

The concept of total footplate removal is a good one as evidenced by the preceding data, providing that the surgical principle of atraumatic footplate removal is adhered to by removing only part of the footplate that comes out easily, and a tissue graft with a self-centering prosthesis is used. A safe stapedectomized ear necessitates a tissue seal of the oval window opening and requires more than a one-cell-layer membrane so that the sudden violent excursions of the prosthesis during extreme barometric changes do not result in a perilymphatic fistula with transient or permanent vertigo or a sensorineural hearing loss.

TABLE 3. COMPARISON OF TOTAL AND PARTIAL FOOTPLATE REMOVAL: RESULTS OF FOOTPLATE SURGERY (N = 4761, 1961-1980)

	Total Removal (N = 3521)		*Partial Removal (N = 1097)*		*Drillout (N = 143)*	
	No.	*%*	*No.*	*%*	*No.*	*%*
A-b Gap Closure to 10 dB	3415	97	1064	96	129	90
A-b Gap Complete closure	2922	83	856	78	92	64

In addition to a safe ear there should be a maximum improvement in hearing as evidenced by *complete* air-bone gap closure, as well as improvement in the frequencies below and above the speech frequencies. Long-term maintenance of the hearing improvement is a requisite for any surgical technique. The fact that 93% of all these patients continued to maintain closure of the air-bone gap to within 10 dB speaks for itself. Other factors such as delayed sensorineural hearing losses due to presbycusis, cochlear otosclerosis, excessive noise exposure, etc, have not been elaborated upon in this paper as they are common to all stapedectomized ears regardless of the surgical technique employed.

REFERENCES

1. Shea JJ Jr. Fenestration of the oval window. Ann Otol Rhinol Laryngol 1958; 67:932-51.

2. Robinson M. A four-year study of the stainless steel stapes. Arch Otolaryngol 1965; 82:217-35.

3. Moon C. Stapedectomy, connective tissue graft and the stainless steel prosthesis. Laryngoscope 1968; 78:798-807.

4. Austin DF. Stapedectomy with tissue seal. In: Snow JB Jr, ed. Controversy in otolaryngology. Philadelphia: WB Saunders Co, 1980.

5. Robinson M. The stainless steel stapedial prosthesis, one year's experience. Laryngoscope 1962; 72:514-20.

6. Robinson M. Six years experience with the stainless steel stapedial prosthesis and vein graft. Rev Panam Otorrinolaringol Broncoesofagol 1968; 2:85.

7. Robinson M. The Robinson stapes prosthesis: a fifteen-year study. Otolaryngol Head Neck Surg 1979; 87:60-5.

COMPARISON OF SMALL FENESTRA AND TOTAL STAPEDECTOMY

T. MANFORD MCGEE, MD
SOUTHFIELD, MICHIGAN

A biostatistical study of the results of 280 consecutive operations for clinical otospongiosis are analyzed over a seven-year period. One hundred forty-one (141) operations were done utilizing the "total stapedectomy" technique, and 139 were done utilizing the "small fenestra" technique. The auditory acuity of the two groups is compared with reference to conductive and sensorineural performance. All the surgery was performed by the authors, the data was collected by a third party and analyzed by a statistician. All audiograms were performed by the same audiologist under the same conditions. The data indicates that the preferred operation for this clinical disease is the small fenestra technique.

The purpose of this paper is to report a statistical study of two methods of managing the oval window in the surgical treatment of otospongiosis. The first and most commonly practiced method of treating oval window disease is to remove the entire footplate and seal the oval window with a tissue graft upon or in which rests the prosthesis used to restore continuity between the long process of the incus and the inner ear. This procedure shall be referred to as the "total stapedectomy" technique (TS). The second method of oval window treatment is to remove only a small portion of the footplate and to insert into the vestibule, through the oval window fenestra, a solid piston prosthesis which restores the continuity of the ossicular chain and the inner ear. The prosthesis is sealed in its circumference with a tissue graft to prevent perilymphatic fistulization. This procedure shall be referred to as the "small fenestra" technique (SF).

For some time the author has had the clinical impression that patients treated with the SF technique perform better over the years than those who had TS surgery. To test this clinical impression, a statistical study is presented.

METHODS AND MATERIALS

A biostatistical study was made of 280 consecutive patients who had surgery for clinical otospongiosis. One hundred forty-one (141) cases were done by the TS technique and 139 by the SF technique. Patients in the TS group received a connective-tissue-fat wire prosthesis. Patients in the SF group received a stainless steel piston (McGee type diameter 0.6 mm). The surgery was performed by the author and all preoperative and postoperative audiograms were done under the same conditions using the same equipment. All tests were performed by the same audiologist. The data was collected and recorded by a third party and given to the statistician for analysis. The statistician stated that the patients studied represented a random sample since each subject had an equal chance of being assigned to either treatment group, and the time period between the start of one treatment group and the start of the other was insignificant.

The patients in the study were not classified by age, sex, preoperative audiograms or pathology since the purpose of the study was to reflect the findings of a random sample of patients with clinical disease. Such a sample by definition contains individuals who exhibit the variables mentioned.

CONDUCTIVE DATA

Revisions. Of 299 primary operations, 19 required a second surgery to correct significant conductive pathology. These 19 patients were excluded from the statistical analysis. Fourteen revisions were from the TS group and five from the SF group. The most common finding at revision surgery in the TS group was that of retraction of the wire prosthesis to the margin of the oval window. The conductive pathology in the five SF patients was related to a loosening of the wire at its attachment to the incus. This loss of continuity was due to notching of the incus as a result of faulty surgical technique and reduction in the circumference of the incus as a result of osteoperosis.[1] There were no cases of perilymphatic fistulization in the 19 revision operations.

Air-Bone Gap Study. Table 1 presents the results of the study of closure of the air-bone gap to within 10 dB or better of the preoperative bone conduction average for the three speech frequencies. It is obvious in measuring this parameter that the SF technique is superior to TS since the statistical trend is in favor of the SF in five of the eight time periods studied. This data supports the postmortem findings and conclusions of Schuknecht and Jones[2] that the prosthesis with tissue seals which overlap the margins of the oval window following TS may result in incomplete closure of the air-bone gap due to improper placement or subsequent migration of the prosthesis. They further suggest that these conductive problems can be avoided by using a SF technique.

SENSORINEURAL DATA

Bone Conduction Study. Table 2 presents the data concerning the study of bone conduction thresholds for the average of the three speech fre-

From the Department of Otolaryngology, Providence Hospital, Southfield, Michigan, and Wayne State University School of Medicine, Detroit.
Presented at the meeting of the American Otological Society, Inc., Vancouver, British Columbia, May 9-10, 1981.
REPRINTS — T. Manford McGee, MD, 22000 Greenfield, Oak Park, MI 48237.

TABLE 1. CLOSURE OF THE AIR-BONE GAP TO 10 dB OR BETTER OF THE PREOPERATIVE BONE CONDUCTION FOR THE THREE SPEECH FREQUENCIES

Follow-up (yr)	*Surgery*	*Criteria Satisfied Yes*	*No*	*Total*	*Percent Improved*	*μ*	*X²(1df)*	*P*	*Trend*
½	SF	134	5	139	96.4				
	TS	121	20	141	85.8				
	Total	255	25	280	91.1		8.61	<.005	SF
1	SF	12	2	14	85.7				
	TS	12	1	13	92.3				
	Total	24	3	27	88.9	0.55	0.30	NS	None
2	SF	24	2	26	92.3				
	TS	14	8	22	63.6				
	Total	38	10	48	79.2	2.44	5.95	.025<p <.01	SF
3	SF	23	3	26	88.5				
	TS	23	8	31	74.2				
	Total	46	11	57	80.7	1.35	1.82	NS	None
4	SF	16	2	18	88.9				
	TS	14	8	22	63.6				
	Total	30	10	40	75.0	1.83	3.35	.05<p <.10	SF
5	SF	18	2	20	90.0				
	TS	13	9	22	61.9				
	Total	31	11	42	75.6	2.30	5.29	.01<p <.025	SF
6	SF	18	6	24	75.0				
	TS	10	16	26	38.5				
	Total	28	22	50	56.0	2.60	6.76	.005<p <.01	SF
7	SF	8	3	11	72.7				
	TS	0	5	5	0.0				
	Total	8	8	16	50.0	Fisher's Exact		p<.025	None

quencies followed over a seven-year period. It is interesting to note that there is very little significant statistical difference between the two techniques with the exception of the first six months and the fifth postoperative year. Bone conduction at 4 kHz in the SF patients averaged 7½ to 10 dB better during the years studied than did the patients in the TS group. These findings concerning 4 kHz are in agreement with and support the data of Smyth and Hassard[3] who reported that 4 kHz was significantly better in patients who received the SF operation as opposed to those that received a large fenestra or TS operation. Their data extended through ten years of follow-up. Smyth and Hassard also reported in long-term studies of bone conduction of the three speech frequencies that the SF technique did not provide better bone conduction at 0.5 kHz and provided less satisfactory thresholds at 1 and 2 kHz than did the TS or large fenestra group. The present study does not support this data when the three speech frequencies are averaged. There is, in fact, a slight trend in favor of the SF technique (six months and five years).

All of the above data, when considered in con-

TABLE 2. PATIENTS WITHIN 10 dB OF THE PREOPERATIVE BONE CONDUCTION AVERAGE OF THREE SPEECH FREQUENCIES

Follow-up (yr)	*Surgery*	*Criteria Satisfied Yes*	*No*	*Total*	*Percent Improved*	*μ*	*X²(1df)*	*P*	*Trend*
½	SF	139	0	139	100.0				
	TS	137	4	141	97.2				
	Total	276	4	280	98.6		4.06	.025<p <.05	SF
1	SF	14	0	14	100.0				
	TS	13	0	13	100.0				
	Total	27	0	27	100.0	Fisher's Exact		NS	None
2	SF	26	0	26	100.0				
	TS	21	1	22	95.5				
	Total	47	1	48	97.9	0.21	0.04	NS	None
3	SF	25	1	26	96.2				
	TS	28	3	31	90.3				
	Total	53	4	57	93.0	1.32	1.74	NS	None
4	SF	17	1	18	94.4				
	TS	19	3	22	86.4				
	Total	36	4	40	90.0	0.84	0.71	NS	None
5	SF	20	0	20	100.0				
	TS	16	6	22	72.7				
	Total	36	6	42	85.7	2.52	6.35	.01<p <.025	SF
6	SF	23	1	24	95.8				
	TS	22	4	26	84.6				
	Total	45	5	50	90.0	1.32	1.74	NS	None
7	SF	9	3	12	75.0				
	TS	3	2	5	60.0				
	Total	12	5	17	70.6	Fisher's Exact		NS	None

TABLE 3. PATIENTS WITH DISCRIMINATION SCORES WITHIN 10% OR BETTER OF THE PREOPERATIVE SCORE

Follow-up (yr)	*Surgery*	*Criteria Satisfied* Yes	No	*Total*	*Percent Improved*	*μ*	*X²(1df)*	*P*	*Trend*
½	SF	129	10	139	92.8				
	TS	118	23	141	83.7				
	Total	247	33	280	88.2		5.69	.01<p <.025	SF
1	SF	12	2	14	85.7				
	TS	12	1	13	92.3				
	Total	24	3	27	88.9			NS	None
2	SF	24	2	26	92.3				
	TS	19	3	22	86.4				
	Total	43	5	48	89.6	1.30	1.69	NS	None
3	SF	24	2	26	92.3				
	TS	27	4	31	87.1				
	Total	51	6	57	89.5	0.64	0.41	NS	None
4	SF	16	2	18	88.9				
	TS	13	9	22	59.1				
	Total	29	11	40	72.5	2.07	4.28	.025<p <.05	SF
5	SF	19	1	20	95.0				
	TS	15	7	22	68.2				
	Total	34	8	42	81.0	2.21	4.88	.01<p <.025	SF
6	SF	22	2	24	91.7				
	TS	16	10	26	61.5				
	Total	38	12	50	76.0	2.49	6.20	.01<p <.25	SF
7	SF	10	1	11	90.9				
	TS	4	1	5	80.0				
	Total	14	2	16	87.5			p<.025	SF

junction with the discrimination studies that follow, suggests that bone conduction changes which affect speech discrimination most likely occur at frequencies above 2 kHz if the average of the three speech frequencies are within 10 dB or better of the patient's norm.

Discrimination Study. Table 3 reflects the most sensitive measure of sensorineural function, which is the ability to discriminate language. The data reveal that there is a strong trend in favor of the superiority of the SF technique with respect to the ability of patients to discriminate words. This trend is present at six months and present consecutively for years four through seven. The discrimination study, coupled with the bone conduction data reviewed above, strongly suggests that 4 kHz is important to good discrimination assuming that 0.500, 1 and 2 kHz are within reasonably normal limits. Since bone conduction thresholds at 4 kHz are consistently lower in the SF technique, it is not unreasonable to assume that 3 kHz is also significantly improved. If this assumption is valid, then another factor favoring the SF operation is present.

COMMENTS ON FOLLOW-UP STUDIES

The mobility of our society, especially in highly industrialized centers, is one factor which contributes to lack of meaningful follow-up studies beyond eight to ten years. There are other contributory factors, such as death, no known address, inability of patients to cooperate due to personal reasons, and finally lack of patient interest. It is dangerous to assume that lack of patient interest is related to the fact that their hearing remains adequate. However, patients frequently report when contacted for follow-up studies that they felt no need to see the doctor because their hearing was unchanged. We do not, therefore, know for certain if these statistics are biased, and if they are, in which direction the bias is slanted. By using a random sample of consecutively operated patients the author hopes to have minimized the problem of sample bias.

The follow-up rate in this study varies from 100% at six months to as low as less than 10% at year 7. With the exception of six months, the highest follow-up rate peaked at year 3, then held fairly steady until year 7. In spite of these variations in follow-up rate, the statistician is confident that the numbers are of statistical significance.

CONCLUSIONS

The data clearly support the author's original impression that the SF technique is the treatment of choice in the surgical management of clinical otospongiosis. This is confirmed by both conductive and sensorineural statistical data. The type of prosthesis used in the TS technique is probably of no significance; however, the SF technique requires a piston type prosthesis by definition. It is of importance to adequately seal the piston and fenestra in its circumference to preclude any perilymphatic fistulization. Speculation as to why the statistical difference between the two techniques exists is in part conjecture. However, there are pathological and experimental studies which suggest that surgical trauma and problems related to overlapping the oval window with tissue grafts in the TS technique may be contributing factors.[2,4]

REFERENCES

1. McGee TM. The loose wire syndrome. Laryngoscope 1981 (in press).

2. Schuknecht HF, Jones DD. Stapedectomy postmortem findings. Ann Otol Rhinol Laryngol 1979; 88 Suppl 55.

3. Smyth G, Hassard TH. Eighteen years experience in stapedectomy. Ann Otol Rhinol Laryngol 1978; 87 Suppl 49.

4. Hayden RC Jr, McGee TM. Traumatized oval window fat grafts. Arch Otolaryngol 1965; 81:243-9.

CONTRAINDICATIONS TO THE SMALL HOLE STAPEDECTOMY

BROWN FARRIOR, MD

TAMPA, FLORIDA

A small hole stapedectomy with an unprotected piston is contraindicated in an ear subjected to excessive pressure changes whether these are excessive fluid pressure changes which occur in the inner ear or excessive air pressure changes in the middle ear. Excessive fluid pressure changes in the inner ear may be the result of an overly patent aqueduct of the cochlea or a permeable internal auditory canal. These excessive fluid pressure changes may produce fistulas or a dilated blister around the piston called a tented piston. Excessive air pressure changes in the middle ear will produce excessive excursions of the tympanic membrane which may result in vertigo or a dislocated piston.

INTRODUCTION

The small hole stapedectomy with an unprotected piston is contraindicated in an ear subjected to excessive pressure changes whether these are excessive fluid pressure changes in the inner ear or excessive air pressure changes in the middle ear. These pressure changes are contraindications for they may produce fistulas, a tented piston, or a dislocated piston, as will be described in a series of 315 mature, small hole stapedectomies performed about 15 years ago.

Perilabyrinthine Hydrops. The excessive fluid pressure changes in the inner ear may be the result of a permeable membrane at the internal auditory canal or an overly patent aqueduct of the cochlea. I have called these positive pressures "perilabyrinthine hydrops." In a true stapes gusher of cerebrospinal fluid as seen in congenital mixed deafness or the permeable internal auditory canal of a true Mondini-Alexander syndrome, the flow of CSF cannot be controlled with a bare piston. In the usual stapes operation, after perforation of the stapedial footplate, the perilabyrinthine fluid repeatedly wells up to fill the oval window. This evidence of positive perilabyrinthine fluid pressure is a contraindication of the use of the bare piston because it will result in an immediate and possibly permanent poststapedectomy oval window fistula. If the oval window fistula does seal with a good mucoendosteal membrane, this mucoendosteal membrane is subjected to the continuous excessive pressure of the

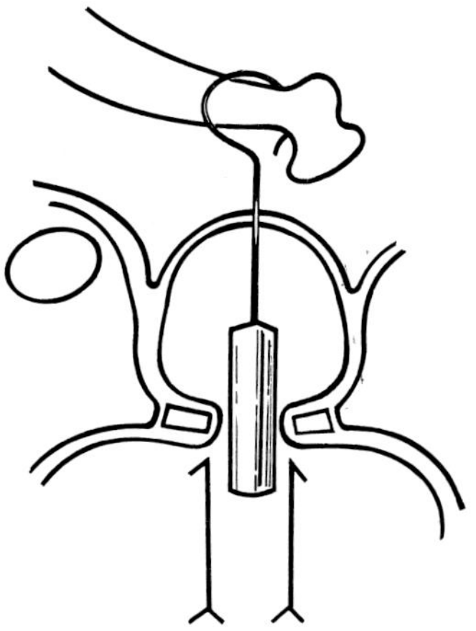

Fig. 1. Excessive inner ear changes will gradually push the mucoendosteal membrane up the shaft of the piston to produce a tented piston. These excessive pressure changes may be produced by a patent aqueduct of the cochlea or a permeable internal auditory canal.

perilabyrinthine hydrops and will eventually result in blister formation in the oval window. The mucoendosteal membrane is gradually pushed outward to the "lips" of the oval window, and with time may be pushed outward up the shaft of the piston so that it hangs over the piston as a tent (Fig. 1).

From these internal pressures a tented piston may develop ten or more years after an apparent and dramatic successful small hole stapedectomy. The patient will present symptoms of slowly progressive hearing loss and distortion of hearing, and although this may be the patient's better hearing ear he does

From the Otolaryngology Service of St. Joseph's Hospital and University of South Florida College of Medicine, Tampa. Supported by Grant 1980-9, The David Falk Foundation.

Presented at the meeting of the American Otological Society, Inc., Vancouver, British Columbia, May 9-10, 1981.

REPRINTS — Brown Farrior, MD, 509 Bay Street, Tampa, FL 33606.

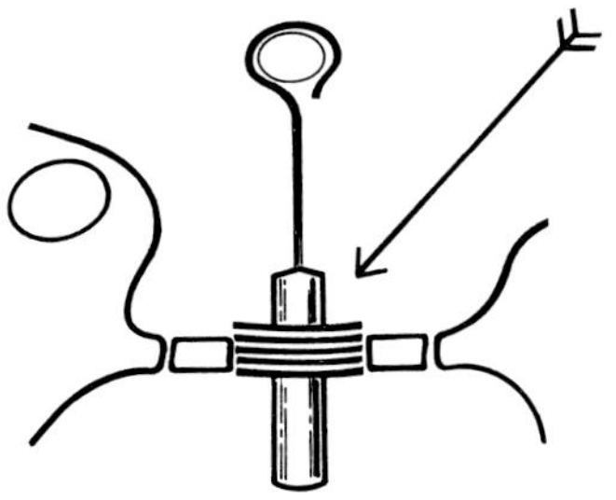

Fig. 2. In a tented piston the elevated mucoendosteal membrane must be stripped from the piston and returned to the normal "lips" of the oval window. Tenting may be prevented by placing a graft under the piston. A graft may be required with the argon laser.

not like the quality of his hearing. I have had three such tented pistons develop more than ten years after I performed small hole stapedectomies in which I stripped the tent from around the piston and returned the stripped membrane to the level of the oval window (Fig. 2). This has resulted in the restoration of hearing to the optimal level. However, in one of these over the past two years there has been a gradual hearing loss apparently from a recurrence of the tented piston.

For 20 years I have taught that the oval window should be sealed with a viable tissue graft to prevent the development of postoperative fistulas. If I return to the use of the small hole stapedectomy, I would seal the oval window with a very thin fascia graft by placing a "sock" of thin fascia over the foot of the piston. Such a socked piston may be fabricated by pressing a small 2 x 2 mm thin fascia graft into a 0.6 mm hole in the DIE with a 0.4 mm piston or simply by pressing the fascia through the hole in the footplate. However, I prefer the former prefabrication to avoid impacting the footplate. Since 1964, I have always sealed the piston with a viable graft, but prefer to have a thin graft under the piston, ie, a socked piston or a "capped" piston.

Middle Ear Pressure Changes. The small hole stapedectomy with the unprotected piston is contraindicated in any patient subjected to high middle ear pressure changes which cause excessive excursions of the tympanic membrane, incus, and piston. These excessive excursions result in the dislocation of a short piston (Fig. 3) or in vertigo in the case of a long piston.

The middle ear pressure changes may be the result of a patulous eustachian tube with hyperventilation of the middle ear and the excessive movement of the drum, incus, and piston. Before performing any stapedectomy one should always have the patient perform the Valsalva maneuver and observe for this excessive movement of the tympanic membrane. Routinely the incus should be elevated to inspect and insure adequate length of the piston.

In patients such as divers, pilots, and patients with a patulous eustachian tube who are subjected to excessive middle ear pressure changes, I will

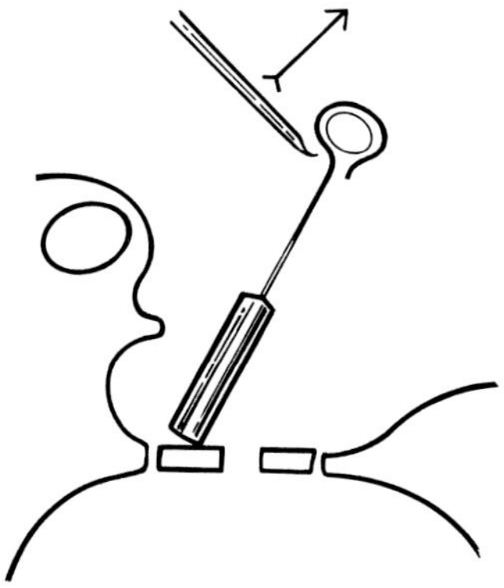

Fig. 3. A dislocated piston may be caused by excessive air pressure changes in the middle ear and the resultant excessive movement of the tympanic membrane, malleus, incus and prosthesis. Excessive middle ear pressure changes occur in pilots, divers and patients with patulous, abnormally patent eustachian tubes.

usually preserve the stapedius tendon in an effort to limit the mobility of the incus. The technique used will be dependent upon its anatomic placement on the lenticular process of the incus, the neck of the stapes or the posterior crus of the stapes. The tendon may be left attached to the incus, to the transposed or repositioned posterior crus, or to a double crurotomy. In these patients subjected to pressure changes, I prefer to have the graft incorporated in the wire rather than use an onlay type of prosthesis laid over the graft material because with excessive movement of the drum, the prosthesis may be dislocated to one side. In one patient with an abnormally patent eustachian tube, I observed an onlay prefabricated wire perforate a perichondrial graft and produce a buttonhole fistula into the oval window.

In stapedectomy for more than 20 years I have routinely used the incorporated tissue wire prosthesis beginning with the Kos vein plug because I believe that the vein tissue has certain advantages over the Schuknecht graft. However, the latter has certain advantages of its own: first, the greatest advantage is the ability to mold the lobule graft so that there is a gentle seal of the oval window; second, the incorporated lobule graft is firmly fixed at the lips of the oval window so that it cannot be dislocated outward or inward; third, in contrast to the onlay oval window graft, the mucosa need be stripped only from the very lips of the oval window and there is therefore minimal incidence of postoperative fistulas. With a lobule graft, a fistula will form only if the graft inadequately fills the window or if the flaps of the mucous membrane are folded into the inner ear.

Of course, with complete removal of the footplate there is a greater risk of trauma to the inner ear, but hopefully this is minimized with experience, as is proven by Robinson's excellent presentation.[1] The poorest results are obtained in those cases in which we have the most surgical problems.

TABLE 1. 1000 STAPEDECTOMIES PERFORMED BETWEEN 1963-1968

Case No.	Year	Drill	Small Hole or Piston
1401 - 1500	1963	9	22
1501 - 1600	1963	14	55
1601 - 1700	1964	13	25
1701 - 1800	1964	9	30
1801 - 1900	1965	10	21
1901 - 2000	1965	10	75
2001 - 2100	1966	11	43
2100 - 2200	1966	7	12
2201 - 2300	1967	8	14
2301 - 2400	1968	7	18
Total		98	315

The 315 small hole stapedectomies started with 34 McGee pistons (0.8 mm), then changed to the telf-wire piston and beginning in 1963, are the 0.6 mm pistons. With the 0.6 mm piston the opening in the footplate is just large enough to permit the free movement of the 0.6 mm piston gauge, an estimated 0.7 mm opening in thin footplates and an estimated 0.8 mm opening in the drill cases. To prevent the formation of a fistula, a lobule graft (fat) seal was placed around the piston beginning in January 1964.

RESULTS

I have reviewed 1,000 stapedectomies performed between 1963 and 1968; among these are included 315 small hole stapedectomies, an incidence of 31.5% (Table 1). Among the latter were 98 drill cases, an incidence of 9.8% with thick footplates or obliterative otosclerosis.

The highest incidence of small hole stapedectomies was 75% performed in the second 1965 series. The percentage decreased rapidly, and the incidence has now decreased to less than 10% because of two reasons: 1) my personal preference for the security of an incorporated wire-lobule graft and 2) the decreasing backlog of long-standing cases of otosclerosis. Therefore, there is now a decreasing incidence of thick or obliterative otosclerosis which requires the use of the hand or power drill. The detailed analysis and comparative statistics are not completed, but I have been impressed with the hearing acuity in these piston cases. In those patients with a small hole stapedectomy and piston in one ear and an incorporated wire-lobule graft (fat) in the other ear, when the pure tone and speech are practically identical, the patient will occasionally complain that the hearing is sharper in the piston ear and they prefer the hearing in the lobule graft ear.

Drill Cases and the Small Hole Stapedectomy. The small hole stapedectomy with the piston and graft seal is the operation of choice in thick footplate otosclerosis and in obliterative otosclerosis that require the use of the hand or power drill to create an opening through the footplate into the inner ear. In these drill cases there appears to be enough irritation at the level of the footplate to produce a good cicatricial ring around the piston and hold the mucoendosteal membrane at the level of the footplate and thus prevent postoperative fistulas or the long delayed tenting of the piston.

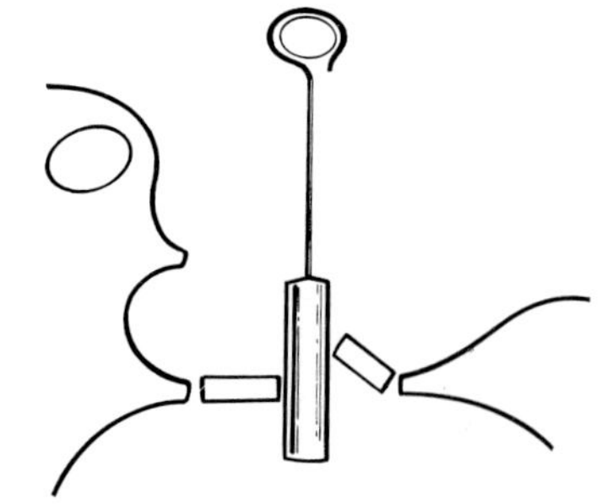

Fig. 4. When a tilted footplate is produced in attempting a small hole stapedectomy, the tilted footplate should be removed and replaced with a graft. The argon laser will reduce the incidence of a tilted footplate but alone it is uncertain whether it will produce an adequate seal at the "lips" of the oval window.

In drill cases, I have not seen a postoperative fistula and I do not know of a surgeon who has seen a fistula in a patient with thick or obliterative otosclerosis. Also, I have not seen the delaying tenting of the piston in such a patient.

In regard to the use of the argon laser in a small hole stapedectomy, I am not certain that the laser will produce enough annular cicatrization to fix the mucoendosteal membrane at the level of the footplate. Therefore, if one is going to perform a laser small hole stapedectomy, I would recommend the use of thin fascia over the foot of the piston, a socked piston, or a capped piston.

With the thick footplate and obliterative otosclerosis which require the use of a drill to create an opening in the oval window, this opening must be of sufficient size to permit the free movement of the piston, ie, it will require a 0.8 mm opening in the oval window to permit the free movement of an 0.6 mm piston and/or an 0.6 mm opening to permit the free movement of an 0.4 mm piston. For this purpose in the early 1960s I developed the piston gauge and oval window elevator to insure and calibrate an adequate opening in the footplate. Now manufactured with a cap diameter of 0.5 and 0.6 mm and the shaft which is calibrated at 5 mm, this instrument has proven very useful in estimating the exact size of the opening in the footplate and also in removing fragments of the footplate in all directions. In total stapedectomies it also permits scarification of the "lips" of the oval window to prevent postoperative fistulas.

With Smyth using an 0.3 mm piston, Fisch an 0.4 mm piston, and McGee using an 0.6 mm and 0.4 mm piston, where we originally started with an 0.8 mm piston, we must define a small hole stapedectomy and propose the following: a small hole stapedectomy should be defined as a stapedectomy with an 0.6 mm piston or less, with the removal of less than 25% of the footplate and with or without a thin tissue graft under the piston.

Tilting of the Footplate. When planning to perform a small hole stapedectomy with a piston, tilting the front or the back half of the footplate (Fig. 4), and inserting the piston thinking free movement will result, one will usually be disappointed in the patients who usually obtain only a partial closure of the air-bone gap. Therefore, if tilting of the remaining portion of the footplate is obtained, I would recommend a contraindication to the small hole stapedectomy that the remaining portion of the footplate be removed and that one proceed with a total stapedectomy and the total graft to the oval window be the technique of choice.

Argon Laser. The "burned hole" stapedectomy may eliminate the problem of the tilted footplate, but the laser stapedectomy may still require a thin tissue graft under the piston to prevent fistulas or internal pressure tenting of the piston.

SUMMARY

1. The small hole stapedectomy with a bare piston is contraindicated when there are excessive fluid pressure changes in the inner ear and when there are excessive air pressure changes in the middle ear.

2. The small hole stapedectomy is the operation of choice in thick footplate or obliterative otosclerosis which requires the use of the hand or power drill to create an opening in the oval window.

3. When a small hole stapedectomy is attempted and there is a tilting of a portion of the footplate, the footplate should be removed and the window sealed with a graft.

4. Complications of a small hole stapedectomy are rare but consist of fistulas, a tented piston, a dislocated piston or a partial closure with a tilted footplate.

5. The argon laser "burned hole" technique will reduce the incidence of the tilted footplate. It may or may not produce an adequate seal of the "lips" of the oval window and thereby prevent fistulas and a delayed tented piston.

6. Complications of a small hole stapedectomy may be reduced by placing a thin tissue graft over the foot of the piston, a socked piston or a capped piston.

REFERENCES

1. Robinson M. Total footplate extraction in stapedectomy. Ann Otol Rhinol Laryngol 1981; 90:630-2.

≈

Ann Otol 90:1981

BIOINERT CERAMIC IMPLANTS IN MIDDLE EAR SURGERY

KLAUS JAHNKE, MD DIETRICH PLESTER, MD

TÜBINGEN, FEDERAL REPUBLIC OF GERMANY

The suitability of different ceramic materials for reconstructive middle ear surgery was examined in extensive animal experiments. Since 1978 we have used more than 250 aluminum oxide ceramic implants for ossicular chain reconstruction. The excellent tolerance of this bioinert material was confirmed. The ease and precision with which these implants can be drilled during the operation is especially advantageous. The indications and techniques for the use of the aluminum oxide ceramic implants are described. Our short-term results stimulated the further development of bioinert ceramic implants and our surgical techniques. The special characteristics of bioactive ceramics are such that they can form a tight bond to osseous bone. They are intended for filling bone cavities (porous tricalcium phosphate ceramic) and for reconstruction of the posterior canal wall.

There is no material in reconstructive middle ear surgery which fits the requirements of all specific situations. Autogenous and allogenous ossicles, which we still use in many well-defined cases, may lead to bony fixation to the wall of the attic when lateralization occurs, or fixation may take place in narrow oval niches. There may be partial resorption or atrophy of the material after extensive shaping or exposure to infection. The same is true of cartilage, which in addition does not exhibit sufficient rigidity. The use of organic alloplastic prostheses often resulted in rejection reactions due to low biocompatibility. Porous plastic prostheses were partially or totally extruded especially when these materials came into contact with the tympanic membrane. This led most surgeons to place cartilage between the implant and the plane of the eardrum.[1] In histological studies of plastic prostheses removed at revision operations of noninfected, closed ears we regularly found a thick fibrous layer covering the porous implant. The pores of the prosthesis were mainly filled with macrophages, giant cells and debris.[2-4]

In the search for better materials for reconstructive middle ear surgery, we examined the following in extensive animal experiments: 1) bioinert highly pure aluminum oxide ceramics (Fig. 1A, B), 2) several bioactive porous and dense tricalcium phosphate ceramics, and 3) bioactive glass ceramic (Macor).

Prior to full acceptance of any prosthetic material we must first convince ourselves of its biocompatibility in various animal tympanoplastic procedures. It is obvious that only a few of the many metals available are applicable for use in middle ear surgery. The same is true of ceramics.

There are striking differences between bioactive and bioinert ceramics, each exhibiting specific advantages for middle ear surgery. The terms bioactive and bioinert are related to the biochemical response induced by the materials at the site of implantation. The tissue reactions caused by relative movements between the implant and the adjacent tissue are not covered by these terms. The special characteristics of bioactive ceramics are such that they can form a tight junction to osseous tissue. It is a purely biochemical phenomenon, due to the dissolution of some ions from the surface of the material into the adjacent tissue.

Porous tricalcium phosphate ceramics are more or less degradable, depending on the various degrees of porosity. They are intended for the filling of bone defects, as the calcium phosphates are rather similar to the mineral composition of bone tissue.[5] We are currently investigating the suitability of porous tricalcium phosphate ceramics for the obliteration of the mastoid air cell system.

The glass ceramic, Macor, which we studied in the rabbit and the guinea pig middle ear, did not show the excellent biocompatibility of the glass ceramics reported by Reck.[6] Since the implantation of this material resulted in new bone formation on its surface, we do not recommend its use in the middle ear.

A highly pure aluminum oxide ceramic* is the prototype of a bioinert material. This means it does not release any trace substances detectable by current analytical methods.[7] It consists of corundum crystals, about 5 μm in size, built into a dense and practically poreless structure. In respect to its chemical composition and its crystal structure, corundum is basically identical to ruby and sapphire.

The outstanding biocompatibility of this material after being implanted into the middle ear has been shown by our animal experiments which included

*Frialit (a trademark of Friedrichsfeld GmbH, Postfach 7, D-6800 Mannheim 71, West Germany).

From the ENT-Department, University of Tübingen, Federal Republic of Germany.

Presented at the meeting of the American Otological Society, Inc., Vancouver, British Columbia, May 9-10, 1981.

REPRINTS — Klaus Jahnke, MD, ENT-Department, University of Tübingen, D7400 Tübingen - 1 Silcherstrasse 5, Federal Republic of Germany.

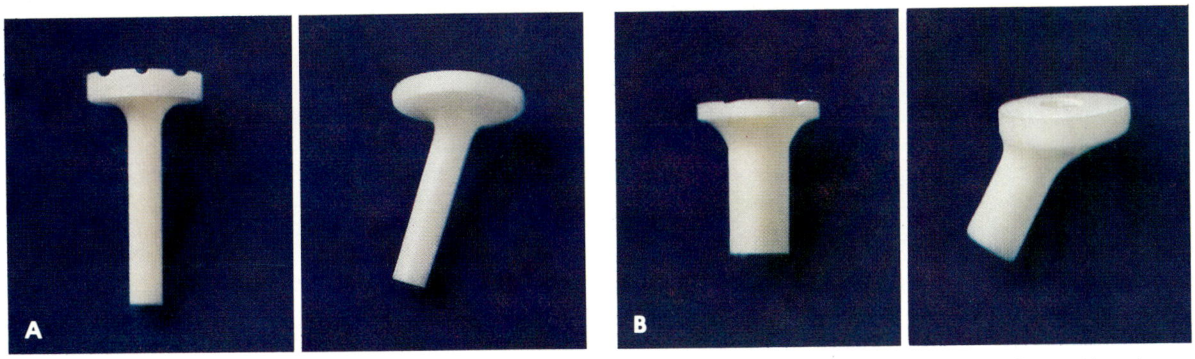

Fig. 1. Straight and angled aluminum oxide ceramic implants. A) Columella type (8 mm); B) hollow shaft type (5 mm).

scanning as well as transmission electron microscopic studies.[8] Within three weeks the implants were covered with a delicate mucous membrane (Fig. 2A). We usually found a cuboidal epithelium with microvilli, occasionally some ciliated cells, both on an intact basement membrane. There was a normal subepithelial cell layer with active fibroblasts, blood vessels and nerve fibers. We observed no encapsulation by connective tissue, and no macrophages or giant cells were detected three weeks postoperatively or thereafter.

Since 1978 we used bioinert aluminum oxide ceramic implants in more than 250 patients for the reconstruction of the ossicular chain. We designed both a columella-type implant and a hollow-shaft implant for interposition between the head of the stapes and the plane of the tympanic membrane (Fig. 1A, B).[9] Almost always the selected implant has to be ground during the operation to the required dimensions with a diamond drill (Fig. 2B). This is the only way a final implant form can be created to achieve exact fit, positional stability and optimal physiological conditions. One groove of the end-plate may be deepened and broadened in order to prevent its slipping off the handle of the malleus (Fig. 2C). In addition we learned from our short-term follow-up studies that the grooves on the end-plate are an important factor in the nutrition of the adjacent tympanic membrane graft. We regularly found blood vessels within the grooves. Furthermore the attachment of the end-plate to the tympanic membrane graft can be improved by drilling small holes into the end-plate. In selected instances a piece of tragal cartilage is interposed between the tympanic membrane graft and the implant for stabilization of atrophic eardrums and in order to prevent the development of retraction pockets. The connection between the rigid implant and the head of the footplate of the stapes results in a joint-like linkage. In addition, the interposition of a fascial or perichondrial graft is recommended especially on the footplate in order to protect it and to help in the development of a joint-like type of articulation. A perichondrial graft with an adjacent, perforated piece of cartilage can increase the positional stability of the implant on the footplate of the stapes. The attachment to the capitulum of the stapes can be improved by drilling notches in such a way that the implant can be placed on the tendon of the stapedius muscle, without any risk of bony fixation at the facial canal.

The main purpose of our short-term follow-up studies, which included the first 150 patients, was to evaluate and improve our techniques. The results were reported elsewhere.[10] They are significantly better than our results obtained previously with other alloplastic materials (eg, porous plastic prostheses). Failures (air-bone gap of more than 30 dB)

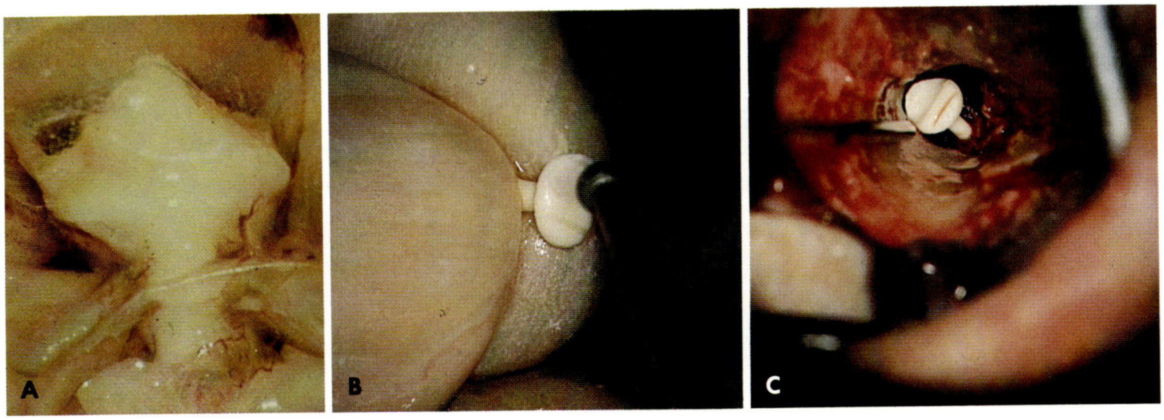

Fig. 2. Aluminum oxide ceramic implant A) 10 months after implantation in rabbit middle ear, covered by normal mucosa (the implant is adjacent to the tympanic membrane); B) shaped with drill; C) inserted.

in our nonstaged tympanoplasties are 10% and were mostly due to tubal dysfunction (3% were due to extrusion). When the malleus lies far anterior in relationship to the stapes, a larger piece of cartilage should be interposed. Especially in such cases, retraction of the entire eardrum and the adjacent implant may cause the end-plate of the implant to turn outwards, resulting in interference with the blood supply of the tympanic membrane. To overcome such problems we also designed two types of angled implants. The advantageous physical properties of these bioinert ceramic implants is demonstrated by the fact that excellent closure of the airbone gap has been achieved in many patients.

REFERENCES

1. Brackmann ED, Sheehy JL. Tympanoplasty: TORPs and PORPs. Laryngoscope 1979; 89:108-14.

2. Belal A, Odnert S. TORPs and PORPs: what happens in the middle ear. Am J Otol 1980; 2:10-4.

3. Galic M, Jahnke K. Kunststoffe in der Mittelohrchirurgie. Presented at the annual meeting of the Deutsche Gesellschaft für Hals-Nasen-Ohren-Heilkunde, Kopf- und Hals-Chirurgie, Wiesbaden, 1981.

4. Kerr AG. Proplast and Plastipore. Clin Otolaryngol 1981; 6:187-91.

5. Koester K, Karbe E, Kramer H, Heide H, König R. Experimenteller Knochenersatz durch resorbierbare Calciumphosphat-Keramik. Langenbecks Arch Chir 1976; 341:77-86.

6. Reck R. Tissue reactions to glass ceramics in the middle ear. Clin Otolaryngol 1981; 6:63-5.

7. Heimke G, Griss P. Ceramic implant materials. Med Biol Eng Comput 1980; 18:503-10.

8. Jahnke K, Galic M, Eitel W, Heumann H. Electron microscope observations of Al_2O_3-ceramic implants in middle ear surgery. In: Advances in biomaterials. Vol. 3. John Wiley and Sons (in press).

9. Jahnke K, Plester D, Heimke G. Aluminiumoxid-Keramik, ein bioninertes Material für die Mittelohrchirurgie. Arch Otorhinolaryngol 1979; 223:373-6.

10. Plester D, Jahnke K. Ceramic implants in otologic surgery. Am J Otol 1981; 2:104-8.

Ann Otol 90:1981

COMPARATIVE STUDY USING COMPUTED TOMOGRAPHIC THIN-SECTION ZOOM RECONSTRUCTIONS AND ANATOMIC MACROSECTIONS OF THE TEMPORAL BONE

CHARLES W. BEATTY, MD
LOWELL D. HARRIS, PhD
KU WON SUH, MD
DAVID F. REESE, MD

ROCHESTER, MINNESOTA

Thin-section (1.5 mm) high-spatial-resolution computed tomography (CT) in combination with computerized high-resolution image reconstruction is an effective, noninvasive means of studying patients with a variety of temporal bone abnormalities. To determine what degree of definition and anatomic accuracy could currently be obtained by using these techniques, we performed thin-section CT and high-resolution image reconstruction with use of two fresh-frozen cadaver head specimens. We then compared these images with the actual anatomic macrosections subsequently obtained from the specimens. We concluded that high-resolution CT scans of the temporal bone can produce accurate, highly detailed, diagnostic images of the internal auditory canal, vestibule, cochlea, vestibular aqueduct, semicircular canals, ossicles, and middle ear space.

Since its introduction[1] and clinical application in 1973[2,3] computed tomography (CT) has made enormous contributions in the areas of diagnostic medicine, treatment planning, and follow-up. During this same period, advances in CT technology and image quality have evolved at a staggering rate.

Two recent innovations in commercial CT have made it possible to obtain exceptionally detailed, magnified, cross-sectional images of the temporal bone. These innovations are the abilities to scan thin (1.5 mm) sections and to perform special high-resolution, magnified, or "zoom" reconstructions of selected regions of a scanned section.

In the past decade, several excellent articles and textbooks have reported correlations of anatomic macrosections[4,5] or histologic sections[6,7] with various conventional multidirectional tomographic images of the temporal bone. In this study, sequential, parallel, 1.5 mm thin-section CT scans were performed covering the extent of the temporal bones in the clinically obtainable coronal and axial planes before the temporal bones were removed from two cadaver head specimens. High-resolution reconstructed images of specified 8 cm-diameter regions encompassing the temporal bones were then generated from the raw data and photographed. The temporal bone blocks were removed from the cadaver head specimens, decalcified, sectioned in the same planes, photographed, and correlated with the reconstructed images to determine what degree of resolution, definition, and anatomic accuracy was possible in a temporal bone.

MATERIALS AND METHODS

Two fresh-frozen cadaver head specimens were used in the study to avoid potential artifacts in the temporal vasculature and middle ear space that might be introduced in the preservation process. The GE 8800 CT/T scanner (General Electric Medical Systems, Milwaukee) was used to scan the two specimens in the clinically obtainable coronal and axial planes. All scans were performed at settings of 600 mA and 120 kVp for 9.6 seconds with a 25 cm elliptical field of view, which produced a 0.8 mm by 0.8 mm pixel.

The axial images were obtained with the specimen positioned so that the supraorbitomeatal line was parallel with the scan planes, that is, rotated approximately 30° from true horizontal (Fig. 1). This orientation of the scan plane was chosen as it is commonly used to exclude the lens of the eye from the scan field when sellar lesions are investigated. It also places the horizontal canals in a plane parallel with the scan. Forty consecutive 1.5 mm thin-section scan images were obtained, 26 images cephalad and 14 images caudal to what was determined to be the midpoint of the internal auditory canals on the scout view, a lateral CT projection image.

The specimen from which the coronal projections were obtained was positioned so that the infraorbitomeatal line was perpendicular to the scan planes (Fig. 2). This allowed scanning of the temporal region without the problem of tooth artifacts. This position can be obtained clinically with reasonable patient comfort in most situations if an angulating or tilting gantry is available. A total of 30 1.5 mm thin-section images were obtained around what was determined from lateral CT projections to be the center of both internal auditory canals, 15 images anterior and 15 images posterior to the midpoint.

The raw data from each scan were stored on magnetic tape. The full-head images were reviewed, and the regions to be reconstructed were selected to include the temporal bone. ReView (General Electric) retrospective image analysis or targeted zoom reconstruction was then performed with use of the stored raw data for each scan. Data from the horizontal projections were also used to generate off-axis sagittal images in some instances.

Photographs of these images were taken directly from the scanner console screen by using a Deardorf professional view camera and Royal Pan ASA 400 black and white film. The window width of the scan display was −1,000 through +3,000 Hounsfield units (HUs) for all images. The window level was adjusted for optimal demonstration of certain features of each section.

Just before the scanning procedure, external ceiling and side-

From the Departments of Otorhinolaryngology, Physiology and Biophysics, and Diagnostic Radiology, Mayo Clinic and Mayo Foundation, Rochester, Minnesota.

Presented at the meeting of the American Otological Society, Inc., Vancouver, British Columbia, May 9-10, 1981.

REPRINTS — C. W. Beatty, MD, ℅ Section of Publications, Mayo Clinic, Rochester, MN 55905.

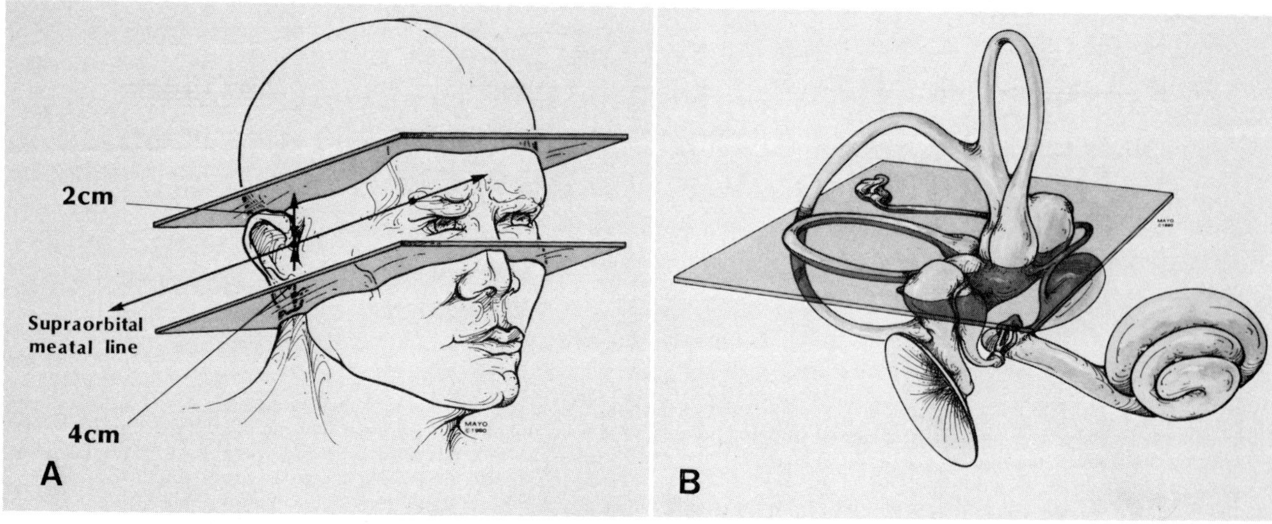

Fig. 1. A) Diagram of region in which axial scans were performed. B) Orientation of planes through temporal bone with regard to right membranous labyrinth, ossicular chain, and tympanic membrane.

mounted laser alignment lights were used to denote the proximal and distal extents of the scan planes. These points were marked on the specimens by using a syringe and 27 gauge needle filled with methylene blue. A scalpel was also used to incise through the soft tissues and periosteum of the skull along the line of the most proximal and distal scan planes.

After scanning was completed, the specimens were refrozen. A band saw was used to cut along the coronal and axial incisional marker lines. The temporal blocks from each specimen were separated by a midsagittal cut.

The blocks were prepared for decalcification by immersion in a phosphate-buffered 10% formaldehyde solution for seven days. The solution was changed five times during that period. The decalcification process was continued for a period of four weeks in 10% trichloracetic acid. The solution was changed five times per week and gently agitated with an ultrasonic washer day and night at a temperature of 40° C.*

The degree of decalcification was monitored radiographically. Because the temporal blocks contained substantial amounts of soft tissue, penetration of the decalcifying solution was partially inhibited. It was necessary to terminate the decalcifying process while there were still some minor calcium deposits deep in the petrous bone to prevent deterioration of the mastoid air cells.

*Sonogen ultrasonic cleaner, model LG-150 with LT-124 M tank, Bronson Instruments, Inc, Stamford, Conn.

The blocks were washed for 8 hours under running tap water and hardened in 10% formaldehyde for 72 to 96 hours before embedding.

The blocks were positioned in a 5% Knox gelatin solution until it gelled. The embedded blocks were then frozen overnight to preserve orientation and to facilitate sectioning. The blocks were sectioned in the appropriate planes by using an adjustable commercial meat slicer (American Slicing Machine Company, Chicago). The sections (1.5 to 2 mm thick) were then placed in a basin of warm water until the gelatin dissolved or was gently dissected free.

Serial photographs of the anatomic macrosections were taken with a Nikon F 35 mm camera and Ektachrome 50 color film with a 1:2.5 setup. The photographs of the macrosections and the reconstructed scan images were then correlated.

RESULTS

In almost every instance, we obtained excellent correlation between the scan images and the anatomic macrosections. Because inclusion of all of the

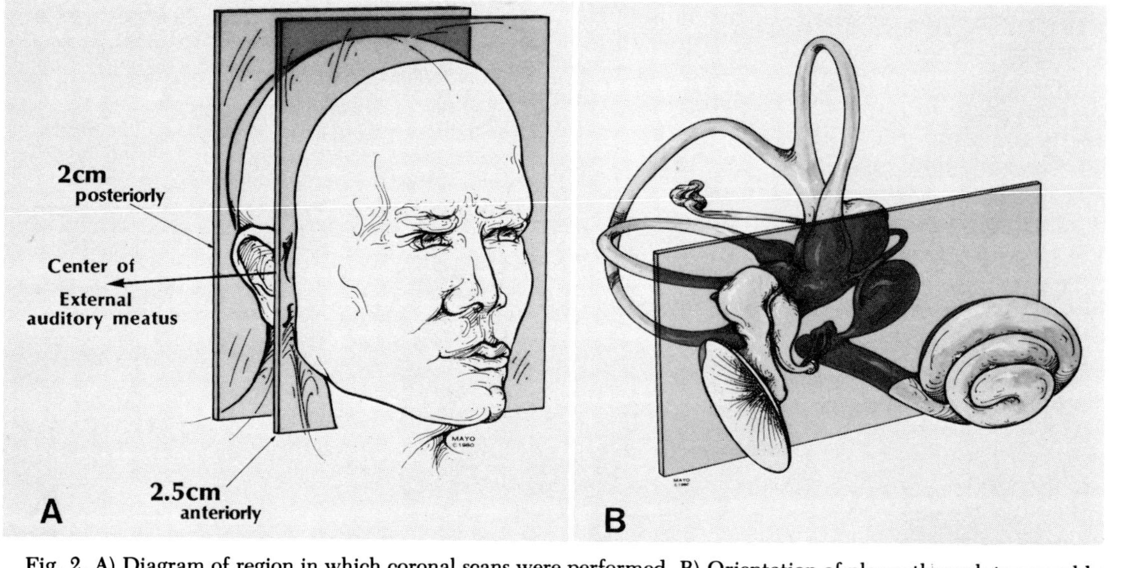

Fig. 2. A) Diagram of region in which coronal scans were performed. B) Orientation of planes through temporal bone with regard to right membranous labyrinth, ossicular chain, and tympanic membrane.

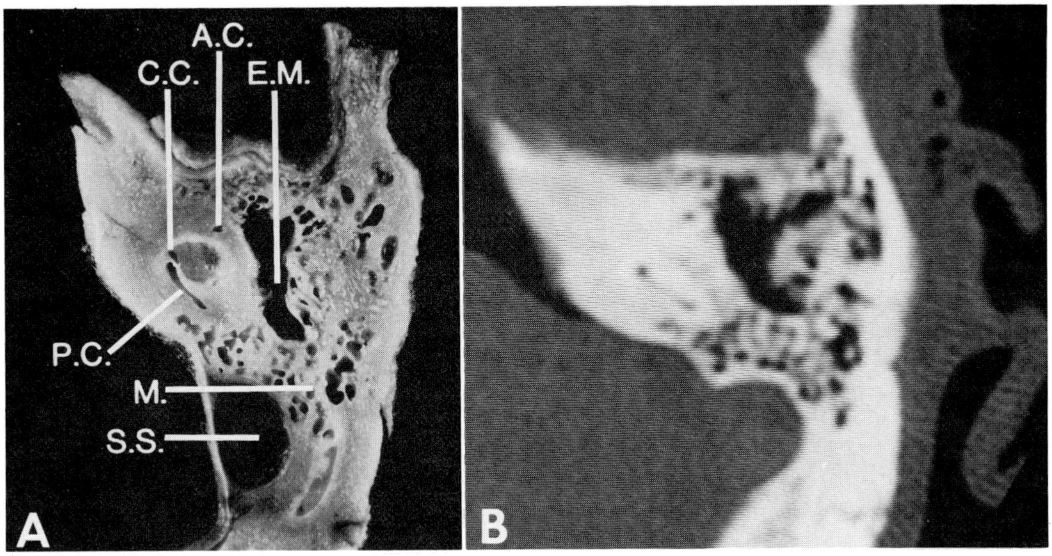

Fig. 3. A) Labeled axial anatomic macrosection through left temporal bone. Note the following structures and their unlabeled correlates in corresponding reconstructed scan image in B): Epitympanum of middle ear space (E.M.), anterior crus of superior canal (A.C.), common crus of superior and posterior canals (C.C.), arch of posterior canal (P.C.), mastoid air cells (M.), and sigmoid sinus (S.S.).

correlated anatomic and scan sections is impossible, a few representative pairs containing middle and inner ear structures of interest are presented.

Figures 3 through 6 show four sequential anatomic and scan pairs obtained in the axial plane through the left temporal bone (see Fig. 1 for orientation); these illustrations reveal the degree of definition and the type of information obtainable with use of serial thin sections. Each consecutive image was made through a plane 1.5 mm inferior to the previous plane. As these were cadaver head specimens, dissection of air up along the brainstem could be seen in the axial sections, similar to what might be seen in an air-contrast study.

Figures 7 and 8 are two representative anatomic and scan pairs obtained in the coronal plane through the right temporal bone (see Fig. 2 for orientation). In addition to the middle and inner ear structures under study, an unsuspected fracture of the squamous portion of the temporal bone in this specimen was easily demonstrated by the scan.

The tissue densities in the temporal bone vary widely from air in the middle ear to dense otic capsular bone. All of the information about bony and soft tissue detail obtained during the scanning process cannot be adequately demonstrated by one particular console density display setting. Similarly, photographs of reconstructed scan images taken

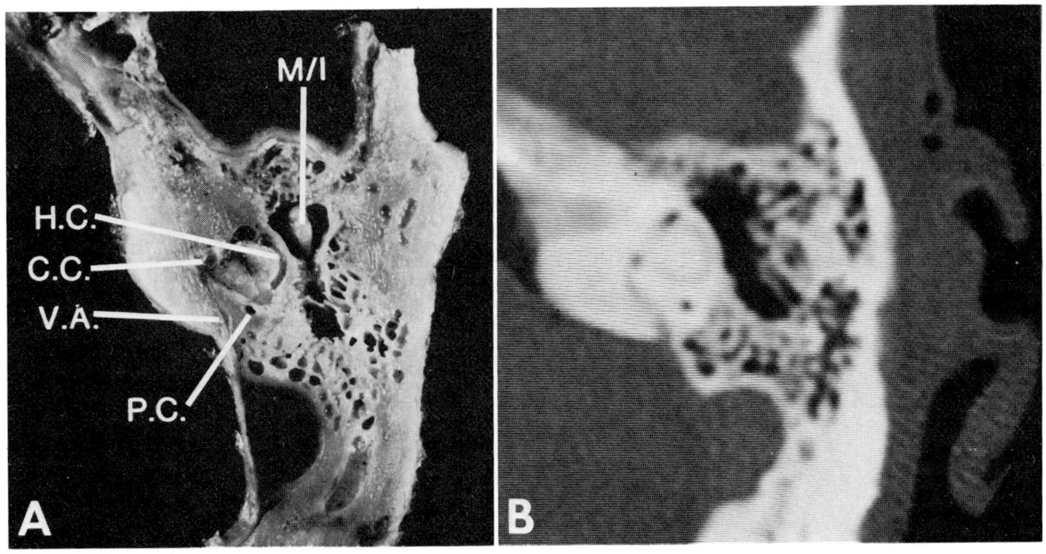

Fig. 4. A) Labeled axial anatomic macrosection ~1.5 mm inferior to section shown in Fig. 3 A. Note the following structures and their unlabeled correlates in corresponding reconstructed scan image in B): Heads of malleus and incus (M/I) (not shown in Fig. 4 B because of slight angulation in anatomic sectioning), horizontal canal (H.C.), common crus (C.C), vestibular aqueduct and endolymphatic sac (V.A.), and posterior canal (P.C.).

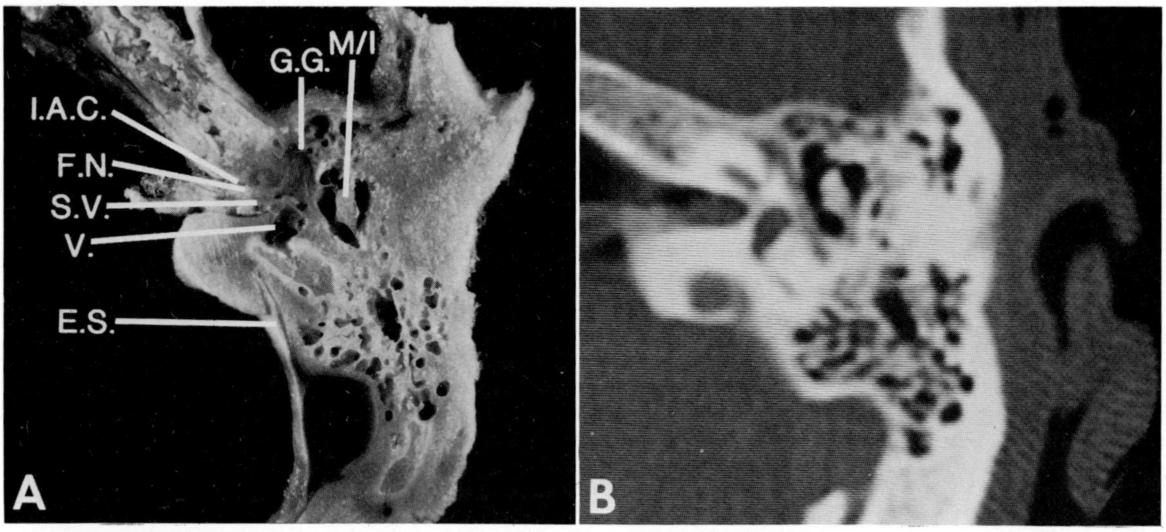

Fig. 5. A) Labeled axial anatomic macrosection ~1.5 mm inferior to section shown in Fig. 4 A. Note the following structures and their unlabeled correlates in corresponding reconstructed scan image in B): Bodies of malleus and incus (M/I), geniculate ganglion (G.G.), internal auditory canal (I.A.C.), facial nerve (F.N.), superior vestibular nerve (S.V.), vestibule (V.), and endolymphatic duct and sac (E.S.) (seen in Fig. 4 B).

from the console screen can reflect only the information displayed for a specific density range, as determined by the particular window level and width chosen by the viewer. We tried to select settings that demonstrated both bony and soft tissue detail to some advantage.

DISCUSSION

Accurate, highly detailed, cross-sectional images of the internal auditory canal, vestibule, cochlea, vestibular aqueduct, semicircular canals, ossicles, and middle ear space are now attainable because of recent advances in CT technology and image quality. Zoom reconstruction and the ability to scan 1.5 mm thin sections are examples of these advances.

Zoom reconstruction allows high-resolution magnified image reconstruction of selected regions of interest without the need for additional radiation exposure or scan time for the subject. This is not merely a magnification process but a larger, more accurate, reconstructed image derived from data that were generated during the original scan and "averaged" to fit the pixel size of the display.

The particular zoom process used in this study (GE ReView) also incorporates an extended CT number scale of density range. This expands the amount of contrast of bone and soft tissue density from a standard scale of −1,000 through +1,000 HUs to a scale of 4,000 CT numbers ranging from −1,000 through +3,000 HUs, with the density of water being equal to zero and that of air equivalent to −1,000 HUs.

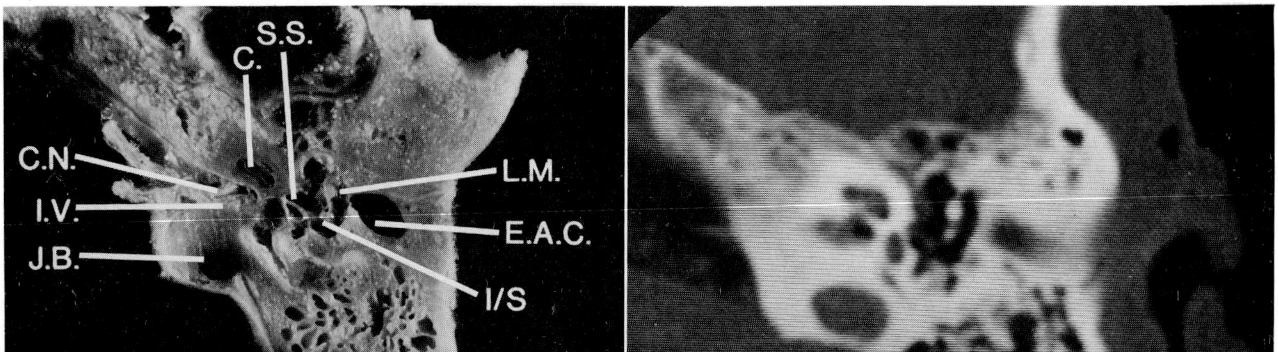

Fig. 6. A) Labeled axial anatomic macrosection ~1.5 mm inferior to section shown in Fig. 5 A. Note the following structures and their unlabeled correlates in corresponding reconstructed scan image in B): Incudostapedial joint (I/S), external auditory canal (E.A.C.), long process of malleus (L.M.), stapes superstructure (S.S.), and footplate in the vestibule, cochlea (C.), cochlear nerve (C.N.), inferior vestibular nerve (I.V.), and roof of jugular bulb (J.B.).

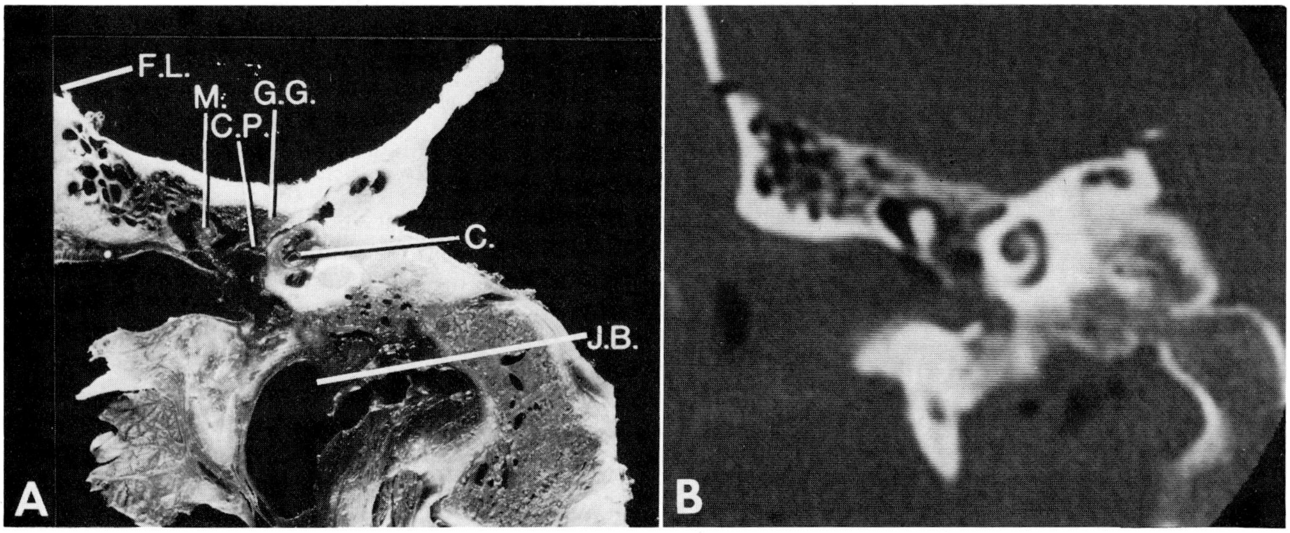

Fig. 7. A) Labeled coronal anatomic macrosection through right temporal bone. Note the following structures and their unlabeled correlates in corresponding reconstructed scan image in B): Fracture line in squamous portion of temporal bone (F.L.), malleus (M.), cochleariform process (C.P.), geniculate ganglion (G.G.), cochlea (C.), and jugular bulb (J.B.). Some clotted blood present in hypotympanum and jugular bulb during scanning was removed during sectioning.

Because no single specific setting of the window width or level can adequately display all the bone and soft tissue information generated during the scanning process and because photographs can represent only the information displayed at the particular settings chosen for each image, in some instances it would be advantageous to have the clinician review the CT studies at the console with the radiologist. This arrangement would help avoid unnecessary invasive diagnostic procedures or additional radiographic studies.

This study was conducted to determine what degree of resolution, definition, and anatomic accuracy was possible in the temporal bone with use of thin-section CT and zoom reconstruction. The following questions might be posed: What advantages do these techniques offer over previous CT imaging, conventional multidirectional tomography, and other radiologic techniques? In what clinical situations might these new techniques be applicable?

It is well known that the methods of CT scanning offer certain innate advantages over multidirectional tomography.[8] The goal of tomography is to display an anatomic plane that sections the body at a given orientation. Conventional multidirectional tomography attempts to accomplish this by blurring unwanted planes through special motions of the ray source and detector while the desired layer is kept in focus. In this process, the emitted rays must pass through all layers before reaching the detecting surface. CT enables complete exclusion of sections not under study by irradiating only the desired sections. Projections of the irradiation detected at multiple angles are then used to reconstruct the anatomic layer with the aid of a computer. By avoiding the lens of the eye and irradiating only the desired sec-

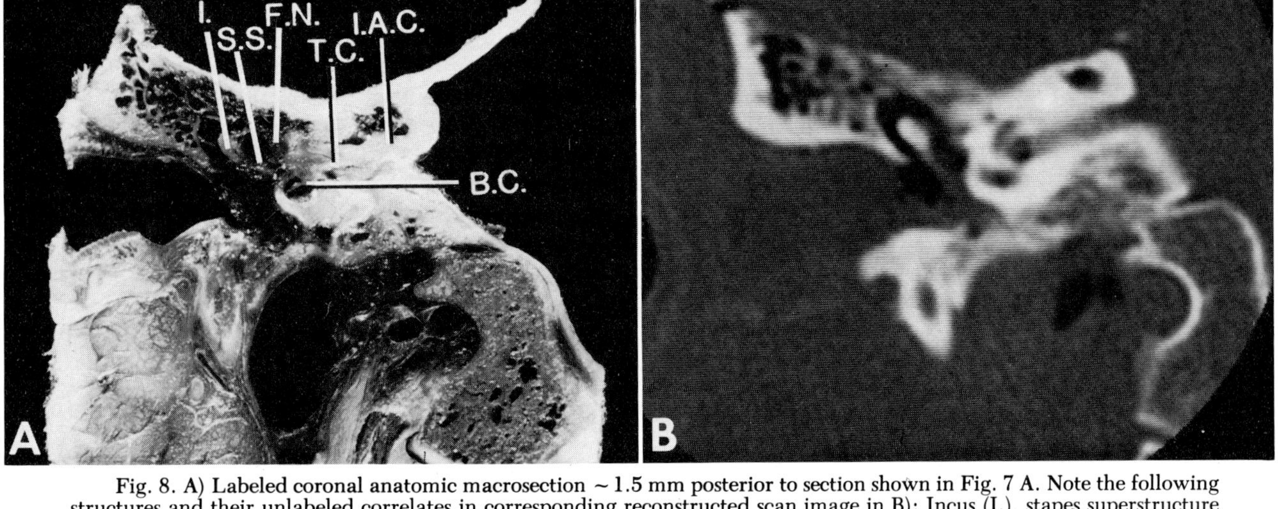

Fig. 8. A) Labeled coronal anatomic macrosection ~ 1.5 mm posterior to section shown in Fig. 7 A. Note the following structures and their unlabeled correlates in corresponding reconstructed scan image in B): Incus (I.), stapes superstructure (S.S.), horizontal portion of facial nerve (F.N.), transverse crest (T.C.), internal auditory canal (I.A.C.), and basal turn of cochlea (B.C.).

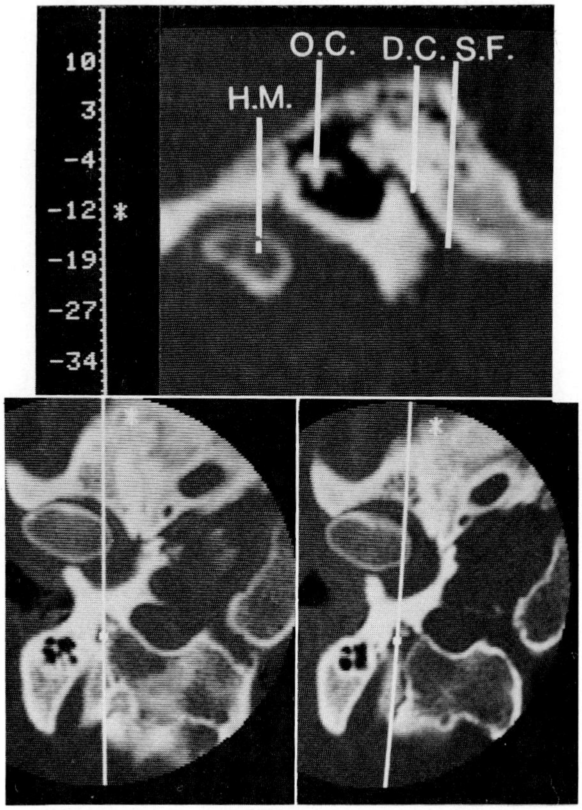

Fig. 9. Off-axis sagittal reconstruction through region of descending portion of facial nerve canal generated from serial axial scan images of right temporal bone. Note the following structures: head of mandible (H.M.), ossicular chain (O.C.), descending portion of facial nerve canal (D.C.), and stylomastoid foramen (S.F.).

tions, the total amount of irradiation received by the subject and the lens of the eye is less than that delivered in similar petrous multidirectional tomographic studies. Inasmuch as the rays pass through only the desired plane, the CT scanner is more sensitive in discriminating minimal differences in tissue densities.

Many of the limitations of CT of the temporal bone region, specifically in detecting lesions of the internal auditory canal and cerebellopontine angle (CPA), have been due to the thickness of the CT scan slices.[9-13] With the minimal slice thickness reduced from 5-10 mm to 1.5 mm, the detection rate of acoustic neuromas and other CPA lesions smaller than 1.5 cm in diameter can be expected to improve considerably.

Shaffer and Haughton[14] recently reviewed their experience with use of thin-section CT in 56 patients. Of these patients, 14 had surgically proved acoustic neuromas that had been scanned preoperatively by using 1.5 mm thin-section CT and contrast. All 14 tumors, including 3 smaller than 1 cm in diameter, had been detected by CT scanning. The manufacturer (General Electric) of the CT unit used in both their study and our own states that the resolving power of the unit is 1 mm by AAPM† pin phantom and 4 mm at 0.4% contrast. It seems reasonable to conclude that thin-section CT images with contrast and zoom reconstruction could frequently obviate the need for invasive studies such as pneumoencephalography and isophendylate (Pantopaque) myelography in detecting small CPA lesions.

It would also appear that thin-section CT and zoom reconstruction could provide important information about the extent and possible labyrinthine involvement of such middle ear processes as cholesteatomas, vascular anomalies, and glomus and other tumors. The definition and resolution of the ossicles suggest that ossicular anomalies and disarticulations might be demonstrated in some cases (Figs. 5-8). The evaluation of temporal bone trauma or fractures by means of CT imaging allows demonstration of fracture lines and assessment of adjacent soft tissues (that is, brain, muscle, and vessels) in one setting. Although no otosclerotic specimens were included in our study, small foci of otosclerosis will probably not be readily apparent with use of these techniques; nonetheless, this will be determined as experience is accumulated.

Another potential application suggested by this study is in the area of diagnosis and treatment planning of some cases of endolymphatic hydrops or Menière's disease. Other investigators have used multidirectional tomography to visualize the vestibular aqueduct in an effort to understand the role it and the endolymphatic sac may play in these diseases.[15-19] In our study, demonstration of the major portion of the vestibular aqueduct was possible in the axial projections (Fig. 4). Even though this was only one specimen and we did not have to contend with movement artifact, we have been able to visualize the vestibular aqueduct in some patients studied subsequently.

An advantage of serial CT imaging is the ability to use the information obtained to perform subsequent off-axis reconstruction, that is, reconstruction in planes other than that in which the subject was originally scanned. For example, sagittal reconstructions can be generated from data obtained during the axial scanning process (Fig. 9). These reconstructions can often show such structures as the facial canal, vestibular aqueduct, and internal auditory canal more advantageously in a different plane. We found that the off-axis reconstructions were of lesser quality but still capable of yielding valuable information. Movement of the subject during scanning will further diminish the quality of off-axis reconstruction.

With thin-section CT scanning and zoom reconstruction, as with any technologic advancement, time and experience will be necessary for appreciation of the full potential and the limitations in the temporal region or other anatomic areas. We believe, however, that the images produced are of ex-

†American Association of Physicists in Medicine.

cellent quality and detail, especially when the difficulties in scanning the dense petrous region are considered. These techniques should contribute vastly to diagnostic imaging and treatment planning. With previous and new methods of CT scanning, to obtain the best-quality, motion-free images, patient comfort and support are imperative and the use of contrast material may be indicated.

ACKNOWLEDGMENT — The authors wish to express their gratitude to Don Volz, General Electric Medical Systems, Milwaukee, and to Dale A. Frank, Mayo Clinic, Rochester, Minn., whose cooperation and assistance made this project possible.

REFERENCES

1. Hounsfield GN. Computerized transverse axial scanning (tomography). I. Description of system. Br J Radiol 1973; 46:1016-22.

2. Ambrose J. Computerized transverse axial scanning (tomography). II. Clinical application. Br J Radiol 1973; 46:1023-47.

3. Baker HL Jr, Campbell JK, Houser OW, Reese DF, Sheedy PF, Holman CB. Computer assisted tomography of the head: an early evaluation. Mayo Clin Proc 1974; 49:17-27.

4. Valvassori GE, Buckingham RA. Microradiography and macrosectioning of the temporal bone. Ann Otol Rhinol Laryngol 1970; 79:738-42.

5. Valvassori GE, Buckingham RA. Tomography and cross sections of the ear. Philadelphia: WB Saunders, 1975.

6. Sesana WE, Senturia BH, Taveras JM, Reyes ET. Correlation of histologic and polytomographic sections of the temporal bone. Ann Otol Rhinol Laryngol 1971; 80:155-70.

7. Wortzman G, Conrad K, Farkashidy J. Temporal bone: a tomographic anatomic study. J Can Assoc Radiol 1977; 28: 95-105.

8. Brooks RA, DiChiro G. Theory of image reconstruction in computed tomography. Radiology 1975; 117:561-72.

9. Davis KR, Taveras JM, Roberson GH, Ackerman RH. Some limitations of computed tomography in the diagnosis of neurological diseases. Am J Roentgenol 1976; 127:111-23.

10. Hoffman JC, Cox GW. Limitations of computerized tomography scanning in acoustic neurinomas. Arch Otolaryngol 1977; 103:594-5.

11. Robbins B, Marshall WH Jr. Computed tomography of acoustic neurinoma. Radiology 1978; 128:367-70.

12. Dubois PJ, Drayer BP, Bank WO, Deeb ZL, Rosenbaum AE. An evaluation of current diagnostic radiologic modalities in the investigation of acoustic neurilemmomas. Radiology 1978; 126:173-9.

13. Palacios E, Valvassori G. Computed axial tomography in otorhinolaryngology. Adv Otorhinolaryngol 1978; 24:1-8.

14. Shaffer KA, Haughton VM. Thin section computed tomography of the temporal bone. Laryngoscope 1980; 90: 1099-1105.

15. Clemis JD, Valvassori GE. Recent radiographic and clinical observations on the vestibular aqueduct (a preliminary report). Otolaryngol Clin North Am 1968; 1:339-46.

16. Stahle J, Wilbrand H. The vestibular aqueduct in patients with Menière's disease: a tomographic and clinical investigation. Acta Otolaryngol (Stockh) 1974; 78:36-48.

17. Gado MH, Arenberg IK. Radiological visualization of the vestibular aqueduct: technique and morphologic features. Radiology 1975; 117:621-6.

18. Valvassori GE, Clemis JD. Abnormal vestibular aqueduct in cochleovestibular disorders. Adv Otorhinolaryngol 1978; 24:100-5.

19. Austin DF. Use of polytomography in Menière's disease. Arch Otolaryngol 1980; 106:377-82.

≈

AUTHOR INDEX

Abel, S.M., Suppl. 79
Andrea, M., 18
Andrews, A.H., Jr., 310
Anniko, M., 25
Apple, D.F., Jr., 323
Aragon, R., 186
Armstrong, B.W., 533
Armstrong, J.R., 339
Armstrong, R.B., 533
Aronson, A.E., 2
Axelsson, A., 281

Babin, R.W., 524
Baim, H., 469
Baker, S.R., 126
Barber, H.O., Suppl. 79
Batsakis, J.G., 190
Beatty, C.W., 643
Becker, G.D., Suppl. 84:8, 23
Benjamin, B., 364, 376, 478
Berci, G., 344, 430
Berg, O., 272
Bergstedt, H., 272
Berliner, K.I., Suppl. 82:4
Biller, H.F., 489; Suppl. 80
Bloch, C.S., 48
Blom, E.D., 498
Bluestone, C.D., 148; Suppl. 84:1, 23, 44, 48, 63, 82, 552
Boberg, R.A., Suppl. 82:25
Bohne, B.A., 412
Boulos, E.J., 181
Brama, I., 387, 475
Brook, I., 261
Brummitt, W.M., 475
Bryson, Y.J., 406
Buncher, C.R., 107
Busby, P.A., 227
Bussen, J., 398

Cabieses, F., 186
Cail, W.S., 619
Caldarelli, D.D., 310
Calearo, C.V., 217
Canalis, R.F., 186
Cantekin, E.I., Suppl. 84:44, 48, 552
Cantrell, R.W., 161, 619
Caparosa, R.J., 109, 535
Carenfelt, C., 272
Carlsson, B., 38
Caroggio, A., 217
Casuccio, J.R., 346
Catlin, F.I., 301
Cherry, J.D., Suppl. 84: 19, 23
Chilis, T., 469
Christian, K.C., 331
Clark, G.M., 227
Cohen, N.L., 67
Cohen, D., 364
Cohen, S.R., 316, 483
Cotton, R.T., 401, 516, 543
Cross, F.S., 383
Cummings, C.W., 396, 413

Davis, G.L., 246
Davis, W.E., 142
Dekker, A., 454
Denneny, J. C., III, 351
DeSanto, L.W., 2
Diven, W.F., 148
Domer, F.R., 255
Donegan, J.O., 495
Dowell, R.C., 227
Dudley, J.P., 406
Duncan, G., 396
Duvall, A.J., III, 584

Eden, A.R., 566
Edens, E.T., 307
Eichenhorn, M.S., 339
Elidan, J., 53
Elverland, H.H., 7
Emery, P.J., 210
Emmett, J.R., 601
Englender, J., 172
Ervin, T.J., 506
Evans, J.N.G., 516

Fabian, R.L., 506
Fairbanks, D.N.F., Suppl. 84:58, 63, 82
Farrior, B., 636
Fearon, B., 387, 475
Fenwick, J.A., Suppl. 82:25
Ferrara, T., 469
Ferwerda, H., 288
Finegold, S.M., Suppl. 84:13, 23
Flach, A.J., 299
Flores, T.C., 383
Fisher, S.R., 331
Fong, M., Suppl. 82:21
Fontana, R.S., 312, 354
Freeman, R.B., 412
Friedman, E.M., 261
Friedman, M., 469
Fujishiro, T., 241
Furuta, M., 80

Gacek, R.R., 423, 581
Gapany-Gapanavicius, B., 42
Garfinkle, T.J., 351
Gay, I., 53
Ge, X.-X., Suppl. 85, Suppl. 88
Geurkink, N.A., 236
Ghorbanian, S.M., Suppl. 84:48
Giebink, G.S., 72
Ginsburg, C.M., Suppl. 84:23, 37, 63
Glasscock M.E., III, 142
Glew, R.H., 148
Gluckman, J.L., 495
Goldman, N.C., 522
Goodhill, V., 99, 607
Goodman, R.S., 67
Gould, W.J., 48
Goycoolea, M., 610
Green, N., 183
Gregg, J.B., 288
Gregg, P.S., 288
Griswold, F.C., 398
Grundfast, K.M., 303
Guth, P.S., 255
Gwaltney, J.M., Jr., Suppl. 84:68, 82

Haar, J.G., 181
Hamaker, R.C., 498
Handler, S.D., 300
Hanks, J.B., 331
Hanson, D.G., 430
Harada, T., 109, 174, 199
Harris, L.D., 643
Harris, M.J., 33
Harrison, D.F.N., 372, 415
Hart, C.W., Suppl. 86:2
Hawrisiak, M.M., 246
Haugeto, O.K., 7
Heffron, T.J., 449
Hemenway, W.G., 186
Henriksson, N.-G., 164
Herzon, F.S., Suppl. 83; Suppl. 84:17, 23
Hinojosa, R., 199
Hirano, M., 48
Hirsh, I.J., 412
Hoffman-Lawless, K., 543
Homick, J.L., 85
Hopla, D.M., 398
House, J.W., 597
House, W.F., Suppl. 82:4
Hubbell, R.N., 465
Hughes, G.B., 142
Hunter-Duvar, I.M., 70
Hyslop, N.E., 251

Igarashi, M., 85, 154
Iizuka, K., 222
Illum, P., 231
Ito, A., 264

Jackson, C.G., 142
Jahnke, K., 640
Jahrsdoerfer, R.A., 161, 619
Jannetta, P.J., 591
Jensen, D.W., 85, 154
Jerger, J., 564
Johns, M.M.E., 161
Johnson, D.W., 89
Johnson, J.T., 454
Jones, R.D., 383
Jones, R.S., 331
Juhn, S.K., 135

Kamio, T., 276
Kammer, R.B., Suppl. 84:79, 82
Kanter, R., 303
Karp, D.D., 506
Keith, R.W., 543
Kenan, S., 42
Kereiakes, J.G., 107
Kileny, P., 194
Kim, J.W., 56
Kishimoto, S., 80
Kitamura, K., Suppl. 78
Klein, J.O., Suppl. 84:23, 30, 63, 82
Konno, A., 222
Konrad, H.R., 398; Suppl. 86:7
Kopolovic, J., 53
Krause, C.J., 126
Kubo, T., 85, 154
Kuczer, A., 198
Kumar, A., 624
Kuritzky, A., 267
Kvale, P.A., 339

Landman, M., 183
Lauter, J., 302
Lawson, W., Suppl. 80; 489
Leake-Jones, P.A., Suppl. 82:6, 19, 27, 30
Lee, C.A., Suppl. 82: 9
Levine, H.L., 409, 492
Lildholdt, T., Suppl. 84:44
Lind, M.G., 272
Lundberg, C., 38

Mair, I.W.S., 7
Maisel, R.H., 89, 460
Malmgren, L.T., 423
Mandel, E.M., Suppl. 84:48
Marshak, G., Suppl. 84:44
Martin, L.F., 227
Mathews, R.G., Suppl. 82:15
Mathog, R.H., Suppl. 86:10
Maxon, H.R., 107
Mays, K., 601
McCabe, B.F., 503
McCracken, G.H., Jr., Suppl. 84:37
McGee, T.M., 633
McLaughlin, C.A., 107
Meikle, M.B., Suppl. 82:9
Merson, R.M., 301
Merzenich, M.M., Suppl. 82:6, 19, 27, 30
Meyerhoff, W.L., 72, 537
Meyers, A., 132
Meyers, W.C., 331
Mikaelian, D.O., 392
Miller, D., 506
Miller, J.M., 281
Millet, V.E., 406
Mitchell, D.P., 70
Mφller, A.R., 591
Mφller, M.B., 591
Montgomery, W.W., 251
Mulvaney, T.J., 169
Mumtaz, A., 303
Murray, H.H., 323
Musiek, F.E., 236
Myers, D., 199
Myers, E.N., 174, 199, 454

Nadol, J.B., Jr., 12, 442
Nakashima, T., 264
Naunton, R.F., 529
Neal, G.D., 396
Neel, H.B., III, 312, 354
Nelson, J.D., Suppl. 84:37
Neu, H.C., Suppl. 84:2, 23, 63
Newton, L., 335
Norris, C.H., 255

Ohlsson, K., 38
Okano, Y., 109
O'Keefe, J.J., 392
Olsen, J.E., Suppl. 86:15
Ono, J., Suppl. 87
Orchik, D.J., 601
O'Reilly, B.F., Suppl. 82:11

Panje, W.R., 116, 503
Paparella, M.M., 610
Paradise, J.L., Suppl. 84:53, 63, 75
Parkin, J.L., 60
Parrish, K.L., 255
Pashley, N.R.T., 287
Patrick, J.F., 227
Peerless, A.G., 512
Peerless, S.A., 512
Perols, O., 272
Phelps, P.D., 210
Pillsbury H.R., III, 512
Pitkin, J., 364
Plester, D., 640
Pollack, M., 303
Pollock, R.A., 323
Popelka, G.R., 302
Popovich, J., Jr., 339
Posner, M.R., 506
Postlethwait, R.W., 331
Potter, W., 281
Prado, S., 135
Proctor, B., 615
Proctor, C., 615
Pulec, J.L., 570
Purvis, J.M., 323
Pyykkö, I., 164

Radke, J.R., 339
Rediano, H., 172
Reese, D.F., 643
Reichert, T.J., 198
Richardson, J.L., 294
Richter, E., 121
Rizvi, S.S., 77
Robinson, M., 630
Rockette, H.E., Suppl. 84:48
Rohn, D.D., Suppl. 84:44
Ruben, R.J., 335, 546
Rubin, W., Suppl. 86:18
Rusnov, M.G., 457, 492
Rybak, L.P., 135

Sadeghi, M.H., 181
Saenger, E.L., 107
Saito, H., 80
Saito, R., 109
Sak, R.J., 546
Sande, M.A., Suppl. 84:68
Sanderson, D.R., 312, 354
Sando, I., 109, 174, 199
Santi, P.A., 584
Schalen, L., 164
Schlenker, R.A., 33
Schreiber, J.T., 401
Schramm, V., Suppl. 84:23, 82
Schrφder, K.E., 7
Schuff, N.R., Suppl. 82:25
Schuit, K.E., Suppl. 84:44
Schuknecht, H.F., Suppl. 78, 527, 618
Sekine, S., 276
Seligman, P.M., 227
Senturia, B.H., 412
Shafer, M.L., 107
Shannon, R.V., Suppl. 82:13
Shea, D., 72
Shea, J.J., 601
Sheehy, J.L., 562
Sheffer, J., 181
Shelton, V., 469
Sherrod, J.L., 406
Shimizu, M., 276
Shugar, J.M.A., 64
Shugar, M.A., 169, 251
Shurin, P.A., Suppl. 84:23, 72, 82
Sia, R.L., 307
Silverman, M., Suppl. 82:19
Simonian, S., 392
Simmons, F.B., Suppl. 82:15
Simpson, R.A., Suppl. 86:26
Singer, M.I., 498
Singh, J., 495
Sismanis, A., 142
Skinner, M.W., 413
Skolnik, E., 469
Slavin, R.G., 300
Smith, C.A., Suppl. 82:25
Smith, L.E., 77
Sobol, S.M., 409
Sofferman, R.A., 465
Som, P.M., 64; Suppl. 80
Spector, G. J., Suppl. 85, Suppl. 88
Spencer, M.J., 406
Steele, J.P., 288
Stennert, E., 577
Stobnicki, M., 469
Stool, S., 94
Strutz, J., 158
Suh, K.W., 643
Sutton, D., 396
Suzuki, M., 346
Sydnor, A., Jr., Suppl. 84:68

Tachibana, M., 255
Takahashi, M., 241
Tapia Acuña, R., 420
Taylor, W.F., 312
Templin, D., Suppl. 86:7
Thomas, D., 267
Thomas, S.R., 107
Thompson, E.G., 161
Thompson, G.E., 328
Thorling, K., 231
Togawa, K., 222
Toglia, J.U., 267
Tong, Y.C., 227
Torok, N., 299, 624
Treyve, E., 328
Troost, B.T., Suppl. 86:29
Tucker, G.F., Jr., 335
Tucker, H.M., 409, 457, 492
Turner, C. W., 584
Turner, J., 454

Uemura, T., 241

Valvassori, G., 624
VanDemark, D., 503
Vermeersch, H., 460
Vivion, M.C., Suppl. 82:19
Vrabec, D.P., 449
Vurek, L.S., Suppl. 82:21, 27

Wald, E., Suppl. 84:82
Walker, M.G., Suppl. 82:15
Walloch, R.S., Suppl. 82:25
Walsh, S.M., Suppl. 82:6, 21, 27, 30
Ward, P.H., 344, 430
Ward, W.D., 584
Watanabe, I., 204
Watanabe, K., 204
Webb, W., 601
Weber, A.L., 169, 192
Weichselbaum, R.R., 506
Weidenbecher, M., Suppl. 81
Weisman, R.A., 351
Welsh, L.W., 413
Wennmo, C., 164
White, M., Suppl. 82:19, 21
White, R.L., Suppl. 82:15
Williams, D.J., 70
Wilson, A.F., 194
Wilson, W.R., 21, 56
Windle-Taylor, P.C., 210
Wolfe, J.W., Suppl. 86:15
Wong-Riley, M.T.T., Suppl. 82:30
Wood, B.G., 409, 492
Woolner, L.B., 312
Wright, W.K., 154
Wroblewski, R., 25
Wu, H.-H., 359

Yagi, T., 276
Yanagisawa, E., 346
Yarington, C.T., Jr., 328
Yocum, P., 261

Zimmerman, L., 288
Zoller, M., 21

SUBJECT INDEX

Accessory Nasal Sinus and Mastoid Cavities; Quantitative Histology of Mucous Membrane of, 33.
Adenoid Hypertrophy; Influence on Secretory Otitis Media, 7.
Adenoma, Pleomorphic, of Hard Palate, 192.
Aerodigestive Tract, Upper; Significance of Positive Bronchial Cytology in Presence of Squamous Cell Carcinoma of, 454.
Aerodigestive Tract of Pediatric Patient, Foreign Bodies in; Unusual Presentations and Problems Created by Mismanagement of, 316.
Allergen, Changes of Nasal Epithelial Cells and Mucus Layer After Challenge of, 204.
Alternaria Sinusitis, 251.
Amoxicillin and Cefaclor for Acute Otitis Media with Effusion, Comparison of, Suppl. 84:48.
Anesthesia for Laryngeal Laser Surgery in Infant and Child, 475.
Anterior Commissure, Vasculature of, 18.
Antibiotics, Oral; Treatment of Otitis Media and Tonsillopharyngitis in Infants and Children, Pharmacology of, Suppl. 84:37.
Antimicrobial Agents; Clinical Pharmacology, for Infections in Ear, Nose and Throat, Suppl. 84:2.
Antimicrobial Prophylaxis for Recurrent Acute Otitis Media, Suppl. 84:53.
Antimicrobial Therapy for Chronic Suppurative Otitis Media, Suppl. 84:58.
  for Infections of the Ear, Nose and Throat — Head and Neck, Recent Advances in, Suppl. 84.
Atresia, Esophageal, and Tracheoesophageal Fistula; Endoscopy in, 376.
Atresia Auris Congenita, Model for Analysis of; Vitamin A-Induced Ear Malformations in Rats. Microsurgical and Histologic Study, Suppl. 81.
Auditory Brainstem and Middle Latency Evoked Response Sensitivity Near Threshold, 236.
Auditory Deprivation for Language and Learning, Temporary; Implications in Recurrent Middle Ear Effusion, 546.
Auditory Nerve, Direct; Electrical Stimulation of, Pitch Correlates of, Suppl. 82:15.
Auditory Processing Abilities in Children with Previous Middle Ear Effusion, 543.
Backflow, Parotolymphatic: A New Sign of Malignancy, 64.
Bacteria, Aerobic and Anaerobic, in Tonsils of Children with Recurrent Tonsillitis, 261.
Bell's Palsy, Early Decompression of Facial Nerve in, 570.
  Panel on Treatment of, 570; Comment, 581.
  Pathomechanisms in Cell Metabolism: A Key to Treatment of, 577.
Blom-Singer Technique for Voice Restoration, Limitations of, 495.
Blood-Brain Circulation, Regional; Central Vestibular Signs, Posterior Fossa Pathology and Computerized Tomography, 624.
Blood-Labyrinth Barrier in Experimental Conditions, Nature of, 135.
Book Reviews
  Aronson, A.E., *Clinical Voice Disorders: An Interdisciplinary Approach*, 301.
  Ballantyne, J., Groves, J., *Scott-Brown's Diseases of the Ear, Nose and Throat*, Fourth Edition, 412.
  Barber, C., *Evoked Potentials*, 302.
  Barr, D.F., Miller, R.K., *Basic Industrial Hearing Conservation*, 301.
  Borden, G.J., Harris, K.S., *Speech Science Primer: Physiology, Acoustics and Perception of Speech*, 412.
  Cooper, J.S., Pizzarello, D.J., *Concepts in Cancer Care*, 413.
  Farb, S.M., *Otorhinolaryngology*, Second Edition, 412.
  García-Ballester, L., Olagüe, G., Ciges, M., *Classics in Modern Otology*, 94.
  Jazbi, B., *Pediatric Otorhinolaryngology*, 198.
  Lockey, R.F., *Allergy and Clinical Immunology*, 300.
  Mawson, S.R., Ludman, H., *Diseases of the Ear: A Textbook of Otology*, Fourth Edition, 94.
  Miller, R., *Guide to Noise Control Literature*, 412.
  Oho, K., Amemiya, R., *Practical Fiberoptic Bronchoscope*, 413.
  Phillips, P.P., *Speech Hearing Pathology and Surgery*, 198.
  Pickett, J.M., *The Sounds of Speech Communication: A Primer of Acoustic Phonetics and Speech Perception*, 302.
  Sadé, J., *Secretory Otitis Media and its Sequelae*, 94.
  Sataloff, J., Sataloff, R.T., Vassallo, L.A., *Hearing Loss*, Second Edition, 413.
Brain, Middle Ear and Eustachian Tube; Neural Connections Between. Implications for Reflex Control of Middle Ear Aeration, 566.
Brainstem, Auditory; Middle Latency Evoked Response Sensitivity Near Threshold and, 236.
Brainstem Evoked Potentials, Neural Generators of. Results from Human Intracranial Recordings, 591.
  Electrically Evoked; Opto-Isolated Stimulators Used for, Suppl. 82:21.
Bronchial Cytology, Positive: Significance in Presence of Squamous Cell Carcinoma of Upper Aerodigestive Tract, 454.
Bronchoscopic Cryotherapy, 354.
Bronchoscopy, Flexible Fiberoptic; Pulmonary Cytology in Evaluation of Patients with Head and Neck Malignancies, 351.
Cancer, Advanced Head and Neck; Role of Chemotherapy in Multidisciplinary Approach. Potentials and Problems, 506.
  Esophageal; Research in the People's Republic of China, 359.
  Head and Neck; Hypothyroidism following Treatment for, 449.
  Head and Neck; Panendoscopy for Second Primaries in, 460.
  Hypopharyngeal and Cervical Esophageal; Surgical Repair in. Analysis of 162 Patients, 372.
  Upper Respiratory Tract; Sputum Cytologic Diagnosis of. Second Report, 312.
Carbon Dioxide Laser, Use in Otology, 70.
Carbon Dioxide Laser Surgery of Larynx, Complications of, 132.
Carcinoid Tumor of Larynx, 42.
Carcinoma, Bilateral Vocal Cord; Bilateral Vertical Partial Laryngectomy for, 489.
  Epiglottis, Treatment of, 442.
  Salivary Glands, Radiation-Associated. A Controlled Study, 107.
  Squamous Cell, of Face; Perineural Metastases from. Therapeutic Considerations, 183.
  Squamous Cell, Upper Aerodigestive Tract; Significance of Positive Bronchial Cytology in Presence of, 454.
Carotid Ligation Complications; Analysis of Factors Affecting, 222.
Cefaclor; Management of Streptococcal Pharyngitis, Otitis Media and Skin Infections, Suppl. 84:79.
  Pharmacokinetics in Chronic Middle Ear Effusions, Suppl. 84:44.
Cefaclor and Amoxicillin for Acute Otitis Media with Effusion, Comparison of, Suppl. 84:48.
Cell Metabolism, Pathomechanisms in. A Key to Treatment of Bell's Palsy, 577.
Cellulitis and Epiglottitis: Invasive *Hemophilus* Infections, Suppl. 84:19.
Cerebellar Dysfunction, New Neurotological Test for Detecting. Vestibulo-Ocular Reflex Changes with Horizontal Vision-Reversal Prisms, 276.
Cervical Esophageal and Hypopharyngeal Cancer, Surgical Repair in. Analysis of 162 Patients, 372.
Cervical Spine Trauma, Esophageal and Hypopharyngeal Injuries in Patients with, 323.
Chemoprophylaxis for Surgery of Head and Neck, Suppl. 84:8.
Chemotherapy, Role of, in Multidisciplinary Approach to Advanced Head and Neck Cancer: Potentials and Problems, 506.
Chondrosarcoma at Skull Base, 53.
Ciliary Ultrastructural Pathology, Upper Respiratory Tract, Suppl. 83.
Cleft, Laryngotracheoesophageal; Management of, 401.
Clerf Lecture, Second Louis H.; Vestibular Neuritis, Suppl. 78.
  Third Louis H.; Legacies of Jefferson Men to Japanese Medicine, Suppl. 87.
Cochlea, Efferent Innervation of, 158.
Cochlear Implant, Multiple-Channel: Evaluation Using Nonsense Syllables, 227.
Cochlear Pathology Following Chronic Intracochlear Electrical Stimulation, Suppl. 82:6.
Cochlear Prosthesis: Histological Examination of Implanted Cats, Suppl. 82:25.
  Model; Electrode Position and Excitation Patterns for, Suppl. 82:19.
  Conference (West Coast), Proceedings of, Suppl. 82.
Computerized Optokinetic Tracking Tests and Sinusoidal Harmonic Acceleration; Proceedings of Seminar on, Suppl. 86.
Contact Granuloma of Vocal Fold; Effect of Voice Therapy on, 48.
Cricoarytenoid Muscle, Posterior; Histochemical Characteristics of Muscle Fiber Types in, 423.
Cryotherapy, Bronchoscopic, 354.
Cytochrome Oxidase Technique, Demonstrating Maintenance of Neuronal Activity by Electrical Stimulation of Unilaterally Deafened Cats, Suppl. 82:30.
Cytology, Pulmonary; Flexible Fiberoptic Bronchoscopy in Evaluation of Patients with Head and Neck Malignancies, 351.
Deafness, Tinnitus and Dizziness, Leaking Labyrinth Lesions, 99.

Dermoid Cyst and Thyroglossal Duct Cyst in Neck, Association of. Case Report, 181.
Dilator, Customized; Treatment of Subglottic Stenosis in Children with, 287.
Diverticulum of Jugular Bulb, Endolymphatic Duct Obstruction from, 619.
Dizziness, Deafness and Tinnitus, Leaking Labyrinth Lesions, 99.
Dysphonia, Adductor Spastic: Following Recurrent Laryngeal Nerve Resection, 2.

Ear, Inner, Developing: Elemental Composition of, 25.
Inner, Fetal Guinea Pig, In Vitro Cultivation of, 246.
Middle; Aberrant Internal Carotid Artery in, 67.
Middle, Chronic Effects of Phasic Pressure Changes, 281.
Middle, Deflation; Pneumococcal Otitis Media Following, 72.
Middle, Effusions; Lysosomal Hydrolases in, 148.
Middle; Pharmocokinetics of Cefaclor in Effusions of, Suppl. 84:44.
Middle, Ventilating Tubes; Panel, 529; Comment, 535.
Ear Deformities Associated with Klippel-Feil Syndrome, 210.
Ear Malformations in Rats, Vitamin A-Induced, as Model for Analysis of Atresia Auris Congenita. Microsurgical and Histological Study, Suppl. 81.
Earplugs for Control of Water-Borne Infection, Objective Evaluation of, 89.
Effusion, Middle Ear, Recurrent, in Childhood: Implications of Temporary Auditory Deprivation for Language and Learning, 546.
Effusions, Middle Ear, Chronic; Pharmacokinetics of Cefaclor, Suppl. 84:44.
Middle Ear. Lysosomal Hydrolases in, 148.
Middle Ear, Previous; Auditory Processing Abilities in Children with, 543.
Middle Ear; Protease Inhibitors in, 38.
Electrical Stimulation of Unilaterally Deafened Cats Demonstrable with Cytochrome Oxidase Technique; Maintenance of Neuronal Activity by, Suppl. 82:30.
Electronystagmographic Study and Pathogenesis of Vestibular Function and Common Migraine, 267.
Electronystagmography, Study of Ventilation Testing with, 56.
Electronystagmography in Congenital and Acquired Syphilitis Otitis, 21.
Endocochlear Potential, Effect of Increased Perilymphatic Pressure on, 264.
Endolymphatic Duct Obstruction from a Jugular Bulb Diverticulum, 619.
Endolymphatic Hydrops, Idiopathic, and Vestibular Aqueduct, 77.
Quantitative Study of Scarpa's Ganglion and Vestibular Sense Organs in, 121.
Endolymphatic Sac Enhancement Surgery for Menière's Disease. An Extension of Conservative Therapy, 610.
Endoscopic Findings in Sarcoidosis. Characteristics and Correlations with Radiographic Staging and Bronchial Mucosal Biopsy Yield, 339.
Endoscopy, Flexible Fiberoptic, in Difficult Intubations, 307.
Endoscopy in Esophageal Atresia and Tracheoesophageal Fistula, 376.
Endotracheal Tubes, Incendiary Characteristics with Carbon Dioxide Laser. An Experimental Study, 328.
ENG of the Month: Periodic Alternating Nystagmus, 524.
Vestibulo-Ocular and Oculomotor Responses Following Brainstem Cerebrovascular Accident, 194.
ENG Test Battery and Optokinetic Test, Suppl. 86:2.
Epiglottic Laryngoplasty for Complicated Laryngeal Stenosis, 409.
Epiglottis, Carcinoma, Treatment of, 442.
Epiglottitis and Cellulitis: Invasive *Hemophilus* Infections, Suppl. 84:19.
Esophageal and Hypopharyngeal Injuries in Patients with Cervical Spine Trauma, 323.
Esophageal Cancer Research in People's Republic of China, 359.
Esophageal Hiatal Hernia in Infants and Children, 387.
Esophagus, Duplication of, 392.
Eustachian Tube, Brain and Middle Ear; Neural Connections between. Implications for Reflex Control of Middle Ear Aeration, 566.
Eustachian Tube Function Testing, Panel, 552; Comment, 564.
Tests; Current Clinical Methods, Indications and Interpretation of, 552.
External Otitis, Necrotizing, Temporal Bone Histopathology of. A Case Report, 109.
Evoked Response Sensitivity (Middle Latency) Near Threshold and Auditory Brainstem, 236.
Eye-Head Coordination and Lateral Canal Block in Squirrel Monkeys, 154.
Eye-Head Coordination in Squirrel Monkeys during Optokinetic Stimulation, 85.
Eye Movement, Compensatory; Gaze Fixation During Active Head Rotation in Patients with Labyrinthine Disorders and, 241.
Facial Nerve, Labyrinthine Segment and Geniculate Ganglion in Fetal and Adult Human Temporal Bones, Suppl. 85.
Facial Nerve Decompression, Early, in Bell's Palsy, 570.
Fascial Stakes with Myringoplasty, 172.
Fenestra, Small; Comparison of Total Stapedectomy and, 633.
Fetal Guinea Pig Inner Ear, In Vitro Cultivation of, 246.
Fetus, Human, and Neonate; Development of Hypotympanum in, Suppl. 88.
Fiberoptic Endoscopy, Flexible, in Difficult Intubations, 307.
Fibroma, Nasopharyngeal, Juvenile, 420.
Fistula (Neoglottis), Tracheopharyngeal, Total Laryngectomy with, 217.
Fistula, Tracheoesophageal, and Esophageal Atresia, Endoscopy in, 376.
Footplate Extraction, Total, in Stapedectomy, 630.
Foreign Bodies in Aerodigestive Tract of Pediatric Patient, Unusual Presentations and Problems Created by Mismanagement of, 316.
Gaze Fixation and Compensatory Eye Movement During Active Head Rotation in Patients with Labyrinthine Disorders, 241.
Geniculate Ganglion and Labyrinthine Segment of Facial Nerve in Fetal and Adult Human Temporal Bones, Suppl. 85.
Gentamicin, Intracisternal, Ototoxicity of, in Cats, 255.
Globus Hystericus, Abnormal Esophageal Manometry in, 383.
Glomus Tumors, Familial, Multiple, and Pheochromocytomas, 60.
Granulomatosis, Wegener's. Long-Term Results of Treatment, 231.
Grassheads in Tracheobronchial Tree: Two Different Outcomes, 406.
Harmonic Acceleration in Patients with Menière's Disease; Comparison of Subjective Symptomatology and Responses to, Suppl. 86:15.
Hearing Loss, Fluctuating, and Sarcoidosis, 161.
Hearing Rehabilitation Research Center Implant Program, Status of, Suppl. 82:4.
Hernia, Esophageal Hiatal, in Infants and Children, 387.
Horseradish Peroxidase Studies in Animals with Neuromuscular Transpositions, 396.
Hypopharyngeal and Cervical Esophageal Cancer, Surgical Repair in. Analysis of 162 Patients, 372.
Hypothyroidism following Treatment for Head and Neck Cancer, 449.
Hypotympanum, Development in Human Fetus and Neonate, Suppl. 88.
Implant, Cochlear, Multiple-Channel: Evaluation Using Nonsense Syllables, 227.
Implants, Ceramic, Bioinert, in Middle Ear Surgery, 640.
Infections, Anaerobic, in Otolaryngology, Suppl. 84:13.
Ear, Nose and Throat; Clinical Pharmacology of Antimicrobial Agents for, Suppl. 84:2.
Ear, Nose and Throat — Head and Neck, Recent Advances in Antimicrobial Therapy for, Suppl. 84.
Invasive *Hemophilus:* Epiglottitis and Cellulitis, Suppl. 84:19.
Postoperative Wound, Suppl. 84:17.
Internal Carotid Artery, Aberrant, in Middle Ear, 67.
Intracochlear Electrical Stimulation, Chronic; Cochlear Pathology following, Suppl. 82:6.
Intracochlear Electrodes, Chronic Electrical Stimulation with. Electrophysiological Results, Suppl. 82:27.
Intracochlear Stimulating Electrodes; Performance Characteristics of, Suppl. 82:9.
Intubations, Difficult; Flexible Fiberoptic Endoscopy in, 307.
Invasive *Hemophilus* Infections: Epiglottitis and Cellulitis, Suppl. 84:19.
Japanese Medicine, Legacies of Jefferson Men to. Third Louis H. Clerf Lecture, Suppl. 87.
Jugular Bulb Diverticulum, Endolymphatic Duct Obstruction from, 619.
Klippel-Feil Syndrome, Ear Deformities Associated with, 210.
Labyrinth-Blood Barrier in Experimental Conditions, Nature of, 135.
Labyrinth Lesions, Leaking, Deafness, Tinnitus and Dizziness, 99.
Labyrinthine Disorders, Compensatory Eye Movement and Gaze Fixation During Active Head Rotation in Patients with, 241.
Labyrinthine Segment and Geniculate Ganglion of Facial Nerve in Fetal and Adult Human Temporal Bones, Suppl. 85.
Laryngeal Cyst: X-Ray Study of the Month, 522.
Laryngeal Dysfunction, Observations on Central Neurologic Etiology for, 430.
Laryngeal Injuries Secondary to Nasogastric Tubes, 469.
Laryngeal Recurrent Nerve Resection: Adductor Spastic Dysphonia following, 2.

Laryngeal Stenosis, Complicated; Epiglottic Laryngoplasty for, 409.
Treatment of. A Conservative New Approach, 512.
Laryngectomee, Voice Button Prosthesis Rehabilitation of. Additional Notes, 503.
Laryngectomy, Bilateral Vertical Partial, for Bilateral Vocal Cord Carcinoma, 489.
Total; Effect on Esophageal Motility, 331.
Total; Further Experience with Voice Restoration after, 498.
Total; Surgical and Radiological Effects upon Development of Speech after, 294.
Total, with Tracheopharyngeal Fistula (Neoglottis), 217.
Laryngectomy and Prosthetic Vocal Rehabilitation: The Voice Button, 116.
Laryngology, Pediatric, Documentation in, 478.
Laryngoscope, Direct; A New Universal Bivalved Speculum, 344.
Laryngoscopy, Video; Using a Rigid Telescope and Video Home System Color Camera. A Useful Office Procedure, 346.
Laryngotracheal Reconstruction in Children. Five-year Follow-up, 516.
Laryngotracheoesophageal Cleft, Management of, 401.
Larynx, Cancer of; Use of Videotape in Diagnosis and Treatment, 398.
Carbon Dioxide Laser Surgery of, Complications, 132.
Carcinoid Tumor of, 42.
Laser, Carbon Dioxide, Incendiary Characteristics of Endotracheal Tubes With. An Experimental Study, 328.
Carbon Dioxide, Treatment of Metatastic Melanoma of Trachea and Bronchi, 310.
CO_2, Use in Otology, 70.
Laser Surgery, Laryngeal, in Infant and Child; Anesthesia for, 475.
Laser Surgery of Larynx, Carbon Dioxide, Complications of, 132.
Lateral Canal Block and Eye-Head Coordination in Squirrel Monkeys, 154.
Ligation, Carotid, Complications of; Analysis of Factors Affecting, 222.
Loudness, Growth of, for Sinusoidal and Pulsatile Electrical Stimulation, Suppl. 82:13.
Lysosomal Hydrolases in Middle Ear Effusions, 148.
Malignancies, Head and Neck, Flexible Fiberoptic Bronchoscopy and Pulmonary Cytology in Evaluation of Patients with, 351.
Manometry, Abnormal Esophageal, in Globus Hystericus, 383.
Mastoid Cavities and Accessory Nasal; Sinus, Quantitative Histology of Mucous Membrane of, 33.
Melanoma, Metatastic, Trachea and Bronchi; Use of Carbon Dioxide Laser in Treatment of, 310.
Menière's Disease; Comparison of. Subjective Symptomatology and Responses to Harmonic Acceleration in Patients with, Suppl. 86:15.
Endolymphatic Sac Enhancement Surgery for. An Extension of Conservative Therapy, 610.
Medical Management of, 142.
Metabolic Management in, 615.
Panel on, 610; Comment, 618.
Metastases, Perineural, from Squamous Cell Carcinoma of Face. Therapeutic Considerations, 183.
Microfissure in Oval Window Area, 174.
Middle Ear, Chronic Effects of Phasic Pressure Changes, 281.
Ventilating Tubes; Panel on Experiences with, 529.
Middle Ear Aeration: Implications for Reflex Control of. Neural Connections Between Middle Ear, Eustachian Tube and Brain, 566.
Middle Ear Surgery; Bionert Ceramic Implants in, 640.
Migraine, Common, and Vestibular Function. Electronystagmographic Study and Pathogenesis, 267.
Möbius Syndrome; Temporal Bone Findings in Patient with, 80.
Motility, Esophageal; Effect of Total Laryngectomy on, 331.
Mucous Membrane of Accessory Nasal Sinus and Mastoid Cavities, Quantitative Histology of, 33.
Mucus Layer and Nasal Epithelial Cells, Changes After Challenge of Allergen, 204.
Multidisciplinary Approach to Advanced Head and Neck Cancer; Role of Chemotherapy in. Potentials and Problems, 506.
Multiplex Congenita (Larsen's) Syndrome, Tracheomalacia in an Infant with, 303.
Muscle Fiber Types in Posterior Cricoarytenoid Muscle, Histochemical Characteristics of, 423.
Myositis Ossificans following Radical Neck Dissection, 169.
Myringoplasty with Fascial Stakes, 172.
Nasal Epithelial Cells and Mucus Layer after Challenge of Allergen; Changes of, 204.
Nasal (Schneiderian) Papillomas, 190.
Nasogastric Tubes, Laryngeal Complications of, 465.
Laryngeal Injuries Secondary to, 469.
Nasopharyngeal Fibroma, Juvenile, 420.
Neonate and Human Fetus; Development of Hypotympanum in, Suppl. 88.
Neoplasms of Head and Neck, Ultrasonic Analysis of. Correlation with Surgical Findings, 126.
Neural Connections between the Middle Ear, Eustachian Tube and Brain. Implications for Reflex Control of Middle Ear Aeration, 566.
Neural Generators of Brainstem Evoked Potentials. Results from Human Intracranial Recordings, 591.
Neuritis, Vestibular. Second Louis H. Clerf Lecture, Suppl. 78.
Neurologic Etiology, Central; Observations on Laryngeal Dysfunction for, 430.
Neuromuscular Transpositions, Horseradish Peroxidase Studies in Animals with, 396.
Neurophysiology, Ocular Motor, Overview of. Suppl. 86:29.
Neurotologic Diagnosis; Developing Computer Laboratory for, Suppl. 86:7.
Noise Damage: Total Energy and Critical Intensity Concepts in, 584.
Nystagmus, Optokinetic; Measurement for Otoneurological Diagnosis, Suppl. 79.
Obituary, Sir Alexander Ewing, 298.
Ocular Motor Neurophysiology, Overview of. Suppl. 86:29.
Optokinetic Nystagmus: Measurement for Otoneurological Diagnosis, Suppl. 79.
Optokinetic Stimulation in Squirrel Monkeys; Eye-Head Coordination during, 85.
Optokinetic Test and ENG Test Battery, Suppl. 86:2.
Orbital Wall, Medial; Surgical Approach to, 415.
Organ of Corti of Man; Reciprocal Synapses at Base of Outer Hair Cells in, 12.
Osteogenesis Imperfecta Tarda and Otosclerosis. Temporal Bone Histopathology Report, 199.
Osteopathology, Otolaryngic, in 14th Century Mid-America, The Crow Creek Massacre, 288.
Otitis, External Necrotizing, Temporal Bone Histopathology of. A Case Report, 109.
Syphilitic, Congenital and Acquired; Electronystagmography in, 21.
Otitis Media, Acute, Recurrent; Antimicrobial Prophylaxis for, Suppl. 84:53.
Acute, with Effusion; Comparison of Cefaclor and Amoxicillin, Suppl. 84:48.
Chronic Nonsuppurative; Comparison of Tympanostomy Tubes and Medication versus Ventilation, 533.
Chronic Suppurative; Antimicrobial Therapy for, Suppl. 84:58.
Microbiology and Antimicrobial Treatment, Suppl. 84:30.
Pneumococcal; Following Middle Ear Deflation, 72.
Secretory; Influence of Adenoid Hypertrophy on, 7.
Streptococcal Pharyngitis and Skin Infections; Cefaclor in Management of, Suppl. 84:79.
Use of Tympanostomy Tubes in, 537.
Otitis Media and Tonsillopharyngitis in Infants and Children, Pharmacology of Oral Antibiotics Used for Treatment of, Suppl. 84:37.
Otolaryngology, Anaerobic Infections in, Suppl. 84:13.
Otology in Today's Medical Setting, 527.
Otoneurological Diagnosis; Measurement of Optokinetic Nystagmus for, Suppl. 79.
Otosclerosis and Osteogenesis Imperfecta Tarda. Temporal Bone Histopathology Report, 199.
Ototoxicity of Intracisternal Gentamicin in Cats, 255.
Oval Window Area, Microfissure in, 174.
Panendoscopy for Second Primaries in Head and Neck Cancer, 460.
Papillomas, Nasal (Schneiderian), 190.
Paranasal Sinusitis in Children; Etiology and Antimicrobial Therapy for, Suppl. 84:72.
Parapharyngeal Space, Tumors of. Preoperative Evaluation, Diagnosis and Surgical Approaches, Suppl. 80.
Parotolymphatic Backflow: A New Sign of Malignancy, 64.
Pathology Consultation: Nasal (Schneiderian) Papillomas, 190.
Pediatric Laryngology, Documentation in, 478.
People's Republic of China, Esophageal Cancer Research in, 359.
Perilymphatic Pressure, Increased; Effect on Endocochlear Potential, 264.
Periodic Alternating Nystagmus; ENG of the Month, 524.
Pharmacology, Clinical; Antimicrobial Agents for Infections in the Ear, Nose and Throat, Suppl. 84:2.
Pharyngitis and Pharyngotonsillitis; Etiology, Diagnosis and Antimicrobial Treatment of, Suppl. 84:75.
Pharyngotonsillitis and Pharyngitis; Etiology, Diagnosis, and Antimicrobial Treatment of, Suppl. 84:75.
Pheochromocytomas and Familial Multiple Glomus Tumors, 60.

Pitch Correlates of Direct Auditory Nerve Electrical Stimulation, Suppl. 82:15.
Postintubation Complication: Pseudolaryngeal Paralysis, 483.
Prophylaxis, Antimicrobial, for Recurrent Acute Otitis Media, Suppl. 84:53.
Prosthesis, Cochlear; Histological Examination of Implanted Cats, Suppl. 82:25.
Proceedings of West Coast Conference on, Suppl. 82.
Prosthesis Rehabilitation (Voice Button), of Laryngectomee. Additional Notes, 503.
Prosthetic Vocal Rehabilitation following Laryngectomy. The Voice Button, 116.
Protease Inhibitors in Middle Ear Effusions, 38.
Pseudolaryngeal Paralysis: A Postintubation Complication, 483.
Pulsatile Electrical Stimulation, and Sinusoidal, Growth of Loudness for, Suppl. 82:13.
Radical Neck Dissection, Myositis Ossificans following, 169.
Rapid Eye Movement, Velocity of; Vertigo of Central Origin and, 164.
Reconstruction, Laryngotracheal, in Children. Five-year Follow-up, 516.
Recurrent Nerve, Laryngeal, Resection of: Adductor Spastic Dysphonia following, 2.
Reinnervation, Laryngeal, for Unilateral Vocal Cord Paralysis. Long-term Results, 457.
Salivary Glands, Carcinoma of, Radiation-Associated. A Controlled Study, 107.
Sarcoidosis, Endoscopic Findings in. Characteristics and Correlations with Radiographic Staging and Bronchial Mucosal Biopsy Yield, 339.
Sarcoidosis and Fluctuating Hearing Loss, 161.
Scala Tympani, Human; Multielectrode Array of 20 mm Long, Model Trauma and Reliability of Placement, Suppl. 82:11.
Scarpa's Ganglion and Vestibular Sense Organs in Endolymphatic Hydrops, Quantitative Study of, 121.
Sinus, Frontal, Prehistoric Trephination of, 186.
Sinusitis, Acute; Etiology and Antimicrobial Treatment, Suppl. 84:68.
Alternaria, 251.
Maxillary, Discrimination of Purulent from Nonpurulent. Clinical and Radiographic Diagnosis, 272.
Paranasal; Etiology and Antimicrobial Therapy in Children, Suppl. 84:72.
Sinusoidal Electrical Stimulation, and Pulsatile, Growth of Loudness for, Suppl. 82:13.
Sinusoidal Harmonic Acceleration, Suppl. 86:10.
and Computerized Optokinetic Tracking Tests, Proceedings of Seminar on, Suppl. 86.
Labyrinthine Test, Clinical Experience, Suppl. 86:26.
Test in Clinical Practice, Suppl. 86:18.
Skin Infections, Streptococcal Pharyngitis and Otitis Media; Cefaclor in Management of, Suppl. 84:79.
Skull Base, Chondrosarcoma at, 53.
Speech, Surgical and Radiological Effects upon Development of, after Total Laryngectomy, 294.
Sputum Cytologic Diagnosis of Upper Respiratory Tract Cancer. Second Report, 312.
Squamous Cell Carcinoma of Face, Perineural Metastases from. Therapeutic Considerations, 183.
Stapedectomy, Small Hole; Contraindications to, 636.
Total; Comparison of Small Fenestra and, 633.
Total Footplate Extraction in, 630.
Stapes Surgery, Panel on, 630.
Stenosis, Acquired Subglottic; Histopathology of. A Documented Case Report, 335.
Congenital Tracheal, 364.
Laryngeal; Treatment of. A Conservative New Approach, 512.
Subglottic, in Children; Customized Dilator for Treatment of, 287.
Stimulators, Opto-Isolated, for Electrically Evoked BSER, Suppl. 82:21.
Streptococcal Pharyngitis, Otitis Media and Skin Infections; Cefaclor in Management of, Suppl. 84:79.
Subglottic Stenosis, Acquired; Histopathology of. A Documented Case Report, 335.
Surgery, Head and Neck; Chemoprophylaxis for, Suppl. 84:8.
Synapses, Reciprocal, at Base of Outer Hair Cells in Organ of Corti of Man, 12.
Syphilitic Otitis, Congenital and Acquired; Electronystagmography in, 21.
Temporal Bone; Comparative Study Using Computed Tomographic Thin-Section Zoom Reconstructions and Anatomic Macrosections of, 643.
Findings in Patient with Möbius Syndrome, 80.
Histopathology in Necrotizing External Otitis. A Case Report, 109.
Thyroglossal Duct Cyst and Dermoid Cyst in Neck, Association of. Case Report, 181.
Tinnitus, Dizziness and Deafness, Leaking Labyrinth Lesions, 99.
Medical Treatment of, 601.
Tinnitus Control, Panel on, 597; Comment, 607.
Tinnitus Patient, Management of, 597.
Tomography, Computed; Thin-Section Zoom Reconstructions and Anatomic Macrosections in Comparative Study of Temporal Bone, 643.
Tomography, Computerized, Posterior Fossa Pathology and Central Vestibular Signs; Regional Blood Brain Circulation, 624.
Tonsillitis, Recurrent; Aerobic and Anaerobic Bacteria in Tonsils of Children with, 261.
Tonsillopharyngitis and Otitis Media in Infants and Children, Pharmacology of Oral Antibiotics Used for Treatment of, Suppl. 84:37.
Tracheal Stenosis, Congenital, 364.
Tracheobronchial Tree, Grassheads in: Two Different Outcomes, 406.
Tracheoesophageal Puncture for Alaryngeal Voice Restoration, 492.
Tracheomalacia, Infant with Multiplex Congenita (Larsen's) Syndrome, 303.
Tracheopharyngeal Fistula (Neoglottis) with Total Laryngectomy, 217.
Trauma, Probability of; Reliability of Placement of 20 mm Long Model Human Scala Tympani Multielectrode Array, Suppl. 82:11.
Trephination, Prehistoric, of Frontal Sinus, 186.
Tumor, Carcinoid, of Larynx, 42.
Tumors, Glomus, Familial, Multiple, and Pheochromocytomas, 60.
Parapharyngeal Space. Preoperative Evaluation, Diagnosis and Surgical Approaches, Suppl. 80.
Tympanostomy Tubes: Medication versus Ventilation in Chronic Nonsuppurative Otitis Media, 533.
The Conservative Approach, 529.
Tympanostomy Tubes in Otitis Media, Use of, 537.
Ultrasonic Analysis of Neoplasms of Head and Neck. Correlation with Surgical Findings, 126.
Upper Respiratory Tract Cancer, Sputum Cytologic Diagnosis of. Second Report, 312.
Upper Respiratory Tract Ciliary Ultrastructural Pathology, Suppl. 83.
Ventilating Tubes, Middle Ear; Panel, 529; Comment, 535.
Ventilation Testing with Electronystagmography, 56.
Vertigo of Central Origin and Velocity of Rapid Eye Movements, 164.
Vestibular Aqueduct and Idiopathic Endolymphatic Hydrops, 77.
Vestibular Function and Common Migraine. Electronystagmographic Study and Pathogenesis, 267.
Vestibular Neuritis. Second Louis H. Clerf Lecture, Suppl. 78.
Vestibular Sense Organs and Scarpa's Ganglion in Endolymphatic Hydrops, Quantitative Study of, 121.
Vestibular Signs, Central, Posterior Fossa Pathology and Computerized Tomography-Regional Blood Brain Circulation, 624.
Vestibulo-Ocular Reflex Changes with Horizontal Vision-Reversal Prisms. New Neurotological Test for Detecting Cerebellar Dysfunction, 276.
Video Laryngoscopy Using a Rigid Telescope and Video Home System Color Camera. A Useful Office Procedure, 346.
Videotape; Use in Diagnosis and Treatment of Cancer of Larynx, 398.
Vitamin A-Induced Ear Malformations in Rats as Model for Analysis of Atresia Auris Congenita. Microsurgical and Histological Study, Suppl. 81.
Vocal Cord Paralysis, Unilateral; Laryngeal Reinnervation for. Long Term Results, 457.
Vocal Fold, Contact Granuloma of; Effect of Voice Therapy on, 48.
Voice Button: Prosthetic Vocal Rehabilitation following Laryngectomy, 116.
Voice Button Prosthesis Rehabilitation of the Laryngectomee. Additional Notes, 503.
Voice Restoration, Alaryngeal; Tracheoesophageal Puncture for, 492.
Limitations of the Blom-Singer Technique for, 495.
Voice Restoration after Total Laryngectomy, Further Experience with, 498.
Voice Therapy, Effect of; on Contact Granuloma of Vocal Fold, 48.
Water-Borne Infection; Objective Evaluation of Earplugs for Control of, 89.
Wegener's Granulomatosis. Long-Term Results of Treatment, 231.
X-Ray of the Month: Pleomorphic Adenoma of Hard Palate, 192.
X-Ray Study of the Month: Laryngeal Cyst, 522.

Second Louis H. Clerf Lecture

VESTIBULAR NEURITIS

Harold F. Schuknecht, MD

Ken Kitamura, MD

Boston, Massachusetts

Vestibular neuritis is a discrete degenerative neuropathy of the vestibular nerve trunks. The clinical manifestations consist of one or more severe prolonged episodes of vertigo, sometimes in association with milder periodic or constant unsteadiness. The atrophic changes in the vestibular nerves are usually sufficiently severe to create vestibular test abnormalities. The clinical and pathological features are consistent with a viral etiology.

The purpose of this paper is to piece together the existing knowledge of a particular disorder of the vestibular system which is known by various terms, the most common of which are vestibular neuronitis, vestibular neuritis, and epidemic vertigo. In 1909 Ruttin[1] provided the first clinical description of the disorder, characterizing it as a sudden unilateral loss of vestibular function without auditory symptoms, occurring in an otherwise healthy patient. Fifteen years later Nylen[2] described an identical case and subsequently many clinical reports of large series of cases have appeared in the literature.

The authors of these reports generally agree that this disease, which we will refer to as vestibular neuritis, is a disorder of the vestibular system without an associated auditory deficit or other disease of the CNS. There is some disagreement, however, as to whether the diagnosis is tenable when there are recurring episodes of vertigo or prolonged dysequilibrium. Hallpike[3] and later Dix and Hallpike[4] preferred the broader definition and included cases with either single or multiple attacks of vertigo, and reported that of 100 cases studied 47 had bilateral canal paresis and 53 had unilateral canal paresis. Harrison[5] studied 67 patients conforming to the description of Dix and Hallpike and found that in 29 of them the attacks of vertigo were repeated over periods of time up to seven years. A more restricted diagnostic criterion limited to a single severe attack of vertigo with subsequent permanent unilateral deficit in caloric response was preferred by Aschan and Stahle[6] and others.[7-10]

We have examined the histological preparations of the temporal bones of four subjects whose clinical course and pathological findings we believe are compatible with the diagnosis of vestibular neuritis. Each showed deficits in the population of peripheral vestibular nerve fibers. The medical histories indicate that the broader concept of the term vestibular neuritis is appropriate. The pathological changes are similar to those occurring in herpes zoster infection of the vestibular system,[11] which suggests that vestibular neuritis may also be attributed to a viral etiology.

CLINICAL MANIFESTATIONS

On the basis of personal clinical experience and a review of the literature it seems quite clear that there are single-attack and multiple-attack forms of vestibular neuritis. The evidence suggests that the disease may affect one or both ears and may involve them concurrently or sequentially. The degree of chronicity may be determined in part by the magnitude of cell death (atrophy) of vestibular neurons caused by the attacks. For example, if an attack of neuritis causes total atrophy of a particular vestibular nerve there would be no further capability for that nerve to cause vertigo. On the other hand, if an attack caused only partial atrophy of a vestibular nerve, or caused a physiological interruption of function of the nerve with subsequent recovery, it would be possible for further episodes of vestibular paralysis to be attributable to that nerve. In this regard Aschan and Stahle[6] have found that after an attack of vertigo some involved ears may subsequently exhibit recovery of depressed caloric sensitivity.

The occurrence of a single acute severe attack of vertigo without associated involvement of the auditory mechanism or CNS has been well documented in the literature. It has been variously referred to as epidemic vertigo[5,12-15] neurolabyrinthitis epidemica,[16] acute labyrinthitis,[17,18] vestibular paralysis,[8] and vestibular neuronitis.[9] The onset is sudden, often occurs during the night, and usually is severe enough to cause nausea and vomiting. In contradistinction to Menière's disease, the vertigo is prolonged and subsides gradually over a period of days or weeks, as would be expected for a disease causing death of vestibular neurons. Coates,[9] after studying a large number of patients with vestibular symptoms, evolved the following diagnostic criteria for this disorder which he termed vestibular neuronitis: 1) an acute unilateral peripheral vestibular disorder

From the Harvard Medical School and the Department of Otolaryngology, Massachusetts Eye and Ear Infirmary, Boston. This study was supported by a research grant from the National Institutes of Health, Public Health Service, NINCDS NS05881.

Presented at the Department of Otolaryngology, Jefferson Medical College of Thomas Jefferson University, Philadelphia, Pennsylvania, May 7, 1980.

without an associated hearing loss, 2) occurrence predominantly in middle age, 3) a single episode of severe prolonged vertigo, 4) decreased caloric response in the involved ear, and 5) complete subsidence of the symptoms within six months.

Limitation of the diagnosis of vestibular neuritis to a single-attack disorder seems, however, to be too restrictive. Several authors conceive of a more chronic form of the disease consisting of recurring episodes of dysequilibrium often associated with persistent or intermittent unsteadiness. The attacks are usually less severe and of shorter duration than those of the single-attack form but may recur over a period of years.[5] Hallpike[3] and later Dix and Hallpike[4] termed the condition vestibular neuronitis (a term Coates used for the single-attack form of the disease) and described the symptomatology as consisting of "sudden and severe transient seizures accompanied by sensations of blackout." On the other hand they also included under the diagnosis of vestibular neuronitis those cases in which there were no severe paroxysms of vertigo, and the dysequilibrium was characterized as "feeling top heavy" or "off balance," particularly when walking or standing. Dix and Hallpike,[4] Pfaltz,[19] and Kattum and Mundnich[20] found a preceding or accompanying infection of the upper respiratory system in a high percentage of patients exhibiting the disorder. Stahle[21] states that there may be decreased vestibular response in one or both ears, or directional preponderance.

Several authors have referred to the epidemic nature of the disease. An editorial[22] referred to the condition as epidemic labyrinthitis. The vertigo was described as being continuous or occurring in waves and disappearing in days or weeks. Worster-Drought[23] published findings of 50 cases of vertigo, some exhibiting nystagmus, lasting for a few days but recurring in some cases. Walford[24] reported four cases who had contact with cases of influenza in the same household. Herberts[25] described a large series of cases associated with upper respiratory infection and Dalsgaard-Nielsen[26] presented 21 cases all of whom had been in contact with other cases of vertigo. Pedersen[13] described 400 cases occurring in a series of epidemics in Denmark.

CLINICAL CASES

The following medical histories of four patients examined in the recent past are compatible with the diagnosis of vestibular neuritis.

Case 1. At age 34 this male had a left stapedectomy and at age 39 a right stapedectomy for otosclerosis with closure of the bone-air gap in each ear. At age 52, while suffering from the "flu," he experienced the sudden onset of severe vertigo with nausea and vomiting. The severe vertigo gradually subsided over a period of two weeks but left him with a feeling of unsteadiness and vertigo when he rolled over on his right side. Examination revealed a spontaneous nystagmus to the left, greatly decreased caloric response in the right ear and positional vertigo of the benign paroxysmal type (cupulolithiasis) in the supine right-ear down position. Audiometric tests showed no change from previous recent tests. Six weeks after the onset of the vertigo he still felt unsteady, positional vertigo could not be elicited, and hearing was unchanged.

Comment. This patient exhibited all of the diagnostic criteria for right vestibular neuritis: 1) an episode of severe prolonged vertigo without auditory manifestations, 2) spontaneous nystagmus to the left, and 3) decreased caloric response in the right ear. Additionally he subsequently had positional vertigo (right cupulolithiasis) for about one month similar to the cases described by Lindsay and Hemenway.[27] The onset occurred while he was suffering from malaise that he assumed was caused by the "flu" and which suggests a probable viral disorder. We doubt a relationship to the otosclerosis or stapes surgery.

Case 2. At the age of 70 this female experienced the sudden onset of severe vertigo associated with nausea, vomiting and diarrhea. She was hospitalized for two weeks during which time the vertigo gradually subsided. Examination revealed a spontaneous nystagmus to the left. All other tests (radiological, blood chemistries, audiological, etc) were reported to be normal. After several months she felt well but continued to have mild unsteadiness. No vestibular tests were done at that time. Two years later at age 72, she experienced another severe attack of vertigo with symptoms identical to the first episode. Again the vertigo gradually subsided over a period of weeks, but the persisting unsteadiness was much more severe than after the first attack of vertigo. At no time did she experience auditory symptoms. Caloric tests done six months after this second attack showed no response to ice water in either ear. Polytomographic radiological studies of the temporal bones were normal. She complained of constant unsteadiness and difficulty walking in the dark, and walked with a wide base. Audiometry revealed a mild bilateral symmetrical sensorineural hearing loss with flat threshold patterns and 100% speech discrimination scores characteristic of the strial atrophy type of presbycusis.

Comment. This patient's vestibular symptoms are consistent with the diagnosis of bilateral sequential vestibular neuritis, involving first the right ear (as evidenced by spontaneous left beating nystagmus) and two years later the left ear.

Case 3. This female was quite well until the age of 34, when during a tennis match she felt unsteady and could not continue. She was confined to her home for three months and spent much of the time in bed because any head movement caused a sensation of vertigo. There were no acute attacks of vertigo and no change in hearing during this period. She then began to have episodes of vertigo about one minute in duration followed in each instance by several days of more severe unsteadiness, occurring at irregular intervals of several weeks. Numerous tests by several otologists included audiometry, ENG, radiologic studies, neurologic evaluation, brainstem evoked response audiometry, etc, and all were negative except for demonstrable intermittent ataxia and nystagmus and a bilateral progressive decrease in caloric response. Eighteen months after the onset of symptoms she still had occasional episodes of vertigo, but the unsteadiness was less severe and she could even play tennis on some "good" days. She now had a mild spontaneous nystagmus to the right, no reaction to ice water caloric testing in either ear and walked with a wide base. Hearing was normal and her general health was excellent.

Comment. The symptoms are consistent with the diagnosis of chronic bilateral vestibular neuritis. It appears that she is experiencing a slowly progressive

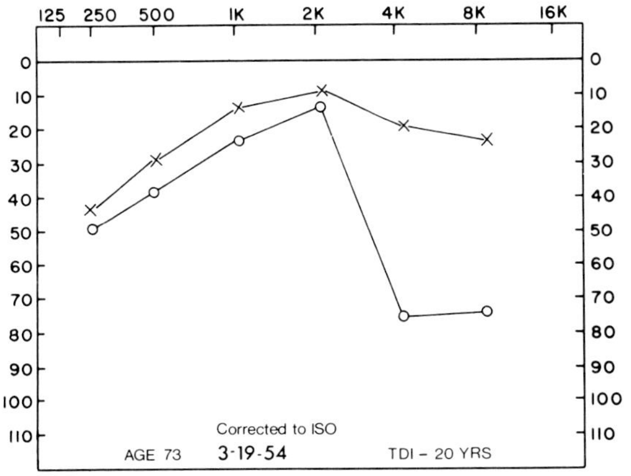

Fig. 1. (Case 5) Air conduction audiogram at 73 years.

somewhat episodic bilateral loss of vestibular function, and it is reasonable to assume that when and if the loss of vestibular function becomes total, the resultant disability will be less severe.

Case 4. This female, while enjoying excellent health and normal hearing, had single acute severe episodes of vertigo at ages 35, 41, and 50. Each attack was associated with nausea and vomiting and confined her to bed for several days. After each attack she experienced ataxia and a sensation of unsteadiness which gradually subsided over a period of several weeks, after which she again felt quite well. Examination three months after the last episode revealed no nystagmus, no response to ice water caloric test in the left ear, normal response to Kobrak minimal test (5 cc, 27 C) in the right ear, normal hearing, and normal polytomographic radiological studies of the temporal bones.

Comment. The symptoms and findings are compatible with the diagnosis of acute recurring left vestibular neuritis.

TEMPORAL BONE CASES

The medical histories and histopathological findings in the temporal bones of the following four subjects are compatible with our concept of vestibular neuritis.

Case 5. The medical records indicate that this female first learned to walk at the age of two years, had difficulty learning to ride a bicycle, exhibited clumsiness and tended to fall frequently. She showed some clumsiness throughout life, was left-handed and could "mirror write," but writing was always difficult. She was otherwise in good general health. At age 72, she described having two episodes of severe dizziness, each lasting two minutes. At age 73 while on a cruise ship in rough seas, she fell in her cabin and sprained her back, but did not hit her head. For several weeks she felt unsteady and had a feeling of fullness in the right ear. Examination at that time revealed normal tympanic membranes. Air conduction audiometry showed moderate low tone hearing losses in both ears and an abrupt high tone loss above 2 kHz in the right ear (Fig. 1). One examiner performed the minimal test of Kobrak (5 cc at 4.4 C) and found no response in the left ear and a normal response in the right ear. One week later another examiner performed bithermal caloric tests (Hallpike method) and recorded normal responses in both ears.

Neurological evaluation revealed limitation of upward gaze, and motor signs which were suggestive of cerebellar and/or pyramidal lesions, possibly resulting from a birth injury. Motor signs noticed by various examiners included walking with a wide base with arms held stiffly and partly flexed, a tendency to drop the

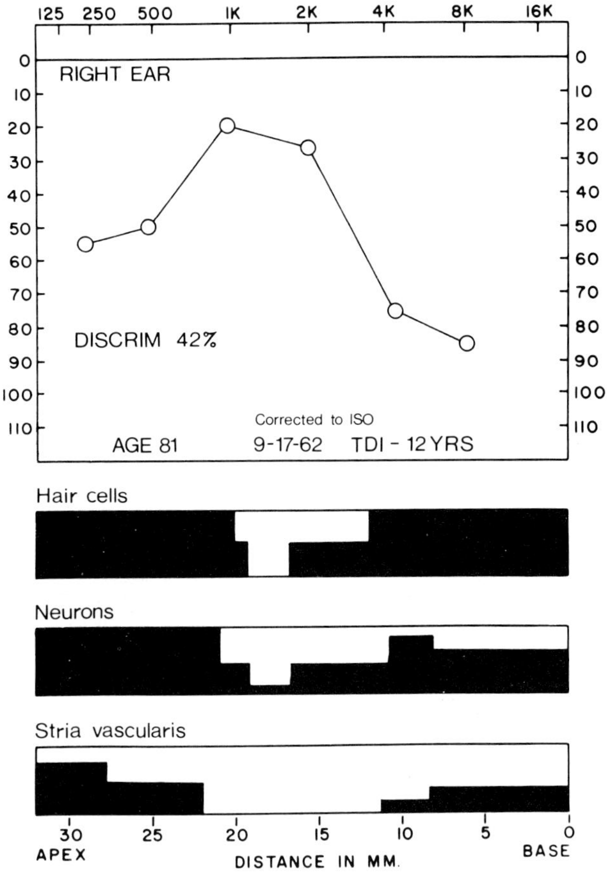

Fig. 2. (Case 5) Right ear. Audiogram at age 81. TDI - Test-death interval was 12 years. The black filling in the bar graphs shows estimated percent of elements missing as a function of distance along the cochlear duct.

right foot, pronation of feet which are small with high arches, weakness of dorsiflexion of the feet and large toes, and a suggestion of sagging of the muscles of the left side of the face.

At the age of 74 she had a sudden attack of vertigo associated with nausea, vomiting and diarrhea. The room seemed to spin to the right. She crawled on her hands and knees to the telephone to summon help. Examination revealed spontaneous nystagmus to the right. The blood pressure was 180/110 and the pupils were small but of equal size. Bithermal caloric tests showed directional preponderance to the right. Ice water caloric tests (5 cc) by another examiner revealed in the right ear an arrest of the spontaneous nystagmus for one minute 12 seconds, and in the left ear no change in the character of the right beating spontaneous nystagmus. The vertigo is reported to have subsided in three days; however, for years both before and after this episode she complained of a constant feeling of unsteadiness.

At the age of 81 she had two episodes in which she suddenly fell to the floor with no loss of consciousness and no vestibular or auditory sensations. She complained of having intermittent tinnitus in the right ear for several years. Air conduction audiograms showed a loss of hearing for high and low tones in the right ear and near normal thresholds in the left ear. Speech discrimination scores (PB Max, live monitored voice) were 42% on the right and 64% on the left ear (Figs. 2 and 4). Cold caloric tests (5 cc at 4.4 C) gave a response of one minute 49 seconds in the right ear and no response in the left ear.

At the age of 93 while suffering from multiple system disorders she died of cardiac arrest. Autopsy revealed severe generalized atherosclerosis. There was a small healed anterior myocardial infarct, but no evidence of ischemic brain disease. Histological

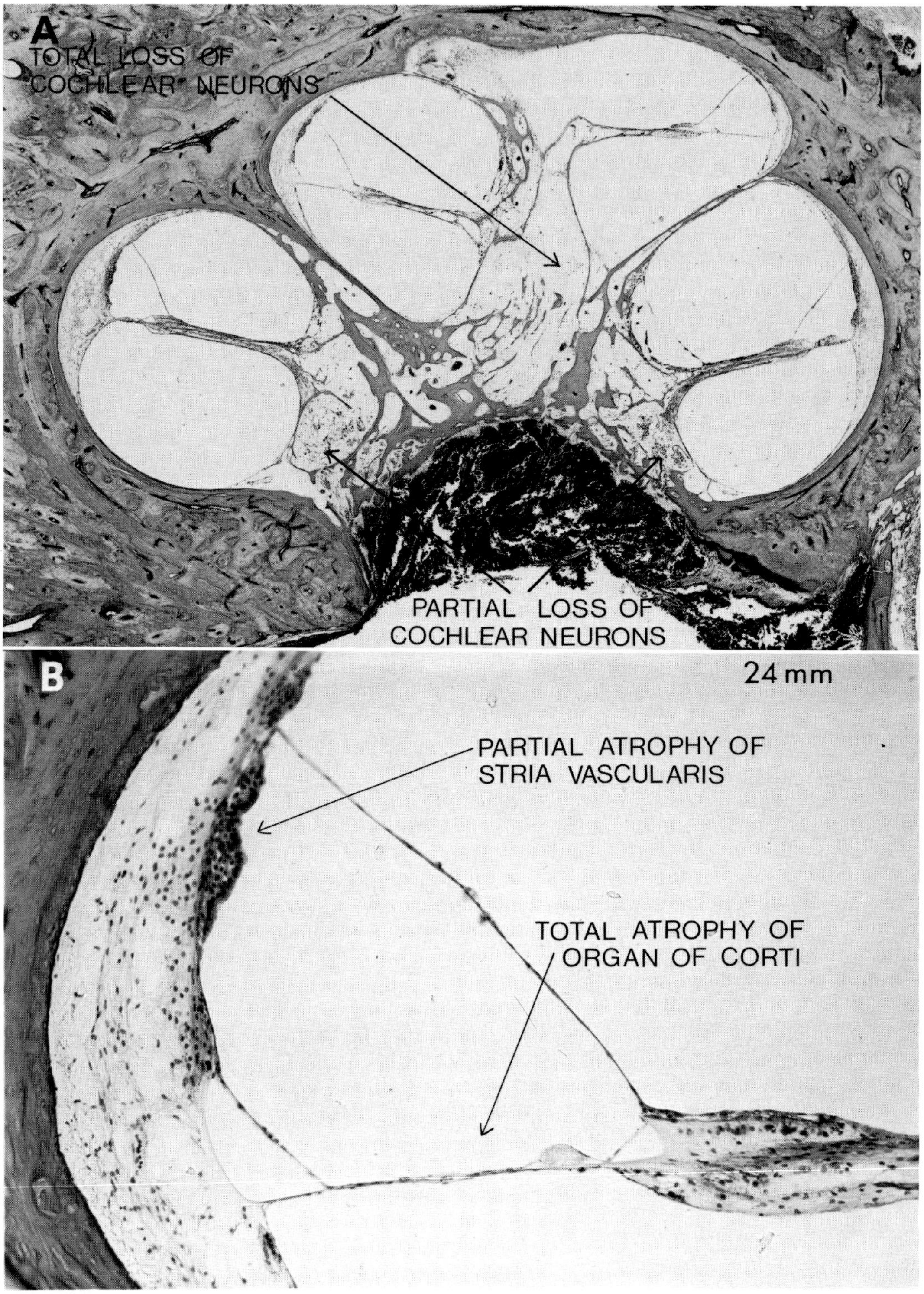

Fig. 3. (Case 5) Right ear. A) Midmodiolar section showing loss of cochlear neurons. B) Cochlear duct in the 24 mm region showing severe atrophy of the organ of Corti and tectorial membrane and partial atrophy of the stria vascularis.

study of the cerebellum and brainstem at the neuropathology department of the Massachusetts General Hospital was reported to show multiple areas of perivascular inflammation of the brainstem, but no evidence of destruction of nervous tissue. The vestibular nuclei and cerebellum appeared normal. The temporal bones were prepared for light microscopic study.

HISTOPATHOLOGY

RIGHT EAR. The tympanic membrane and ossicles are intact and the middle ear, bony labyrinth, and mastoid appear normal. In the basal and apical regions of the cochlea there is severe atrophy of the

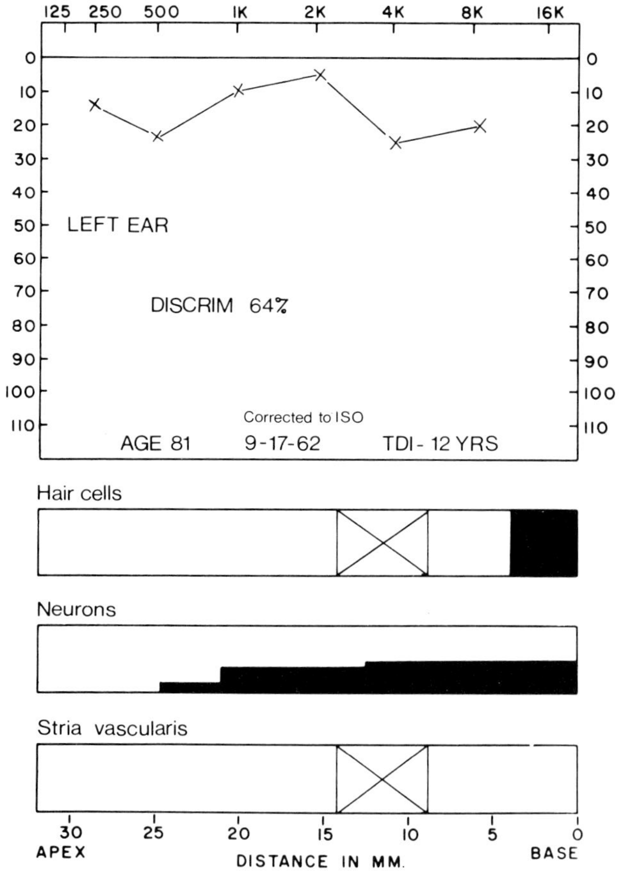

Fig. 4. (Case 5) Air conduction audiogram, left ear. For description of graphs see legend Fig. 2.

organ of Corti and cochlear neurons, and lesser atrophy of the stria vascularis. In the 0 to 12 mm and 21 to 32 mm regions the organ of Corti is either missing or consists of a small mound of undifferentiated cells. In the middle region of the cochlea (12 to 21 mm) hair cells are present, and in the 17 to 20 mm region the organ of Corti is normal. There is a loss of at least 50% of the cochlear neurons in the 0 to 17 mm area and a total loss in the 21 to 32 mm area. The neuronal population is near normal in the 17 to 19 mm regions. The tectorial membrane and stria vascularis show mild atrophy in the 0 to 12 mm area and severe atrophy in the 22 to 32 mm area. Reissner's membrane appears normal (Fig. 3 A, B). The vestibular sense organs appear normal and the vestibular nerve bundles as seen in the various cribrose areas appear normal. The vestibular, cochlear and facial nerve trunks have been avulsed from the internal auditory canal.

LEFT EAR. The tympanic membrane and ossicles are intact and the middle ear, bony labyrinth and mastoid appear normal. The medial part of the basal turn of the cochlea (9.5 to 14.5 mm) has been opened and destroyed by the bone saw during removal of the temporal bone; however, the remainder of the cochlea is well preserved (Fig. 5A). The organ of Corti is missing in the basal 4 mm but is normal in the remainder of the cochlea. There is a loss of about 50% of the cochlear neurons throughout the basal 22 mm. The tectorial membrane, Reissner's membrane and stria vascularis are normal.

There is a severe loss (90%, estimated) of nerve fibers to the macula of the utricle and to the cristae of the lateral and superior semicircular canals (Figs. 5B and 6). This judgment is based on a comparison with the opposite ear of nerve fiber densities of the peripheral part of the nerve extending from the cribrose areas to the sense organs as seen on routine serial sections stained with hematoxylin and eosin. It cannot be determined, of course, whether these remaining fibers are afferent or efferent types. The utricular and ampullary branches of the anterior vestibular artery are patent and appear normal (Fig. 7). The nerves to the macula of the saccule and to the crista of the posterior semicircular canal appear to have normal population densities. The utricular and saccular maculae and the cristae of all three semicircular canals appear normal.

Deposits of pigment (possibly melanin) are seen in the walls of the utricle and ampulla of the posterior semicircular canal. There are also scattered small pale basophilic staining bodies having round, oval, or irregular shapes lying in both endolymphatic and perilymphatic spaces, possibly representing staining artifact.

Comment. From birth this patient exhibited motor deficits such as lateness in learning to walk, clumsiness, frequent falling, sensations of unsteadiness, awkward gait, weakness of dorsiflexion of feet, tendency to drag the right foot, suggestion of drooping of left side of face, and intolerance to being abroad ship. These signs and symptoms are best explained as manifestations of a birth injury to the brain. She first experienced vertigo at age 72 and continued to complain of dysequilibrium until the time of her death 21 years later at age 93. At the age of 74 she experienced a sudden severe episode of vertigo with nausea, vomiting and diarrhea with the severe symptoms subsiding in three days. Examination at that time showed a spontaneous nystagmus to the right and diminished caloric responses on the left. Seven years later caloric tests (5 cc at 4.4 C) revealed a normal response in the right ear and no response in the left ear. The histological findings of degeneration of the superior division of the vestibular nerve in the left ear, without involvement of the auditory system is compatible with acute vestibular neuritis.

It is quite clear that degeneration of the organ of Corti is responsible for the hearing loss in the opposite (right) ear. The loss of cochlear neurons reflects quite accurately the spatial distribution of loss of supporting elements in the organ of Corti, making it reasonably certain that the loss of cochlear neurons is secondary to the lesion of the

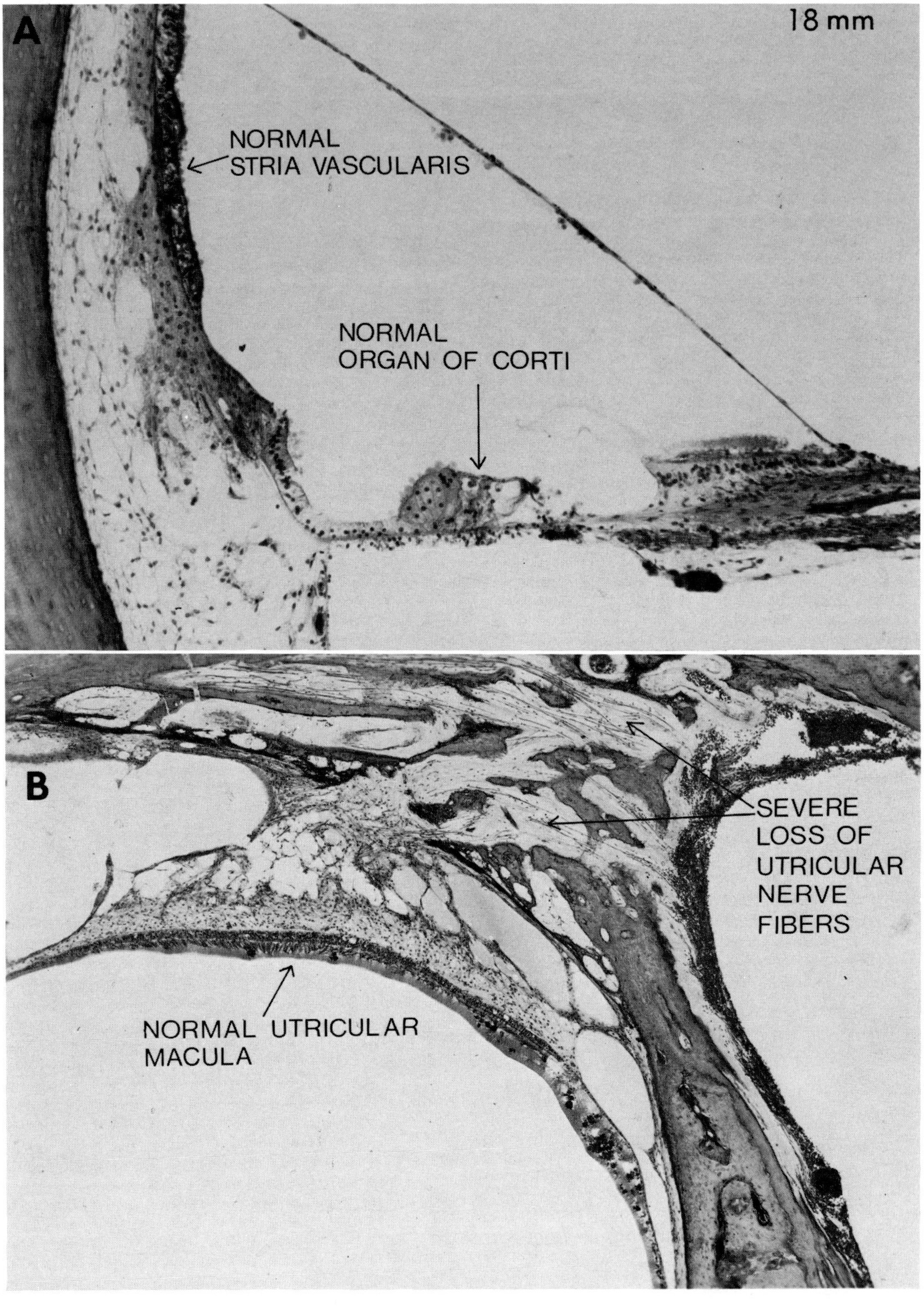

Fig. 5. (Case 5) Left ear. A) Normal cochlear duct in the 18 mm region. B) Atrophy of the utricular branch of the superior division of the vestibular nerve with normal utricular macula.

organ of Corti. The audiometric configuration of threshold losses for high and low tones with better hearing for middle tones was already present 20 years prior to death. There are no clues in the medical record or on histological study to indicate the etiology of this unusual basal-apical lesion. It seems improbable that there is an etiological relationship between the left vestibular lesion and the right cochlear lesion because the former involves the neural structures and the latter involves primarily the sensory structures.

Case 6. This female was in good general health all of her life and at age 75 was treated for minor nose and throat complaints.

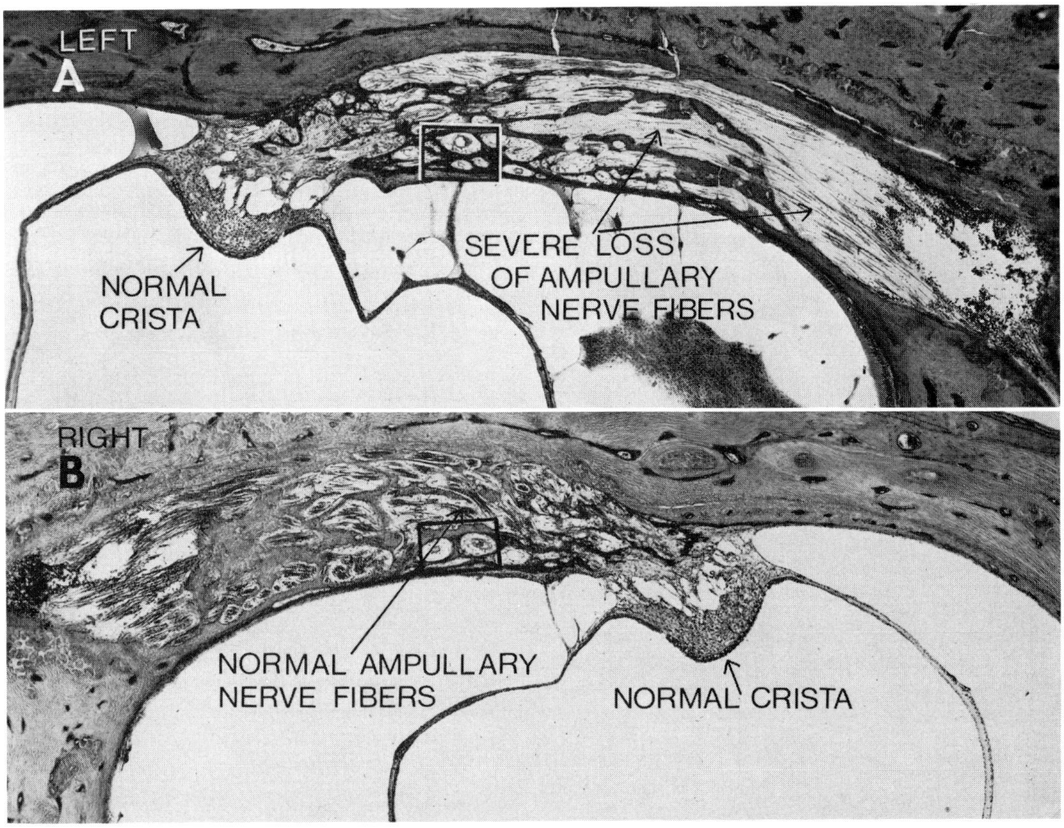

Fig. 6. (Case 5) A, B) Photomicrographs showing cristae and nerves of the lateral semicircular canals. There is severe atrophy of the left ampullary branch of the vestibular nerve. High power view of arteries in rectangles are seen in Fig. 7.

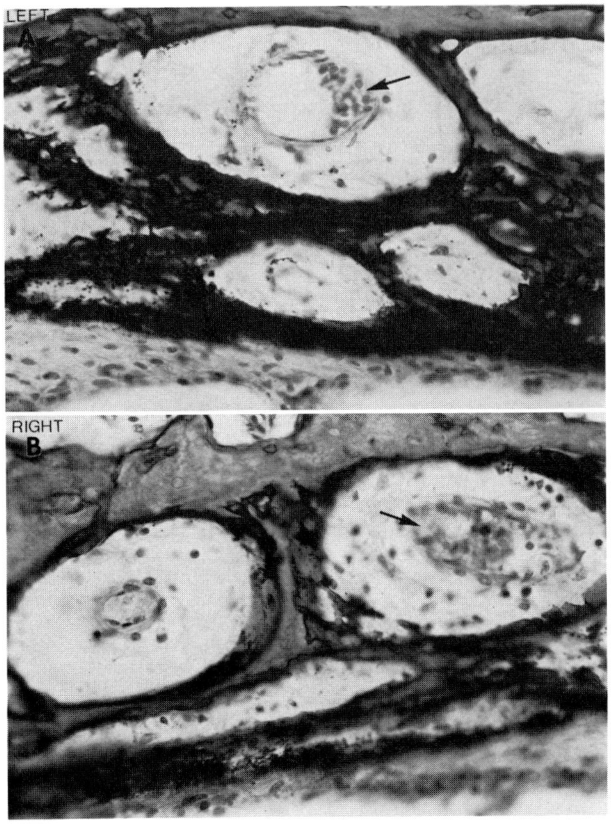

Fig. 7. (Case 5) A, B) High power views of areas shown in rectangles in Fig. 6. The ampullary branches of the anterior vestibular arteries are normal in both ears (arrows).

An audiogram at that time revealed a bilateral symmetrical sensorineural hearing loss characterized by descending threshold patterns (Fig. 8). At the age of 76 she complained of left-sided tinnitus, unsteadiness and a sensation of tilting to the left. She then began digitalis therapy for mild cardiac decompensation. Blood pressure was 165/95. At age 79, she had a small bowel resection for strangulated hernia and received penicillin and streptomycin. Streptomycin was given in an initial dosage of 500 mg followed by 250 mg every six hours given intramuscularly for a total of $6^1/_2$ g in seven days. The feeling of constant unsteadiness which was present before the streptomycin therapy continued unchanged. At age 83, she began taking nitroglycerine for angina. At the age of 84 she had a left mastectomy and radiotherapy for a lesion which was diagnosed histologically as fibroadenoma. At age 85, she had an acute severe episode of vertigo. The onset occurred without

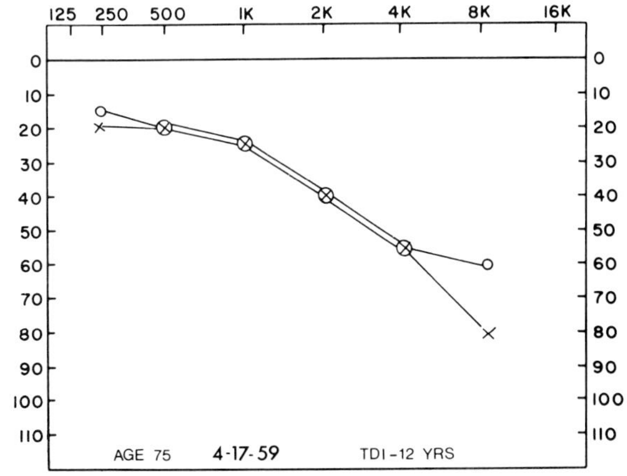

Fig. 8. (Case 6) Audiogram at age 75 years, 12 years before death.

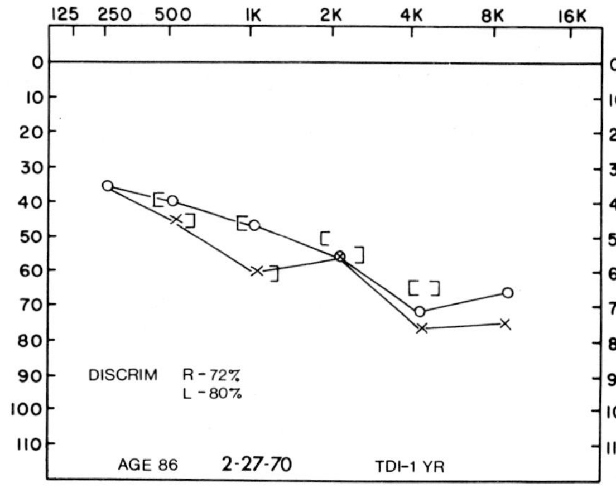

Fig. 9. (Case 6) Audiogram at age 86, one year before death.

warning while she was sitting reading. She was thrown to the right, felt cold and nauseated, and vomited. She reached her bed with difficulty, slept, and awoke the next morning feeling "fine," except for the constant unsteadiness previously noted. Several months later audiometry showed a progression of the sensorineural hearing loss. Caloric tests with 20 cc of ice water showed no response on the right and an active response for two minutes, 30 seconds on the left.

At age 86 she underwent extensive otoneurological evaluation for continuing dysequilibrium and progressive hearing loss. Audiometry revealed a bilateral sensorineural hearing loss with symmetrical descending threshold patterns. Speech reception thresholds were 42 dB in the right ear and 50 dB in the left ear. Speech discrimination scores were 72% on the right and 80% on the left (Fig. 9). Tone decay was tested at 2000 Hz and was negative in both ears. Bithermal caloric tests showed no responses on the right and normal responses on the left. There was also no response to 5 cc of ice water in the right ear. There was no spontaneous nystagmus. Positional tests for nystagmus were positive in the supine, right ear down position. Facial movements were symmetrical, and extraocular motion was full and normal. Corneal sensation was bilaterally equal, pinprick sensation was normal in the face and limbs, and the ocular fundi were normal. The Rhomberg test showed falling to the right. Gait was characterized by short shuffling steps. Tandem walking showed a tendency to fall to the right. Ankle and knee jerks were normal and rapid and alternating movements of the hands were normal.

One year later at the age of 87 she died rather suddenly of complications of coronary atherosclerosis. Autopsy was performed nine hours after death and showed cardiac hypertrophy and dilatation, pulmonary edema, bilateral pleural effusions, mural thrombi of the atria, and embolic infarcts of brain, spleen, both kidneys, and small bowel. The temporal bones were prepared for light microscopic study.

HISTOPATHOLOGY

RIGHT EAR. There are scattered small tears and disruptions of the soft tissue structures as well as of bone, and moderately severe postmorten autolysis in the form of compression artifact. The middle ear and mastoid contain small pools of acidophilic fluid with scattered polymorphonuclear leukocytes. The tympanic membrane, ossicles, bony labyrinth and mastoid are otherwise normal. There is severe atrophy of the spiral ligament in the apical half of

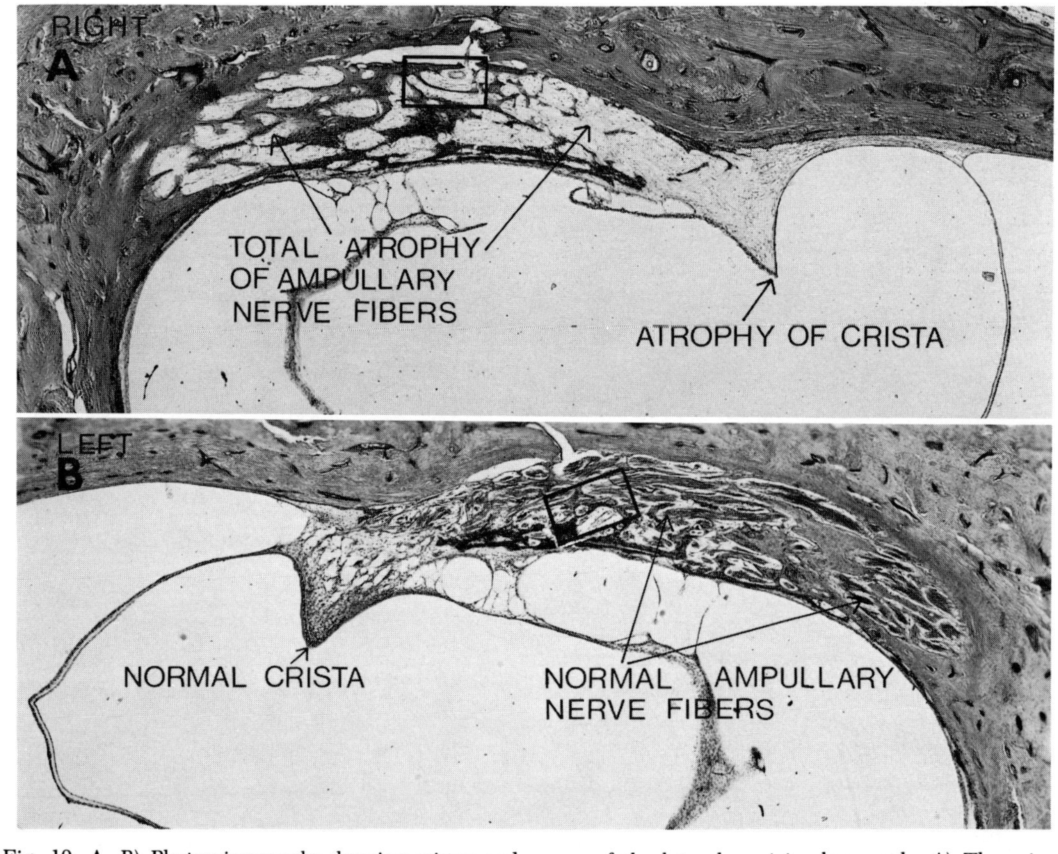

Fig. 10. A, B) Photomicrographs showing cristae and nerves of the lateral semicircular canals. A) There is severe atrophy of the right ampullary branch of the vestibular nerve. High power views of arteries in rectangles are seen in Fig. 12.

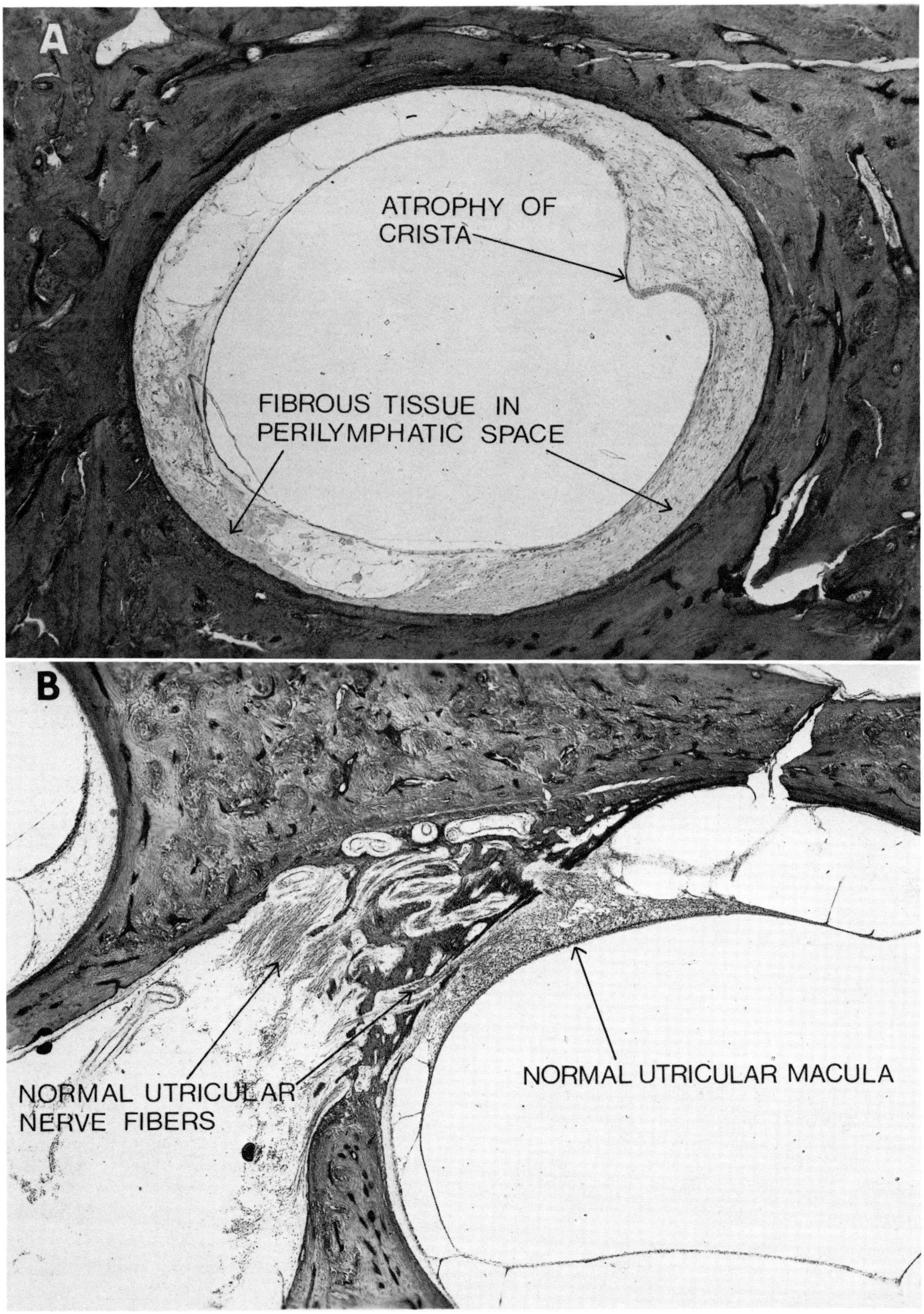

Fig. 11. (Case 6) Right ear. A) Atrophied crista and fibrous tissue in the perilymphatic space of the superior semicircular canal. B) Normal utricular macula and utricular nerve.

the cochlea. Hair cells can be seen throughout the organ of Corti. There is a loss of about 50% of the neurons in the basal turn of the cochlea. The vestibular nerve trunks have been avulsed from the internal auditory canal. Examination of the nerve bundles in their course from the cribrose areas to the sense organs reveals total atrophy of the ampullary branch of the superior division of the vestibular nerve and severe loss of cellularity of the associated cristae of the superior and lateral semicircular canals (Figs. 10 and 11A). The cristae consist of pale staining stroma with scattered small fibrocytes, and

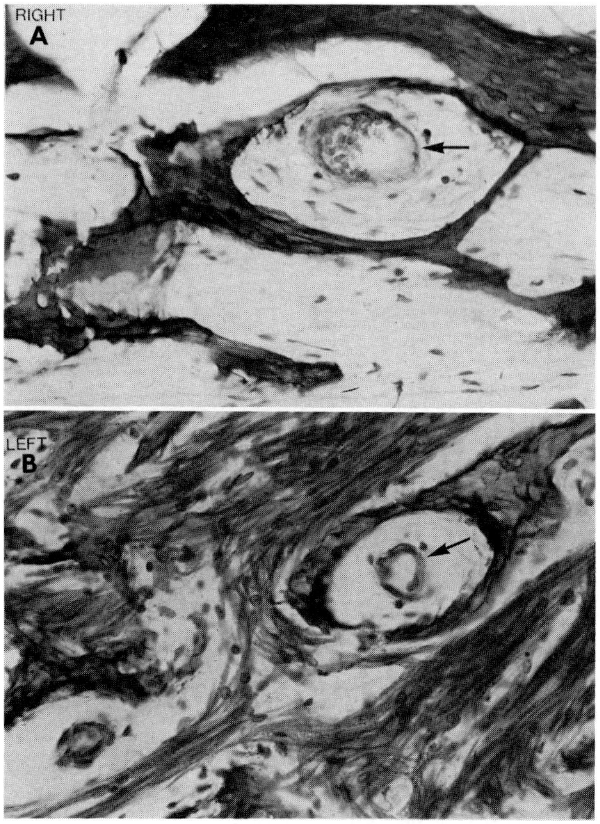

Fig. 12. (Case 6) A, B) High power views of areas shown in rectangles in Fig. 10. The ampullary branches of the anterior vestibular arteries are normal in both ears (arrows).

the sensory epithelia are reduced to a single layer of flat undifferentiated cells. There is a rupture of the ampullary wall of the lateral semicircular canal which may be an artifact of preparation. The perilymphatic space of the ampulla of the superior semicircular canal is partly obliterated by dense fibrous tissue of low cellularity (Fig. 11A). The utricular branch of the superior division of the vestibular nerve and the utricular macula are normal (Fig. 11 B). The inferior division of the vestibular nerve and its associated sense organs (saccule and crista of the posterior semicircular canal) are normal. The ampullary branch of the anterior vestibular artery which accompanies the ampullary nerve is patent, contains blood cells and appears morphologically similar to the same vessel of the opposite ear (Fig. 12).

LEFT EAR. The state of preparation artifact and autolytic change are similar to the opposite ear. The atrophic changes in the spiral ligament and loss of neurons in the basal turn of the cochlea parallels that of the opposite ear. The vestibular nerves and sense organs appear normal.

Comment. This patient complained of a constant sensation of unsteadiness from age 76 until the time of her death 11 years later at age 87. She experienced one short-lasting episode of severe vertigo with vomiting at age 85. Caloric tests which had been performed only subsequent to that episode showed no response to ice water in the right ear. On numerous occasions it was demonstrated that she had a tendency to fall to the right. The histological finding of degeneration of the ampullary branch of the superior division of the vestibular nerve and its associated sense organs (cristae of the lateral and superior semicircular canals) is compatible with right vestibular neuritis with extension to the sense organs.

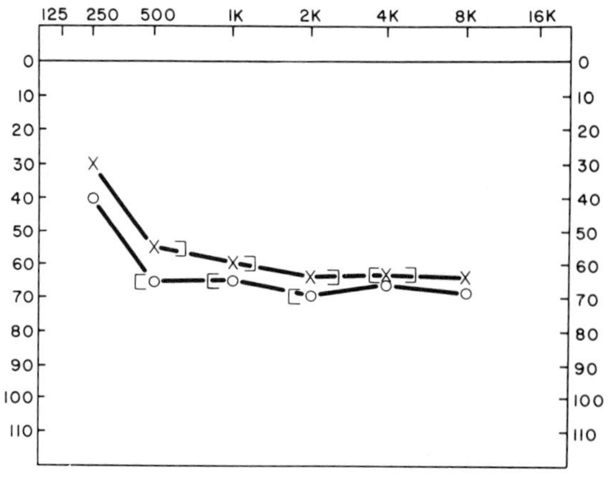

Fig. 13. (Case 7) Audiogram at age 85 years. (Published with permission of *Archives of Otolaryngology*[28])

Case 7. This case, previously reported by Naufal and Schuknecht,[28] concerns a female who first discovered she had diabetes mellitus at the age of 40. Glycosuria and blood sugar levels were controlled by dieting until the age of 80 at which time she took oral hypoglycemic agents (250 mg of tolbutamide [Orinase®] three times each day) until the time of her death at age 86.

Between the ages of 54 and 85, she experienced a series of acute paralytic episodes involving the third, seventh, and eighth cranial nerves. The attacks of third cranial nerve palsy occurred at the ages of 54, 58, 79, and 81, all on the left side. These were of acute onset with total recovery over a period of several months. Attacks of facial palsy occurred at the ages of 56 and 80 on the right side and at the age of 81 on the left. They were of acute onset with complete recovery in six months to one year on each occasion. Severe episodes of vertigo were recorded at ages 67, 69, and 85. The attacks were of acute onset associated with nausea, aggravated by head movement, and required bed rest for several days. Dysequilibrium of mild degree was present for some months following each episode but recovery was complete. Although the patient had noted a slowly progressive bilateral hearing loss for many years, there were no auditory symptoms associated with the attacks of vertigo. Audiometry at ages 62 and 85 showed bilateral symmetrical sensory neural hearing losses exhibiting flat audiometric patterns (Fig. 13). She died at the age of 86 of congestive heart failure.

The temporal bones show almost identical pathological changes. The hearing losses may be attributed to atrophy of the striae vasculares. Both ears show partial degeneration of the vestibular nerve fibers and neurons. Counts of the number of ganglion cells in the superior divisions were 3,390 on the right and 3,700 on the left, which is about 45% of the mean value established for a control group (Fig. 14). The number of ganglion cells in the inferior divisions was 9,040 on the right and 7,210 on the left which is 88 and 71% respectively of the mean normal value. The vestibular sense organs appear normal. The facial nerves appear normal. The walls of the arteries of both inner ears appear to

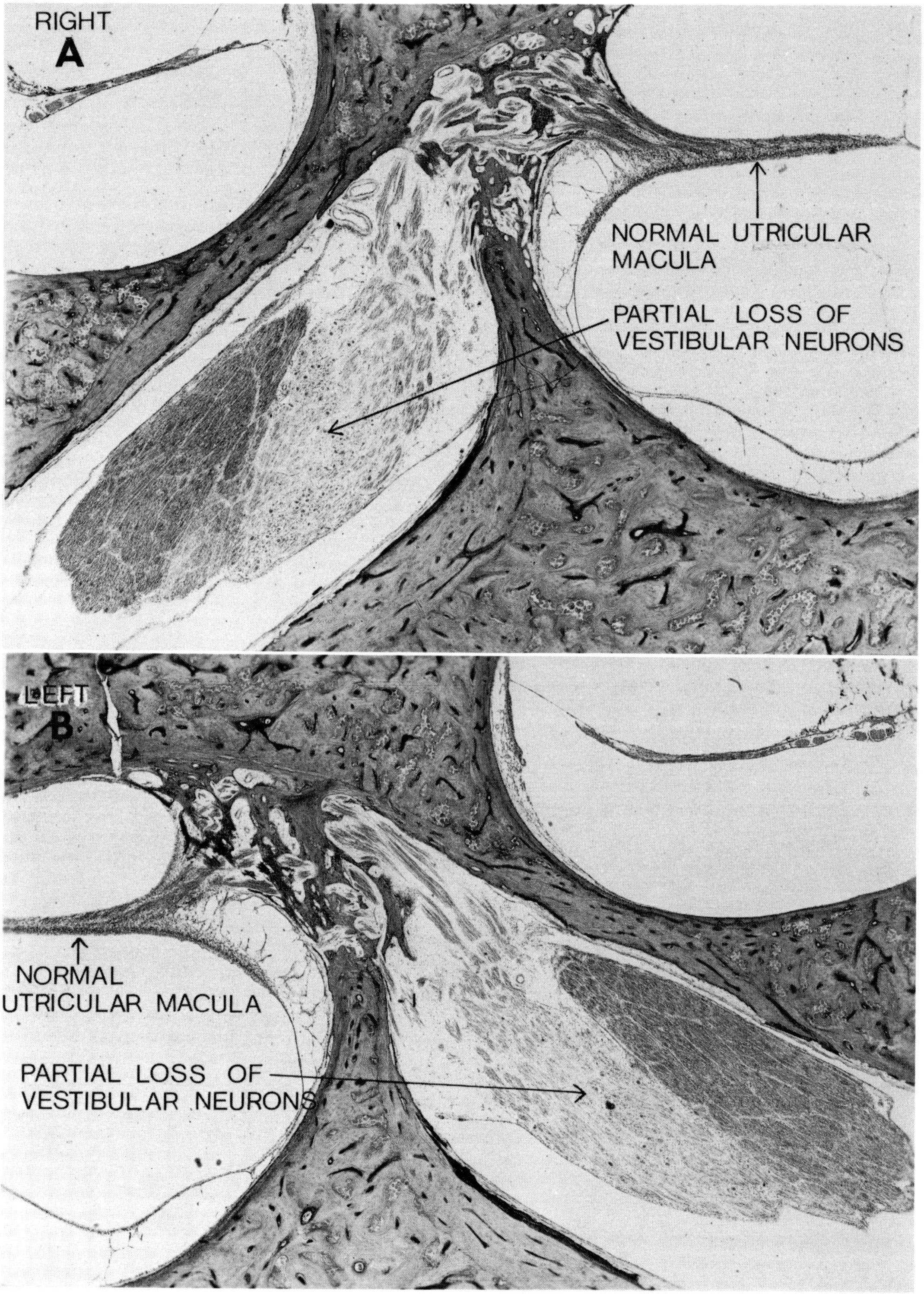

Fig. 14. (Case 7) A, B) The superior divisions of the vestibular nerves contain 3,390 Scarpa's ganglion cells on the right and 3,700 on the left (45% of normal). (Published with permission of *Archives of Otolaryngology*[28])

be somewhat thickened; however all arteries, including the anterior vestibular artery and its branches, appear to be patent and functional.

Comment. The most specific major vascular change that occurs in diabetes mellitus involves the small blood vessels, the arterioles, capillaries, and venules. The lumina of the vessels become narrowed because of hypertrophy and proliferation of the intimal endothelium and deposition of lipids. The etiology is not known but probably is related to excessive deposits of polysaccharides and lipids. This type of pathologic process constitutes the major alteration in the small blood vessels of nerves, skin, skeletal muscle, myocardium, kidney, retina, and placenta.

Another major vascular change in diabetes mellitus, though less specific than the microangiopathies, is arteriolosclerosis. It is more common in diabetics than in nondiabetics, possibly because of the increased incidence of hypertension in diabetes, and thus is not a direct consequence of the metabolic disorder. It involves the small arteries and arterioles through the body and is characterized by intimal fibrosis without endothelial proliferation.

The third major vascular change in diabetes is atherosclerosis. It occurs more often in diabetics than in nondiabetics and affects the larger blood vessels. There is an increased incidence of coronary artery disease, cerebrovascular accidents, and peripheral vascular disease in diabetics. There is usually no endothelial proliferation but the intima becomes thickened and hyalinized. Neuropathies are a common occurrence in diabetes mellitus and involve the central, peripheral, and autonomic nervous system. It has been generally assumed that the underlying pathological changes in the nervous system occurring in subjects with diabetes mellitus are related to the associated vascular disease. We believe, however, that there is reasonable doubt that a vascular etiology can account for the vestibular disease in this patient for the following reasons: 1) histological examination shows that the anterior vestibular artery and its branches are patent and 2) the existence of histologically normal vestibular sense organs indicates a functionally adequate blood supply.

Case 8. This male was first examined at the Massachusetts Eye and Ear Infirmary at the age of 34 years with a history of bilateral suppurative otitis media since childhood. Examination revealed a huge aural polyp in the left ear and infected cholesteatoma in the right middle ear. Roentgenograms showed bilateral sclerosis of the mastoids. At the age of 55 he related having three attacks of dizziness associated with sweating, nausea and vomiting. The first attack occurred while he was driving an automobile. He felt lightheaded, sweated profusely and felt weak for the rest of the day. The second attack occurred while he was walking to work; again the onset of the attack was sudden and he vomited several times. The third attack was much like the previous ones but occurred while he was watching television and again he vomited five or six times. He felt much better two hours later. Audiogram at the age of 55 revealed bilateral combined sensorineural and conductive hearing loss. Bone conduction thresholds were of the descending type and the bone-air gap was 40 to 50 dB. Examination revealed cholesteatoma of both middle ears and granulation tissue in the right middle ear.

Radiological studies showed underdeveloped mastoids, destruction of ossicles on both sides and an enlarged mastoid antrum on the left. He was admitted to the hospital for surgery and it was discovered that he had diabetes mellitus. A left radical mastoidectomy was performed and the operation sheet states as follows: "The epitympanum was lined by squamous epithelium which was open to the external auditory canal — the dura was exposed in one area and granulations were removed from it — care was taken not to endanger the lateral and superior semicircular canals — the facial nerve was identified and noted to be dehiscent — no ossicles were present — the entire middle ear was covered with

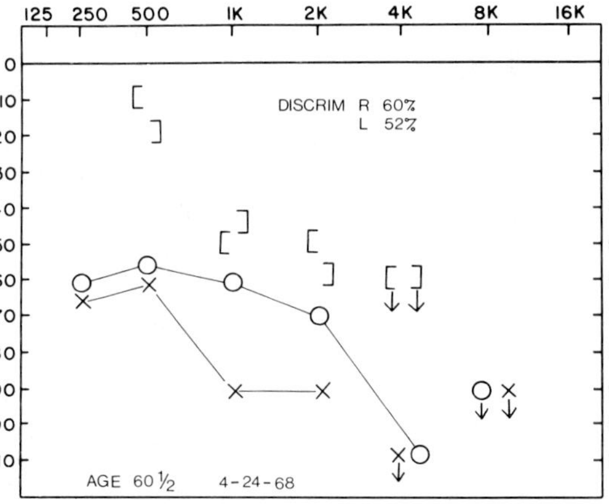

Fig. 15. (Case 8) Audiogram at age 60 showing a bilateral combined sensorineural and conductive hearing loss characterized by descending threshold patterns.

squamous epithelium which was carefully elevated from the promontory and round window — the posterior canal wall was removed to the level of the facial nerve — the patient withstood the procedure well and left the operating room in good condition." He was discharged from the hospital one week later and the mastoid cavity was skin-grafted two weeks after surgery. There is no indication in the hospital record that he experienced vertigo in the immediate postoperative period.

At the age of 60 he again complained of vertigo; he stated that one hour after breakfast he became dizzy. He felt that things were moving back and forth and he became nauseated and vomited. Examination revealed no spontaneous nystagmus or ataxia. The left middle ear and mastoid cavity were clean and dry. The right tympanic membrane was totally missing and the middle ear was lined by skin which extended superiorly into the epitympanum; however there was no suppuration. Audiometry showed a bilateral combined sensorineural and conductive hearing loss, slightly worse on the left side. Bone conduction thresholds showed a descending threshold pattern. Discrimination was 60% on the right and 52% on the left (Fig. 15).

The patient stated that he felt as if his vision were blurred if he bent over and then stood up and things also seemed to appear double at times after this maneuver. He stated that at times he felt like he was walking on high ground or like wearing someone else's glasses. He stated that the dizziness is exactly the same sensation as when doctors probe his right ear.

An otoneurological consultation was acquired from Dr. A Weiss who reported as follows:

"The patient has had recurrent episodes of dizziness which he describes as a feeling of imbalance and feeling wobbly in the legs. Accompanying this is nausea and marked diaphoresis. This may last from a half hour to an hour after which he feels very tired. He has no tinnitus, change of hearing or fullness in the ears accompanying these attacks. He does not have diplopia. What he calls double vision is more accurately described as a blurring of vision in that there is no doubling of images. There are no other neurologic symptoms accompanying these spells. Examinations show full extraocular movements without nystagmus. The fistula test is negative bilaterally. Tandem walking, gait and turning tests are negative. Positional test shows a type III positional nystagmus. Cold air caloric tests with eyes open gave responses of 81 seconds on the right and 57 seconds on the left. The reduced response on the left is confirmed by a right directional preponderance on rotation tests. My impression is that the patient has vertigo on a labyrinthine basis probably associated with bilateral labyrinthine degeneration, perhaps of the type that is seen frequently with chronic middle ear disease. I see no neurologic basis for this complaint. I see no basis for assuming that this represents erosive disease, particularly since vestibular testing implicates the left rather than the right ear."

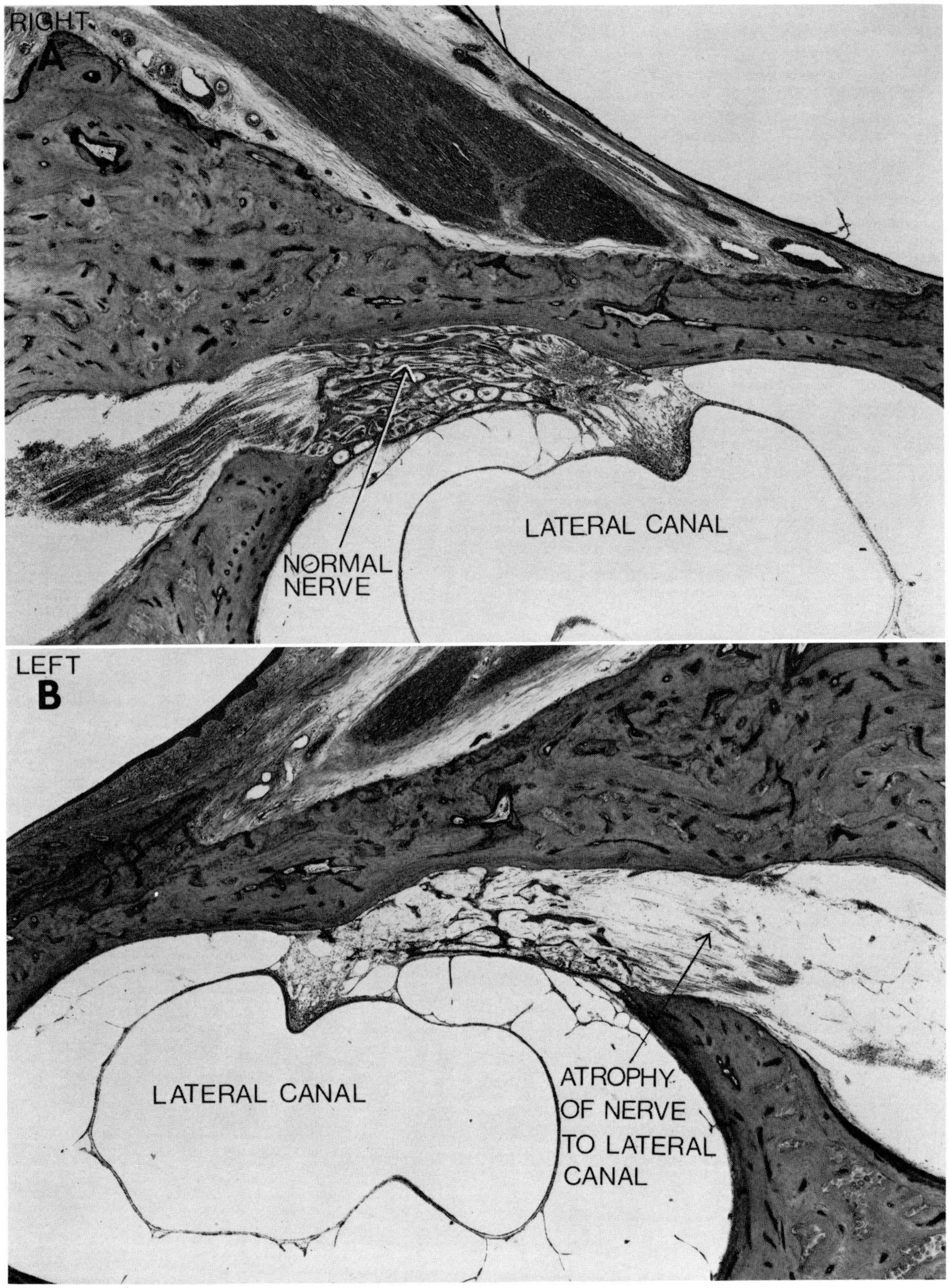

Fig. 16. (Case 8) A) Right ear. Lateral semicircular canal showing normal nerve and crista for comparison with left ear shown below. B) Left ear. Lateral semicircular canal showing severe atrophy of the nerve and partial atrophy of the crista.

Radiologic studies show an underdeveloped right mastoid with destruction of ossicles and a normal appearing lateral semicircular canal, unchanged from the examination of five years previously, and a normal appearing left radical mastoid cavity.

One of us (HFS) concurred with the impression of Dr. Weiss and recommended that no surgery be performed on the right ear but that it should be cleaned frequently. Subsequently he developed an itching discharge from the left ear which was treated with antifungal agents and frequent cleaning with some success.

At the age of 68 he complained again of unsteadiness and mild nausea. His blood sugar was controlled with diet and small dosages of insulin. He was wearing a hearing aid in his right ear. At age 69, he complained of dizziness, sweating and vomiting which subsided in a few days.

At the age of 70 he suffered a cerebrovascular accident with left hemiparesis and aphasia. Otologic examination revealed a purulent discharge from the right ear with granulations in the attic region and an epithelialized middle ear. On the left side there was keratin debris in the middle ear and mastoid. A right brachial angiogram revealed delayed flow through the superior division of the right middle cerebral artery with an associated intraluminal defect. The findings were considered compatible with embolus. Polytomographic reports were as follows: "On the right there is increased density of the external auditory canal, tympanic cavity, epitympanic recess and mastoid antrum. The scutum is eroded and ossicles are almost completely destroyed. The aditus and antrum is enlarged. The tegmen tympani is intact. There is adequate coverage of bone about the lateral aspect of the lateral semicircular canal and cochlea. There is a large bony cavity on the left due to radical mastoidectomy."

At the age of 71 he was admitted to the hospital because of severe chest pain. He was diagnosed as having an anterior myocardial infarction and died five days later. Both temporal bones were removed for histological study.

HISTOPATHOLOGY

RIGHT EAR. The external auditory canal is widened by erosion of its walls. Anteriorly there is a 5 mm defect of the bony wall near the annulus. Posteriorly there is an irregularity of the bony wall characterized by erosions which are filled with fibrous tissue. The tympanic fibrous annulus is visible, however, and pars tensa is missing. The malleus is missing. A remnant of the body of the incus is seen fibrosed to the lateral epitympanic wall and part of the short process remains in the fossa incudis. There are stumps of the crura of the stapes and the footplate is intact. The middle ear and epitympanum are lined by a layer of dense fibrous tissue, and surface of which is partly covered with squamous epithelium. Mucous membrane is seen in the protympanum and posterior mesotympanum. The protympanum is widely patent. The mastoid including the antrum and aditus are totally obliterated by fibrous tissue, bone, and scattered small cystic spaces.

There is moderate postmortem autolysis of the membranous labyrinth; however, all cell types can be readily identified. The hair cell population of the cochlea is normal throughout. The stria vascularis shows small areas of atrophy near the apex of the cochlea. There is a loss of about 50 to 80% of the neurons in the basal turn of the cochlea. The saccular macula, utricular macula and all cristae appear normal and the vestibular nerves appear normal (Fig. 16A). There are small tears of the membranous walls of the utricle and saccule. The facial nerve is intact, however, it is dehiscent of bone throughout a large part of its intratympanic segment.

LEFT EAR. There is a large surgically created mastoid bowl. The external auditory canal, middle ear and mastoid bowl are filled with the keratin-fungus mass and the entire area except for the anteroinferior mesotympanum is lined with epidermis which shows intense infiltration with inflammatory cells, ulceration and collection of pus cells beneath the overlying debris. There is severe erosion of the anterior wall of the external auditory canal with total dehiscence of bone anteroinferiorly. There is resorption osteitis of the lateral cochlear wall and a small bony fistula of the promontory. The adjacent spiral ligament shows an intense infiltrate of inflammatory cells and there is total atrophy of the organ of Corti in this region of the basal turn. There is a thick fibrous membrane bridging and blocking the mouth of the eustachian tube. The round window niche is obliterated with fibrous tissue and cystic spaces. There is partial erosion of the footplate of the stapes but no invasion of the vestibule. There is a surgical lesion of the wall of the lateral semicircular canal with fragments of bone slightly depressed into the canal lumen. There is mild surrounding fibrosis without evidence of fistulization (Fig. 17A).

The organ of Corti is degenerated in the basal 10 mm of the cochlea. There is moderately severe postmortem autolysis of the membranous labyrinth, however, all cell types can be identified. There is a loss of 50 to 80% of the cochlear neurons in the basal turn. The utricular macula and its nerve are normal. The saccular macula and nerve are normal. There is a partial loss of hair cells in the crista of the lateral semicircular canal. The neurons (cell bodies and fibers) to the crista of the lateral semicircular canal are severely atrophied (Figs. 16B, left ear, and 17B, left ear). The anterior vestibular artery and its branches appear patent and histologically similar to the same vessel in the opposite ear. The crista as well as the nerve fibers to the superior canal appear normal. The posterior canal crista and its nerve appear normal. The facial nerve is dehiscent of bone throughout a large part of its intratympanic segment.

Comment. This patient had bilateral otitis media beginning in childhood which continued in chronic form throughout his adult lifetime. At age 55 he complained of having had three recent episodes of severe vertigo with nausea and vomiting. A radical mastoidectomy was performed in the left ear. At this time he was found to have diabetes mellitus which was successfully treated with insulin and diet. Throughout the remainder of his life he had numerous visits to the ear, nose, and throat clinic for cleaning of his ears. On many occasions he complained of having episodes of mild dysequilibrium, sometimes with nausea.

Audiometry on several occasions revealed a combined sensorineural and conductive hearing loss, worse on the left, and 50 to 60% speech discrimination scores. Fistula tests were consistently negative. Cold air caloric tests showed responses in both ears but somewhat diminished in the left ear.

Histological studies reveal atrophy of the nerve to the crista of the lateral semicircular canal of the left ear. The episodic vertigo is most logically attributed to this lesion. The question is whether this lesion is related to the chronic infection, the surgical insult to the lateral semicircular canal or to an unrelated

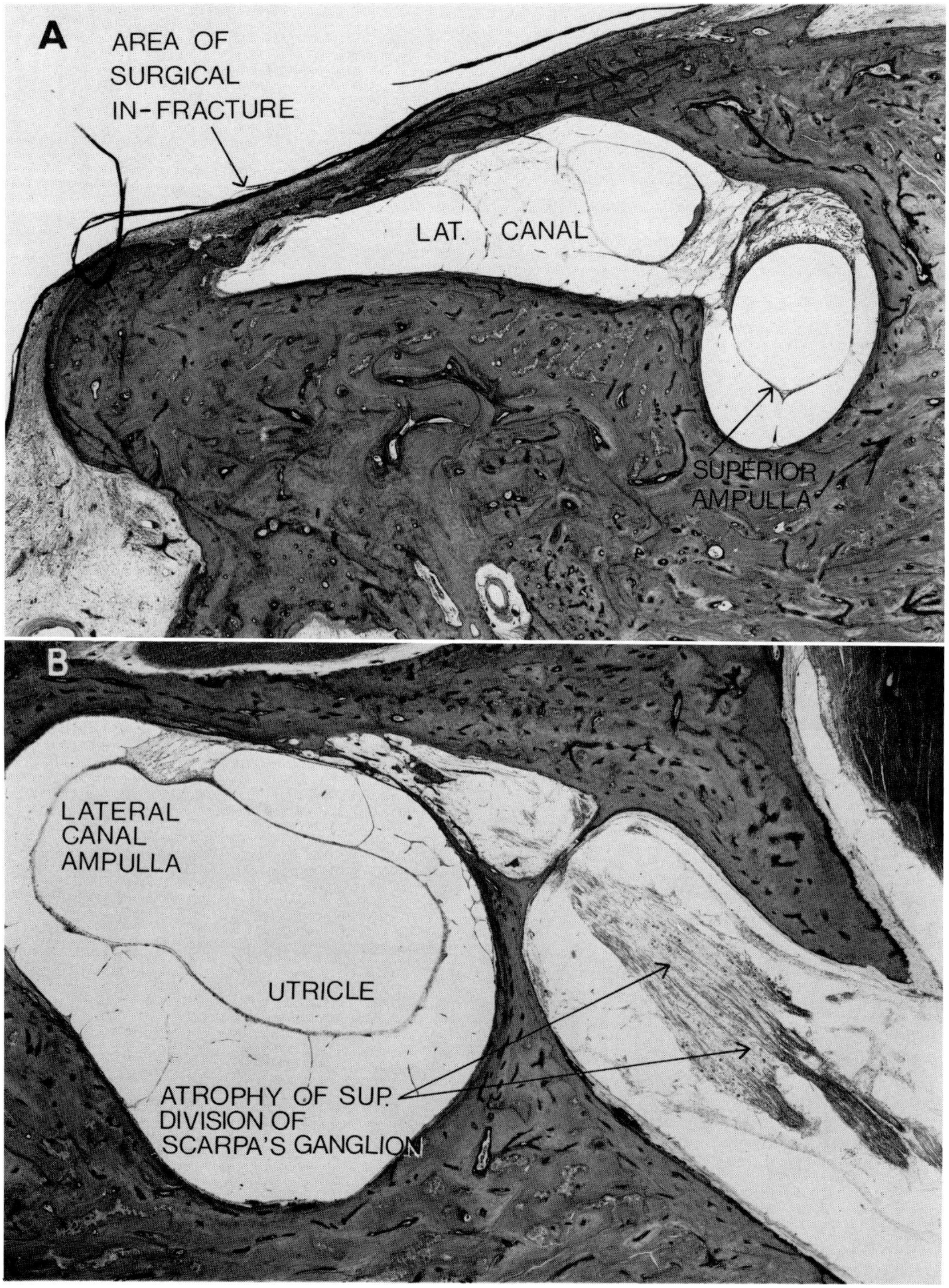

Fig. 17. (Case 8) A) Left ear lateral semicircular canal showing slightly depressed fracture caused by surgery. B) Left ear. View showing severe loss of neurons in the superior division of the vestibular nerve and atrophy of the ampullary branch of the lateral crista.

disorder of the nerve trunk. The most reasonable explanation would seem to be vestibular neuritis, unrelated to the infection or the surgical procedure. There is no histological evidence of encroachment of the infectious inflammatory otitis on the sensory or neural structures of the lateral semicircular canal. The iatrogenic infracture of the bony wall of the lateral semicircular canal is an improbable cause for the nerve atrophy for several reasons: 1) the vertigo began before the surgery was performed, 2) there was no vertigo immediately following surgery indicating minimal vestibular insult, 3) the sense organ (crista) shows only slight atrophic change which would mitigate against "secondary" neural degeneration, and 4) both animal and human temporal bone studies show that surgi-

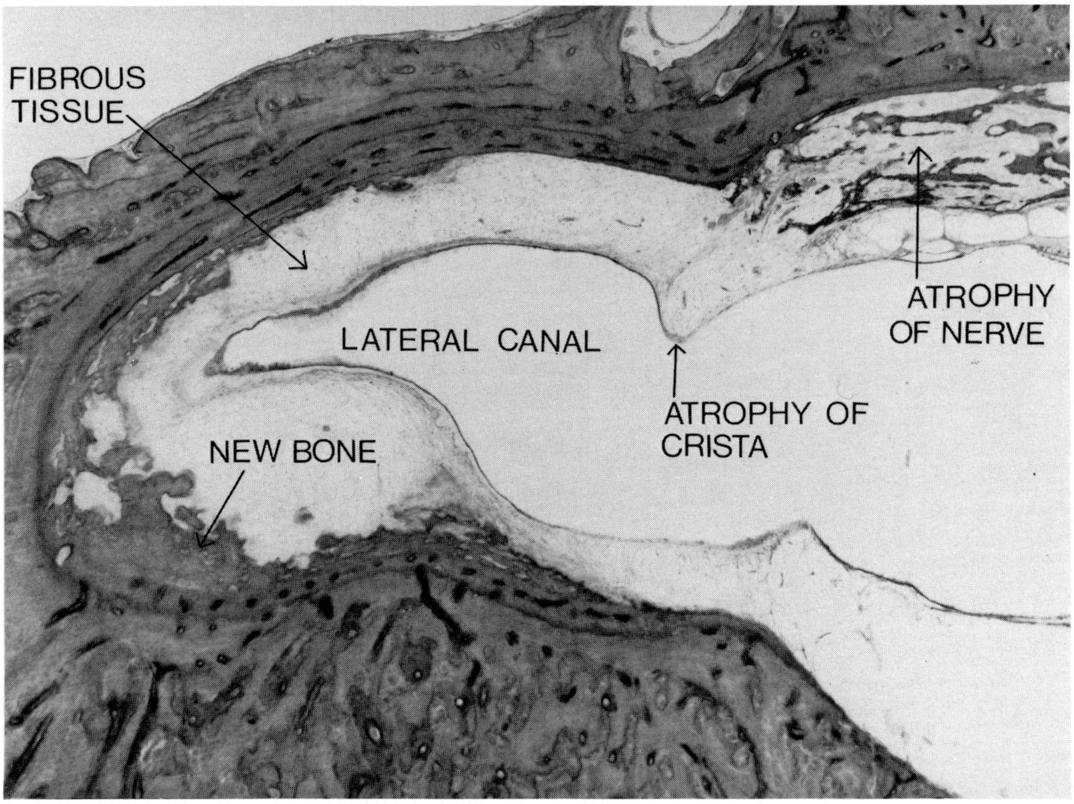

Fig. 18. Case of herpes zoster oticus. (Bone processed by Temporal Bone Laboratory of the University of Chicago) Case published by Zajtchuk et al[11] and republished with their permission. There is atrophy of ampullary branch of the superior division of the vestibular nerve and the lateral canal crista of the left ear. There is fibrous tissue in the perilymphatic space similar to our case 6, Fig. 11 A.

cal fistulization of the bony semicircular canal does not cause neural atrophy.

DISCUSSION

The medical histories and histopathological findings of cases 5, 6 and 8 are remarkably similar. All had protracted dysequilibrium during the latter years of life, one for 21 years (case 5) another for 11 years (case 6) and the third for 13 years (case 8). All three subjects had one or more episodes of vertigo which were sufficiently severe to induce nausea and vomiting, although the duration of dysequilibrium related to these attacks was of short duration. All subjects had protracted periods of lesser dysequilibrium either before or after the single attacks. The histories suggest prolonged active phases of their diseases rather than single insults. All three subjects had decreased cold caloric responses in one ear, and histopathological studies show that each of these ears have total atrophy of a branch of the vestibular nerve: the superior division in case 5, the ampullary branch in case 6, and the branch to the lateral canal only in case 8. The associated sense organs are normal in case 5, severely atrophied in case 6 and partially atrophied in case 8.

The patient in case 7 who had mild diabetes mellitus, experienced three discrete severe episodes of vertigo at ages 67, 69, and 85. She also had recurring neuropathies of the third and seventh cranial nerves. Histopathological studies of the temporal bones show a partial loss of peripheral vestibular neurons in both ears, most severe in the superior divisions in association with normal vestibular sense organs.

We believe the etiology for the isolated atrophy of the vestibular nerves in these cases is viral infection rather than vascular occlusion for the following reasons:

1. Histological studies of the temporal bones of these four cases show no evidence of occlusive vascular lesions. The arterial branches of the anterior and posterior vestibular arteries which accompany the vestibular nerves to the sense organs appear patent.
2. Laboratory studies have shown the improbability of vascular spasm as a cause for vestibular symptoms. It has been shown that neither section of the sympathetic trunk at the stellate ganglion, cervical trunks, or nerves accompanying the vertebral, basilar or anterior inferior cerebellar artery has any visible effect on blood flow in the stria vascularis.[29] Similarly the intravenous injection of pressor agents (adrenaline, noradrenaline) fails to alter the caliber of the strial vessels although there is an increase in blood flow which parallels the increase in carotid blood pressure.[30,31] The arterial supply to the inner

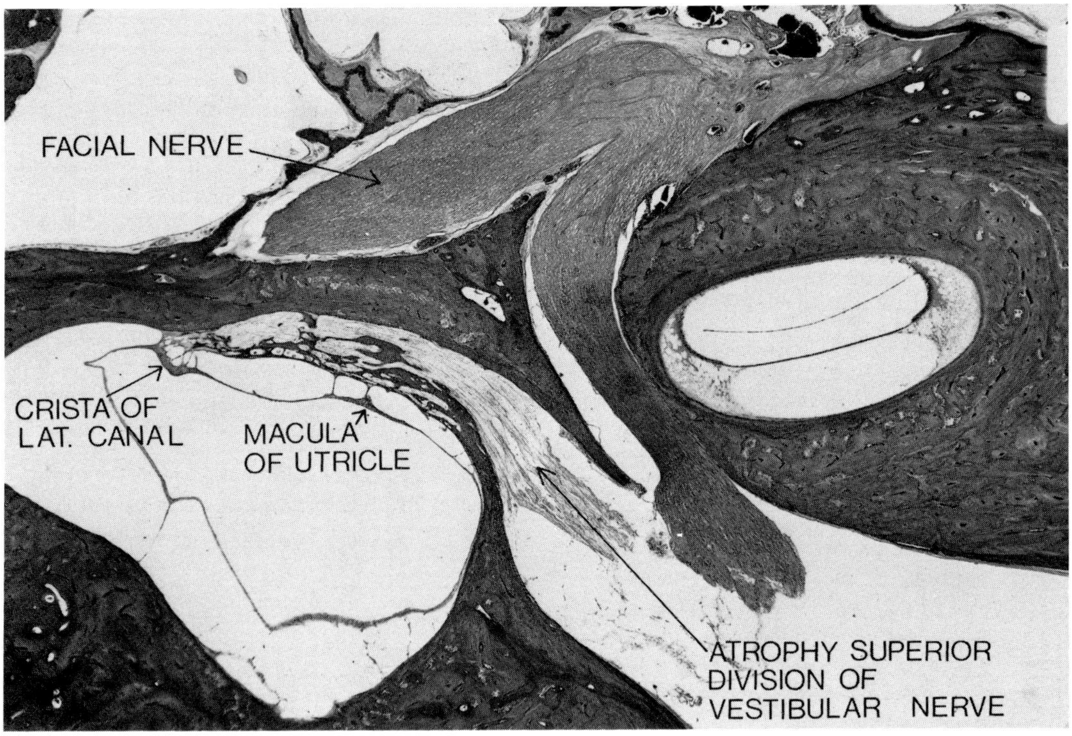

Fig. 19. Case of sudden severe prolonged vertigo. Published by Lindsay and Hemenway[27] and republished with their permission. There is atrophy of the superior division of the vestibular nerve and associated sense organs (utricular macula and superior and lateral canal cristae).

ear, like that to the brain, is not subject to wide fluctuations in flow for very obvious physiological reasons. Stated simply, there are no conditions in which the organism can allow permutation of the oxygen supply to its CNS; therefore vasomotor control of the cerebral vessels (and labyrinthine vessels) is minimal.

3. The pathological findings in cases 5, 6, and 8 are similar to those described and illustrated by Zajtchuk et al[11] in a case of herpes zoster oticus. This patient developed cervical Hodgkin's disease at age 25 years for which she received 4,000 rads of radiotherapy. Nine years later she received 2,300 rads to the abdomen for an enlarged liver and spleen, and during the course of therapy developed herpes simplex infection of the lip. Soon thereafter she noted mild vertigo and a vesicular eruption on the left auricle. Two days later she experienced the onset of severe vertigo with nausea and vomiting. There was spontaneous nystagmus to the right, and normal hearing by auditory tests in both ears. One week later vestibular examination showed a continuing spontaneous nystagmus to the right and no response to ice water caloric in the left ear. Vertigo gradually subsided and she left the hospital 16 days after the onset of vertigo. Two months later she appeared to be totally recovered. She died 21 months after the attack of herpes zoster oticus. Histological study of the temporal bones revealed severe degeneration of the ampullary branch of the superior vestibular nerve and atrophy of the crista of the lateral semicircular canal of the left ear. There was fibrous tissue and new bone in the perilymphatic space surrounding the ampulla of the lateral canal. All other structures were normal (Fig. 18).

A paper by Lindsay and Hemenway[27] is of special interest. They described a symptom complex, occurring in nine patients, most of whom were in the latter years of life, who experienced the sudden onset of severe vertigo with nausea and vomiting without evidence of involvement of the auditory organs or CNS. The vertigo gradually subsided over a period of weeks as would be consistent with an acute destructive insult to the vestibular system. A further manifestation of the syndrome was the development of positional vertigo several weeks following the original attacks of vertigo and persisting for weeks or years. Schuknecht,[32-34] has previously suggested that the positional vertigo in these cases might be caused by the implantation on the cupula of the posterior semicircular canal of otoconia released from a degenerating utricular macula. Lindsay and Hemenway acquired the temporal bones of a patient with this syndrome (acute attacks of vertigo followed by positional vertigo) and found severe atrophy of the superior division of the vestibular nerve and associated sense organs (utricular macula and cristae of the lateral and superior canals) in one ear (Fig. 19). They attributed the disorder to occlusion of the vessel that supplies the labyrinth but made no mention of the histological appearance of the arteries. In a previous report of our case 6, we had also attributed the atrophic changes to probable vascular occlusion; however, further study shows all vessels to be patent and intact. Thus it seems possible that the cases described by Lindsay and Hemenway[27] are of viral rather than vascular etiology.

DIFFERENTIAL DIAGNOSIS

The following disorders must be considered in the differential diagnosis of vestibular neuritis:

Menière's Disease. Menière's disease is characterized histologically to be endolymphatic hydrops and usually can be differentiated from vestibular neuritis by the presence of the characteristic hearing loss. However, when Menière's disease presents only the vestibular symptoms, as may occur early in the course of the disease, it may be confused with vestibular neuritis. The differentiation can usually be made on the following bases: a) Frequent and numerous episodes of vertigo are characteristic of Menière's disease, while vestibular neuritis more often presents as one episode or as several episodes occurring over a period of months or years. b) The vertiginous attacks in Menière's disease are of limited duration, often no longer than three or four hours, after which the patient usually feels well, while in vestibular neuritis the acute episode may persist for a period of days. c) Early in the course of Menière's disease the caloric response may be normal, while in vestibular neuritis it is frequently reduced or absent. d) A positive Hennebert's sign (fistula test) is indicative of vestibular fibrosis and when it occurs, is diagnostic for endolymphatic hydrops, thus favoring the diagnosis of Menière's disease.

Vestibular Schwannoma. Vertigo caused by an expanding mass in the internal auditory canal or cerebellopontine angle, such as vestibular schwannoma, may stimulate vestibular neuritis. The differentiation can usually be made on the following bases: a) The vestibular schwannoma usually causes a hearing loss which of course does not occur with vestibular neuritis. b) A single severe attack of vertigo or recurring severe attacks over a period of months or years as commonly seen in vestibular neuritis is unusual for vestibular schwannoma. c) Signs of involvement of the fifth and seventh cranial nerves (abnormalities in corneal sensitivity, taste, stapedial muscle reflex, blink reflex, etc) are common with vestibular schwannoma but absent in vestibular neuritis.

In some cases it will be necessaary to perform CT scan and polytomography, and possibly posterior fossa myelography to assist in the differentiation of these disorders.

Fenestral Fistula. While the frequency of occurrence of spontaneous fistulae of the oval and round windows is probably exaggerated in the current literature, these do occur and must be considered in the differential diagnosis. The following features will usually serve to differentiate a fenestral fistula from vestibular neuritis: a) With the fenestral fistula there is often a history of a precipitating incident (sudden changes in air pressure as in air flight, scuba diving, and nose blowing, straining, head blow or blast in air, stapes surgery). b) Positional vertigo and a positive fistula test often occur with a fenestral fistula, possibly caused by an air bubble in the labyrinth. c) Hearing loss, often fluctuating, is common in the presence of a fenestral fistula but absent in vestibular neuritis. d) The caloric response is usually normal with fenestral fistula and usually diminished or absent in vestibular neuritis.

Cerebellar Infarction. A small cerebellar infarct may present symptomatically as a sudden severe attack of vertigo with nausea and vomiting.[35] When it occurs without hearing loss or other neurological symptoms, it can mimic the single-attack type of vestibular neuritis. Predisposing factors for cerebellar infarction appear to be hypertension, arteriosclerotic cardiovascular disease, estrogen replacement therapy and blood dyscrasias. The infarction may be characterized by either occlusion or hemorrhage of a branch of either the anterior-inferior or posterior-inferior cerebellar arteries. Such a lesion may cause compression or destruction of part of the vestibular nuclei and/or vestibular connections in the cerebellum (flocculus, nodulus, uvula). Computed tomography is the most sensitive method of detecting cerebellar infarction. Nonhemorrhage infarcts appear as low density areas and hemorrhage infarcts as high density areas.

For neuroanatomical reasons it seems highly improbable that the isolated peripheral vestibular nerve degenerations occurring in our cases 5 -8 were caused by cerebellar infarctions. A lesion involving any of the vestibular nuclei, were it to cause anterograde degeneration of vestibular nerve fibers, would necessarily involve segments of both superior and inferior divisions of the vestibular nerve.

Multiple Sclerosis. In unusual cases vertigo can occur as the initial symptom of multiple sclerosis. It may present as acute severe vertigo or protracted unsteadiness. All signs may be identical to vestibular neuritis, including nystagmus, diminished caloric response and normal hearing. Onset after the age of 40 rules out multiple sclerosis. In rare cases it may be impossible to differentiate multiple sclerosis from vestibular neuritis until further CNS involvement becomes evident.

Dysequilibrium of Aging. The dysequilibrium of aging[34] is caused by degenerative changes in the peripheral vestibular labyrinth which interfere with the motion mechanics of the sense organs. The symptoms consist of momentary or prolonged unsteadiness following stimulation of the vestibular system such as occurs with sudden head movements (turning, stooping, rolling over in bed, rising from the bed, etc).

SUMMARY

The histopathological evidence in the temporal bones of four subjects who had prolonged symptoms of vertigo, as well as our clinical experience and literature review, supports the existence of a discrete degenerative neuropathy of the vestibular nerve. The characteristic features are severe vertigo without hearing loss, accompanied by objective evidence of vestibular abnormality (nystagmus, diminished or absent caloric response). The vertigo may occur as a single severe prolonged episode or as recurring severe episodes, either of which may be associated with milder periodic or constant unsteadiness. One or both ears may be involved either concurrently or sequentially.

The pathological correlate as determined by temporal bone studies is atrophy of one or more vestibular nerve trunks, with or without their associated sense organs. Because the disorder usually occurs as an isolated neuropathy, sometimes in the presence of an upper respiratory infection, and because of its pathological similarity to a reported case of herpes zoster oticus, we suspect a viral etiology and recommend that it be known by the term vestibular neuritis.

The differential diagnosis includes Menière's disease, vestibular schwannoma, fenestral fistula, cerebellar infarction, multiple sclerosis, and dysequilibrium of aging.

REFERENCES

1. Ruttin B. Zur Differentialdiagnose der Labyrinth-u. Hornerverkrankungen Z Ohrenheilkd 1909; 57:327-31.

2. Nylen C. Some cases of ocular nystagmus due to certain positions of the head. Acta Otolaryngol (Stockh) 1924; 6:106-123.

3. Hallpike C. The pathology and differential diagnosis of aural vertigo. London: 4th International Congress on Otolaryngology 1949; 2:514.

4. Dix M, Hallpike C. The pathology, symptomatology and diagnosis of certain common disorders of the vestibular system. Ann Otol Rhinol Laryngol 1952; 61:987-1016.

5. Harrison M. Epidemic vertigo-vestibular neuronitis, a clinical study. Brain 1962; 85:613-20.

6. Aschan G, Stahle J. Vestibular neuritis. J Laryngol Otol 1956; 70:497-511.

7. Cawthorne T. Otological aspects in the differential diagnosis of vertigo. In: Fields W, Alford B, eds. Neurological aspects of auditory and vestibular disorders. Springfield: Charles C. Thomas, 1964:271-82.

8. Hart C. Vestibular paralysis of sudden onset and probably viral etiology. Ann Otol Rhinol Laryngol 1965; 74:33-47.

9. Coates A. Vestibular neuronitis. Trans Am Acad Ophthalmol Otolaryngol 1969; 73:395-408.

10. Meran A, Pfaltz C. Der akute vestibulcrisausfall. Arch Otorhinolaryngol (NY) 1975; 209:229-44.

11. Zajtchuk J, Matz G, Lindsay J. Temporal bone pathology in herpes oticus. Ann Otol Rhinol Laryngol 1972; 81:331-8.

12. Charters A. Epidemic vertigo in Kenya. E African Med J 1957; 34:7-14.

13. Pedersen E. Epidemic vertigo. Clinical picture and relations to encephalitis. Brain 1959; 82:566-80.

14. Pedersen E. Epidemic vertigo in Denmark. World Neurol 1961; 2:212.

15. Merfield D. Self-limited idiopathic vertigo (epidemic vertigo). Arch Otolaryngol 1965; 81:355-8.

16. Meulengracht E. Correspondence. Br Med J 1950; 2:1493.

17. Burrowes W. Acute labyrinthitis. Br Med J 1952a; 2:408.

18. Burrowes W. Acute labyrinthitis. Br Med J 1952b; 2:1182-3.

19. Pfaltz C. Diagnose und Therapie der vestibularen Neuronitis. Pract Otorhinolaryngol 1955; 17:454-61.

20. Kattum F, Mundnich K. Kristische Betrachtungen zur Neuritis vestibularis (Hallpike). Z Hals-Nas-Ohrenheilkd 1957; 6:232.

21. Stahle J. Vestibular neuritis. In: Wolfson RJ, ed. Vestibular system and its diseases. Philadelphia: University of Pennsylvania Press, 1966:459-70.

22. Walford P. Editorial comment. Lancet 1952; 1:415.

23. Worster-Drought C. Editorial comment. Lancet 1952; 1:371-2.

24. Walford P. Correspondence. Br Med J 1949; 1:821-2.

25. Herberts G. Post-infections meningo-encephalitis as etiological factor in certain cases of vertigo. Acta Otolaryngol (Stockh) 1954; 118:109-13.

26. Dalsgaard-Nielsen T. Further clinical studies on epidemic vertigo, nevroxite vertig ineuse. Acta Psychiatr Neurol 1953; 28:263-7.

27. Lindsay J. Hemenway W. Postural vertigo due to unilateral sudden partial loss of vestibular function. Ann Otol Rhinol Laryngol 1956; 65:692-706.

28. Naufal P, Schuknecht H. Vestibular facial and oculomotor neuropathy in diabetes mellitus. Arch Otolaryngol 1972; 96:468-74.

29. Perlman H, Kimura R. Observations of the living blood of the cochlea. Ann Otol Rhinol Laryngol 1955; 64:1176-92.

30. Nomura Y. Observations on the microcirculation of the cochlea. Ann Otol Rhinol Laryngol 1962; 70:1037-54.

31. Perlman H, Tsunoo M, Spence A. Cochlear blood flow and function: effect of pressor agents. Acta Otolaryngol (Stockh) 1963; 56:587-98.

32. Schuknecht H. Positional vertigo: clinical and experimental observations. Trans Am Acad Ophthalmol Otolaryngol 1962; 66:319-32.

33. Schuknecht H. Cupulolithiasis. Arch Otolaryngol 1969; 90:765-8.

34. Schuknecht H. Pathology of the ear. Cambridge: Harvard University Press, 1974.

35. Rubenstein R, Norman D, Schindler R, Kaseff L. Cerebellar infarction — a presentation of vertigo. Laryngoscope 1980; 90:505-14.

MEASUREMENT OF OPTOKINETIC NYSTAGMUS FOR OTONEUROLOGICAL DIAGNOSIS

SHARON M. ABEL, PhD HUGH O. BARBER, MD, FRCS(C)

TORONTO, ONTARIO, CANADA

Optokinetic nystagmus was recorded and measured in 101 subjects comprising six diagnostic categories: 1) normal, screened for otologic disease, 2) chronic unilateral labyrinthectomy, 3) unilateral Menière's disease, 4) neurologically confirmed focal brainstem lesion, 5) brainstem-cerebellar syndrome, and 6) focal unilateral supratentorial lesion. For the OKN test, each subject looked at a translucent screen onto which a field of parallel black and white bars was back-projected. The array of bars could be projected vertically or horizontally to allow for study of nystagmus beating right and left or up and down. The speed of movement of the bars varied over a range from 20 to 140°/sec of visual angle, in each axis for both directions.

An analysis of the slow phase velocity of OKN indicated that patients with brainstem disease produced significantly lower eye speeds than did normal subjects or patients with chronic peripheral vestibular disease. The latter groups could not be distinguished. The responses of patients with cortical lesions fell midway between these two extremes and were significantly different from those of the brainstem group. Directional preponderance of nystagmus proved to be significantly related to the side of lesion for both the labyrinthine and cortical groups. However, the absolute value of the difference in slow phase velocity for nystagmus beating toward or away from the side of lesion was no greater than the difference between right and left-beating nystagmus in normal subjects. While the results provide statistical confirmation for the findings of earlier investigations, it is noted that for purposes of clinical diagnosis, the test is of value only in the context of the otoneurological test battery. Distribution of results for individuals in the various groups overlap considerably. The designation of a numerical cutoff for differential diagnosis leads to error rates far in excess of what may be confidently attributed to chance.

Observation of optokinetic nystagmus (OKN) has been included in both neuro-opthalmologic and otoneurologic examinations for the past 50 years.[1-3] The response has been used to assess higher cortical function, as well as the integrity of a variety of systems, including the peripheral and central oculomotor and vestibular pathways; abnormalities have been reported in the presence of lesions throughout the brain.[4]

The examination is easily performed. One method is to use a small drum, about 30.5 cm in diameter, with alternating black and white stripes, which is held about 46 cm in front of the patient's eyes and slowly rotated. In place of the drum, many clinicians use a tape consisting of a series of colored patches sewn on a strip of white cloth. The strip is moved slowly to the right or left, up or down. The patient is instructed to gaze straight ahead at the stripes (or visual targets) without deliberate fixation. Typically, if the targets move continuously from left to right, the eyes will alternately move slowly to the right and quickly return to the midline position. The speed of the slow phase is generally related to the speed of movement of the targets, increasing to about 50°/sec for a target speed of 80°, and then slowly decreasing as adjacent targets begin to fuse.[5-9]

The eye movement may be evaluated using qualitative description. For example, Smith[10] rates the response on a categorical scale from brisk to nil. Alternately one may use the techniques of electronystagmography.[8,9,11] The former method is entirely subjective and relies wholly on the impression of the examiner. The latter method gives an objective analogue representation of the eye movements on a polygraph recorder. The response appears as a triangular wave for each cycle of nystagmus (slow plus quick phase). The slope of the slow component gives the velocity of movement of the eyes in relation to the movement of the targets. One may also calculate the frequency of the response, ie, the number of beats (quick phases) per second, and the amplitude of response, ie, the maximum excursion of the eyes from the midline position.

SYNOPSIS OF THEORY OF CLINICAL FINDINGS

Several proposals have been made to describe the neurologic pathways subserving optokinetic nystagmus. The most widely popularized views are those of Cords[3] and Ling and Gay.[12]

Cords' hypothesis,[3] published in 1926, has been well described by Carmichael et al.[13] Briefly, the theory states that for targets moving from left to right, impulses from the right halves of the two retinae are projected to an optomotor center in the right peristriate cortex. Way stations include the right external geniculate body, optic radiation and visual cortex. For the efferent leg of the reflex, fibers from the peristriate area join the posterior part of the optic radiation and move forward, leaving the optic radiation at its anterior third to join the cerebral peduncle. From here fibers cross the midline to the posterior longitudinal bundle on the opposite side and go to the center for conjugate gaze in the pons.

From the Departments of Otolaryngology at Sunnybrook Medical Centre and the University of Toronto. This research was supported by grant No. MA-5209 from the Medical Research Council of Canada.

Cords' system predicts that a lesion anywhere along the path from the optomotor center in the cortex to the pontine gaze center will result in the abolition of OKN beating left. If the lesion occurs in that part of the path associated with optic radiation, then the added feature of homonymous hemianopia will appear. This syndrome of unilateral OKN deficit together with field blindness should be evident primarily in cases of deep parietal lesions. On the other hand, lesions involving the optic tracts, lateral geniculate body, temporal or occipital lobes might produce hemianopia but OKN should be brisk bilaterally.

Evidence in support of Cords' hypothesis has been given by Smith[10] and Cogan and Loeb.[14] Smith describes the findings of Kestenbaum[15] for a series of 59 cases of homonymous hemianopia. The data, based on visual inspection of the eyes by the examiner, indicate that in 28 instances of a positive optokinetic sign (ie, clear asymmetry in horizontal OKN) 10 were associated with lesions close to and 17 within the parietal region. For 24 instances of negative optokinetic sign, (ie, brisk response bilaterally) there were 10 patients with lesions distant from, and 5 with lesions close to the parietal region.

Smith's own observation of OKN in 100 patients with homonymous hemianopia are also reported in his monograph. Again the response was elicited using a strip of cloth and described on a four-point rating scale. An asymmetry in response, right-beating versus left-beating, was observed in 28 of 33 cases of parietal lesion. In the presence of a temporal lobe lesion, either proven or judged clinically, 19 of 24 patients showed negative OKN signs. For 39 occipital lobe lesions the OKN sign was negative in 31 instances, positive in 7, and absent in 1. In the presence of an occipital field defect, a negative OKN sign usually signified a vascular lesion, whereas a positive OKN sign was associated with a mass lesion (Cogan's Rule). Details of this research and autopsy study are given in Smith[16] and Smith and Cogan.[17,18]

Cords' predictions appear to be supported. Smith emphasizes that the hypothesis applies specifically to cerebral lesions and not to brainstem disease. He notes that in cases of brainstem involvement there may be a generalized depression or total absence of OKN. The latter finding may also be due to sedation or low vision.

Evidence against Cords' hypothesis has also been reported. Davidoff et al[19] studied OKN for a variety of cerebral lesions in a series of 37 patients. Each patient was placed for testing inside a rotating drum 91 cm in diameter and 61 cm in height. Normal OKN was defined as regular, rhythmical, symmetrical, well-sustained nystagmus with readily identifiable quick and slow components for both directions of the drum. An attempt was made to correlate the site of major brain damage and defects in horizontal OKN, although as the authors point out, strict anatomic correlation is often precluded by the multiplicity of lesions and extent of involvement. Other parts of the brain may be implicated by the pathological process.

The results showed that of the patients with abnormal OKN, 13 had tumors limited to cortex and underlying white matter of cerebral hemisphere. The OKN was "defective" when the drum was rotated toward the side of the lesion. Three patients had predominantly frontal lobe lesions, two temporal and four parieto-occipital lesions. The rest had lesions involving more than one lobe. Normal responses were found in patients with extensive lesions in the parietal lobe, hypothalamus, the lateral and anterior parts of the brainstem, and in patients with unilateral, bilateral, or diffuse lesions. Thus, the conclusion reached by the authors was that no correlation was possible between any specific type of optokinetic dysfunction and pathology involving any specific anatomic area. However, the claim was made that the test had use in lesion lateralization. The authors stated that, "In general, the more massive the disturbance in motor, somato-sensory and visual function, the more probable a defect in optokinetic nystagmus would be elicited."[19] This was especially true if a decrease in the state of alertness was also present. The results showed that normal OKN bilaterally was observed in cases of severe visual field deficit. Patients with gaze palsy showed defective OKN when the direction of defective gaze movement and direction of defective optokinetic response coincided.

A second major theory, not widely popularized, is that there are two centers for OKN, one in the frontal lobe and the second in the occipital lobe.[20] Recently, Ling and Gay[12] have attempted an expansion of this view. According to these investigators, any proposal for an OKN pathway must take into account the following facts:

1. The afferent limb of OKN is the same as that for visual afferents. Only one occipital lobe is required; thus, unilateral occipital lesions do not affect OKN.

2. The slow phase of OKN is mediated through the optomotor field of the occipital lobe. The mechanism is the same as that for ocular pursuit; the efferent path leads directly from the occipital lobe to the brainstem.

3. The fast phase depends on frontal lobe activity. The assumption is made that the pathway from frontal lobe to brainstem nuclei is identical to that for the fast phase of vestibular nystagmus and voluntary gaze.

4. Most patients with asymmetric OKN due to cerebral lesions have involvement deep in the parietal lobe. The abnormality is seen as a loss of the fast phase to the side opposite the lesion.

These facts suggest the following mechanisms:

> "Afferent impulses for the optokinetic reflex travel the visual pathway to the occipital lobe. This initiates the slow phase of the reflex, causing the eyes to deviate conjugately to the side toward which the target is moving. The efferent impulses for the slow phase travel directly to the brainstem from the occipital lobe. At the completion of the slow phase, the frontal lobe on the side toward which the eyes are deviated initiates the fast corrective phase of the reflex. This frontal lobe is activated by impulses from both the ipsilateral, and by way of the corpus callosum, the contralateral occipital lobe. The impulses from the frontal lobes in optokinetic nystagmus travel to the brainstem in the same pathway as the impulses for voluntary gaze and the fast phase of vestibular nystagmus."[21]

Thus, if optokinetic targets move from the patient's left to right, the left occipital lobe will be activated and cause the eyes to deviate right. The right frontal lobe will then initiate the fast phase left to bring the eyes back to midline. Impulses travel from both occipital lobes to the frontal lobe via a pathway deep in the parietal lobe. There is anatomical evidence for such a pathway.[22] The predictions that follow and receive support are that:

1. For unilateral occipital lesions OKN will be normal. In cases of bilateral occipital lesions, OKN will be normal so long as some vision remains.

2. For both deep parietal lobe and diffuse frontal lobe lesions, OKN will be impaired to the side opposite the lesion. Lesions anywhere along the frontomesencephalic pathway from the frontal lobe to the brainstem may produce a deficit of the fast phase to the opposite side.

SUPPORT FROM ANIMAL RESEARCH

Detailed, scholarly discussion of the vestibular and oculomotor pathways in animal models are presented in Bender,[23] and Bach-Y-Rita et al.[24] We will not attempt a review of the literature in this section but will describe briefly a few investigations illustrating the effects of central lesions on OKN.

The role of both the cortex and thalamus on the integrity of OKN has been demonstrated by Neverov et al.[25] These investigators used the technique of spreading depression through microinjection of drugs into the parietal cortex or superior colliculus to blockade the functions of these structures during OKN or after-nystagmus. The subjects were eight rabbits placed securely in the center of an OKN drum (80 cm high by 140 cm in diameter) for testing. OKN was elicited during clockwise rotation of the drum at six revolutions per minute for 90 minutes. Frequency of OKN was markedly decreased by spreading depression in either the right hemisphere or right superior colliculus. By contrast, reduction in the activity of the left hemisphere or thalamus affected after-nystagmus.

Cohen[26] has shown the importance of the paramedian zone of the pontine reticular formation (PPRF) for normal OKN. Electrolytic lesions to the right PPRF resulted in changes in right-beating OKN. The quick phase was of relatively small amplitude, high frequency and low maximum velocity. There was a strong tonic deviation of the eyes to the left.

TABLE 1. DISTRIBUTION OF SUPRATENTORIAL LESIONS

Type	*No.*
Frontal mass lesion	3
Frontal-parietal mass lesion	2
Parietal infarction	5
Middle cerebral artery occlusion	5
Parietal-occipital infarction	2
Occipital pole infarction	1
Occipital mass lesion	1
Temporal mass lesion	4
Pontine infarction	1
Total	24

PRESENT INVESTIGATIONS

Rationale. While evidence may exist to support correlations between theoretical prediction and observation of eye movements in patients with well-documented lesions, the strength of OKN as a test for clinical diagnosis is not clear. Specifically, given a unilateral deficit of OKN, one may question the extent to which the result distinguishes two clinical groups with different sites of lesion. The data published are usually qualitative in nature, and the judgement of abnormality depends on a subjective evaluation by the examiner. To some extent his decision will reflect his knowledge of the results of clinical tests administered concurrently, and his own theoretical bias.

An attempt to collect quantitative data for various clinical groups was made by Morissette et al.[9] Their particular interest was the usefulness of OKN measurements for distinguishing peripheral from central vestibular lesions. Horizontal and vertical OKN in normal subjects and in patients with chronic unilateral labyrinthectomy and confirmed brainstem lesions were compared. The techniques of electronystagmography were used for documentation and analysis of response. Statistically significant differences between the normal and labyrinthectomy groups on the one hand and the brainstem group of the other suggested the value of the test for clinical otoneurological diagnosis.

The present study is a continuation of this work. The OKN of subjects in six groups are compared: normal subjects screened for vestibular disease, and patients with unilateral labyrinthectomy, Menière's disease, neurologically confirmed focal brainstem lesions, diffuse brainstem disease and radiologically confirmed supratentorial lesions. The focus of the work is an attempt to establish quantitative criteria for evaluating OKN in the diagnosis of peripheral vestibular and central nervous system lesions.

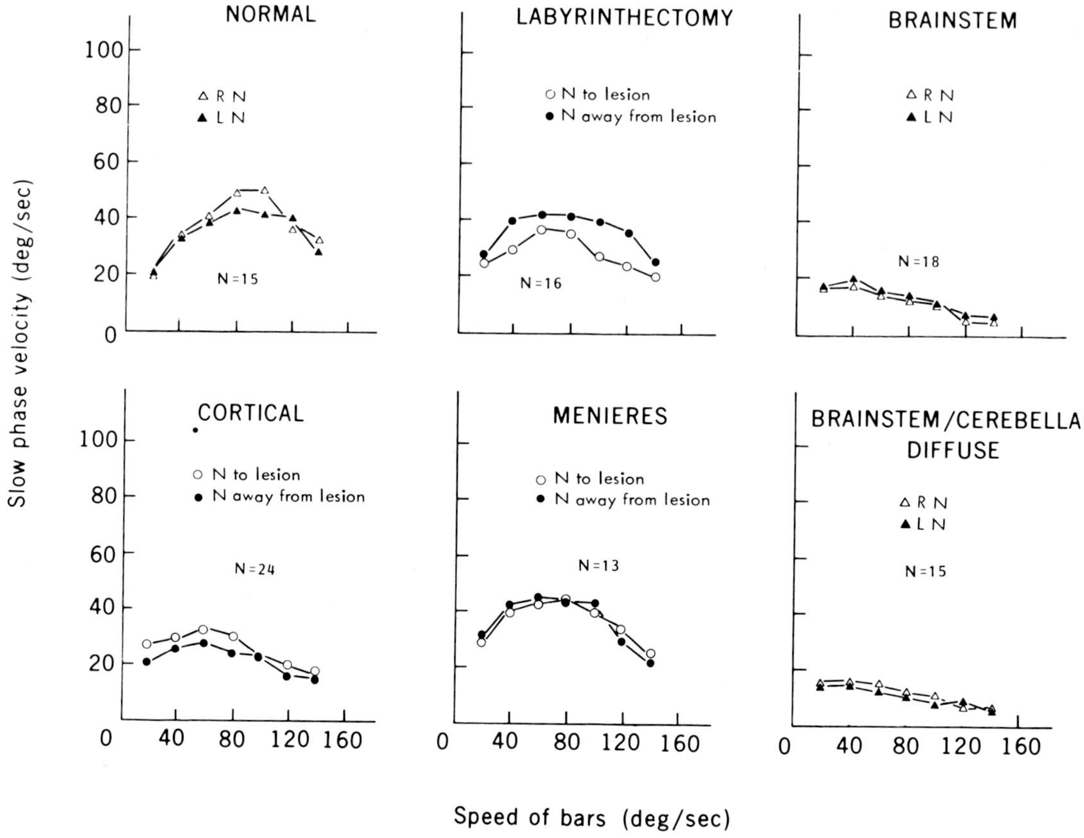

Fig. 1. Horizontal OKN.

METHODS

Subjects. One hundred and one paid volunteers served as subjects. All had normal vision, in some cases obtained with corrective lenses. They comprised six experimental groups:

1. Fifteen normal subjects, aged 18 to 39 years screened for otologic disease by routine audiometric and vestibular testing.

2. Sixteen patients with unilateral labyrinthectomy (11 right ear, 5 left), aged 31 to 72 years. The time lapse between surgical procedure and OKN test ranged between 1 and 52 months.

3. Thirteen patients with unilateral Menière's disease (6 right ear, 7 left), aged 33 to 72 years. In all cases the clinical diagnosis was based on unilateral vestibular reduction, fluctuating sensorineural hearing loss and severe episodic vertigo.[27]

4. Eighteen patients with neurologically confirmed brainstem lesions, 11 with infarction, 5 with multiple sclerosis, 1 with intrinsic neoplasm, and 1 with Arnold Chiari malformation, aged 27 to 85 years.

5. Fifteen patients with brainstem-cerebellar syndrome (eg, diffuse cerebellar degeneration, parkinsonism, encephalopathy of thiamine deficiency, neurofibromatosis) aged 27 to 90 years.

6. Twenty-four patients with focal unilateral supratentorial lesions with localization evident on radiologic examination, aged 25 to 76 years.

The distribution of lesions is given in Table 1.

Vestibular function was evaluated in each subject using a routine, standardized test battery. The battery included caloric testing, ie, irrigation of the two ears using hot (44 C) and cold (30 C) water, search for gaze nystagmus with lateral deviations of the eyes of 30° and vertical gaze directions of 10° from the primary eye position, examination of ocular tracking of a moving pendulum, and posture tests.[28] Eye movements were monitored and recorded using ENG.

Apparatus. The apparatus used for the experiment has been described previously.[9] During the OKN test, the subject was seated in a darkened room facing a translucent white screen at a distance of 80 cm. A circular field of parallel black bars covering 60° of visual angle was back-projected onto the screen. The bars were 5 cm wide and the distance between bars was 8.1 cm. The luminance of the ground was 1.75 foot-candles and the luminance gradient between the ground and bars was in the ratio of about 10:1.

The field of bars was produced by placing an opaque spiral drawn on a transparent disc between the condensor of a slide projector and a 35 mm wide angle lens. The disc was placed in the optical path of the projector in such a way that the rotary movement of the spiral would result in movement of the bars in a horizontal or vertical direction.

The speed of rotation of the disc was controlled by a feedback system in which the output from a potentiometer controlled by the experimenter and a tachometer were fed to a comparator. The speed of the motor driving the disc was increased or decreased depending on the voltage response of this comparator. A milliammeter connected to the tachometer was calibrated to read the speed of movement of the bars in degrees of visual angle per second ranging from 20 to 400. To avoid a stroboscopic effect, the projector was modified to work on direct current.

Eye movements were recorded using electronystagmography (AC coupling, time constant of five seconds), eyes separately and together in the horizontal axis and one eye in the vertical axis.

Procedure. Subjects were instructed to gaze at the surface of the screen. They were told to look at each bar as it passed the center point and to try not to follow any one bar as it moved from the center to the periphery of the visual field. In cases of response inhibition, subjects were instructed repeatedly to maintain a high level of attention.

The bars were projected successively at speeds ranging from 20

TABLE 2. MAXIMUM RESPONSE FOR HORIZONTAL OKN

Group		No.	Mean*	SD	Lowest Value	Highest Value
Normal	RN	15	59	25	22	122
	LN	15	55	20	28	101
Labyrinthectomy	N→L	16	46	17	25	77
	N←L	16	53	21	31	102
Menière's disease	N→L	13	49	12	31	70
	N←L	13	50	10	32	67
Brainstem	RN	18	20	11	3	38
	LN	18	22	9	7	43
Brnstm-cereb diffuse	RN	15	22	10	10	39
	LN	15	21	13	4	49
Cortical	N→L	24	38	14	7	67
	N←L	24	34	18	3	70

*Slow phase velocity in °/sec.

SD - Standard deviation; Brnstm-cereb - Brainstem-cerebellar; RN - Right-beating nystagmus (bars move left); LN - Left-beating nystagmus (bars move right); N→L - Nystagmus beating toward side of lesion; N←L - Nystagmus beating away from side of lesion.

to 140°/sec, in steps of 20°. Movement to the right and left of bars projected vertically were alternated for each speed. The procedure was repeated for the vertical axis, with a display of horizontal bars moving upwards and downwards.

At each speed (by direction) the display was presented for 20 to 30 seconds, the time required to observe at least one strong burst of nystagmus. If for any stimulus (speed by direction) no nystagmus was seen within 30 seconds, that presentation was discontinued and a zero recorded.

RESULTS

The response for each combination of direction of movement of the bars (right, left, up, and down) and bar speed (20°, 40°, 60°, 80°, 100°, 120°, 140°) was evaluated by measuring the slow phase velocity of OKN. The average value of the slope for the three fastest beats in the most easily identified group of beats persisting for at least five seconds was tabulated as the response.

HORIZONTAL OPTOKINETIC NYSTAGMUS

Figure 1 shows the average response plotted against bar speed for patients in the six groups. We have taken the liberty of labelling the supratentorial group as cortical, since in only one case was the lesion nonhemispheric. For normal subjects and those with brainstem lesions or diffuse brainstem-cerebellar disease the results are given separately for right-beating (RN) (bars move left) and left-beating (LN) (bars move right) OKN. For the other groups, labyrinthectomy, Menière's disease and supratentorial lesion, the laterality of the lesion was taken into account and the results are plotted separately for nystagmus beating toward (N → L) and away from (N ← L) the affected side, irrespective of the direction of movement of the bars.

Two distinct trends are apparent in these data. For normal subjects and those with chronic unilateral labyrinthectomy or Menière's disease, eye speed is a curvilinear function of bar speed, reaching a maximum for values of about 80°/sec. On the other hand, the brainstem and brainstem-cerebellar groups show a steady and gradual decline in eye speed for increases in stimulus speed. The data for patients with cortical lesions are midway between these two trends.

In order to compare the groups statistically, in a way which might prove useful for clinical diagnosis, we examined 1) the maximum value of slow phase velocity achieved by each subject, regardless of bar speed; 2) the bar speed giving the maximum response; and 3) the slow phase velocities obtained for relatively high and low bar speeds of 80° and 20°/sec, respectively.

Maximum Response. Table 2 shows the mean maximum response observed for subjects in each of the six groups. The standard deviation as well as the lowest and highest values of maximum response observed for the subjects in each group are given. Statistical comparison of the maximum response ob-

TABLE 3. RESULTS OF STATISITCAL COMPARISON OF MAXIMUM VALUES OF RESPONSE

	t	df	α
Within-group comparisons			
Labyrinthectomy			
N→L vs N←L	2.93	15	.050
Between-group comparisons			
Normal vs brainstem			
RN vs RN	6.03	31	.001
LN vs LN	6.29	31	.001
Normal vs cortical			
RN vs N→L	3.45	37	.010
N←L	3.77	37	.001
LN vs N→L	3.09	37	.010
N←L	3.45	37	.010
Labyrintectomy vs brainstem			
N→L vs RN	5.31	32	.001
LN	5.25	32	.001
N←L vs RN	5.99	32	.001
LN	5.93	32	.001
Labyrinthectomy vs cortical			
N→L vs N→L	NS		
N←L	2.17	38	.050
N←L vs N→L	2.86	38	.010
N←L	3.26	38	.010
Brainstem vs cortical			
RN vs N→L	4.32	40	.001
N←L	2.82	40	.010
LN vs N→L	4.10	40	.001
N←L	2.57	40	.050

NS - Not significant; N→L - Nystagmus beating toward side of lesion; N←L - Nystagmus beating away from side of lesion. Other abbreviations same as Table 2.

TABLE 4. DISTRIBUTION OF OBSERVED MAXIMUM SPEEDS

Maximum Slow Phase Velocity (°/sec)	*Normal* RN	LN	*Labyrinthectomy* N→L	N←L	*Menière's Disease* N→L	N←L	*Brainstem* RN	LN	*Brnstm-Cereb Diffuse* RN	LN	*Cortical* N→L	N←L
1- 10							4	2	1	3	1	1
11- 20							7	6	7	6	2	4
21- 30	2	1	3				3	7	3	3	4	9
31- 40	2	3	5	5	3	2	4	2	4	1	6	2
41- 50	0	3	1	3	5	3		1		2	7	3
51- 60	3	3	5	2	3	7					3	2
61- 70	4	2		4	2	1					1	3
71- 80	3	2	2									
81- 90				1								
91-100												
101-125	1	1		1								
Total No.	15	15	16	16	13	13	18	18	15	15	24	24

N→L - Nystagmus beating toward side of lesion; N←L - Nystagmus beating away from side of lesion. Other abbreviations same as Table 2.

served for left and right-beating nystagmus or for nystagmus beating to and away from the side of lesion within each group shows a significant difference only in the case of subjects with chronic unilateral labyrinthectomy. For this group the eye speed is higher when the nystagmus beats away from the side of the lesion.

Pairwise comparisons between the various groups show that the maximum response of patients with chronic unilateral labyrinthectomy or unilateral Menière's disease are not significantly different from those of normal subjects. On the other hand, the maximum response for patients with brainstem lesions or diffuse brainstem-cerebellar disease was significantly less than those for normals. The result for patients with cortical lesions fell midway between and was significantly different both from those of normal subjects and patients with brainstem findings.

In making the pairwise comparisons, the groups were compared on the basis of right-beating and left-beating nystagmus, taken separately. If lesion laterality was a factor for both groups then all four possible matches were made: nystagmus beating toward and away from the side of lesion in one group was compared with nystagmus beating toward and away from the side of lesion in the other group. If lesion laterality was known for only one of the two groups under comparison, then right and left beating nystagmus in the one group were each compared with nystagmus beating toward and away from the side lesion in the second group. The details of the *t*-tests are given for significant outcomes in Table 3. It should be noted that patients with Menière's disease and diffuse brainstem-cerebellar syndrome were included in the experiment to provide clinical controls for patients with chronic labyrinthectomy and focal brainstem lesions, respectively, and were compared only with these groups in this and subsequent analyses.

Table 4 shows the distribution of observed maximum speeds for all subjects. While significant differences were noted (see above) between the average values for the various groups, it is evident from this analysis that the ranges of values overlap considerably. Any choice of cut-off for decision making along the maximum slow phase velocity axis will be associated with some probability of error in diagnosis. Thus, for example, if a response of 30°/sec were to be chosen, 13% of normal subjects would be classified as abnormal (maximum less than 31°/sec) and 42% of cortical (N←L) and 22% of brainstem pa-

TABLE 5. BAR SPEED GIVING THE MAXIMUM RESPONSE FOR HORIZONTAL OKN

Group		*No.*	*Mean**	*SD*	*Lowest Value*	*Highest Value*
Normal	RN	15	81.3	29.7	20	120
	LN	15	89.3	28.1	40	140
Labyrinthectomy	N→L	16	65.0	33.1	20	140
	N←L	16	76.3	31.2	40	120
Menière's disease	N→L	13	70.7	24.0	40	120
	N←L	13	64.6	24.7	20	100
Brainstem	RN	18	40.0	25.7	20	100
	LN	18	43.3	25.0	20	100
Brnstm-cereb diffuse	RN	15	45.3	24.5	20	100
	LN	15	34.7	17.7	20	80
Cortical	N→L	24	50.8	22.8	20	100
	N←L	24	50.8	29.5	20	140

*Slow phase velocity in °/sec.

N→L - Nystagmus beating toward side of lesion; N←L - Nystagmus beating away from side of lesion. Other abbreviations same as Table 2.

TABLE 6. RESULTS OF STATISTICAL COMPARISON OF BAR SPEEDS GIVING THE MAXIMUM RESPONSE

	t	df	α
Within-group comparisons			
Labyrinthectomy			
N→L vs N←L	2.76	15	.050
Between-group comparisons			
Normal vs brainstem			
RN vs RN	4.29	31	.001
LN vs LN	4.97	31	.001
Normal vs cortical			
RN vs N→L	3.61	37	.010
N←L	3.13	37	.010
LN vs N→L	4.68	37	.001
N←L	4.04	37	.001
Labyrinthectomy vs brainstem			
N→L vs RN	2.48	32	.050
LN	2.17	32	.050
N←L vs RN	3.72	32	.001
LN	3.42	32	.010
Labyrinthectomy vs cortical			
N→L vs N→L	1.61	38	NS
N←L	1.42	38	NS
N←L vs N→L	2.98	38	.010
N←L	2.61	38	.050

NS - Not significant; N→L - Nystagmus beating toward side of lesion; N←L - Nystagmus beating away from side of lesion. Other abbreviations same as Table 2.

tients (RN or LN) would be called normal (maximum greater than 30).

Position of Maximum Response. The average value of bar speed for which the maximum response occurred is presented in Table 5. A summary of significant differences within and between groups is given in Table 6. The normal subjects and patients with labyrinthectomy are not different from each other in this analysis and the bar speed giving the maximum is between 65° and 90°/sec on the average for the two groups. For the brainstem group the maximum response occurs at a much slower bar speed of about 40°/sec. Patients with cortical lesions show a maximum response at a relatively higher speed of 50°. This is significantly different from the outcome for normal subjects but not from that observed for patients with brainstem disease.

OKN at Relatively High and Low Bar Speeds. In the last section, we demonstrated that normal subjects show a maximum slow phase velocity for a bar speed close to 80°/sec. A statistical comparison of the response was made both within and between subjects specifically for this bar speed. The data for a bar speed of 80° are given in Table 7 and the significant differences between groups are shown in Table 8. The trends observed are similar to those for maximum response given in Table 3.

To contrast the response for the various groups at high bar speeds, we compared the groups for the lowest bar speed. The significant comparisons are presented in Table 9. These data indicate that for a bar speed of 20°/sec the laterality of the lesion is important for patients with chronic unilateral labyrinthectomy and cortical lesions. For the former group the slow phase velocity is higher when the nystagmus beats faster away from the lesion and for the latter group, when the nystagmus beats in the direction of the lesion. An unexpected finding is the relatively greater response for these patients, when compared with that of normal subjects, regardless of the direction of nystagmus. By comparison, patients with brainstem lesions showed responses well within the normal range.

The distribution of results for the bar speed of 20°/sec are given for each of the groups in Table 10. Examination of right-beating nystagmus in normal subjects indicates that 11 of 15 give speeds between 16° and 25°/sec. Of the 13 patients with Menière's disease, 11 give speeds greater than 25° both for nystagmus beating to and away from the side of lesion. For 16 patients with labyrinthectomy 10 give slow phase velocities greater than the range when the nystagmus is beating away from the side of lesion.

Direction Preponderance of Maximum Response. In investigation of the peripheral vestibular system directional preponderance (DP) of eye movements in response to caloric stimuli is often used as a method for within-subject comparison of the two ears. Applying this logic to OKN[29] we calculated the difference in maximum slow phase velocity between right and left-beating nystagmus or between the maximum response for nystagmus beating toward

TABLE 7. RESPONSE FOR BAR SPEED OF 80°/SEC

Group		No.	Mean*	SD	Lowest Value	Highest Value
Normal	RN	15	49	21	11	72
	LN	15	43	19	9	77
Labyrinthectomy	N→L	16	36	21	3	77
	N←L	16	42	22	11	83
Menière's disease	N→L	13	44	16	19	70
	N←L	13	44	14	12	63
Brainstem	RN	18	12	9	0	30
	LN	18	13	9	2	43
Brnstm-cereb diffuse	RN	15	13	11	1	39
	LN	15	13	13	1	49
Cortical	N→L	24	30	16	3	58
	N←L	24	25	18	2	70

*Slow phase velocity in °/sec.

N→L - Nystagmus beating toward side of lesion; N←L - Nystagmus beating away from side of lesion. Other abbreviations same as Table 2.

TABLE 8. SIGNIFICANT DIFFERENCES IN RESPONSE FOR BAR SPEED OF 80°/SEC

	t	*df*	α
Within-group comparisons	No significant differences		
Between-group comparisons			
Normal vs brainstem			
RN vs RN	6.97	31	.001
LN vs LN	6.09	31	.001
Normal vs cortical			
RN vs N→L	3.32	37	.010
N←L	3.78	37	.001
LN vs N→L	2.45	37	.050
N←L	2.98	37	.050
Labyrinthectomy vs brainstem			
N→L vs RN	4.34	32	.001
LN	4.11	32	.001
N←L vs RN	5.35	32	.001
LN	5.11	32	.001
Labyrinthectomy vs cortical			
N→L vs N→L	1.02	38	NS
N←L	1.62	38	NS
N←L vs N→L	2.02	38	.050
N←L	2.56	38	.050
Brainstem vs cortical			
RN vs N→L	4.12	40	.001
N←L	2.88	40	.010
LN vs N→L	3.84	40	.001
N←L	2.64	40	.050

NS - Not significant; N→L - Nystagmus beating toward side of lesion; N←L - Nystagmus beating away from side of lesion. Other abbreviations same as Table 2.

and away from the side of lesion, whichever was appropriate to the group. The mean differences are plotted for the six groups in Table 11, and it is evident that the values obtained are fairly similar. In the case of chronic unilateral labyrinthectomy, 12 of 16 patients show a higher maximum for nystagmus beating away from the side of lesion. For patients with Menière's disease, 8 of 13 show a DP favoring the side opposite the lesion. In contrast, 16 of 24 patients with cortical lesions show a higher maximum response for nystagmus beating toward the side of lesion.

CORTICAL LESIONS

Since much of the literature on OKN concerns the effect of the location of a cortical lesion, we attempted to subdivide our group of 24 patients with supratentorial lesions in terms of both locus and type of lesion. As indicated in Table 1, our sample consisted of 14 cases of infarction and 10 cases of mass lesion. Of the former group, 12 involved some area of the parietal cortex. In the latter group, two were anterior parietal. The location and type of lesion are highly related for our sample and thus, may not be evaluated separately.

Table 12 shows the range of maximum slow phase velocities observed for nystagmus beating toward (N→L) and away from (N←L) the side of lesion for the mass and infarction groups respectively. The median values are shown to allow a rough comparison. For the group of infarctions, the median value of maximum slow phase velocity for nystagmus beating away from the lesion has a value of 25. This is relatively low in comparison with the other values

TABLE 9. SIGNIFICANT DIFFERENCES IN RESPONSE AT BAR SPEED OF 20°/SEC

	t	*df*	α
Within-group comparisons			
Labyrinthectomy			
N→L vs N←L	2.59	15	.050
Cortical			
N→L vs N←L	3.28	23	.010
Between-group comparisons			
Normal vs labyrinthectomy			
RN vs N→L	3.17	29	.010
N←L	3.83	20	.001
LN vs N→L	3.24	29	.010
N←L	3.89	29	.001
Normal vs Menière's			
RN vs N→L	5.82	26	.001
N←L	5.70	26	.001
LN vs N→L	6.29	26	.001
N←L	5.92	26	.001
Normal vs cortical			
RN vs N→L	2.76	37	.010
LN vs N→L	2.67	37	.050
Labyrinthectomy vs Menière's			
N→L vs N→L	2.96	27	.010
Labyrinthectomy vs brainstem			
N→L vs RN	3.22	32	.010
LN	3.71	32	.001
N←L vs RN	3.88	32	.001
LN	4.36	32	.001
Labyrinthectomy vs cortical			
N←L vs N←L	2.77	38	.010
Brainstem vs cortical			
RN vs N→L	3.51	40	.010
LN vs N→L	3.81	40	.001

N→L - Nystagmus beating toward side of lesion; N←L - Nystagmus beating away from side of lesion. Other abbreviations same as Table 2.

shown. However, a statistical comparison of the maximum values observed for individuals using the Mann-Whitney U test for unrelated samples shows no differences between mass and infarction groups either for nystagmus beating toward or away from the side of lesion.

A measure of directional preponderance (DP) was calculated for each subject using the difference between the maximum value of slow phase velocity observed for nystagmus beating toward and away from the side of lesion. The range of DP is given in Table 12 for the two groups. In the case of mass lesions, (nonparietal lobe) the value of DP is equally likely to be positive or negative and fairly symmetric about zero. On the other hand, for infarctions, (parietal lobe) in 12 of 14 cases the nystagmus beating away from the lesion is relatively diminished. Of the two exceptions, DP = 0 and − 13, the latter value was obtained for the one patient who had sustained a stroke to the pons. Statistical evaluation of these data using the Wilcoxon test indicates that the average DP is significantly different from zero in the case of infarctions. The test takes into account the sign of relative magnitude of the difference observed for each subject. Under the null hypothesis of no directional bias the probability of the obtained outcome is 0.005. For mass lesions the probability was 0.5, ie, the results were highly likely given no expectation of a DP.

TABLE 10. DISTRIBUTION OF RESPONSE FOR BAR SPEED OF 20°/SEC

Slow Phase Velocity (°/sec)	*Normal*	*Labyrinthectomy*		*Menière's Disease*		*Brainstem*	*Cortical*	
	RN	*N→L*	*N←L*	*N→L*	*N←L*	*RN*	*N→L*	*N←L*
1-5						1		1
6-10						4	1	0
11-15	3					3	2	3
16-20	4	2	3		1	3	1	8
21-25	7	9	3	2	1	3	8	7
26-30	1	4	6	5	2	3	3	2
31-35		0	2	4	5	1	5	2
35-40		1	1	2	3		3	0
41-45			1	0	1		1	1
Total No.	15	16	16	13	13	18	24	24

N→L - Nystagmus beating toward side of lesion; N←L - Nystagmus beating away from side of lesion. Other abbreviations same as Table 2.

VERTICAL OPTOKINETIC NYSTAGMUS

Figure 2 shows the average slow phase velocity as a function of bar speed for vertical OKN. Values for upbeating and downbeating nystagmus were analyzed separately.

Maximum Response. As for horizontal OKN, the maximum response observed across bar speeds was tabulated for each subject. Mean values of the maximum are shown for the six groups in Table 13. The significant statistical differences are given in Table 14. Within-group and between-group analyses were based on comparison of maximum slow phase values for up and down-beating nystagmus respectively. In making between-group comparisons lesion laterality was ignored.

These results show that for vertical OKN normal subjects give responses that are statistically greater than those for patients with brainstem or cortical lesions. The range of values for these groups, given by the lowest and highest scores in Table 13, indicate considerable overlap in response. For upward beating nystagmus, 9 of 17 subjects with localized brainstem disease fell below the range for normals and 8 within. For downward beating nystagmus only 6 subjects give values below the range and 11 give values comparable to those of normal subjects.

Vertical OKN at Low Speeds. The slow phase velocity observed for a bar speed of 20° was also examined. The average values for upward and downward beating nystagmus are presented in Figure 2. Significant comparisons are given in Table 15. Normal subjects give higher values for upbeating nystagmus than do patients with brainstem lesions. However, only 5 of 17 in the latter group are clearly below the normal range.

DISCUSSION AND CONCLUSIONS

The focus of interest of the present research has been the measurement of OKN for use in otoneurological diagnosis. In this regard the effect of a wide range of optokinetic target speeds on the slow phase velocity of OKN has been investigated both for horizontal and vertical target arrays. The groups tested were normal subjects and patients with well-defined peripheral vestibular lesions (chronic unilateral labyrinthectomy), focal brainstem lesions, and supratentorial tumor or infarction. Two additional groups, patients with Menière's disease and diffuse brainstem-cerebellar syndromes, were included on grounds of clinical relevancy. The etiology for these is often less clearly defined and we wondered how similar their performance would be to the patients with circumscribed lesions in the same areas, ie, labyrinthine and lower brainstem focus respectively.

We chose to isolate several features of the data for statistical analysis, with a view to defining quantitative criteria for routine clinical diagnosis. These were 1) the maximum slow phase velocity observed over the range of bar speeds used; 2) the bar speed at which the maximum response occurred; 3) the response at very low (20°/sec) and relatively high (80°/sec) bar speeds; and 4) the directional preponderance, or the difference in maximum response observed for nystagmus beating toward and away from the side of lesion. In an attempt to evaluate current theories of the neurological

TABLE 11. DIRECTIONAL PREPONDERANCE IN MAXIMUM SLOW PHASE VELOCITY

Group	*No.*	*Mean Difference (°/sec)*	*SD*	*Lowest Value*	*Highest Value*	*No. of Subjects with No Difference*
Normal	15	10	7	1	21	0
Labyrinthectomy	16	11	8	1	28	1
Menière's disease	13	9	7	1	20	0
Brainstem	18	9	8	1	26	4
Brnstm-cereb diffuse	15	6	4	2	13	1
Cortical	24	11	7	0	27	0

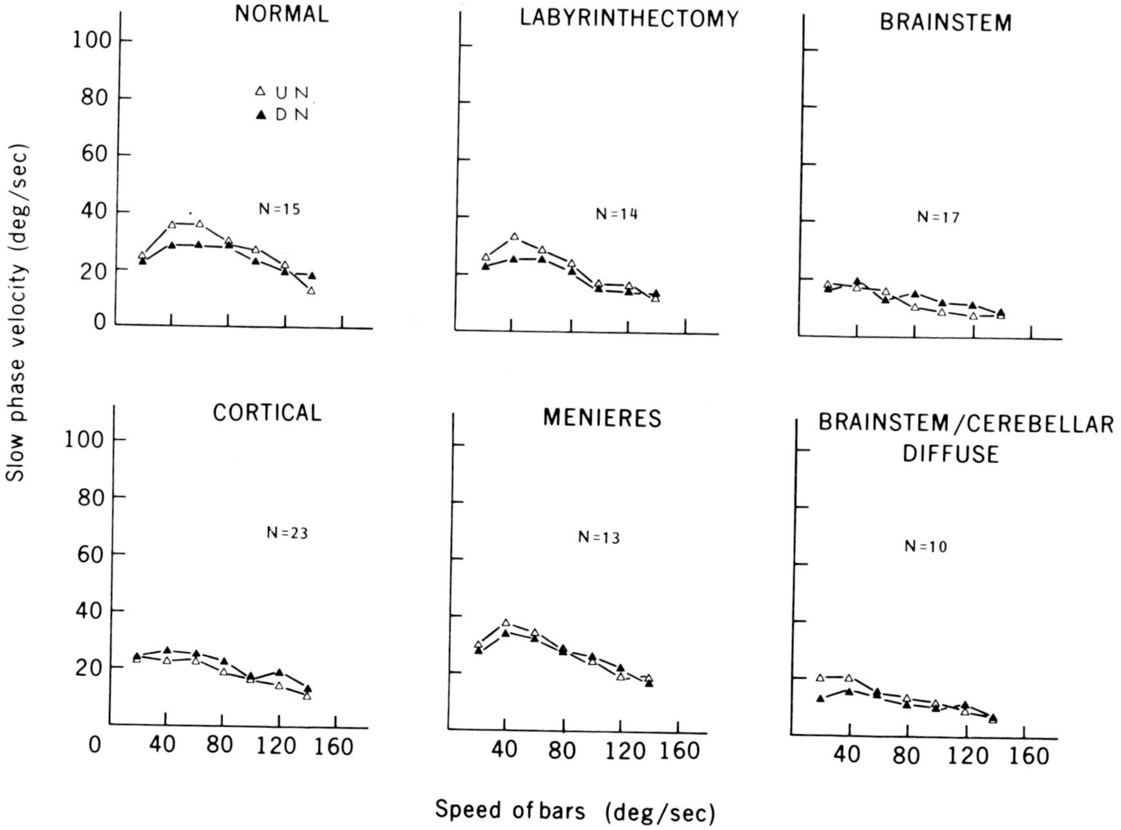

Fig. 2. Vertical OKN.

pathways subserving OKN we subsequently subdivided the cortical group for the purpose of studying the effect of the location (hemispheric lobe) and nature of the lesion (mass vs infarction) on OKN. Our findings indicate that for *horizontal* OKN:

1. The maximum slow phase velocity allows us to differentiate normal subjects and patients with unilateral labyrinthectomy on the one hand, from patients with focal brainstem lesions on the other. On the basis of this index, patients with Menière's disease were not unlike those with labyrinthectomy, nor could we distinguish brainstem-cerebellar syndromes from focal brainstem lesions. The average maximum slow phase velocity for patients with cortical lesions fell midway between the averages computed for normal subjects and patients with brainstem disease and was significantly greater than the value for the latter of these two groups.

2. The distributions of maximum response (ie, values observed in individuals) for groups which give significantly different results overlap considerably. We attempted to establish a cut-off value for use in the detection of abnormality and noted that the probability of false positives and negatives would be relatively high. Nevertheless, a maximum slow phase velocity of 30°/sec provides a crude yardstick. By this criterion, we find that 13% of normal subjects would be judged abnormal and 22% (about 1 in 5) of patients with brainstem disease would be judged normal.

3. Patients with chronic unilateral labyrinthectomy show a significantly lower maximum response for nystagmus beating toward the side of the lesion. However, the magnitude of the difference in each patient is 11° on the average and is similar to that observed for the difference between right and left-beating nystagmus in normal subjects.

4. The average bar speed at which the maximum response occurs is significantly greater for normal subjects (85°/sec) and patients with labyrinthectomy (70°/sec) than those with brainstem and cortical lesions. The position of maximum response for cortical lesions was 50°/sec on the average and this

TABLE 12. MAXIMUM RESPONSE FOR CORTICAL LESIONS

	No.	*N→L* *Range of Max. Resp.**	*Median*	*N←L* *Range of Max. Resp.*	*Median*	*Range of DP*
Mass lesion	10	24-58	42	20-70	38	− 22 to 19
Infarction	14	7-67	38	3-55	25	− 13 to 27

*°/sec.

N→L - Nystagmus beating toward side of lesion; N←L - Nystagmus beating away from side of lesion.

TABLE 13. MAXIMUM RESPONSE FOR VERTICAL OKN

Group		No.	Mean*	SD	Lowest Value	Highest Value
Normal	UN	15	41.3	12.6	24	78
	DN	15	36.9	9.6	15	50
Labyrinthectomy	UN	13	37.6	18.0	12	67
	DN	13	29.2	13.4	6	48
Menière's disease	UN	13	42.6	22.2	14	86
	DN	13	37.6	15.5	17	74
Brainstem	UN	17	20.9	12.4	6	40
	DN	17	21.4	8.5	6	31
Brnstm-cereb diffuse	UN	10	22.7	10.4	8	38
	DN	10	19.6	11.0	0	37
Cortical	UN	23	28.2	10.1	15	56
	DN	23	31.2	10.1	7	52

*Slow phase velocity in °/sec.

SD - Standard deviation; UN - Upbeating nystagmus; DN - Downbeating nystagmus.

was not significantly different from the value of 40° observed in the presence of brainstem lesions.

5. Analysis of the results obtained at a bar speed of 80°/sec yielded the same conclusions as those for analysis of the maximum responses (see Item 1 above).

6. At the slowest bar speed, 20°/sec, patients with lower brainstem lesions are not different from normal. However, patients with either peripheral vestibular disorders (labyrinthectomy or Menière's disease) or cortical lesions give eye speeds which are significantly greater than those of normal subjects and patients with focal brainstem lesions. This finding was unexpected and to our knowledge has not been previously reported. For both labyrinthectomy and cortical cases, lesion laterality is a significant factor. Specifically, for the former group eye speeds are higher for nystagmus beating away from the lesion (bars moving toward the side of lesion). For the latter group the eye speeds are higher for nystagmus beating toward the lesion. These data confirm the earlier findings of Davidoff et al.[19] In Menière's disease there were no significant within-group differences due to laterality.

7. While we find directional differences to be related to lesion laterality, the average value of 10° to 11°, as well as the highest and lowest value, are similar to normal. In patients with brainstem disease the average difference across patients as well as the highest observed value are smaller by a factor of two. These data suggest that on its own DP would not provide a good diagnostic index of abnormality. The range of values of DP for cortical lesions, both mass and infarctions (or parietal versus nonparietal lobe) are not different in absolute value from those of the other groups. However, in the case of infarctions we note that the direction of difference is significantly related to the laterality of the lesion (beating more strongly toward the lesion). In mass lesions it is unrelated.

For *vertical* OKN, lesion laterality was not taken into account and in all statistical comparisons the direction of nystagmus was held constant, either upbeating or downbeating.

The values observed for normal subjects are on the average 20° less than those for horizontal OKN. For brainstem subjects horizontal and vertical OKN are comparable. In terms of the maximum response observed for vertical OKN, normal subjects produce significantly higher values than do patients with focal brainstem lesions. Cortical lesions result in significantly lower values for upbeating but not downbeating nystagmus. A comparison of results between groups for a bar speed of 20° shows that the only group different from normal was the brainstem, but for upbeating not downbeating nystagmus.

TABLE 14. STATISTICAL COMPARISON OF MAXIMUM VALUES OF RESPONSE FOR VERTICAL OKN

	t	*df*	α
Within-group comparisons			
Labyrinthectomy			
UN vs DN	2.27	12	.050
Between-group comparisons			
Normal vs brainstem			
UN vs UN	4.61	30	.001
DN vs DN	4.87	30	.001
Normal vs cortical			
UN vs UN	3.56	36	.010
DN vs DN	1.76	36	NS
Brainstem vs cortical			
UN vs UN	2.03	38	NS
DN vs DN	3.24	38	.010

NS - Not significant. Other abbreviations same as Table 13.

TABLE 15. SIGNIFICANT DIFFERENCES IN VERTICAL OKN OBSERVED FOR A BAR SPEED OF 20°/SEC

	t	*df*	α
Within-group comparisons	No significant differences		
Between-group comparisons			
Normal vs brainstem			
UN vs UN	2.28	30	.05
DN vs DN	No significant differences		
Labyrinthectomy vs brainstem			
UN vs UN	2.13	29	.05
DN vs DN	No significant differences		
Brainstem vs cortical			
UN vs UN	2.16	38	.05
DN vs DN	2.16	38	.05

Abbreviations same as Table 13.

SUMMARY

The experimental results discussed above provide statistical confirmation for OKN findings previously reported in the literature. In summary, we find that compared with any other diagnostic category, the maximum slow phase velocity of OKN for the range of bar speeds studied is significantly reduced in patients with brainstem lesions. Patients with cortical lesions fall midway between the normal and brainstem groups and give significantly higher values on the average than the latter. Directional differences were investigated as an alert to the laterality of lesion and it was noted that in the case of chronic unilateral peripheral vestibular disease, nystagmus beat less strongly when the targets moved toward the lesion. The opposite was true for cortical infarctions located in the parietal region. An unexpected finding was the elevation in eye speed for very low target speeds in the case of patients with chronic unilateral labyrinthectomy and Menière's disease.

While the above conclusions are statistically significant, by itself the measurement of OKN is of limited use for purposes of clinical diagnosis. The distributions of observed maximum slow phase velocities for individuals in the various patient groups overlap considerably. The optimum criterion or cut-off value for decision-making leads to high error rates in predicting the presence of a lesion. While DPs were found to be related to the side of lesion for patients with either peripheral vestibular or cortical disease, the absolute size of the difference between the maximum slow phase velocity for nystagmus beating toward and away from the side of lesion was not different from the difference between left and right beating nystagmus in normal subjects.

ACKNOWLEDGMENTS — We are indebted to the vestibular technologists at Sunnybrook Medical Centre for their assistance in the testing of patients and analysis of ENG records, and wish to thank in particular Grace Wright, Antje Slessor, Lynn McIlmoyl and Carlos Dioknos. Special thanks are due to the staff of the Department of Neurosciences for making their patients available to us.

REFERENCES

1. Barany R. Zur Klinik und Theorie des eisenbahn-Nystagmus. Acta Otolaryngol (Stockh) 1922; 3:261.

2. Ohm J. Die klinische Bedeutung des optischen Dreyhnystagmus. Klin Monatsbl Augenheilkd 1922; 68:323.

3. Cords R. Optisch-motorisches Feld und optisch-motorische Bahn. Arch Ophthalmol 1926; 117:58.

4. Tos M, Adser J, Rosborg J. Horizontal optokinetic nystagmus in cerebral disease. Acta Neurol Scand 1972; 48:607-20.

5. Honrubia V, Scott BJ, Ward PH. Experimental studies of optokinetic nystagmus. I. Normal cats. Acta Otolaryngol (Stockh) 1967; 64:388-402.

6. Honrubia V, Downey WL, Mitchell DP, Ward PH. Experimental studies of optokinetic nystagmus. II. Normal humans. Acta Otolaryngol (Stockh) 1968; 65:441-8.

7. Honrubia V, Jenkins HA, Downey WL, Ward PH. Experimental studies in optokinetic nystagmus. III. Modifications produced by labyrinthectomy and hemidecortication in cats. Ann Otol Rhinol Laryngol 1971; 80:97-110.

8. Morissette Y, Abel SM, Barber HO. Optokinetic nystagmus: its value in the diagnosis of certain vestibular lesions. In: Guedry FE Jr, ed. The use of nystagmography in aviation medicine. AGARD Conf Proc No. 128, May 1973.

9. Morissette Y, Abel SM, Barber HO. Optokinetic nystagmus in otoneurological diagnosis. Can J Otolaryngol 1974; 3:348-62.

10. Smith JL. Optokinetic nystagmus: Its use in topical neuro-ophthalmologic diagnosis. Springfield: Thomas, 1963.

11. Baloh RW, Honrubia V, Sills A. Eye-tracking and optokinetic nystagmus: results of quantitative testing in patients with well-defined nervous system lesions. Ann Otol Rhinol Laryngol 1977; 86:108-14.

12. Ling W, Gay AJ. Optokinetic nystagmus: a proposed pathway and its clinical application. In: Smith JL, ed. Neuro-opthalmology. Vol. 4. St. Louis: Mosby, 1968.

13. Carmichael EA, Dix MR, Hallpike CS. Lesions of the cerebral hemispheres and their effects upon optokinetic and caloric nystagmus. Brain 1954; 77:345-71.

14. Cogan DG, Loeb DR. Optokinetic response and intracranial lesions. AMA Arch Neurol Psychiatry 1948; 61:183-7.

15. Kestenbaum A. Clinical methods of neuro-ophthalmologic examination. 2nd ed. New York: Grune and Stratton, 1961.

16. Smith JL. Homonymous hemianopia — A review of 100 cases. Am J Ophthalmol 1962; 54:616-23.

17. Smith JL, Cogan DG. Optokinetic nystagmus: a test for parietal lobe lesions. Am J Ophthalmol 1959; 48:187-93.

18. Smith JL, Cogan DG. Optokinetic nystagmus in cerebral disease — A study of 14 autopsied cases. Neurology 1960; 10:127-37.

19. Davidoff RA, Atkin A, Anderson PJ, Bender MB. Optokinetic nystagmus and cerebral disease. Arch Neurol 1966; 14:73-81.

20. Fox JC, Holmes G. Optic nystagmus and its value in the localization of cerebral lesions. Brain 1926; 49:333-71.

21. Gay AJ, Newman NM, Keltner JL, Stroud MH. Eye movement disorders. Saint Louis: Mosby, 1974.

22. Crosby E. Correlation anatomy of the nervous system. New York: Macmillan, 1962.

23. Bender MB, ed. The oculomotor system. New York: Harper and Row, 1964.

24. Bach-Y-Rita P, Collins CC, Hyde JE, eds. The control of eye movements. New York: Academic Press, 1971.

25. Neverov VP, Ueda M, Bures J. The effect of cortical and collicular spreading depression on the optokinetic and reversive postoptokinetic nystagmus in rabbits. Brain Res 1976; 115: 318-23.

26. Cohen B. Vestibulo-ocular relations. In: Bach-Y-Rita P, Collins CC, Hyde JE, eds. The control of eye movements. New York: Academic Press, 1971.

27. Alford BR. Report of subcommittee on equilibrium and its measurements. Menière's disease: criteria for diagnosis and evaluation of therapy for reporting. Trans Am Acad Ophthalmol Otolaryngol 1972; 76:1462-4.

28. Barber HO, Stockwell CW. Manual of electronystagmography. Saint Louis: Mosby, 1976.

29. Coats AC. Central and peripheral optokinetic asymmetry. Ann Otol Rhinol Laryngol 1968; 77:938-48.

TUMORS OF THE PARAPHARYNGEAL SPACE
PREOPERATIVE EVALUATION, DIAGNOSIS AND SURGICAL APPROACHES

PETER M. SOM, MD
HUGH F. BILLER, MD
WILLIAM LAWSON, MD
NEW YORK, NEW YORK

TUMORS OF THE PARAPHARYNGEAL SPACE
PREOPERATIVE EVALUATION, DIAGNOSIS AND SURGICAL APPROACHES

PETER M. SOM, MD

HUGH F. BILLER, MD WILLIAM LAWSON, MD

NEW YORK, NEW YORK

This report demonstrates that preoperatively the radiologist can provide the surgeon with the size, extent, origin and probable histology of a parapharyngeal space tumor. Using this information, the surgeon can then determine the best surgical approach for complete and safe tumor excision.

Neoplasms involving the paraphargeal space present a formidable challenge to the clinician with regard to both their preoperative diagnosis and the specific technique of their surgical removal. Improved preoperative evaluation now allows a more accurate assessment of the tumors involving this space. The purpose of this paper is to present a technique for the systematic preoperative evaluation of these lesions. This process has provided a method which allows one not only to accurately map the extent of the tumor, but in addition, to correctly establish the histologic diagnosis preoperatively in many cases. From this information, a rational surgical approach for the tumor removal can be selected. This method of management has evolved from the authors' experience in assessing and treating 30 patients with tumors involving the parapharyngeal space.

ANATOMY

An understanding of the anatomy of both the parotid gland and the parapharyngeal space is essential to appreciate the findings upon which the radiologist bases his diagnosis and the surgeon plans his operative approach.

The major portion of the parotid gland (80%) rests primarily upon the outer surface of the masseter muscle and the mandibular ramus (Fig. 1). It is situated above a line drawn between the mastoid process tip and the angle of the mandible and lies below the zygomatic arch. The posterior margin can have identations from the adjacent external acoustic meatus, the mastoid process and the anterior border of the sternocleidomastoid muscle (SCM). The deep lobe, or retromandibular portion of the parotid gland, extends medially between the posterior border of the mandible and the anterior margin of the SCM muscle. It then proceeds to course in front of the posterior belly of the digastric muscle, rests lateral to the styloid muscle group and abuts upon the posterior surface of the internal pterygoid muscle and the mandibular ramus.

The facial nerve descends from the stylomastoid foramen and courses laterally to lie between the posterior belly of the diagastric muscle and the SCM muscle. It then enters the posterior surface of the parotid gland. After it penetrates the parotid, it divides within the substance of the gland into its major divisions. The main parotid vessels are the external carotid artery and the posterior facial vein, both of which traverse the gland in its immediate

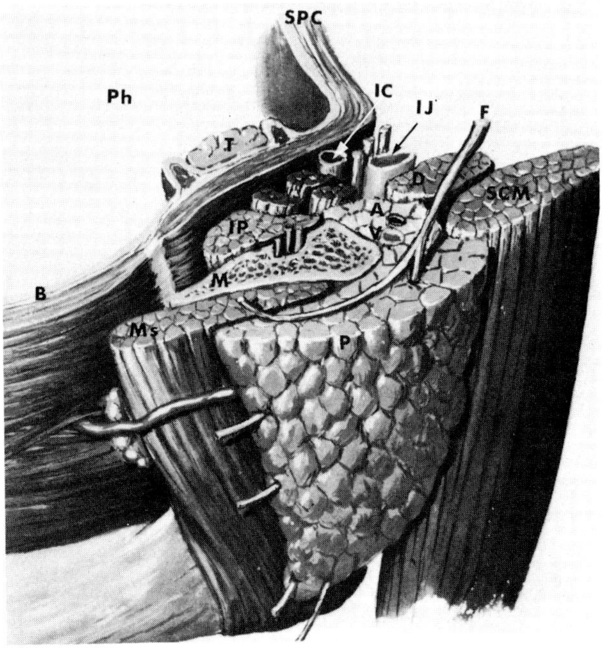

Fig. 1. Normal anatomy of the left parotid gland and parapharyngeal space viewed obliquely and from above. Ph - Pharynx; SPC - Superior pharyngeal constrictor muscle; T - Tonsil; B - Buccinator muscle; Ms - Masseter muscle; SCM - Sternocleidomastoid muscle; D - Posterior belly of digastric muscle; IP - Internal pterygoid muscle; M - Mandible; IC - Internal carotid artery; IJ - Internal jugular vein; P - Parotid gland; F - Facial nerve; A - External carotid artery; V - Posterior facial vein. (Reprinted with permission from Som and Biller.[3])

From the Departments of Radiology and Otorhinolaryngology, The Mount Sinai Hospital and School of Medicine of the City University of New York.

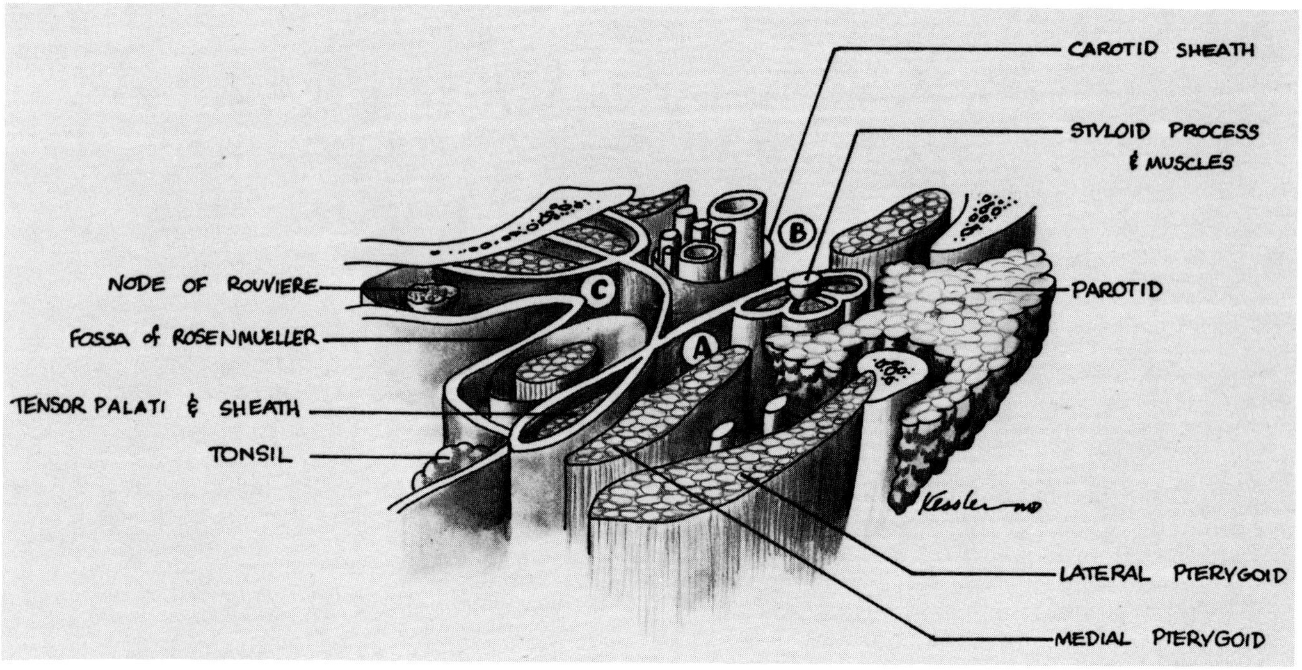

Fig. 2. Normal anatomy of the left parotid gland and parapharyngeal space viewed obliquely and from above. The fascial planes have been emphasized to demonstrate the three compartments of the parapharyngeal space. A - Prestyloid space; B - Retrostyloid space; C - Retropharyngeal space.

retromandibular region or its narrow waist-like isthmus. The parotid gland is not divided into anatomically separate superficial and deep lobes. Rather, this division is an artificial one and is established by a plane between the site of the facial nerve trunk's entrance into the posterior portion of the parotid gland and the posterolateral margin of the mandibular ramus anteriorly. Any parotid tissue lying medial to this plane is considered to be in the deep lobe of the gland. The external carotid artery and the posterior facial vein are in this deep lobe.

The entire gland is enclosed within a fibrous capsule which is continuous with the deep cervical fascia. There are two separate groups of lymph nodes that are in relationship to the gland: a superficial group which is under the outer parotid fascia and a deep group which is both within the substance of the gland and on its undersurface. They all drain into the superior deep cervical nodal chain.

The main parotid duct (Stensen's duct) exits the gland at its anterior border, usually under the body of the zygoma. It crosses the masseter muscle and buccal fat pad before it turns sharply medially to pierce the buccinator muscle and buccal mucosa, then opens intraorally opposite the second upper molar tooth. Stensen's duct lies at a topographic level approximated by a line drawn between the lower margin of the external auditory meatus and a point just above the commissure of the lips. A small accessory parotid gland is present in about one fifth of the cases. It usually rests above Stensen's duct and lies anterior to the main parotid gland.[1-3]

The parapharyngeal space is roughly in the shape of an inverted pyramid whose base is the base of the skull and whose apex is the greater cornu of the hyoid bone. The medial border of this potential space is the superior pharyngeal constrictor muscle and the tonsillar fossa. The lateral boundary is formed respectively from anteriorly to posteriorly by the internal pterygoid muscle, the inner surface of the ramus of the mandible, the deep lobe of the parotid gland and the posterior belly of the diagastric muscle. The posterior boundary is the vertebral column and the paravertebral muscles. Within the fibro-fatty supporting connective tissue matrix of this space are the internal carotid artery, the internal jugular vein, the styloid group of muscles, cranial nerves IX, X, XI, XII, the sympathetic nerve chain and lymph nodes.

Since the base, posterior and lateral walls are bony, masses arising within this space enlarge medially and downward where the boundaries are only

TABLE 1. HISTOLOGY OF PARAPHARYNGEAL SPACE TUMORS (N = 30)

Mixed tumor of the deep lobe of the parotid		5
Mixed tumor of the palate		3
Paraganglioma		5
Schwannoma		6
Miscellaneous		11
Metastatic tumor	2	
Branchial cleft cyst	1	
Liposarcoma	1	
Meningioma	1	
Lymph node	2	
Chordoma	1	
Fibrosarcoma	1	
Hemangioma	1	
Lymphangioma	1	

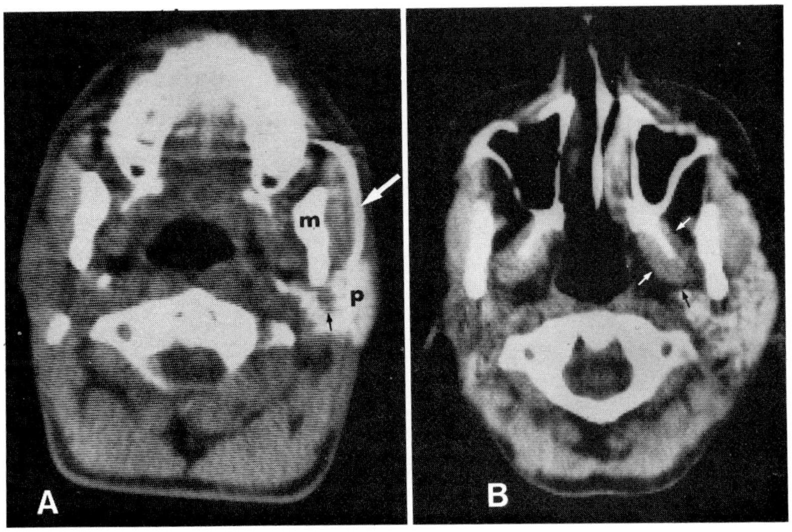

Fig. 3. A) Normal CT sialogram taken parallel to the IOM plane. Contrast is seen in Stensen's duct (white arrow) and the left parotid gland (p). The lucency in the immediate retromandibular region of the gland (black arrow) represents the area of the normal external carotid artery and the posterior facial vein. m - Mandible. B) Normal CT sialogram taken parallel to SOM plane. Normal fat tissue planes (dark areas) are seen adjacent to the internal pterygoid muscle (white arrows) and the medial extent of the parotid deep lobe (black arrow).

composed of soft tissue structures and are thus pliable. Because of this, the most common physical findings are medial bulging of the lateral pharyngeal wall and tonsillar fossa as well as a downward and medial displacement of the palate and/or a mass just below the angle or body of the mandible, near the greater cornu of the hyoid bone.

The parapharyngeal space can be divided into three compartments by its fascial planes (Fig. 2). The fascia enveloping the styloid process and its muscles extends anteromedially to merge with the fascia surrounding the tensor veli palatini muscle. This divides the parapharyngeal space into an anterior (prestyloid) and posterior compartment. Fascia from the carotid sheath extends from this plane posterolaterally to the prevertebral fascia and so divides the posterior compartment into the lateral (retrostyloid) and medial (retropharyngeal) compartment. The convergence of these fascial spaces takes place just below and lateral to the apex of the fossa of Rosenmüller.

These compartments are important primarily in relation to spread of nasopharyngeal neoplasms; however, certain diagnostic criteria and surgical relationships are made clearer by reviewing their anatomy.

The prestyloid space contains the internal and external pterygoid muscles, the mandibular condyle and ramus, and the deep lobe of the parotid gland. The internal maxillary artery and the lingual, inferior dental and auriculotemporal nerves also pass through this space. The lateral nasopharyngeal wall and the fossa of Rosenmüller superiorly and the tonsillar fossa inferiorly relate to the medial wall of the prestyloid space. Directly above lies the greater wing of the sphenoid bone with the foramen ovale and foramen spinosum as well as access into the temporal fossa. The floor of this compartment is related to the submaxillary gland. Disease in this space can cause trismus (pterygoid muscle involvement), bulging of the tonsillar fossa and depression of the soft palate, as well as sensory and motor involvement of the third division of the trigeminal nerve. The facial nerve rarely can be involved via disease extension in the parotid gland.

The retrostyloid space contains the internal carotid artery, internal jugular vein, the four caudal cranial nerves and the cervical sympathetic chain. It also contains numerous lymph nodes. Involvement of this compartment can be either by direct extension or by metastatic lymph node disease. Clinically, symptoms relate primarily to involvement of cranial nerves IX, X, XI, XII and the cervical sympathetic nerves.

The retropharyngeal space is near the midline by position and separates the nasopharynx from the prevertebral muscles and nodes. The node of Rouviere in particular may be involved by metastatic disease. Symptoms are uncommon, but disease extension can progress posteriorly into the spine or anterolaterally into the retrostyloid space.[3-5]

ANALYSIS OF CASES

Thirty patients presenting with a parapharyngeal mass were admitted and operated upon by the Otolaryngology Service of The Mount Sinai Hospital between 1972 and 1980. Most patients were asymptomatic and their mass was either discovered by the patient or by an examining physician. All patients exhibited a bulge of the lateral pharyngeal wall. Most patients had a visible or palpable mass, or fullness at the angle of the mandible. When present, symptoms varied with the size of the tumor and its histologic character. These included aural fullness, sore throat, difficulty in swallowing, voice change, nasal obstruction and symptoms secondary to paralysis of cranial nerves IX, X, XI or XII. The histology of the tumors is shown in Table 1.

RADIOLOGIC PREOPERATIVE EVALUATION

A parotid sialogram is performed first. Ethio-

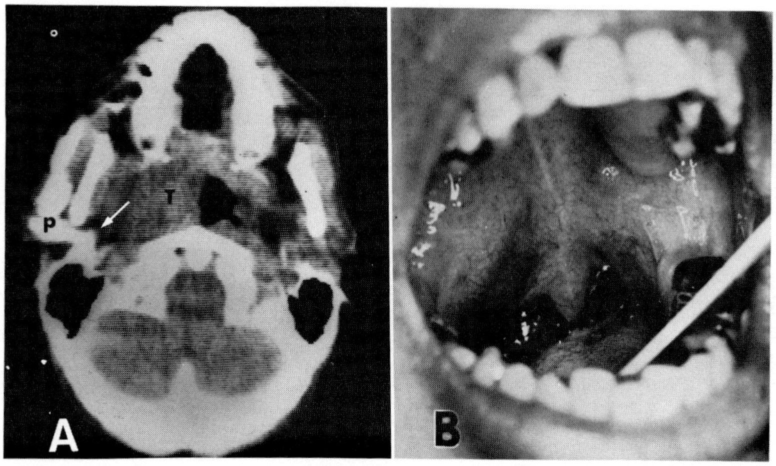

Fig. 4. A) CT sialogram of a nonenhancing extraparotid minor salivary gland benign mixed tumor (T). Note the lucent line (arrow) between the tumor and the contrast-filled parotid deep lobe (p). B) Open mouth picture of same patient showing fullness of the right soft palate and lateral pharyngeal wall.

dal® is used as the contrast medium, but a water-soluble contrast material (Sinografin®) can also be used. After filming, the patient is moved to the CT scanner with the sialographic cannula still in position. This step is important because the in-place cannula inhibits the rapid emptying of the contrast material from the parotid gland. This in turn insures the maximum visualization of the parotid gland on the CT scan.

One of the difficulties with the water-soluble contrast agents is that if the patient cannot be placed on the scanner immediately, the contrast material may resorb by the time the scan is performed. A reinjection at the time of the scanning is then necessary to eliminate this problem.

Before the scan is started, intravenous contrast is administered either by a bolus (50 cc Renographin 60®) or an IV drip (300 cc Reno-M-Dip®). The scan is then preferably performed parallel to the inferior orbital-meatal line (IOM), from the lowermost palpable margin of the mass (usually just below the angle of the mandible) up to the level of the temporomandibular joint.

An alternate scheme is to start the scan and if the mass is seen to be parotid in origin, no intravenous contrast need be given. If the mass is extraparotid, then the contrast is administered. Although this technique may be slightly more time-consuming, it avoids giving intravenous contrast to patients who will not benefit from it.

Many times patients may have considerable scan artifacts caused by metal fillings in the mandibular and/or maxillary teeth. If these artifacts degrade images of particular interest, realigning the scan parallel to the superior orbital-meatal line (SOM) usually allows visualization of the desired levels, albeit with a slightly altered anatomical appearance due to the scan angle (Fig. 3). On those patients with an enhancing extraparotid parapharyngeal mass, a carotid angiogram via femoral catheterization is performed prior to surgery.[3,6]

INTERPRETATION OF THE RADIOGRAPHIC STUDIES

The purpose of the combined CT sialogram is twofold. First, to allow differentiation of a deep lobe parotid tumor from an extraparotid parapharyngeal space mass, and second, to evaluate whether the tumor is an enhancing or nonenhancing mass. The sialographic contrast allows maximal visualization of the parotid gland margins. If a lucent line (zone of decreased attenuation) is seen on the CT scan between the posterolateral margin of the parapharyngeal mass and the contrast-filled parotid gland, then the mass is extraparotid in origin (Figs. 4 and 5). This line need not be seen on all scans, but if present it should be seen on most cuts through the main body of the tumor. A line usually will be seen at the extreme upper and lower margins

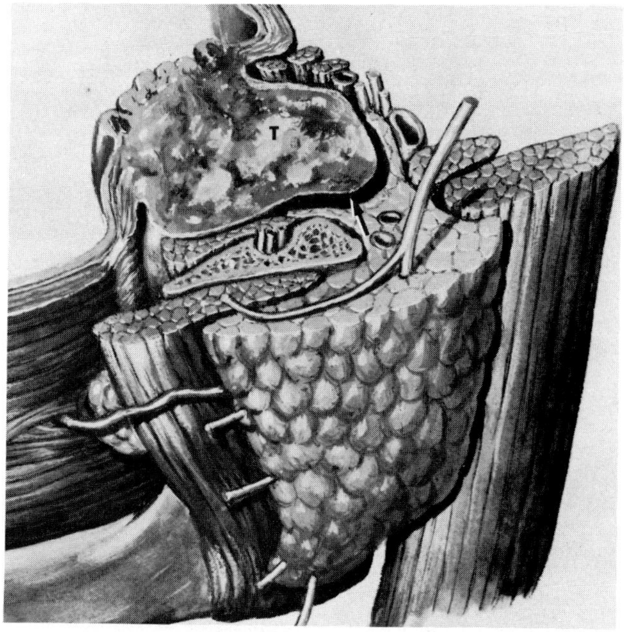

Fig. 5. The parapharyngeal space seen obliquely and from above illustrates a minor salivary gland tumor (T) growing from the lateral pharyngeal wall. The arrow points to the fibro-fatty tissue of the parapharyngeal space compressed between the mass and the parotid gland. This gives the lucent line seen on CT scanning.

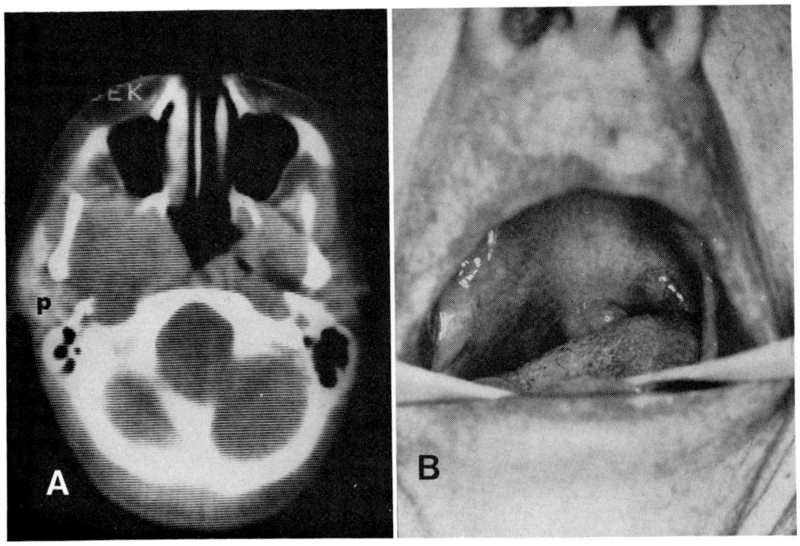

Fig. 6. A) CT sialogram reveals a right parapharyngeal space nonenhancing mass with no lucent line between the mass and the contrast-filled parotid gland (p). Deep lobe parotid mixed tumor. B) Open mouth picture of same patient showing a bulging of the right soft palate and lateral pharyngeal wall. Clinically it is similar to Fig. 4B.

of the mass, but it is not diagnostic in these regions. This line represents the fibro-fatty supporting matrix of the parapharyngeal space as it is compressed between the mass and the deep lobe of the parotid gland. If no line is seen on the midtumor scans, then the mass is a deep lobe parotid tumor (Figs. 6 and 7).[3,6]

As each generation of new scanners brings better resolution, it is now possible to outline the parotid gland without first doing a sialogram. However, one cannot obtain routine sialographic information about the tumor (abrupt ductal cutoff or ductal displacement) and one will not be able to consistently localize the lucent line against the normal decreased attenuation of the parotid gland. Since this is a crucial point in the workup, a sialogram is performed routinely to allow the greatest accuracy, reliability and return of information from this study.

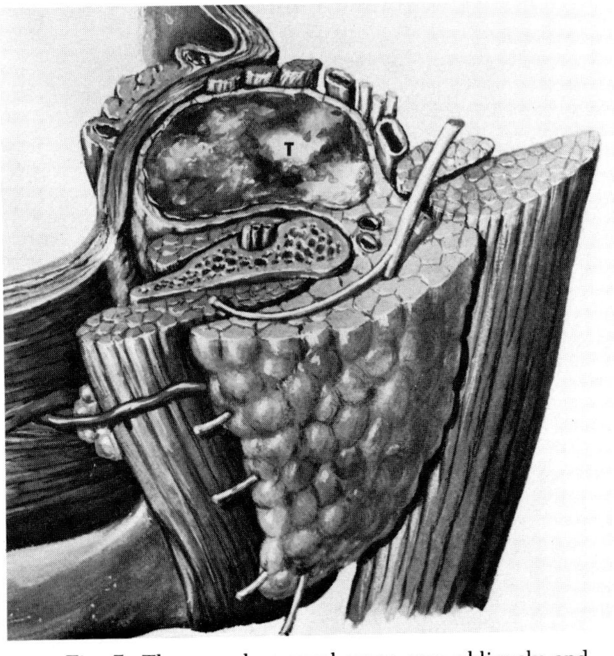

Fig. 7. The parapharyngeal space seen obliquely and from above illustrates a deep lobe parotid gland tumor (T). Since the mass originates from the parotid gland, there is no intervening compressed fibro-fatty tissue (compare to Fig. 5).

NONENHANCING PARAPHARYNGEAL SPACE MASSES

Less than 10% of all parotid tumors are located in the deep lobe. Of these deep lobe tumors, 80-90% are benign mixed tumors and the remaining lesions of significance are acinic cell, adenoid cystic and mucoepidermoid carcinomas. If the sialogram does not detect the malignant nature of the carcinoma, malignant tumors of the deep lobe cannot be differentiated preoperatively. Symptomatically, malignant deep lobe parotid tumors can be suspected if pain and facial paresis are present.[7]

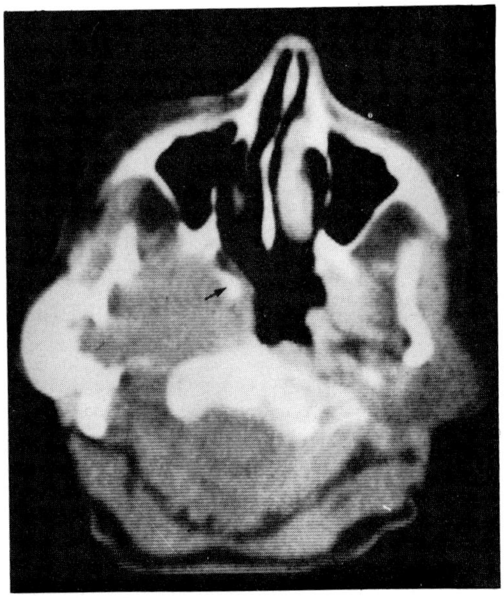

Fig. 8. CT sialogram reveals a dumbbell-shaped mixed tumor of the parotid deep lobe. It is a nonenhancing mass. Contrast material from the sialogram is seen lying on the medial surface of the mass (arrow) in displaced parotid ducts.

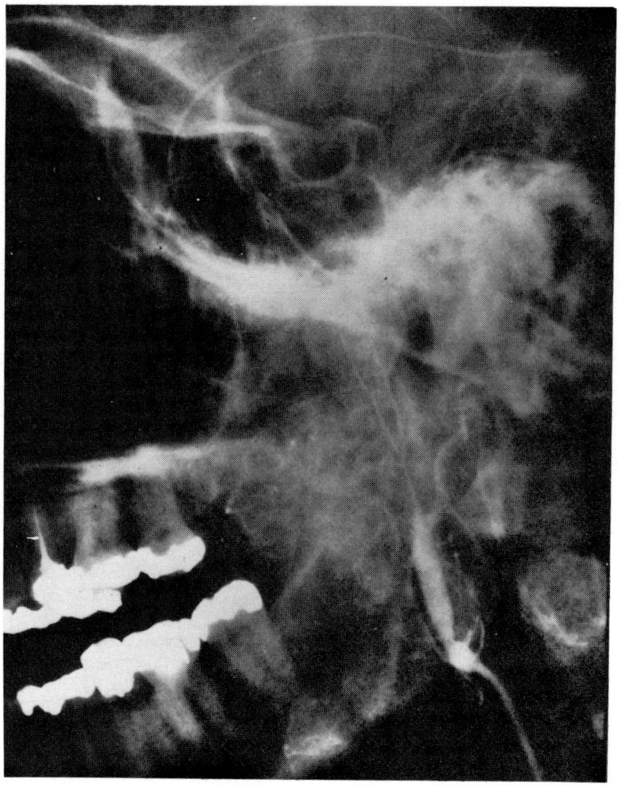

Fig. 9. Lateral film from subselective carotid angiogram reveals very minimal tumor vascularity. This was a benign mixed tumor of minor salivary gland origin and did not enhance on the CT scan.

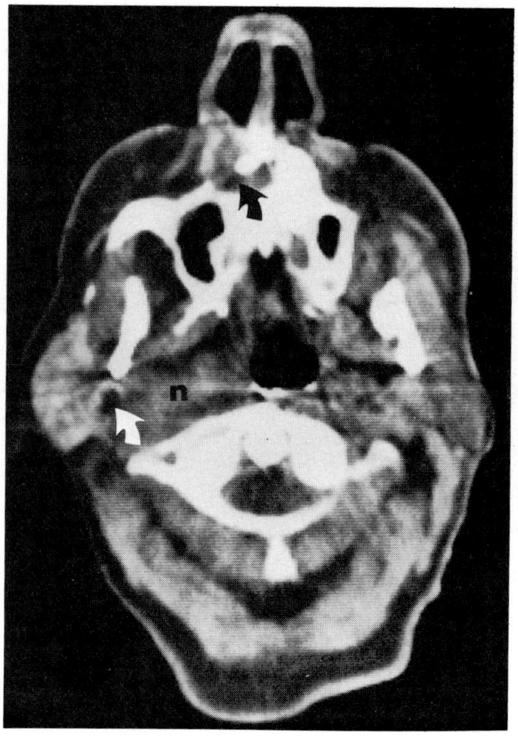

Fig. 10. CT sialogram reveals a slightly nodular right parapharyngeal mass (n) with a lucent line between it and the contrast-filled parotid gland (white arrow). In addition, there is osseous destruction of the right anterior maxilla (black arrow). Metastatic squamous cell carcinoma to bone and pharyngeal space nodes.

A special comment should be made about the configuration of deep lobe parotid tumors. There are two shapes, the dumbbell and the round (Figs. 6-8). Most have the hourglass or dumbbell configuration which results from the tumor arising in the deep lobe lateral to the stylomandibular tunnel. As the mass grows medially, its growth is physically restricted by this tunnel and further expansion only can occur deep to this area. Thus a mass is seen on each side of the stylomandibular tunnel with its waist marking the location of this structure.[8]

If the tumor arises deep to the stylomandibular tunnel, it grows as a rounded mass. This appearance is less common than the dumbbell shape and may be more easily clinically confused with an extraparotid pharyngeal mass.

Most parapharyngeal tumors are salivary in origin, arising in the parotid gland or from minor salivary glands. All of the minor salivary gland lesions in our series were benign mixed tumors and occurred either in the palate or the lateral pharyngeal wall (Fig. 5). None of these tumors enhanced and since carotid angiograms performed on several of our cases failed to reveal a significant vascular blush or tumor vascularity, we no longer believe it is necessary to do angiograms on nonenhancing masses (Fig. 9). No significant additional information was gained from this invasive procedure.

Lymphomatous and metastatic nodal involvement of the parapharyngeal space also appeared as a nonenhancing mass. No large solitary mass was identified as with minor salivary gland lesions and in most cases the slightly nodular contour suggested a nodal lesion (Fig. 10).

A variety of miscellaneous lesions have been reported in the parapharyngeal space. There is nothing unique or specific about their appearance on the scan. It is only the rarity of these lesions that makes them an unlikely diagnosis.[7-9]

LOW DENSITY PARAPHARYNGEAL MASSES

Lipomas, liposarcomas and hibernomas rarely involve the parapharyngeal space. Their fat content should allow identification as a low attenuation mass on CT scan (Fig. 11). Dermoids and teratomas have been reported to occur in the parapharyngeal space. In addition to low density areas, these lesions may have areas that are either isodense or calcified, suggesting their diagnosis.

ENHANCING PARAPHARYNGEAL MASSES

The only deep lobe parotid tumor that significantly enhances is the hemangioma. The most common enhancing extraparotid lesion is the schwannoma which accounts for nearly 20% of all parapharyngeal space lesions. The sites of origin are primar-

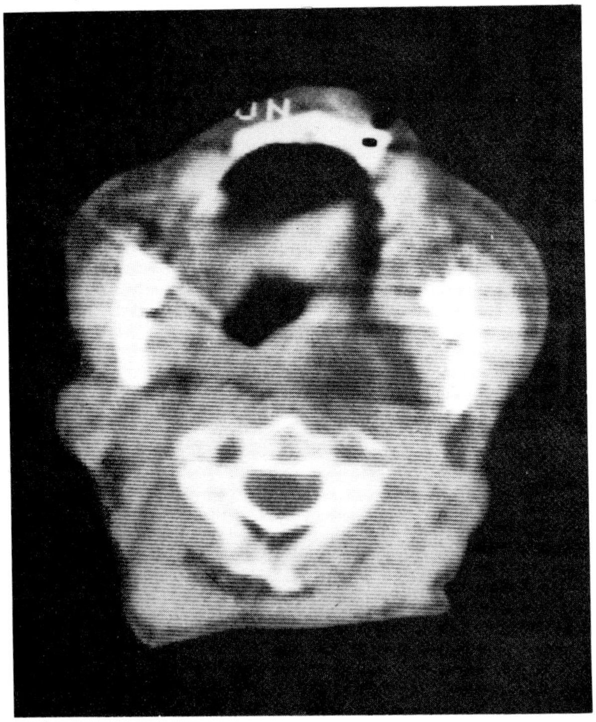

Fig. 11. Nonenhanced CT scan reveals a left parapharyngeal space mass of decreased attenuation. (Liposarcoma.)

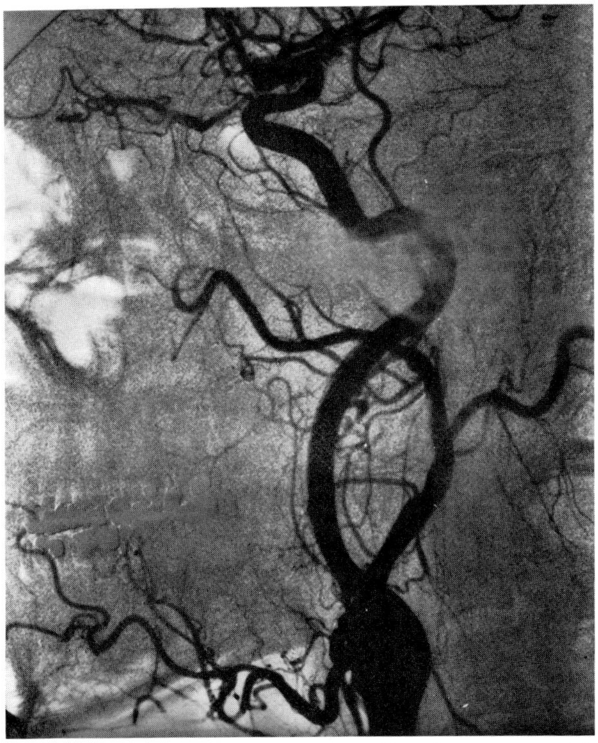

Fig. 13. Lateral subtraction film from a carotid angiogram reveals an avascular mass bowing and displacing the internal and external carotid arteries. (Schwannoma.)

ily the vagus nerve and the sympathetic chain. Usually they occur as solitary masses which may or may not cause symptoms referable to the nerve of origin. Often symptoms are produced by adjacent nerves which are stretched over the tumor mass. Almost all are benign and enhance with contrast. Since areas of hemorrhage or cystic degeneration can occur, some tumor areas may not enhance, with this irregular enhancement actually suggesting the specific diagnosis (Fig. 12A,B).

An angiogram will usually show anteromedial displacement of the internal carotid artery although because of the variable location and level of occurrence within the retrostyloid space this anteromedial displacement is not constant (Fig. 13). These are basically avascular lesions and the contrast enhancement appears to be on the basis of extravascular accumulation of the contrast medium.

Neurofibromas are rare and usually occur as multiple lesions. There need not be an association with neurofibromatosis. Roentgenographically, they are indistinguishable from schwannomas.

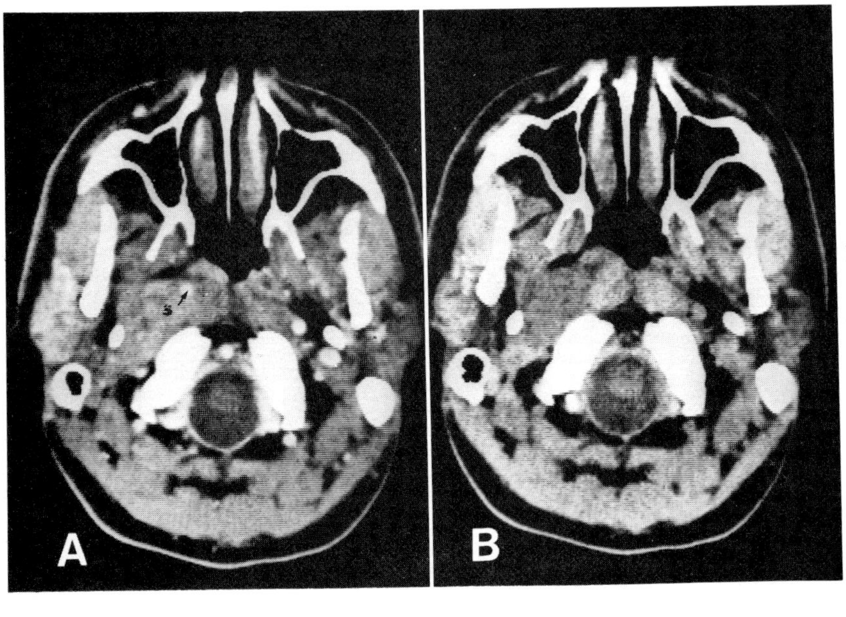

Fig. 12. A) CT sialogram reveals a slightly enhanced extraparotid right parapharyngeal space mass (s). The internal carotid artery is pushed anteriorly (arrow). B) CT sialogram at slightly different level reveals the mass to have a decreased attenuation. (Schwannoma.)

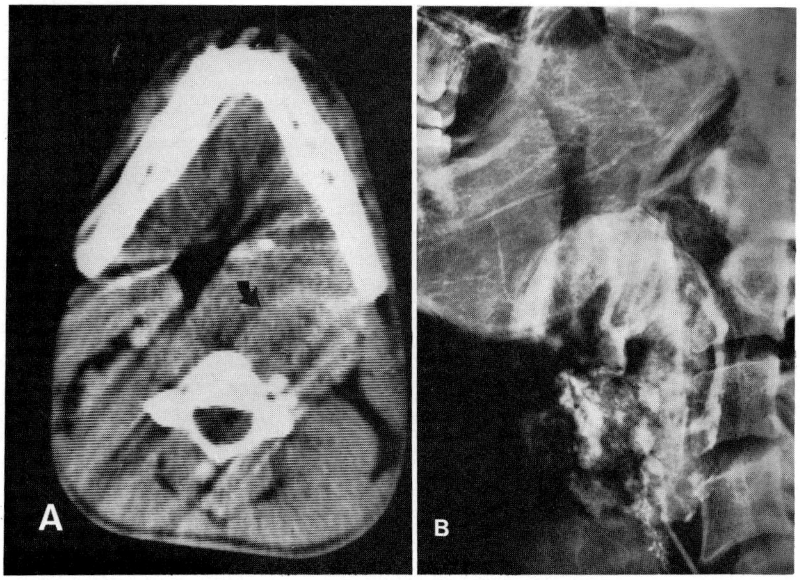

Fig. 14. A) Contrast-enhanced CT scan of the lower parapharyngeal space reveals an enhancing mass deep to the pharyngeal musculature (arrow). B) Lateral film from the end of a subselective carotid angiogram reveals the typical vascular pattern of a paraganglioma. (Carotid body tumor.)

Paragangliomas of the parapharyngeal space represent tumors arising from the carotid body or from glomic tissue associated with the ganglion nodosum of the vagus nerve. Usually the carotid body lesions are located lower in the neck and only 8% extend into the parapharyngeal space (Fig. 14). On the other hand, two thirds of the glomus vagale tumors are parapharyngeal in position (Figs. 15 and 16). These lesions uniformly enhance and show a characteristic pattern of vascularity on carotid angiography. The tumor vasculature is maximally distended with the angiogram, consequently the paragangliomas always appear larger arteriographically than at surgery. The CT scan gives a more accurate assessment of the actual tumor size.

Meningiomas and metastases can extend downward into the parapharyngeal space from the skull base. Our case of meningioma was diagnosed preoperatively because of the detection of an intracranial component of the tumor (Fig. 17). At the time the CT scan is performed, the person monitoring the examination must continue taking scans upwards through the base of the skull and intracranially if the parapharyngeal tumor is seen to extend up to the skull base. In this way, destruction of the skull or intracranial disease will not be overlooked.

SELECTION OF SURGICAL EXPOSURE FOR TUMOR RESECTION

The ability to accurately assess preoperatively both tumor size and in most cases the tumor histology allows selection of an appropriate surgical exposure. This exposure should enable total tumor extirpation with the least incidence of morbidity and tumor recurrence.

The approaches to the parapharyngeal space include 1) peroral, 2) cervical with or without angle mandibulotomy, 3) transparotid-cervical with or without angle mandibulotomy, and 4) cervical-transpharyngeal with midline mandibulotomy.

Peroral Excision. This approach can be utilized

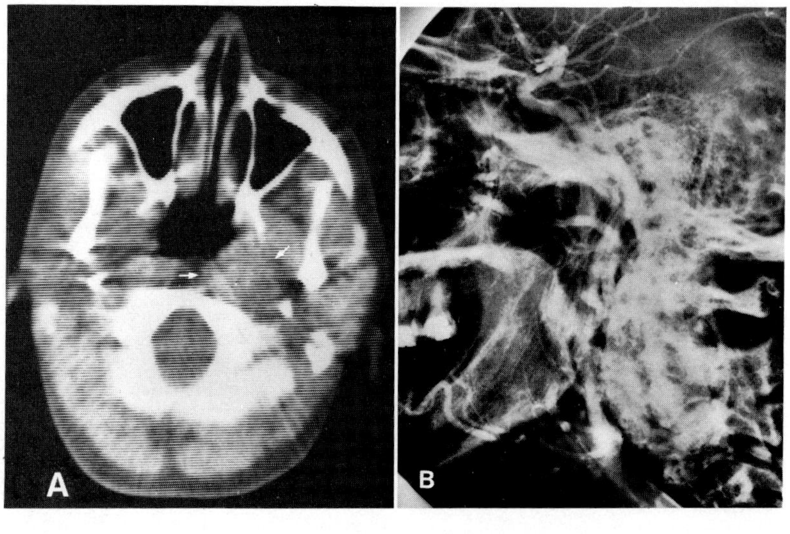

Fig. 15. A) CT sialogram reveals an enhancing extraparotid parapharyngeal space mass (arrows). B) Lateral carotid angiogram film reveals typical paraganglioma vascular stain. (Glomus vagale tumor.)

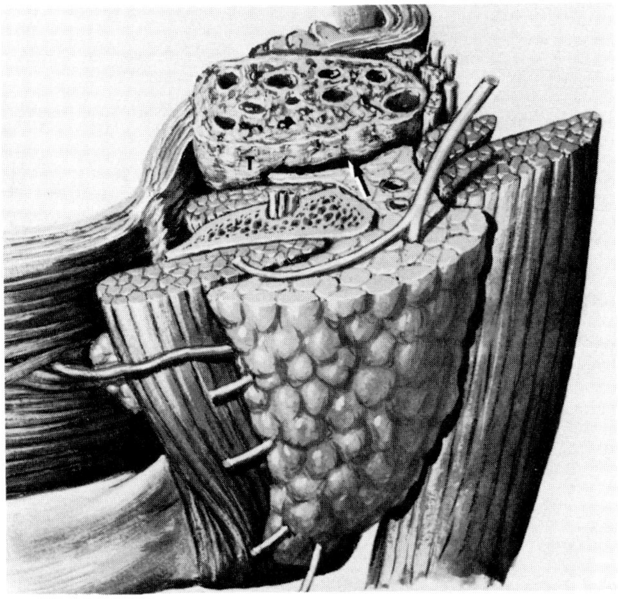

Fig. 16. The parapharyngeal space seen obliquely and from above illustrates a vascular tumor mass (T) arising from within the parapharyngeal space. The compressed fibro-fatty tissue (arrow) is seen between the mass and the parotid deep lobe. (Paraganglioma.)

for small mixed tumors arising from the palate or lateral pharyngeal wall. The size of the tumor and the fact that it is most likely a mixed tumor are determined by the preoperative evaluation. Peroral removal alone should be reserved for tumors which do not as yet extend to the area of the styloid process. When the tumor is large and extends up to the styloid process, a combined technique is preferred. This consists of a cervical approach with separation of the tumor by blunt dissection followed by tumor removal perorally. The resulting space available for tumor removal is larger when utilizing a peroral approach than it is when using the cervical approach. Therefore, tumor rupture is more likely to occur when using the cervical approach alone. In addition, the peroral technique allows excision of the mucosa if a prior transoral biopsy has been performed.

Cervical Approach. The cervical approach involves a transverse incision at the level of the hyoid bone. The submaxillary gland and the fascia are incised and the gland is reflected superiorly. The digastric tendon is followed posteriorly until the styloglossus muscle and the stylohyoid ligament are identified. These structures are severed and the parapharyngeal space is entered. Exposure is limited, but blunt finger dissection is possible and a parapharyngeal space tumor of small size can be removed. This technique, therefore, is reserved for small extraparotid tumors. Its disadvantage is the limited exposure medially, superiorly and posteriorly. This necessitates finger dissection and results in poor control of vascular structures at the skull base. In addition, there is limited room for extraction of the tumor mass. The operative field may be improved by dislocating the mandible anteriorly. If there is still insufficient room, an osteotomy may be performed at the angle of the mandible without facial nerve exposure (Fig. 18).

Transparotid-Cervical Approach. This approach is utilized for deep lobe parotid tumors. Routine isolation of the facial nerve is necessary to avoid its injury. A superficial lobectomy is then performed and the branches of the facial nerve are retracted. If necessary, the styloid process is sectioned, the mandible is dislocated anteriorly and then the tumor is removed by blunt dissection (Fig. 19). If the tumor is so large that there is insufficient exposure to avoid the possibility of tumor rupture during removal, an osteotomy is performed at the angle of the mandible. This osteotomy transects the inferior alveolar

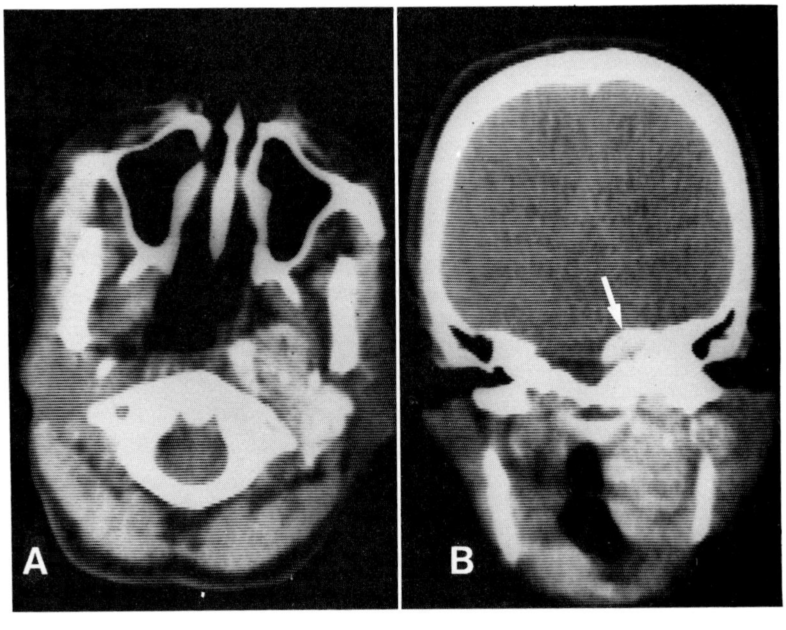

Fig. 17. A) Axial CT enhanced study reveals a partially calcified enhancing parapharyngeal space mass. B) Coronal CT scan reveals the extent of the calcified enhancing mass not only in the parapharyngeal space, but also intracranially (arrow). (Meningioma.)

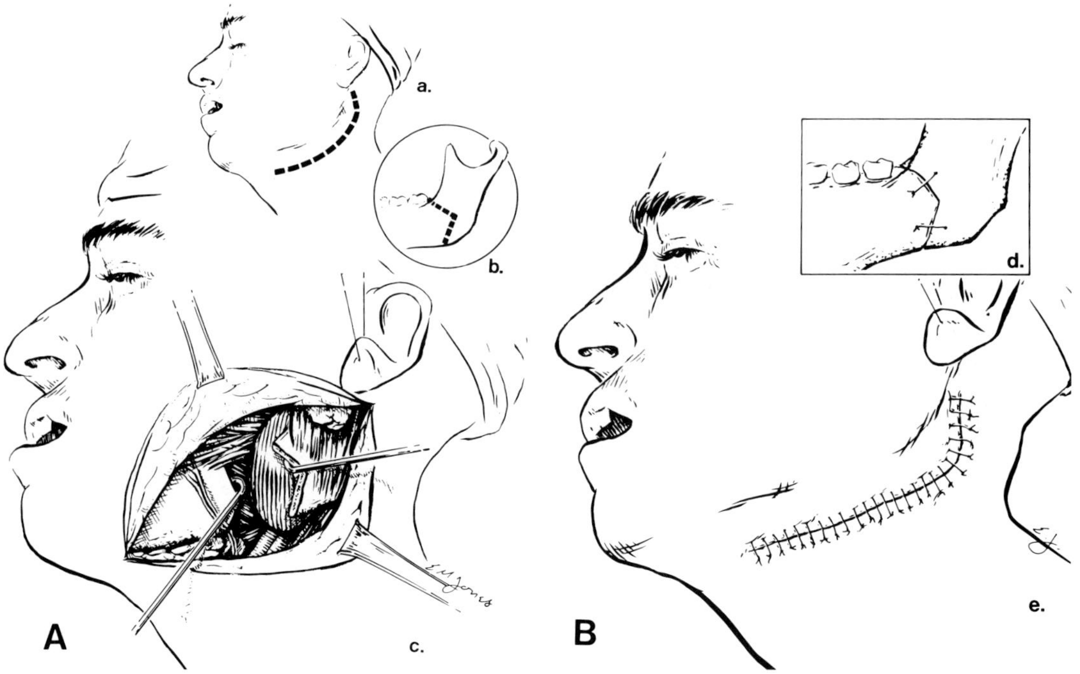

Fig. 18. Diagram of the transcervical approach with an osteotomy. A) a - Incision; b - Osteotomy outline; c - Exposure. Note that the facial nerve is not exposed. B) d - Rewiring osteotomy; e - Closure.

nerve. The resulting exposure is limited at the base of the skull medially and posteriorly. Extraction of the tumor is usually accomplished by blunt finger dissection and injury to the lingual nerve is likely.

Cervical-Transpharyngeal with Midline Mandibulotomy. This approach is primarily reserved for the large extraparotid parapharyngeal space tumors which are vascular and for which maximum exposure at the base of skull is required both for control of bleeding and tumor removal. However, its wide exposure is also excellent for removal of large tumors involving the parotid deep lobe and for deep lobe lesions which are thought to be malignant.

A tracheotomy is required. Exposure is accomplished via a transverse incision at the level of the hyoid bone, the medial limb of which extends superiorly to split the lip in the midline (Fig. 20A). A midline osteotomy is performed with a Gigli saw after drill holes are made (Fig. 20B). The osteotomy cut is beveled both in the vertical and horizontal planes. The floor of the mouth is incised along the lateral gutter midway between the alveolus and the tongue. The incision is extended to the superior aspect of the anterior tonsillar pillar (Fig. 20C). The lingual and hypoglossal nerves are identified and preserved. The mandible is retracted laterally after severing the floor of the mouth musculature (Fig. 20D). The internal and external carotid arteries are identified and secured with tapes. The submaxillary gland is retracted superiorly and the external carotid artery is ligated and divided. Exposure is now adequate for tumor excision. If this approach is used for deep lobe parotid tumors, then the facial nerve is isolated. Interdental wiring is not required at closure (Fig. 20E). The disadvantages of this exposure are the necessity of tracheotomy, a temporary lingual nerve deficiency, and a minimal cosmetically detracting scar.

DISCUSSION

The symptoms relating to a parapharyngeal

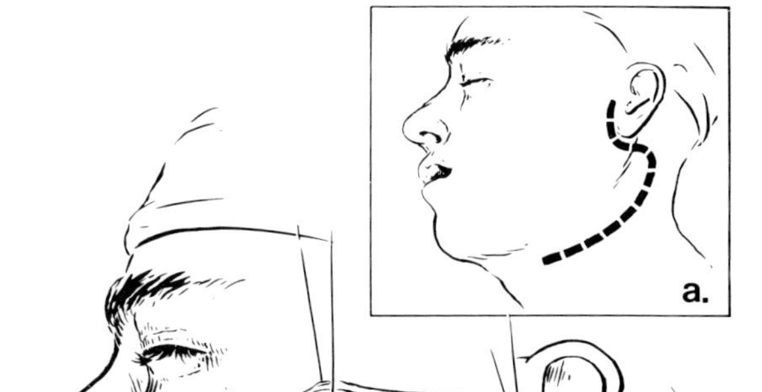

Fig. 19. Diagram of the transparotid approach. a) Incision. b) The facial nerve is identified and a superficial parotidectomy is performed. The tumor is then extracted inferior to the facial nerve. An osteotomy can also be performed.

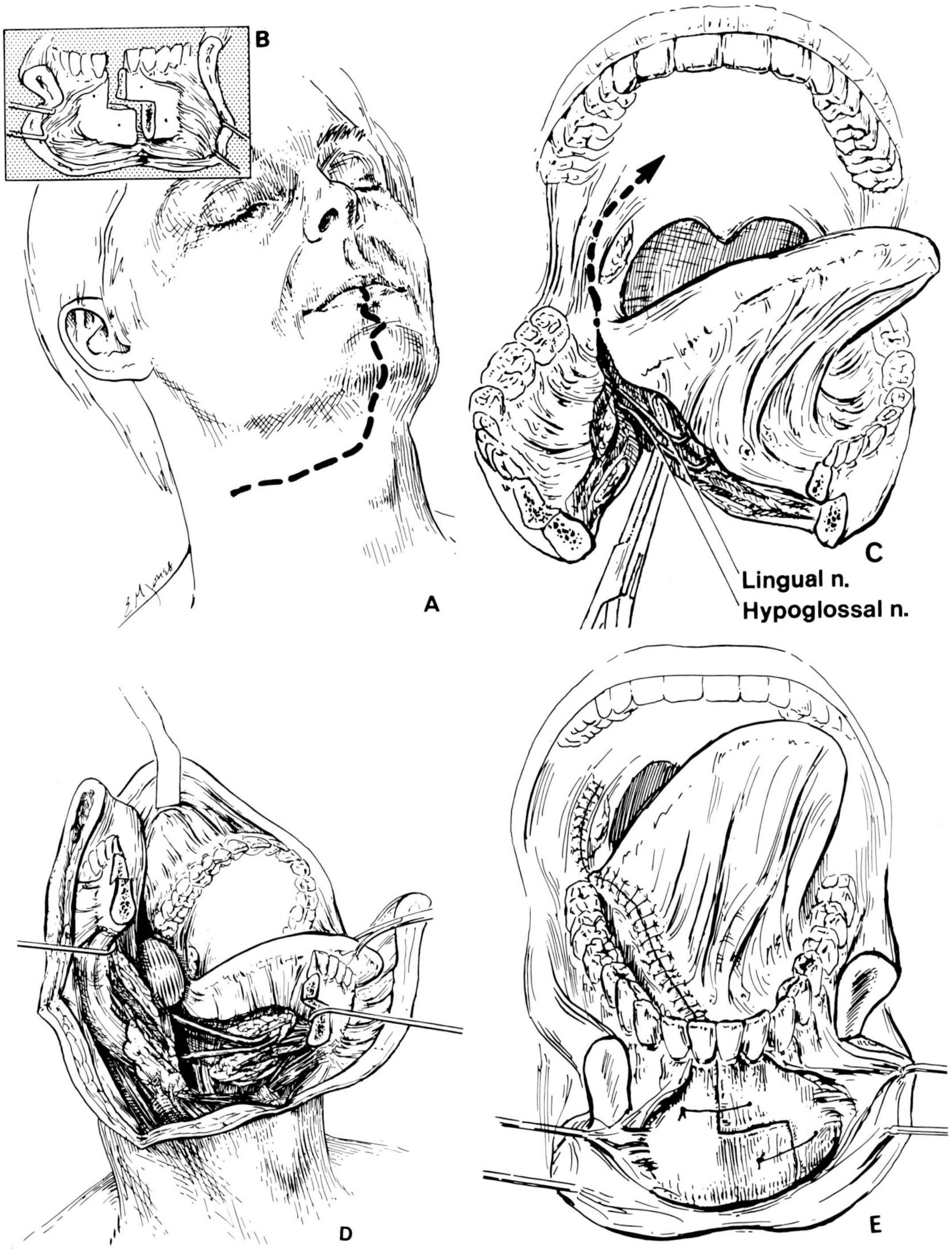

Fig. 20. Diagram of the cervical transpharyngeal approach. A) Incision; B) Osteotomy — midline; C) Following mandibulotomy, the floor of the mouth is incised preserving the lingual and hypoglossal nerves. The mucosal incision is then extended upward to the anterior tonsillar pillar and the palate. D) Retraction of the mandible yields an excellent exposure of the parapharyngeal space. E) Mucosal closure is with interrupted sutures, with wires closing the mandibulotomy. Interdental wiring is not required.

space tumor are usually minimal. In most cases, the patient is incidentally noted to have a bulge in the lateral pharyngeal wall on routine examination, or the patient notices a mass at the angle of the mandible. Involvement of the four caudal cranial nerves, or the sympathetic chain, may be present with tumors that are large or malignant, most commonly schwannomas, or paragangliomas. Facial nerve paralysis is always related to malignant tumors of the deep lobe. Eustachian tube obstruction resulting in hearing loss may be present. Throat discomfort, dysphagia, nasal obstruction, or a change in voice may also occur.

Physical diagnosis establishes that the parapharyngeal space is expanded, a bulge of the lateral pharyngeal wall being present. If the tumor is large enough, a mass at the angle of the mandible will also be palpable. Smaller masses may require bimanual palpation to diagnose any parapharyngeal space involvement. A preauricular discrete mass associated with lateral pharyngeal wall bulging indicates a bilobed tumor of the parotid gland. Involvement of the retromandibular extension of the parotid gland will result in a mass which cannot be differentiated on physical examination from any other parapharyngeal space tumor. Similarly, minor salivary gland tumors which originate in the pharynx and enlarge sufficiently to extend into the parapharyngeal space cannot be distinguished clinically from any other parapharyngeal space tumor. Although some surgeons[10] feel that the character of the oral mass permits differentiation between a deep lobe parotid and a tumor of minor salivary gland origin, the authors are of the opinion that this differentiation is not possible. In addition, it is difficult to differentiate even at surgery whether a large mixed tumor arises from a major or minor salivary gland. This is because the usual mode of tumor removal is one of blunt dissection and therefore the attachment to the parotid may not be discernible.

Palpable pulsations over the mass are inaccurate for evaluating intrinsic tumor vascularity. Frequently the pulsations are transmitted, or conversely, vascular tumors may not cause pulsations. Physical examination alone, therefore, is only diagnostic of an expanded parapharyngeal space and does not reveal the specific tumor type. Multidirectional tomograms and conventional sialograms, likewise, do not aid in distinguishing the type of tumor present. It was the advent of the CT scan and the CT sialogram that has allowed a more systematic preoperative evaluation which gives the following information: 1) determines which tumor requires preoperative angiography, 2) determines the size and extent of the tumor, 3) differentiates between parotid and extraparotid origin, and 4) suggests in many cases the probable histology.

Initially, angiography was advocated in selected cases in which the tumor was thought to be vascular.[9] Later, it was employed routinely in all cases of parapharyngeal space tumors.[11-14] This allowed a preoperative diagnosis of vascular lesions which were usually either carotid body or glomus vagale tumors. Rarely, fibrosarcomas and malignant histiocytomas demonstrate a vascular stain. Displacement of the internal carotid artery anteriorly by an avascular mass was frequently diagnostic of schwannomas arising primarily from the vagus nerve or sympathetic chain.

Angiography is of no diagnostic value with the mixed tumor, which represents the majority of parapharyngeal space tumors. If the tumor does not enhance on the CT scan, angiography is noncontributory in virtually all cases. Exceptions would be related to a huge tumor size, or the suspicion of a malignancy with vascular encasement or invasion. Thus, using these criteria, an invasive procedure with a low but recognized morbidity can be avoided in the majority of cases.

The CT scan also allows accurate assessment of the extent of tumor involvement. This is particularly important in establishing whether intracranial extension and/or pterygopalatine space involvement has occurred. Either of these situations requires additional surgical exposure.

The ability to preoperatively differentiate between a parotid and an extraparotid mass is critical if the correct surgical approach is to be planned. Until the present time all parapharyngeal space tumors were excised through either a cervical or transparotid approach with isolation of the facial nerve.[8-14] Although peroral excision has been used extensively in the past,[15,16] recent authors have condemned it because of the risk of hemorrhage and inability to control bleeding, the chance of tumor rupture or subtotal removal, the possibility of facial nerve injury, and wound contamination with subsequent infection.[8-14] A transparotid approach with facial nerve dissection is essential for all deep lobe tumors. However, a superficial parotidectomy and facial nerve exposure is not necessary if the lesion is extraparotid in origin. In these cases, a transcervical approach can be utilized with anterior displacement of the submaxillary gland. The tumor removal is usually by blunt finger dissection. However, the medial, posterior and superior dissection is not performed under direct vision because of the limited exposure. If the tumor is too large to extract, with the danger of capsular rupture, anterior dislocation of the mandible and fracture of the styloid process can be performed to increase the size of the operative field. All attempts should be made to avoid rupture of a mixed tumor's capsule because of the associated high recurrence rate. If tumor rupture is still imminent, an osteotomy at the angle of the mandible will further widen the field. Unfortunately, this osteotomy does not enhance the exposure medially, posteriorly, or superiorly; it also severs the inferior alveolar nerve and frequently the lingual nerve. Once an extraparotid mixed tumor is mobilized and there still appears to be limited space for removal inferior to the mandible, another route of extraction is possible. Although transoral tumor removal is dangerous because of the possibility of poor control of bleeding and the greater incidence of capsular rupture while trying to free the tumor laterally, peroral extraction can be safely combined with transcervical mobilization of the tumor. The resulting space for extraction is greater via the oral cavity than it is through the neck incision without an angle osteotomy. This alternative to osteotomy should be considered especially if a previous transoral biopsy has been performed which requires excision of the biopsy site.

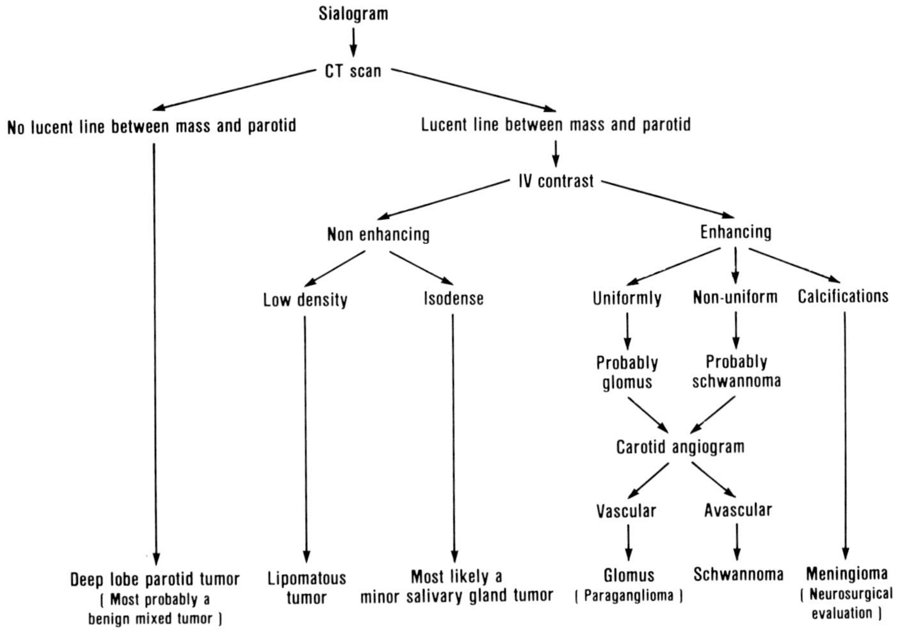

Fig. 21. Flow chart summarizing preoperative evaluation of parapharyngeal space tumors.

Tumors which extend to the skull base are usually schwannomas or paragangliomas and require greater exposure than that provided by the transcervical or transparotid approach with angle osteotomy. The cervical-transpharyngeal approach with a midline osteotomy provides complete exposure medially, posteriorly and at the skull base. It thus provides maximal vascular control. The carotid artery is covered with prevertebral fascia or a dermal graft at the end of the procedure to prevent carotid rupture in the event of a postoperative infection secondary to oral suture line dehiscence. This latter approach has proven to be more advantageous than the previously cited methods and the cosmetic deformity is minimal. In addition, there is no functional deficiency or injury to the lingual or inferior alveolar nerves.

The flow chart shown in Figure 21 summarizes our preoperative evaluation of parapharyngeal space tumors. By utilizing it, mixed tumors, paragangliomas and schwannomas can be clinically identified with a high degree of confidence. Since these tumors comprise 70-85% of all tumors involving this space, obtaining a presumptive histologic diagnosis preoperatively permits selection of the best surgical approach for tumor removal.

REFERENCES

1. Johns ME. The salivary glands: anatomy and embryology. Otolaryngol Clin North Am 1977; 10:261-71.

2. Gray H. Anatomy of the human body. 27th ed. Goss CM, ed. Philadelphia: Lea & Febiger, 1963:1237-9.

3. Som PM, Biller HF. The combined CT sialogram. Radiology 1980; 135:387-90.

4. Heeneman H, Gilbert JJ, Rood SR. The parapharyngeal space: anatomy and pathologic conditions with emphasis on neurogenous tumors. Rochester, Minn: Am Acad Otolaryngol, 1980.

5. Lederman M. Cancer of the nasopharynx. Its natural history and treatment. Springfield, Ill: Charles C Thomas, 1961:7-27.

6. Som PM, Biller HF. The combined computerized tomography-sialogram. A technique to differentiate deep lobe parotid tumors from extraparotid pharyngomaxillary space tumors. Ann Otol Rhinol Laryngol 1979; 88:590-5.

7. Batsakis J. Tumors of the head and neck. Clinical and pathological considerations. 2nd ed. Baltimore: Williams and Wilkins, 1979: 1-120; 240-380; 448-91.

8. Work WP. Parapharyngeal space and salivary gland neoplasms. Otolaryngol Clin North Am 1977; 10:421-6.

9. Work WP. Tumors of the parapharyngeal space. Trans Am Acad Ophthalmol Otolaryngol 1969; 73:389-94.

10. Baker D, Conley J. Surgical approach to retromandibular parotid tumors. Ann Plast Surg 1979; 3:304-12.

11. Work WP, Hybels R. A study of tumors of the parapharyngeal space. Laryngoscope 1974; 84:1748-55.

12. McLean WC. Differential diagnosis and management of deep lobe parotid tumors. Laryngoscope 1976; 86:28-33.

13. Lawson V. Unusual parapharyngeal lesions. J Otolaryngol 1979; 8:241-50.

14. Heeneman H, Maran A. Parapharyngeal space tumors. Clin Otolaryngol 1979; 4:57-66.

15. Havens FZ, Butler LC. Mixed tumors of the posterior pharyngeal wall. Ann Otol Rhinol Laryngol 1955; 64:457-65.

16. McIlrath DC. Tumors of the parapharyngeal region. Surg Gynecol Obstet 1963; 116:88-94.

CONTENTS

Introduction 3
Goals
Atresia Auris Congenita

Methods 4

Results 4
Incidence of Experimentally Produced Malformations
Types of Ear and Skull Malformations
Observations on Experimentally Produced Atresia Auris Congenita in Rat Fetuses
Formation of the Atresia Plate
Observations on Experimentally Induced Atresia Auris Congenita in Adult Animals

Discussion 7
Suspected Mode of Action of Teratogenic Substances
Deformed Ears and Neighboring Regions
Clinical Meaning of the Experimental Results

VITAMIN A-INDUCED EAR MALFORMATIONS IN RATS AS A MODEL FOR ANALYSIS OF ATRESIA AURIS CONGENITA

A MICROSURGICAL AND HISTOLOGICAL STUDY

MANFRED WEIDENBECHER, MD

ERLANGEN, GERMANY

Teratogenic damage was induced in pregnant Wistar rats with an overdose of vitamin A to clarify the genesis of the atresia plate, the behavior of the facial nerve, and the rotation of the middle ear. Results suggested that contradictory statements in the literature concerning the atresia plate could be explained in the following way: the plate does not arise from a single branchial arch. The os tympanicum, the pars squamosa of the temporal bone, and the hyperplastic labyrinthine capsule share in its formation. Findings similar to the human atresia auris congenita, such as malformation of the auricle, atresia of the external ear canal, and changes in the ossicles and lumen of the middle ear space, were obtained. A cranial and labyrinthine dysmorphia leads to rotation of the middle ear and a walling-in of the facial nerve, which explains its functional disturbance. Extreme variations in the course of the facial nerve were not found. In 62 cases of severe human ear malformation, the operative findings corresponded to the experimentally produced ear malformations.

INTRODUCTION

GOALS

Until now, no successful explanation of the genesis of ear atresia has resulted from histological investigation of human temporal bone pathology.[1-3] The creation of similar malformations in an animal model was undertaken by inducing teratogenic damage in rats with overdoses of vitamin A. The following questions were posed:

1. From what structures does the atresia plate arise?

2. Is the bony deformity and displacement of the external auditory canal related to excessive or inhibited bony development?

3. What causes the rotation of the middle ear seen in human ear malformation?

4. Is the observed atypical course of the facial nerve in the temporal bone an exceptional or common occurrence?

5. Is complete or incomplete facial nerve paralysis caused by a dysplasia of the facial nerve due to a mechanical disturbance of the nerve's course through the temporal bone?

ATRESIA AURIS CONGENITA

Atresia auris congenita includes a group of congenital ear dysplasias of different forms and severity. Malformations occur when damage takes place before the end of the second fetal month. Virchow[4] stated that the cause is not only simple suppression, but "active, irritating, locally active, irreversible exogenic proceedings." Often aplasia or hypoplasia of the os tympanicum is found, and the mandible articulates with the anterior part of the mastoid process. Furthermore, the pyramid is changed in its orientation to surrounding structures; it is rotated medially and downward.[5]

Atresia Plate. The atresia plate is 2-12 mm thick, bony, partly homogeneous, and partly spongy. Lüscher[6] states that it is divided by fibrous tissue into a medial and lateral lamella. The atresia plate is the border between the external canal and the middle ear. The tympanic membrane is usually absent or rudimentary.[7] The plate is reported to lie medial to the position where the eardrum is normally located and is united with the tegmen tympani. The plate continues downwards into a network of bony trabeculae, which extend to the middle ear spaces.

The genesis of the plate is unclear, as indicated by the many hypotheses in the literature:

1. Proliferation of the styloid processes in combination with the os tympanicum.[8] The end of the styloid process projects from below like a club into the middle ear space, forming a morphologic unity with the tegmen tympani.

2. Hypertrophy of the styloid process in combination with hypoplasia of the os tympanicum.[9,10] In these cases the os tympanicum is found as a rudimentary structure in the form of an arch or plate.

3. Hyperplasia of the os tympanicum.[11] The hyperplastic, concentrically growing os tympanicum narrows or closes the external auditory canal against which the hyperplastic styloid process rests.

4. Hyperplasia of the pars mastoidea.[12] Because of hypoplasia of the os tympanicum, the pars mastoidea undergoes compensatory hyperplasia.

5. Process of the pars squamosa. Some investigators saw the atresia plate as a caudally directed process of the squama of the temporal bone.

6. Concentric narrowing of surrounding structures. Deutsch[13] considered the genesis of the atresia plate to be a concentric constriction of all surround-

From the Department of Otolaryngology, University of Erlangen-Nürnberg, West Germany.

TABLE 1. PATHOLOGICAL CHANGES IN FETUSES

Change	% of Animals
Malformation and malposition of the auricle and atresia of the external ear canal	12
Malformation of the extratemporal course of the facial nerve	4
Hypoplasia of the tympanic portion of the facial nerve	8
Thickening and changes in the form of the os tympanicum	10
Absent tympanic membrane and absent annulus	12
Prominent supratympanic bulging	3
Rotation of the pyramid	17
Malformation of the mandible	16

TABLE 2. PATHOLOGICAL CHANGES IN ADULT ANIMALS

Change	% of Animals
Atresia and blind-ending external ear canal	46
Changes of the middle ear space	21
Replacement of the eardrum by bone or fibrous tissue	42
Aplasia or malformation of the ossicles	14
Atypical intratympanic course of the facial nerve	8
Hypoplasia of the facial nerve	21
Atresia of the foramen ovale	2
Displacement and hypertrophy of the middle ear muscles	17

ing structures of the ear. Through bone resorption and following bone apposition a plate-like formation could be created.

METHODS

Wistar rats weighing from 140 to 160 g were chosen as experimental animals. After determination of the menstrual cycle by vaginal smears, the females in estrus were paired with male rats. By vaginal smear the presence of sperm was verified and the date of the smear was designated as day one of the 21-day pregnancy term. Overdoses of vitamin A were used as the teratogenic agent.[14]

Schedule and Dose of Vitamin A. The most sensitive time for teratogenic damage to embryonic structures is between the 8th and 14th day of pregnancy.[15] No determination point specific for ear malformation is known. Therefore 120 pregnant rats were divided equally into four groups (8th, 9th, 10th and 11th day of pregnancy).

The 30 animals in each group were subdivided into groups of ten. Each animal in the subgroup received 50,000, 80,000, or 100,000 units of vitamin A in oil (Arovit®) via a nasogastric tube under anesthesia (Nembutal® 1 mg/kg intraperitoneally). Thus 12 x 10 animals received different doses of vitamin A on different days of pregnancy. The fetuses could be regarded as being damaged to different extents. Two hundred twenty-nine fetuses and 75 adult animals were examined. Litter numbers were low because of intrauterine resorption of approximately 51%. In addition many of the deformed animals were eaten by the mother. In order not to loose valuable material, caesarian sections were performed on the 21st day in a portion of the animals.

The term "fetus" includes all animals which could be acquired by caesarian section on the 20th day of pregnancy and those which could be examined one day after spontaneous delivery. The term "adult" includes rats which were raised to a weight of 160 g (six weeks postpartum).

Microsurgical Preparation. Under the operating microscope, using microsurgical instruments and technique, the specimens were dissected (from outside to inside) taking special notice of the auricle, the external auditory canal, the tympanic membrane, the middle ear, the ossicles, the facial nerve, the mandible, the hyoid, and the temporal bone. Important findings were photographed. Cross sections 5-7 μ thick were prepared for histologic examination.

In order to analyze the relationship of different parts of the ear to each other and to the surrounding structures (ie, mandible, squama, Meckel's cartilage, os tympanicum, the tympanic course of the facial nerve, and the relationship of the ossicles to the atresia plate), the heads were dissected differently. Parts of the deformed heads were sectioned frontally, some vertically and the rest horizontally. Altogether 1,280 sections were analyzed.

RESULTS

INCIDENCE OF EXPERIMENTALLY PRODUCED MALFORMATIONS

Of the 229 fetuses and the 75 adult animals microsurgically prepared and histologically examined, 49 fetuses and 28 adult animals showed suspicious changes in the ear regions and surrounding areas.

The majority of malformed fetuses were found in animals receiving vitamin A on the eighth or ninth day of pregnancy. There was no difference in the nature and extent of malformations of the ear region. Higher dosage of vitamin A is correlated with an increasing rate of fetus malformations.

TYPES OF EAR AND SKULL MALFORMATIONS

Microsurgical and histological examination revealed pathological abnormalities in fetuses (Table 1) and in adult animals (Table 2). In fetuses, malformations of the ear occurred bilaterally in 3% and unilaterally in 26%, while in adults they occurred bilaterally in 21% and unilaterally in 42%.

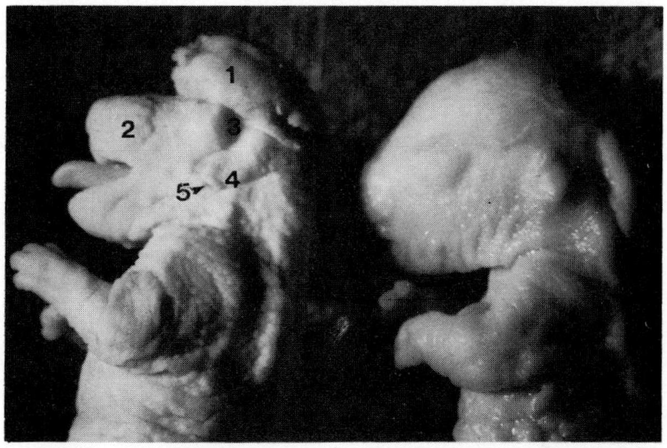

Fig. 1. In comparison to a normal rat fetus (right), the following abnormalities are present in the deformed animal (left). 1 - The cranium is absent, the brain sits like a mushroom on the base of the skull. 2 - The upper and lower jaws are greatly reduced, the tongue is hypertrophied. 3 - The left eye is prominent. 4 - The movement of the auricle backwards and superiorly did not occur. 5 - The auricle itself is malformed.

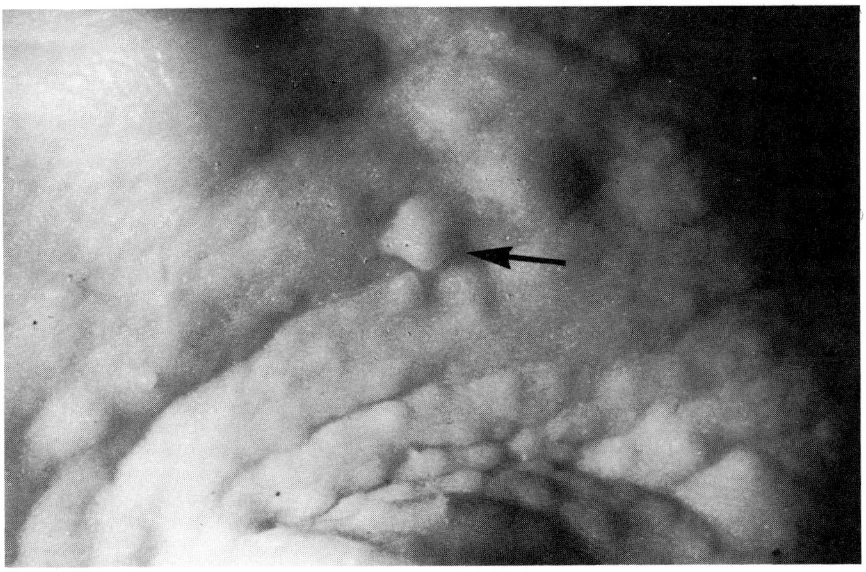

Fig. 2. The left auricle of the damaged fetus is malformed. The fusion of the left auricle hillocks did not occur. The external ear canal is not present.

OBSERVATIONS ON EXPERIMENTALLY PRODUCED ATRESIA AURIS CONGENITA IN RAT FETUSES

Malformation of the Auricle. The auricle was present unilaterally in four of six fetuses and bilaterally twice as a rudiment or as a small protuberance. The normal movement of the auricle upwards and backwards did not occur (Figs. 1 and 2).

Atresia of the External Ear Canal. In six fetuses no external ear canal could be found (Figs. 2 and 3). These cases were combined with hypoplasia or aplasia of the middle ear.

Rotation of the Plane of the Eardrum. Through chondrohyperplasia and malformation of the base of the skull, and especially the labyrinthine capsule, the middle ear was rotated so that the plane of the eardrum was almost parallel to the base of the skull (Figs. 4 and 5).

FORMATION OF THE ATRESIA PLATE

ROLE OF THE OS TYMPANICUM. The anlage of the os tympanicum was cartilaginous in the fetus (Fig. 6). The thin arch of the annulus in a normal ear (Fig. 4) was plump (Fig. 7); the os tympanicum was enlarged from below and irregularly thickened; it replaced the bottom half of the eardrum (Fig. 8).

ROLE OF THE SQUAMA. The pars squamosa contributed to the development of the supratympanic tuberosity (Fig. 9).

SUPRATYMPANIC TUBEROSITY. Almost all malformed ears showed a cartilaginous tuberosity (Fig. 6) in the upper portion of the eardrum. It was like a protuberance pushed in front of the eardrum and directed forward and downward. The supratympanic tuberosity corresponded histologically either to a caudally directed process of the squama or to a hyperplastic cartilaginous labyrinthine wall (Fig.

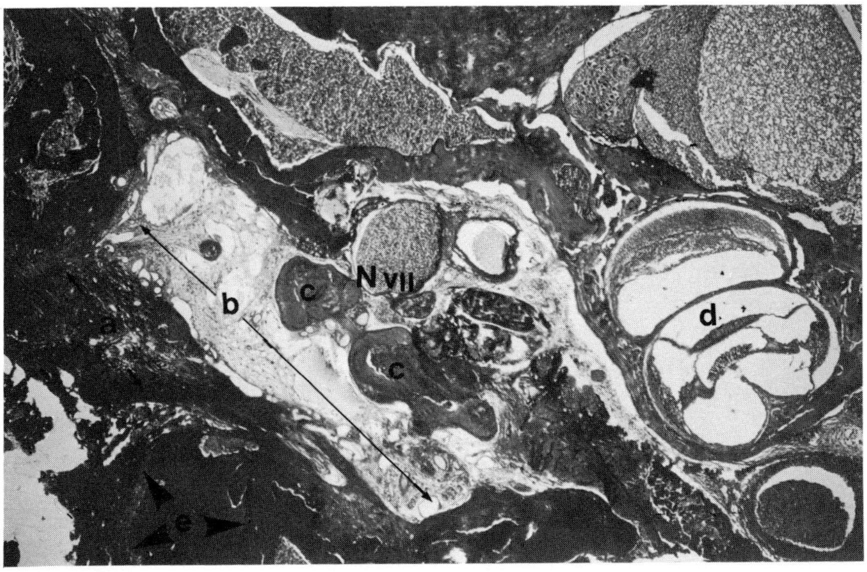

Fig. 3. Histological section of the malformed ear of an adult rat. Instead of the eardrum a fibrous plate is present (a). The middle ear space is shrunken and not air-filled (b). The ossicles are deformed and dislocated (c). The inner ear is dislocated (d). e - Os tympanicum; N_{VII} - Seventh nerve.

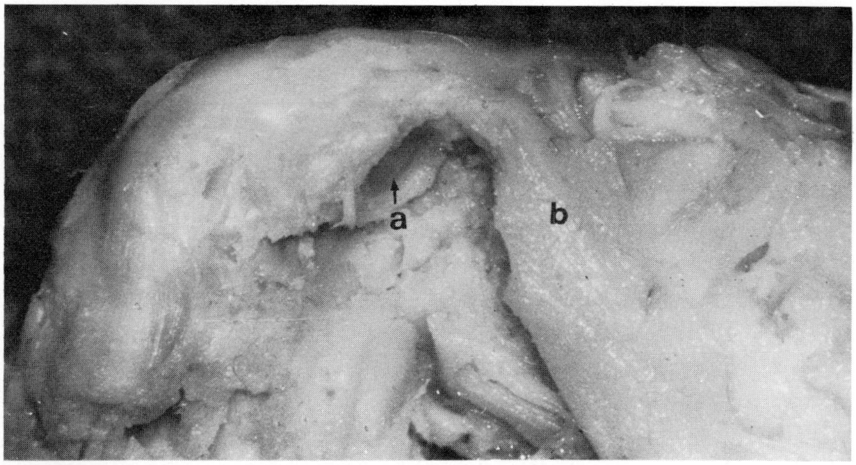

Fig. 4. Microsurgical demonstration of a newborn whose skull was bitten off by the mother animal, showing an atypical ramus of the mandible (b). Note also that the middle ear is rotated so that the eardrum (a) lies almost parallel to the skull base.

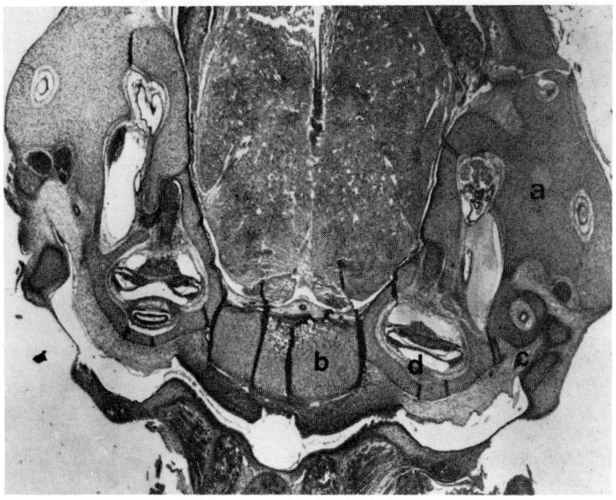

Fig. 5. Frontal section of the skull of a rat fetus showing the topographic relationship of the middle ear to the floor of the skull. Because of the chondrohyperplasia of the labyrinth (a), both middle ears (c) were rotated around their sagittal axes. The base of the skull (b) is included in the cartilaginous hyperplasia. d - Inner ear.

9), which pushed the middle ear downward and inward toward the base of the skull.

Chondrohyperplasia of the Base of the Skull. The malformed fetuses showed massive cartilaginous proliferation. The base of the skull, the labyrinthine capsule and the os tympanicum all were involved. The result of this diffuse dysplasia is a walling-in of the facial nerve and rotation of the middle ear around the sagittal axis (Fig. 10).

Observations on the Facial Nerve. In malformed ears the facial nerve was in the typical position in the middle ear. Striking was that in 8% of the cases histologically examined it was walled in by masses of cartilage of the hyperplastic labyrinthine capsule. The diameter of the facial nerve was a quarter of its normal thickness (Fig. 11).

OBSERVATIONS ON EXPERIMENTALLY INDUCED ATRESIA AURIS CONGENITA IN ADULT ANIMALS

Atresia of the External Ear Canal. This condition in adult rats is similar to human atresia. A small groove indicates the external ear canal (Fig. 12).

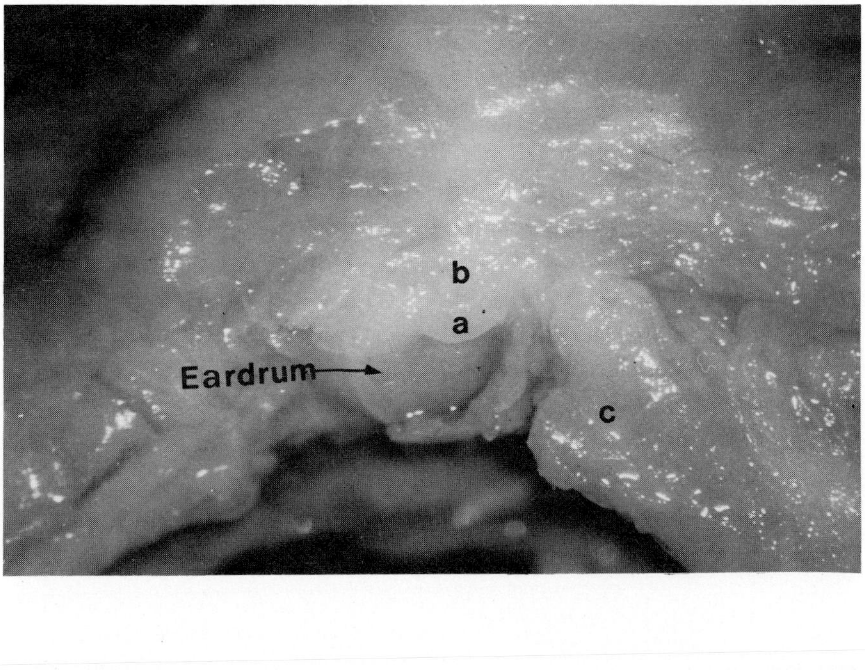

Fig. 6. Microsurgically prepared fetal ear shows diffuse cartilaginous hyperplasia, which includes the supratympanic tuberosity (a), the cranially lying bone (b), and the end of the mandible (c).

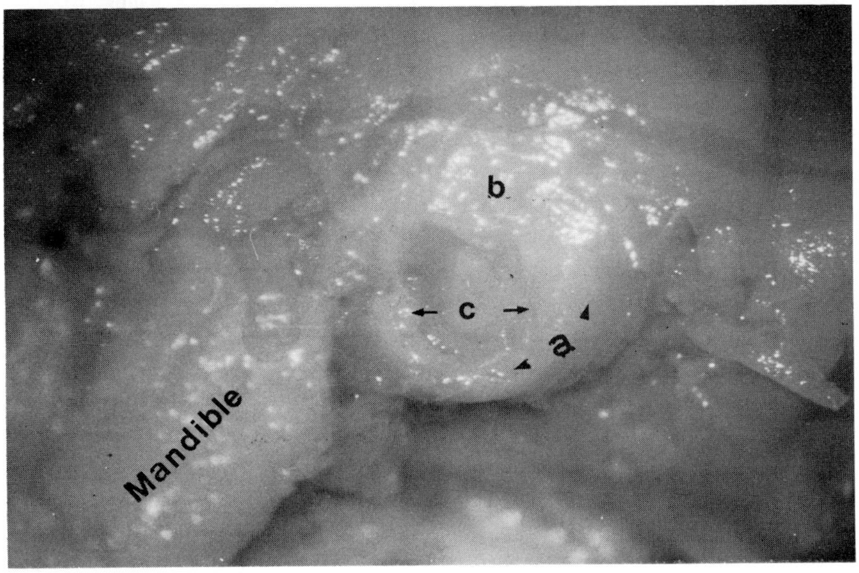

Fig. 7. Microsurgically prepared fetal head shows a massive proliferation of cartilage, which includes the os tympanicum (a), the supratympanic tuberosity (b), and the bone of the cranium. This proliferation extends to the eardrum (c) which is therefore thickened and less transparent than a normal eardrum.

Malformation of the Tympanic Membrane. The anomalous eardrum was located in a normal position in the deformed external ear canal. It was either thickened by fibrous tissue, or partially or completely replaced by bone (Figs. 13-15).

Formation of the Atresia Plate. The os tympanicum was cartilaginous in the fetus (Fig. 8), but fibrous (Fig. 16) or bony in adults (Figs. 13-15). The hyperplastic os tympanicum either replaces the lower part of the eardrum (Fig. 14), or is found lateral to the eardrum (Fig. 15) in contact with the temporal bone.

Middle Ear Space. A complete aplasia of the middle ear was seen twice. Slight and moderate deformities or reduction in size were seen more often. The middle ear space was like a cleft, shrunken in all directions, and in an atypical position in the temporal bone (Fig. 3). The ossicles were sometimes absent or fused, and the middle ear muscles were hypertrophic and displaced (Fig. 14).

Facial Nerve. In adult animals with deformed middle ears, there were some variations in the course of the facial nerve: 1) dehiscence of the fallopian canal (Fig. 16); 2) hypoplasia of the nerve with development from a tenth to a half of its normal diameter (Fig. 17); 3) atypical position of the geniculate ganglion; and 4) atypical position of the stylomastoid foramen.

DISCUSSION

A single large dose of vitamin A (50,000, 80,000, or 100,000 units) given at different times (8th, 9th, 10th, or 11th day of pregnancy) to Wistar rats, resulted in severe deformities in the fetus of the outer and middle ear and the facial nerve, as well as in contiguous areas of the skull. The deformities visi-

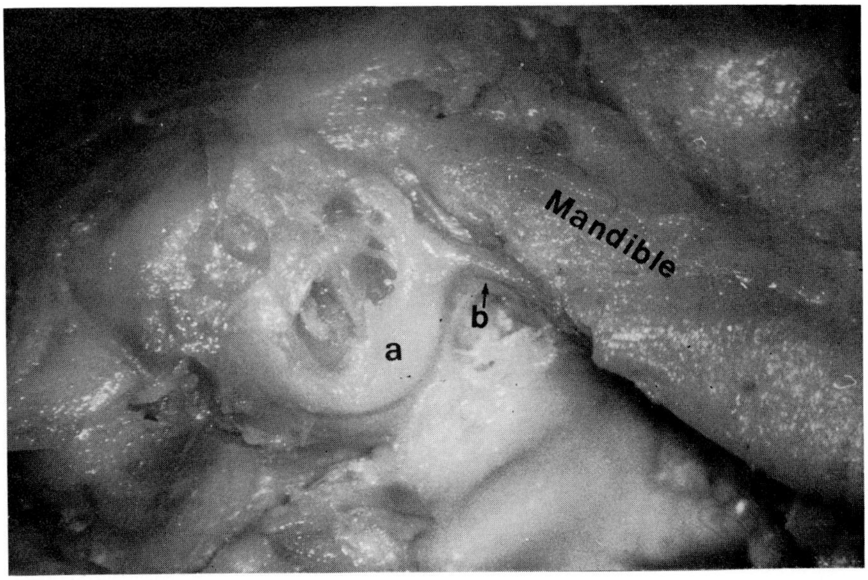

Fig. 8. Microsurgically prepared ear of a fetus shows the enlarged os tympanicum (a), which grows from below and replaces the bottom of the eardrum. The upper part of the eardrum is normal. b - Meckel's cartilage.

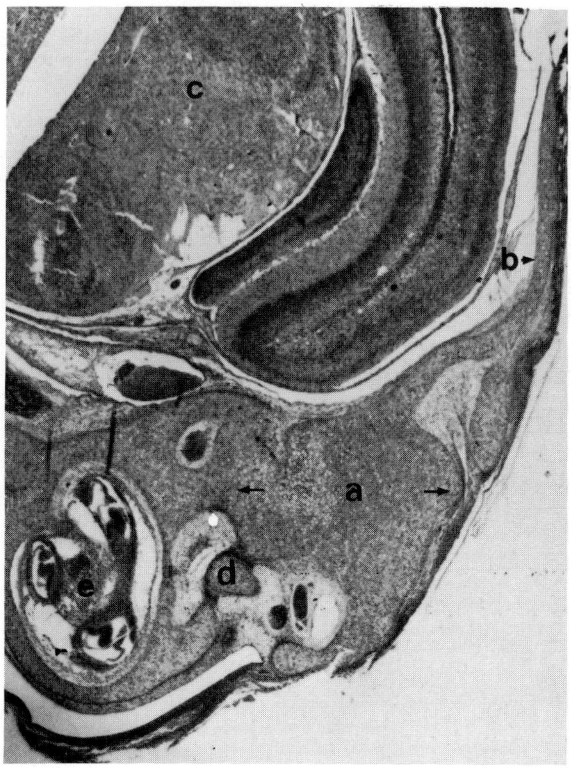

Fig. 9. Histological section of a left fetal ear shows the hyperplastic labyrinthine wall (arrows) appearing as the protuberance. In contrast to Fig. 5, the labyrinthine capsule forms a morphologic union with the squama (b) of the temporal bone. a - Labyrinthine capsule; c - Brain; d - Stapes; c - Inner ear.

ble in histological sections are similar to the human atresia auris congenita seen in great numbers during the thalidomide era in Germany.

SUSPECTED MODE OF ACTION OF TERATOGENIC SUBSTANCES

The precise role of vitamin A in developmental malformations is not known. The literature suggests three possible mechanisms: 1) vitamin A may act directly on the fetus to produce abnormalities; 2) vitamin A may block the chorionic villi; 3) vitamin A may affect the adrenal cortex of the mother.

The question of why normal and deformed animals occur in the same litter has not been clarified. McLarren and Michie[16] suggest that not all eggs implant at the same time; Hertwig[17] discusses the possibility that the placentas do not become attached to the maternal circulation at the same time.

DEFORMED EARS AND NEIGHBORING REGIONS

Induced malformations in this series (in both fetuses and adult rats) included aplasia and dysplasia of the auricle, the external ear canal, the middle ear space, the ossicles, the muscles, and the course of the facial nerve. Other areas of the first branchial arch also severely damaged included the mandible (Fig. 4) and the zygomatic arch.

Formation of the Atresia Plate. In the microsurgically examined animals the atresia plate seemed to develop from several different components.

OS TYMPANICUM. The widening and shield-like bulging of the os tympanicum (Figs. 7 and 8) was regarded as a part of the atresia plate. This displacement into the tympanic membrane occurred mainly from the caudal and lateral areas.

SUPRATYMPANIC TUBEROSITY. In 8% of the animals the labyrinthine capsule evidenced a huge proliferation of cartilage: the supratympanic tuberosity (Figs. 6 and 9), which pushed the middle ear around its sagittal axis. In six animals the squama of the os temporale (Fig. 9) was a component of this cartilaginous hyperplasia. These findings are consistent with operative techniques used in humans. When opening the middle ear the ossicles are uncovered from above and not from the side.

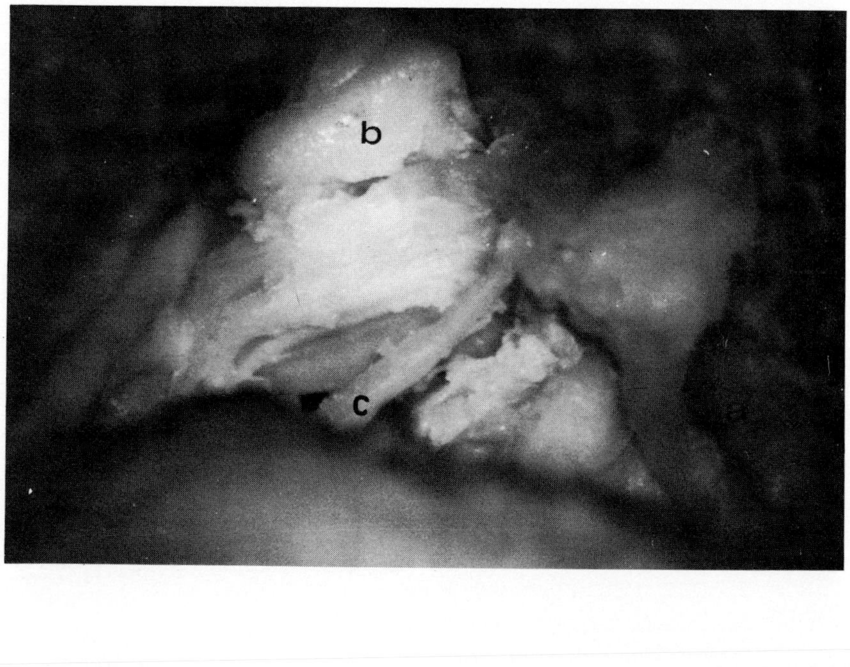

Fig. 10. Prepared malformed fetal head after removal of the brain, showing a severely deformed base of the skull with a proliferation of cartilage in the posterior fossa (a). The left eye (b) is prominent and deformed. After removal of a portion of the mandible a persisting Meckel's cartilage (c) can be seen.

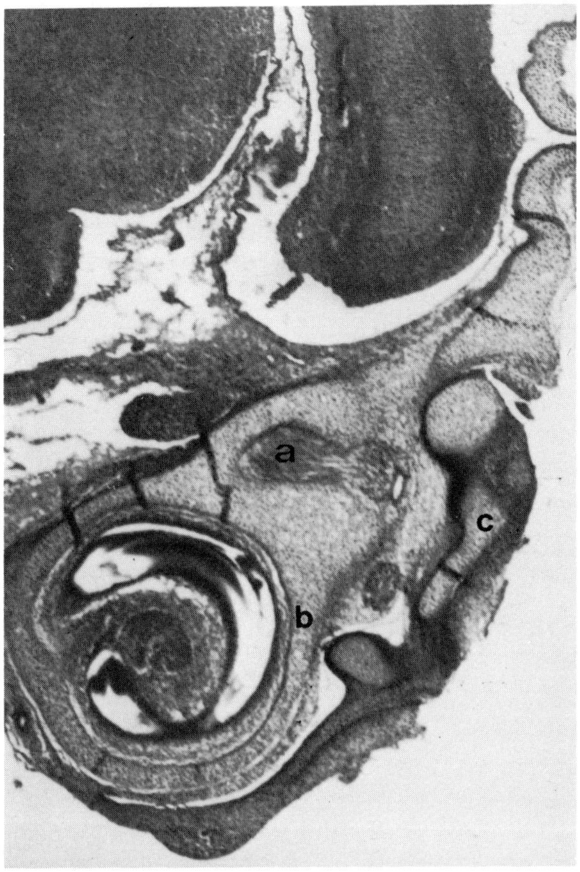

Fig. 11. Histological section of a fetal rat showing the facial nerve (a) walled in by masses of cartilage of the labyrinthine capsule (b). In contrast, in a normal ear the facial nerve is covered by fibrous tissue and less cartilage. c - Malleus.

External Auditory Canal. The bony malformation of the external auditory canal seems to be caused by a compensatory enlargement of a part of the first branchial arch producing hyperplasia of the os tympanicum.

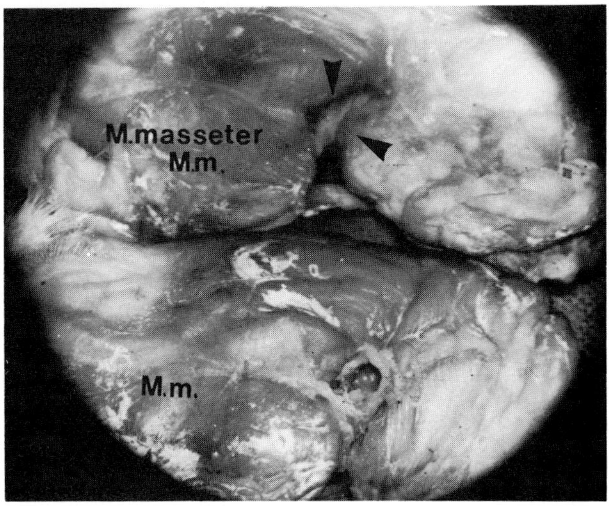

Fig. 12. In the upper half of the picture is an adult rat skull microsurgically prepared. The external auditory canal is not present (arrows). The lower half of the picture is a normal rat ear. M.m. - Musculus masseter.

Rotation of the Middle Ear. As mentioned above, the rotation of the middle ear is caused by a proliferation of cartilage. When opening the middle ear, the surgeon is forced to perforate either the hyperplastic os tympanicum and/or the ossified supratympanic tuberosity.

Malformation of the Fallopian Canal. The course of the facial nerve is of considerable interest to otologists. Many investigators describe an extremely atypical course from the entrance of the nerve into the middle ear to its exit from the styloid foramen. Extreme variations in the course were not observed in this series, although dehiscence of the fallopian canal was frequently seen. These experimentally produced observations correspond with those of Wigand[18] who found in 62 severe human ear malformations none in which the course of the facial

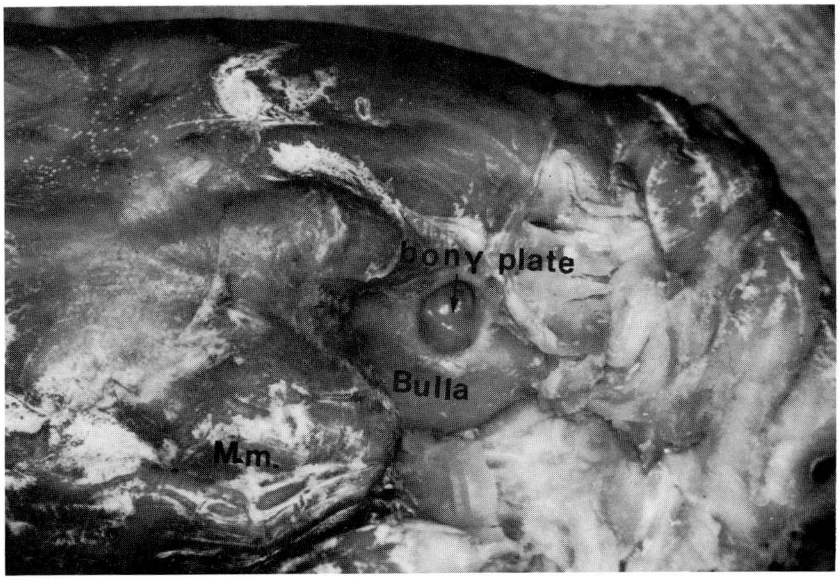

Fig. 13. In the depth of a microsurgically prepared left rat ear, a massive bony plate is present instead of the eardrum. M.m. - Musculus masseter.

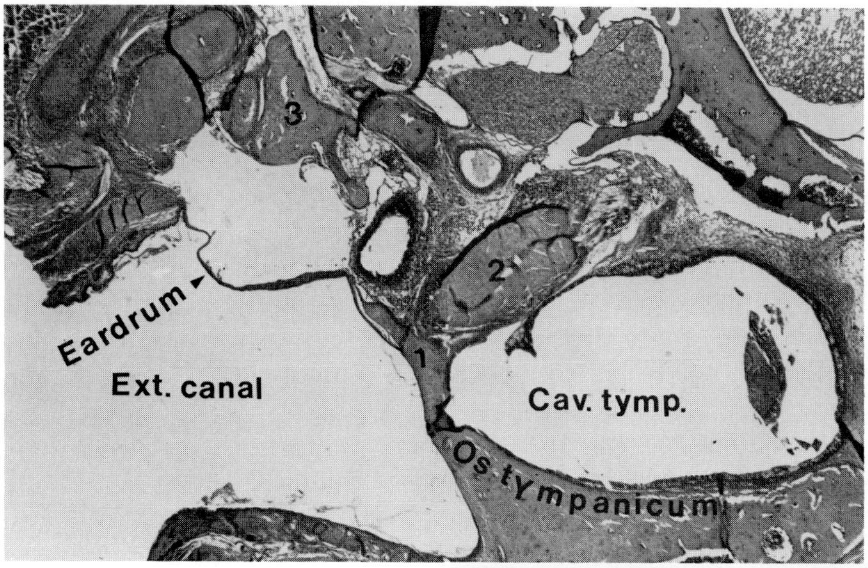

Fig. 14. Histological section of an adult rat right ear. 1 - The lower part of the eardrum is replaced by proliferation of the os tympanicum. 2 -The middle ear space is deformed and divided by a bony septum. 3 - The ossicles are hypoplastic and dislocated, without contact with the eardrum or the proliferated os tympanicum. Cav. tymp. - Cavum tympani; Ext. canal - External ear canal.

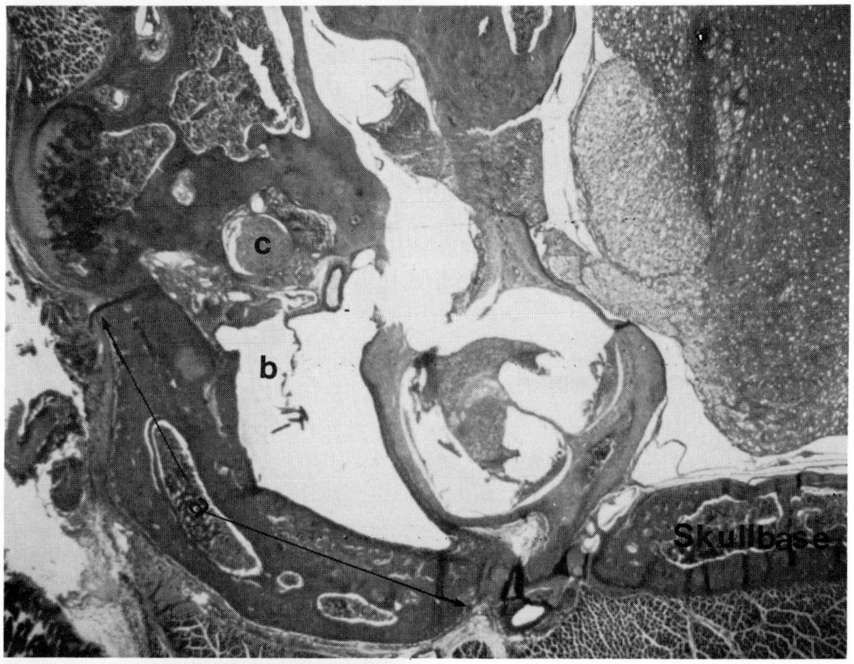

Fig. 15. Histological section through an adult rat right ear showing hyperplasia of the os tympanicum (a), which reaches from below to the roof of the external ear canal. The os tympanicum is plate-like and lies lateral to the eardrum (b). The upper half remains as a remnant. c - Facial nerve.

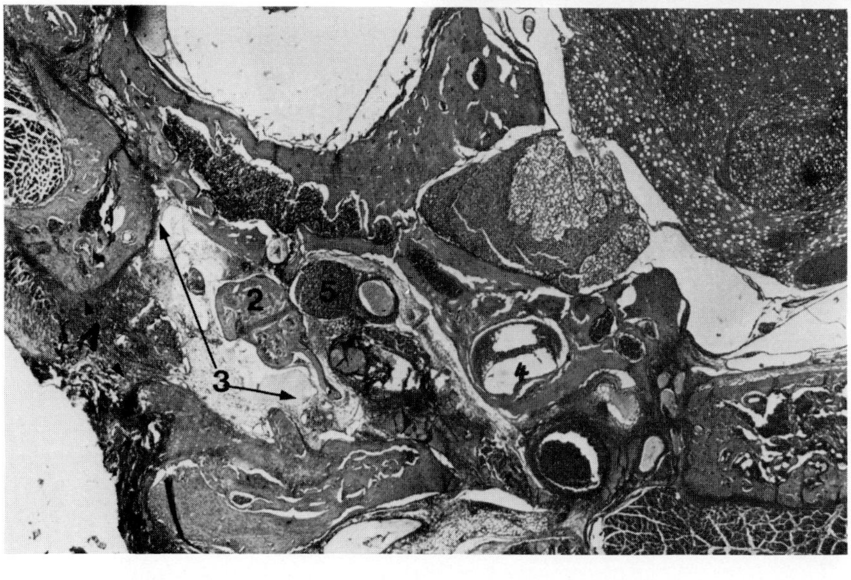

Fig. 16. Histological section of a malformed right ear of an adult rat shows the following special features: 1 - Instead of the eardrum, a thick fibrous plate. 2 - The ossicles are malformed and/or fused. 3 - The tympanic cavity is narrowed and deformed. 4 - The inner ear lies in a displaced position. 5 - The facial nerve is not covered by bone.

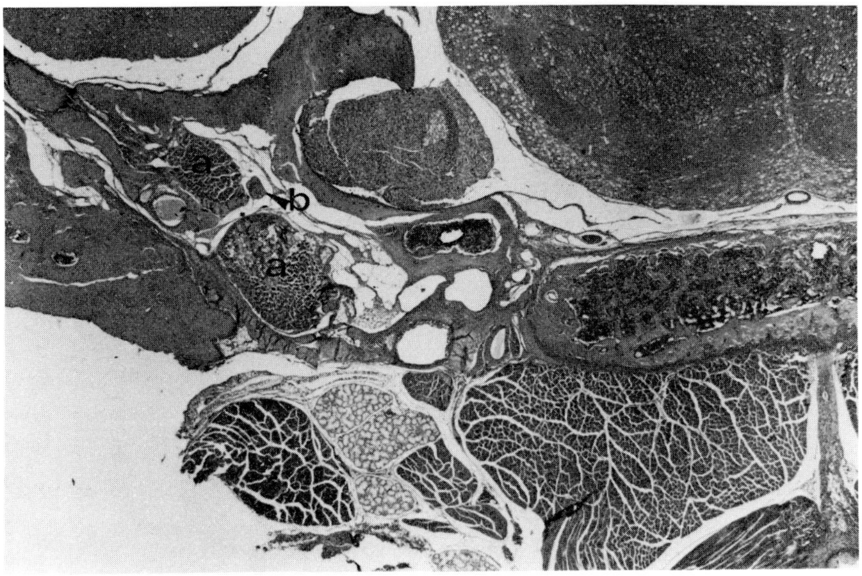

Fig. 17. Histological section of an adult rat ear showing a hypoplastic facial nerve (b) running uncovered through the tympanic cavity. The diameter of the nerve is reduced to one tenth of its normal thickness. Further anomalies are: atypical position of the middle ear muscles (a); the cavum tympani is narrowed to a cleft.

nerve within the temporal bone was grossly abnormal.

Malformation of the Facial Nerve. In the histologically examined fetal rat ears the nerve was found in its usual position in the middle ear, although often hypoplastic and walled-in by masses of cartilage. This walling-in could explain the hypoplasia of the nerve seen in adult animals. Hypoplasia can result in complete or incomplete facial nerve paralysis.[19] Miehlke and Partsch[20] do not agree that the functional disturbance is caused by the walling-in process but rather results from damage to the nucleus of the nerve. To clarify this latter point, further investigation was undertaken. Pregnant Wistar rats received high doses (15-20 mg) of pure thalidomide. The nucleus of the nerve showed the same structures and the same cell pattern as normal control rats.

Facial nerve malformation was never seen as an isolated finding in an *adult* rat. It was always combined with malformations of the outer and middle ear. A striking finding was that in 4% of the adult animals the nerve was hypoplastic and in extreme cases, only one tenth of its normal diameter.

CLINICAL MEANING OF THE EXPERIMENTAL RESULTS

In what ways can this study help clarify atresia auris congenita in humans? There were many parallels: auricular malformations, atresia of the external ear canal, the atresia plate, changes in the ossicles, the course of the facial nerve, and changes in the size of the middle ear space. These anomalies, typical of the Franceschetti syndrome, could be found alone or in combination with malformations of the surrounding structures, as, for example, in the mandible.

For the first time, the enormous chondrohyperplasia and dysplasia of the middle ear, the labyrinthine capsule, surrounding structures, and the base of the skull were demonstrated. Hyperplasia of cartilage causes a rotation of the middle ear (which is always found in human atresia auris congenita) and a walling-in of the facial nerve which reduces its diameter, and may be the reason for the functional disturbance.

The study showed that the atresia plate arises from more than one anlage. In most animals the plate was formed by a hyperplastic os tympanicum, which grew from below into the tympanic membrane. Other structures contributed to the development of the atresia plate; these include the ossified supratympanic tuberosity, the labyrinthine capsule and the squama of the temporal bone (Fig. 18). In the presence of polymorphic damage to the entire ear region it seems unlikely that the atresia plate could arise from a single part of the branchial arch. From a practical standpoint, the following conclu-

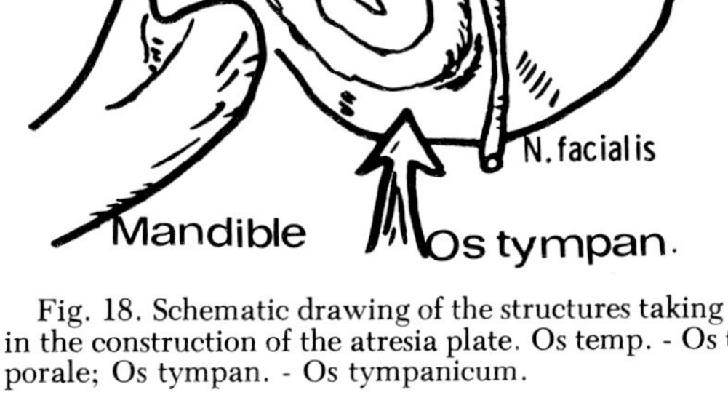

Fig. 18. Schematic drawing of the structures taking part in the construction of the atresia plate. Os temp. - Os temporale; Os tympan. - Os tympanicum.

sions are relevant for the treatment of this malformation:

1. The facial nerve shows only slight variation from its normal course, so that the risk of damaging the nerve is not great.

2. Because the middle ear is rotated, it will be opened from above when the approach is from the lateral surface of the temporal bone.

3. The atresia plate is found in the position of the normal eardrum.

REFERENCES

1. Altmann F. Malformations of the auricle and the external auditory meatus. Arch Otolaryngol 1951; 54:115-39.

2. Altmann F. Zur Anatomie und formalen Genese der Atresia auris congenita. Monatsschr Ohrenheilkd 1933; 67:756-822.

3. Nager F, Reynier J. Das Gehörorgan bei den angeborenen Kopfmissbildungen. New York: Karger, 1948.

4. Virchow R. Über Missbildungen am Ohr und im Bereich des 1. Kiemenbogens. Virchows Arch Pathol Anat 1864; 30:221-45.

5. Terrahe K. Missbildungen des Innen- und Mittelohres als Folge der Thalidomid-Embryopathie. Fortschr auf dem Gebiet der Roentgenstr und der Nuklearmedizin Diagnostik, Physik, Biologie, Therapie Erganzüngsbände 1965; 102:14-29.

6. Lüscher E. Zwei Fälle von kongenitaler Atresie des menschlichen Ohres. Arch Ohrenheilkd 1929; 123:136-52.

7. Alexander G. Benesi O. Zur Kenntnis der Entwicklung und Anatomie der kongenitalen Atresie des menschlichen Ohres. Monatsschr Ohrenheilkd 1921; 55:195-230.

8. Reichert C. Über die Visceralbogen der Wirbeltiere im Allgemeinen und deren Metamorphosen bei den Vögeln und Säugetieren. Arch Anat Physiol Wissensch Med 1837; 120-2.

9. Marx A. Beitrag zur Morphologie und Genese der Mittelohrmissbildungen mit Gehörgangsatresie. HNO 1922; 2:230-46.

10. Marx H. Die Missbildungen des Ohres. In: Henke F, Lubarsch O, eds. Handbuch der speziellen pathologischen Anatomie und Histologie. Berlin: Springer, 1926:609.

11. Politzer A. Lehrbuch der Ohrenheilkunde. Bd. II. Stuttgart: Enke, 1882:863.

12. Meyer W. Ein Beitrag zu den Missbildungen im Bereich der ersten Kiemenspalte und des ersten Kiemenbogens. Arch Klin Chir 1883; 29.

13. Deutsch L. Zur Morphologie und Genese der angeborenen Gehörgangsatresie. Monatsschr Ohrenheilkd 1925; 59:993-1001.

14. Cohlan SQ. Congenital anomalies in the rat produced by excessive intake of vitamin A during pregnancy. Pediatrics 1954; 13:556-67.

15. Hamburgh M. Malformation in mouse embryo induced by trypian blue. Nature 1952; 169:27.

16. Cohlan SQ, Stone SM. Observations on the effect of experimental endocrine procedures on the teratogenic action of hypervitaminosis A in the rat. Biol Neonate 1961; 3:330-42.

17. Hertwig P. Die Genese der Hirn- und Gehörgangsmissbildung bei Röntgenmutierten Kreisler-Mäusen. Z Menschl Vererb Konstitutionslehre 1944; 28:327-54.

18. Wigand ME. Tympano-mèatoplasie endaurale pour les atrèsies congènitales sèvères de l'oreille. Rev Laryngol Otol Rhinol (Bord) 1978; 99:15-28.

19. Sugàr M. Rudimentär entwickelte, missgebildete Ohrmuschel mit Atresie des Gehörganges, Fistulae auriculae congenitae und Hemiatrophia facialis, wahrscheinlich in Folge congenitaler Hypoplasie des paralytischen N. facialis. Arch Ohrenheilkd 1902; 58:216-25.

20. Miehlke A, Partsch EJ. Ohrmissbildung, Facialis und Abduzenzlähmung als Syndrom der Thalidomidschädigung. Arch Ohren Nasen Kehlkopfheilkd 1963; 181:154-74.

PROCEEDINGS OF THE WEST COAST COCHLEAR PROSTHESIS CONFERENCE

UNIVERSITY OF CALIFORNIA AT SAN FRANCISCO

February 23-24, 1979

PAPERS PREVIOUSLY PUBLISHED

*Estimates of Essential Neural Elements for Stimulation Through a Cochlear Prosthesis.
B.M. Clopton, PhD, F.A. Spelman, PhD, J.M. Miller, PhD, Department of Otolaryngology, University of Washington, Seattle

*Brainstem Histopathology Following Chronic Scala Tympani Implantation in Monkeys.
J.M. Miller, PhD, D. Sutton, PhD, D.B. Webster, PhD, Department of Otolaryngology, University of Washington, Seattle, and Louisiana State University Medical Center, New Orleans

†Speech Perception with Hearing Aids and Cochlear Implants.
E. Owens, PhD, C.C. Telleen, MA, Department of Otolaryngology, University of California at San Francisco

*Operating Ranges for Cochlear Implants.
B.E. Pfingst, PhD, F.A. Spelman, PhD, D. Sutton, PhD, Department of Otolaryngology, University of Washington, Seattle

*Design of the Cochlear Prosthesis: Effects of the Flow Current in the Implanted Ear.
F.A. Spelman, PhD, B.M. Clopton, PhD, B.E. Pfingst, PhD, J.M. Miller, PhD, Department of Otolaryngology, University of Washington, Seattle

*Comparison of Cochlear Histopathology Following Two Implant Designs for Use in Scala Tympani.
D. Sutton, PhD, J.M. Miller, PhD, B.E. Pfingst, PhD, Department of Otolaryngology, University of Washington, and Virginia Mason Research Center, Seattle

----

*Animal Studies of a Cochlear Prosthesis. Ann Otol Rhinol Laryngol 1980; 89 Suppl 66.

†Arch Otolaryngol 1981; 107:160-3.

CONTENTS

Status of Hearing Rehabilitation Research Center Implant Program.
W.F. House, MD, K.I. Berliner, PhD 4

Cochlear Pathology Following Chronic Intracochlear Electrical Stimulation.
P.A. Leake-Jones, PhD, S.M. Walsh, PhD, M.M. Merzenich, PhD 6

Performance Characteristics of Intracochlear Stimulating Electrodes.
M.B. Meikle, PhD, C.A. Lee, BA 9

Probability of Trauma and Reliability of Placement of a 20 mm Long Model Human Scala Tympani Multielectrode Array.
B.F. O'Reilly, MBChB, FRCS 11

Growth of Loudness for Sinusoidal and Pulsatile Electrical Stimulation.
R.V. Shannon, PhD 13

Pitch Correlates of Direct Auditory Nerve Electrical Stimulation.
F.B. Simmons, MD, R.L. White, PhD, M.G. Walker, PhD, R.G. Mathews, PhD 15

Electrode Position and Excitation Patterns for a Model Cochlear Prosthesis.
M.C. Vivion, PhD, M.M. Merzenich, PhD, P.A. Leake-Jones, PhD, M. White, PhD, M. Silverman, BS 19

Opto-Isolated Stimulators Used for Electrically Evoked BSER.
L.S. Vurek, M. White, PhD, M. Fong, MS, S.M. Walsh, PhD 21

Cochlear Prostheses: A Histological Examination of Implanted Cats.
R.S. Walloch, PhD, C.A. Smith, PhD, J.A. Fenwick, BS, N.R. Schuff, BS, R.A. Boberg, BS 25

Chronic Electrical Stimulation with Intracochlear Electrodes: Electrophysiological Results.
S.M. Walsh, PhD, P.A. Leake-Jones, PhD, L.S. Vurek, M.M. Merzenich, PhD 27

Maintenance of Neuronal Activity by Electrical Stimulation of Unilaterally Deafened Cats Demonstrable with Cytochrome Oxidase Technique.
M.T.T. Wong-Riley, PhD, S.M. Walsh, PhD, P.A. Leake-Jones, PhD, M.M. Merzenich, PhD 30

STATUS OF HEARING REHABILITATION RESEARCH CENTER IMPLANT PROGRAM

W. F. HOUSE, MD

K. I. BERLINER, PhD

LOS ANGELES, CALIFORNIA

Since our meeting in December 1977, the Hearing Rehabilitation Research Center (HRRC) cochlear implant research program has continued to grow. The number of implanted subjects has increased and so has the staff responsible for dealing with those subjects. Our facilities have been expanded and new equipment has been obtained.

Subjects. To date (February 1979), 43 subjects at HRRC have undergone cochlear implant surgery to receive a single-electrode induction coil implant. One of these subjects is now deceased. Five of these are recent operations and are awaiting return to HRRC to be fitted with the external device.

Five subjects currently have nonfunctioning internal coils. One of these is scheduled for replacement surgery in March. Three have had nonfunctioning coils for some time and have not chosen to have reimplantation.

Of the remaining 32 subjects, 3 are known to be not using their devices at all. Two of these, however, have expressed some recent interest in perhaps beginning use again, following some lifestyle changes. Another two or three subjects are suspected of using their implants only infrequently, if at all, at present. All other subjects use their implants on a routine basis, some as much as 16-17 hours per day.

Three of the subjects now have a functioning implant in both ears. One of these is currently wearing bilateral stimulator units. A second just recently had her second operation and only has one external unit as yet. The third bilateral subject has worn two units at different time periods but is currently using only one on a regular basis since one ear is much "weaker" than the other.

In summary, 43 subjects have received implants as part of the HRRC program. Approximately 27 of these are currently using their device daily, while another 5 are awaiting their external device and training in its use. One subject is deceased and another is scheduled for surgery to replace a nonfunctioning internal coil. Nine other subjects are not regularly using the implant, either by choice or due to malfunction. In addition to the HRRC subjects, US coinvestigators working in conjunction with HRRC have recently implanted several subjects. Of four subjects implanted by our coinvestigators, one is currently wearing an implant on a regular basis and three are still awaiting their external devices.

Engineering. HRRC now has its engineering laboratory and engineering staff on the premises, and does its own construction of the external stimulators. The engineering lab has been relocated in larger quarters and has been provided with substantial test equipment. Protocols for engineering testing of research subjects are currently being developed. Construction of the stimulator has been simplified by use of printed circuit boards. Development of a multiple electrode system is in the initial planning phase with the first subject tentatively scheduled.

FACILITIES AND MATERIALS

In order to more efficiently handle the large amounts and wide variety of data being gathered on our implant subjects among others, the Ear Research Institute has installed a computer sciences laboratory and two computers, and added to its staff a biomedical computer expert and a computer programmer. In conjunction with the use of the computer, all data acquisition forms have been redesigned for ease of computer entry. The critical analysis of these forms has also led to content modifications. We are in the process of combining the data acquisition forms and the instructions for their use with a detailed description of the procedures which produce the data, thus yielding a procedural package that could be used by others interested in research dealing with profoundly deaf adults using an auditory prosthesis.

RESULTS

Audiological. Patient performance with the single electrode cochlear implant has been measured on a variety of audiological tasks. Results have been reported elsewhere.[1-3] To briefly reiterate, subjects using the implant score significantly above chance on a number of specific forced-choice discrimination tasks, including a rhyme test for phoneme discrimination, a spondaic words test, and an environmental sounds test. As a group, they also score significantly better on these tests than do like subjects using powerful hearing aids.

Vestibular. At our prior meeting, there was some discussion of possible effects of cochlear electrical stimulation on the vestibular system. Since then,

From the Hearing Rehabilitation Research Center, a nonprofit corporation affiliated with the Ear Research Institute, Los Angeles.

some of our studies on this topic have reached completion. A report on these studies and the results will be available in detail at a later date.* However, we will briefly summarize some of the findings here.

Implant subjects were evaluated for vestibular function with ENG measurements prior to implant surgery and postoperatively and with the Ataxia Test Battery with and without implant activated. Electronystagmography results prior to implantation were compared to those at two intervals postoperatively. One group of subjects had a short-term follow-up, having received electrical stimulation for an average of six months at the time of posttesting. A second group had long-term follow-up, with an average of five years of electrical stimulation at the time of posttesting.

Only one of nine subjects on short-term testing showed a reduction in caloric response as compared to presurgery. Three of seven showed a reduction on long-term follow-up. In all four cases of reduced response, the decrease was bilateral rather than localized to the ear receiving electrical stimulation.

Eight subjects also were given the Sono-Postural test, derived from the Ataxia Test Battery, both presurgery and postsurgery. Eight subtest scores were combined to yield a total score for each subject. There was no significant difference between the presurgery and postsurgery scores ($p \geq 0.1$). In order to further validate the Ataxia Test Battery as a measure of vestibular function, a small sample size, nonparametric statistical test was performed comparing ENG and Ataxia Test Battery results. A significant positive relationship was found (Fisher's test, $p \leq .05$).

The Sono-Postural test was also used to measure vestibulospinal function with and without the implant activated, since the possibility exists that the implant might cause an increase in postural instability by stimulating the vestibular system. Total score for the unaided condition was compared to total score for the implant-activated condition on 16 subjects, including both short and long-term users. There was a statistically significant increase in postural *stability* with the implant activated ($t = 1.94$, $p \leq .05$), had the hypothesis been stated in this direction!

In summary, objective test results to date confirm the subjective observations of the subjects that the implant does not make their vestibular problems any worse. Computerized posturography data has also been collected and is in the process of being analyzed. All results and further details on individual subject's vestibular status will be prepared for publication at a later date.

*Eisenberg LS, Nelson JR, House WF. Effects of the single-electrode cochlear implant on the vestibular system of the profoundly deafened adult. In preparation.

REFERENCES

1. Eisenberg LS, Norton NB. Consonant discrimination with the cochlear implant. Paper presented at XIV International Congress of Audiology, Acapulco, Mexico, 1978.

2. House WF, Berliner KI, Eisenberg LS. Present status and future directions of the Ear Research Institute cochlear implant program. Acta Otolaryngol (Stockh) 1979; 87:176-84.

3. Norton NB, Berliner KI. Cochlear implants and hearing aids: a comparison study. Paper presented at XIV International Congress of Audiology, Acapulco, Mexico, 1978.

COCHLEAR PATHOLOGY FOLLOWING CHRONIC INTRACOCHLEAR ELECTRICAL STIMULATION

P. A. LEAKE-JONES, PhD
S. M. WALSH, PhD
M. M. MERZENICH, PhD
SAN FRANCISCO, CALIFORNIA

The feasibility and application of multichannel cochlear prostheses is critically dependent on the ability of the cochlea to withstand long-term electrical stimulation without developing pathological changes which might eventually render these devices ineffective. Therefore, a principal objective of current research in the Coleman Laboratory is to define "safe" limits of intracochlear electrical stimulation; ie, to determine the maximum current level at which electrical stimulation of the auditory nerve can be effected with bipolar intracochlear electrodes for long periods without damage to cochlear structures. An initial step in our experimental strategy has been to define stimulus levels at which damage is clearly induced and to examine, histologically, the nature and extent of that damage.

Electrical "overstimulation" studies were conducted in cats with bipolar elements of chronically implanted ($3^1/_2$ to 7 months) scala tympani electrodes. The multielectrode arrays embedded in Silastic® carriers were models of those designed for use in human prostheses. Brainstem evoked responses to electrical stimulation were monitored to determine the functional status of the auditory nerve. Charge-balanced biphasic pulses, (100-200 μs/phase) were delivered at a rate of 20-25 pulses/sec. Long periods of continuous stimulation at high current levels (4 to 8 mA) induced elevations in evoked response thresholds, apparently indicating destructive changes within the cochlea.[1]

These overstimulated cats were allowed to survive 8 to 20 days after cessation of stimulation. Their cochleas were preserved by perilymphatic perfusion of fixative and prepared for histological examination. Surface preparations and 1-2 μm toluidine blue stained sections (radial sections of the organ of Corti and spiral ganglion, and tangential sections through the osseous spiral lamina) were included in the light microscopic analysis.

The major histopathological consequences of

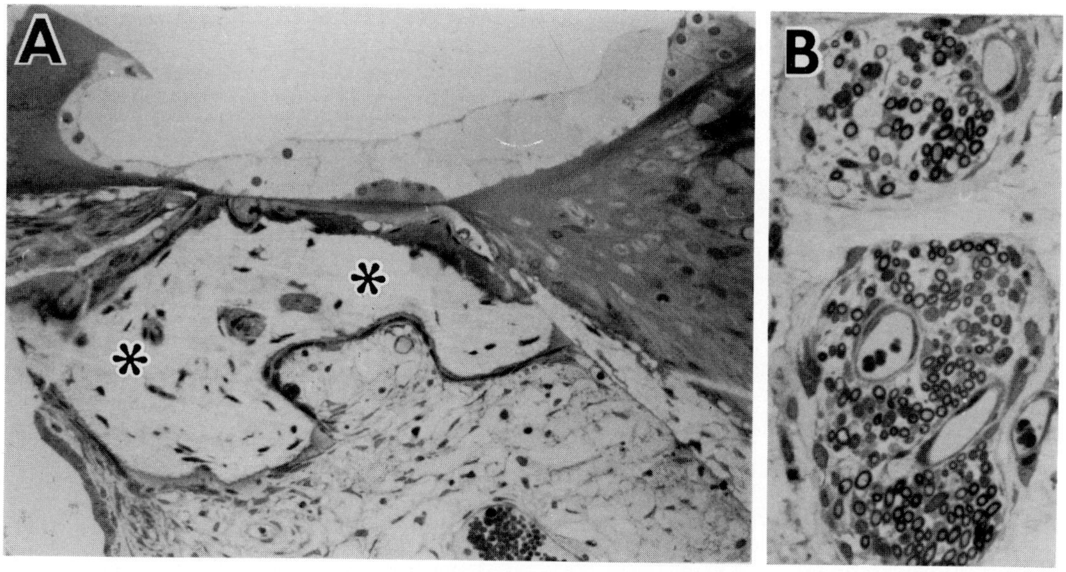

Fig. 1. Sections through A) organ of Corti and B) osseous spiral lamina taken 4 mm from the basal end of a cochlea which received over 300 hours of continuous stimulation (approximately half at 8 mA). A plate of newly formed bone (asterisks) extended between the osseous spiral lamina and the secondary spiral lamina over the stimulating electrode pair. A transition in nerve survival occurred in this region with about 70% loss basal to the 4 mm position (upper portion of B) and close to normal numbers apical to this level (lower portion of B; also see Fig. 3).

From the Coleman Laboratory, University of California at San Francisco. Supported by NIH Contract NS-7-2364, NIH Grant NS-11804 and Hearing Research, Inc.

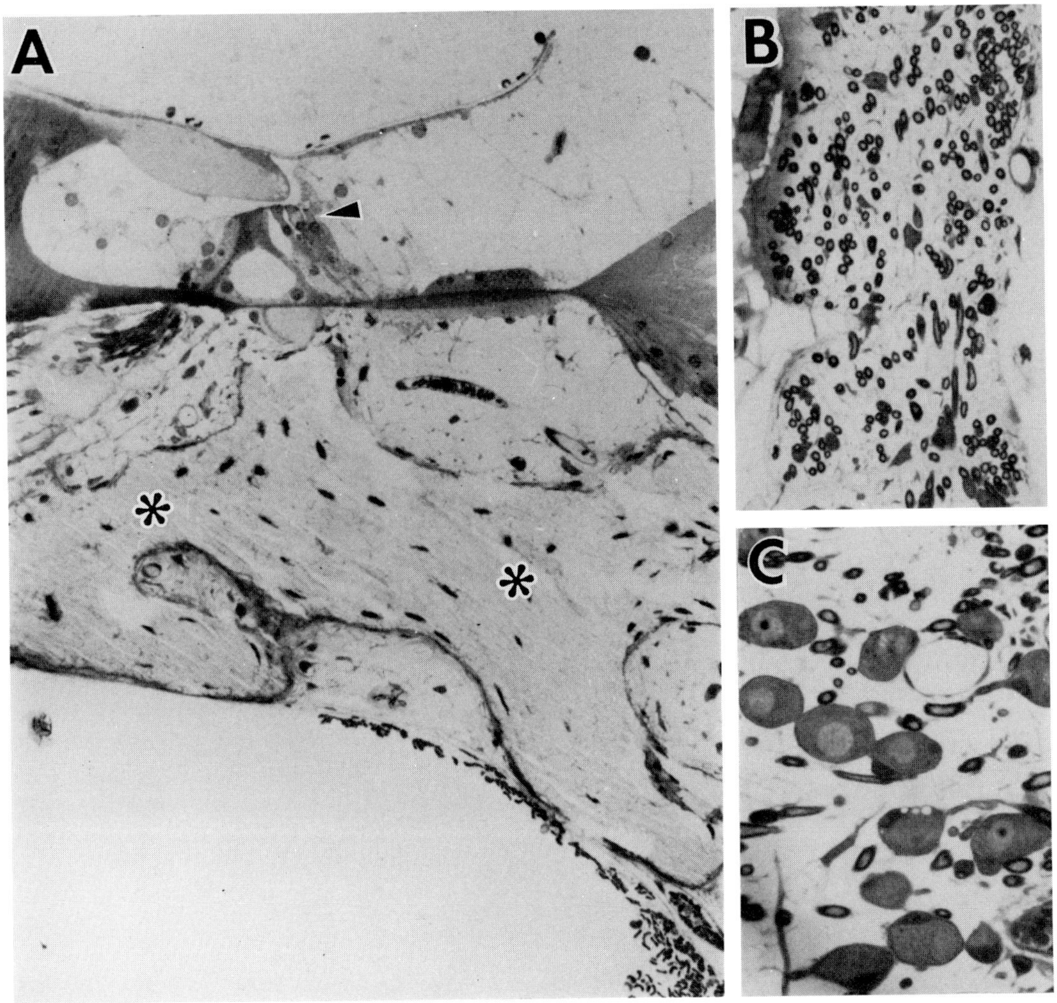

Fig. 2. Chronically implanted for seven months, this cochlea was stimulated for more than 120 hours at a 4 mA current level. A) Pillar cells and the reticular lamina were largely intact and some outer hair cells (arrow) were recognizable in the region of osteogenesis (asterisks) overlying the electrode. Survival of B) myelinated laminar nerve fibers and C) spiral ganglion cells was approximately 60%.

chronic implantation and electrical overstimulation with these intracochlear electrodes included: 1) osteogenesis within the scala tympani, 2) breakdown of the reticular lamina and resorption of the organ of Corti, and 3) degeneration of the first order auditory neurons.

Osteogenesis occurred over a short distance (1 to 4 mm) in the basal cochlear turn and was restricted to an area within the scala tympani above and immediately adjacent to the implant. The conformation of ectopic bone varied, but in all cases at some point a continuous plate formed between the osseous spiral lamina and the secondary spiral lamina (Fig. 1A). Chronic implantation of these electrodes, studied in many previous cases in which there was little or no electrical stimulation, demonstrated that damage due to the implantation itself (if any) was always restricted to the extreme cochlear base ("hook" region).[2,3] That is, osteogenesis was never induced by the passive presence of the implant unless severe trauma resulted in basilar membrane rupture and/or if damage to the bony spiral lamina occurred. The basilar membrane was intact in all cochleae examined in the present series. Bone formation in these cases was restricted to a region overlying the stimulating electrode elements and was considered to be stimulus induced. The deposition of bone probably led to a significant displacement of the electrode carrier within the scala. This could account for the elevations of evoked response thresholds which occurred only after many hours or days of stimulation. However, other long-term processes (eg, the accumulation of toxic platinum salts dissolved from electrode surfaces) could also be consistent with the time course of observed physiological changes.

In regions of bone growth the status of the sensory epithelium ranged from total resorption of the organ of Corti to preservation of the tunnel of Corti and even some surviving hair cells (Fig. 2A). In one case, severe degeneration of Corti's organ was evident throughout the most basal 8 mm and total resorption of the sensory epithelium was observed 2 mm apical to the upper end of the implant. The

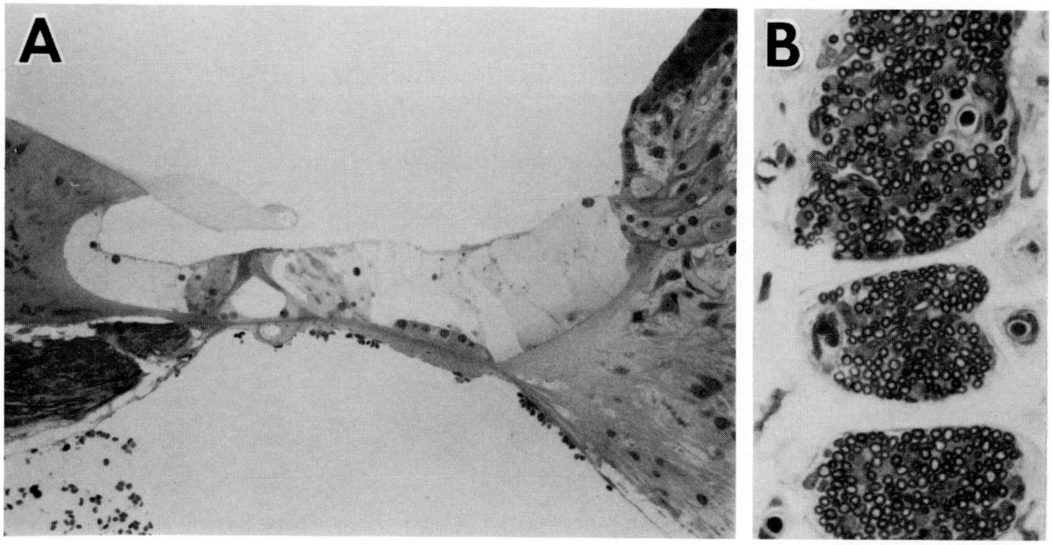

Fig. 3. Sections taken from the 6 mm position (ie, at the upper end of the electrode carrier) of the same cochlea illustrated in Fig. 1. The reticular lamina is intact although hair cells are lost or degenerating (A). The nerve is apparently normal (B) even though this region was subjected to extremely intense stimulation.

pattern of destruction in that animal which received over 500 hours of continuous stimulation (with more than half of this period at 8 mA), indicated that at very high current levels, electrical overstimulation may result in a breakdown of the reticular lamina, and in very significant degeneration of auditory nerve fibers.

It is not clear which specific factor(s) account for the variable loss of ganglion cell dendrites in the examined cochleas. There is some question whether the degeneration was related to direct trauma from the electrical stimulation, since survival of dendrites was excellent in some heavily stimulated regions (Fig. 3). Profound loss was always observed in regions where resorption of the organ of Corti occurred; yet significant nerve destruction was also noted in some regions with good preservation of the reticular lamina (Fig. 2). Data is inadequate at this time to correlate current levels and length of stimulation with the observed variations in extent of damage. Changes in pH concomitant with the osteogenic process must also be considered as a possible factor which might be toxic to neurons. The loss of myelinated laminar dendrites was closely correlated with loss of spiral ganglion cells in Rosenthal's canal (Fig. 2 B, C).

It is important to remember that the described histopathology was induced with current levels considerably greater than those required to excite the auditory nerve with proposed prosthetic devices. Additional data on long-term stimulation at appropriate current levels (ie, 1.5 to 2 mA) must be collected.

REFERENCES

1. Walsh SM, Leake-Jones PA, Vurek LS, Merzenich MM. Chronic electrical stimulation with intracochlear electrodes: electrophysiological results. Ann Otol Rhinol Laryngol 1981; 90 Suppl 82:27-9.

2. Schindler RA, Merzenich MM. Chronic intracochlear electrode implantation: cochlear pathology and acoustic nerve survival. Ann Otol Rhinol Laryngol 1974; 83:202-16.

3. Schindler RA, Merzenich MM, White MW, Bjorkroth B. Multielectrode intracochlear implants: nerve survival and stimulation patterns. Arch Otolaryngol 1977; 103:691-9.

PERFORMANCE CHARACTERISTICS OF INTRACOCHLEAR STIMULATING ELECTRODES

M. B. MEIKLE, PhD

C. A. LEE, BA

PORTLAND, OREGON

At present the cochlear implant techniques used in this country have concentrated on stimulation of the basal turn. However in some implant candidates the basal turn may not retain sufficient nerve fibers to permit usable sensations from basal turn stimulation. Furthermore the attempt to achieve multiple-channel stimulation may necessitate appealing to a more widely distributed population of cochlear nerve fibers. It is thus of interest to know whether stimulation techniques developed for the basal turn will produce the same, or different, results when applied more apically.

Data from intracochlear stimulation in the guinea pig are relevant to this question. In anesthetized guinea pigs we have used direct stimulation of the cochlear nerve for the purpose of mapping the cochlear projections to the auditory cortex. The cochlear capsule is opened widely to permit direct application of a bipolar pair of stimulating electrodes to the osseous spiral lamina in one or more turns. The stimulus is a symmetrically biphasic rectangular current pulse lasting 2 msec (1 msec in each direction), repeated once per second. In each case the resulting cortical responses are localized to particular locations within the auditory cortex, consistent with the cochleotopic organization of the primary auditory regions.[1,2*] All response characteristics described here were based on averages of ten responses each and were measured at the appropriate cortical response focus (cortical location at which responses to the particular cochlear stimulation site were maximal).

Figure 1 illustrates intensity functions for electrical stimulation in the various cochlear turns of three representative animals. A tendency is evident for the basal turn intensity functions to rise more steeply than intensity functions obtained with stimulation in turns 2, 3, or 4. This difference in slope is apparently due to several factors. Table 1 presents data from a number of different animals, indicating that threshold currents are in general lower in turn 1 than in the higher turns. In addition, Table 2 shows that response maxima tend to be greatest for turn 1 stimulation. Table 3 summarizes these observations in terms of the slopes of all intensity functions obtained so far during stimulation of the various cochlear turns. All but four of the turn 1 slopes are greater than 1.5. The arctan transformations show the angles (in degrees) corresponding to each of these slopes. Comparison of these means

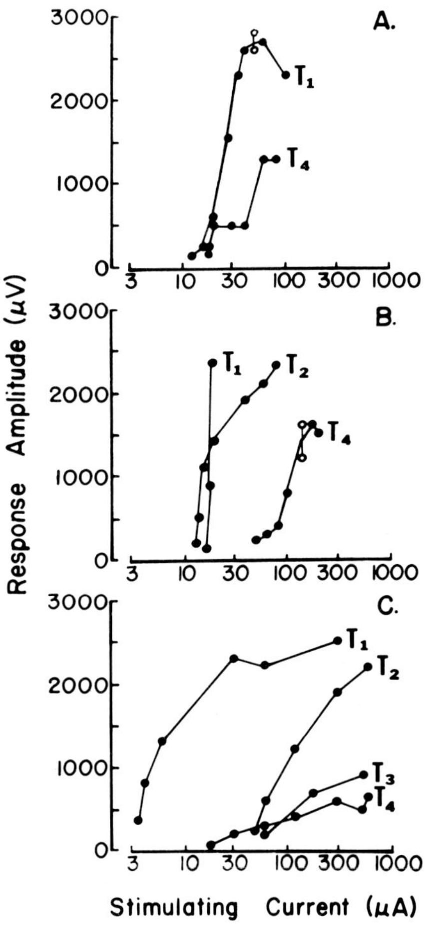

Fig. 1. Intensity functions of cortical responses elicited by bipolar electrical stimulation of the osseous spiral lamina. Data from three different guinea pigs are shown in A, B, and C. In each case the individual intensity functions were obtained at the appropriate cortical response focus for the cochlear turn in question. Order of recording was from apex to base (T_4 first, T_1 last).

*Meikle MB, Lee CA, Gillette RG. Cochleotopic organization of the guinea pig auditory cortex. In preparation, 1980.

From the Kresge Hearing Research Laboratory, Department of Otolaryngology, University of Oregon Health Sciences Center, Portland. This work was supported by the Deafness Research Foundation.

TABLE 1. RESPONSE THRESHOLDS FOR BIPOLAR STIMULATION OF OSSEOUS SPIRAL LAMINA IN VARIOUS COCHLEAR TURNS

	(Threshold current, μA)	
	Turn 1	*Turns 2, 3, and 4*	
	1.0	3	T_2: Mean = 18.5
	1.2	8	
	3.6	15	
	4.0	48	
	4.0	6	T_3: Mean = 26.7
	10.0	32	
	12.0	42	
	14.0	8	T_4: Mean = 23.4
	20.0	16	
	78.0	18	
		25	
		50	
Mean	14.8	22.6	

supports the generalization that there is a systematic difference between intensity functions in the base vs the higher cochlear turns.

The tendency for basal turn intensity functions to rise more steeply and reach greater response maxima than do intensity functions in more apical cochlear locations might reflect variations in innervation

TABLE 2. MAXIMUM RESPONSE AMPLITUDES FROM BIPOLAR STIMULATION OF OSSEOUS SPIRAL LAMINA IN VARIOUS COCHLEAR TURNS

	(Response Amplitude, μV)			
	Turn 1	*Turn 2*	*Turn 3*	*Turn 4*
	3000	2400	990	1400
	2800	1500	900	1300
	6300	2200		1180
	4200			600
	4300			1600
	4200			
	5000			
	2300			
	4100			
	1555			
Mean	3776	2033	945	1216

TABLE 3. SLOPES OF INTENSITY FUNCTIONS IN VARIOUS COCHLEAR TURNS

	Turn 1		*Turn 2*		*Turn 3*		*Turn 4*	
	Slope	*Tan⁻¹**	*Slope*	*Tan⁻¹**	*Slope*	*Tan⁻¹**	*Slope*	*Tan⁻¹**
	16.60	87.6	1.80	61.0	1.42	54.8	1.50	59.7
	12.75	86.5	1.34	53.3	0.21	11.9	1.40	56.3
	6.32	81.0	1.29	52.2	0.16	9.8	1.16	49.3
	4.89	78.5	1.11	48.0			0.76	37.3
	2.56	68.7	0.88	38.7			0.69	34.7
	1.73	60.0	0.33	18.3				
	1.70	59.7						
	1.27	51.8						
	0.86	40.8						
	0.72	35.9						
	0.65	33.0						
Mean		62.1		45.2		25.5		47.5

Slopes calculated from log-log plots, response amplitude (μV) vs current strength (μA).

*Angles expressed in degrees.

density within the cochlea.[3,4] However there is evidence that in the guinea pig the afferent innervation is relatively constant throughout the cochlear turns.[5] It is possible that the differences between the slopes of the intensity functions from the different cochlear turns reflect differences between turn 1 and the other turns in regard to cross-sectional area, radius of curvature, or other structural features.[6] If so, such differences might also influence the intensity functions to be obtained in different regions of the human cochlea, although the quantitative relationships between morphology and electrode performance would of course be different in the different species.

The present results suggest that cochlear prostheses involving both basal and apical stimulation sites may require different gain controls for the different channels. These data were obtained using bipolar stimulating electrodes. We have yet to determine whether similar relationships apply to monopolar stimulation in the various cochlear turns.

REFERENCES

1. Kayser D, Libouban S. Representation au niveau de l'aire auditive du cobaye des differentes spires de la cochlee. J Physiol (Paris) 1963; 55:153-6.

2. Walloch RA. A study of the auditory cortex in the guinea pig with implications for the development of an electrical prosthesis for the hard of hearing. Dissertation, University of Oregon Medical School, Portland, 1971.

3. Guild SR, Crowe SJ, Bunch CC, Polvogt LM. Correlations of differences in the density of innervation of the organ of Corti with differences in the acuity of hearing. Acta Otolaryngol (Stockh) 1931; 15:269-308.

4. Spoendlin H. The afferent innervation of the cochlea. In: Naunton R, Fernandez C, eds. Evoked electrical activity in the auditory nervous system. New York: Academic Press, 1978: 21-41.

5. Morrison D, Schindler RA, Wersäll J. A quantitative analysis of the afferent innervation of the organ of Corti in guinea pig. Acta Otolaryngol (Stockh) 1975; 79:11-23.

6. Fernandez C. Dimensions of the cochlea (guinea pig). J Acoust Soc Am 1952; 24:519-23.

PROBABILITY OF TRAUMA AND RELIABILITY OF PLACEMENT OF A 20 MM LONG MODEL HUMAN SCALA TYMPANI MULTIELECTRODE ARRAY

B. F. O'REILLY, MBChB, FRCS

SAN FRANCISCO, CALIFORNIA

Tests in animals have revealed that control of excitation of discrete sectors of the auditory nerve array can be effected with stimulation with appropriately positioned, bipolar stimulating elements of multiple electrode arrays. To achieve optimal spatial control of excitation, bipolar electrode elements must be apposed to the upper surface of the scala and the electrode position and orientation on that surface is of fundamental importance.

Thus, the mechanical characteristics of multielectrode arrays with potential application in man must insure 1) apposition of electrode contact surfaces with the upper surface of the scala, 2) acceptable electrode element placement reliability and 3) acceptably low risk of cochlear trauma when they are introduced 20-25 mm into the cochlea.

Model human multielectrode arrays have been constructed. Systematic testing of these arrays is required to direct changes in the mechanical design in order to meet the above criteria. In this preliminary report, the basic approach to evaluate these mechanical properties of multielectrode arrays will be described, along with initial data documenting electrode placement reliability and the probability of trauma.

The multielectrode arrays were hand fabricated with medical grade Silastic®. The wires were a platinum/rhodium alloy (90:10), 3 mil in diameter and insulated with Pyre-ML®. The wires were stacked into a vertical central band in order to minimize flexion in the vertical plane but to allow flexion in the axis of curvature of the cochlea.

The length of the intracochlear portion of the electrode was 20 mm and the pairs of electrodes were positioned on the apical 13.5 mm of the electrode with approximately 2 mm longitudinal separation between pairs. The horizontal distance between each electrode of a pair was approximately 0.5 mm.

Human cadaver temporal bones were removed as soon as possible after death and then stored in a deep freeze. They were defrosted for 48 hours in 10% formalin. The round window niche was opened up, the membrane exposed and removed.

The opening of the round window was enlarged anteriorly and inferiorly. The multielectrode array was then inserted. The cochlea was then uncapped and any damage to the basilar membrane assessed. After drying the specimen, the basilar membrane becomes brittle and can be easily removed without damaging the bony spiral lamina.

Longitudinal measurements were taken by laying a thread along the edge of the bony spiral lamina from the beginning of the basilar membrane in the vestibule to the first pair and then from the first pair to the eighth pair. The length of thread and the distance of each electrode from the edge of the bony spiral lamina were measured with a micrometer.

The incidence of trauma to the cochlea was assessed in ten implantation procedures using the same electrode. In eight uses there was no apparent damage to either the bony spiral lamina or the basilar membrane. In one of the two cases with traumatic insertions the electrode perforated the basilar membrane and the most apical 3.7 mm of the electrode entered the scala vestibuli. Rather surprisingly the bony spiral lamina was not fractured. In the other traumatic insertion case the basilar membrane was damaged at about 1.5 mm basal to the front electrode pair and also at the third electrode pair. There was a fracture of the bony spiral lamina joining these two points and extending about three quarters of the distance to the modiolus.

In studies preliminary to this test series the behavior of several kinds of electrode arrays was observed as they were inserted into previously dissected cochleas. There were three characteristic ways in which damage to the basilar membrane could be relatively easily effected. The first was as the tip reaches about 13 mm from the base instead of rotating around in the axis of curvature of the cochlea it turns upwards and perforates the basilar membrane. This is a special problem in electrode arrays with a relatively firm tip. The second mode of damage was found when the whole electrode array was too stiff. The tip of the electrode would start to rotate normally but stop about 16 mm from the base. Further insertion of the electrode array results in the midportion moving away from the

From the Coleman Laboratory, University of California at San Francisco.

TABLE 1. LONGITUDINAL MEASUREMENTS

	Base to 1st Pair (mm)	*Base to 8th Pair (mm)*
	6.90	19.70
	7.60	20.20
	7.20	19.95
	7.10	19.60
	7.05	19.50
	6.85	19.25
	7.30	19.70
	8.10	20.70
	6.80	19.20
	6.70	19.00
Average	7.16 (SD 0.62)	19.68 (SD 0.67)
Freq. stim.	7.5 kHz	1.2 kHz

bony spiral lamina, rotating vertically and rupturing a long segment of the basilar membrane. The third mode of damage was that already described in which there was a longitudinal fracture of the basal aspect of the bony spiral lamina. This was caused both by the buckling of the basal portion of the electrode array which was too flexible and by overrotating the electrode in an attempt to prevent the tip from perforating the basilar membrane.

The distances from the base to the first pair and to the apical eighth pair are shown in Table 1. It can be seen that the placement is fairly reproducible with an average distance from base to front pair of 7.16 mm with a standard deviation of 0.62 mm. The average distance from the base to the eighth pair was 19.68 mm with a standard deviation of 0.67 mm. These measurements correspond to the frequency "places" for 7.5 kHz and 1.2 kHz. For speech discrimination an acceptable range would be from 3 kHz to 400 Hz. These frequencies correspond to distances of 13.6 and 26.1 mm from the base of the basilar membrane. Thus the distance between the first and eighth pair would seem to be ideal but all the pairs should be moved a further 6.5 mm towards the apex. This would require the electrode array to be about 26.5 mm in length.

From the radial measurements shown in Table 2

TABLE 2. MEASUREMENTS OF DISTANCE FROM LATERAL EDGE OF BONY SPIRAL LAMINA TO OUTER ELECTRODE

Pair	*Distance (mm)*	*SD (mm)*
1st	0.125	0.09
2nd	0.220	0.17
3rd	0.420	0.23
4th	0.575	0.20
5th	0.680	0.10
6th	0.665	0.16
7th	0.666	0.16
8th	0.255	0.13

there would seem to be fairly good reproducibility of electrode distance from the lateral margin of the bony spiral lamina. The electrode array was designed so that the radial pairs would be centered along this line and therefore the ideal distance from the lateral margin of the bony spiral lamina to the outer electrode would be 0.25 mm. In fact only the second, third and eighth pairs were consistently in a good position. The first pair were consistently too medial while the fourth, fifth, sixth and seventh pairs were consistently too lateral. The fourth pair had the poorest results and in most cases the inner electrode was lateral to the lateral margin of the bony spiral lamina.

One fact that has become clear is that these hand fabricated electrode arrays behave in an individual but predictable manner. There would appear to be good reproducibility of both longitudinal and lateral placement of the electrodes. However, some alteration in the lateral positioning of the pairs of electrodes would help to center them on the lateral edge of the bony spiral lamina. We have gained some insight into the mechanical characteristics that are important in minimizing the risk of trauma during the insertion of the electrode array. *Systematic testing* of electrode arrays with a variety of mechanical characteristics would enable us to direct changes which would facilitate the insertion of longer electrode arrays covering the frequency "places" necessary for speech discrimination.

GROWTH OF LOUDNESS FOR SINUSOIDAL AND PULSATILE ELECTRICAL STIMULATION

R. V. SHANNON, PhD
SAN FRANCISCO, CALIFORNIA

The perception of loudness produced by electrically stimulating a cochlear prosthesis is different for different electrical waveforms. The two waveforms studied in the present experiment were biphasic pulses and sinusoids. In general, the growth of loudness curves are steeper for biphasic pulses than for sinusoids, when the two waveforms are equated for equal charge per unit time. The growth of loudness curves are steeper for low frequencies than for high frequencies, for both pulsatile and sinusoidal stimulation.

The implant was a Silastic® mold of the scala tympani containing 16 wires. These wires were positioned so that they would contact the superior surface of the scala tympani on insertion. The present results were obtained from stimulating wires 5 and 6 as a bipolar pair. These two wires were oriented radially within the cochlea and were approximately 10-12 mm from the round window.

The patient had a progressive, profound loss of hearing. The implant had been in place for over six months and thresholds were stable for a period of three months preceding the present measurements.

The stimulator was a custom-designed current source that could produce either sinusoidal or biphasic pulse output at various frequencies (or pulse rates). Each phase of the biphasic pulse was 200 μs in duration.

The data were collected using a simplified magnitude estimation procedure. A stimulus was presented and the patient was instructed to assign a value of 0 to 100 cents to the loudness of the sound. He was instructed to assign twice as large a value to a sound that was twice as loud as another. Note, however, that magnitude estimations, obtained in conditions where the end-points of the response scale are fixed, are biased near those end-points. In the following data it should be noted that the exact shape of the loudness growth curves is influenced by the nature of the task. The standard deviation of the data is typically ± 15 cents.

Figure 1 presents the loudness estimation data for both biphasic (Fig. 1A) and sinusoidal (Fig. 1B) stimulation. The slope of the growth of loudness curves decreases with increasing stimulus frequency or pulse rate. For a given stimulus rate, biphasic stimulation produces a steeper growth of loudness than sinusoidal stimulation. For sinusoid frequencies between 500 Hz and 4 kHz there is little change in the slope of the loudness growth curves. The 8

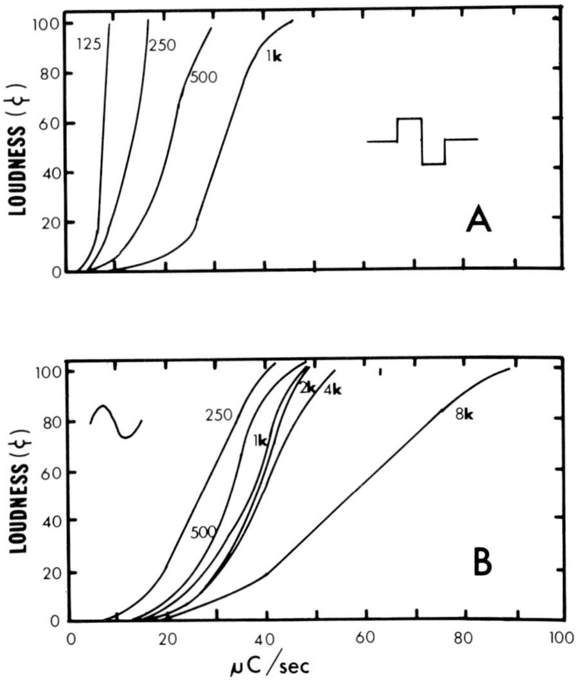

Fig. 1. Loudness estimates for A) pulsatile and B) sinusoidal electrical stimulation in terms of charge (μC) per second.

From the Coleman Laboratory, University of California at San Francisco.

kHz sinusoid produces a considerably shallower growth of loudness curve than lower frequencies.

The data of Figure 1A, B are replotted in Figure 2A, B, respectively, as equal loudness contours. Note that all thresholds are approximately the same for both biphasic and sinusoidal stimulation, and that threshold is independent of stimulating frequency. This suggests that the threshold is determined by a constant amount of charge. The threshold data of Eddington et al[1] are also presented in Figure 2A.

Suprathreshold loudness depends on frequency of stimulation differently for biphasic pulses and sinusoids. As the frequency of a sinusoid is increased, the charge per unit time remains constant. In Figure 2B the equal loudness curves are nearly flat for frequencies between 500 and 4 kHz, ie, a constant charge per second yields approximately the same loudness.

Our results suggest a slower growth of loudness and a larger dynamic range at all frequencies than the data of Eddington et al. This is perhaps due to the fact that Eddington et al used monopolar stimulation. The present data were collected with bipolar stimulation, shown by Merzenich et al[2] to produce more local stimulation than monopolar.

In summary, pulsatile stimulation becomes relatively more effective at producing loudness as pulse rate increases. The loudness produced by a sinusoid is nearly independent of stimulation frequency. Sinusoid and pulsatile stimuli, equated for charge, do not produce the same loudness, except at threshold.

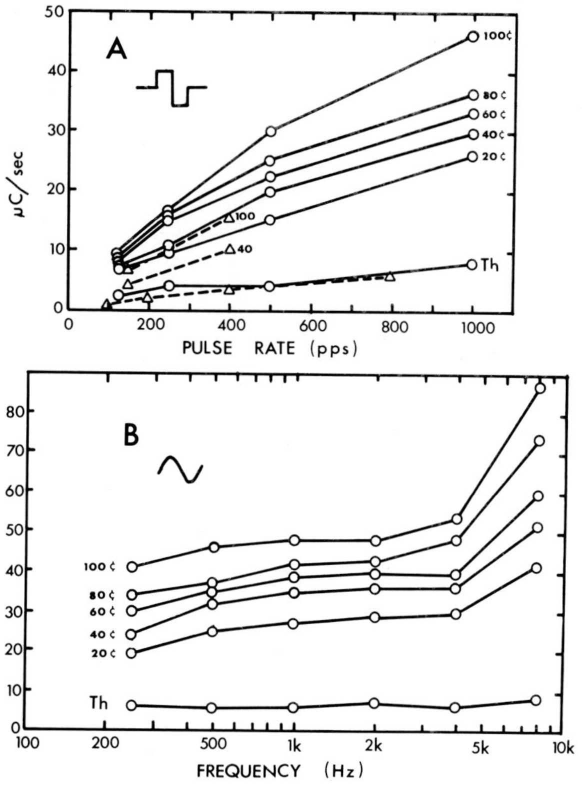

Fig. 2. Equal loudness contours for A) pulsatile and B) sinusoidal stimulation as a function of frequency. Data from Eddington et al[1] are presented by triangles and dashed lines in A for comparison.

REFERENCES

1. Eddington DK, Dobelle WH, Brackman DE, Mladejovsky MG, Parkin JL. Auditory prosthesis research with multiple channel intracochlear stimulation in man. Ann Otol Rhinol Laryngol 1978; 87 Suppl 53.

2. Merzenich MM, Schindler DN, White MW. Symposium on cochlear implants. II. Feasibility of multichannel scala tympani stimulation. Laryngoscope 1974; 84:1887-93.

PITCH CORRELATES OF DIRECT AUDITORY NERVE ELECTRICAL STIMULATION

F. B. SIMMONS, MD
M. G. WALKER, PhD
R. L. WHITE, PhD
R. G. MATHEWS, PhD
STANFORD, CALIFORNIA

INTRODUCTION

The most important question for multichannel stimulation is its capacity to transfer enough additional information to the auditory nerve (and brain) to justify its use instead of a single electrode. If true, and we suspect it is, it will shortly be time to decide on how to do this best. Important criteria are the location of the electrodes, merits of the scala tympani, and the auditory nerve approaches. We hope this conference will make a beginning in comparing data, both in those parameters which seem the same and in identifying those which, at this point, seem different.

This paper summarizes our observations on the perception of pitch by stimulating the auditory nerves of two volunteers who have had four electrodes placed permanently in their nerves for the last 18 months. The percepts reported were all produced using charge-balanced biphasic pulses of 0.25 ms. The amplitudes between threshold and "maximum loudness" covered a range of 5 to 50 nC and were delivered at rates between 1 and 1000 Hz. There has been no evidence of nerve injury or performance deterioration to date.

PITCH

In theory, there are two known determinants for differences in pitch, the nerve fibers which are being stimulated (place pitch) and the periodicity of the stimulation (rate pitch). The separation between these two was not always clear except at the extremes: ie, the pitch of a single pulse and *perhaps* the pitch of a brief burst of pulses at rates above the presumed limits for perceiving differences in rate pitch. In between, all sounds had components of both pitches.

Other features of the stimuli had important influences upon the perceptions of pitch, some probably related to the experiential backgrounds of the two subjects. Like the Eskimos who have more than 30 nouns for snow, we have probably learned to distinguish an equal number of differences among "buzzing or buzzer-like" percepts. Stimulus intensity had more than a modest (occasionally profound) effect on pitch. For example, a "low-pitched buzzer" could be changed to a "ring," and a "high-pitched buzzer" changed to a "bell" or "screech" by increasing intensity. Pitch percepts were also affected by frequency modulation, irregular interpulse intervals, and perhaps by stimulus duration.

PLACE PITCH

Both subjects 1 and 2 reported on or were able to rank "pitch or quality" differences among many single and two-electrode combinations when the same stimulus was used. These high-to-low rankings were stable only with single pulses or very slow repetition rates, and high rates (500-1000 Hz) in short bursts of 12 ms. Longer bursts, say 24-50 ms, began to change ranking and steady state stimulations were unrankable. We assume the character of the sounds on each E* (or combination) was, however, fundamentally the same in any set of stimuli since neither subject was able specifically to identify which electrode was being stimulated; ie, 1E had no consistently special sound quality which was uniquely different from 2E or 3E, etc. (Subject 1 could identify 2E by the associated "pressure" sensation or tipsiness.) Thus, while some elements of place pitch were clearly present, the percepts resulting from stimulation of 1E, eg, were not heavily colored by the unique pitchiness of the electrode.

Being more specific first requires some philosophical hunches on our subjects' understanding of pitch. Both had great difficulties inventing imaginative "what-it-sounds-like" pitch information, especially from steady-state inputs: A 10 Hz, "tick, tick, tick . . ." was more difficult to rank (for us) than, "horses running on concrete" (the same 10 Hz with every fourth pulse missing) when compared to 10 Hz on another electrode described as a "woodpecker" (bird) at work in a tall, thin tree about 30 m distant. Neither understood the concept of a musical octave. Subject 1 was accused by his friends

*Abbreviations used are: E - Electrode; $E_1 + E_2$ - Any combination of 2 Es; 1E, 2E, 3E, 4E - Specific electrodes; A,B,C - Different stimuli; AE_1 - Stimulus A to E_1; ABE_1 - Two different but simultaneous stimuli to E_1; A,BE_1 - A and B alternate.

From the Stanford University Medical Center, Division of Otolaryngology, Stanford, California. This research was sponsored by NIH NINCDS Grant No. NS10532-08.

REPRINTS — F. Blair Simmons, MD, Stanford University Medical Center, 300 Pasteur Drive, Stanford, CA 94305.

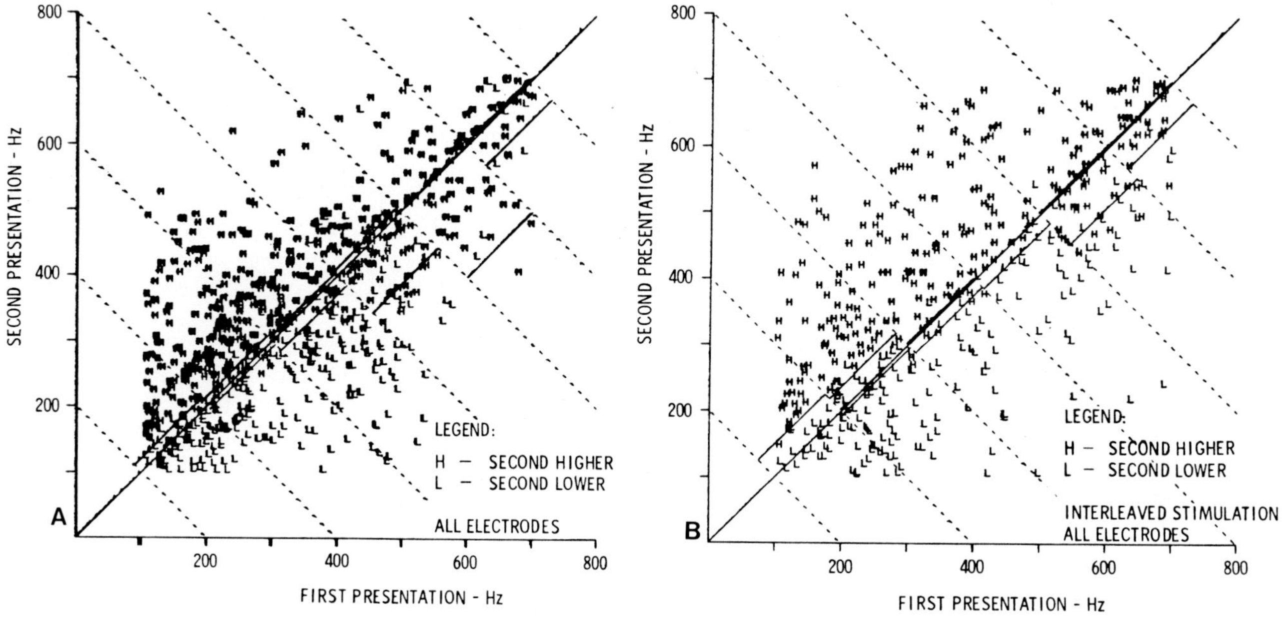

Fig. 1. (Subject 1) A) Forced-choice rate DLs. Data were plotted to 700 Hz. B) Interleaved stimulation rate DL data. The forced-choice paradigm was used.

as having a "tin ear" before his deafness. Subject 2 once wanted to know, "Is a 'tick' higher than a 'tink'?," and how was he to rank a "psst"? Thus, the place-pitch sounds seemed rich in "harmonics," sometimes musical, sometimes not, but still predictably rankable.

Subject 1 was more consistent than subject 2. For individual electrodes, subject 1 always ranked 4E highest and 2E lowest while the in-between ranking of 1E and 3E varied. Stimulus intensity changes probably affected the comparative rankings of 1E and 3E because whichever electrode acquired the greater increment during pretest loudness balances was judged higher-pitched than the other in at least 75% of judgments which followed. Subject 1 consistently ranked 14 (of 28) single and bipolar combinations higher or lower in pitch. Subject 2 was definitely not as adept at abstract ranking of pitches from pulses. Of the 16 possible 1 and 2-electrode combinations, he was completely consistent for only 5, and in all tests identified 3E as the lower-pitched. Electrode 1E (from anecdotal data and daily experience) was higher-pitched than 2E, but in formal competition between 1E and 2E, 2E was higher-pitched. Subject 2 ranked (high to low) $1E > 13 > 12 \geq 2 \equiv 3$, with 13E and 23E combinations variable. Subject 1 ranked $4E > (34 \text{ or } 14) > (1 \text{ or } 3) > 13 > 12 > 23 > 24 > 2$.

The sounds described during very slow stimulus rates (circa 1/s) produced the most consistent agreements with abstract pitch rankings. The pitch range of sounds heard with single pulses and less than 10/s stimuli extended from "thuds" and "knocking on a large board" to, "the altar boys' bell during Mass" (a strike tone of at least 2,000 Hz). We collected a similar range of sounds, "thuds" (from subject 1's lowest-pitched E) and "clear, bell-like" (small hammer on anvil) sounds (his highest-pitched E), with brief (12 ms) bursts at 500 Hz. Longer (and therefore louder) pulses created higher-pitched sounds and in one session actually caused a change in the rankings of two bipolar pairs when the duration was extended to 24 and 50 ms from 12 ms.

Stimulus Intensity and Place Pitch. Stimulus magnitude had an important impact on place pitch for most electrodes. An increase in intensity *always* caused an increase in the pitch of single-electrode sounds, and never a decrease in pitch. Thus five of seven electrodes typically produced "thuds," "tinks," or dull "tapping" sounds near threshold. The same stimuli at medium intensities caused "bells," "ringings," and "high-pitched buzzers." At higher intensities the sounds became small or large "triangles," "steady high-pitched sounds," and occasionally, unpleasant "screeches" and "howls." However, both subjects each reported that with one of their electrodes, loudness increased at least modestly without a pitch increase. In no instance did the pitch ever decrease with increasing intensity or loudness during either single or bipolar stimulations. Pitches did drop and loudness increased only in other stimulus modes (see section on rate pitch).

Harmonic Coloring. In our view, none of the sounds described by the subjects were even close to being pure tones, though many had "musical qualities." Most of the sounds seemed jagged or rough, many times leading to predictable confusions perhaps caused by these "harmonics." Subject 1, for example, ranked place pitch for pulses: $4E > 34$ $13 \equiv 1 > 3 > 14$ . . ., wherein 34 and 13 were many times called "the same." We used this 34-13 similarity to construct a continuously downward pitch ramp: 4E→*13*→1→3→34→13→1̣→3→34 . . ., which seemed to subject 1 to be getting continuously lower pitched.

RATE PITCH

Figure 1A shows representative difference limens (DL) for the detection of stimulus rate change. These data were collected using a random number generator. The subjects were asked if the second sound was higher or lower in pitch. A judgment of "same" was allowed only if they listened to the two rates a second time. The DL averaged around 5% at low rates and became almost infinitely large at rates above 350 Hz. (This electrode difference is in itself interesting and unexplained, but is in good agreement with earlier data.[1]) We assume that the character of these sounds did not change radically between the individual pairs of compared rates since this same paradigm using the instruction, "tell us if the two sounds are the same or different" produced much larger DLs.

The rate-related percepts were strikingly nonlinear. As rates increased from about 50 Hz to 150-200 Hz the pitch increased gradually from a low- to a higher-pitched "buzz" which roughly corresponded with our own perceptions from the auditory monitor. As the rates increased further, the anecdotal pitch descriptions rose rapidly to sound corresponding with frequencies between 2 and 4 kHz at 350 pulses per second.

Figure 1B shows the rate DLs when pulses were alternated between two electrodes at equal interpulse intervals: $^{E_1\,\cdot\,\cdot\,\cdot\,\cdot\,\cdot}_{E_2\,\cdot\,\cdot\,\cdot\,\cdot\,\cdot}$. The figure shows the combined rate, $E_1 + E_2$. Note that this extends the upper limit to about 700 Hz, just about twice the single E rate. Also note that the DLs themselves are poorer by about a factor of two than with single E stimulation. We confirmed the single vs two E DL difference in other experiments using fixed rates rather than the random number generator. We thus gain no better resolution by alternating pulses. These observations strongly suggest that the two nerve fiber populations stimulated retain at least some of their separate perceptual identities during multichannel stimulation.

Pitch matching experiments using alternating pulses seem to confirm this. We asked the subjects to compare the pitches of: $^{E_1\,\cdot\,\cdot\,\cdot\,\cdot\,\cdot}_{E_2\,\cdot\,\cdot\,\cdot\,\cdot\,\cdot}$ with E_1 . . . . . or E_2 . . . . . $E_1 + E_2$ was always lower-pitched (and louder) than the total rate to a single E, below 500 Hz. At rates between 500 and 700 Hz, the $E_1 + E_2$ stimulations were *usually* higher-pitched. Our undocumented (but strong) impression from these results is that the "pitchiness" of each alternated channel corresponded roughly to the same pitchiness when stimulated singly; ie, E_1 at 150 Hz + E_2 at 150 Hz (combined alternated stimulation) compared to 300 Hz on either E_1 or E_2 retained much of the individual 150 Hz percepts. The perceptual gestalt, however, probably lies in between complete separateness of two channels and complete fusion.

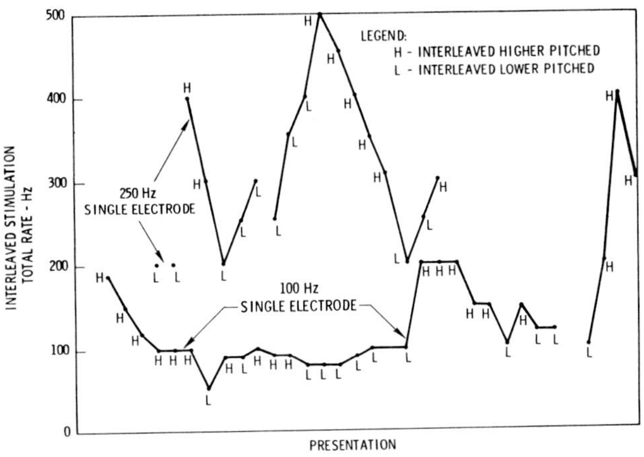

Fig. 2. (Subject 2) Pitch-matching responses. For each set, the single-electrode stimulation rate was constant. The ordinate is the total multielectrode stimulation rate which was compared to the single-electrode reference. Responses are noted next to each point.

The suspicion that some fusion and some separateness occur is probably best documented by the fact that we could not achieve a pitch match between alternating pulses to two electrodes and any rate on a single electrode. Figure 2 shows one try in which the E_1 rate was fixed at 100 and 200 Hz and the $E_1 + E_2$ rate was systematically increased or decreased until a "higher" or "lower" judgment was expressed. Note, for example, that the first (left hand side) lower to higher pitch change from $E_1 + E_2$ required more than a 250% rate increase. Then, the judgment of higher was retained until the $E_1 + E_2$ rate descended below 350 Hz.

CONCLUSIONS

Both place and rate pitch sensations were created by electrical stimulation. Convincing evidence for place pitch, however, could only be demonstrated for nonsteady state stimuli (single pulses, slow repetition rates, or brief bursts at very high rates). There seemed to be no special perceptual characteristic, by either place or rate stimulation, which seemed unique for an individual electrode; ie, that would allow the subjects to know specifically which electrode was being stimulated.

Rate pitch DLs were limited to a maximum of about 350 Hz, excepting one electrode with a 450 Hz limit. Simultaneous alternating stimulation of two electrodes did not extend the useful range of rates, even though the combined rate extended to 700 Hz, the DLs were roughly twice as large. These stimulations did, however, clearly demonstrate that simultaneous stimulations on two electrodes do remain at least partially separate in their perception. This observation, along with others not mentioned here, provide good evidence that multichannel stimulation does transfer more information than single-channel stimulation.

REFERENCES

1. Simmons FB. Electrical stimulation of the auditory nerve in man. Arch Otolaryngol 1966; 84:2-54.

ELECTRODE POSITION AND EXCITATION PATTERNS FOR A MODEL COCHLEAR PROSTHESIS

M. C. VIVION, PhD
MADISON, WISCONSIN

M. M. MERZENICH, PhD
M. WHITE, PhD
SAN FRANCISCO, CALIFORNIA

P. A. LEAKE-JONES, PhD
M. SILVERMAN, BS
SAN FRANCISCO, CALIFORNIA

Electrophysiological experiments were conducted to determine "optimum" intracochlear locations for bipolar elements of a multichannel cochlear prosthesis. Brainstem evoked response (BSER) mapping procedures were used to define the spread of excitation across the auditory nerve array as a function of stimulus current level for different bipolar electrode locations and configurations.

The mapping experiments were conducted in two different deaf animal populations: a) cats which were deafened just prior to being studied in an acute mapping experiment, by slow infusion of neomycin sulfate into the cochlea via the round window; and b) cats which were deafened by daily intramuscular administration of neomycin sulfate. These animal models were differentiated on the basis of the histological consequences of both deafening procedures and were classified on the basis of the extent of auditory nerve survival into high and low nerve-survival groups.

Experiments were conducted in the dissected cochleas of the anesthetized cats. Electrodes were positioned on the superior surface of the most basal (approximately 13 mm) part of the scala tympani. A bipolar pair of elements, which were platinum-iridium balls of 100-500 μ in diameter (typically 200), were positioned using micromanipulators, and a BSER intensity series was derived for each position. Stimuli were biphasic pulses, 100 μs per phase, and were presented 500 or 1000 times at a rate of 20/s to derive each BSER.

Since previous experiments had indicated a monotonic relationship between relative BSER amplitude and number of nerve fibers excited,[1] rate of growth of BSER amplitude as a function of stimulus current level was considered to be indicative of the spread of excitation across the nerve array. Using relative RMS amplitude functions derived from the BSERs, three kinds of electrode placement effects were studied in these cats: a) orientation of a bipolar pair, b) interelectrode separation or distance within an electrode pair, and c) mediolateral placement over the upper surface of the scala tympani.

On a first level of understanding, studies of electrode pair orientation indicated that "ideal" electrode elements should be positioned longitudinally, ie, parallel to the long axis of the basilar membrane, or at least at an angle away from the radial. Effect of interelectrode separation is generally described by the root mean square (RMS) functions in Figure 1, which shows the effect of increasing interelectrode distance of a longitudinally-oriented pair from a minimum of 0.3 mm (curve 1) to a maximum of about 7 mm (curve 8). Merzenich et al give a more detailed description of some of these effects.[2]

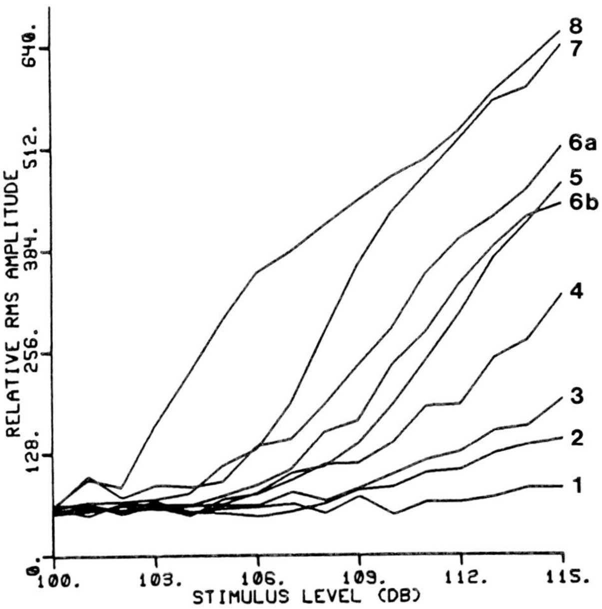

Fig. 1. Relative RMS amplitudes of cat BSERs (N = 1000) as a function of stimulus current level and electrode placement. Ipsilateral BSERs were recorded during biphasic electrical stimulation, as described earlier. Electrodes were positioned parallel to the long axis of the basilar membrane. Interelectrode distance was systematically increased, from a minimum of 0.3 mm (curve 1) to a maximum of about 7 mm (curve 8).

From the Coleman Laboratory, University of California at San Francisco. Work supported by NIH Grant No. NS-11804, NIH Contract No. N01-NS-7-2367, and Hearing Research, Inc.

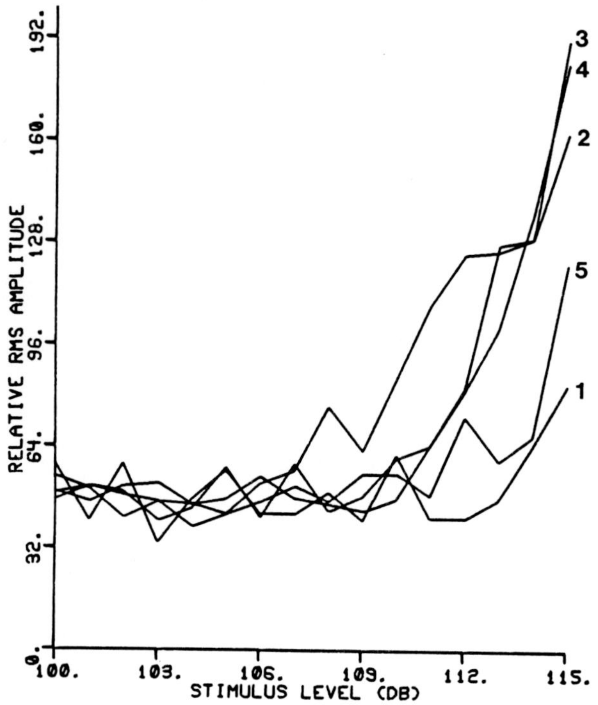

Fig. 2. Relative RMS amplitude of cat BSERs (N = 1000) as a function of stimulus current level and mediolateral electrode placement on the superior surface of the scala tympani. Ipsilateral BSERs were recorded during biphasic electrical stimulation (100 μs each phase, 20/s, 113 dB = 1 mA). These five electrode pairs were all oriented parallel to the long axis of the cochlea. Interelectrode separation was a constant 1.2 mm. Curve 5 was derived with the electrodes positioned over the basilar membrane. Curve 4 was derived over the bony spiral lamina, midway between the basilar membrane and the medial edge of the bony spiral lamina. Curve 3 was derived with the electrodes along the medial edge of the bony spiral lamina. Curves 2 and 1 were derived with the electrodes positioned in two equal steps farther medialward. In this cochlea, lowest threshold and largest amplitude responses were consistently recorded along the medial edge of the bony spiral lamina.

In low nerve-survival cats, thresholds decreased and growth rates of BSER amplitudes increased as interelectrode distance was increased. In high nerve-survival cats, thresholds and growth rates of BSER amplitudes were only nominally affected until interelectrode distance exceeded 1 mm.

Given the findings that indicated a longitudinally-oriented electrode pair with a relatively narrow interelectrode separation produces a low threshold and a slow growth of BSER amplitude, and therefore a slow spread of excitation across the nerve array, the effect of mediolateral placement of an electrode pair was then investigated. Figure 2 shows RMS amplitude functions for a low nerve-survival cat that were derived using a longitudinally-oriented electrode pair having a constant separation of 1.2 mm. The functions represent successive mediolateral placements progressing from over the basilar membrane (curve 5) to maximally medialward (curve 1). In low nerve-survival cats, optimal excitation was observed with electrode placements over Rosenthal's canal. In high nerve-survival cats, discrete low-threshold excitation was effected with the electrode positioned anywhere across the spiral lamina.

In summary, the results of these mapping experiments, to date, indicate that appropriate discrete stimulation of the auditory nerve array can be achieved using bipolar electrode pairs and that such electrode elements are suitable for the development of a multielectrode array. It is clear that orientation, separation, and mediolateral placement of the elements of the electrode pair are critical for effecting discrete stimulation of the auditory nerve array.

REFERENCES

1. Merzenich MM, White MW. Cochlear implant: the interface problem. In: Resnick J, Hambrecht T, eds. Functional electrical stimulation. New York: M. Dekker, 1977.

2. Merzenich MM, Leake-Jones PA, Walsh S, Vivion MC. Development of multichannel electrodes for an auditory prosthesis. NIH Contract N01-NS-7-2367. Neuroprosthesis Contract Program, Washington, NINCDS. Q Prog Rep 1978-79.

OPTO-ISOLATED STIMULATORS USED FOR ELECTRICALLY EVOKED BSER

SOME OBSERVATIONS ON ELECTRICAL ARTIFACT

L. S. VUREK
M. FONG, MS
M. WHITE, PhD
S. M. WALSH, PhD

SAN FRANCISCO, CALIFORNIA

This lab uses optically isolated voltage controlled constant current stimulators in its animal experiments. The stimulators are an "in house" design and are normally used in conjuction with the D/A output on our Nova computer; in most of our work a 100 μs per phase biphasic pulse is used. The principal advantages of these stimulators in the research environment are 1) ability to produce a relatively high isolated current — up to 17.2 mA peak to peak into a 10 kΩ load (with an overall dynamic range of 85 dB), 2) ability to take any shape waveform and produce a constant current output of the same shape, 3) simplicity of design and construction, 4) relatively low artifact operation in electrically stimulated BSER experiments, and 5) a high output impedance — approximately 10 Meg.

Operation. The calibration procedure will serve to illustrate the operation of the stimulator (Figs. 1 and 2): A digital to analog converter (D/A) is driven by the computer, the output of the D/A goes to a digital attenuator, the output of the attenuator is connected to the stimulator. The stimulator input is 600 Ω to match the impedance of the attenuator; the input to the unisolated side of the Burr Brown 3652 is differential (for common mode noise rejection); the 3652 provides a gain of 10 and an isolated output, which drives the analog devices 171j, which is configured as a voltage controlled constant current source; the 5kΩ pot is adjusted until a 10 V drop is measured across the precision 10kΩ calibrate resistor, at this point, the current source is calibrated for 1 mA for a given attenuator setting. It can be seen, that the load is in series with the 5kΩ pot to ground; the voltage drop across the pot will always try to seek the voltage present at the noninverting input of the AD 171j. The stimulator exhibits a 1 V in to 10 mA out linear transfer characteristic. The series capacitors serve as added protection against direct current potentials. The limitation of this stimulator circuitry is the frequency response of the opto-isolators (3652), which is 3 dB down at 15kc.

Measurements Performed on Stimulators. The input to the stimulators was shorted with a 1.8 m piece of wire to ground, the observed output noise was measured across a 10kΩ load, 10 mV peak to peak of wide-band high frequency noise was observed (0.5 μA peak); the stimulators were driven with a 10 kc sine wave, the output reached 130 V (13 mA peak to peak) before clipping would occur with 67.5 V batteries and the output reached 172 V (17.2 mA) with 90 V batteries; this equates to an 82 dB and 85 dB dynamic range.

Electrical Artifact During Electrically Stimulated BSER Experiments. In this instance, "electrical artifact" is defined as a component of the electrical stimuli, which appears to extend in time past the end of the biphasic pulse (Fig. 3).

A few observations have been made, which consistently correlate with the time after stimulation of the artifact is present. 1) On the evoked response monitoring amplifier or preamplifier a setting of = 100 Hz high pass and/or a = 10 kc low pass filter setting will increase the duration of the artifact. 2) In a linear type electrical stimulator a flat frequency response below 10 kc, decreases the artifact. 3) Due to the low level of the BSER signal (microvolt and submicrovolt) the settling time *measured to a microvolt level* is important and should be closely observed when evaluating digital (pulse only) stimulators or linear stimulators used in pulse modes.

Generally, construction techniques which minimize any type of coupling between unisolated and isolated stages appears to reduce artifact. Being cognizant of these factors doesn't assure artifact-free BSERs, and other factors not easily able to be correlated also contribute to electrical artifact.

From the Coleman Laboratory, University of California at San Francisco. Work supported by NIH Grant NS-11804, NIH Contract NO 1-NS-7-2367 NINCDS.

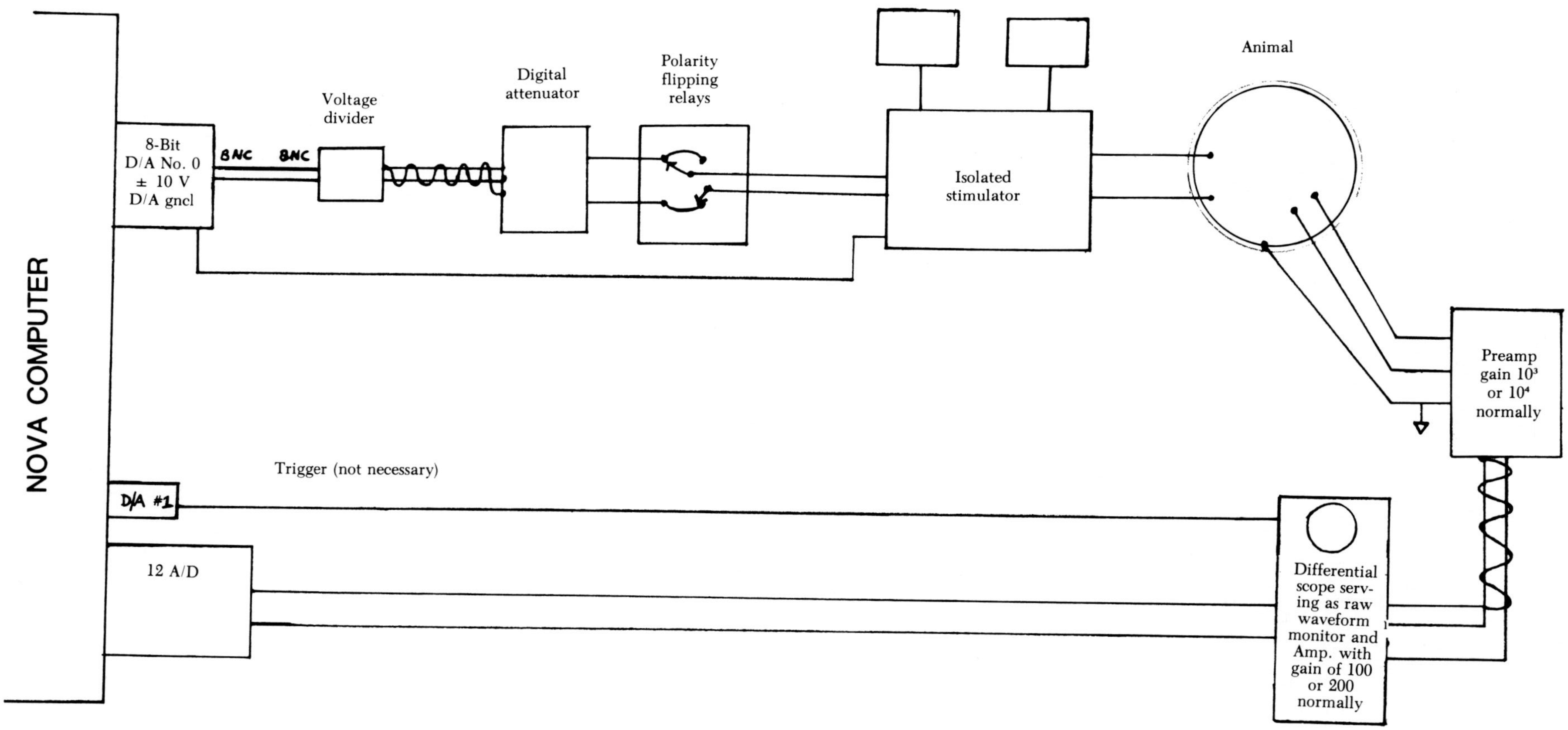

Fig. 1. Typical connection diagram for the Coleman Laboratory's one channel electrical stimulation-evoked response experiments. The typical output of the D/A is a 100 μsec per phase biphasic pulse, whose polarity is flipped every other trail. Dependent upon the software and speed of the system, the voltage divider, digital attenuator and polarity flipping relay could be eliminated.

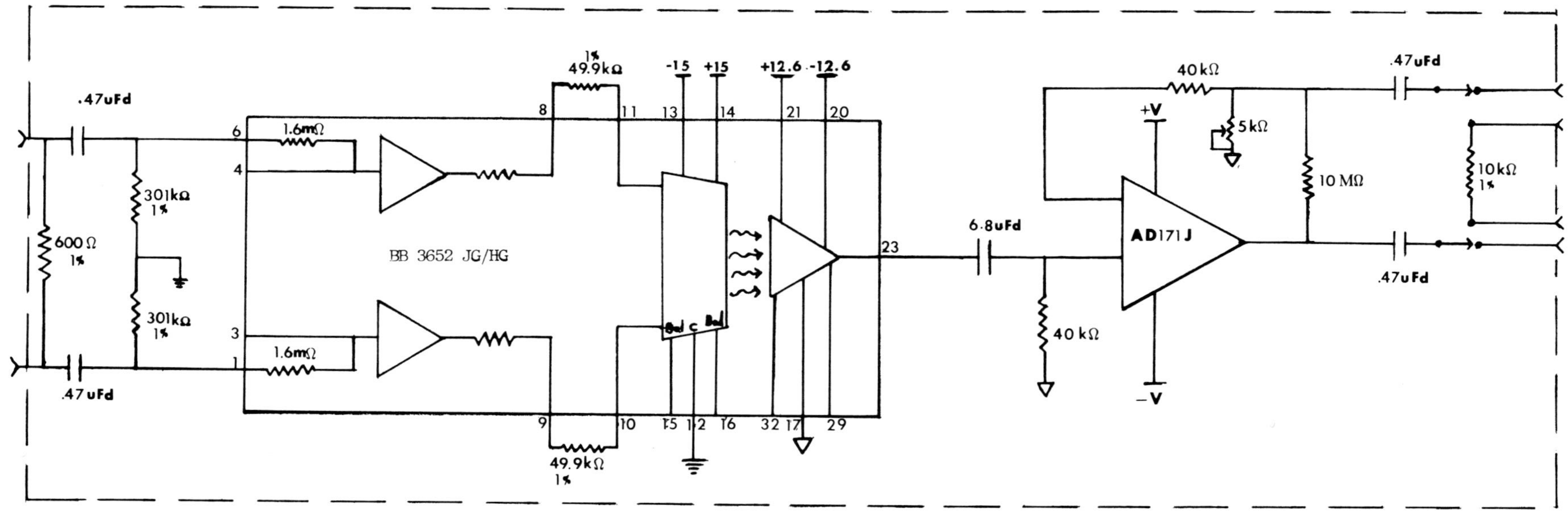

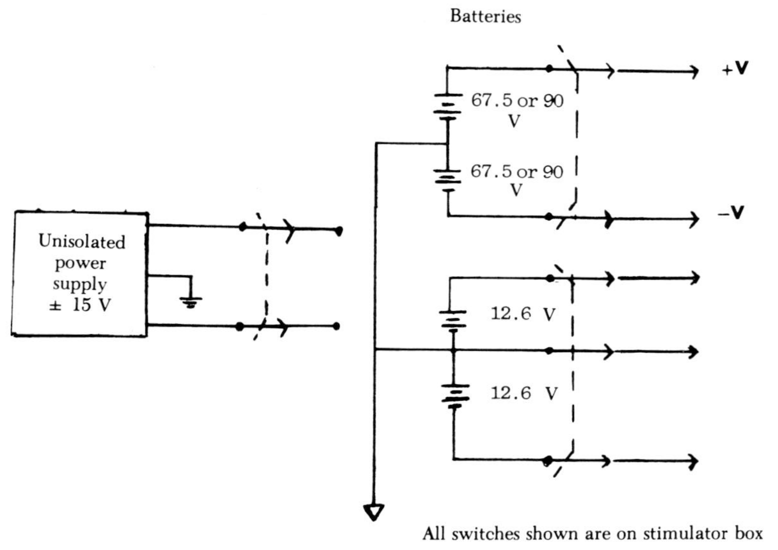

Fig. 2. Complete schematic and parts diagram of Opto-isolated stimulator. Isolated-stimulator enclosures are plastic “vero” boxes No. 65-2522K. Dimensions 18.7 x 10.8 x 6 cm. Battery pack is a “freezette” plastic container. Dimensions 10.1 x 10.1 x 13.3 cm. All connections are female banana jacks, except the power connector, spaced to accept a banana to BNC plug. Power connectors are 5-pin “DIN” connectors.

Unisolated Side Pin	Isolated Side Pin
1 = gnd	1 = gnd
2 = − 15	2 = − 12.6
3 = + 15	3 = + 12.6
4 = not used	4 = − 67.5 (− 90)
5 = not used	5 = + 67.5 (+ 90)

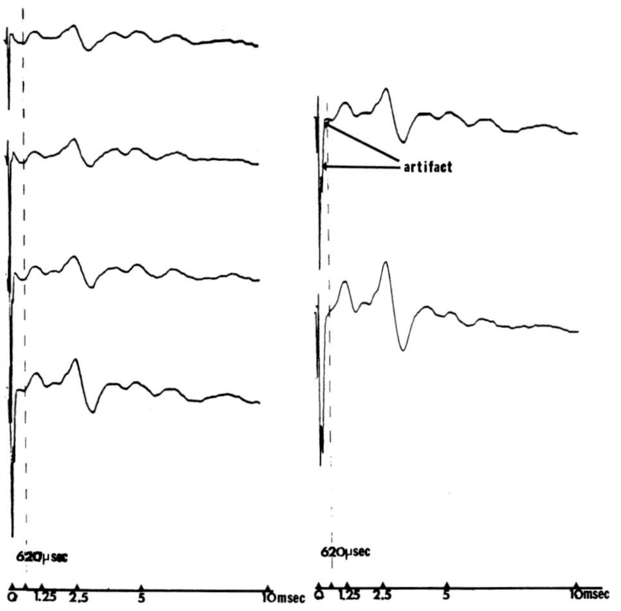

Fig. 3. Growth of electrical artifact as intensity of stimulation grows is illustrated. The plots are of a cat BSER with a maximum stimulus intensity of 2 mA.

COCHLEAR PROSTHESES

A HISTOLOGICAL EXAMINATION OF IMPLANTED CATS

R. A. WALLOCH, PhD

C. A. SMITH, PhD
N. R. SCHUFF, BS

J. A. FENWICK, BS
R. A. BOBERG, BS

PORTLAND, OREGON

Within recent years, the cochlear implants have provided the sensation of hearing to a number of the totally deaf. Despite this impressive progress in development of the cochlear implant, many significant questions remain. Among these is the potential damage to the cochlea and auditory nerve fibers.

To study the effects of chronic implantation and electrical stimulation of the cochlea, five behaviorally trained cats were implanted with multielectrode arrays (Table 1). Four of the cats received implants similar to those developed by Dr. R. Michaelson and the fifth cat received an implant of the type designed by Dr. W. House.

Immediately after implantation, the cats had relatively high electrical thresholds which decreased about 60-70% within the following three months. This drop in thresholds within the first few months of stimulation had been mentioned by other investigators at this Cochlear Prosthesis Conference. When the thresholds appeared stabilized (Table 1, column 5), the behavioral study was begun.[1] That study demonstrated that pulse width but not pulse repetition rates affect reaction times. Throughout the study the cats were stimulated for one hour daily, five days a week.

After a period of consistent threshold recording (column 5), the thresholds began to increase in the three cats with Michaelson-type electrodes. This increase in thresholds was not observed in the single cat with the House-type electrode. In a few weeks, these thresholds had increased to the point where behavioral data could no longer be obtained. At that point, the cats were sacrificed and histology performed. Interestingly, a higher amount of current was used in the three cats with the Michaelson-type implant.

Cat 1 actually had both ears implanted. The head plug became dislodged only a few days after receiving the first implant. At that time, the contralateral ear was implanted. Therefore, cat 1 had a Michaelson-type electrode in each cochlea, however, only the left cochlear implant was stimulated.

When the cats were sacrificed, gross inspection was made of their bullae. All electrodes appeared properly oriented in the round window. Cat 2 had considerable stenosis of the bulla with concomitant obliteration of the external auditory meatus.

Microscopic examination of the ears revealed changes similar to those described by other investigators[2-5] (Table 2). The basal turns of all implanted ears showed some sensory cell loss which ranged from a few scattered missing hair cells (cat 1, right ear) to almost complete degeneration of the organ of Corti in cat 3. Nerve fiber and ganglion cell degeneration varied from place to place and was least in cat 1, right ear.

There was considerable variation between animals in the apical turns. Ears of cat 1, right, and cat 4, right, had normal apical turns, whereas the left ear of cat 1, had considerable outer hair cell loss. In most cats, the ganglion cell loss fit in with the sensory cell degeneration. In the exception, cat 5, only

TABLE I. SUMMARY OF CHRONIC ELECTROCOCHLEAR STIMULATION IN CATS

Cat	*Implant Date*	*ET*	*Sacrifice Date*	*Sacrifice Reason*	*BT (μA)*	*Length of Stimulation (mo)*
1R	8-3-77	M	6-29-78	Head plug pulled out	NS	NS
1L	8-22-77	M	6-29-78	HT	300	4
2	7-28-77	M	6-29-78	HT	300	1
3	7-27-77	M	5-14-78	HT	175	5
4	8-18-77	H	6-29-78	End of Study	50	6
5	1-13-77	M	3-24-77	Head plug pulled out	175	NA

ET - Electrode type; M - Michaelson; H - House; HT - High threshold; BT - Best thresholds; NS - Not stimulated; NA - Not applicable.

From the Kresge Hearing Research Laboratory, Department of Otolaryngology-Maxillofacial Surgery, University of Oregon Health Sciences Center, Portland. This work was supported by grants from the National Institutes of Health (No. NS12864), Deafness Research Foundation and the Medical Research Foundation of Oregon.

REPRINTS — Richard A. Walloch, PhD, Kresge Hearing Research Laboratory, Dept. of Otolaryngology-Maxillofacial Surgery, University of Oregon Health Sciences Center, Portland, OR 97201.

TABLE 2. HISTOLOGICAL EXAMINATION OF IMPLANTED COCHLEA.

	1R	*1L*	*2*	*3*	*4*	*5*
Stimulating current	NS	300 μA	300 μA	175 μA	50 μA	NS
Basal turn						
Hair cells	Few scattered OHC lost	Some degen. IHC; some missing OHC	Many hair cells degen.	Almost complete degen.	Many hair cells lost	Complete degen.
Spiral ganglion	Some sl. loss, most at RW	1/4-1/2 lost	1/4-3/4 lost	1/4-3/4 lost	1/4-3/4 lost	1/4-3/4 lost
Apical turn						
Hair cells	OK	Most OHC lost	Some loss of OHC	Some loss of OHC	OK	Almost complete degen.
Spiral ganglion	OK	1/3-1/2 lost	Sl. loss	1/4-3/4 lost	Probably OK	Sl. loss
Bone growth or deposit at round window	Slight	Large	Large	Slight	Slight	Extensive up into basal turn
Debris in scalae in basal turn	sc t. & sc v.	Slight	No	Yes	Yes	Yes
Apical turn bone	No	No	No	No	No	No
Debris in apical turn	Yes	No	No	No	Yes	Yes
Penetrated basilar membrane	No	No	No	No	Yes	Yes
Other observations		Hydrops throughout			Elec. broke through sp. lam. & Reissner's in T_1 RW	

NS - Not stimulated; Sl. - Slight; Degen. - Degeneration; RW - Round window; sc t. - Scala tympani; sc v. - Scala vestibuli; elec. - Electrode; sp. lam. - Spiral lamina.

slight loss of the apical spiral ganglion was observed, although the hair cells were almost completely degenerated.

All cats showed some new bone formation but this was limited to a small area at the round window and was probably related to injury or infection. Except for cat 5, extensive new bone growth was not seen in the scalae for the remainder of the cochlea as described by Leake-Jones et al.[2]

Cat 5 was the first animal implanted and new bone had formed near the tip of the electrode where it had penetrated the spinal lamina.

REFERENCES

1. Walloch RA, Fenwick JA, Boberg R. A reaction-time analysis of electrocochlear stimulation in cats. Laryngoscope 1980; 90:861-6.

2. Leake-Jones PA, Walsh MA, Merzenich MM. Chronic electrical stimulation with intracochlear electrodes: stimulus induced cochlear pathology. Association for Research in Otolaryngology, Second Midwestern Research Meeting, January 22-24, 1979.

3. Sutton D, Pfingst BE, Miller JM, Webster DB. Cochlear and CNS histopathology in monkeys with chronic cochlear implants. Association for Research in Otolaryngology, Second Midwestern Research Meeting, January 22-24, 1979.

4. Schindler RA, Merzenich MM, White MM, Bjorkroth B. Multi-electrode intracochlear implants. Arch Otolaryngol 1977; 103:691-9.

5. Schindler RA, Merzenich MM. Chronic intracochlear electrode implantation: cochlear pathology and acoustic nerve survival. Ann Otol Rhinol Laryngol 1974; 83:202-14.

CHRONIC ELECTRICAL STIMULATION WITH INTRACOCHLEAR ELECTRODES: ELECTROPHYSIOLOGICAL RESULTS

S. M. WALSH, PhD
L. S. VUREK
P. A. LEAKE-JONES, PhD
M. M. MERZENICH, PhD
SAN FRANCISCO, CALIFORNIA

The insertion of an array of bipolar electrode pairs (embedded in a molded Silastic® carrier) into the scala tympani of the cochlea has been proposed as a means of effecting multichannel stimulation of the eighth nerve in profoundly deaf patients. Since electrical stimulation can destroy as well as activate neural tissue,[1,2] use of such multielectrode arrays depends on an empirical definition of long-term stimulus conditions resulting in cochlear damage.

Cats were implanted with two channel (4-wire) bipolar electrode arrays having PtRh (90:10) electrodes with spherical tips (200-300 μ in diameter) and interelectrode separations of 1-2 mm. The brainstem evoked response (BSER) was recorded to monitor physiological responses to biphasic pulsatile stimulation in these chronic preparations. Baseline data (ie, threshold of BSER, growth of magnitude of BSER as a function of increase in stimulus current intensity level, electrode impedance measurements) were collected over a two-week to six-month period following surgery. During this period a single electrode pair was selected for test. Animals were then exposed to long periods (120-1,000 hours) of continuous high level stimulation: 40-200 μC/phase/cm² real surface area, 100 μs/phase in duration at 20-25 pulses/s. Stimuli were delivered through a portable constant-current stimulating system designed to ensure delivery of charge-balanced biphasic waveforms.

The animals were tested frequently during the period of stimulation and for 8 to 20 days following cessation of stimulation with a standard intensity series. Since extensive neural changes in the cochlea are not induced by the presence of an electrode array of this type[3] an elevation in the threshold of BSER and/or a change in the magnitude of response at a given level of current, were interpreted as indication of *stimulus induced* damage to the cochlea. Stable electrode impedances would indicate whether observed changes were physiological rather than mechanical in nature, eg, breaks or leaks resulting in diminished current flow. Additional control studies insured that electrophonic activation of the contralateral cochlea did not contribute to the elec-

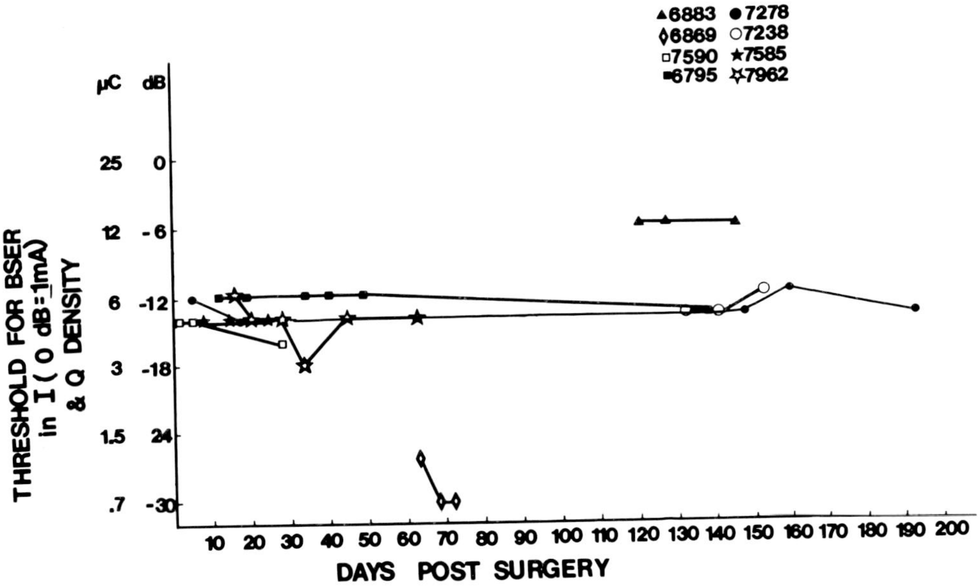

Fig. 1. Threshold of BSER recordings during the baseline period. During this time implanted animals are periodically monitored awaiting initiation of chronic stimulation. Data from eight animals indicate that thresholds are stable for periods as great as six months postimplantation. Data re growth of magnitude of response of BSER reflect the same stability in responsiveness of eighth nerve during the prestimulation period.

From the Coleman Laboratory, University of California at San Francisco.

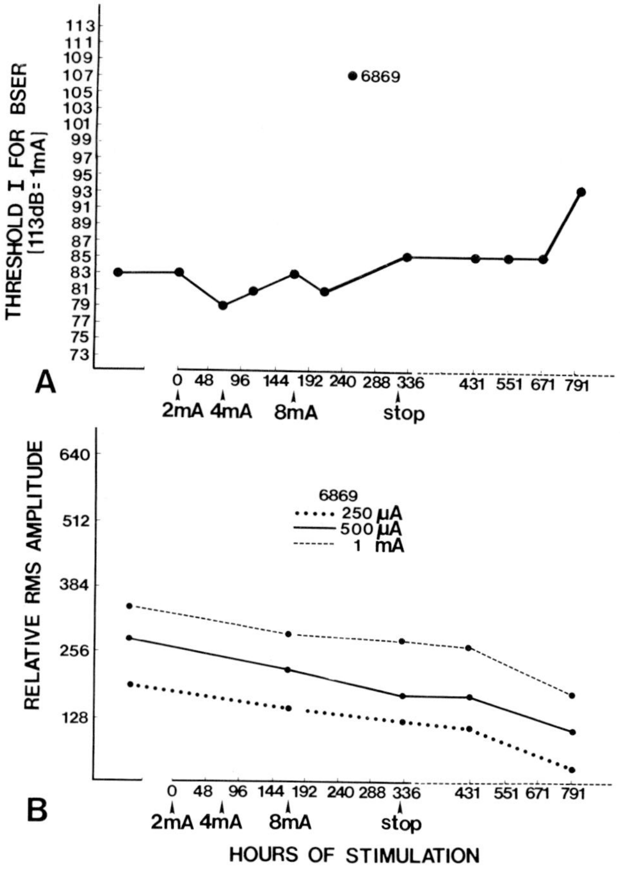

Fig. 2. A) Threshold of BSER recordings over the total time of study for one representative case. No significant change in response occurs during periods of 2mA (50 μC/phase/cm²r) or 4mA (100 μC/phase/cm²r) stimulation. Only a slight elevation follows introduction of 8mA (200 μC/phase/cm²r) stimulation. The major shift in threshold occurs following the cessation of stimulation. B) The growth of magnitude of response as a function of increase in stimulus current intensity level is displayed for the same case. Some change is indicated during the period of 4mA (100 μC/phase/cm²r) stimulation. Most dramatic changes occur following the administration of 8mA (200 μC/phase/cm²r) stimulation and following the cessation of stimulation. In several of the cases studied changes in responsiveness appeared in the growth of magnitude of response functions before they were manifested as changes in threshold.

trically evoked response. Results are based on data obtained from nine animals studied over periods of two to nine months.

Despite the individual differences in stimulus regimes, several features are common to all animals which showed a change in response. Electrode impedances in all animals were stable throughout the entire period of testing, ie, baseline through poststimulation periods. In prior-normal cases, no change in physiological response was seen during the baseline period, ie, during the time in which electrodes were in situ but not subjected to significant stimulation (Fig. 1). These data demonstrate that nontraumatic insertion and a significant period of indwelling (six months) are not sufficient to elicit physiological changes.

Cases which were treated with neomycin prior to implantation had gradually diminishing physiological responses during the prestimulation period. Since changes in baseline data occurred only within this subgroup, these can be correlated with degenerative changes associated with ototoxically induced cochlear pathology.

No change in physiological response was seen following periods of 50 μC (48-800 hours) and 100 μC (96 hours) stimulation. When the stimulus level was adjusted to 200 μC, changes were finally observed, but these did not appear immediately after the increase. Evidence of an elevation in BSER threshold emerged slowly and in some cases was seen only after the cessation of stimulation. Significant changes in the growth of magnitude of response of BSER were observed concurrent with changes in threshold. Figure 2 illustrates threshold measurements and the magnitude of response (at three specified intensity levels) over the total time course of stimulation for one representative case. Preliminary data suggest that by limiting stimulation to levels below 40 μC/phase/cm² real surface area, the extensive damage which resulted from exposure to the very high charge densities employed in this study, may be prevented.

In all damaged cases studied, two effects were evident in the cochlear material examined: 1) presence of new bone growth within the scala tympani and 2) degeneration of auditory nerve fibers and spiral ganglion cells. Both of these effects were most prominent in the region of the cochlea corresponding to the stimulated electrode pair.[4]

These data have significant implications for the application of scala tympani prostheses. Indications of damage to the cochlea following electrical stimulation emerge very slowly, even when the stimulus level is set purposely high in an attempt to ensure damage. In fact, had our protocol been modeled on investigations of safe limits for other applications (stimulus exposure usually less than two days) we would not have observed any physiological indications of detrimental effects to the cochlea following electrical stimulation representing charge densities as great as 200 μC. Furthermore, results of monitoring BSER following the cessation of stimulation demonstrate that the active process(es), once evoked, have continuing effects, ie, effects which do not reverse, nor cease following a lengthy recovery period.

The complement of physiological and histological results suggest several mechanisms for the damage elicited in these cases: 1) Bone growth may displace the electrode, situating it further away from its target structures or may provide an additional impedance barrier within the cochlea. 2) Nerve damage could result when reaction products are released in electrochemical activity occurring at the electrode-tissue interface. Some of these reactions are prevented by the use of balanced biphasic pulses which allow charge injection to occur via double-layer charging.[5] Prevention of oxidation of saline, metal and organics, however, requires that charge densities be restricted according to empirically defined limits. 3) Nerve damage could result from electrical and/or chemical changes brought about by the presence of new bone within the cochlea. 4) Damage to nerve could result from interference with the vasculature supplying that area.

It is not clear which process or combination of processes are active in this damage model. There is little likelihood that rapid onset etiologies are responsible for the effects we have observed. The delayed emergence and the progressive nature of physiological changes are most compatible with hypotheses related to deposition of new bone and/or accumulation of toxic ions at the nerve.

REFERENCES

1. Roland V, MacIntyre WJ, Bidder TG. The production of brain lesions with electrical currents. II. Bidirectional currents. J Neurosurg 1960; 17:55-69.
2. Pudenz RH, Bullara, LA, Jacques S, Hambrecht T. Electrical stimulation of the brain. III. The neural damage model. Surg Neurol 1975; 4:389-400.
3. Schindler RA. The cochlear histopathology of chronic intracochlear implantation. J Laryngol Otol 1976; 90:445-7.
4. Leake-Jones PA, Walsh SM, Merzenich MM. Cochlear pathology following chronic intracochlear electrical stimulation. Ann Otol Rhinol Laryngol 1981; 1981; 90 Suppl 82:6-8.
5. Brummer SB, Turner MJ. Electrochemical considerations for safe electrical stimulation of the nervous system with platinum electrodes. IEEE Trans Biomed Eng 1977; 24:59-63.

MAINTENANCE OF NEURONAL ACTIVITY BY ELECTRICAL STIMULATION OF UNILATERALLY DEAFENED CATS DEMONSTRABLE WITH CYTOCHROME OXIDASE TECHNIQUE

M. T. T. WONG-RILEY, PhD
P. A. LEAKE-JONES, PhD
S. M. WALSH, PhD
M. M. MERZENICH, PhD

SAN FRANCISCO, CALIFORNIA

When cats are implanted with a Silastic® scala tympani insert introduced nontraumatically via the round window, nearly all the auditory nerve fibers survive the long-term implantation.[1] However, numerous physiological studies reveal that these cats are profoundly deaf in the implanted ear.[2,3] This deafness leads to a "silencing" of brainstem auditory nuclei (from the cochlear nuclei to the inferior colliculi) that receive excitatory input mainly from the deafened ear. This prolonged inactivity, in turn, can cause morphological and functional changes that have classically been regarded as "degenerative" in the affected nuclear groups. An index of functional changes can be derived histochemically by determining the level of cytochrome oxidase activity. Normally, functioning auditory neurons have high levels of cytochrome oxidase activity, presumably reflecting a high rate of energy utilization.[4] Subsequent to chronic unilateral deafness, the level of cytochrome oxidase activity within the "silenced" auditory relay nuclei is dramatically reduced.[4]

In order to test for the effect of reactivating "silenced" neuronal populations by elecrical stimulation, we have examined cytochrome oxidase activity in the brainstem auditory nuclei of two cats that were unilaterally deafened for five to six months, and then continuously stimulated for about one month.

Stimuli were biphasic pulses delivered at a rate of 20 pps. The animals were monitored physiologically throughout the experiment by recording brainstem evoked responses. The evoked potentials indicated that *all* (or nearly all) cochlear nerve fibers were excited by the applied electrical stimuli, throughout the stimulation period. After cessation of continuous stimulation, several additional brief periods of stimulation were given during interim survival times of 8 days for one cat and 15 days for the other.

Serial frozen sections through the brainstem were cut and incubated for cytochrome oxidase, using the technique as described before.[5] In examining those nuclear groups that received their excitatory

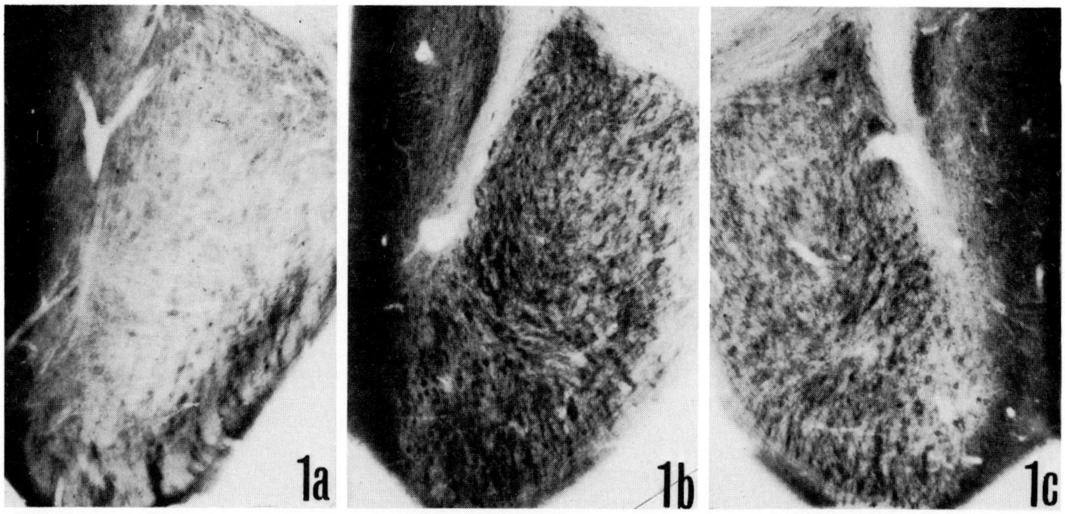

Fig. 1. Coronal sections through the level of the posterior ventral cochlear nuclei (PVCN) incubated for cytochrome oxidase activity without any counterstaining. Compare the b) normal with the c) experimentally-deafened and stimulated sides from the same section. By contrast, the PVCN from a representative deafened and nonstimulated case (a) shows a much lowered level of cytochrome oxidase activity. (x20)

From the Department of Anatomy, Coleman Laboratory and Department of Physiology and Otolaryngology, University of California at San Francisco.
This work was supported by NIH Grant NS 12995, NIH Grant NS 11804, NIH Contract N01-NS-7-2367 and Hearing Research Institute.
REPRINTS — M. T. T. Wong-Riley, PhD, Dept. of Anatomy, School of Medicine, University of California, San Francisco, CA 94143.

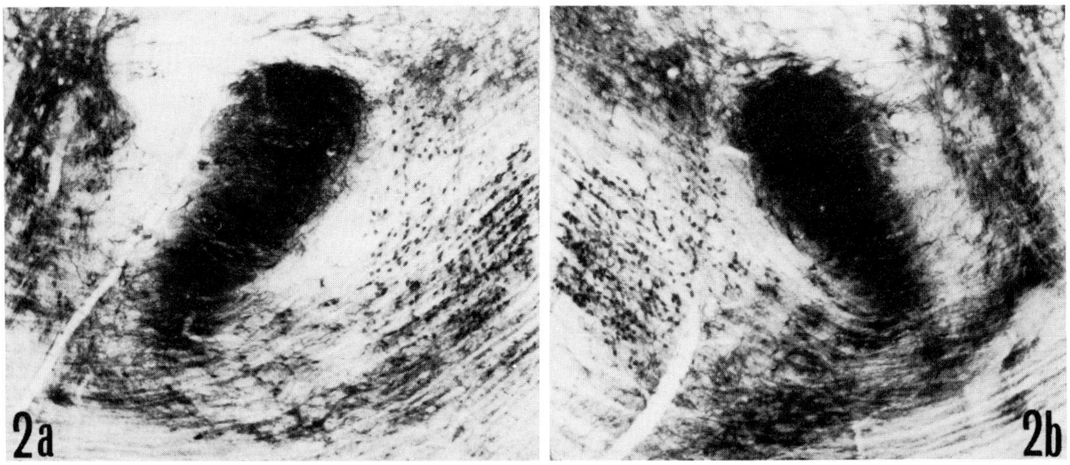

Fig. 2. Coronal section through the level of superior olivary complex from the sides a) contra- and b) ipsilateral to the stimulated implant, incubated for cytochrome oxidase activity without counterstaining. Little difference is detectable between the medial nuclei of the trapezoid body, the medial superior olive and the lateral superior olive of the two sides at this level. (x20)

input directly and/or indirectly from the experimental ear, it was found that their levels of cytochrome oxidase activity had almost reached those of the control sides. Within the ipsilateral ventral cochlear nuclei (Fig. 1b, c), the contralateral medial nuclei of the trapezoid body (Figs. 2a, b; 3b, c), the ipsilateral lateral superior olive and periolivary nuclei (Fig. 2a, b), the contralateral nuclei of the lateral lemnisci and the contralateral caudal inferior colliculi, the levels of enzyme staining were moderately decreased in the high frequency representational aspect. The levels increased in the lower-frequency representational regions, and became closely comparable (if not identical) to the control sides through one third to one half of the extent of each nucleus. As with unilaterally deafened, unstimulated cats, there was little difference between the dorsal cochlear nuclei and the medial superior olive of the two sides.

In comparison to chronically implanted, nonstimulated cases described previously,[4] the present data indicated that, within the parameters of the programmed stimulation employed, the level of cytochrome oxidase activity was significantly higher than in nonstimulated cats, and approached that

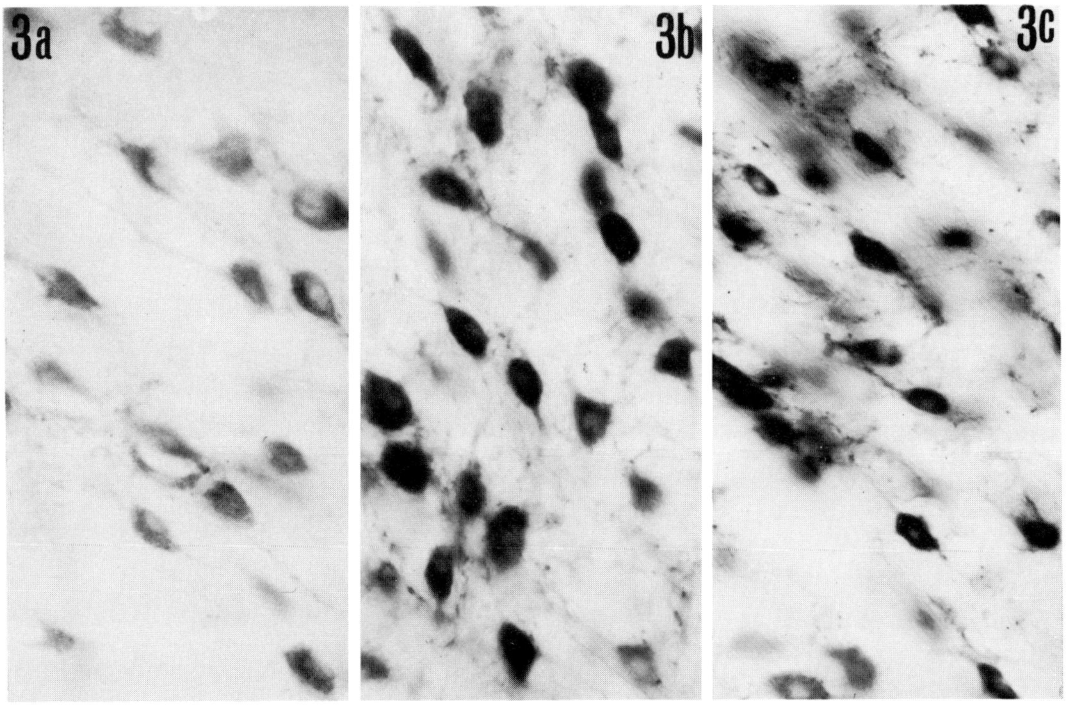

Fig. 3. Higher magnification of neurons within the medial nucleus of the trapezoid body, incubated for cytochrome oxidase activity without counterstaining. The levels of cytochrome oxidase activity are comparable between the one receiving input from b) the normal ear and those from c) the deafened and stimulated ear. a) Representative neurons from a deafened and nonstimulated case, for comparison (x200)

of the normal (see Figs. 1a-c and 3a-c for comparisons). The regions of lowest level of staining were zones of high frequency representation, and therefore received input mainly from the basal turn of the cochlea. This lower level of staining was probably accounted for by some damage to the auditory nerve array near the site of implantation. The portions of nuclear groups representing middle and low frequencies (middle and apical parts of the cochlea) appeared to have benefited from the effect of electrical stimulation, when compared to unstimulated implanted cochleas. The levels of enzyme activity reached in auditory relay nuclei in these cats reflect the consequences of continuous stimulation at relatively low rates (20 pps) for a relatively short time (about one month), following five to six months of profound deafness. With longer periods and/or higher rates of stimulation, the activity of oxidative enzymes in the affected nuclei might be further enhanced. The time lapse between the cessation of stimulation and sacrifice may have also been a factor in determining the level of enzyme activity seen histochemically.

Thus, our preliminary results demonstrate that auditory neurons deprived of normal input may be functionally quiescent, but they retain their ability to respond to subsequent stimulation. The re-activation of "silenced" auditory nerve fibers by intracochlear electrical stimulation appears to result in at least partial restoration and maintenance of the level of oxidative enzyme activity close to that of the normal. Such plastic changes in the functional state of neurons are detectable histochemically by the cytochrome oxidase technique.

REFERENCES

1. Schindler RA, Merzenich MM. Chronic intracochlear electrode implantation: cochlear pathology and acoustic nerve survival. Ann Otol Rhinol Laryngol 1974; 83:202-16.

2. Merzenich MM. Studies on electrical stimulation of the auditory nerve in animals and man; cochlear implants. In: Tower DB, ed. The nervous system, vol 3. Human communication and its disorders. New York: Raven Press, 1975:537-48.

3. Merzenich MM, White M. Cochlear implants: the interface problem. In: Hambrecht T, Reswick JB, eds. Biomedical engineering and instrumentation, vol 3. Functional electrical stimulation. Application in neruronal prostheses. New York: Marcel Dekker, Inc, 1977:321-40.

4. Wong-Riley MTT, Merzenich MM, Leake PA. Changes in endogenous enzymatic reactivity to DAB induced by neuronal inactivity. Brain Res 1978; 141:185-92.

5. Wong-Riley M. Changes in the visual system of monocularly-sutured or enucleated cats demonstrable with cytochrome oxidase histochemistry. Brain Res 1979; 171:11-28.

UPPER RESPIRATORY TRACT CILIARY ULTRASTRUCTURAL PATHOLOGY

FRED S. HERZON, MD

ALBUQUERQUE, NEW MEXICO

Nasal and sinus ciliary ultrastructure was evaluated in 16 patients with various pathologies of the upper respiratory tract including sinusitis, nasal polyposis, purulent rhinitis, and rhinitis medicosa. Ultrastructural findings include absent dynein arms, central tubule disorientation, radial spoke defects, atypical microtubule patterns and ciliary membrane abnormalities. Examples of each condition are presented and the implications of these findings are discussed.

INTRODUCTION

Cilia perform an effective and vital protective function in the upper and lower respiratory tract. Much of the early clinical research on cilia focused on their involvement in moving the mucus blanket within the nose.[1] In the early 1960s observations of aberrant ultrastructural patterns of cilia were reported.[2-4] Afzelius[2] described cilia and flagella in normal animal populations that did not conform to expected ultrastructural patterns. Although these findings were isolated, they fostered interest in ultrastructural pathology of cilia. With the findings of absent dynein arms within sperm tails, further research in the last decade was geared toward infertility and immotile sperm.[5,6] As ciliary structure is consistent throughout the body this work was redirected to the respiratory tract and led to the initial ciliary ultrastructural pathologic observations.[7-16] This paper will present ciliary ultrastructural pathology found in various upper respiratory tract diseases and review the present knowledge concerning this pathology.

METHODS

Ciliary biopsies were taken from the posterior and middle one third of the inferior turbinate of 16 patients. The biopsies were obtained with a biting forceps or by curettage with small sinus and buck ear curets. Both the biopsied and the curetted material were fixed in 2.5% glutaraldehyde in an 0.075 M calcium hydrochloride buffer for 24 hours. The curetted material was centrifuged and the resulting pellet was processed. After rinsing in cacodylate buffer the biopsy was fixed for one hour in 1% osmium tetroxide and block stained in uranyl acetate for three hours and then dehydrated in graded series of alcohol. The biopsies were embedded in Epon 812®. Silver-to-grey thin sections were cut on an ultramicrotome and stained with uranyl acetate and lead citrate, and photographed in a Hitachi HS75 electron microscope.

CILIA STRUCTURE AND PHYSIOLOGY

A cilium is composed of a sheath of microtubules called an axoneme. The microtubules are in a 9 + 2 pattern which is consistent for all cilia in the body (Fig. 1). The nine outer doublet microtubules are composed of two subfibers, A and B. Two arms and a radial spoke are attached to subfiber A. The arms are dynein molecules which exhibit adenosine triphosphatase (ATPase) activity. The entire axoneme is surrounded by a cell membrane.[17]

The basic motion of cilia is thought to be caused by the microtubules in the outer ring of doublets sliding past one another (Fig. 2). Energy for this is derived from dynein breaking down adenosine triphosphate (ATP). The actual bending of a cilium is thought to be caused by the radial spokes detaching and reattaching at specific intervals along the sheath surrounding the central doublet and thus creating a shearing force which in turn causes the bending.[18]

Cilia of the respiratory tract have a metachronal rhythm in which cilia in successive rows beat sequentially so that each row starts at a slightly different time and a wave is produced which can move mucus. The direction of the beat is always along the axis (Fig. 1). The exact mechanism of control of the beat, however, is not known. Some of the factors which are known to affect frequency and its coordination are ATP concentration, temperature, dynein, calcium and magnesium concentration, and the viscosity of the medium in which the cilia beat.[19]

RESULTS

Dynein. Figure 3B shows a cilium from a nasal biopsy of a 12-year-old female with sinusitis and chronic inflammatory pulmonary disease. The patient does not have situs inversus. The figure illustrates an absence of dynein arms on the A subfiber.

Radial Spokes. Two cilia from a 72-year-old male with rhinitis medicosa are presented in Figure 4. The cilium on the bottom shows a 9 + 4 pattern and no observable radial spokes. A clear area can be seen surrounding the two central doublets in which

From the Division of Otolaryngology, University of New Mexico School of Medicine, Albuquerque. Supported in part by Veteran's Administration grant 000-949-04-6 and NIH grant RR-00997.

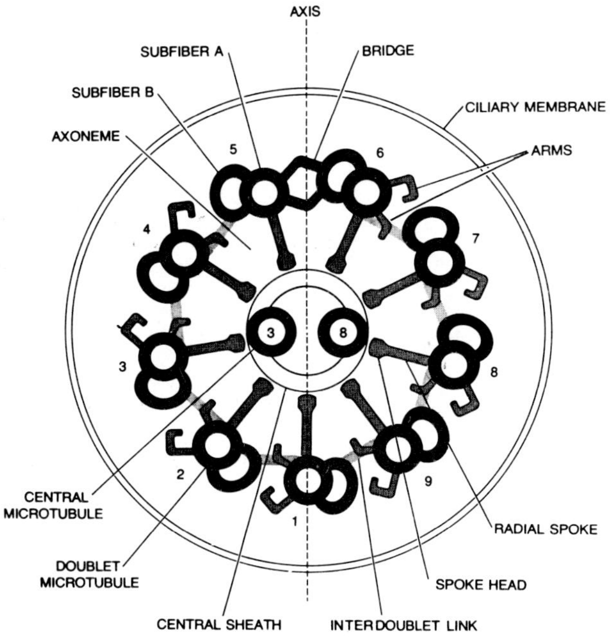

Fig. 1. Individual cilium cross section. Each doublet microtubule has two subfibers, A and B; arms project from subfiber A toward the next microtubule's subfiber B (see doublet 6). The axis is an imaginary line defining the plane of the cilium's effective stroke, bisecting the bridge, the central microtubule pair and the doublet designated No. 1. Cilium is viewed here from base toward tip. (From Satir P.[17] Reprinted with permission.)

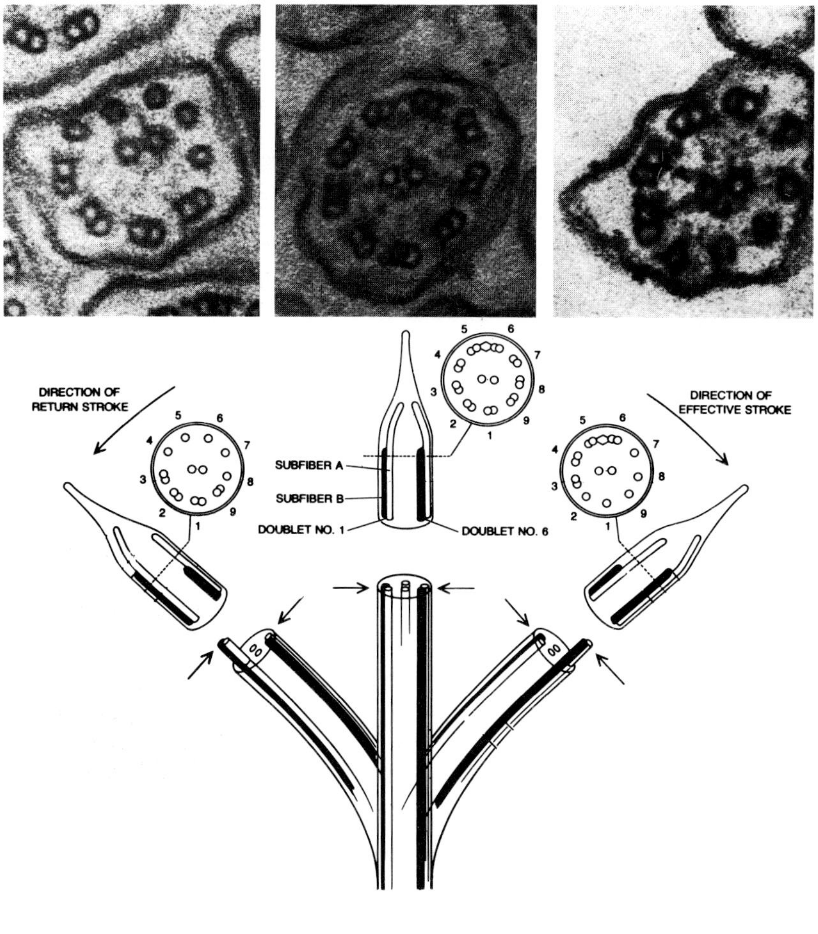

Fig. 2. Sliding of microtubules. The sliding is manifested by differences in the pattern of subfibers near the tip of the cilium. Here the relations among sliding, bending, and tip pattern are shown for two doublets, nos. 1 and 6, in the three stroke positions: straight up, bent in the effective-stroke direction (right), and bent in the return stroke direction (left). The arrows mark equal distances along the microtubules from the beginning of the bend. Because the microtubules are flexible but of constant length the doublet on the inner, concave side of a bend must slide tipward. As the three base-to-tip cross section diagrams of the indicated part of each cilium show, in the straight position all subfiber Bs should be present but in the bent positions subfiber B of the doublets on the outer side of the bend will be missing. The expectation is confirmed by the three electron micrographs (top, x100,000 approx.). When the dynein arms cause microtubules to slide past one another sheer resistance (thought to be the result of radial spokes detaching and reattaching along the central sheath) in the cilium changes sliding to bending. (From Satir P.[17] Adapted with permission.)

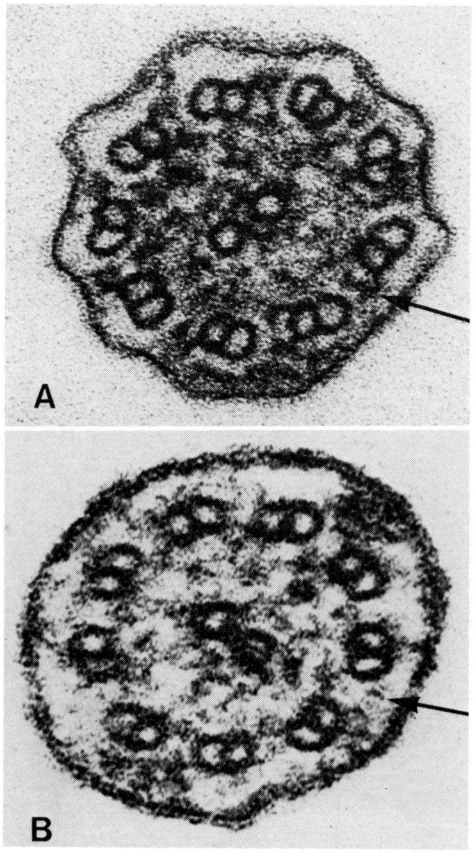

Fig. 3. Cross section of cilium without dynein arms. Arrows point to A) normal dynein arms and B) where they are missing. (x75,000)

no radial spoke material can be seen. This is contrasted with the cilium above it in which the radial spokes can be made out leading to a normal single central doublet.

Pathology of Microtubules. Many variations of microtubule pathology were observed. A 9 + 3 pattern is clearly seen in the cilium in Figure 5 from a patient with rhinitis medicosa. A maxillary sinus biopsy from a 17-year-old female with systemic rheumatoid arthritis and subacute maxillary sinusitis is shown in Figure 6. A cluster of three cilia is observed with an 8 + 4 pattern. The single subfibers in the cilium in the lower part of the figure probably represent a normal cross section near the tip of the cilium. Figure 7, a nasal biopsy from a 15-year-old with severe nasal polyposis, reveals two fiber abnormalities, an extra subfiber on the outside of the 9 + 2 configuration and an absent B subfiber within the standard 9 + 2 pattern. Incomplete subfibers are more clearly demonstrated in Figure 8, from a $3^1/_2$-year-old with asthma and sinusitis. It is impossible to tell whether it is the A or B subfibers that are incomplete. This extensive subfiber anomaly has not been previously described.

Orientation. The nasal biopsy of a 2-year-old with rhinitis and middle ear effusion (Fig. 9) il-

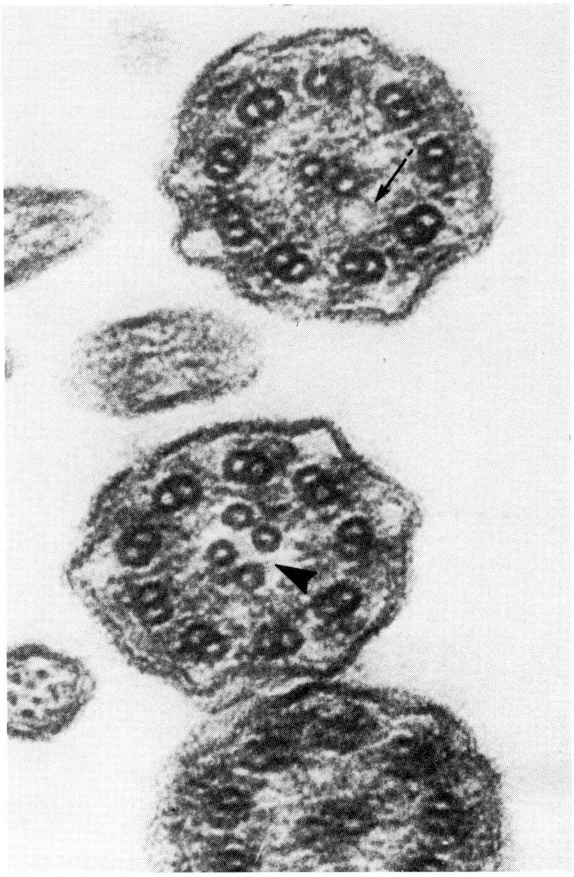

Fig. 4. Radial spoke abnormality, 9 + 4 pattern. Arrowhead points to the clear area in which no radial spoke material can be seen. The arrow in the upper cilia points to a normal spoke. (x140,000)

lustrates a marked variation in the axis through the central doublet between various adjacent cilia. Orientation abnormalities are also revealed by examining the foot processes of cilia as seen in Figure 10 in which virtually a 90° angle can be observed between two adjacent cilia.

Membrane Abnormalities. Compound cilia are those which have a single cell membrane but con-

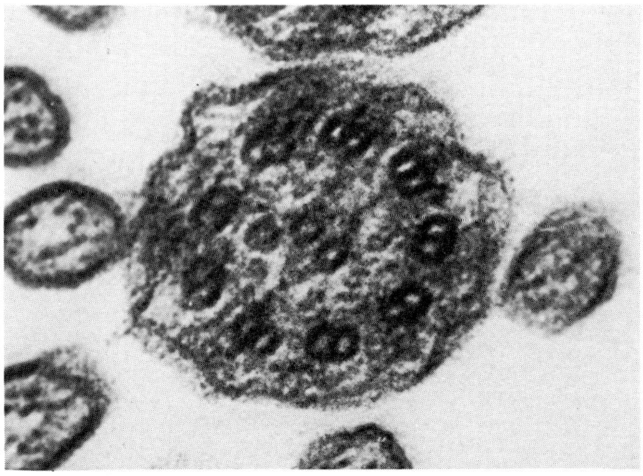

Fig. 5. Cross section of cilia with a 9 + 3 pattern. (x140,000)

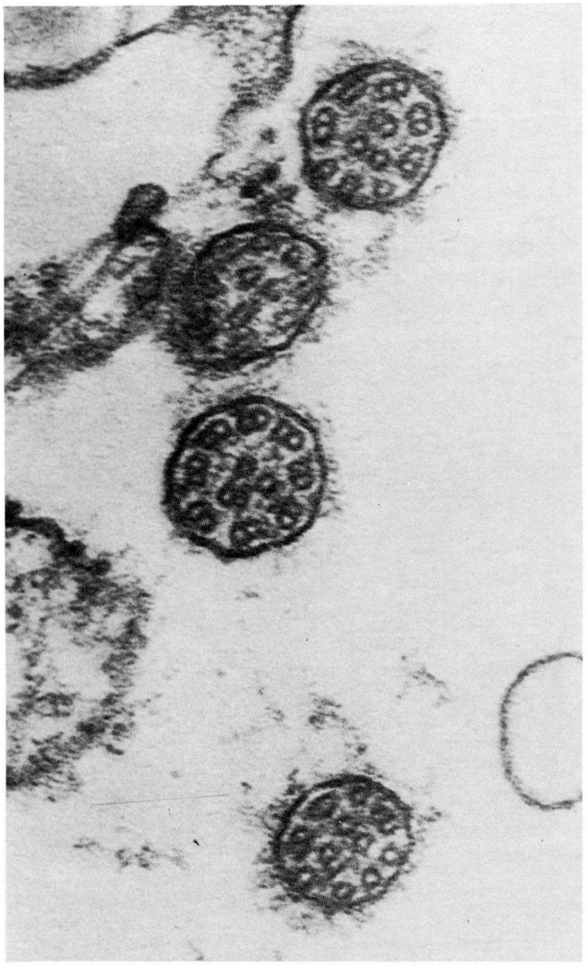

Fig. 6. Multiple cilia with 8 + 4 pattern. (x100,000)

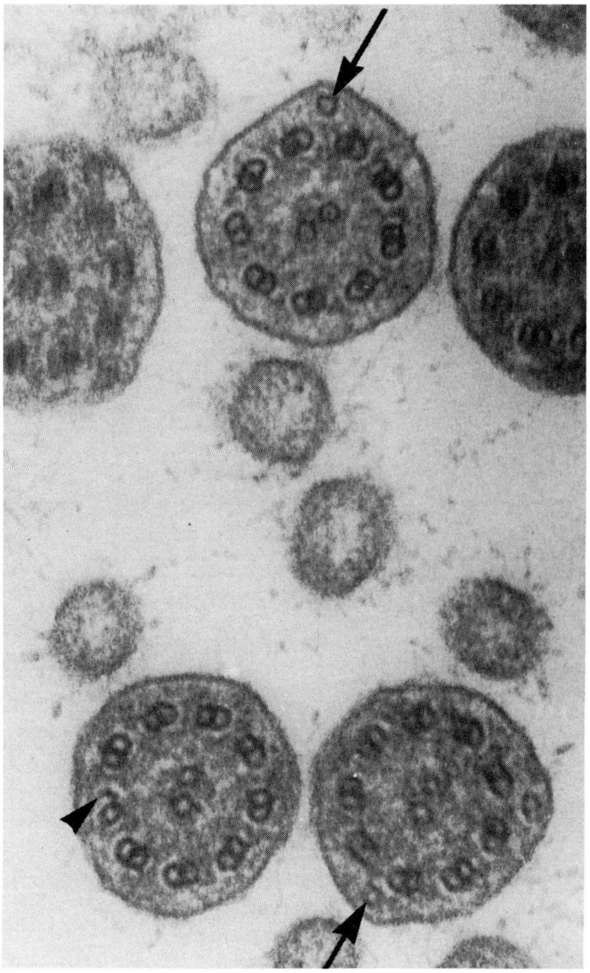

Fig. 7. 1 + 9 + 2 pattern. Arrows point to extra tubules. The arrowhead points to a missing A subfiber. (x150,000)

tain, in varying degrees, multiple axonemes immersed in greater or lesser amounts of cytoplasm. Figure 11 illustrates a cross section of such a cilium. Figure 12 reveals a longitudinal section of a smaller but similar type of adhesive compound cilium.[14] A second kind of compound cilium is the bulging type (Fig. 13) in which there is a much greater amount of cytoplasm and a few irregular axial filaments either in whole or in part seen within the cell membrane.

Although not previously described, Figure 14 represents what is felt to be essentially a fused cilium rather than a microtubule abnormality. The figure illustrates a central normal-appearing axoneme with multiple doublets surrounding it. Figure 15 illustrates what might be the predecessor of such a cilium in which there is a partial fusing of two adjacent cilia with their component microtubules.

Table 1 represents a summary of the 16 patients whose cilia were examined for ultrastructural defects. Abnormal cilia were found in 11. Two, one with Kartagener's syndrome[20] and another with chronic sinusitis, had what appeared to be normal ciliary ultrastructure. In three patients with various diagnoses no cilia could be found on the biopsies. Nine had ultrastructural defects other than compound cilia. In two others the ultrastructure was normal except for the finding of multiple compound cilia. In seven patients, compound cilia were noted either alone or in conjunction with other ultrastructural abnormalities.

DISCUSSION

In 1975[5,6,15] the lack of dynein arms on the A subfiber of human spermatazoa and the cilia of the respiratory tract were described. Further observations[9] characterized the "immotile cilia syndrome" which affected the entire respiratory tract. Additionally, disorientation of the central tubules was also proposed as contributing to this syndrome.

As the ATPase activity of dynein is thought to be necessary for ciliary motility, the lack of that activity has been proposed as the pathophysiology of Kartagener's syndrome. It was proposed that this was a congenital anomaly compatible with an autosomal recessive mode of inheritance.[21] Afzelius,[7] in his initial discussion of this syndrome, postulated that the

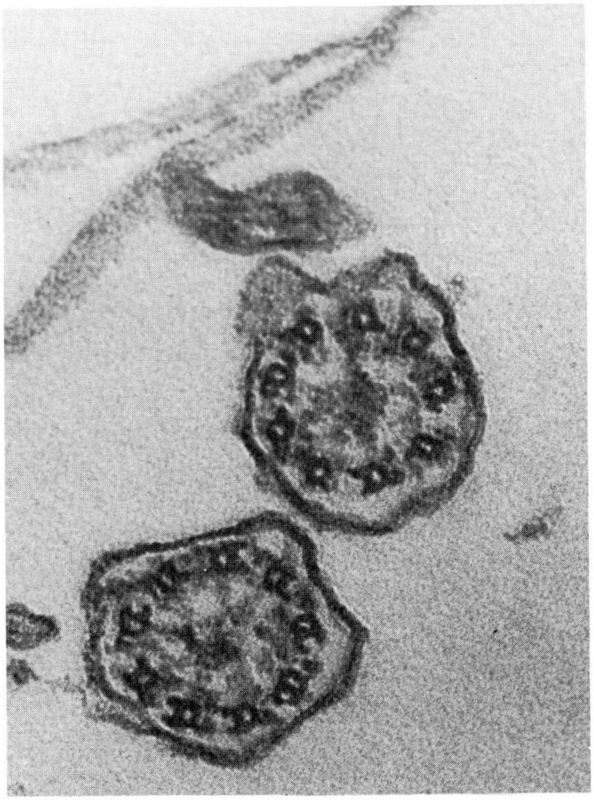

Fig. 8. Multiple subfibers are missing throughout the outer nine doublets. (x125,000)

defect could be either that the subject could not produce dynein or that the dynein could not attach to the A subfiber. Additionally, he felt that because of the embryological need for motile cilia causing rotation of organs during development that immotile cilia might also be responsible for the situs inversus. Recent data by Forrest et al,[22] where viable cilia from patients with Kartagener's syndrome were removed and activated by adding ATPase, would seem to indicate that the defect in the syndrome is an inability to produce the dynein rather than one of attachment.

Only one patient with a dynein defect has been followed. After the diagnosis was established very aggressive and radical sinus surgery was performed in order to promote drainage and clear the upper respiratory tract of infection. For a short time this was successful; however, even with adequate "mechanical" drainage, purulent rhinitis and sinusitis persisted in association with a chronic middle ear effusion. The significance of the Forrest study is that it not only suggests the specific problem in Kartagener's syndrome but also leaves hope that people with dynein defects may be helped by specific biochemical correction.

In 1962 Satir[4] described what in effect was a radial spoke and fused cilium abnormality in a clam gill. Sixteen years later Sturgess et al[11] described a family in whom radial spoke abnormalities were detected in the upper and lower respiratory tract. They describe and make the case for a congenital defect. Cilia described showed eccentric and multiple central tubules with 6 + 2, 9 + 4, etc, patterns. Clear spaces around the central tubules were interpreted to be abnormalities in the radial spokes. In the present study, similar cilia were found in a more isolated fashion. Figures 4 and 5, from the patient with rhinitis medicosa and no lower respiratory pathology, have identical abnormal patterns to that described by Sturgess et al. Cilia from the sinus of a 16-year-old female with maxillary sinusitis also manifest similar changes (Fig. 4). These data would suggest that similar findings may be the result of acquired disease.

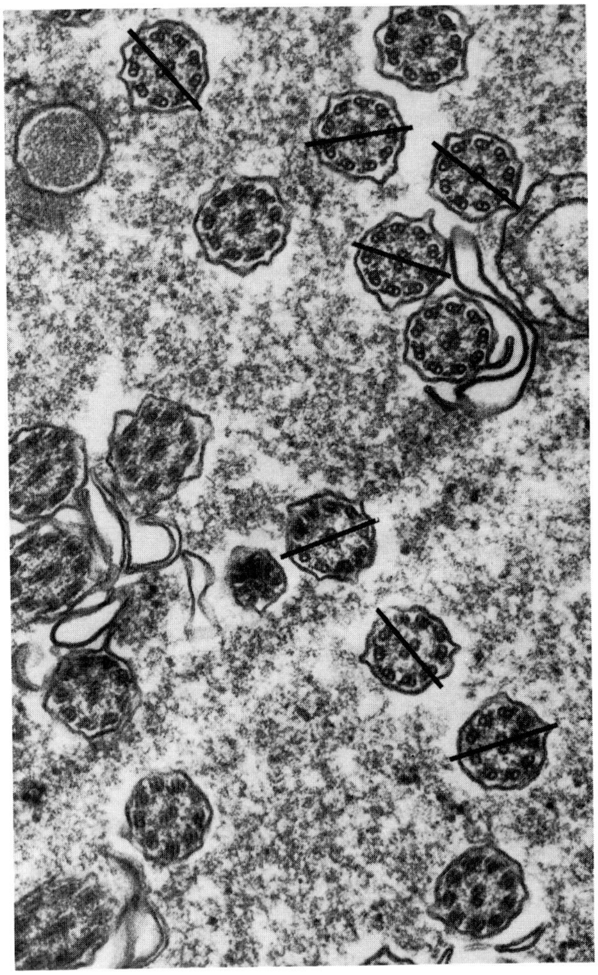

Fig. 9. Cilia cross sections with central tubule axes varying beyond 25°. (x45,000)

Microtubule patterns other than the normal 9 + 2 have been described by Afzelius[2] and Pitelka[3] in various lower animals. These patterns, among them 2 + 9 + 2, 5 + 8 + 2, 9 + 4 and 10 + 4, were found in normal populations of sea urchins, mussels, and worms. Takasaka et al[14] described six cilia found in three patients from some 25 studied with upper respiratory pathology with atypical microtubule patterns. Konradova et al[23] observed 140 anomalous

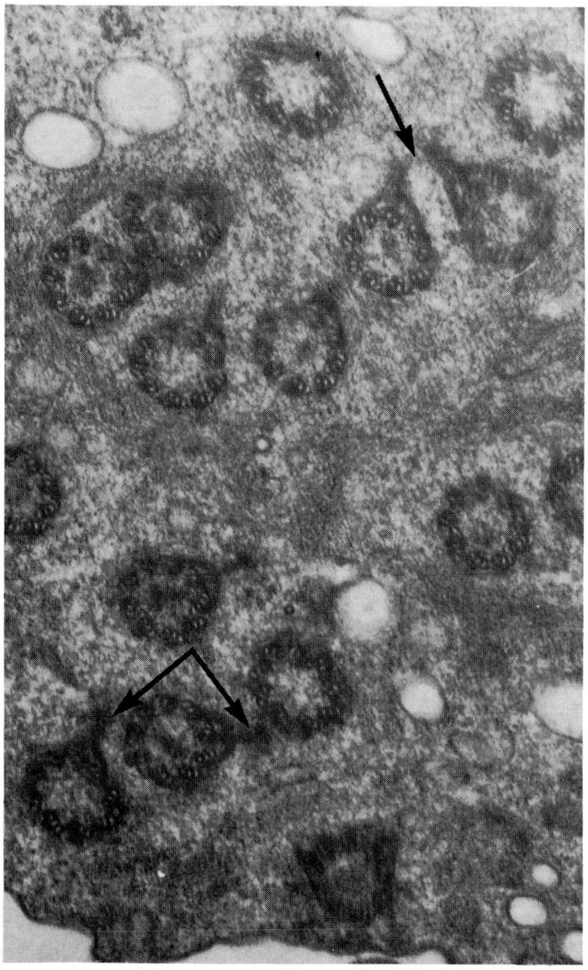

Fig. 10. Basilar feet of cilia. Arrows point to basilar feet of separate cilia and show virtually a 90° angle between them. (x50,000)

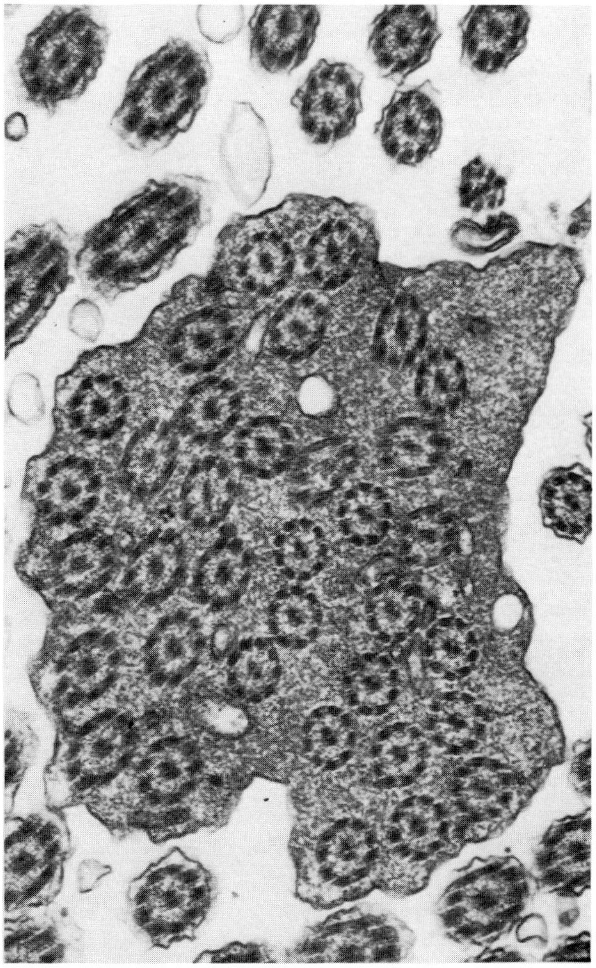

Fig. 11. Cross section through a large compound cilia with multiple axonemes. (x30,000)

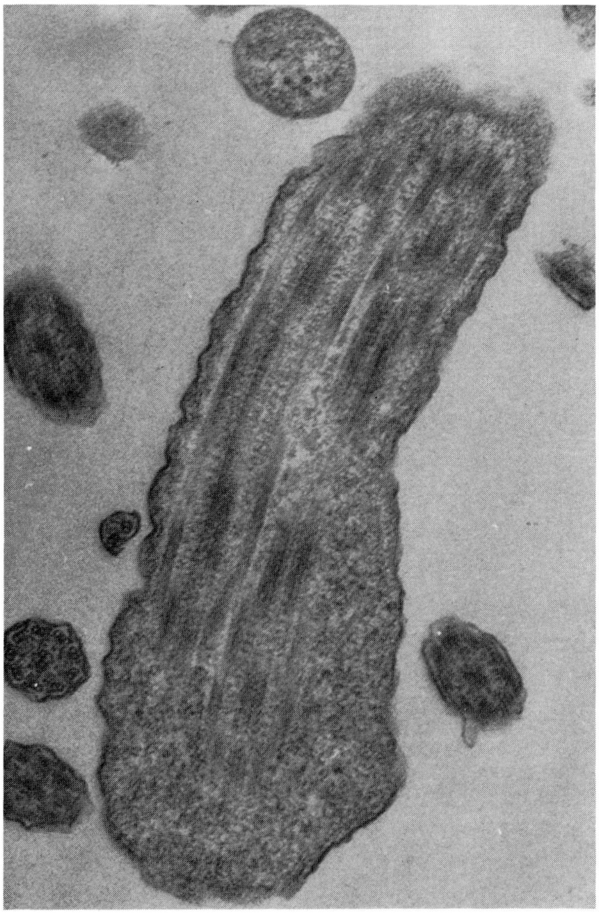

Fig. 12. Longitudinal section of a smaller but similar type of compound cilium. (x42,000)

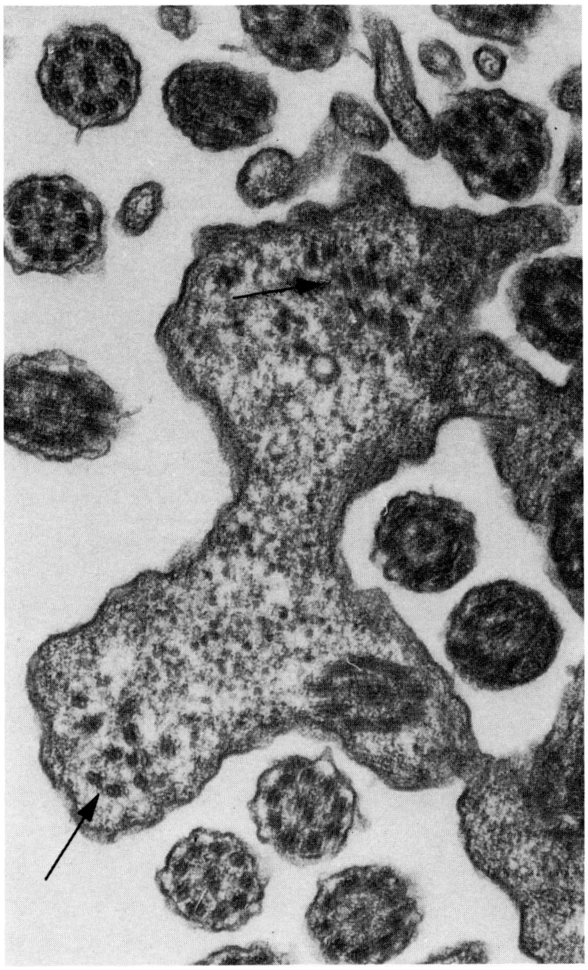

Fig. 13. Bulging compound cilia. Arrows note limited and sometimes irregular microtubules.

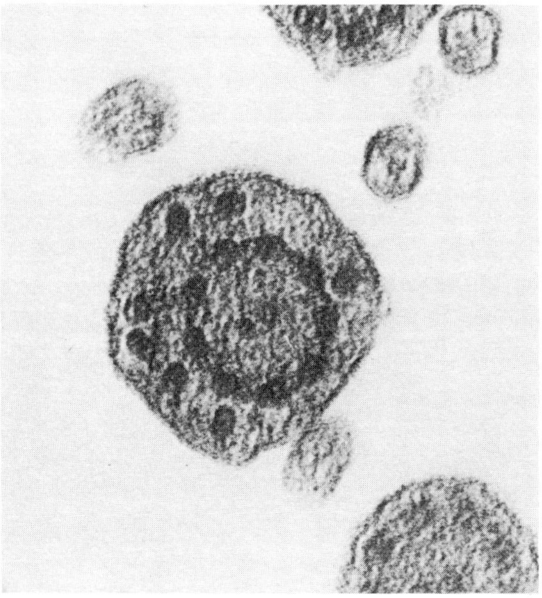

Fig. 14. Fused cilia. There are multiple extra doublets surrounding a normal 9 + 2 axonome. (x124,000)

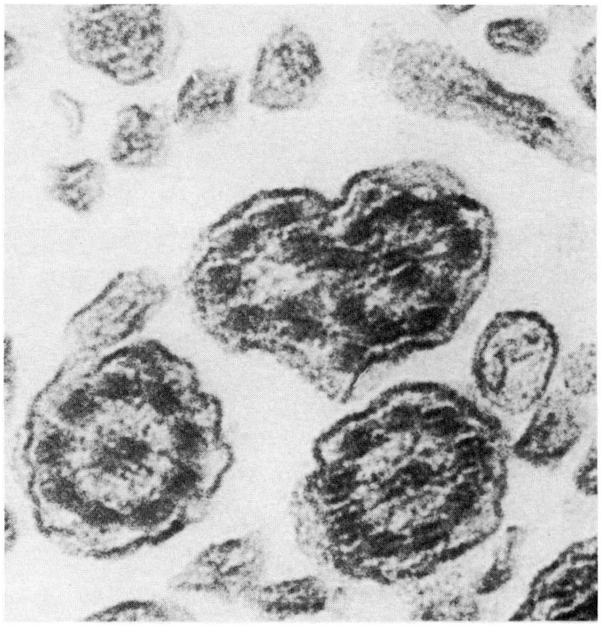

Fig. 15. Partial fusing of two adjacent cilia. Possible predecessor of fused cilia in Fig. 14. (x134,000)

cilia with patterns such as 8 + 2 and 9 + 0. Virtually all of the variations described have been observed in the present material (Figs. 4-7, 13). One of the major issues is the significance of these findings as these cilia have been observed within normal animal populations[2-4] and the amounts seen have been limited.

It seems possible that major microtubule changes such as an 8 + 4 or a 9 + 3 would interfere with ciliary function by interfering with radial spoke detaching and reattaching along the central sheath and interfering with the axis of motion. It is also likely that unless these abnormal cilia made up a significant proportion of the cilia that no major respiratory tract dysfunction would occur. Figures 16 and 17 show a wide field of cilia from two patients with chronic sinusitis and rhinitis medicosa

TABLE 1. RESULTS OF ULTRASTRUCTURAL ANALYSIS

Patient	*Age*	*Diagnosis*	*Biopsy*	*Ultrastructure Results*	*Figure*
1	15	Nasal polyposis	IT	Extra microtubules Missing B subfibers Compound cilia	7
2	50	Nasal polyposis Chronic MS	IT	Multiple microtubule defects Compound cilia	14,15,16
3	2	Kartagener's syndrome	IT	Normal ultrastructure[20]	3
4	3½	Asthma MS	IT	Absent A and B subfibers Compound cilia	8
5	2	Rhinitis Serous otitis	IT	Central tubule disorientation	9
6	2	Cystic fibrosis	IT	No cilia found	
7	72	Rhinitis medicosa	IT	Multiple microtubule defects Disorientation	4,5,10,17
8	7	Rhinitis	IT	Compound cilia	
9	17	Subacute MS Rheumatoid arthritis	MA	8 + 4 Microtubule defects	6
10	25	Chronic MS Deviated nasal septum	MA	Normal ultrastructure	
11	40	Chronic MS	IT MA	No cilia found	
12	12	Kartagener's syndrome	IT	Absent dynein arms Compound cilia	
13	3	Rhinitis MS	IT	Multiple compound cilia	11,12,13
14	70	MS	IT	No cilia found	
15	12	Chronic pansinusitis Multiple lobe syndrome	IT	Absent dynein arms Compound cilia	3
16	5	Rhinitis MS	IT	Basilar foot disorientation 4 + 9 + 2, 2 + 9 + 2 microtubule defects	

MS - Maxillary sinusitis; IT - Inferior turbinate; MA - Maxillary antrum.

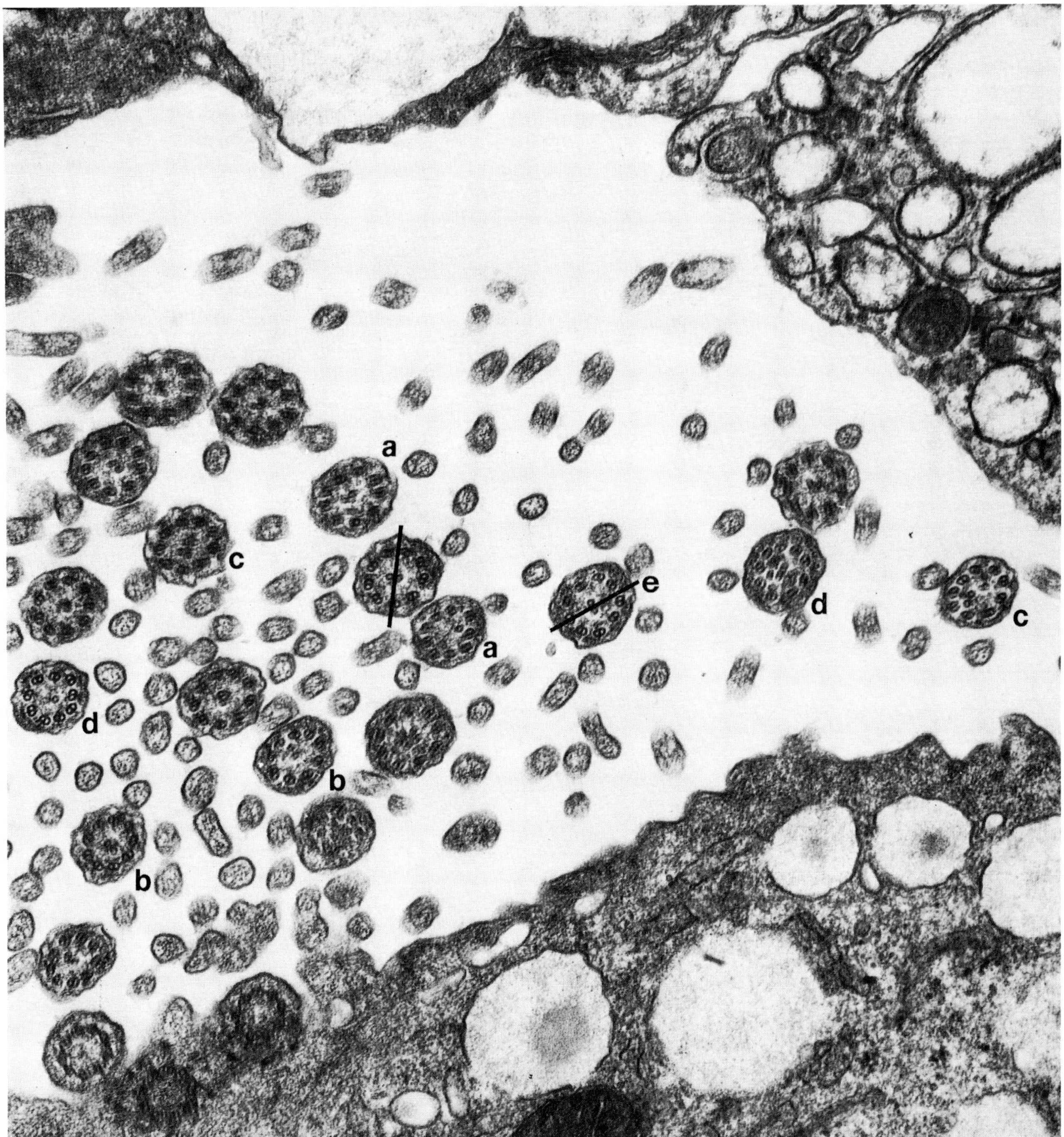

Fig. 16. A wide field of cilia with multiple defects. a - 9 + 1; b - Eccentric central microtubules — radial spoke abnormality; c - 9 + 4; d - Multiple central microtubules; e - Axis disorientation. (x48,000)

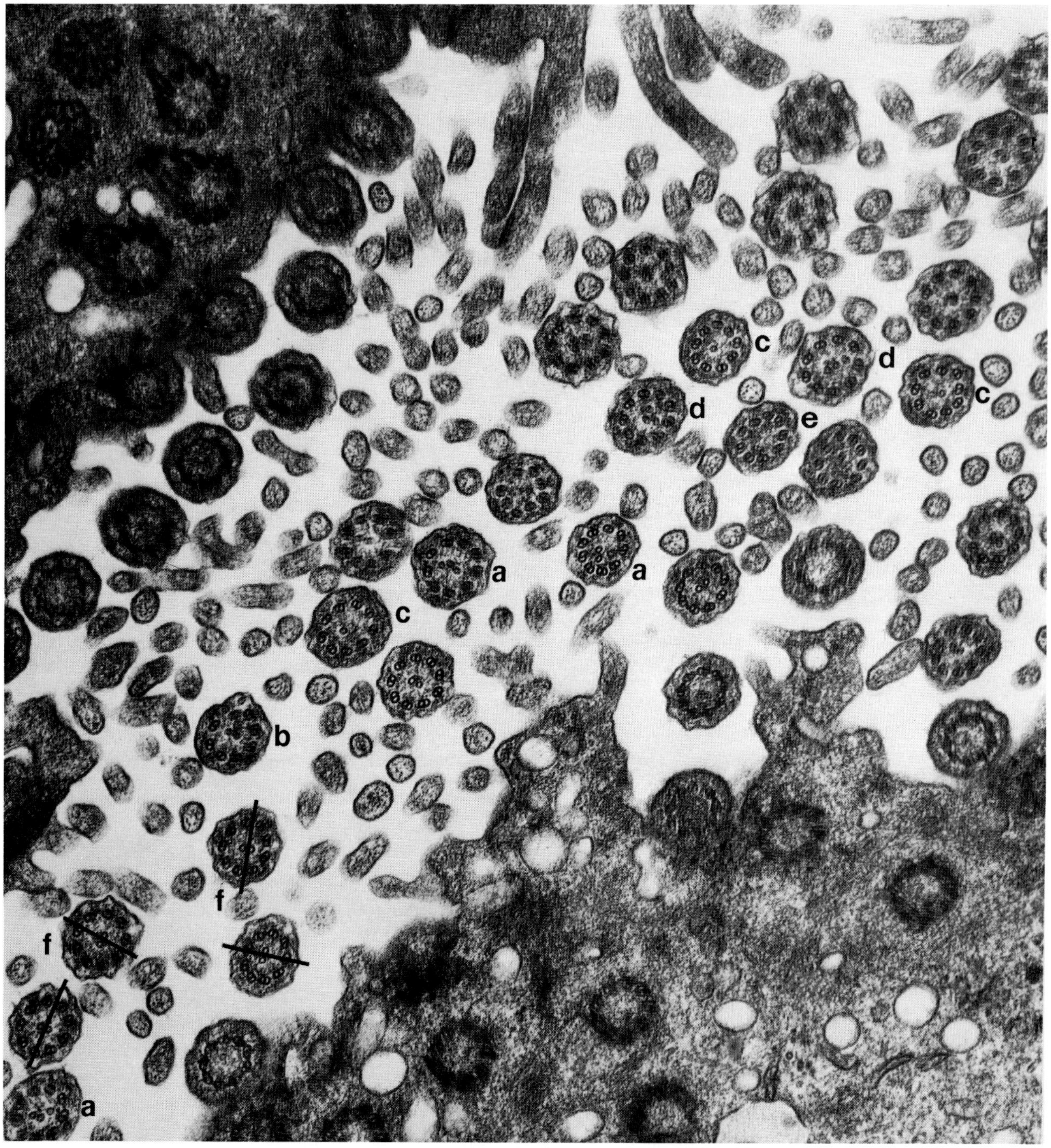

Fig. 17. Wide field of cilia with multiple abnormalities. a - 9 + 3; b - 8 + 3; c - 9 + 1; d - 9 + 4; e - 9 + 0; f - Axis disorientation. (x48,000)

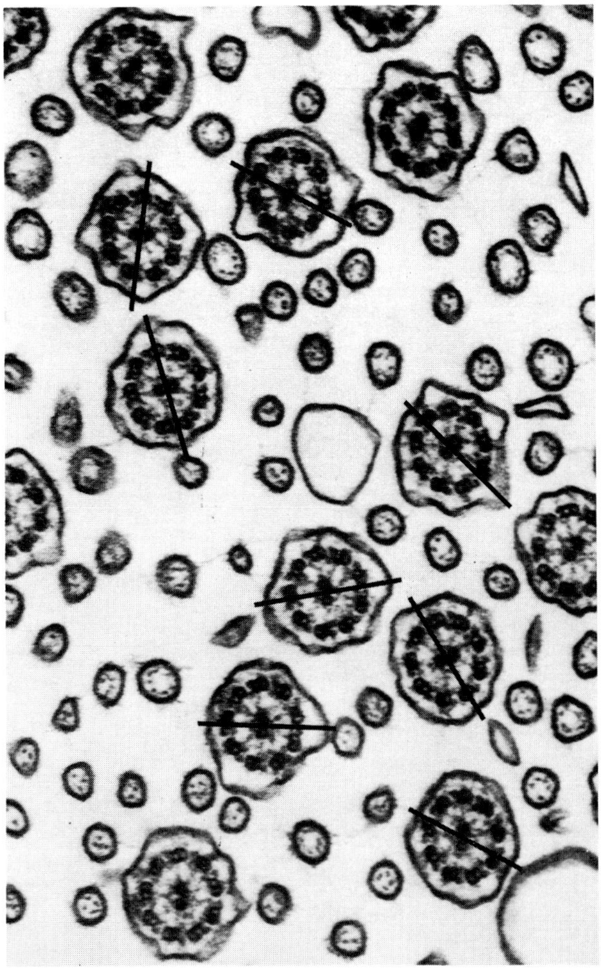

Fig. 18. Cross section of cilia from a mouse. Note the central axis deviations beyond 25°. (x55,000)

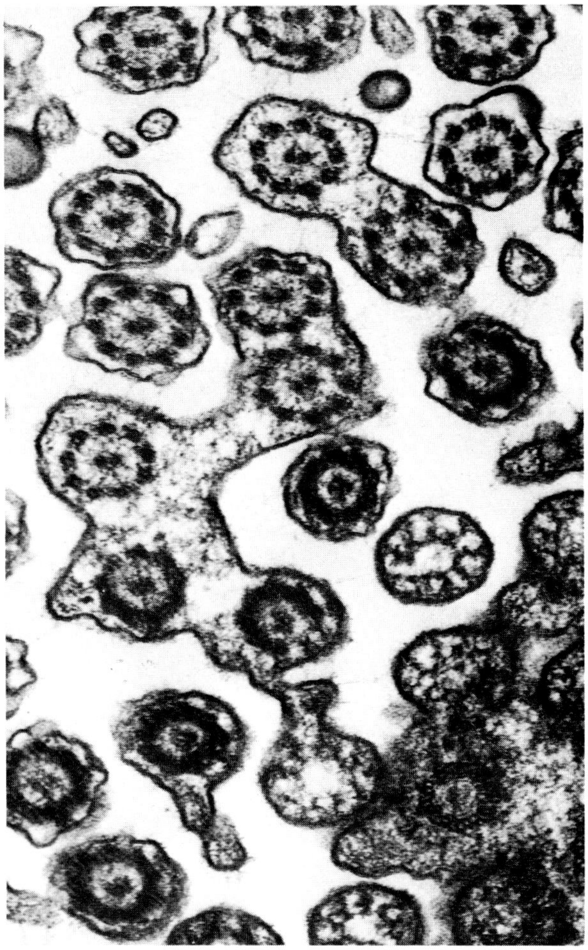

Fig. 19. Nasal cilia from a mouse with a compound cilia present. (x28,000)

respectively. As there is significant microtubule pathology throughout the fields there would be a question concerning its effect on the disease. These observations do not represent a quantitative ultrastructural evaluation of these patients' cilia but they do show that the microtubule defects observed were not isolated phenomena.

A line drawn through and perpendicular to the two central microtubules of a cilium is assigned as the axis through which it moves.[17] The accepted variation of the axis between adjacent cilia is from 5 to 26°.[9] The variation in Figures 9 and 10 clearly approaches 90°. There is, however, some question that the disorientation is pathological if it is an isolated finding.

In Satir's[24] study of the normal metachronal wave, differences in axes between adjacent cilia were measured up to 90°. Additionally, Omoto and Kung[25] describe rotation of central tubules of paramecium of up to 360°. Depending, therefore, on when a biopsy is taken and a fixation occurs, it is conceivable that an orientation of up to 90° could be seen between adjacent cilia.

One of the controls in the Jahrsdoerfer et al[13] study of middle ear cilia had "poor central tubule orientation." Figure 18 represents a ciliary field from a mouse without respiratory disease in which the orientation is far greater than 5 to 25°. It would seem then that unless orientation is irregular throughout a large field of cilia and is associated with other abnormalities (Figs. 16 and 17), that one cannot make the assumption that disorientation alone is the cause of ciliary dysfunction.

Much has been made of the pathologic significance of compound cilia in both the upper and lower respiratory tract and middle ear mucosa.[8,12,14,15] These cilia were found in seven of the patients studied here, with that being the sole "abnormality" found in two. Figure 19 represents a field from a mouse without any known respiratory pathology which clearly shows some compound cilia. Although Lupin and Misko[15] imply that these compound and "megacilia" may be the fundamental pathology in Kartagener's syndrome it would seem possible that they are the result of an acquired process. If there were enough of these cilia they might contribute to cilia dysfunction. This, however, has not been proven.

In 3 of the 16 patients no cilia were found on biopsies taken from the posterior two thirds of the inferior turbinate. It is unlikely that these patients have no cilia but rather for some reason it was technically difficult to find the cilia in the biopsy material.

One has to be extremely careful in suggesting that ciliary ultrastructural abnormalities cause specific disease states. Available quantifying methods cannot measure the extent to which these abnormalities interfere with normal function. The only ciliary defect which can directly cause respiratory pathology is dynein absence. Although Sturgess et al imply that there is a primary radial spoke abnormality causing respiratory disease, similar findings in the present material indicate that some acquired process could be involved. Careful prospective and quantitative studies are necessary in order to clarify the meaning of the other observed cilia variations. I propose to examine this question by studying the results of infectious and chemical injury on the cilia of animals.

ACKNOWLEDGMENT — I would like to thank Jeffrey Huser and Ms. Judith B. DeLongo for their fine technical assistance in preparing this material and Drs. Linda C. Saland and Aaron J. Ladman for their advice and encouragement.

REFERENCES

1. Hilding A. The physiology of drainage of nasal mucous. Arch Otolaryngol 1932; 15:92-100.

2. Afzelius BA. Cilia and flagella that do not conform to the 9 + 2 pattern. J Ultrastruct Res 1963; 9:381-92.

3. Pitelka DR. Observations on normal and abnormal cilia in *Paramecium*. Proceedings of the 5th International Congress of Electron Microscopy. In: Breese SS Jr, ed. New York: Academic Press, 1962.

4. Satir P. On the evolutionary stability of the 9-2 pattern. J Cell Biol 1962; 12:181-4.

5. Pedersen H, Rebbe H. Absence of arms in the axoneme of immobile human spermatozoa. Biol Reprod 1975; 12:541-4.

6. Afzelius BA, Eliasson R, Johnson ϕ, Lindholmer C. Lack of dynein arms in immotile human spermatozoa. J Cell Biol 1975; 66:225-32.

7. Afzelius BA. A human syndrome caused by immotile cilia. Science 1976; 193:317-9.

8. Ailsby RL, Ghadially FN. Atypical cilia in human bronchial mucosa. J Pathol 1973; 109:75-8.

9. Eliasson R, Mossberg B, Camner P, Afzelius BA. The immotile-cilia syndrome. N Engl J Med 1977; 297:1-6.

10. Camner P, Mossberg B, Afzelius BA. Evidence for congenitally nonfunctioning cilia in the tracheobronchial tract in two subjects. Am Rev Respir Dis 1975; 112:807-9.

11. Sturgess JM, Chao J, Wong J, Aspin N, Turner JAP. Cilia with defective radial spokes. N Engl J Med 1979; 300:53-6.

12. Kawabata I, Paparella M. Atypical cilia in normal human and guinea pig middle ear mucosa. Acta Otolaryngol (Stockh) 1969; 67:511-5.

13. Jahrsdoerfer R, Feldman PS, Rubel EW, Guerrant JL, Eggleston PA, Selden RF. Otitis media and the immotile cilia syndrome. Laryngoscope 1979; 89:769-77.

14. Takasaka T, Sato M, Onodera A. Atypical cilia of the human nasal mucosa. Ann Otol Rhinol Laryngol 1980; 89:37-45.

15. Lupin AJ, Misko CJ. Kartagener syndrome with abnormalities of cilia. J Otolaryngol 1977; 7:95-102.

16. Camner P, Mossberg B, Afzelius BA. Evidence for congenitally nonfunctioning cilia in the tracheobronchial tract in two subjects. Am Rev Respir Dis 1975; 112:807-9.

17. Satir P. How cilia move. Sci Am 1974; 231:44-52.

18. Warner FD, Satir P. The structural basis of ciliary bend formation. J Cell Biol 1974; 63:35-63.

19. Gibbons IR. Structure and function of flageller microtubules. In: Brinkley BR, Portor KR, eds. International cell biology. New York: Rockfeller University Press 1976-7:348-57.

20. Herzon FS, Murphy S. Normal ciliary ultrastructure in children with Kartagener's syndrome. Ann Otol Rhinol Laryngol 1980; 89:81-3.

21. Holmes LB, Blennerhasset JB, Austen KF. A reappraisal of Kartagener's syndrome. Am J Med Sci 1968; 255:13-28.

22. Forrest JB, Rossman CM, Newhouse MT, Ruffin R. Activation of nasal cilia in immotile cilia syndrome. Am Rev Respir Dis 1979; 120:511-5.

23. Konradova V, Hlouskova Z, Tomanek A. Atypical cilia in human epithelium from large bronchus. Folia Morphal (Praha) 1975; 23:293-5.

24. Satir P. Studies on cilia: the fixation of the metachronal wave. J Cell Biol 1963; 18:345-65.

25. Omoto CK, Kung C. The pair of central tubules rotates during ciliary beat in paramecium. Nature 1979; 279:532-4.

RECENT ADVANCES IN ANTIMICROBIAL THERAPY FOR INFECTIONS OF THE EAR, NOSE AND THROAT—HEAD AND NECK

Editors

Ben H. Senturia, MD
Charles D. Bluestone, MD

SYMPOSIUM PARTICIPANTS

Charles D. Bluestone, MD, Symposium Moderator
Professor of Otolaryngology
University of Pittsburgh School of Medicine
Director, Department of Otolaryngology
Children's Hospital of Pittsburgh

Gary D. Becker, MD
6200 Wilshire Blvd., Suite 1710
Los Angeles

James D. Cherry, MD
Professor, Department of Pediatrics
Center of the Health Sciences
UCLA School of Medicine
Los Angeles

David N. F. Fairbanks, MD
Chairman, Division of Otolaryngology
George Washington University Hospital
Associate Professor of Clinical Otolaryngology
George Washington University School of Medicine
Washington, DC

Sydney M. Finegold, MD
Chief, Infectious Diseases Section
VA Wadsworth Medical Center
Professor of Medicine
UCLA School of Medicine
Los Angeles

Charles M. Ginsburg, MD
Director, Ambulatory Services
The University of Texas Health Science Center at Dallas
Southwestern Medical School
Dallas

Jack M. Gwaltney, Jr., MD
Professor of Internal Medicine
Head, Division of Epidemiology and Virology
University of Virginia School of Medicine
Charlottesville

Fred S. Herzon, MD
Chief, Division of Otolaryngology
Associate Professor of Surgery
University of New Mexico School of Medicine
Albuquerque

Robert B. Kammer, MD
Clinical Investigator
Lilly Research Laboratories
Indianapolis

Jerome O. Klein, MD
Professor of Pediatrics
Boston University School of Medicine
Associate Director, Department of Pediatrics
Boston City Hospital

Torben Lildholdt, MD*
Odense University Hospital
DK 5000 Odense C
Denmark

Harold C. Neu, MD
Professor of Medicine and Pharmacology
Head, Division of Infectious Diseases
College of Physicians and Surgeons of Columbia University
New York

Jack L. Paradise, MD
Medical Director, Ambulatory Care Clinic
Children's Hospital of Pittsburgh
Professor of Pediatrics and Community Medicine
University of Pittsburgh School of Medicine

Jack S. Remington, MD†
Chief, Division of Allergy, Immunology, and Infectious Disease
Palo Alto Medical Research Center
Professor of Medicine
Stanford University School of Medicine
Stanford, California

Victor L. Schramm, Jr., MD§
Associate Professor of Otolaryngology
School of Medicine — Eye and Ear Hospital
University of Pittsburgh

Paul A. Shurin, MD
Assistant Professor of Pediatrics
Case Western Reserve University
Associate Director, Pediatric Infectious Disease Service and Pediatric Ambulatory Service
Cleveland Metropolitan General Hospital

Philip M. Sprinkle, MD†
Professor and Chairman
Division of Otolaryngology
West Virginia School of Medicine
Morgantown

Ellen R. Wald, MD§
Assistant Professor of Pediatrics
University of Pittsburgh
Division of Ambulatory Pediatrics
Children's Hospital of Pittsburgh

---

*Dr. Lildholdt was a Visiting Fellow in Pediatric Otolaryngology in the Department of Otolaryngology, University of Pittsburgh School of Medicine and Children's Hospital of Pittsburgh, from January through June 1979.

†Manuscript not available for publication.

§Panelist.

THESE PAPERS WERE PRESENTED AT A MEETING SPONSORED BY ELI LILY AND COMPANY
HELD IN SAN FRANCISCO, JUNE 11-12, 1979.

CONTENTS

Introduction. C. D. Bluestone, MD 1

Clinical Pharmacology of the Antimicrobial Agents for Infections in the Ear, Nose and Throat. H. C. Neu, MD 2

Chemoprophylaxis for Surgery of the Head and Neck. G. D. Becker, MD, FACS 8

Anaerobic Infections in Otolaryngology. S. M. Finegold, MD 13

Postoperative Wound Infections. F. H. Herzon, MD 17

Invasive *Hemophilus* Infections: Epiglottitis and Cellulitis. J. D. Cherry, MD 19

Panel Discussion — Moderator, Dr. Bluestone 23

Microbiology and Antimicrobial Treatment of Otitis Media. J. O. Klein, MD 30

Pharmacology of Oral Antibiotics Used for Treatment of Otitis Media and Tonsillopharyngitis in Infants and Children. C. M. Ginsburg, MD; G. H. McCracken, Jr., MD; J. D. Nelson, MD 37

Pharmacokinetics of Cefaclor in Chronic Middle Ear Effusions. T. Lildholdt, MD; E. I. Cantekin, PhD; G. Marshak, MD; C. D. Bluestone, MD; D. D. Rohn, BA; K. E. Schuit, MD 44

Comparison of Cefaclor and Amoxicillin for Acute Otitis Media with Effusion. E. M. Mandel, MD; C. D. Bluestone, MD; E. I. Cantekin, PhD; S. N. Ghorbanian, MD; H. E. Rockette, PhD 48

Antimicrobial Prophylaxis for Recurrent Acute Otitis Media. J. L. Paradise, MD 53

Antimicrobial Therapy for Chronic Suppurative Otitis Media. D. N. F. Fairbanks, MD 58

Panel Discussion — Moderator, Dr. Bluestone 63

Etiology and Antimicrobial Treatment of Acute Sinusitis. J. M. Gwaltney, Jr., MD; A. Sydnor, Jr., MD; M. A. Sande, MD 68

Etiology and Antimicrobial Therapy of Paranasal Sinusitis in Children. P. A. Shurin, MD 72

Etiology, Diagnosis, and Antimicrobial Treatment of Pharyngitis and Pharyngotonsillitis. J. L. Paradise, MD 75

Cefaclor in Management of Streptococcal Pharyngitis, Otitis Media, and Skin Infections. R. B. Kammer, MD 79

Panel Discussion — Moderator, Dr. Bluestone 82

INTRODUCTION

CHARLES D. BLUESTONE, MD
PITTSBURGH, PENNSYLVANIA

Otolaryngologists teach all phases of medical education to students and house staff officers and are often involved in continuing education programs. Because of this academic interest in otolaryngology, we have asked some of the leading authorities in this country in infectious diseases to speak to us and share their ideas, concepts and facts concerning the use of antimicrobials.

It has been brought to my attention by infectious disease experts that surgeons in general need to know more about antimicrobial therapy as well as the basis of the infectious disease process. Depending on which aspect of otolaryngology you are in, you may prescribe antimicrobial agents with every patient or only infrequently. As a pediatric otolaryngologist, I find myself prescribing antimicrobials not just daily but with almost every patient I see.

So often meetings I attend deal with complicated surgical procedures while failing to address the more general question of which antimicrobial agents are best for which infections. Eli Lilly and Company has a new antimicrobial drug which they have been working with for many years. Ceclor® is the trade name and cefaclor is the generic name. We are not here to discuss cefaclor specifically, but to discuss antimicrobial therapy for infections of the ear, nose and throat and the head and neck.

This is not intended to be a rigid, formal meeting. I hope that there will be a free exchange of ideas through the panel discussions and question and answer periods, and I hope there will be many questions. This is not a meeting limited to cephalosporins, although we anticipate that they will be mentioned frequently as they come up during the natural course of the discussions by the speakers. At the end of the meeting we have asked Dr. Robert Kammer, who has been working on cephalosporins for Eli Lilly and Company, to review their data on some of the cephalosporins and some of the most recent information which they have accumulated about cefaclor.

So I think we here are blessed with an invitation to learn, and I hope that by the end of this meeting we will have all gained something in terms of the treatment of our patients, the education of our students and the education of physicians who are responsible for continuing education.

CLINICAL PHARMACOLOGY OF THE ANTIMICROBIAL AGENTS FOR INFECTIONS IN THE EAR, NOSE AND THROAT

HAROLD C. NEU, MD

NEW YORK, NEW YORK

Knowledge of which microorganisms cause infection in the ear, nose and throat must be coupled with an understanding of the susceptibility patterns of these bacteria as well as knowledge of the pharmacokinetic properties of antimicrobial agents. Even though many of the bacteria which produce community-acquired infection are susceptible to the older agents, specific problems have developed with regard to species such as *Hemophilus influenzae* and to *Staphylococcus aureus*. Hospital-acquired infections due to Enterobacteriaceae may be resistant to the penicillin drugs and to some of the older cephalosporins and aminoglycosides. Use of the new agents often requires an understanding of how rapidly the compounds are cleared from the body or if they will accumulate to toxic levels in the elderly patient with decreased renal function. This article reviews the antimicrobial activity and clinical pharmacology of agents commonly used to treat infections of the ear, nose and throat.

The proper use of antimicrobial agents in the treatment of infections of the head and neck supposes that the otolaryngologist has an appreciation of both the microorganisms involved in infections in his area of the body and that he also understands the aspects of the pharmacokinetics of the agents he uses to treat these infections. This discussion will review in brief some of the antibacterial mechanisms of antibacterial agents and will put in perspective when it may be necessary to change old patterns of antibiotic use to most effectively eradicate infection.

Unlike the situation which exists with most pharmacologic agents, there is an added factor in the usual host-drug interaction; namely the infecting microorganism, as well as the effect of the hospital or community environment upon both the patient and the microorganism (Fig. 1). This interaction of the environment upon the selection of antimicrobial agent can be illustrated by the need to consider whether the *Hemophilus influenzae* in a community are β-lactamase-producing bacteria, and hence resistant to ampicillin.

Selection of an antimicrobial agent is based upon the area of the body in which the infection exists, the host defense capabilities of the patient, the degree of seriousness of the infection, and the suspected bacterial etiology (Table 1). Once these factors have been considered, there are further considerations about the degree of bacterial resistance to be expected, the absorption (whether oral or parenteral) of the agent selected, the agent's distribution to various tissues in the body in the presence of health and disease, and finally, any potential toxic side effects which could be anticipated and avoided by judicious adjustment in the dosage program of that particular agent.

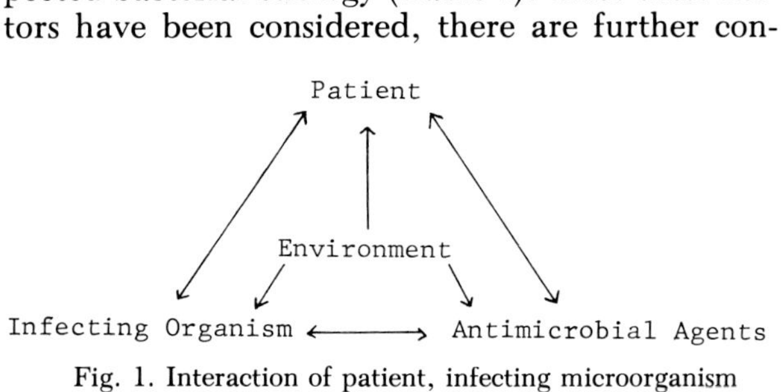

Fig. 1. Interaction of patient, infecting microorganism and antimicrobial agent.

The current antimicrobial agents which are available for use in the treatment of otolaryngological infection span all of the classes of agents. The antibiotics can attack microorganisms from various different approaches[1] (Table 2). Penicillins and cephalosporins are β-lactam antibiotics which interfere with the synthesis of bacterial cell wall. Bacteria possess an outer cell wall which protects them from lysing when they divide during growth. β-Lactam antibiotics bind to specific receptor sites important for cell wall integrity which are present in both Gram-positive and Gram-negative bacteria. The activity of β-lactams, penicillins and cephalosporins is based on their ability to reach receptor sites in the bacterial cell, to evade β-lactamases that most bacteria possess and to bind firmly to the receptor.

The organisms involved in head and neck infection (Table 3) which penicillin G inhibits are *Streptococcus pneumoniae*, *Streptococcus pyogenes* group A, *Neisseria meningitidis*, and anaerobic mouth flora, ie, peptostreptococci, fusobacteria and *Bacteroides melaninogenicus*. Ampicillin and amoxicillin also inhibit streptococci, but also inhibit

TABLE 1. BASIS FOR THE SELECTION OF AN ANTIMICROBIAL AGENT

1. Area of the body in which infection is present
2. Host defenses
3. Seriousness of the infection
4. Suspected bacterial etiology

From the Departments of Medicine and Pharmacology, College of Physicians and Surgeons, Columbia University, New York.

TABLE 2. MECHANISM OF ACTION OF ANTIMICROBIAL AGENTS

Agents	Type of Action	Site of Action
1. β-Lactam antibiotics penicillins cephalosporins	Bactericidal	Cell wall
2. Vancomycin	Bactericidal	Cell wall
3. Aminoglycosides gentamicin tobramycin amikacin	Bactericidal	Protein synthesis
4. Erythromycin	Bacteriostatic	Protein synthesis
5. Clindamycin	Bacteriostatic	Protein synthesis
6. Tetracyclines	Bacteriostatic	Protein synthesis
7. Chloramphenicol	Bacteriostatic	Protein synthesis
8. Trimethoprim-sulfamethoxazole	Together bactericidal	Folic acid synthesis
9. Rifampin	Bactericidal	RNA synthesis

many *Hemophilus* organisms, except those which produce β-lactamases. Carbenicillin and ticarcillin inhibit the mouth anaerobic flora and also inhibit *Pseudomonas aeruginosa* and *Enterobacter cloacae.*

Cephalosporins such as cephalothin and cefazolin inhibit *Staphylococcus aureus*, *S pneumoniae* and β-streptococci. They also inhibit most *Escherichia coli* and *Klebsiella*. Cefamandole inhibits these organisms but it also inhibits anaerobic mouth flora and *Hemophilus* and enterobacters. Cefoxitin inhibits staphylococci as well as β-lactamase-producing Enterobacteriaceae and *Bacteroides*.

Cephalexin, cephradine and cefaclor all inhibit staphylococci, pneumococci and streptococci, but cefaclor also inhibits *H influenzae* at concentrations less than the other agents do.[2]

The other antibiotic class which interferes with cell wall structure is vancomycin.

Aminoglycoside antibiotics — gentamicin, tobramycin, amikacin — interfere with protein biosynthesis. They are bactericidal agents. These agents are active only against Gram-negative organisms of the Enterobacteriaceae (*E coli, Klebsiella, Proteus*) and *P aeruginosa*. Although the aminoglycosides inhibit *S aureus*, they should not be considered agents of choice to inhibit these organisms.

Erythromycin is a bacteriostatic agent which inhibits most of the organisms of the oral cavity such as staphylococci, streptococci, and to some extent *Hemophilus*. Clindamycin has a similar spectrum of activity, but it does not inhibit *Hemophilus*. Both of these agents inhibit the anaerobic, oral flora involved in infections of the head and neck and are very useful in oral-facial infections. Tetracyclines are also bacteriostatic agents whose in vitro spectrum of activity covers bacteria prominent in head and neck infections. Anaerobic species, *Hemophilus*, streptococci and pneumococci are inhibited. But many Gram-negatives such as *E coli* and *Klebsiella* are resistant, as are *Pseudomonas*. There are some suggestions that minocycline is more active against

TABLE 3. MICROORGANISMS INVOLVED IN OTOLARYNGOLOGICAL INFECTIONS AND AGENTS WHICH INHIBIT THEM

Organism	Agents of Choice
S pneumoniae	Penicillins, cephalosporins, erythromycin
S pyogenes	Penicillins, cephalosporins, erythromycin
S aureus	Nafcillin, oxacillin, cloxacillin, cephalosporins
N meningitidis	Penicillin
H influenzae	Ampicillin, amoxicillin, cefaclor, cefamandole, trimethoprim-sulfamethoxazole
E coli	Cephalosporins
Klebsiella	Cephalosporins, aminoglycosides
Pseudomonas	Carbenicillin, ticarcillin, tobramycin
B fragilis	Clindamycin, chloramphenicol, cefoxitin
Anaerobic streptococci	Penicillins
Fusobacteria	Penicillins
B melaninogenicus	Penicillins, erythromycin, clindamycin, cephalosporins

staphylococci than are other tetracyclines and doxycycline is more active against anaerobic species.

The combination agent trimethoprim-sulfamethoxazole (TMP-SMX) has an in vitro spectrum which includes *S pneumoniae, Hemophilus*, staphylococci and most Gram-negative enteric bacteria. It does not inhibit *S pyogenes* as well as penicillin or cephalosporins, so should not be used for those infections. TMP-SMX also does not inhibit enterococci nor *Pseudomonas*. Polymyxins which interfere with Gram-negative cytoplasmic membranes have no activity against Gram-positive bacteria nor anaerobic bacteria, and are really only effective topically or in the kidney. They do not have a role in the systemic therapy of infection but are locally effective against *P aeruginosa*.

An agent which has not been used to any extent in ENT infection is rifampin. It is of use against *Mycobacterium tuberculosis* and currently is being evaluated as an ancillary agent in some staphylococcal infections.

Chloramphenicol remains an important agent because of its activity against *S pneumoniae, N meningitidis* and *Hemophilus*, as well as Enterobacteriaceae, and thus it is an alternative agent to use in the penicillin-allergic patient.

With such a group of antibiotics, the physician may logically ask why new ones are continually being introduced. The reason is bacterial resistance (Table 4). Bacteria can inactivate many of these agents because bacteria can contain extrachromosomal pieces of DNA which confer on the microorganisms the ability to produce enzymes which protect the microorganisms.[3] The most common form of resistance of bacteria to β-lactam antibiotics is the production of a β-lactamase. Virtually all staphylococci today possess β-lactamases, making them resistant to penicillin G, ampicillin and carbenicillin. Fortunately the semisynthetic parenteral

TABLE 4. MECHANISMS OF PLASMID-DETERMINED ANTIBIOTIC RESISTANCE

Antibiotic	Mechanism	Bacteria Which Can Be Resistant
Penicillins Cephalosporins	β-Lactamases	Staphylococci, *Hemophilus*, Enterobacteriaceae, *Pseudomonas*
Aminoglycosides		
kanamycin	Adenylation	Staphylococci, enterococci, Enterobacteriaceae, *Pseudomonas*
gentamicin	Phosphorylation	
tobramycin	Acetylation	
amikacin		
Chloramphenicol	Acetylation	Staphylococci, Enterobacteriaceae
Tetracycline	Decreased entry of drug	Staphylococci, Enterobacteriaceae
Erythromycin	Altered 23S methylase	Staphylococci
Clindamycin	Altered 23S methylase	Staphylococci

penicillins — nafcillin, oxacillin, methicillin — and the oral cloxacillin and the cephalosporins — cephalothin, cefazolin, cefamandole — are resistant to staphylococcal β-lactamase. Among the Gram-negative bacteria *Hemophilus* in some communities have acquired a plasmid from *E coli* which allow the *Hemophilus* to produce a β-lactamase.

Plasmid resistance is of importance to the head and neck surgeon since the open, purulent area that may be present after radical operations is in some ways analogous to a burn. This type of area is one in which bacteria can mate with one another and exchange genetic information. Thus a *Pseudomonas* can mate with an *E coli* or *Klebsiella* providing these latter bacteria with genes which make them resistant to common antibiotics. This form of plasmid resistance is of particular concern since unlike a mutational event in which resistance to one antibiotic develops, in this situation it is possible for the organism to become resistant simultaneously to five or six first-line agents. Inappropriate use of antibiotics in the hospital or community can act as a selection pressure to cause the emergence of multiresistant bacteria. As the foregoing would indicate, it is useful for the surgeon to have an idea of the particular resistance patterns of his hospital so as to be able to select the most appropriate agent when his patient develops an infection. Table 5 is an example of such a sensitivity profile.

The pharmacokinetics of antibiotics are similar to the properties of other drugs.[4] When an antibiotic is given orally, intramuscularly or intravenously, it becomes mixed in the plasma where it is bound to varying degree to protein and then distributed to various extravascular tissues in which it may be free or bound. The distribution of an antibiotic results in a rapid fall in plasma concentration from the peak level which occurs at the end of an intravenous infusion, 30-60 minutes after an intramuscular injection and one to two hours after oral ingestion.[5] Subsequent decreases in serum levels are related to renal and biliary excretion and to a minor extent for antibiotics to biotransformation. Extravascular tissue concentrations are dependent upon the concentration gradient from serum to tissue fluid, the degree of protein binding, and the diffusibility of the antibiotic which is determined by molecular size, pK and lipid solubility.

Most antibiotics follow fairly linear kinetics after absorption and distribution so that it is possible to calculate the half-life of the drugs in the body. Half-life is a measure of how rapidly the drug is removed from the body. The half-life of many antibiotics is increased when there is a change in the renal clearance mechanisms because so many of the antibiotics are removed from the body by renal excretion or glomerular filtration. Knowledge of the half-life of an antibiotic is important in some infections, particularly life-threatening infections, since a more frequent mode of administration may be necessary to achieve optimal therapeutic results. Similarly, a drug with a longer half-life and one which provides adequate serum and tissue concentrations for a long period can be given less frequently, perhaps only two or three times a day. This latter factor can be of great importance when considering whether the patient will show reasonable compliance with the program selected.[6]

Although concentrations of antibiotics may at certain points in time exceed the serum levels, in

TABLE 5. TYPICAL SUSCEPTIBILITY PATTERNS OF COMMON ORGANISMS

	% Susceptible									
Organism	*TMP-SMX*	*Penicillin*	*Ampicillin*	*Chloramphenicol*	*Erythromycin*	*Tetracycline*	*Cephalosporins*	*Gentamicin/ Tobramycin*	*Amikacin*	*Clindamycin*
S pneumoniae	90	100	100	99	98	95	100	—	—	95
S pyogenes	50	100	100	90	95	90	100	—	—	95
H influenzae	98	—	90	99	80	80	50*	—	—	—
S aureus	90	15	15	95	90	90	98	95	95	—
E coli	95	—	80	90	—	70	85	95	98	—
Klebsiella	95	—	5	80	—	70	85	90	98	—
P mirabilis	95	—	95	85	—	0	95	95	98	—
Pseudomonas	0	—	0	—	0	0	90	95	—	
Serratia	95	—	0	50	—	5	0	50	90	—
Bacteroides	20	50	10	95	80	50	0†	0	0	95

*Susceptible to cefaclor and cefamandole.

†Susceptible to cefoxitin (90%).

— Not an appropriate agent.

TABLE 6. CONCENTRATIONS OF ANTIMICROBIAL AGENTS IN ENT TISSUES

Tissue or fluid		Dose	Route	Concentration µg/ml
Maxillary sinus	Penicillin V	400 mg	Oral	<0.2
	Penicillin G	1.2 mega U	IM	0.2
	Doxycycline	200 mg	Oral	0.5 - 6
	Amoxicillin	500 mg	Oral	0.3 - 1.3
Tonsillar	Ampicillin	250 mg	Oral	0.02 - 0.09
	Ampicillin	500 mg	Oral	2 -
	Benzathine penicillin G	1.2 mega U	IM	0 - 0.04
	Penicillin V	250 mg	Oral	0 - 0.17
	Amoxicillin	250 mg	Oral	0.2 - 0.27
	Erythromycin estolate	250 mg	Oral	0.3 - 1.35
Middle ear	Ampicillin	34 mg/kg	Oral	9.5*
	Penicillin V	13 mg/kg	Oral	2.1*
	Penicillin V	26 mg/kg	Oral	6.3*
	Procaine penicillin G +	300,000	IM	1.3*
	Aqueous penicillin G	100,000		
	Erythromycin succinate	12.5 mg/kg	Oral	0.8*
	Erythromycin estolate	12.5 mg/kg	Oral	4.2*
	Erythromycin estolate	8 mg/kg	Oral	1.3*
	Oxytetracycline	100 mg	IM	0.6*
	Penicillin V	12 mg/kg	Oral	0.2*
	Amoxicillin	10 mg/kg	Oral	2.2*
	Amoxicillin	1000 mg	Oral	6.2
	Ampicillin	1000 mg	Oral	1.5*
	Sulfonamide	30 mg/kg	Oral	8.3

*Mean levels.

general tissue concentrations of antibiotics are lower than serum levels except in the case of certain highly lipid-soluble compounds. Most antibiotics are bound to serum proteins to varying degrees. Only a drug which is free can exert its antibacterial action. However, protein binding is a dynamic equilibrium, and it is only when a drug is 90% or more protein-bound that protein binding becomes important.[6] Only the antistaphylococcal penicillins — oxacillin, cloxacillin, dicloxacillin — are more than 90% protein-bound. Cephalosporins range in protein binding from 15% for cephalexin to 85% for cefazolin. Aminoglycosides are not protein-bound and protein binding does not affect the activity of erythromycin, clindamycin or the tetracyclines.

Other factors which may affect the activity of antibiotics at the site of infection are the pH, anaerobic or aerobic conditions, degree of purulent material, osmolality and concentrations of divalent cations. For example, aminoglycosides are not active at acid pH, in anaerobic conditions, and high concentrations of cellular DNA-RNA material will reduce their activity against organisms such as *Pseudomonas, E coli*, etc. Some bacteria are dormant in purulent material, and β-lactam antibiotics, penicillins and cephalosporins will not kill bacteria unless the bacteria are actively growing. These factors explain to some extent why antibiotics must be given over a long period in deep tissue infections since the antibiotic must not only diffuse to the site of the infection, but must attack the organisms when they are in a state that allows the antibiotic to affect the cellular process it inhibits.

TISSUE DISTRIBUTION OF ANTIBIOTICS

Florey and associates[7] in 1946 showed that penicillin could be measured in wound exudates eight hours after an intramuscular injection of a small amount of penicillin G. Weinstein and colleagues[8] showed that antibiotics persisted in sterile fibrin clots several hours after injection. Numerous other workers have developed models to study the concentration of antibiotic in wound fluid and the kinetics of its movement in and out of wounds. In general, older wounds have less antibiotic, and rapidly excreted drugs produce less drug in tissue cages set up to measure antibiotics. It is interesting that fairly protein-bound drugs still can enter wound tissue to yield therapeutically effective concentrations.[9] Although there have been extensive studies of the concentrations of antibiotics in pulmonary, cardiac, bone and biliary areas, the studies of levels of antibiotics in the tissues of the head and neck have been fewer and often unsatisfactory. Levels of penicillins, cephalosporins, erythromycin and sulfonamides have been measured in sinus tissue, lacrimal and salivary secretions and tonsillar tissue[10-16] (Table 6). No satisfactory correlation of such tissue levels with clinical cures is available, and the results of assay often are open to question since there is contamination with blood at the time of sampling. Tonsillar tissue levels of penicillin, erythromycin, amoxicillin and ampicillin all have been obtained and in general exceed the usual inhibitory levels of the antibiotics against group A streptococci and against *S pneumoniae*. Concentrations of ampicillin, amoxicillin, cefaclor and TMP-SMX in middle ear fluid are adequate to inhibit both *S pneumoniae* and *H influenzae*. Concentrations of erythromycin often are not adequate to inhibit a number of *H influenzae* strains, whereas ear concentrations of sulfonamide have been adequate. Although European studies of chronic sinusitis have demonstrated higher levels of ampicillin when given as pivampicillin, these studies have not correlated with clinical cures. Levels of penicillin V in sinus tissue after doses of 400 mg have been disappointing.

The aforementioned examples of tissue and secretion analysis of antibiotics of ENT infections probably are of minor significance since the volume of infections seen clinically has permitted good clinical studies which in the long run are more significant than tissue levels of the antibiotics. In some ENT infections, however, tissue levels may be critical. The prime example would be a condition such as necrotizing otitis due to *P aeruginosa*. Cure rates of this serious infection have improved with the ability to

TABLE 7. TOXIC REACTIONS TO ANTIMICROBIAL AGENTS

Agent	Mechanism	Signs
Hematologic		
Chloramphenicol	Inhibit protein synthesis	Reversible anemia, leukopenia
	Damage stem cell	Aplastic anemia
Sulfonamides	G6PD deficiency	Hemolytic anemia
Carbenicillin	Platelet aggregation inhibited	Bleeding
Nervous System		
Aminoglycosides	Binding hair cells or organ of Corti	Deafness
	Binding vestibular cells	Vertigo
	Competitive neuromuscular blockade	Respiratory paralysis
Polymyxins	Noncompetitive neuromuscular blockade	Respiratory paralysis
Penicillins and cephalosporins	Cortical stimulation	Myoclonic seizures
Gastrointestinal		
Rifampin Isoniazid Tetracycline	Liver cell damage	Hepatitis
Neomycin	Villi damage	Malabsorption
Clindamycin Lincomycin	Altered bowel flora - overgrowth *C difficile*	Diarrhea, pseudomembranous colitis
All agents	Altered bowel flora - overgrowth *C difficile*	Diarrhea, pseudomembranous colitis
Renal		
Penicillins	Interstitial nephritis	Fever, eosinophilia, azotemia
Cephaloridine	Tubular necrosis	Azotemia
Aminoglycosides	Tubular necrosis	Cylinduria, azotemia
Polymyxins	Tubular necrosis	Azotemia
Metabolic		
Penicillins Carbenicillin Ticarcillin	Nonabsorbable anion	Hypokalemia
Allergic		
Penicillins	IgE	Anaphylaxis
	IgM	Rash
Cephalosporins	?	Rash
Tetracyclines	?	Rash
Miscellaneous		
Cephalosporins		False-positive glucose tests

utilize antibiotics which act synergistically and with use of higher concentrations of the drugs — both the aminoglycosides, tobramycin or gentamicin, and the anti-*Pseudomonas* penicillins, carbenicillin and ticarcillin. It is in infections of this type that the otolaryngologist should know the actual inhibitory concentrations required to inhibit the infecting organism and also should know what serum levels actually could be achieved using the program selected.

SAFETY FACTORS TO BE CONSIDERED IN USE OF ANTIBIOTICS

Antimicrobial use is associated with some degree of untoward side effects in a small number of patients.[17] It is not possible in this brief review to consider all of the possible reactions about which the ENT expert should be concerned. But several toxic reactions bear mentioning. Table 7 lists many adverse effects. The most common reaction to penicillins is an allergic reaction. These are fairly infrequent considering the overall use of penicillins. Anaphylaxis occurs to any of the penicillins and seems to be due to minor determinants of breakdown of the penicillin nucleus. Patients who have had anaphylaxis should not be retreated with penicillins. In contrast, allergic reactions of the rash type can be of two types. In one the reaction probably is IgM mediated. Patients will repeat a rash if rechallenged. But there is another skin rash, namely that associated with ampicillin use, which is not antibody-mediated. It occurs most often if the patient has a viral illness and does not preclude reuse of ampicillin, penicillin G or other penicillins. This rash occurs in almost all patients who receive penicillin while they have infectious mononucleosis.

Less frequent reactions to penicillins are the neutropenia, allergic interstitial nephritis and antibiotic-associated enterocolitis. The physician should realize that diarrhea due to ampicillin can be either due to nonspecific factors or to overgrowth of *Clostridium difficile* in the colon. Stopping the antibiotic will stop the reaction. A side effect associated with high dose therapy with carbenicillin or ticarcillin is hypokalemia due to the large load of nonreabsorbable anion delivered to the distal renal tubule. Potassium supplementation is necesary when these antibiotics are used.

Cephalosporins are associated with few major adverse reactions. Phlebitis at intravenous (IV) sites is common, but can be avoided by frequent IV changes and greater dilution of the antibiotic. Excessive use of cephalosporins will result in overgrowth of *Candida* and *Pseudomonas* in severe wounds and should be watched for in the debilitated patient. One reaction the elderly diabetic patient should be advised of is that the compounds will give false positive tests for glucose with the Benedict's test.

Minocycline, because of its good activity against both anaerobic mouth organisms and staphylococci, may be used in some chronic oral infections. The drug can cause vertigo, in females more than in males. If a tetracycline has to be used in a patient with decreased renal function, only doxycycline should be used.

The otolaryngologist is clearly aware of the vestibular hazards of therapy with aminoglycosides as well as the hearing loss associated with this class of compounds. However, knowledge of the nephrotoxicity of aminoglycosides may not be as well appreciated. These antibiotics produce a nonoliguric renal failure with loss of urinary concentrating ability followed by development of proteinuria, renal casts and rise in BUN and serum creatinine. This change in renal function can occur after therapy has ended. It is essential that the physician realize that a normal serum creatinine value cannot be equated with normal renal function. A serum creatinine of 1.4 mg/dL in a 120 kg male of 22 reflects a creatinine clearance of 100 ml/min. But a serum creatinine of 1 mg/dL in a 70-year-old, 45 kg female reflects a clearance of only 45 ml/min. Thus adjustments in dosage of aminoglycosides are necessary when the drugs are used in the elderly patient. We currently prefer to use tobramycin when dealing with serious *Pseudomonas* infection requiring long therapy.

The pseudomembranous colitis which followed therapy with clindamycin is well known. It is now realized that this is due to overgrowth of *C difficile* in the colon with production of a toxin affecting the colonic mucosa. Stopping the drug will usually solve the problem, but if the diarrhea persists, use of oral vancomycin at 125 mg every six hours will eradicate the *Clostridium* and indeed allow one to continue using the clindamycin if it is necessary in treating a serious anaerobic infection of the neck.

SUMMARY

This article has been an attempt to pull together some of our current understanding about mechanisms of antibacterial agents, the resistance of bacteria to antibiotics and concepts of the pharmacology of antibiotics. As more agents become available it will be no less difficult to choose the most appropriate to treat an infection. Thus minor differences in antibacterial activity, differences in pharmacology, as well as factors of safety will play a more important role. Better utilization of currently available agents is possible if more attention is given to proper administration. Keeping the factors discussed in this paper in mind will improve cure rates and reduce unwanted side effects.

REFERENCES

1. Neu HC. Perspectives on antibiotics. In: Weinstein L, Fields BN, eds. Seminars in infectious diseases, vol 1. New York: Stratton Medical Book Corp, 1978:97-121.

2. Sinai R, Hammerberg S, Marks MI, Pai CH. In vitro susceptibility of *Haemophilus influenzae* to sulfamethoxazole-trimethoprim and cefaclor, cephalexin and cephradine. Antimicrob Agents Chemother 1978; 13:861-4.

3. Davies J, Smith DI. Plasmid determined resistance to antimicrobial agents. Am Rev Microbiol 1978; 32:469-518.

4. Greenblatt DJ, Koch-Wieser J. Clinical pharmacokinetics. N Engl J Med 1973; 293:702-5, 964-9.

5. Gibaldi M, Levy G. Pharmacokinetics in clinical practice. JAMA 1976; 235:1864-7, 1987-92.

6. Neu HC. Clinical pharmacokinetics in preventive antimicrobial therapy. S Med J 1977; 70(S):14-23.

7. Florey ME, Turton EC, Duthe ES. Penicillin in wound exudates. Lancet 1946; 2:405-9.

8. Weinstein L, Daikos GK, Perrin TS. Studies on the relationship of tissue fluid and blood levels of penicillin. J Lab Clin Med 1951; 38:712-8.

9. Alexander JW, Sykes NS, Michell MM, et al. Concentrations of selected intravenously administered antibiotics in experimental surgical wounds. J Trauma 1973; 13:423-34.

10. Eneroth CM, Lundberg C, Wretlind B. Antibiotic concentrations in maxillary sinus secretions and in sinus mucosa. Chemotherapy 1975; 21(S):1-7.

11. Lungberg C, Malmberg AS. Concentrations of penicillin V and tetracycline in maxillary sinus secretions after repeated doses. Scand J Infect Dis 1973; 5:123-8.

12. Kaplan JM, McCracken GH Jr, Culbertson MC. Penicillin and erythromycin concentrations in tonsils. Am J Dis Child 1974; 127:206-11.

13. Klimek JJ, Nightingale C, Lehmann WB, Quintiliani R. Comparison of concentrations of amoxicillin and ampicillin in serum and middle ear fluid of children with chronic otitis media. J Infect Dis 1977; 135:999-1002.

14. Silverstein H, Bernstein JM, Lerner PI. Antibiotic concentrations in middle ear effusions. Pediatrics 1966; 38:33-9.

15. Bass JW, Steele RW, Wiebe RA, Dierdoff EP. Erythromycin concentrations in middle ear exudates. Pediatrics 1971; 48:417-22.

16. Lahikainen E. Penicillin concentrations in middle ear secretions in otitis. Acta Otolaryngol (Stockh) 1970; 70:358-62.

17. Neu HC. Toxicity of antimicrobial agents. In: Neu HC, Caldwell ADS, eds. Problems in antibiotic therapy. London: Academic Press, 1979:71-82.

CHEMOPROPHYLAXIS FOR SURGERY OF THE HEAD AND NECK

GARY D. BECKER, MD, FACS
LOS ANGELES, CALIFORNIA

A prospective study of patients undergoing major head and neck cancer surgery was undertaken to 1) define the value of cefazolin prophylaxis in reducing the incidence of wound infection, 2) define the value of preoperative and intraoperative (perioperative) cultures in identifying the patient at high risk of wound infection and in predicting the bacteriology of subsequent wound infection, and 3) demonstrate the most common aerobic and anaerobic flora of infected wounds. Preoperatively, the neck skin, oropharynx and anterior nares were swabbed for aerobic cultures. An intraoperative wound culture was obtained after the mucosal defect was sutured and the wound irrigated with water and sent for aerobic culture. All infected wounds were cultured for aerobic and anaerobic flora. Cefazolin, 1 g, was given intramuscularly (IM) about two hours before the skin incision, and continued in 0.5 g doses IM or intravenously (IV) every six hours for four doses. Cefazolin prophylaxis significantly reduced the incidence of postoperative wound infection. Isolation of aerobic pathogens perioperatively was not correlated with a greater risk of wound infection and did not accurately predict the flora of subsequent wound infection. The most common pathogenic aerobes isolated from infected wounds were *Staphylococcus aureus* and *β-Streptococcus* not group A, as well as a variety of Gram-negative organisms. The most common anaerobic isolate was *Bacteroides melaninogenicus*.

INTRODUCTION

Wound infection is a common complication of head and neck cancer surgery, especially if the upper aerodigestive tract is opened from the neck, thereby contaminating the operative wound with oropharyngeal flora.

Identifying the patient likely to develop a wound infection and predicting the flora of subsequent wound infection would allow a rational approach to antibiotic prophylaxis or initiation of treatment at the first sign of infection, pending definitive culture and sensitivity. While perioperative cultures may be of predictive value in this setting, data from abdominal surgery[1-4] is conflicting and from head and neck surgery virtually nonexistent.[5] Also, antibiotics are often given prophylactically under these circumstances even though there has been little valid evidence from prospective double-blind clinical trials supporting their use.

Since the operative wound requires a minimum bacterial contamination to become infected,[6] we reasoned that culturing the likely sources of contamination, ie, the patient's skin and oropharynx, may be of predictive value. The purpose of this article is 1) to define the prophylactic value of cefazolin in reducing the incidence of wound infection, 2) to establish the value of perioperative cultures in identifying the patient at high risk of wound infection and in predicting the bacteriology of subsequent wound infection, and 3) to document the flora of subsequent wound infection.

TABLE 1. COMPARISON OF RATE OF FISTULA FORMATION BETWEEN PLACEBO AND CEFAZOLIN GROUPS

	Number of Patients			
	Treated	*Infected*	*Local Wound Infections*	*Fistula Formations*
Placebo	25	21	4 (16%)	17 (68%)
Cefazolin	32	10	4 (13%)	6 (19%)

METHODS

In this prospective, randomized, double-blind study, patients underwent major head and neck cancer surgery in which the upper aerodigestive tract was opened from the neck. The study was conducted at the Veterans Administration, Wadsworth Hospital Center, in Los Angeles. Aerobic cultures of the skin of the neck and oropharynx were obtained one or two days before surgery. Many patients also had swab cultures of the anterior nares and intraoperative wound. All infected wounds were cultured for aerobic as well as anaerobic organisms. Patients received 1 g cefazolin or a placebo with the preoperative medications (approximately two hours before skin incision). This was continued in 0.5 g doses, either IM or IV, every six hours for four doses. Details of the study design, cefazolin prophylaxis results, and some bacteriologic data have been previously reported.[7,8] This paper evaluates unreported bacteriologic data obtained in this study.

RESULTS

Table 1 summarizes the types of infections encountered in 57 determinate patients. The distribution of surgical procedures in the placebo and cefazolin groups was similar. The most common procedures were laryngectomy with radical neck dissection and composite resections (tongue-jaw-neck). The incidence of fistula formation was 68% and 19% in the placebo and cefazolin groups respectively. This represents a statistically significant reduction, suggesting that the use of cefazolin

TABLE 2. INFECTION RATE AMONG THE CEFAZOLIN AND PLACEBO GROUPS

	Cefazolin	*Placebo*
Patients	32	23
Infected	12 (38%)	20 (87%)
P value	$P<0.001$	—

From the Section of Head and Neck Surgery, Veterans Administration, Wadsworth Hospital Center, Los Angeles.
REPRINTS — Gary D. Becker, MD, 1320 Pacific Street, Santa Monica, CA 90405.

TABLE 3. INCIDENCE OF ISOLATION OF AEROBIC PATHOGENS PERIOPERATIVELY IN PATIENTS WITH INFECTED AND NONINFECTED WOUNDS

	Number of Patients					
	Treated	*Infected*	*With Perioperative Pathogens*	*Infected with Perioperative Pathogens*	*Not Infected*	*Not Infected with Perioperative Pathogens*
Cefazolin	32	10	21	6 (60%)	20	15 (75%)
Placebo	25	21	13	11 (52%)	4	2 (50%)
Total	55	31	34	17 (55%)	24	17 (68%)

results in a less serious type of wound infection. Of 55 determinate patients in the prophylaxis study, 32 received cefazolin and 23 placebo (Table 2). The infection rate was 38% (12/32) and 87% (20/23) respectively, which is a statistically significant reduction in infection. There were two nonwound (sinusitis and pneumonia) infections in the cefazolin group.

Table 3 compares the frequency of isolation of aerobic pathogens perioperatively with the subsequent development of wound infection. Pathogens were isolated from the majority of patients whether they subsequently became infected or not. Table 4 summarizes the distribution of perioperative isolation of pathogens from subsequently infected and noninfected patients. In this study, a pathogen was defined as an isolate other than *Staphylococcus epidermidis*, *Candida* and yeast species, *Acinetobacter calcoaciticus*, *Corynebacterium* species, γ-streptococci, α-hemolytic streptococci, *Hemophilus* species (other than *H influenzae* or *H parainfluenzae*) and *Neisseria* species (other than *N meningitidis*). The most common isolate cultured preoperatively in either group of patients was α-hemolytic streptococci from the pharynx and *S epidermidis* from the skin. A variety of aerobic Gram-positive and Gram-negative pathogens were isolated from perioperative cultures in subsequently infected as well as noninfected patients. The infected group did not harbor more pathogens perioperatively compared to noninfected patients. Thirty pathogens were isolated perioperatively from 17 noninfected patients (1.8 pathogens/patient) and 28 pathogens from 17 subsequently infected patients (1.7 pathogens/patient). A separate analysis of patients with nasal carriage of *S aureus* was made (Table 5) to determine if this group was at greater risk of developing wound infection. The wound infection rate between carriers and noncarriers is not statistically significant. It does not appear from any of these data that a patient at high risk of wound infection may be defined on the basis of perioperative aerobic bacteriology.

A pathogen isolated preoperatively or intraoperatively was subsequently recovered from 56% and 86% of infected wounds, respectively (Table 6). In the majority of patients, however, either the perioperative culture or infected wound culture grew one or more additional pathogens. Because of this variability in bacteriology, the choice of antibiotic for prophylaxis or initial therapy of wound infection is difficult to define. Table 7 summarizes the frequency of isolation of aerobic pathogens cultured from subsequently infected wounds. The most common wound pathogens in the placebo group were *β-Streptococcus* not group A and *S aureus*. In the cefazolin group, a dramatic decrease in the incidence of *S aureus* resulted in the emergence of *β-Streptococcus* not group A as the most common pathogenic isolate. A wide variety of Gram-negative pathogens were isolated from both groups. As may be anticipated, the incidence of isolation of cefazolin-sensitive bacteria was reduced in the cefazolin group, but there appeared to be no definite emergence of resistant or unusual pathogens.

TABLE 4. FREQUENCY OF PERIOPERATIVE ISOLATION OF AEROBIC PATHOGENS FROM INFECTED AND NONINFECTED PATIENTS

	Placebo Group		*Cefazolin Group*	
	Isolates Obtained from Infected Patients	*Isolates Obtained from Noninfected Patients*	*Isolates Obtained from Infected Patients*	*Isolates Obtained from Noninfected Patients*
Gram-positive:				
S aureus	4	1	7	6
β-Streptococcus (not group A)	3	—	3	2
β-Streptococcus (group A)	—	—	1	—
S pneumoniae	2	—	—	3
Gram-negative:				
K pneumoniae	3	—	—	6
H influenzae	1	—	2	—
E cloacae	—	—	1	3
P maltophelia	—	—	1	—
P aeruginosa	—	1	—	1
P vulgaris	—	—	—	1
N meningitidis	—	—	—	3
E coli	—	2	—	1

TABLE 5. COMPARISON OF POSTOPERATIVE WOUND INFECTION RATE WITH PREOPERATIVE NASAL CARRIAGE OF *S AUREUS*

	Placebo	*Cefazolin*	*Combined*
Patients screened with preoperative nasal cultures	14	20	34
Nasal *Staphylococcus* isolated	3 (21%)	6 (33%)	9 (26%)
Postoperative infection	3 (100%)	2 (33%)	5 (56%)
Staphylococcus isolated in wound	1 (33%)	0 (0%)	1 (11%)
Nasal *Staphylococcus* not isolated	11	14	25
Postoperative infection	9 (82%)	6 (43%)	15 (60%)
Staphylococcus isolated in wound	2 (22%)	0 (0%)	2 (13%)

Table 8 summarizes the anaerobic flora cultured from infected wounds. The majority of isolates were Gram-negative rods, mainly *Bacteroides melaninogenicus* and *Fusobacterium nucleatum*. *Bacteroides fragilis* was never isolated. Table 9 summarizes the number of aerobic and anaerobic isolates (pathogens and nonpathogens) from infected wounds. Virtually every wound was infected by a variety of aerobes and anaerobes. The average number of different bacterial isolates totaled 8.1 and 7.5 in the placebo and cefazolin groups respectively. This ranged from as few as two to as many as 13 different isolates from a single infected wound. An average of 1.6 commonly recognized aerobic pathogens/wound were isolated from both the placebo and cefazolin groups. These data support the concept of polymicrobial wound infections in head and neck cancer surgery, involving both aerobic and anaerobic bacteria.

DISCUSSION

Cefazolin was chosen for prophylaxis because of its known effectiveness against aerobic pathogens most commonly isolated from infected wounds and anaerobic bacteria normally resident in the oropharynx. In this study, cefazolin was administered so that appropriate tissue levels were present at the time of bacterial intraoperative wound contamination, and maintained until bacterial contamination was presumably over. This study established the effectiveness of the perioperative use of cefazolin in reducing the incidence of wound infection in general and fistula formation in specific. We feel that an important variable contributing to wound infection in the cefazolin group was continued bacterial seeding through an incontinent mucosal suture line after cefazolin levels had decreased. Future studies should evaluate the benefit of more prolonged antibiotic prophylaxis.

The major variable contributing to postoperative wound infection is contamination of the operative wound by bacteria.[9] We therefore reasoned that patients at high risk of wound infection would likely be those who carried pathogenic bacteria on the skin of the incision site or oropharynx, and that these pathogens would emerge in the wound infection. As any bacteria may become pathogenic in another site or in a compromised host or tissue, our definition of pathogen is arbitrary, but, we feel, appropriate for this study. While this study demonstrated that the vast majority of wound infections after head and neck cancer surgery involve anaerobic as well as aerobic bacteria, the value of perioperative isolation of anaerobes was not investigated. Other investigators have demonstrated that in patients undergoing transperitoneal surgery the isolation of mixed anaerobic and aerobic

TABLE 7. FREQUENCY OF ISOLATION OF AEROBIC PATHOGENS FROM INFECTED WOUNDS

	Isolates Obtained	
	Placebo Group	*Cefazolin Group*
Gram-positive:		
S aureus	8	1
β-Streptococcus (not group A)	10	5
β-Streptococcus (group A)	2	1
Gram-negative:		
K pneumoniae	4	1
H influenzae	3	0
H parainfluenzae	2	0
E aerogenes	1	1
E cloacae	1	1
P mirabilis	1	1
P aeruginosa	1	1
E corrodens	1	0
Capnocytophaga sp	0	1
E coli	0	1
S liquifaciens	0	1
S marcescens	0	1

TABLE 6. COMPARISON OF PERIOPERATIVE ISOLATION OF PATHOGENS WITH THEIR SUBSEQUENT RECOVERY IN WOUND INFECTION

	Placebo		*Cefazolin*		*Combined*	
	Preoperative	*Intraoperative*	*Preoperative*	*Intraoperative*	*Preoperative*	*Intraoperative*
Cultures obtained from subsequently infected patients	21	9	10	7	31	16
Patients with positive perioperative cultures	11	4	7	3	18	7
Isolation of same pathogen in wound	5 (45%)	4 (100%)	5 (71%)	2 (66%)	10 (56%)	6 (86%)
Identical isolation of pathogens from perioperative and infected wound cultures	0 (0%)	1 (25%)	2 (29%)	1 (14%)	2 (11%)	2 (29%)

TABLE 8. FREQUENCY OF ISOLATION OF ANAEROBIC BACTERIA FROM INFECTED WOUNDS

	Isolates Obtained	
	Placebo Group	*Cefazolin Group*
Gram-positive cocci		
Pc asaccharolyticus	1	2
Pc magnus	1	2
Pc prevotii	6	1
Pc variabilis	1	0
Ps anaerobius	3	1
Ps micros	7	2
Gram-positive rods		
Actinomyces sp	1	0
A viscosus	1	0
Bifidobacterium sp	1	0
Eubacterium sp	3	1
L catenaforme	1	0
L delbraeckii	1	0
L minutus	1	1
Lactobacillus sp	4	1
P acnes	1	1
Propionibacterium sp	2	0
Gram-negative rods		
B amylophilus	1	0
B capillosus	1	0
B disiens	2	0
B melaninogenicus sp	4	2
B melaninogenicus (ss *intermedius*)	8	3
B melaninogenicus (ss *melaninogenicus*)	9	6
B oralis	7	3
B ruminicola (ss *brevis*)	5	3
Bacteroides sp	6	2
F aquatili	1	0
F necrophorum	1	0
F nucleatum	8	4
Gram-negative cocci		
V alcalescens	3	1
A fermantans	1	1
V parvula	5	5

bacteria from the operative wound is associated with a much higher incidence of subsequent wound infection than if aerobes or anaerobes are isolated alone.[9] In this study, a variety of Gram-positive and Gram-negative aerobic pathogenic bacteria were isolated perioperatively from both subsequently infected and noninfected patients with no definite trend toward more frequent isolation in the infected group. In addition, a separate analysis of patients with nasal carriage of *S aureus* did not reveal a higher incidence of wound infection. For these reasons, we do not feel that a bacteriologic definition of a patient at high risk of wound infection can be made on the basis of preoperative aerobic cultures.

In more than one half the patients, a pathogen isolated perioperatively subsequently emerged in the wound infection. However, in most patients, additional pathogens were isolated from either the perioperative swab or infected wound culture, limiting its value as a guide to antibiotic prophylaxis or initial therapy of wound infection.

TABLE 9. AEROBIC AND ANAEROBIC BACTERIA ISOLATED FROM INFECTED WOUNDS

	Average Number and Range		
	Aerobic Isolates	*Anaerobic Isolates*	*Combined Isolates*
Placebo	3.7 (1-6)	4.4 (0-8)	8.1 (5-13)
Cefazolin	3.1 (1-5)	4.4 (1-9)	7.5 (2-13)

Wound infection following major head and neck cancer surgery is polymicrobial, evidenced by the variety of Gram-positive and Gram-negative anaerobic and aerobic bacteria isolated from subsequently infected wounds. While the most common aerobic Gram-positive pathogens isolated from infected wounds were *β-Streptococcus* not group A and *S aureus*, the variety of Gram-negative aerobic pathogens recovered discourage the use of a single antibiotic for prophylaxis or initial therapy of infection.

More anaerobes were isolated from infected wounds than aerobes. Numerically, the most important anaerobes were Gram-negative rods, consisting mainly of *B melaninogenicus* and *F nucleatum*. *B fragilis*, an anaerobe universally resistant to the penicillins and cephalosporins, was not isolated in this study. Cefazolin prophylaxis did not lead to a definite reduction in total number of aerobic or anaerobic isolates in general, or in aerobic pathogenic isolates in specific. The reason for this lack of suppression of susceptible organisms in the presence of a definite reduction in wound infection is speculative. Inhibition of phagocytosis of some pathogenic aerobic bacteria by *B melaninogenicus* and other obligate anaerobes in vitro has been demonstrated by others,[10] and represents one possible mechanism of polymicrobial bacterial interaction in the causation of wound infection. Metronidazole, an agent with broad spectrum anaerobic bactericidal effects, has been used unsuccessfully on patients in this study for treatment of established infections. A more logical approach would be to use metronidazole prophylactically, perhaps in combination with an antibiotic effective against the most common aerobic pathogens encountered in wound infections.

CONCLUSIONS

On the basis of clinical and bacteriologic data obtained in this study, we conclude that in the setting of head and neck cancer surgery in which the upper aerodigestive tract is opened from the neck, 1) the perioperative use of cefazolin results in a significant reduction in wound infection and fistula formation, 2) a bacteriologic definition of a patient at high risk of wound infection cannot be made on the basis of preoperative aerobic bacteriology, 3) the flora of a wound infection cannot be accurately predicted on the basis of preoperative or intraoperative aerobic cultures, and 4) wound infections are polymicrobial, involving both aerobic and anaerobic bacteria.

REFERENCES

1. Polk HC Jr. Postoperative wound infection: prediction of some responsible organisms. Am J Surg 1973; 126:592-4.

2. Delikaris PG, Michail PO, Klonis GD, Haritopoulos NC, Golematis AC, Dreiling DA. Biliary bacteriology based on intraoperative bile cultures. Am J Gastroenterol 1977; 68:51-5.

3. Bartlett JG, Condon RE, Gorbach SL, Clarke JS, Nichols RL, Ochi S. Veterans Administration Cooperative study on bowel preparation for elective colorectal operations: impact of oral antibiotic regimen on colonic flora, wound irrigation cultures and bacteriology of septic complications. Ann Surg 1978; 188:249-54.

4. Scheibel JH, Lykkegaard N, Wamberg T. Septic complications in colo-rectal surgery after 24 hours versus 60 hours of preoperative antibiotic bowel preparation, II. Significance of bacterial concentrations in the bowel for contamination of the operative field and subsequent wound infection. Acta Chir Scand 1978; 144:527-32.

5. Ketcham AS, Bloch JH, Crawford DT, Lieberman JE, Smith RR. The role of prophylactic antibiotic therapy in control of staphylococcal infections following cancer surgery. Surg Gynecol Obstet 1962; 114:345-52.

6. Cruse P. Infection surveillance: identifying the problems and the high risk patient. South Med J 1977; 70 Suppl 1:4-8.

7. Becker GD, Parell GJ. Cefazolin prophylaxis in head and neck cancer surgery. Ann Otol Rhinol Laryngol 1979; 88:183-6.

8. Becker GD, Parrell GJ, Busch DF, Finegold SM. Anaerobic and aerobic bacteriology in head and neck cancer surgery. Arch Otolaryngol 1978; 104:591-4.

9. Kelly MJ, Warren RE. The value of an operative swab sent in transport medium in the prediction of later clinical wound infection: a controlled clinical and bacteriological evaluation. Br J Surg 1978; 65:81-8.

10. Ingham HR, Tharagonnet D, Sisson PR, Selkon JB, Codd AA. Inhibition of phagocytosis in vitro by obligate anaerobes. Lancet 1977; 2:1252-4.

ANAEROBIC INFECTIONS IN OTOLARYNGOLOGY

SYDNEY M. FINEGOLD, MD

LOS ANGELES, CALIFORNIA

The role of anaerobes in head and neck infections is discussed. Data from several key studies are presented. It is emphasized that the source of anaerobic organisms in otolaryngological infections is the indigenous flora of the upper respiratory tract.

By way of background information, I would like to show you the incidence of anaerobes present as normal flora (Table 1). Notice that in the mouth and upper respiratory tract there are large numbers of anaerobic cocci and anaerobic Gram-negative bacilli, but relatively few other anaerobic types. Thus these two groups of organisms can be commonly expected in infections in the head and neck area.

Some of the major infections in this area involve anaerobic organisms: chronic otitis media and mastoiditis and certain complications of these, such as epidural abscess and brain abscess; chronic sinusitis; Vincent's angina, which is a membranous tonsillitis caused by *Fusobacterium necrophorum*, a Gram-negative anaerobic rod (this is a very serious infection complicated frequently by bacteremia and metastatic sepsis); peritonsillar abscess; Ludwig's angina, a very serious infection involving the submandibular and sublingual spaces in the neck; other neck space infections; infections of the head and face; and finally, actinomycosis.

In a study of acute otitis media performed by Brook et al,[2] anaerobes played a relatively minor role (Table 2). In this group of 62 patients there were 35 who had infections with aerobic bacteria only; there were nine cases in which anaerobes were isolated and eight in which both aerobes and anaerobes were isolated. But most of the anaerobes that were isolated were really not significant in these patients. The majority of anaerobes were *Propionibacterium*, the so-called anaerobic diphtheroid, which is essentially nonpathogenic and certainly nonpathogenic in this particular setting. There were a few infections where anaerobic cocci were involved. However, for the most part acute otitis media is primarily an aerobic infection.

TABLE 1. INCIDENCE OF VARIOUS ANAEROBES AS NORMAL FLORA IN THE HUMAN

	Anaerobic Cocci	*Anaerobic Gram-Negative Bacilli*	*Clostridia*	*Gram-Positive Non-Sporulating Anaerobic Bacilli*
Skin	+*	− −	− −	+ to + +
Upper respiratory tract†	+ + +	+ +	− −	+
Mouth	+ + + +	+ + + +	Rare	+ to + +
Intestine	+ + + +	+ + + +	+ + + +	+ + + +
Genitourinary tract§	+ + +	+ +	+	+ to + +

*The ranking, + to + + + +, reflects both consistency of occurrence and density of numbers.

†Includes nasal passages, nasopharynx, oropharynx and tonsils.

§Includes vagina, external genitalia and urethra.

Adapted from Finegold.[1] Reprinted with permission.

Chronic otitis media, on the other hand, does involve anaerobic bacteria quite frequently.[3] In a group of 50 patients with chronic otitis media there were 48 isolates of anaerobic bacteria (Table 3). Anaerobic cocci and streptococci predominated, but there was also quite a large number of anaerobic Gram-negative bacilli.

TABLE 2. BACTERIOLOGY OF ACUTE OTITIS MEDIA (N = 62)

Patients with aerobes only		35
Patients with anaerobes only		9
Peptococcus	4	
Propionibacterium	6	
Patients with aerobes and anaerobes		8
Peptococcus + aerobes	3	
Propionibacterium + aerobes	5	
Negative cultures		10

To keep this in perspective, we see in Table 4 that the aerobic flora in these patients still predominated, ie, a total of 68 isolates compared to 48 anaerobic isolates; and we see *Pseudomonas* as the predominant organism numerically.

The data from Frederick and Braude[4] on chronic

TABLE 3. ANAEROBIC BACTERIAL ISOLATES IN 50 PATIENTS WITH CHRONIC OTITIS MEDIA

Gram-positive cocci	24
Bifidobacterium sp	2
Propionibacterium acnes	3
Clostridium sp	1
Fusobacterium nucleatum	2
Bacteroides melaninogenicus	6
B fragilis	3
B distasonis	4
B corrodens	1
Bacteroides sp	2
Total	48

From the Veterans Administration, Wadsworth Hospital Center, and the UCLA School of Medicine, Los Angeles.

REPRINTS — Sydney M. Finegold, MD, Infectious Disease Section (691/111F), V.A. Wadsworth Medical Center, Wilshire and Sawtelle Blvds., Los Angeles, CA 90073.

TABLE 4. AEROBIC BACTERIAL ISOLATES IN 50 PATIENTS WITH CHRONIC OTITIS MEDIA

S pneumoniae	2
α-Hemolytic streptococci	2
Group A, β-hemolytic *Streptococcus*	1
S aureus	6
Proteus sp	7
P aeruginosa	36
K pneumoniae	2
E coli	2
Miscellaneous	3
Total	68

sinusitis (Table 5) probably is the best available implicating anaerobes in this situation. Of a total of 83 specimens, one fourth were sterile, about one third yielded only anaerobes, and there were comparable numbers that were mixed infections with anaerobes plus aerobes or that involved aerobes only (about 20% in each of these latter two groups). On the other hand, if we concentrate on 28 of these specimens in which heavy growth was obtained, and clearly these must have been the most reliable specimens, it is interesting to note that 82% of these yielded only anaerobic bacteria and an additional 7% yielded anaerobes along with aerobes. So this data suggests that chronic sinusitis is primarily an anaerobic process.

TABLE 5. BACTERIOLOGY OF CHRONIC SINUSITIS

	No. Specimens	*No. Specimens with Heavy Growth*
Total	83	28
Anaerobes only	26 (31%)	23 (82%)
Aerobes only	19 (23%)	3 (11%)
Anaerobes + aerobes	17 (20%)	2 (7%)
Sterile	21 (25%)	—

Adapted from Frederick and Braude[4]. Reprinted with permission.

Let us consider some examples of these types of infections. First is a young girl with a retropharyngeal abscess as a complication of membranous tonsillitis (Vincent's angina) which started out

TABLE 7. BACTERIOLOGY OF FIFTEEN SPACE INFECTIONS*

Aerobes		
Streptococci		18
α-Hemolytic	10	
β-Hemolytic (nongroup A or D)	3	
Enterococci	4	
Group D (nonenterococci)	1	
S epidermidis		1
S aureus		1
E coli		1
P aeruginosa		1
E corrodens		2
Neisseria sp		2
Lactobacillus		1

Anaerobes		
Peptostreptococci		8
Ps intermedius	4	
Ps micros	2	
Ps parvulus	1	
Ps productus	1	
Peptococci		6
Pc prevotii	4	
Pc morbillorum	2	
Unidentified Gram-positive cocci		2
Bacteroidaceae		12
B melaninogenicus	9	
B oralis	1	
B fragilis	1	
B pneumosintes	1	
Fusobacteria		5
F nucleatum	4	
F necrophorum	1	
Unidentified Gram-negative bacilli		3
Actinomyces		3
A naeslundii	2	
Actinomyces sp	1	
Eubacteria		6
E lentum	3	
E limosum	1	
E alactolyticum	1	
Eubacterium sp	1	
Lactobacillus		4
Propionibacterium acnes		2
Veillonella		2

*Includes space infections along the mandible (12 cases) and three anterior visceral space infections (thyroid abscess, paratracheal abscess, and laryngeal crepitant cellulitis).

on a Friday afternoon with a sore throat and temperature of 102 C. She was brought into the hospital on a Monday morning, acutely ill with a temperature of 105 C, and was found to have sepsis with *F necrophorum*. She developed a fistula between the retropharyngeal space and the subarachnoid space

TABLE 6. SPACE INFECTIONS OF THE LOWER HEAD AND NECK

Location	*Space*	*Common Portal of Entry*	*Anticipated Bacteriology*
Mandible	Mental	Dental — low anterior teeth	Oral anaerobes
	Buccal	Dental — upper second and third molars	Oral anaerobes
	Submandibular	Dental — lower first and second molars	Oral anaerobes
	Sublingual	Dental — lower bicuspids	Oral anaerobes
	Masticator	Dental — third molars	Oral anaerobes
	Mandibular	Dental — bicuspids, first and second molars	Oral anaerobes
	Parotid	Stensen's duct	*S aureus*
Upper jaw	Canine	Dental — anterior, upper teeth and bicuspids	Oral anaerobes
Posterior pharynx	Peritonsillar	Pharynx	*S pyogenes* and oral anaerobes
	Retropharyngeal	Pharynx	*S pyogenes* and oral anaerobes
	Pharyngomaxillary	Pharynx, mastoiditis, lower molars, extension from other space infections	*S pyogenes* and oral anaerobes
Neck	Superficial	Skin	*S aureus*
	Anterior visceral space	Pharynx, trauma to esophagus or larynx	Oral anaerobes
	Carotid sheath	Extension from infections of deep cervical fascia, especially posterior pharyngomaxillary space	Oral anaerobes and *S pyogenes*

From Bartlett and Gorbach.[5] Reprinted with permission.

	1	2	3	4	5	6	7	8	9	10	11	12	13	14	15	16	17	18	19	20	21
GRAM-POSITIVE COCCI																					
Peptococcus asaccharolyticus							●														
P magnus		●																			
P prevotii	●		●				●		●						●	●					
P variabilis									●												
Peptostreptococcus anaerobius			●					●										●			
P micros					●			●				●		●			●		●	●	
GRAM-POSITIVE RODS																					
Actinomyces sp							●														
A viscosus	●																				
Bifidobacterium sp							●														
Eubacterium sp			●							●			●								
Lactobacillus catenaforme										●											
L delbrueckii		●																			
L minutus			●																		
Lactobacillus sp			●			●	●		●												
Propionibacterium acnes									●												
Propionibacterium sp		●			●																
GRAM-NEGATIVE RODS																					
Bacteroides amylophilus											●										
B capillosus															●						
B disiens											●						●				
B melaninogenicus sp							●	●		●	●										
B melaninogenicus (ss *intermedius*)					●						●	●	●	●		●	●	●			
B melaninogenicus (ss *melaninogenicus*)					●	●		●		●				●	●	●			●	●	
B oralis			●		●	●		●					●	●						●	
B ruminicola (ss *brevis*)					●					●				●		●	●				
Bacteroides sp							●	●		●	●					●	●				
Fusobacterium aquatili																	●				
F necrophorum	●																				
F nucleatum			●		●			●		●			●		●	●			●		
GRAM-NEGATIVE COCCI																					
Veillonella alcalescens			●															●		●	
Acidaminococcus fermentans															●						
V parvula		●									●						●	●			●

Fig. 1. Anaerobic flora cultured from infected wounds. Closed circles indicate wounds; ss - subspecies. From Becker et al.[6] Reprinted with permission.

and then *Fusobacterium* meningitis. She also developed purulent arthritis of the sternoclavicular joint and both hip joints, and many other types of metastatic disease.

Data from a study by Bartlett and Gorbach[5] (Table 6) point out that the anticipated bacteriology in these various space infections primarily involves anaerobes of the normal oral flora. The one exception is *Staphylococcus aureus* in parotid infection. But even here, on occasion, anaerobic bacteria may also be involved. We can also see in Table 6 that group A β-hemolytic streptococci may be involved in infections related to the pharynx. In addition, one sees oral anaerobes and in other cases only oral anaerobes. The major exception here would be infections related to the skin; in superficial infections *S aureus* would be the primary pathogen.

Table 7 presents bacteriologic data from a study of 15 neck space infections, again by Bartlett and Gorbach;[5] this shows a clear predominance of anaerobic bacteria. The aerobic organisms that were recovered were chiefly streptococci, especially of the α-hemolytic variety. The list of anaerobes is much more impressive. We see many anaerobic cocci and many Gram-negative anaerobic bacilli, as well as occasional anaerobes of other types.

Figure 1 shows some of the data from a study done at Wadsworth VA Hospital[6] on infection following radical head and neck surgery for cancer. Note the large number of Gram-negative anaerobic rods recovered. *Bacteroides fragilis* was not recovered at all in this study and, indeed, is seldom encountered in head and neck infections. The importance of this is the fact that the *B fragilis* group is much more resistant to antimicrobial agents than other anaerobic organisms, including those that we are particularly concerned with here. This is particularly true of cell-well active agents such as penicillins and cephalosporins. Figure 1 also contains data from this study showing the involvement of anaerobic cocci and some Gram-positive anaerobic rods.

A second example is a submandibular space infection and cellulitis of the jaw in which the underly-

TABLE 8. MISCELLANEOUS HEAD AND NECK INFECTIONS INVOLVING ANAEROBES

Salivary gland infection
Para-, retropharyngeal infection
Paratracheal abscess
Laryngeal infection
Suppurative thyroiditis
Nasal infections

ing process is Vincent's gingivitis, itself an important anaerobic process. A third example is cervicofacial actinomycosis in which woody swelling of the jaw and chronic draining sinuses occur.

Table 8 lists a number of miscellaneous head and neck infections in which anaerobes may be involved. In recent years most paratracheal abscesses have been complications of transtracheal aspiration; these abscesses are usually relatively minor infections that respond well to simple drainage, with or without antimicrobial therapy.

In summary, I would emphasize that anaerobes are clearly important in a wide variety of head and neck infections. The source of these organisms is the indigenous flora of the upper respiratory tract.

REFERENCES

1. Finegold SM. Anaerobic bacteria in human disease. New York: Academic Press, 1977.

2. Brook I, Anthony BF, Finegold SM. Aerobic and anaerobic bacteriology of acute otitis media in children. J Pediatr 1978; 92:13-5.

3. Brook I, Finegold SM. Bacteriology of chronic otitis media. JAMA 1979; 241:487-8.

4. Frederick J, Braude A. Anaerobic infection of the paranasal sinuses. N Engl J Med 1974; 290:135-7.

5. Bartlett JG, Gorbach SL. Anaerobic infections of the head and neck. Otolaryngol Clin North Am 1976; 9:655-78.

6. Becker GD, Parell GJ, Busch DF, Finegold SM, Acquarelli MJ. Anaerobic and aerobic bacteriology in head and neck cancer surgery. Arch Otolaryngol 1978; 104:591-4.

POSTOPERATIVE WOUND INFECTIONS

FRED S. HERZON, MD
ALBUQUERQUE, NEW MEXICO

Postoperative wound infection represents a serious complication of any surgical procedure. Prevention is the cornerstone when approaching this problem. Host factors, prophylactic antibiotics and meticulous surgical technique are key elements in achieving normal wound healing. These are discussed, as is wound infection in various types of surgery of the head and neck.

A postoperative wound infection is one of the most important of the various major postoperative complications. No matter what the surgical procedure, severe infection in the postoperative period almost always gives a poor result. Not only will the probable result of the procedure be significantly affected but the morbidity and sometimes the mortality may be markedly increased.

Prevention is the real basis of management of postoperative infection. Three factors must be considered in prevention: 1) prophylactic antibiotics, 2) host conditions, and 3) basic surgical principles. As prophylactic antibiotics are considered elsewhere in this symposium, I will only look at the last two conditions.

Both the general condition and local surgical site of the patient influence the possibility of postoperative infection. Local radiation and its effect on wound healing need not be recounted here. Nutrition in a debilitated patient must not be ignored prior to surgery. Every effort must be made to achieve an anabolic state.

Meticulous surgical technique is still perhaps the most important factor affecting postoperative infection. In 1936 Reed[1] said, "It is questionable if bacteria assume a role of greater importance in wound healing than do necrosis, debris and devitalized tissue or granulation tissue or fibrin or other factors which must be taken into consideration." Two more recent scientific studies[2,3] would seem to prove that statement. In both, two types of experimental wounds were compared; one in which meticulous atraumatic technique was used in opening and closure and the other where traumatic and rough tissue handling was the norm. Bacteria were added to the wound utilizing the first technique. It was the second wound which had the overwhelming number of infections.

Many if not most of the surgical procedures in the head and neck involve interruption of nonsterile mucosal surfaces, and additionally may be specific therapeutic modalities for chronic infectious diseases such as sinusitis or tympanomastoiditis. This places an added emphasis on following meticulous atraumatic surgical technique.

OTOLOGIC SURGERY

Wound infection in clean, otologic surgery, ie, stapedectomy, seventh nerve decompression, etc, is not a major problem (the reported incidence is less than 2%).[4,5] Although one report[6] gives a 10% figure for tympanomastoid procedures, continued postoperative drainage is not necessarily a postoperative infection.

The most commonly performed otologic procedure today is the myringotomy with ventilation tube insertion. In the literature and in our experience at the University of New Mexico, it also has the greatest incidence of immediate and later postoperative infection.

Of the 140 patients reviewed at the University of New Mexico, 7.8% had otorrhea within seven to ten days after surgery and 21% had drainage sometime during intubation. Others[7-9] have reported 15, 25, and 68% incidence of ventilation tube drainage. Our experience indicates a single course of antibiotics will clear the infection with only a small percentage extruding the tubes.

HEAD AND NECK TRAUMA

Host and environmental factors play an important role here as the type and condition of the injury will often influence whether a wound infection will occur. The reported wound infection rate is 8 to 10%.[6,10] Meticulous wound care when patients are injured is the surest way of controlling postoperative wound infections in this area.

RHINOLOGIC AND SINUS SURGERY

It is difficult to find statistics on the postoperative infection rate in functional rhinologic and sinus operations. As most sinus procedures are essentially incision and drainage, the incidence of "postoperative infections" cannot be very accurately determined. In functional operations on the nose, submucous resection of the nasal septum and the like, the incidence of infection is extremely small, probably under 1%.

From the Division of Otolaryngology, University of New Mexico School of Medicine, Albuquerque.

REPRINTS — Fred S. Herzon, MD, Center for Otolaryngology and Communicative Disorders, University of New Mexico, 2211 Lomas Blvd., NE, Albuquerque, NM 87131.

TABLE 1. HEAD AND NECK SOFT TISSUE INFECTIONS

Type of Case	*No.*	*Infections*
Open,* no radiation	16	1
Open, radiation (5-7000R)	25	3
Closed,† radiation (5-7000R)	10	1
Closed, no radiation	23	0

*Open - Mucosal surface cut.
†Closed - No mucosal surface cut.

FACIAL PLASTIC SURGERY

Perhaps in no other area is the problem of postoperative infection more greatly feared than in rhinoplasty, blepharoplasty, rhytidectomy, or other elective cosmetic procedures in the head and neck. The incidence however, when reported, is extremely small, under 1%.[11] So with sound basic surgical techniques, it is unlikely that a major problem should occur.

HEAD AND NECK SURGERY

The incidence of postoperative infection in a major, clean head and neck surgery (thyroidectomy, simple radical neck dissection, cyst removal, etc) is extremely small, less than 1 or 2%. With basic concepts being applied, major problems should be avoided.

However, in major head and neck cancer surgery wound breakdown from infection and/or fistula is common. Incidence varies from 5 to 80%[6,12-14] and our experience at the University of New Mexico with 74 consecutive cases showed a wound infection/fistula rate of under 7% (Table 1). Whether it is infection or fistula which occurs first is frequently difficult to determine.

Much has been written about the cause and prevention of these problems. However, an area which has not been looked at is the large variation reported in incidence. This should probably be examined further.

Though not a problem in all areas of the head and neck, postoperative wound infection remains a disturbing factor in major head and neck cancer surgery and on occasion, in otologic surgery and maxillofacial trauma. Prevention through basic surgical practices and indicated prophylactic chemotherapy should be encouraged. When a surgical infection does occur cultures and appropriate local and systemic therapeutic regimens are indicated.

REFERENCES

1. Reid MR. Some considerations of the problem of wound healing. N Engl J Med 1936; 215:753-66.

2. Condie JD, Ferguson DJ. Experimental wound infections: contamination versus surgical technique. Surgery 1961; 50: 367-71.

3. Dunphy JE, Jackson DS. Practical applications of experimental studies in the care of the primarily closed wound. Am J Surg 1962; 104:273-82.

4. Leonard JR. Prophylactic antibiotics in human stapedectomy. Laryngoscope 1967; 77:663-80.

5. Strong MR. Wound infection in otolaryngologic surgery and the inexpediency of antibiotic prophylaxis. Laryngoscope 1961; 73:165-84.

6. Eschelman LT, Schleuning AJ II, Brummett RE. Prophylactic antibiotics in otolaryngologic surgery: a double-blind study. Trans Am Acad Ophthalmol Otolaryngol 1971; 75:387-94.

7. Birck HG, Mravec JJ. Myringostomy for middle ear effusions. Ann Otol Rhinol Laryngol 1976; 85 Suppl 25:263-7.

8. Kokko E. Chronic secretory otitis media in children. Acta Otolaryngol (Stockh) 1974; Suppl 327:7-44.

9. Paradise JL, Bluestone CD. Early treatment of the universal otitis media of infants with cleft palate. Pediatrics 1974; 53:48-54.

10. Paterson JA, Cardo VA Jr, Stratigos GT. An examination of antibiotic prophylaxis in oral and maxillofacial surgery. J Oral Surg 1970; 28:157-65.

11. Dykes ER, Anderson R. Atraumatic technic-the sine qua non of operative wound infection prophylaxis. Cleve Clin Q 1961; 28:157-65.

12. Dor P, Klastersky J. Prophylactic antibiotics in oral, pharyngeal and laryngeal surgery for cancer (a double-blind study). Laryngoscope 1973; 83:1992-8.

13. Gall AM, Sessions DG, Ogura JH. Complications following surgery for cancer of the larynx and hypopharynx. Cancer 1977; 39:624-31.

14. Becker GD, Parell GJ, Busch DF, Finegold SM, Acquarelli MJ. Anaerobic and aerobic bacteriology in head and neck cancer surgery. Arch Otolaryngol 1978; 104:591-6.

INVASIVE *HEMOPHILUS* INFECTIONS: EPIGLOTTITIS AND CELLULITIS

JAMES D. CHERRY, MD

LOS ANGELES, CALIFORNIA

Epiglottitis, along with other infectious croup syndromes (laryngotracheitis and spasmodic croup), are illnesses which cause acute upper airway obstruction. They are discussed in terms of etiology, symptoms, diagnosis and treatment. Cellulitis and the role of *Hemophilus influenzae* and antibiotic therapy are also described.

INTRODUCTION

For this symposium, I've been asked to start with an infectious agent, *Hemophilus influenzae*, and work backwards to the illnesses. In clinical infectious diseases, we usually begin with the anatomical site of infection, eg, otitis media or sinusitis, then work up a differential diagnosis and therapy, frequently based on several organisms at first, then narrowing it down to one or two. Since many mistakes are made in therapy by employing the organism-first approach, I would like to consider the topics from the perspective of illness rather than etiology.

CROUP SYNDROMES INCLUDING EPIGLOTTITIS

Epiglottitis is only one of several clinical entities reacting with acute upper airway obstruction. In the classification of the illnesses that cause upper airway obstruction (Table 1), there are three categories, only one of which is an infectious diseases group. Serious mistakes can be made if allergic disease or mechanical problems are overlooked. In the infectious group, acute membranous laryngotracheitis due to *Corynebacterium diphtheriae* is always a possibility which must be considered.

ACUTE EPIGLOTTITIS

Acute epiglottitis is usually due to *H influenzae*, type B. The age range is from two to seven years, which is slightly older than the age range of viral croup. There is rapid onset and progression, so that a person can be virtually well and nine hours later be in dire distress. Illness initially is sore throat followed by difficulty in swallowing, drooling, retching and difficulty in breathing. There is no hoarseness but muffled or thick-sounding speech. A croupy barking cough should be absent and virtually always there is high fever. It occurs more commonly in boys. In almost 800 cases, over half were in two- to four-year-olds. In contrast, 57% of the cases of laryngotracheitis occurred in children under the age of two years.

TABLE 1. CLASSIFICATION OF CROUP

Infectious
Acute epiglottitis
Acute laryngotracheitis
Acute membranous laryngotracheitis
Spasmodic croup
Mechanical
Foreign body
Secondary to surgical procedure
Extrinsic tumor
Allergic (angioneurotic edema)

Although acute epiglottitis is predominantly an illness of children, there are many case reports of adults with similar acute fulminating disease. Agents other than *H influenzae* are rarely associated etiologically and some authors have pointed out that these organisms may be contaminants and not causative. The agents which are listed in Table 2 were all isolated from the blood of patients who were ill. The pneumococcus and other *Hemophilus* sp are noted in both children and adults, and one child had a *Staphylococcus aureus* bacteremia associated with epiglottitis.

The pathology of epiglottitis is familiar to otolaryngologists. The classic finding is a cherry-red epiglottis which is swollen and boggy. But the point to emphasize is that there is also involvement of the aryepiglottic folds and perhaps also the false cords.

Table 3 summarizes several papers.[1-4] In all cases, fever and respiratory distress were present; but sore throat was only noted in 60%, perhaps because of the young age of some patients; dysphagia and stridor were found in only about 50%;

TABLE 2. AGENTS OTHER THAN *H INFLUENZAE* ASSOCIATED WITH EPIGLOTTITIS

Children
S pneumoniae
S aureus
H paraprophilus
Adults
H parainfluenzae
S pneumoniae

From the Division of Infectious Diseases, Department of Pediatrics, Center for the Health Sciences, UCLA School of Medicine, Los Angeles.

REPRINTS — James D. Cherry, MD, Dept. of Pediatrics, Div. of Infectious Diseases, UCLA School of Medicine, 22-442 MDCC, Los Angeles, CA 90024.

TABLE 3. SYMPTOMS AND SIGNS OF ACUTE EPIGLOTTITIS

Symptoms	
Fever	100%
Respiratory distress	100%
Sore throat	60%
Dysphagia	60%
Stridor	50%
Irritability/restlessness	50%
Drooling	40%
Cough (often barking)	35%
Hoarseness/aphonia	25%
Signs	
Cyanosis	25%
Retractions	20%

irritability, restlessness and drooling in even less. What I want to emphasize, however, is that in about 33% of the cases a barking cough was noted, leading to some difficulty in diagnosis. Maybe all these cases were not epiglottitis, or perhaps in some cases in addition to involvement of the epiglottis, there was some subglottic involvement as well.

In the literature, there is a great deal of discussion regarding diagnosis, much of which is confusing. But the clinical picture of most children with epiglottitis should be diagnostic from 20 feet away. In epiglottitis you will not find a child lying down. He or she will sit up, frequently in tripod fashion with the arms and head back, the mouth open and the jaw protruding. If the child is anxious and having difficulty getting air, this behavior is about all you need for the diagnosis; you proceed immediately to therapy.

The question is often asked, in the child who is not in particularly severe distress, is it safe to look at the epiglottis? I think the answer is yes, provided that the child is not forced to lie down. Some time ago, I reviewed cases that did get in trouble and had cardiorespiratory arrest. In every instance, the children were forced to lie down.

Another aspect of diagnosis is the use of the lateral neck x-ray. Most of the time this is a useless test. If you can make the diagnosis from 20 feet away, go on to therapy. I am personally aware of several patients who died in the x-ray department, never having received therapy. Although there are some situations where an x-ray helps, in the majority of clear-cut cases of epiglottitis, x-ray need not and probably should not be obtained.

The studies which should be done are blood culture and culture of the epiglottis at the time of the therapeutic surgical procedure. A white count can be helpful; the majority demonstrate a shift to the left with counts over 15,000/mm^3.

The primary aspect of treatment is not the use of antibiotics, but the establishment of an airway. In the past most of us felt that tracheostomy was the procedure of choice. Hospital services that have a planned team approach to management of children with epiglottitis have consistently better results than services in which the approach to epiglottitis has not been organized in advance.

Recently published studies have recommended the more frequent use of endotracheal intubation as satisfactory therapy for epiglottitis.[4] Cantrell and Bell recently reviewed approximately 800 cases.[5] In that group, those who got tracheostomy had about a 0.9% mortality rate, and those who had endotracheal intubation had a similar mortality rate. The important point to emphasize, though, is that in those who had no intubation or tracheostomy, the mortality rate was 6%. Therefore, I do not believe there is any place for conservative therapy in this illness.

Initial antibiotic therapy for epiglottitis must take into consideration the fact that a significant number of strains of *H influenzae* are resistant to ampicillin and an occasional strain has been found to be resistant to chloramphenicol. All patients should receive both ampicillin (300 mg/kg/day q4h) and chloramphenicol (100 mg/kg/day q6h) by the intravenous route.

LARYNGOTRACHEITIS AND SPASMODIC CROUP

Laryngotracheitis and spasmodic croup are distinctive viral illnesses that differ considerably from epiglottitis.

Laryngotracheitis. Three viruses are most important in this illness. The most common cause of laryngotracheitis is parainfluenza 1 virus and the second most common cause is parainfluenza type 2. Influenza A is important because it causes particularly severe croup. The age prevalence ranges from six months to three years and is generally younger than that for epiglottitis. Generally the causative viruses are prevalent in the winter and spring. The onset of illness is gradual and builds up, usually over a two-day period, initially with upper respiratory infection (URI) and then progressing to gradual inspiratory stridor, hoarseness and the typical croupy, barking, seal-like cough and mild to moderate fever. The duration of illness is three to seven days.

The child with laryngotracheitis will not be disturbed by lying down, which is quite different from the patient with epiglottitis. This is important because a child with acute laryngotracheitis can have retractions to the extent that the xiphoid looks like it is hitting the vertebral column, and yet not be in particularly great distress.

Spasmodic Croup. Spasmodic croup is an illness that occurs in children who are otherwise well and frequently have had a mild URI, with normal temperature. The onset is always at night. It comes on suddenly, with hoarseness, stridor, and barking cough. If untreated, there will be repeated episodes the same night and perhaps the next night. There is a strong family history either in siblings or in the parents. The illness is apparently due to laryngeal spasm. When the subglottic area is looked at there is no evidence of exudate or any damage to the epithelium. This is in contrast to acute laryngotracheitis, where there is severe destruction of the ciliated epithelium, inflammatory exudate and edema. There is a marked difference in pathogenesis and pathology in this illness compared to laryngotracheitis. The major component of therapy consists of taking the child from the bedroom into the bathroom and turning on the shower. This usually does the trick. Mild sedation will prevent further attacks.

Therapy of Laryngotracheitis. In therapy for acute laryngotracheitis, the mainstay is moist air. Moist air will clearly reach the subglottic level and will liquify secretions and help remove desquamated ciliated epithelial cells. If you do blood gas studies, most patients with acute laryngotracheitis will be found to be mildly hypoxic even if they do not appear so, so that oxygen is reasonable to give, along with the moist air. Fluids for hydration are important, as they also will help liquify secretions. A single dose of paraldehyde or phenobarbital in certain children when they first come in may help allay their fears and prevent a tracheostomy.

The use of steroids I thought was obsolete, but a recent report[6] suggested that they have some benefit. However, the number of cases and the period of observation in the study leads me to question whether steroids do any good at all in this particular illness. On the other hand, I don't think there is any evidence that steroids have done any particular harm.

The newest addition to therapy is the use of aerosols and particularly racemic epinephrine by IPPB. This method was studied in Utah first.[7] Some 400 consecutive patients received this therapy, and recovered without tracheostomy or other difficulty. In a St. Louis study, we found we could do just as well with aerosolized saline.[8] Looking back both at the Utah data and our own, I think spasmodic croup was not ruled out very carefully. In Denver a racemic epinephrine study was conducted and fortunately very good viral studies were done, confirming the presence of severe croup due to parainfluenza viruses in most of their cases.[9] Their patients did show a transitory benefit which was clearly related to racemic epinephrine as compared to the administration of saline alone. So, perhaps in some instances racemic epinephrine will tide a patient over a critical period until the other aspects of therapy can become effective.

Laryngotracheobronchitis. In Table 1 laryngotracheobronchitis has been omitted. This was done intentionally because it has been my past impression that this entity rarely occurs. But recently two things have caused me to reconsider. First, I went over the literature very carefully, and second, I went through the records for two years at Cardinal Glennon Memorial Hospital for Children in St. Louis. I discovered that things were not as clear as I have tried to make them in this presentation.[10] The St. Louis chart review data indicated that in many cases the physician had difficulty in differentiating epiglottitis from laryngotracheitis, and many cases of croup in addition had lower respiratory complaints. There were many patients with signs of subglottic distress who had elevated white counts with a shift to the left in which the physician on examination saw a red epiglottis that was not swollen. Cultures in these cases often revealed *H influenzae* and other pathogens in the blood as well as in high concentrations in subglottic region.

In reviewing the literature from 1920 to 1940, I found there was another disease, bacterial croup, which was not epiglottitis. Those patients frequently started out with acute laryngotracheitis, probably a viral disease, but had superimposed infection with either the group A *Streptococcus* and/or *S aureus* and *Hemophilus*. Very recently, a paper from Utah with eight cases had reconfirmed this.[11] They reported *S aureus* in six patients and *Hemophilus* and group A *Streptococcus* in the other two.

H INFLUENZAE CELLULITIS

I also want to discuss briefly *H influenzae* cellulitis. This cellulitis can occur anywhere in the body, but the primary site of infection is respiratory. There is some question about how it gets to other sites, but it seems to be hematogenous in nonfacial lesions. The buccal surface is a common site of *H influenzae* cellulitis. Nelson and Ginsburg have suggested that this surface infection is secondary to otitis media and lymphatic spread.[12] My own feeling is that it is more likely due to trauma and direct local invasion by the organism.

In most cases the main lesions are on the face with buccal orbital or periorbital involvement. Most cases with periorbital involvement have maxillary and/or ethmoidal sinusitis. Characteristically, the majority of cases occur from age 6 months to 24 months. The period prior to seeking medical attention is very short, less than two days. The temperature is greater than 39.4 C in 70% of the cases. The major location is the cheek in 59% and the orbit in 22%; the other locations are systemic sites. A bluish color of the cellulitis is noted in about half of the cases, particularly those with buccal involvement. The white count is greater than 20,000 cells/mm^3 in 67% of the cases. Cultures of the blood are positive in 74%, and response to therapy is very rapid so that 67% of the cases are afebrile in 24 hours.

In nonfacial cellulitis, *H influenzae* generally accounts for a relatively small percentage of the cases;

S aureus is much more common, and group A streptococci and pneumococci are second and third in prevalence. But in facial lesions a much greater percentage are due to *H influenzae*.

When you are dealing with facial lesions in children, a culture from the anterior nasal fossa is very useful in detecting *H influenzae*, the pneumococcus and the group A *Streptococcus*, because these organisms are not part of the nasal flora. If these organisms are in the anterior nose, it means that there is a treatable infection present; the presence of *H influenzae* correlates very nicely with cellulitis. A throat culture is not very useful, but blood studies are.

In aspirating a local lesion you do not need fluctuance as an indication to insert a needle. Many people have recommended entering the edge of the lesion. But I don't really think that that is important. Going in just slightly tangentially, injecting 0.1 ml of saline (being sure that it is a nonbacteriostatic preparation), the cultures are quite likely to be positive.

The therapy of facial cellulitis depends on the clinical status of the particular patient. In the average patient with cellulitis, our main therapy in the past has been ampicillin or amoxicillin; in patients who are toxic, the systemic administration of ampicillin and chloramphenicol is recommended. We need to be sure that a particular lesion is not due to *S aureus*. That is why it is so important to do the needle aspiration and perform both a smear and culture. When we have a severely ill patient in which we cannot definitely rule out staphylococcal disease, we need to include staphylococcal coverage by using oxacillin and chloramphenicol.

SUMMARY

Let me conclude by reminding you first that epiglottitis is one of the real pediatric emergencies. Proper therapy (mechanical management first and antibiotics second) make the difference between life and death. Secondly, we can say that *H influenzae* cellulitis responds very rapidly and dramatically to proper antibiotic therapy.

REFERENCES

1. Berenberg W, Kevy S. Acute epiglottitis in childhood: a serious emergency, readily recognized at the bedside. N Engl J Med 1958; 258:870-4.

2. Bass JW, Steele RW, Wiebe RA. Acute epiglottitis: a surgical emergency. JAMA 1974; 229:671-5.

3. Johnson GK, Sullivan JL, Bishop LA. Acute epiglottitis. Review of 55 cases and suggested protocol. Arch Otolaryngol 1974; 100:333-7.

4. Battaglia JD, Lockhart CH. Management of acute epiglottitis by nasotracheal intubation. Am J Dis Child 1975; 129:334-6.

5. Cantrell RW, Bell RA, Morioka WT. Acute epiglottitis: intubation versus tracheostomy. Laryngoscope 1978; 138:994-1005.

6. Leipzig B, Oski FA, Cummings CW, Stockman FA, Swender P. A prospective randomized study to determine the efficacy of steroids in treatment of croup. J Pediatr 1979; 94:194-6.

7. Adair JC, Ring WH, Jordan WS, Elwyn RA. Ten-year experience with IPPB in the treatment of acute laryngotracheobronchitis. Anesth Analg 1971; 50:649-55.

8. Gardner HG, Powell KR, Roden VJ, Cherry JD. The evaluation of racemic epinephrine in the treatment of infectious croup. Pediatrics 1973; 52:68-71.

9. Westley CR, Cotton EK, Brooks JG. Nebulized racemic epinephrine by IPPB for the treatment of croup. Am J Dis Child 1978; 132:484-7.

10. Cherry JD. The treatment of croup: continued controversy due to failure of recognition of historic, ecologic, etiologic and clinical perspectives. J Pediatr 1979; 94:352-4.

11. Jones R, Santos JI, Overall JC Jr. Bacterial tracheitis. JAMA 1979; 242:721-6.

12. Nelson JD, Ginsburg CM. An hypothesis on the pathogenesis of Hemophilus influenzae buccal cellulitis. J Pediatr 1976; 88:709-10.

PANEL DISCUSSION

DR. BLUESTONE (Moderator): Dr. Cherry, you stated that in acute epiglottitis, which is almost invariably caused by type B *H influenzae*, the treatment of choice is chloramphenicol and ampicillin. I think this is right out of the Red Book from the American Academy of Pediatrics. Should we give both antibiotics initially, or should we wait until the blood culture comes back to see if the organism is sensitive to ampicillin? Should we use chloramphenicol and ampicillin for the entire course of the treatment? If the organism is not sensitive to ampicillin, should we stop the ampicillin? Are there any other antimicrobials that might be indicated?

DR. CHERRY: I should have emphasized that with proper therapy in epiglottitis rapid improvement is seen, so that a total duration of seven days of antibiotic is all that is usually necessary. The odds on the organism being resistant to both chloramphenicol and ampicillin are virtually zero. My own preference is chloramphenicol if the organism is sensitive to it. Therefore I would discontinue ampicillin once I knew the organism was sensitive to chloramphenicol. You only need to give one antibiotic or the other. If the organism is sensitive to ampicillin, many infectious diseases experts would discontinue the chloramphenicol.

DR. BLUESTONE: Would you stop the chloramphenicol as soon as you receive laboratory confirmation that the organism is not resistant to ampicillin?

DR. CHERRY: As I said, I prefer chloramphenicol to ampicillin, but either drug can be stopped once sensitivity of the organism to the drug to be continued has been demonstrated.

DR. BLUESTONE: There was an article this month on ampicillin-resistant organisms in epiglottitis being treated with very large doses of ampicillin. Do you think there is any place for this type of therapy?

DR. CHERRY: In general, I don't think that is the right approach to the problem. For epiglottitis I would use chloramphenicol. Whenever you start using drugs for organisms with high minimum inhibitory concentrations (MIC), you are bound to have difficulty. This is true for *Staphylococcus* where you have MICs in the 3 μg/ml range, and for *Hemophilus* with high MICs. Using ampicillin would not make sense to me if another drug is available.

DR. SCHRAMM: I would like to ask for an opinion regarding the efficacy of doing aspirations of areas involved with cellulitis. It has been my experience based on a review of 40 children who had orbital cellulitis that there is little correlation between blood cultures and, in this particular example, lid aspirates. In fact, 70% of this group had positive blood cultures but only two had the same organism isolated from the lid aspirant. There were, however, frequently organisms other than *H influenzae* or *S pneumoniae* cultured.

DR. BLUESTONE: Dr. Schramm is questioning the efficacy of needle aspiration. I think he has reference to false negative aspirants. This is precisely one of the reasons that we are here today, since there are some otolaryngologists who feel that aspiration is not indicated or that it has not been satisfactory. Where the technique has been used routinely the needle aspiration may be very effective in helping us arrive at the proper diagnosis.

DR. SHURIN: Dr. Cherry has reviewed the current recommendations as to the use of ampicillin and chloramphenicol for the treatment of *H influenzae* type B infections, and I think there are two issues that we should raise here. One is that although this has not yet been a problem, we may in the near future see multiple drug-resistant strains of this organism, so we need to anticipate what therapy would be useful. The more immediate concern is that in our area, many physicians have begun using other drugs, particularly the newer cephalosporins such as cefamandole. The published literature is not yet complete enough to support this change in routine therapy of *H influenzae* type B infections. I am speaking with the exception, of course, of meningitis. I want to ask Dr. Cherry what his view of the current state of these drugs is; and if he shares mine, what studies should we be doing to confirm or deny the place of such drugs in these infections?

DR. CHERRY: Our experience with ampicillin in *H influenzae* cellulitis and periorbital cellulitis has been good. The only failure I have ever seen in *H influenzae* periorbital cellulitis was a patient we treated initially with cefazolin. His fever came down in 24 hours and his cellulitis improved dramatically. We then switched to cephalexin, and he had a return of symptoms. When we looked at the sensitivity of the organism the result was predictable: the MIC of cephalexin for the organism was 5 μg/ml.

FLOOR COMMENT: I have always been very reluctant to use chloramphenicol initially for epiglottitis, because I have never seen or spoken to anyone who has seen a patient who has subsequently developed meningitis. I would be very interested if anyone has had a clinical situation where he really was obliged to use chloramphenicol first because of meningitis.

It was mentioned that certain antibiotics will impair the T-cell ability to recognize an invading microorganism and thus impair the immunological response. This is certainly something which is repeated in the literature, particularly in regard to otitis media. It has been suggested by some that one delay antibiotics for two to five days in order to get an established T-cell response. Investigators I have asked feel that the T-cells should be able to recognize an organism promptly, rather than taking five or six days.

DR. BLUESTONE: Dr. Cherry, why are you giving chloramphenicol? Is it to prevent meningitis?

DR. CHERRY: No, I hope I did not give that impression. We use ampicillin and chloramphenicol in life-threatening *Hemophilus* infections; one of those is meningitis and the other is epiglottitis. One reported patient who, I believe, had epiglottitis, did get ampicillin but failed, and went on to die of septicemia.

FLOOR COMMENT: There is no question about the resistance to ampicillin; in fact, we are now running 5 to 10% resistance rates. Has anyone had the experience in a patient with epiglottitis where it was not the airway that was the problem, but the meningitis? In my personal experience, with airway problems you have all the time you need to get your cultures back. Moreover, having had the experience of a death from chloramphenicol, I am gun-shy.

DR. CHERRY: I am also aware of one death in spite of a satisfactory airway in a patient who got ampicillin. I think his death was due to septicemia.

DR. NEU: I know of a child with epiglottitis with a resistant strain of *H influenzae* who died in New York City with septicemia. So it does occur.

There is a misconception. I don't believe that there is a clearly established case in the world literature of a patient who died following the use of chloramphenicol intravenously. There are two patients described in the literature, one following the use of eye drops, another following oral therapy, but other than these two cases which are questionable, there are no cases of aplastic anemia following intravenous chloramphenicol. There has not been one case seen in the last decade and a half following intravenous use.

FLOOR COMMENT: That of course is what is commonly stated; it is said in the textbooks that aplastic anemia does not occur after parenteral chloramphenicol. However, in the latest information letter by Parke-Davis Co. they recommend that the patient be given an oral chloramphenicol as soon as feasible. I cannot believe that any drug company would make a recommendation like that while the scientific literature is saying that the only way we can get aplastic anemia is to give a patient an oral medication. Maybe they know something we don't.

DR. KLEIN: I think that this is a very important issue to clarify. We reviewed the literature at the time that the American Academy of Pediatrics Committee on Infectious Disease made its recommendation regarding ampicillin-resistant strains. There are five cases reported since the drug was introduced in 1954 where parenteral chloramphenicol alone was used and aplastic anemia followed.[1-4] Of the five cases, three had another possible etiology for the aplastic process. It is very difficult to know how much parenteral chloramphenicol alone (without oral chloramphenicol) has been used over the years. But even if you took a very conservative figure of 50,000 to 100,000 courses per year in a 25-year period, the data suggest a record of safety rather than a liability for the parenteral drug. And we are talking about use of parenteral chloramphenicol for potentially life-threatening disease.

The Parke-Davis drug recommendation in terms of oral use is a very separate issue. The drug is used extensively in an oral form in many parts of the world as an over-the-counter product. We really have no idea of the number of courses of oral drug administered. The best information suggests that aplastic anemia occurs in 1 case per 20,000 courses. Thus, the parenteral appears to be a safe product whereas the oral form has a limited but definite potential for causing aplastic anemia.

DR. BLUESTONE: If you do find that the organism is sensitive to ampicillin, do you think it is worthwhile to continue the chloramphenicol, or should we give the ampicillin?

DR. KLEIN: That is a judgment issue, because if only the parenteral drug is used, then the concern for its usage in terms of the aplastic process is very limited; and what happens subsequently (when you know there is a sensitive strain) is of relatively limited importance. My choice would be to change to ampicillin, but I would have no argument with those who wanted to continue the parenteral chloramphenicol.

DR. BLUESTONE: Would the panel like to discuss anything further related to the antimicrobial treatment of epiglottitis?

DR. GINSBURG: I don't think that under any circumstances that cefamandole is an alternative for chloramphenicol in a condition such as buccal cellulitis. Our experience has been that approximately 10% of children with buccal cellulitis have an associated meningitis and some may not have a CSF

1. Domart A, Hazard J, Husson R. Fatal bone marrow aplasia after intramuscular chloramphenicol administration in two adults. Sem Hop Paris 1961; 37:2256-8.

2. Grilliat J-P, Streiff F, Hua G. Fatal cytopenia after chloramphenicol hemisuccinate therapy. Ann Med Nancy 1966; 5:754-62.

3. Restrepo MA, Zambrano F. II. Late-onset aplastic anemia secondary to chloramphenicol. Report of ten cases. Antioquia Medica 1968; 18: 593-606.

4. Wallerstein RO, Condit PK, Kasper CK, et al. Statewide study of chloramphenicol therapy and fatal aplastic anemia. JAMA 1969; 208: 2045-50.

pleocytosis, initially. I think that chloramphenicol is the initial drug of choice.

FLOOR QUESTION: First, in the preoperative preparation of the head and neck cancer patient, does Betadine® gargle or something similar have any usefulness? Secondly, do topical agents have any usefulness in clearing the draining tympanostomy tube problem?

DR. HERZON: I am unaware of any data in the nasal surgery field which suggests that the topical preparation of mucosal surfaces had any statistical effect in reducing postoperative wound infections, all other things being equal.

FLOOR COMMENT: At the ACS Surgical Forum last fall, there was a report of a study that showed a marked decrease in the number of bacteria as well as subsequent wound infection where GI surgery was performed after the area to be resected had been clamped and then treated with Betadine. We can extrapolate, perhaps, from that and say that in some areas it has been shown that preoperative topical exposure with an antiseptic agent will have some positive effects.

DR. HERZON: I did a study once on nasal packs and the incidence of bacterial infection. I compared the effectiveness of topical antibiotics on the gauze on one side with no medication on the other side; there was an advantage to the antibiotic-impregnated gauze. However, whether or not it will truly decrease the number of bacteria in head and neck cancer where there are so many other facets involved, I don't know.

In answer to the second question, I did not examine the question of the drops. They were given in a totally arbitrary fashion; one day they were given and another day they were not. To the best of my knowledge, drops had no effect on the course of any of those tube infections. I am not sure how one can put drops through a 2 mm lumen anyway.

DR. BLUESTONE: You stated that the biggest problem in infectious disease was the tympanostomy tube and the otorrhea that occurred following its insertion. How do you get a culture of the middle ear when a tympanostomy tube is in place, and how do you know if what you find from the culture is causing the infection?

DR. HERZON: In four of the serious infections presented previously, the tubes were removed from the middle ear at surgery and cultures were taken from the middle ear space. Two sets of instruments with traps were used, as was described previously. Any attempt to culture directly from the tympanostomy tube in a 2- to 3-year-old patient is going to be difficult except under a general anesthetic.

DR. BLUESTONE: When you used two sets of instruments, did you culture the ear canal first?

DR. HERZON: No.

DR. BLUESTONE: We try to get an external canal culture first. You can do it in a 2- or 3-year-old by wrapping or restraining the child before taking the canal culture. Then with a blunt-nose needle with a Senturia trap, we aspirate the middle ear contents. This is effective when you have a draining ear through a tympanostomy tube or for that matter through a perforation (which we will discuss this afternoon). Admittedly this is not the best of techniques, because we are dealing with a contaminated area. This was discussed to some extent this morning. It was said that there were anaerobes in the middle ear effusions but no external canal cultures were obtained. Therefore the anaerobic organisms found in the middle ear effusion were probably contaminants from the external canal. I think the same problem exists when there is drainage through a tympanostomy tube. You must culture the external canal and then assess what is found in the middle ear, but it is difficult, admittedly.

FLOOR QUESTION: Dr. Herzon, how do you prepare your surgical field before inserting tympanostomy tubes?

DR. HERZON: I don't.

DR. BLUESTONE: If we have established the idea that there are potential pathogens in the external ear canal, then why do we not use aseptic surgical techniques in preparing our operative field for tympanostomy tubes?

DR. HERZON: First, the incidence of serious infections is extremely small. Secondly, there is the question of time in the operating room. Now the data may suggest that you should use general surgery principles in preparing the operative field for tympanostomy, but obviously a controlled study should be done. I should like to review the incidence of otorrhea after insertion of posttympanostomy tubes. Dr. Bluestone reported a 68% incidence in cleft palate patients. Another study from the Scandinavian countries reported a 25% incidence of otorrhea, most of which occurred some time after insertion. In other words, failure to prepare the canal has nothing whatsoever to do with infections that occur three and four months later. It is a very small percentage, so I am not sure it is worth it.

DR. BLUESTONE: You mean that these ears begin to drain after a quiescent period?

DR. HERZON: Yes, in fact there were only 11 draining ears in the whole study that occurred immediately postoperatively.

FLOOR COMMENT: I think you are talking about two different things: there are draining tubes, and then there are tubes that drain; and my clinical experience is that tubes that drain respond very nicely to topical application of a medication. Now, draining tubes might not. There is a child who has tubes inserted and is bad with them but worse without them; he has only a draining ear with the tube in.

But if you take a child who reacts to tubes, he gets an immediate postoperative infection. I cannot allow that. In my clinical experience, such patients respond to topical instillation of ear drops. Sometimes the parents may not get the drops in but if I bring the patient into the office, and suction out the ear and blow in the drops, I uniformly hear that within about two days the drainage is gone.

DR. NEU: Pharmacologically there may be an explantion why the drops work. When the physician instills drops, it is not actually the same as when the parent does. When you remove all the debris, you eliminate a significant amount of calcium, magnesium and other material which inactivates the polymyxin B or the polymyxin E, that is, the colistimethate. With these drugs you can get *Pseudomonas* and other Gram-negatives to grow by just dropping in some calcium or magnesium. Indeed, if you could maybe wash the ear with a 10^{-3} or 10^{-4} molar solution of ethylene diaminetetraacetic acid (EDTA) initially, which would not damage the tissue but chelates the debris, and then use polymyxin, it would be much more efficacious.

DR. BLUESTONE: Dr. Finegold, what is the significance of anaerobes being cultured from the sinuses and middle ears? There was some discussion recently as to whether anaerobes are really present in acute or chronic otitis media with effusion.

DR. FINEGOLD: We have to examine the question in perspective. Regardless of the type of organism, aerobic or anaerobic, one must decide on clinical grounds and other information available what the significance of the isolate is. This is particularly true in many head and neck infections where mixed infections occur very commonly, often involving six or seven organisms. Does one have to treat for all of these organisms? I would say in general, no. The majority of the organisms in head and neck infection, as you have seen from the data presented, are susceptible to cell-wall-active agents such as penicillins and cephalosporins. The major exceptions would be *S aureus* and Gram-negative facultative bacilli, neither of which are commonly encountered unless a patient has received prior antimicrobial therapy.

It is clear that the anaerobes are really present, but it is somewhat difficult to establish their significance in mixed infections of this sort. One cannot depend on Koch's postulates, as we typically have done in the past. There is evidence that the anaerobes are important, and, in selected cases, if one fails to take them into account in designing antimicrobial therapy, the patient will not respond until an appropriate agent is added. In general I would say that penicillins and cephalosporins represent valuable agents in this group of infections.

FLOOR QUESTION: In the prophylaxis study, if you had a group like you described, would penicillin have worked as well as a cephalosporin?

DR. FINEGOLD: To a large extent it would have, but a certain number of the infections did involve *S aureus*, and those particular ones would not have responded. But for the other types of organisms, penicillin would have been a good choice.

DR. NEU: I was surprised that you had so few *Klebsiella* considering a VA population. Data like that of Drs. Fuxench-Lopez and Ramirez-Ronda and several other groups have shown the heavy colonization of *Klebsiella* in the patient with alcoholism. I always associate alcoholism with nasopharyngeal carcinomas and similar diseases. Have you not seen that heavy concentration of *Klebsiella* in such patients?

DR. FINEGOLD: As a matter of fact, *Klebsiella pneumoniae* is the major nosocomial pathogen at Wadsworth, and I cannot imagine why in our VA population, where alcoholism is so widespread, we did not see more.

DR BLUESTONE: Dr. Klein, I know you have some new data from Boston about anaerobic organisms in otitis media with effusion. Would you share that with us?

DR. KLEIN: The data are that of Drs. Teele, Healy, and Tally.[5] They found no isolates of anaerobic organisms in persistent middle ear effusions of 30 children (51 ears) who came for insertion of ventilating tubes or a myringotomy. Cultures of the surface of the tympanic membrane also failed to yield anaerobic bacteria.

This is a new technology, a new area of investigation. The reader must look very carefully at the materials and methods and be certain that the investigator is appropriately cleansing the external canal before aspirating material from the middle ear, so that there is a clear distinction between the organisms obtained from that fluid and organisms that might have been contaminants from the external canal.

These data will no doubt be refined as the technology extends from Dr. Finegold's laboratory to other laboratories, and more studies are performed. Right now the data are quite mixed, and the more recent studies of both acute otitis media and chronic otitis media from different laboratories seem to show a very limited incidence of anaerobic organisms.

Dr. Finegold's point was very well taken, that in acute otitis media the data seem to show very few anaerobes while in chronic otitis media there is a discrepancy. The more recent studies from Boston[5] show no anaerobic organisms, whereas the study done in Los Angeles[6] showed a very significant proportion of anaerobic bacteria.

5. Teele DW, Healy GB, Tally FP. Persistent middle ear effusions in young children; cultures for anaerobic bacteria. Ann Otol Rhinol Laryngol 1980; 89 Suppl 68:102-3.

6. Brook I, Anthony BF, Finegold SM. Aerobic and anaerobic bacteriology of acute otitis media in children. J Pediatr 1978; 92:13-5.

FLOOR QUESTION: Dr. Neu, you were talking about carbenicillin and gentamicin in the treatment of severe external otitis. Were those two agents for systemic *Pseudomonas* infection?

DR. NEU: I think that they are very useful in the systemic treatment of those conditions. We have switched over pretty much to using ticarcillin, because it is slightly more active and effective in lower doses. Many of these people are older and have the problem of congestive heart failure. We also have tended to use tobramycin. The studies from our own group, at least, comparing the ticarcillin-tobramycin regimen versus carbenicillin-gentamicin have shown a greater degree of synergy. Usually, because of the length of time that you have to treat the patient, you probably have less chance of nephrotoxicity. There is a lower degree of ototoxicity, probably, with tobramycin than with gentamicin.

DR. FINEGOLD: I think that there basically is very little difference between gentamicin-tobramycin and carbenicillin-ticarcillin; therefore, it probably does not make a great deal of difference which one you use. There are certain situations in which one might be preferable. Tobramycin, I think, does have somewhat better activity against *Pseudomonas*; on the other hand, gentamicin has somewhat better activity against *Klebsiella*. Ticarcillin also has an advantage in terms of the sodium load.

FLOOR QUESTION: In diabetic people with external infections, what would you use as your drug of choice? They are usually infected with Gram-negative bacilli.

DR. BLUESTONE: First of all, are you satisfied with the terminology? I know that you did not use the term malignant otitis media. Dr. Neu, would you like to clarify the terminology for us who are in otolaryngology?

DR. NEU: I do not think that the condition is an otitis. I think it is really a disease of the mastoid bone, a mastoiditis, that has caused pressure and involved the lining of the brain in most of the cases. We now have treated about 15 people with the disease, so we have a fairly good experience. We have used most of the aminoglycosides and most of the semisynthetic penicillins.

There are several things that are important. One is regulation of the diabetes. In somebody who is going to have to receive 30-40 g carbenicillin or 18-24 g ticarcillin and a great deal of either gentamicin or tobramycin, you really cannot use an indwelling intravenous catheter for extended periods. We have gone to these heparin-lock IV devices so that we do not have to have a glucose "keep open" situation which tends to throw off the diabetes. We have made a major attempt to have the diabetologist, otolaryngologist, and dietician work with us on these patients, to make sure that we can get the diabetes in good control.

It has been our experience initially that some otolaryngologists use the same instruments throughout the whole operative procedure; we now ask them to have two sets of instruments. For culture purposes we would like to have bone that they remove from the inner part of the ear. One of my Fellows picks up the specimens in the OR during the procedure. We request that the first bone specimen not have been in contact with the initial skin incision; and we ask that a last specimen be an inner piece of bone that is obtained by chipping, so that we may determine if it is indeed *Pseudomonas*. If it is an anaerobe, we take the specimens to the laboratory immediately and they are immediately ground with the glass pestle and handled aerobically and anaerobically. On occasion we have found anaerobes, but that is not a problem, obviously, if you are using carbenicillin or ticarcillin, since they have a fair degree of anaerobic activity. But you would like to be sure that they would be active against those organisms. The other problem is that treatment must extend for a six-week period.

I think the concern about the aminoglycosides causing ototoxicity to the contralateral good ear or damaging the kidney has resulted often in underdosing and so we follow the blood level, and we very carefully do creatinine clearances, usually at six-hour intervals. I realize that you cannot get a 24-hour creatinine clearance in a patient who does not have an indwelling urethral catheter. We do a partial clearance, and we also calculate on the basis of age and body weight. Because of these things, our success in the last four or five patients has been excellent.

DR. BLUESTONE: I would like to ask Dr. Neu to review the bacteriology in the cases where he had an opportunity to get really good specimens. How many of them yielded *Pseudomonas* and how many of them yielded other kinds of organisms? What has been your overall mortality?

DR. NEU: The overall mortality in the total series runs about 30%. We have tended to see the patients quite early because of our interest in the disease, and maybe we are seeing a slightly different population. They are not older alcoholics, but they are diabetic. Most of them are fairly affluent.

We have been surprised at our microbiologic findings recently since we have been doing anaerobic cultures: there are, in addition to the *Pseudomonas*, anaerobes as well. We have cultured *B fragilis*, *Fusobacterium*, peptococci and other organisms, when my Fellow has been present during the operative procedure to take the specimen to the lab immediately; unless someone immediately processes the culture, they are missed. A patient with necrotizing external otitis is always done as the last case of the day because it is a dirty case and the specimens frequently never get to the laboratory. Therefore, I do not know what the original bacteriology was in such cases. We always grew the *Pseudomonas* because they are there. Now there is some question in my mind whether *Pseudomonas* is the only pathogen.

DR. BLUESTONE: So we should name the disease *necrotizing external otitis* or *mastoiditis* or *necrotizing osteomyelitis* of the temporal bone and possibly base of the skull.

FLOOR QUESTION: I noticed, Dr. Neu, that on your slide dealing with the sinuses you listed various antibiotics but you left out the erythromycins. Would you comment on the use of erythromycins for sinus infections?

DR. NEU: I think that erythromycin does provide good concentrations. The difficulty with erythromycin in the adult is the poor tolerance to the drug. There has been a real problem from its oral use in this kind of population: older individuals who have chronic disease and on whom mainly tetracyclines and the penicillins have been used.

DR. BLUESTONE: From the data that are presently available, is chemoprophylaxis effective in surgical cases like the routine stapedioplasty, tympanoplasty, tympanomastoidectomy, and following a rhinoplasty in which intranasal packing has been employed? There is much controversy in otolaryngology over whether we should use antimicrobial prophylaxis. Dr. Becker pointed out in his paper that he feels a cephalosporin is effective for preventing postoperative wound infections.

DR. KLEIN: I think there has been a marked change in the attitude toward chemoprophylaxis. Just a few years ago, apart from usage of penicillin G for patients who had rheumatic heart disease or for patients who had underlying heart disease at the time of procedures such as dental surgery, chemoprophylaxis was frowned upon. Now use of antimicrobial agents for prevention has many approved uses. This change has come because of the presentation of excellent double-blind studies demonstrating a difference in results in those patients who had short preoperative courses of prophylaxis.

I think the major criticism that I would have of the way prophylactic antimicrobial agents are used now by our surgeons is that they are extended far too long. What we are talking about is the use of the drug at the time of the infectious challenge. This requires a concentration of drug in the tissues at the time of operation and for a very brief period afterwards. I think that perhaps Dr. Becker might comment on this and whether even the extension of the drug for 24 hours is necessary.

DR. FINEGOLD: In general, I would agree. In situations where it is truly clean surgery and where there is no normal flora involved at the site of operation, prophylaxis is not indicated. I would emphasize the short duration of prophylaxis but also recommend that therapy be started just an hour or two prior to surgery, so that one does not have a chance to modify the flora and select out more resistant organisms.

DR. NEU: I feel fairly strongly that in much of the clean surgery performed, antibiotics are not indicated. In specific operations, their use is reasonable. I think that in the alcoholic patient with poor protoplasm who is debilitated and similar cases, it is probably very reasonable to administer antibiotics because of bad tissues. But I am not sure that someone needs antibiotics who lives on the 80th floor of an apartment overlooking Park Avenue and who is to have an ear operation.

DR. BECKER: Someone had mentioned that *Klebsiella* was seldom seen. This organism was our most common Gram-negative aerobe cultured preoperatively, as well as the common Gram-negative cultured in infected wounds. Secondly, as far as ear infection goes, Dr. Eugene Derlacki told me some years ago, I believe, that among some 17,000 ear cases he did not observe many infections. So why use prophylactic antibiotics? He thought there were some surgical procedures which were clearly benefited by the use of chemoprophylaxis, but other surgical procedures which clearly were not benefited. In the future, we will need to look at individual procedures as well as duration of antibiotic prophylaxis.

FLOOR QUESTION: Dr. Becker, your rate of fistula formation was quite high; higher than we see in Michigan. I just wondered if you have analyzed your statistics as to the training of residents who are doing the surgery, or the difficulty of the surgery? Can you explain your high rate of fistula formation?

DR. BECKER: No, I cannot. Most of our patients were alcoholic, malnourished, with poor dental hygiene, and had been radiated preoperatively. All the surgery was done by residents, and took longer than most private practitioners. Among other circumstances which could lead to this higher incidence is salivary leakage through an incontinent mucosal suture line after effective antibiotic tissue levels had ceased.

FLOOR QUESTION: Dr. Neu, you mentioned osteomyelitis in describing mastoiditis. I wondered if in the treatment of either acute or chronic mastoiditis, one needs the length of therapy used, six to eight weeks, for example, as in long bone infection. Do you have some suggestions on infections of the mastoid bone?

DR. NEU: I now treat those patients for six to eight weeks. I think that it is very important to get the exact microbiology if you possibly can, because it will give you an idea whether you might be able to use an oral agent. With some of those patients, particularly if the anaerobes are involved, you might be able to proceed with high concentrations of oral penicillin or with a drug like clindamycin or metronidazole.

If you truly have the Gram-negatives, which is what one encounters from the outside of tracts, particularly in those people who have been operated on several times, you usually will never be able to use oral therapy. The reason we follow this procedure is that we have had several patients come back to us with brain abscesses three or four months after getting a two-week course in the hospital. I view mastoiditis in the present era as just as severe a complication as it was prior to the development of the antibiotics.

MICROBIOLOGY AND ANTIMICROBIAL TREATMENT OF OTITIS MEDIA

JEROME O. KLEIN, MD
BOSTON, MASSACHUSETTS

Appropriate choice of antimicrobial agents for therapy of otitis media (OM) is based on an understanding of the microbiology of the acute and chronic diseases. The results of studies of bacteriology of OM are very similar: ***Streptococcus pneumoniae*** and ***Hemophilus influenzae*** are the most important pathogens; Gram-negative enteric bacilli are isolated from middle ear fluids (MEF) of approximately 20% of infants to 6 weeks of age; group A β-hemolytic ***Streptococcus*** and ***Staphylococcus aureus*** are infrequent causes of otitis. Preliminary results suggest that anaerobic bacteria are responsible for some episodes of OM. Viruses and mycoplasma are infrequently isolated from MEF but *Chlamydia trachomatis* appears to be a significant cause of OM in young infants. Recent studies of asymptomatic children with persistent MEF indicate that bacterial pathogens are present in some of these fluids. The significance of these results is uncertain, but they suggest that the persistent effusion may be a result of prolonged infection or may be an immune response to bacterial antigens. Based on the bacteriology, amoxicillin or ampicillin are the currently preferred drugs for initial treatment of otitis media. For the child who is allergic to penicillins, cefaclor or erythromycin combined with a sulfonamide or trimethoprim-sulfamethoxazole are satisfactory alternatives. The current incidence of ampicillin-resistant *H influenzae* responsible for OM is low but if the patient does not respond to initial therapy with ampicillin or amoxicillin, infection with a resistant strain of *H influenzae* should be considered and a change in therapy to include a sulfonamide, trimethoprim-sulfamethoxazole or cefaclor is appropriate.

Appropriate choice of antimicrobial agents for otitis media is based on an understanding of the microbiology of the acute and chronic diseases. The bacteriology of acute otitis media has been well documented, but only recently are data available about bacteria associated with the chronic disease. The purpose of this report is to review the results of microbiologic studies of acute and chronic middle ear infection, to review data about the in vitro activity and clinical and microbiologic efficacy of antimicrobial agents of value in otitis media, and to consider therapeutic plans for prophylaxis and treatment.

MICROBIOLOGY OF ACUTE OTITIS MEDIA

The microbiology of otitis media has been defined by culture of middle ear fluids obtained by needle aspiration. Many studies of the bacteriology of acute otitis media have been performed, and the results are remarkably consistent in demonstrating the importance of *Streptococcus pneumoniae* and *Hemophilus influenzae* as pathogens. Although epidemiologic evidence associates virus infection with otitis media, viruses are isolated infrequently from middle ear fluids. Similarly, *Mycoplasma* are seldom associated with otitis media. *Chlamydia* may be important in the etiology of otitis media in young infants.

Bacteria. Studies of the bacteriology of otitis media conducted in Sweden, Finland, and the United States all gave similar results[1] (Fig. 1). *S pneumoniae* is the most common agent in all age groups, and *H influenzae* is second in importance. Group A *Streptococcus* was the pathogen in a significant number of cases studied in Scandinavia, but this was not the case in the United States. *Staphylococcus aureus* and Gram-negative enteric bacilli are infrequent causes of acute otitis media in children and adults but are responsible for about 25% of cases in newborn infants. These bacteria may be the agents of infection in patients with chronic perforation of the tympanic membrane.

Because *S pneumoniae* is the most important cause of otitis media, investigators have carefully studied the types responsible for infections of the middle ear. The results of studies of approximately 2,000 children indicate that relatively few types are responsible for most disease.[2-4] The most common types in order of decreasing frequency are 19, 23, 6, 14, 3, 18, 4, 15, 9, 7, and 1 (Table 1). All are included in the currently available 14 type pneumococcal vaccines (Pneumovax®, Merck Sharp & Dohme; and Pnu-Immune®, Lederle Laboratories).

Most cases of otitis media due to *H influenzae* are attributable to nontypable strains. Type B strains are present in about 10% of cases of otitis media due to *H influenzae*. Children with infection due to type B *H influenzae* appear toxic, and about one quarter of these children have concomitant bacteremia or meningitis.[5] Until recently *H influenzae* appeared to be limited in importance to preschool children; however, new information indicates that this organism is a significant cause of otitis media in older children, adolescents, and adults.[1]

Group A β-hemolytic *Streptococcus* has been a significant pathogen in some studies from Scandi-

From the Departments of Pediatrics, Boston University School of Medicine and Boston City Hospital. This work was supported in part by the National Institute of Allergy and Infectious Diseases, Contract No. N01-A1-5235, and a grant from the Mancini Charitable Foundation.

REPRINTS — Jerome O. Klein, MD, Maxwell Finland Laboratory for Infectious Diseases, Boston City Hospital, Boston, MA 02118.

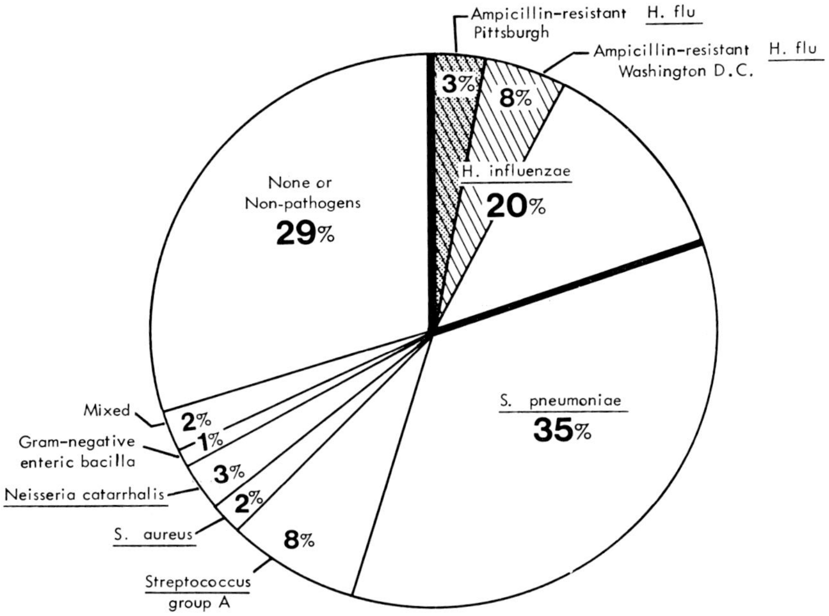

Fig. 1. Bacteriology of acute otitis media with effusion based on reports from centers in the United States, Finland and Sweden, 1953-1975, including 3,583 children. Incidence of ampicillin-resistant strains of *Hemophilus influenzae* are noted.[1] (From Klein JO. Management of acute and chronic otitis media. In: Remington JS, Swartz MN, eds. Current clinical topics in infectious diseases — 2. New York: McGraw-Hill, 1980. Adapted with permission.)

navia but has been less frequent in published reports from the United States.

Gram-negative enteric bacilli are responsible for about 20% of otitis media in young infants, but these organisms are rarely present in middle ear fluids (MEF) of older children with acute otitis media.[6-9] Other than the increase in otitis due to Gram-negative bacilli and the presence of other organisms responsible for neonatal sepsis such as group B *Streptococcus* and *S aureus*, the bacteriology of otitis in the infant to 6 weeks of age is similar to that in older children.

The role of *Branhamella* (formerly *Neisseria*) *catarrhalis* and coagulase-negative staphylococci in acute otitis media is uncertain. These organisms are considered commensals and are part of the skin flora of the external ear canal. But some investigators have reported isolation of pure cultures of *B catarrhalis*[10] or coagulase-negative staphylococci[11] from cases of purulent middle ear effusions after adequate cleansing of the external canal. Organisms are seen in Gram-stained material both free and engulfed by polymorphonuclear leukocytes. The findings suggest that in some cases, these bacteria may be responsible for suppurative otitis media.

TABLE 1. DISTRIBUTION OF SEROTYPES OF 1,837 STRAINS OF *S PNEUMONIAE* ISOLATED FROM MIDDLE EAR FLUIDS OF CHILDREN WITH ACUTE OTITIS MEDIA[2-4]

Serotype	*No. of Strains (%)*
*1**	38 (2.1)
3	157 (8.5)
4	63 (3.4)
6	220 (12.0)
7	43 (2.3)
8	28 (1.5)
9	54 (2.9)
10	27 (1.5)
11	34 (1.9)
14	189 (10.3)
15	59 (3.2)
18	106 (5.8)
19	423 (23.0)
22	32 (1.7)
23	230 (12.5)
35	20 (1.1)
Others†	114 (6.2)
% in 14 type vaccine	(84.7)

*Serotypes in 14 type vaccine italicized.

†Serotype (number) - *2* (1), 5 (4), *12* (6), 13 (2), 16 (17), 17 (12), 20 (5), 21 (5), 24 (6), *25* (0), 27 (1), 29 (3), 31 (11), 33 (17), 34 (4), 37 (1), 38 (10), 46 (1), 48 (1), nontypable (7).

Recent studies of Brook et al suggest that anaerobic bacteria may cause otitis media.[12] *Peptococcus*, an organism that colonizes the upper respiratory tract and may cause lower respiratory tract disease, and *Propionibacterium acnes*, a component of the normal skin flora, were the most frequently isolated anaerobic organisms. In some studies, the external canal was not cleansed prior to aspiration of the middle ear fluid; therefore, it is possible that the organisms isolated represent contaminants from the external canal rather than pathogens causing otitis media. In a study of children with persistent middle ear effusion, Teele et al used appropriate methods of cleansing the canal and failed to isolate anaerobic bacteria from the middle ear.[13]

Disparate results of bacterial cultures of middle ear fluid obtained by needle aspiration from children with bilateral otitis media have been reported by several investigators. In most cases culture of the effusion from one ear is sterile but a bacterial pathogen is isolated from the other ear. In some cases, a different bacterial pathogen is isolated from each of the two ears. Pelton et al[14] cultured middle ear fluid from both ears of 122 children with bilateral acute otitis media; disparate results were found in 27 (22%) of the children. These data indicate that investigative studies of the microbiology of bilateral

TABLE 2. ISOLATION OF VIRUSES IN PATIENTS WITH OTITIS MEDIA[16] (N = 663)*

Virus	No. of Patients
Respiratory syncytial virus	22
Influenza viruses	4
Coxsackievirus B4	1
Adenovirus 3	1
Parainfluenza 2	1
Totals	29 (4.4%)
No growth	634

*622 patients had acute and 41 had chronic otitis media.

otitis media must include aspiration of both ears to determine the efficacy of methods of treatment (ie, trials of antimicrobial agents) or prevention (ie, evaluation of vaccines or drugs).

Viruses. Epidemiologic data suggest that virus infection is sometimes associated with acute otitis media. In a longitudinal study of respiratory illnesses and complications in children six weeks to 11 years of age, Henderson and colleagues[15] demonstrated a correlation between isolation of viruses from the upper respiratory tract and the clinical diagnosis of otitis media. Outbreaks of viral infection coincided with epidemics of otitis media. In contrast to this epidemiologic association are the results of studies of fluid obtained for viral culture from middle ear effusions of children and adults with acute and chronic otitis media. Viruses were infrequently isolated from the middle ear effusions: a virus was isolated from only 29 (4.4%) of 663 fluids.[16] (Table 2) Respiratory syncytial virus and influenza virus were the most common isolates, and they were most likely to be present in middle ear fluid during periods of epidemic infection in the community. The low frequency of isolation of viruses from middle ear fluids does not support the belief that these agents play a direct role in the etiology of acute otitis media. However, it is possible that 1) viruses present early in the course of the disease were no longer present when the patients sought medical attention, 2) the viruses were present in low concentrations and were not readily isolated from the ear fluids, or 3) inhibitory material, such as antibody, interferon, or lysozyme, prevented successful isolation of the virus.

Mycoplasma. A report of a study with adult volunteers suggested a role for *Mycoplasma pneumoniae* in otitis media. Myringitis, associated with hemorrhage and bleb formation, was observed in nonimmune volunteers inoculated with this organism.[17] However, when specimens of the middle ear fluid of a large number (771) of patients were cultured for isolation of *M pneumoniae*, this organism was isolated from the fluid of only one patient.[16] Thus results of this study suggest that mycoplasmas do not play a significant role in the vast majority of cases of acute otitis media. Some cases of respiratory infection due to *M pneumoniae* are accompanied by inflammation of the tympanic membrane, either alone or in association with middle ear effusion.

Chlamydia. Chlamydia trachomatis causes a mild but prolonged pneumonitis in young infants. This organism has been isolated from middle ear fluids of some infants with pneumonitis.[18] Dawson and colleagues isolated *C trachomatis* from the middle ear fluid of a patient with inclusion cell conjunctivitis[19] and produced otitis in adults experimentally infected with the organism by the ocular route.[20] These studies suggest a significant role for *C trachomatis* as a cause of otitis media.

MICROBIOLOGY OF CHRONIC OTITIS MEDIA

The results of recent studies of the bacteriology of chronic otitis media with effusion suggest that the middle ear fluids of asymptomatic children with persistent effusion harbor bacterial pathogens. At the time of myringotomy or the placement of tympanostomy tubes, cultures of middle ear fluid revealed bacteria in about half of the children; *S pneumoniae, H influenzae*, and group A *Streptococcus* were isolated from 10 to 20% of these asymptomatic children. There were only minimal differences in the rates of isolation of bacteria from serous, mucoid, or purulent fluids.[21-23] The significance of this finding is, at present, uncertain. The bacteria may colonize the persistent fluid without producing pathologic changes, or the organisms may be responsible for a low-grade or subclinical infection that may be a factor in the development and persistence of the middle ear fluid.

MICROBIOLOGIC DIAGNOSIS

The correlation between bacterial cultures of the nasopharynx and the oropharynx and cultures of middle ear fluids is poor. Thus, cultures of the upper respiratory tract are of limited value in specific bacteriologic diagnosis of otitis media. In contrast, the consistent results of microbiologic studies of middle ear fluid of children with acute otitis media provide an accurate guide to the most likely pathogens. If the patient is toxic or has a localized infection elsewhere, culture of the blood and of the focus of infection should be performed.

Needle aspiration of middle ear effusion of patients with acute otitis media provides immediate and specific information about bacterial pathogens and should be considered in the following circumstances: if the patient is critically ill when first seen, if the patient fails to respond appropriately to initial therapy for acute otitis media, or if the patient has altered host defenses. The latter group includes the newborn infant and the patient with malignancy or immunologic disease since these patients may be infected with unusual agents.

MANAGEMENT OF ACUTE OTITIS MEDIA

In Vitro Activity of Antimicrobial Agents of Value in Otitis Media. The antimicrobial agent

TABLE 3. CONCENTRATION OF ORALLY ADMINISTERED ANTIMICROBIAL AGENTS IN SERUM AND MIDDLE EAR FLUIDS OF CHILDREN WITH ACUTE OTITIS MEDIA

Agent	Dosage (mg/kg)	Concentration (μg/ml)* S†	MEF§	MEF/S	Reference
Penicillin V	13.0	8.1	1.8	0.22	26
Ampicillin	10.0	4.3	1.2	0.28	27
Amoxicillin	10.0	4.8	2.2	0.46	28
Erythromycin estolate	7.5	3.9	1.3	0.33	28
Sulfonamide (trisulfapyrimidine)	30.0	13.4	8.3	0.62	28

*Measured at 0.5-2 hours after administration.

†Serum.

§Middle ear fluid.

prescribed for the patient with otitis media must be active against *S pneumoniae* and *H influenzae*. The penicillins, cephalosporins, erythromycin, clindamycin, and trimethoprim-sulfamethoxazole (TMP-SMZ) are effective against *S pneumoniae*. Only the aminoglycosides are relatively ineffective against this organism. Ampicillin, amoxicillin, carbenicillin, ticarcillin, TMP-SMZ, chloramphenicol, and the aminoglycosides are active against *H influenzae* but relatively high concentrations of penicillin V, the penicillinase-resistant penicillins, cephalothin, erythromycin, and clindamycin are required for inhibition of this organism. Penicillin G is intermediate in activity between ampicillin and penicillin V and may be sufficiently active against *H influenzae* to be efficacious for therapy of otitis media due to some strains of this species.

Recent reports of multiresistant strains of *S pneumoniae* in South Africa[24] and of the isolation of a penicillin G-resistant strain of type 14 in Minnesota[25] suggest the possibility of a major change in the pattern of antimicrobial susceptibility of *S pneumoniae*. The South African strains are remarkable in being not only significantly resistant to penicillin G but also resistant to most of the other antimicrobial agents considered as alternatives including erythromycin, tetracycline, clindamycin, and TMP-SMZ. These strains have a minimal inhibitory concentration (MIC) of ≥ 4 μg/ml, which is far greater than the usual MIC of 0.005 to 0.05 μg/ml. Of equal importance has been the identification of strains intermediate in susceptibility to penicillin G with MICs of 0.1 to 1.0 μg/ml.

We studied 173 strains of *S pneumoniae* obtained from middle ear fluids and nasopharyngeal secretions of children with acute otitis media during the period 1975-1980; three had MICs of 0.1-0.4 μg/ml, but all the others were more susceptible to penicillin G. Thus, at present, the highly resistant strains noted in South Africa have not been identified in Boston, and the strains of intermediate susceptibility are of low incidence in that location.

Strains of *H influenzae* resistant to ampicillin were first isolated in 1973. At present, approximately 15% of nontypable strains of *H influenzae* isolated from the middle ear fluid of children with otitis media in our clinic are resistant to ampicillin (Teele DW, Norton C, Klein JO, unpublished data). A similar incidence was noted by investigators in Pittsburgh but in Washington, D.C., approximately 30% of strains of *H influenzae* isolated from MEF of selected children were ampicillin-resistant (Fig. 1). Resistance to ampicillin is attributable to production of a penicillinase that hydrolyzes ampicillin, amoxicillin, penicillin G and V, and, to a lesser extent, carbenicillin. Sulfonamides, TMP-SMZ, and the new cephalosporins, cefamandole and cefoxitin (both administered parenterally) and cefaclor (administered orally) are effective *in vitro* against these strains of ampicillin-resistant, nontypable *H influenzae*.

Diffusion of Antimicrobial Agents into Middle Ear Fluids. Although studies of concentrations of various drugs in serum and middle ear fluid (Table 3) used different dosage schedules, times of collection, and methods of assay, the results all indicate that most antimicrobial agents of value for treatment of acute otitis media achieve significant concentrations in middle ear fluid.[26-29] Penicillin G and V produce concentrations in middle ear fluid that are 13 to 22% of levels in serum. Approximately half of the concentration in serum is present in middle ear fluid after oral administration of ampicillin, amoxicillin, erythromycin, and sulfonamides. Concentrations of ampicillin in middle ear fluid of patients with serous otitis media are lower than concentrations in fluid of patients with acute disease, but concentrations of amoxicillin are similar in acute suppurative and serous effusions. Thus, usual dosage schedules of penicillins and erythromycin produce concentrations of antimicrobial activity in middle ear fluid that are sufficient to inhibit *S pneumoniae*, but concentrations in middle ear fluid produced by intramuscular administration of benzathine penicillin G, penicillin V, and erythromycin are not adequate to inhibit most strains of *H influenzae*.

The "In Vivo Sensitivity Test." Drs. Virgil Howie and John Ploussard, pediatricians in practice in Huntsville, Alabama, have contributed significant information about the epidemiology, diagnosis, and management of otitis media (Table 4). The "in vivo sensitivity test" is one of their most valuable studies.[30] The middle ear fluid of children with acute otitis media was aspirated and cultured before commencement of therapy with antimicrobial agents. All drugs were prescribed in their usual dosage schedules, and patients were advised to return in two to five days. If fluid was still present at the second visit, a culture of the fluid was again obtained. The results of these studies are consistent with results expected on the basis of data from in vitro studies and achievable concentrations of drug in middle ear fluid (Table 3). Penicillins G and V,

TABLE 4. RESULTS OF ANTIMICROBIAL THERAPY IN OTITIS MEDIA: THE "IN VIVO SENSITIVITY TEST"[30]

Drug	No. of Patients with Organism Recovered*/No. of Patients with Bacterial OM	
	S Pneumoniae	*H Influenzae*
Phenoxymethyl penicillin	0/2	7/7
Phenoxymethyl penicillin with sulfonamides	0/17	2/6
Ampicillin	1/20	0/17
Benzathine, procaine, aqueous penicillin (intramuscular)	1/9	7/7
Erythromycin ethyl succinate	1/15	17/20
Erythromycin ethyl succinate — triple sulfonamide suspension	3/8	2/7
Triple sulfonamide suspension	8/18	3/8

*Two to 10 days after beginning therapy.

benzathine penicillin G (administered intramuscularly as a single dose), and erythromycin were all successful in eradicating *S pneumoniae* from middle ear fluid. Sulfonamides and tetracyclines did not sterilize middle ear fluid infected with *S pneumoniae. H influenzae* was eradicated by ampicillin but not by penicillin V, intramuscular benzathine penicillin G, or erythromycin. None of the strains of *H influenzae* possessed β-lactamase activity. The high MIC of penicillin V for *H influenzae* and the relatively low concentrations of benzathine penicillin G achieved in serum (and by extrapolation in middle ear fluid) probably explain the failure of these two penicillins to eradicate *H influenzae* from middle ear fluid. An oral form of penicillin G was not studied.

New Antimicrobial Agents. Although few data are available regarding the efficacy of the new antimicrobial agents TMP-SMZ and cefaclor, both appear to be effective in treatment of acute otitis media. Both agents have a spectrum of activity that includes the major pathogens responsible for otitis media, ie, *S pneumoniae* and *H influenzae* (including both β-lactamase-negative and -positive strains).

There is a paucity of published information on the clinical efficacy of TMP-SMZ for middle ear infection. In a randomized trial in which TMP-SMZ was compared with ampicillin, Shurin and colleagues[31] treated 132 children with acute otitis media. The antibacterial efficacy of the drugs was assessed from results of cultures of middle ear aspirates obtained during or after therapy. The number of microbiologic failures (including persistent, recurrent, and new infections of the middle ear) was similar for both groups. The drug regimens were well accepted by the patients and were not associated with significant side effects. Schwartz and colleagues evaluated TMP-SMZ for otitis media and found that the combination was effective against strains due to ampicillin-resistant *H influenzae*; resolution of the infection occurred promptly after therapy with TMP-SMZ.[32] These data indicate that TMP-SMZ is an effective alternative to ampicillin for initial treatment of acute otitis media and may be recommended when the presence of ampicillin-resistant strains of *H influenzae* is known or suspected. TMP-SMZ is also useful for patients who are allergic to penicillins. The combination can be given twice daily as compared with three times per day for amoxicillin and four times per day for ampicillin. However, TMP-SMZ would not be expected to be effective for otitis media due to group A *Streptococcus* since the combination drug is, like other sulfonamides, inadequate for treatment of streptococcal tonsillopharyngitis.

Cefaclor, an orally administered cephalosporin with stability to β-lactamases, was introduced in 1979. Until that time oral cephalosporins, including cephalexin and cephradine, had poor activity against most strains of *H influenzae* and only limited effectiveness in therapy of acute otitis media. Nelson and colleagues found that cefaclor was similar in efficacy for treatment of acute otitis media to amoxicillin or a combination of a sulfonamide plus erythromycin or penicillin B.[33]

Recommendations for Initial Choice of Antimicrobial Therapy for Patients with Acute Otitis Media. Amoxicillin or ampicillin are the currently preferred drugs for initial treatment of otitis media since they are active both in vitro and in vivo against *S pneumoniae* and *H influenzae.* Other regimens that are satisfactory include combinations of a sulfonamide with benzathine penicillin G (administered by the intramuscular route as a single injection) and with oral penicillin G or V, erythromycin, TMP-SMZ, and cefaclor. For the child who is allergic to penicillins, cefaclor or erythromycin combined with a sulfonamide or TMP-SMZ provides equivalent antimicrobial coverage.

With appropriate antimicrobial therapy, most children with acute bacterial otitis media are significantly improved within 48 to 72 hours. The physician should be in contact with the patient (or the patient's parents) to ascertain that improvement has occurred. If the patient remains toxic or his/her condition worsens, he/she must be re-evaluated and a change in antimicrobial therapy, myringotomy for drainage, or needle aspiration for diagnosis should be considered.

The current incidence of strains of ampicillin-resistant *H influenzae* is low (only 3 to 8% of all cases of acute otitis media) and does not require a change in these recommendations for initial therapy (Fig. 1). However, if the patient does not respond to initial therapy with ampicillin or amoxicillin, infection with a resistant strain of *H influenzae* should be considered. If the patient is not toxic, a change in therapy to include a sulfonamide, TMP-SMZ, or cefaclor is appropriate.

The bacteriology of middle ear infections in children who have recurrent episodes of acute otitis media is similar to that found in first episodes; the predominant pathogens are *S pneumoniae* (though of different serotypes) and nontypable strains of *H influenzae*. Thus, the child with a recurrent episode of otitis media should be treated initially with the same antimicrobial regimens as the child with a first episode of middle ear infection.

MANAGEMENT OF CHRONIC OTITIS MEDIA

The term chronic otitis media includes recurrent episodes of acute infection and prolonged effusion of the middle ear resulting from acute infection. For prevention of recurrent episodes of acute otitis media, management should include consideration of chemoprophylaxis (use of antimicrobial agents for prolonged periods) or immunoprophylaxis (use of pneumococcal vaccine). For management of persistent middle ear effusions, four methods are considered: myringotomy, adenoidectomy, placement of tympanostomy tubes, and use of steroids. Although there is evidence for the support of each method for management of chronic otitis media, the data are incomplete. Management of chronic otitis media is a subject of current interest in many centers in the United States, Canada, Western Europe, and Japan and new information is expected to clarify some of the unresolved issues.

Management of Recurrent Episodes of Acute Otitis Media by Chemoprophylaxis. Recent studies of children in Alaskan Eskimo villages[34] and in Rochester, New York,[35] suggest that chemoprophylaxis may be of value in prevention of acute illness in children who have suffered from recurrences of middle ear infections. Eskimo children treated with a course of ampicillin (four times daily for ten days) had a smaller number of episodes of otorrhea as compared with controls. The children in the Rochester study were enrolled in a randomized, double-blind control trial in which sulfisoxazole and a placebo were used. After three months, children who received the antimicrobial agent had significantly fewer episodes of otitis media than did children who received the placebo. The groups were switched for the following three months, and the results again indicated efficacy of sulfisoxazole in prevention of new clinical episodes. Although these data are persuasive, there are significant limitations in the design of each study, including failure to evaluate persistence of middle ear effusion.

The currently licensed pneumococcal vaccine contains purified polysaccharide antigens of 14 types. Although 85 immunologically distinct capsular types of pneumococci are known, the strains incorporated into the vaccine have been responsible for more than 85% of cases of otitis media. Studies in children have indicated that, as with the polysaccharide vaccines prepared from capsular materials of *H influenzae* type B and *Neisseria meningitidis* groups A and C, children younger than 2 years exhibit low and irregular serologic responses to the vaccine. Children over 2 years respond satisfactorily.

Preliminary results of three studies of use of pneumococcal vaccine for prevention of recurrences of otitis media in children have been presented.[36] Studies of Boston, Massachusetts, and Huntsville, Alabama, children used an octavalent vaccine whereas study of children in Oulu and Tampere, Finland, used the available 14 type vaccine. Some of the antigens were better immunogens and more likely to be associated with protection than others. Each study showed some protection against pneumococcal otitis due to types present in the vaccine. The overall effect on experience with otitis media was not different in vaccinees and controls in the American studies whereas a protective effect of about 50% was apparent in the Finnish study. Based on these data, no firm recommendation for use of the vaccine to prevent otitis media in children can be made. Further studies are in progress that will define the value of the vaccine for prevention of pneumococcal otitis media.

REFERENCES

1. Klein JO. Microbiology of acute and chronic otitis media. Ann Otol Rhinol Laryngol 1980; 89 Suppl 68:98-101.

2. Austrian R, Howie VM, Ploussard JH. The bacteriology of pneumococcal otitis media. Johns Hopkins Med J 1977; 141:104-11.

3. Gray BM, Converse GM III, Dillon HC Jr. Serotypes of *Streptococcus pneumoniae* causing disease. J Infect Dis 1979; 140:979-83.

4. Kamme C, Ageberg M, Lundgren K. Distribution of *Diplococcus pneumoniae* types in acute otitis media in children and influence of the types on the clinical course in penicillin V therapy. Scand J Infect Dis 1970; 2:183-90.

5. Harding AL, Anderson P, Howie VM, Ploussard JH, Smith DH. *Hemophilus influenzae* isolated from children with otitis media. In: SHW Sell, DT Karzon, eds. *Hemophilus Influenzae*. Nashville: Vanderbilt University Press, 1973:21-8.

6. Berman SA, Balkany TJ, Simmons MA. Otitis media in infants less than 12 weeks of age: differing bacteriology among inpatients and out-patients. J Pediatr 1978; 93:453-4.

7. Bland RD. Otitis media in the first six weeks of life: diagnosis, bacteriology, and management. Pediatrics 1972; 49:187-97.

8. Shurin PA, Howie VM, Pelton SI, et al. Bacterial etiology of otitis media during the first six weeks of life. J Pediatr 1978; 92:893.

9. Tetzlaff TR, Ashworth C, Nelson JD. Otitis media in children less than 12 weeks of age. Pediatrics 1977; 59:827.

10. Coffey JD Jr, Martin AD, Booth HN. *Neisseria catarrhalis* in exudative otitis media. Arch Otolaryngol 1967; 86:403-6.

11. Feigin RD, Shackelford PD, Campbell J, et al. Assessment of the role of *Staphylococcus epidermidis* as a cause of otitis media. Pediatrics 1973; 52:569-75.

12. Brook I, Anthony BF, Finegold SM. Aerobic and anaerobic bacteriology of acute otitis media in children. J Pediatr 1978; 92:13-5.

13. Teele DW, Healy GB, Tally FP. Persistent middle ear effusions in young children: cultures for anaerobic bacteria. Ann Otol Rhinol Laryngol 1980; 89 Suppl 68:102-3.

14. Pelton SI, Teele DW, Shurin PA, Klein JO. Disparate cultures of middle ear fluids in bilateral otitis media. Am J Dis Child 1980; 134:951-3.

15. Henderson FW, Collier AM, Clyde WA Jr, et al. The epidemiology of acute otitis media in childhood. Program and Abstracts of the 16th Interscience Conference on Antimicrobial Agents and Chemotherapy. Washington, DC: American Society for Microbiology, 1976 (Abstract No. 188).

16. Klein JO, Teele DW. Isolation of viruses and mycoplasmas from middle ear effusions. A review. Ann Otol Rhinol Laryngol 1976; 85 Suppl 25:140-4.

17. Rifkind DR, Chanock R, Kranetz H, Johnson K, Knight V. Ear involvement (myringitis) and primary atypical pneumonia following inoculation of volunteers with Eaton agent. Am Rev Respir Dis 1962; 85:479-89.

18. Tipple MA, Beem MD, Saxon EM. Clinical characteristics of afebrile pneumonia associated with *Chlamydia trachomatis* infections in infants less than 6 months of age. Pediatr 1979; 63:192-7.

19. Dawson C, Schacter J. TRIC agent infections of the eye and genital tract. Am J Ophthalmol 1967; 63:1288-98.

20. Dawson C, Wood TR, Rose L. Experimental inclusion conjunctivitis in man. III. Keratitis and other complications. Arch Ophthalmol 1967; 78:341-9.

21. Liu YS, Lim DJ, Lang RW, Birck HG. Chronic middle ear effusions. Immunochemical and bacteriological investigations. Arch Otolaryngol 1975; 101:278-86.

22. Healy GB, Teele DW. The microbiology of chronic middle ear effusions in children. Laryngoscope 1977; 57:1472-8.

23. Riding KH, Bluestone CD, Michaels RH, Cantekin EI, Doyle WJ, Poziviak CS. Microbiology of recurrent and chronic otitis media with effusion. J Pediatr 1978; 93:739-43.

24. Jacobs MR, Koornhof HJ, Robins-Browne RM, et al. Emergence of multiply resistant pneumococci. N Engl J Med 1978; 299:735-40.

25. Cates KL, Gerrard JM, Giebink GS, et al. A penicillin-resistant pneumococcus. J Pediatr 1978; 93:624-6.

26. Kamme C, Lundgren K, Rundcrantz H. The concentration of penicillin V in serum and middle ear exudate in acute otitis media in children. Scandinav J Infect Dis 1969; 1:77-83.

27. Lahikainen EA, Vuori M, Virtanen S. Azidocillin and ampicillin concentrations in middle ear effusions. Acta Otolaryngol (Stockh) 1977; 84:227-32.

28. Howard JE, Nelson JD, Clahsen J, Jackson LH. Otitis media of infancy and early childhood. Am J Dis Child 1976; 130:965-70.

29. Lundgren K, Ingvarsson L, Rundcrantz H. The concentration of penicillin-V in middle ear exudate. Int J Pediatr Otorhinolaryngol 1979; 1:93-6.

30. Howie VM, Ploussard JH. The "in vivo sensitivity test" — bacteriology of middle ear exudate during antimicrobial therapy in otitis media. Pediatrics 1969; 44:940-4.

31. Shurin PA, Pelton SI, Donner A, Finkelstein J, Klein JO. Trimethoprim-sulfamethoxazole compared with ampicillin in the treatment of acute otitis media. J Pediatr 1980; 96:1081-7.

32. Schwartz R, Rodriguez WJ, Ross S, Kahn WN. Treatment of otitis media with trimethoprim-sulfamethoxazole. Letter to editor. J Pediatr 1979; 95:666-7.

33. Nelson JD, Ginsburg CM, Clahsen JC, Jackson LH. Treatment of acute otitis media of infancy with cefaclor. Am J Dis Child 1978; 132:992-6.

34. Maynard JE, Fleshman JK, Tschopp CF. Otitis media in Alaskan Eskimo children. Prospective evaluation of chemoprophylaxis. JAMA 1972; 219:597-9.

35. Perrin JM, Charney E, MacWhinney JB, McInerny TK, Miller RL, Nazarian LF. Sulfisoxazole as chemoprophylaxis for recurrent otitis media. A double-blind crossover study in pediatric practice. N Engl J Med 1974; 291:664-7.

36. Klein JO, Teele DW, Sloyer JL Jr, et al. Use of pneumococcal vaccine for prevention of recurrent episodes of otitis media. In: Robbins JB, Hill JC, Sadoff JC, eds. Bacterial vaccines. New York: Thieme-Stratton, Inc (in press).

PHARMACOLOGY OF ORAL ANTIBIOTICS USED FOR TREATMENT OF OTITIS MEDIA AND TONSILLOPHARYNGITIS IN INFANTS AND CHILDREN

CHARLES M. GINSBURG, MD
GEORGE H. MCCRACKEN, JR., MD
JOHN D. NELSON, MD
DALLAS, TEXAS

Data are presented from pharmacologic evaluations of major oral antibiotics used in treatment of acute otitis media and tonsillopharyngitis in children. Information is included on serum and middle ear specimens obtained almost simultaneously following administration of many of these antibiotics. Discussion covers ampicillin and amoxicillin, penicillin G and V, erythromycin estolate, erythromycin ethylsuccinate and the orally administered cephalosporins.

Acute otitis media is not only one of the more frequent but, undoubtedly, one of the more perplexing of the infectious conditions that affects infants and young children. Depending on the season of the year, it accounts for between 10 and 25% of all visits to a pediatrician's office (Ginsburg CM, Kramer RI, unpublished data). In general pediatric practice, only well baby visits and URIs are seen with greater frequency. Although the true incidence of this condition is not known, recent studies indicate that anywhere from 40 to 60% of children will have experienced at least one episode of acute otitis media by their first birthday.[1] With few exceptions, the majority of children with acute otitis media receive at least one and, occasionally, two or three oral antimicrobial agents.

Despite the widespread use of these agents there is a paucity of information on the pharmacology of these drugs in infants and young children, particularly with regard to their ability to achieve concentrations at the local site of infection, the middle ear. Additionally, it is important to remember that in the majority of instances we are administering these drugs, in the form of suspensions, to infants and young children. Despite the pharmaceutical industry's efforts to produce formulations which are palatable, it is sometimes not possible to get little Johnny or Susie to take his or her medication. Parents frequently resort to disguising the various oral preparations in milk, formula, or other food substances. This practice is far more common than we would like to believe, and occurs regardless of the physician's advice concerning proper administration. It is extremely important, therefore, to consider whether these vehicles will effect the absorption of the antibiotic which you have prescribed.

During the past four years, my coauthors, George McCracken and John Nelson, and I have performed pharmacologic evaluations in infants and young children with the majority of the oral antibiotics used for the treatment of acute otitis media and tonsillopharyngitis in children. We have also obtained almost simultaneous serum and middle ear specimens from other children after single and multiple doses of many of these antibiotics. These data, some of which have been published previously, serve as the basis for this communication.[2-4]

AMPICILLIN AND AMOXICILLIN

Figure 1 shows serum concentration-time curves for ampicillin and amoxicillin after administration orally to infants in dosages of 25 and 15 mg/kg, respectively. These curves provide a means for comparing bioavailability, or the amount of administered drug which enters the systemic circulation. Mean peak serum concentrations of 4.1 to 5.0 μg/ml were observed one hour after administration of ampicillin. Infant formula did not adversely effect the absorption of ampicillin. Although the peak level is slightly blunted, there are no substantial differences when the drug is administered with milk or formula. The drug was present in the serum of all patients at six hours; the mean concentrations were 0.2 to 0.3 μg/ml.

Also shown in Figure 1 are serum concentration-time curves for amoxicillin (15 mg/kg dose). It is important to remember that although the antimicrobial spectrum for amoxicillin is virtually identical to that of ampicillin, they are different drugs. In advertisements it is stated that the major advantage of amoxicillin over ampicillin is that the former is more completely absorbed after oral administration; therefore, you need to administer less of the drug to achieve serum levels comparable to those of ampicillin. Additionally, diarrhea is less frequent following amoxicillin than ampicillin. After 15

From the Department of Pediatrics, Southwestern Medical School, Dallas. These studies were funded by grants from Eli Lilly Research Laboratory and Mead Johnson Pharmaceuticals.

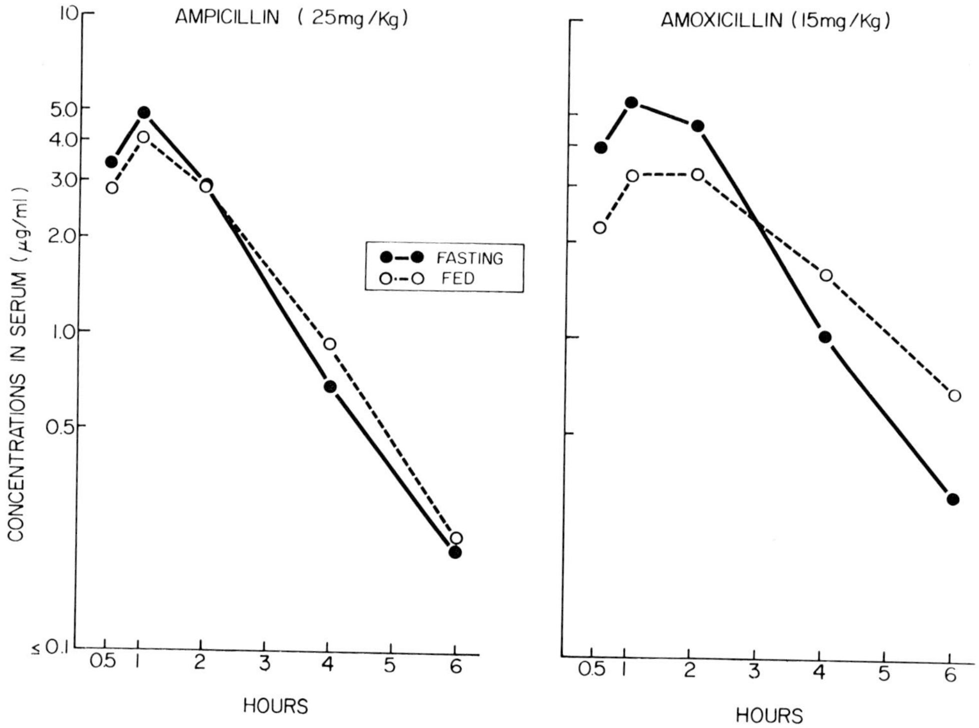

Fig. 1. Serum concentration-time curves for ampicillin (25 mg/kg) and amoxicillin (15 mg/kg) in infants and children.

mg/kg doses, amoxicillin is well absorbed and levels with this dose are comparable to those achieved with a 25 mg/kg dose of ampicillin. Like ampicillin, amoxicillin serum concentrations are substantially greater than the minimum inhibitory concentrations (MIC) for group A *Streptococcus*, *Streptococcus pneumoniae* and, in most instances, are in excess of those required to eradicate most non-β-lactamase-producing strains of *Hemophilus influenzae*.

How well does this drug get into middle ear fluid? There is very little information available to answer this question. For example, in one study middle ear concentrations of amoxicillin were measured in patients who were undergoing myringotomy for chronic middle ear effusions.[5] The concentrations in the middle ear were large but so was the dose of medication: 1 g. If prescribed on a weight basis this would be the dose for a patient weighing 66 pounds, obviously, a very large infant!

Serum and middle ear fluid concentrations from 12 infants who received 15 mg/kg doses of amoxicillin for acute otitis media are shown in Figure 2. All serum samples and approximately 60% of middle ear fluid specimens contained concentrations of drug in excess of the MIC for 90% of ampicillin-susceptible strains of *H influenzae*. Additionally, the concentrations in both body fluids were far in excess of the MICs for group A *Streptococcus* and strains of *S pneumoniae*.

PENICILLIN G AND PENICILLIN V

Penicillin G and penicillin V are the two penicillin preparations most frequently prescribed for infants and young children. Penicillin G has been available for years but it has been said that its ab-

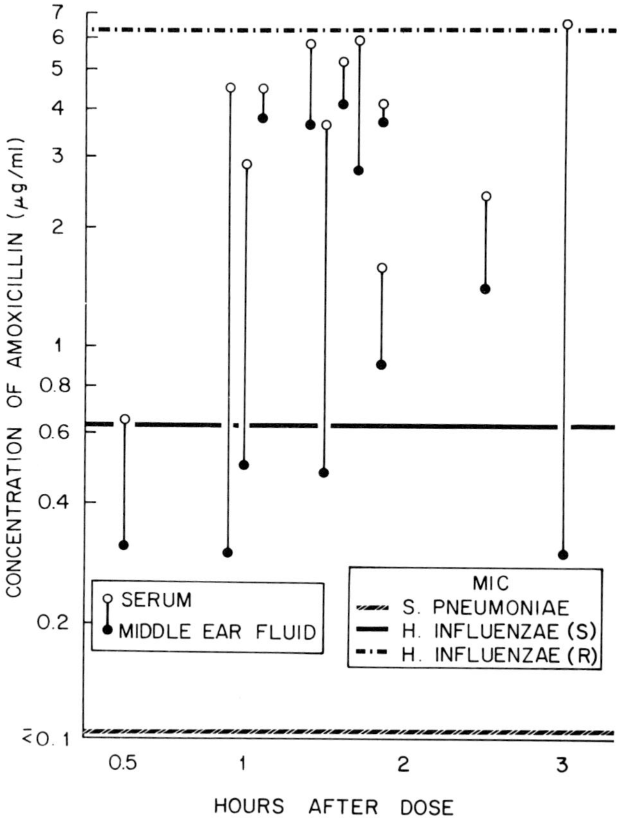

Fig. 2. Concentrations of amoxicillin in serum and middle ear fluid from children with acute otitis media after 15 mg/kg doses of amoxicillin.

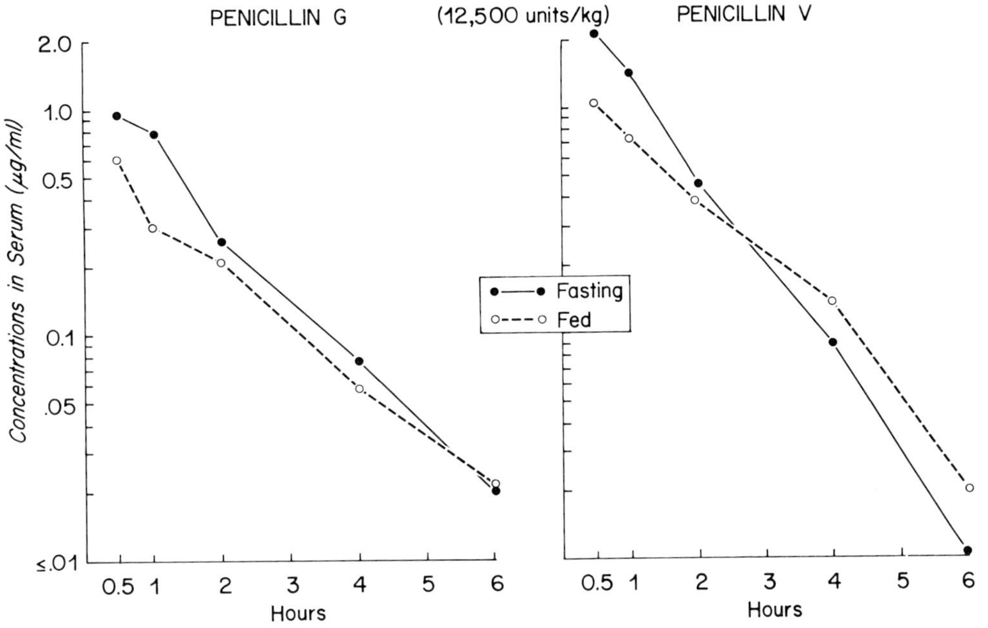

Fig. 3. Serum concentration-time curves for penicillin G (8 mg/kg) and penicillin V (8 mg/kg) in infants and children.

sorption from the gastrointestinal tract was unreliable and, therefore the drug would not be as efficacious as the more reliably absorbed penicillin V. At one time, a major advantage of penicillin G was its lower cost, but this is no longer true. The cost is comparable for the liquid formulations of both drugs.

Serum concentration-time curves for penicillin G and penicillin V in infants and children are shown in Figure 3. Both drugs were administered in an 8 mg/kg or 12,500 units/kg dosage. The serum levels after penicillin V were approximately twice those obtained after penicillin G. Although this is not surprising, it should be pointed out that only mean values are displayed and that the scatter around the mean was similar for both drugs. In other words, there were poor absorbers in each group of children, not only in those who received penicillin G. Additionally, the absorption of both drugs was decreased approximately 50% when administered with milk or infant formula.

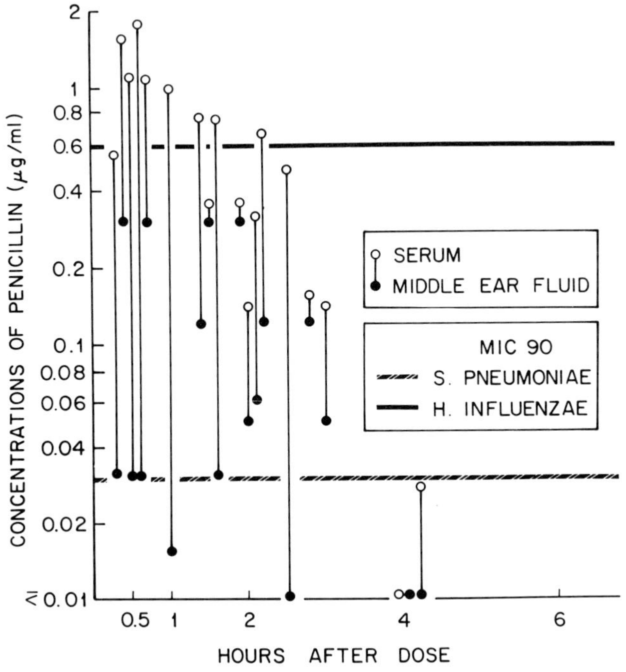

Fig. 4. Concentrations of penicillin in serum and middle ear fluid from children with acute otitis media after 8 mg/kg doses of penicillin V.

Figure 4 shows simultaneous serum and middle ear fluid concentrations of penicillin in patients with acute otitis media who received 8 mg/kg doses of penicillin V. During the first 2½ hours after administration, all serum and 14 of 16 middle ear fluid specimens (87%) contained concentrations of penicillin that would be inhibitory for *S pneumoniae* and group A *Streptococcus*. By contrast, only 20% of middle ear fluid specimens contained concentrations of drug that would inhibit approximately 50% of non-β-lactamase-producing strains of *H influenzae*. These data demonstrate why penicillin has not been highly efficacious for treatment of acute otitis media caused by strains of *H influenzae*.

ERYTHROMYCIN

Erythromycin has been used for many years for treatment of acute otitis media. Serum concentration-time curves for erythromycin estolate administered in a 10 mg/kg dose are displayed in Figure 5. This dosage may be somewhat lower than used in clinical practice; more frequently, a dose of 15 to 20 mg/kg is used. Also shown are the curves for erythromycin ethylsuccinate administered in a 15

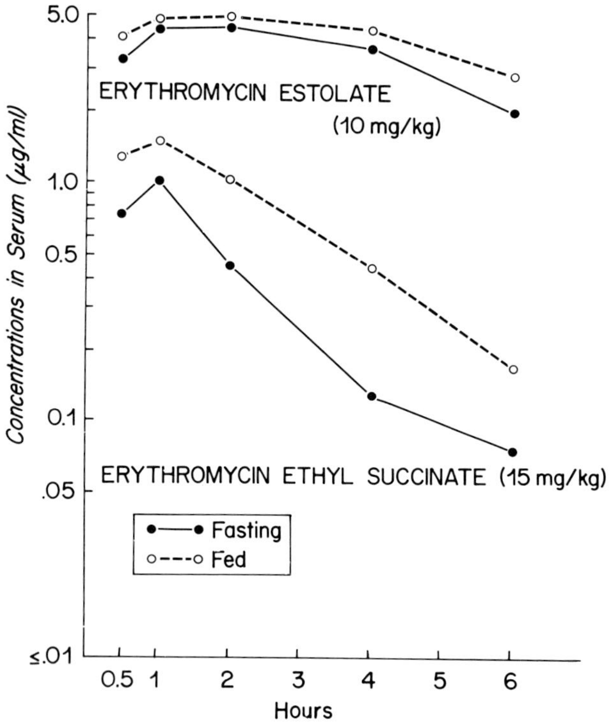

Fig. 5. Serum concentration-time curves for erythromycin estolate (10 mg/kg) and erythromycin ethylsuccinate (15 mg/kg) in infants and children.

mg/kg dose. Although this dose of the ethylsuccinate was 30% larger than that of the estolate, the serum concentrations following the estolate were three to five times larger than those following the ethylsuccinate. Additionally, unlike most other antibiotics, erythromycin ethylsuccinate is better absorbed when coadministered with milk. These differences in pharmacology between the two oral erythromycin esters have been previously noted.[6] It is important to point out, however, that despite the superior bioavailability of the estolate, there are no data to indicate that this formulation has superior efficacy over the other forms of erythromycin. It is unlikely that this controversy will ever be settled.

What about other body fluids? Serum and tonsil concentrations of erythromycin after administration of single and multiple doses of erythromycin estolate and erythromycin ethylsuccinate are shown in Figure 6. Although the concentrations in tonsils were larger and more sustained in the patients who received estolate, the majority of levels after the ethylsuccinate were in the range required to kill strains of group A *Streptococcus.* Furthermore, clinical studies have failed to demonstrate superiority of one preparation over the other for treatment of tonsillopharyngitis caused by group A *Streptococcus.*[6]

Figure 7 shows serum and middle ear fluid concentrations from patients with acute otitis media who received erythromycin ethylsuccinate or erythromycin estolate. Both drugs achieved concentrations in serum and middle ear fluid that were in excess of the MIC_{90} for strains of *S pneumoniae* but not for *H influenzae*.

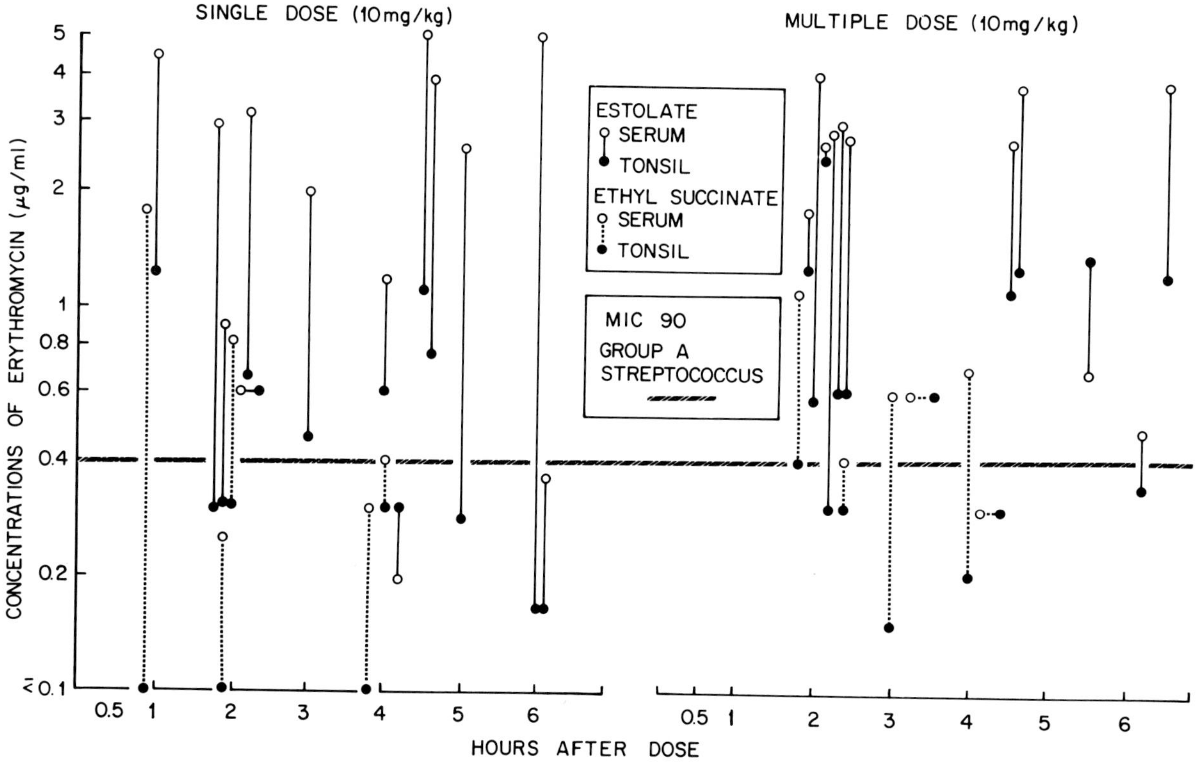

Fig. 6. Serum and tonsil concentrations of erythromycin after erythromycin estolate (10 mg/kg) and erythromycin ethylsuccinate (15 mg/kg).

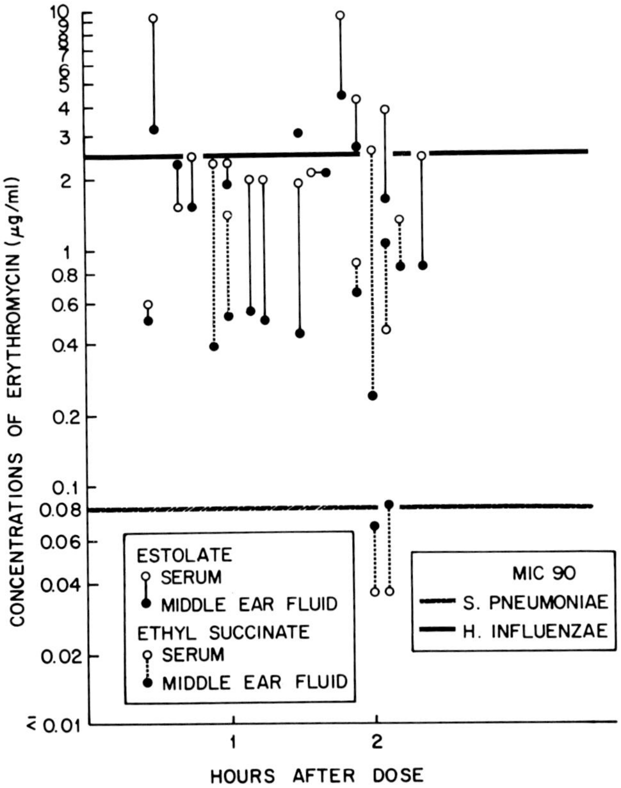

Fig. 7. Concentrations of erythromycin in serum and middle ear fluid from children with acute otitis media after erythromycin estolate (15 mg/kg) and erythromycin ethylsuccinate (15 mg/kg).

What does this mean to the practicing physician? For tonsillopharyngitis the answer is fairly simple: penicillin is the drug of choice. In the penicillin-allergic patient erythromycin is an acceptable alternative. Although pharmacokinetic data suggest that the estolate should offer an advantage over the ethylsuccinate, this has not been born out in clinical studies. One possible exception is that the estolate is effective for therapy of group A streptococcal pharyngitis when administered on a twice daily basis.[7] This has not been demonstrated for the other erythromycin formulations.

What about management of acute otitis media? Based on in vitro susceptibility data, pharmacokinetic data, and on the results of several therapeutic efficacy studies, erythromycin should not be used alone, unless there is evidence that the pneumococcus or group A *Streptococcus* is causing the middle ear disease. To obtain optimal coverage for *H influenzae*, erythromycin should be combined with a sulfonamide. The pharmacologic justification for this is shown in Figure 8. Serum and middle ear concentrations of sulfa were measured in six children. Following administration of trisulfapyrimidine (30 mg/kg) serum and middle ear fluid were in excess of the MIC for *H influenzae*, pneumococcus and *Streptococcus pyogenes*. These data suggest that a sulfonamide alone would be the ideal candidate for the treatment of otitis media. However, it is important to emphasize that the sulfonamides have not proven clinically effective against pneumococcus and strains of group A *Streptococcus*. The reason for this is unknown. Recently the combination of erythromycin ethylsuccinate-sulfasoxazole in a 1:3 ratio has been marketed and should be very useful for initial therapy of acute otitis media.

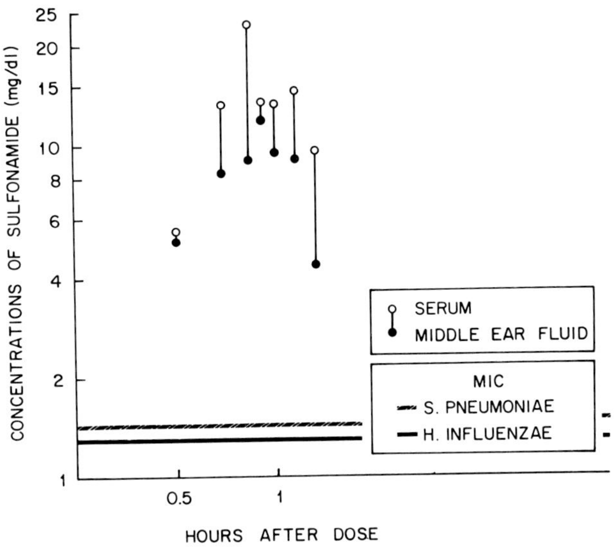

Fig. 8. Concentrations of sulfonamide in serum and middle ear fluid from children with acute otitis media after 80 mg/kg doses of trisulfapyrimidine.

CEPHALOSPORINS

Until relatively recently there has been little interest in this class of drugs as first-line agents for treatment of respiratory infections in children. The basis for this was that, although effective in treating infections caused by group A *Streptococcus* and *S pneumoniae*, these agents have inferior in vitro activity against most strains of *H influenzae*. Therefore, they offer no advantage over penicillin or erythromycin, and are usually far more expensive.

The pharmacokinetics of four orally administered cephalosporins (cephalexin, cephradine, cefaclor and cefadroxil) are compared in Figure 9. Cephloglycine is not shown because of its limited usefulness in pediatric patients. A dose of 15 mg/kg was administered to all infants. Analysis of the serum concentrations-time curves shows that the coadministration of infant formula substantially reduces the bioavailability of cephalexin and cephradine but not that of cefadroxil or cefaclor. Additionally, the half-life of cefadroxil was approximately 30 minutes longer than those of the other preparations.

Do these drugs have a place in the otitis media treatment armamentarium? Cefadroxil has not yet been approved by the FDA for use in children, but when marketed for pediatric use, it will not be recommended for otitis media. Cephradine has not

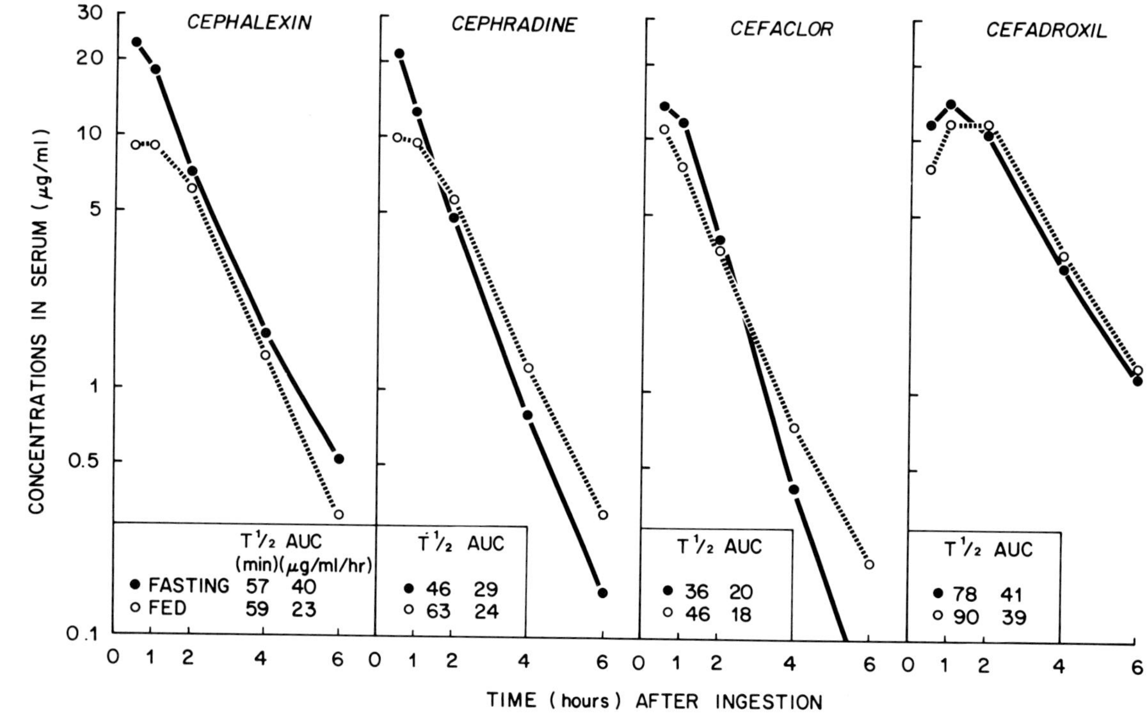

Fig. 9. Serum concentration-time curves and pharmacokinetics for cephalexin, cephradine, cefaclor and cefadroxil after 15 mg/kg doses.

been studied extensively in this condition, but because of its similarity to cephalexin, the two drugs can be considered together. There have been several studies which have evaluated the efficacy of cephalexin for treatment of acute otitis media and, with one exception, the drug has not been found to be effective in infections caused by *H influenzae*.[8,9] The probable explanation for this is its inability to attain concentrations in middle ear fluid that are bactericidal for *Hemophilus*. In one study, a daily dosage of 100 mg/kg, two times that routinely recommended, was shown to be effective.

What about cefaclor, the newest of the cephalosporin derivatives? Cefaclor has substantially greater in vitro activity against pneumococci, β-lactamase-positive and negative strains of *H influenzae* and certain of the Enterobacteriaciae than do cephalexin or cephradine. Its activity against Gram-negative enteric bacilli may be important because these organisms cause acute otitis media in 10-20% of infants who are less than six weeks of age. Many of these organisms are resistant to the antimicrobial agents used to treat this condition.

The concentrations of cefaclor in the middle ear fluid of infants and children in relation to the levels in serum and saliva are presented in Figure 10. Although we did not measure salivary or tear concentrations of cefaclor in the 30- to 120-minute period after administration, the levels of drug in these body fluids appear to be comparable to those collected in middle ear fluid. Approximately 75% of middle ear fluid specimens obtained during the first two hours after the dose contained concentrations of cefaclor that were equal to or greater than 0.63 μg/ml, a concentration that should inhibit all pneumococci, group A streptococci, and most strains of *H influenzae*. Although limited, these pharmacologic data and the results of clinical efficacy studies indicate that cefaclor should be an ef-

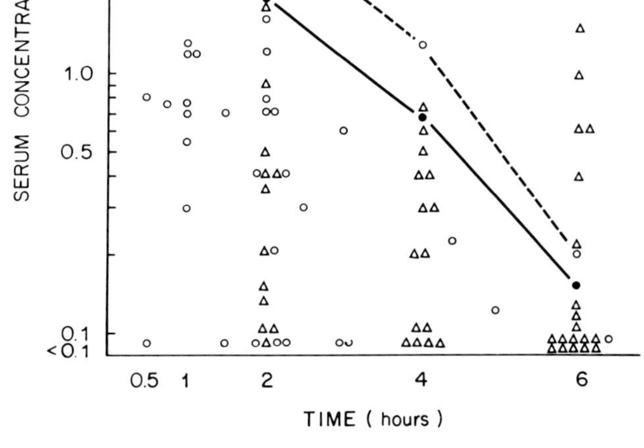

Fig. 10. Middle ear fluid and salivary concentrations of cefaclor from children with acute otitis media after 10 mg/kg doses of cefaclor.

fective agent for initial therapy of acute otitis media in infants and young children.

EPILOGUE

Although these data provide a pharmacologic rationale for the use of the various orally administered antimicrobials for treatment of otitis media and tonsillopharyngitis, it is important to recognize that antibiotics alone are not the sole determinants of effective therapy. The epidemiology and characteristics of the various offending pathogens, the child's host defenses, and the presence of underlying anatomic or functional abnormalities, as well as a number of less well defined factors, are all important.

REFERENCES

1. Howie VM, Ploussard JH. The "otitis-prone" condition. Am J Dis Child 1975; 129:676-8.

2. McCracken GH Jr, Ginsburg CM, Clahsen JC, Thomas ML. Pharmacologic evaluation of orally administered antibiotics in infants and children: effect of feeding on bioavailability. Pediatrics 1978; 62:738-43.

3. Ginsburg CM, McCracken GH, Thomas ML, Clahsen J. Comparative pharmacokinetics of amoxicillin and ampicillin in infants and children. J Pediatr 1979; 64:627-31.

4. Ginsburg CM, McCracken GH, Culbertson MC. Concentrations of erythromycin in serum and tonsil: comparison of the estolate and ethylsuccinate suspensions. J Pediatr 1976; 89:1011-3.

5. Klimek JJ, Nightingale C, Lehmann WB, Quintiliani R. Comparison of concentrations of amoxicillin and ampicillin in serum and middle ear fluid of children with chronic otitis media. J Infect Dis 1977; 135:999-1001.

6. Ginsburg CM, Eichenwald HF. Erythromycin: a review of its uses in pediatric practice. J Pediatr 1976; 89:872-84.

7. Breese BB, Disney FA, Talpey WB, Green J, Tobin MD. Streptococcal infections in children. Comparison of penicillin V, clindamycin and erythromycin treatment. Am J Dis Child 1974; 128:457-61.

8. Stechenberg BW, Anderson D, Chang MJ, et al. Cephalexin compared to ampicillin treatment of otitis media. Pediatrics 1976; 58:532-6.

9. McLinn SE, Daly JF Jr, Jones JE. Cephalexin monohydrate suspension. JAMA 1975; 235:171-4.

PHARMACOKINETICS OF CEFACLOR IN CHRONIC MIDDLE EAR EFFUSIONS

TORBEN LILDHOLDT, MD
ODENSE, DENMARK

ERDEM I. CANTEKIN, PhD
PITTSBURGH, PENNSYLVANIA

GABRIEL MARSHAK, MD
REHOVOT, ISRAEL

CHARLES D. BLUESTONE, MD
PITTSBURGH, PENNSYLVANIA

DALE D. ROHN, BA
PITTSBURGH, PENNSYLVANIA

KENNETH E. SCHUIT, MD
PITTSBURGH, PENNSYLVANIA

Fifty children aged 1 to 13 years with chronic or recurrent otitis media with effusion received a single dose of cefaclor (15 mg/kg body weight) by the oral route 30 minutes to seven hours before the removal of middle ear effusion and insertion of tympanostomy tubes. Serum and middle ear aspirate concentrations of the antibiotic were determined employing a microbiological assay technique by a disk diffusion method. Middle ear specimens were also cultured for aerobic bacteria. The mean peak serum concentration level (8.49 ± 7.89 µg/ml) was observed after 30 minutes, whereas the middle ear peak level (0.47 ± 0.78 µg/ml) occurred after one hour. Of the 87 middle ear specimens, 37 had cefaclor concentrations which were detectable within the resolution of the bioassay method (>0.16 µg/ml). There was no correlation between the type of middle ear effusion (mucoid or serous) and the concentration of cefaclor in the middle ear. Only 18% of the middle ear cultures were positive for aerobic bacteria; *Hemophilus influenzae* was the most common organism.

INTRODUCTION

Chronic otitis media with effusion (OME) is characterized by an accumulation of liquid in the middle ear cavity. In contrast to acute OME, bacteria have been considered in the past to be of minor importance in the pathogenesis of chronic OME. Nevertheless, antibiotics have been used in the treatment of this chronic condition, often as the primary choice. No controlled double-blind clinical trials of the efficacy of antibiotics for the management of chronic OME have been reported and according to the few uncontrolled studies published, efficacy was not demonstrated.[1] Despite these observations, bacterial involvement in chronic OME is of growing concern, as refined culture techniques have shown bacteria to be present in up to 45% of ears with a chronic effusion.[2-4] The significance of these findings remains to be demonstrated, but they provide a rationale for the clinical use of antibiotics prior to surgical intervention. The efficacy of antibiotics in eliminating chronic middle ear effusions (MEE) may be related to the concentration of specific antimicrobial agents in the middle ear. Unfortunately, there are very few studies that have evaluated middle ear concentrations of these agents.[5-9] This study was part of an evaluation of a new oral cephalosporin, cefaclor (Eli Lilly Co., Indianapolis). The object was to determine the kinetics of this antibiotic in the blood and MEE after a single oral dose administration.

METHODS

Fifty children (87 ears) with chronic OME or with recurrent OME who had myringotomy and tympanostomy tube insertion constituted the study population. The age and sex distribution of the subjects are shown in Table 1. Many of the patients had been treated previously with decongestants, antihistamines, or antibiotics. Only children who had not received antibiotic treatment during the week prior to the surgery were qualified to participate in the study. After informed consent was obtained, each child was given a single oral dose of cefaclor (15 mg/kg) at intervals from 30 minutes to seven hours before myringotomy. The drug administration was directly supervised by one of the investigators (TL or GM). All children were fasting prior to the administration of the antibiotic.

With the patient under general anesthesia (oxygen, nitrous oxide, and halothane) applied by oropharyngeal airway and mask, the otomicroscope was used to inspect each ear. The ear canal was debrided of cerumen and cultured with Calgiswab® (Falton, Oxnard, Calif). The canal was then filled with 70% ethyl alcohol, which remained in the external ear for 60 seconds and was then removed by aspiration. Tympanocentesis was performed in the anterosuperior quadrant using an Alden-Senturia trap with a No. 18 needle attached. Occasionally a counterincision had to be made in the inferior portion of the tympanic membrane in order to allow very viscous, mucoid material to be removed by suction. If an effusion was not found, nonbacteriostatic, freshly sterilized, isotonic saline was introduced into the middle ear with a syringe and needle through the tympanocentesis, and aspirated into the collection trap.

Based on the findings at myringotomy, the effusions were classified as *serous* — pale, usually yellow liquid with low viscosity, or *mucoid* — thick, usually gray liquid. No purulent effusions were found and some middle ears were dry. After collecting the specimen, the needle and trap were rinsed by suctioning 250 µl of nonbacteriostatic saline through the system; in some cases, this rinsing was necessary in order to obtain a sample of adequate size.

TABLE 1. AGE AND SEX DISTRIBUTION OF THE STUDY POPULATION

	Age (years)				
	1-3	*4-6*	*7-9*	*10-13*	*Total*
Male	9	8	8	2	28
Female	3	9	8	3	22
Total	12	17	16	5	50 (87 ears)

From the Departments of Otolaryngology and Infectious Diseases, University of Pittsburgh School of Medicine and Children's Hospital of Pittsburgh.
This study was supported in part by the Eli Lilly Company, Indianapolis.
REPRINTS — Erdem I. Cantekin, PhD, Department of Otolaryngology, Children's Hospital of Pittsburgh, 125 DeSoto St., Pittsburgh, PA 15213.

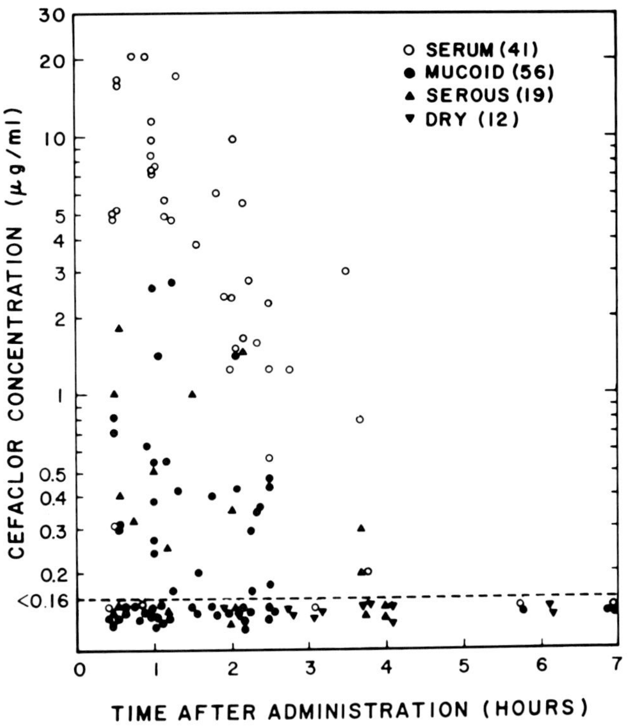

Fig. 1. Serum and middle ear aspirate concentrations of cefaclor as a function of time after administration of a single dose of 15 mg/kg.

A venous blood sample was drawn at the time of the myringotomy, and the serum was separated by centrifugation without adding anticoagulant.

The serum and middle ear specimens were instantly placed on ice and processed within one to two hours. Concentrations of cefaclor were measured by bioassay using *Sarcina lutea* (ATCC 9341). On the day of the assay, antibiotic assay medium (Difco) at 50 C was mixed with a standardized suspension of the bacteria and poured into 150 mm Petri plates. Samples consisting of 20 μl of middle ear fluid or cefaclor standards (in phosphate buffer, pH 4.5) were dropped onto 6 mm cellulose disks which were then placed on the inoculated agar. Antibiotic standards were prepared daily and the inoculated plates were incubated for 16 to 18 hours at 35 C and the resulting zones of inhibition measured in duplicate with a Fisher-Lilly zone reader to the nearest 0.1 mm. A standard curve was constructed using the zones of inhibition around each of the reference disks. The concentration of antibiotic in each sample was calculated from the standard curve; concentrations ranging from 0.16 to 20 μg/ml could be measured reliably.

Because the myringotomy procedure frequently caused bleeding, contamination of the middle ear specimen with blood could not always be avoided, and in these cases a correction was made. Spectrophotometry measuring the absorption of light of wavelength 540 nm was used to determine the concentration of hemoglobin in the contaminated middle ear specimens. Prior to the measurement, each specimen was completely hemolyzed employing the Unopette system.* The concentration of hemoglobin in whole blood was found from standard tables and by comparison the concentration of blood in the middle ear specimen was calculated. Accordingly, the measured concentration of cefaclor in the blood of the child was used to adjust the concentration in the middle ear specimen.

The culture materials from the external ear canal and from the middle ear effusion were inoculated onto chocolate agar, 5% sheep blood agar, MacConkey agar, and Columbia CNA agar with sheep blood, and also onto trypticase soy broth and thioglycolate broth. The plates were placed in a CO_2 jar and incubated for 18 to 48 hours. If there was no growth on agar after 48 hours the plates were discarded, but the two broth cultures were kept for a total of ten days each.

*Becton-Dickinson, Rutherford, NJ.

RESULTS

Of the 87 middle ear aspirates, 56 were classified as mucoid and 19 were serous; the remaining 12 specimens were obtained from dry middle ears by saline washings. Bacterial cultures were performed on 83 of these specimens, where 68 showed no bacterial growth in ten days. Of the remaining 15 aspirates, 9 contained *Hemophilus influenzae* (7 were untypable), 3 had *Staphylococcus epidermidis*, 1 had *Streptococcus pyogenes*, 1 had *Corynebacteria*, and 1 had *Pseudomonas*. These organisms were found only in the middle ear specimens, thus excluding the contamination possibility due to external ear canal bacterial flora.

The serum and the middle ear aspirate concentrations of cefaclor at the various time intervals after the administration of the drug are shown in Figure 1. The peak serum levels were observed after 30 minutes and the peak middle ear levels were around one hour after the administration of the drug. After four hours, there were no detectable levels of cefaclor, both in serum and middle ear specimens. The middle ear concentration of cefaclor did not seem to depend on the type of effusion. There were no apparent differences in concentrations for mucoid and serous types of effusions, but none of the 12 specimens obtained from dry middle ears by saline washings contained detectable drug levels.

Table 2 shows the mean concentrations of cefaclor in serum and in middle ear aspirate at different time intervals. Overall, 36 of the 41 serum samples showed detectable levels of cefaclor and 37 of the 87 middle ear specimens had measurable concentrations of the drug. No correlation could be found between the serum and the middle ear concentrations when these samples were matched for the individual subject. There were 76 specimens of MEE which were obtained from 38 patients with bilateral MEE. Of these bilateral cases, 17 pairs had no detectable concentrations for both ears, 15 pairs showed very large differences in concentrations between left and right ears, and only 6 pairs had approximately the same concentration levels for both ears, suggesting that penetration of the drug through the middle ear mucosa was dependent on local conditions.

In this study, 82% of the middle ear cultures were sterile for aerobic bacteria, which was significantly different from previous findings.[2-4] *H influenzae* was the predominant microorganism found in the nonsterile cultures. The nine middle ear specimens with *H influenzae* had high cefaclor

TABLE 2. MEAN CONCENTRATIONS* OF CEFACLOR IN SERUM AND IN MIDDLE EAR ASPIRATE AFTER A SINGLE DOSE (15 mg/kg)

		Time after administration (hours)								
		$^1/_2$	1	$1^1/_2$	2	$2^1/_2$	3	$3^1/_2$	>4	Total
Serum	$\overline{X}$	8.49	7.95	-	3.69	1.36	-	1.31	0	
	S.D.	7.89	5.02	-	2.85	0.62	-	1.45	-	
	+	7	10	2	9	5	0	3	0	36
	N	8	11	2	9	5	1	3	2	41
Middle ear	$\overline{X}$	0.36	0.47	0.28	0.18	0.18	-	0.10	0	
	S.D.	0.51	0.78	0.35	0.36	0.20	-	0.14	-	
	+	8	12	4	6	5	0	2	0	37
	N	16	22	7	16	10	2	5	9	87

*Concentrations in μg/ml.

+ Number of specimens with detectable levels of cefaclor.

concentrations (1.13±1.04 μg/ml). Of interest is that the top five highest cefaclor concentrations were measured in middle ear specimens which had this bacteria, evidencing a better mucosal penetration of the antibiotic in such cases.

DISCUSSION

Contamination of middle ear specimens with blood and dilution of the specimens with saline were the two methodological problems encountered during this study. The measured concentrations of cefaclor in such samples were corrected according to the volume ratio of blood and saline to middle ear aspirate. But in several cases, the accurate determination of the middle ear aspirate volume was almost impossible because of the high viscosity and the small volume (around 100 μl). When saline dilution was required, always a standard volume of 250 μl was added on the sample. In some cases, this would amount to more than two-fold dilution possibly rendering the concentration of the drug in the specimen below the sensitivity of the bioassay method. The viscous mucoid aspirates presented a considerable difficulty during pipette use to spot 20 μl samples onto diffusion disks. Such specimens were processed by dipping the disks in the aspirate and estimating the volume from the dry and wet weight of the disk. Consequently, the measurement of the concentration of cefaclor in the middle ear employing this technique may not be an accurate assessment.

Penetration of different antibiotics into chronic MEE were reported only in a few previous studies.[5-9] Silverstein et al[5], Lahikainen[6] and Lahikainen et al[7] found small amounts of antibiotics (penicillin, oxytetracycline, azidocillin, and ampicillin) in the middle ear after a single dose administration. They contrasted these findings with the concentration levels of antibiotics in acute MEE which were also included in their studies. In the absence of an acute inflammatory process, antibiotic concentrations were generally very low, and unlike the acute cases, the middle ear levels did not correlate with the serum concentrations. In Lahikainen's study[6] of chronic MEE penicillin concentrations, 9 of the 22 specimens (41%) had detectable levels of the antibiotic, which is similar to the findings of the present study of cefaclor (42.5%). Fourfold standard single oral dose[8] and multiple dose[9] studies of antibiotic penetration into chronic effusions showed high levels of concentration, and serum levels were correlated with middle ear levels.

In a recent study, Ginsburg and coworkers[10] measured the concentrations of cefaclor in the MEE of infants and young children with acute otitis media. They reported that approximately 75% of middle ear specimens collected in the first two hours after a 10 mg/kg dose contained more than 0.63 μg/ml of cefaclor. In the present study, six of the nine middle ear specimens from which *H influenzae* was cultured contained more than 0.5 μg/ml of cefaclor.

The clinical implications of the pharmacokinetics and microbiological findings of this study remain to be shown. However, it is significant that cefaclor can penetrate rapidly into the MEE. The efficacy of cefaclor in the treatment of chronic OME can only be established following a controlled double-blind clinical trial.

Dr. Lildholdt is at present at the Odense University Hospital, DK 5000 Odense C, Denmark. Dr. Marshak is at Kaplan Hospital, Rehovot, Israel.

REFERENCES

1. Podoshin L, Persico M, Fradis M. Otitis media with effusion — a steroid and antibiotic therapeutic trial before surgery. Ann Otol Rhinol Laryngol 1978; 87:191-6.

2. Liu YS, Lim DJ, Lang RW, Birck H. Chronic middle ear effusions: immunological and bacteriological investigations. Arch Otolaryngol 1975; 101:278-86.

3. Healy GB, Teele DW. The microbiology of chronic middle ear effusions in children. Laryngoscope 1977; 87:1472-9.

4. Riding KH, Bluestone CD, Michaels RH, Cantekin EI, Doyle WJ, Poziviak CS. Microbiology of recurrent and chronic otitis media with effusion. J Pediatr 1978; 93:739-43.

5. Silverstein H, Bernstein JM, Lerner PI. Antibiotic concentrations in middle ear effusions. Pediatrics 1966; 38:33-9.

6. Lahikainen E. Penicillin concentration in middle ear secretion in otitis. Acta Otolaryngol (Stockh) 1970; 70:358-62.

7. Lahikainen E, Vuori M, Virtanen S. Azidocillin and ampicillin concentration in middle ear effusion. Acta Otolaryngol (Stockh) 1977; 84:227-32.

8. Klimek JJ, Nightingale C, Lehmann WB, Quintiliani R. Comparison of concentrations of amoxicillin and ampicillin in serum and middle ear fluid of children with chronic otitis media. J Infect Dis 1977; 135:999-1002.

9. Sundberg L, Eden T, Ernstson S, Pahlitzsch R. Penetration of erythromycin through respiratory mucosa — a study using secretory otitis media as a model. Acta Otolaryngol (Stockh) 1979; Suppl 365:1-17.

10. Ginsburg CM, McCracken GH, Nelson JD. Pharmacology of oral antibiotics used for treatment of otitis media and tonsillopharyngitis in infants and children. Ann Otol Rhinol Laryngol, 1981 Suppl 84;37-43.

COMPARISON OF CEFACLOR AND AMOXICILLIN FOR ACUTE OTITIS MEDIA WITH EFFUSION

ELLEN M. MANDEL, MD

CHARLES D. BLUESTONE, MD ERDEM I. CANTEKIN, PhD

S. NASRIN GHORBANIAN, MD HOWARD E. ROCKETTE, PhD

PITTSBURGH, PENNSYLVANIA

A double-blind randomized clinical trial was conducted comparing cefaclor and amoxicillin for the treatment of acute otitis media with effusion in 110 children (150 ears). Each child underwent unilateral or bilateral tympanocentesis and then randomly received a 14-day course of either amoxicillin or cefaclor. Of 57 children in the cefaclor group, only 3 children (5.3%) had persistent or recurrent symptoms during the 14-day course of treatment, as compared to 5 of 53 children (9.4%) in the amoxicillin group, but this difference is not significant. After completion of the 14 days of therapy, 45 of 76 ears (59.2%) of the children in the cefaclor group were effusion-free, as compared to only 28 of 64 ears (43.7%) of the children in the amoxicillin group. When adjusted for age and race, this difference is statistically significant ($p = .03$). However, the difference between the effect of the two antimicrobials is not statistically significant in children. Cefaclor is a reasonable choice for antimicrobial therapy for acute otitis media with effusion, and from these study findings, it appears that cefaclor may be more effective than amoxicillin in resolving the middle ear effusion at the completion of 14-day therapy.

INTRODUCTION

Otitis media with effusion (OME) is one of the most common infectious diseases of infants and children. In fact, OME was the most frequent illness reported in a survey of office visits to pediatricians.[1]

Rational therapy for acute OME depends upon the physician having some knowledge of the bacteria that have been isolated from middle ear effusions. In a review of the literature Bluestone and Shurin[2] found that *Streptococcus pneumoniae* has been cultured from about 50% of effusions and is the most common causative agent in all age groups. *Hemophilus influenzae* causes approximately 20% of cases, while β-hemolytic *Streptococcus pyogenes* causes less than 5%, and *Staphylococcus aureus* has been isolated from only a small percentage of cases. *Branhamella catarrhalis*, isolated in from 1 to 8% of cases, has been considered by some to be a pathogen.[3,4] In about 25% of cases, the effusion is sterile.

The clinician is rarely certain of the causative organism before initiating therapy for acute OME. Therefore, ampicillin (or its analog, amoxicillin) has been the single most popular drug since it usually is effective against the three most commonly encountered bacteria, *S pneumoniae, H influenzae*, and *S pyogenes*. However, an increasing incidence of acute OME due to ampicillin-resistant strains of *H influenzae* has been reported. Schwartz et al[5] found that at least 8% of all cases of acute OME in the Washington DC area were caused by ampicillin-resistant strains of *H influenzae*. The combined problem of the increasing incidence of ampicillin-resistant *H influenzae* cases and the ineffectiveness of ampicillin against the occasional *S aureus* cases has led to the search for a more effective antimicrobial agent, primarily among the cephalosporins. When cephalexin monohydrate was tested for ear disease, it was found to be relatively ineffective against *H influenzae*.[6,7]

Cefaclor, however, appears to be effective in the management of acute OME. In vitro studies have shown *H influenzae* to be more sensitive to cefaclor than to the older cephalosporins.[8] With the increasing development of resistance of *H influenzae* and *S pneumoniae* to the penicillins, cefaclor could increasingly become useful in the treatment of acute OME. It would be more advantageous than trimethoprim-sulfamethoxazole, which may not be efficacious when *S pyogenes* is the etiologic agent.[9]

In an attempt to determine the efficacy of cefaclor in treating infants and children who have acute symptomatic OME, a double-blind, randomized, clinical trial of cefaclor compared with amoxicillin has been conducted at Children's Hospital of Pittsburgh.

METHODS

Children who were between 7 months and 16 years of age and who were suspected of having acute OME by the house staff in the ambulatory care facilities were evaluated by pneumatic otoscopy and tympanometry. Otoscopic criteria for the diagnosis of acute OME were the presence of erythema, white opacification (other than scarring), or both, of the tympanic membrane, accompanied by fullness or bulging and impaired mobility of the membrane. At least one of the associated symptoms of acute OME, such as otalgia or irritability or fever, was also present.

Subjects were excluded from the study for any of the following reasons: 1) underlying serious disease, 2) concomitant infection

From the Department of Otolaryngology, University of Pittsburgh School of Medicine and Children's Hospital of Pittsburgh, and the University of Pittsburgh Graduate School of Public Health. This study was supported in part by a grant from Eli Lilly and Company, Indianapolis.

REPRINTS — Ellen M. Mandel, MD, Department of Otolaryngology, Children's Hospital of Pittsburgh, 125 DeSoto Street, Pittsburgh, PA 15213.

TABLE 1. POPULATION CHARACTERISTICS

	Cefaclor		Amoxicillin		Total	
	Children	Ears	Children	Ears	Children	Ears
Total with acute OME	57	78	53	72	110	150
Age of patients						
7-23 mo	18 (31.6)	25 (32.1)	18 (34.0)	28 (38.9)	36 (32.7)	53 (35.3)
2- 5 yr	28 (49.1)	40 (51.3)	22 (41.5)	25 (34.7)	50 (45.5)	65 (43.3)
6-12 yr	10 (17.5)	12 (15.4)	12 (22.6)	18 (25.0)	22 (20.0)	30 (20.0)
13-16 yr	1 (1.8)	1 (1.3)	1 (1.9)	1 (1.4)	2 (1.8)	2 (1.3)
Sex						
Male	31 (54.4)		32 (60.4)		63 (57.3)	
Female	26 (45.6)		21 (39.6)		47 (42.7)	
Race						
Black	27 (47.4)		17 (32.1)		44 (40.0)	
White	30 (52.6)		36 (67.9)		66 (60.0)	
Laterality of disease						
Unilateral	36 (63.2)		34 (64.2)		70 (63.6)	
Bilateral	21 (36.8)		19 (35.8)		40 (36.4)	

Numbers in parentheses indicate percentage.

that might interfere with evaluation of drug efficacy, 3) vomiting which might preclude the use of oral medications, 4) need for concurrent use of a second systemic antimicrobial agent, 5) known allergy to the cephalosporins or penicillins, 6) prior tonsillectomy or adenoidectomy or both, 7) medical conditions with a predisposition for OME (eg, cleft palate, Down's syndrome). Previously unsuccessful antimicrobial therapy (other than with amoxicillin or cefaclor) did not exclude the patient from the study. If the clinical history and results of the otoscopic examination qualified the child for the study, the details of the study were described to the child's parents and informed written consent for the child to participate in the study was obtained.

Method of Tympanocentesis. All children with unilateral acute OME underwent a diagnostic tympanocentesis. Those subjects with bilateral acute OME were randomly assigned to have either a unilateral or a bilateral middle ear aspiration at the physician's discretion.

Tympanocentesis was performed in most children without general anesthesia or sedation. With the aid of an otomicroscope or an otoscope with an operating head, the external auditory canal was debrided of cerumen and then a culture of the external canal was obtained with a Calgiswab®* which had been moistened with trypticase soy broth. The canal was then filled with a 70% alcohol solution for one minute,[10] after which the alcohol was removed by aspiration. Using an Alden-Senturia trap† with a No. 18 needle attached, a tympanocentesis was performed in the inferior portion of the tympanic membrane. Care was taken not to close the suction hole in the trap before entering the middle ear. No attempt was made to aspirate any more effusion than was necessary for microbiological assessment. If no effusion was aspirated, the child was excluded from the trial.

Following tympanocentesis, the middle ear aspirate in the collection trap was removed with a sterile cotton swab and placed in the trypticase soy broth.

Bacteriologic Methods. Each of the external and middle ear swabs was inoculated onto chocolate agar, 5% sheep blood agar, Columbia CNA agar, and MacConkey's agar, and also into trypticase soy broth and thioglycolate broth. The plates were incubated in a CO_2 incubator for 18 to 48 hours. If there was no growth on agar after 48 hours the plates were discarded, but the two broth cultures were kept for a period of ten days. Sensitivities of the organisms isolated were tested by the standard Kirby-Bauer disc method. If the organism was found to be resistant to penicillin or ampicillin, it was then tested for β-lactamase.[11]

Antibiotics. Subjects who qualified for the study were randomly assigned to receive either cefaclor or amoxicillin, 40 mg/kg/day

*Falton, Oxnard, Calif.

†Storz Instrument Co., St. Louis.

in three divided doses, for 14 days. No other medication was administered. The drug was to be discontinued if 1) significant adverse effects occurred, 2) the original pathogen(s) was not susceptible to the drug as shown by the results of microbiologic testing, in association with an unsatisfactory clinical response, or 3) an unsatisfactory clinical response necessitated a second tympanocentesis which revealed the presence of a pathogen.

Subsequent Management. Children were re-examined 14 days after entering the study. They also returned whenever the clinical course of the OME warranted follow-up visits. Each examination included an interval history, physical examination with pneumatic otoscopy, and a tympanogram. Positive response to therapy was separated into two types: 1) satisfactory symptomatic or clinical response, and 2) resolution of the OME. A satisfactory clinical response was defined as relief of otalgia and defervescence. If the child had persistent or recurrent otalgia or fever or both after three days of treatment, a repeat tympanocentesis was performed when possible in the manner described previously. The middle ear effusion was then re-examined for organisms.

Resolution of the OME was defined as the absence of OME at the 14-day visit as determined by otoscopy, and tympanometry when possible.

Tympanometry. Tympanograms were obtained using an electroacoustic impedance bridge* and were plotted with an X-Y plotter.† Tympanogram patterns were classified according to the system suggested by Cantekin and Bluestone.[12] The tympanometric variants were based on the degree of tympanic membrane compliance, the air pressure at peak tympanic membrane compliance, and the gradient of the tympanogram curve. The otoscopic diagnosis and tympanometric variants were then combined from which the probability of OME being present could be determined.

Statistical Methods. Proportions were compared using the usual chi-square statistics unless the sample size was too small, in which case Fisher's Exact Test was used. When comparing proportions while adjusting for confounding variables, the Mantel-Haenzel Chi-Square Test with one degree of freedom was used.

RESULTS

One hundred twenty-four patients with acute OME entered the study and underwent tympanocentesis. However, only 110 children returned for the 14-day follow-up visit and it is this group which comprises this report.

As shown in Table 1, the two treatment groups

*Model Z073, Madsen Electronics, Oakville, Ontario, Canada.

†Model 7010A, Hewlett-Packard Medical Instruments, Waltham, Mass.

TABLE 2. CLINICAL (SYMPTOMATIC) RESPONSE OF 110 CHILDREN (150 EARS) DURING 14-DAY ANTIBIOTIC TREATMENT

	Cefaclor		Amoxicillin	
	Children	Ears	Children	Ears
Success	54	74	48	65
Failure	3 (5.3)	4 (5.1)	5 (9.4)	7 (9.7)
Total	57	78	53	72

Numbers in parentheses indicate percentage.

were similar in age and sex. Seventy-eight percent of the children were between 7 months and 5 years of age. Race, however, was unequally distributed; 52.6% of the children in the cefaclor-treated group were white, as compared to 67.9% of the amoxicillin-treated group. The two groups were comparable in the age of onset of first episode of acute OME and frequency of episodes, and allergy history. At the time they entered the study, 48% of the children in the cefaclor group had symptoms of an upper respiratory infection as did 59% of those in the amoxicillin group.

Table 2 compares the clinical responses of the two treatment groups. Of the 57 children who received cefaclor, only 3 children (4 ears) remained symptomatic or had recurrence of symptoms after the first three days of treatment. No organisms had been isolated initially from these four ears and these ears were again sterile when the tympanocenteses were repeated. However, of the 53 children who received amoxicillin, 5 (7 ears) remained symptomatic or had recurrence of symptoms while on the drug, and in 4 children (6 ears), tympanocentesis was repeated; this difference is not statistically significant ($p>0.2$). At the time of initial tympanocentesis pathogenic bacteria had been isolated from these ears but none had bacteria isolated on repeat tympanocentesis although symptomatic. One child in the amoxicillin group with recurrence of symptoms did not have a repeat tympanocentesis. This child had *S pneumoniae* isolated initially from one ear and had an intact tympanic membrane three days after initial tympanocentesis. She returned ten days after entry into the trial and was found to have a spontaneously perforated tympanic membrane and purulent otorrhea, from which *H influenzae* type B, resistant to ampicillin, was isolated. Her treatment was then changed to cefaclor and she remained asymptomatic. In no child was either amoxicillin or cefaclor discontinued because of side effects.

In addition to symptomatic response, the two treatment groups were compared as to presence or absence of OME at the end of antibiotic treatment. Presence or absence of OME at 14 days related to the initial middle ear aspirate is shown in Table 3. The organisms initially isolated from the two groups are comparable with the exception that all the ampicillin-resistant organisms (*H influenzae* in three ears, *S aureus* in one) were isolated from middle ear aspirates in the cefaclor group. No cefaclor-resistant organisms were found, but one child had ampicillin-resistant *H influenzae* bilaterally which was only intermediately sensitive to cefaclor. More than one pathogen was isolated from four ears. Of 16 children undergoing bilateral tympanocentesis, 8 had the same culture result in both ears; 7 had a pathogen isolated from one ear while the other ear was sterile, and one child had two pathogens in one ear but only one of these pathogens in the other ear. Twenty-four ears were diagnosed as having acute OME but tympanocentesis was not performed on these ears. When grouped by middle ear isolate, most groups are too small to make any meaningful comparisons. The larger groups (those with *S pneumoniae* and those that were sterile or contained

TABLE 3. PRESENCE OR ABSENCE OF OME AFTER 14 DAYS OF TREATMENT RELATED TO INITIAL MIDDLE EAR ISOLATE AND ANTIBIOTIC RECEIVED

	Cefaclor				Amoxicillin				
	OME	No OME	P or E*	Total	OME	No OME	P or E*	Total	Total Ears
Isolate									
S pneumoniae	10	14	1	25	11	12	2	25	50 (39.7)
H influenzae (S)†	4	2	0	6	7	2	3	12	18 (14.3)
H influenzae (R)§	1	2	0	3	0	0	0	0	3 (2.4)
S pyogenes	1	2	0	3	2	3	1	6	9 (7.1)
S aureus (R)	0	1	0	1	0	0	0	0	1 (0.8)
B catarrhalis	0	4	0	4	2	0	0	2	6 (4.8)
H influenzae (S) & *S pneumoniae*	0	1	0	1	1	0	0	1	2 (1.6)
B catarrhalis & *S pneumoniae*	1	0	0	1	0	0	0	0	1 (0.8)
S pyogenes & *S pneumoniae*	0	1	0	1	0	0	0	0	1 (0.8)
Sterile or nonpathogen	11	7	1	19	7	9	0	16	35 (27.8)
All ears receiving tympanocentesis	28 (45.2)	34 (54.8)	2	64	30 (53.6)	26 (46.4)	6	62	126 (100.0)
Ears with acute OME not receiving tympanocentesis	3	11	0	14	6	2	2	10	24
Total all ears	31 (40.8)	45 (59.2)	2	78	36 (56.3)	28 (43.7)	8	72	150

*Perforation or excluded.

†S - Ampicillin sensitive.

§R - Ampicillin resistant.

Numbers in parentheses indicate percentage.

TABLE 4. PRESENCE OR ABSENCE OF OME AT 14 DAYS RELATED TO AGE, RACE, AND ANTIBIOTIC RECEIVED IN 140 EVALUABLE EARS*

	White				*Black*				*Total*				
	Cefaclor		*Amoxicillin*		*Cefaclor*		*Amoxicillin*		*Cefaclor*		*Amoxicillin*		
	OME	*No OME*	*OME*	*No OME*	*OME*	*No OME*	*OME*	*No OME*	*OME*	*No OME*	*OME*	*No OME*	*Significance*†
7-23 mo	4	5	12	2	11	3	8	1	15(65.2)	8(34.8)	20(87.0)	3(13.0)	p = .17
2-5 yr	7	16	8	6	5	12	5	4	12(30.0)	28(70.0)	13(56.5)	10(43.5)	p = .08
6-16 yr	2	7	3	14	2	2	0	1	4(30.8)	9(70.0)	3(16.7)	15(83.3)	p>0.2
Total	13 (31.7)	28 (68.3)	23 (51.1)	22 (48.9)	18 (51.4)	17 (48.6)	13 (68.4)	6 (31.6)	31 (40.8)	45 (59.2)	36 (56.3)	28 (43.7)	p = .07§

*Nonevaluable ears are those with a perforation, or those that required a tympanocentesis or change in antibiotic treatment prior to 14-day visit.

†For age groups only.

§When adjusted for both age and race, then p = .03.

Numbers in parentheses indicate percentage.

nonpathogenic organisms) are similar in the numbers of ears with OME present after 14 days of treatment. Interestingly, all four ears with *B catarrhalis* of the children receiving cefaclor were effusion-free at 14 days but the two ears with this organism in the amoxicillin group had the persistent effusion.

When the ears receiving tympanocentesis are compared in regard to treatment, a higher percentage of ears of children in the cefaclor-treated group were effusion-free, but the difference between the two treatment groups is not statistically significant. When the ears with acute OME that did not receive tympanocentesis are compared, a significant proportion of ears of children in the cefaclor-treated group had no effusion after treatment ($p = 0.04$). Overall, 59.2% of the evaluable ears* in the cefaclor group were effusion-free at 14 days as compared to 43.7% of ears in the amoxicillin group, but this difference is not statistically significant. Table 4 shows the OME status at 14 days as related to antibiotic received, age, and race. When age only is considered, there is no statistically significant difference between the two antibiotics for any individual age group or for total ears ($p = 0.07$). When race alone is considered, more ears of the white children in both treatment groups had no OME at 14 days ($p = .10$). Adjusting for race, there was a significantly higher percentage of ears without OME in the cefaclor-treated group ($p = .05$). When the 14-day status in regard to presence or absence of effusion is adjusted for both age and race, the difference between the cefaclor- and amoxicillin-treated groups is significant ($p = 0.03$).

*Ears with perforations at the 14-day visit were excluded from analysis as to the presence or absence of OME, as were ears that received a tympanocentesis or a change in antibiotic treatment before the 14-day visit due to persistent or recurrent symptoms.

Table 5 summarizes the middle ear status of the children after 14 days of treatment, separated into whether they had unilateral or bilateral OME upon entry into the study. Nineteen of 34 patients (55.9%) with unilateral acute OME who received cefaclor treatment were effusion-free as compared to only 14 of 32 patients (43.8%) on amoxicillin who were effusion-free after treatment. Of those children with bilateral disease, 15 of 21 (71.4%) on cefaclor had no effusion in either ear or only one ear with persistent OME as compared to only 8 of 16 children (50%) on amoxicillin; however, these differences are not statistically significant.

Information regarding the recurrence of symptomatic acute OME during the 28-day period following the end of antibiotic treatment was available on 49 children in the cefaclor-treated group and 35 children in the amoxicillin-treated group. Four children in each group had a recurrence.

CONCLUSIONS

Microbiologically, our study population is representative of acute OME; the percentages of isolates are consistent with those reported in the literature.[2] We found that cefaclor was at least as effective as amoxicillin in relieving the clinical symptoms of the disease; although there were fewer persistently symptomatic children in the cefaclor-treated group as compared to the amoxicillin group, the difference is not statistically significant. When the mid-

TABLE 5. PRESENCE OR ABSENCE OF OME AT 14 DAYS RELATED TO LATERALITY OF DISEASE AND ANTIBIOTIC RECEIVED (N = 103 CHILDREN)*

	Status at 14 Days							
	Cefaclor				*Amoxicillin*			
	Bilateral OME	*Unilateral OME*	*No OME*	*Total Children*	*Bilateral OME*	*Unilateral OME*	*No OME*	*Total Children*
Status at entry								
Unilateral	—	15	19	34	—	18	14	32
Bilateral	6	4	11	21	8	2	6	16
Total children	6	19	30	55	8	20	20	48

*Excluded from analysis are 2 children in the cefaclor-treated group with unilateral disease and 5 children in the amoxicillin-treated group, 2 with unilateral disease and 3 with bilateral disease.

dle ear status following antimicrobial therapy was examined, there were fewer ears with OME in the children in the cefaclor-treated group; when adjusted for age and race, the difference between the two antimicrobials is statistically significant. Of interest is the consistent difference in OME status at 14 days between white and black children regardless of treatment. The reasons for this difference are not clear; among those to be considered are differences in anatomy,[13] drug compliance (which was not measured in the present study) and socioeconomic status.

Also encouraging is the fact that cefaclor was effective in the cases of acute OME in which ampicillin-resistant organisms had been isolated; none of the children was persistently symptomatic after the third day of treatment and three of the four ears of these children were also effusion-free after 14 days of treatment. From this clinical trial, cefaclor is a reasonable choice for the treatment of acute OME. Fewer children were symptomatic after three days of treatment, and significantly fewer ears had residual effusion after a 14-day course of cefaclor as compared to children treated with amoxicillin.

ACKNOWLEDGMENT — The authors wish to thank Richard H. Michaels, MD; Dale D. Rohn, BA; M. Christine Wright, RN; and Mary Ann Fagan, RN, for their clinical assistance, and Suzanne Stewart and Bibi Hill for their assistance in the preparation of the manuscript.

REFERENCES

1. Koch H, Dennison NJ. Office visits to pediatricians. National Ambulatory Medical Care Service, National Center for Health Statistics, Washington, DC, 1974.

2. Bluestone CD, Shurin PA. Middle ear disease in children: pathogenesis, diagnosis, and management. Ped Clin North Am 1974; 21:379-400.

3. Coffey JD Jr, Martin AD, Booth HN. *Neisseria catarrhalis* in exudate otitis media. Arch Otolaryngol 1967; 86:403-6.

4. Halstead C, Lepow ML, Balassanian N, Emmerich J, Wolinsky E. Otitis media: clinical observations, microbiology, and evaluation of therapy. Am J Dis Child 1968; 115:542-51.

5. Schwartz RH, Rodriguez W, Khan W, Ross S. The increasing incidence of ampicillin-resistant *Haemophilus influenzae*. A cause of otitis media. JAMA 1978; 239:320-3.

6. McLinn SE, Daly JF Jr, Jones JE. Cephalexin monohydrate suspension. Treatment of otitis media. JAMA 1975; 234:171-3.

7. Stechenberg BW, Anderson D, Chang MJ, et al. Cephalexin compared to ampicillin treatment of otitis media. Pediatrics 1976; 58:532-6.

8. Sinai R, Hammerberg S, Marks MI, Pai CH. "In vitro" susceptibility of *Haemophilus influenzae* to sulfamethoxazole-trimethoprim and cefaclor, cephalexin and cephardine. Antimicrob Agents Chemother 1978; 13:861-4.

9. Trickett PC, Dineen P, Mogabgab W. Trimethoprim-sulfamethoxazole versus penicillin G in the treatment of group A beta-hemolytic streptococcal pharyngitis and tonsillitis. J Infect Dis 1973; 128:693-5.

10. Riding KH, Bluestone CD, Michaels RH, Cantekin EI, Doyle WJ, Poziviak CS. Microbiology of recurrent and chronic otitis media with effusion. J Pediatr 1978; 93:739-43.

11. Rosen IG, Jacobson J, Rudderman R. Rapid capillary tube method for detecting penicillin resistance in *Staphylococcus aureus*. Appl Microbiol 1972; 23:649-50.

12. Cantekin EI, Bluestone CD. Identification of otitis media with effusion in children. Ann Otol Rhinol Laryngol 1980; 89 Suppl 68:190-5.

13. Doyle WJ. A functiono-anatomic description of eustachian tube vector relations in four ethnic populations: an osteologic study. Doctoral Dissertation, University of Pittsburgh, 1977.

ANTIMICROBIAL PROPHYLAXIS FOR RECURRENT ACUTE OTITIS MEDIA

JACK L. PARADISE, MD

PITTSBURGH, PENNSYLVANIA

Antimicrobial prophylaxis for children who have frequently recurring, severe episodes of acute otitis media appears to constitute a reasonable management option, even though it is not yet clear whether the advantages outweigh the disadvantages and risks. It remains for well-designed and well-executed studies that extend over relatively long periods to indicate whether this approach to management is the best of the available options, and if so, which of the available drugs is preferable.

The attempt to prevent otitis media by administering antimicrobial drugs involves certain principles, concerns, and unanswered questions which deserve review.

WHY PREVENT OTITIS MEDIA?

The potential benefits to children to be derived from preventing otitis media are summarized in Table 1, and most of them are self-evident. Specifically with regard to long-range sequelae, while suppurative forms of otitis media still sometimes result in permanent middle ear damage, the frequency of this occurrence has of course declined markedly since antimicrobial treatment for ear infection has become routine. Of greater interest currently is the question whether the hearing impairment that accompanies persistent *nonsuppurative* (secretory or serous) otitis media early in life can result in developmental impairments that persist into later childhood, long after normal hearing has been recovered.[1] The evidence favoring this proposition is in my judgment insubstantial, and much research will be required in order eventually to clarify the issue. In the meantime, I would suggest extreme skepticism about assertions to the effect that if an infant or young child experiences two or three months of middle ear effusion he is thereby at risk of becoming learning-disabled or language-impaired.

TABLE 1. REASONS FOR ATTEMPTING TO PREVENT EPISODES OF ACUTE OTITIS MEDIA

Reduce pain, fever
Shorten duration of hearing impairment
Reduce cost
MD visits
Surgical procedures
Drugs
Reduce inconvenience
Allay parental anxiety
Prevent long-range sequelae
Middle ear damage
Developmental impairments ?

APPROACHES TO PREVENTING OTITIS MEDIA

A number of approaches to the prevention of otitis media are in current use, and these are summarized in Table 2. Regarding the efficacy of either adenoidectomy or T&A in the prevention of otitis media, we are currently involved in studies designed to answer some aspects of that question,[2,3] but no clear-cut answers are yet available. Regarding ventilating tubes for recurrent acute otitis media, support for their use stems entirely from personal experience rather than published data. Whether recurrences of otitis might be prevented by more liberal use of myringotomy for acute episodes remains an untested hypothesis. Antimicrobial prophylaxis is the principal subject of the present report and will be considered in detail below. Finally, there is hope that polyvalent pneumococcal vaccine will prove efficacious in reducing episodes due to the most commonly responsible pathogen, *Streptococcus pneumoniae*. This question is currently being tested in a number of separate studies.

POTENTIAL CANDIDATES FOR PREVENTION

If we think about trying to prevent recurrent acute otitis media, who might be potential candidates for such an endeavor? The landmark study of Kessner et al reminds us that otitis media is a very common disease whose prevalence in the winter months reaches the range of 25 to 30% in the younger age groups.[4] Obviously, prophylaxis should not be considered for such large proportions of the childhood population, but rather for children with

TABLE 2. CURRENT APPROACHES TO THE PREVENTION OF RECURRENT OTITIS MEDIA

Adenoidectomy or T&A
Ventilating tubes
Myringotomy more liberally for acute otitis media
Antimicrobial prophylaxis
Polyvalent pneumococcal vaccine

From the Departments of Pediatrics and Community Medicine, University of Pittsburgh School of Medicine, and the Ambulatory Care Center, Children's Hospital of Pittsburgh.

REPRINTS — Jack L. Paradise, MD, Children's Hospital of Pittsburgh, Pittsburgh, PA 15213.

TABLE 3. CIRCUMSTANCES IN WHICH ANTIMICROBIAL PROPHYLAXIS IS INDICATED OR REASONABLE

1.	Rheumatic heart disease	
2.	Gonococcal ophthalmia	
3.	Prevention of subacute bacterial endocarditis	
4.	Tuberculosis	
5.	Syphilis exposure	
6.	Gonorrhea exposure	
7.	Diphtheria exposure	susceptibles only
8.	Pertussis exposure	susceptibles only
9.	Meningococcal disease exposure	
10.	*H influenzae* type B disease exposure	
11.	Splenectomy/sickle-cell disease	
12.	Compound fractures	
13.	Skull fractures with CSF leak	
14.	Recurrent urinary tract infection	
15.	Contaminated injuries and bites	controversial
16.	Burns	controversial
17.	Intestinal surgery	controversial

frequent recurrences in the recent past. Reasonable criteria might be three episodes of acute suppurative otitis media in the preceding six months or four episodes in the preceding year.

Also presenting as reasonable candidates for prevention are particular populations, such as Eskimo and American Indian children, who are very prone to develop severe recurrent disease. In a survey of British Columbia Indians of all ages, 45% were found to have had previous otitis media, and 16% had currently active infection.[5] Of a group of Baffin Island Eskimo children under 10 years of age, 31% were found to have actively draining ears.[6] In a group of Western Alaskan Eskimo infants, 38% had developed at least one episode of draining ears within the first year of life, and 19% had experienced their initial episode prior to four months of age[7] — extraordinary statistics when compared with those of populations most of us are accustomed to dealing with. And, in a group of South Dakota Indian school children, those with either acute or chronic otitis media comprised about 30% of the population studied.[8]

Finally, we might include a group of children who for one reason or another had received tympanostomy tubes, and who then develop frequent episodes of purulent otorrhea — indicating middle ear infection — through the tubes. Especially susceptible in this category are infants with cleft palate.

ESTABLISHED OR REASONABLE INDICATIONS FOR ANTIMICROBIAL PROPHYLAXIS

Although in pediatric circles antimicrobial prophylaxis has a rather dubious reputation in general, it is important to recall that in a number of circumstances antimicrobial prophylaxis is accepted as either standard or at least reasonable procedure (Table 3). Some of these circumstances are well established and require no comment here. Regarding tuberculosis, while there may be some controversy, most authorities consider it advisable to administer isoniazid (INH) to the patient who converts from a negative to a positive tuberculin test, not in order to treat the infection underlying that phenomenon, but rather to prevent the development of tuberculous complications such as meningitis or miliary tuberculosis. Antimicrobial prophylaxis is appropriately administered to patients exposed to syphilis or gonorrhea, particularly to individuals who have been raped, and also to susceptible patients (those not previously immunized fully) who have been exposed to either diphtheria or pertussis. In patients who have sickle-cell disease, or who have received splenectomy, antimicrobial prophylaxis in an effort to prevent pneumococcal infection is standard. Finally, there is a group of conditions in which, allowing for some controversy, there is reason to believe that antimicrobial prophylaxis might be appropriate. These conditions include recurrent urinary tract infection, contaminated injuries and bites, severe burns, and intestinal surgery.

Of the 17 items listed in Table 3, the first 11 involve protection against infection with a single organism, rather than the multiple organisms capable of causing otitis media. This difference may or may not be important, but seems worthwhile to keep in mind.

NONINDICATIONS FOR ANTIMICROBIAL PROPHYLAXIS

There are a number of circumstances in which antimicrobial prophylaxis has been found to be ineffective, specifically in common viral respiratory infections and in measles.[9]

POTENTIAL PROBLEMS OF ANTIMICROBIAL PROPHYLAXIS FOR OTITIS MEDIA

Potential problems of long-term prophylaxis include, of course, the emergence of resistant strains of bacteria on the one hand, and the occurrence of adverse drug reactions on the other. However, an issue that has probably not received sufficient attention is the possibility that, as a result of antimicrobial agents having been administered, symptoms of otitis media may be suppressed and the disease masked rather than having been eliminated or reduced. We would like to be confident that the main effect of prophylaxis is not to generate a population of children with middle ear effusion that is asymptomatic and therefore not likely to be detected.

REPORTED STUDIES OF PROPHYLAXIS FOR OTITIS MEDIA

In considering what might be accomplished with antimicrobial prophylaxis, it seems important to consider carefully the four studies reported to date.[7,10-12]

TABLE 4. SUMMARY RESULTS OF THE ENSIGN ET AL STUDY[10] OF SULFAMETHOXYPYRIDAZINE PROPHYLAXIS

History of Otorrhea in Previous Years	Antimicrobial Reportedly Administered	N	Proportion of Children Who Developed Earache Only	Otorrhea
No	Regularly	34	0%	0%
(N = 91)	Irregularly	15	7%	0%
	Little or none	42	14%	10%
Yes	Regularly	18	11%	6%
(N = 29)	Irregularly	3	0%	0%
	Little or none	8	25%	38%

The Ensign et al Study.[10] This study was carried out among Indian children under 11 years of age in Montana. The drug used was one no longer commercially available, sulfamethoxypyridazine, a long-acting sulfonamide popular at the time for treating urinary tract infection. A single dose was administered three times a week to older children, and twice a week to infants weighing less than 20 pounds. The study was not controlled; rather, every accessible child in the population was advised to take the drug. The subsequent occurrence of otitis was not monitored directly, but was based on parental accounts.

The authors divided the population into two groups (Table 4). The first group contained 91 children who had not had a history of otorrhea in previous years, while the second group consisted of 29 children who had had a history of otorrhea in previous years, and who were therefore considered to be at greater risk. In each group, some children reportedly took the drug regularly, some reportedly took it irregularly, and some apparently stopped the drug after a short period or did not take it at all. In both groups, among those who reportedly took the drug regularly or irregularly, there was relatively little middle ear disease, whereas among those who essentially failed to take the drug, much larger proportions developed earache or otorrhea or both.

The Maynard et al Study.[7] This study involved a group of Western Alaskan infants and children less than 7 years of age. Children $2^1/_2$ years of age or older were given 250 mg of ampicillin once daily; those younger were given half that amount. The design involved a one-year-long, double-blind trial of drug versus placebo. The subjects in the two treatment groups were carefully matched for family size, age, sex, and prior otitis history. An episode of otitis media was defined as the occurrence of otorrhea as reported by parents, after a two-week-free interval. Of interest was the fact that, prior to entry into the trial, the tympanic membranes were deemed normal in only 15% of the ampicillin group and only 12% of the placebo group. The study group as a whole thus already had been severely affected with middle ear disease before entry into the study.

Table 5 summarizes the study's findings. Of those

TABLE 5. SUMMARY RESULTS OF THE MAYNARD ET AL STUDY[7] OF AMPICILLIN PROPHYLAXIS

No. of Episodes in 1 Yr	Proportion of Subjects Experiencing Episodes of Otitis Media, Treatment Group: Ampicillin (N = 173)	Placebo (N = 191)	P
≥ 1	24%	40%	< .005
≥ 3	4%	11%	< .05

who received ampicillin only 24% (42 of 173) developed at least one new episode of otorrhea, as compared with 40% of those receiving placebo. Three or more episodes of otorrhea were experienced by only 4% of the ampicillin-treated group compared with 11% of the placebo-treated group.

The Perrin et al Study.[11] This study involved 54 children, ranging in age from 11 months to 8 years, who were enrolled in a suburban Rochester, New York, practice conducted by four pediatricians. Eligibility for entering the study consisted of at least three episodes of otitis media in the preceding 18 months, or at least five episodes at any time in the course of a lifetime. This entry criterion seems not very stringent — five episodes of otitis media over a period of eight years is probably not a great deal more than average — and therefore allows for considerable heterogeneity in the study population. The antimicrobial used was sulfisoxazole (Gantrisin®); 0.5 g was administered, irrespective of age, twice daily. The study extended over a six-month period from December to May, and the method involved a double-blind comparison between sulfisoxazole and placebo, in a cross-over design. Thus during the first three months of the study half the subjects received sulfisoxazole and the other half, placebo; during the second three months the treatments were reversed. The subjects were examined every six weeks. An episode of acute otitis media was defined by whatever criteria each individual physician used for making that diagnosis; the criteria were not specified.

Table 6 summarizes the results of the study. Of the 54 children, 4 experienced one or more episodes of acute otitis media during the combined three-month periods while receiving sulfisoxazole, compared with 21 children who experienced one or more episodes while receiving placebo. With regard to the otitis media attack rate, there was a sevenfold advantage favoring the sulfisoxazole group. The reduction in attack rate was, however, significant only in the children less than 6 years of age. Above that age there was no substantial difference, per-

TABLE 6. SUMMARY RESULTS OF THE PERRIN ET AL STUDY[11] OF SULFISOXAZOLE PROPHYLAXIS

	Sulfisoxazole	Placebo	P
Children with ≥ 1 episode in 3 mo period	4/54	21/54	< .02
Attack rate: Episodes/child/6 mo	0.15	1.05	< .001

TABLE 7. SUMMARY RESULTS OF THE BIEDEL STUDY[12] OF SULFONAMIDE PROPHYLAXIS

Symptomatic Otitis Recurrence Rate with New URI, Weeks 2-8		
Sulfonamide	*Decongestant*	*P*
4/71 (5.6%)	15/76 (20%)	<.001

haps because, for such older children, the dose of sulfisaxazole had not been adequate.

The Biedel Study.[12] The fourth reported study dealt with children recently recovered fully from an attack of acute otitis media. Diagnostic criteria involved the use of pneumatic otoscopy. A sulfonamide, in most instances sulfisoxazole, was compared with an oral decongestant, considered a "control" drug. The period of study extended for eight weeks. The design involved treating each child at the onset of symptoms of a new episode of upper respiratory infection (URI) with either sulfonamide or decongestant for the duration of respiratory symptoms and for a minimum of six days. The treatment regimens were alternated with succeeding subjects: one sulfa, one control, etc. The study was neither single- nor double-blind: ie, both the parents and the physician knew which drug was being taken. Children who developed symptoms that appeared indicative of middle ear disease were brought for examination, but otherwise no systematic examinations were carried out.

The results of the study are shown in Table 7. The first week after the initiation of treatment was excluded from consideration because of the possibility that otitis found during this period might represent a flare-up of prior infection rather than a new episode. Among the 71 children for whom sulfonamide was prescribed at the onset of URI there were 4 symptomatic otitis recurrences; by contrast, among the 76 children in the decongestant group, there were 15 otitis recurrences.

LIMITATIONS OF THE STUDIES

The limitations common to all of these studies can be summarized as follows. First, since the studies were designed to detect only symptomatic episodes, they do not provide data concerning the possible occurrence of episodes of acute suppurative otitis media that were not accompanied by symptoms. Certainly such cases are a matter of common experience. Secondly, the studies provide no data directly or indirectly about middle ear effusion, and there is concern that the antimicrobial agents used might have served merely to suppress symptoms without actually preventing infection or inhibiting inflammation. Finally, the longest period of follow-up in any of the studies was one year, a period much shorter than the duration of risk for most children severely affected by recurrent otitis media, and therefore too short a period on which to base estimates of the risks and problems deriving from prophylaxis, particularly the emergence of resistant strains of bacteria, and the potential toxicity of drugs.

TABLE 8. PRINCIPAL UNTOWARD REACTIONS TO SULFONAMIDES

Fever
Rash
Granulocytopenia
Aplastic anemia
Stevens-Johnson syndrome
Urticaria
Nausea
Hepatitis
Headache
Behavior or mood disorders
Vasculitis
Nephrosis
Hemolysis in patients with glucose-6-phosphate-dehydrogenase deficiency

CURRENT RECOMMENDATIONS

Despite the limitations of the data available, antimicrobial prophylaxis currently appears to constitute a reasonable management option for children who have extraordinary difficulty with recurrent acute infection, ie, who may recover from one severe episode, often slowly or incompletely, only to develop another. (For such children, myringotomy and tympanostomy tube insertion is sometimes undertaken, but that method remains unsupported by data and is attended by risks of other types, and in any case is beyond the scope of the present discussion). If the physician decides to embark on prophylaxis, which children are proper candidates, and which drug should be used? As mentioned earlier, three episodes of acute otitis in six months or four episodes in one year seems a reasonable minimum criterion. The drugs that have been tested most are the sulfonamides, but sulfonamides are by no means entirely innocuous. Although side-effects occur relatively infrequently, they include some that are serious and some that may be fatal; a partial listing is shown in Table 8. An alternative drug that seems worthy of consideration is penicillin G. While some bacteria are resistant to penicillin G and others may develop resistance, penicillin G when administered orally has the advantages of being 1) relatively free of serious side effects, 2) inexpensive, and 3) probably relatively efficacious against most strains of *Hemophilus influenzae* — in vitro six or eight times as efficacious as penicillin V.[13] Pending further studies, either sulfisoxazole or penicillin G or ampicillin would appear to be acceptable agents to try.

REFERENCES

1. Paradise JL. Review article: otitis media in infants and children. Pediatrics 1980; 65:917-43.

2. Paradise JL. Clinical trials of tonsillectomy and adenoidectomy: limitations of existing studies and a current effort to

evaluate efficacy. South Med J 1976; 69:1049-53.

3. Paradise JL, Bluestone CD. Toward rational indications for tonsil and adenoid surgery. Hosp Practice 1976; 11(2):79-87.

4. Kessner DM, Snow CK, Singer J. Assessment of medical care for children: contrasts in health status. Vol. 3. Washington, DC: Institute of Medicine, National Academy of Sciences, 1974:38-54.

5. Cambon K, Galbraith JD, Kong G. Middle ear disease in Indians of the Mount Currie Reservation, British Columbia. Can Med Assoc J 1965; 93:1301-5.

6. Ling D, McCoy RH, Levinson ED. The incidence of middle ear disease and its educational implications among Baffin Island Eskimo children. Am J Public Health 1969; 60:385-90.

7. Maynard JE, Fleshman JK, Tschopp CF. Otitis media in Alaskan Eskimo children. Prospective evaluation of chemoprophylaxis. JAMA 1972; 219:597-9.

8. Gregg JB, Steele JP, Clifford S, et al. A multidisciplinary study of ear disease in South Dakota Indian children. SD J Med 1970; 23:11-20.

9. Davis SD, Wedgwood RJ. Antibiotic prophylaxis in acute viral respiratory disease. Am J Dis Child 1965; 109:544-53.

10. Ensign PR, Urbanich EM, Morgan M. Prophylaxis for otitis media in an Indian population. Am J Public Health 1960; 50:195-9.

11. Perrin JM, Charney E, MacWhinney JB Jr, et al. Sulfisoxazole as chemoprophylaxis for recurrent otitis media: a double-blind crossover study in pediatric practice. N Engl J Med 1974; 291:664-7.

12. Biedel CS. Modification of recurrent otitis media by short-term sulfonamide therapy. Am J Dis Child 1978; 132:681-3.

13. Klein JO, Finland M. The new penicillins. N Engl J Med 1963; 260:1019-25.

ANTIMICROBIAL THERAPY FOR CHRONIC SUPPURATIVE OTITIS MEDIA

David N. F. Fairbanks, MD
Washington, D. C.

In chronic draining ear associated with a tympanic membrane perforation and/or cholesteatoma, the infection is that of bacterial contamination. Both aerobic and anaerobic organisms are found, notably *Pseudomonas*, *Staphylococcus*, and enteric organisms, particularly *Bacteroides*. The disease exists because of a structural defect in the middle ear cleft, which requires surgery as definitive treatment. Medical therapy is valuable as a temporary measure, in preoperative preparation, and in prevention and management of intracranial extension. Topical therapy with antibiotic ear drops is often helpful, but also important is local care with cleansing, drying, and antiseptic solutions or powders. Therapy is usually directed against the *Pseudomonas* organism with aminoglycosides and polymyxins, but *Bacteroides fragilis* now looms as an important pathogen in 13% of affected patients, requiring chloramphenicol. Since drugs directed against *Bacteroides* are ineffective against *Pseudomonas*, and vice versa, there is no one agent we can rely upon for treatment of both. What we are all looking for, of course, is that brand new antibiotic the FDA hasn't released yet: "panaceamycin." It hasn't even been developed yet. None of the ones we have are a panacea; and until we get one, we will have to stick with what we have, exercise clinical judgment, and base our antibiotic selections on, if not proven culture results, then at least established microbial probabilities.

INTRODUCTION

In a 1928 report from the University Clinic in Basel recounting 25,000 clinic visits for acute and chronic otitis media in a 30-year period,[1] eighty-six patients died of intracranial complications. That figures to almost three deaths per year from otitis media. Today, of course, this situation has changed dramatically. The impact of antibiotics has been tremendous on the practice of otolaryngology and on the course of diseases in our patients.

However, if we are to maximize the benefits available to us with such drugs, we need to choose between them with discrimination, with an understanding of the microbial population, and with a knowledge of their indications and limitations.

This is especially true in the chronic draining ear, where the offending organisms can be quite unpredictable, may be difficult to culture, and may be resistant to all acceptable antimicrobials.

PREVALENCE

The incidence of this problem varies considerably, depending on socioeconomic status and race. Eskimos and American Indians have a well-known high incidence. Tschopp's survey of Alaskan native children[2] showed prevalence as high as 12% in the 16-year-old group.

Similar prevalence rates are seen in Australian aboriginal children.[3] But this is not simply a racial problem, since the prevalence of draining ears in poor whites in Appalachia (Kentucky) is more like that of the American Indians than that of their middle-class American white contemporaries. Even among our affluent patients, this is not a rare disease.

CLINICAL ENTITIES

Two distinctly different anatomical defects in the tympanic structures predispose the patient to chronic suppurative otitis media.

1. Perforation of the tympanic membrane, which exposes the middle ear mucosa to external contamination through the external ear canal.

2. Penetration of the tympanic and mastoid spaces by keratin-producing epithelium (eg, epidermis), which allows accumulation of keratin, which is subject to contamination through the external ear canal. Some 120 years ago, Virchow looked at one of these epidermal inclusion cysts in the mastoid. He saw cholesterol crystals in it and named it "cholesteatoma." Better terms would be "keratoma" or "keratosis of the mastoid and middle ear spaces."

Chronic suppurative otitis media is most often a recurrent rather than a constant infection. Chronicity describes its time of onset and the effects of tissue destruction and scarring rather than the activity level of bacterial invasion.

Although the disease may be quiescent for long periods, it is only a matter of time before contamination occurs, and the exposed middle ear mucosa, or the accumulated cheesy debris of the cholesteatoma, becomes a culture medium for opportunistic bacteria.

MICROBIOLOGY

Occasionally an infection may ascend the eustachian tube from the nose, sinuses, adenoids, or

From the Department of Otolaryngology, George Washington University School of Medicine, Washington, D.C.
Reprints — David N. F. Fairbanks, MD, 2141 K St., N.W., Washington, DC 20037.

TABLE 1. BACTERIOLOGY OF CHOLESTEATOMA[5]

Culture Results	Number	Percent
No growth	4	13
Anaerobes present	20	67
Aerobes present	21	70
Both present	15	50
Aerobes		
P aeruginosa	11	
P fluorescens	2	
Proteus species	4	
E coli	4	
Klebsiella-Enterobacter-Serratia	4	
Streptococcus		
β-hemolytic	2	
α- or μ-hemolytic	5	
faecalis	1	
Alcaligenes-Achromobacter	3	
S aureus	1	
S epidermidis	2	
CDC group F	2	
Anaerobes		
Bacteroides	13	
Peptococcus-Peptostreptococcus	11	
Propionibacterium acnes	8	
Fusobacterium	4	
Bifidobacterium	3	
Clostridium	2	
Eubacterium	2	

pharynx. It will then drain out an open perforation. These will be the usual pneumococcal, streptococcal, or *Hemophilus* organisms. But such is an *acute* infection. The *chronic* draining ear is an infection of contamination from the outside through the external ear canal into the middle ear through the perforation or into the mastoid. Whatever bacteria are available in the outside world can become the invading pathogen. For example, Brooks cultured chronic draining ears of residents in a home for the mentally retarded. The microbiology was characteristically that of fecal contamination.*

The ubiquitous *Pseudomonas aeruginosa* has traditionally been blamed for chronic draining ears, although Friedmann's cultures of 1,500 ears put *Staphylococcus* higher on the list.[4] *Proteus* and *Escherichia coli* are noted in every survey. Until recently these were the organisms generally considered responsible for the chronic draining ear, despite the common observation that the secretions are foul smelling, and smelly pus usually means anaerobic infection. Furthermore, intracranial extension of chronic otitis media, specifically otitic brain abscess, is almost invariably an anaerobic infection. These are compelling reasons to suspect anaerobic organisms in chronic otitis and mastoiditis.

In 1975, Harker and Koontz[5] sampled thirty cholesteatoma ears with both aerobic and strict anaerobic methods (Table 1). Most of the patients were young people. Over 50% of the infections were mixed, with two to five organisms typically present. In nine cases, five or more organisms were identified. Aerobes and anaerobes were present in two thirds of the cases, almost in equal proportions, and half of the cultures had both aerobic and anaerobic growth.

P aeruginosa was the most frequent aerobic organism identified. The rest of the aerobes represent a mixed flora of enteric organisms and numerous others. For anaerobes, *Bacteroides* was most frequently encountered, and this is probably the circumstance in head and neck infections where *B fragilis* can be most frequently cultured. Varieties of the anaerobic *Staphylococcus* and *Streptococcus* were the next most frequent, in various differing colony types. By and large, the organisms identified, both aerobic and anaerobic, are known as aggressive pathogens. When a foul smell was noted preoperatively, multiple organisms were identified, including anaerobes. Pure cultures of *Pseudomonas* in the laboratory do not have a foul smell, whereas anaerobic infections characteristically do. But only 50% of anaerobic strains produce odors. The smell of anaerobic streptococci has been described as foul and putrid. (Other bacterial odors, not from ear infections, include clostridial myonecrosis, which has the sweetish smell like a steak first put on a grill, and diphtheria, which smells like mouse feces.)

MANAGEMENT

Structural defects in an organ interfere with its ability to maintain a normal environment. Just as renal stones predispose the kidney to infections and bronchiectasis to constant contamination of the lung, so do anatomic defects in the ear create an invitation for bacterial propagation. Typically, antibiotics only suppress the organism, or if it is eradicated, a new strain appears. Permanent cure is unlikely as long as the defect remains. Therefore, the definitive care is a surgical correction. Nevertheless, surgery is most successful if the infection is brought under control by medical means. And in patients for whom surgery is unavailable or inadvisable, the ear, chronically draining through a large tympanic perforation, can usually be rendered dry with topical medications. That is not true, however, of cholesteatomas.

The first objective of treatment is to make the environment less hospitable to the organism. Cleansing the area by aspiration helps remove secretions and debris that serve as culture media. Most organisms prefer an alkaline medium; therefore, irrigating solutions and medications should be slightly acidic. Most otic preparations have an acid pH (they contain boric acid or acetic acid) such as Domeboro®, VoSol® and the like. Sultzberger's powder is iodine and boric acid. It provides nonspecific antiseptic activity against bacteria and fungi.

*Brooks I. Personal communication, May 1979.

Gentian violet and Cresylate® are similar nonspecific antiseptics.

Do-it-yourselfers can mix their own ear drops: vinegar as the acid and alcohol as the antiseptic. Alcohol also absorbs the water and dries out the ear. Through an open perforation this may be too painful to use, but it is great for preventing swimmer's ear.

Many otic preparations contain antibiotics. The popular ones are formulated with the aerobic organisms in mind — particularly *Pseudomonas*. Cortisporin® suspension contains polymyxin B and neomycin as antibiotics, hydrocortisone as an antiinflammatory agent, and alcohol in the carrier vehicle. Colymycin® is only slightly different; it contains colistin — which is polymyxin E. It has, again, neomycin and hydrocortisone. It has acetic acid in the carrier. Other preparations such as Otocort® and Otobione® are variations on the same theme. The acetic acid and alcohol sometimes cause burning when they are applied through a perforation, and patients may refuse to use such drops, especially the clear solution of Cortisporin®, which contains hydrochloric acid. An alternative is the ophthalmic preparation of Cortisporin®, which doesn't contain alcohol. Another is ophthalmic gentamicin (Garamycin®), which is, of course, good against *Pseudomonas*.

Neomycin, as the single antibiotic, is found in several preparations (Neo-Cort-Dome®, Otobiotic®). Neomycin has been implicated as a cause of contact dermatitis, but the incidence is much less than it is commonly thought to be. In one study[6] only two patients out of 2,000 who received neomycin-containing ear drops suffered such a reaction, and these were patients whose chronic otitis had required ear drop treatments for many years, so that they had probably experienced considerable prior exposure to neomycin topically.

We also have otic drops with polymyxin as the single antibiotic (Pyocidin®, Lidosporin®). Polymyxin B and colistin (polymyxin E) are bactericidal to most Gram-negative organisms, notably *P aeruginosa*, *E coli*, *Klebsiella*, and *Enterobacter*. But the spectrum does not include *Proteus* or *B fragilis* or Gram-positive organisms such as *Staphylococcus*, which are often present.

Neomycin, on the other hand, is a broad spectrum antibiotic bactericidal to many pathogens, both Gram-positive and Gram-negative, notably *S aureus* and *Proteus* species. It is an aminoglycoside, like gentamicin, except that most *Pseudomonas* have, by now, become resistant to neomycin. Furthermore, aminoglycosides are notably ineffective against anaerobic bacteria. In fact, they may be added to the very medium used to culture anaerobes, to suppress overgrowth of aerobes so that anaerobes will grow. If one remembers that, he will remember how ineffective the aminoglycosides are against anaerobes.

TABLE 2. TOPICAL ANTIBIOTIC THERAPY FOR CHRONIC OTITIS MEDIA

Polymyxin B
Colistin (Polymyxin E)
Bactericidal to Gram− organisms
Pseudomonas
E coli
Klebsiella
Enterobacter
Resistances: Gram+ organisms
Proteus
B fragilis
Renal and CNS toxicity
Neomycin
Bactericidal to many Gram+ and Gram− organisms
eg, *S aureus*, *Proteus* species
Resistances: All anaerobes
Many *Pseudomonas*
Ototoxicity and nephrotoxicity
Chloramphenicol
Bactericidal to
Staphylococcus, coagulase positive, 99%
Staphylococcus, coagulase negative, 95%
Group A *Streptococcus*, 100%
E coli, 96%
P mirabilis, 90%
Proteus sp, 60%
Klebsiella, 92%
Enterobacter, 93%
Pseudomonas, 5%

So, the popular antibiotic-containing otic drops are for treatment of the well-known aerobes (Table 2). The combination preparations are preferable, using polymyxin for *Pseudomonas* and neomycin for *Staphylococcus*, *Streptococcus*, *Proteus* and the rest, with acid and alcohol carriers for antisepsis. However, anaerobic bacteria may not be covered by that combination. *B fragilis*, found in 13% of cholesteatomas, is resistant to both polymyxin and neomycin.

For years the Otologic Medical Group has used chloramphenicol as a dusting powder for the ear. Chloramphenicol otic drops are also available in an acid carrier, but they are quite painful when they go through an open perforation into the middle ear.

Chloramphenicol exerts a bacteriostatic effect on a wide range of Gram-negative and Gram-positive bacteria, such as *Staphylococcus*, *Streptococcus*, *E coli*, *Klebsiella*, and *Proteus*; the most pertinent for our purposes is the notorious anaerobe *B fragilis*. This would seem to be a first-rate otic preparation for chronic draining ears except that *P aeruginosa* is resistant to it. Once again, there is no single preparation that can be used in all cases.

In clinical practice, treatment can be initiated with the neomycin-polymyxin combination and cleansing procedures. Treatment failures, especially those with foul-smelling secretions not cultured as *P aeruginosa*, might be candidates for chloramphenicol drops. Anaerobic culturing, if available, relieves one of the uncertainties of such empirical therapy. Anaerobic bacteria are slow growers, however, and the Gram stain affords more prompt information.

Topical therapy raises two important questions. We are using drugs well known for their neurotoxic and ototoxic potentials. Are they, in topical preparations, absorbed to the extent that they cause ototoxicity in the treated ears? And secondly, do they reach any significant therapeutic concentration at the site of infection? As to the first question, these drugs are, in fact, absorbed from otic preparations; they are recoverable in the urine of dogs when applied to the ears, especially if the tympanic membrane is perforated.[7]

In 1957 Schuknecht[8] applied streptomycin to the middle ear in animals and subsequently in live patients, hoping to destroy the vestibular apparatus to treat Menière's disease. It worked, but unfortunately hearing was damaged. So, round window membrane absorption into the inner ear can certainly occur. Proud[9] dusted the round window of guinea pigs with chloramphenicol powder and showed cochlear damage from a drug otherwise thought not to be ototoxic. The well-known ototoxic drugs, neomycin, gentamicin, and polymyxin, have all been shown to produce damage to cochlear function (electrocochleography) and to the sensory epithelium (histopathology), again in guinea pigs.[10] In Brummett's studies[11] the concentrations used were those of our clinical commercial preparations of ear drops.

Despite these warnings which have been with us for more than a decade, these drops continue to be popular in the treatment of otitis media, even when perforations are present. And we have yet to see reports of adverse effects on hearing. Dr. Brummett and his group in Oregon have postulated three possible reasons for this.

1. There is a significant difference in the anatomy of the round window in man and in the guinea pig. In the animal the window is prominently exposed to the tympanic cavity. In man it is at the apex of a deep, narrow, round window niche. Perhaps the drops just do not make it all the way in there or are blocked from it by mucus or extra sheets of membrane.

2. Since early damage occurs in high frequencies, over 8000 Hz, and these are not detectable with the clinical audiometer, damage may be present but not observed.

3. Chronic otitis media by itself, untreated, also causes deterioration of cochlear function. Yet most chronic otitis shows a mixed loss with a mild nerve type component as well as the expected conductive loss. This was noted in the literature as early as 1941 (in the preantibiotic era even before we had the ear-

TABLE 3. SYSTEMIC ANTIBIOTIC THERAPY FOR CHRONIC OTITIS MEDIA

Aerobic Organisms	*Systemic Antibiotics*
Pseudomonas	Aminoglycoside ± carbenicillin
P mirabilis	Ampicillin or cephalosporin
P morganii } *P vulgaris* }	Aminoglycoside ± carbenicillin (some totally resistant)
E coli	Ampicillin or cephalosporin
Klebsiella	Cephalosporin or aminoglycoside
Enterobacter	Aminoglycoside
S aureus	Anti-*Staphylococcus* penicillin
	Cephalosporin
	Erythromycin
	Aminoglycoside
Streptococci	Penicillin or any of above
Anaerobic Organisms	*Systemic Antibiotics*
B fragilis	Clindamycin
All others	Penicillin
	Cephalosporins, etc.

drops in question). It has been confirmed by Paparella and Brady in 1970.[12] They postulate that bacterial and inflammatory toxins are absorbed across the round window membrane and damage the cochlea. So, if ototoxicity also occurs from the drops, what proportion is attributable to the disease as opposed to the treatment? We are obviously more comfortable blaming it on the disease.

To summarize the risks of the use of ototoxic antibiotic ear drops, we can probably accept the idea that they are risky to apply in the middle ear during surgery, especially if the labyrinth has been opened. But in chronic otitis media, their widespread clinical use with virtually no reported complications suggests that the risk cannot be very large. And if it is present at all, it is obscured by the effects of the disease itself. In fact, the risk must be weighed against probably the greater risk of nontreatment.

The second question is, are they effective at all? Topically administered antibiotics are placed on the exuding surface of a lesion. The active infection is deeper in the tissue, and it is advancing in the opposite direction of its discharge. It is difficult to show that a topically applied agent would penetrate to that area in adequate amounts, which is probably why the FDA has recently questioned the need for these preparations. Nevertheless, clinicians who use them all the time think that they work just fine, and we are waiting for someone to come up with a well-controlled study to prove it.[13]

This brings us to the question of systemic antibiotics (Table 3). Admittedly, they are not often required but could be in uncontrolled infection, in the diabetic, the leukemic, the elderly, or the debilitated. Reviewing the aerobic organisms, we note that *Proteus mirabilis* responds to ampicillin or a cephalosporin. The other strains of *Proteus* are unpredictable; some are resistant to all available agents, but gentamicin and carbenicillin can be tried. *E coli* needs ampicillin or a cephalosporin;

Klebsiella, a cephalosporin; *Enterobacter*, an aminoglycoside such as gentamicin. Many agents are available for staphylococci: the anti-*Staphylococcus* penicillins such as nafcillin or oxacillin-cloxacillin, the cephalosporins, old-fashioned erythromycin, and even the aminoglycosides. For streptococci, try penicillin or practically all of the above. *Pseudomonas* is the difficult and stubborn actor here. An aminoglycoside with or without carbenicillin is the correct choice. A few strains are becoming resistant to gentamicin but are handled by newer agents such as tobramycin or amikacin.

Aminoglycosides do not reach therapeutic levels in the serum unless given by the parenteral route. But parenteral therapy means an expensive, lengthy hospitalization. And these drugs are nephrotoxic and ototoxic, and again they fail in treatment of anaerobes.

For the anaerobic organisms, all are susceptible to penicillin (or cephalosporins for penicillin-allergic patients) except *B fragilis*, which requires clindamycin or chloramphenicol. Clindamycin is, of course, the safer drug; and it will effectively manage all of the anaerobes listed here plus most aerobes except for *Pseudomonas*. It has the highly publicized disadvantage of causing a fulminating diarrheal disorder that can be fatal. When the drug was at its peak of popularity, several outbreaks occurred in patients taking the drug — notably in St. Louis where it occurred in 10% of the patients. It also occurred in a few other communities but not nationwide in any uniform pattern. It is known now that the cause was overgrowth of an enteric clostridial organism probably endemic in those communities, which produced a toxin that led to the enterocolitis. It can be effectively managed with vancomycin.

The other disadvantage of clindamycin is that it crosses the blood-brain barrier poorly. Therefore, when intracranial spread of chronic otitis is suspected, treat with chloramphenicol. It attains cerebrospinal fluid concentrations of at least 50% of serum concentrations. It is effective against Gram-positive and Gram-negative organisms and against both anaerobic and aerobic organisms except for *Pseudomonas*.

What of combinations for an emergency, such as otitic meningitis or brain abscess or intracranial contamination during ear surgery when the dura is penetrated? The obvious choice is chloramphenicol to cover *B fragilis*, plus an aminoglycoside to cover *Pseudomonas*. Remember, aminoglycosides cross the blood-brain barrier poorly, so they require intrathecal administration; but carbenicillin crosses it and can be given parentally. In such a combination, chloramphenicol and gentamicin cover most other organisms that might be present, but we often see anti-*Staphylococcus* penicillins added in to cover the occasional *Staphylococcus* that is resistant to gentamicin.

REFERENCES

1. Ruegg K. Frequency of otitic complications of the brain. In: Small CP, Andrews AH, Shambaugh GE, eds. The practical medical series: the eye, ear, nose, throat. Chicago: Year Book 1928:268.

2. Tschopp CF. Chronic otitis media and cholesteatoma in Alaskan native children. In: McCabe BF, Sadé J, Abramson M, eds. Cholesteatoma, First International Conference. Birmingham: Aesculapius, 1977:290.

3. McCafferty GJ, Coman WB, Shaw E, Lewis N. Cholesteatoma in Australian aboriginal children. In: McCabe BF, Sadé J, Abramson M, eds. Cholesteatoma, First International Conference. Birmingham: Aesculapius 1977:293.

4. Friedmann I. The pathology of otitis media. J Laryngol Otol 1957; 71:313.

5. Harker LA, Koontz FP. The bacteriology of cholesteatoma. In: McCabe BF, Sadé J, Abramson M, eds. Cholesteatoma, First International Conference. Birmingham: Aesculapius, 1977:264-7.

6. Leyden JJ, Kligman AM. Contact dermatitis to neomycin sulfate. JAMA 1979; 242:1276-8.

7. Weinstein MJ, Oden EM, Zeman WV, Wagman GH. Antibiotic absorption after otic administration in dogs. Antimicrob Agents Chemother 1965; 5:239-44.

8. Schuknecht HF. Ablation therapy in the management of Meniere's disease. Acta Otolaryngol (Stockh) 1957; Suppl 132:1-42.

9. Proud GO, Mittelman H, Seiden GD. Ototoxicity of topically applied chloramphenicol. Arch Otolaryngol 1968; 87:580-7.

10. Kohonen A, Tarkanen J. Cochlear damage from ototoxic antibiotics by intratympanic application. Acta Otolaryngol (Stockh) 1969; 68:90-7.

11. Brummett RE, Harris, RF, Lindgren JA. Detection of ototoxicity from drugs applied topically to the middle ear space. Laryngoscope 1976; 86:1177-87.

12. Paparella MM, Brady DR. Sensorineural hearing loss in chronic otitis media and mastoiditis. In: Morrison WH, Shambaugh GE Jr, Williams HL. Trans Am Acad Ophthalmol Otolaryngol 1970; 74:108-15.

13. Mittelman H. Ototoxicity of "ototopical" antibiotics: past, present, and future. In: Morrison NH, Williams HL, Cody DTR. Trans Am Acad Ophthalmol Otolaryngol 1972; 76:142-3.

PANEL DISCUSSION

DR. BLUESTONE (Moderator): It has been suggested by some people that antimicrobial therapy may not be indicated at all, but rather that just doing a myringotomy is indicated. Perhaps the antimicrobial therapy is causing the problem in certain children, and we should resort to antimicrobial therapy only for those patients who don't "respond well" in the natural course of events. Maybe the reason we are having these so-called "otitis prone" children is because we are treating them with antimicrobials as soon as they have the first sign of an earache.

DR. KLEIN: We should consider that suppurative acute otitis media is an abscess, and that in some patients the abscess drains spontaneously, either through a perforation in the tympanic membrane, or because the eustachian tube opens up temporarily and the pus is evacuated. In such children antimicrobial agents may not be necessary. Many children who had otitis media in the preantibiotic era did not go on to have an extension of the infection or generalized sepsis, and many recovered; but our hospitals were filled with children with mastoid disease and chronic suppurative drainage. There are some recent data on children who were treated alternately with placebo or an antimicrobial agent; about a third of the placebo children had spontaneous resolution. However, you cannot predict that any given child will resolve spontaneously.

The majority of children continue to have signs and symptoms of the suppurative event, and require the specific antimicrobial agent for that pathogen. Simply because some children recover without antimicrobial agents, we should not be deluded into limiting the great benefit that comes from antimicrobial therapy.

DR. PARADISE: We would all agree that if we could safely get by with treating some episodes of acute otitis media without antibiotics, the problems of the emergence of resistant strains of bacteria, adverse reactions to antibiotics, and perhaps other problems such as persistence of effusion or recurrence of infection might be ameliorated. However, what we need is not opinion but data. There are no studies as yet directed to the question of whether certain patients could be identified by their minor clinical characteristics and singled out for more conservative management *without* antimicrobial treatment, reserving antimicrobials for those who have more severe clinical features such as fever, pain, toxicity, etc.

It might be possible to separate what is perhaps a large majority of patients with relatively mild acute otitis media from the more severe cases for an analysis of treatment versus no treatment. The problem with previous studies that compared antimicrobial treatment with placebo is that there was no attempt to distinguish between more severe and less severe cases. The possibility therefore exists that the better outcome in the treated group as a whole was attributable solely to effects in the subgroup of severely affected patients. Investigation of such a possibility is very much needed.

DR. BLUESTONE: Let me remind you that the Diamant/Diamant study reported several years ago considered some 10,000 cases done in Sweden. All patients received myringotomy initially. There was surgical drainage of the ear. The study compared those who had antimicrobial therapy and myringotomy with those who had myringotomy alone. But there were flaws in that study, as Dr. Paradise has pointed out.

Let us discuss the possibility of timing: allowing a certain number of days to go by to see how the patient is progressing; and if he is not doing well, then starting antimicrobial therapy. In this manner the immunodefense system is allowed to operate and create antibodies, as was suggested by Professor Laurell at the Second International Symposium on Otitis Media in Columbus three weeks ago. She suggested that it is possible that we are stifling the immune mechanism by giving children antimicrobial therapy immediately.

DR. NEU: I think we ought to put the immunological question to rest. There is a lot of controversy currently whether our protection against these organisms is in any way related to the organisms that were present in the first place. The question may actually be whether or not we should be colonized with certain strains of *E coli*, *Bacillus cereus*, *Neisseria lactamicus* or other organisms which have at their surfaces a cross-reacting polysaccharide, which may actually protect us. I think it is becoming more and more questionable whether these kinds of infections actually protect us against reinfection. This possibility is, in fact, under study in great detail at NIH, both in animal and human models.

There were a couple of things in the previous discussion that bothered me a little. One was the use of penicillin G as a drug. I would be quite concerned about that, because the children in whom we have used penicillin G orally (such as those who are receiving rheumatic fever prophylaxis) are in fact the kinds of children and the young adults out of whom Dr. K. Sprunt at Columbia was able to grow these fairly resistant strains of *S viridans*. And you can move the pneumococci up in their MIC. It is very selective. It is actually the technique that

Harry Eagle used in 1943-44. I am not very worried about sulfa being in the environment, because it is there all the time. These children are small, and their mothers very sexually active young women who have a large number of urinary tract infections. These women often have *E coli* in their gut and have flora that have been exposed to sulfa. So the whole family has been exposed to sulfa.

The other thing is the question about the meninges. We feel fairly strongly about meningococcal prophylaxis. (We had two families in one year in which three members in a family developed meningococcal meningitis. Furthermore, many of the group B meningococci strains are again sulfonamide-susceptible, so we may be able to go back to sulfonamide prophylaxis.) Next, if you have a child who had *H influenzae* in a family, should you consider prophylaxis of *H influenzae* meningitis for the rest of the family? We are moving to prophylaxis in the immediate family.

One thing that intrigued me as I heard the last presentation was the question of why we haven't used another drug, one which has not been mentioned as yet: metronidazole. We are using it presently in the treatment of brain abscesses. It has been tremendously successful in the treatment of infections in England and in the Scandinavian countries. It is really a fantastic drug. With Dr. Abramson, the Chairman of our Department of Otolaryngology, we have just treated some chronic ears with the drug, orally. It is not approved by the FDA for this, but it penetrates in tremendous concentration.

Although we've had mixed infections with *Pseudomonas* and anaerobes, once we have cleared up the anaerobes with metronidazole, sometimes the *Pseudomonas* has gone away. It is a little unfortunate that nobody in this country has looked at this drug. There is the question of its being a mutagenic agent, but it is only mutagenic in one strain of mice. If a quarter of their entire food intake for two of the three years of their life consists of metronidazole, then it becomes a mutagen. It does nothing to rabbits, rats or similar animals. It does mutate *Salmonella*. But so far, in man (at least in Europe and in England where it has been used extensively) there has been no problem, and it can be given orally. I think that this is something that perhaps otolaryngologists ought to look into, because maybe if you actually eradicated the anaerobes, the *Pseudomonas* might fade off.

DR. PARADISE: On the penicillin G question, my suggestion was one of desperation, because I don't know a good drug that can be administered safely over a long period of time. I am concerned about sulfa from the standpoint of exposure to a large population, because of the risk that occasional patients may develop severe idiosyncratic reactions. If it were administered to relatively small numbers of patients, it might be relatively safe and effective. But I share a lot of apprehension about its widespread use.

DR. BLUESTONE: Dr. Klein, you published the data to which Dr. Paradise alluded. What do you think about penicillin G as a prophylactic agent, or for that matter, as an antimicrobial for otitis media?

DR. KLEIN: It is of interest that it has not been studied. The figures of in vitro susceptibility are very close for *H influenzae* (the non-β-lactamase producers), for ampicillin, and for penicillin G. I think there is every reason to consider the possibility that in most cases penicillin G might be just as effective for those strains of *H influenzae* that are not β-lactamase producers.

Dr. Neu did not mention an issue that I think we should bring up, and that is the concern for developing resistance among pneumococci. We have heard about the increasing incidence of *H influenzae* that are β-lactamase producers and have a specific reason for their resistance, ie, the production of this enzyme which inactivates penicillin G, penicillin V, ampicillin, and amoxicillin. But the reported penicillin resistance of the pneumococcus is a different story. What we are concerned about is not only those unique strains that were identified in South Africa in May of 1977 that are completely resistant.[1] There is also another problem: the phenomenon of moderately resistant strains. First, let us consider a few statistics on MIC regarding what we mean by sensitive, moderately resistant, and resistant. The usual MIC of penicillin G necessary to inhibit the pneumococcus has a median value of 0.01 μg/ml. Now, for the resistant strains in South Africa, the median is about 4 μg/ml; a 400% increase. We are now seeing in the United States an intermediate group, those that are moderately resistant, significantly more resistant than has been previously noted, with an MIC of 0.1 to 1.0 μg. The incidence of these moderately resistant strains is still low; about 2% of strains of *S pneumoniae* recently tested in our laboratory have MICs in this range. The moderately resistant group may not be amenable to our usual dosage schedules, and we may have to start adjusting dosage schedules to a higher range. We may see failures when the usual course of penicillin G is given for pneumococcal disease, and it may be associated with these moderately resistant strains.

DR. BLUESTONE: Dr. Richard Michaels, who is the Chief of our Department of Infectious Diseases, has just reported two cases from Children's Hospital of Pittsburgh. So it is in the United States.

Dr. Ginsburg, you said that you thought that when acute otitis media is present in adolescents and adults you wouldn't worry about *H influenzae*. Do you feel that we can give agents other than those

1. Jacobs MR, Koornhof HJ, Robbins-Browne RM et al. Emergence of multiply resistant pneumococci. N Engl J Med 1978; 299:735-43.

we have been talking about for younger children to adolescents or adults?

DR. GINSBURG: I don't know. Several years ago we were told that after the age of two years we did not need to worry about *H influenzae*. Then it went to three, then four, and now it is ten years. I don't really know where *H influenzae* ends as a cause of otitis media. However, I am aware that it has been shown to be a pathogen in older children. Certainly Dr. Sande's group has shown that it is incriminated in acute sinusitis in adults. So it is conceivable, therefore, that it is a pathogen in older children with otitis. The question I have is: how frequently does one see the adolescent with acute otitis media? In our experience it is relatively uncommon. Now it may be that they are seen by the internist or go directly to the otolaryngologist.

DR. KLEIN: I think Dr. Ginsburg is right. It is less frequent in older children and adolescents. But when it does occur, what is the microbiology? I am familiar with data of Dr. Richard Schwartz who recently reported a study of 18 cases of otitis media in patients 8 to 17 years of age. Six were *Hemophilus*. And there was Herberts's study prior to that.[2]

DR. BLUESTONE: Herberts's study is nine years old and has been buried in the literature, but it shows that there are numerous cases of *H influenzae* otitis media in adults. So I think that we have to be very careful about prescribing antimicrobials that are not effective against *H influenzae*, eg, giving penicillin V to an adult with an acute otitis media, even though *H influenzae* is less frequent in adults than it is in children.

The next question is epidemiology. Dr. Schwartz has us all frightened that the disease is going to move like a gale from Washington to Pittsburgh and points west; that we are going to start seeing huge numbers of resistant *H influenzae*. Dr. Klein has told us that he likes to use ampicillin as his drug of choice in Boston because he doesn't have a high percentage of β-lactamase-producing *H influenzae*, and we in Pittsburgh would agree with him. How do you in Washington DC feel about this since that area has been shown to have a high incidence?

DR. FAIRBANKS: In patients who come to us with a primary infection, we usually use amoxicillin for initial treatment, and we think your figures are correct. Only 8% of all otitis media walking through our office door in Washington DC would be ampicillin-resistant *H influenzae*, so we will usually prescribe it. But if it is a referral case that has already been treated, most of us use erythromycin/sulfa combinations.

DR. PARADISE: If you are thinking about using erythromycin and sulfonamides, you should at the same time think about using as an alternative trimethoprim-sulfamethoxazole (TMP/SMX), because the toxicity inherent is that of the sulfonamide rather than the erythromycin. The efficacy is probably about the same unless one is dealing with a β-hemolytic streptococcal infection, in which efficacy remains questionable. The issue that argues in favor of TMP/SMX over erythromycin/sulfa is that of parental compliance in administering medications. Giving a medication twice a day is a lot easier for parents than giving it four times a day, and especially at six-hour intervals, which is really the ideal way to give sulfisoxazole.

FLOOR COMMENT: That is a fallacy. Sulfisoxazole probably could be given twice a day rather than three times a day. The reason I know that is I was just checking the original data. Probably we overtreat them.

DR. PARADISE: If that is true I stand corrected.

DR. BLUESTONE: Dr. Klein, if the initial treatment with ampicillin has failed, what would you advise?

DR. KLEIN: I have my own question. What is the microbiology of the children who have multiple episodes of acute otitis media? They have a suppurative episode, they're treated, they recover, the effusion goes away. Then they come down with another case, and this occurs repeatedly during the first few years of life. The microbiology for those repeated episodes is identical to that of the child who has one episode. It is still disease due to the pneumococcus and *H influenzae*. The upper respiratory tract flora does not shift to Gram-negatives or to anaerobes. In the child with acute, recurrent episodes, the recurrences are due to these two organisms and the strains do not shift in their resistance pattern. We have looked at this in children where we have isolated the organisms after multiple episodes, and where the children have had repeated courses of therapy, and the MICs are virtually the same. I think this is a host problem and not a problem of increasing drug resistance.

DR. BLUESTONE: If your first drug failed, what would you prescribe then?

DR. KLEIN: If we are talking about the child with an acute episode who is treated with ampicillin, we expect to see some resolution of signs and symptoms by 72 hours. After that time if the child is still toxic or is febrile, the ampicillin-resistant strains of *Hemophilus* must be considered. If the child continues to be sick, then you must define the microbiology, and I think tympanocentesis should be performed. It is important to know the microbiology to be sure that it is not an *S aureus* or some other unusual organism. If the child is not toxic, then switch to one of the drugs that would include coverage for the ampicillin-resistant *Hemophilus* such as cefaclor or TMP/SMX or erythromycin combined with a sulfonamide.

2. Herberts G, Jeppson PH, Nylen O. Acute otitis media. Pract Otorhinolaryngol 1971; 33:191.

DR. BLUESTONE: Dr. Ginsburg, how long should we treat our patients who have acute otitis media? And how do we get the patients to take their medications for the recommended period?

DR. GINSBURG: We recommend a period of 10-14 days. I have surveyed the practicing pediatricians in Dallas, and the vast majority of them treat between 12 and 14 days. Some have the patient return on the ninth day and look at the ear and see how it is doing, and others see them at 12 days. I think that otitis media is analogous to many other diseases in that there are really no good data on duration of antimicrobial therapy.

DR. NEU: Why don't we ever grow rhinoviruses or coronaviruses, which are the major cause of upper respiratory disease? Is it that the ear infection has occurred afterwards, and there is such a high concentration of interferon there? Interferon does inhibit these viruses. Has anybody looked at this?

DR. KLEIN: The last study with significant data was about 1971.[3] The methods that were used were adequate for isolation of rhinoviruses. They used WI 38 tissue cultures. But nobody has used techniques adequate for coronaviruses, so these remain an open question. Such studies are expensive and have not been performed in recent years, so there is no conclusive answer.

DR. NEU: Have any of you used counterimmunoelectrophoresis in the diagnosis? If you have gone to the trouble to do an ear tap and you have this material, you can know in 20 minutes whether or not you have group A *Streptococcus* and *H influenzae*, or a pneumococcus.

DR. KLEIN: The question has been looked at by a group studying middle ear effusions in Israel.[4] In fact, there are antigens present that can be identified using counterimmunoelectrophoresis. I think the numbers were not large, but the paper demonstrated that it was a promising technique. In some cases the organism was not isolated but the antigen was present. Certainly where patients had recently received antimicrobial agents, it would be a very fruitful mode of diagnosis.

FLOOR QUESTION: Would it be getting too far off the subject to consider the importance of treating prophylactically with an antimicrobial and an antihistamine-decongestant?

DR. BLUESTONE: There has not been a study reported that satisfies critical clinicians that using an antimicrobial agent or decongestants or antihistamines, either singly or in combination, is effective. There have not been conclusive studies as far as I'm concerned.

3. Klein JO, Teele DW. Isolation of viruses and mycoplasmas from middle ear effusions: a review. Ann Otol Rhinol Laryngol 1976; 85:140-4.

4. Ostfeld E, Altmann E. Evaluation of countercurrent immunoelectrophoresis as a diagnostic tool in bacterial otitis media. Ann Otol Rhinol Laryngol 1980; 89 Suppl 68:110-4.

FLOOR COMMENT: Those of us who have relatively large surgical practices see populations somewhat different from those in universities. Several things puzzle me. I am bothered by the fact that we are about to consider undertaking a number of studies about a disease that we describe as chronic otitis media with effusion; this seems to be a wastebasket term, about on a par with, perhaps, dementia praecox. I wonder if we ought to define what disease we are studying before we attempt to figure out how we should control it. I would like some comments on this.

And I wonder how the panel feels about the use of corticosteroids in an attempt to relieve the effusion after perhaps five or ten days of antibiotic therapy when the disease is, in terms of the infection, reasonably under control.

DR. BLUESTONE: We have two experts on definitions, Dr. Paradise and Dr. Klein, who were on Dr. Senturia's ad hoc panel on definitions. Could you define chronic otitis media with effusion and the etiology thereof?

DR. PARADISE: I think that all you can say is that otitis media is an inflammatory disease. Middle-ear effusion is the presence of liquid in the middle ear cavity. When it gets down to more refined definitions than that, more exact diagnostic techniques are needed, ranging from culture to biopsy with electron microscopy.

There is a variety of ways of classifying disease — otitis media and a host of others — that become, in the end, arbitrary. My own view is that if you simply describe as much as you know and no more than that, and try to identify as many features of the illness as you can, that is the best you can do with classification.

FLOOR COMMENT: Some of these children, perhaps, simply have wide-open eustachian tubes and everything that rolls out of the backs of their noses rolls straight into their ears. Others seem to have a nonfunctioning eustachian tube. In others, perhaps the adenoid has something to do with it, or perhaps allergies, and in some perhaps it is a reaction to a specific organism. What I am concerned with is not so much the definition of what is a chronic otitis media, but the fact that until the classification of some of the underlying conditions is made, we're always going to have people who fall out on both ends of the spectrum, who do extremely well and extremely poorly, and it really is not a fair evaluation whether or not the therapy was effective.

DR. BLUESTONE: Chronic otitis media with effusion possibly has multiple pathogenic mechanisms. In an individual child it may be one mechanism such as the in vivo model which was presented at the Columbus Symposium two weeks ago. That study involved American Indians in whom low resistance (semi-patulous) to the air flow through the eustachian tube was described. It was postulated that they have "reflux of otitis media," causing perforation of tympanic membrane and discharge. They also have a low incidence of cholesteatoma. At the other end of the spectrum is the cleft palate child in whom the eustachian tube actually constricts. They have a high incidence of cholesteatoma. As was said, it is very difficult to do studies on the whole gamut of chronic otitis media with effusion without knowing something of the pathogenesis.

FLOOR COMMENT: I would like to get the panelists' ideas on the relative and absolute indications for tympanocentesis.

DR. KLEIN: Tympanocentesis is a diagnostic technique which is available when the microbiology of the disease is critical to appropriate management. This is not necessary for the vast majority of cases of children who present with acute otitis media. The microbiologic data that I presented from the 11 studies are so consistent that the physician can initiate therapy with the information from those studies, without data from the individual child. However, there are circumstances where the microbiologic data are critical in appropriate management. For instance, we have found cases of otitis media in newborn infants, where the signs simulate neonatal sepsis. This is an abscess where the organisms may be different from those seen in older children. They may include Gram-negative organisms, group B *Streptococcus* as well as *Hemophilus* and pneumococcus. In order to provide rational therapy to that newborn, you have to know the etiology of the disease. That is one situation. The second situation involves children who are critically ill at onset, who are very septic, and for whom the etiology is not apparent. You may not have time to wait for the results of the cultures to come back to provide the most appropriate therapy. When the child is critically ill, I think tympanocentesis has a role. Third, tympanocentesis should be considered for the child who fails on therapy and is very sick. For that child, the microbial etiology is important in defining the rational therapy. Finally, tympanocentesis is appropriate for those who are immunocompromised, where they may have unusual organisms. One cannot rely on the data that has been accumulated about the etiology of otitis media for the abnormal host.

I think these four circumstances require tympanocentesis. We do about three or four procedures per week in a busy children's service, so this is a relatively small percentage.

DR. BLUESTONE: I would like to add to the list, regarding suppurative complications. If a child has an acute otitis media and an associated facial paralysis, I would perform a tympanocentesis/myringotomy. I would probably also perform a myringotomy in all the cases that Dr. Klein spoke about. As an otolaryngologist, I would initially perform a tympanocentesis to obtain a middle ear aspirate and then enlarge the opening for adequate drainage. Another example of a suppurative complication would be mastoid periostitis, with acute infection of the middle ear space and mastoid. We believe that immediate myringotomy (and culture) is very important in the prevention of subperiosteal abscess and subsequent mastoidectomy.

DR. KLEIN: There is a point in regard to culture technique that we should note. After having done a myringotomy and having an outpouring of the purulent material from the middle ear, I have seen our otolaryngologists then take a cotton-tipped wire loop, put it into the external canal, mop up the purulent material and send it off to the laboratory. That is inadequate because you are culturing the contaminants in the canal in addition to the agent present in the middle ear fluid. Myringotomy, rather than needle aspiration, as Dr. Bluestone has said, is fine, if you maintain purity of the material from the middle ear.

DR. BLUESTONE: You certainly will not get a satisfactory culture if only the tip of the myringotomy knife makes contact with the middle ear fluid.

We did not answer the question about corticosteroids for chronic otitis media with effusion. I will take this opportunity to attempt to answer that question. There is a double-blind study that Dr. Schwartz performed in Washington DC which looks promising. He has compared steroids versus placebo in chronic otitis media with effusion, and he has seen improvement in those patients put on systemic corticosteroids over a short period of time. We need further studies that show whether or not this can be replicated in other centers with larger numbers of patients.

FLOOR QUESTION: Dr. Neu mentioned metronidazole, and I would like to ask him what advantage it would have over clindamycin. We feel that clindamycin is effective against *Bacteroides*, and it has the advantage of having bone concentration where the cholesteatoma is advancing and eroding bone.

DR. NEU: It has been used for treatment of facial osteomyelitis with good success. For osteomyelitis there are about a dozen groups around the country studying its use.

You mentioned one thing that is very important: the *Clostridium difficile* is the cause of the necrotizing enterocolitis due to clindamycin. We have not seen a case due to metronidazole. The last three cases we have had in our institution from whom we have isolated the organism and found the toxin were due to TMP/SMX, to ampicillin, and to cephalexin. Actually, any antibiotic, except probably erythromycin, or vancomycin given orally, can cause this.

ETIOLOGY AND ANTIMICROBIAL TREATMENT OF ACUTE SINUSITIS

JACK M. GWALTNEY, JR., MD

AUSTIN SYDNOR, JR., MD MERLE A. SANDE, MD

CHARLOTTESVILLE, VIRGINIA

Acute maxillary sinusitis is a disease of varied etiology. Over half of the cases are caused by *Streptococcus pneumoniae* and *Hemophilus influenzae.* Anaerobic bacteria account for another 10% of cases and these are usually of dental origin. The rest of the cases are caused by several other bacteria, each of which cause a small proportion. Rhinoviruses, influenza, and parainfluenza viruses also invade the sinuses and probably lead to secondary bacterial infection. Diagnosis of acute sinusitis on clinical grounds is difficult. Sinus transillumination and x-ray are the most valuable routine tests available. Ampicillin, amoxicillin, trimethoprim-sulfamethoxazole, and cefaclor have been shown to be effective treatment for most cases of acute sinusitis. Infection persists when there is inadequate or inappropriate treatment. The patient may become relatively asymptomatic in the face of persistent active infection. Follow-up clinical and x-ray examinations are indicated, when possible, to detect treatment failures. Although not a routine diagnostic procedure, sinus puncture and aspiration may be of value in the seriously ill patient or one who has not responded to treatment.

Approximately 0.5% of common colds are complicated by sinus infection.[1] As adults average two to three colds per year and children six to eight, sinusitis is one of the most common infectious problems seen in outpatient practice. Despite the frequency of the disease, progress has been slow in the development of satisfactory methods for its diagnosis and treatment. Also, while the bacterial etiology of acute maxillary sinusitis in adults is now well established, this knowledge has not been widely disseminated among physicians. *Streptococcus pneumoniae* and *Hemophilus influenzae* cause over half of all cases of acute maxillary sinusitis, and yet, when treating the disease, physicians often fail to prescribe an antimicrobial which is effective against both of these bacteria.

Knowledge about the etiology of sinus infections comes from studies in which the culture specimens were obtained by direct puncture and aspiration of the sinus cavity.[2-8] This method of sampling avoids contamination of the specimens with the bacterial flora of the nasal fossae. This is important, since a culture of the nose or throat is not an accurate way to determine which bacteria are growing in the sinus cavity. There has been good agreement among the findings of the various studies of patients with acute maxillary sinusitis in which puncture and aspiration were used. The causes of acute infection of the other sinuses and of the disease in children have not been well established but are presumably similar.

Because of the importance of the pneumococcus and *H influenzae*, ampicillin has been recommended as the drug of choice for the treatment of acute sinusitis. Three newer antimicrobials are now available which have activity against these two bacteria. These are amoxicillin, trimethoprim-sulfamethoxazole, and cefaclor. This paper compares the results of an earlier trial using ampicillin, amoxicillin, and trimethoprim-sulfamethoxazole[8] to a more recent study of cefaclor. It also includes findings relating to the diagnosis and microbial etiology of acute maxillary sinusitis observed in this and earlier studies.[7,8]

METHODS

Population. The study was conducted with 113 patients, ages 18-62, who presented to otolaryngologists. This group was selected on the basis of the otolaryngologists' impression that the patients might have acute bacterial sinusitis. The patients' complaints included facial pain, purulent nasal discharge, and less commonly headache and fever. No patient had received antimicrobial treatment in the two weeks before enrollment in the study.

Clinical Evaluation. Transillumination and x-rays of the sinuses were performed on some patients. Puncture and aspiration of one or both maxillary antra were performed on all patients prior to antimicrobial treatment. Seven to ten days after institution of therapy, patients returned for clinical evaluation and repeat sinus aspiration and culture.

Specimen Collection and Testing. The area of the nares below the inferior turbinate was cleansed by action suction and swabbing and then treated with Betadine®. The site was then anesthetized with 10% cocaine solution. The medial wall of the antrum was then punctured with a 12-gauge needle and any fluid present in the sinus was aspirated with a syringe. If fluid could not be obtained, 1 ml of normal saline, without preservative, was instilled into the cavity and then aspirated back into the syringe. After the air was expelled, the syringe was capped and delivered to the laboratory.

Portions of the sample of the undiluted specimen were inoculated into blood and chocolate agar for aerobic bacterial cultures and into roll tubes under CO_2 for anaerobic bacterial cultures. In addition, hundredfold dilutions of the specimen were inoculated into the media to quantify the bacteria present in the aspirate. A sample of the aspirate was also tested in human embryonic lung cells (WI-38) and Rhesus monkey kidney cells for viruses.

From the Department of Internal Medicine, University of Virginia School of Medicine, and the Department of Otolaryngology, University of Virginia and Martha Jefferson Hospitals, Charlottesville.

REPRINTS — Jack M. Gwaltney, MD, Dept. of Internal Medicine, Box 473, Univ. of Virginia School of Medicine, Charlottesville, VA 22908.

TABLE 1. COMPARISON OF RESULTS OF SINUS TRANSILLUMINATION AND SINUS ASPIRATION IN PATIENTS WITH ACUTE MAXILLARY SINUSITIS

Transillumination	*Number of Sinuses*	*Abnormal Aspirate**
Normal	18	1 (6%)
Dull	26	7 (27%)
Opaque	23	23 (100%)

*The presence of fluid on direct aspiration and/or > 1000 WBC/mm^2, and/or ≥ 10^4 CFU of bacteria/ml in the aspirate.

Antimicrobial Treatment. Patients were treated orally with antimicrobials on one of the following schedules: 1) ampicillin — 2 g/day in four divided doses; 2) amoxicillin — 1.5 g/day in three divided doses; 3) trimethoprim — 80 mg, sulfamethoxazole — 400 mg, two tablets twice a day; 4) cefaclor — 1 g/day in two divided doses. (For reasons given below, this dose was later increased to 2 g/day given in four divided doses.) The patients were treated with ampicillin and trimethoprim-sulfamethoxazole in random assignment and with the amoxicillin and cefaclor in consecutive order. The antimicrobials were initially given for seven days. When an infection was found to have persisted until the time of the repeat puncture, treatment was extended for an additional seven to ten days.

RESULTS

Diagnosis. The clinical features of the patients' illnesses were of little help in making the diagnosis of acute sinusitis. The history of purulent nasal discharge and of facial discomfort or pain, the two most common complaints, did not correlate well with puncture results. Fever occurred in only half of puncture-positive cases and other objective signs, such as facial tenderness, were too infrequent to be useful. A history or objective evidence of periapical dental infection was helpful in recognizing the approximately 10% of patients whose sinus infection was of dental origin. In these patients, mixed anaerobic infections were the rule.

Transillumination of the sinuses was of value in the hands of some but not all otolaryngologists participating in the study. It appeared most helpful when the results were placed into three categories: normal, dull, and opaque. Normal light transmission correlated well with the absence of evidence of infection, as determined by puncture (Table 1). Conversely, a finding of complete opacity was a reliable indicator of active infection. Approximately one third of the patients examined by transillumination were judged to have partial reduction of light transmission ("dull") and only a third of these patients had an abnormal aspirate. It should be emphasized that all of the patients examined were thought to have had previously normal sinuses. In patients with chronic sinus disease, the results of transillumination are less helpful because of persistent mucosal abnormalities.

Forty-eight aspirates were obtained from sinuses that were considered to be abnormal by x-ray examination (Table 2). Thirty-four (71%) of these were found to be infected by puncture. The abnormalities seen on x-ray were air-fluid level, present in 18 (37%); complete opacity in 18 (37%); and mucosal thickening in 12 (25%). Of the 34 sinuses with positive cultures, 16, 10, and 8 had air-fluid level, opacity, or mucosal thickening, respectively. Two of the 10 sinuses with a normal radiograph also had a positive culture.

TABLE 2. COMPARISON OF RADIOGRAPHIC FINDINGS WITH CULTURE RESULTS IN 43 PATIENTS (58 SINUSES) WITH ACUTE MAXILLARY SINUSITIS

Radiograph	*Number of Sinuses*	*Positive Culture**
Abnormal	48	34
Air-fluid level†	18	16
Opacity	18	10
Mucosal thickening (≥5 mm)	12	8
Normal	10	2

*Bacteria (≥ 10^4 CFU/ml) and/or virus.

†Mucosal thickening also present in three cases.

The measurements of mucosal width were taken near the lateral angle of the sinus between the air interface and the bone, using the Water's view. A mucosal thickness of approximately 5 mm tended to discriminate between those with a positive puncture and those in whom the puncture was negative. Above 5 mm, the puncture was usually positive.

Bacterial and Viral Cultures. One hundred-forty aspirates were obtained from the 113 patients. Some patients had aspirates obtained from both antra, and some of the specimens contained more than one organism. All of the bacteria reported were present in titers of equal to or greater than 10^4 colony-forming units per ml. There was a strong correlation between bacterial titers of this magnitude and the presence of white cells in the aspirate. Cultures containing fewer organisms (most often aerobic Gram-negative bacteria) were thought to have been contaminated during handling.

The most common isolate was the pneumococcus, with 37 strains, or 43% (Table 3). Next in frequency were unencapsulated strains of *H influenzae*, 27 strains (31%). Nine percent of the bacterial isolates were anaerobes; these were usually in mixtures (eg, fusobacteria, anaerobic streptococci, and *Bacteroides*). *Branhamella catarrhalis* accounted for 5%

TABLE 3. BACTERIA AND VIRUSES ASSOCIATED WITH ACUTE MAXILLARY SINUSITIS (86 POSITIVE ASPIRATES*)

Microorganism	*No. (%)*
S pneumoniae	37 (43)
H influenzae	27 (31)
Anaerobic bacteria	8 (9)
B catarrhalis	5 (5)
α-Streptococcus	3 (3)
S aureus	3 (3)
S pyogenes	2 (2)
Non-group A β-hemolytic *Streptococcus*	2 (2)
P aeruginosa	2 (2)
E coli	1 (1)
Rhinovirus	7 (8)
Influenza type A	3 (3)
Parainfluenza	2 (2)

*The culture was negative in 63 (42%) of 149 aspirates tested.

TABLE 4. COMPARISON OF SIMULTANEOUS NASAL SWAB AND SINUS ASPIRATE CULTURES IN PATIENTS WITH ACUTE MAXILLARY SINUSITIS

	Recovery Site		
Bacteria	Nose Alone	Sinus Alone	Nose and Sinus
S epidermidis	24	0	0
Diphtheroids	14	0	0
S aureus	9	1	0
H influenzae	6	1	5
α-hemolytic *Streptococcus*	3	0	1
B catarrhalis	3	0	1
S pneumoniae	2	2	1
Micrococcus species	2	0	0
Proteus species	2	0	0
S pyogenes	1	0	1

of infections. Alpha-hemolytic streptococci and *Staphylococcus aureus* each were associated with 3%. Beta-hemolytic streptococci (4%) and aerobic Gram-negative bacteria (3%) accounted for the rest. Viruses were recovered from 12 specimens, sometimes in association with bacteria. Seven rhinoviruses, three influenza type A, and two parainfluenza viruses were identified. No microorganisms were recovered from 63 aspirates (42% of the total).

Nasal swab cultures obtained prior to sterilization of the puncture site did not correlate well with cultures done on the sinus aspirate (Table 4). *Staphylococcus epidermidis* and diphtheroids were frequently present in the nose but never recovered from the sinus. *S aureus* was found in the nose on nine occasions but in the sinus aspirate only once. This reflects the relatively frequent nasal carriage of this organism which has lead to its overdiagnosis as a cause of acute sinusitis. *H influenzae* was obtained six times from the nose alone, once from the sinus alone, and five times from both the sinus and the nose. Likewise, pneumococci, α-streptococci, *B catarrhalis*, and *Streptococcus pyogenes* were sometimes implicated as pathogens and other times found only in the nasal carrier state. A patient might have one potential pathogen (eg, *H influenzae*) in the nose while another (eg, *S pneumoniae*), which was the true cause of that patient's disease, was recovered from the sinus.

Antimicrobial Treatment. A total of 25 patients received ampicillin. Of these, 13 had positive cultures (Table 5). Fifteen sinuses were studied in these 13 patients. *H influenzae* was recovered from six of the patients and seven of the sinuses. On follow-up examination, five of the six patients were improved clinically. On repeat puncture, four of the six sinuses were sterile. The patient with no improvement gave a history of discontinuing ampicillin treatment after two days because of diarrhea. At this time, there were 10^5 and 10^7 CFU of *H influenzae* in the sinus aspirates, indicating persistence of active infection. Five patients (six sinuses) had pneumococcal infection and all improved with treatment. Repeat punctures were negative. Two

TABLE 5. RESULTS OF ANTIMICROBIAL TREATMENT* OF PATIENTS WITH ACUTE MAXILLARY SINUSITIS

Therapy, Bacterial Isolates	No. Pts.	No. Sinuses	No. Patients Improved	No. Sinuses Sterile after Therapy/ No. Tested
Ampicillin				
H influenzae	6	7	5	4/6
S pneumoniae	5	6	5	4/4
α-Streptococci	2	2	2	2/2
Total	13	15	12	10/12
Amoxicillin				
H influenzae	6	8	6	4/6
S pneumoniae	2	3	2	2/3
S pyogenes	2	2	2	ND†
Anaerobic bacteria	1	1	1	ND
B catarrhalis	1	1	1	1/1
E coli	1	1	1	1/1
P aeruginosa	1	1	1	ND
Total	14	17	14	8/11
Trimethoprim-sulfamethoxazole				
S pneumoniae	8	10	8	7/8
Anaerobic bacteria	5	5	5	4/5
H influenzae	2	3	2	2/2
B catarrhalis	2	2	2	2/2
S aureus	1	1	1	1/1
Non-group A β-hemolytic *Streptococcus*	1	1	0	0/1
Total	19	22	18	16/19
Cefaclor				
S pneumoniae	12	17	9	8/12
H influenzae	6	10	4	8/10
α-Streptococcus	1	1	1	ND
F necrophorum	1	1	1	ND
S aureus	1	2	1	2/2
P aeruginosa	1	1	1	1/1
Total	22	32	17	19/25

*After initial 7-10 days of treatment.

†ND - Not done.

patients had infection with α-streptococci. Both improved and repeat punctures were negative.

A total of 22 patients received amoxicillin; 14 had positive cultures, and they accounted for 17 sinuses studied. *H influenzae* was cultured from six patients (eight sinuses). Six of the eight patients were improved on follow-up and four of six sinuses had negative cultures. In both of the sinuses with positive cultures, the bacterial titers had fallen to low levels (10^2 CFU/ml). Two patients (three sinuses) had infections with pneumococci. Both patients showed clinical improvement. Two of the three sinuses were negative on repeat culture, but in one the titer was still 10^6 CFU/ml. Two patients (two sinuses) yielded a group A β-hemolytic *Streptococcus*. Both of the patients improved clinically, but follow-up punctures were not done. Anaerobic bacteria, *B catarrhalis*, *Escherichia coli*, and *Pseudomonas aeruginosa* were present in one patient each. All of these patients improved, and the two sinuses in which punctures were done had become sterile.

Thirty patients received trimethoprim-sulfamethoxazole. Nineteen (22 sinuses) had evidence of infection on puncture. Eight patients (10 sinuses) had pneumococci. Eight patients were improved and seven of eight sinuses were sterile on repeat culture. A low bacterial titer (10^2 CFU/ml) was present in the aspirate from the one sinus in which infection was still present. Five patients had mixed anaerobic infections. All five patients improved; four of five sinuses were negative. In one there was still a low titer of a *Bacteroides* species. Two patients each had *H influenzae* and *B catarrhalis*; both patients improved and their sinuses were negative on repeat culture. *S aureus* and a non-group A β-hemolytic *Streptococcus* was present in one patient each. The clinical and bacteriologic response was satisfactory with the *S aureus*, but the patient with the streptococcal infection remained symptomatic and had a positive culture (10^5 CFU/ml).

A total of 33 patients received cefaclor, 22 (32 sinuses) of whom had proven infection. Twelve patients (17 sinuses) had pneumococcal infection. Nine of the patients were improved when they returned for follow-up examination, and eight of the 12 sinuses had negative cultures. Sinus aspirates from four patients still contained high titers of bacteria. Three of these four patients were placed on 2 g/day of cefaclor for an additional six or seven days and repeat punctures were found to be negative. Six patients (10 sinuses) had *H influenzae* infections. Four of these patients had a satisfactory response. Two patients remained symptomatic, and the repeat cultures were still positive ($\geq 10^7$ CFU/ml). One of these individuals was on 1 g/ day of cefaclor; the dose was increased to 1.5 g/ day for an additional 10 days, and the repeat puncture was then found to be negative. The other patient was on a 1.5 g/day dose of cefaclor. (When the repeat puncture was positive, the patient was placed on amoxicillin, 1.5 g/day following which repeat aspiration was negative.) In one patient with α-streptococcal and another with *Fusobacterium necrophorum* infection, clinical responses were satisfactory; punctures were not repeated. One patient (two sinuses) had a *S aureus* and another a *P aeruginosa* infection. Clinical responses were satisfactory, and on repeat puncture the sinuses were sterile.

DISCUSSION

The clinical improvement and bacteriologic responses seen with the four antimicrobials were similar. Most patients improved during the period of treatment, and cultures of the sinus aspirates became negative. The dosage of cefaclor which was initially used did not appear to be adequate. A higher dose (30 mg/kg) which is similar to that used for the treatment of otitis media (30-40 mg/kg) should probably be used for the treatment of acute sinusitis.

The above results were combined with findings from an earlier small study using clindamycin. In 73 patients who were judged to be adequately treated (the patient gave a history of taking the drug for the prescribed course and the bacterium showed in vitro sensitivity to the antimicrobial used), there were 66 (90%) bacteriologic "cures."* In contrast, in the six instances where patients gave a history of not taking the full course of the antimicrobial as directed or in vitro resistance of the bacterium was present, there were no cures at the time of repeat puncture. Thus, these findings are further evidence for the effectiveness of antimicrobics in the treatment of acute sinusitis.

*Sterile culture or titer decrease $\geq 10^5$ CFU/ml on repeat puncture.

REFERENCES

1. Dingle JH, Badger GF, Jordan WS Jr. Patterns of illness. In: Illness in the home. Cleveland: Western Reserve University, 1964:347.

2. Urdal K, Berdal P. The microbial flora in 81 cases of maxillary sinusitis. Acta Otolaryngol (Stockh) 1949; 37:20-5.

3. Bjorkwall T. Bacteriological examinations in maxillary sinusitis: bacterial flora of the maxillary antrum. Acta Otolaryngol (Stockh) 1950; Suppl 83:33-58.

4. Lystad A, Berdal P, Lund-Iversen L. The bacterial flora of sinusitis with an in vitro study of the bacterial resistance to antibiotics. Acta Otolaryngol (Stockh) 1964; Suppl 188:390-9.

5. Rantanen T, Arvilommi H. Double-blind trial of doxicycline in acute maxillary sinusitis: a clinical and bacteriological study. Acta Otolaryngol (Stockh) 1973; 76:58-62.

6. Axelsson A, Brorson JE. The correlation between bacteriological findings in the nose and maxillary sinus in acute maxillary sinusitis. Laryngoscope 1973; 83:2003-11.

7. Evans FO, Sydnor JB, Moore WEC, et al. Sinusitis of the maxillary antrum. N Engl J Med 1975; 293:735-9.

8. Hamory BH, Sande MA, Sydnor A Jr, et al. Etiology and antimicrobial therapy of acute maxillary sinusitis. J Infect Dis 1979; 139:197-202.

ETIOLOGY AND ANTIMICROBIAL THERAPY OF PARANASAL SINUSITIS IN CHILDREN

PAUL A. SHURIN, MD
CLEVELAND, OHIO

Paranasal sinusitis in children is discussed in terms of pathogenesis, diagnosis, etiology and antimicrobial therapy.

GENERAL CONSIDERATIONS

Sinusitis is generally considered to occur frequently in children. However, objective diagnostic techniques to establish the presence or etiology of the disease have not been widely used. For instance, the validity of specific clinical findings in differentiating sinus infection from uncomplicated rhinitis has not been well established, and some of the radiographic findings which are thought to be indications of sinusitis are very frequently found in radiographs of normal children.[1] Because of these diagnostic difficulties, adequate information concerning the incidence of the disease and its optimal therapy is not yet available.

PATHOGENESIS

Sinusitis appears most frequently to be a complication of a viral upper respiratory infection. Suggested mechanisms for this relationship include a) local vascular congestion, b) narrowing and obstruction of the sinus ostia, c) alterations in the local milieu for bacterial growth, and d) reduction in the effectiveness of mucociliary action.

Disease entities which have been associated with sinusitis in children are listed in Table 1. Nasal allergy is thought to be a major cause of sinus disease in children. Sensitivity to environmental allergens, to foods, and to drugs such as aspirin have all been incriminated. The various malformations and traumatic defects presumably affect the sinuses by obstructing their ostia. Clouding of the sinuses and mucosal thickening have frequently been identified radiologically in children with cleft palate,[2] but the clinical significance of this is not clear. Radiologic signs of sinusitis have been reported to be seen especially frequently in children with cyanotic congenital heart disease.[3] The sinus alterations may be due to vascular engorgement and proliferation of venous channels. Chronic sinus infection might contribute to the frequent occurrence of such complications as brain abscess in these children. Sinus disease in children with cystic fibrosis is generally identified in conjunction with the nasal polyps which are a frequent manifestation of the disease; the highly viscous mucus secretions may also play a role in sinus disease. The manifestations of Kartagener's syndrome (situs inversus, bronchiectasis, and sinusitis) appear to result from a structural defect in cilia throughout the body.[4] The ciliary abnormality in Kartagener's syndrome has recently been termed the "immotile cilia syndrome." Since approximately half the reported cases have not had situs inversus, this defect should be considered in the differential diagnosis of children with chronic or recurrent respiratory infections. The diagnosis can be suggested by physiologic tests of ciliary clearance and documented by ultrastructural examination of the respiratory epithelium. Sinus infection may occur in immunodeficiency disorders of all types. However, these disorders are uncommon in comparison to the frequency of sporadic cases of sinusitis; it is in general necessary to consider immune defects only when the sinusitis is unusually severe or persistent or when there has been significant infection of other organs as well.

DIAGNOSIS

The diagnosis of sinusitis in infants and children is suggested by the presence of purulent rhinorrhea and nasal obstruction in conjunction with systemic signs such as fever and irritability. Other manifestations include headache or a sense of fullness, tenderness over the involved sinus, or a disturbed sense

TABLE 1. DISORDERS ASSOCIATED WITH PARANASAL SINUSITIS

1. *Anatomic*
   a. Nasal malformations
   b. Nasal trauma
   c. Tumors and polyps
   d. Cleft palate
   e. Foreign bodies
   f. Dental infection
   g. Cyanotic congenital heart disease
2. *Physiologic*
   Barotrauma
3. *Abnormalities of Local Defense Mechanisms*
   a. Allergy
   b. Cystic fibrosis
   c. Immotile-cilia syndrome and Kartagener's syndrome
4. *Abnormalities of Systemic Defense Mechanisms*
   Immunodeficiency, primary or secondary

From the Department of Pediatrics, Case Western Reserve University School of Medicine, and Cleveland Metropolitan General Hospital, Cleveland.
REPRINTS — Paul A. Shurin, MD, Department of Pediatrics, 3395 Scranton Rd., Cleveland, OH 44109.

TABLE 2. BACTERIAL SPECIES IDENTIFIED IN SINUS EXUDATES IN ACUTE MAXILLARY SINUSITIS[5-9]

Bacterial Species	Percent of Cases
S pneumoniae	25-45
H influenzae	13-30
Group A β-hemolytic streptococci	2- 6
Neisseria sp.	0- 1
S aureus	0-10
Enteric Gram-negative bacilli	1- 9
None (sterile exudates)	20-30

of smell. Because these signs are nonspecific, in pediatric practice the diagnosis is often considered only when local or systemic spread of infection has occurred.

ETIOLOGY

Specific identification of the causative organisms in sinusitis requires culture of aspirated sinus secretions by appropriate methods. Because potentially pathogenic bacteria are found in the nasal passages of most or all normal children, culture of nasal secretions is not helpful and may give misleading results.[5] Sinus aspiration is indicated when accurate bacteriologic diagnosis is needed. Specific indications for sinus aspiration include 1) sinusitis in children who are seriously ill or who appear toxic, 2) the presence of a sinus infection which has not responded to initial antimicrobial drug therapy, 3) the onset of sinusitis in a patient who is receiving antibiotics, 4) the presence of suppurative complications, and 5) sinusitis in debilitated or immunologically deficient patients. In each of these instances, both specific identification of the causative organism or organisms and in vitro antibiotic susceptibility tests may be essential to proper patient management. The procedure may be performed by cannulation of the ostium of the affected sinus or by antral or frontal puncture. Care is required to avoid contamination of the secretions by nasal material. Examination of Gram-stained smears is necessary to provide a rapid presumptive diagnosis and to help exclude consideration of bacteria which may later appear as contaminants in the cultures. Children who are ill enough to require these procedures should have cultures of blood and usually of such other potentially infected sites as the cerebrospinal fluid. Few systematic investigations of the bacterial etiology of sinusitis in children have been performed. Thus, much of the available information is derived from studies in which adequate cultures have been obtained from adults with acute maxillary sinusitis (Table 2).[5-9] *Streptococcus pneumoniae* and *Hemophilus influenzae* are the predominant bacterial pathogens, one of these two organisms having occurred in 50 to 75% of cases in various studies. It should be emphasized that infection due to *H influenzae* occurs frequently at all ages although it may be most common in young children. The majority of *H influenzae* strains isolated from infected sinuses are nontypable and thus differ from the strains causing such serious infections as meningitis. Group A β-hemolytic streptococci have been involved in a small proportion of cases. Many early investigations have incriminated *Staphylococcus aureus* as an important pathogen in sinusitis. However, this organism is rarely identified if care is used to avoid contamination of the sinus specimens with nasal material. A major problem in interpreting reports of the bacterial etiology of acute sinusitis is the large number of additional bacterial species which have been incriminated in a small proportion of patients. Because of the difficulty of obtaining satisfactory culture material, particularly from young children, the importance of bacteria other than *S pneumoniae* and *H influenzae* as agents of acute sinus infection cannot be evaluated at present. Unusual or drug-resistant bacterial infection might be suspected when an acute infection does not respond to antibacterial therapy. Further attempts at obtaining a specific diagnosis would be indicated in such cases. Aspirated sinus exudates have been bacteriologically sterile in approximately 25% of cases. A few such cases have yielded respiratory viruses when appropriate tissue culture techniques were used;[5] the relation of infectious agents to most such cases is unknown.

TABLE 3. ANAEROBIC BACTERIA ISOLATED FROM SURGICAL SPECIMENS OF PATIENTS WITH CHRONIC MAXILLARY SINUSITIS[10]

Bacterial Species	Percent of Cases
Anaerobic streptococci	57
B funduliformis	14
B fragilis	14
B melaninogenicus	4
Veillonella	11
Corynebacteria sp	4
Micrococcus	4

Chronic sinusitis is unusual in children. Recent studies of this disorder have shown that anaerobic bacteria can frequently be isolated from sinus secretions obtained at the time of surgery (Table 3).[10] This finding is of importance in that such anaerobic infections may require different antibacterial therapy from that given for the common agents of acute sinusitis. Moreover, the potential clinical importance of anaerobic infection is shown by the fact that the bacteria involved are the same as those generally isolated in brain abscesses and other intracranial complications of chronic sinus infection. Thus, anaerobic cultures are required to define the bacterial etiology of cases of chronic sinusitis. Several bacterial species are often present and the organisms are those which are part of the normal oral and upper respiratory flora. Therefore, in suspected anaerobic infection, culture material should be obtained surgically with strict attention to avoid contamination from nonsterile areas. Anaerobic infection is suggested clinically by a) the presence of a foul-smelling discharge, b) the occurrence of infection following surgical procedures or dental infection, c) the presence of tissue destruction and abscess formation, and d) by a mixed flora seen in Gram stains or aerobic cultures which are negative.[11] Most reported cases of anaerobic sinusitis have been of long duration. *Bacteroides* sp and anaerobic streptococci are the most common bacterial isolates in such cases, but a variety of other organisms may be present.

THERAPY

Attention to anatomic abnormalities and their surgical correction, investigation of allergies and removal of potentially significant allergens, and therapy of any underlying disorders are utilized when indicated. Local and systemic decongestants are widely used in the therapy of sinus disease; there is, however, no documentation that they provide more than transient, symptomatic relief.[12,13]

Many investigations have shown that systemic, orally administered antibiotics provide symptomatic and objective improvement in acute sinus infections. In uncomplicated cases in which the causative organism is not known at the time of diagnosis, antibiotics active against both pneumococci and *H influenzae* are required; the drugs and dosages used are the same as those employed for children with acute otitis media. Based upon the available evidence, these considerations are the same for all age groups beyond the neonatal period. In the first weeks of life, sinus infection with group B *Streptococcus* and enteric Gram-negative bacilli has been reported. For such infections, broad-spectrum antibiotic therapy, usually including an aminoglycoside (gentamicin or kanamycin) plus a penicillin (ampicillin or penicillin G) is required initially; modifications may be made when culture results are available. At all ages, organisms other than *S pneumoniae* and *H influenzae* have been isolated from a considerable proportion of cases. Therefore, in unusually severe cases parenteral administration of broad-spectrum antibiotics in high doses is required until culture reports are available and a favorable clinical response has occurred. The therapy of sinus infection due to less common bacterial species is dependent upon identification of the organism and its antibiotic susceptibility. Surgical drainage is most important in chronic infection with anaerobic bacteria. For the majority of such infections, penicillin G or ampicillin provide effective antibacterial therapy and should be used in high doses. Alternative drugs for treatment of anaerobic infections include chloramphenicol and clindamycin, and these should be considered when penicillin-resistant bacteria have been identified.

REFERENCES

1. Shopfner CE, Rossi JO. Roentgen evaluation of the paranasal sinuses in children. Am J Radiol 1973; 118:176-86.

2. Jaffe BF, DeBlanc B. Sinusitis in children with cleft lip and palate. Arch Otolaryngol 1971; 93:479-82.

3. Rosenthal A, Fellow KE. Acute infectious sinusitis in cyanotic congenital heart disease. Pediatrics 1973; 52:692-6.

4. Eliasson R, Mossberg B, Camner P, Afzelius BA. The immotile cilia syndrome. A congenital ciliary abnormality as an etiologic factor in chronic airway infections and male sterility. N Engl J Med 1977; 297:1-6.

5. Evans FO, Snydor JB, Moore WEC, et al. Sinusitis of the maxillary antrum. N Engl J Med 1975; 293:735-9.

6. Urdal K, Berdal P. The microbial flora in 81 cases of maxillary sinusitis. Acta Otolaryngol (Stockh) 1949; 37:20-5.

7. Axelsson A, Chidekel N. Symptomatology and bacteriology correlated to radiological findings in acute maxillary sinusitis. Acta Otolaryngol (Stockh) 1972; 74:118-22.

8. Rantanen T. Clinical function tests of the maxillary sinus ostium. Acta Otolaryngol (Stockh) 1974 Suppl 328:1-38.

9. Chapnik JS, Bach MC. Bacterial and fungal infections of the maxillary sinus. Otolaryngol Clin North Am 1976; 9:43-54.

10. Frederick J, Braude AI. Anaerobic infection of the paranasal sinuses. N Engl J Med 1974; 290:135-7.

11. Bartlett JG, Gorbach SL. Anaerobic infections of the head and neck. Otolaryngol Clin North Am 1976; 9:655-78.

12. Roth RP, Cantekin EI, Bluestone CD, Welch RM, Cho YW. Nasal decongestant activity of pseudoephedrine. Ann Otol Rhinol Laryngol 1977; 86:235-42.

13. Lampert RP, Robinson DS, Soyka LF. A critical look at oral decongestants. Pediatrics 1975; 55:550-2.

ETIOLOGY, DIAGNOSIS, AND ANTIMICROBIAL TREATMENT OF PHARYNGITIS AND PHARYNGOTONSILLITIS

JACK L. PARADISE, MD

PITTSBURGH, PENNSYLVANIA

This review focuses on clinically important aspects of the etiology, diagnosis, and antimicrobial treatment of pharyngitis and pharyngotonsillitis. Most episodes of throat infection are of viral etiology, and accordingly are not susceptible to antimicrobial drugs currently available. By contrast, streptococcal and other varieties of bacterial pharyngitis do call for appropriate antimicrobial treatment. The review encompasses a discussion of clinical, bacteriological, and serological diagnosis; an algorithm for decision-making about antimicrobial treatment that is based on both clinical findings and culture results; and a summary of treatment regimens, emphasizing the management of streptococcal throat infection.

ETIOLOGY

Microorganisms of many kinds cause pharyngitis. Those most familiar, of course, are bacteria and viruses; but *Mycoplasma*, and *Toxoplasma* — which can be acquired from pet cats — also can cause pharyngitis. *Monilia* infections of the mouth, especially in infants but sometimes in older, immunocompromised patients, can by direct spread lead to pharyngitis as well.

Of bacteria, three organisms that we know of are important agents in the etiology of pharyngitis: the Group A β-hemolytic *Streptococcus*, *Corynebacterium diphtheriae*, and, apparently more commonly of late, *Neisseria gonorrhoeae*. There exists the possibility — not yet investigated fully — that pharyngitis may be caused also by other respiratory pathogens, particularly the prevalent *Streptococcus pneumoniae*, *Hemophilus influenzae*, and *Staphylococcus aureus*; occasional cases unquestionably due to Group B or C β-hemolytic streptococci have been reported. Rarely, exudative pharyngitis may be the principal manifestation of tularemia.[1]

Among the viruses, I have singled out those that seem to be the most prominent causes of pharyngitis, based on a review of the literature. While they all can cause pharyngitis, some of them tend to cause other infections more frequently and more importantly.

Adenovirus may be responsible for the common cold and for conjunctivitis, but its most important manifestation probably is pharyngitis. The illness may or may not be accompanied by exudate, and from a clinical standpoint is not distinguishable from β-hemolytic streptococcal pharyngitis or other varieties of exudative pharyngitis.

Parainfluenza virus, the principal cause of croup in infants, can sometimes cause instead the common cold or bronchiolitis or viral pneumonitis, and also pharyngitis, usually without an exudate.

Rhinovirus, the principal cause of the common cold, also can cause pharyngitis, again usually without an exudate; less commonly, *coronavirus* has been implicated as a cause of pharyngitis.

Herpes simplex virus most commonly causes the adult "cold sore," or, in infants and young children before a degree of immunity has been established, gingivostomatitis. In other instances the virus can cause exudative or nonexudative pharyngitis, mainly in older children and adults.

Respiratory syncytial virus is the principal agent of bronchiolitis in infants, but like the aforementioned respiratory viruses, it also can cause a spectrum of upper and lower respiratory infections, included among which is pharyngitis, with or without exudate.

The *Epstein-Barr virus* may cause — apart from the characteristic mononucleosis syndrome with its range of possible complications — simple pharyngitis with or without exudate.

Influenza virus causes not only influenza, but on occasion, simple pharyngitis.

Coxsackie A virus. The best known and most common manifestation of infection with this virus is the disease herpangina. This variety of pharyngitis is characterized by small vesicles with erythematous bases, soon becoming ulcers, scattered over the anterior pillars, tonsils, palate, and posterior pharynx. Another much less common type of Coxsackie A infection is known as acute lymphonodular pharyngitis; the lesions are similar to those of herpangina, but less ulcerated and more nodular in appearance.

Cytomegalovirus infection is often asymptomat-

From the Departments of Pediatrics and Community Medicine, University of Pittsburgh School of Medicine, and the Ambulatory Care Center, Children's Hospital of Pittsburgh.

REPRINTS — Jack L. Paradise, MD, Children's Hospital of Pittsburgh, Pittsburgh, PA 15213.

ic, but also may cause a wide range of illnesses in patients of all ages, including pharyngitis. The pharyngitis occurs as one component of an infectious mononucleosis-like illness, in which the pharyngitis tends to be less prominent and milder than in infectious mononucleosis itself.

Much of our epidemiologic information about the etiology of pharyngitis and tonsillitis comes from a study reported by Glezen and colleagues in 1967[2] involving 715 patients with throat infection seen in two pediatric practices in Chapel Hill, N.C. Most of the subjects were in preschool and elementary school age groups, but a few were adolescents and young adults. In the age group below two years of age, only 3.4% of the patients were found to have positive throat cultures for group A β-hemolytic streptococci. However, apparent streptococcal infection became much more common after age two: positive cultures were found in 29.4% of the 2- to 5-year age group, 51.7% of the 6- to 8-year age group, 37.6% of the 9- to 11-year age group, and 45.5% of the 12- to 14-year age group. Among patients 15 years of age or older, the frequency was considerably lower, but the total number of such patients studied was small. In the study population as a whole, slightly more than one third had positive cultures for group A streptococci.

Although this study was completed over ten years ago, and isolation techniques for some types of viruses were probably not adequate, nonetheless respiratory viruses were recovered from 50% of all subjects under two years of age with pharyngitis. The proportion fell off sharply in older children.

Mycoplasma also was looked for in all of these patients. The organism was virtually absent in younger infants and children, but became increasingly prevalent in the latter years of childhood and early adolescence.

DIAGNOSIS

STREPTOCOCCAL PHARYNGITIS

Since from the standpoint of treatment it is streptococcal pharyngitis that is of principal concern, its diagnosis deserves detailed consideration. The most characteristic clinical features are fever, sore throat that may or may not be severe, difficulty in swallowing, exudate, enlarged tender anterior cervical lymph nodes, and in children a scarlatiniform rash. It is important to recall in this connection the phenomenon in infants known as *streptococcosis*, characterized not by pharyngitis but by chronic rhinitis, often with excoriation of the skin at the margins of the nares, cervical lymphadenopathy, and failure to "do well." Often these infants, rather than being investigated and treated properly with penicillin, tend to be either overlooked or misdiagnosed as having "colds" or "allergy."

The sudden onset, in association with a sore throat, of coryza, hoarseness, or cough, should lead one away from a clinical diagnosis of streptococcal disease, although by no means excluding the possibility.

For a specific diagnosis of streptococcal infection, cultures are helpful but cannot be relied upon exclusively. In about half the patients from whom streptococci are cultured it is not possible to detect a rise in antistreptococcal antibodies, and it is reasonable to conclude that such patients are probably carriers of streptococci who are experiencing associated viral infections. Offsetting and complicating this observation is the fact that a significant minority of patients who have symptoms of pharyngitis and who prove to be culture-negative subsequently do develop rises in antistreptococcal antibody titers indicating that the episodes in question had indeed been streptococcal. The culture is thus far from a perfect instrument for detecting streptococcal throat infection. In reviewing the problems of precise diagnosis, Wannamaker concluded that attempts to identify in advance patients at risk of developing nonsuppurative complications (ie, rheumatic fever and glomerulonephritis) result in a vast margin of error.[3] Depending on clinical findings, the clinician can often guess with fair accuracy whether patients have streptococcal infections, and can certainly refine the guesses by obtaining cultures. However, even when the results of culture are available, diagnosis is not certain without antibody studies, and such studies under ordinary circumstances of practice hardly seem justifiable.

PHARYNGITIS DUE TO EPSTEIN-BARR VIRUS INFECTION

I will not review Epstein-Barr (EB) virus infection except to point out that in instances when infectious mononucleosis is suspected, and the clinical findings seem at odds with the heterophile antibody or Monospot® test results, a battery of EB virus antibody tests can help determine whether or not EB virus infection is currently active.[4]

TREATMENT

STREPTOCOCCAL PHARYNGITIS

For a number of reasons it is advisable to treat all patients with streptococcal pharyngitis with an appropriate antimicrobial drug. There is first of all more certain improvement and more rapid relief of symptoms in treated than in untreated patients, although the difference is not dramatic, usually in the range of 24 to 36 hours. Next, there is the likelihood that with treatment we can prevent various local suppurative complications, particularly peritonsillar or retropharyngeal abscess, or cervical lymphadenitis, cellulitis, or abscess. Whether there is efficacy in preventing the development of otitis media or sinusitis is questionable.

As for the prevention of nonsuppurative complications, the one of greatest concern is of course rheumatic fever. Herein lies the most important reason for treating with penicillin or an equivalent drug, for reasonably prompt treatment should virtually eliminate the possibility that rheumatic fever will develop. Unfortunately, however, such is not the case with acute glomerulonephritis, which appears not to be preventable by early antistreptococcal treatment.

Whether antibiotic treatment of a single episode of streptococcal pharyngitis lowers the risk of recurrent streptococcal episodes is not known; it seems a fair inference but has never been established. Early treatment probably can effectively prevent the spread of streptococcal infection to others — a goal that seems particularly worthwhile if the infection involves a nephritogenic strain of *Streptococcus.*

A number of regimens for treating streptococcal pharyngitis are acceptable. The most certain involves administering a single injection of 900,000 units of benzathine penicillin G combined with 300,000 units of procaine penicillin G. Equally effective, but considerably more painful, is to give an injection of benzathine penicillin G only, 1,200,000 units to patients 10 years of age and older, and 600,000 units to younger patients.

An alternative to these intramuscular regimens is to prescribe phenoxymethyl penicillin (penicillin V) orally, 250 mg three or four times daily, irrespective of age, for a ten-day period. One can afford to be generous with the dose because the drug is relatively inexpensive and nontoxic, and using large doses may perhaps help compensate for occasional lapses in compliance.

Valid arguments can be made both for and against administering penicillin intramuscularly. The overriding advantage of the intramuscular route is that treatment is both certain and completed immediately, and the problem of poor compliance with oral regimens is bypassed. On the other hand, there are disadvantages, not the least of which is pain. Children become very upset about injections, and subsequent rapport becomes more difficult. Moreover, intramuscular administration is more likely than oral to result in penicillin sensitization, especially if the drug used is procaine penicillin G, which quickly breaks down to component substances that are probably more allergenic than the penicillin itself. Finally, in treating patients who may previously have been sensitized unknowingly, the risk of inducing anaphylaxis is much greater if penicillin is administered intramuscularly.

On balance, intramuscular injection would appear preferable if a) the patient is very ill and vomiting and it seems doubtful that he or she will be able to retain oral medication; or b) it seems unlikely that the drug is going to be administered by the family as prescribed; or c) the patient has had repeated recurrences of streptococcal infection despite high-dose oral penicillin treatment with each episode; or d) the patient has rheumatic heart disease and the most certain method of administration is a necessity in order to minimize the risk of a rheumatic recurrence.

If the patient is allergic to penicillin, currently acceptable alternatives would consist of erythromycin or a cephalosporin, 40 to 50 mg/kg/day in divided doses.

PRESUMABLY NONSTREPTOCOCCAL PHARYNGITIS

I would like to call attention to a study by Merenstein and Rogers that is not often quoted, but reminds us that we have much to learn about treating throat infection.[5] The study was begun as an investigation of the functions of nurse-practitioners in family physicians' offices. In the course of the study, the investigators established an algorithm based on clinical symptoms and signs — eg, the presence of high fever, toxicity, severe pain, exudate, and lymphadenopathy — to indicate whether or not an individual episode of pharyngitis was probably streptococcal. The study protocol involved identifying all patients who, according to the algorithm, probably had streptococcal pharyngitis, and assigning each of them randomly and in double-blind fashion to either a penicillin- or a placebo-treated group. All subjects received throat cultures initially; those in the penicillin group who subsequently proved to be culture-negative had penicillin discontinued at that point, while those who proved to be culture-positive were continued on penicillin.

In examining the clinical results after the first 24 hours, the investigators found, not to their surprise, that among the culture-positive subjects those who had been treated with penicillin fared better symptomatically than those receiving placebo; of 17 on penicillin 14 (78%) were definitely improved within 24 hours, as compared with only 5 of 14 (35%) on placebo — a significant difference. They next examined results among the patients who proved to be culture-negative, and now much to their surprise, found that after 24 hours there had been definite improvement in 8 of the 16 (50%) treated with penicillin, but in only 1 of 14 (7%) treated with placebo, again a statistically significant difference.

Several possible explanations of those findings come to mind. First of all was the possibility that bacteriological technique had been faulty and that there had been a high proportion of false-negative cultures. However the technique used was a standard one that has been well established. Another possibility, alluded to above, was that penicillin-sensitive organisms other than Group A streptococci had been involved etiologically in some of the patients' episodes. Finally was the possibility that, despite the apparent statistical significance, the findings had occurred by chance, and a repeat study with larger numbers of subjects might show differing findings. This study has apparently not been replicated, but it raises the question whether the only variety of pharyngitis that responds to penicillin is β-hemolytic streptococcal pharyngitis.

Based on their findings, Merenstein and Rogers proposed the following algorithm for systematic decision-making regarding penicillin or other antibiotic treatment of an individual episode of pharyngitis. We use this algorithm in our current study of indications for tonsillectomy:[6]

> If a streptococcal infection seems likely on the basis of clinical findings, obtain a throat culture and begin treatment. If the culture proves to be positive, continue treatment for a total of ten days. If the culture proves to be negative, inquire about the patient's course. If there has been marked improvement within 24 hours, continue treatment for a total of ten days despite the negative culture. If, on the other hand, the patient is little or not at all improved, stop treatment.
>
> If a streptococcal infection seems unlikely — ie, the patient has acute coryza, or lacks most of the symptoms and signs mentioned above as characteristic of streptococcal pharyngitis — obtain a culture but refrain from treating. If the culture proves negative, continue to withhold treatment. If the culture proves positive, proceed to treat, even though in perhaps half the instances the patient will have been a *Streptococcus* carrier who does not have a streptococcal infection.

Treatment of other known bacterial causes of pharyngitis is as follows. For diphtheria the principal treatment is of course specific antitoxin, supplemented by intramuscularly administered penicillin, or in penicillin-sensitive patients, orally administered erythromycin. For gonoccocal pharyngitis, the treatment of choice is penicillin intramuscularly, or in penicillin-sensitive patients, tetracycline orally. For all forms of tularemia the drug of choice is streptomycin, of necessity administered intramuscularly.

REFERENCES

1. Levy HB, Webb CH, Wilkinson JD. Tularemia as a pediatric problem. Pediatrics 1950; 6:113-23.

2. Glezen PW, Clyde WA Jr, Senior RJ, et al. Group A streptococci, mycoplasmas, and viruses associated with acute pharyngitis. JAMA 1967; 202:455-60.

3. Wannamaker LW. Perplexity and precision in the diagnosis of streptococcal pharyngitis. Am J Dis Child 1972; 124:352-8.

4. Fleisher G, Lennette ET, Henle G, Henle W. Incidence of heterophil antibody responses in children with infectious mononucleosis. J Pediatr 1979; 94:723-8.

5. Merenstein JH, Rogers KD. Streptococcal pharyngitis: early treatment and management by nurse practitioners. JAMA 1974; 227:1278-82.

6. Paradise JL, Bluestone CD, Bachman RZ, et al. History of recurrent sore throat as an indication for tonsillectomy: predictive limitations of histories that are undocumented. New Engl J Med 1978; 298:409-13.

CEFACLOR IN MANAGEMENT OF STREPTOCOCCAL PHARYNGITIS, OTITIS MEDIA, AND SKIN INFECTIONS

ROBERT B. KAMMER, MD
INDIANAPOLIS, INDIANA

Cefaclor, a semisynthetic cephalosporin antibiotic for oral use, was studied by 62 clinical investigators in six countries in 3,084 adult and pediatric patients. The pooled data reveal that satisfactory clinical responses were obtained in 96% of the streptococcal pharyngitis cases, 93% of the cases of otitis media, and 97% of skin infections. Administration of this antibiotic was associated with a low incidence of adverse reactions, including 73 gastrointestinal and 34 hypersensitivity reactions. Of particular clinical interest were the outstanding results obtained in the treatment of otitis media.

INTRODUCTION

Since most oral cephalosporins have only limited activity against strains of *Hemophilus influenzae*, a pathogen commonly seen in ear, nose, and throat infections, these drugs have not been widely used in otolaryngology practice. However, a new oral cephalosporin, cefaclor, offers good activity against not only *H influenzae* but also *Streptococcus pneumoniae* and many other species of Gram-positive and Gram-negative bacteria.[1-8]

Preclinical toxicology studies showed that the drug has a low order of toxicity in animals. Several investigators evaluated the clinical pharmacology of the compound.[9-13] Peak serum levels after oral administration were one half to three fourths those of cephalexin administered in equal dosage. Fifty-five to 80% of the drug was recovered unchanged in the urine, indicating that it is excreted primarily by the kidneys. As a result of these promising preclinical evaluations, a large-scale efficacy testing program was implemented, eventually involving 62 investigators from six countries.

MATERIALS AND METHODS

Four hundred forty-five patients were treated for upper respiratory infections (mostly streptococcal pharyngitis). An additional 263 patients, mostly children, were treated for otitis media and 532 patients with skin infections were also treated with cefaclor. The data on these patients were collected and pooled.

TABLE 1. CRITERIA FOR SYMPTOMATIC CLINICAL EVALUATION

Satisfactory	Disappearance or improvement during therapy of the patient's signs and symptoms due to the infection
Satisfactory with recurrence	Same as above, only the signs and symptoms recurred after completion of the treatment period
Unsatisfactory	No improvement of signs and symptoms
Unable to evaluate	Protocol not followed, poor patient cooperation, noncompliance, etc

The incidence of side effects was evaluated in 3,084 patients who received the drug. These studies utilized the protocol and criteria described below.

The therapeutic effectiveness and safety of cefaclor were evaluated in various types of bacterial infections including streptococcal pharyngitis, otitis media, and skin infections. For each type of infection, evaluation of the effectiveness of cefaclor was based on strict clinical (Table 1) and bacteriologic criteria. In all cases, history and physical examination were required to document the diagnosis before therapy. Dosages employed in these trials differed slightly with the diagnosis and are summarized in Table 2. Follow-up clinical evaluation was carried out in all patients at the end of cefaclor therapy. Only cases meeting all of the clinical and bacteriologic requirements were judged evaluable in these studies. In addition, specific bacteriologic and clinical requirements pertinent to the particular diagnosis are listed below.

Streptococcal Pharyngitis. Throat cultures (swabs) were taken within 3 days before therapy, within 48 hours after therapy (early posttherapy), and again 12 to 16 days after therapy (late posttherapy). Isolates were kept for typing should a posttherapy culture again be positive for a group A *Streptococcus*. Typing was then performed in an attempt to differentiate failures from reinfections.

Otitis Media. Tympanocentesis and culture of aspirated middle ear fluid were undertaken within 24 hours before cefaclor therapy. Repeat tympanocentesis and culture were done in most cases, if there was a poor clinical response.

Skin Infections. Pretherapy culture of the lesion was undertaken including aspiration of abscesses and tissue biopsy when appropriate. Cultures were repeated if the infection persisted.

CLINICAL RESULTS

Upper Respiratory Infections. Pharyngitis was diagnosed in 442 cases. Sixty-four of these patients

TABLE 2. CEFACLOR DOSAGE

Streptococcal pharyngitis
- Adults — 250 mg every 6 or 8* hr
- Children — 20 mg/kg/day every 6 or 8* hr
- Duration — 10 days

Otitis media — children
- 40 mg/kg/day every 6 or 8* hr
- Duration — 10 to 14 days

Skin infections
- Adults — 250 mg every 6 or 8* hr
- Children — 20 mg/kg/day every 6 or 8* hr
- Duration — 5 to 14 days

*Usual dosage employed.

From Lilly Research Laboratories, Eli Lilly and Company, Indianapolis.

TABLE 3. UPPER RESPIRATORY TRACT INFECTIONS

Bacteriologic Response	*No. of Patients*
Early posttherapy	
Cure	427
Failure	18
Late posttherapy	
Sterile culture	378
Reinfection, new pathogen	13
Reinfection, original serotype	36
Patients failed to return	18

also had tonsillitis. Group A *Streptococcus* was the pathogen encountered in 442 of these cases. There were also 3 additional patients treated for sinusitis, making a total of 445 patients. The symptomatic response was either satisfactory, recurrent, or unsatisfactory. At the early posttherapy culture, there were 427 cures and 18 bacteriologic failures. At the late posttherapy culture, there were 378 cures; 13 patients had been infected with a new organism, and there were 36 who were reinfected with the original serotype. These data have been summarized in Table 3.

Otitis Media. Two hundred sixty-three children with otitis media were treated with cefaclor. Approximately equal numbers of boys and girls participated in the trial, although their age distribution was not uniform. There was a small group of children under 6 months of age, a substantial group 7 to 12 months of age, and smaller numbers of older children (Table 4).

S pneumoniae, the most frequent organism obtained at tympanocentesis, was seen in 127 cases including 11 cases where there were multiple organisms, usually found with *H influenzae*. Group A streptococci were found in 12 cases. *Staphylococcus aureus* was recovered in 22 cases. These clinical isolates were not contaminants from the external auditory canal. Sterile cultures from the canal were obtained prior to tympanocentesis. *H influenzae*, also a frequently encountered organism, was isolated in 83 cases, of which there were nine treatment failures. A total of 276 organisms were isolated from these 263 cases (Table 5). There were 19 treatment failures. Thus, there were 244 cures in 263 patients (93%).

Skin Infections. There were 532 skin infections. Table 6 shows the diagnosis and symptomatic response for these infections. There were 515 satisfactory responses (97%), 8 recurrences, and 9 failures.

TABLE 4. SEX AND AGE DISTRIBUTION OF OTITIS MEDIA CASES EVALUATED FOR EFFICACY

Age	*Male*	*Female*	*Total Patients*
2-6 mo	19	16	35
7-12 mo	62	57	119
1.1-3 yr	26	33	59
3.1-14.9 yr	26	28	54
Totals	133	134	267

TABLE 5. PATHOGENS ISOLATED BY TYMPANOCENTESIS FROM OTITIS MEDIA CASES

	Single Isolates	*Multiple Isolates*	*Total Isolates*
S pneumoniae	127 (6)	11	138 (6)
Streptococcus group A	11	1	12
S aureus	21 (2)	1	22 (2)
S epidermidis	4 (1)	3 (1)	7 (2)*
H influenzae†	74 (8)	9 (1)	83 (9)
Hemophilus sp	6		6
H parainfluenzae	1		1
N catarrhalis	2	1	3
Neisseria sp	3	1	4
Totals	249 (17)	27 (2)	276 (19)

Number of total isolates classified as failures shown in parentheses.

*Not present in tympanic membrane culture prior to tympanocentesis.

†Of 83 strains, 7 were resistant to ampicillin in vitro. No clinical failures were encountered in this group.

S aureus accounted for the largest number of microorganisms encountered, followed by group A *Streptococcus*; when they occurred, multiple-pathogen infections were almost invariably *S aureus* mixed with group A *Streptococcus*.

ADVERSE EXPERIENCES

Among the 3,084 patients who received cefaclor, 135 had adverse reactions or abnormal lab values that their physician felt were drug related. In an additional 205 patients, adverse experiences of uncertain etiology occurred and the role of the test drug, if any, could not be established.

The major adverse effect categories and their observed incidence are summarized in Table 7. No serious adverse effects were seen during these trials. Mild gastrointestinal upsets were the most common type of adverse reaction reported. These included 40 reports of diarrhea and 21 of nausea, some of which occurred in the same patients. Mild hypersensitivity reactions were seen infrequently (34 reactions). The reactions observed included rash (17) and pruritus (6).

Hematopoietic reactions were encountered, although none were serious and all were promptly reversible upon discontinuance of therapy. These in-

TABLE 6. SKIN INFECTIONS — PRIMARY DIAGNOSIS AND CLINICAL RESPONSE

Primary Diagnosis	*Symptomatic Response* S*	R†	U§	Total
Impetigo	249	7	5	261
Pyoderma	114	1	1	116
Cellulitis	52		1	53
Abscess, subcutaneous	59			59
Wound infection, traumatic	19			19
Wound infection, postoperative	9		1	10
Skin ulcer, infected	5		1	6
Miscellaneous	8			8
Totals	515	8	9	532

*S - Satisfactory.

†R - Recurrent.

§ - Unsatisfactory.

TABLE 7. ADVERSE EXPERIENCES ENCOUNTERED DURING CEFACLOR TRIALS

Gastrointestinal	
Diarrhea	40
Nausea	21
Dyspepsia	7
Miscellaneous	5
Hypersensitivity	
Rash	17
Pruritus	6
Miscellaneous	11
Hematopoietic	
Eosinophilia	67
Lymphocytosis	35
Leukopenia	12
Leukocytosis	5
Miscellaneous	2
Total	121

cluded 67 instances of eosinophilia and 35 of lymphocytosis, mostly in small children. There were also 12 reports of leukopenia, between 3000 and 4000 WBC/cu mm. In all cases, a definite relationship to drug therapy could not be established.

Elevated SGOT values were found in 22 patients and elevated SGPT in 10. No evidence of overt hepatic disease was noted in any patient. Enzyme abnormalities were all transient and mild.

DISCUSSION

Cefaclor is readily absorbed from the gastrointestinal tract, and is active against those pathogens commonly found in infections of the upper respiratory tract and skin and skin structures.

Of particular interest in the studies reported here are the excellent results obtained with cefaclor in the treatment of otitis media. The continued isolation of *H influenzae* resistant to ampicillin in this disease lends particular importance to the development of a new oral agent for its treatment.

Therapy with cefaclor was associated with a low incidence of adverse effects. In fact, no serious side effects were encountered. In 58 penicillin-allergic patients treated with cefaclor, one skin rash was the only reaction reported.

In this summary of data collected from 62 investigators, it is clear that cefaclor is safe and effective in the treatment of a variety of infections due to susceptible organisms. It can be concluded, therefore, that cefaclor is a promising new oral antibiotic, particularly effective in the treatment of infectious diseases like otitis media and streptococcal pharyngitis encountered frequently by ear, nose, and throat specialists.

REFERENCES

1. Bill NJ, Washington JA. Comparison of in vitro activity of cephalexin, cephradine, and cefaclor. Antimicrob Agents Chemother 1977; 11:470-4.

2. Jorgensen JH, Alexander GA. Comparative activities of selected beta-lactam antibiotics against Haemophilus influenzae. Antimicrob Agents Chemother 1978; 13:342-3.

3. Meyers BR, Hirschman SZ. Antimicrobial activity in vitro of cefaclor, a new oral cephalosporin. J Clin Pharmacol 1978; 18:85-90.

4. Neu HC, Fu KP, Cefaclor: in vitro spectrum of activity and beta-lactamase stability. Antimicrob Agents Chemother 1978; 13:584-8.

5. Sanders CC. In vitro studies with cefaclor, a new oral cephalosporin. Antimicrob Agents Chemother 1977; 12:490-7.

6. Santoro J, Levison ME. In vitro activity of cefaclor, a new orally administered cephalosporin antibiotic. Antimicrob Agents Chemother 1977; 12:442-3.

7. Shadomy S, Wagner G, Carver M. In vitro activities of five oral cephalosporins against aerobic pathogenic bacteria. Antimicrob Agents Chemother 1977; 12:609-13.

8. Sinai R, Hammerberg S, Marks MI, Pai CH. In vitro susceptibility of Haemophilus influenzae to sulfamethoxazole-trimethoprim and cefaclor, cephalexin and cephradine. Antimicrob Agents Chemother 1978; 13:861-4.

9. Bloch R, Szwed JJ, Sloan RS, Luft FC. Pharmacokinetics of cefaclor in normal subjects and patients with chronic renal failure. Antimicrob Agents Chemother 1977; 12:730-2.

10. Korzeniowski OM, Scheld WM, Sande MA. Comparative pharmacology of cefaclor and cephalexin. Antimicrob Agents Chemother 1977; 12:157-62.

11. Meyers BR, Hirschman SZ, Wormser G, Gartenberg G, Srulevitch E. Pharmacologic studies with cefaclor, a new oral cephalosporin. J Clin Pharmacol 1978; 18:174-9.

12. Santoro J, Agarwal BN, Martinelli R, Wenger N, Levison ME. Pharmacology of cefaclor in normal volunteers and patients with renal failure. Antimicrob Agents Chemother 1978; 13:951-4.

13. Spyker DA, Thomas BL, Sande MA, Bolton WK. Pharmacokinetics of cefaclor and cephalexin: dosage nomograms for impaired renal function. Antimicrob Agents Chemother 1978; 14:172-7.

PANEL DISCUSSION

DR. BLUESTONE (Moderator): Drs. Ellen Wald and Victor Schramm have joined our panel. Dr. Schramm has recently published an article on orbital cellulitis. Dr. Schramm, do we have any new information on the etiology of sinusitis?

DR. SCHRAMM: My information is derived from a review of 140 children with a complication of sinusitis, specifically orbital cellulitis with or without meningitis. One fourth of the patients had been treated with an orally administered antibiotic prior to hospitalization. These patients had experienced progression of their disease while on oral therapy. It is apparently psychologically difficult for physicians to obtain cultures by maxillary sinus aspiration in children. Cultures of conjunctival drainage or soft tissue aspirates had little correlation with blood or sinus cultures. Nasal cultures were inaccurate as compared to sinus or blood cultures except when they grew *S pneumoniae* or *H influenzae*. In this series, *Staphylococcus* infections were extremely rare and no ampicillin-resistant *H influenzae* were identified.

DR. BLUESTONE: So, you will agree with the percentages of organisms that were presented by both Dr. Gwaltney and Dr. Shurin.

DR. WALD: Studies that I am familiar with were performed on youngsters who were having ventilation tubes inserted, and in which sinus aspirates were obtained at the time of tube placement. About a third of them at that time were found to be colonized with the same organisms that we associate with acute middle ear disease and acute sinusitis, ie, *Hemophilus* and pneumococcus.

DR. FAIRBANKS: Before someone decides to go out to initiate the definitive study on sinus aspirates, I will remind you that the maxillary sinus does not reach the level of the floor of the nose until (on the average) age 8 to 10 years. So in some very young children, if the inferior meatus approach to the sinus is used, you will not be able to get the needle through the thick nasal bone no matter how hard you push. One of the reasons we do not see studies of sinus aspirates for cultures is the difficulty of performing the procedure.

DR. BLUESTONE: Let us consider the list of indications for aspiration in acute sinusitis. We agree that the organisms that were listed by both Dr. Gwaltney and Dr. Shurin are the ones we are seeing and are the same organisms, essentially, which have been found in acute otitis media.

Now, since you brought up the subject of aspiration of the maxillary sinuses, Dr. Shurin, will you answer Dr. Fairbanks's concern about aspiration of sinuses in children? Do you think that his concern is well-founded?

DR. SHURIN: I think it is. But I really do not have any experience since I personally do not do this procedure. I would like to return with a question. Can x-rays help you delineate the margins of the sinus, when you are planning a procedure of this sort in a child?

DR. FAIRBANKS: Yes, they can, because the sinuses grow differently in different children. In 50% of the children it takes to age 8 to 10 for the maxillary sinus to reach the level of the floor of the nose. So some children will be good candidates for aspiration while others will not.

DR. WALD: Other objections that have been raised, at least in the literature, concern damage to the teeth and the fear of osteomyelitis. I do not know if these are legitimate objections, and I would ask your opinion.

DR. SCHRAMM: We have reviewed the sinus radiographs of 100 patients with orbital cellulitis and compared them with 100 age-matched patients who had facial x-rays following trauma. We looked specifically at the radiographic development of the paranasal sinuses and attempted to determine what was "normal" mucosal thickening and opacification at various ages. The maxillary sinus is developed adequately in 3-year-old children to allow sinus aspiration, and in many 2-year-old children this could be done.

Under age 2, where orbital complications of sinusitis are most common, maxillary sinus aspiration would generally not be clinically practical though the sinus outline can be well defined. I do not think there will be any problem with the dentition because the teeth are anterior and lateral to the location of the aspiration in the inferior meatus. The bone in this area may be slightly thicker in small children and this should be kept in mind when entering the sinus. Osteomyelitis should not be a problem in a patient concurrently treated with an appropriate antibiotic.

Regarding the appearance of the mucosal lining of the maxillary and ethmoid sinuses there is no thickening, opacity or asymmetry in appearance after age 2 years in normal sinuses. Less than 40% of children under age 2 will have clouding or opacification and only 7% will be asymmetrically involved.

DR. BLUESTONE: We appear to have a "non-consensus." Some of the panel are concerned that aspiration should probably be performed in patients who are acutely ill or toxic so we can learn more about etiologic factors, and also to aid in determining in those patients who have sinus radiographs that show opacification whether they have the disease or not. We are concerned about the full development of the sinuses, but Dr. Schramm has suggested that with care in getting preaspiration films, you can do the procedure quite safely. I think we are not doing aspirations frequently enough.

DR. SCHRAMM: I personally feel that sinus aspirations are indicated only when there is a complication of sinusitis. I think that we can obtain enough bacteriologic information to treat sinusitis in everyday practice. Personally, I do not recommend a sinus aspiration during routine therapy for my younger patients or for anyone else.

DR. WALD: I am not sure we know when children have sinusitis because I do not think we have really defined it, except clinically; and there is no agreement that radiographs are helpful in interpretation. So, I think we need a study similar to that done by Dr. Gwaltney and his colleagues, to obtain correlation between clinical presentation, radiographic findings, aspirate bacteriology and perhaps ultrasound. There has been some suggestion recently in the literature that ultrasound may be a helpful adjunct to the diagnosis of a fluid-filled sinus.

DR. BLUESTONE: Dr. Shurin, are you satisfied that the etiology of sinusitis in infants and children which you presented is correct?

DR. SHURIN: Yes. One point that might be made is that in children with orbital complications, there is a difference. The *H influenzae* are not the relatively untypable avirulent strains that are predominant in uncomplicated sinusitis, but are almost entirely type B strains. These have great invasive potential and ability to cause lethal complications. A number of such cases, some of which were due to ampicillin-resistant organisms, have been reported.

DR. WALD: I would like to comment that the evidence that periorbital or orbital cellulitis is related to ethmoiditis is all radiographic, and I think there has been some doubt cast on whether radiography is the absolute measure of sinus disease.

DR. SCHRAMM: It no longer is. In the patients with clinical orbital cellulitis and clinical sinusitis, less than 10% of them did not have radiographic evidence of sinus abnormality. The abnormality may either be ipsilateral opacification or asymmetrical mucosal thickening or clouding. So a child with an immediately antecedent upper respiratory infection and a complication such as orbital cellulitis with a unilateral sinusitis, I think, probably suggests that pus in the nose is not coming from a buccal cellulitis or vice versa.

FLOOR COMMENT: In my prior practice, I irrigated hundreds of sinuses in children, and noticed, clinically, that the children who came to the otolaryngologist were primarily those who pediatricians were unable to cure with repeated doses of ampicillin. On examination, almost all of these children had a very milky exudate along the floor of the nose. You will find that as many as 60 or 70% of those children will have abnormal Waters radiographic views of the sinuses.

I was disturbed that most radiologists would read the film as underdeveloped maxillary sinuses. That simply indicates to me that the radiologist does not know that children are born with maxillary sinuses; and opacification of the maxillary sinuses in small children is so common that rendering of a correct x-ray diagnosis has been delayed for many years. But I will assure you that you can aspirate the maxillary sinus fairly easily in children, even at the age of 12 months, and you can obtain pus from them.

One thing I have gained from this meeting is that in future studies I must take cultures in a different way. While doing irrigations, we recovered a high percentage of *S pneumoniae* and *H influenzae*. Also I have become aware of almost a typical appearance of staphylococcal rhinitis in which almost all of the cases are penicillin-resistant.

It is curious that children with *S pneumoniae* and *H influenzae* who received repeated, prolonged high doses of ampicillin drugs come to the otolaryngologist and many have penicillin-resistant staphylococci in their noses. Perhaps the staphylococcal rhinitis produces some blockage of the nose and causes obstruction of sinus drainage. We grow the same organism out of the ear a significant number of times, and those children almost all improve on a cephalosporin. That is what I prescribe entirely for the patient who has pus in the nose, who has repeatedly infected ears and has an opacification of the maxillary sinus. We are able usually to clear up their most recent acute infection. We stop the antibiotic two days before we insert tubes and do a sinus irrigation and then start them back on postoperatively. And we do not see recurrences in these children.

DR. BLUESTONE: Dr. Gwaltney, if a patient has acute sinusitis, what is your drug of choice, without an aspiration?

DR. GWALTNEY: Ampicillin or amoxicillin for the usual case.

FLOOR QUESTION: In the *H influenzae* that you found, what were the sensitivities and the type? Were these really the typable *H influenzae*, or were they nontypable bacteria?

DR. GWALTNEY: They were not group B, and they were not typable. They were all unencapsulated strains. We had one strain that was ampicillin-resistant.

The amoxicillin-ampicillin drugs have advantages and disadvantages. They are bactericidal for most of the causative agents, and they are relatively inexpensive. They have the disadvantage of being ineffective for ampicillin-resistant *H influenzae*. Likewise, they are *not* satisfactory for the unusual case due to penicillin-resistant *S aureus* or resistant Gram-negative bacteria.

Trimethoprim sulfa has the advantage of activity against *S pneumoniae* and ampicillin-resistant *H influenzae*. It probably has less activity against the β-hemolytic *Streptococcus*. It may present the problem of sulfa allergy, so it also has its pros and cons.

Cefaclor has some very desirable characteristics in terms of spectrum, particularly with coverage of ampicillin-resistant *H influenzae* and penicillin-resistant *S aureus*. However, the cost will certainly be a consideration in its selection.

DR. BLUESTONE: Dr. Gwaltney, what percentage of the bacteria that you isolated were penicillin-resistant?

DR. GWALTNEY: I don't know the exact percentage. Most, except for many *H influenzae* and penicillin-resistant *S aureus*, are sensitive. These are important exceptions, however.

FLOOR QUESTION: It has been my experience in culturing sinuses in adults who have orbital cellulitis that *H influenzae* or staphylococci that were penicillin-resistant were not present. So, as far as I am concerned, the first line drug in adults is still plain penicillin, before you go on to ampicillin or certainly to more expensive medications.

DR. BLUESTONE: Dr. Fairbanks, what is your drug of choice for adults with acute sinusitis, without a previous aspirate?

DR. FAIRBANKS: I share the concern about *S aureus*. I remember Dr. Mark Rafferty used to say that we are prisoners of our own experience. I remember a 23-year-old nurse who came into Johns Hopkins with a sinusitis from which an *S aureus* was cultured, and she developed meningitis. We routinely use erythromycin and sulfa as the empirical therapy while we are awaiting the cultures.

DR. BLUESTONE: So, you are concerned about Dr. Gwaltney's 2% *S aureus* problem, and you are going to treat with erythromycin and sulfa. Dr. Shurin, what is your treatment of choice for acute sinusitis in children?

DR. SHURIN: In the complicated cases, certainly those with orbital involvement, the initial treatment would be ampicillin and/or chloramphenicol. I think in simple cases amoxicillin would be a reasonable enough choice at the present time.

DR. BLUESTONE: How would you deal with the problem of *S aureus* in children when amoxicillin is not adequate? Will you wait to see if the infection responds, as we do in ear disease, and switch if the child does not improve?

DR. SHURIN: That would depend on the clinical circumstance. The common concerns in pediatrics are children who fail on many courses of antibiotic therapy, or cases in which sinusitis appears in leukemic or otherwise compromised children. In these cases, I think, you need to be much more aggressive than sometimes we are in obtaining a bacteriologic diagnosis.

DR. BLUESTONE: Dr. Wald, what would you prescribe as the antimicrobial drug of choice for acute sinusitis in a child?

DR. WALD: In acute life-threatening infections like orbital complications, I would begin with ampicillin and chloramphenicol. In the outpatient management of acute sinus disease, similar to the situation for acute otitis media, I would begin with ampicillin. We are saying that some 20% of these cases are probably caused by *Hemophilus*. Even in the geographic areas where ampicillin resistance is 15%, that will result in approximately 3% of patients having a resistant organism. If you follow the patient carefully, you can judge a clinical failure and get an aspirate and change therapy.

DR. BLUESTONE: Dr. Gwaltney, do we know the concentration of cefaclor in the sinus mucosa and the exudate in adults?

DR. GWALTNEY: We don't have that information. As far as I know, it is not available and information available on other antibiotic concentrations in sinus aspirates is somewhat conflicting and confusing to me. That is one of the reasons I am concerned about treating with penicillin alone. Perhaps we should observe a group of patients treated with penicillin to see if it eradicates *H influenzae* satisfactorily. I am concerned about the antibiotic levels that can be achieved in the maxillary sinus with the various antibiotics.

DR. BLUESTONE: Dr. Gwaltney, could you tell us if there is any benefit from taking a nasopharyngeal culture in an adult or child? Is there any correlation between nasopharyngeal cultures and what is found in the sinuses?

DR. GWALTNEY: No. Most of the time you will be misled by nasopharyngeal cultures. It is better to know what the agents are that are likely to cause sinusitis and to base your treatment on that knowledge. I think nasopharyngeal cultures are a waste of the patient's money and, more importantly, may lead to improper therapy.

DR. BLUESTONE: Do you agree with that, panelists?

DR. WALD: I think nasal cultures are a waste of money. However, there was a study that appeared last month from the Children's Hospital National Medical Center which tried to correlate nasopharyngeal cultures with middle ear isolates. By doing semiquantitative bacteriology, they have shown some correlation between the nasopharyngeal flora and the middle ear effusion isolate. Perhaps with that technique, there may be some correlation between surface cultures (nasopharyngeal) and cultures of sinus aspirates.

DR. BLUESTONE: The studies to determine whether or not nasopharyngeal cultures really do correlate with what is inside the sinuses, especially in children, are yet to be done.

DR. KLEIN: The considerations that we have for antimicrobial therapy and for diagnosis aspiration are almost identical, with a couple of modifiers. In orbital cellulitis, one has to consider that these may be invasive type B strains of *H influenzae*. It would be an extraordinary situation, I think, if the problem of ampicillin-resistant *H influenzae* did not appear in sinusitis in the same degree as it did in otitis media.

One note to underline is that when we talk about penicillin resistance or penicillin sensitivity or resistance in relation to *Hemophilus*, we have to be sure to distinguish which penicillin is considered. There are only minor differences of in vitro efficacy between ampicillin and penicillin G, but too often physicians consider penicillin G and penicillin V to be comparable products. They possess comparable activity against the pneumococcus but penicillin V is significantly less effective than penicillin G against *H influenzae*.

Now the question I would have for the panel and, perhaps, for those in the audience, is a tough diagnostic problem for pediatricians. Are there any investigations now under way using the most recent radiologic techniques, ultrasound or radionucleoid studies, that can define for us more precisely the presence of fluid in the sinuses of children? I know that, at present, we don't have such techniques, but are you aware of any investigations that would have some promise of more specific techniques in the future?

DR. WALD: There was a brief note in the *Lancet* earlier this year about ultrasound being used in children with clinical diagnoses of acute sinusitis. The author was comparing the sensitivity of ultrasound to x-ray in detecting fluid within the maxillary sinus. At this time, ultrasonography may not be an adequate definition or measure of sinus disease, but the appeal is that it is a noninvasive procedure that utilizes nonionizing radiation.

FLOOR QUESTION: We have talked about "the drug of choice," but actually all we have talked about is the *antimicrobial* choice. I would like to ask Dr. Gwaltney if in his study any adjunctive treatments with systemic decongestants, topical vasoconstrictors and so forth were employed. Also, I would like an opinion on the use of enzymes, which have been advocated by some people for sinusitis.

DR. GWALTNEY: These adjunctive measures were used at Dr. Sydnor's discretion. We did not control for these measures alone. However, we learned that if we used them "alone," that is, in the patients who had resistant organisms or who did not take their antibiotics, adjunctive measures did not result in sterilization of the sinus cavity. So as the only form of treatment they did not seem to be effective. Now, whether they would be effective in preventing sinusitis in the first place is an interesting question as yet unanswered.

DR. BLUESTONE: Dr. Klein, what would be your drug of choice for cervical adenitis, when you haven't inserted a needle for diagnostic purposes?

DR. KLEIN: Initial therapy must cover the possibilities of group A *Streptococcus* and β-lactamase-producing strains of *S aureus*. So a penicillinase-resistant penicillin would be appropriate. If the patient is allergic, you have a choice of cephalosporin, erythromycin or clindamycin.

DR. BLUESTONE: Dr. Klein, you have seen the data on cefaclor used for the ear, nose and throat. Is it promising for the ENT clinician?

DR. KLEIN: I think the major feature that interests pediatricians who are concerned with infections of the upper respiratory tract, otitis media, sinusitis and also lower respiratory tract and pneumonias, is the efficacy of the drug against the pneumococcus, but also aganist *H influenzae*, both ampicillin-sensitive and resistant strains. As the various speakers have noted, the incidence of ampicillin-resistant strains of *H influenzae* in terms of the microbiology of sinusitis or otitis media indicates that the incidence of β-lactamase-producing *H influenzae* is relatively low today, in June 1979. If this problem becomes more significant, then the importance of the drug will increase.

The other consideration would be choice for initial therapy if the patient fails. Since at least one of the possibilities of that failure is β-lactamase-producing strains of *H influenzae*, then cefaclor could be a candidate drug for such a patient. Our interest should focus on its efficacy as the first oral cephalosporin that has such efficacy for β-lactamase-producing strains of *H influenzae*. However, it goes into the marketplace in competition with other drugs such as trimethoprim-sulfa and erythromycin in combination with sulfa, which are also effective for the same range of organisms. Not only is cefaclor active against β-lactamase-producing strains, it is considerably more active against all *Hemophilus* than previously available oral cephalosporins.

FLOOR COMMENT: I have found occasionally when I treated a patient with otitis media or pharyngitis with Keflex® and I did not get a response, I could put him on cephradine, and for some reason he would clear up. So I think there may be a synergistic effect in these drugs that probably has not been discussed at all.

Now, in my town an anaerobic culture costs $96, especially if it is a mixed bacterial infection. I am not as liberal with my patients' money as a lot of people may be.

DR. BLUESTONE: That is a very important point. We could say that for most patients with otitis media, initial cultures may not be cost-effective. The microbiologic data are so consistent that you can begin therapy on the basis of what you know about the incidence of bacteria in your community.

The same may be said of the majority of patients with sinusitis or cervical adenitis. So, for those three conditions I agree we should begin with drugs that are effective against the known agents. However, if the patient doesn't respond to the initial antibiotic, then a culture would be helpful. In fact, you may be saving your patient money in the long run by avoiding the expenses of hospitalization. We need to select and be very specific in terms of what the culture information has to offer.

I am not sure what to say about your comment about cephradine following Keflex, except that I think neither drug is appropriate for otitis media that is due to *Hemophilus*. Both would be effective for pneumococcal otitis. Without the microbiologic information, we have no way of evaluating what that means.

FLOOR QUESTION: Dr. Kammer, can you give us information in regard to the anaerobic activity of cefaclor?

DR. KAMMER: The anaerobic activity of cefaclor is very much like that of the penicillins and the rest of the cephalosporins, excluding, of course, cefoxitin. It has the good activity against most of the upper respiratory tract Gram-negative anaerobes that penicillin does. Most strains of *B fragilis* will be resistant to it; more than 60% will be.

DR. KLEIN: We are still dealing with the susceptibility pattern for anaerobes in the upper respiratory tract where they are susceptible to penicillins and selected cephalosporins. We have to be alert to the concern for *B fragilis* and a few strains of *B melaninogenicus* that are resistant to penicillins, but these are relatively uncommon. So for the most part, invasions by anaerobes in the upper respiratory tract, be it local head and neck infections or pulmonary disease, are susceptible to penicillins and cephalosporins. *B fragilis* should be kept in mind, but it is still an uncommon agent responsible for disease in the upper respiratory tract.

LABYRINTHINE SEGMENT AND GENICULATE GANGLION OF FACIAL NERVE IN FETAL AND ADULT HUMAN TEMPORAL BONES

XIAN-XI GE, MD GERSHON J. SPECTOR, MD

ST. LOUIS, MISSOURI

The later stages of development (15-40 weeks in utero) of the geniculate ganglion and labyrinthine segment of the facial nerve in the human fetus demonstrate minimal neuronal growth. The vascular supply is well established. The major changes occur in the perineural ossification pattern. The canal of the labyrinthine facial nerve segment ossifies first via the petrous apex and periotic capsule. The narrowest portion of the canal is at the geniculate ganglion in the earlier stages and at the fundus of the internal auditory canal at term. The geniculate ganglion area ossifies by means of two bony plates. The medial plate is a derivate of the periosteal growth of the petrous apex and the lateral plate is an extension of membranous bone from the squama. The major relationships to the middle ear do not change. The hiatus of the facial canal diminishes in size during gestation, but remains patent at birth.

INTRODUCTION

Clinical studies on facial nerve paralysis have suggested that the proximal portion of the facial nerve, ie, the labyrinthine and meatal segments, may be the major sites of pathological lesions.[1-9] Fisch and Esslen noted pathologic nerve fiber changes (following total intratemporal nerve VII exposure for Bell's palsy) in the labyrinthine segment in 11 of 12 cases and in the proximal meatal facial nerve segment in 8 of 11 cases.[10] Many authors have noted lesions in the labyrinthine segment, geniculate ganglion, and in the proximal part of the internal auditory canal in herpes zoster oticus and other viral diseases.[11-18] In addition, a vast variety of other lesions have been attributed to this area.[19-27]

The purposes of this paper are:

1. To observe the ossification pattern surrounding the geniculate ganglion and labyrinthine segment of the facial nerve in human fetal temporal bones.

2. To measure the labyrinthine segment and geniculate ganglion in the fetal and adult temporal bones.

3. To measure the critical anatomic distances and relationships of the labyrinthine segment and geniculate ganglion to the neighboring anatomic structures.

4. To elucidate the clinical and surgical significance of the developmental and anatomic features of the geniculate ganglion and the labyrinthine segment of the facial nerve.

MATERIALS AND METHODS

FETAL STUDIES

Forty consecutive temporal bones were obtained from fetuses and neonates who died of various medical disorders. Complete autopsies were performed in all cases. The autopsy information on these temporal bones has been previously reported.[28,29] All temporal bones which were used for this light microscopic study were cut adequately for direct measurements. These included 13 pairs of temporal bones from fetuses and neonates for comparison of one ear to another.

A fixative consisting of 4% glutaraldehyde in a sodium phosphate buffer (pH 7.4), brought to tonicity (Osmette A® digital osmometer, Precision Systems, Inc., Sudbury, Mass.) with sucrose (280 mOsm), was prepared just prior to use. Temporal bones were injected with fixative by the transtympanic route and then removed with a Stryker saw. After fixation overnight, the temporal bones were decalcified with RDO® (DuPage Kinetic Labs, Inc., Downers Grove, Ill.). The bones were trimmed, care being taken to preserve the neural elements attached to the cranial surface, then dehydrated in graded ethanols, and embedded in colloidin. After embedding, the bones were oriented in the microtome so that sectioning was parallel to the labyrinthine segment of the facial nerve. The temporal bones were cut in the classic vertical sectional plane. Sections were taken every 20 μ, mounted in serial order, labeled and stained with hemotoxylin and eosin. Some sections were stained with a nuclear stain.

Only temporal bones with the entire length of the labyrinthine segment of facial nerve and geniculate ganglion on a single tissue section were used for the measurements. A slide projector with a magnification ratio of 45:1 was used. The critical parameters were drawn on grid paper for accurate measurements.

The fetal measurements of gross body length, weight, and gestational age were determined by the pathologist by direct measurements and acceptable gestational criteria and correlated with the maternal history.[28] The following measurements were performed:

1. Length and width of geniculate ganglion at different gestational ages.

2. Entire length of labyrinthine segment from the vertical crest (in the fundus of the internal auditory canal) to the geniculate ganglion.

3. Widths at the narrowest and widest portions of the labyrinthine segment.

4. Relationship between the size of the labyrinthine facial nerve segment and its bony canal at the entrance and exit of the Fallopian canal; also the narrowest diameter of the bony canal was determined.

5. Distance from geniculate ganglion to middle ear.

6. Ossification pattern around the geniculate ganglion, the

From the Department of Otolaryngology, Washington University School of Medicine, St. Louis. This research was supported by a grant from the EAR Foundation, Nashville, Tennessee.

Dr. Ge is a visiting scholar from the Department of Otolaryngology, 6th People's Hospital, Shanghai, China.

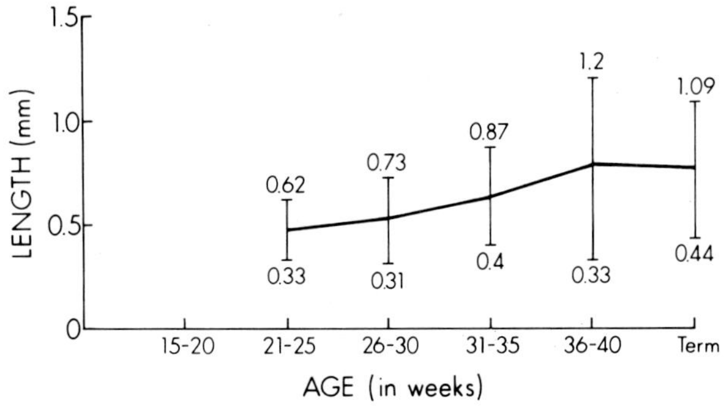

Fig. 1. Geniculate ganglion length vs gestational age. Geniculate ganglion length does not increase significantly with the later stages of gestation.

labyrinthine segment and the middle fossa plate were also determined.

ADULT STUDIES

Ten human temporal bones (five pairs) were removed at autopsy from adults. The dura was attached to the bone and the nerve endings were preserved in the internal auditory canal. The temporal bones were freshly frozen in saline. A simple mastoidectomy was performed. The mastoid cells were exenterated and the semicircular canals were skeletonized. The facial nerve was identified and skeletonized. Removal of the bony cover from the fallopian canal allowed for exposure of the nerve sheath to the anterior portion of the geniculate ganglion. It was necessary to identify and preserve the cochleariform process just below the anterior part of the tympanic segment of the facial nerve.

A labyrinthectomy was begun by opening the semicircular canals. The vestibule was opened widely and the internal auditory canal was exposed. The vertical and transverse crest was exposed. Posterior to the vertical crest the superior vestibular nerve was identified and removed. Anterior to the crest the facial nerve was identified and preserved. Further dissection removed the bony cover and exposed the labyrinthine segment and geniculate ganglion of the facial nerve. In some cases a middle fossa dissection was performed for better visualization and measurement.

Measurements were taken within a dissecting microscope (at 10x and 16x magnification) which was fitted with a microruler within one eyepiece. The following measurements were performed:

1. Length of labyrinthine segments.

2. Width at the narrowest and widest portions of the labyrinthine segment.

3. Distance from the geniculate ganglion to the end of the labyrinthine segment at the fundus of the internal auditory meatus.

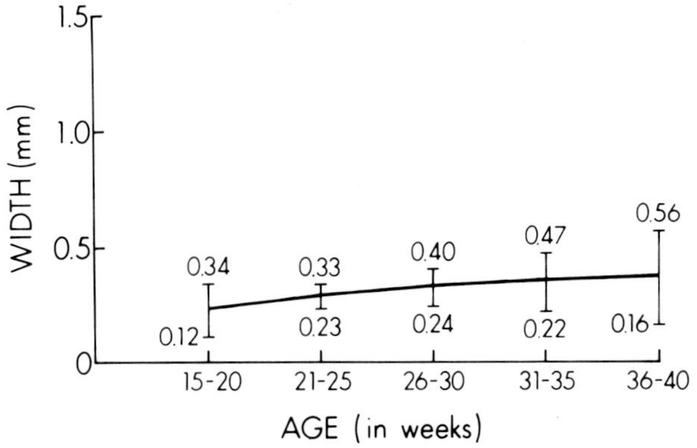

Fig. 2. Geniculate ganglion width vs gestational age. Geniculate ganglion width does not increase significantly with the later stages of gestation.

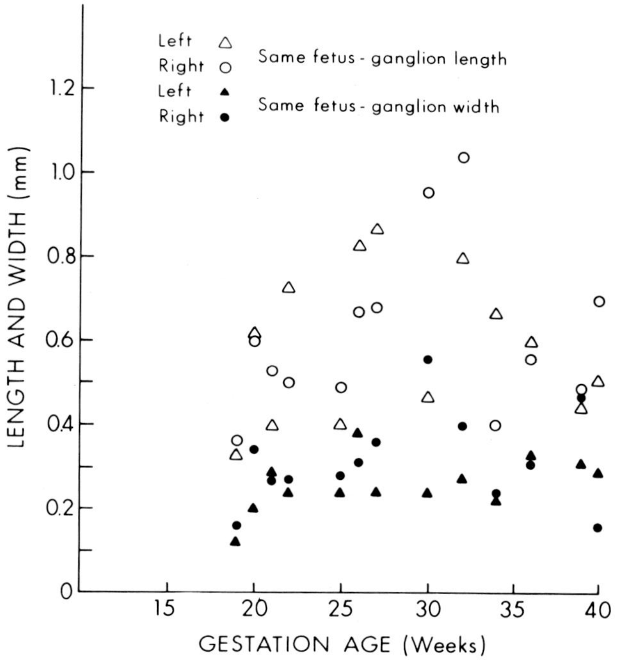

Fig. 3. Comparison of the geniculate ganglion on both sides of the same fetus. A wide variation of readings with a significant degree of asymmetry is shown. However there is no progressive enlargement during 20-40 weeks of gestation.

4. Length and width of the geniculate ganglion.

5. Sizes of the bony entrance of the fallopian canal and the meatal fundus.

6. Distances from cochleariform process to the anterior part of the geniculate ganglion.

RESULTS

FETAL TEMPORAL BONES

Geniculate Ganglion.

MEASUREMENTS. The length and width of the geniculate ganglion were measured at various gestational ages of the fetus (15-40 weeks in utero) and also correlated with fetal weight and length. At each age group no statistically significant differences in the

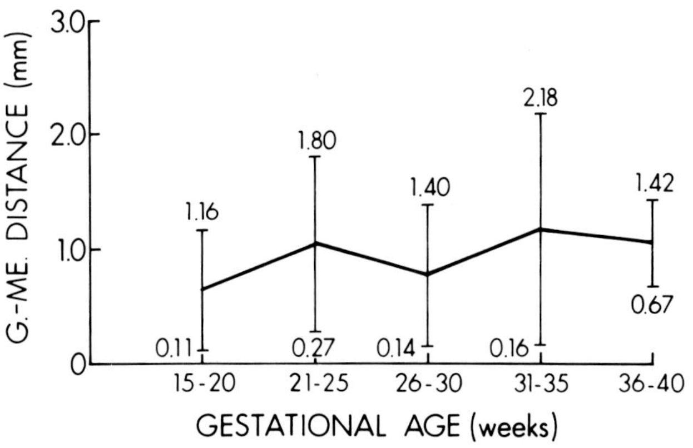

Fig. 4. Distance from ganglion to middle ear (G.-ME.) vs gestational age. Distance from the anterior border of the geniculate ganglion to the middle ear does not change during the later stages of gestation.

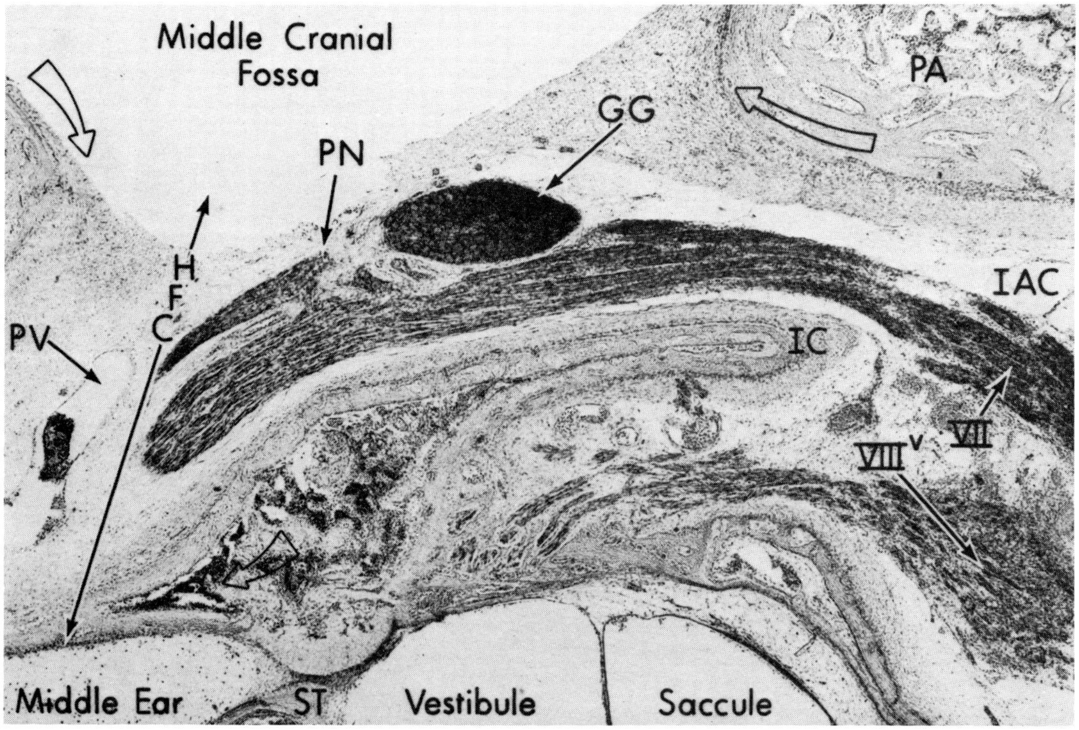

Fig. 5. At 15 weeks gestation the primitive hiatus of the facial canal (HFC) communicates the middle cranial fossa with the middle ear. The canal of the labyrinthine segment of the facial nerve (VII), otic capsule, vertical crest (IC), petrous apex (PA), and stapes (ST) are not ossified. The geniculate ganglion (GG) and distal labyrinthine nerve segment are dehiscent. Clear arrows denote bone development. PN - Petrosal nerve, IAC - Internal auditory canal, VIII^{V} - Superior vestibular nerve, PV - Petrosal vein. (PTAH stain)

length and width of the geniculate ganglion were observed (Figs. 1 and 2).

The length of the ganglion ranged from 0.33 to 1.2 mm with an average of 0.97 mm. Generally the smaller ganglia were noted at earlier gestational ages, lower fetal weights and shorter lengths. The width of the geniculate ganglion ranged from 0.12 mm to 0.56 mm with an average width of 0.32 mm. Generally the widest ganglia are associated with increased gestational age, higher fetal weight and larger fetuses.

A comparison with fetal weight and length showed a similar correlation. This indicates that the growth of the geniculate ganglion in the later stages of development in the human fetus is minimal. There is a slight increase (statistically insignificant) in geniculate ganglion parameters from 15 weeks until 35 weeks in utero and then the slope of the curve flattens out until term is reached at 40 weeks in utero (Figs. 1 and 2).

Comparison of ganglion measurements (length and width) on both sides of the same fetus demonstrates statistically significant apparent differences (Fig. 3). Both sides in the same fetus tend not to be symmetrical between 20-35 weeks in utero. However, there is no progressive enlargement of the geniculate ganglion size with gestational age. Thus it appears that the geniculate ganglion is formed prior to 15 weeks in utero to a stage of development which is seen at term or delivery.

The distance from the geniculate ganglion to the epitympanum is similar at all stages of fetal development. This constant parameter is approximately 1 mm during the entire gestational period. It does not vary with fetal weight and length (Fig. 4).

OSSIFICATION PATTERN. Unlike the ossification pattern of the canal of the labyrinthine segment of the facial nerve (which forms in the petrous bone), the geniculate ganglion area is ossified partially in the membranous bone (squama of the temporal bone) of the middle fossa plate, ie, the floor of the middle cranial fossa.

At 15 weeks in utero the geniculate ganglion and its blood supply (the superficial petrosal branches from the middle meningeal artery which is derived from the internal maxillary artery) lie in the dural condensation on top of the anterior epitympanum. At this stage the middle fossa is continuous with the middle ear spaces via the epitympanum (Fig. 5). This constitutes the primitive hiatus of the facial canal. At 20 weeks in utero medial and lateral bony plates begin to form in the squama and petrosa along the floor of the middle fossa (Fig. 6). These two plates of bone begin to approximate each other during the later part of gestation. At 35 weeks in utero the undersurface of the geniculate ganglion is separated from the epitympanum by bone (Fig. 7). This closes the primitive hiatus of the facial canal and separates the epitympanum from the middle cranial fossa. However the cranial surface is still

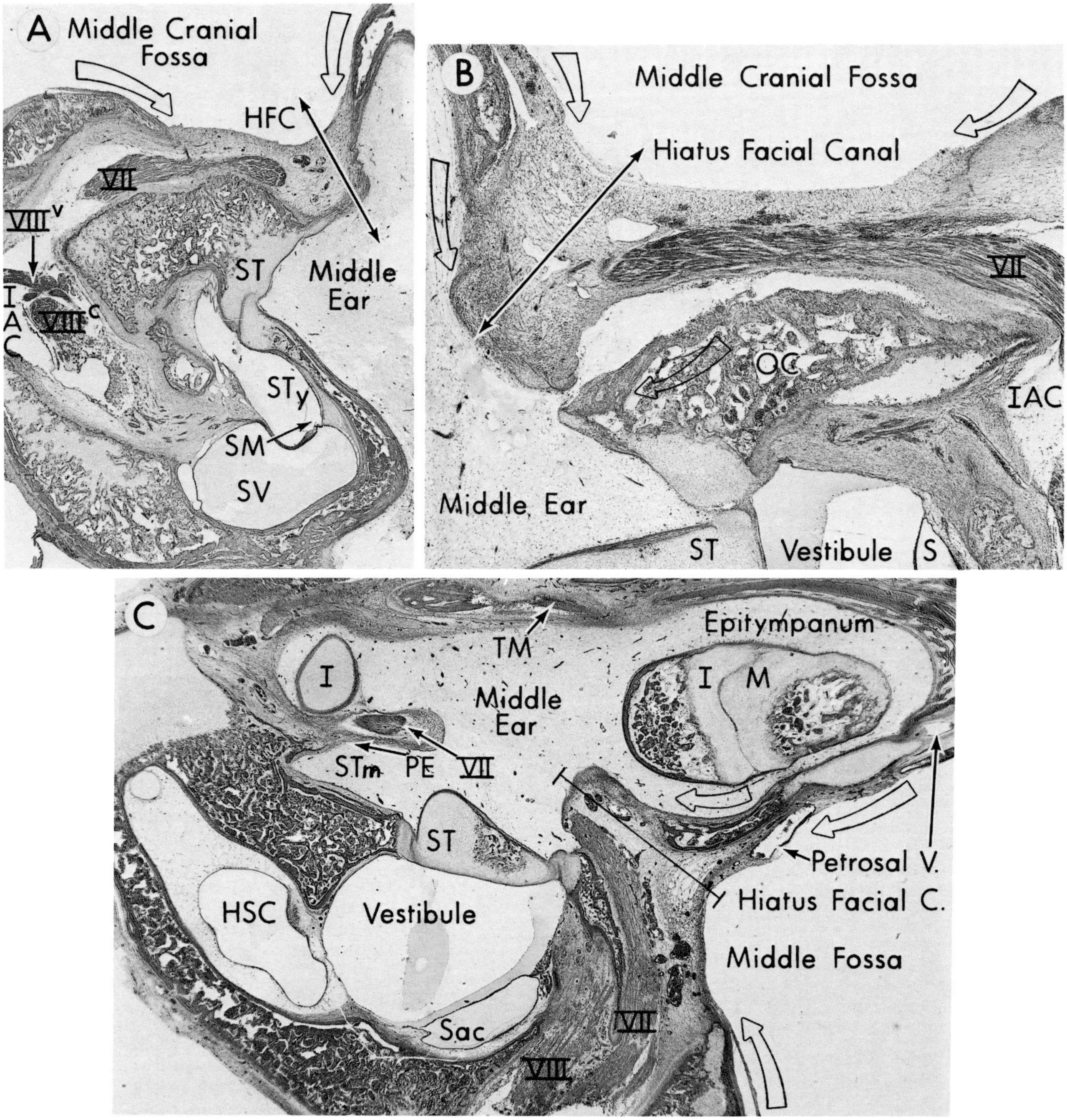

Fig. 6 A-C). Development of medial and lateral bony plates (clear arrows) between 15-20 weeks gestation. The primitive HFC is still patent, communicating middle ear with middle cranial fossa. A) SM - Scala media, SV - Scala vestibuli, VIII^{c} - Cochlear nerve, STy - Scala tympani. B) OC - Otic capsule, S - Saccule. C) M - Malleus, I - Incus, HSC -Horizontal semicircular canal, STm - Sinus tympani, PE - Pyramidal eminence.

dehiscent with direct dural attachment to the geniculate perineural tissues. A portion of this dehiscence persists into adulthood as the hiatus of the facial canal (hiatus facialis) (Fig. 8).

All of the cases (including the infants from term until one month postpartum), except for three later stage fetuses, had persistent dehiscences of the bony covering over the dural surface of the geniculate ganglion. Thus the geniculate ganglion was in direct communication with the middle fossa dura. Nevertheless the size of the middle fossa dehiscence decreased in direct relation to increasing gestational age. The size of the middle fossa plate dehiscence over the geniculate ganglion is similarly related to increasing fetal weight and length (Fig. 9).

From our study it appears that the bony middle fossa plates (medial and lateral) form at 20 weeks in utero and fuse by 35 weeks in utero. The vast majority of ganglia are dehiscent at birth (ergo the surgeon must be aware of this fact while elevating

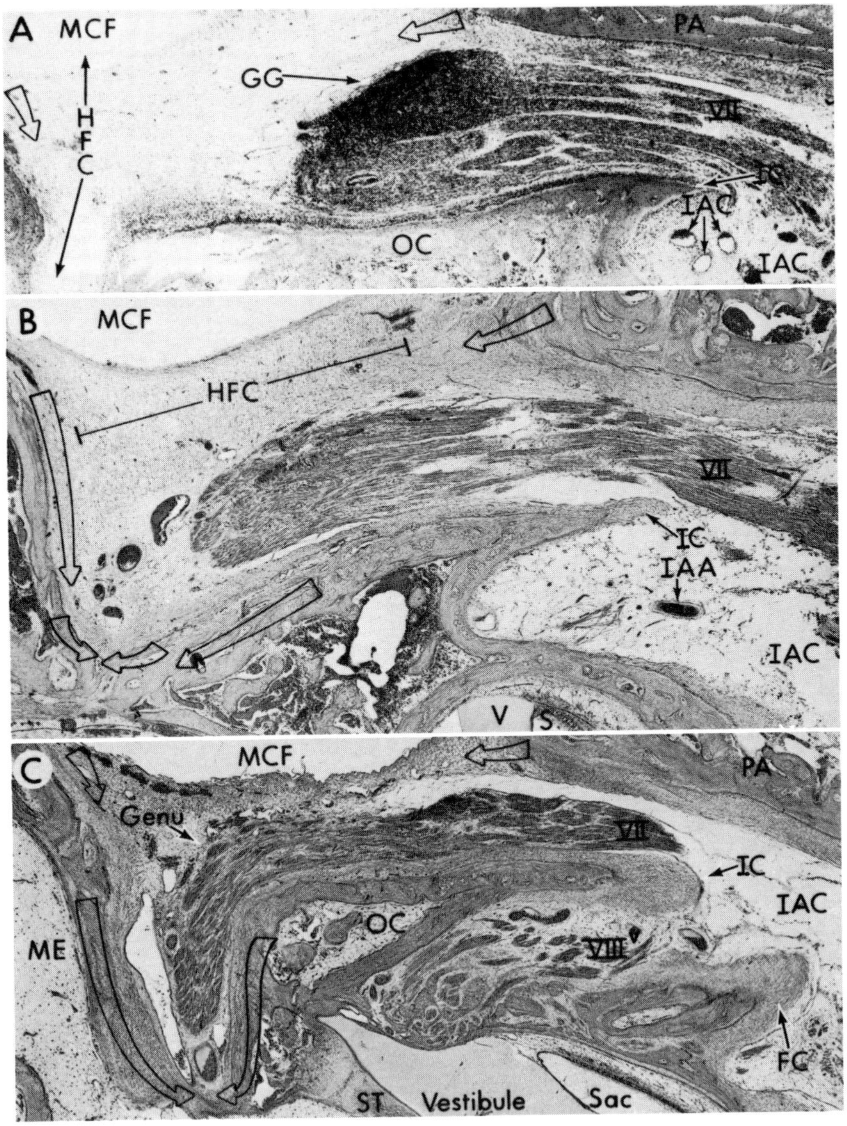

Fig. 7 A-C). Closure of the primitive HFC separating middle cranial fossa (MCF) from the middle ear (ME) between 20 and 35 weeks in utero. Clear arrows depict the growth of the bony plates. IAA - Internal auditory artery, FC - Falciform crest. (A - PTAH stain, B and C - H & E)

the middle fossa dura so as not to damage the geniculate ganglion in infants and young children). A comparison of the ossification of the middle fossa plate on both sides in the same fetus demonstrates an asymmetrical ossification pattern. Thus both geniculate ganglia may not be similarly covered with bone (Fig. 3).

As bone covers the geniculate ganglion, the surrounding dura and its blood supply (petrosal branches of the middle meningeal artery) are encompassed simultaneously. Thus the blood supply which arises from the middle meningeal artery enters the geniculate at the middle fossa plate dehiscence, ie, the hiatus of the facial canal. Then the vessels divide to supply the distal labyrinthine segment (anastomosing with branches from the internal auditory artery which is usually a division from the anterior inferior cerebellar artery) and follow the facial nerve in the fallopian canal into the middle ear (anastomosing with the stylomastoid artery which is a division of the occipital or posterior auricular arteries) (Fig. 10).

Labyrinthine Segment.

MEASUREMENTS. The length and narrowest width of the labyrinthine segment of the facial nerve were measured at various gestational ages (15-40 weeks in utero) and also correlated with fetal weight and length. At all age groups no statistically significant differences were noted in the length of the labyrinthine segments (Fig. 11). Generally the larger fetuses (longer and heavier) had longer labyrinthine segments. Thus the length of the labyrinthine segment remains constant during the later stages of gestation (15-40 weeks in utero).

There is a slight tendency on the average to note an increase in the labyrinthine segment of the facial nerve in the 2500-3000 g fetal stages (0.6-0.7 mm) and at 40 mm fetal length (Fig. 11). The labyrinthine segment ranged from 0.71 mm to 2.13 mm with an average of 1.67 mm in length.

The narrowest width of the labyrinthine segment is not constant along the nerve (as measured from the fundus of the internal auditory meatus to the

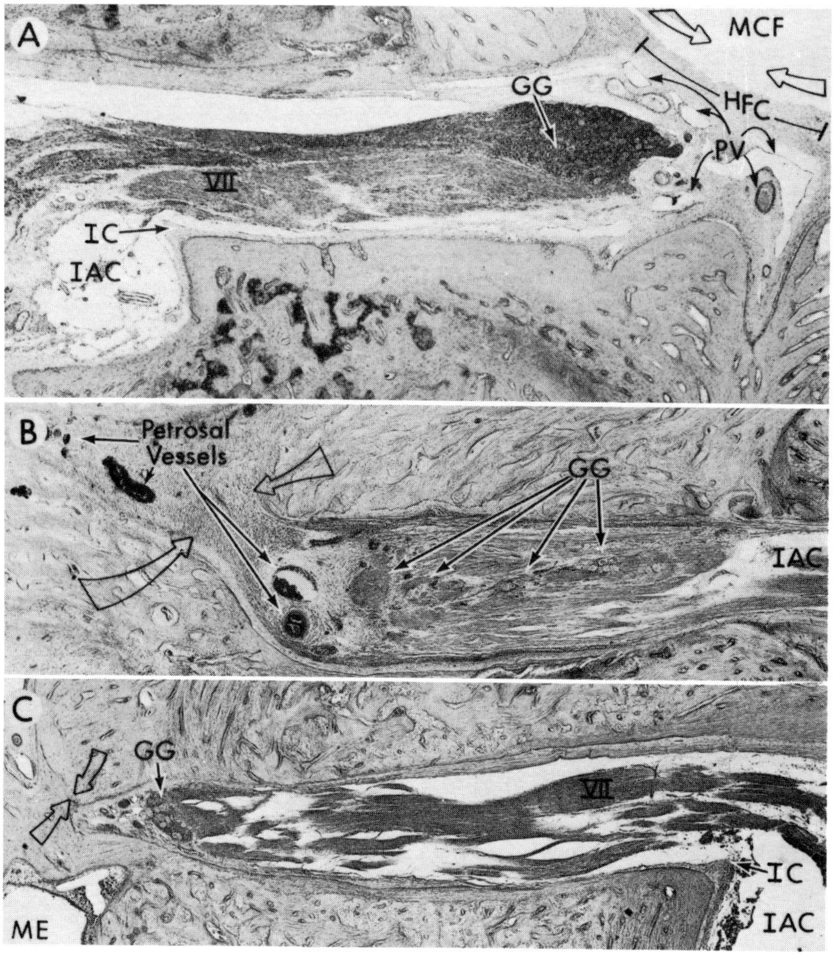

Fig. 8 A-C). Progressive narrowing of the HFC. Narrowing is indicated by the clear arrows at 35 weeks to one month postpartum. Geniculate ganglion is partially covered with bone. Note in B) that the geniculate cell bodies are not localized in a ganglion but are dispersed throughout the labyrinthine segment of the facial nerve. (A - PTAH stain, B and C - H & E)

geniculate ganglion). Thus the narrowest portion can be located near the geniculate ganglion or near the vertical crest or in the middle of the segment. The same is true for the widest portion of the segment (Tables 1 and 2). Generally over half of the narrowest diameters of the segment are near the geniculate ganglion. The widest diameter of the labyrinthine segment ranged from 0.16 mm to 0.78 mm with an average of 0.4 mm. The narrowest diameter ranged from 0.08 mm to 0.3 mm with an average of 0.24 mm.

OSSIFICATION PATTERN. The ossification pattern for the bony canal which encases the labyrinthine segment of the facial nerve is intimately associated with the ossification of the petrous bone and the otic capsule surrounding the apical turn of the cochlea. The ossification of the petrous pyramid occurs in a cartilaginous framework as a preexisting mold. In addition there are contributions from Reichert's cartilage to the formation of the fallopian canal.

At 20 weeks in utero we note ossification along the luminal surface of the bony canal. The vertical crest is still cartilaginous (Fig. 5). The otic capsule is still filled with vascular channels. The petrous apex is filled with vascular channels, bone marrow spaces and still has cartilaginous rests. The stapes and footplate are cartilaginous. There is early ossification beginning in the heads of the malleus and incus (Fig. 6). The facial canal is wide open and short with a nerve to canal width ratio of 1:5 (Fig. 5). There is some ossification beginning on the superior luminal surface of the internal auditory meatus (Fig. 12).

With progressive ossification the bony canal lengthens and narrows. The distal end fuses with the middle fossa bony plate. The superior border ossifies in continuation with the superior lip of the

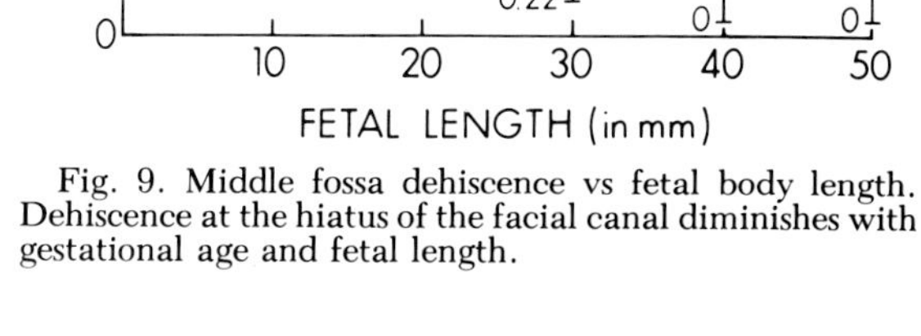

Fig. 9. Middle fossa dehiscence vs fetal body length. Dehiscence at the hiatus of the facial canal diminishes with gestational age and fetal length.

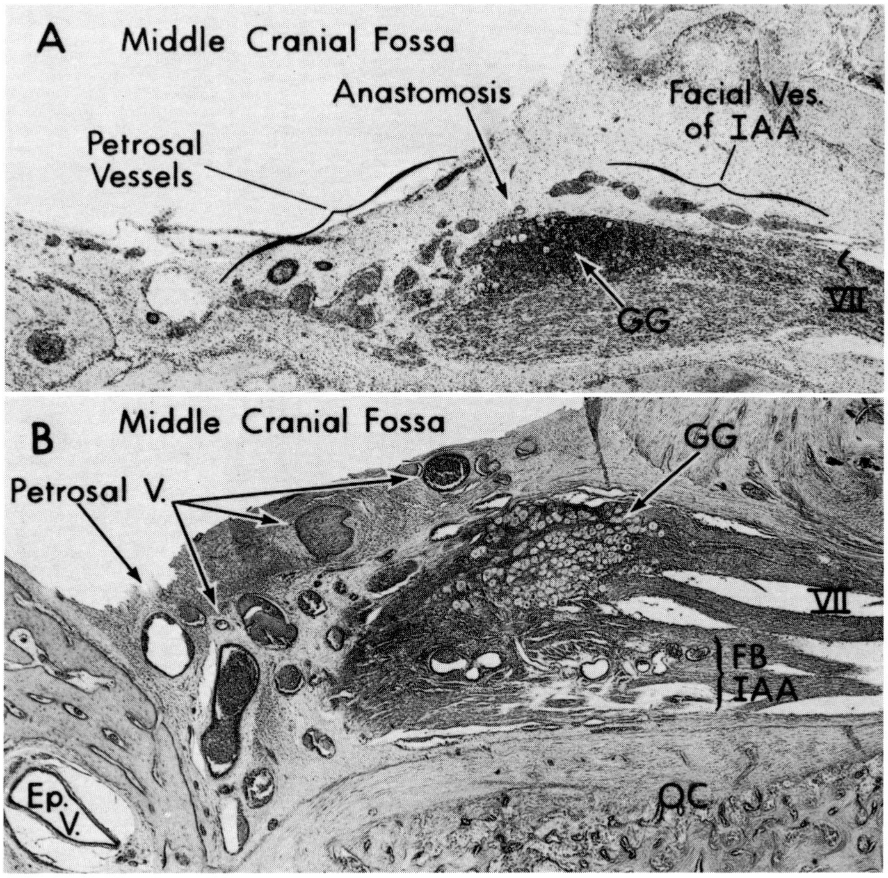

Fig. 10 A,B). Vascularity of the geniculate ganglion and labyrinthine segment. Note that temporal bones were cut in a transverse plane. The petrosal vessels are cut in cross-section (ie, they run in a horizontal plane) and facial branches (FB) from the internal auditory artery run parallel. EP.V. - Epitympanic vessel. Also note Figs. 7 B,C and 12.

internal auditory canal. The inferior border ossifies with the otic capsule of the cochlear apex. At 25 weeks in utero the nerve-to-canal width ratio is 1:3.9, by 30 weeks it is 1:2.9 and at 35 weeks the ratio is 1:1.9. The overall ratio of nerve-to-canal width at 35-40 weeks in utero is 1:1.9 or less. In some term fetal temporal bones the ratio is almost 1:1.

We have noted a few variations in the relationship of the labyrinthine segment of the nerve to its bony canal. The most common pattern is that of a long bony canal which is twice as large as the nerve in width (17 cases). In three cases the bony canal was almost the same width as the nerve. The perineurium is closely attached to the bony canal wall. In two cases the entrance to the bony canal was quite small. In these the vertical crest protruded into the canal and was fixed tightly against the labyrinthine segment of the facial nerve (Fig. 13B). In six cases we noted a constriction along the bony canal, distally, near the geniculate ganglion (Fig. 13A). Thus the ossification pattern, which is not symmetrical in both temporal bones of the same fetus, produces variations in bony canal conformation to the shape of the labyrinthine segment of the facial nerve. This, of course, may have a bearing on the clinical manifestations of facial nerve disorders.

An interesting observation is the comparison of the data from Tables 1 and 2 which signifies that the greatest variation in size occurs in the proximal portion of the bony canal, ie, near the vertical crest of the internal auditory canal. Thus the widest and narrowest diameters occur in this region. These may reflect the ossification pattern of the vertical crest at the canal inlet (fundus) (Fig. 13).

ADULT TEMPORAL BONES

Five pairs (10 bones) of temporal bones were studied. These were obtained randomly at autopsy. It should be noted that a comparison of measurements from the fetus to the adult is not possible in these experiments since the temporal bones were

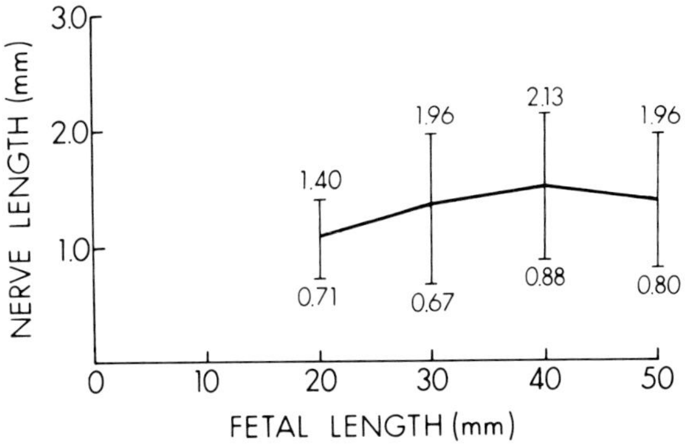

Fig. 11. Labyrinthine segment length vs fetal body length. Labyrinthine segment of the facial nerve does not elongate with gestational age.

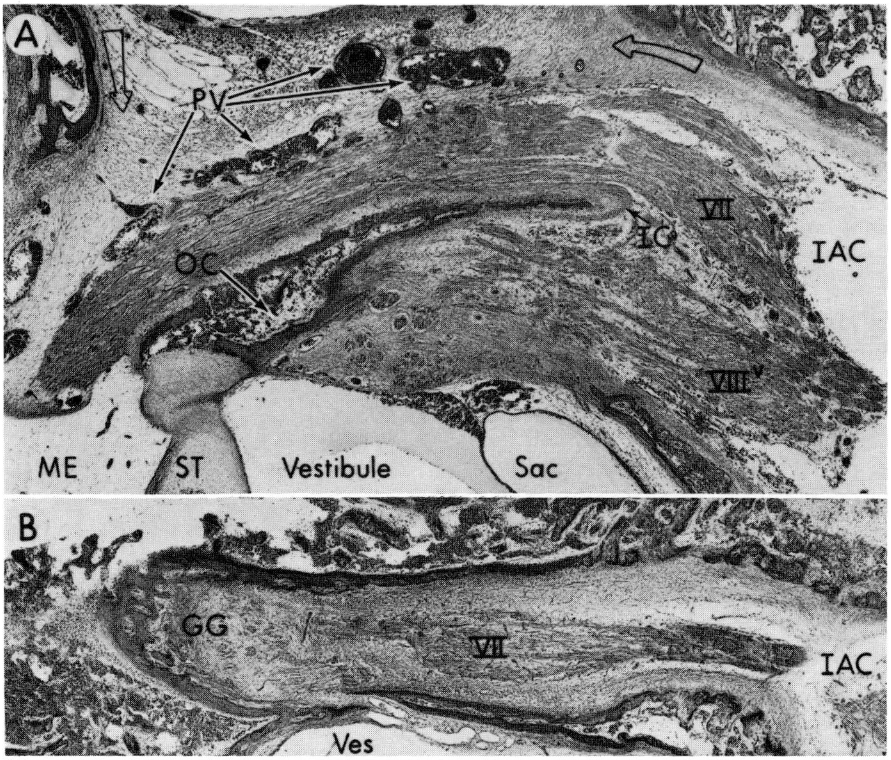

Fig. 12 A,B). Ossification pattern of the labyrinthine segment of the facial nerve (VII). Clear arrows indicate the medial and lateral bony plates. A) Ossification of the otic capsule. The vertical crest is still cartilaginous as is the stapes. The falciform crest is not formed. B) Ossification of the bony canal surrounding the labyrinthine segment starts from the luminal surface.

processed differently. The fetal bones were fixed for prolonged periods of time, embedded and processed. The adult bones were freshly frozen and dissected. In addition the variation of tissue responses of shrinkage to fixation is variable and different for fetal and adult tissues. Nevertheless, labyrinthine segments and geniculate ganglia in adults have been previously measured and reported.[30]

Geniculate Ganglion.

MEASUREMENTS. The length of the geniculate ganglion varied from 1.2 mm to 2.25 mm with an average length of 1.76 mm. The width of the ganglion ranged from 0.9 mm to 1.95 mm with an average width of 1.29 mm. Generally the sizes of the geniculate ganglia were similar in most temporal bones except for two cases (Table 3).

OSSIFICATION PATTERN. In all cases the geniculate ganglion area was completely ossified on the dural surface with a small hiatus of the facial canal persistent for the exit of the petrosal nerve. Nevertheless in two cases the bony plate was thin enough to visualize the geniculate ganglion pinkish-yellow discoloration beneath.

The distance from the cochleariform process to the anterior border of the geniculate ganglion ranged from 1.05 mm to 3.75 mm with an average distance of 2.1 mm (Table 3).

Labyrinthine Segment.

MEASUREMENTS. The length of the labyrinthine segment varied from 2.25 mm to 3 mm with an average of 2.82 mm. The width of the narrowest portion of the labyrinthine segment ranged 0.6 mm to 0.9 mm with an average of 0.7 mm. The narrow width was on the average 2.55 mm from the geniculate ganglion, ie, near the internal auditory meatal fundus or proximal portion of the bony canal. The widest portion of the nerve ranged from 0.9 mm to 1.5 mm with an average of 1.12 mm. The widest area was on the average of 0.9 mm from the geniculate ganglion, ie, near the distal portion of the canal or near the ganglion.

OSSIFICATION PATTERN. In all the adult cases the narrowest part of the bony canal was near the fundus of the internal auditory meatus and the widest part was near the geniculate ganglion. However in the fetal bones in half of the cases the narrowest part of the canal was near the geniculate ganglion (Fig. 13).

The adult bony canal at the meatus (just beyond the vertical crest) ranged in width from 0.6 mm to 0.9 mm with an average of 0.75 mm. The widest area ranged from 1.5 mm to 2.9 mm with an average of 1.9 mm. Thus the nerve canal ratio of 1:1.9 which is noted in the fetus is also maintained in the adult temporal bone.

In all our cases the labyrinthine segment was entirely covered with bone. There were not areas of dehiscences.

DISCUSSION

GENERAL COMMENTS

The anatomic studies of Rabl[31] and Gegenbaur[32] on the embryonic development of the seventh nerve

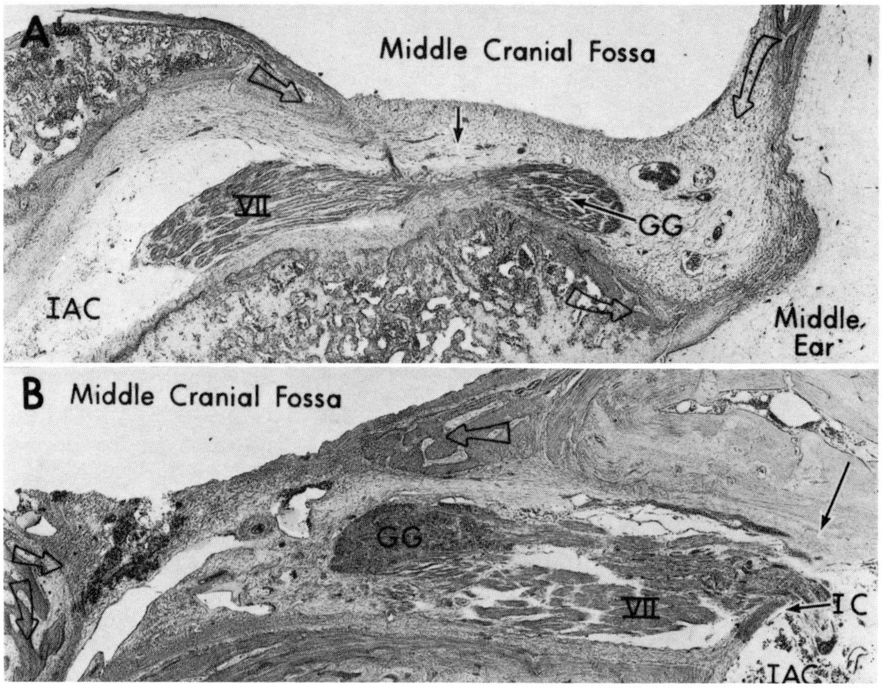

Fig. 13 A,B). Comparison of the narrowest portions (dark arrow) of the labyrinthine nerve segments at A) 20 weeks and B) 35 weeks in utero. Note that early in gestation the narrowest part is near the geniculate ganglion and at later stages near the internal auditory canal and vertical crest. Clear arrows indicate bony plates.

lead to its association with the second branchial or hyoid arch.[33,34] The close proximity of the developing geniculate ganglion to the second arch placode has suggested an intimate relationship between these two structures. It has been demonstrated that the developing ganglion enlarges as the otic placode disappears. The facial nerve develops from its facio-acoustic primordium of the second branchial arch preceding the 4 mm stage.[35] By the 8 - 10.6 mm stage the facial nerve separates from the acoustic division.

Since the nervus intermedius arises from the geniculate ganglion it is possible to study the formation of the ganglion cells by analyzing the facial nerve roots. His did not see fibers from the geniculate ganglion until the third month in utero.[36] Streeter, however, found the nervus intermedius and geniculate ganglion primordia in a 3 mm embryo.[37] Gasser noted a well-developed ganglion in the 11 mm embryo and a discrete, although smaller, nervus intermedius at a slightly later time.[35]

Both Rabl[31] and Futamura[38] noted that the greater petrosal nerve is the second branch to develop. It is preceded by the chorda tympani nerve at the 4.8 mm embryonic stage. Streeter noted that at this stage the nervus intermedius, which carries the sensory fibers of the chorda tympani, is well developed at the 4.5 mm embryo state.[37] Early the nerve gives off the posterior auricular and a branch to the posterior belly of the digastric muscle. Then it ends peripherally as a meshwork of intermingling fibers. At 14-20 weeks in utero the chorda tympani joins the lingual nerve. The muscular branches follow the formation of the facial muscle masses and usually lie deep to them.[39] The lesser petrosal nerve is noted at the 16.5 mm stage and at 22 mm the tympanic plexus is delineated. At 26 mm the peripheral facial nerve divisions are present. At 80 mm all the common facial nerve communications exist except with the trigeminal nerve. This develops later at the 146 mm stage. The last communications are those with the second and third cervical ganglia which establish the greater auricular, transverse cervical and lesser occipital nerves.[40]

Our studies begin at this late stage of fetal development (approximately 15 weeks in utero and 167 mm fetal length stage). Our concern is with the anatomic parameters, ossification patterns and critical associated anatomic landmarks of the geniculate ganglion and labyrinthine segment which may be of importance to the otologic surgeon.

Von Spee[41] noted that a bony covering was missing over the geniculate ganglion in the first year of life. He named this defect which may persist occa-

TABLE 1. LOCATION OF NARROWEST PART OF LABYRINTHINE SEGMENT IN FETAL TEMPORAL BONE (mm)

Distance to Ganglion	*0.08 ~ 0.10*	*0.11 ~ 0.15*	*0.16 ~ 0.20*	*0.21 ~ 0.25*	*0.26 ~ 0.29*	*Total No.*
0.01 ~ 0.50	2	2	7	6	3	20
0.51 ~ 1.00	1	3	4	3	3	14
1.01 ~ 1.50		1	2	1		4
1.51 ~ 2.00				2		2
Total No.	3	6	13	12	6	40

TABLE 2. LOCATION OF THE WIDEST PART OF THE LABYRINTHINE SEGMENT IN FETAL TEMPORAL BONE (mm)

Distance to Ganglion	*0.16 ~ 0.20*	*0.21 ~ 0.30*	*0.31 ~ 0.40*	*0.41 ~ 0.50*	*0.51 ~ 0.78*	*Total No.*
0.01 ~ 0.50	2	6	6	1	1	16
0.51 ~ 1.00	1	5	5	1	1	13
1.01 ~ 1.50		2	5	1		8
1.51 ~ 2.00		1	1			2
2.01 ~ 2.50			1			1
Total No.	3	14	18	3	2	40

sionally in adults as the spurious hiatus of the facial canal. Batson[42] stated that the geniculate ganglion is uncovered by bone throughout early childhood. Dandy[43] noted protrusion of the geniculate ganglion via congenital defects of the roof of the temporal bone. House and Crabtree[44] noted a dehiscent geniculate ganglion in 5% of their middle cranial fossa surgical cases. Hall et al in a study of 100 adult temporal bones at autopsy noted a 15% incidence of dehiscence with a 50% bilateral proclivity (this was a symmetrical finding).[30]

Bartholdy[45] initially described in detail the blood supply to the facial nerve. Since that time various authors have defined the gross anatomic and fine detail observations of the vascularity and anastomosis of the facial nerve.[46-51] Our interest is with the pattern of incorporation of the intrinsic facial nerve blood supply into the fallopian canal and geniculate ganglion.

PRESENT OBSERVATIONS

The present study deals with the facial nerve at a stage when all major communications are established both centrally and peripherally. Morphologically the nerve is equivalent to the postpartum configuration. This is evident from the microscopic measurements of the labyrinthine segment and geniculate ganglion, which show no statistically significant changes. In other words there is no enlargement of the geniculate ganglion or lengthening of the labyrinthine facial nerve segment after 20 weeks in utero. However, the ossification pattern surrounding the facial nerve and the incorporation of its vascular supply do alter in the latter stages of development.

The vascularity surrounding the labyrinthine segment of the facial nerve is primarily derived from the internal auditory artery. These vessels reach to the level of the geniculate ganglion. There they anastomose with the geniculate circulation. The facial branches of the internal auditory artery enter the bony canal of the labyrinthine segment via the fundus of the internal auditory meatus. They persist in this canal during the ossification (Figs. 10A, B and 12A).

The petrosal branches of the middle meningeal artery travel superficial to the dura on top of the middle fossa plate. They enter the geniculate ganglion area from the cephelad direction. There these vessels form a plexus and intercommunicate with the facial branches of the internal auditory artery. As this primitive facial hiatus is closed by progressive ossification the vessels are incorporated into the geniculate ganglion area from above. In addition epitympanic and middle ear branches are established prior to completion of the ossification of the epitympanum (Fig. 10B).

Early in gestation the middle meningeal artery lies just anterior and lateral to the geniculate ganglion. With progressive ossification these two structures are separated by bone. Nevertheless the middle meningeal artery leaves a trail behind it via the petrosal and superior tympanic vessels. The internal auditory artery branches lie in the plane of the bony canals for the labyrinthine segment of the seventh nerve. However, the petrosal vessels lie in a horizontal plane almost at 90° to the former. These anastomose near the posterior border of the geniculate ganglion. In addition, the petrosal vessels send vascular branches variable distances beyond the facial genu (Fig. 10).

The ossification of the canal of the labyrinthine facial nerve segment occurs in conjunction with the ossification of the otic capsule and petrous apex. It precedes the ossification of the stapes footplate and round window niche.[29] The ossification begins in the luminal surface of the canal on both the dorsal and ventral surfaces at 20 weeks in utero. The last structure to be ossified is the vertical crest (Fig. 12).

After completion of the ossification, while vascular channels are still present in the otic capsule, a

TABLE 3. MEASUREMENTS IN ADULT TEMPORAL BONES (mm)

Dimensions	*Ganglion* *L*	*W*	*CP-G*	*Labyrinthine Facial Nerve* *L*	*N*	*D-G (N)*	*WN*	*D-G (WN)*	*Bony Canal Diameter*
Maximum	2.25	1.95	3.75	3.00	0.90	3.00	1.50	1.56	1.50-2.9
Minimum	1.20	0.90	1.05	2.25	0.60	1.50	0.90	0.30	0.60-0.9
Average	1.76	1.29	2.10	2.82	0.69	2.55	1.10	0.89	0.75-1.9

L - Length; W - Width; CP-G - Distance from cochleariform process to anterior geniculate ganglion; N - Narrowest width; D-G - Distance from internal auditory canal to geniculate ganglion; WN - Widest width.

periosteal ledge of bone begins to grow from the superior lip of the roof of the internal auditory canal. This medial bony plate covers the distal labyrinthine nerve segment and the posterior aspect of the geniculate ganglion (Figs. 6-8). At the same time ossification of the membranous bone from the squama proceeds from the lateral aspect of the middle fossa. This forms a lateral bony plate which covers the epitympanic roof separating the middle meningeal artery and its branches from the geniculate ganglion. As these two bony plates begin to approach each other, superficial to the dura, they effectively close the primitive hiatus under the geniculate ganglion and separate the epitympanum from the middle cranial fossa (Fig. 7). However this closure is not complete on the superior surface of the geniculate ganglion at birth; in only 3 of 40 temporal bones was the geniculate ganglion covered by bone. The epitympanum is closed, however, and separated from the middle cranial fossa. This process stops at 35 weeks in utero. Further growth and ossification proceeds postpartum with further skull development and growth (Fig. 8).

It is interesting to note that at 20 weeks in utero the size of the labyrinthine segment and geniculate ganglion is similar to the adult stage. In fact the width of the nerve to canal ratio in the labyrinthine segment, 1:1.9, remains constant from 35 weeks in utero through adult age. In addition the relationship of the anterior border of the geniculate ganglion to the processus cochleariformis remains constant from late gestation to adult life, ie, approximately 2 mm. However, the ossification alters the shape of the bony canal. In the fetus the narrowest portion of the bony canal is near the geniculate ganglion in 50% of the cases while in the adult it is universally at the fundus of the internal auditory canal in the region of the vertical crest (Fig. 13). Since the latter region ossified last it shows the greatest variability in luminal diameters. Thus it appears that in the adult, if constriction of the facial nerve is postulated as a cause for facial nerve paralysis, the most likely area is at the junction of the fundus of the internal auditory canal and the bony canal for the labyrinthine segment (ie, in the region of the vertical crest).

SUMMARY

This paper presents the microscopic anatomy and relations of the geniculate ganglion and the labyrinthine segment of the facial nerve in the human fetus. Regarding the later stages of development, the following observations were made:

1. The vascularity of the geniculate ganglion and labyrinthine segment of the facial nerve are well-established at 20 weeks in utero and precede the ossification of this region (Figs. 5 and 6).

2. The labyrinthine segment is primarily supplied by the facial branches of the internal auditory artery (Fig. 10A).

3. The geniculate ganglion is supplied by the petrosal branches of the middle meningeal artery (Fig. 10B).

4. The later two blood supplies anastomose at the medial border of the geniculate ganglion (Fig. 10).

5. The facial branches of the internal auditory artery follow the facial nerve via the fundus of the internal auditory canal (Fig. 10A).

6. The petrosal vessels enter via the primitive facial hiatus. In addition these send branches to the superior epitympanum and middle ear. These vessels travel in a horizontal plane at 90° to the facial vessels from the internal auditory artery (Figs. 6C, 10B and 12A).

7. The canal for the labyrinthine segment is ossified in cartilage via the petrous apex and otic capsule. The luminal surface is ossified first and the vertical crest last (Fig. 12).

8. The geniculate ganglion area is ossified incompletely by two plates of bone, ie, the medial plate is a periosteal derivative of the petrous bone and the lateral plate is a membranous bone derivate from the squamous portion of the temporal bone (Figs. 7 and 8).

9. The ossification pattern, which starts at 20 weeks in utero, is completed by 35 weeks in utero. Further ossification of the geniculate ganglion area region occurs postpartum.

10. These anatomic relationships, during the later stages of development, do not vary with the adult configuration: a) the nerve-canal ratio remains 1:1.9; b) the geniculate ganglion distance to the middle ear and cochleariform process remains 2 mm (Fig. 6); c) the dimensions of the labyrinthine nerve segment and geniculate ganglion remain the same (Figs. 1, 2, and 11).

11. The only variations noted at these stages of development deal with the pattern of ossification: a) the hiatus of the facial canal becomes smaller with increasing gestational age (Fig. 9); b) there is progressive narrowing of the fundus of the internal meatus at the inlet to the facial canal (Tables 1 and 2); c) the epitympanum is separated from the middle fossa by membranous bone formation (Fig. 7); d) the ossification pattern may not be symmetrical in both temporal bones of the same fetus.

12. In adult temporal bones the fetal parameters and configuration persist. However, in our specimens the geniculate ganglion region was completely ossified. All petrosal nerves had areas of bone dehiscence.

REFERENCES

1. Miehlke A. Surgery of the facial nerve. Philadelphia: WB Saunders Co, 1973.

2. Fisch U. Facial paralysis in fractures of the petrous bone. Laryngoscope 1974; 89:2141-54.

3. Fisch U. Transtemporal surgery of the internal auditory canal. Adv Otorhinolaryngol 1970; 17:203.

4. House WF. Surgical exposure of the internal auditory canal and its contents through the cranial middle fossa. Laryngoscope 1961; 71:1363-85.

5. House WF. Middle cranial fossa approach to petrous pyramid. Arch Otolaryngol 1963; 78:460-9.

6. House WF. Surgery of the petrous portion of the VIIth nerve. Ann Otol Rhinol Laryngol 1963; 72:802-7.

7. Cawthorne T. The geniculate ganglion and facial palsy. Arch Otolaryngol 1965; 81:502-3.

8. Cawthorne T, Wilson T. Indications for intratemporal facial nerve surgery. Arch Otolaryngol 1963; 78:429-34.

9. Cawthorne T. Intratemporal facial palsy. Arch Otolaryngol 1969; 90:789-99.

10. Fisch U, Esslen E. Total intratemporal exposure of the facial nerve. Arch Otolaryngol 1972; 98:335-41.

11. Denny-Brown DE, Adams RD, Fitzgerald PJ. Pathologic features of herpes zoster. Arch Neurol 1944; 51:216-31.

12. Devriese PP. Facial palsy in cephalic herpes zoster. Ann Otol Rhinol Laryngol 1968; 77:1101-19.

13. Doering G. Uber ein Ganglion geniculi-Syndrom als parasympathische Funkionsstorung. Acta neurochir (Wien) 1950; 1:502.

14. Glaninger J. Uber den Herpes zoster oticus und ein Beitrag zur Likalisationsbestimmung des Krankheitsherdes im Gehororgan mittels Audiometrie. Monatschr Ohrenhkld 1955; 89:81-8.

15. Hunt JR. On herpetic inflammations of the geniculate ganglion; a new syndrome and its complications. J Nervment Dis 1907; 34:73-90.

16. Hunt JR. A further contribution to the herpetic inflammations of the geniculate ganglion. Am J Med Sci 1908; 136:226-41.

17. Findely JP. Facial paralysis: a clinical review with an autopsy report of histopathology in a case of infection of the geniculate ganglion by the virus of cephalic herpes zoster. Med J Aust 1952; 2:810-5.

18. Wallace DS. Persistent facial paralysis associated with chickenpox. Can Med Assoc J 1960; 82:198-9.

19. Kettel K. Repair of intratemporal lesions of the facial nerve due to traumas. Ann Otol Rhinol Laryngol 1963; 72:756-73.

20. Jongkees LBW. The treatment of traumatic intratemporal palsy. Pract ORL (Basel) 1962; 24:203.

21. McHugh HE. Facial paralysis in birth injury and skull fractures. Arch Otolaryngol 1963; 78:443-55.

22. Sheridan MR, Banham TM. Progressive facial nerve palsy due to temporal epidermoid. J Laryngol Otol 1948; 62:170-2.

23. Jefferson G, Smalley AA. Facial palsy produced by intratemporal epidermoids. J Laryngol Otol 1938; 53:417-43.

24. Miehlke A. Normal and anomalous anatomy of the facial nerve and an embryonal study of the thalidomide catastrophe in Germany. Trans Am Acad Ophthalmol Otolaryngol 1964; 68: 1030-44.

25. Tremble EG, Penfield W. Operative exposure of the facial canal with removal of a tumor of the greater superficial petrosal nerve. Arch Otolaryngol 1936; 23:573-9.

26. Spector GJ, Druck N, Gado M. Neurologic manifestations of glomus tumors in the head and neck. Arch Neurol 1976; 33:270-4.

27. House WF. Monograph II. Acoustic neuroma. Arch Otolaryngol 1968; 88:575-715.

28. Spector GJ, Pettit JW, Davis G, Strauss M, Ranchbach E. Fetal respiratory distress causing inner ear and CNS hemorrhage. Laryngoscope 1976; 88:764-86.

29. Spector GJ, Lee D, Carr C, et al. Later stages of development of the periotic duct and its adjacent area in the human fetus. Laryngoscope 1980; Suppl 20:1-31.

30. Hall GM, Pulec Jl, Rhoton AL Jr. Geniculate ganglion anatomy for the otologist. Arch Otolaryngol 1969; 90:567-71.

31. Rabl K. Uber das Gebiet des Nervus facialis. Anat Anz 1887; 2:219-27.

32. Gegenbaur C. Lehrbuch der Anatomie des Menschen. Aufl 4 Band 2. Leipzig: Engelmann, 1890:448-9.

33. Bast BJ, Anson BJ, Richany SF. The development of the second branchial arch (Reichert's cartilage), facial canal and associated structures in man. Northwestern Univ Med Sch Q Bull 1956; 30:235-49.

34. Harper DG, Anson BJ. Development relationships of Reichert's cartilage to the wall of the facial canal. Northwestern Univ Med Sch Q Bull 1962; 36:144-50.

35. Gasser RF. The development of the facial nerve in man. Ann Otol Rhinol Laryngol 1961; 76:37-56.

36. His W. Zur Entwicklungsgeshichte des Acoustico-Facialgebietes beim Menschen. Z Anat Entwicklungsgesch 1889:1-28.

37. Streeter GL. On the development of the membranous labyrinth and the acoustic and facial nerves in the human embryo. Am J Anat 1907; 6:139-65.

38. Futamura R. Uber die Entwicklung der Facialsmuskulatur des Menschen. Anat Heft 1906; 30:433-516.

39. Popowsky I. Zur Entwicklungsgeschichte des N Facialis beim. Menschen Morphol Jahrb 1895; 23:329-74.

40. Pearson AA. The roots of the facial nerve in human enbryo and fetuses. J Comp Neurol 1947; 87:139-59.

41. Von Spee FG. Skeletlehre: Kopf. In: von Bardeleben K, ed. Handbuch der Anatomie des Menschen. Vol 1. Jena, Germany: G Fisher Verlag 1896:93-372.

42. Batson OU. Applied anatomy of the temporal bone. In: Schenck HP. Otolaryngology. Vol 1. Hagerstown: WF Prior, 1966:11.

43. Dandy WE. An operation for the cure of tic douloureux: Partial section of the sensory root at the pons. Arch Surg 1929; 16:687-734.

44. House WF, Crabtree JA. Surgical exposure of the petrous portion of the VII nerve. Arch Otolaryngol 1965; 81:506-7.

45. Bartholdy K. Die Arterien der Nerven. Morphol Arbeiten 1897; 7:393-458.

46. Nager GT. Origins and relations of internal auditory artery and subarcuate artery. Ann Otol Rhinol Laryngol 1954; 63:51-61.

47. Blunt MJ. The blood supply of the facial nerve. J Anat 1954; 88:520-6.

48. Blunt MJ. The possible role of vascular changes in the etiology of Bell's palsy. J Laryngol Otol 1956; 70:701-13.

49. Bosatra A. Some observations on the vascularization of the VII nerve. J Laryngol Otol 1956; 70:605-13.

50. Clarke JA. An x-ray microscopic study of the arterial supply to the facial nerve. J Laryngol Otol 1965; 79:987-94.

51. Anson BJ, Donaldson JA, Warpeha LR, Rensink MJ. The facial nerve, sheath and blood supply in relation to the surgery of decompression. Ann Otol Rhinol Laryngol 1970; 79:710-27.

PROCEEDINGS OF THE SEMINAR ON SINUSOIDAL HARMONIC ACCELERATION AND COMPUTERIZED OPTOKINETIC TRACKING TESTS

CONTENTS

The Optokinetic Test and the ENG Test Battery. Cecil W. Hart, MD 2

Developing a Computer Laboratory for Neurotologic Diagnosis. Horst R. Konrad, MD; Don Templin 7

Sinusoidal Harmonic Acceleration. Robert H. Mathog, MD 10

Comparison of Subjective Symptomatology and Responses to Harmonic Acceleration in Patients with Menière's Disease. James E. Olson, Lt Col, MC, USAF; James W. Wolfe, PhD 15

Sinusoidal Harmonic Acceleration Test in Clinical Practice. Wallace Rubin, MD 18

Sinusoidal Harmonic Acceleration Labyrinthine Test: Clinical Experience. Roger A. Simpson, MD 26

An Overview of Ocular Motor Neurophysiology. B. Todd Troost, MD 29

THE OPTOKINETIC TEST AND THE ENG TEST BATTERY

CECIL W. HART, MD

CHICAGO, ILLINOIS

The importance of including optokinetic nystagmus as part of a more comprehensive visual test battery in ENG testing is discussed. Useful clinical information may be obtained which not only may confirm the presence of peripheral disease, but also may reveal evidence of disturbed central vestibular function. The technique and some of the diagnostic possibilities are described.

INTRODUCTION

The optokinetic test is well established as a neurologic and neuro-ophthalmic investigative tool, but its importance in the conventional ENG test battery performed by the otologist or neurotologist is still being debated. Obviously, in its own right, it can reveal very significant evidence of brain disease. As the neurotologist's horizons of interest penetrate deeper into the realm of brain function, so will his interest in optokinetic testing increase.

From a more practical point of view, however, the optokinetic test, as part of the visual test battery, serves as a very useful baseline assessment of part of the cristo-ocular reflex arc. In particular, both reflex arcs share in common the final oculomotor pathways from the oculomotor nuclei to the eye muscles, and also the fixation reflex arc, which is usually evaluated for the fixation effect upon spontaneous or induced vestibular nystagmus. If one has not tested the integrity of the visual-oculomotor system, how can one be sure whether the abnormal eye movements that are recorded, either spontaneously or induced by vestibular stimulation, are indeed due entirely to a labyrinthine dysfunction? If the visual test battery is normal, then the conclusions regarding labyrinthine function drawn from the vestibular test battery are on much firmer ground.

OPTOKINETIC METHODOLOGY

The choice of the stimulus to employ is critical, and in order to keep the test short and simple, it is necessary to make a number of compromises. Many variables need to be controlled.

The physical size of the visual stimulus is important. A choice must be made between a full-visual field stimulus, which tests the entire retina, and a pinpoint light source, which mainly stimulates the fovea. These are two very different stimuli, which in turn may reveal different clinical information.

The induced eye speed is important. If the stimulus speed is constant, and if it is too fast, the "fail rate" will be too high, and vice versa. An accelerating optokinetic drum is a useful compromise.

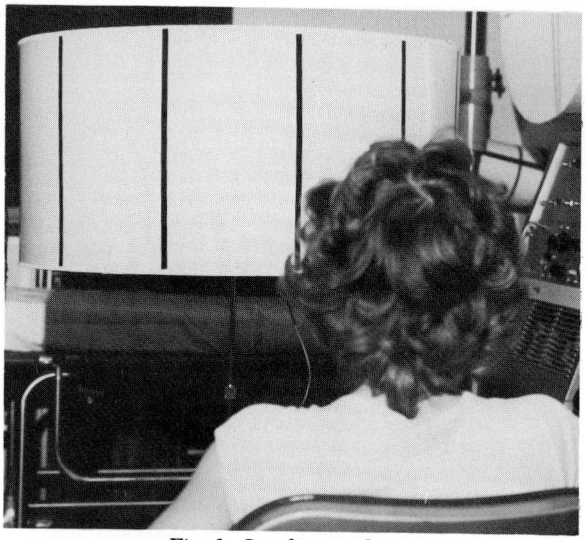

Fig. 1. Optokinetic drum.

The number of stripes should be chosen such that at the desired drum speed a clearly defined saw-tooth ENG signal is generated. The width of the stripes also has some relevance, in that with a wide stripe the subject may tend to look back and forth from, for example, the leading black/white margin to the following white/black margin, and if these saccades are large enough they will appear on the ENG recording.

Most testing is done in the horizontal visual field, although vertical testing is at times very important. Oblique or rotatory testing has not been extensively studied.

The instruction to the patient is another variable to be controlled. The reflex arc is modified depending upon whether the patient is instructed to follow visually each stripe as it passes in front of the field of vision, or whether the patient should gaze straight ahead and ignore the stripe ("follow" or "stare" modes).

Finally, on a more immediate level, patient drug

From the Department of Clinical Otolaryngology and Maxillofacial Surgery, Northwestern University Medical School, Chicago.

REPRINTS — Cecil W. Hart, MD, Vestibular Research Laboratory, Northwestern University Medical School, 320 E. Superior Street, Chicago IL 60611.

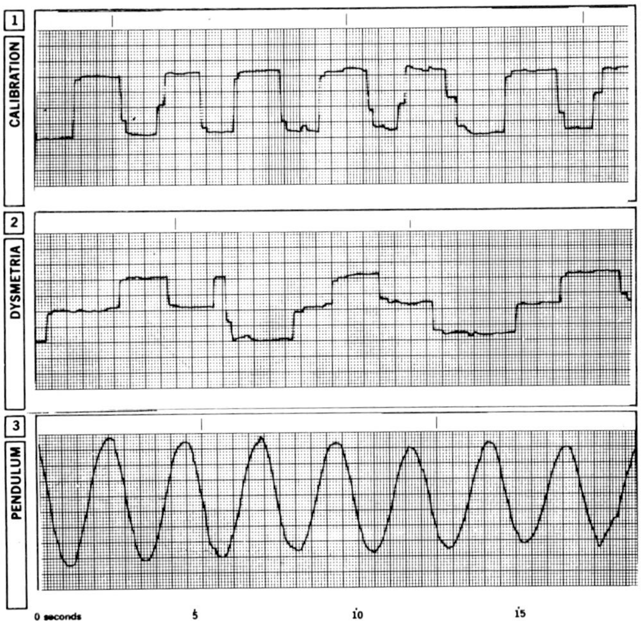

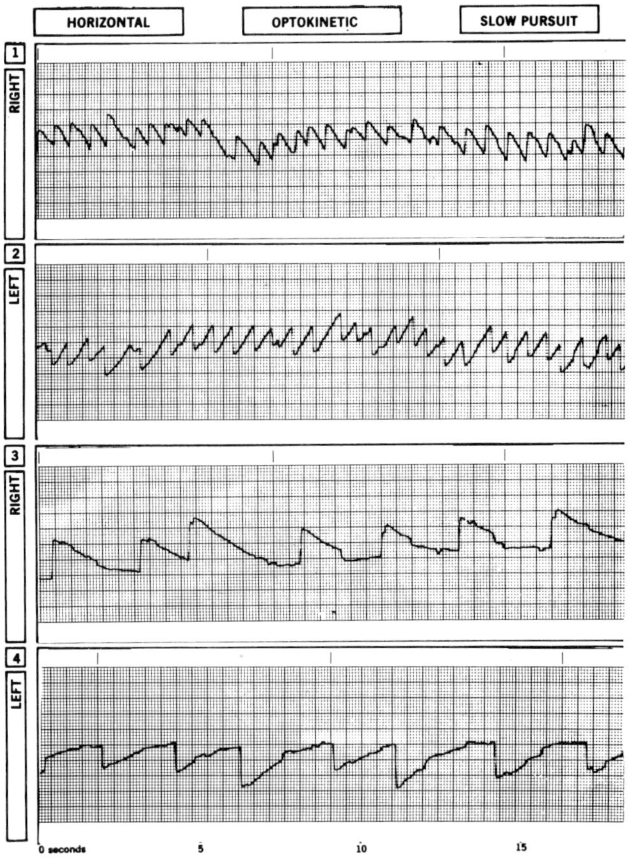

Fig. 2. (Patient 1, male, March 15, 1980) Routine visual test battery. 1) Calibration — 20° saccades. 2) Dysmetria — 10° saccades in both directions, both centrifugal and centripetal. 3) Pendulum — Sinusoidal stimulus. Optokinetic test — 1) Nystagmus to the right; 2) nystagmus to the left. Slow pursuit — 3) Saccades to the right, slow pursuit to the left; 4) saccades to the left, slow pursuit to the right.

intake should be controlled as much as possible. Many drugs may degrade the optokinetic response.

Current Practice. The optokinetic drum used at the Northwestern University Vestibular Research Laboratory for the past 12 to 15 years is shown in Figure 1. The diameter of the drum is 75 cm, the distance from the surface of the drum to the nasion is the same, and the stripe width is 0.63 cm, which is sufficient just to overfill the fovea. The drum speed is set such that the expected induced pursuit eye speed is 10°/s, and the patient is instructed actively to follow the stripes as they pass across the field of vision. The routine visual test battery performed at this time is shown in Figure 2. The left tracings show 1) 20° calibrations, 2) a saccade dysmetria test, and 3) a pendulum tracking test, simply performed with a yellow golf ball suspended by string from the ceiling.

The right side tracings are performed with a 1 m diameter optokinetic drum, with the patient seated 1 m distance from the surface. The two upper tracings are induced by a white optokinetic drum with 14 black stripes of 1.25 cm width, with an expected induced eye speed of 10°/s. The lower two tracings are obtained with a similar drum but with only six stripes, and with an expected induced eye speed of 5°/s.

Signal Analysis. The most simple evaluation is to watch the patient's eyes during the test, and determine whether "the response is normal or nearly so in one direction, and either nil or definitely impaired in the other direction."[1] A judgment can also be made whether it is symmetrically impaired or not, and whether both eyes are responding in the same manner.

ENG recording of optokinetic nystagmus (OKN) allows a much more precise signal analysis, but it opens the door to overinterpretation of the findings. The most simple analysis is a visual evaluation of the recordings. Mathematic analysis, eg, the manual measurement of the slow phase velocity, nystagmus frequency or amplitude, may allow a more accurate evaluation. Computer analysis of the signal may make the findings more objective. Mathematical reduction also allows more accurate comparative measures, eg, of the signal with the stimulus, or of one signal with another. Direct current (DC) OKN recording may demonstrate induced deviation of the direction of gaze. Recording with the eyes closed may elicit optokinetic afternystagmus (OKAN).

Using the routine methodology described above, the following are some of the useful clinical deductions which can be made from such a test procedure. Obviously, optokinetic testing generally is capable of revealing much more, but this would necesitate additional changes in the equipment and procedures.

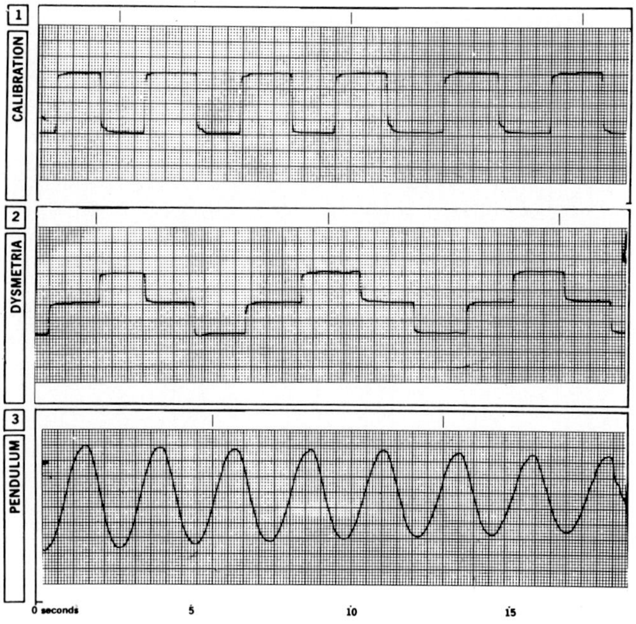

Fig. 3. (Patient 2, female, March 28, 1980) Extremely precise visual pursuit test sometimes found in anxious patients.

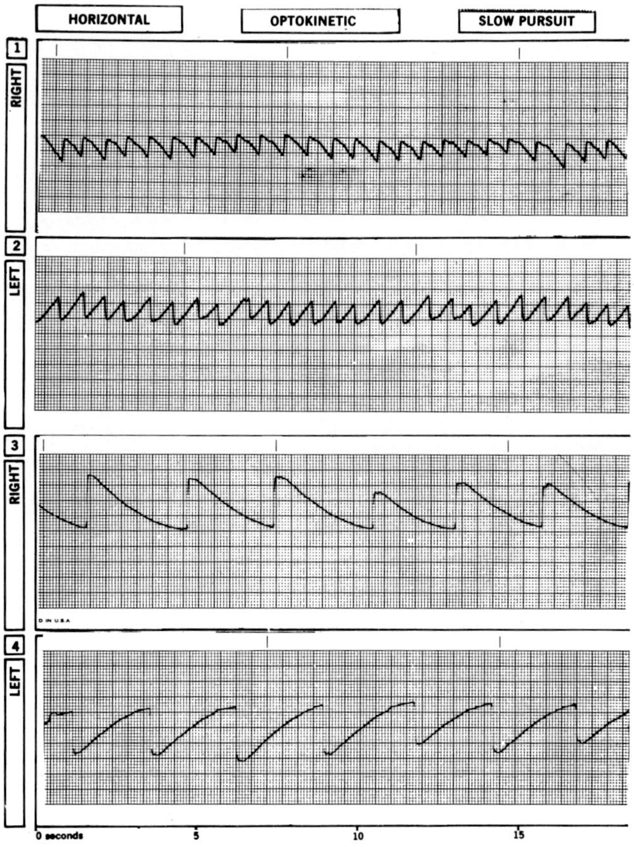

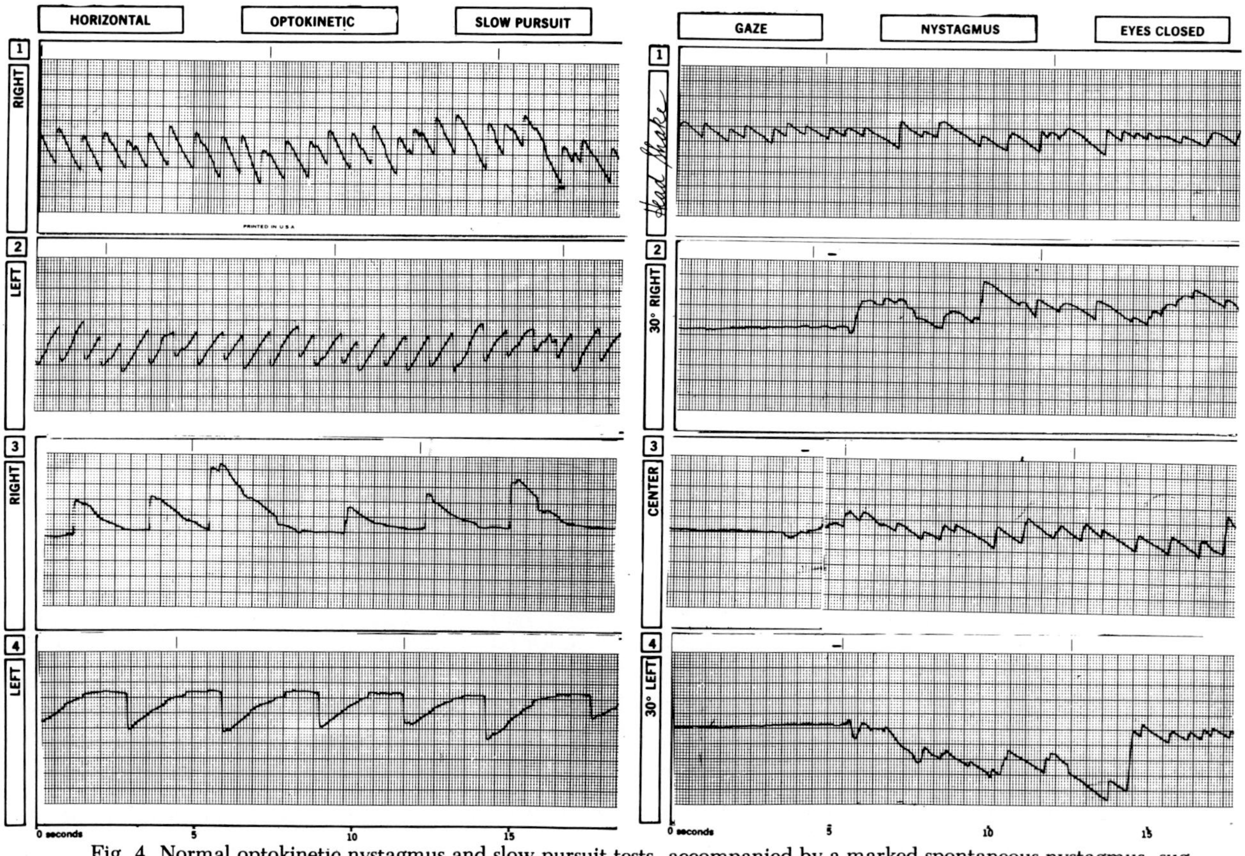

Fig. 4. Normal optokinetic nystagmus and slow pursuit tests, accompanied by a marked spontaneous nystagmus, suggestive of a central vestibular disturbance.

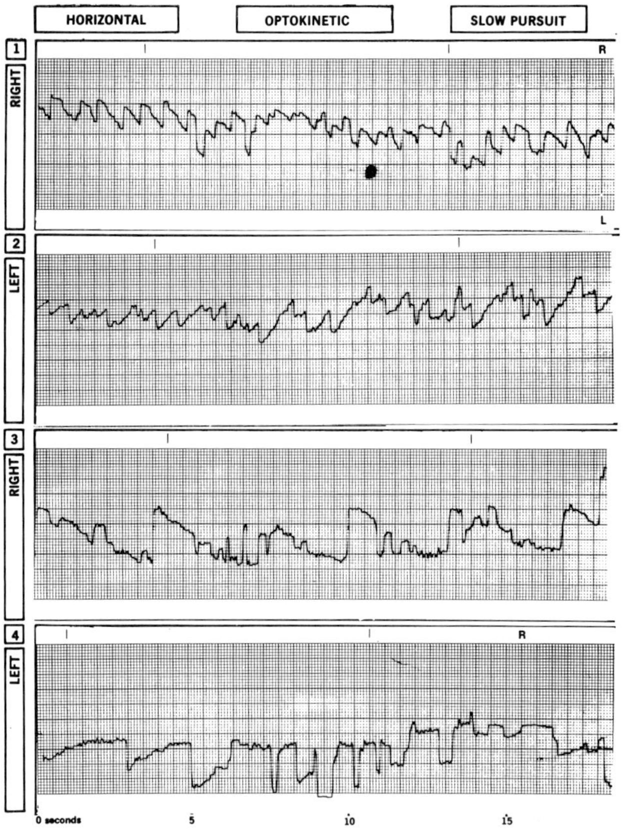

Fig. 5. Dysrhythmic optokinetic nystagmus and slow pursuit, suggestive of a central vestibular disturbance.

CLINICAL FINDINGS

The evaluation of the OKN response should be based upon the best recording obtainable. Lack of effort or interest on the part of the patient causes the signal to degrade, which may in turn be misdiagnosed as being indicative of disease. The signal also degrades with age, such that allowance should be made for this factor. Some irregularity of the signal is permissible at any age, but more so with advancing years. The exact permissible amount of degradation at a given age requires considerable clinical experience and judgment.

The opposite phenomenon is the anxious and/or neurotic patient. The OKN signal has the appearance of emanating from a function generator, it is so precise (Fig. 3)! In addition, this patient frequently complains that the stimulus produces a sensation of dizziness, or even frank vertigo, and may state that the sensation is exactly like, and possibly even more intense than, his own complaint.

A bidirectional reduced OKN response, symmetric or asymmetric, indicates central disease, usually in the brainstem or the cerebellum. An asymmetric response, but normal in one direction, may be of either peripheral or central origin. Comparison of the OKN with the spontaneous nystagmus (SN), eyes closed (EC), will often distinguish the two. In the presence of a vigorous SNEC, in the

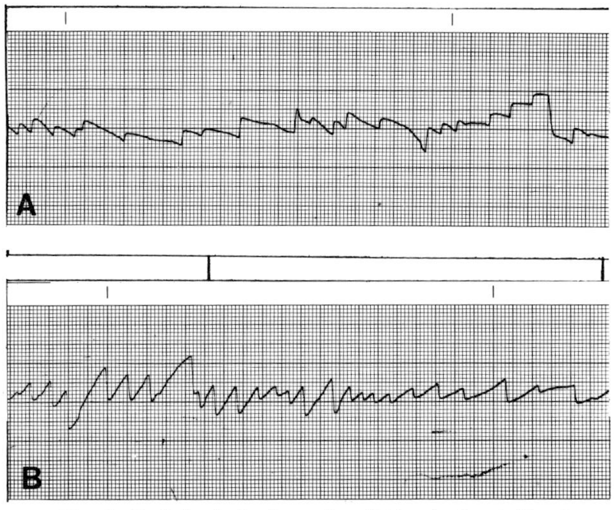

Fig. 6. Pathological adaptation (fatigue) of optokinetic nystagmus. The stimulus should induce a response of 20°/s. A) The right beating response simply shows some dysrhythmia and reduced slow phase velocity. B) Adaptation is better seen in the lower trace response.

same direction as the normal OKN response, the etiology is probably peripheral. In the absence of a SNEC, or with a SNEC in the direction of the smaller OKN response, the etiology is probably central. Similarly, a normal OKN response with an intense SNEC also suggests a central cause (Fig. 4).

Two other central signs which may be elicited are dysrhythmia and "fatigue." Dysrhythmia is hard to define in mathematical terms, and its detection is essentially a visual pattern recognition task. The saccades are of varying amplitude, the intersaccade interval is irregular, and the slow phase of varying speed (Fig. 5). Fatigue is the clinical term used to indicate pathological adaptation of the response (Fig. 6).

Finally, comparison of the OKN saccade with the caloric nystagmus saccade may suggest brainstem disease. Normally, the caloric nystagmus saccade is slightly slower and of longer duration than the OKN saccade. Comparisons should be made between OKN and caloric nystagmus signals of the same slow phase velocity. With central disease, the caloric nystagmus saccade may be of abnormally slow velocity and long duration (Fig. 7).

CONCLUSION

The optokinetic test, as part of the visual test battery, is an essential part of the ENG test battery. Not only does it assess the central portion of the cristo-ocular reflex, and thus avoid the pitfall of mistaking a central disturbance for a peripheral one, but also in its own right, it may be the source of much useful clinical information. Taken in isolation, it may show various abnormalities indicative of central disease, and, in addition, comparison of the OKN with other portions of the ENG test battery may give other evidence of central and/or peripheral disease.

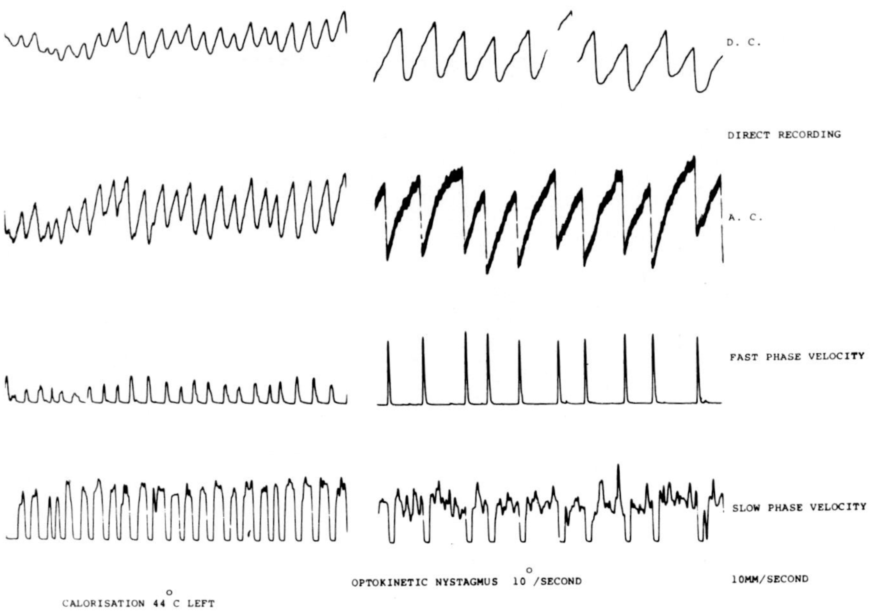

Fig. 7. (Patient 3, male, August 4, 1969) Slowed caloric nystagmus saccade in patient with brainstem lesion. The caloric and optokinetic nystagmus slow phase velocities are approximately equal (channel 4), but the caloric saccade speeds (channel 3 peak height) are slower and the durations longer (peak width) than the optokinetic saccades.

REFERENCES

1. Smith J. Optokinetic nystagmus. Springfield: Charles C Thomas, 1963.

DEVELOPING A COMPUTER LABORATORY FOR NEUROTOLOGIC DIAGNOSIS

HORST R. KONRAD, MD DON TEMPLIN

SPRINGFIELD, ILLINOIS

The authors, with the help of a community hospital engineering staff, constructed a modern neurotological testing facility capable of performing on-line computer measurements of vestibulo-oculomotor, visual vestibulo-oculomotor, smooth pursuit, saccade, and optokinetic reflexes. The laboratory was built from component parts and uses a Digital Corporation laboratory computer. Programs from the UCLA Human Vestibular Laboratory were modified to work with the new laboratory. Construction and program modification cost $60,000 and was completed in seven months. The laboratory was working at full capacity six months after construction testing patients with suspected neurotologic and neurologic disorders. The procedures of construction as well as the financial and safety problems are discussed.

Recent developments in small computers, combined with advances in the understanding of the eye tracking and vestibulo-oculomotor reflexes, have made the development of a computer neurotologic laboratory possible even for a smaller regional medical center. This paper is a description of our development of such a laboratory at a regional hospital in Springfield, Illinois, a community of 100,000 population.

In the past, the costs of computers, the difficulties of finding competent programmers, mechanical or engineering personnel, and basic and clinical scientists with a background in vestibular system physiology and disorders forced development of such systems into large university complexes. Although our understanding of many of the basic processes is just in its infancy, there are already significant clinical applications from earlier investigations which give the clinician who uses such a laboratory a significant advantage in diagnosis. In order to provide this advantage to the patients of our community, we made the decision to build such a laboratory.

Plans for construction were made in December 1978. Construction began in April 1979 and was completed in November 1979 at a cost of $60,000. The laboratory is capable of measuring eye movement and vestibular reflexes including pursuit, saccade, optokinetic, vestibulo-oculomotor reflexes, and visual vestibular interactions. It is an integral unit of the sensory and neurological testing facility which includes audiology, auditory, visual, somatosensory evoked response testing, peripheral neural, electroencephalography, and electromyography laboratories.

FINANCIAL CONSIDERATIONS

In August 1978, we approached one of the hospitals in the community and asked them to consider financial commitment to develop the laboratory. In December, the commitment was made, space allocated, and planning begun. Budget was estimated at $50,000 with six months' time estimated for building.

COMPUTER, RECORDING, AND STIMULATING DEVICES

The choice of computer must go hand in hand with the choice of software and plans for future development. Completed devices, including software, are available now (Contraves Goerz Corp., Pittsburgh, Pa.), but we decided to build our own system for several reasons:

1. Initial cost is less.

2. By having the hospital personnel participate in the construction, they would be in a better position to provide maintenance.

3. Flexibility of the system for future development is higher since we worked from component parts and our personnel knew the components of the system.

4. By using software from universities actively engaged in research, we would be in a better position to work with their future developments and eventually develop our own research programs. The Division of Head and Neck Surgery at UCLA kindly provided us with their programs.

Since we were most familiar with the system at UCLA,[1-4] we decided to stay with Digital Equipment Company machines.

An LS-11 microprocessor with floppy disks would have sufficed for our initial needs but would not have given us as much flexibility for future developments as we wanted. For this reason, a minicomputer with two disks (MINK-11) was purchased.

In addition, a 4-channel paper recorder (Beck-

From the Division of Otolaryngology, Southern Illinois University School of Medicine, Springfield.

REPRINTS — Horst R. Konrad, MD, Division of Otolaryngology, Southern Illinois University School of Medicine, Springfield, IL 62702.

man polygraph R511A) and an FM tape recorder (Tanberg series 115 4-channel), a digital VT-105CRT, and a Diablo hard copy printer (Model No. 1620) were purchased.

CONSTRUCTION

Space was chosen to be low in ambient noise, vibrations, and radiofrequency transmissions. A hospital safety engineer was consulted at the beginning of planning and periodically as equipment was installed, and at completion. Although the testing does not produce significant illness, the testing of sick patients requires that medical personnel and resuscitation equipment is nearby. The layout was sketched and the parts ordered. Room modifications were begun, dividing the room into testing and control areas. Four months later, the parts had all arrived and construction was started.

Eye Tracking. The eye tracking stimulator was built from a laser projecting to a galvonometer mounted mirror to a back screen projector. The galvonometer is controlled from a function generator or the computer.

Optokinetic Drum. The drum is a 150 cm diameter, 175 cm high black cloth drum with 24 2.5 cm wide vertical white stripes spaced 15° apart. It is driven by a DC Servo motor with velocity feedback (static torque 120 cm kg) mounted in the ceiling. In operation, it completely surrounds the chair and patient, but can be retracted up or down. The drum can be controlled from a function generator or computer or outside control panel, and produces constant velocity or sinusoidal stimulation.

Rotary Chair. The chair is a contoured chair with a head restraining device mounted coaxially with the optokinetic drum driven by a DC Servo motor with velocity feedback (static torque 420 cm kg). The chair is driven from an outside function generator either separately or with the optokinetic drum or from the computer.

Caloric Testing. Caloric stimulating devices are standard 30°, 44° C thermostat controlled with timed irrigation. Signals are recorded with electronystagmography silver silver chloride electrodes and amplified by a 3-channel preamplifier attached to the patient with a gain of 200. The preamplified signal is them passed to the amplifier of the paper and FM recorder, and to the computer.

CAPABILITIES

In addition to spontaneous, gaze, positional, and caloric nystagmus, the system can record and measure the following:

Pursuit at 0.2 and 0.4 Hz. Gain (defined as eye velocity divided by target velocity) is measured for movements to the left and right separately. The entire response is graphically displayed.

Saccade. Saccade accuracy for each eye, mean saccade velocity, saccade velocity vs amplitude, mean delay between target movement and eye movement.

Optokinetic. Constant velocity or sinusoidal stimulation may be tested. For constant velocity, the mean and standard deviation, minimum and maximum velocities of the slow component of nystagmus can be obtained. For sinusoidal stimulation, the mean (also a measure of asymmetry) minimum and maximum slow component velocity of nystagmus (SCV) are obtained. Gain to clockwise vs counterclockwise stimulation is also given.

Rotational — Vestibulo-Oculomotor Reflex (VOR). Constant acceleration, series of impulses of change in table velocity and sinusoidal stimulation can be delivered. The maximum SCV can be obtained for constant acceleration and impulsive stimulation. For sinusoidal stimulation, gain to clockwise and counterclockwise stimulation are given. Analyses of phase relationship between stimulus and response are also calculated.

Vestibular, Visual Interactions. The chair may be rotated within the stationary optokinetic drum with lights on to produce both vestibular and optokinetic stimulation. The chair can be rotated in the dark with a central placed light on rotating with the patient to give visual fixation. For both forms of visual vestibular stimulation, gain and phase can be calculated.

UTILIZATION

Initially, most patients referred for testing came from otolaryngologists' offices; however, there is a gradual change to more referrals now originating from neurologists', internists', and ophthalmologists' offices. The most common reason for referral is to help differentiate between central nervous system and peripheral vestibular abnormalities. Recently, patients have been referred to answer specific questions such as eye muscle involvement in Grave's disease, specific oculomotor weakness or paralysis, tensilon tests with documentation of saccade velocity to more objectively measure changes in myasthenia gravis. Six months after the laboratory's completion, it was utilized at full capacity.

DISCUSSION

The effectiveness of such a laboratory in diagnosis is difficult to estimate. Its cost effectiveness is even more difficult to quantify. The laboratory has provided better measurement of eye movement reflexes and thereby aids in the differential diagnosis of central vs peripheral disorders effecting the vestibular and oculomotor systems. It has also provided for better evaluation of changes in these systems over time. An actual evaluation of cost effectiveness has to not only consider the hardships and costs of patient's medical diagnosis and management, disability and loss due to incorrect or late diagnosis, but also the cost of transportation of the patient to another institution where such services are available. At the completion of this laboratory, there were no clinical facilities for computer measurements of eye movements available in Illinois, Missouri or Indiana. To obtain such measurements would have required sending the patient over great distances.

The development and maintenance of such a laboratory in a smaller medical center has demonstrated the feasibility of bringing sophisticated medical technology to regional centers where patients and physicians can have better access to the fruits of such technology.

ACKNOWLEDGMENTS — This laboratory was constructed by Memorial Medical Center, Springfield, Illinois, during the period April to November 1979, with assistance from the following:

1. System design and construction supervision by: Don Templin, Laytonville, Calif.

2. Basic concepts and computer programming by: Paul Ward, MD, Vicente Honrubia, MD, Robert Baloh, MD; Lauren Langhofer, Programmer, UCLA Human Vestibular Laboratory, NIH Grant from NINCDS No. NS09823, Los Angeles, Calif.

3. Computer program modifications by: Robert W. Fox, Capital Computer Systems, Springfield, Ill.

REFERENCES

1. Honrubia V, Strelioff D, Ward PH. Computer analysis of induced vestibular and optokinetic nystagmus. Ann Otol Rhinol Laryngol 1971; 80: Suppl 3.

2. Honrubia V, Strelioff D, Ward PH. Computer analysis of nystagmus induced by constant angular accelerations in normal and labyrinthectomized cats. Adv Otorhinolaryngol 1973; 19: 254.

3. Sills AW, Honrubia V, Kumley WE. Analysis of nystagmus using a digital computer. Aviat Space Environ Med 1975; 46:934-42.

4. Baloh RW, Langhofer L, Honrubia V, Yee RD. On-line analysis of eye movements using a digital computer. Aviat Space Environ Med 1980; 51:563-7.

SINUSOIDAL HARMONIC ACCELERATION

ROBERT H. MATHOG, MD

DETROIT, MICHIGAN

The need for accurate and reliable diagnostic tests for the evaluation of vestibular function has stimulated investigation of rotational methods and more recently, an evaluation of harmonic angular acceleration. Initial studies, using these techniques in humans, demonstrated a linear input-output function from 0.24 to 0.04 cycles/s at 0.4 radians/s^2, but a reduction in the increase of response with an increase of acceleration or a decrease of frequency from this range. Nystagmic responses were symmetrical in these same normal individuals. In patients with vestibular disease, input-output functions, as well as symmetry, were altered, and appeared related to the degree of pathology. Evaluation of the test system in animals, rendered ototoxic with streptomycin, showed a depression in response similar to caloric tests. All data suggested that harmonic angular acceleration provided a reliable and sensitive method for evaluation of vestibular function, and a useful and important confirmation to the other methods that are available for these evaluations.

During the past ten years there has been much interest in the development and investigation of new tests for the evaluation of vestibular function. Modern goals have been to find techniques that are easy to perform, accurate in identifying pathology and reliable on a test-retest basis.

In 1965, Niven et al[1] described a sinusoidal angular acceleration system and stimulus-response characteristics for normal individuals. Several years later, Mathog[2] and Mathog and Cramer[3] applied the stimulus to individuals with vestibular disorders. At that time, the test appeared to have much potential, expecially since the angular acceleration could be quantified and the test performed rapidly enough to minimize changes in the mental status of the patient. Moreover, the test stimulus appeared physiologic, resembling a movement of the head often used by individuals to maintain visual contact and spatial orientation.

Initial studies[2,3] utilized a yaw axis device, consisting of an encapsulated chair and torque motor (Inland Motors). Electronystagmographic responses were hand-scored according to the methods of Cassel and Mathog.[4] Information was also collected on the subjective responses of subjects to this type of manipulation.

Data were evaluated for stimulus-response characteristics, particularly the gain in nystagmic response as a function of stimulus frequency and acceleration. Responses were also evaluated for symmetry (as the subject was turned in a right or left direction) and for any habituation that occurred from repetitive testing.

Responses in Normal Human Subjects. Initial studies utilized 16 normal airmen. The responses of these subjects to sinusoidal angular acceleration are shown in Table 1 and Figure 1, where the nystagmic velocity (maximum velocity of the right-beating nystagmus) was evaluated with regard to a changing frequency (or period) of stimulation. Such data showed that variability of the response was low at the higher frequencies and became increased at the lower frequencies. Moreover, there was a linear relationship between frequency and nystagmic velocity throughout the entire test frequencies, except that at a period of 25 seconds (0.04 cycles/s) or longer the gain was substantially decreased.

Upon evaluation of the changes in nystagmic response that occurred with a stimulus of constant frequency, but with varying angular acceleration, one could observe shifts in the stimulus-response curves. In Figure 2, six normal subjects were evaluated for different accelerations at 0.2, 0.4, and 0.6 radians/s^2. As the stimulus was increased to a greater ac-

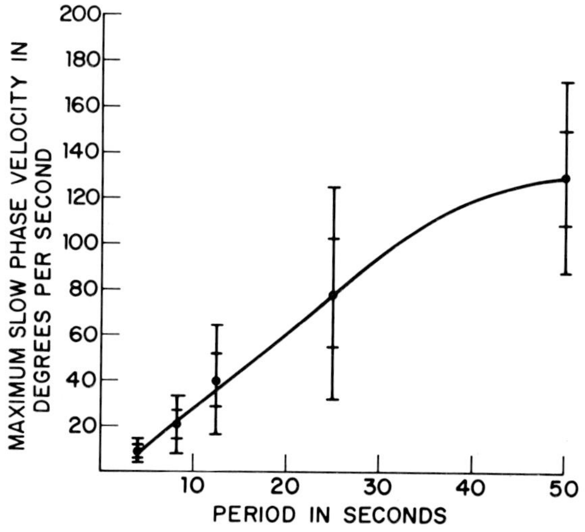

Fig. 1. Maximum average peak velocity of the slow component of nystagmus as a function of period. The plotted values are an average of the peak nystagmus developed in a clockwise or counterclockwise rotation. (From Mathog RH, Cramer RL.[3] Published with permission.)

From the Department of Otolaryngology, Wayne State University School of Medicine, Detroit.

REPRINTS — Robert H. Mathog, MD, Department of Otolaryngology, Wayne State University School of Medicine, 540 East Canfield Street, Detroit, MI 48201.

TABLE 1. PEAK VELOCITY OF NYSTAGMUS IN RESPONSE TO SINUSOIDAL STIMULI (N = 16)

Stimulus parameters					
Frequency (Hz)	0.24	0.12	0.08	0.04	0.02
Period (s)	4.2	8.3	12.5	25.0	50.0
Peak velocity (rpm)	2.6	5.4	8.0	16.0	32.0
Peak acceleration (rad/s²)	0.4	0.4	0.4	0.4	0.4
Peak velocity of nystagmus					
Average (°/s)	9.6	20.9	40.9	78.8	130.3
Range of values (°/s)	15.5-14.1	10.6-32.0	23.4-64.4	42.0-132.0	83.0-155.0
SD (°/s)	2.6	6.5	11.9	23.4	21.0

From Mathog RH.[2] Published with permission.

celeration, the system showed signs of overdrive with a decrement in gain.

In comparing right to left preponderance the nystagmic velocity to the right was approximately equal to the nystagmic velocity to the left (Fig. 3). The directional or labyrinthine preponderance was determined by a modification of Jongkees's formula in which the preponderance was equal to the difference of the nystagmic velocity to the right and to the left, over the sum of the nystagmic velocity to the right and to the left. This calculation allowed for the directional preponderance to vary between 0 and 1 or 0 and 100% if the data were multiplied by 100%. As shown in Figure 3, the subjects were not only "symmetrical" but these calculations showed minimum variability.

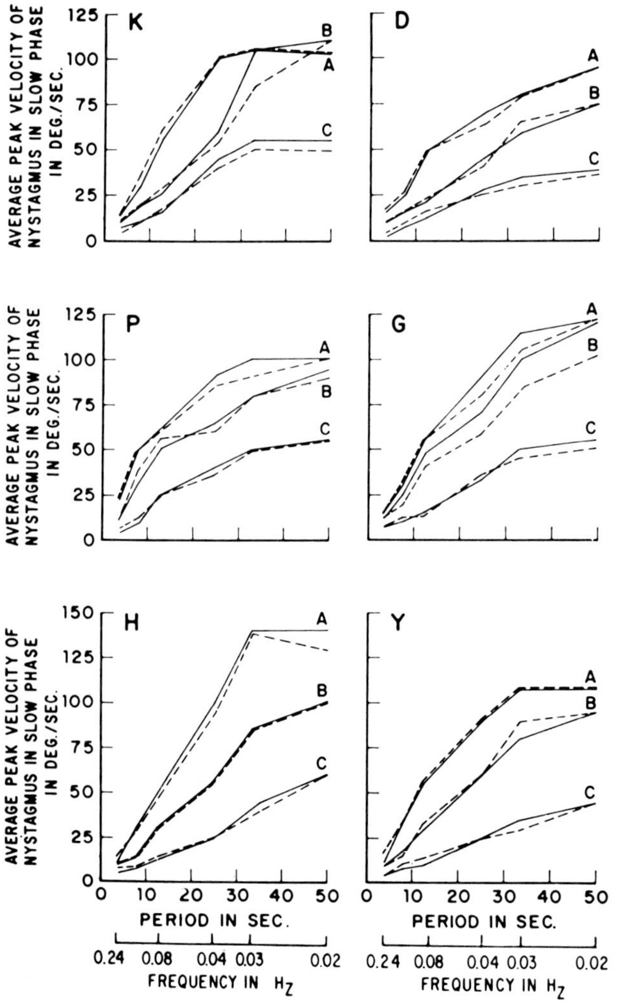

Fig. 2. Nystagmic responses of six normal subjects as a function of peak acceleration and cyclic periods or frequency. Plots of A, B, and C represent, respectively, accelerations of 0.6, 0.4 and 0.2 rad/s² with calculations of left-beating (—) and right-beating (- - -) nystagmus. (From Mathog RH.[2] Published with permission.)

The phase shifts, measuring the relationship of the change in direction of the eyes to the chair, as described by Niven et al[1] were also evaluated by the handscoring techniques. These early analyses were difficult to perform and it was not easy to determine the exact point of phase shift, thus creating a great deal of variability in the data. There was no attempt at computer analysis of the data which apparently has been successful for phase determination in more recent investigation.[5]

Responses in Disease Conditions. Following completion of analysis of normative data, the sinusoidal angular acceleration test was administered to several patients. Figure 4 demonstrates a typical stimulus and response in a patient with an acoustic neuroma. As exemplified by this patient, the velocity of the

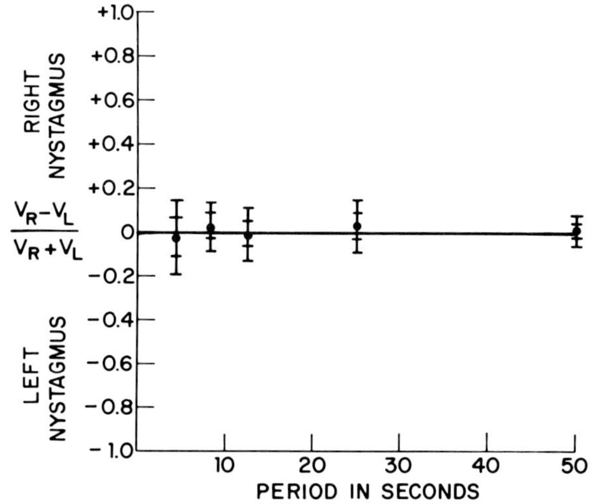

Fig. 3. Relative direction of response (preponderance) with respect to the maximum velocity of the slow component of nystagmus. V_R is the maximum velocity of the slow component of nystagmus to the right. V_L is the maximum velocity of the slow component of nystagmus to the left. (From Mathog RH, Cramer RL.[3] Published with permission.)

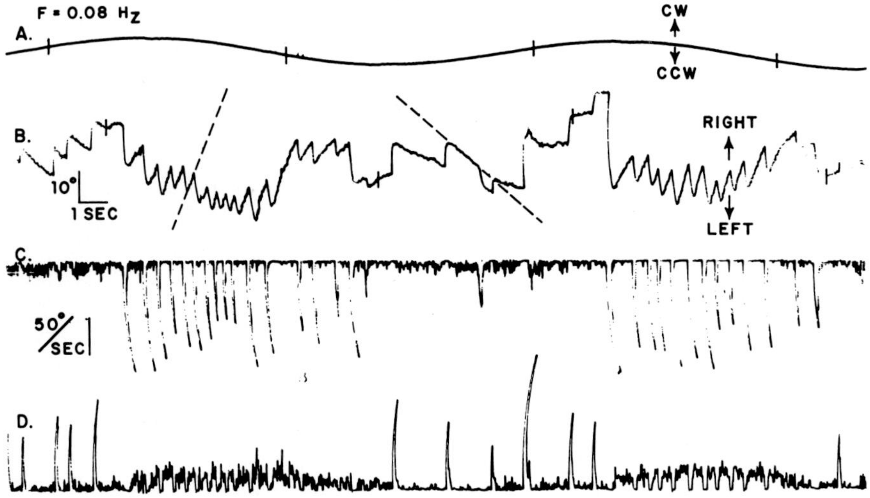

Fig. 4. Nystagmic responses in an individual with a cerebellopontine angle tumor. Line A represents the recording of the accelerometer and demonstrates the frequency, direction and magnitude of oscillation. Line B shows the slope method of determining the maximum slow-phase velocity of nystagmus, while lines C and D define the clamped derivative in two directions. (From Mathog RH.[2] Published with permission.)

response in one direction was very much diminished as compared to the velocity of the response in the other direction. In observing patients following removal of the acoustic neuroma, the patients did better clinically and showed a decrease in the amount of asymmetry of response.

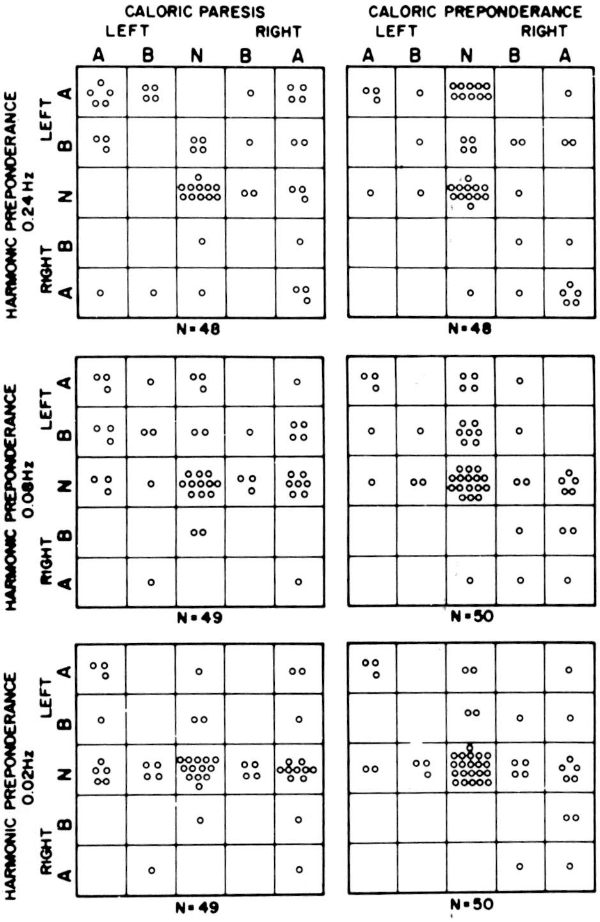

Fig. 5. Frequency distribution comparing the degree and direction of abnormality from caloric and sinusoidal stimulations. All patients were not included in every category. Normal (N), borderline (B), and abnormal (A), responses are defined in the text. (From Mathog RH.[2] Published with permission.)

The sinusoidal stimulus was also evaluated in 52 patients representing various diseases of the vestibular system (Fig. 5). The scattergram shown in Figure 5 compares the preponderance of an angular acceleration test to that of a caloric stimulus. For these purposes directional preponderance or labyrinthine preponderance was classified according to Jongkees's formula as normal, borderline, or abnormal using normal as 0-20% and abnormal as 30% or greater preponderance. With stimuli at high frequency (ie, 0.24 cycles/s) the preponderance from the sinusoidal acceleration was more to the left side signifying the possibility of an impulse artifact of the system. At the midfrequencies (ie, 0.08 cycles/s) preponderance resulting from sinusoidal acceleration was similar to that resulting from caloric stimulation. At a low frequency (ie, 0.02 cycles/s) patients with abnormal responses to sinusoidal acceleration distinguished themselves by having significant pathology. It was at this particular frequency of stimulation that patients with Menière's disease had abnormal responses for sinusoidal acceleration and normal responses to caloric stimulation. Other investigators[6,7] have also observed different sensitivities of the system at lower frequencies of stimulation, but the low frequency stimulus has not

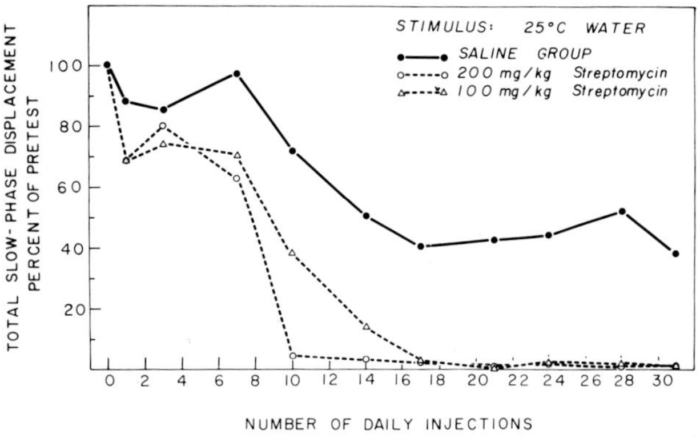

Fig. 6. Total slow-phase displacement of the eyes induced by caloric stimulation in the saline, 200 mg/kg streptomycin and 100 mg/kg streptomycin treated groups. (From Reder et al.[8] Published with permission.)

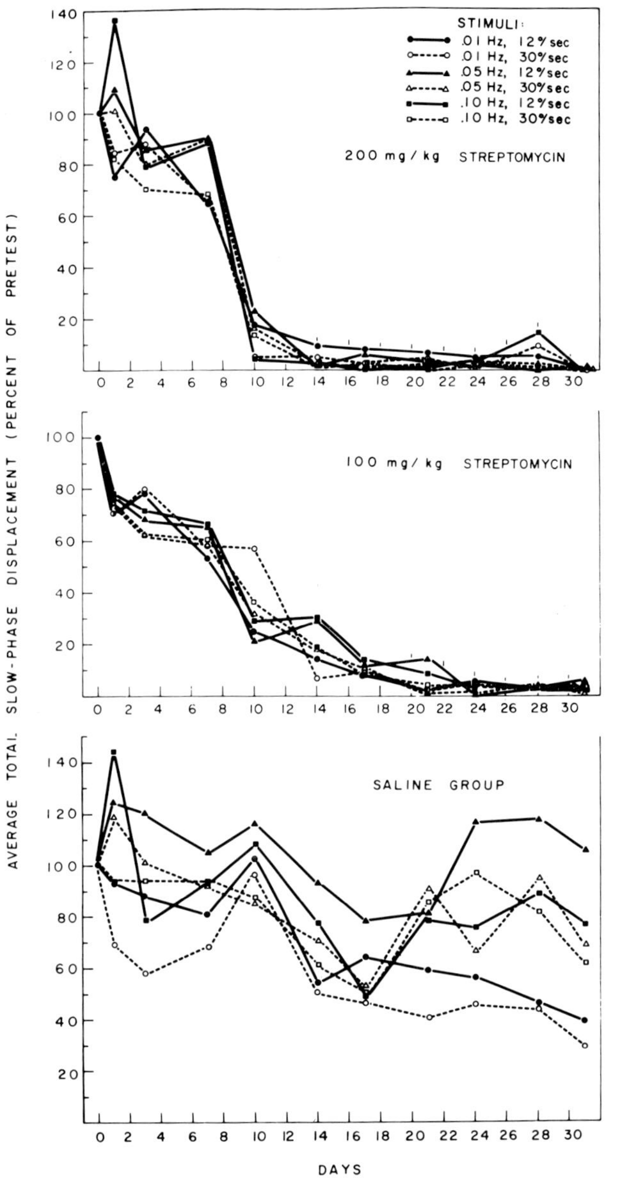

Fig. 7. Total slow-phase displacement of the eyes induced by various frequency-acceleration combinations of sinusoidal angular acceleration in the saline, 200 mg/kg streptomycin and 100 mg/kg streptomycin treated groups. (From Reder et al.[8] Published with permission.)

proven particularly beneficial in these later studies for identifying the unilateral lesion.

Animal Studies. In an attempt to evaluate sinusoidal angular acceleration as a method for investigating disease in man, several animal models were also studied. It was observed that the cat responded well to sinusoidal acceleration and that the animal could be calibrated with standard optokinetic techniques.[8] The cat was also suited for comparative caloric tests.

After initial studies had established normative data in cats, Reder et al[8] investigated sinusoidal stimulation and responses in cats that were rendered ototoxic. In these experiments, groups of cats were stimulated with repetitive caloric or sinusoidal acceleration stimuli. Peer groups were then treated similarly following injections of streptomycin. As shown in Figure 6, animals receiving caloric stimulation following saline injections showed habituation of approximately 60% in three weeks. In animals receiving 100 mg/kg streptomycin, responses disappeared completely at 16 days, while in animals receiving 200 mg/kg of streptomycin, responses disappeared in 10 days. Animals stimulated with sinusoidal angular acceleration demonstrated a 30% habituation during the three-week time period (Fig. 7). These animals, when administered streptomycin at 200 mg/kg, lost responses at 10 days and, when given 100 mg/kg of streptomycin, lost responses at 16 days. It was concluded from these experiments that the sinusoidal angular acceleration was as sensitive as the caloric test in determining ototoxicity and that these acceleration tests could be also used to follow toxicity in patients receiving drug therapy.

SUMMARY

The experience with sinusoidal angular acceleration demonstrated a potential application of a new system for the analysis of human vestibular disorders. Normative data were established and in several individuals limits for stimulation were obtained. Symmetry of response appeared very consistent suggesting that an analysis of symmetry could be used in observing imbalance in the vestibular system as well as providing a method to follow continued imbalance or recovery to normal. It could thus be determined whether an individual's condition was improving or worsening, depending upon the degree of labyrinthine preponderance from one testing session to another. The test was also useful in selecting abnormal vestibular conditions especially at lower frequencies of acceleration.

Additional studies on ototoxicity demonstrated that the test was as sensitive as caloric testing in evaluating deficits of the vestibular system. Since stimulation could be provided in a very short period of time, it was possible to perform a rapid testing of the vestibular system with potentially minimal discomfort to the patient.

These studies also showed that sinusoidal acceleration had limits in detecting a site of lesion of vestibular dysfunction. It was also not possible to determine which ear had sustained damage; and with this consideration it would be unlikely that this stimulus would ever replace the caloric test. Yet, in spite of these limitations, the studies appeared to indicate that the sinusoidal stimulus added another useful and important dimension to the evaluation of the function of the vestibular system.

REFERENCES

1. Niven JI, Hixon C, Correia MJ. An experimental approach to the dynamics of the vestibular organs in the exploration of space. Pensacola: NASA AP-77, 1965; 43-56.

2. Mathog RH. Testing of the vestibular system by sinusoidal angular acceleration. Acta Otolaryngol (Stockh) 1972; 74:96-103.

3. Mathog RH, Cramer RL. Testing of the vestibular system. Aerosp Med 1971; 42:741-5.

4. Cassel JC, Mathog RH. A variable slope plotter of nystagmic velocity. Arch Otolaryngol 1972; 96:185.

5. Wolfe JW, Engelkem E, Kos CM. Low frequency harmonic acceleration as a test of labyrinthine function: basic methods and illustrated cases. Trans Am Acad Opthalmol Otolaryngol 1978; 86:130-42.

6. Jenkins HA, Lau CGY, Baloh RW, Honrubia V. Implication of Ewald's second law for diagnosis of unilateral labyrinthine paralysis. Otolaryngol Head Neck Surg 1979; 87:459-62.

7. Kim YS, Lau CGY, Jenkins HA, Honrubia V. Implications of Ewald's second law for the evaluation of vestibular function. Otolaryngol Head Neck Surg 1979; 87:453-8.

8. Reder MS, Mathog RH, Capps MJ. Comparison of caloric and sinusoidal tests in the vestibulotoxic cat. Laryngoscope 1977; 87:2008-15.

COMPARISON OF SUBJECTIVE SYMPTOMATOLOGY AND RESPONSES TO HARMONIC ACCELERATION IN PATIENTS WITH MENIÈRE'S DISEASE

JAMES E. OLSON, LT COL, MC, USAF

JAMES W. WOLFE, PhD

SAN ANTONIO, TEXAS

Vestibular function testing employing caloric stimulation has been of limited value in the evaluation of patients with Menière's disease, with its cardinal shortcoming being poor repeatability. This modality has not been useful in determining appropriate treatment for these individuals. We have used low frequency harmonic acceleration to study patients with vestibular pathology and have noted a high level of repeatability of responses to this type of stimulation. This study was designed to determine if the clinical status of patients with Menière's disease could be correlated with their responses to harmonic acceleration. Thirty-six patients with typical symptoms of Menière's disease were evaluated and divided into four groups based on severity of symptoms. Analysis of variance of the phase shifts in asymmetry (or preponderance) showed a significant difference between the groups. Responses to this type of stimulation correlated with the clinical status of the patients to a significant degree. These data indicate that harmonic acceleration can be of value to the otologist in the evaluation of patients with Menière's disease.

Vestibular function testing employing caloric stimulation has been of limited value in the evaluation and treatment of Menière's disease. In several series of patients with Menière's disease, it has been noted that many of the patients (30-50%) have normal caloric responses.[1,2] We have used low frequency harmonic acceleration to study patients with vestibular pathology and have noted a high level of sensitivity and repeatability of responses with this type of stimulation. The purpose of this study was to determine if the clinical condition of patients with Menière's disease could be correlated with their responses to harmonic acceleration. They were divided into clinical groups and their responses compared to normals and to each other.

METHODS

All patients with Menière's disease (diagnosed by AAOO criteria)[3] seen between September 1977 and July 1978 were clinically categorized according to what we have elected to refer to as "stage" and "status." The "stage" of the disease is essentially a time categorization, indicating to some degree the length of time the patient has had the disease and the type of symptoms present. "Status" refers to the current activity level of the disease. Although arbitrary, these classifications divide the patients into clinically recognizable groups and allow us to analyze the rotational data from several points of view. The following criteria were utilized to differentiate groups in each category.

STAGES OF DISEASE

Early. The patient has had only one or two classic attacks; usually he has noted fullness, tinnitus and intermittent mild unsteadiness. He may be unsure of hearing fluctuation, but it can be documented audiometrically. If the patient goes into remission, he often neglects to return for follow-up thinking the disease has cured itself. The arbitrary limit for this stage is two years.

Mid. The patient has had several classic attacks and is well aware of his disease. He may be in remission or may be having frequent exacerbations, but the diagnosis of Menière's disease is clear. This stage may last from several months to 20 to 30 years; most patients are in this stage for at least several years.

Late A. A patient in the late A stage has violent attacks of vertigo with no warning and will often be unsteady most of the time. He has made (or is considering making) drastic changes in his lifestyle.

Late B. The patient has no more attacks of vertigo. His hearing is depressed and no longer fluctuates. He is not really bothered by his disease unless there is involvement of the other ear.

CURRENT STATUS OF PATIENT

Mild. This patient knows that some problem is present. He usually has occasional unsteadiness, pressure and a change in tinnitus or hearing. He has had only one classic attack or has been in remission for at least six months. He may have minor motion intolerance. If he has been treated he meets the AAOO criteria for control of vertigo.

Moderate. Although the patient may have regular minor attacks, he has had no classic attack for three months. He remains concerned that one of these may become a major attack. The patient's minor attacks usually consist of intermittent fullness, pressure, a change in tinnitus or hearing and mild unsteadiness, or a combination of these.

Severe. The patient is very concerned about his disease. He has regular minor attacks and occasional classic attacks. He is constantly concerned about another major attack and has had one within three months. Most importantly, he has been through enough remissions and exacerbations to know the disease will persist for many years. Medicine is regularly sought by the patient, and he will seriously consider, and may ask for, surgery.

Very Severe. A major change in lifestyle has taken place or is imminent. He may have stopped driving and may be unable to work. He wants immediate treatment to eliminate his regular classic attacks. He may be unsteady most of the time and will consider any treatment no matter how irrational.

After these arbitrary categories were established, each patient was evaluated and placed in the appropriate group on each clinic visit or hospitalization. Thirty-six patients were evaluated receiving a complete otoneurologic evaluation as well as special vestibu-

From the Department of Otolaryngology, Wilford Hall USAF Medical Center, Lackland Air Force Base and the USAF School of Aerospace Medicine, Brooks Air Force Base, San Antonio, Texas.

REPRINTS — James E. Olson, Lt Col, MC, USAF, Wilford Hall USAF Medical Center/SGHSO/STOP 84, Lackland Air Force Base, TX 78236.

TABLE 1. PATIENT CATEGORIES

Stage	*No. Patients*
Stage of Disease	
Early	4
Mid	26
Late	6
Status of Patient	
Mild	4
Moderate	8
Severe	19
Very Severe	5

lo-oculomotor tests including sinusoidal (harmonic) acceleration and are the subjects of this study.

The vestibulo-oculomotor tests consisted of pursuit tracking optokinetic stimulation, testing for spontaneous and positional nystagmus (including the Dix-Hallpike maneuvers), bithermal caloric stimulation and harmonic acceleration. A detailed description of these procedures has been previously presented;[2,4] only a summary of the harmonic acceleration method will be provided. Each subject was seated in a chair which was encapsulated by a lightweight drum and driven by a torque-motor turntable system (Contraves-Goerz DP-300). The head was positioned so that the horizontal canals were in the plane of rotation. The patient was tested in the dark with eyes opened while arithmetic problems and questions were employed to maintain adequate alertness. The electronystagmogram (ENG) was obtained for the summated horizontal and the left and right eyes independently. However, only the summated ENG was evaluated in the present study.

The patients were tested at frequencies of 0.01, 0.02, 0.04, 0.08 and 0.16 Hz at a maximum velocity of 50°/s. Acceleration thus varied from 3°/s^2 to 50°/s^2. Analog and digital computer techniques were utilized to analyze the data. Output measures were the phase relationships between the input stimulus and the eye movements and asymmetry (labyrinthine preponderance). Phase relationships (referenced to velocity) were obtained by cross-correlating the tachometer input signal with the inverted slow-phase derivative. Labyrinthine preponderance (LP) was determined by separately integrating the total slow-phase output to the left and right and converting the differences to percentages. These parameters were obtained at each test frequency.

RESULTS

The patients had a mean age of 39, ranging from 10 to 67. Twenty of the 36 patients were males. Twenty-three (59%) had caloric responses that were within normal limits, ie, unilateral weakness and directional preponderance (caloric) of less than 20%.

Four patients were in the early stage, 26 in midstage and 6 were late. Of those in the late stage, three were classified at Late A (decompensated) and three were Late B (burned out). When grouped according to status, 4 were mild, 8 were moderate, 19 were severe, and 5 were very severe (Table 1).

Initially, data from the patients were pooled and compared with our normal data. Analysis of variance of the phase measures showed the Menière's groups to be significantly different from normals at 0.01 and 0.02 Hz (Fig. 1). When the LP of all patients was compared with normals, there was no significant difference.

The phase measurements of the stage groups (early, mid and late) and the status groups (mild,

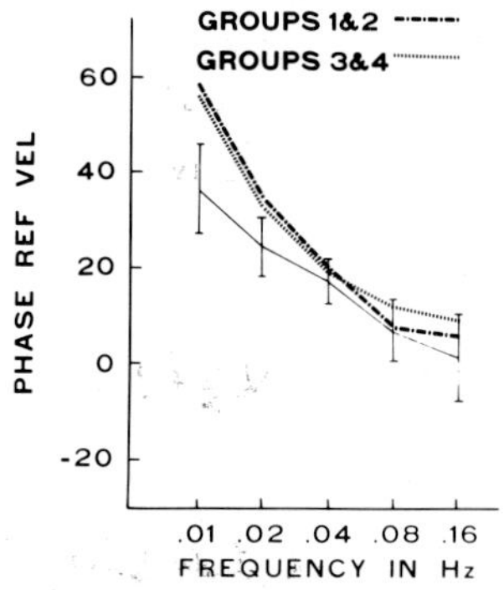

Fig. 1. Phases of status of patient groups 1 & 2 and 3 & 4 plotted for each frequency of rotation. Each group and combined groups are significantly different from normals at frequencies 0.01 and 0.02.

moderate, severe, very severe) were then compared individually, in combination to each other, and to normals. Most of the comparisons yielded no significant differences and will not be discussed.

However, when a comparison of the LP of status groups, mild and moderate versus severe and very severe, was carried out, the LP was significantly different between groups at all five frequencies of stimulations (Fig. 2). There were also significant differences between the moderate versus severe group and between the moderate versus very severe group. On examination we noted there appeared to be a significant clinical division between the moderately symptomatic patients and those with severe symptoms. It appears as though close proximity (within three months) to a classical attack will convert a moderately symptomatic patient to a severe one both clinically and on rotational testing.

On examination of the Late A stage (decompensated) and Late B stage (burned out), the Late A patients had a labyrinthine preponderance indicating increased output on the diseased side; whereas, the "burned out" patient had a diseased ear which was depressed.

DISCUSSION

Although each patient's data are unique, the above statistical results permit some conclusions.

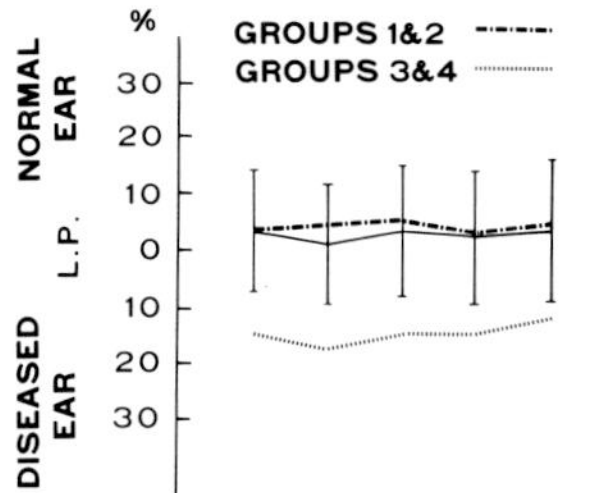

Fig. 2. Labyrinthine preponderance of status of patient groups 1 & 2 and 3 & 4 plotted for each frequency of rotation. Combined groups 3 & 4 are significantly different from normals at all frequencies while groups 1 & 2 are not.

The phase measure is highly repeatable and appears to be quite sensitive for peripheral disorders. The phase was abnormal in all of our patients with clinical Menière's disease and appears to be resistant to CNS compensation. Once the disturbance is initially manifest clinically, the phase measures at the very low frequencies will show an abnormality regardless of the clinical status of the patient. Thus, phase relationships at the 0.01 Hz stimulus frequency appear to be a consistent and sensitive indicator of peripheral end-organ disease.

Comparison of phase and labyrinthine preponderance parameters between patients of differing clinical status showed some interesting findings. When patients began having regular (more often than every three months) attacks, their preponderance markedly changed. This was usually shown by an asymmetry indicating irritation (increased output) of the vestibular system with utriculopetal movement on the diseased side. In the "burned out" patients, the preponderance indicated depression of the involved ear. The patients with depression of the involved ear were usually less symptomatic than those with irritation.

Those patients with a marked asymmetry indicating irritation of the involved ear are much more liable to a classic attack than those who are symmetrical or depressed. Thus, the preponderance reflects the clinical status of the patient as indicated by the presence or absence of classical attacks. This may enable the clinician to more accurately advise the patient concerning medical or surgical treatment. Certainly the patient severely asymmetric to the side of the involved ear (irritation) should be treated and followed closely in an attempt to reduce the irritation even though the patient has not had a recent attack.

CONCLUSIONS

Harmonic acceleration was employed in the evaluation of 36 patients with classical Menière's disease and certain conclusions can be made.

1. Low frequency sinusoidal (harmonic) acceleration provides phase and directional preponderance measures which are sensitive for peripheral labyrinthine disorders.

2. The phase change is resistant to CNS compensation.

3. The labyrinthine preponderance or asymmetry measurements reflect the clinical status of the patient as indicated by the classic attack.

4. When the asymmetry shows that the involved ear is irritable, the patient is more likely to have classic attacks.

5. Sinusoidal (harmonic) acceleration produces quantitative data which may be correlated with pathophysiologic changes in the inner ear.

ACKNOWLEDGMENTS — The authors wish to express appreciation to Mrs. Jo Kast for typing and proofreading the manuscript and to John W. Docken, Daniel E. Dreher, Norwood E. Gray, Jr., and TSgt Lloyd J. Loup for their technical assistance.

REFERENCES

1. Silverstein H. The effect of the endolymphatic subarachnoid shunt operation on vestibular function. Laryngoscope 1978; 88:1603-11.

2. Wolfe JW, Engelken EJ, Olson JE, Kos CM. Vestibular responses to bithermal caloric and harmonic acceleration. Ann Otol Rhinol Laryngol 1978; 87:861-7.

3. Alford BR. Report of subcommittee on equilibrium and its measurement. Trans Am Acad Ophthalmol Otolaryngol 1972; 76:1462-4.

4. Wolfe JW, Engelken EJ, Kos CM. Low frequency harmonic acceleration as a test of labyrinthine function: basic methods and illustrative cases. Trans Am Acad Ophthalmol Otolaryngol 1978; 86:130-42.

SINUSOIDAL HARMONIC ACCELERATION TEST IN CLINICAL PRACTICE

WALLACE RUBIN, MD
METAIRIE, LOUISIANA

The author's experience during the first year of use of the Sinusoidal Harmonic Acceleration test in clinical practice is presented. The advantages of this test both in the diagnostic and monitoring areas are illustrated with patient evaluation summaries. Further, use of this test on a daily basis in the office practice of neurotology will define its role in the evolution and follow-up of neurotologic problems.

Barany[1] introduced the concept of the clinical usefulness of rotational tests for vestibular evaluation in 1907. Since that time there has been a great deal of interest in the development and improvement of rotational techniques for testing. The trend has been to use more sophisticated methods which employ precise stimuli and sophisticated recording equipment. The technique of cupulometry was introduced by van Egmond and Groen in 1953.[2] The subliminal rotation test of Montadon[3] was introduced in 1954 and the vestibulometry tests of Torok were introduced in 1971.[4]

Several investigators, Niven et al,[5] Cramer et al,[6] and Eviatar and Goodhill,[7] described methods of continuous harmonic or sinusoidal oscillation. Such techniques provided an efficient and quantitative acceleration stimulus. They also suggested simple methods of evaluating the nystagmic response. Preliminary reports suggested an application to the clinical evaluation of patients, although the tests were initially restricted to laboratory animals and normal subjects.

Mathog made some significant observations in 1972.[8] He stated that he found that sinusoidal stimulation, as defined at a specific frequency and peak acceleration, proved useful in the evaluation of the vestibular system. When applied to abnormal cases, he found that it was possible to determine directional preponderance and that it was also possible to distinguish severe pathology. The rotational techniques did not delineate the particular pathologic ear but did provide a method for following a changing disease state. In conjunction with caloric tests, the sinusoidal rotational stimulus did allow for a more complete understanding of the vestibular system.

Mathog[8] and others have since attempted to utilize and analyze the diagnostic value of the sinusoidal stimulus. My remarks will be limited to the utilization of such a technique in the clinical environment of my office practice during the past year. The data derived from these determinations were then applied to a variety of clinical problems, comparing results from sinusoidal stimulation to those of other vestibular tests. It was anticipated that this study would clarify some of the difficulties in rotational testing, as well as provide new methods for differentiating and monitoring vestibular pathology.

My involvement in this effort was stimulated by the work of Wolfe et al[9,10] and by the personal consultation with and encouragement of V. Honrubia. My continued search for the "better mousetrap" with which to evaluate the dizzy patient was further propelled with W. Wolfe's and Honrubia's stimulation and the technological assistance of J. Parmentier.

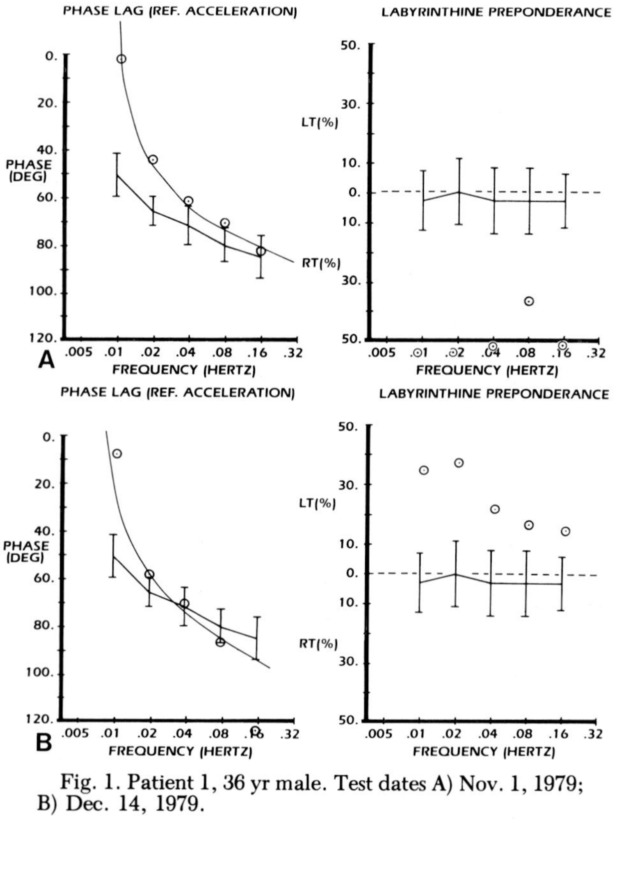

Fig. 1. Patient 1, 36 yr male. Test dates A) Nov. 1, 1979; B) Dec. 14, 1979.

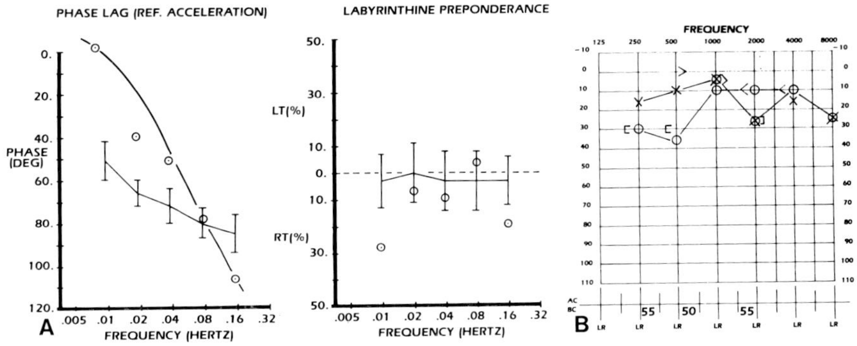

Fig. 2. Patient 2, 34 yr female. A) Test date: April 27, 1979. B) Audiogram: April 27, 1979.

This presentation will be confined to excerpted material from patient evaluations. These patients have been selected to illustrate the value of the Sinusoidal Harmonic Acceleration (SHA) test as first, a means of rapidly solving subtle diagnostic dilemmas; second, as a more accurate method of differentiating central from peripheral abnormalities; and third, and probably most important, as a modality for monitoring patient progress. These changes over time probably occur as a result of the presence or absence of central vestibular compensation.

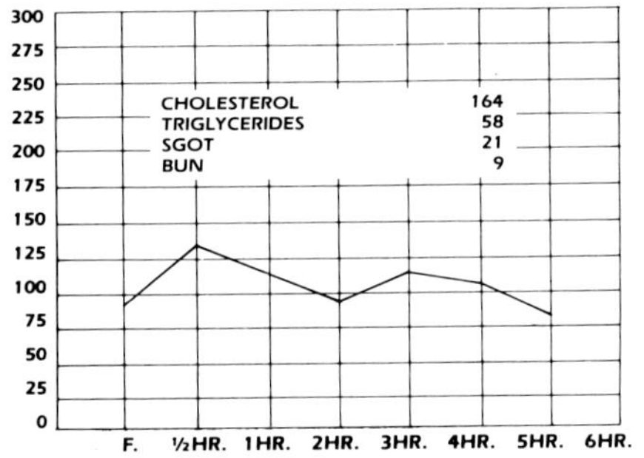

Fig. 3. Patient 2. Blood fat studies and glucose tolerance curve: Aug. 6, 1979.

TECHNIQUE CONCEPTS

Evaluation of symmetry in the abnormal group of subjects revealed different patterns developing with changes in stimulus frequency. The analysis demonstrated: 1) distortion at high frequency from stimulus artifact; 2) directional preponderance similar to the results of caloric tests at midfrequency; and 3) what appeared as a separation of severe from lesser pathology at the lower frequency stimulation. Although the pattern of response for each individual throughout an entire frequency range of 0.24 to 0.02 Hz was useful, the clinical application was

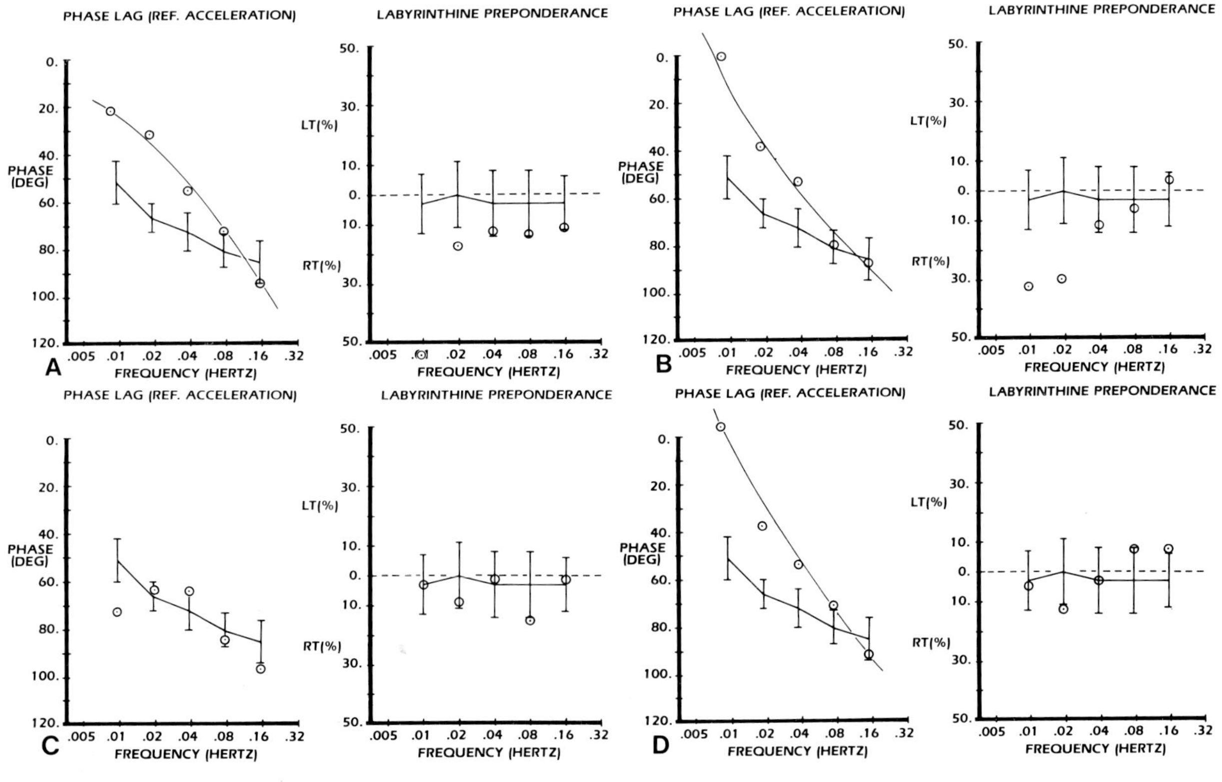

Fig. 4. Patient 2. Test dates A) Aug. 6, 1979; B) Dec. 14, 1979; C) March 21, 1980; D) Aug. 21, 1980.

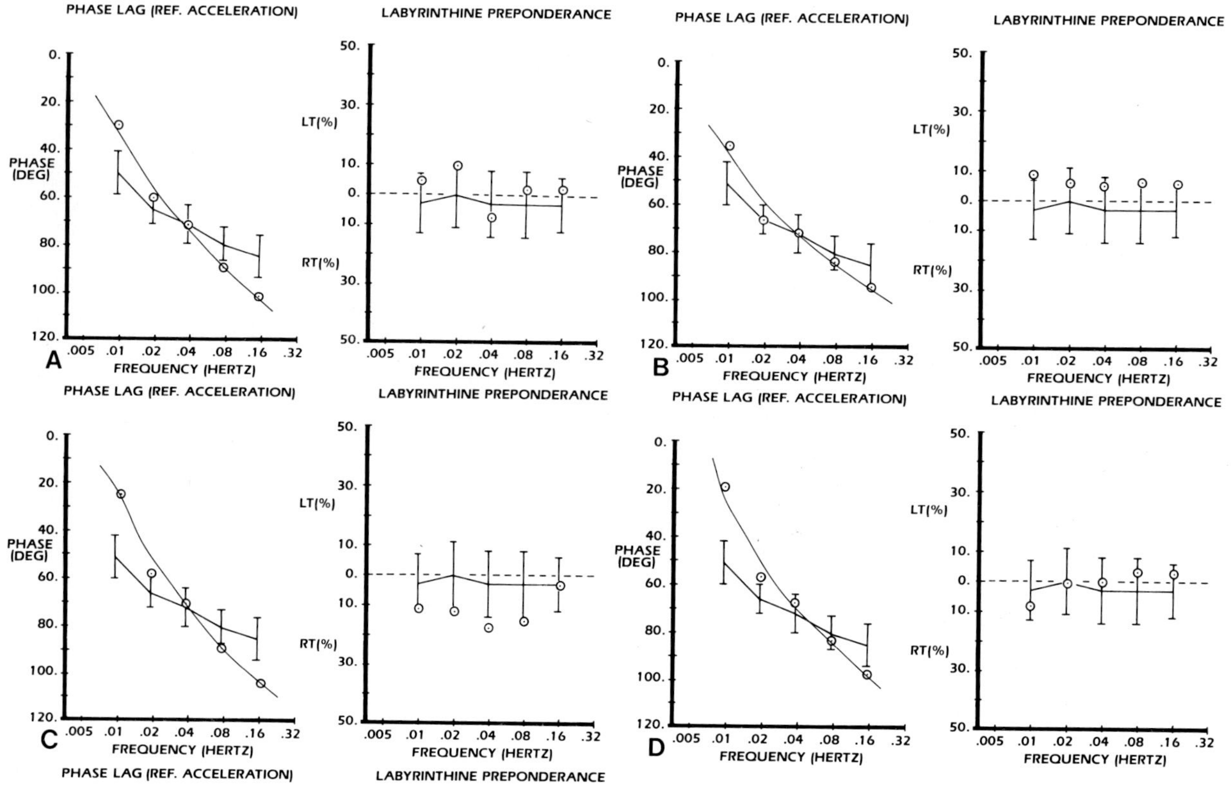

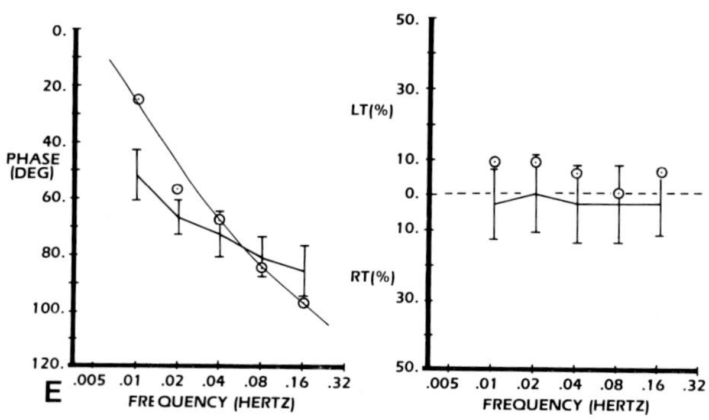

Fig. 5. Patient 3, 51 yr male. Test dates A) Jan. 31, 1980; B) Feb. 13, 1980; C) March 24, 1980; D) April 28, 1980; E) Aug. 14, 1980.

most valuable at the greater stimulation (0.02 Hz), employing the longer period of lower frequency.

In addition to these general relationships of stimulus and response, other information derived from individual cases demonstrated the possibility of evaluating changing pathology. Usually, the directional preponderance elicited by sinusoidal stimulation remained constant for at least 24 hours, but in some patients, evaluation at a later time demonstrated a change in direction and a tendency toward symmetry. The phenomenon was particularly characteristic of those few patients where there was recovery following injury to the vestibular system; ie, head injury and destructive labyrinthectomy.

On the basis of such information, changes of symmetry of response were used to determine the extent of healing processes. If the directional preponderance remained constant over a period of time, it was possible to assume a lack of compensation and the likelihood of an active or progressive lesion.

CASE REPORTS

The following patient summaries illustrate the use of the SHA to advantage: 1) A better discriminator of abnormality; 2) to monitor progress; 3) to show patient inprovement in spite of continuing complaints; and 4) to confirm lack of patient improvement.

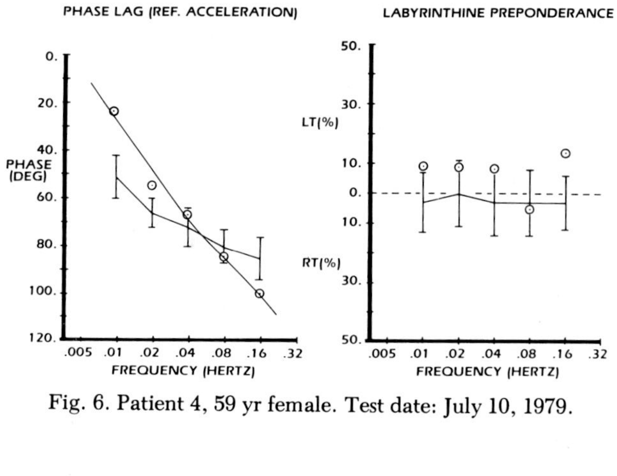

Fig. 6. Patient 4, 59 yr female. Test date: July 10, 1979.

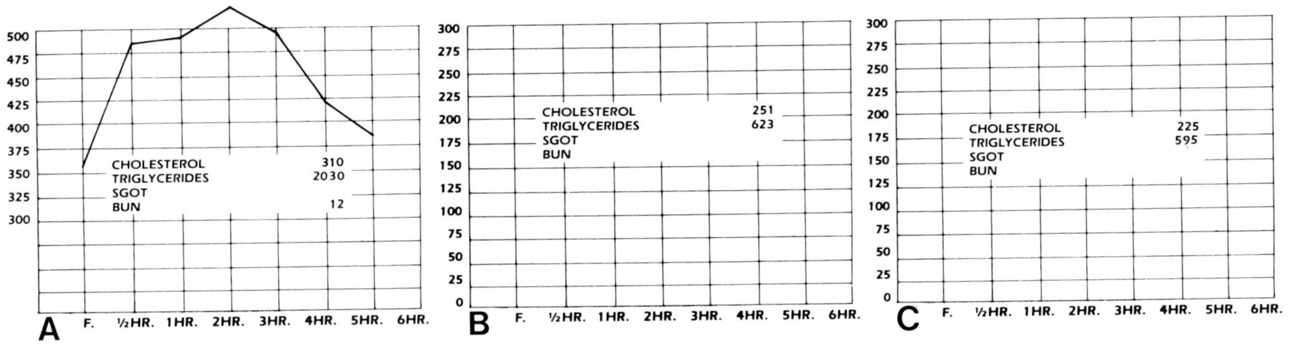

Fig. 7. Patient 4, 60 yr female. A) Glucose tolerance curve: July 23, 1979. B) Blood fat studies: Sept. 10, 1979. C) Blood fat studies: Oct. 30, 1979.

Following is an outline of the work-up of all patients seen in this study:

1. Physical examination.

2. Hearing evaluation including conventional hearing tests and brainstem evoked response (ABR).

3. Conventional electronystagmography (ENG), including alternate and simultaneous binaural bithermal testing (ABB and SBB).

4. Sinusoidal Harmonic Acceleration testing (SHA) including phase lag and preponderance.

5. Radiography.

As a Better Discriminator. Patient 1, a 36-year-old male construction worker was first seen November 23, 1979, having suffered from dizziness for 20 hours. He was extremely nervous, only able to navigate with help, and was slightly nauseated. He was in excellent general health, and after the work-up admitted to taking moderate-to-large amounts of at least two psychotropic drugs daily. The evaluation performed revealed the following:

1. Physical examination: Romberg positive, gait and cerebellar tests normal.

2. Hearing evaluation:

   a. Conventional hearing tests, bilateral high-tone mild loss.

   b. ABR abnormal bilaterally.

3. Conventional ENG:

   a. Left spontaneous nystagmus.

   b. Left directional preponderance on ABB and SBB.

4. SHA: phase lag, central abnormality; preponderance, right (marked) (Fig. 1A).

5. Radiography: polytomes normal.

6. Biochemistry: normal.

A second evaluation on December 14, 1979, after cessation of drug ingestion showed marked improvement on SHA which correlated with the symptomatic improvement. There was, however, no change on the conventional ENG (Fig. 1B).

To Monitor Progress. Patient 2, a 34-year-old female was seen first on April 27, 1979, because of recurrent dizzy episodes accompanied by fullness, diplacusis and hearing loss in the right ear. There were no other general medical problems of significance. None of the so-far tried medical regimens had been of benefit in controlling her rather obvious problem with endolymphatic hydrops. She was an intense, hard-working individual (both at home and in industry), and admitted to poor eating habits over a long period of time.

The evaluation revealed the following:

1. Physical examination: normal.

2. Hearing evaluation:

   a. Conventional hearing evaluation, right mild sensorineural hearing loss (low tone primarily) (Fig. 2).

   b. ABR abnormal right.

3. Conventional ENG:

   a. Right spontaneous nystagmus.

   b. ABB — right reduced response.

   c. SBB — peripheral right reduced response.

4. SHA: Phase lag — peripheral abnormality; preponderance — right (marked) (Fig. 2).

5. Radiography: polytomes normal.

6. Biochemistry: normal except for flat glucose tolerance test (Fig. 3).

The serial SHAs correlated exactly with the remission and exacerbations of the symptoms related by the patient (Fig. 4), but the hearing evaluations and the conventional ENGs from April 27, 1979, through July 21, 1980, did not at all correlate with the reported remissions and exacerbations of the patients symptoms.

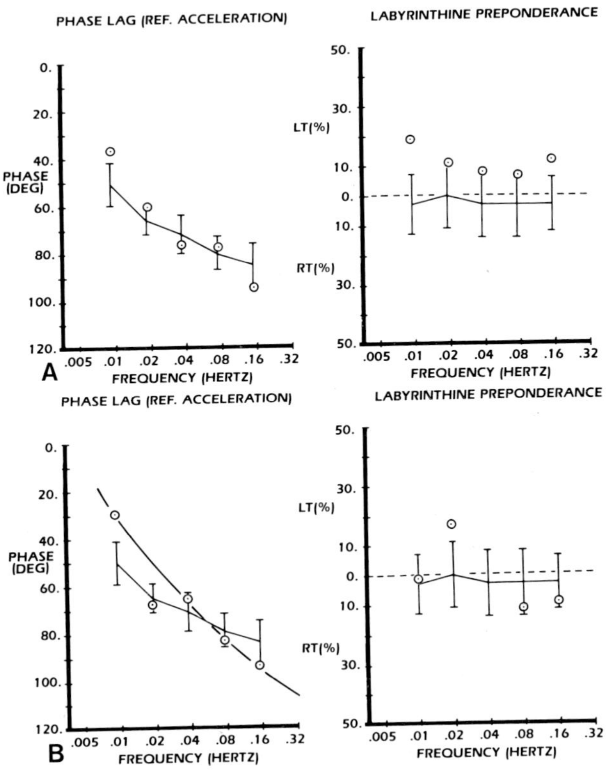

Fig. 8. Patient 4. Test dates A) Sept. 10, 1979; B) Oct. 30, 1979.

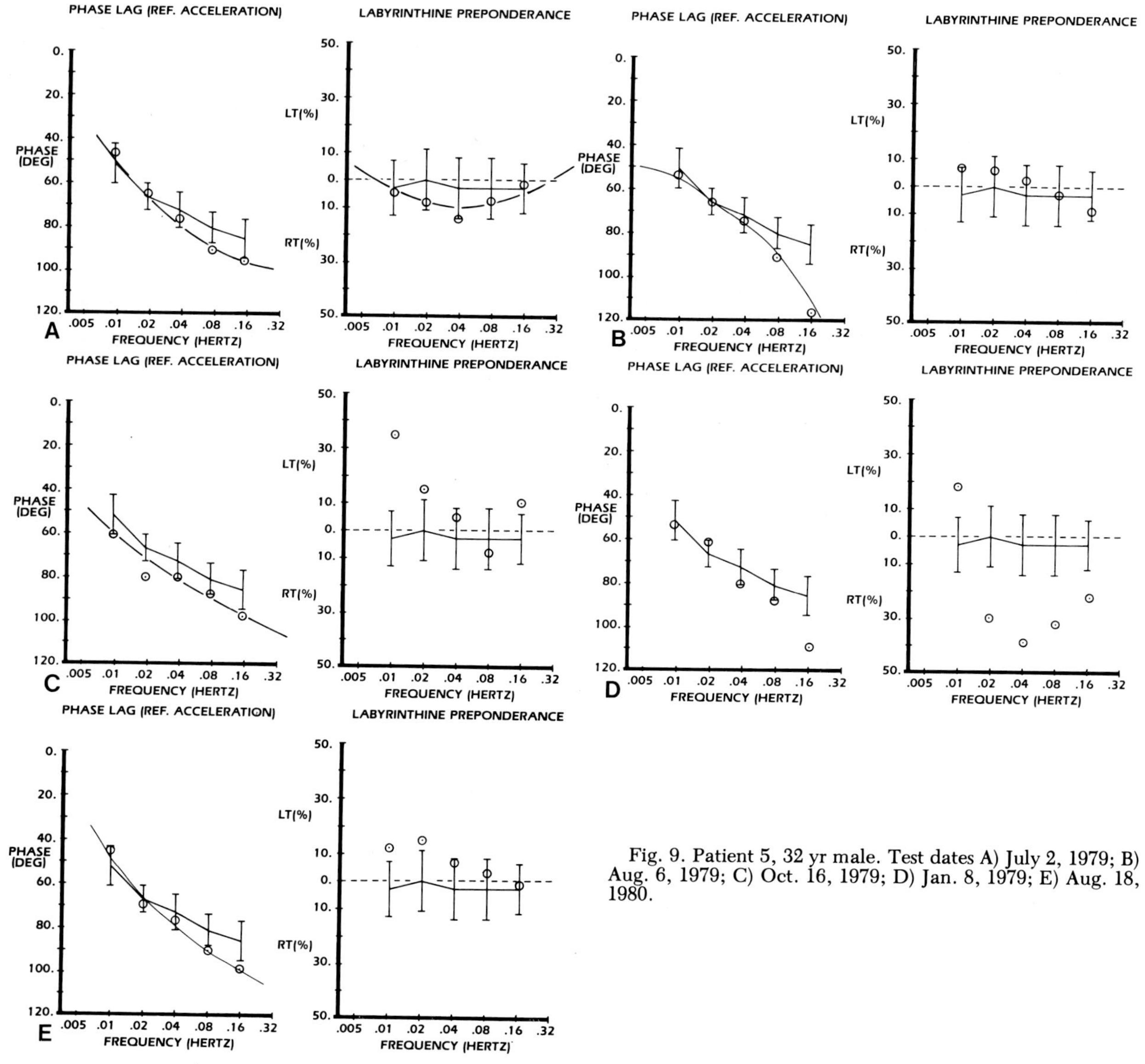

Fig. 9. Patient 5, 32 yr male. Test dates A) July 2, 1979; B) Aug. 6, 1979; C) Oct. 16, 1979; D) Jan. 8, 1979; E) Aug. 18, 1980.

To Monitor Progress Following Trauma. Patient 3, a 50-year-old male, became wobbly and had a staggered gait immediately following an injury on board a barge on November 13, 1979. The barge was struck by a boat and the patient was thrown against a stove in the galley, pinned against a wall, struck the left side of his head, and was knocked unconscious for about five minutes. He was treated at a local hospital and sent home. He reported being lethargic for a couple of days and since that time he complained of staggering and dizzy episodes daily.

Evaluation on January 31, 1980, revealed the following:

1. Physical examination: no abnormalities.
2. Hearing evaluation:

   a. Conventional hearing tests, flat bilateral sensorineural loss with excellent discrimination.

   b. ABR — bilateral abnormality but especially left side.
3. Conventional ENG:

   a. No spontaneous or positional nystagmus.

   b. ABR — right directional preponderance.

   c. SBB — 30° right beating (type IV).
4. SHA: phase lag — peripheral; preponderance — none.
5. Radiography: normal polytomes and scan.
6. Biochemistry: normal.

He has improved gradually and his SHA tests confirmed his progress objectively (Fig. 5).

As A Better Discriminator and to Monitor Progress (Metabolic). Patient 4, a 59-year-old female, was first seen on July 10, 1979, because of a week-long period of weakness, dizziness, vomiting, confusion and episodes of falling. She had been hospitalized for treatment of similar symptomatology on May 19, 1979. She had not improved on the previous treatment regimen (she probably did not follow the prescribed regimen).

Evaluation on July 10, 1979, revealed these significant findings:

1. Physical examination: obese female in obvious distress as a result of nausea and dizziness. She exhibited an abnormal Romberg, gait and cerebellar function.
2. Hearing evaluation:

   a. Conventional — normal except for bilateral high-tone loss (8,000 Hz).

   b. ABR — abnormal bilaterally.

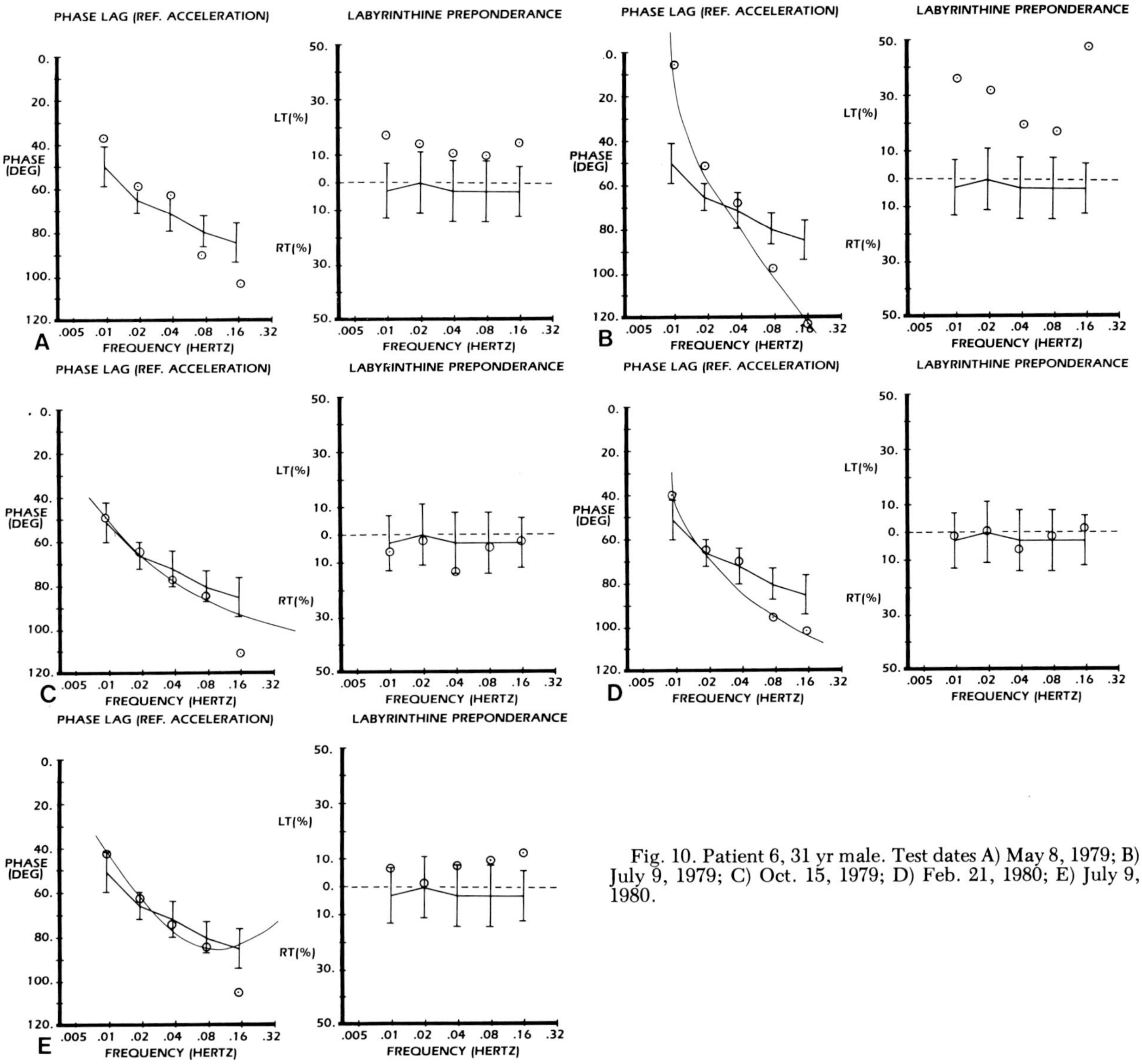

Fig. 10. Patient 6, 31 yr male. Test dates A) May 8, 1979; B) July 9, 1979; C) Oct. 15, 1979; D) Feb. 21, 1980; E) July 9, 1980.

3. Conventional ENG:

   a. Direction changing positional nystagmus.

   b. ABB — left reduced response.

   c. SBB — left reduced response.

4. SHA: Phase lag — peripheral abnormality; preponderance — left (Fig. 6).

5. Radiography: polytomes normal.

6. Biochemistry: elevated sugar (357), cholesterol (310), triglyceride (2030), type IV phenotype, HDL was unreadable (Fig. 7A).

She improved markedly over the next 90 days but never did achieve the anticipated improvement because she followed instructions erratically. Her SHA tests did (Fig. 8A, B), however, correlate completely with her biochemical surveys and her erratic performance (Fig. 7B, C).

To Monitor Fluctuating Symptoms Following Trauma. Patient 5 , a 22-year-old male oil worker, was hit by a drill pipe over the right eye while working on a rig on May 12, 1978. He was dazed but not unconscious and did not see a physician until July 19, 1978. He complained of headache, nausea, floating feeling and dizziness since the time of the accident. He was first seen by me on February 13, 1979, after being under the care of at least five different physicians in multiple specialties. He had not worked at any occupation since the date of the accident. There was no history of any prior significant medical problem. Evaluation revealed:

1. Physical examination: no abnormalities.

2. Hearing evaluation:

   a. Conventional hearing tests — normal.

   b. ABR — normal.

3. Conventional ENG:

   a. Left spontaneous nystagmus.

   b. Direction changing positional nystagmus.

   c. ABB — left reduced response.

   d. SBB — left reduced response.

4. SHA: phase lag — peripheral abnormality; preponderance — none.

5. Radiography: polytomes normal.

6. Biochemistry: normal.

He improved gradually with symptomatic therapy but in spite of objection SHA improvement into the normal range, he never has admitted to subjective improvement (Fig. 9A-E).

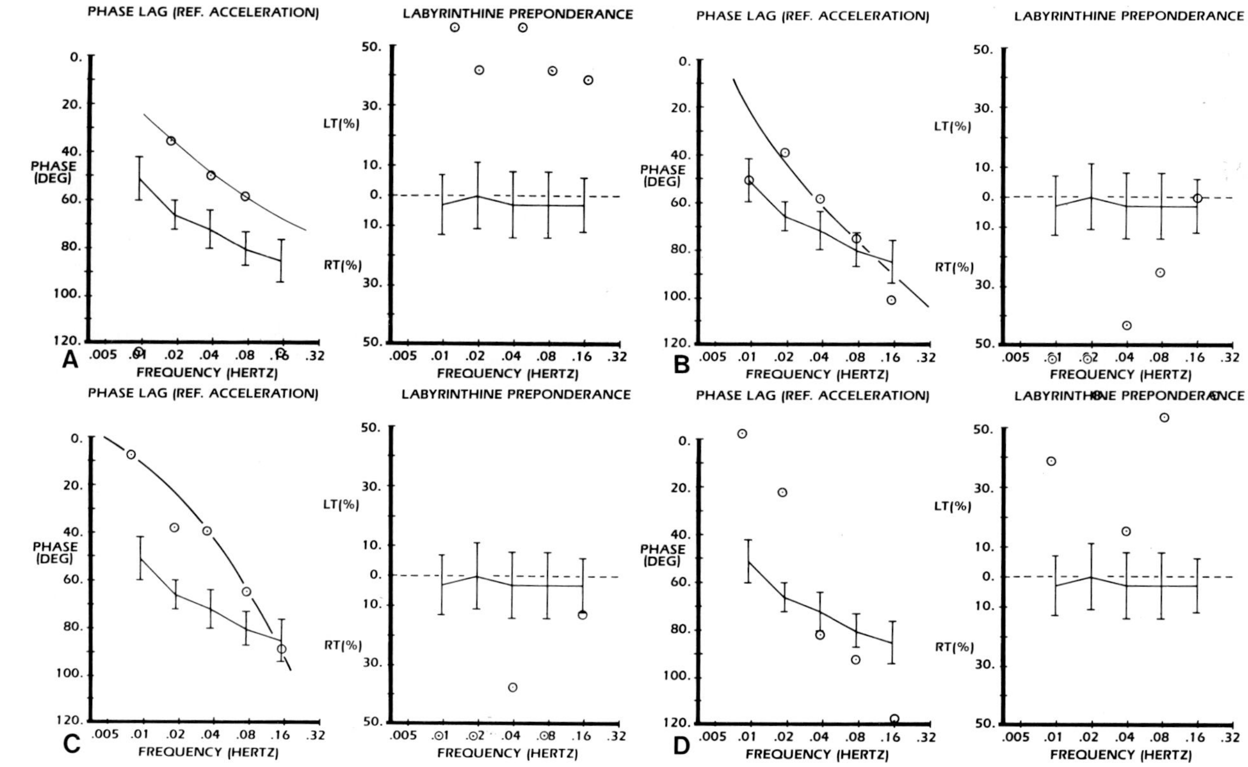

Fig. 11. Patient 7, 55 yr male. Test dates A) May 14, 1979; B) July 12, 1979; C) July 23, 1979; D) Oct. 22, 1979.

To Confirm Improvement Despite Complaints. Patient 6, a 31-year-old male industrial diver, suffered a "hit" at 59 m (194 ft) on May 23 and May 25, 1978. From that time until he was seen on November 8, 1978, he complained of irritability, forgetfulness, dizzy episodes, and hearing loss. He had been a commercial diver for ten years prior to the incident and had been "bent" on at least two prior occasions, once in 1974 and once in January 1978. Both of these episodes were limb "hits." He was otherwise in excellent health.

Evaluation and findings on November 8, 1978, were as follows:

1. Physical examination: normal.

2. Hearing tests: high-tone sensorineural hearing loss (3,000, 4,000, 6,000, and 8,000 Hz); good discrimination bilaterally.

3. Conventional ENG:

   a. Left spontaneous nystagmus.

   b. Direction changing positional nystagmus.

   c. ABB — left reduced response.

   d. SBB - normal.

4. SHA: Phase lag — peripheral; preponderance — left.

5. Radiography: polytomes normal.

6. Biochemistry: CBC — 7% eosinophilia; flat glucose tolerance test, otherwise normal.

Patient's SHA improved gradually to complete recovery but he never did quit complaining of dizziness and lightheadedness (Fig. 10A-E).

Lack of Improvement Following Use of Ototoxic Drug. Patient 7, male, age 55, was first seen on May 14, 1979, because of complaints of staggering gait, wobbly posture, foggy head and dizziness since April 29, 1979. These symptoms followed a prostatectomy procedure done on April 25, 1979. He received 240 mg per day of gentamicin for seven days starting April 5, 1979. Other than being a heavy smoker and drinker, his health was good.

Evaluation on May 14, 1979, revealed the following:

1. Physical examination: positive Romberg, abnormal gait and abnormal cerebellar function.

2. Hearing evaluation:

   a. Conventional hearing — right sensorineural hearing loss, mild, flat.

   b. ABR — not done.

3. Conventional ENG:

   a. Right spontaneous nystagmus.

   b. ABB — right reduced response.

   c. SBB — right preponderance.

4. SHA: Phase lag — central abnormality; preponderance — left.

5. Radiography: polytomes normal.

6. Biochemistry: normal.

An SHA monitor over a 15-month period confirmed the negative progress for almost the first year after gentamicin therapy. The improvement which has now begun, is confirmed by the correlation of the patient's symptom and the SHA tests (Fig. 11A-G).

CONCLUSIONS

The case histories are illustrative of the aforementioned advantages of SHA utilization.

Patient 1 illustrates the ability to quickly and accurately differentiate between peripheral and central vestibular abnormality in an individual whose conventional ENG testing was completely useless because of the heavy ingestion of psychotropic drugs. The SHA test done at the same sitting as the conventional ENG was not affected by the drug use. It clearly and precisely defined the abnormality which was central in origin.

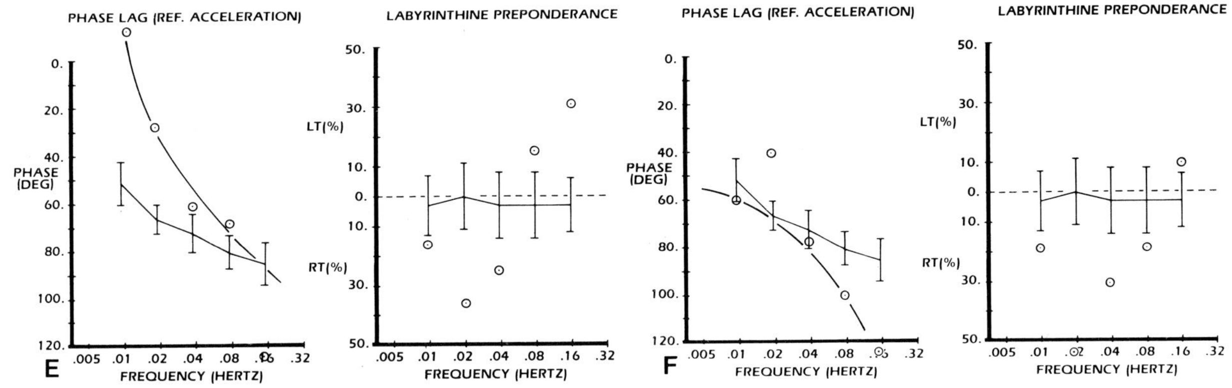

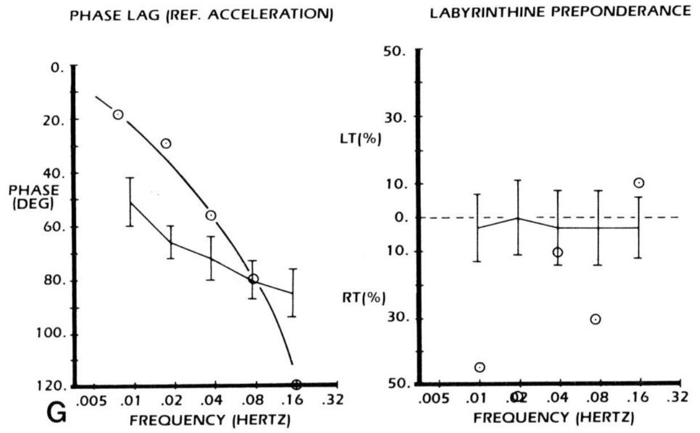

Fig. 11 (cont'd). E) Dec. 17, 1979; F) Feb. 18, 1980; G) April 28, 1980.

Patient 2 clearly demonstrates the effectiveness of the use of the SHA test for accurately monitoring and comparing test results and patient symptoms. It is well established that conventional ENGs rarely change at all in spite of marked patient symptom change.

Patient 3 reveals the effective use of SHA in monitoring patient progress following trauma. In this particular instance, the patient was an honest, accurate historian and in spite of the fact that the follow-up conventional ENG showed no change from the original evaluation, the SHA monitor tests correlated accurately with patient symptom-reporting. In this kind of patient, the physician can document and confirm the exact time for safe return to full employment.

Patient 4 illustrates the effective utilization again of the SHA test in patient monitoring. In this instance, the test was helpful in monitoring progress in a patient with obesity, hypertension and elevated blood fats. The patient's lack of cooperation in following the prescribed dietary regimen was confirmed on the SHA monitor follow-ups.

Patients 5 and 6 show the utilization of the SHA test for confirmation that vestibular compensation had occurred in spite of the fact that both patients continued to complain of dysequilibrium.

Patient 7 illustrates the complete lack of improvement in a patient with vestibular involvement due to hypertension or diabetes. Conventional ENG showed no change at all but the question of vestibular compensation was answered with the use of the SHA test.

REFERENCES

1. Barany R. Physiologie und Pathologie des Bogengangsapparates. Vienna: Deuticke, 1907.

2. van Egmond AAJ, Groen JJ. Cupulometry. Pract Otorhinolaryngol (Basel) 1953; 17:206.

3. Montadon A. A new technique for vestibular investigation. Acta Otolaryngol (Stockh) 1954; 44:594.

4. Torok N. An attempt to integrate various physical stimuli in vestibulometry. Confin Neurol 1961; 21:412.

5. Niven JI, Hixon C, Correia MJ. An experimental approach to the dynamics of the vestibular mechanisms. Symposium on the role of the vestibular organs in the exploration of space. Pensacola, Florida: NASA SP-77, 1965;43-65.

6. Cramer RL, Dowd PJ, Helms DB. Vestibular responses to oscillations about the yaw axis. Aerospace Med 1963; 34:1031.

7. Eviatar A, Goodhill V. Comparative sequential studies of effects of drugs on the vestibular system iof laboratory animals. Acta Otolaryngol (Stockh) 1968; Suppl 237.

8. Mathog RH. Testing of the vestibular system by sinusoidal angular acceleration. Acta Otolaryngol (Stockh) 1972; 74:96-103.

9. Wolfe JW, Engelken EJ, Kos CM. Low frequency harmonic acceleration as a test of labyrinthine function: basic methods and illustrative cases. ORL Digest 1978; 86:130-42.

10. Wolfe JW, Engelken EJ, Olson JW, Kos CM. Vestibular responses to bithermal caloric and harmonic acceleration. Ann Otol Rhinol Laryngol 1978; 87:861-7.

SINUSOIDAL HARMONIC ACCELERATION LABYRINTHINE TEST
CLINICAL EXPERIENCE

ROGER A. SIMPSON, MD

IOWA CITY, IOWA

Responses of 135 patients subjected to Sinusoidal Harmonic Acceleration Labyrinthine Test are reported. These patients are categorized into four clinical impression disease groups: 1) classic Menière's disease; 2) labyrinthine ischemia; 3) neurological diseases; 4) no labyrinthine or neurological disease. A case report in each category is presented. We find Sinusoidal Harmonic Acceleration Labyrinthine Test to be a useful tool in evaluation of the dizzy patient.

Sinusoidal Harmonic Acceleration (SHA) Labyrinthine testing was carried out by our group on 135 patients between May 1979 and March 1980. In this test group patients with peripheral labyrinthine disease show lag phase distortion in the low frequencies, and responses within the expected range of normal subjects in the higher frequencies. J. W. Wolfe has reported the same experience (unpublished observations).

CASE REPORTS

Twenty-eight of the patients tested exhibited the classic Menière's disease triad of fluctuating hearing loss, episodic vertigo, and tinnitus. These patients' SHA tests exhibited distortion in the two frequencies of the lag phase portion of the test. They usually also exhibited a predominance of the contralateral labyrinth.

Patient 1. A 65-year-old male presented with a three-month history of vertigo associated with fluctuating hearing loss and right tinnitus. His physical examination was normal throughout except for audiometry showing high-tone sensorineural loss and a mild right low-tone sensorineural loss (Fig. 1A). The SHA test revealed a mild lag phase shift and left labyrinthine preponderance (Fig. 1B). He responded well to medical management of his Menière's disease.

Sixteen of the 135 patients tested also had low frequency lag phase distortion in the SHA test with higher frequency lag phase. These people, however, had a constant unsteadiness on motion or had waves of vertigo in certain head positions. Their hearing loss was sensorineural, high tone, without fluctuation. Most exhibited high tone tinnitus. These people also underwent electronystagmography and were found to have positional nystagmus. They tended to be in the older age group of the 135 people tested. Our clinical impression is these people suffer from inner ear circulatory insufficiency or labyrinthine ischemia.

Patient 2. A 64-year-old female had a two-month history of lightheadedness on motion and on lifting her head to look upward. She had no tinnitus and complained of no hearing loss. Her physical examination was normal throughout except for a mild sensorineural hearing loss (Fig. 2A). Electronystagmography revealed positional nystagmus of fleeting duration. Her SHA tests were abnormal, revealing low frequency lag phase and a definite right

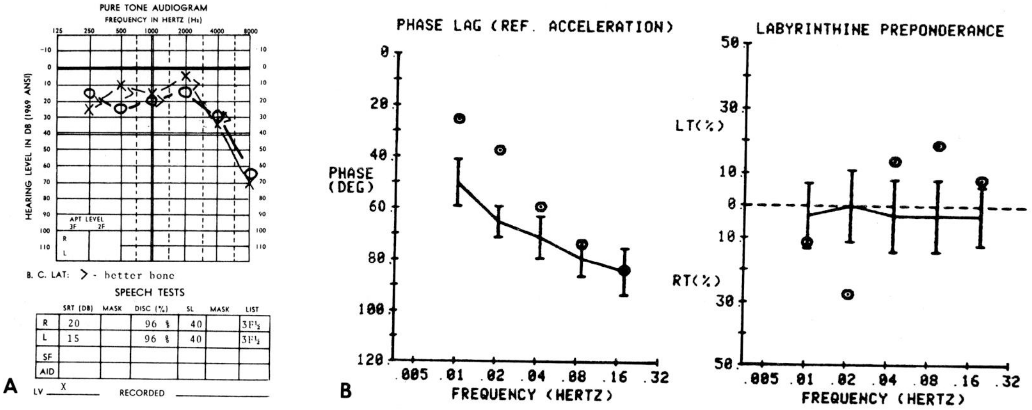

Fig. 1. (Patient 1, aged 65 yr, Sept 27, 1979) A) Audiologic examination. B) SHA test.

From the Otologic Medical Services, P.C., Iowa City.

REPRINTS — Roger A. Simpson, MD, Otologic Medical Services, P.C., Iowa City, IA 52240.

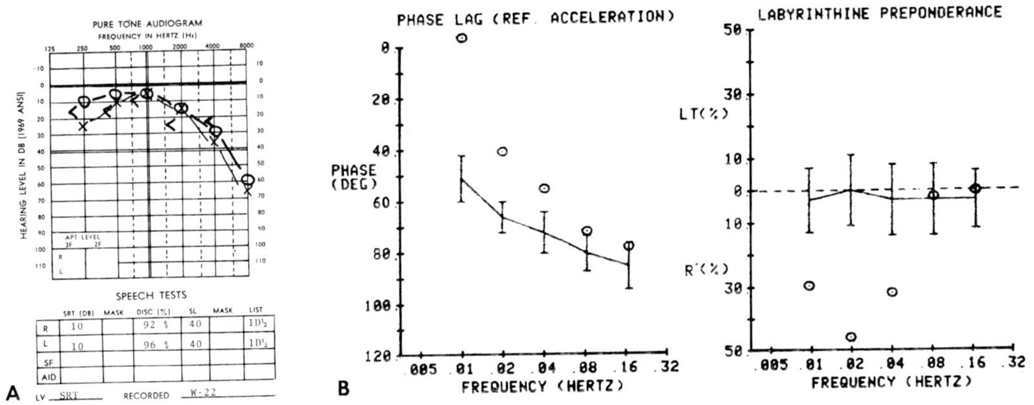

Fig. 2. (Patient 2, aged 64 yr) A) Audiologic examination, Feb 26, 1980. Impedance: Normal tympanograms AU; normal reflex and no decay. B) SHA test Feb 28, 1980.

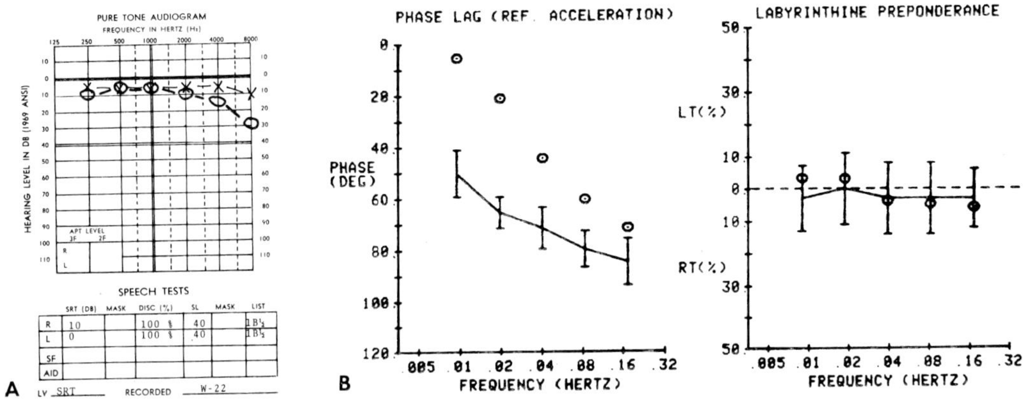

Fig. 3. (Patient 3, aged 47 yr) A) Audiologic examination, Sept 12, 1979. Impedance: Normal tympanograms AU; normal reflexes and no decay. B) SHA test Sept 13, 1979.

labyrinthine preponderance (Fig. 2B). This patient responded nicely to vasodilators and head exercises for labyrinthine accommodations.

Twenty-six patients complaining of dizziness had a variety of neurological histories, signs and symtoms which lead to diagnosis of central nervous system disease. Head trauma, headache, numbness, paralysis and paresthesia are such signs and symptoms. Diagnosis of acoustic neuroma, cerebral concussion, encephalitis and multiple sclerosis are representative. This group of patients' SHA tests demonstrated lag phase shifts in all frequencies. Sensorineural hearing loss was usually present.

Patient 3. A 47-year-old female presented with a six-week history of unsteadiness on motion and postional change. At the onset of her disorder, she had temporary right facial weakness which cleared within two days. She had no right ear pain or hear-

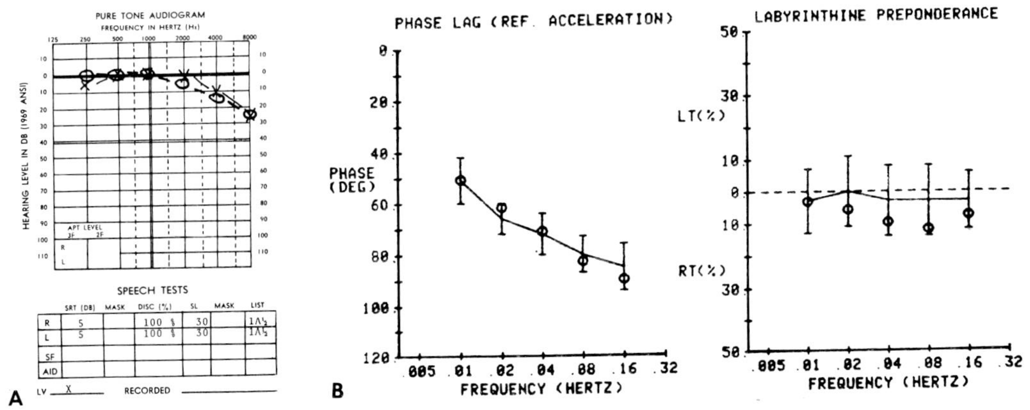

Fig. 4. (Patient 4, aged 50 yr, Nov 26, 1979). A) Audiologic examination. Impedance: Flacid tympanograms AU; reflex present, no decay AU. B) SHA test.

ing loss. At initial presentation, her physical examination was normal. Audiometry revealed a slight high tone sensorineural hearing loss on the right (Fig. 3A). Electronystagmography showed a right unilateral labyrinthine weakness. Her SHA test revealed a very marked phase lag shift in all frequencies, with no specific labyrinthine preponderance (Fig. 3B). Later neurological manifestations helped to establish the diagnosis of multiple sclerosis for this patient.

There was a large group of patients (65) who came for our services complaining of dizziness whose examination was normal, hearing was normal and the SHA testing was normal.

Patient 4. A 50-year-old male was hospitalized with acute unsteadiness for approximately 12 hours. At the time of our evaluation, he had no complaints of tinnitus or hearing loss, ear pain or drainage. Our physical examination was normal throughout with hearing audiometry revealing normal hearing (Fig. 4A). The SHA test was normal (Fig. 4B). Using these tests, we were able to reassure this man that he had no evidence of labyrinthine or central nervous system disease.

CONCLUSIONS

I believe the SHA test has a high degree of sensitivity and is repeatable. If the patient has a normal or abnormal SHA test and has a change of symptoms, this will usually be reflected in the repeated test results.

I believe this is a useful clinical and research tool and when used in association with other labyrinthine tests and other neurological evaluations, is useful for diagnosis and prognosis of otoneurological disease.

AN OVERVIEW OF OCULAR MOTOR NEUROPHYSIOLOGY

B. TODD TROOST, MD

CLEVELAND, OHIO

A review of current concepts in ocular motor neurophysiology is presented. Four separate subsystems of eye movements are recognized: saccadic, smooth pursuit, vergence, and vestibular. Each subsystem is characterized by different physiologic characteristics and different anatomic substrates which may be selectively affected in different pathologic states. A further eye movement response, optokinetic nystagmus, is complex and may be considered a separate system. To regard the horizontal optokinetic response as merely a combination of pursuit and saccades is an oversimplification but one which may be useful in clinical localization.

The purpose of this review is to provide a brief update of recent advances in ocular motor neurophysiology and anatomy particularly as they relate to horizontal eye movements and the optokinetic response. More extensive reviews of various aspects of eye movements are found in a number of reviews.[1-8] Four distinct classes of ocular motor behavior may be defined: saccadic, pursuit, vestibular, and vergence. To regard optokinetic nystagmus (OKN) as just composed of saccades and smooth pursuit eye movements is an oversimplification. Such an approach may be useful for initial clinical localization[2] but the complexity of the optokinetic response justifies its consideration as a separate system. Nonetheless an understanding of the saccadic and smooth pursuit eye movement systems provides a basis for the study and interpretation of investigations concerning the optokinetic system. Particularly, knowledge of the interrelationship of the saccadic and pursuit system during conscious tracking of moving objects provides a clue to the interactions of the optokinetic and vestibular systems during head movements. The subtypes of eye movements have specific physiologic characteristics which may be altered collectively or separately by disease and experimental conditions.[1,2]

Saccades are rapid eye movements used during voluntary refixations or in response to reflex visual or auditory stimuli. They possess certain velocity-amplitude relationships which allow them to be characterized clinically and physiologically.[3] Bahill and Troost[4] have reviewed the different types of saccadic eye movements and their correlation with clinical conditions. Other authors have provided an overview of the general processes which generate saccades[9,10] and the concept of neural plasticity within the system.[11] *Smooth pursuit* or tracking eye movements are those produced by following a moving target or its perceived path. Actually human visual tracking uses two types of eye movements: smooth pursuit and saccadic. Typical velocities for pursuit movements range from 1-30°/s, depending on the speed of the target; in contrast, velocities for saccadic eye movements can be over 900°/s, depending on the size of the movement.[12,13] The two subsystems may be differentially affected by cerebral lesions[14-19] or by drugs.[20,21]

There have been several quantitative studies of human saccadic eye movements. However, there have been relatively few quantitative studies of human smooth pursuit eye movements. While there may be many reasons for this difference, the basic one is that the smooth pursuit system is more difficult to study. Conceptually, there has been greater change in the understanding of the mechanisms which control smooth pursuit in recent years. It was once believed that a visible, moving target was necessary to elicit a pursuit eye movement leading to reports of slow "pursuit" eye movements which paradoxically occurred in the absence of moving visual stimuli such as afterimages, imagined targets, proprioceptive inputs and seemingly at will. Additional understanding of these seeming paradoxes occurred when it was realized that tracking or pursuit movements might occur not just in response to a retinal velocity error signal, but in response to an internal idea or "percept" of target motion.[22-24]

Quantitative parameters for saccades have been defined such as amplitude, peak velocity and duration.[25-29] These parameters yield a quantitative measure of saccadic eye movement quality.

However less quantitative data is available for smooth pursuit. A subjective visual analysis of electro-oculographic records has been used for qualitative assessment of tracking attempts.[30-36] Previous investigators have also attempted to assess the effects of drugs using qualitative impressions of the efficacy of pursuit tracking.[20,21,37,38] In recent years further attempts have been made to quantitate pursuit function by a variety of methods such as counting the number or amplitude of saccades which occur during each sinusoidal cycle[19,39-41] or by determining the number of times eye velocity

From the Neurology Service, Veterans Administration Medical Center and the Department of Neurology, Case Western Reserve University School of Medicine, Cleveland.

REPRINTS — B. Todd Troost, MD, Neurology Service, Veterans Administration Medical Center (127), 10701 E. Boulevard, Cleveland, OH 44106.

drops to zero.[42-44] The methodology of the last studies has been criticized because of the recording system employed and artifacts introduced.[45] Further analyses have employed methods to determine a *gain* for the pursuit system, either by determining the ratio of the eye velocity to target velocity[46,47] or by determining how often the eye velocity approached or matched target velocity.[48] Two problems with such studies are that limited frequencies were used and/or that the target waveforms had very predictable paths.

More theoretical analyses of the pursuit subsystem have also been performed to define the nature of the control system and provide models to aid its understanding.[24,49,50] These investigators used sinusoidal targets and calculated gain and phase relationships at various frequencies. Two problems associated with using such analyses for the smooth pursuit subsystem are: 1) the interaction of the saccadic subsystem with the pursuit subsystem and 2) the learning process. There is an intimate, functional relationship between the pursuit subsystem and the saccadic subsystem. The combined effect of the two subsystems when tracking moving targets is to maintain the target image on the fovea. When the velocity of the eye movement is not equal to the velocity of the target, an error accumulates which triggers a corrective or "catch-up" saccade. With target velocities above 30°/s, the tracking eye movements are comprised almost entirely of saccades. This type of tracking is termed saccadic pursuit. An interaction between the saccadic and smooth pursuit subsystems can occur when tracking sinusoidally moving targets with interspersed saccadic and pursuit segments. To generate the transfer function for the ocular motor tracking mechanism, the gain of the system must be calculated at discrete frequencies over the system bandwidth (0-2.5 Hz). As the target frequency increases, the number of corrective saccades per cycle also increases. Above 2 Hz, the tracking is almost entirely saccadic.[41] At such frequencies any analysis really is describing the combined response of the two subsystems.

In summary, it is almost impossible to construct any test stimulus that will elicit only smooth pursuit eye movements. Moreover, it is the interaction between the smooth pursuit subsystem and the saccadic subsystem that is demonstrated when one attempts to induce smooth pursuit eye movements using slowly moving targets.

The second problem with investigating the smooth pursuit subsystem is the influence of the learning process, described by Dallos and Jones.[51] This process is especially prominent when tracking periodic targets such as repetitive sinusoids or ramps. When tracking a simple, periodic target, the pattern is learned and this results in an improvement in gain and a reduction of phase lag as a function of time. Such learning or adaptation eliminates the actual visual input and replaces it with "perceived target velocity," which is then tracked.[22,23,51-53] This process makes it difficult to study the smooth pursuit system with periodic targets since a change in observed eye movement response could be the result of a change in prediction strategy. Psychological inputs decrease the likelihood of reproducible responses when periodic targets are used. It is believed that a subject primarily employs visual, rather than percept, tracking in response to random target motion. To reduce the effects of long-term learning or prediction, the target motion must be random. The realization that prediction may be involved in pursuit tracking has stimulated us to use aperiodic targets in studying smooth pursuit.[54,55] We used pseudorandom target motion (PRTS) which provided a rapid reliable measure of tracking ability by comparing *pure* pursuit movements with the *combined* saccadic and pursuit attempts as the target speed increased.

ANATOMY AND PHYSIOLOGY

Recent advances in the understanding of supranuclear eye movement control are reviewed in the following sections.

Cortical Influences. Despite the fact that the existence of the frontal eye fields was first described over a century ago, the precise nature of their role in the control of eye movements is still unclear. Clinical observations often prove difficult to reconcile with anatomical and electrophysiological findings. One problem has been that few investigators have been able to identify cortical cells that fire prior to the onset of voluntary, nonvisually induced, eye movements. For this reason, anatomic studies are particularly important. A recent investigation of the efferent pathways of the frontal eye fields was performed in the macaque by Kunzle and Akert,[56] using autoradiography. They found projections to frontal, temporal and parietal association cortex, and to the contralateral frontal eye field. These investigators also reported ipsilateral connections of area 8 with the basal ganglia and pretectum, a brainstem region known to be involved in both horizontal and vertical eye movement control. The authors also reported projections to the superior colliculus. These latter areas also receive retinal afferents and projections from visual cortex.[57] The connections with the lower portion of the brainstem were concentrated in the tegmental and basilar pontine nuclei. No projections were found to the oculomotor nuclei, "accessory oculomotor" nuclei, or the pontine paramedian reticular formation (PPRF), the latter region being particularly important for the control of horizontal eye movements. Guitton and Mandl[58] reported a possible exception to the absence of cell activation prior to eye movements. They found cells in the cat frontal eye fields that fired before and during upward saccadic tracking of visual stimuli.

Lynch et al[59-61] examined neural activity in the inferior parietal lobule (area 7) of monkeys before and during certain ocular motor behavior. They found three classes of visuomotor cells: fixation neurons, which fire during fixation or smooth pursuit of a desired object; tracking neurons, which only fire during pursuit; and saccade neurons, which fire before and during visually evoked (but not spontaneous) saccades. In all cases the monkey had to be actively interested in the object being viewed in order for these parietal lobe cells to fire. Spontaneous saccades were not preceded by any such firing. These investigators suggested that one function of area 7 was to compare the neural code representing the external environment with that which describes an organism's internal state. The comparison would then be used to inititate saccadic refixations or to maintain fixation, depending on which was needed for the desired direction of visual attention.

Goldberg and Robinson[62] reported that electrical stimulation of occipital cortex also elicits eye movements. It does not appear, however, that this area serves a direct motor function itself but that its visual processing is involved in visually evoked eye movements. Hence, stimulation of the occipital cortex may produce an intense phosphene which serves an an apparent visual target.

Most investigators believe that lesions involving subcortical parietal and occipital regions have an effect on the generation of ipsilateral visual tracking which is apparent clinically when testing pursuit function with moving targets or with optokinetic stimuli.[2,63] Some postulate an "optomotor" area in the parieto-occipital region which generates ipsilateral smooth pursuit movements, but experimental evidence in support of a direct connection to ocular motor nuclei is lacking. Updyke suggested that any influence on eye movement is probably mediated via the superior colliculus and/or pretectal region.[64] Both of these regions receive inputs from cortical areas 17, 18, and 19. The clinicopathologic observations of Sharpe and Deck[17] suggest that normal pursuit is possible even when the internal sagittal striatum is disrupted.

Subcortex and Thalamus. Stimulation of thalamic neurons can produce saccades,[5] but the exact role of the thalamus in eye movement control remains unclear. Ungerleider and Christenen[65] examined the effect of ablation of the pulvinar on visual discrimination training in monkeys and found a paucity of saccades to involve visual field regions and abnormally long fixations. Schlag and Schlag-Rey[66,67] found that many cells in the thalamic internal medullary lamina in the cat fired before and during spontaneous saccades in both light and darkness. In most cases the units were directionally selective. Many of the cells had a firing pattern resembling that seen in PPRF neurons, but with an additional visual component. The precise ocular motor role of this region has still to be defined.

Brainstem. An extensive review of brainstem eye movement anatomy and physiology has appeared[6] and some of this information is summarized.[1]

The paramedian zone of the PPRF plays a vital role in the generation of all types of saccadic[68] and probably smooth pursuit, vestibulo-ocular, and optokinetic eye movements in the horizontal plane.[3] This is the region which was once referred to as the parabducens nucleus or the "center" for the conjugate gaze. The PPRF lies ventral to the medial longitudinal fasciculus (MLF) and rostral to the abducens nucleus within about 2 mm of the midline. The PPRF exerts a strong excitatory influence on the ipsilateral lateral rectus via motoneurons within the abducens nucleus and upon the contralateral medial rectus via a subgroup of motoneurons lying within the oculomotor nucleus. In addition, the PPRF establishes connections with several other brainstem nuclei (ig, perihypoglossal nuclei and the rostral intersitial nucleus of the medial longitudinal fasciculus which have been shown to influence eye movement,[6] particularly in a vertical direction.[69] A number of investigations have defined the characteristics of neuronal groups in the PPRF.[70-74] Recent electrophysiological[75] and clinical[76,77] reviews document the importance of the PPRF in gaze.

The final common pathway to the extraocular muscles from the CNS begins in the motoneurons of the oculomotor (III), trochlear (IV) and abducens (VI) nuclei situated in a paramedian location in the midbrain (III and IV) and pons (VI). Classically all the neurons arising within these nuclear groups were believed to project to specific extraocular muscles: the IV nucleus cells to the superior oblique, VI to the lateral rectus and III to medial, inferior, and superior recti and to the inferior oblique. While this is true for the majority of the large ocular motor neurons, recent anatomic and physiologic evidence has disclosed more complex interconnections of the nuclei than was previously realized.[1,78-81] The cell bodies whose axons are destined for the various ocular muscles, are admixed in the third and sixth cranial nerve nuclei with smaller neurons, "oculomotor internuclear neurons," which have projections linking the two nuclei and additional brainstem regions.

The MLF has long been a brainstem region of interest to ocular motor physiologists and clinicians because of the syndrome of internuclear ophthalmoplegia. Recent investigations have further defined the role of the MLF and other premotor pathways of the brainstem in the regulation of eye movements.[81] Some of these anatomic connections unknown only a decade ago will undoubtedly become more important clinically as more clinicopathologic data is carefully analyzed.

Several investigators[80-85] have identified reciprocal connections within the MLF between groups of interneurons found within and around the nuclei of III and VI. These cells are smaller than motor neurons and have different staining characteristics. The rostrally directed projection from the interneurons associated with the sixth nerve nucleus is contralateral, crossing at the level of the sixth nerve and ascending via the MLF to ocular motor neurons in the nucleus of III while the reciprocal projection (nuc. III to nuc. VI) is bilateral.[79,81] Steiger and Buttner-Ennever[83] estimate that approximately one half of the cells within, and immediately around, the sixth nerve nucleus are interneurons, while only 3% of cells in the third nerve nucleus fall into this category. There is thus a marked asymmetry of the reciprocal III/VI connections within the MLF in favor of the ascending counterpart.

Highstein[80] physiologically demonstrated that the projection to the medial rectus component of the nucleus III was an excitatory one and might function as a "final common pathway" rostrally, relaying information for all saccadic eye movements (vestibular, voluntary or optokinetic) as well as pursuit and fixation movements.[84] Interruption of this internuclear connection may be important in generating the deficits observed clinically in internuclear ophthalmoplegia, deficits which have been generally attributed to disruption of direct vestibulo- or reticulo-oculomotor fibers. However, secondary vestibular or reticular fibers which terminate on the medial rectus motonuerons have never been convincingly demonstrated.[85] Other brainstem regions which have attracted considerable interest in recent years are the perihypoglossal nuclei.[86,87] The nuclei play a role in cerebellar and vestibular regulation of eye movements but may even be responsible for the deficits in vertical eye movements that follow lesions in the MLF.[86]

Vestibular System. Baloh and Honrubia[88] have recently detailed the clinical neurophysiology of the vestibular system. Only some of the information relating to ocular motor control is reviewed here. In view of the importance of the vestibulo-ocular reflex it is appropriate to discuss those vestibular pathways involved in the control of eye movements. The convergence of visual and vestibular stimuli can be demonstrated electrophysiologically in the vestibular nuclei.[89] Many cells in these nuclei respond to rotation either of the subject or of the environment around a stationary observer. The response to two forms of stimulation provides a physiological explanation to phenomena such as circularvection, the illusion of rotation experienced while watching a full visual field of moving optokinetic stripes (see Optokinetic System).

During operation of the vestibulo-ocular reflex (VOR), the pathways connecting the vestibular nuclei to the third, fourth, and sixth nerve nuclei are activated to produce the compensatory eye movements needed to maintain fixation on a stationary object during head movement. Although the VOR is a function of brainstem and cerebellar activity, it appears that in man, at least, it is subject to modification by cortical influences. Barr et al[90] reported that, with training, subjects rotated in darkness could significantly raise or lower their VOR gain, depending on whether an imagined fixation point was thought to be stationary or moving with the observer. The clinical effects of vestibular lesions and their complex interconnections have been recently reviewed.[1,88]

The trochlear nuclear motoneurons project crossed axons which emerge dorsally unlike any other cranial nerve to cross in the anterior medullary velum and innervate the contralateral superior oblique. Therefore the motoneurons of both the superior rectus and the superior oblique supply contralateral muscles. Zee[91] has offered a possible explanation of this "seeming anatomic quirk" which lies in the functional organization of the VOR. Ocular rotations caused by stimulation of the vertical semicircular canal or utricle are primarily caused by various actions of the superior recti and oblique as well as reciprocal action of the inferior oblique and rectus. The appropriate ocular motor subnuclei subserving these muscles all lie on the same side of the brainstem and it may be that the organization of the subnuclei evolved from the anatomic requirements for appropriate vestibulo-ocular reflexes.

Cerebellum. It is well known that cerebellar system abnormalities not only produce abnormalities of posture and coordination but a variety of eye movement disturbances as well.[2] ". . . Many if not most of the cell groups participating in direct premotoneuronal pathways of the oculomotor system are affiliated by afferent or efferent connections with particular subdivisions of the cerebellum."[68] Llinas and Wolfe found that stimulation of the cerebellar vermal cortex could produce both saccadic and smooth pursuit eye movements.[92] One cerebellar region that has received considerable attention in recent years is the vestibulocerebellum, including all those folia which receive a direct projection from the vestibular component of the eighth nerve. The vestibulocerebellum has long attracted attention with regard to its involvement in visuomotor tasks. Experiments by Lisberger and Fuchs[93] indicate that the flocculus plays a major role in modulating smooth pursuit eye movements of nonvestibular origin. The anatomical basis for interaction between the vestibulocerebellum and nuclei in the brainstem involved in control of eye movement has been reviewed by Alley.[94] A projection from the inferior olive is believed to be the final link for the relay of afferent input from the visual system to the cerebellum.[95] This pathway begins in the retina with a projection to the contralateral pretectal area. Visual information is then passed on to the ipsilateral inferior olivary nucleus and finally to the cerebellar flocculus.

One exciting area in ocular motor neurophysiology is the discovery of a modifiable reflex, the VOR. The vestibulocerebellum has been implicated in the gain control of the VOR (gain = slow phase eye velocity/head velocity). In humans,[96] cats,[97] and rabbits,[98] alterations in retinal slip caused by the wearing of prisms or lenses have been compensated for by changes in the VOR gains. Robinson[97] found that cats in which this adaptive process had already taken place completely lost all of these plastic changes after removal of the vestibulocerebellum. He contended that these compensatory changes in VOR gain were probably carried out via modifiable synapses in the cerebellum, possibly those between the T-fibers and Purkinje cells, with the climbing fibers providing the input for the modification. In general, this adaptive activity is in keeping with the idea of the cerebellum as a "repair shop," compensating for changes elsewhere in the motor pathways which would otherwise produce dysmetria. The search for the precise region of cerebellum or brainstem which is the site of the "modifiable" synapses is continuing.

Optokinetic System. As pointed out by Enoksson,[99] it was Purkinje who introduced the scientific study of the optokinetic response when he noted the patterned eye movements of spectators watching a parade in Vienna in 1825.[100] Barany[101] termed the phenomenon he noted in train passengers "Eisenbahnnystagmus." Since that time innumerable studies have investigated different aspects of OKN only a few of which are cited here.[102-109] Many factors determine the magnitude and character of the response including the instructions, nature of the target, area of visual field subtended and region of retina stimulated, duration of the stimulus and concomitant input particularly from the vestibular and smooth pursuit systems. Two general types of OKN are believed to occur in animals with foveal vision (including man): termed "Stiernystagmus" and "Schunystagmus."[102-107] These have been anatomically translated as subcortical and cortical respectively or according to the region of stimulation as "field" and "object" OKN.[110] Subcortical or field OKN depends upon the stimulation of most of the visual field (also called peripheral OKN), is inhibited by the presence of stationary contours, is followed by afternystagmus (OKAN), survives decortication in experimental animals but is impaired by brainstem and peripheral labyrinthine injury.[108,111-113] Cortical or object OKN is most closely allied with visual smooth pursuit tracking, and occurs with small field stimulation, is not inhibited by surround stationary contours, is not followed by OKAN, and is clearly dependent upon attention and disappears following decortication in animals. Cortical and subcortical OKN summate when both the peripheral and central retina are stimulated in the same direction, but when oppositely directed optokinetic stimuli are produced on central and peripheral retinal regions, the central component is dominant. The intense activity in the vestibular nuclei during full field optokinetic stimulation has emphasized the role of these nuclei in OKN slow phase generation and provided insight into visual-vestibular interactions during head rotation.[89,114-117] A definite interaction, if not algebraic summation, of visual and vestibular information takes place in the region of the vestibular nuclei.[110,113,116-118] The same vestibular neurons which are activated by horizontal head rotations in one direction are also excited by horizontal rotations of the visual surround in the opposite direction. This in part explains the fact that when humans sit inside a full field optokinetic environment they experience an illusion of self-rotation, circularvection, which is indistinguishable from the vestibular sensation of true rotation.[15,119] The knowledge of visual-vestibular interactions has given rise to a number of models explaining the interrelationships and the optokinetic response.[16,89,118,120]

What then might be the role of the optokinetic response in the freely moving animal? The earlier pragmatic suggestion which identified slow phase OKN with smooth pursuit is oversimplified. Foveal smooth pursuit and OKN slow phases are not identical: OKN is present in infants prior to smooth pursuit; afoveate animals may have OKN but no clear smooth pursuit; and the gain of OKN slow phases (OKN slow phase velocity/stimulus velocity) depend upon stimulus size while smooth pursuit gain depends primarily upon actual retinal slip velocity.[107] However, pursuit gain, as alluded to in the earlier discussion also depends upon the predictability of the target waveform which may be a less important factor in OKN slow phase gain. Simply put, the optokinetic system functions along with the vestibulo-ocular reflex in man to provide retinal image stability.

Various anatomical schema have been proposed to explain observed responses with a variety of CNS disorders in man but most of these have been based upon limited clinical observations under poorly controlled conditions and have suffered from lack of consistent clinicopathologic correlation. It is not sufficient to have gross clinical localization or a clinical diagnosis of "multiple sclerosis" or "spinocerebellar degeneration" to define the nature of the neurologic dysfunction. And as pointed out by Zee et al,[113] "Even in intact foveate animals, the slow phases of nystagmus induced during optokinetic stimulation may be, in part, produced by the pursuit system. Many optokinetic stimuli, such as hand drums that do not induce circularvection or prolonged OKAN, may not appreciably excite the optokinetic system." Newer methods of OKN stimulation and their correlation with specific pathologic entities are areas for further investigation.

REFERENCES

1. Pedersen RA, Abel LA, Troost BT. Anatomy of eye movements. In: Jacobiec F, eds. Biomedical foundations in ophthalmology.Hagerstown: Harper and Row (in press).

2. Daroff RB, Troost BT. Supranuclear disorders of eye movements. In: Glaser JS, ed. Neuro-ophthalmology. Hagerstown: Harper and Row, 1978: 201-18.

3. Troost BT, Dell'Osso LF. Fast eye movements (saccades): Basic science and clinical correlations. In: Thompson HS, ed. Topics in neuro-ophthalmology. Baltimore: Williams and Wilkins, 1979: 246-65.

4. Bahill AT, Troost BT. Types of saccadic eye movements. Neurology 1979; 29:1150-2.

5. Carpenter RHS. Movements of the eyes. London: Pion Press, 1977.

6. Baker R, Berthoz A. Control of gaze by brain stem neurons, developments in neuroscience. New York: Elsevier/North-Holland Biomedical Press: vol 1, 1977.

7. Brooks BA, Bajandas FJ. Eye movements, ARVO symposium. New York: Plenum Press, 1977.

8. Thompson H. Topics in neuro-ophthalmology. Baltimore: Williams and Wilkins, 1979.

9. Becker W, Jurgens R. An analysis of the saccadic system by means of double step stimuli. Vision Res 1979; 19:967-83.

10. Hou RL, Fender DH. Processing of direction and magnitude by the saccadic eye-movements system. Vision Res 1979; 19:1421-6.

11. Abel LA, Schmidt D. Dell'Osso LF, Daroff RB. Saccadic system plasticity in humans. Ann Neurol 1978; 4:313-8.

12. Bahill AT, Clark MR, Stark L. The main sequence, a tool for studying human eye movements. Math Biosciences 1975; 24:191-204.

13. Boghen DA, Troost BT, Daroff RB, Dell'Osso LF, Birkett JE. Velocity characteristics of normal human saccadic eye movements. Invest Ophthalmol 1974; 13:619-23.

14. Troost BT, Daroff RB, Dell'Osso LF. Hemispheric control of eye movements. II. Quantitative analysis of smooth pursuit in a hemispherectomy patient. Arch Neurol 1972; 27:449-52.

15. Brandt T, Dichgans J, Koenig E. Differential effect of central versus peripheral vision on egocentric and exocentric motion perception. Exp Brain Res 1973; 16:476-91.

16. Raphan T, Cohen B, Matsuo V. A velocity-storage mechanism responsible for optokinetic nystagmus (OKN), optokinetic afternystagmus (OKAN), and vestibular nystagmus. In: Baker R, Berthoz A, eds. Control of gaze by brain stem neurons, developments in neuroscience. New York: Elsevier/North-Holland Biomedical Press: vol 1, 1977: 37-47.

17. Sharpe JA, Deck H. Destruction of the internal sagittal stratum and normal smooth pursuit. Ann Neurol 1978; 4:473-6.

18. Sharpe JA, Lo AW, Rabinovitch HE. Control of the saccadic and smooth pursuit systems after cerebral hemidecortication. Brain 1979; 102:387-403.

19. Hartje W, Kerschensteiner M. A quantitative analysis of saccadic pursuit eye movements in patients with unilateral hemispheric lesions. Z Neurol 1973; 203:299-310.

20. Rashbass C. The relationship between saccadic and smooth tracking eye movements. J Physiol 1961; 159:326-38.

21. Norris H. The action of sedatives on brain stem oculomotor systems in man. Neuropharmacology 1971; 10: 181-91.

22. Yasui S. Nystagmus generation, oculomotor tracking and visual motion perception. PhD thesis, Massachusetts Institute of Technology, 1976.

23. Yasui S, Young LR. Perceived visual motion as effective stimulus to pursuit eye movement system. Science 1975; 190:906-8.

24. Yasui S, Young LR. Eye movements during after-image tracking under sinusoidal and random vestibular stimulation. In: Lennerstrand G, Bach-y-Rita P, eds. Basic mechanism of ocular motility and their clinical implications. New York: Pergamon Press, 1975b:509-13.

25. Cook G, Stark L. Horizontal eye movements studied with the online computer. Arch Ophthalmol 1966; 76:589-96.

26. Bahill AT, Stark L. Overlapping saccades and glissades are produced by fatigue in the saccadic eye movement system. Exp Neurol 1975; 48:95-106.

27. Bahill AT, Stark L. The trajectories of saccadic eye movements. Sci Am 1979; 240:108-17.

28. Baloh RW, Sills AW, Kumley WE, Honrubia V. Quantitative measurement of saccadic amplitude, duration, and velocity. Neurology 1975; 25:1065-70.

29. Baloh RW, Konrad HR, Sills AW, Honrubia V. The saccade velocity test. Neurology 1975; 25:1071-6.

30. Benitz JT. Eye-tracking and optokinetic tests: diagnostic significance in peripheral and central vestibular disorders. Laryngoscope 1970; 80:834-48.

31. Von Noorden GK, Preziosi TJ. Eye movement recordings in neurological disorders. Arch Ophthalmol 1966; 76:162-71.

32. Corvera J, Torres-Courtney G, Lopez-Rios G. The neurotological significance of alterations of pursuit eye movements and the pendular eye tracking test. Ann Otol Rhinol Laryngol 1973; 82:1-13.

33. Larmande AM, Delplace MP. L'epreuve de poursuite pendulaire. Principe et technique. Arch Ophthalmol 1973; 33:269-78.

34. Rodin EA. Impaired ocular pursuit movements. Arch Neurol 1964; 10:327-30.

35. Bogacz J, Mendilaharsu C, De Mendilaharsu SA. Electro-oculographic study of saccadic pursuit eye movements in patients with brain lesions. Electroencephalogr Clin Neurophysiol 1977; 42:23-30.

36. Vedel-Jensen N. Pathological ocular fixation instability. Acta Ophthalmol (Kbh) 1966; 44:481-92.

37. Frank MC, Kuhlo W. Die Wirkung des Alkohols auf die raschen Blickzielbewegungen (Saccaden) beim Menschen. Arch Psychiatr Nervenkr 1970; 213:238-45.

38. Wilkinson IMS, Kime R, Purnell M. Alcohol and human eye movement. Brain 1974; 97:785-92.

39. Yamazaki A. Electrophysiological study on saccades during fixation and small smooth pursuit movement in neurological disorders. Acta Soc Ophthalmol Jpn 1970; 74:244-52.

40. Yamazaki A, Ishikawa S. Horizontal and vertical smooth pursuit eye movements. Jpn J Ophthalmol 1973; 103:103-12.

41. Hartje W, Steinhauser D, Kerschensteiner M. Diagnostic value of saccadic pursuit eye movement in screening for organic cerebral dysfunction. J Neurol 1978; 217:253-60.

42. Holzman PS, Proctor LR, Hughes DW. Eye-tracking patterns in schizophrenia. Science 1973; 181:179-81.

43. Holzman PS, Levy DL, Proctor LR. Smooth pursuit eye movements, attention, and schizophrenia. Arch Gen Psychiatry 1976; 33:1415-20.

44. Shagrass C, Roemer RA, Amadeo M. Eye-tracking performance and engagement of attention. Arch Gen Psychiatry 1976; 33:121-5.

45. Troost BT, Daroff RB, Dell'Osso LF. Eye tracking patterns in schizophrenia. Science 1974; 184:1202-3.

46. Troost BT, Weber RB, Daroff RB. Hemispheric control of eye movements. I. Quantitative analysis of refixation saccades in a hemispherectomy patient. Arch Neurol 1972; 27:441-8.

47. Troost BT, Daroff RB. The ocular motor defects in progressive supranuclear palsy (PSP). Ann Neurol 1977; 2:397-403.

48. Baloh RW, Kumley WE, Sills AW, Honrubia V, Konrad HR. Quantitative analysis of smooth pursuit eye movements. Ann Otol Rhinol Laryngol 1976; 85:111-8.

49. Stark L, Vossius G, Young LR. Predictive control of eye tracking movement. Inst Radio Eng Trans Hum Factors Electron 1962; 3:52-7.

50. Shirachi DK, Monk DL, Black JH. Head rotational spectral characteristics during two dimensional smooth pursuit tasks. IEEE Trans Systems, Man and Cybernetics 1978; SMC-8:332-41.

51. Dallos PJ, Jones RW. Learning behaviour of the eye fixation control system. IEEE Trans on Automatic Control 1963; AC-8:218-27.

52. Young LR. Pursuit eye movement — what is being pursued? In: Baker R, Berthoz A, eds. The control of gaze by brainstem neurons. New York: Elsevier/North-Holland Biomedical Press, 1977: 29-36.

53. Steinback MJ. Pursuing the perceptual rather than the retinal stimulus. Vision Res 1976; 16:1371-6.

54. Iandolo MJ, Bahill AT, Troost BT. Quantitative study of human smooth pursuit tracking. Soc Neurosc Abs 1978; 4:163.

55. Bahill AT, Iandolo MJ, Troost BT. Smooth pursuit eye movements in response to unpredictable target waveforms. Vision Res 1980; 20:923-31.

56. Kunzle H. Akert K. Efferent connections of cortical area 8 (frontal eye field) in Macaca fascicularis. A reinvestigation using the autoradiographic technique. J Comp Neurol 1977; 173: 147-53.

57. Ogren M, Hendrickson A. Pathways between striate cortex and subcortical regions in Macaca mulatta and Saimiri sciureus: evidence for a reciprocal pulvinar connection. Exp Neurol 1976; 53:780-800.

58. Guitton D, Mandl GR. The frontal eye field in cat. In: Baker R, Berthoz A, eds. Control of gaze by brain stem neurons. New York: Elsevier/North-Holland Biomedical Press: vol 1, 1977: 463-7.

59. Lynch JC, Mountcastle VB, Talbot WH, Yin TCT. Parietal lobe mechanisms for directed visual attention. I. J Neurophysiol 1977; 40:362-70.

60. Lynch JC, Mountcastle VB, Talbot WH, Yin TCT. Parietal lobe mechanisms for directed visual attention. II. J Neurophysiol 1977; 40:371-89.

61. Lynch JC. The functional organization of posterior parietal association cortex. Behav Brain Sci 1980; 3:485-534.

62. Goldberg ME, Robinson DL. Visual mechanisms underlying gaze: function of the cerebral cortex. In: Baker R, Berthoz A, eds. Control of gaze by brain stem neurons, developments in neuroscience. New York: Elsevier/North-Holland Biomedical Press: vol 1, 1977: 469-76.

63. Baloh RW, Honrubia V, Sills A. Eye-tracking and optokinetic nystagmus. Results of quantitative testing in patients with well-defined nervous system lesions. Ann Otol Rhinol Laryngol 1977; 86:108-14.

64. Updyke BV. Topographic organization of the projections from cortical areas 17, 18, and 19 onto the thalmus, pretectum, and superior colliculus in the cat. J Comp Neurol 1977; 173:81-7.

65. Ungerleider LG, Christensen CA. Pulvinar lesions in monkeys produce abnormal eye movements during visual discrimination training. Brain Res 1977; 136:189-91.

66. Schlag J, Schlag-Rey M. Visuomotor properties of cells in cat thalmic internal medullary lamina. In: Baker R, Berthoz A, eds. Control of gaze by brain stem neurons, developments in neuroscience. New York: Elsevier/North-Holland Biomedical Press: vol 1, 1977: 453-62.

67. Schlag-Rey M, Schlag J. Visual and presaccadic neuronal activity in thalamic internal medulary lamina of cat: a study of targeting. J Neurophysiol 1977; 40:156-73.

68. Graybiel AM. Organization of oculomotor pathways in the cat and rhesus monkey. In: Baker R, Berthoz A, eds. Control of gaze by brain stem neurons, developments in neuroscience. New York: Elsevier/North-Holland Biomedical Press: vol 1,, 1977: 79-88.

69. Kompf D, Pasik T, Pasik P, et al. Downward gaze in monkeys. Stimulation and lesion studies. Brain 1979; 102:527-58.

70. Van Gisenbergen JAM, Robinson DA. Generation of micro- and macrosaccades by burst neurons in the monkey. In: Baker R, Berthoz A, eds. Control of gaze by brain stem neurons, developments in neuroscience. New York: Elsevier/North-Holland Biomedical Press: vol 1, 1977:301-8.

71. Buttner U, Hepp K, Henn V. Neurons in the rostral mesencephalic and paramedian pontine reticular formation generating fast eye movements. In: Baker R, Berthoz A, eds. Control of gaze by brain stem neurons, developments in neuroscience. New York: Elsevier/North-Holland Biomedical Press: vol 1, 1977: 309-18.

72. King WM, Fuchs AF. Neuronal activity in the mesencephalon related to vertical eye movements. In: Baker R, Berthoz A, eds. Control of gaze by brain stem neurons, developments in neuroscience. New York: Elsevier/North-Holland Biomedical Press: vol 1, 1977: 319-26.

73. Keller EL. Control of saccadic eye movements by midline brain stem neurons. In: Baker R, Berthoz A, eds. Control of gaze by brain stem neurons, developments in neuroscience. New York: Elsevier/North-Holland Biomedical Press: vol 1, 1977: 327-36.

74. Fuchs AF. Role of the vestibular and reticular nuclei in the control of gaze. B: reticular prepositus and other internuclear neuronal activity. In: Baker R, Berthoz A, eds. Control of gaze by brain stem neurons, developments in neuroscience. New York: Elsevier/North-Holland Biomedical Press: vol 1, 1977: 341-8.

75. Raphan T, Cohen B. Brainstem mechanisms for rapid and slow eye movements. Ann Rev Physiol 1978; 40:527-44.

76. Ash PR, Keltner JL. Neuro-ophthalmic signs in pontine lesions. Medicine 1979; 58:304-15.

77. Pedersen RA, Troost BT. Abnormalities of gaze in cerebrovascular disease. Stroke 1981 (in press).

78. Akagi Y. The localization of the motor neurons innervating the extraocular muscles in the oculomotor nuclei of the cat and rabbit, using horseradish peroxidase. J Comp Neurol 1978; 181:745-55.

79. Maciewicz RJ, Spencer RF. Oculomotor and abducens internuclear pathways in the cat. In: Baker R, Berthoz A, eds. Control of gaze by brain stem neurons, developments in neuroscience. New York: Elsevier/North-Holland Biomedical Press: vol 1, 1977: 99-108.

80. Highstein SM. Abducens and oculomotor internuclear neurons: relation to gaze. In: Baker R, Berthoz A, eds. Control of gaze by brain stem neurons, developments in neuroscience. New York: Elsevier/North-Holland Biomedical Press: vol 1, 1977: 153-62.

81. Graybiel AM. Direct and indirect preoculomotor pathways of the brainstem: an autoradiographic study of the pontine reticular formation in the cat. J Comp Neurol 1977; 175:37-45.

82. Buttner-Ennever JA. Pathways from the pontine reticular formation structures controlling horizontal and vertical eye movements in the monkey. In: Baker R, Berthoz A, eds. Control of gaze by brain stem neurons, developments in neuroscience. New York: Elsevier/North-Holland Biomedical Press: vol 1, 89-98.

83. Steiger HJ, Buttner-Ennever J. Relationship between motoneurons and internuclear neurons in the abducens nucleus: a double retrograde tracer study in the cat. Brain Res 1978; 148:181-9.

84. King WM, Lisberger SG, Fuchs AF. Responses of fibers in medial longitudinal fasciculus (MLF) of alert monkeys during horizontal and vertical conjugate eye movements evoked by vestibular or visual stimuli. J Neurophysiol 1976; 39:1135-49.

85. Highstein S. Abducens to medial rectus pathway in the MLF: a possible cellular basis for the syndrome of internuclear ophthalmoplegia. In: Brooks BA, Bahandas FJ, eds. Eye movements, ARVO symposium. New York: Plenum Press, 1977: 127-35.

86. Baker R, Berthoz A, Delgado-Garcia J. Monosynaptic excitation of trochlear motoneurons following electrical stimulation of the prepositus hypoglossi nucleus. Brain Res 1977; 121:157-60.

87. Baker R. The nucleus prepositus hypoglossi. In: Brooks BA, Bahandas FJ, eds. Eye movements, ARVO symposium. New York: Plenum Press, 1977: 145-56.

88. Baloh RW, Honrubia V. Clinical neurophysiology of the vestibular systems. Philadelphia: FA Davis, 1979.

89. Robinson DA. Linear addition of optokinetic and vestibular signals in the vestibular nucleus. Exp Brain Res 1977; 30:447-50.

90. Barr CC, Schultheis LW, Robinson DA. Voluntary, nonvisual control of the human vestibulo-ocular reflex. Acta Otolaryngol (Stockh) 1976; 81:365-70.

91. Zee DS. The organization of the brainstem ocular motor subnuclei. Ann Neurol 1978; 4:384.

92. Llinas R, Wolfe JW. Functional linkage between the electrical activity in the vermal cerebellar cortex and saccadic eye movements. Exp Brain Res 1977; 29:1-4.

93. Lisberger SG, Fuchs AF. Role of the primate flocculus in smooth pursuit eye movements and rapid behavioral modification of the vestibulo-ocular reflex. In: Baker R, Berthoz A, eds. Control of gaze by brain stem neurons, developments in neuroscience. New York: Elsevier/North-Holland Biomedical Press: vol 1, 1977; 381-9.

94. Alley K. Anatomical basis for interaction between cerebellar flocculus and brainstem. In: Baker R, Berthoz A, eds. Control of gaze by brain stem neurons, developments in neuroscience. New York: Elsevier/North-Holland Biomedical Press: vol 1, 1977: 109-17.

95. Mackawa K, Takeda T. Afferent pathways from the visual systems to the cerebellar flocculus of the rabbit. In: Baker R, Berthoz A, eds. Control of gaze by brain stem neurons, developments in neuroscience. New York: Elsevier/North-Holland Biomedical Press: vol 1, 1977: 187-95.

96. Gonshor A, Melvill Jones G. Extreme vestibulo-ocular adaptation induced by prolonged optical reversal of vision. J Physiol 1976; 256:381-92.

97. Robinson DA. Adaptive gain control of the vestibulo-ocular reflex by the cerebellum. J Neurophysiol 1976; 39:954-65.

98. Collewijn H. The modifiability of the adult vestibulo-ocular reflex. Trends Neurosc 1979; 1:98-105.

99. Enoksson P. Optokinetic nystagmus. Ophthalmologica 1974; 169:176-83.

100. Purkinji J. Beobachtungen und Versuche zur Physiologie der Sinne. Neue Beitrage zur Kenntnis des Sehens in subjectiver Hinischt. Berlin: G. Reimer, 1825; 2:60-1.

101. Barany R. Zur Klinik und Theorie des Eisenbahn-Nystagmus. Arch Augenheilk 1921; 88:139-42.

102. Ter Braake JWC. Untersuchungen uber optokinetischen Nystagmus. Arch Neurol Physiol 1936; 21:309-76.

103. Hood JD. Observations upon the neurological mechanism of optokinetic nystagmus with special reference to the contribution of peripheral vision. Acta Otolaryngol (Stockh) 1967; 63:208-15.

104. Honrubia V, Scott BJ, Ward PH. Experimental studies on optokinetic nystagmus. I. Normal cats. Acta Otolaryngol (Stockh) 1967; 64:388-402.

105. Honrubia V, Jenkins H, Downey W, et al. Experimental studies on optokinetic nystagmus. III. Modifications produced by labyrinthectomy and cerebral hemidecortication in cats. Ann Otol Rhinol Laryngol 1971; 80:97-110.

106. Honrubia V, Downey W, Mitchell DP, et al. Experimental studies on optokinetic nystagmus. II. Normal humans. Acta Otolaryngol (Stockh) 1968; 65:441-8.

107. Dichgans J. Optokinetic nystagmus as dependent on the retinal periphery via the vestibular nuclei. In: Baker R, Berthoz A, eds. Control of gaze by brain stem neurons, developments in neuroscience. New York: Elsevier/North-Holland Biomedical Press, vol 1, 1977: 261-7.

108. Cohen B, Matsuo V, Raphan T. Quantitative analysis of the velocity characteristics of optokinetic nystagmus and optokinetic afternystagmus. J Physiol 1977; 270:321-44.

109. Baloh RW, Yee RD, Honrubia V. Optokinetic nystagmus and parietal lobe lesions. Ann Neurol 1980; 7:269-76.

110. Wallace M, Blair SM, Westheimer G. Neural pathways common to vestibular and optokinetic eye movements. Exp Brain Res 1978; 33:19-25.

111. Cheng M, Outerbridge JS. Optokinetic nystagmus during selective retinal stimulation. Exp Brain Res 1975; 23:129-39.

112. Dubois MF, Collewijn H. Optokinetic reactions in man elicited by localized retinal motion stimuli. Vision Res 1979; 19:1105-15.

113. Zee DS, Yee RD, Robinson DA. Optokinetic responses in labyrinthine-defective human beings. Brain Res 1976; 113:423-8.

114. Henn V, Young LR, Finley C. Vestibular nucleus units in alert monkeys are also influenced by moving visual fields. Brain Res 1974; 71:144-9.

115. Allum JHJ, Graf W, Dichgans J, et al. Visual-vestibular interactions in the vestibular nuclei of goldfish. Exp Brains Res 1976; 26:463-85.

116. Waespe W, Henn V. Neuronal activity in the vestibular nuclei of the alert monkey during vestibular and optokinetic stimulation. Exp Brain Res 1977a; 27:523-39.

117. Waespe W, Henn V. Vestibular nuclei activity during optokinetic after-nystagmus (OKAN) in the alert monkey. Exp Brain Res 1977b; 30:323-30.

118. Robinson DA. Vestibular and optokinetic symbiosis: an example of explaining by modelling. In: Baker R, Berthoz A, eds. Control of gaze by brain stem neurons, developments in neuroscience. New York: Elsevier/North-Holland Biomedical Pres: vol 1, 1977: 49-58.

119. Brandt T, Dichgans J, Buchele W. Motion habituation: inverted self-motion perception and optokinetic after-nystagmus. Exp Brain Res 1974; 21:337-52.

120. Schmid R, Zambarbarbieri D, Sardi R. A mathematical model of the optokinetic reflex. Biol Cybernetics 1979; 34:215-25.

THIRD LOUIS H. CLERF LECTURE

Presented

at the

Department of Otolaryngology

Jefferson Medical College

Thomas Jefferson University

Philadelphia, Pennsylvania

May 1, 1981

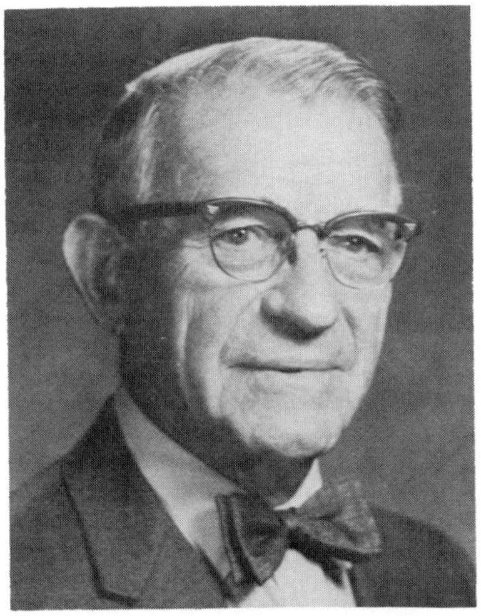

LOUIS H. CLERF, MD
Emeritus Professor of Laryngology
and Bronchoesophagology
Jefferson Medical College, Philadelphia

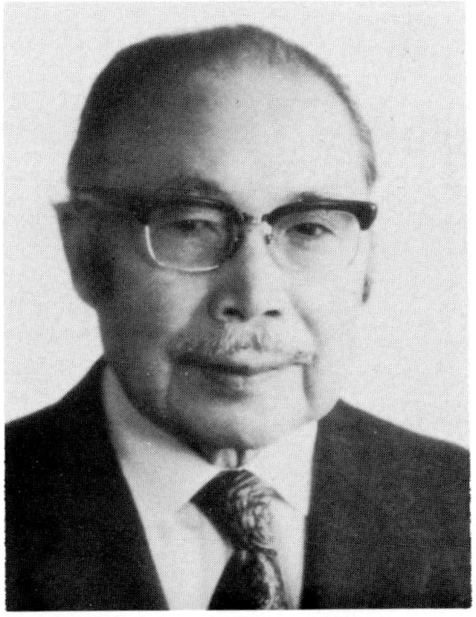

JO ONO, MD
Visiting Professor of Bronchoesophagology
Keio University School of Medicine, Tokyo

THIRD LOUIS H. CLERF LECTURE

LEGACIES OF JEFFERSON MEN TO JAPANESE MEDICINE

JO ONO, MD

TOKYO, JAPAN

The legacies of Jefferson men to Japanese medicine are portrayed in early and recent contacts: 1) Japanese physicians attended the Gross Clinic in 1860. The significant fact is that this was the very first visit made in over 240 years during which time Japan had been in self-imposed seclusion from foreign countries. 2) Dr. John C. Berry, a Jefferson alumnus, came to Japan in 1872 and served as a doctor, teacher, prison reformer, and founder of a hospital and a training school for nurses. He dedicated himself for 22 years to the service of religious and humanitarian fields in Japan. 3) A group of 104 Jeffersonians visited Japan in 1975, and programs of medical seminars, visits to hospitals and institutions were featured. 4) The influence of Drs. Chevalier Jackson and Louis H. Clerf contributed greatly toward development and growth of bronchoesophagology in Japan. A gratifying fact is that bronchoesophagology was legally sanctioned as a full-fledged specialty in 1953.

It was indeed a wholly unexpected surprise to be invited to give the Clerf Lecture today. I felt I could not do justice to this honor, but I accepted as I hold Dr. Clerf in very high esteem. Since leaving his clinic in 1934 I have kept in touch with him in a close, friendly relationship for 46 years. Dr. Clerf (Fig. 1) has been my mentor and inspiration all through the trying years I experienced after returning to Japan, attempting to teach bronchoesophagology and to have it recognized by the Japanese government as a specialty in its own right. At the end of this talk, I would like to expand a little more on bronchoesophagology in Japan.

In talking to you about the legacies of Jefferson men to Japanese medicine, it is not generally known that there were a number of contacts even as far back as 1860. These legacies relate to two phases of medicine during the last century, both of which were linked with Jefferson Medical College.

However, first I need to tell you a bit of the historical background which led to Japanese doctors visiting the Samuel D. Gross Clinic.

EARLY CONTACTS

Background. The first Westerners to reach the shores of Japan were Portuguese who arrived towards the middle of the 16th century.[1(pp 117-25)] They were followed by the Spaniards, the Dutch and the English. The Portuguese and the Spaniards were mainly interested in the promotion of Christianity, although trade motives were also a factor, whereas the Dutch and the English came solely for trade.

Following the arrival in 1549 of St. Francis Xavier, the Jesuit missionary, Christianity made remarkable progress and by the end of the century, Christians in Japan reached some 300,000 in number. For various reasons, however, the missionaries were subjected to severe persecution in the latter part of the century.[1(pp 140-1)] During the time from 1622 to 1661, when Iemitsu Tokugawa was Shogun (that is, the military ruler), all Westerners except a stipulated few were expelled and the doors of Japan closed to foreigners. Thus, the Tokugawa clan established over the country an iron rule of self-imposed seclusion-exclusion from foreign countries which endured until their overthrow and the restoration of Emperor Meiji in 1868. During this

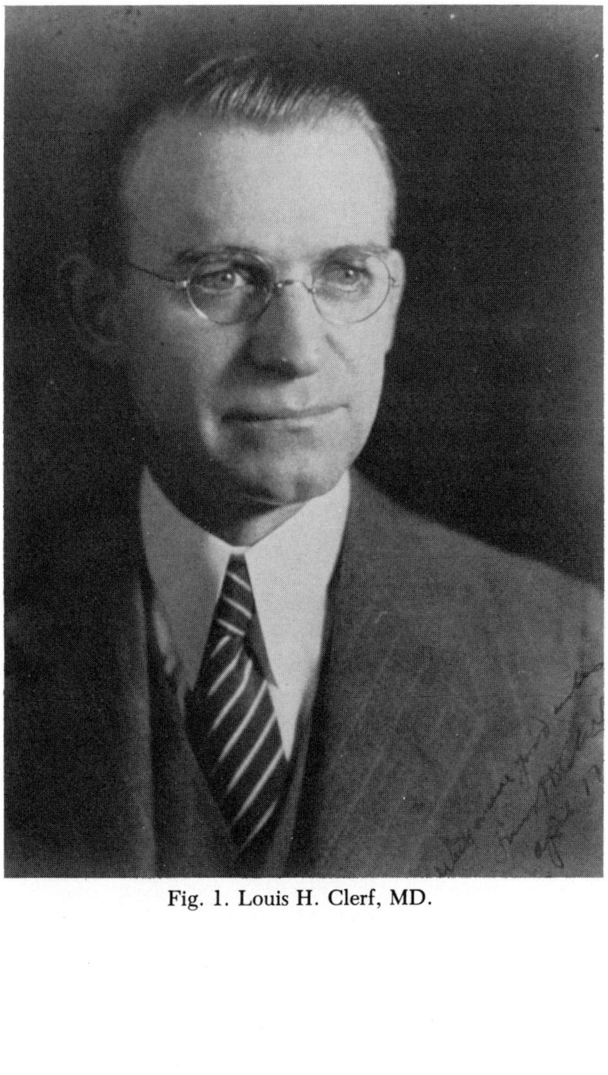

Fig. 1. Louis H. Clerf, MD.

relatively long period of more than 240 years, Japan was ruled under a dual system of government. The actual power rested in the hands of Tokugawa, a military government with its capital in Edo, now known as Tokyo. The nominal power, however, rested in the hands of the Emperor residing in the ancient capital of Kyoto, who in effect remained only as the symbol of divine authority.

During the Tokugawa period, Japan was a hermit nation committed to a policy of isolation from the rest of the world. The only foreigners permitted in Japan were a limited number of Dutch and Chinese who were authorized to carry on restricted commercial operations from prescribed bases in the Nagasaki area. The Dutch, however, exercised a function of significant value to the Tokugawa, namely that of a "window" so to speak, through which information came concerning the outside world.

As for the American contacts with Japan, an American ship may have entered Japanese water as early as 1790. I shall, however, skip all the accounts of that event and limit myself to Commodore M.C. Perry's so-called "United States - Japan Expedition" and its related history.

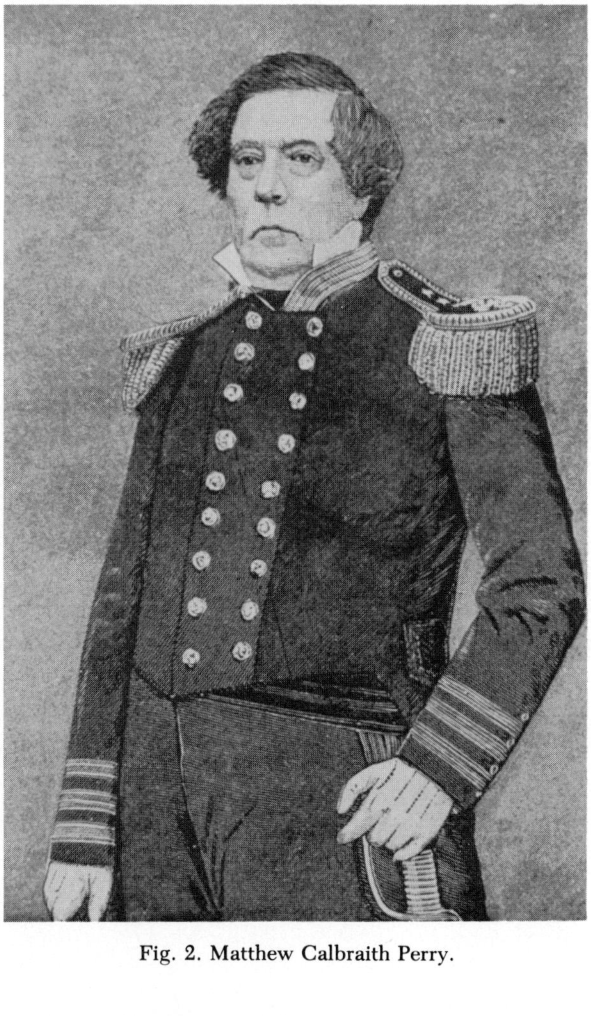

Fig. 2. Matthew Calbraith Perry.

The Opening of Japan to the World. In need of a steppingstone to her trade with China, the United States wanted Japan to open her country to foreign intercourse.[2] In 1853, the American government called upon Commodore Perry to command the Far Eastern squadron in order to make a proposal to Japan (Fig. 2).

In the following year the Japanese government acceded to the American demand and the historic treaty of Kanagawa was signed. The treaty was a simple one, stipulating that there would be established between the two countries "a perfect, permanent, universal peace and sincere and cordial amity." The treaty was a historic milestone, since it definitely ended the long period of Japanese seclusion. Other Western nations shortly after followed suit and concluded similar treaties.

In accordance with the provisions of the Treaty of Kanagawa, the US government commissioned Townsend Harris as the first American consul-general to reside in Shimoda. Harris was successful in 1859 in concluding the first treaty of commerce by Japan since the beginning of the 17th century, which served as a model for treaties subsequently negotiated by the other powers such as the Netherlands, Russia, England and France. The Harris treaty provided for the exchange of ratifications in Washington.

To accomplish this purpose of exchanging ratification, the Japanese mission, consisting of 77 persons headed by two principal ambassadors was dispatched[3(pp 1-2)] (Fig. 3). It was the first embassy ever sent by Japan to a world power under mutual agreement. They left Yokohama on February 13, 1860, on board the US frigate "Powhatan" which was sent by the US government. After having touched at Hawaii and San Francisco and passing through the isthmus of Panama, they reached Washington DC, where they stayed 24 days.

After their audience with President James Buchanan and the exchange of ratifications of the treaty, they were received with a royal welcome at the White House[3(pp 45-71)] (Fig. 4). On their way home they also were warmly welcomed in Philadelphia and New York where they were given one of the most brilliant receptions in the history of the then young United States. The magnificent welcome inspired Walt Whitman to write *A Broadway Pageant.* It begins:

Over the western sea hither from Niphon
come,
Courteous, swart-cheeked, two-sworded
envoys,
Leaning back in their open barouches,
bare-headed, impassive
Ride today through Manhattan.

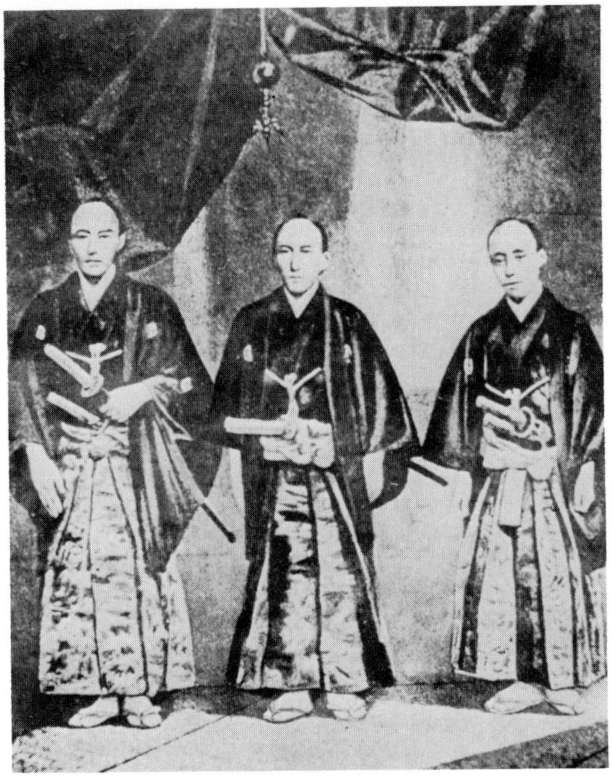

Fig. 3. Japanese envoys to United States, 1860.

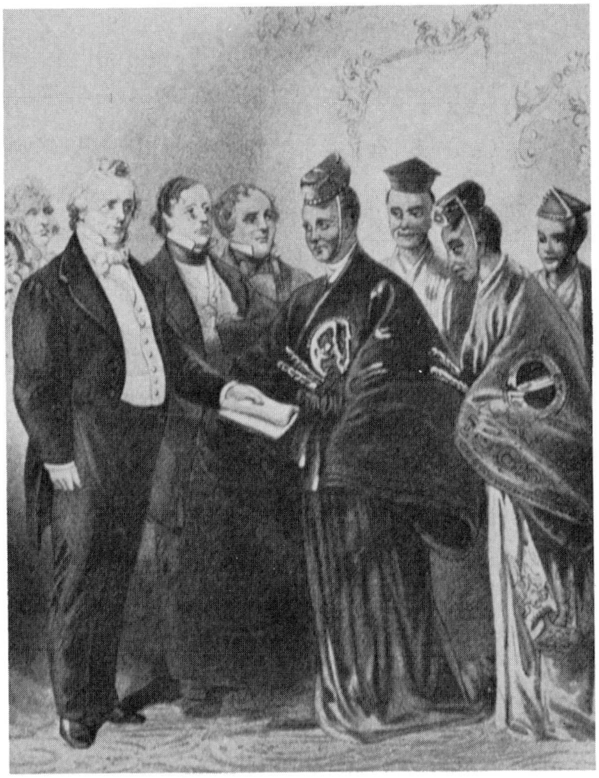

Fig. 4. Meeting of Japanese envoys with President James Buchanan.

JAPANESE PHYSICIANS' FIRST VISIT TO THE GROSS CLINIC

While in Philadelphia, the three physicians attached to the embassy, Drs. Ritsugen Miyazaki, Hakugen Murayama and Domin Kawasaki, together with Governor Naruse and the interpreter, attended a bladder stone operation performed by the distinguished Dr. Samuel D. Gross (Fig. 5) at the patient's residence.[3(pp 297-301)] The anesthetic was administered by no less a personage than the famous William Morton, the discoverer of sulphuric ether for this use. The whole performance was a revelation to the Japanese. They poured ether on their hands and smelled it, astonished at the coldness resulting from its evaporation. After the operation they carefully examined the instruments and showed so much interest in the whole subject that they were invited to visit the Jefferson Medical College where Dr. Gross was Professor of Surgery.

Among the gifts which members of the embassy received were medical instruments, artificial dentures on a gold plate, and books on surgery. It can easily be assumed that the Japanese doctors received from Jefferson Medical College Dr. Gross's first edition of *The System of Surgery* which was published only the year before in 1859.

Forty-six years later, in 1906, just after the Russo-Japanese War, Admiral Baron Takagi (Fig. 6), Surgeon General of the Imperial Japanese Navy, visited Jefferson Medical College and gave an address to the students. He said, "Japanese surgery is founded on the teaching of Dr. Samuel D. Gross who for so many years was a surgeon in this splendid medical college in which we are gathered. Dr. Gross's *The System of Surgery*, translated into German, was taken by my countrymen and retranslated into Japanese and upon that has been built Japanese surgery as practiced today." The Baron said that the Japanese nation was indebted to the medical profession of the United States and added, "The United States has been our teacher. We have tried our best to prove our faith in your teachings and doctrines by effective application of your principles in safeguarding the health of our people."

Incidentally, in Gross's *The System of Surgery* there is included a chapter on otology. This chapter was rendered into Dutch and then retranslated into Japanese in 1877 as *Principles of Otology* which became the very first book in the realm of otolaryngology published in Japan. It was my privilege about 40 years ago to donate a copy of the Japanese edition of this book to the Jefferson Medical College Library. I hope it is still there if anyone is interested in reading it in Japanese.

In retrospect, the days of Japanese doctors' visits to the Gross Clinic in 1860 were stirring times. At the presidential election a politically strong candidate, William Henry Seward, was defeated by the unknown Abraham Lincoln. Those were the days of Browning, Tennyson, Hawthorne and Oliver Wendell Holmes. Those also were the days of Darwin who wrote *The Origin of Species* and Virchow who

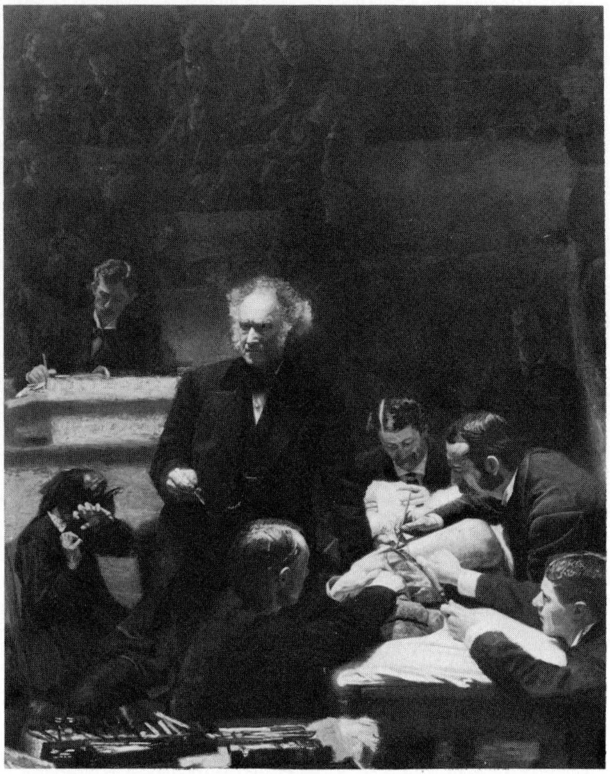

Fig. 5. Samuel D. Gross, MD, in the operating theatre. (Detail of painting by Thomas Eakins. Reproduced with permission from Jefferson Medical College, Philadelphia.)

wrote *Cellular Pathology*. Broca discovered the speech center in the brain; Pasteur demonstrated the presence of bacteria in the air. Those were highly exciting days, not only because of the advances in medicine but because of progress in all branches of human endeavor. Japan was fortunate, thanks to the thoughtful consideration of the United States, in arousing herself from the lethargy of centuries of secluded life.

BERRY'S MISSION TO JAPAN

Another Jefferson graduate who contributed greatly to Japanese medicine was John C. Berry (Fig. 7). A little more than 100 years ago, in 1872 to be exact, a young man of 25 and his even younger bride left a comfortable home in a small New England town to travel to the other side of the world, the unknown and remote country of Japan.[4(p 26)] The two young people were John C. Berry, a Jefferson alumnus, and his wife who had set out from Bath, Maine, in order for Dr. Berry to become a physician to the Japan Mission of the American Board of Boston.

It was while Berry was rooming with a friend who was serving an apprenticeship with a physician in Brunswick that the former began to think seriously about his career.[4(pp 22-3)] At the advice of a local physician he entered Jefferson Medical College, "rated the best school for study." In 1871 Berry, at age 24, was graduated with honors. During his studies at Jefferson, he came under the instruction of such professors as W.W. Keen, S. Wier Mitchel, well-known novelist and physician, and other world-renowned men of medicine at Jefferson. (Incidentally, our class, perhaps, was the last to hear Dr. Keen lecture.)

Dr. Berry was one of the first medical missionaries to arrive in the Far East at a crucial and opportune period in the history of Japan. It was only 18 years before that Commodore Perry had come to Japan and succeeded in opening its door to the world. The year 1872 is considered to be a year of progress: the railway service between Tokyo and Yokohama was started and also in that year the calendar of the western world was adopted and the post office organized. Another important and significant change which took place the following year was the imperial proclamation withdrawing the public notice against Christianity which for more than 200 years had been posted in every town. This meant that now it was permissible to openly teach Christianity.

Despite language difficulties and differences in customs and concepts, Dr. Berry found that as far as his activities were concerned, it was fertile ground in which to work. Medical science in Japan then was far behind compared to Western standards; the Chinese school of medicine introduced in the sixth century still flourished.

Aside from the American doctor's responsibility for the health of the mission members and care of the Japanese patients who came to him, for a year he gave medical service at the International Hospital in Kobe. His concern and interest were not limited to medicine alone.[4(pp 50-61)] They were surprisingly diverse. In 1873, he founded a Sunday school which was the first one for the Japanese in the country. The following year he was the first to compile a Japanese hymnbook.

A year after his arrival, Dr. Berry was called into the city prison because of an epidemic of beri-beri among the inmates, thereby unexpectedly throwing him into another phase of humanitarian reform. He drew up a detailed outline of reforms, including better hygiene requirements, disinfection, proper care of the sick, introduction of manual labor and industrial employment, and appointment of a prison chaplain. He even drew plans for the new prison buildings.

His interest in prisons was to result in another "first" for him. He asked the governor for permission to use unclaimed bodies of executed criminals for postmortem examinations and dissection to aid in teaching the study of anatomy to the hospital staff and student physicians. Permission was granted by the central government in Tokyo, a drawing plan of a dissecting room was given to the governor and the facility was duly built. Thus, this energetic young American started in central Japan the first classroom in the study of human anatomy by dissection. During his second furlough, Dr. Berry took a refresher course in his specialty of otolaryngology in London and Vienna. Upon his return to Japan, he took his family to Kyoto, where he spent the last, eventful nine years of his residence in Japan.[4(pp 149-59)] Here it was that his dream of building a hospital and nurses' training school attached to Doshisha University was realized. In November 1887, a formal opening of the Hospital Nurses' Training School took place, the culmination of the doctor's dream and a great day, indeed, for him.

MODERN EXCHANGES

1975 SEMINAR AND TOUR

A little more than 100 years after Dr. and Mrs. Berry came to Japan, a group of Jeffersonians visited my country, this time a group of 104 doctors and accompanying members, in April 1975 to be exact. This was the "Orient Paradise Tour" which John Killough, Associate Dean of Jefferson Medical College, had organized.

Between the first letter from Dr. Killough dated August 1, 1974, announcing this intended tour, to the day of their arrival at the Imperial Hotel in Tokyo on April 7, 1975, more than 250 letters, telegrams and other communications were exchanged with President Peter A. Herbut, Drs. Killough and Takeda, the travel agent, myself, and speakers at the scientific meeting as well as others concerned. Fortunately, all the preparations were duly made by noon of the arrival of the Jefferson guests.

That evening under the auspices of President and Mrs. Herbut, a reception with approximately 150 doctors and their accompanying members and guests was held at the Imperial Hotel. This was followed by a formal dinner, a very gala affair. A number of Japanese doctors and their wives were invited to this dinner which was an opportunity for meeting old friends and making new ones.

On April 8, there was a scientific meeting from 9 am to 1 pm. The following was the program for the Jefferson Medical Seminar.

OPENING REMARKS

Peter A. Herbut, MD, President, Thomas Jefferson University

RELATIONSHIP BETWEEN JEFFERSON MEDICAL COLLEGE AND JAPAN IN THE EARLY DAYS

Jo Ono, MD, Visiting Professor of Bronchoesophagology, Keio University School of Medicine

MAN'S RESISTANCE TO INFECTION: A REVIEW OF IMMUNE AND OTHER RESISTANCE MECHANISMS

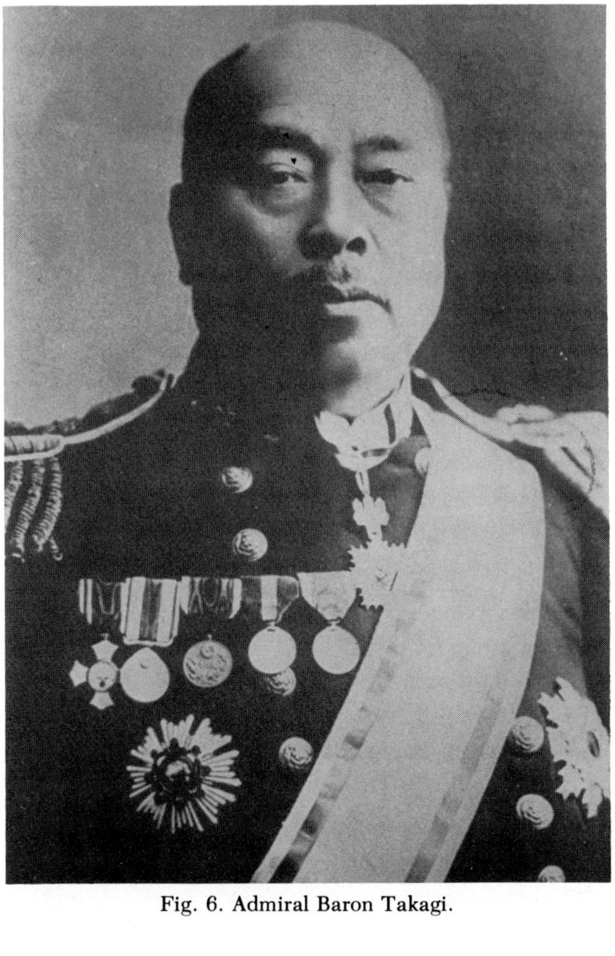

Fig. 6. Admiral Baron Takagi.

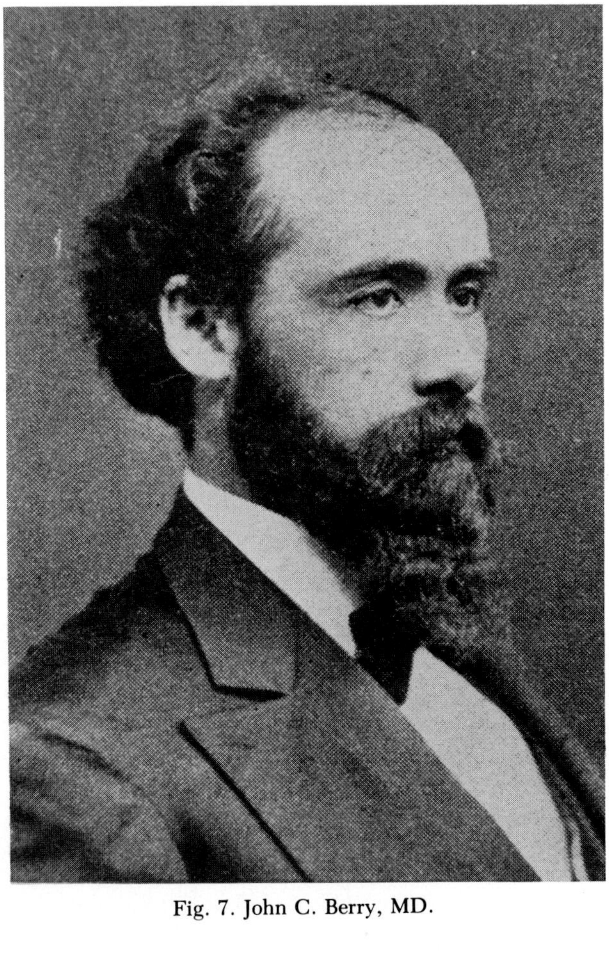

Fig. 7. John C. Berry, MD.

J.J. Saukkonen, MD, Professor of Microbiology, Jefferson Medical College

THE ROLE OF THE PHYSICIAN CONCERNING ENVIRONMENTAL POLLUTION IN JAPAN

Kensaburo Tsuchiya, MD, Professor of Preventive Medicine and Public Health, Keio University School of Medicine

DIAGNOSTIC CYTOLOGY OF PULMONARY DISEASES

Misao Takeda, MD, Assistant Professor, Director of School of Cytotechnology, Thomas Jefferson University

THE MEDICAL INSURANCE IN JAPAN

Akio Tanaka, MD, Chief of Medical Service Section, Health Insurance Bureau, Ministry of Health and Welfare

Each of the 30-minute talks was stimulating and rewarding.

On April 9, a program of hospital visits was arranged to the National Cancer Center, Kitazato University Medical School, the Women's Medical College with the Japan Heart Center and the Japanese Red Cross Medical Center which had recently been rebuilt. Each doctor was allowed to choose where he wished to go. A remark was made by one of the doctors after the visit that he had "learned more at this visit than in four years of pathology class."

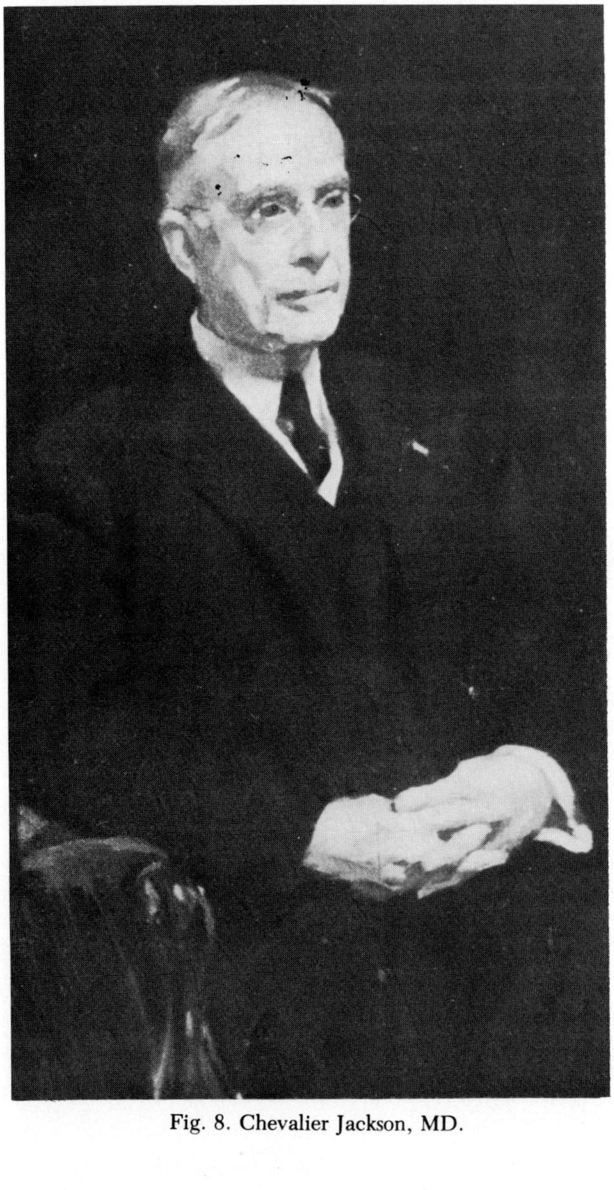

Fig. 8. Chevalier Jackson, MD.

From April 10-14, the group went sightseeing in different parts of Japan including the world-famous Temple of Nikko, the 700-year-old Giant Buddha of Kamakura, the snow-covered cone that is Mt. Fuji, the ancient capital city of Kyoto, and Nara by bullet train.

In this 7-day sojourn in Japan, the participating doctors and their families exchanged not only scientific knowledge and enjoyed scenic and cultural beauties but they contributed towards promotion of good will and understanding through meeting of the minds between the two countries. We sincerely appreciate this Jefferson legacy leading towards world peace.

THE INFLUENCE OF JACKSON AND CLERF

Finally I will discuss the two illustrious doctors, Chevalier Jackson (Fig. 8) and Louis H. Clerf, their specialty of bronchoesophagology, and how they contributed toward development of bronchoesophagology in Japan.

It would be presumptuous of me, I am sure, to try to tell you about Dr. Jackson, for every one of you must know of him and his work. However, very few, if any, I believe, had direct contact with him or saw him perform endoscopy. Dr. Clerf must be the only living person who was fortunate enough to work with Dr. Jackson.

In this respect, I can say I was fortunate too in being able to attend his bronchoscopic course in 1933, nearly half a century ago (Fig. 9).

One of the deepest impressions Dr. Jackson left in me was his remarkable spirit of persistent practice.[5] He said the bronchoscopic course is to teach the technique of peroral endoscopy; but the knowledge of how to do it is only a start. He said, "Facility can be obtained only by educating the eye and the fingers in repeated exercise until 'nerve cell habit' is formed." He further said, "Efficient use of forceps requires practice in handling of the forceps until it has become as natural and free from thought as the use of knife and fork."

Here I would like to recite a few of Dr. Jackson's aphorisms.

Educate your eye and your fingers.
Be sure you are right, but not too sure.
Follow your judgment; never your impulse.
Cry over spilt milk enough to memorize how you spilt it.
Let your mistakes worry you enough to prevent repetition.

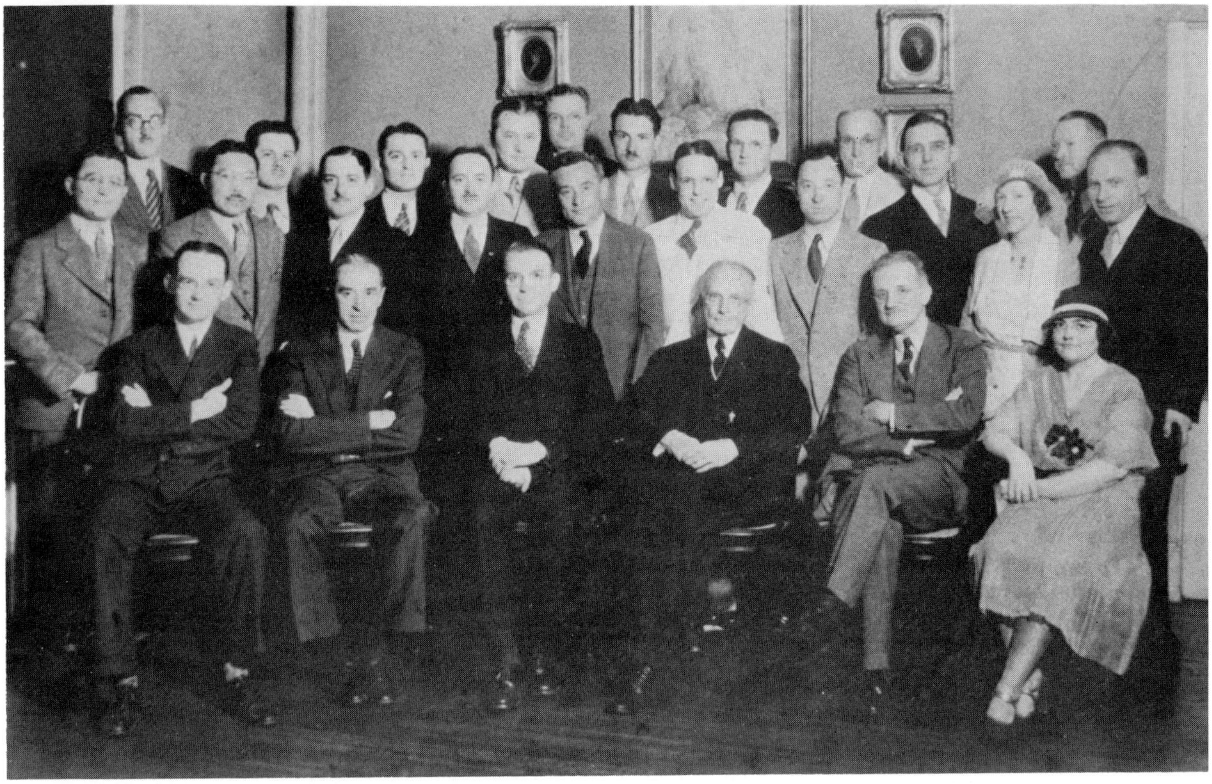

Fig. 9. Jackson Bronchoscopic Course, 1933. Seated, left to right: C. L. Jackson, W. F. Moore, L. H. Clerf, C. Jackson, G. Tucker, Sr., and E. L. Van Loon. (*Ed:* Author standing second from left.)

These aphorisms still stand as golden rules among the endoscopists who read Dr. Jackson's book entitled *Bronchoscopy, Esophagoscopy and Gastroscopy* which I translated into Japanese. While it is now out of print, this book is still widely read, not because I did the translation but because the original was written by Chevalier Jackson.

When I started internship at Jefferson Hospital in the summer of 1928, I was spellbound by the uncanny skill in endoscopy performed by Clerf in the then Fourth Annex operating room. I quickly gave up my intention of specializing in internal medicine and decided to study bronchoscopy so that I might practice and teach it in Japan where this branch of specialty was yet unknown.

However, in order to study bronchoscopy, the basic study of the chest was indispensable in the days when tuberculosis was rampant, and at the suggestion of Dr. Clerf and Dean Ross V. Patterson, I obtained a position as physician at Pennsylvania State Sanitarium at Mont Alto. I obtained good experience in tuberculosis among 800 inpatients, studying pneumothorax treatment since no antibiotics as yet were available in those days. After 1½ years study at the Mont Alto sanitarium, I returned to Jefferson to study bronchoscopy under Dr. Clerf. I stayed at his clinic until April 1934 when I returned to Japan.

You all know Dr. Clerf who graciously came all the way from Florida to attend this meeting. The fact that Dr. Clerf is a member and/or officer of 25 local, national and foreign medical societies attests to his prominence and importance. One should also remember that he was the first person to receive the Alumni Achievement Award of Jefferson Medical College and also the Chevalier Jackson Award from the American Broncho-Esophagological Association, among other awards.

Dr. Clerf attended the Eighth International Congress of ORL, held in Tokyo in October 1965, at which he gave invaluable guidance and suggestions to the hosting officers, particularly to me as I happened to be the Secretary-General of the Congress. More than 4,600 otolaryngologists and their families from 60 countries registered at that meeting. Dr. Clerf has been Honorary Advisor of the Japan Bronchoesophagological Society since its founding in 1949.

BRONCHOESOPHAGOLOGY IN JAPAN

Finally, as mentioned at the beginning of my talk, I should like to tell you something about bronchoesophagology in Japan.

For all practical purposes, bronchoesophagology was nonexistent in Japan until 1934. Returning from the United States at the invitation of Rudolf Teusler, director of St. Luke's International Hospital in Tokyo, I was to be the bronchoscopist at this hospital. However, because bronchoesophagology was unknown and not listed as a legally recognized specialty, I had to be known as an internist or otolaryngologist. After more than 19 years of effort on my part as well as some of my colleagues, it was possible to have my specialty receive an official sanction from the Japanese government in April 1953. Between 1949 and 1959, I arranged and taught 3-day bronchoesophagology courses to interested practitioners. A total of 53 sessions were given, with 1,500 participants coming from as far as Hokkaido in the north and Okinawa in the south.

We were also working on organizing the Japan Bronchoesophagological Society and on November 20, 1949, the first general meeting was held. In spite of an unseasonable blizzard, nearly 100 doctors came to this meeting. In those days it was necessary to obtain permission to hold a meeting from the Supreme Commander of Allied Powers by applying for it in writing in English as well as in Japanese.

The charter members of the Society numbered 80; it has grown now to more than 2,100 members including endoscopists, otolaryngologists, internists, pediatricians, thoracic surgeons, anatomists, roentgenologists, physiologists, pathologists and anesthesiologists.

Some of the activities of the Japan Bronchoesophagological Society, of which I served as president for 25 years, are as follows:

1. Annual administrative and scientific meetings are held regularly with as many as 100 to 140 papers presented at each meeting.

2. The Journal of the Japan Bronchoesophagological Society which was published quarterly in the beginning has been expanded to six issues annually since 1963.

3. The Society has published five books including one entitled *Bronchoesophagology* which has 643 pages with 559 illustrations and tables.

4. The Society hosted the Seventh International Congress of Bronchoesophagology in Kyoto in 1958.

5. The Society hosted the 11th International Congress of Bronchoesophagology in Hakone in 1965 after the Eighth International Congress of ORL held in Tokyo.

6. The Society has been conducting a campaign through publications, radio, television and lectures for prevention of foreign body accidents. As part of this program, in 1971 a 24-minute sound-color motion picture film entitled *Foreign Body Accidents — You May be the One Involved* was produced in both English and Japanese versions. As of March 3, 1981, the film has been shown 251 times to the general public as well as at medical meetings throughout the country. It was also shown at the Tenth World Congress of ORL, at Venice, Italy, in 1973, and received favorable comments.

7. For educational purposes for the members, the Society obtained numerous medical movie films from foreign countries, the first one being Clerf's *Surgery for Esophageal Diverticulum*, 1934. Also, we had Paul H. Holinger's *Endoscopy of Air and Food Passages*, 1953; C.L. Jackson's *Nomenclature of Bronchial Trees;* Dr. Jude's *External Cardiac Massages;* Dr. Cooley's *Human Heart Surgery* and more recently in 1980, Dr. Heimlich's *How to Save a Choking Victim.*

8. Notable contributions in the development of flexible endoscopes and other instruments have been made by such members of the Japan Bronchoesophagological Society as Shigeto Ikeda and others.

Needless to mention, these activities have been accomplished through the cooperation of the members of the Society.

CONCLUSION

It has been my pleasure and privilege to introduce some of the Jefferson legacies to Japan. It is hoped that they may not easily be dismissed or forgotten.

I wish to express deep gratitude for the honor accorded me to present a Clerf Lecture before distinguished Jefferson men. On this day, I look with ever-increasing admiration upon Dr. Clerf's distinguished services. Few men at Jefferson have been privileged to serve in so many important capacities as he has. As one of his students I am proud of my chief. May we continue to derive the benefit of his wise counsel and guidance. May he have many more years of health and happiness.

REFERENCES

1. Ienaga S. History of Japan. Tokyo: Japan Travel Bureau, 1954.

2. Reischauer O. The United States and Japan. Cambridge, Mass: Harvard University Press, 1954: 9-10.

3. Shibama C. The first Japanese embassy to the United States. Tokyo: The America-Japan Society, 1920.

4. Berry KF. A pioneer doctor in old Japan. New York: Fleming H. Ravell Co, 1940.

5. Jackson CL. Bronchoscopy, esophagoscopy and gastroscopy: a manual of peroral endoscopy and laryngeal surgery, 3rd ed. Philadelphia: W. B. Saunders Co, 1934: 149-50.

THE ANNALS PUBLISHING COMPANY
4949 FOREST PARK BLVD.
ST. LOUIS, MISSOURI 63108

DEVELOPMENT OF THE HYPOTYMPANUM IN THE HUMAN FETUS AND NEONATE

Gershon J. Spector, MD

Xian-Xi Ge, MD

DEVELOPMENT OF THE HYPOTYMPANUM IN THE HUMAN FETUS AND NEONATE

GERSHON J. SPECTOR, MD   XIAN-XI GE, MD

ST. LOUIS, MISSOURI

The human hypotympanum develops over a 10-week period in utero (22-32 weeks) as a triphasic osseous mosaic. The tympanic bone ossifies as a membranous bone (8-36 weeks in utero). The canalicular otic capsule ossifies in cartilage by 26 weeks in utero. A petrosal ledge of bone ossifies as periosteal bone at 24-29 weeks in utero. The fusion of these three bony structures closes the hypotympanum and forms two persistent hypotympanic fissures. The medial hypotympanic fissure forms between the canalicular otic capsule and petrosa at 24 weeks in utero. It transmits the medial hypotympanic artery and vein (from the posterior CNS circulation) and Jacobson's nerve (from the ninth nerve). The lateral hypotympanum fissure forms between the tympanic bone and the petrosa at 29 weeks in utero. It transmits the lateral hypotympanic artery and vein from the external carotid circulation. The two vascular supplies form a rich hypotympanic plexus on the floor of the middle ear. The fibrous annulus and middle layer of the tympanic membrane form an avascular plane.

INTRODUCTION

The precise steps in the formation of the hypotympanum of the fetal human temporal bone are not elucidated in the literature.[1-16] Universally two developmental factors are mentioned. 1) There is a consensus of opinion that the hypotympanum ossifies by the 34th week in utero. 2) Both surgical specimen and temporal bone histologic studies confirm the common occurrence of bony dehiscences in this region.[1-16]

The purposes of this study are:

1. To describe the embryologic formation and ossification pattern of the hypotympanum,
2. To delineate and measure the fissures in the hypotympanum,
3. To describe the major neural and vascular structures that pass near or through this region, and
4. To elucidate the clinical and surgical significance of the developmental and anatomic features of the hypotympanum.

MATERIALS AND METHODS

Fifty-four consecutive pairs of temporal bones were obtained from fetuses (16 weeks in utero and older) and neonates (up to one month postpartum) who died of various medical disorders. Complete autopsies were done on all cases. The autopsy information has been previously published.[17] Only 52 temporal bones were adequately cut for the study of the hypotympanum. These included 23 pairs and 6 single temporal bones. There were 29 left and 23 right bones. Twenty-four bones were from fetuses (16-38 weeks in utero) and 18 from neonates (39 weeks in utero until one month postpartum).

The fixation, decalcification, cutting and section preparation of the temporal bones have been previously described.[17] All temporal bones were cut in the classical vertical plane, perpendicular to the long axis of the temporal bone, stained with hematoxylin and eosin (H&E), and mounted in serial order. Some sections were stained with a phosphotungstic acid-hematoxylin (PTAH) stain for nuclear and neural detail.[18]

High power (under oil) and low power resolution by light microscopy were used for the detailed histology and serial reconstructions. A slide projector with a magnification ratio of 45:1 and an appropriately scaled grid was used for accurate measurements.[17] The critical parameters were drawn on grid paper for accurate representation and measurement.[17] The drawing and measurements were done in a double-blind fashion so that the slide number and age of the fetus or neonate were not known. The graphic representation and measurements were alternated between two observers in a double-blind fashion. The two sets of data were compared to each other. The statistical error in measurements was less than $\pm 2\%$. In addition, black and white photographs were obtained at 18 and 32 times magnification for a permanent record.

For each temporal bone, sections were viewed from the anterior to the posterior borders of the hypotympanum.

HYPOTYMPANIC BORDERS

The hypotympanum is a crescent-shaped space with the concave surface facing inferiorly. Although for the otologic surgeon the borders may be quite variable depending on the specific anatomy of the particular surgical temporal bone, for the purposes of this study more definite landmarks were needed. Therefore the roof on the jugular bulb was used as the inferior border. The superior border was a horizontal plane projected from the inferior fibrous annulus towards the basal turn of the cochlea or canalicular otic capsule. The anterior border was a vertical line projected from the eustachian tube orifice or processus cochleariformis towards the internal carotid artery as it enters the temporal bone inferiorly. The posterior border was a vertical line drawn from the posterior bony rim of the round window or the posterior semicircular canal ampulla to the origin of the sigmoid sinus.

MEASUREMENT PARAMETERS

Measurements of the histologic temporal bone sections were taken at 45 times magnification in a serial fashion starting from the anterior border of the hypotympanum (Fig. 1). The distance from the medial edge of the tympanic bone to the lateral edge of the canalicular otic capsule (T-CO) in the region of the posterior canal ampulla was used to measure the ossification and growth of the posterior hypotympanum at different gestational ages. The anterior hypotympanum width was measured from the medial edge of the tympanic bone to the cochlear otic capsule in the region of the internal carotid artery at various gestational ages. These distances represent the ossification and growth of the tympanic bone and otic capsule.

From the Department of Otolaryngology, Washington University School of Medicine, St. Louis; and the Department of Otolaryngology, 6th People's Hospital, Shanghai, China.

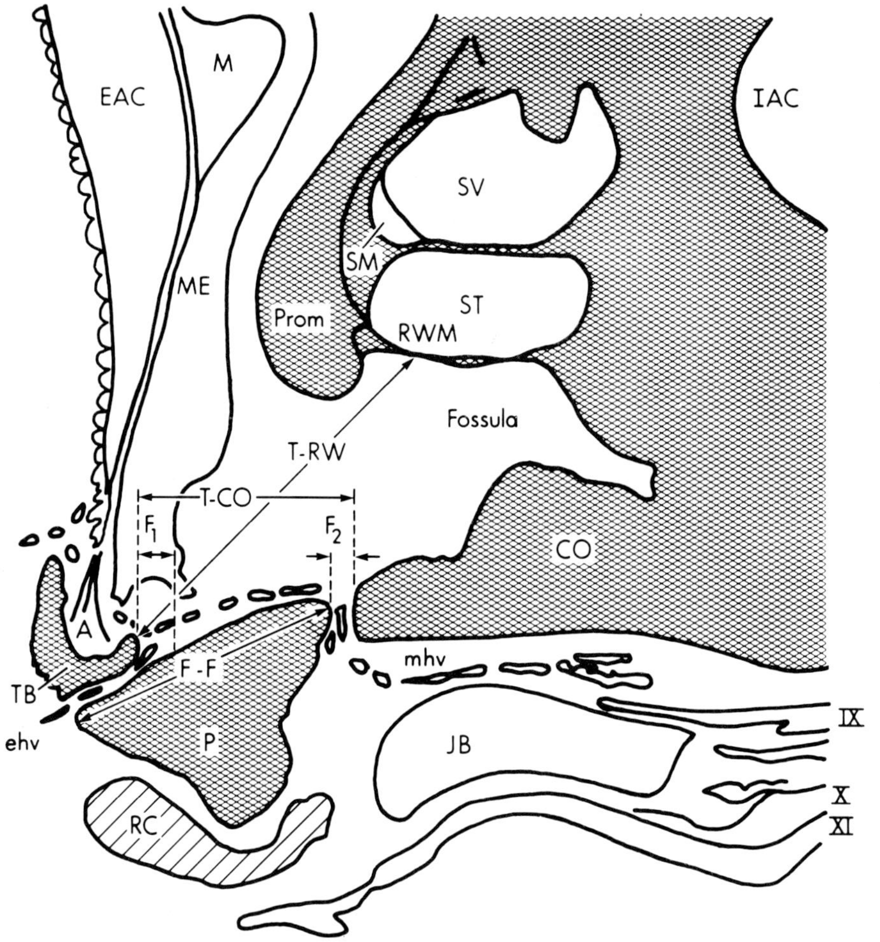

Fig. 1. Schematic representation of the posterior hypotympanum of a right temporal bone denoting the measured parameters: F_1 - Lateral hypotympanic fissure; F_2 - Medial hypotympanic fissure; T-CO - Distance from the tympanic bone to canalicular otic capsule (CO); T-RW - Distance from tympanic bone to round window membrane (RWM); and (F-F) - Interfissure distance; and P - Petrosal growth. EAC - External auditory canal; M - Malleus; ME - Middle ear; TB - Tympanic bone; ehv - Lateral hypotympanic vessels; A - Fibrous annulus; mhv - Medial hypotympanic vessels; JB - Jugular bulb; RC - Reichert's cartilage; IAC - Internal auditory canal; Prom - Promontory; IX, X and XI - Cranial nerves; SV - Scala vestibuli; SM - Scala media; ST - Scala tympani.

The distance from the medial edge of the inferior tympanic bone to the round window membrane (T-RW) was used to measure the overall growth of the posterior hypotympanum. This distance represents the combined growth of the tympanic bone, otic capsule and petrosa. The difference between the former and latter readings represents the petrosal component of the hypotympanum.

An alternative and more direct way to determine the ossification and growth of the periosteal petrosal ledge of bone is to measure the interfissure distance (F-F). Since the medial fissure (F_2) is between the canalicular otic capsule and petrosa, and the lateral fissure (F_1) is between the tympanic bone and petrosa, the interfissure distance is a direct measure of the petrosal periosteal elongation. A comparison of the two sets of data demonstrated less than $\pm 8\%$ error.

The medial (F_2) and lateral (F_1) hypotympanic fissures are measured directly from bone to bone. The lateral fissure is the distance from the medial border of the tympanic bone to the lateral edge of the petrosa at the level of the hypotympanum. The medial fissure is the distance from the lateral edge of the otic capsule to the medial edge of the petrosa. The anterior and posterior hypotympanic measurements were taken at the level of the internal carotid artery and posterior semicircular canal ampulla respectively.

A comparison of the measurements of the two temporal bones in the same fetus was performed in a double-blind random fashion (see below).

RESULTS

EMBRYOLOGY

The development and ossification of the hypotympanum occurs late in the gestational period (22-32 weeks in utero). At 16 weeks in utero the otic capsule is cartilaginous. The cartilaginous structures of the ossicles are present without ossification centers. The fetal structures exist in their normal anatomic locations. The vascular structures of the middle ear are rudimentary. The middle ear "potential" space is filled with embryonal mesenchyme (Fig. 2). Extending from the inner layer of the tympanic membrane are epithelial grooves (composed of cuboidal cells) which are centers for liquification necrosis and mesenchymal resorption. These grooves eventually lead to removal of the embryonal middle ear mesenchyme and formation of an air-containing middle ear space which is lined with epithelium and retains some of the mesenchyme as a thin subepithelial connective tissue layer (Fig. 3).

The earliest area of mesenchymal resorption occurs in the protympanum and hypotympanum, ie, the pneumatization pattern of the middle ear is crescent-shaped with the concave surface facing superiorly. The pneumatization originates from the eustachian tube orifice and extends along the anterior wall of the protympanum to the hypotympanum. The last area of resorption of the primitive mesenchyme is the round window niche. At 16 weeks in utero the tympanic bone is rudimentary and incomplete. However, the tympanic membrane

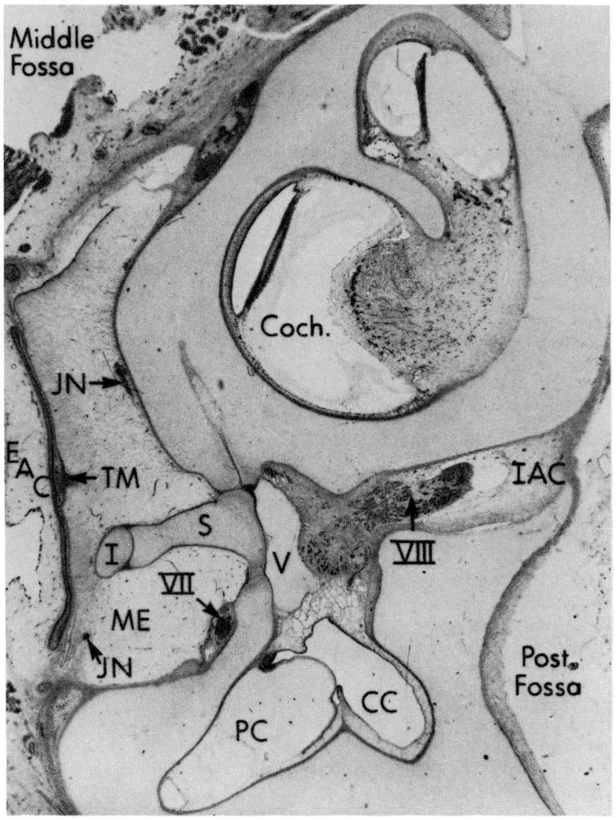

Fig. 2. Right temporal bone of 16-week fetus demonstrating middle ear (ME) filled with mesenchyme. Jacobson's nerve (JN) is present in the hypotympanum and on the promontory. The otic capsule is not ossified; the hypotympanum is not formed. VII - Facial nerve; I - Incus; S - Stapes; V - Vestibule; VIII - Cochlear nerve; CC - Crus commune; PC - Posterior canal; Coch. - Cochlea; and TM - Tympanic membrane. (H&E, x12)

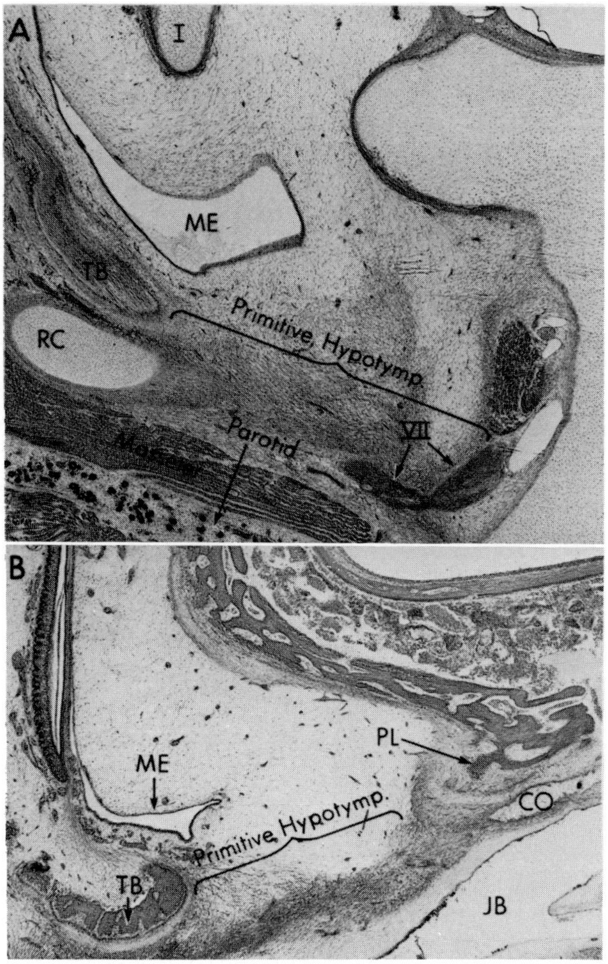

Fig. 3. Primitive hypotympanum in right temporal bones of fetuses denoting pneumatization of the middle ear (ME). A) 16 weeks; B) 20 weeks. Note in A the exit of facial nerve (VII) through primitive hypotympanum (future stylomastoid foramen). PL - Petrosal ledge of bone; CO - Cartilaginous canalicular otic capsule. (H&E, x25)

and fibrous annulus are well-formed (Fig. 3B).

During the 16-19-week-in utero interval the main developmental change is the completion and ossification of the tympanic bone. The petrous apex and otic capsule are incompletely ossified. The primitive hypotympanum is in continuity with the posterior cranial fossa and the rudimentary parotid ductal system. Thus the entire hypotympanum is uncovered and widely open. The anterior hypotympanum is wider than the posterior region (3.25 mm vs 2 mm). The styloid process anlage (Reichert's cartilage) is not fused with the hypotympanum (Fig. 3).

At 19 weeks in utero the neural structures are in their final anatomic location. The posterior cranial nerves (IX-XII) and major venous sinuses are in their normal anatomic position. Jacobson's nerve has entered the primitive (16-week fetus) hypotympanum (anteriorly near the internal carotid artery) and formed a plexus on the cartilaginous promontory (Fig. 2). The facial nerve and its first major division (chorda tympani) are in the middle ear. The former exits through the wide primitive hypotympanum (Fig. 3A). The fallopian canal is not formed (Figs. 2 and 3A). A rudimentary pyramidal eminence and stapedius muscle are present (Fig. 4A, B). The vascular supply to the hypotympanum is rudimentary and incomplete.

During the 19-22 weeks in utero there is a progressive widening of the posterior hypotympanum. The main ossification feature at this time is the completion of ossification of the canalicular otic capsule (Figs. 4 and 5). The middle ear is further pneumatized, but primitive mesenchyme is still present in the fossula of the round window. The hypotympanum is widely open and continuous with the posterior cranial fossa (Fig. 3B).

During the 22-32-weeks-in utero stage, the major closure of the hypotympanum occurs. This staged process transforms the primitive widely open hypotympanum to the adult configuration and sequesters it into the middle ear. The sequestration of the hypotympanum depends on three interrelated events, ie, the ossification and further enlargement of the tympanic bone, completion of the ossification of the canalicular otic capsule, and progressive periosteal ossification and growth of the petrosa.

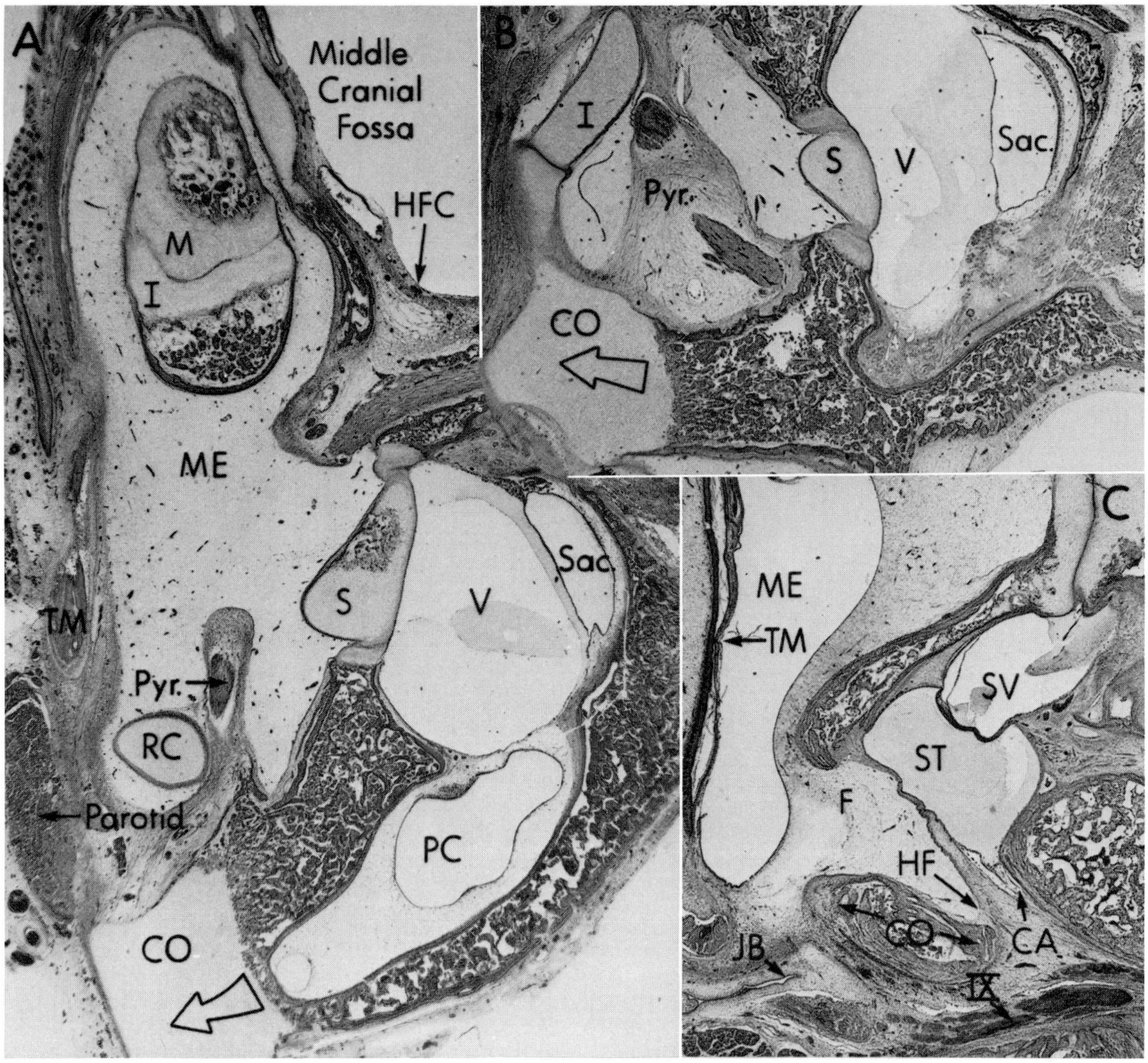

Fig. 4. Ossification of the canalicular otic capsule cartilage (CO) covering the posterior semicircular canal (PC) of three right temporal bones A, B) at 19-22 weeks in utero (clear arrows). C) At a later stage there is progressive growth of posterior otic capsule (arrows). Pyr. - Pyramidal eminence; Sac. - Saccule; HFC - Hiatus of facial nerve; HF - Hyrtl's fissure; CA - Cochlear aqueduct; F - Round window niche. (H&E: A, x35; B, C, x12)

The tympanic bone continues to enlarge, ossify and grow during the entire period of 16-36 weeks in utero. It enlarges four times in size from 16-36 weeks in utero. Further growth continues postpartum. By the end of the 36th week in utero the tympanic bone forms a ring which is incomplete superiorly. The cross section of the tympanic bone in the hypotympanum shows that it is concave superiorly. This concavity is filled with the fibrous annulus. These developmental parameters are described in the literature.[19] Thus the tympanic bone is the first structure to ossify in the hypotympanum. Its ossification pattern is that of membranous bone.

The canalicular otic capsule ossifies at 18-26 weeks in utero. The ossification is complete by 26 weeks in utero with the final event being the ossification of the round window niche and posterior canal ampulla (Fig. 5).

In a previous report we demonstrated that the ossification of the medial border of the canalicular otic capsule obliterates Hyrtl's fissure and forms the definitive cochlear aqueduct by 24 weeks in utero.[17] At the same time the lateral border of the canalicular otic capsule ossifies the ampulla of the posterior semicircular canal. Eventually this portion of the otic capsule fuses with the periosteal petrosal growth centers which leads to ossification of the hypotympanum. The latter occurs at 26 weeks in utero or two weeks after obliteration of Hyrtl's fissure (Fig. 6).

The ossification of the lateral canalicular otic capsule is the second hypotympanic structure to develop. Its formation narrows the anterior hypotympanum to a much greater extent than the posterior hypotympanum. The ossification pattern is that of enchondral bone or ossification in cartilage.

Between 24-26 weeks in utero a ledge of bone forms as a periosteal growth from the petrosa under

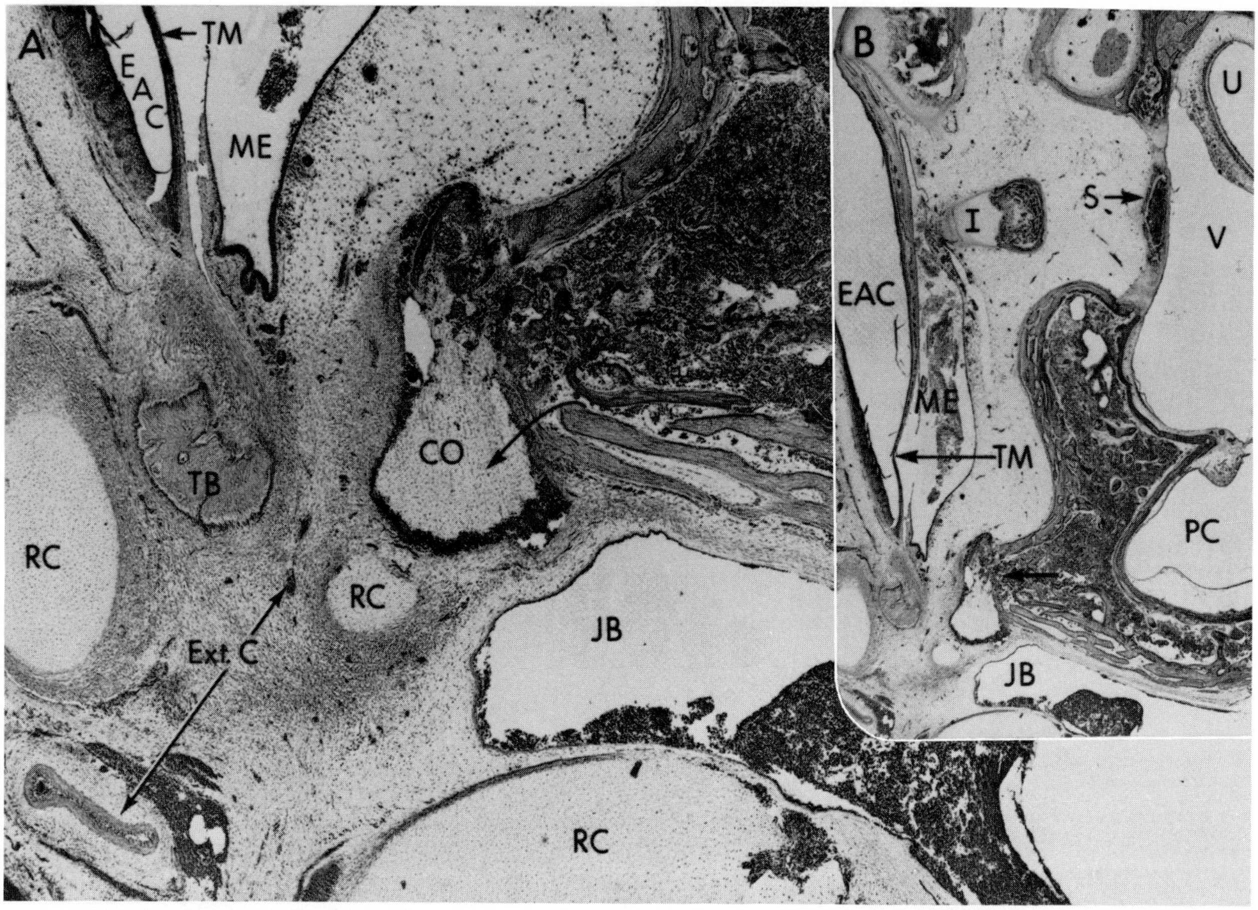

Fig. 5. Final ossification of canalicular otic capsule (CO) in a 26-week right temporal bone B) over the posterior semicircular (PC) canal (arrow) at low power (x12). A) High power (x35). Note the proximity of the external carotid vessels (Ext. C) to the hypotympanum and Reichert's cartilage (RC). U - Utricle.

the canalicular otic capsule, ie, beneath the posterior canal ampulla (Fig. 3). This ledge lies superior to Reichert's cartilage which it follows as a template (Fig. 6B). The periosteal petrosal ledge of bone grows in the future hypotympanic region towards the tympanic bone, ie, medially to laterally. In addition it enlarges from the posterior towards the anterior border of the hypotympanum (Fig. 7). During the 29-32-weeks-in utero period the growth of the petrosal ledge almost meets the tympanic bone. This process effectively closes the hypotympanum and isolates it from the posterior fossa. Nevertheless, during the entire gestational period, all temporal bones have persistent dehiscences which communicate the hypotympanum with the posterior cranial fossa (Fig. 8).

The petrosal ledge of bone is the third developmental structure to form in the hypotympanum. It completes the formation of this region. Its growth and ossification pattern is that of periosteal bone formation.

In summary, the hypotympanum forms by ossification of three structures by three different bone-forming patterns. The tympanic bone forms as a membranous bone with a growth pattern which is progressive until 36 weeks in utero. The canalicular otic capsule ossifies in cartilage by 26 weeks in utero. The petrosa forms as a periosteal growth of bone which forms a ledge to bridge the hypotympanum (from the canalicular otic capsule to the tympanic bone) by 29-32 weeks in utero (Fig. 9).

HYPOTYMPANIC FISSURES

As the petrosa grows from the canalicular otic capsule region towards the tympanic bone, it separates the hypotympanum from the posterior cranial fossa. At the same time it forms two fissures in the regions of osseous fusion with the otic capsule and tympanic bone. These areas allow the neurovascular structures to enter the hypotympanum. These fissures are crescent-shaped and run in an antero-posterior axis. We have named these the medial (F_2) and lateral (F_1) hypotympanic fissures (Fig. 10).

The medial hypotympanic fissure lies in the region of fusion between the canalicular otic capsule and the petrosal ledge of bone. It transmits the tympanic branch of the glossopharyngeal nerve (IX) or Jacobson's nerve, and an artery and vein which originate from the CNS (posterior cranial fossa) cir-

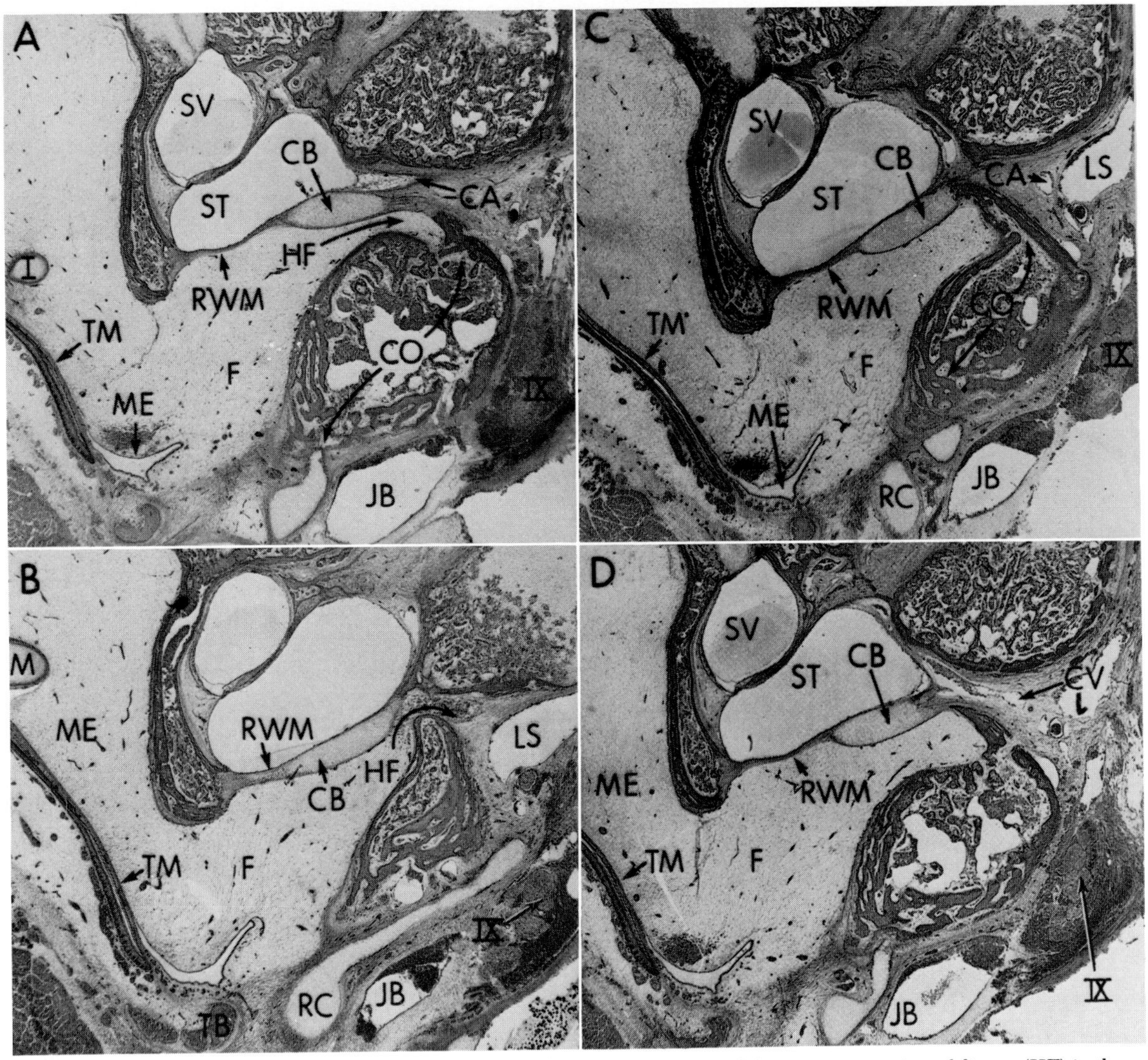

Fig. 6. Growth of canalicular otic capsule (CO with arrows) and closure of the tympanomeningeal fissure (HF) in three 24-week right temporal bones. A, B) The hypotympanum is widely open. Note the relationship of Reichert's cartilage (RC) to the otic capsule and to the jugular bulb (JB) in B. C) The medial ossification of the otic capsule fuses with the round window cartilaginous bar (CB) two weeks prior to lateral ossification of the otic capsule in C, D, above the glossopharyngeal nerve (IX) and lateral sinus (LS). A-D) The middle ear, except for the hypotympanum is filled with mesenchyme. D) The hypotympanum is widely open and Hyrtl's fissure is closed. (H&E, x18).

culation. These vessels provide circulation to the medial hypotympanum and round window niche. They accompany Jacobson's nerve to the cochlear promontory. In addition, these vessels anastomose with the vessels which enter the hypotympanum via the lateral hypotympanic fissure.

The medial hypotympanic fissure first appears in the anterior hypotympanum, near the internal carotid artery at 18 weeks in utero and it elongates posteriorly by 24 weeks in utero. At 22 weeks in utero the medial fissure is complete with a uniform width in the anterior and posterior region. As the fissure grows posteriorly, Jacobson's nerve and the accompanying vessels and nerves move posteriorly towards the anterior rim of the round window. As this occurs the nerves and vessels leave a trail of neural and vascular branches from Jacobson's nerve and caroticotympanic sympathetic nerves (from the internal carotid artery) on the promontory of the cochlea.

The lateral hypotympanic fissure lies in the fusion plane between the petrosal ledge of bone and the tympanic bone. It is the passageway for an artery and vein from the external carotid circulation. These supply the lateral hypotympanum and the medial surface of the tympanic membrane. The vessels anastomose with those vessels from the medial hypotympanic fissure region.

The lateral fissure first forms at 22 weeks in utero. It is much wider anteriorly than posteriorly. This lateral fissure narrows initially in the posterior hypotympanum and later in the anterior hypotympanum with a 2-week time separation for completion (see below).

The hypotympanic fissures are formed over a

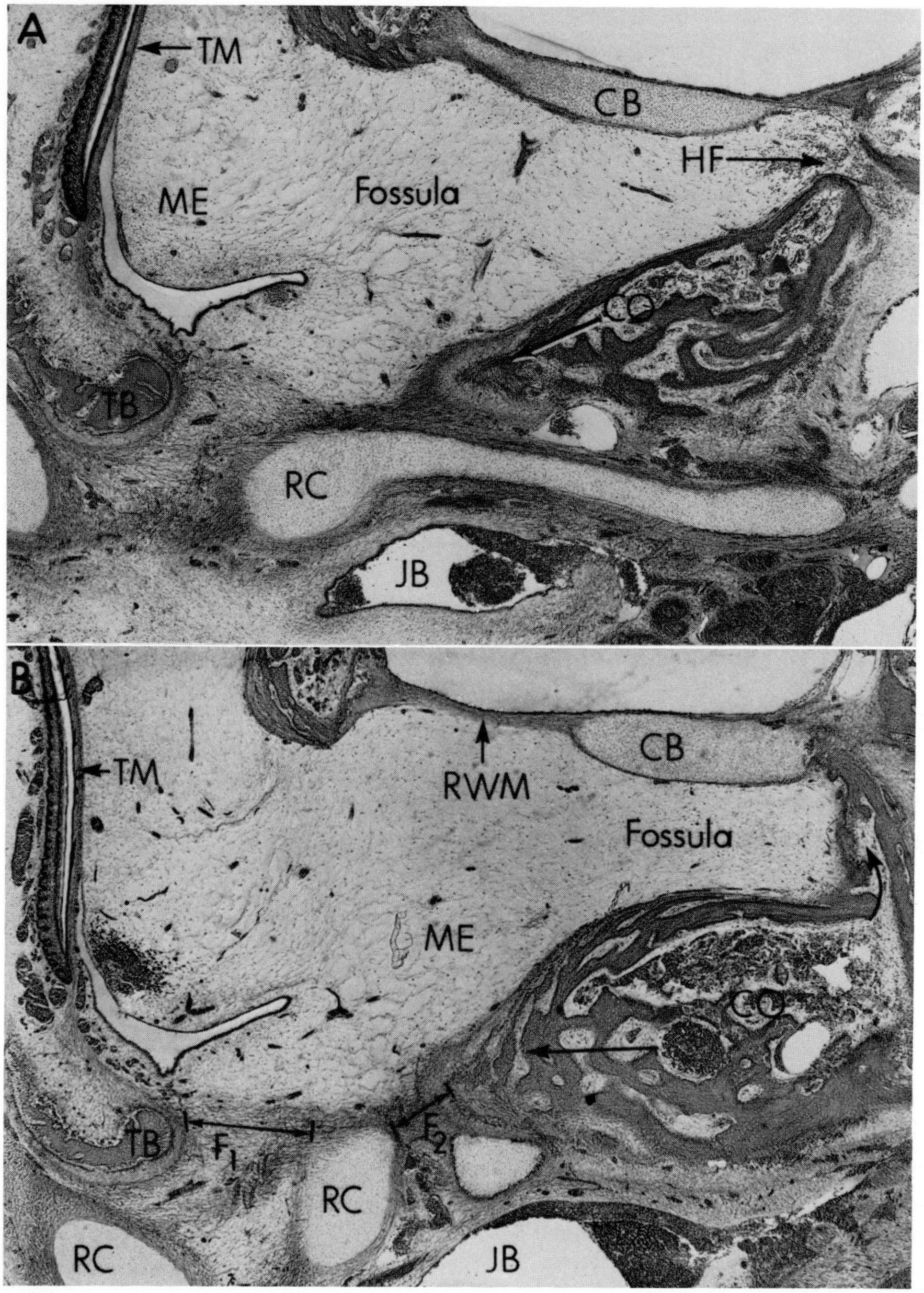

Fig. 7. High power magnification of canalicular otic capsule ossification in two right temporal bones at A) 24 and B) 26 weeks in utero. Initially Hyrtl's fissure (HF in A) is closed in B; then the lateral ossification closes the hypotympanum in B. Reichert's cartilage is the template on which the otic capsule and petrosa grows (RC in A). This is the earliest stage of medial (F_2) and lateral (F_1) hypotympanic fissure delineation in B. (H&E, x60)

4-week period and are well-developed by the 26-28th week in utero. The remaining four weeks (28-32 weeks in utero) until completion of the hypotympanum are devoted mainly to progressive ossification of the petrosa, narrowing of the fissures, and closure of the hypotympanum. At the end of 32 weeks in utero, the hypotympanum assumes an adult configuration.

From the 32nd week in utero until term, no major new ossification patterns occur. The major events are the progressive widening of the hypotympanum, enlargement of the tympanic bone, and persistence of the two hypotympanic fissures (see below). All temporal bones (except one bone from a 1½-day-old neonate) had persistent patent hypotympanic fissures and dehiscences. The distance between the fissures correlated well with the gestational age of the fetus (see below). In older fetuses the interfissure distance is larger. This correlation existed in both the anterior and posterior regions of the hypotympanum.

NEUROVASCULAR STRUCTURES

From 16 weeks in utero until ossification of the canalicular otic capsule at 22-26 weeks in utero the major neurovascular structures assume the usual adult anatomic relationship to the hypotympanum. From the 26th-32nd week in utero the major altera-

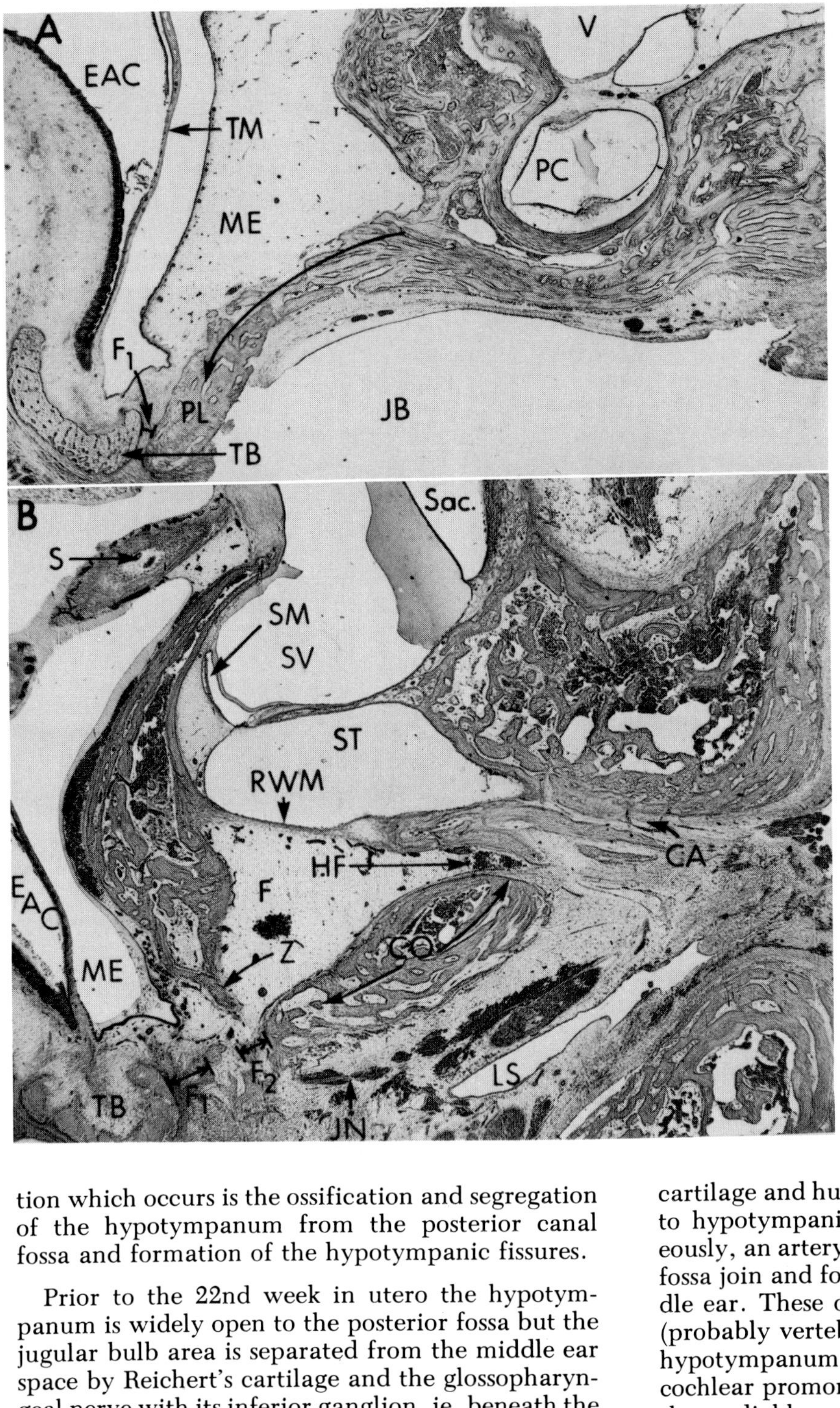

Fig. 8. Comparison of a right A) postpartum and B) 26-week fetal hypotympanum. Note the bony coverage of the hypotympanum in the neonate in A. In the fetus there are three fissures: the lateral (F_1) and medial (F_2) hypotympanic fissures, and the tympanomeningeal fissure (HF). Z - Subiculum. (H&E, x18)

tion which occurs is the ossification and segregation of the hypotympanum from the posterior canal fossa and formation of the hypotympanic fissures.

Prior to the 22nd week in utero the hypotympanum is widely open to the posterior fossa but the jugular bulb area is separated from the middle ear space by Reichert's cartilage and the glossopharyngeal nerve with its inferior ganglion, ie, beneath the hypotympanum lie the following structures from a superior sequential order — Reichert's cartilage, the inferior ganglion and nerve of the ninth cranial nerve and the jugular bulb (Fig. 11B). Beneath the jugular bulb lie the 10th and 11th cranial nerves (Fig. 11A). At this time there is no interjugular process. Jacobson's nerve is seen to take origin from the cephalic portion of the inferior (petrosal) glossopharyngeal ganglion at 16 weeks in utero (Fig. 11B). It enters the middle ear anterior to Reichert's cartilage and hugs the canalicular otic capsule prior to hypotympanic ossification (Fig. 12). Simultaneously, an artery and vein from the posterior cranial fossa join and follow Jacobson's nerve into the middle ear. These originate from the CNS circulation (probably vertebral vessels) and supply the medial hypotympanum, round window niche area and cochlear promontory. We have named these vessels the medial hypotympanic artery and vein (Fig. 13).

At the same time, an artery and vein originating from the external carotid circulation (most probably the ascending pharyngeal artery) travel beneath the tympanic bone to enter the hypotympanum through the lateral fissure (Fig. 5). These supply the lateral floor of the hypotympanum and the inner surface of the tympanic membrane. We have named these vessels the lateral hypotympanic artery and vein. In the literature these vessels are

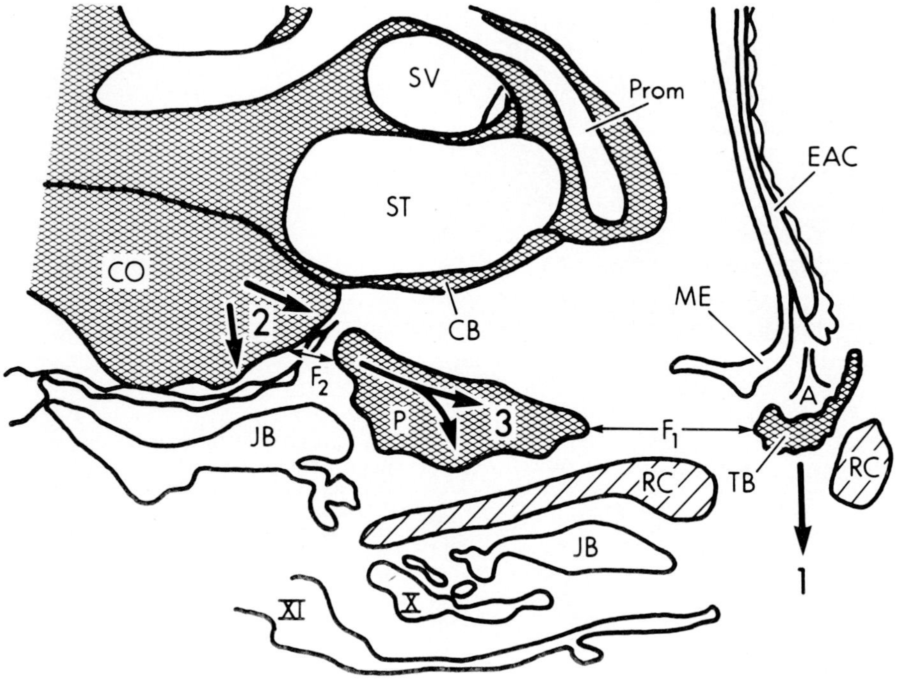

Fig. 9. Schematic representation of the hypotympanic triphasic pattern of ossification in a left temporal bone. Initially the tympanic bone (TB) forms in membrane (1), then the canalicular otic capsule (CO) ossifies in cartilage (2) and finally periosteal petrosal bone (P) closes the gap between the former two structures (3). This forms two fissures, ie, medial (F_2) and lateral (F_1) hypotympanic fissures. Reichert's cartilage (RC) lies beneath these ossifications and forms a template as well as determines the height of the hypotympanum and the jugular bulb.

called the inferior tympanic vessels[9,20] (Fig. 14).

The medial and lateral hypotympanic vessels form a rich vascular anastomosis along the floor of the primitive hypotympanum. However, the enlarging tympanic bone, fibrous annulus, and middle layer of the tympanic membrane prevent vascular anastomosis between the lateral hypotympanic vessels and those vessels which enter the external auditory canal (Figs. 13 and 14). Thus the fibrous annulus forms an avascular plane separating the lateral hypotympanic blood supply from the external auditory canal circulation (Fig. 15).

After the 24th week in utero, these neurovascular relationships remain constant, and the main event is the ossification of the hypotympanum and narrowing of the medial and lateral hypotympanic fissure. Reichert's cartilage is resorbed and incorporated into the fallopian canal and styloid process (Figs. 4A, 7B, and 11A). The canalicular otic capsule is ossified and the petrosal periosteal ledge of bone begins to close the hypotympanum. The latter lies cephalad to Reichert's cartilage which it follows as a template (Fig. 7A).

MEASUREMENTS

Hypotympanum. The size of the hypotympanum varies with the gestational age of the fetus. The growth and development of the area has a 3-phase pattern. This can be demonstrated by various direct measurements as illustrated in Figures 16 and 17.

At 16 weeks in utero the distance from the inferior tympanic bone to the lateral aspect of the cochlear otic capsule is approximately 3.27 mm. This represents the anterior width of the hypotym-

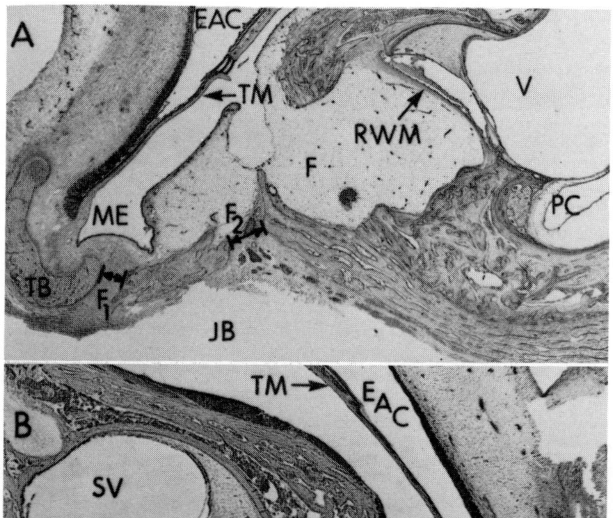

Fig. 10. Two different neonatal temporal bones. A) Usual adult pattern in a right temporal bone with two hypotympanic fissures. The medial fissure (F_2) transmits Jacobson's nerves. B) Three fissures in a left temporal bone; the medial (F_2), lateral (F_1), and tympanomeningeal (HF) or Hyrtl's fissures. MHA - Medial hypotympanic vessels. (H&E: A, x11; B, x12)

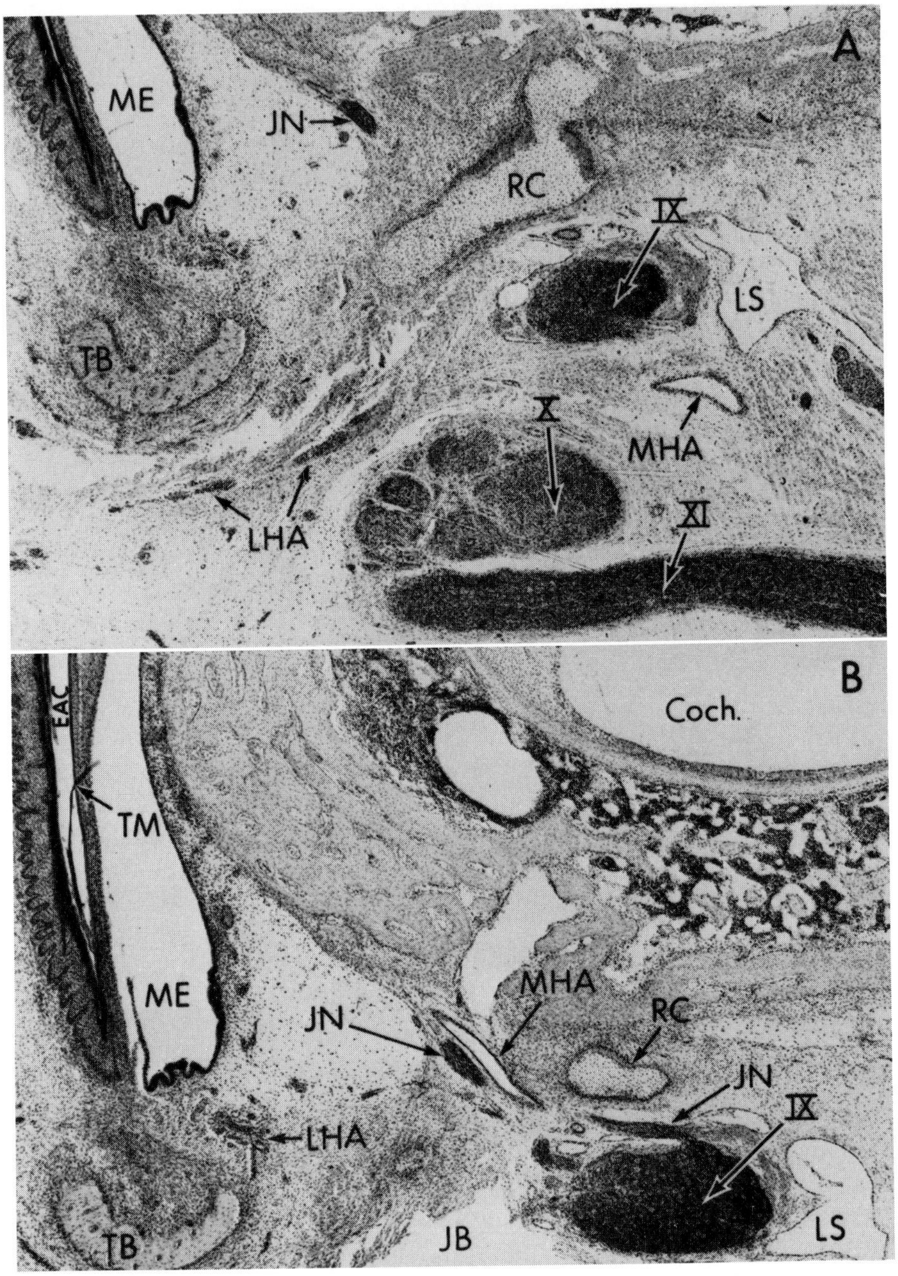

Fig. 11. Neural structures below an 18-week right hypotympanum. A) Relationship of nerves IX (glossopharyngeal), X (vagus), and XI (spinal accessory) to Reichert's cartilage (RC). B) Origin of Jacobson's nerve (JN) from the cephalic portion of the inferior glossopharyngeal ganglion (IX) and its accompanying medial hypotympanic vessels (MHA). The lateral hypotympanic vessels (LHA) enter the hypotympanum under the tympanic bone (TB). (PTAH stain, x90)

panum. At 22 weeks in utero the width of the anterior hypotympanum begins to diminish (3.05 mm) until the 28th week in utero. At this time the anterior hypotympanum is 1.25 mm in width. This first phase of growth represents primarily the ossification of the otic capsule and the enlargement of the tympanic bone (Fig. 16).

From the 28th week in utero until term there is a progressive enlargement of the anterior hypotympanum from 1.25 to 3 mm in width. However, between the 28th week and 32nd week in utero there is a lag phase in growth of the hypotympanum (1.25 to 1.5 mm in width). At this time the petrosal periosteal bone ledge invades the anterior hypotympanum. This process segregates the hypotympanum to the middle ear. After the 34th week in utero there is a rapid enlargement of the hypotympanum until term. This is primarily due to the expansion of the middle ear cavity, growth of the tympanic bone, and the periosteal overgrowth of the petrosa. From birth until the first month postpartum there is no enlargement of the anterior hypotympanum (Fig. 16).

The development of the posterior hypotympanum defines the three growth phases more clearly. This can be delineated by measuring the distance from the posterior edge of the tympanic bone to the round window membrane. At 16-19 weeks in utero the posterior hypotympanum is 1.97-2.04 mm in width and is static in size. At 19 weeks in utero there is rapid enlargement of the posterior hypotympanic diameter. This phase ends at 24 weeks in utero with

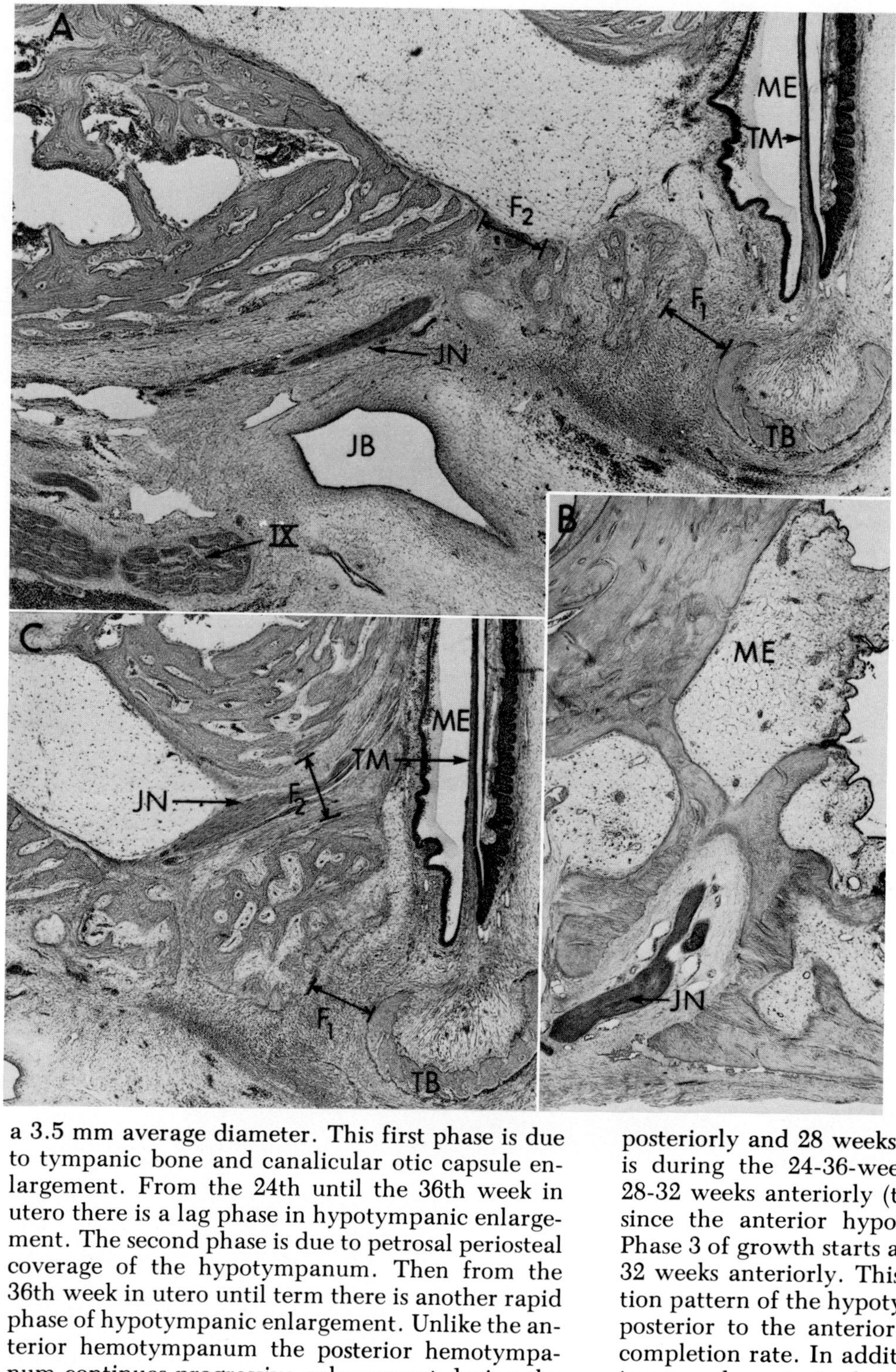

Fig. 12. The course of the tympanic branch of the glossopharyngeal nerve (Jacobson's nerve) in two left postpartum temporal bones. A) Jacobson's nerve enters the medial hypotympanum fissure (F_2) cephalad to the jugular bulb (JB). B) Tympanic branch is accompanied by vessels in the medial hypotympanic fissure. C) Nerve traverses the hypotympanum to lie on the cochlear promontory. (H&E, x90)

a 3.5 mm average diameter. This first phase is due to tympanic bone and canalicular otic capsule enlargement. From the 24th until the 36th week in utero there is a lag phase in hypotympanic enlargement. The second phase is due to petrosal periosteal coverage of the hypotympanum. Then from the 36th week in utero until term there is another rapid phase of hypotympanic enlargement. Unlike the anterior hemotympanum the posterior hemotympanum continues progressive enlargement during the first months postpartum (Fig. 17). The last phase is due to petrosal overgrowth and expansion.

Both anterior and posterior hypotympanum show the three phases of the growth patterns. However, the posterior hypotympanic curve precedes the anterior curve by four weeks in utero (compare Figs. 16 and 17). Thus phase 1 starts at 19 weeks in the posterior hypotympanum and 22 weeks in the anterior hypotympanum. Phase 2 starts at 24 weeks posteriorly and 28 weeks anteriorly. The lag phase is during the 24-36-week period posteriorly and 28-32 weeks anteriorly (the latter period is shorter since the anterior hypotympanum is narrower). Phase 3 of growth starts at 36 weeks posteriorly and 32 weeks anteriorly. This implies that the ossification pattern of the hypotympanum proceeds from a posterior to the anterior direction with a 4-week completion rate. In addition, although at 16 weeks in utero the anterior hypotympanum is wider than the posterior hypotympanum (3.25 mm vs 2 mm), by term the posterior hypotympanum becomes wider (3 mm vs 4.15 mm). Furthermore, the posterior hypotympanum continues to enlarge at a dramatic rate during the first postpartum month (3 mm to 5.58 mm) while the anterior hypotympanum does not enlarge.

Another way to assess the growth pattern of the hypotympanum is to measure the distances between

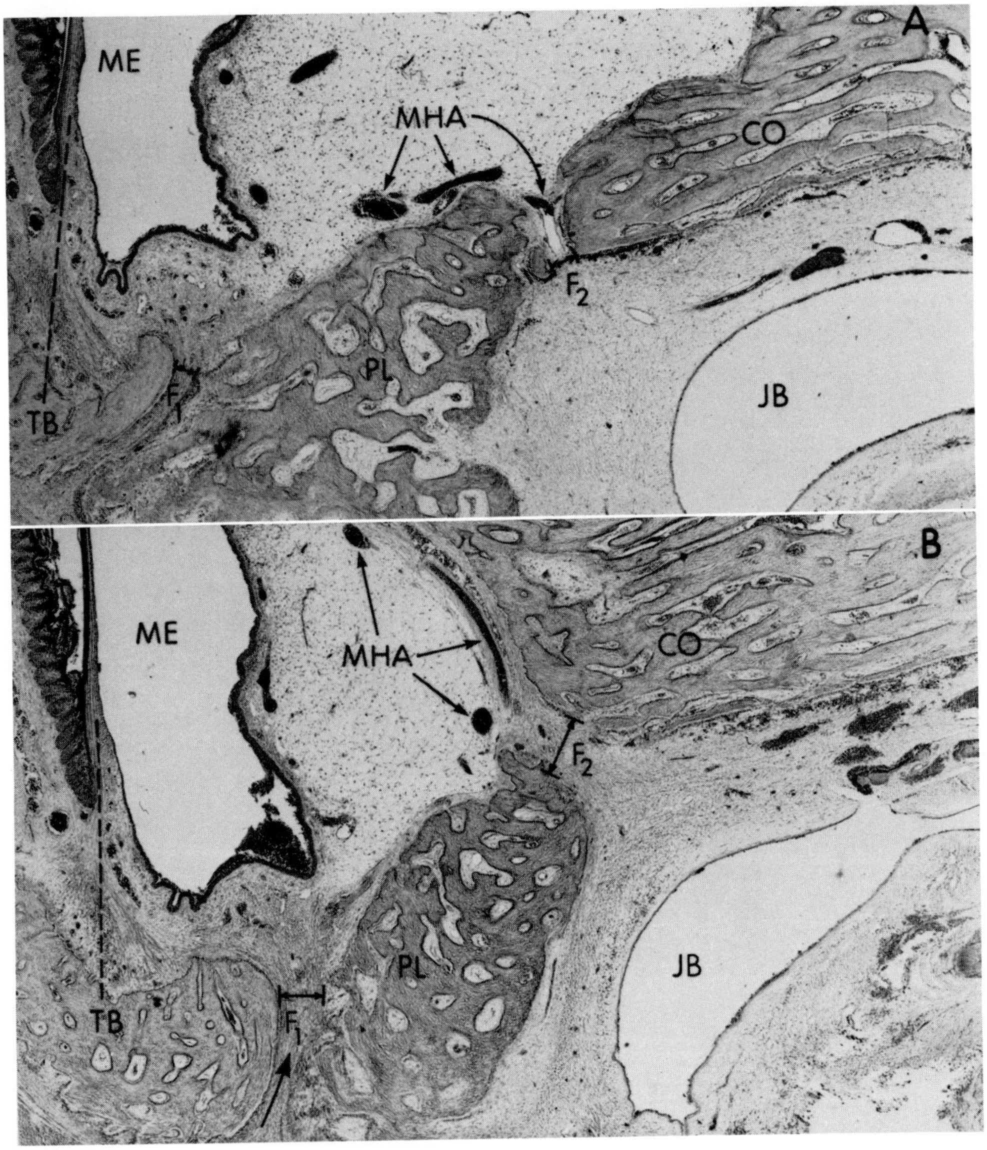

Fig. 13. Medial hypotympanic fissure (F_2) in a right postpartum temporal bone transmits the medial hypotympanic vessels (MHA). A) One branch traverses above the hypotympanum; B) another branch hugs the otic capsule. Note the lateral hypotympanic vessels enter the middle ear anteriorly and are not seen at this level. Dashed lines denote the avascular plane created by the fibrous annulus and middle fibrous layer of the tympanic membrane. (H&E, x35)

the medial and lateral hypotympanic fissures at various gestational ages. This is best done at the round window niche area where the round window membrane is visible, or in the region which is just anterior to the round window niche where Jacobson's nerve enters the middle ear. This is a direct measurement of the actual width of the petrosal ledge of bone and is unlike the former two measurements which are based on nonfixed hypotympanic landmarks (Fig. 18).

The growth of the petrosa in the hypotympanum as measured by the interfissure distance also has a 3-phase pattern. There is a rapid growth from 20 to 26 weeks in utero, a lag phase from 26-32 weeks in utero, and a rapid growth phase from 32 weeks in utero until term. The time pattern of petrosal growth is intermediate between that for the anterior and posterior hypotympanum and fits well with the previous data (Figs. 16-18). In addition there is a dramatically rapid growth pattern from term until one month postpartum. The postpartum petrosal growth is associated with the development of the osseous external auditory canal (Fig. 18).

From these data we can define more fully the phases of hypotympanic development. The initial phase is due primarily to ossification and growth of the canalicular otic capsule and tympanic bone. Phase 2, or lag phase, is due to the growth of the periosteal petrosal ledge of bone which closes the primitive hypotympanum between the tympanic bone and otic capsule. This petrosal growth closes the primitive hypotympanum without expanding its width, by simply bridging the gap between the canalicular otic capsule and the tympanic bone. Phase 3 is due to progressive overgrowth and ossification of the petrosal ledge of bone pushing the tympanic bone further away from the canalicular otic capsule. A final growth phase occurs during the first month postpartum (and later) when the petrosa continues to grow and ossify in the posterior hypotympanum (Figs. 17 and 18). This last phase (not covered in this paper) aids in the formation of

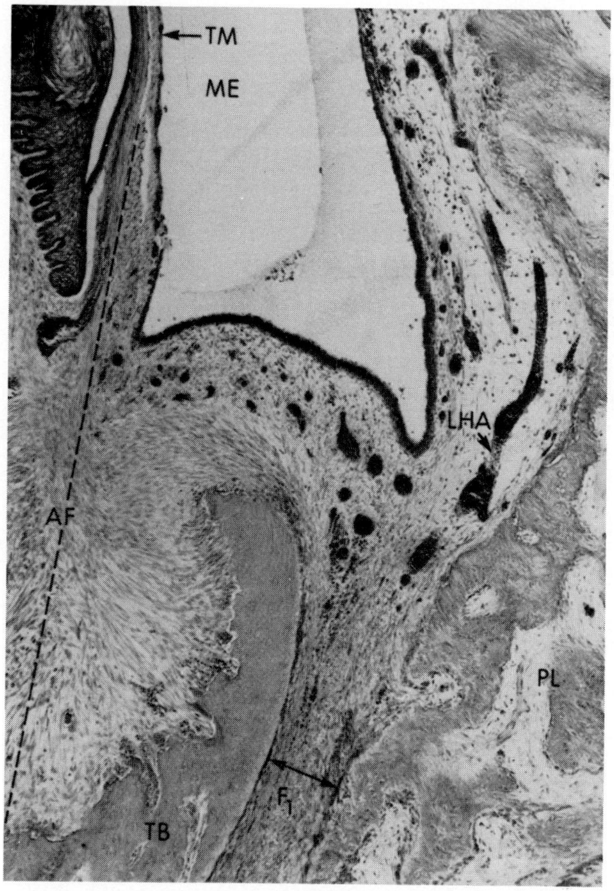

Fig. 14. Lateral hypotympanic fissure (F_1) in a right postpartum temporal bone transmits the lateral hypotympanic vessels (LHA). One branch follows the hypotympanum and another the inner surface of the tympanic membrane (TM). Dashed line represents the avascular plane which is created by the fibrous annulus (AF). (H&E, x90)

the external auditory canal and closes the canal of Huschke.

To further delineate the second or lag phase of hypotympanic development as related to the periosteal petrosal bone growth we can measure the widths of the medial and lateral hypotympanic fissures in relation to gestational age.

Hypotympanic Fissures. In all temporal bones prior to 22 months in utero there exist three fissures which communicate the middle ear space to the posterior cranial fossa. These are the lateral hypotympanic fissure (F_1), the medial hypotympanic fissure (F_2), and the tympanomeningeal fissure (Hyrtl's fissure) (Figs. 6, 8B, and 10B).

Hyrtl's fissure, which we described in a previous publication,[17] closes by fusion of the medial ossification center of the canalicular otic capsule to the cartilaginous bar which forms the medial lip of the round window rim (Figs. 6, 7, and 8B). This occurs at 24 weeks in utero. The two hypotympanic fissures remain patent at least until one month postpartum (Figs. 8A, 13, and 15A). These fissures are narrowed by progressive enlargement and ossification of the three temporal bone components, ie, the ossification of the cartilaginous canalicular otic capsule, the periosteal growth of the petrosa and the membranous ossification of the tympanic bone.

LATERAL HYPOTYMPANIC FISSURE. The lateral hypotympanic fissure (F_1) can be clearly delineated at 22 weeks in utero. The fissure is wider anteriorly with an average width of 1.84 mm (0.91 - 3.02 mm range) (Fig. 19). Posteriorly the width is 1.4 mm with a range of 0.66 to 1.57 mm. The lateral fissure narrows rapidly at 24 weeks. The average anterior width is 0.67 mm (range of 0.35 - 1.51 mm). By the 29th week the width is 0.37 mm with a range of 0.11 - 1.13 mm. After the 29th week in utero the anterior width remains uniform at least until the first month postpartum. Posteriorly the lateral fissure narrows at a 2-week-faster rate. At 22 weeks the fissure is 0.45 mm and at 24 weeks 0.4 mm wide. The fissure continues to narrow until the 26th week in utero to a 0.21 mm width. Thereafter it remains constant until one month postpartum.

The narrowing of the lateral fissure is due primarily to petrosal and tympanic bone ossification. The fissure tends to narrow to an adult configuration from a posterior to an anterior direction. It is interesting to note that prior to 32 weeks in utero there is asymmetrical ossification of the hypotympanum and narrowing of the lateral fissure, and thereafter both temporal bones tend to develop in a similar fashion (Fig. 20).

MEDIAL HYPOTYMPANIC FISSURE. The medial hypotympanic fissure (F_2) lies between the canalicular otic capsule and the petrosal ledge of bone. It first appears anteriorly at 18 weeks in utero. Its width is on the average 0.64 mm. The posterior aspect of the fissure is noted at the 22nd week in utero stage. At the 21-22-week stage the anterior width ranged from 0.31 mm to 1.02 mm with an average width of 0.59 mm. By the 24th week in utero the final postpartum width dimensions are achieved (an average width of 0.32 mm) (Fig. 21).

After the 22nd week in utero the medial fissure is constantly seen in all fetuses and neonates. The fissure is wider anteriorly and ossifies in a posteroanterior direction. Its width is initially one third of the lateral hypotympanic fissure. The width narrows to the postpartum dimensions five weeks prior to narrowing of the lateral fissure (Figs. 19 and 21). This defines the growth of the periosteal petrosal ledge of bone to a period between the 24th and 29th week in utero. The maximal narrowing of the medial hypotympanic fissure occurs at 24 weeks in utero (medial approximation of petrosa to canalicular otic capsule) and the maximal narrowing of the lateral fissure occurs at 29 weeks in utero (lateral approximation of the petrosa to the tympanic bone). These data correlate well with the delineation of the lag phase (periosteal petrosal growth) as determined previously.

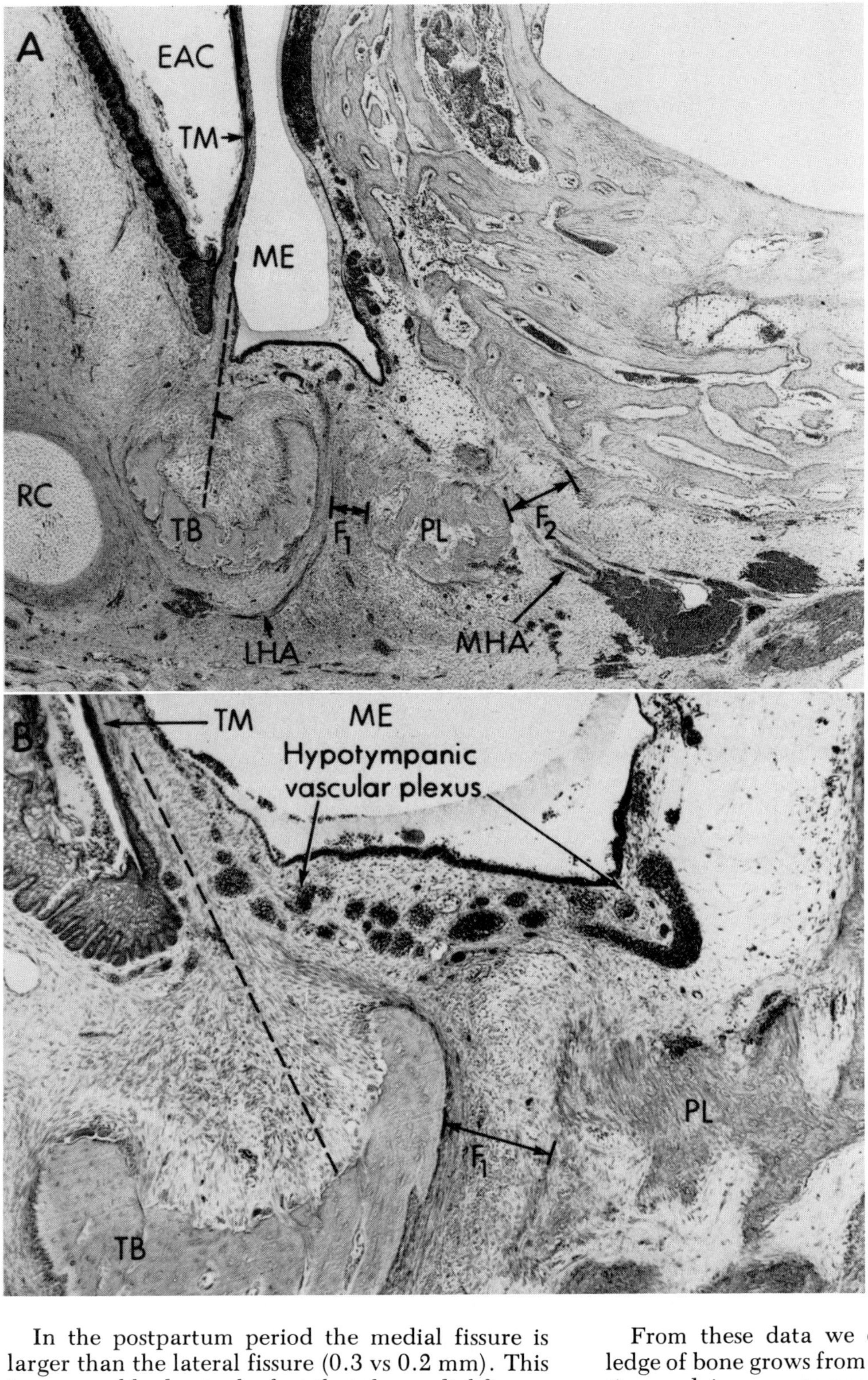

Fig. 15. A) Blood supply of the hypotympanum is composed of two different vascular systems. Lateral hypotympanic vessels (LHA) from the external carotid system enter via the lateral hypotympanic fissure (F_1), and the medial hypotympanic vessels (MHA) from the vertebral circulation enter the medial hypotympanic fissure (F_2). B) These vessels form a vascular hypotympanic plexus along the floor of the hypotympanum. Note the avascular plane (dashed line) separating the blood supply from the external auditory canal (EAC) and the lateral hypotympanic vessels. (H&E: A, x35; B, x90)

In the postpartum period the medial fissure is larger than the lateral fissure (0.3 vs 0.2 mm). This is presumably due to the fact that the medial fissure transmits Jacobson's nerve and the medial hypotympanic artery and vein. The lateral fissure transmits mainly the lateral hypotympanic artery and vein. Asymmetric ossification of the medial fissure occurs until the 32nd week in utero. Thereafter both temporal bones tend to be similar (Figs. 20 and 21).

From these data we can see that the petrosal ledge of bone grows from a medial to a lateral direction and in a posteroanterior axis over a 5-week period (24-29 weeks in utero). The medial fissure narrows five weeks prior to the narrowing of the lateral fissure. Both temporal bones ossify asymetrically until the 32nd week in utero; thereafter they tend to be similar. This process of fissure formation and narrowing occurs during the lag phase of hypotympanic growth and is primarily a function of per-

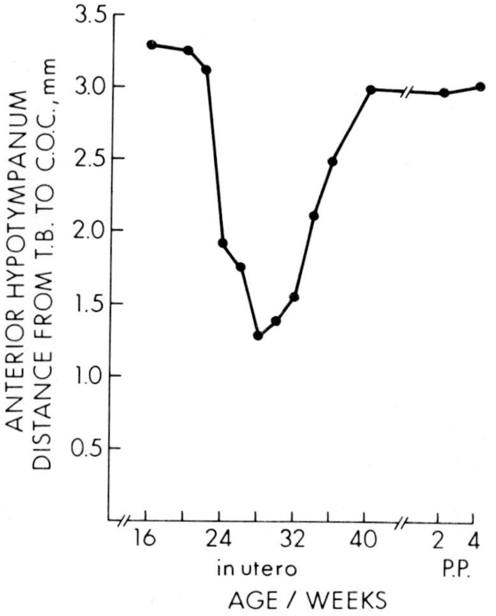

Fig. 16. Ossification of the anterior hypotympanum as measured by the distance from the tympanic bone (TB) to the cochlear otic capsule (COC). There is a triphasic growth pattern. Phase 1 (tympanic bone and otic capsule growth) starts at 18 weeks in utero and is completed at 28 weeks in utero. Phase 2 (petrosal ledge growth) occurs at 28-32 weeks in utero. The third phase starts at 34 weeks in utero and is completed at term (expansion of the middle ear). P.P. - Postpartum.

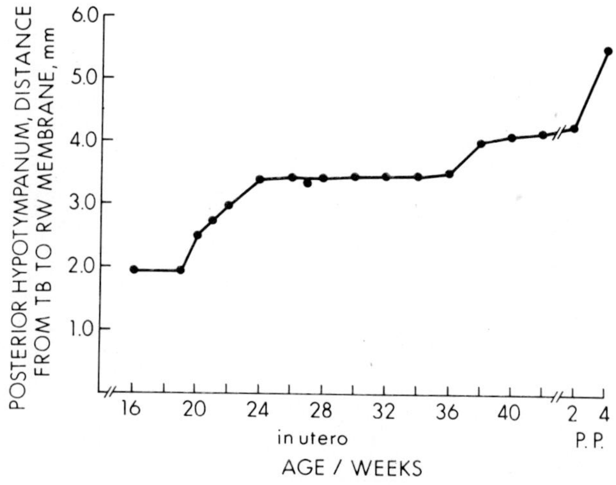

Fig. 17. Growth of the posterior hypotympanum has a triphasic pattern. The first phase occurs from 18-24 weeks in utero and denotes growth of the otic capsule and tympanic bone. The second phase occurs 24-36 weeks in utero and denotes petrosal bone growth. The third phase starts at 36 weeks in utero and continues until at least one month postpartum (petrosal overgrowth and formation of external auditory canal).

iosteal petrosal bone growth. During this time the hypotympanum is sequestered into the middle ear and separated from the jugular bulb and posterior cranial fossa.

DISCUSSION

OSSIFICATION

The temporal bone is composed of three major divisions: petrous, squamous and tympanic. However, the hypotympanum develops in relation to two of these, ie, the petrous and tympanic portions. Furthermore, the petrous ossification is composed of two different patterns: canalicular otic capsule ossification and periosteal petrosal ossification (Fig. 9).

The ossification pattern of the hypotympanic regions can be divided into three patterns. These are the membranous bone formation of the tympanic ring, the cartilaginous ossification of the canalicular otic capsule and the periosteal growth of the petrosa (Fig. 9). Initially the tympanic bone is formed at eight weeks in utero as a mesenchymal condensation beneath the squama. At nine weeks in utero the first ossification center is noted and at ten weeks all four ossification centers appear. By 12 weeks in utero the ossification centers fuse to form a tympanic ring. The tympanic bone quadruples in size by 22 weeks and quintuples by 35 weeks in utero.[19] Therefore, the tympanic bone is the first structure to ossify as a membranous bone (Figs. 2, 3, 5-7, 11-15).

The canalicular otic capsule ossification starts at 18-20 weeks in utero. Then it progresses in two directions. The medial ossification fuses the canalicular otic capsule to the cartilaginous medial rim of the round window and obliterates Hyrtl's fissure at 24 weeks in utero[17] (Figs. 6 and 7). The lateral ossification progresses at a 2-week slower rate to ossify the cartilaginous covering over the ampulla of the posterior semicircular canal. It partially covers the medial border of the hypotympanum (Figs. 4 and 5). The canalicular otic capsule ossifies in cartilage (enchondral ossification). It is the second bony structure to ossify (Fig. 9).

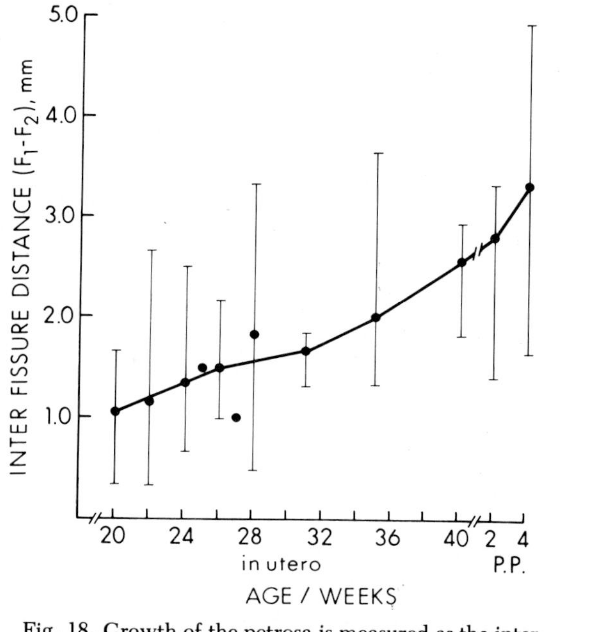

Fig. 18. Growth of the petrosa is measured as the interfissure distance (F - F). This demonstrates a triphasic growth pattern. Phase 1, 22-26 weeks; phase 2, 26-32 weeks; and phase 3, 32 weeks until one month postpartum.

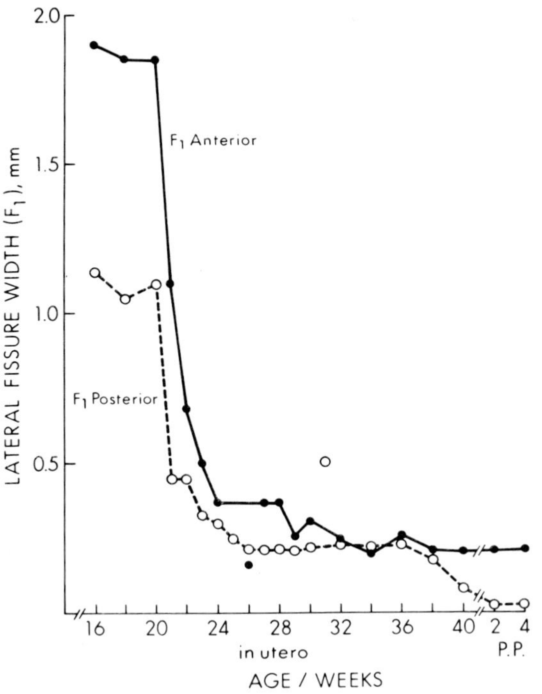

Fig. 19. Narrowing of the lateral fissure (F_1) proceeds from the posterior towards the anterior axis with a 2-week delay. The fissure narrows from 20-24 weeks posteriorly and 22-26 weeks anteriorly. The final size is achieved at 29-32 weeks in utero.

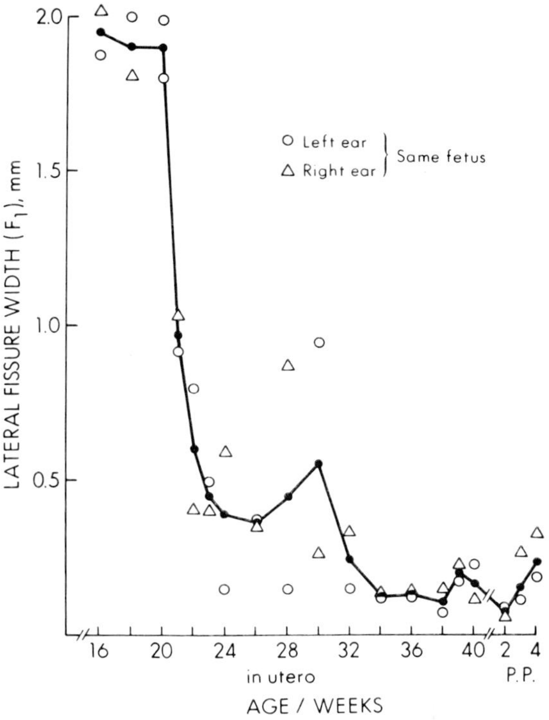

Fig. 20. Comparison of the narrowing of the lateral hypotympanic fissures in both temporal bones of the same fetus. The ossification tends to be asymmetrical until 32 weeks in utero; thereafter both temporal bones tend to be similar.

The lateral periosteal petrosal bony ledge is initially seen at 24 weeks as a small bony projection beneath the canalicular otic capsule (Fig. 3B). During the 24-29-weeks-in utero interval the periosteal ledge grows laterally to almost meet the enlarging tympanic bone (Figs. 10, 13, and 18). This effectively occludes the hypotympanic communication with the posterior cranial fossa and sequesters the hypotympanum to the middle ear. The petrosal ossification is the third bony structure to ossify and its bony formation is that of periosteal bone growth (Fig. 9).

Prior to 24 weeks in utero there are two major communications from the middle ear to the posterior cranial fossa. These are Hyrtl's fissure and the primitive hypotympanum (Figs. 6B, C, and 7A). In some instances after 24 weeks in utero, when Hyrtl's fissure remains patent, the hypotympanic communication is divided into a medial and lateral hypotympanic fissure by the petrosal ledge of bone. Thus there may be three persistent communications from the hypotympanum to the posterior cranial fossa (Figs. 8B and 10B). Starting medially and progressing laterally these are Hyrtl's fissure, medial hypotympanic fissure, and lateral hypotympanic fissure (Fig. 8B).

During the entire period of ossification of the hypotympanum Reichert's cartilage forms the postero-inferior boundary of the hypotympanum (Figs. 6, 7A, and 11A). It lies cephalad to the jugular bulb region and beneath the petrosal ledge (Fig. 7A). A portion of Reichert's cartilage forms the facial fallopian canal. Since the petrosal periosteal growth extends on top of Reichert's cartilage and follows it towards the tympanic bone, and since the periosteal petrosal ledge of bone grows from a posterior towards an anterior direction, therefore Reichert's cartilage forms a template for the hypotympanum. Thus Reichert's cartilage predetermines the jugular bulb height and the level of the hypotympanic floor.

From our study we can see that the hypotympanum is not a single region but a mosaic of three different bone formations (membranous, periosteal, and enchondral), and three different structures (tympanic bone, canalicular otic capsule, and petrosa). Each has its own pattern of growth. This fact is reflected by the triphasic ossification curves for the hypotympanum and the fissures. It is our contention, therefore, that the hypotympanum is more likely to have malformation, malfusions, and dehiscences because of inappropriate bony approximations. In addition we postulate that these dehiscences must occur prior to the 32nd week of gestation. Also malformations in Reichert's cartilage may lead to major dehiscences or total malformations of the hypotympanic floor. Since hypotympanic ossification prior to 32 weeks in utero tends not to be symmetrical in both temporal bones of the same fetus, we propose that hypotympanic dehiscences in the adult population may be asymmetrical.

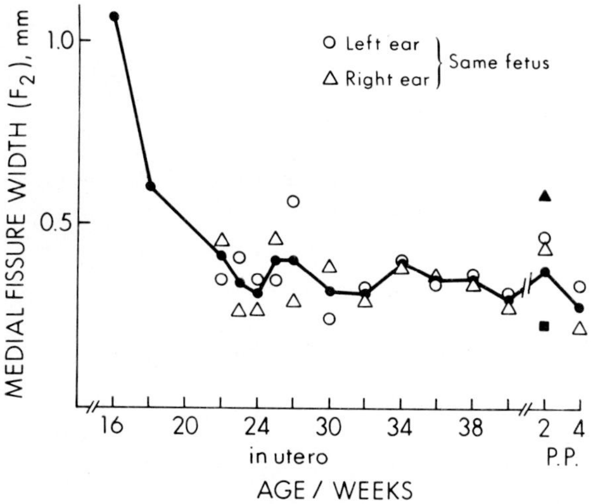

Fig. 21. Narrowing of the medial hypotympanic fissure occurs from 16-24 weeks; thereafter, the diameter of the fissure remains constant until birth. Both medial fissures ossify asymmetrically until 32 weeks in utero; thereafter they tend to be similar. At two weeks postpartum there were two sets of temporal bones, one denoted by clear and the other by black symbols.

Korner and Grunberg found gross anatomic dehiscences in the jugular bulb dome in 30 of 449 skulls.[21] They concluded, as others had after them, that jugular bulb and hypotympanic dehiscences were not uncommon.[21] Many authors have described similar observations of dehiscent jugular bulbs.[22-27] Overton and Ritter noted a 6% incidence of jugular bulb dehiscence with extension to the middle ear in 257 temporal bones.[27] Furthermore, jugular bulb thrombophlebitis is a well-known complication of otitis media and mastoiditis.[28-31] A direct extension by contiguous or continuous pathways are generally the main pathologic events. Dehiscences of the jugular bulb are therefore a higher risk for septic thromboembolization.[28-31]

An interesting observation is that those bones which had persistent Hyrtl's fissures (malfusion of the medial canalicular otic capsule to the inferior round window rim) had persistently larger hypotympanic fissures (malfusions of the lateral petrosal ledge of bone to the lateral canalicular otic capsule or to the tympanic bone) (Figs. 8B and 10B). Thus in general hypotympanic dehiscences reflect either an inappropriate ossification of the petrosa, a malfusion of the three hypotympanic osseous components or malformation of Reichert's cartilage. In addition they would tend to be asymmetrical in both temporal bones of the same individual.

HYPOTYMPANIC FISSURES

The ossification of the hypotympanic periosteal petrosal ledge of bone progresses from a medial (canalicular otic capsule) to a lateral (tympanic bone) direction. The axis of growth is from the posterior (round window niche area) towards the anterior (carotid canal) direction. The approximation of the petrosa to the other two bony structures forms two fissures. These have not been clearly described in the literature (Figs. 10A, 12A, 13A, B, and 15A).

The malfusion of the petrosa to the tympanic bone forms the lateral hypotympanic fissure (Figs. 13-15A). This fissure has occasionally been called the inferior tympanic canaliculus. The malfusion of the petrosa to the canalicular otic capsule is called the medial hypotympanic fissure or Jacobson's nerve canal (Figs. 12, 13A, B, and 15B).

These fissures form during the lag phase of hypotympanic expansion when the petrosal ossification catches up with the ossification of the tympanic bone and canalicular otic capsule. The medial fissure narrows to the adult configuration at 22-24 weeks in utero and the lateral fissure at 29-32 weeks in utero. Since they determine the medial and lateral edges of the petrosa, the fissure demarcates the period of petrosal growth that is needed to cover the hypotympanum to a 10-week period (22-32 weeks).

Our study indicates that the primitive hypotympanum is segregated from the posterior cranial fossa to form the adult configuration at a much earlier date than mentioned in the literature.[1-16] Our data further indicate that between the 29-32 weeks in utero the hypotympanum is covered by bone except for the two persistent fissures. In addition, except for one postpartum bone, all temporal bones from 16 weeks in utero until one month postpartum had persistent dehiscences in the hypotympanum (Figs. 8A, B, and 10A, B).

NEUROVASCULAR STRUCTURES

In a previous report we demonstrated that the superior (jugular) ganglion of the glossopharyngeal nerve (IX) lies at the meningeal opening of the cochlear aqueduct (Fig. 6).[17] The inferior (petrosal) ganglion of the ninth nerve lies on the medial surface of the jugular bulb region beneath the posterior semicircular canal ampulla (Fig. 11). Although there is some confusion as to the origin of Jacobson's nerve, our data indicate that it arises from the cephalic border of the inferior (petrosal) glossopharyngeal ganglion (Fig. 11B). The latter usually lies cephalad to the jugular bulb. The nerve enters the future medial hypotympanic fissure (prior to hypotympanic ossification) anterior to the round window and forms the tympanic plexus (with the sympathetic caroticotympanic nerves) on the cochlear promontory (Fig. 12).

Initially, at 19 weeks in utero, the tympanic nerve enters the middle ear anteriorly and close to the internal carotid artery. However the formation of the medial fissures (anteriorly initially then progressing posteriorly) and the growth of the petrosa pushes the nerve posteriorly towards the anterior rim of the round window. As the nerve moves backward it pulls with it the branches of the caroticotympanic plexus and the associated blood supply. This spreads the neural and vascular supply over the entire promontory. The final location is determined at 24-26 weeks when the medial fissure assumes the adult configuration and diameter (Fig. 12).

In one of our bones the tympanic branch of the ninth nerve traversed in the subiculum.

The tympanic nerve supplies the parasympathetic fibers to the parotid gland through the otic ganglion and sensory fibers to the mucous membrane of the middle ear. Later it leaves the ear to form the lesser (superficial) petrosal nerve.

A most important observation of our study is the nature of the hypotympanic circulation. It has been universally accepted that the inferior tympanic artery, a branch of the ascending pharyngeal artery of the external carotid system is the main blood supply to this region (Fig. 5).[9,32] The inferior tympanic vein returns the blood from the middle ear to the pterygoid venous plexus. In addition it is stated that these vessels and Jacobson's nerve enter the middle ear via the inferior tympanic canaliculus. Our observations indicate that this is not the case.

Our study indicates that there are two separate arteries and veins involved in the circulation of the hypotympanum (Fig. 15A). The lateral vessels are the inferior tympanic artery and vein (which we have renamed the lateral hypotympanic artery and vein) (Figs. 14 and 15A, B). They enter the middle ear via the lateral hypotympanic fissure, and supply the lateral hypotympanum and the inner mucosal surface of the tympanic membrane (Fig. 14). There is an avascular plane formed by the fibrous annulus and middle fibrous layer of the tympanic membrane which prohibits further anastomosis with external auditory canal vessels (Figs. 13-15). Medially, however, the lateral hypotympanic vessels form a rich anastomatic plexus with the medial hypotympanic vessels (Figs. 13A and 15B).

The medial vessels accompany the tympanic branch of the ninth nerve (Figs. 11B, 12B, 13A, B, and 15). These vessels arise from the CNS circulation of the posterior cranial fossa, probably from the vertebral artery and vein system. The artery and vein enter the middle ear through the medial hypotympanic fissure (Figs. 13 and 15A). We have named these the medial hypotympanic artery and vein. They supply the medial hypotympanum, round window niche, cochlear promontory and medial wall of the middle ear (Fig. 13). In addition, the medial hypotympanic vessels anastomose with the lateral hypotympanic vessels along the floor of the hypotympanum just above the petrosal ledge of bone. Thus there is an external carotid-vertebral anastomosis in the hypotympanum. We have named this the hypotympanic vascular plexus (Fig. 15).

ACKNOWLEDGMENTS — We wish to acknowledge and thank Mrs. Jean Mayo for the preparation of the manuscript and Ms. Alice I. Clark for the preparation of the illustrations.

REFERENCES

1. Fitzgerald MJT. Human embryology: a regional approach. Hagerstown, Md: Harper & Row, 1978.

2. Harrison RG. Clinical embryology. London: Academic Press, 1978.

3. Langman J. Medical embryology. 2nd ed. Baltimore: Williams & Wilkins, 1969.

4. Allan FD. Essentials of human embryology. 2nd ed. New York: Oxford University Press, 1969.

5. Arey LB. Developmental anatomy. Philadelphia: WB Saunders, 1965.

6. Anson BJ, Davies J. Embryology of the ear. Developmental anatomy of the ear. In: Paparella MM, Shumrick DA, eds. Otolaryngology. 2nd ed. Vol. 1. Philadelphia: WB Saunders, 1980: 3-25.

7. Ballantyne J. Anatomy of the ear. In Scott-Brown's diseases of the ear, nose and throat, 3rd ed. Vol. I. Philadelphia: JB Lippincott, 1971: 1-60.

8. Pearson AA, Developmental anatomy of the ear. In: English GM, ed. Otolaryngology. Rev. ed. Hagerstown, Md: Harper & Row, 1979: 68.

9. Wolff D, Bellucci RJ, Eggston AA. Surgical and microscopic anatomy of the temporal bone. New York: Hafner, 1971.

10. Hamilton WJ. Human embryology. 3rd ed. Cambridge, England: Heffer & Sons, Ltd, 1962.

11. Steffen TN. Vascular anomalies of the middle ear. Laryngoscope 1968; 78:171-97.

12. Marovitz WF, Porubsky ES. The embryological development of the middle ear space — a new concept. Ann Otol Rhinol Laryngol 1971; 80:384-9.

13. Proctor B. The development of the middle ear spaces and their surgical significance. J Laryngol Otol 1964; 78:631-48.

14. Proctor B. Surgical anatomy of the posterior tympanum. Ann Otol Rhinol Laryngol 1969; 78:1026-40.

15. Schuknecht HF. Pathology of the ear. Cambridge, Mass: Harvard University Press, 1974: 79-92.

16. Graham MD. The jugular bulb: its anatomic and clinical considerations in contemporary otology. Laryngoscope 1977; 87:105-25.

17. Spector GJ, Lee D, Carr C, et al. Later stages of development of the periotic duct and its adjacent area in the human fetus. Laryngoscope 1980; 90 Suppl 20: 1-31.

18. Ge X-X, Spector GJ. The development of the labyrinthine segment and geniculate ganglion of the facial nerve in human fetal and neonatal temporal bones. Ann Otol Rhinol Laryngol 1981; 90 Suppl 85.

19. Anson BJ, Bast TH, Richany SF. The fetal and early postnatal development of the tympanic ring and related structures in man. Ann Otol Rhinol Laryngol 1955; 64:802-23.

20. Anson BJ, Donaldson JA. Surgical anatomy of the temporal bone and ear. 2nd ed. Philadelphia: Saunders, 1973.

21. Korner O, Grunberg K. Die Otitischen Erkrankungen des Hirns, der Hiruhäute und der Blutleiter, Wiesbaden, Germany, 1908.

22. Beyer H. Abnorme Ausdehnung der Fossa Jugularis am Boden der Paukenhohle mit Verlagerung des Schneckenfensters. Passow Schaefer's Beitr 1910-1; 4:397.

23. Page JR. Injury to the jugular bulb following myringotomy. Ann Otol Rhinol Laryngol 1914; 23:161-3.

24. Gejrot T. Retrograde jugularography in the diagnosis of abnormalities of the superior bulb of the internal jugular vein. Acta Otolaryngol (Stockh) 1964; 57:177-80.

25. Smythe GD, Black JHA. A case of protruding jugular bulb. Laryngoscope 1965; 75:669-72.

26. Steffen TN. Vascular anomalies of the middle ear. Laryngoscope 1968; 78:171-97.

27. Overton SB, Ritter FN. A high placed jugular bulb in the middle ear: a clinical and temporal bone study. Presented at the AMA meeting, San Francisco, California, 1972.

28. Voss F. Operation der Sinusthrombose ohne Eroffrung des Antrum nach ausgehilter acuter Mittelohrentzundung. Z Ohrenheilkd 1903; 45:45-56.

29. Grunert K. Weiterer Beitrag zur Infektiosen Thrombose des Bulbus Venae Jugularis und zur Frage ihrer Operativen Behandlung. Arch Klin Exp Ohren Nasen Kehlkopfheilkd 1902-3; 57:23.

30. Piffel O. Zur operativen Freilegung des Bulbus der Vena Jugularis Interna. Arch Klin Exp Ohren Nasen Kehlkopfheilkd 1903; 58:76-81.

31. Whiting F. A contribution to the symptomatology and treatment of pyaemic sinus thrombosis based upon three successfully operated cases. Arch Otolaryngol 1898; 27:26-7.

32. Barrett JH, Lawrence VL. Aneurysm of the internal carotid artery as a complication of mastoidectomy. Arch Otolaryngol 1960; 72:366-8.